SURGERY OF THE SPINE

To Andrea and Meg

SURGERY OF THE SPINE

A COMBINED ORTHOPAEDIC AND NEUROSURGICAL APPROACH

Edited by

GORDON FINDLAY
BSc MB ChB FRCS
Consultant Neurosurgeon
Department of Medical and Surgical Neurology
Walton Hospital, Liverpool

and

ROBERT OWEN
DL, MB BS MCh(Orth) FRCS
Emeritus Professor of
Orthopaedic and Trauma Surgery
University of Liverpool

With an Introduction by

HENK VERBIEST

IN TWO VOLUMES

VOLUME 1

OXFORD
BLACKWELL SCIENTIFIC PUBLICATIONS
LONDON EDINBURGH BOSTON
MELBOURNE PARIS BERLIN VIENNA

Editorial offices:
Osney Mead, Oxford OX2 0EL
25 John Street, London WC1N 2BL
23 Ainslie Place, Edinburgh EH3 6AJ
3 Cambridge Center, Cambridge
Massachusetts 02142, USA
54 University Street, Carlton
Victoria 3053, Australia

Other editorial offices:
Librairie Arnette SA
2, rue Casimir-Delavigne
75006 Paris
France

Blackwell Wissenschafts-Verlag
Meinekestrasse 4
D-1000 Berlin 15
Germany

Blackwell MZV
Feldgasse 13
A-1238 Wien
Austria

First published 1992

Set by Excel Typesetter Ltd, Hong Kong
Printed and bound by Kin Keong, Singapore

DISTRIBUTORS

Marston Book Services Ltd
PO Box 87
Oxford OX2 0DT
(*Orders*: Tel: 0865 791155
Fax: 0865 791927
Telex: 837515)

USA
Blackwell Scientific Publications, Inc.
3 Cambridge Center
Cambridge, MA 02142
(*Orders*: Tel: 800 759-6102
617 225-0401)

Canada
Times Mirror Professional Publishing, Ltd
5240 Finch Avenue East
Scarborough, Ontario M1S 5A2
(*Orders*: Tel: 800 268-4178
416 298-1588)

Australia
Blackwell Scientific Publications
(Australia) Pty Ltd
54 University Street
Carlton, Victoria 3053
(*Orders*: Tel: 03 347-0300)

A catalogue record for this book is available from the British Library

ISBN 0–632–03021–6 (The Set)
0–632–03246–4 (Vol. 1)
0–632–03247–2 (Vol. 2)

Contents

List of Contributors

G.M. BEDBROOK, Kt, OBE, OStJ, MS(Melb), HonMD(WA), HonFRCS(Ed), HonDTech(Curtin), FRCS, FRACS, DPRM(Syd), HonFCRM, *Emeritus Orthopaedic Surgeon, Royal Perth Rehabilitation Hospital, Perth, Australia*

S.H. BIGNER, MD, *Professor of Pathology, Duke University Medical Center, PO Box 3712, Durham, NC 27710, USA*

L.D. BLUMHARDT, BSc, MD, FRACP, *Reader in Clinical Neurology, Department of Neurological Science, Faculty of Medicine, Liverpool University; Honorary Consultant Neurologist, Walton Centre for Neurology Walton Hospital, Rice Lane, Liverpool, L91AE, UK*

H.H. BOHLMAN, MD, FACS, *Professor and Vice Chairman of Orthopaedics, Case Western Reserve University School of Medicine, Department of Orthopaedics, University Hospitals of Cleveland, 2074 Abington Road, Cleveland, Ohio 44106-2602 USA; Chief, Spinal Cord Injury Service, Department of Veterans Affairs, 10701 East Blvd., Cleveland, OH 44106, USA*

M.J. BOLESTA, MD, FACS, *Assistant Professor of Orthopaedics, Case Western Reserve University School of Medicine, Department of Orthopaedics, University Hospitals of Cleveland, 2074 Abington Road, Cleveland, Ohio 44106-2602, USA; Administration Chief, Spinal Cord Injury Service, Department of Veterans Affairs, 10701 East Blvd., Cleveland, OH 44106, USA*

R.E.M. BOWDEN, OBE, MB, BS, DSc, FRCS, *Emeritus Professor of Anatomy, University of London; formerly Sir William Collins Professor of Humanities and Comparative Anatomy, Department of Anatomy, Royal College of Surgeons of England, Lincoln's Inn Fields, London WC2A3PN, UK*

D.R. BOWSHER, MA, MD, Ph.D, MRCP(Ed), MRCPath, *Director of Research, Pain Research Institute, Walton Hospital, Liverpool L91AE, UK; Honorary Consultant Neurologist, Mersey Regional Centre for Pain Relief*

I.M. BOYD, FFARCS, MB, BS, BSc, DCH, *Consultant Anaesthetist, Department of Anaesthesia, Royal Liverpool Children's Hospital, Alder Hey, Eaton Road, Liverpool L122AP, UK; Honorary Lecturer, Liverpool University*

R. BRAAKMAN, MD, PhD, *Professor of Neurosurgery, Department of Neurosurgery, Erasmus University Rotterdam, University Hospital Rotterdam-Dijkzigt, Dr. Molewaterplein 40, 3015 GD, The Netherlands*

M. BROCK, MD, *Professor and Chairman, Department of Neurosurgery, Universitaetsklinikum Steglitz/Free University of Berlin, Hindenburgdamm 30, W-1000, Berlin 45, Germany*

R.G. BURWELL, BSc, MD, FRCS, *Professor of Human Morphology and Experimental Orthopaedics, Department of Human Morphology, University of Nottingham, Queen's Medical Centre, Nottingham NG72UH; Honorary Consultant in Orthopaedics, Nottingham Health Authority*

H. CARTY, FRCPI, FRCR, *Consultant Radiologist and Lecturer in Radiodiagnosis, Department of Radiology, Royal Liverpool Children's Hospital, Alder Hey, Eaton Road, Liverpool L122AP, UK*

V. CHACKO, MB, BS, MS(Orth), *Consultant Orthopaedic Surgeon, 'Illampallil, Tiruvalla-689 101, Kerala, India; Formerly Director/Professor and Head of Orthopaedics, Kasturba Medical College, Manipal; President of Indian Orthopaedic Association*

R.C.M. COOK, MA, BM, BCh, FRCS, *Consultant Paediatric Surgeon, Royal Liverpool Children's Hospital, Alder Hey, Eaton Road, Liverpool L122AP, UK*

P.R. COOPER, MD, *Professor of Neurosurgery, Department of Neurosurgery, New York University Medical Center 550 1st Avenue, New York, USA*

R.A. COWIE, BSc, MB, ChB, FRCS(Ed), FRCS(Ed) (SN), *Consultant Neurosurgeon, Department of Neurosurgery, Hope Hospital, Eccles Old Rd., Salford M68HD, UK; Department of Neurosurgery, Royal Manchester Children's Hospital, Hospital Road, Pendlebury, Swinton, Manchester M271HA, UK*

H.A. CROCKARD, FRCS(Ed), FRCSE, *Consultant Neurosurgeon, Department of Surgical Neurology, The National Hospital for Neurology and Neurosurgery, Maida Vale, London W91TL, UK; Honorary Senior Lecturer, Institute of Neurology*

P.H. DANGERFIELD, MD, *Lecturer in Human Anatomy and Cell Biology, Clinical Lecturer in Orthopaedic Surgery, Department of Human Anatomy and Cell Biology, University of Liverpool, PO Box 147, Liverpool, L693BX, UK*

J. DOVE, FRCS, *Director, Stoke-on-Trent Spinal Service, 31 Quarry Avenue, Hartshill, Stoke on Trent ST47EW, UK*

J. DVORAK, MD, *Head of Neurology Department, Spine Unit, Schuethese Hospital, 8008 Zurich, Switzerland*

M.A. EDGAR, MA, M.Chir, FRCS, *Consultant Orthopaedic Surgeon, 149 Harley St., London W1N2DE, UK; The Middlesex and University College Hospital, London W1; The Royal National Orthopaedic Hospital, Stanmore, Middlesex, UK; Civilian Consultant Adviser in Orthopaedics to the RAF*

R.H.T. EDWARDS, BSc, PhD, MB, FRCP, *Professor of Medicine, Director of Magnetic Resonance Research Centre, Director of Muscle Research Centre, Department of Medicine, University of Liverpool, PO Box 147, Liverpool L693BX, UK*

S.M. EISENSTEIN, MB, BCh, PhD, FRCS(Ed), *Director, Centre for Spinal Studies, Department for Spinal Disorders, The Robert Jones and Agnes Hunt Orthopaedic Hospital, Oswestry Hospital, Oswestry, Shropshire SY107AG, UK*

F.J. EPSTEIN, MD, *Director of Pediatric Neurosurgery, Professor of Neurosurgery, Department of Neurosurgery, New York University Medical Center, 550 1st Avenue, New York, USA*

J.A. EPSTEIN, MD, FACS, *Professor of Neurosurgery, Cornell University Medical College, 410 Lakeville Road, Ste #100, New Hyde Park, NY 11042, USA; Associate Clinical Professor of Neurosurgery, Albert Einstein College of Medicine; Attending Neurosurgeon, North Shore University Hospital and Long Island Jewish Medical Center*

N.E. EPSTEIN, MD, FACS, *Associate Clinical Professor of Neurosurgery, Cornell University Medical College, 410 Lakeville Road, Ste #100, New Hyde Park, NY 11042, USA; Assistant Attending Neurosurgeon, North Shore University Hospital and Long Island Jewish Medical Center*

H.S.Y. FANG, CBE, MB, BS, MCh(Orth), LLD(Hon), HKU, CUHK, FRCSE, FFACS, FACS, FRCPE, JP, *Consultant Orthopaedic Surgeon, Room 306, TakShing House, 20 Des Voeux Road, Hong Kong*

G.F.G. FINDLAY, BSc, MB, ChB, FRCS, *Consultant Neurosurgeon, Department of Neurosurgery, Walton Hospital, Rice Lane, Liverpool L91AE, UK*

P.M. FOY, MB, CHB, FRCS, *Consultant Neurosurgeon, Mersey Regional Department of Medical and Surgical Neurology, Department of Neurosurgery, Walton Hospital, Liverpool L91AE, UK; Clinical Lecturer, University of Liverpool*

R.D. FRASER, MB, BS, MD, FRACS, *Head of Spinal Unit, Department of Orthopaedic Surgery and Trauma, Royal Adelaide Hospital, Adelaide 5000, South Australia; Senior Clinical Lecturer, University of Adelaide*

C.S.B. GALASKO, MSc, MB, ChM, FRCS(Eng), FRCS(Ed), *Consultant Orthopaedic Surgeon, Department of Orthopaedic Surgery, Clinical Sciences Building, Hope Hospital, Eccles Old Road, Salford M68HD, UK; Consultant Orthopaedic Surgeon, Royal*

Manchester Children's Hospital; Professor of Orthopaedic Surgery, University of Manchester

A.D.H. GARDNER, MB, BS(Lond), FRCS(Eng), *Consultant Orthopaedic Surgeon, Basildon Hospital, Nethermayne, Basildon, Essex S16SNL, UK and Black Notley Hospital, Braintree, Essex*

M. GLANTZ, MD, *Assistant Professor of Neurooncology, University of Minnesota, Box 295, 420 Delaware Street, South-East Minneapolis, MN 55455, USA*

D.I. GRAHAM, MB, BCh, PhD, FRCPath, *Professor of Neuropathology, The University of Glasgow; Department of Neuropathology, Institute of Neurological Sciences, Southern General Hospital, Glasgow G514TF, UK*

R.D. GRIFFITHS, BSc, MD, MRCP, *Muscle Research Centre, Department of Medicine, University of Liverpool, PO Box 147, Liverpool L693BX, UK*

K.B. HEITHOFF, MD, *Medical Director, Center for Diagnostic Imaging(CDI), 2800 Chicago Avenue, Minneapolis, MN 55407, USA; CDI 5775 Wayzata Blvd., St Louis Park, MN 55416; 910 Sibley Memorial Highway, St Paul, MN 5518; CDI, 9247 North Meridian Street, Indianapolis, IN 46260, USA; Abbott Northwestern Hospital, 28th and Chicago Avenue, Minneapolis, MN 55407, USA*

N.J. HENDERSON, BM, BCh, FRCS, *Consultant Orthopaedic Surgeon, Stoke Mandeville Hospital, Aylesbury, Bucks HP218AL*

R.J. HERZOG, MD, *Medical Director, San Francisco Neuroskeletal Imaging Center, 1850 Sullivan Avenue, Suite 100, Daly City, California 94015, USA; Assistant Clinical Professor, Musculoskeletal Section, Department of Radiology, University of California, San Francisco*

E.K.W. HO, MB, BS, FRCSG, FRACS, *Senior Lecturer, Department of Orthopaedic Surgery, University of Hong Kong; Medical Director, The Duchess of Kent Children's Hospital, 12 Sandy Bay Road, Hong Kong*

H.J. HOFFMAN, MD, BScMed, FRCSC, FACS, *Neurosurgeon-in-Chief, The Hospital for Sick Children, 555 University Avenue, Toronto M5G1X8, Canada; Professor of Surgery, University of Toronto*

P.R.D. HUMPHREY, DM, FRCP, MA, BM, BCh, *Consultant Neurologist, Mersey Regional Department of Medical and Surgical Neurology, Walton Hospital, Rice Lane, Liverpool L91AE, UK*

M.I.V. JAYSON, MD, FRCP, *Professor of Rheumatology and Director of University Centre for Study of Chronic Rheumatism, Rheumatic Diseases Centre University of Manchester, Hope Hospital, Salford M68HD, UK*

T.E. JEFFREYS, FRCS(Ed), FRCS(Eng), *Emeritus Consultant Orthopaedic Surgeon, The Robert Jones and Agnes Hunt Orthopaedic Hospital, Oswestry, Shropshire SY107AG, UK*

J.R. JOHNSON, MB, BS, FRCS(Eng), *Consultant Orthopaedic Surgeon, Department of Orthopaedic Surgery, St Mary's Hospital and Medical College, Praed Street, London W2, UK*

R.A. JOHNSTON, BSc, MD, FRCS, *Consultant Neurosurgeon, Department of Neuorosurgery, Institute of Neurological Sciences, Southern General Hospital, Glasgow G514TF, Scotland, UK*

J.A. KANIS, MD, FRCP, *Professor in Human Metabolism and Clinical Biochemistry, World Health Organisation Centre for Metabolic Bone Disease, University of Sheffield Medical School, Sheffield S102DU, UK*

J.P. KOSTUIK, MD, FRCS(C), *Professor, Departments of Orthopaedics and Neurosurgery, Chief, Division of Spinal Surgery (Orthopaedics), John Hopkins Hospital, John Hopkins University, Baltimore, Maryland, USA*

J.C.Y. LEONG, FRCS, FRCSE, FRACS, *Professor and Head, Department of Orthopaedic Surgery, University of Hong Kong, 5/F Professorial Block, Queen Mary Hospital, Hong Kong*

M.C. LYNCH, MB, ChB, MChOrth, FRCS, *Consultant Orthopaedic Surgeon, Broadgreen Hospital, Liverpool L143LB, UK*

J.A. McCULLOCH, MD, FRCSC, *Professor of Orthopaedics, North-eastern Ohio Universities, College of Medicine, 75 Arch Street, 501 Akron, Ohio 44304, USA*

M.J. McMASTER, MD, FRCS, *Consultant Orthopaedic Surgeon, Princess Margaret Rose Orthopaedic Hospital, Edinburgh EH107ED, Scotland, UK*

T. McSWEENEY, MB, BCh, BAO(NUI), MCh, MChOrth, FRCS(Eng), FACS, *Emeritus Consultant Traumatic and Orthopaedic Surgeon, The Robert Jones and Agnes Hunt Orthopaedic Hospital, Oswestry, Shropshire SY107AG, UK*

H.M. MAYER, MD, *Assistant Professor, Department of Orthopaedic Surgery, Free University of Berlin, Oskar-Helene-Heim, Clay Allee 229, W-1000, Berlin 33, Germany*

P. MERTENS, MD, DSc, *Department of Neurosurgery, University of Lyon, Hospital Neurologique, 59 Blvd. PINEL, 69003 Lyon, France*

J.B. MILES, MB, ChB, FRCS, *Consultant Neurosurgeon, Walton Hospital, Rice Lane, Liverpool L91AE, UK*

R.M. MORAN, MCh(Orth), FRCSI, *Consultant Orthopaedic Surgeon, Beaumont Hospital, Beaumont Road, Dublin 9, Ireland*

R.C. MULHOLLAND, MB, BS, FRCS(Eng), *Consultant Orthopaedic Surgeon, Harlow Wood Orthopaedic Hospital, Mansfield; Queen's Medical Centre, Nottingham University Hospital, Nottingham, UK*

J.W. OGILVIE, MD, *Associate Professor, Department of Orthopaedic Surgery, University of Minnesota; Director, Twin Cities Scoliosis Spine Center, 2737 Chicago Ave So. LL-200, Minneapolis, Minnesota, USA*

A.K. OMMAYA, MA, MD, FRCS, FACS, *Professor of Neurosurgery, George Washington University, 8006 Glenbrook Road, Bethesden Md. 20814, Washington DC, USA*

O.L. OSTI, MD, PhD, *Orthopaedic Registrar, Royal Adelaide Hospital, Adelaide 5000, South Austrailia*

R. OWEN, DL, MB, BS, MChOrth, FRCS, *Emeritus Professor of Orthopaedic and Trauma Surgery, University of Liverpool, UCD Block, 4th floor, Royal Liverpool Hospital, Prescot Street, Liverpool L693BX, UK*

K.F. PARSONS, MB, ChB, FRCSE, FRCS, *Consultant Urological Surgeon and Director of Urological Studies, The 92 Link Unit, University of Liverpool, Royal Liverpool Hospital NHS Trust, Prescot Street, Liverpool L78XP, UK; Mersey Regional Spinal Injuries Centre, Town Lane, Kew, Southport*

R.W. PORTER, MD, FRCS, FRCSE, *Professor of Orthopaedics, Aberdeen University, University Medical Buildings, Foresterhill, Aberdeen A392ZD, Scotland, UK*

R.G. PRINGLE, FRCS, *Consultant Orthopaedic Surgeon, The Robert Jones and Agnes Hunt Orthopaedic Hospital, Oswestry, Shropshire SY107AG, UK; Consultant Orthopaedic Surgeon to Midlands Spinal Injury Unit and Royal Shrewsbury Hospital*

A.O. RANSFORD, BA(Hons), MB, BChir(Cantab), FRCS(Eng), *Orthopaedic Department, University College Hospital, 107 Harley Street, London W1, UK; Royal National Orthopaedic Hospital, Brockley Hill, Stanmore, Middlesex*

R. REID, BSc, MB, ChB, MRCPath, *Senior Lecturer in Osteoarticular Pathology and Honorary Consultant Pathologist, Osteoarticular Unit, University Department of Pathology, Western Infirmary, Glasgow G116NT, Scotland, UK*

E.B. RISKA, MD, *Professor and Head, Orthopaedic Department, Dextra Medical Centre, Rumantie La, 00350 Helsinki, Finland; Associate Professor, Department of Orthopaedics and Traumatology, Helsinki University Central Hospital, Helsinki, Finland*

T. RUSSELL, BSc(Hons), MB, ChB, FRCS(Ed), FRCS(Glas), *Consultant Neurosurgeon (Lothian Health Board), Department of Clinical Neurosciences, Western General Hospital, Crewe Road, Edinburgh EH42XU, Scotland, UK; Part-time Senior Lecturer in Neurosurgery, University of Edinburgh*

R.A. SAVAGE, MCSP, BSc, PhD, *Magnetic Resonance Research Centre, University of Liverpool, PO Box 147, Liverpool L693BX, UK*

S.C. SCHOLD, MD, *Professor of Neurology, Duke University Medical Center, PO Box 3963, Durham, NC 27710, USA*

R.J. SCOTHORNE, BSc, MD(Leeds and Chicago), FRCS(Glas), FRS(Ed), *Regius Professor of Anatomy (Emeritus), Department of Anatomy, University of Glasgow, G128QQ, Scotland, UK*

J.R. SILVER, MB, BS, FRCP(Ed and Lond), *Consultant Physician in Spinal Injuries, National Spinal Injuries Centre, Stoke Mandeville Hospital, Mandeville Road, Aylesbury, Bucks HP218AL, UK*

M.P. SINDOU, MD, DScBiol, *Professor of Neurosurgery, Department of Neurosurgery, University of Lyon, Hospital Neurologique, 59 Blvd PINEL, 69003 Lyon, France*

E.T.S. SMITH, MB, ChB, DMRD, FFR, RCSI, FRCR, *Consultant Radiologist, Walton Hospital, Rice Lane, Liverpool L91AE, UK*

M.F. SULLIVAN, MA, MB, BChir, FRCS, *Consultant Orthopaedic Surgeon, Royal National Orthopaedic Hospital, Bolsover Street, London W1, UK; Consultant Orthopaedic Surgeon, Institute of Orthopaedics, University of London; President of the European Spinal Society*

J.F. TAYLOR, MD, MChOrth, FRCS, DTM&H, *Consultant Orthopaedic Surgeon, Royal Liverpool Children's Hospital, Alder Hey, Eaton Road, Liverpool L122AP, UK*

M.J. TORRENS, BSc, MB, BS, MPhil, ChM, FRCS, *Consultant Neurosurgeon, Department of Neurosurgery, Iatriko Kentro (Athens Medical Centre), Maroussi, Athens, Greece*

N.J. TREBLE, MChOrth, FRCS, *Consultant Orthopaedic Surgeon, Department of Orthopaedics, North Devon District Hospital, Raleigh Park, Barnstaple, Devon UK; Consultant Orthopaedic Surgeon, Princess Elizabeth Orthopaedic Hospital, Wonford Road, Exeter, Devon*

H. VERBIEST, MD, PhD, Hon FRCS(Eng), *Emeritus Professor, Utrect University, Wilhelminapark 32, 3581 NH Utrecht, The Netherlands*

J.K. WEBB, FRCS, *Consultant Orthopaedic Surgeon, Harlow Wood Orthopaedic Hospital, Mansfield, Nottingham, UK*

A.I. WEIR, BSc, MSc, MB, ChB, FRCP(Glas), *Consultant Clinical Neurophysiologist, Department of Clinical Neurophysiology, Institute of Neurological Sciences, Southern General Hospital, Glasgow G514TF, Scotland, UK; Honorary Senior Clinical Lecturer, University of Glasgow*

J.C.D. WELLS, MB, ChB, FFRACS, *Director, Centre for Pain Relief, Walton Hospital, Liverpool L91AE, UK*

B. WILLIAMS, MD, ChM, FRCS, *Midland Centre for Neurosurgery and Neurology, Holly Lane, Warley, W. Midlands B677JX, UK*

S.J. WILLIAMS, FRCP, *Consultant Physician, Chest Unit, Stoke Mandeville Hospital, Mandeville Road, Aylesbury, Bucks HP21 8AL, UK*

P.J. WITHEROW, MB, ChB, FRCS, *Consultant Orthopaedic Surgeon, United Bristol Healthcare Trust, Bristol Royal Hospital for Sick Children, St Michael's Hill, Bristol BS28BJ, UK*

P.M. YEOMAN, MA, MB, BChir, MD, FRCS, *Consultant Orthopaedic Surgeon (Hon), The Royal National Hospital for Rheumatic Diseases, Bath BA1 1RL, UK*

Preface

The history of spinal surgery as we know it today extends back to the early years of this century when Sir Robert Jones established the surgical practice of Orthopaedics in Liverpool and Britain. In the years that followed, interest in all aspects of the human spine caught the imagination of many specialities, though the majority of developments occurred in the fields of orthopaedics and neurosurgery. However, it was regrettable that those disciplines showed a tendency to develop in relative isolation. Fortunately, in recent years the gap between these two specialities has begun to close with reference to the spine.

Cooperation between orthopaedists and neurosurgeons has been developing in many centres around the globe. In some of these units, the level of involvement may be restricted to certain areas but in others all aspects of spinal disease are cared for by multidisciplinary teams. These teams have arrived from different paths of training; be it orthopaedics, neurosurgery, radiology, rheumatology, rehabilitation or other allied disciplines. However, it is clear that spinal surgery has become established as a speciality in its own right and is here to stay.

With the growing interest in spinal surgery many textbooks have been published. The vast majority deal only with specific areas, such as the cervical or lumbar spine, within the greater compass of the many diseases which afflict the spine. Very few have attempted to address all those disease processes from a truly multidisciplinary approach.

For several years, we have run an annual instructional training programme which has brought together eminent orthopaedic surgeons and neurosurgeons in equal numbers from across the world to teach on the programme. The syllabus has been designed to cover every aspect of spinal disease in detail on the premise that the increased knowledge and awareness which this gives to individuals heightens their ability to practice in whatever sphere of spinal surgery is their chosen area. It also helps to lay the foundations for the training of the true spinal surgeons of the future.

The origins of this textbook of spinal surgery lie in this programme. Therefore, within this book will be found a truly comprehensive account of the most current thoughts on the nature of all conditions which affect the spinal column and its neurological contents, including their surgical management. Each chapter is written by an acknowledged expert in that field, many of whom have been actively involved in the Liverpool Spine Course over the years. To them we express our most grateful thanks, not only for their outstanding contributions but also for their continuing friendship.

GORDON FINDLAY
ROBERT OWEN
Liverpool

SIR GEORGE BEDBROOK

It was with great regret that the news of the death of Sir George Bedbrook in October of 1991 was received. One of the great pioneers of both the treatment and rehabilitation of spinal disorders, he will be sadly missed by his friends, colleagues and his many grateful patients.

SECTION 1
INTRODUCTION

1 · History and Development of Spinal Surgery

By H. VERBIEST

The organs contained in this region are: (1) the spinal cord with the spinal meninges; (2) the vertebral column from atlas to tip of coccyx included; and (3) the muscles both great and small which are attached to the vertebrae, together with the integuments that cover them. The welfare of these organs is a subject of extremely great importance, inasmuch as their integrity, considering them as a unit, is essential to the very existence of man as an animal. (John Lidell, 1884)

It was a great pleasure to receive the editors' honourable invitation to write the introductory chapter to this book.

Looking through the list of authors and the subject-matter of their contributions, one of the first thoughts which comes to mind is whether the title of this book is a forerunner of a new speciality called: spinal surgery, eventually accompanied, according to the old tradition, by its medical partner, 'spinology', in analogy to, among other things, neurology. Another question is whether spinal surgery may become a mono-speciality or be bound to teams of specialists limiting at least a great deal of their activities to particular surgical conditions of the spine.

Medical journals, books and societies may, apart from distributing new knowledge and technology, elicit chain reactions by creating a forum for research in new fields of interest. The forum in turn may provide fertile soil for the evolution of new mono- or team-specialist activities and organizations.

The two architects of this book deserve great appreciation for the achievement of their objective, especially so in our times where rumours of the impending death of the scientific book are being spread. As a matter of fact medical journals display a greater vitality than books. They are more widely distributed in libraries, and with limited budgets the libraries tend to reduce the purchase of books rather than interrupting subscriptions to their journals. Journals present a smaller lag-time in transmitting new knowledge than do books, and new knowledge is rarely first published in books. Papers in medical journals are therefore much more frequently cited than are books. Finally, authors in medical journals may have their name listed in scientific citations and other indexes that have become, rightly or wrongly, a measure of the authors' scientific dimensions. Authors of books do not benefit from these privileges, although their intellectual efforts may be greater than required for writing valuable scientific papers.

Yet medical books may have some superior qualities. They may distribute knowledge more in depth and extent, and particularly indicate its value and place in the framework of pre-existing knowledge. Findlay and Owen's book on spinal surgery presents the state and subject-matter of spinal surgery in the 1990s in full magnitude, accompanied by references to the pertinent literature of the period. In terms of Boolean logic and Venn diagrams the book presents the 'universal set' of spinal surgery, with its subsets and intersections with the sets of other specialities. Papers in journals on spinal surgery are by their nature limited to subsets. The presentation of this 'universal set' of spinal surgery is due to the multidisciplinary spectrum of the professions of the authors and to my knowledge, makes this all-inclusive book on spinal surgery the most complete volume available in this field.

Apart from its primary function as a source of orientation about the present state of theory and practice which, hopefully, will maintain this function in the future with updated new editions, the present edition will in later years become an important historical source. Readers who have access to books on spinal surgery written in different periods may obtain a better impression of the currents of ideas, their parentage, interplay, results and changes in time. Not infrequently lists of references of papers in medical journals incorrectly give the impression that the history of its authors' subject-matter covers only a few years, or has no history at all. Few readers may know, for instance, that the first techniques of laminectomy at the end of the 19th century included the placing back of the laminae and spinous processes, a method called osteoplastic laminectomy (Abbe, 1890; Dawbarn, 1889; Urban, 1892; Bickham, 1905). This technique was intended to prevent postoperative spinal instability. In later years this method became obsolete, to be recently described by some modern authors as an entirely new method.

Other such signs of collective amnesia are caused by the absence or disuse of memory systems. In addition, even modern databases are not all-inclusive, so that consulting textbooks which appeared in the period of interest may remain important in retrieving printed memory.

For future planning of spinal surgery a historical study of the determinants of its development such as parentage, field of interest, means, output, fostering needs and the national health care systems involved, may be of interest. The first three of these six determininants are primary, whereas the other three are of enhancing or inhibiting nature and vary with time and place.

An introduction cannot enter into details of the history of spinal surgery without touching upon some aspects of its origins and trends. From the beginning of modern spinal surgery until the present time its evolution was generated by both orthopaedic- and neurosurgically minded surgeons and therefore includes influences from two different fields of interest. The question arises whether orthopaedic surgery and neurosurgery will continue dominating the field of spinal surgery or give up their rights to spinal surgeons. The history of the founders of modern spinal surgery shows interesting combinations. Orthopaedic surgery is the oldest parent. It borrowed its name from the title of the book *L'Orthopédie ou l'art de prévenir et de corriger dans les enfants les difformités du corps* (1741), written by Nicholaus Andry (1658–1742), Professor of Medicine at the University of Paris. The Greek roots of the term 'orthopedia', and the title of Andry's book, indicated that prevention and care of abnormalities of bones and joints should begin at an early age.

Autonomous orthopaedic institutes were already founded in the late 18th and early 19th centuries: at the Swiss town of Orbe (1790), in Birmingham (1817), and the Royal Orthopaedic Hospital in London (1837). The only early succesful spinal operations were tenotomies of the sterno-cleido-mastoid muscles for torticollis, first practised by an open approach in 1651 by the Dutchman Isaac De Minne, also called Isacius Minnius. It concerned the 12-year-old son of a burgomeister of Middelburg. His head was 'stiff' and kept inclined towards the left shoulder. Willem van der Straeten, the court physician of William II, Prince of Orange, advised that the 'tight band that pulled the head to the shoulder' should be interrupted from the ear unto the trachea. Minnius first applied a caustic solution upon the skin in this area, and when it had changed into a crust he inserted a knife above the clavicle. Minnius remarked that the interruption of the muscles was performed by stabbing rather than by cutting. After the operation the head could be moved in all directions. The patient survived the operation. This case was reported by Nicolaas Tulp (1593–1674) in his *Observationes Medicae* (1652), well known because they also contained the first descriptions of beri-beri disease and Tulp's valve, as well as the first illustration of rachischizis. Nicolaas Tulp is the dissector in Rembrandt's 'The lesson in anatomy'.

The more modern subcutaneous tenotomies for torticollis were developed in the first half of the 19th century by the German Stromeyer (1833) and introduced to England by Little (1839). Guérin, a French orthopaedic surgeon, who shared Andry's view that spinal scoliosis had a myogenic aetiology, performed subcutaneus myotomies of the posterior spinal muscles on the concave side of the curvature (1839). Malgaigne (1844) performed a similar technique but the results were disappointing.

The outcome of other operations upon the spine, with the exception of rare reports on successful removal of sequesters or evacuation of abscesses in cases of Pott's spondylitis, and of very rare cases of improvement of traumatic spinal cord deficit following 'trephining' of the laminae, were not rewarding and often were disastrous. The most characteristic therapeutic means of spinal orthopaedics in that early period were various mechanical devices for external application in cases of spinal deformity or instability.

In the second half of the 19th century societies were founded for the care of the crippled and the deformed in many countries. The first real orthopaedic journals were founded in France in 1880 (*Revue illustré de Polytechnique médical et de Chirurgie orthopédique*, Paris, Labellond et Chanet); in Germany in 1884 (*Zentralblatt für orthopedische Chirurgie*, Von Beely, Bern); in Italy in 1884 (*Archivio di Ortopedia*, Panzeri e Margery, Milan); and in the USA in 1889 (*Transactions of the American Orthopedic Association*). Hoffa and Blenckes' book (1905) of references to the orthopaedic 'world' literature, mainly of the 19th century and the first three years of the 20th century, covers 70 of its 446 pages with references to spinal papers and books, but among their authors there were also general surgeons and neurologists.

These data show that orthopaedics was well established when, in the modern era of surgery, the first spinal operations were performed. According to the old tradition, the first orthopaedic spinal operations consisted of treating spinal instability, such as occurred in various types of scoliosis, spinal fractures, poliomyelitis and Pott's disease. The first operations to this purpose consisted of immobilizing the unstable spinal portion with the use of foreign material, initially through wiring (Hadra, 1891; Chipault, 1896). In later years Lange described the use of celluloid plates combined with metal bars in some cases combined with wiring (1910, 1924). The effects of these operations were disappointing. Better results were obtained in the early 20th century with the use of autologous bone grafts (Albee, 1911; Hibbs, 1911; MacKenzie, 1920).

In later years, when the occurrence of Pott's disease and poliomyelitic paralysis of spinal muscles diminished considerably, traumatic and degenerative spinal conditions became the most frequent fields of activity for both orthopaedic surgeons and neurosurgeons but the treatment of scoliosis and kyphoscoliosis remained, true to Andry's message, the inalienable field of orthopaedics.

Neurosurgery is a much younger speciality than orthopaedics. It was only after the development of knowledge of the external and internal anatomy of the nervous system in the 17th and 18th century, and of the function of various nervous structures in the 19th century, complemented by the introduction of asepsis, antisepsis and anaesthesia, that the Scottish surgeon Macewen, in 1883 and 1884, performed the first decompressive laminectomies in two paraplegic patients with Pott's disease with good results (Macewen, 1884, 1885). The English surgeon, Victor Horsley, was the first (in 1887) to remove a dural spinal fibromyxoma, with equally good results (Gowers & Horsley, 1888).

Both surgeons also performed brain surgery, Macewen even six years earlier (1881) than Horsley (1887). Horsley's research (1892, 1908, 1909) and the development of surgical techniques, such as the use of antiseptic wax for arresting haemorrhage from cancellous bone (Horsley, 1892) and the development of a stereotactic apparatus (Horsley, 1908) for the nervous system, allowed the development of the prototype of the neurosurgeon. Macewen's practice, on the contrary, also included osteotomies for treating bony deformities of the extremities, laboratory research on osteogenesis, bone growth, auto-, homo- and heterologous transplantation of bone in animals, and reparative surgery of bones with auto- and homologous, particularly cancellous, bone grafts (Macewen, 1878, 1912). Macewen not only combined orthopaedic surgery and neurosurgery, he also performed the first pneumectomy for tuberculosis (1895), the patient surviving for at least 40 years. In addition, he introduced chromic catgut as suture material and endotracheal intubation as an alternative of tracheostomy (Macewen, quoted by Earl Walker, 1951, and by Jennett, 1985).

The merits of Macewen and Horsley are still cited, but at the turn of the 19th century there was a third impressive pioneer in spinal surgery, whose name was frequently cited during his lifetime but became almost completely forgotten in later years. This may be due to the fact that all his writings were in French, and also to his own decision to leave no trace of the last 15 years of his short life. His name was Antonie Maxime Chipault (1866–1920), and he was born in Orléans, France. His father was a surgeon. He graduated at Paris University in 1890 and had training in surgery, neurology, obstetrics, gynaecology, otology and facial surgery. He worked as an assistant in the anatomical laboratory and was elected a member of the French anatomical society in 1891. His doctoral thesis (1894a) on the anatomical relationship between the spinous processes and the spinal nerve roots was important at a time when radiology was not yet available, so that levels of spinal cord lesions were localized by means of disturbances observed in myotomal or dermatomal areas, and determination of the levels of entrance into the vertebral canal of the spinal nerves involved.

In the period between 1890 and 1894 Chipault had already published 40 papers, 13 of them on spinal surgery, four on cranial surgery and the others mainly on affections of bones and joints other than of the spine and skull. In 1894 he published his book on spinal surgery: *Etudes de Chirurgie Médulaire. Historique, Chirurgie Opératoire, Traitement*, that in 400 pages, presented the most complete survey of past and present spinal surgery at that time (Chipault, 1894b). In 1896 he started a specialistic yearbook, *Travaux de Neurologie Chirurgicale*, that from 1898 became a quarterly journal, and the first neurosurgical journal in the world. In 1897 he described with the radiologist Londe their first roentgenographic experiences with the skull and spine. The exposure times varied between 20 and 50 minutes, during which period the patients had to remain absolutely still. In 1904 his book: *Manuel d'Orthopédie Vertébrale* was published. It is a textbook that begins with the orthopaedic physiology and anatomy of the spine, followed by chapters on Pott's disease, traumatic deformities, adolescent scoliosis and all sorts of other causes of spinal deviations or deformities. He distinguished a separate entity, the 'scoliose souplé' as a consequence of muscular–ligamentous laxity. He also described wiring of spinous processes, laminae and of transverse processes as stabilizing operations (Chipault, 1896) Finally, in 1902–03 three large volumes on the actual state of *Chirurgie nerveuse* were published under the supervision of Chipault, where in 2826 pages neurological surgeons of all developed countries of the world reported on the state of neurosurgery in their homeland in that period (for Great Britain: Mr Ch. A. Ballance, surgeon at St Thomas and the National Hospital in London; Mr R. Kennedy of the Western Infirmary and St Andrew's University Hospital in Glasgow; Mr A. Thomson, Royal Infirmary in Edinburgh; and Mr Rodocanachi, who worked with Sir William Thorburn at the Royal Infirmary of Manchester). At the end of the third volume is a subject index that facilitates, for instance, finding descriptions of the state of vertebral surgery in the various countries with references to pertinent literature. It is interesting to read in Londe's contribution (1902) that the exposure time of a radiograph of the spine was 3 minutes instead of the 20–50 minutes exposure 15 years earlier. This series contains historical treasures for spinal surgeons. Of Chipault's 90 papers published in various journals a fair number involved non-spinal orthopaedic subjects. In addition he published a textbook on surgery of the nervous system (Chipault, 1894c/1895).

Chipault was a very extraordinary person. He held no official position in any Paris hospital but seems to have operated in various hospitals. In all his books and papers he mentions his name as 'Chipault de Paris'. For authors in his yearbook and later quarterly he mentions his home address, 24 Rue Hallé in Paris, as the editorial office. When he published with co-authors they were always renowned medical specialists. He produced this tremendous activity, while he was a bachelor, in a period of 14 years, as if he sensed that soon, in 1905 at the age of 39, he would develop a slowly progressive paraplegia of unknown origin that caused his disappearance from the medical scene. On 31 December 1907, he married Mrs Janine Poiret, and adopted a son. The family retired to Orchamps in the Jura where Antonie died in 1920. No trace of relatives of Chipault could be detected by Professor Petit Dutaillis or by Patric Baduel (1980, 1981) who wrote his thesis on Antonie Chipault.

Neurosurgery as a speciality in its own right began with the foundation of the first neurosurgical societies: the Society of Neurological Surgeons in the USA (1920) and the British Society of Neurological Surgeons (1926).

A milestone in spinal surgery between the two world wars was the joint publication of the neurosurgeon W. J. Mixter and the orthopaedic surgeon J. S. Barr, in the *New England Journal of Medicine* (1934), that established the relation between traumatic or degenerative lumbar disc herniations and sciatica.

The desire to remove caries of the vertebral body or pus in its vicinity in Pott's disease had already induced the general surgeon Sir Frederick Treves to approach the lumbar vertebral bodies through a paravertebral approach with resection of transverse processes (1884, 1892), while the orthopaedic surgeon Vincent (1892) approached the diseased thoracic vertebral bodies bilaterally and extrapleurally via the intercostal spaces or, if necessary, after resection of one or more ribs.

Another orthopaedic surgeon, Ménard (1894, 1895) developed an extrapleural approach via a method called costotransversectomy. In this pre-radiographic period the top of the gibbus was the localizing landmark. In 1954 the orthopaedic surgeon Capener performed costotransversectomy plus ipsilateral laminectomy and removal of the posterolateral joints at two levels for removing protruding posterior bony ridges of vertebral bodies that produced paraplegia as a result of kyphosis in Pott's disease. In order to prevent resulting instability following this type of operation it was modified by the neurosurgeons Norman Dott (1947) and G. L. Alexander (1946) by limiting it to an extrapleural exposure only, after performance of a sufficient number of costotransversectomies.

These experiences encouraged the approach of tumours of the vertebral bodies. Boudreaux, who was trained in general, orthopaedic and neurosurgery described in 1936 a number of direct approaches to the vertebral bodies in the various spinal regions, but reported on only one case of a surgical approach, without laminectomy, of a vertebral body tumour in the cervical region. This operation was performed by the neurosurgeon Petit Dutaillis. No mention was made of reparative surgery after tumour removal from the body. Guleke, in 1935, described similar approaches without comment on repair or replacement of the vertebral body, and no case reports were presented.

I still have a vivid memory of our first efforts in this field. In 1942 (Verbiest, 1947, 1965) we removed a giant cell tumour from the body of L5 in a 35-year-old female by means of laminectomy, leaving only the posterolateral joints, the transverse processes and the very thinned endplates of the body of L5 intact. The residual upper and lower endplates of the L5 body fused with each other without producing kyphotic deformity. Twenty years later the alignment of the lumbosacral junction was normal and there was no tumour recurrence.

In a second case, a 40-year-old male, a chordoma of the 12th thoracic vertebral body had invaded the epidural space. Encouraged by previous experience the tumour was removed from the epidural space and curetted from the vertebral body via laminectomy. An Albee fusion was performed (July 1945). The patient was free from signs and symptoms until April 1946 when he developed severe back pain. The X-rays showed fracture of the Albee grafts and cuneiform collapse of the body of T12 with resulting kyphosis. There was abnormal movement at this level. Via left and right costotransversectomies in two stages (April and May 1946) the entire body of T12 was removed. After this operation the anterior inferior border of the body of T11, that was already near to the anterior superior border of the body of L1, was seen to fuse with this body. At the last check-up, eight months later, the patient was pain-free, the kyphosis was stabilized but he needed the support of a brace because of low back ache. The patient did not return for further follow-up.

In 1952 we performed complete vertebrectomy of C5, in a quadriplegic 29-year-old female (Verbiest, 1970, 1986). The X-rays showed osteolysis of the body of C5 and 8° kyphosis above that level. First the body was removed via an anterolateral approach, and six months later the other vertebral structures were removed through a posterior approach, followed by an Albee fusion from C3 to C7. The pathology was a solitary plasmocytoma. After the operation the kyphosis had increased to 13°. The quadriplegia disappeared completely and at the last check-up, 27 years later, the patient was free from signs and symptoms.

Our first experience of good vertebral alignment following corporectomy of L5 was not confirmed by these two cases of corporectomy at higher vertebral levels. Therefore, in 1958, we were more careful with our fourth case, a 23-year-old girl, in whom the third lumbar vertebral body was removed by means of a right anterolateral extraperitoneal approach because it was invaded by a giant-cell tumour. The postoperative alignment of the lumbar spine was regularly checked radiologically while the patient was nursed in a plaster cast. When it was found that the gap between the L2 and L4 bodies diminished, with some anterior angulation, the empty space was occluded via a left retroperitoneal approach by means of tibial cortical grafts anteriorly and posteriorly while the space between these grafts was obliterated with cancellous bone. The patient was immobilized in plaster for six months, resulting in good fusion with only minor anterior angulation. Preoperative paralysis of toes and feet recovered within one month. At last follow-up, 22 years later, the fusion had not changed and the patient was free from signs and symptoms. One year after this operation Sicard (1959) described in his book, *Chirurgie du Rachis*, various approaches to tumours of the vertebral bodies, but still did not pay attention to the repair of destroyed, or replacement of removed, vertebral bodies.

In 1960 we corrected a cervical kyphosis due to collapse of the sixth cervical vertebral body involved in malignant degeneration of a giant-cell tumour by replacement of that body with tibial cortical grafts. It was a much easier performance than in the lumbar area. In the same year Boling *et al.* reported on partial or total replacement of vertebral bodies by bone grafts. With one exception the follow-ups were only a few months. The neurosurgeon Cloward (1960) replaced the C3 and C4 bodies invaded by a neurofibroma by an iliac graft obtained from a cadaver. The follow-up was also short, seven months only, but the surgery of vertebral bodies had entered the field of interest of spinal surgeons.

In 1961 Cloward reported on his anterior burrhole and dowel bone anterior fusion for the treatment of fractures and fracture dislocations of the spine. In 1962 and 1969, we reported on three different methods of anterior operations upon the cervical spine for the repair of various types of traumatic deformities. Senning *et al.* (1962) developed a telescoping metallic vertebral body prosthesis, and in 1967 the neurosurgeon Scoville and co-workers (1967) reported on the use of acrylic in replacing vertebral bodies.

The orthopaedic surgeons Robinson and Smith (1955) performed the first anterolateral cervical intervertebral disc surgery with interbody fusion, followed by Dereymaeker and Mulier, neurosurgeon and orthopaedic surgeon respectively (1956). Whereas these surgeons limited their intervention to the disc space Cloward (1958) introduced a larger but more destructive access to the disc space, that allowed a more radical excision of posterior protrusions and osteophytes. Whereas Robinson and Smith were of the opinion that the treatment of spondylotic myelopathy could be limited to interbody fusion, the osteophytes protruding from the posterior rims of the vertebral body disappearing spontaneously after this procedure, we could not confirm this view, and removed the posterior osteophytes by means of an anterior transdiscal approach (Verbiest & Paz y Geuze, 1966). Since this approach carried a risk of damaging the spinal cord, we extended the method of uncusectomy, first developed by Jung (1963), for the removal of uncal osteophytes to a lateral transdiscal approach for the removal of central posterior osteophytes (Verbiest, 1968). This brings to a close the story of the milestones of pioneer spinal surgery.

Since 1960 some surgical techniques have been refined but it has been the ancillary sciences which have subsequently promoted the evolution of spinal surgery, especially imaging techniques, clinical neurophysiology and biomechanics. The early evolution of radiographic imaging methods of the spine and its neural contents, such as: tomography (Vallebona, 1930; Ziedses des Plantes, 1932, 1934, 1973); radiographic subtraction (Ziedes des Plantes, 1934, 1961); and spinal angiography (Djindjian *et al.*, 1968) presented no major problems in interpretation for either orthopaedic surgeons or neurosurgeons. However, the evolution of more recent methods—such as bone scanning, computerized tomographic (CT) scanning and three-dimensional reconstruction, digital subtraction imaging and magnetic resonance imaging (MRI)—demand high-quality radiological interpretation. This has resulted in a much closer relationship between radiologists with a spinal interest and spine surgeons.

The basic principles of the methods of modern clinical neurophysiological examination of the spinal cord and nerve roots, such as electromyography (EMG) (Adrian & Bronk, 1929), nerve conduction (Hodes *et al.*, 1948), F responses (Maglarady & McDougal, 1950), H reflexes (Hoffmann, 1918) and somatosensory evoked potentials (Dawson, 1947), were already established between 1925 and 1950. It was the introduction of the computer, allowing for more exact quantitative processing of a great number of various data and automatic analysis of the findings, combined with refinements in electrodes and stimulators, that prepared the field of the new speciality of neurophysiology. It also lured the orthopaedic spinal surgeons to the field of the neurosciences.

It is not the only field of the neurosciences that is of interest to the spinal surgeon. Other topics are the body-posture regulating neural systems and, particularly, problems in distinguishing between nociceptive, referred and deafferentation pains in spinal disorders. The treatment of chronic vertebrogenic and radicular pain had to liberate itself from the idea that transmission of the painful message is only determined by nerve tracts and synapses, but that chemical transmission has an important share. An ever-growing number of neuroactive peptides, such as neurotransmitters, modulators or other function types of neuromediators, are being identified. The same holds for corresponding responsive postsynaptic receptors. There is some system in the distribution of these various neuroactive substances involved in the chemical transmission of information so that they may be mapped as a sort of chemical anatomy of the central nervous system (Nieuwenhuys, 1985). The new findings shattered oversimplified conceptions and the resulting treatment of vertebrogenic and so-called radicular pains.

Biomechanics, initiated in the 17th century by Borelli (1680, 1681, 1989) became the scientific basis of orthopaedics. Fick, in 1911, wrote an early and extensive contribution to spinal biomechanics. Gilles de la Tourette and Chipault (1898) had already discovered the relation between spinal and spinal cord biomechanics by demonstrating that flexion of the spine produced lengthening of the spinal cord. In later years Breig (1960, 1978) made major contributions to the interrelation between biomechanics of the spine, spinal cord and nerve roots. The present author reported on improvement of chronic or late onset of spinal cord function by relieving traction and anterior compression of the cord through reduction of vertebral displacement or correction of traumatic kyphosis (Verbiest, 1962, 1969).

This short historical review demonstrates the evolution of the practice of spinal surgery as it was influenced by the development of scientific research, and differences of interest that resulted in the evolution of orthopaedic and neurosurgical approaches to the spine.

The increase in factual knowledge has also generated concepts on a more abstract level. Physicists have, for a long time, been far ahead of medical professionals in approaching the most basic scientific aspects of their science, namely the analysis of empirical knowledge and of the logic of their reasoning. In modern medicine similar attention is being given to methods of longitudinal prospective and retrospective studies of the natural history of disease, methods of clinical trials and systems of diagnostic logic as guides in clinical decision-making.

Basic writings on the explosive influence of imaging methods of the spine in diagnostic thinking are still limited (Verbiest, 1983; Wackenheim, 1986). Imaging methods in the diagnosis of diseases of the spine itself led to the development of new concepts on vertebral anatomy at a macrolevel. This may appear amazing, since it concerns visible anatomy that is supposed to have been exhaustively described in previous years. Examples are the concept of the vertebral motion segment, introduced in 1952 by Junghanns (1968), and the concepts of the cervical intertransverse space (discussed in Chapter 46).

The explanation of changes in macro-anatomical concepts of the spine involve the psycho-philosophical differences between looking and seeing. Seeing is different from looking, in that seeing is subject to experience and learning processes. Before entering into details of this particular subject a short excursion in some theories of human knowledge, demonstrated with practical examples concerning medical aspects of the spine, is justified.

The anatomists of the Graeco-Roman and Mediaeval periods were not worried by questions about whether the objects perceived in the external world exist and act independently of our knowledge or only exist in the human mind. Their anatomical descriptions manifested a certain naivety mixed with idealistic interpretations of unseen mechanisms of functions and teleological views about their purposes. The philosopher Immanuel Kant (1724–1804) was the first to make a distinction between the existence of objects in the external world and the way they become objects of our senses. He stressed that it is impossible to acquire knowledge of what things are 'in themselves' ('Ding an sich'). We can only know the appearance of objects as determined by their influence upon our sense organs. In Kant's view the human mind is provided with principles, called categories, which order sensory data into perceptions as subjects of thought processes and judgements.

The physicist Ernst Mach (1838–1916) was impressed by Kant's theories but he approached the mechanism of human knowledge free from philosophical considerations (Mach, 1886, 1959). He was of the opinion that the physiological processes involved in knowledge are not different from the physical processes in dead nature. In comparison with chemistry Mach called the primitive sensory data, such as colour or sound, the sensory elements. Our perception of things is more complex than a sum of sensory data. Perception involves arrangements of sensory input into some order, making an impression of objects, situations or occurrences that Mach called 'Gestalten' (plural of the German 'Gestalt'). This word has been assimilated into the English language. In present-day terms 'Gestalt' perception would be interpreted as resulting from cerebral modulation of the input of sensory data. Experience and memory have a part in this modulating activity. Mach's theories initiated the development of 'Gestalt psychology' by, amongst others: von Ehrenfels (1892); Koffka (1912, 1935); and Köhler (1947, 1971). The Gestalt theories have been criticized for their holistic views

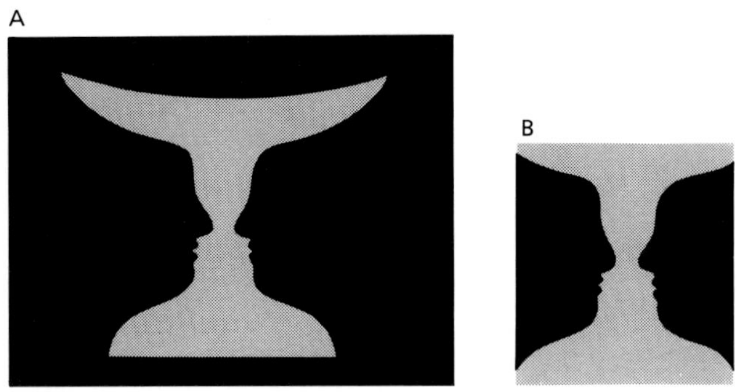

Fig. 1.1 A test figure demonstrating a Gestalt phenomenon. The observer of A may either perceive the bowl or the profiles of two opposite human faces, detailed in B.

stating that the Gestalt is more than the sum of its parts.

Sherrington (1951) clearly criticized this holistic theory by writing that the Gestalt is not 'more than' but 'other than' the sum of its constituents, and that the Gestalt has a function that none of its parts possesses. In addition, later research demonstrated that the Gestalt theories do not hold for all sorts of perceptions. Some of its concepts, however, are interesting in the study of the development of imaging methods of the spine. The Gestalt psychologies added, for instance, to Mach's theory of Gestalt perception that it is impossible to perceive a Gestalt without a (back)ground; the property of this (back)ground being that it is less distinct even when it contains other Gestalten. The occurrence of the latter mechanism is demonstrated by the well-known test figure allowing the perception of either the 'Gestalt' of a vase or the Gestalten of two opposite profiles of faces (Fig. 1.1). It is never possible, however, to perceive both the vase and the profiles of faces at the same time. Either of them may alternate as a 'figure' or vanish in a 'ground' when the other one assumes Gestalt function. Most observers of the test figure detect only one of the two possible Gestalten. It raises the question about what determines the selection between the two possible Gestalt perceptions. An explanation may be that one of the two alternative Gestalten represents qualities of a more obvious Gestalt, but personal experience may equally determine the unconscious selection. With one of the two alternative Gestalten perceived, the perception of the other one is suppressed for the need of its background function. This means that a voluntary effort is needed to analyse whether the background may contain other Gestalten.

These facts explain possible pitfalls in the interpretation of CT spinal images, as may be illustrated by the following example. In our experience most radiological records of CT scans of stenotic vertebral canals contain descriptions of the conditions of its walls without mentioning measurements of diameters or of the cross-sectional surface areas of the vertebral canal, although only the latter measurements provide direct proof of the presence of stenosis. The description of the walls is equally important for a diagnosis of the cause(s) of the stenosis. Neglected analysis of the canal may be due to the fact that CT scans with window level and width on hard tissue level do not present a structure of the canal that borrows its shape from the outlining bony structures. With window setting on soft tissue level the structures of the dural theca or nerve roots draw the attention as Gestalten at the expense of the background function of the remaining hypodense portions of the vertebral canal. Therefore the Gestalt of the canal is much weaker, and lends itself more readily to background function in the diagnostic analysis of CT scans.

Another pitfall is that perception of the whole of the Gestalt may lead to neglecting the analysis of its parts. This neglect may be enhanced by the so-called 'closure phenomenon'. A striking example of this fact in the interpretation of spinal CT images has been published by van Schaik *et al.* (1985). During morphometric studies of the lower lumbar vertebral bodies in CT scans it was concluded that because of the frequent wedge shape of the L5 body, it does not present an interface for the orthogonal X-rays in AP views. Consequently it was to be expected that AP views of the L5 body usually do not visualize its lateral borders. This postulated finding was verified by examining AP views of L5 vertebral bodies. Up to that time we had been completely unaware of this fact. Interviewing a number of radiologists in our own country and other countries revealed that this fact was equally unknown to them. This is an example of the 'closure phenomenon'. With this phenomenon an incomplete Gestalt pattern showing much similarity to a known Gestalt tends to be perceived as if it is completed into that Gestalt. Since all vertebral bodies, with the exception of C2 and L5, present lateral borders in AP views they tend to represent the prototype of the normal Gestalt of vertebral bodies. Through the closure phenomenon the missing lateral borders of the L5 body in AP X-ray view are 'filled in' during the process of perception. It is obvious that this mechanism may be reinforced by the well-known propensity to neglect the analysis of all parts forming the Gestalt, that is, in the present case, of all borders of each vertebral body visualized in the AP view.

If radiologists or other specialists interested in the spine had systematically analysed all parts of the L5 body in AP X-ray views, the frequent non-visualization of its lateral borders would not have passed unnoticed.

Teaching is an important extra-observer influence in avoiding pitfalls in Gestalt perception such as discussed above. Radiological diagnostic protocol prescribing the various steps in the making of a diagnosis might be helpful, although it does not promote creative 'seeing' in radiology.

A particular property of the Gestalt is that it induces the observor to think of its function, and that on the other hand functions may induce new Gestalt perception. Discoveries of new functions may alter the structure of a previously admitted Gestalt. The development of a new surgical approach to the cervical spine (Verbiest, 1968) led to the concept of the cervical intertransverse space (see Chapter 46) and a review of the definition of the intervertebral foramen.

The sensory data composing perception are volatile when the corresponding object is removed from the field of the sense organs. There remains, however, a more permanent core, that Russell (1980) called the 'perceptive experience'. It is less distinct than the perception. It is a product of empirical knowledge and judgements about its reality. Humans report on their perceptions, judgements and other thought products verbally and react with behavioural responses. Knowledge, language and behaviour are mutually dependent variables. Erroneous use of each of the three affects the other two, and each of the three may control errors in the functions of the other two.

The value of these general principles applied to the study of the spine may be demonstrated with the following examples. Vertebrae are very complex Gestalten that may be decomposed into a number of more elementary Gestalten, such as the body, the posterolateral joints, the intervertebral disc. From another point of view Junghanns (1952, 1968) divided the spine into vertebral segments and motion segments. The vertebral segments consist of the bony structures. Motion segments form the connections between the vertebrae allowing for the mobility of vertebrae upon their neighbours. With the exception of the C1–C2 motion segment that contains no intervertebral disc, each of the other 23 motion segments consists of an intervertebral disc, capsules and ligaments connecting the bony structures of adjoining vertebrae.

Penning (1968), in his monograph that appeared before the introduction of CT body imaging, wrote that the vertebral segments are radiographically visible while the motion segments manifest themselves as the empty spaces between the vertebral segments. The mobility in the motion segments could be measured by means of ranges of displacement between adjacent vertebral segments by comparing profile X-rays with the spine in flexion and extension, and AP views with the spine in left and right lateral flexion or with rotation to the left and the right. In that period disease of the motion segment could be visualized through flattening of, and vacuum phenomena inside, the disc space, shift of facet joints and reactive changes of skeletal structures. With modern imaging through CT and MRI the motion segments are no longer represented by empty spaces, since pathological changes and abnormal displacement of the soft tissue structrues of the motion segments are visualized. The components of the motion segment can be perceived but the motion segment itself is conceptual rather than perceptional. Yet, with the concept of the motion segment, the question arises whether the term intervertebral disc disease is based upon logical and practicable inferences. The structures of the motion segment are regularly interacting and interdependent. Pathological changes of the intervertebral disc always disturb the function of the structures of the motion segment, and may do this through production of shifts between the posterolateral facets and through reactive osteophyte formation at the borders of the vertebral bodies and of the posterolateral joint spaces. Replacing the term 'disc disease' by 'motion segment disease' is no wordmongering, since languages influence precepts and concepts in diagnostic thinking.

Some effects of disc disease such as reactive osteophytes or protrusions may interfere with neural functions. After Mixter and Barr's paper disc protrusions became recognized as a frequent cause of radicular pains. The cause (disc protrusion) to effect (radicular signs and symptoms) relationship had to be reviewed with the demonstration of large asymptomatic disc protrusions. It might be an indication that discogenic radicular pathology also depends upon 'causes' inside the nerve roots. CT scans after chymopapain treatment or percutaneous nucleotomy in cases of disc protrusions with radicular pain have demonstrated that in some of the cases the radicular pains may disappear while the size of the disc protrusion did not change. It is through imaging methods that we learn that the pathology of the disc is more directly determinant in producing disturbances of the motion segment than in the production of neural pathology.

When I had reported my first cases of stenosis of the vertebal canal it appeared to me that, in addition to the condition of the vertebral and the motion segments advanced by Junghanns as the two basic categories in the diagnosis of spinal disease, the condition of the capacity of the vertebal canal is equally important and completes a triad of basic categories (Verbiest, 1954).

Language is an important carrier of thoughts. Creeping careless use of language and definition is, for instance, encountered in a classification of stenosis of the vertebral canal where stenosis as a disease and stenosis as a symptom of another disease are listed under a common denominator. With the explosive growth of medical terminology, nomenclature committees have been active in the past years in purifying terminology and defining their meanings. It is a difficult task that should not freeze living language but prevent its careless use. Cooperation with linguists may be needed. The remarkable fact remains that, for instance, when speaking of vertebral instability everyone seems to understand what it means, but no satisfactory definition of vertebral instability has been generally accepted at the present time.

Who will be the future leaders of spinal surgery? The responses of medical society to the evolution of spinal surgery may be divided into unifying and diversifying trends. This is actually most evident in the housing of spinal surgery. There already exist spinal units in some hospitals in modern countries, usually as subdivisions of orthopaedic or surgical clinics. In other areas traumatic spinal lesions are treated in trauma centres and rehabilitation centres; neoplastic affections in oncological institutes; and scoliosis in specifically adapted centres. Spinal surgery requires the formation of teams in units where all-inclusive surgical and/or medical treatment of spinal diseases can be practised.

As to future health planning the question arises whether these different patterns of evolution or more unifying trends in organization of spinal surgery should be facilitated by the national health authorities. The pace of prominent surgeons in the field of spinal disorders has been cautious, and has not yet resulted in the birth of the prototype of the specialist in all-inclusive spinal surgery of both spinal column and its neural contents. The differences in vocation between orthopaedists and neurosurgeons are determined by moving spirits that are difficult to analyse. For the time being it is highly improbable that the average neurosurgeon would desire to treat kyphoscoliosis because it resulted in spinal cord deficit, or that an orthopaedic surgeon would wish to treat an intramedullary tumour since it has caused scoliosis. Such attitudes, whatever their origin may be, are prime movers in self-limitation of fields of interest.

In general there is a greater interest of orthopaedic surgeons than of neurosurgeons in spinal surgery. All neurosurgeons count the treatment of the neural content of the vertebral column within the field of their activities, but relatively few of them are genuinely interested in treating pathological conditions of the spine. The orthopaedic surgeons have maintained their superiority in the field of biomechanics, the use of foreign materials and of internal or external instrumentation. The treatment of scoliosis and kyphoscoliosis has remained their untransferable domain.

In a speculative paper (Verbiest, 1989) the author demonstrated that among members of multidisciplinary spine societies, or authors of books on spinal disorders, the orthopaedic surgeons outnumbered neurosurgeons. Such facts may be of influence in the development of spinal surgery. Training programmes have a similar role. In earlier years orthopaedic surgeons and neurosurgeons had received full training in general surgery. In later years it was rightly observed that training in visceral surgery is not needed for making good orthopaedic surgeons or neurosurgeons, so that general surgery was very much reduced or almost disappeared from their curriculum. I have encountered orthopaedic surgeons and neurosurgeons from various countries who had not learned how and where to open a thorax or abdomen, or to approach the cervical spine for an adequate exposure of the vertebral bodies. This was the reason they limited their surgery to posterior approaches of the spine.

Both editors of the present book can look back on a great history of their home town in the fields of neurosciences and orthopaedic surgery. Hugh Owen

Thomas (1834–91) and his nephew Robert Jones (1858–1933) were internationally known founders of modern orthopaedic surgery in Liverpool, and they prepared the cradle of the famous Robert Jones and Agnes Hunt Orthopaedic Hospital at Oswestry. The history of Liverpool neurosurgery is more recent, but years earlier, from 1895 to 1913, Sherrington did his remarkable neurophysiological research in Liverpool, where he was visited by the father of neurosurgery, Harvey Cushing, and the Utrecht Professor Rudolf Magnus, widely known because of his book on body posture *Körperstellung* (1924).

Both editors organize annual multidisciplinary courses on spinal disorders in the Liverpool Medical Institution (more than 150 years old) that harbours the famous Medical Library, founded in 1779. Professor Robert Owen became the first president of the British Cervical Spine Society and his successor was the neurosurgeon Philip Harris. Gordon Findlay is a founder member of the European Spine Society, which is a multidisciplinary society encompassing interests in all aspects of spinal disease. The cooperation between orthopaedic surgeons, neurosurgeons and practitioners of the auxiliary sciences, that was initiated in Liverpool and laid down in the present book, seems for the time being the best mechanism for guiding future spinal surgery through its complicated development.

REFERENCES

Abbe, R. (1890) Spinal surgery—a report of eight cases. *Med. Rec.*, **38**, 85.

Adrian, A.D. & Bronk, D.W. (1929) The discharge of impulses in motor nerve fibres. Part II. *J. Physiol.*, **67**, 119.

Albee, F.H. (1911) Transplantation of a portion of the tibia into the spine for Pott's disease: a preliminary report. *J. Am. Med. Assoc.*, **57**, 885.

Alexander, G.L. (1946) Neurological complications of spinal tuberculosis. *Proc. Roy. Soc. Med.*, **39**, 730.

Baduel, P. (1980) L'oeuvre neuro-chirurgicale d'Anthonie Chipault 1866–1920, Thèse pour le Doctorat en Médecine, Université de Rennes.

Baduel, P. & Bucy, P.C. (1981) Antony Chipault, 1860–1920. *Surg. Neurol.*, **16**, 165.

Bickham, W.S. (1905) Technique of exposure of the spinal cord and canal; osteoplastic resection and laminectomy. *Ann. Surg.*, **41**, 372.

Boling, M.D., Taxdal, D. & Robinson, R.A. (1960) Six case histories demonstrating the feasibility of partial or total replacement of vertebral bodies by bone grafts. *Am. Surg.*, **26**, 236.

Borelli, J.A. (1680, 1681) *De Motus Animalium*. Bernado, Rome.

Borelli, J.A. (1989) *On the Movement of Animals* (transl. by P. Maquet). Springer, London.

Boudreaux, J. (1936) *Les tumeurs primitives du rachis*. Vigot, Paris.

Breig, A. (1960) *Biomechanics of the Central Nervous System*. Almqvist, Stockholm.

Breig, A. (1978) *Adverse Mechanical Tension in the Central Nervous System*. Almqvist, Stockholm; John Wiley, New York.

Capener, N. (1954) The evolution of lateral rachotomy. *J. Bone. Jt. Surg.*, **36B**, 173.

Chipault, A. (1894a) Les rapports des apophyses épineuses avec la moëlle, les racines médullaires et les méninges. Thèse pour le doctorat en médecine, Université de Paris.

Chipault, A (1894b) *Etudes de Chirurgie Médullaire*. Alcan, Paris.

Chipault, A. (1894c, 1895) *Chirurgie Opératoire du Système Nerveux*, 2 vol s. Rueff, Paris.

Chipault, A. (1896) L'Orthopédie rachidienne opératoire: ligature et suture des vertèbres; quatre interventions, l'une contre une luxation cervicale ballante, trois autres contre des gibbosités pottiques rapidement croissantes. *Trav. Neurol. Chir.*, **1**, 222.

Chipault, A. (1896–1907) *Travaux de Neurologie Chirurgicale*. Vigot Frères, Paris.

Chipault, A. (1904) *Manuel d'Orthopédie Vertébrale*. Maloine, Paris.

Chipault, A. (1902, 1903) *L'État Actuel de la Chirurgie Nerveuse*. Rueff, Paris. I, 1902; II, 1903; III, 1903.

Chipault, A. & Londe, A. (1897) Des applications de la radiographie à la chirurgie du système nerveux. *Travaux de Neurologie Chirurgicale*, 2ème Année, 1–14.

Cloward, R.B. (1958) The anterior approach for removal of ruptured cervical disks. *J. Neurosurg.*, **15**, 602.

Cloward, R.B. (1960) Destruction of cervical vertebrae by solitary neurofibroma. *J. Neurosurg.*, **17**, 511.

Cloward, R.B. (1961) Treatment of acute fractures and fracture-dislocations of the cervical spine by vertebral body fusion. *J. Neurosurg.*, **18**, 201.

Dawbarn, H.M. (1889) A successful case of spinal resection. *NY Med. J.*, **49**, 713.

Dawson, G.D. (1947) Cerebral responses to electrical stimulation of peripheral nerve in man. *J. Neurol., Neurosurg., Psychiatry*, **10**, 134.

Dereymaeker, A. & Mulier, J. (1956) Nouvelle cure chirurgicale des discopathies cervicales. *Neurochirurgie*, **2**, 233.

Djindjan, R., Hurth, M. & Julian, H.J. (1968) Artériographie de la moelle épinière dorsale et dorso-lombaire par aortographie sélective. *J. Radiol.*, **49**, 289.

Dott, N.M. (1947) Skeletal traction and anterior decompression in the management of Pott's paraplegia. *Edin. Med. J.*, **54**, 620.

Ehrenfels, von Ch. (1892) Uber Gestaltqualitäten. *Viertelljahresschr. Phil.*, **14**, 249.

Fick, R. (1911) *Handbuch der Anatomie und Mechanik der Gelenke*, Vol. III, pp. 35–113. Gustav Fischer, Jena.

Gilles de la Tourette, G. & Chipault, A. (1898) Le traitement de l'ataxie par l'élongation vraie de la moelle. *Trav. Neurol. Chir.*, **3**, 204.

Gowers, W.R. & Horsley, V. (1888) A case of tumour of the spinal cord: removal, recovery. *Med. Chir. Trans.*, **53**, 377.
Guérin, J.R. (1839) Traitement des déviations latérales de l'épine par la myotomie rachidienne. *Gaz. Méd.*, **13**, 413.
Guleke, N. (1935) In Kirschner, M. (ed.) *Operationslehre*, Vol. 3, Part I, pp. 943–954. Springer, Berlin.
Hadra, B.E. (1891) Wiring the spinous processes in Pott's disease. *Trans. Am. Orthop, A*, **4**, 206.
Hibbs, R.A. (1911) An operation for progressive spinal deformities. A preliminary report of three cases from the service of the Orthopaedic Hospital. *NY Med. J.*, **93**, 1013.
Hodes, R., Larrabee, M.G. & German, W. (1948) The human electromyogram in response to nerve stimulation and the conduction velocity of motor axons. Studies on normal and injured peripheral nerves. *Arch. Neurol. Psychiatry*, **60**, 340.
Hoffa, A. & Blencke, A. (1905) *Die Orthopädische Literatur*. Enke, Stuttgart.
Hoffmann, P. (1918) Uber die Beziehung der Sehnenreflexe zur willkürlichen Bewegung und zum Tonus. *Z. Biol.*, **68**, 351.
Horsley, V. (1887) Remarks on ten consecutive cases of operations upon the brain and cranial cavity to illustrate the details and safety of the methods employed. *Br. Med. J.*, **1**, 863.
Horsley, V. (1892) Antiseptic wax. *Br. Med. J.*, **1**, 1165.
Horsley, V. (1892) The origin and seat of epileptic disturbance. *Br. Med. J.*, **1**, 696.
Horsley, V. (1908) The structure and function of the cerebellum examined by a new method. *Brain*, **31**, 45.
Horsley, V. (1909) The function of the so-called motor area of the brain. Linacre Lecture. *Br. Med. J.*, **2**, 125.
Jung, A. (1963) Résection de l'articulation unco-vertébrale et ouverture du trou de conjugaison par voie antérieure dans le traitement de la névralgie cervicobrachiale. Technique opératoire. *Mém. Acad. Chir.*, **89**, 361.
Junghanns, H. (1952) Funktionelle Röntgenuntersuchung der Halswirbelsäsule. *Fortschr. Roentgenstr.*, **76**, 391.
Junghanns, H. (1968) *Die gesunde und kranke Wirbelsäule in Röntgenbild und Klinik*. Thieme, Stuttgart.
Koffka, K. (1912) Perception: an introduction to the Gestalt theory. *Psychol. Bull.*, **19**, 521.
Koffka, K. (1935) *Principles of Gestalt Psychology*, Harcourt Brace, New York.
Köhler, W. (1947) *Gestalt Psychology*. Liveright, New York.
Köhler, W. (1971) *Selected Papers* (ed. Henle, M.). Liveright, New York.
Lange, F. (1910) Support for the spondylitic spine by means of buried steel bars attached to the vertebrae. *Am. J. Orthop. Surg.*, **8**, 344.
Lange, F. (1924) Die operative Schienung der spondylitischen Wirbelsäulen mit Zelluloid-Staben. *Z. Orthop. Chir.*, **45**, 492.
Lidell, J.A. (1884) *The International Encyclopedia of Surgery* (ed. Ashurst, J.) Vol. IV, p. 667. Macmillan, London.
Little, W.J. (1839) *Treatise on the Nature of Club-foot and Analogous Distortions*: London.
Londe, A. (1902) Remarques Techniques sur l'Application des Sciences Photographiques à la Chirurgie Nerveuse. In Chipault, A. (ed.) *Etat Actuel de la Chirurgie Nerveuse*, Vol. I, p. 23. Rueff, Paris.
Macewen, W. (1881) Intracranial lesions illustrating some points in connection with the localisation of cerebral affections and the advantage of antiseptic trephining, III. Tumor of the dura mater; IV. Abscess of brain. *Lancet*, **2**, 581.
Macewen, W. (1884) Trephining of the spine for paraplegia. *Glasgow Med. J.*, **22**, 55.
Macewen, W. (1885) Two cases in which excision of the laminae of portions of the spinal vertebrae had been performed in order to relieve pressure on the spinal cord causing paraplegia. *Glasgow Med. J.*, **25**, 210.
Macewan, W. (1912) *Growth of Bone: Observations on Osteogenesis*. J. Maclehose and Sons, Glasgow.
Macewen, W. (1878) On antiseptic osteotomy of the genu valgum, genu varum, and other osseous deformities. *Lancet*, **1**, 912.
Macewen, W. Mentioned by A. Earl Walker (1951) In *A History of Neurological Surgery*, p. 179. Williams & Wilkins, Baltimore, MD.
Macewen, W. Mentioned by B. Jennet (1985) In his biography of Macewen in Bucy, P. (ed.) *Neurosurgical Giants: Feet of Clay and Iron*, p. 33. Elsevier, New York.
MacKenzie Forbes, A. (1920) The operative treatment of scoliosis. *J. Bone Jt. Surg.*, **4**, 1922.
Mach, E. (1886) *Die Analyse der Empfindungen und des Verhältnis des Psychischen zum Physischen*. Gustav Fischer, Jena.
Mach, E. (1959) *The Analysis of Sensation*. Dover Publications, New York.
Maglarady, J.W. & McDougal, D.B. (1950) Electrophysiological studies of nerve and reflex activity in normal man. I. Identification of certain reflexes in the electromyogram and the conduction velocity of peripheral nerves. *Bull. Johns Hopkins Hosp.*, **86**, 265.
Magnus, R. (1924) *Körperstellung*. Springer, Berlin.
Malgaigne, J.F. (1844) Mémoire sur la valeur reëlle de l'orthopédie et spécialement de la myotomie rachidienne dans le traitement des déviations latérales du rachis. *C.R. Acad. Sci.*, **13**, 15.
Ménard, V. (1895) Traitement de la paraplégie du mal de Pott dorsal par le drainage latéral. Costo-transversectomie. Ass. Franç. Chir. 1894, 8ème congres, Lyon, 1894. *Proces-verbaux, Mémoires et discussions*, p. 645. Paris.
Ménard, V. (1894) Causes de paraplégie dans le mal de Pott. Son traitement chirurgical par ouverture directe du foyer tuberculeux des vertèbres. *Rev. Orthop.*, **5**, 47.
Mixter, J.W. & Barr, J.S. (1934) Rupture of the intervertebral disk with involvement of the spinal canal. *N. Engl. J. Med.*, **211**, 240.
Nieuwenhuys, R. (1985) *Chemoarchitecture of the Brain*. Springer, Berlin.
Penning, L. (1968) *Functional Pathology of the Cervical Spine*. Excerpta Medica, Amsterdam.
Robinson, R.A. & Smith, G. (1955) Anterolateral cervical disk removal and interbody fusion for cervical disk syndrome. *Bull. Johns Hopkins Hosp.*, **96**, 223.
Russell, B. (1980) *An Inquiry into Meaning and Truth*. Unwin, London.

Schaik, J.J.P. van, Verbiest, H. & Schaik, F.D.J. van. (1985) Morphometry of lower lumbar vertebrae as seen on CT scans. Newly recognized characteristics. *Am. J. Roentgenol.*, **145**, 327.

Scoville, W.H., Palmer, A.H., Samra, K. & Chong, G. (1967) The use of acrylic plastic for vertebral replacement or fixation in metastatic disease of the spine. *J. Neurosurg.*, **27**, 274.

Senning, A., Weber, G. & Yasargil, M.G. (1962) Zur operativen Behandlung von Tumoren der Wirbelsäule. *Schweiz. Med. Wochensch.*, **92**, 1574.

Sherrington, Ch. (1951) *Man on his Nature*, 2nd edn. Cambridge University Press, Cambridge.

Sicard, A. (1959) *Chirurgie du Rachis*. Masson, Paris.

Stromeyer, G.F.L. (1833) Beitrag zur operativen Orthopädie oder Erfahrungen über die subcutane Durchschneidung verkürtzer Muskeln. Hannover, 1838, see also: *Mag. Ges. Heilkunde, Berlin*, **34**, 195.

Treves, F. (1884) The direct treatment of psoas abscess with caries of the spine. *Med. Chir. Trans.*, **67**, 113.

Treves, F. (1892) On the treatment of spinal and other tuberculous abscesses. *Lancet*, **1**, 1122.

Tulp, N. (1652) *Observationes Medicae, Editio nova, libro quarto auctior et sparsium multis in locis emendiator*. Book IV, observation 49, ap. L. Elsevirium, Amstelredami.

Urban, J. (1892) Ueber operative Eingriffe bei Compression des Rückenmarkes durch Verschiebung der Wirbelkörper. *Verh. Deutsch. Ges. Chir.*, **21**, 211.

Vallebona, A. (1930) Una modalita di technica per la dissociazione radiografica delle ombre applicata allo studio del cranio. *Radiol. Med.*, **17**, 1090.

Verbiest, H. (1947) Le traitement neurochirurgical dans les tumeurs bénignes des corps vertébraux avec compression de la moelle. *Rev. Neurol.*, **79**, 528.

Verbiest, H. (1954) Moderne overwegingen over compressio medullae. *Ned. T. Geneesk.*, **98**, 2972.

Verbiest, H. (1962) Anterior operative approach in cases of spinal cord compression by old irreducible displacement or fresh fracture of the cervical spine. *J. Neurosurg.*, **19**, 389.

Verbiest, H. (1965) Giant-cell tumors and aneurysmal bone cysts of the spine. *J. Bone Jt. Surg.*, **47B**, 699.

Verbiest, H. (1968) Technique and indications of a lateral approach to the cervical spine. *J. Neurosurg.*, **28**, 191.

Verbiest, H. (1969) Anterolateral operations for fractures and dislocations of the middle and lower parts of the cervical spine. *J. Bone Jt. Surg.*, **51A**, 1489.

Verbiest, H. (1970) *La Chirurgie antérieuere et latérale du Rachis Cervical*, Ch. V, pp. 171–203. *Neurochirurgie*, Tome 16, suppl. 2. Masson, Paris.

Verbiest, H. (1983) Words, images, knowledge and reality. Reflections from the neurosurgical perspective. Fourth European Lecture. *Acta Neurochir.*, **69**, 163.

Verbiest, H. (1983, 1989) Benign tumors of the cervical spine. In Cervical Spine Research Society (eds) *The Cervical Spine*, 1st edn, pp. 430–477; 2nd edn, pp. 723–774. Lippincott, Philadelphia.

Verbiest, H. (1986) Future role of neurosurgery in the care of spinal disorders. *Neurosurg. Rev.*, **9**, 89.

Verbiest, H. & Paz y Geuze, H.D. (1966) Antero-lateral surgery for cervical spondylosis in cases of myelopathy or nerveroot compression. *J. Neurosurg.*, **25**, 611.

Vincent, E. (1892) Contribution à la chirurgie rachidienne du drainage vertébral dans le mal de Pott. *Rev. Chir. Paris*, **12**, 273.

Wackenheim, A. (1986) *Les radiologists imagiers de la médecine*. Axone, Montpellier.

Ziedses des Plantes, B.G. (1932) Eine neue Methode zur Differenzierung in der Roentgenographie (Planigraphie). *Acta Radiol.*, **13**, 182.

Ziedses des Plantes, B.G. (1934) Planigraphie en Subtractie. PhD thesis, Utrecht University.

Ziedses des Plantes, B.G. (1961) *Subtraction*. Thieme, Stuttgart.

Ziedses des Plantes, B.G. (1973) *Selected Works of Ziedses des Plantes*. Excerpta Medica, Amsterdam.

SECTION 2
ANATOMY AND FUNCTION OF THE SPINE

2 · Embryology of the Human Spine

By R.J. SCOTHORNE

This account of the development of the neurovertebral axis concentrates upon topics likely to be of interest and importance to the clinician. Attention is focused upon the events and their chronology in the human embryo and fetus, but understanding of the mechanisms involved in normal and abnormal development requires reference also to experimental investigations.

Surgeons need no reminder of the clinical significance of the close topographical relationship between the two components of the neurovertebral axis, which reflects the outcome of a long series of mutual interactions between the ectodermal, neural component and the mesodermal, vertebral component. Because the neurovertebral axis is the first major organ system to be established, the search for the origin of both dysraphic and non-dysraphic disorders must begin with a consideration of the earliest developmental events, which include:

1 the initial formation of the notochord and paraxial mesoderm, precursors of the vertebral column;
2 induction, by this chordamesoderm, of the neural plate, forerunner of the spinal cord and spinal nerves;
3 formation of the neural tube—neurulation—and of the neural crest;
4 the origins of segmentation, both in the mesodermal precursors of the vertebral column and in the neural tube and spinal nerves;
5 harmonization of segmentation in the vertebral column and spinal cord to provide, for example, for the normal emergence of spinal nerves through intervertebral foramina.

Once these basic patterns have been considered, the later stages of normal development and the possible genesis of abnormality will be reviewed.

The sequence and timing of developmental events

Since 'a fundamental principle in speculating on the pathogenesis of any malformation is the correct interpretation of the sequence of normal events' (Lemire, 1969), it is important to place a series of different embryos in their correct order, and to establish a timetable for major developmental changes. For human embryos the Carnegie system of staging (O'Rahilly & Muller, 1987) is widely used. An embryo is assigned to a particular stage if it possesses most of the structural features characteristic of that stage. Events will be referred to the Carnegie stage, supplemented by reference to the more familiar, but less discriminative, parameters of the postovulatory age and length of the embryo or fetus (Table 2.1).

Formation of primitive streak, notochord and embryonic mesoderm

Towards the end of the third postovulatory week the embryo is a pear-shaped disc, with the three primary germ layers—ectoderm, mesoderm and endoderm—already established (Fig. 2.1). In the midline of the embryonic disc, towards its caudal end, is the *primitive streak*, formed mainly by cells of the ectodermal layer, which migrate ventrally through the streak, and spread out on either side of it to form embryonic mesoderm. From the cranial end of the streak there extends forwards, between ectoderm and endoderm, the *notochordal process*, the axial structure around which the vertebral column will be built.

Overlying the notochordal process, and coextensive with it, the ectoderm shows a shallow midline groove, the *neural groove*, 'the first visible indication of the

Table 2.1 Chronology of development. Based on data of O'Rahilly & Meyer (1979), Muller & O'Rahilly (1986), O'Rahilly & Muller (1987), Sensenig (1949)

Spinal cord and nerves	Age (days)	Length (mm)	Carnegie stage	Notochord, somites vertebral column
	16	0.4	7	Notochordal process appears
Neural plate, groove, folds	18–20	1.0–2.5	8/9	Somites: 1–3 pairs
First fusion of folds: neural crest first visible	22	2.0–3.5	10	Somites: 4–12 pairs; migration of sclerotomic cells begins
Cranial neuropore closes	24	2.5–4.5	11	Somites: 13–20 pairs
Caudal neuropore closes; secondary neurulation begins	26	3–5	12	Somites 21–29 pairs; sclerotomic migration continues
Ventral roots of spinal nerves appear	28	4–6	13	Cranial and caudal sclerotomites appear
Full complement of dorsal root ganglia present	32	5–7	14	Perichordal centra and discs distinguishable
	33	7–9	15	Full complement of somites
	41	11–14	17	Chondrification of centra begins
Secondary neurul-lation completed	44	13–17	18	Chondrification of laminae begins
Regression of caudal neural tube	56	27–31	23	Cartilaginous arches extend to dorsal roots of spinal nerves
		30–35	—	Cartilaginous arches extend medially, dorsal to cord
	63	50	—	Cartilaginous arches unite dorsal to cord; ossification starts

nervous system in the human embryo' (O'Rahilly & Muller, 1981).

Induction of the neural plate

The notochord, and the paraxial mesoderm flanking it on each side, together constitute the *chordamesoderm* which, through its close proximity to the overlying ectoderm, induces the formation of a thickened *neural plate.* This is now irrevocably committed to form nervous tissues, while the rest of the ectoderm will form epidermis. Neural induction is therefore an early, and fundamental, dichotomy in development. The nature of the inducing agent is not known, but it is thought to be chemical, and to act over a short distance, involving proximity, but not actual cellular contact, between the two tissues. Thickening of the neural plate involves elongation of its constituent cells, while those of the epidermis flatten (Fig. 2.2). There is substantial evidence that axially orientated microtubules—part of the cytoskeleton—are actively involved both in producing and maintaining the elongated form of the neuroepithelial cells, as they are in cell elongation in other systems.

Induction determines not only the formation of a neural plate, but also the establishment of patterns

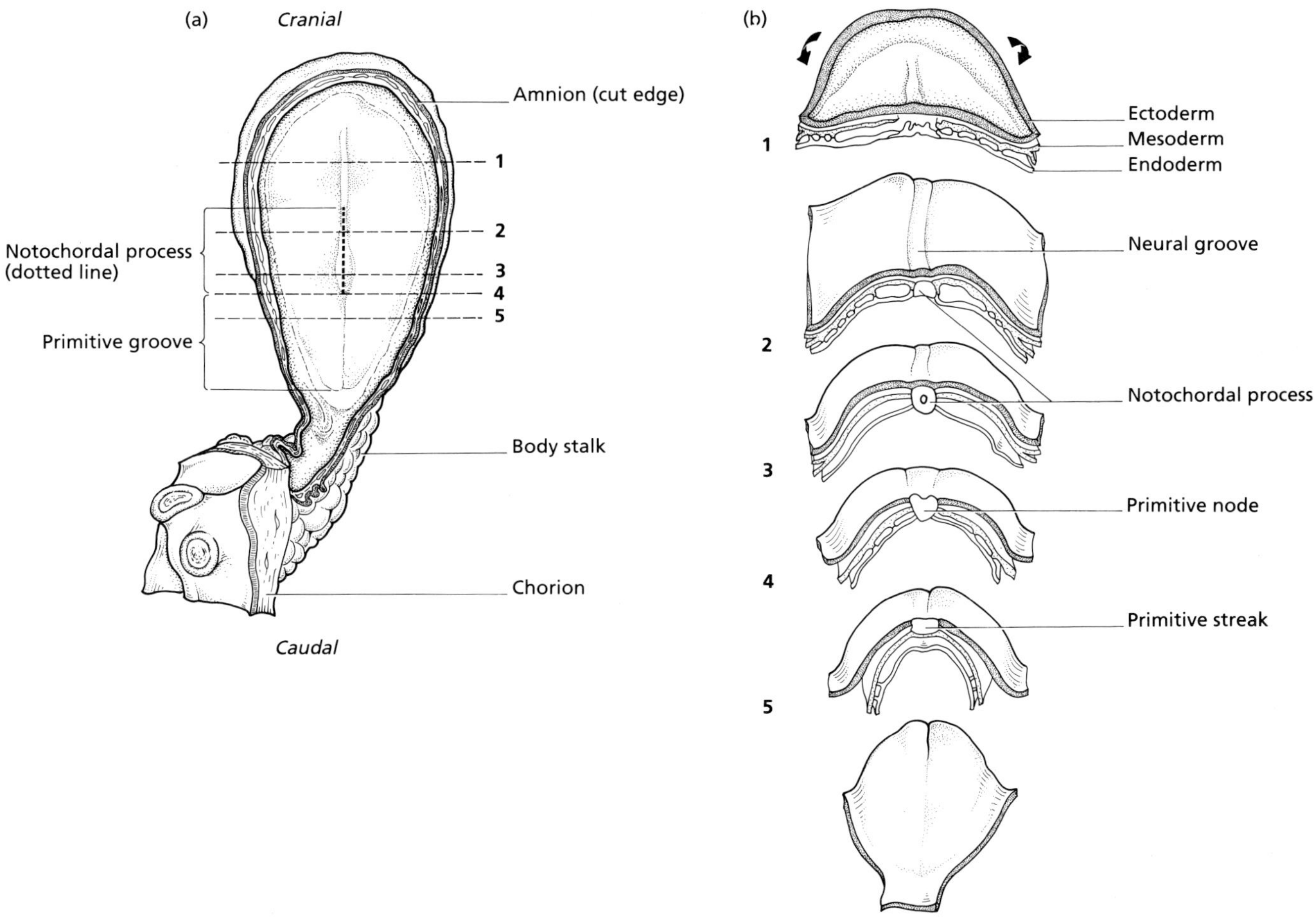

Fig. 2.1 Human embryo, Stage 8, approximately 18 days, approximately 1.5 mm long. (a) Dorsal view of pear-shaped embryonic disc, seen after removal of amnion. Primitive groove marks position of primitive streak. Dotted line marks position of notochord, overlain by neural groove, which is first indication of formation of neural plate. (b) 'Exploded' diagram, showing cross-sections at levels 1, 2, 3, 4 and 5 marked on (a). Based on Heuser (1932), and O'Rahilly & Muller (1987).

within the plate, and the programming of its cells to differentiate into neurones and glia. By using various chemical treatments of amphibian embryos, Warner (1988) has shown that these three fundamental events —neurulation, pattern formation and cell differentiation—can be separately interfered with. Separation of these inductive events is also evident in some cases of human myeloschisis, in which maturation of the neuroepithelium, i.e. its histogenesis, can occur normally, despite the failure of the morphogenetic events for closure of the neural tube.

The inductive interaction between chordamesoderm and neural ectoderm is not one-way only, but reciprocal: the neural plate and tube will presently be principally responsible for inducing the segmental subdivision of the paraxial mesoderm, into somitomeres and somites, and therefore, ultimately, for the segmented pattern of the vertebral column.

Formation of the neural tube: primary neurulation

This includes all the events from the initial folding of the neural plate to the closure of the caudal neuropore. The newly formed plate is a pseudo-stratified columnar epithelium; all its cells extend throughout the thickness of the layer, but their nuclei are arranged at various levels, giving an appearance of stratification.

FOLDING OF THE PLATE

This begins about a midline hinge-like axis, in close proximity to the notochord, and is followed by further

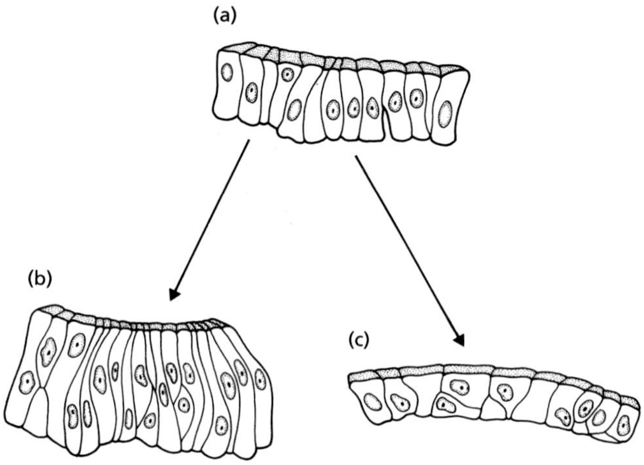

Fig. 2.2 Changes in cell shape which occur in the primitive ectoderm (a) (simple columnar), to produce the pseudo-stratified columnar epithelium of the neural plate (b) and the simple cubical epithelium of the primitive epidermis (c). Based on Burnside (1973).

bending of each lateral plate about a dorsolateral axis, bringing the edges of the folds close together (Fig. 2.3a).

The mechanism of neurulation has been a matter for investigation—and speculation—for more than 100 years (reviewed by Gordon, 1985; Campbell *et al.*, 1986). Of the many plausible models proposed, the following are currently the more favoured.

1 The neural plate behaves as a viscoelastic system that, when stretched along its length by the rapid elongation of the 'notoplate' (i.e. the notochord and the firmly adherent neural plate), rolls up into a tube, like a stretched sheet of rubber (so-called 'Eulerian buckling').

2 Lateral pressure is exerted on the neural plate by the paraxial mesoderm, as the glycosaminoglycans of its interstitial connective tissue become hydrated and swell (Schoenwolf and Fisher, 1983).

3 There are active changes in the shape of neural plate cells (particularly those at the main sites of folding) which become wedge-shaped (Fig. 2.3b), through contraction of microfilaments at their apical ends, acting like a purse-string, and movement of cytoplasm towards their basal ends, through the agency of microtubules. These changes in cell shape are probably reinforced by the fact that the nuclei of neuroepithelial cells spend much of their cycle of interkinetic migration (see later) in the basal end of the cell.

Each of these possible mechanisms must be considered in evaluating the hypothesis of 'failure-to-close' as an explanation of the pathogenesis of neural tube defects.

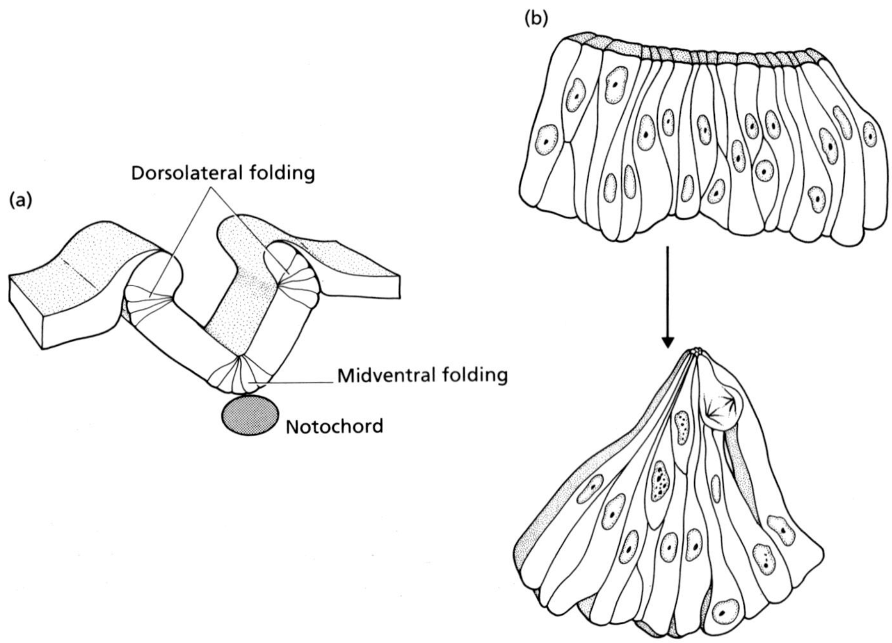

Fig. 2.3 (a) Mechanism of folding of neural plate, produced, in part, by changes in shape of neuroepithelial cells, in midventral line and dorsolateral lines. (b) Along lines of folding, neuroepithelial cells become narrower at their apices, broader at their bases. Based on studies on chick embryo (Schoenwolf & Franks, 1984). Changes in mammals are similar, but the dorsolateral folds are less conspicuous.

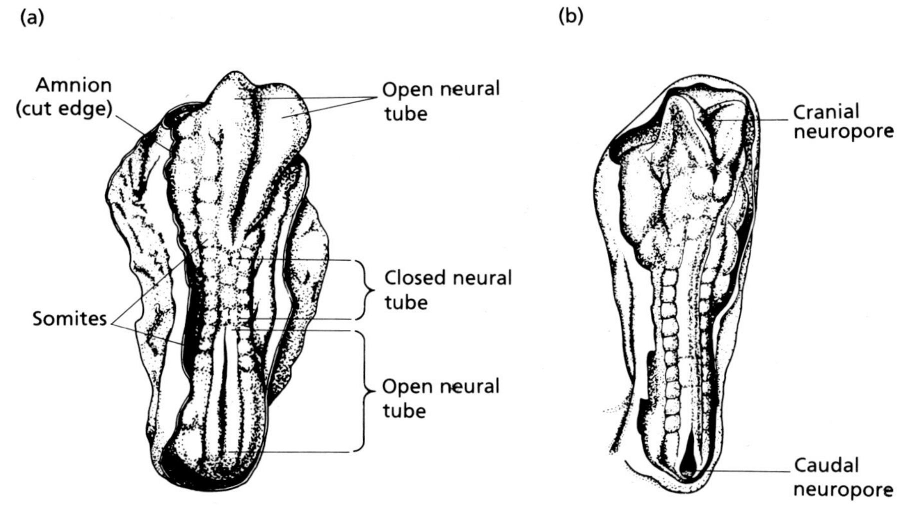

Fig. 2.4 Closure of the neural tube in human embryos. Stage 10, about 22 days. (a) Eight-somite embryo. After Payne (1925). (b) Ten-somite embryo. After Corner (1929).

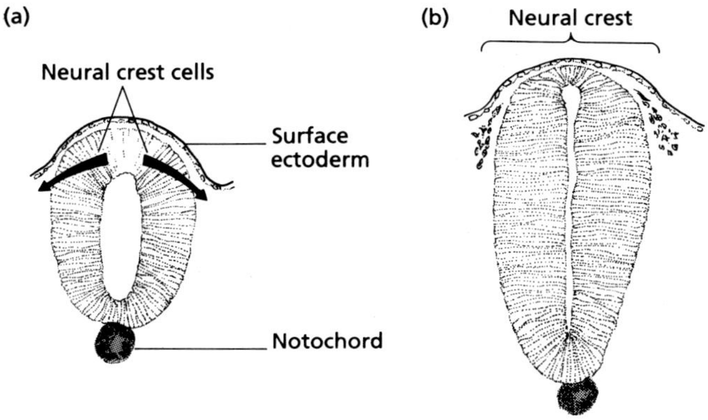

Fig. 2.5 Transverse sections of neural tube, 17-somite human embryo (Stage 11, about 24 days). (a) At a more caudal level, showing the neural crest as an integral part of the dorsal wall of the tube before migration (arrows). (b) At a more cranial level (more advanced in development) neural crest cells have migrated from the wall of the tube and formed a dorsolateral column of cells on each side of the tube. Redrawn after O'Rahilly & Muller (1987).

FUSION OF NEURAL FOLDS

This process begins, in embryos of Stage 10 (about 22 days old), at the junction between hind brain and cervical spinal cord (Fig. 2.4). From here it extends cranially and caudally, somewhat like a double zip fastener, although closure may occur in several places independently. In the spinal region the first contact is between surface ectoderm at the apices of the two folds, followed by fusion of the neurectoderm. Within the dorsal wall of the newly closed tube lies a wedge of *neural crest* cells (Fig. 2.5), which will presently free themselves and begin to migrate in two streams —one dorsolaterally, beneath the surface ectoderm, the other ventrolaterally through the developing somites. Their fate is described later.

The phase of primary neurulation ends with the closure of the caudal neuropore. It is an important event, because of its possible significance in the genesis of defects at the caudal end of the neural tube. In a most detailed study of the process, Muller & O'Rahilly (1987) established that closure occurs in a craniocaudal direction and is generally completed in embryos with about 25 pairs of somites (Stage 12, Day 26). The site of final closure lies adjacent to *non-segmented* paraxial mesoderm (Fig. 2.6). By 'counting-down' from the last-formed somite (the 25th), Muller & O'Rahilly (1987) estimated that the level of closure corresponded approximately with the future somites 30–31, i.e. with the first to second sacral vertebral level. This would mark the boundary between that part of the neural tube formed by folding of a neural plate—primary neurulation—and that part formed by secondary neurulation (see below). It should be noted that this is substantially further caudally than some other estimates (e.g. Lemire, 1974), which indicated a level of the twenty-fifth pair of somites, i.e. of lumbar vertebrae 1 and 2.

There are several features of the caudal neuropore which might predispose to failure of its closure: no tissue intervenes between the surface ectoderm and

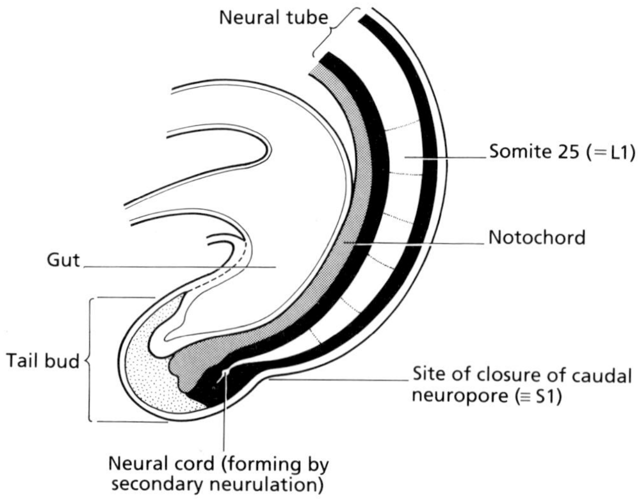

Fig. 2.6 Midsagittal section of caudal end of 25-somite human embryo (Stage 12, about 26 days). The caudal neuropore has just closed (arrow). The most recently formed somite is No. 25 (= first lumbar). The site of closure is estimated to lie opposite the future fist to second sacral somites. Redrawn after Muller & O'Rahilly (1987).

the neuroepithelium and 'neural crest cannot be detected at the site of closure' (Muller & O'Rahilly, 1987); at the level of the caudal neuropore the neural groove is very shallow; and the caudal neuropore lies immediately adjacent to the complex events of secondary neurulation, which lead to the formation of sacral and coccygeal segments of the spinal cord.

Secondary neurulation and the tail bud

At about the time that the caudal neuropore closes, the tail end of the embryo consists of *the tail bud*, a mass of undifferentiated (pluripotent) cells, 'mesenchymal' in appearance, covered by surface ectoderm. It is derived from, and replaces, the primitive streak and gives rise directly to structures which, at more cranial levels, develop from defined germ layers: centrally and dorsally, a *neural cord*, which will form sacral and coccygeal segments of the neural tube and the corresponding dorsal root ganglia; on either side of the neural cord, a block of cells, which will form sacral and coccygeal somites; and, ventrally to the neural cord, the notochord and the tail end of the gut tube (Fig. 2.7a).

The neural cord is initially solid. Its peripheral cells become radially arranged, as a pseudo-stratified neuroepithelium, around a neural canal. There are important species differences in the method of formation of the neural canal. In the chick, Schoenwolf (1978) described the coalescence of a number of spaces, arising independently of one another, to form a single lumen which overlapped, and subsequently became

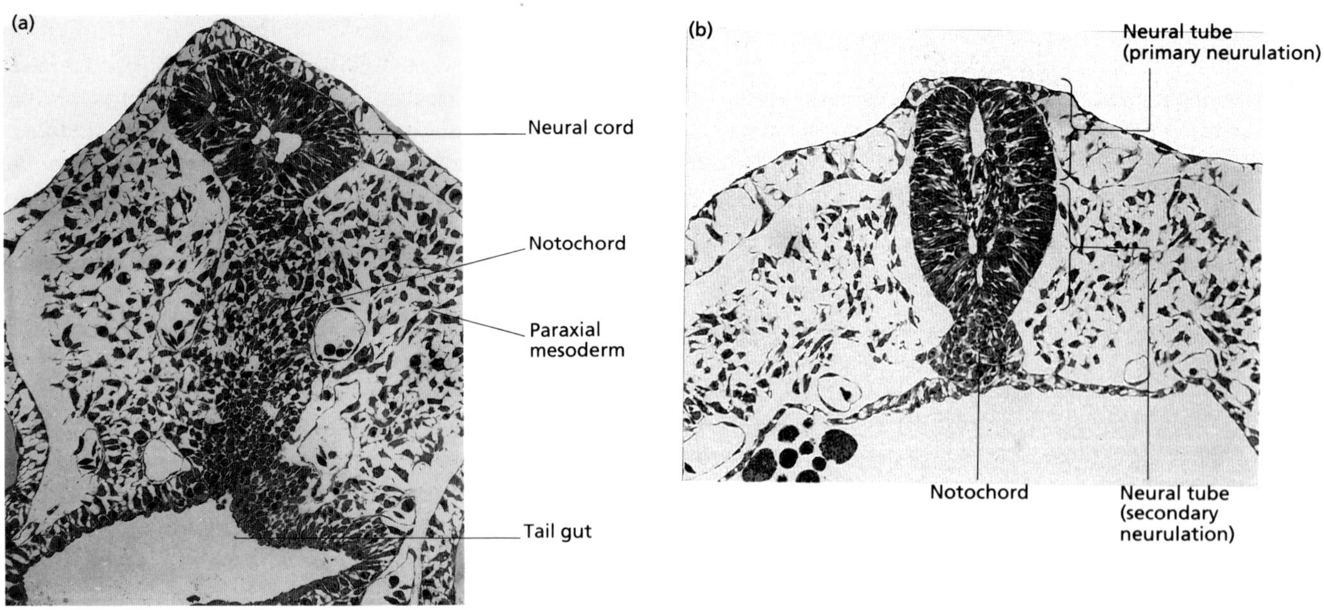

Fig. 2.7 Process of secondary neurulation (in chick). (a) Transverse section through tail bud, chick embryo, showing neural cord, with multiple lumina developing notochord and paraxial mesoderm (×169). (b) Same, at a more cranial level, showing overlap zone between neural tube produced by folding (primary neurulation) and that produced by cavitation (secondary neurulation) (×188). Photomicrographs from preparations by John Farrow.

continuous with, the neural canal formed by primary neurulation (Fig. 2.7b). In humans the mechanism is not certainly known. Both Lemire (1969) and Hughes & Freeman (1974) found accessory lumina in the neural cord of several human embryos, otherwise apparently normal, and felt that this indicated irregular coalescence of initially separate cavities, as in the chick. Hughes & Freeman (1974) attached teratological significance to this method of 'canalization', pointing to the high incidence of defects of the caudal end of the neural tube, appearing either spontaneously, as in humans, or produced experimentally by a wide range of teratogens, as in chick. In tailed mammals (e.g. pig, sheep, rodents), on the other hand, they found that the neural canal extended caudally in a more even manner, and correlated this with the rarity of developmental abnormalities of the caudal neural tube in this group of animals. The validity of this correlation is supported by the high incidence of spontaneous neural tube defects in the (tail-less) hamster, and by the association of genetically determined short or curly-tail defects with spina bifida in mice. Hughes & Freeman's (1974) idea that evolutionary reduction of the tail in humans and chick makes them more liable to caudal neural tube defects deserves more attention.

Both Schoenwolf (1984) in the mouse, and Muller & O'Rahilly (1987) in humans, describe the origin of the secondary neural canal as different from that in the chick, claiming that it arises as a caudal extension of the primary neural canal. In both species, caudal extension of the cavity may require fluid pressure (cf. expansion of the cerebral ventricles—see later).

Because of its developmental fate the tail bud has significance in the genesis of several malformations. Its defective development may result in sacral agenesis (Tondury, 1944) (see Chapter 16). Spinal cord abnormalities at levels below the second sacral segment may result from defective secondary neurulation. Seven of eight human embryos studied by Lemire (1969) had accessory lumina at the caudal end of the neural tube, which he thought might be attributable to a process of cavitation similar to that seen in the chick (cf. Fig. 2.7b). Duplication of the neural tube has also been reported, in otherwise normal human embryos, by Kunimoto (1918), Streeter (1919) and Kernohan (1925). Of particular interest is the finding that, in 100 cases of meningomyelocele in children, the spinal cord *caudal* to the lesion was either duplicated locally or showed double or multiple central canals (Emery & Lendon, 1973). They speculated that 'these defects may result from faulty canalisation of the tail-bud tissue'.

Occlusion of the neural canal

Some reference must be made to the phenomenon of occlusion of the spinal neural canal, because of its significance in the response of the neural tube to experimental incision of the roof plate (and therefore to the 'failure-to-close' v. 'secondary reopening' controversy—see later) and because of its wider importance for the growth of the brain. Occlusion refers to the temporary obliteration of the neural canal, through adhesion of the ependymal lining of its lateral walls. In human embryos (Desmond, 1982) it first occurs at Stage 11 (24 days), when the cranial neuropore is closed, the caudal neuropore is closing, and the neural canal is becoming a closed system. Occlusion is most prominent at Stages 11 and 12 (24–26 days), and is absent by Stage 14 (32 days). Although it is a transient phenomenon it appears in a regular pattern, involving the cord more or less without interruption between somites 3 and 9—essentially the cervical region of the cord. The mechanism of occlusion, and of subsequent reopening, of the neural canal is not certainly known, but the evidence from experimental animals indicates: (a) that occlusion is not an artifact; (b) that it provides a physiological seal in the cervical cord, sufficiently strong to resist the flow of early cerebrospinal fluid caudally from the IVth ventricle; and (c) that, as a consequence, there is a temporary build-up of intraventricular pressure which has been shown experimentally, in the chick embryo, to be important in the early expansion of the brain, and presumably serves the same purpose in humans (Desmond & Schoenwolf, 1986).

Histogenesis and growth of the spinal cord

From the time of its first appearance the neural plate shows a characteristic pattern of cell division. All its cells extend throughout the thickness of the neuroepithelium, and all are capable of division. The nucleus lies towards the basal end of the cell when DNA replication begins; it then migrates towards the apical end, and the cell retracts its basal process and rounds up. Cell division is completed while the cell lies in the future ependymal layer; the daughter cells extend their cytoplasm to make contact again with

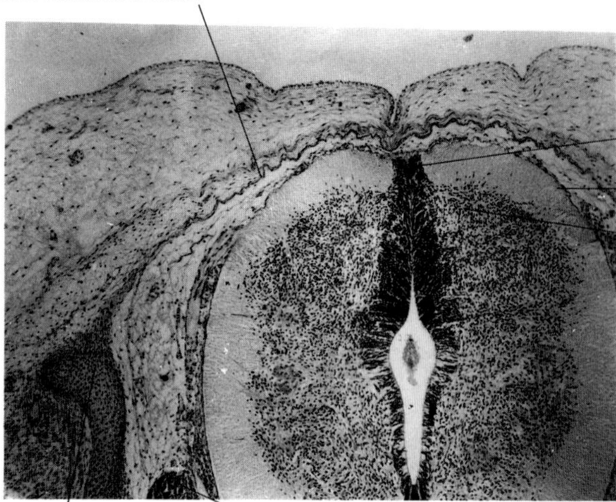

Fig. 2.8 Transverse section of neural tube of human embryo 17 mm (Stage 18–19, seventh week). Shows ependymal, mantle and marginal zones; note also: dorsal tip of cartilaginous neural arch; membrana reuniens dorsalis; dorsal root ganglion; loose paraneural mesenchyme—future pia-arachnoid (×50). Author's collection.

the basal lamina, and their nuclei also retreat basally. This rising and falling 'dance of the nuclei' is called *interkinetic nuclear migration.* It is repeated many times until, at an unknown signal, the daughter cells withdraw their apical and basal processes; some migrate to a middle position in the neuroepithelium and differentiate into young nerve cells, which are postmitotic, or into astroglia or oligodendroglia, which retain the capacity to divide, even into adult life. Others remain near the free (apical) surface of the neuroepithelium and form the definitive *ependymal zone* whose cells, in higher vertebrates, cease to divide during embryonic life.

The intermediate layer, in which postmitotic neurones differentiate, constitutes the *mantle zone* of the neural tube, the future grey matter. The *marginal zone,* the outermost layer of the neural tube, consists at first of the outer cytoplasmic parts of the neuroepithelium. It forms the matrix through which run the processes of neurones entering or leaving the spinal cord, and running to or from higher centres. This zone becomes the white matter of the adult cord (Fig. 2.8).

Growth of the spinal cord involves many events: proliferation of neuroepithelial precursors of neurones and glial cells and the continuing proliferation of glia; growth of neurones, as they differentiate and send out axons and dendrites; the formation of investing sheaths, particularly myelin, around axons and dendrites.

A striking feature of all neural development is that, of all the neurones generated, a significant proportion —commonly 40–50%—die, a process called *physiological* (or 'programmed') *cell death.* It affects groups of cells at a time when their synaptic connections are being established, and its extent depends upon the size of the projection field in which their axons terminate. Reduction of the size of the projection field is followed by increased cell death, while increasing the size of the target may save some neurones from premature death. It seems that neuronal development—both in the central and peripheral nervous systems—involves an initial overproduction, followed by a selective elimination of the surplus, thereby matching the size of neuronal groups to the size of their target tissues (for review see Cowan, 1982).

The most familiar expression of this phenomenon is the association of the cervical and lumbar enlargements of the spinal cord with the origin of the limb plexuses; its most complete manifestation is the 'regressive differentiation' of the coccygeal segments of the cord (see below).

Development of spinal nerves and the origin of their segmental arrangement

What determines the segmental pattern of the spinal nerve roots, which is the most obvious sign of segmentation of the nervous system?

There is abundant experimental evidence that when the spinal nerves develop, their segmental pattern is determined by that of the somites. The ventral

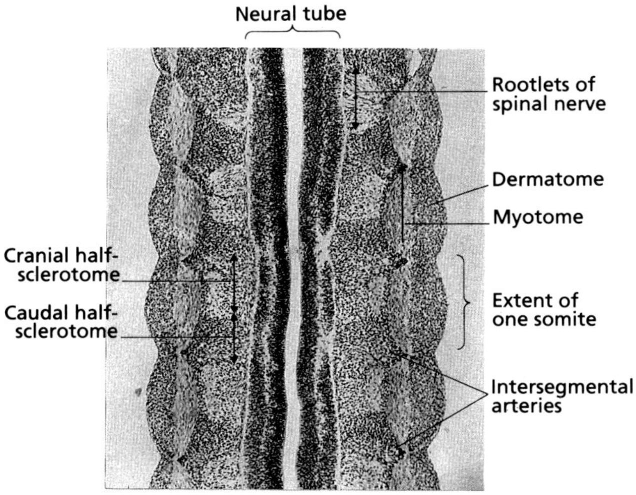

Fig. 2.9 Coronal section of neural tube and somites. Shows subdivision of each somite into dermatome, myotome and sclerotome. Each sclerotome shows a more darkly stained cellular ('condensed') caudal half and a paler, looser, cranial half, through which run the rootlets of spinal nerves. Note: 'intersclerotomal fissures' are defined only by intersegmental arteries; 'intrasclerotomal fissures' are not present. Sheep embryo, 10 mm. Anatomy Departmental Collection, University of Glasgow.

rootlets of a spinal nerve develop first, through the outgrowth of axons from the perikarya of motor neurones in the ventral part of the mantle zone, which forms the ventral grey column of the cord. The first ('pioneering') axons leave the cord where it lies adjacent to the cranial half of the corresponding sclerotome, through which they grow. They are followed by groups of axons which leave the cord opposite the caudal half of the sclerotome, but soon deviate and grow along the pioneering fibres, by a process called selective fasciculation, so that they too traverse the cranial half of the sclerotome (Fig. 2.9). The developing axons of the dorsal rootlets of the spinal nerve, arising from young neurones in the segmentally arranged neural crest, behave similarly, so that the entire spinal nerve runs through the cranial half of the corresponding sclerotome. This preference of outgrowing motor and sensory axons for the cranial half-sclerotome seems to rest on differences in molecular markers on the cell surface and/or the extracellular matrix in the two halves of the sclerotome (for a review, see Keynes & Stern, 1988).

These events, which determine at an early stage of development that the dorsal root ganglion and the spinal nerve and its roots lie in register with the cranial half of the sclerotome, have important consequences for the definitive relationship between spinal nerves and vertebrae.

The neural crest and dorsal roots of spinal nerves

The neural crest arises at the lateral edges of the neural plate, at its junction with the future epidermis. When the tube closes, the crest cells form a wedge-shaped mass in its dorsal wall, from which they migrate extensively along two principal pathways: dorsolaterally, between the somite and the surface ectoderm, and ventrolaterally through the cranial half of the sclerotome. Neural crest cells give rise to a wide variety of cell types. We are concerned here only with those which start out on the ventrolateral pathway, but become arrested within the cranial half of the sclerotome, where they form segmental clusters of neuroblasts and satellite cells, the future dorsal root ganglia. As the primary sensory neurones differentiate, they send central axonal processes into the neural tube, and peripheral axons to sensory terminations. These axons collectively form the dorsal root of the spinal nerve.

When it first separates from the future spinal cord the neural crest forms a more or less continuous cord of cells, lying medial to the somites. It becomes segmented, in register with the somites (Fig. 2.10), and the segmental pattern, size and position of the dorsal root ganglia is determined primarily by inductive influences from the somites. Experimental analysis (in the chick) showed that when a block of somites was replaced by a strip of mesoderm made up of the cranial halves of several somites, the adjacent neural crest gave rise to a single unsegmented ganglion, about twice the total size of the contralateral (control) ganglia. By contrast, when faced with mesoderm made up of caudal halves of several somites, the neural crest formed ganglia, but their segmentation was disturbed and their final size reduced (Kalcheim & Teillet, 1989). Other experiments have shown that the neural tube is also involved, by producing a neurotrophic factor which supports the survival of developing cells of the dorsal root ganglia.

Regression of caudal end of neural tube and formation of filum terminale

The first two stages in development of the neural tube—primary and secondary neurulation—are pro-

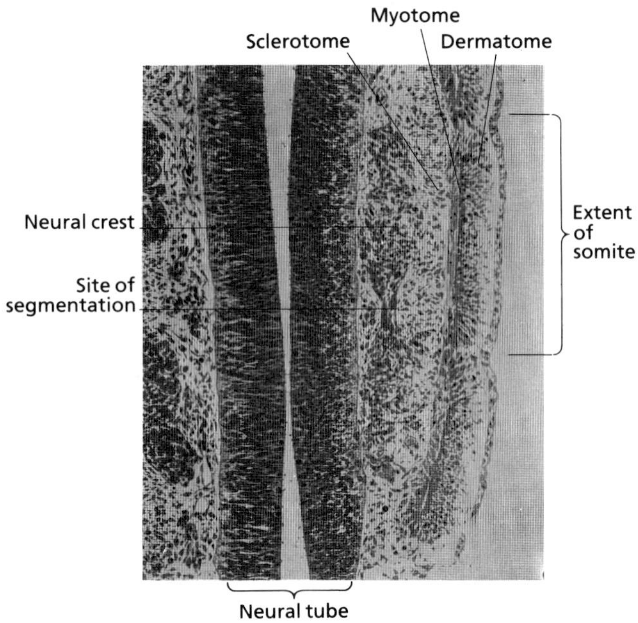

Fig. 2.10 Coronal section of neural tube, neural crest and somites. On (reader's) right, shows segmentation of originally unsegmented column of neural crest cells. Each segmental clump is coming to lie in the *cranial* half-sclerotome. Chick embryo. Photomicrograph from a preparation by John Farrow (×50).

gressive. They are followed by a third, which is regressive, and involves degeneration of the most caudal (coccygeal and postcoccygeal) segments of the neural tube.

In an embryo of 11.5 mm (Stage 17), Streeter (1919) described the neural tube as extending beyond the tip of the vertebral column (coccygeal vertebra 9 or 10). There were five coccygeal ganglia, of which only the first two were well developed and, opposite the ganglia, the cord showed characteristic ependymal, mantle and marginal zones. Further caudally it was poorly differentiated.

At the end of the embryonic period (Stage 23, eight weeks, about 30 mm), the spinal cord and vertebral column are coterminous and there are about five coccygeal vertebrae. The caudal end of the neural tube—essentially the coccygeal segments—is much narrowed and tapering, and its wall is made up only of ependyma and a thin marginal zone. The future conus medullaris lies opposite the first coccygeal vertebra. (Fig. 2.11b).

Thereafter, in the fetal stage, the vertebral column elongates more rapidly than does the spinal cord, whose cranial end is anchored to the brain. There occurs, therefore, a (relative) cranial migration of the caudal end of the spinal cord and of the attachments to it of the sacral nerves. Since the dorsal root ganglia are held in the intervertebral foramina, the dorsal roots become elongated, by a process of interstitial

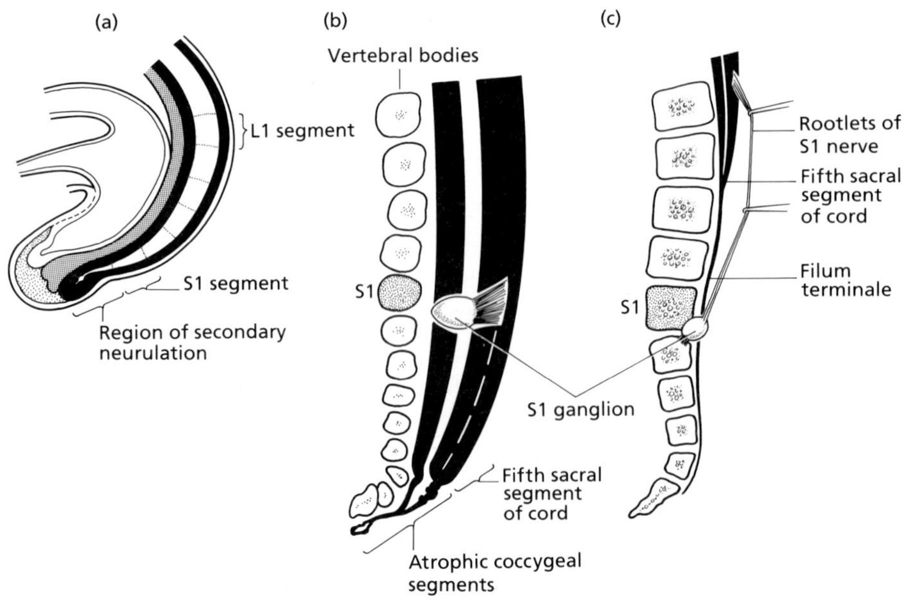

Fig. 2.11 Regression of coccygeal segments of spinal cord, formation of filum terminale and 'ascent' of conus medullaris. (a) Stage 12, 25 somites, about 26 days (cf. Fig. 1.6). After Muller & O'Rahilly (1987). (b) Stage 23, 30 mm, age eight weeks. The coccygeal segments have regressed; conus medullaris lies at level of first coccygeal vertebra; first sacral dorsal root ganglion lies at level of S1 vertebra. (c) 221 mm, age about 21 weeks. Conus medullaris lies at level of L3–L4. Atrophic coccygeal segments of cord drawn out to form filum terminale. S1 ganglion remains at S1–S2 intervertebral foramen. (b) and (c) after Streeter (1919). To allow comparison between three specimens, S1 somite (or derivatives) are aligned at same horizontal level.

growth rather than simple stretching. The filum terminale, which is formed from the atrophic coccygeal segments of the spinal cord, with its pial covering, is similarly elongated between its fixed caudal end and its continuity with the 'migrating' sacral region of the cord (Fig. 2.11c).

The relative 'ascent' of the termination of the cord is greatest between nine weeks and 19 weeks, when it lies at the level of the fourth lumbar vertebra. At birth it has reached the lower border of second lumbar vertebra and it attains its 'adult' level, between the first and second lumbar vertebrae, two months after birth (Barson, 1970a).

Three further points are worthy of note:

1 The retrogressive changes in the cord are confined to its coccygeal segments, which are formed by secondary neurulation (although they spare the lower sacral segments, which are similarly derived).

2 There is a high incidence of duplication of the central canal in the filum terminale of apparently normal children (Lendon & Emery, 1970), reflecting no doubt the frequency of duplication of the central canal of the coccygeal cord in apparently normal human embryos.

3 Differential growth of the vertebral column and the spinal cord affects the angulation of the roots of spinal nerves, which originally run directly laterally from their attachment to the cord to their exit through the intervertebral foramina. Because the cervical cord is fixed to the brain, the differential growth of vertebral column and spinal cord is manifest in caudal angulation of the spinal nerve roots, which increases progressively as one descends the series, being greatest in the sacral nerve roots (for details see Barry, 1956).

This normal pattern of 'ascent' of the spinal cord and the associated caudal angulation of the spinal nerve roots is commonly disturbed in cases of lumbar myelocoele (see later).

Somitomeres and somites

SOMITOMERES

So far we have considered development only of the neural component of the neurovertebral axis. We must now look at events in the mesodermal component, the paraxial mesoderm. Segmentation of paraxial mesoderm is expressed overtly by the formation of mesodermal somites, but, as first shown by Meier (1979), segmentation is already occurring in the paraxial mesoderm *before* somites appear. These presomitic segments are called somitomeres. They are formed, as paired two-layered discs of loosely arranged mesenchymal cells, beneath the still-open neural plate. They develop, in craniocaudal sequence, at the time of initial formation of the paraxial mesoderm from cells of the epiblast which ingress through the primitive streak.

Somitomeres become transformed into somites, as their constituent mesenchymal cells become epithelial (see review by Jacobson, 1988).

The factors which control somite formation have been analysed experimentally in amphibia and birds, and it seems likely that they are similar for mammals, including humans (reviewed by Nieuwkoop *et al.*, 1985). The neural plate is the principal inductor of somitomeres (and hence of somites) but the notochord also plays an important part. Continued intimate contact between axial structures and presomitic mesoderm is necessary for the formation of new somites, the maintenance of existing ones, and their further differentiation.

SOMITES

The somites form in pairs, in craniocaudal sequence (Fig. 2.12) starting at about three weeks postovulatory age. Although the maximum number in humans is normally said to be about 42–44, made up of four

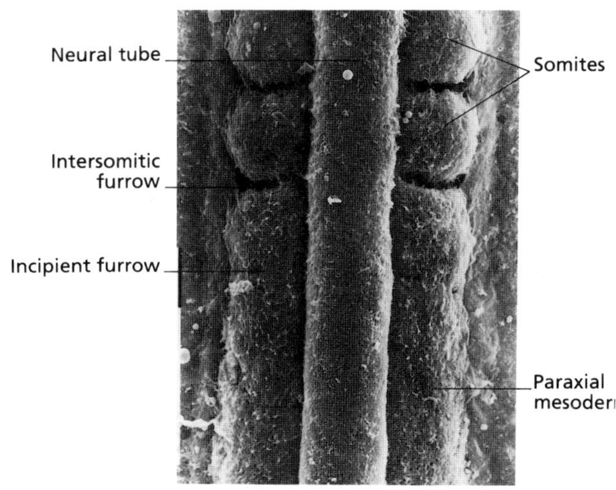

Fig. 2.12 Dorsal view of neural tube, flanked by paraxial mesoderm, exposed by removal of surface ectoderm. Somites are developing in craniocaudal sequence. Scanning electron micrograph of a preparation by John Farrow.

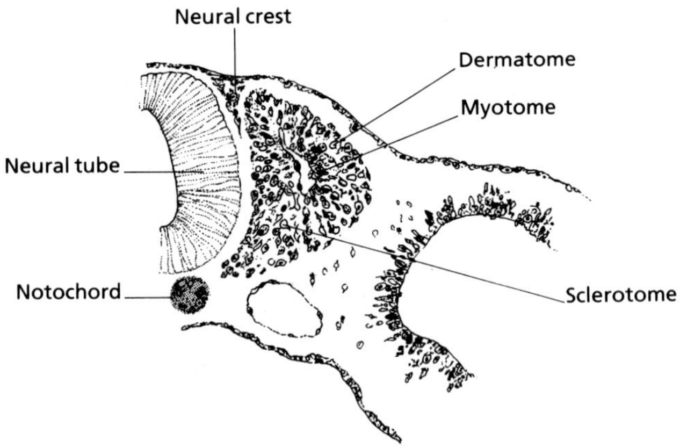

Fig. 2.13 Transverse section of a 15-somite human embryo (Stage 11, about 24 days). The somite is a clearly circumscribed, wedge-shaped structure flanking the neural tube. The positions of dermatome, myotome and sclerotome are indicated, but they are not yet clearly demarcated. Note the cell-free zone around the notochord. Drawing based on a photomicrograph by Mizoguti (1989).

occipital, eight cervical, twelve thoracic, five lumbar, five sacral and a variable number of coccygeal, the largest number present at any one time is about 38, due to loss of occipital and coccygeal somites (see O'Rahilly and Meyer, 1979; Muller & O'Rahilly, 1986).

FATE OF THE SOMITES

The epithelial somite, originally a ball of cells, with a small lumen (the myocele), becomes wedge-shaped and differentiates into three components: dermatome, myotome and sclerotome (Fig. 2.13).

The *dermatome* is the epithelial outer wall of the somite. Its cells will later migrate, in a delimited group, under the ectoderm, to form the dermis and subcutis. The *myotome* will give rise to myoblasts, precursors of the skeletal muscle fibres of limbs and trunk. Both dermatome and myotome are induced by the adjacent epidermis; the neural tube is essential for the maintenance of the myotomes, and it enhances muscle differentiation. The *sclerotome* forms the ventromedial part of the wedge. Its development is dependent upon the proximity of the notochord, of the ventral part of the neural tube and of the neural crest. Its cells lose their compact epithelial arrangement and form a loose-meshed embryonic connective tissue—mesenchyme. Sclerotomic cells are usually said to migrate medially into the extracellular matrix which surrounds the notochord and the neural tube. This 'migration' may be more apparent than real: Gasser (1979) suggested that the dermatomyotome component of the somite moves laterally as the embryo grows, trailing behind it cells which proliferate and form a condensed mass, the membranous precursor of the centrum, neural arch and costal element of the vertebra.

Development of the vertebral column

Three stages may be recognized, although there is considerable overlap between them:

1 the mesenchymal stage: formation of a blastema of condensed mesenchyme;

2 cartilaginous transformation of the blastema; and

3 ossification of the cartilage model.

The mesenchymal stage

This follows almost immediately upon the formation of somites in the paraxial mesoderm and proceeds in craniocaudal sequence as new somites are added caudally in the series. As cells migrate from the sclerotome their loss is made good by cell proliferation in the somites, which therefore serve as growth centres for the early vertebral column.

The mesenchymal stage may be said (somewhat arbitrarily) to end in embryos of 8–10 mm (Stage 16; 37 days) which show the latest stage in mesenchymal condensation, prior to cartilage formation. A mesenchymal component of the vertebrae is still seen, however, in embryos of 50 mm (about nine weeks) which also show advanced chondrification, and even the start of ossification.

The early part of the mesenchymal stage is of importance to the clinician because it is then that the patterns in the future vertebral column—of segmentation, of regional specialization and of the relationship of vertebrae to spinal nerves—are being established.

Although there have been various views about the relationship between the segmental pattern of the somites and that of the definitive vertebrae to which they give rise, they are mostly variations on a theme, common to most textbooks, and usually illustrated by coronal sections, which cut the notochord along its length and show it flanked on each side by a series of sclerotomes (Fig. 2.14). The sclerotomic portions of adjacent somites are shown as demarcated from one

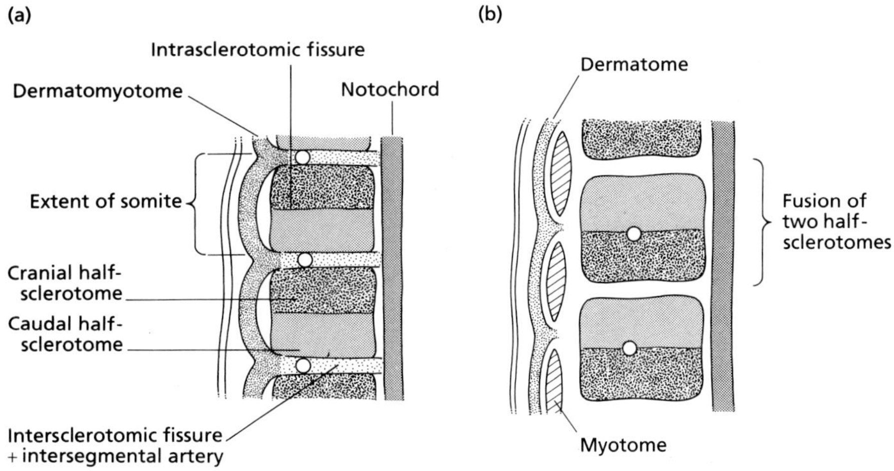

Fig. 2.14 Scheme of traditional view of vertebral development, as seen in coronal section through notochord and somites of one side of body. (a) Each sclerotome shows loosely cellular cranial half and dense ('condensed') caudal half. Sclerotomes are demarcated by 'intersclerotomic fissure', containing intersegmental artery. (b) After 'resegmentation', caudal half of one sclerotome fuses with cranial half of one caudal to it, to form an (intersegmental) vertebral body. Based on Arey (1965).

another by *intersegmental fissures*, occupied by intersegmental arteries. Each sclerotome is bisected horizontally, by an *intrasclerotomic fissure*, into cranial and caudal halves, a process called *resegmentation*. Each half is called a *sclerotomite*. Resegmentation is visibly reinforced when the caudal sclerotomite becomes more densely cellular ('condensed') while the cranial one remains loosely cellular and palely stained. The mesenchymal blastema of a single vertebra is said to be formed by the migration of the condensed (caudal) sclerotomite, and its fusion with the looser (cranial) sclerotomite lying caudally to it; i.e. each vertebra receives contributions from two sclerotomes; one sclerotome contributes to two adjacent vertebrae. This means, of course, that the mesenchymal blastema is *intersegmental*, an arrangement which conveniently allows for the exit of *segmental* spinal nerves through the intervertebral foramina. The mesenchymal blastema so formed consists of a continuous mass, within which there will eventually develop the future centrum (only roughly equivalent to the body of a vertebra), two neural processes, which together will form the neural arch, and two costal processes, which will form ribs in the thoracic region and the costal elements (rib-equivalents) elsewhere in the vertebral column. The nucleus pulposus of the intervertebral disc is derived from the notochord, which normally disappears where it runs through the centra of the vertebrae.

The variations on this classical view of vertebral development were based on differing assessments of the relative contribution of caudal and cranial portions of a sclerotome to the centrum, neural and costal processes. In so far as a generalization can be made, it is perhaps that expressed by Arey (1965): 'the denser portion is the dominant part of the vertebral primordium. It shares in the formation of the centrum and, almost unaided, gives rise to the processes that become the vertebral arch and ribs.'

This general consensus, such as it is, was challenged most recently and most cogently, by Verbout (1985), whose main contentions were these (Fig. 2.15):

1 That the term 'sclerotome', as used above, was inappropriate, since the mesenchyme arising by loosening of the medial walls of adjacent somites, formed at first a single uninterrupted longitudinal block of tissue, and that the intersegmental fissures were either artifacts, or represented sectional profiles of intersegmental vessels which happened to fall in the plane of section.

2 That, while agreeing that the 'region bounded by two successive intersegmental vessels' (i.e. the 'sclerotome' of traditional accounts) *did* show a loosely cellular cranial half and a condensed caudal half; it did *not* become divided along the boundary between these two halves. The so-called intrasclerotomic fissure was an artificial split or tear along the boundary between the dense caudal half and the loose cranial half, whose cells were becoming orientated concentrically around the developing roots of the associated spinal nerve.

3 That the neural arch and the costal process both developed *in situ* from the *caudal* condensed mesenchyme. 'The question whether the cranial half of the same segment contributes . . . is not relevant' (Verbout, 1985, p. 71).

4 That the axial column of vertebral bodies arose principally from an initially unsegmented *perichor-*

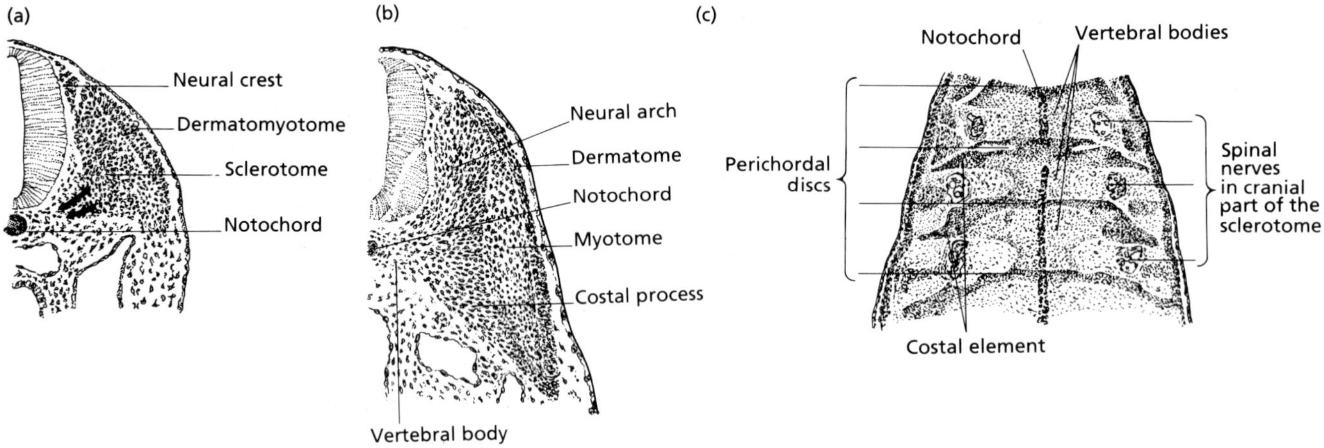

Fig. 2.15 Contribution of sclerotome to formation of mesenchymal vertebra. (a) Transverse section of somite in 25-somite embryo, showing beginning migration of sclerotomal cells medially, (arrows) to contribute to loosely cellular perichordal mesenchyme. (b) Transverse section of 7 mm embryo, passing through condensed caudal half of a sclerotome, whose cells contribute to vertebral body, neural arch and costal process. (c) Coronal section through notochord with surrounding vertebral and intervertebral structures. Based on illustrations in Arey (1965) and Verbout (1985).

dal tube, formed of layers of cells arranged concentrically around the notochord, and derived from a loose column of *axial* mesenchyme, not solely of somitic origin, although probably reinforced by medially migrating somitic cells.

5 That within the axial column, condensations appeared which would form the annuli fibrosi of the intervertebral discs: two adjacent discs defined between them the membranous precursor of the vertebral body.

The traditional view, and Verbout's (1985) denial of most of its tenets, were both based on microscopic study of histological sections, with all the attendant hazards of reconstructing a dynamic process from a series of static pictures. Disagreements of this magnitude between the findings of skilled observers probably point to the inherent limitations of the techniques used. Recent experimental studies have thrown new light on an old problem and, perhaps surprisingly, have tended to support certain features of the traditional view. That they were, of necessity, carried out on avian embryos should not lead one to discount their relevance for mammalian development; Verbout (1985) himself stressed that his concepts were equally applicable to birds and mammals.

Bagnall *et al.* (1988) replaced a single somite in a chick embryo with a single somite from a quail embryo, and followed the fate, in the resultant chick–quail chimaera, of the quail cells, which carried a readily identifiable, and permanent, nuclear marker. In general, the results supported the concept of resegmentation. Cells from a *single* somite were found to migrate, and to contribute to the caudal half of one vertebral body, the intervening disc and the cranial half of the next vertebral body. This division was also found in the neural arch: a single somite contributed to the caudal and cranial portions of adjacent arches, but the major contribution was to the caudal arch.

This experimental evidence of the different fate of cranial and caudal halves of the sclerotome reinforces other evidence that the two halves differ from one another, quite apart from the obvious difference in their cellular density: (a) when like somite halves (cranial or caudal) are placed adjacent to each other their cells mix, while those from unlike halves do not (Stern & Keynes, 1987); (b) cranial somite halves selectively determine segmentation of the neural crest and the migration pathway of dorsal and ventral roots of developing spinal nerves (see above).

Bagnall *et al.* (1989) also provided experimental proof that, in addition to its contribution to the vertebrae, the sclerotome gave rise to other components of the vertebral column: the annulus fibrosus of the intervertebral disc, the meninges, the endothelium of some meningeal blood vessels, and the ligaments and general connective tissue of the column. In short, all the tissues within a segment (defined by a pair of somites) were formed from somitic cells, except for the notochord, neural tube, epidermis and gut epithelium. They found little mixing of cells from a particular somite with similar cells of adjacent somites, even during their migration. Of particular interest is their suggestion that even cells from the cranial and caudal halves of the *same* sclerotome do not mix during migration, but stay in their segmental position.

The controversy over resegmentation is not, of course, purely 'academic': its resolution is essential to clear thinking about several vertebral abnormalities. Can we, therefore, reconcile the conflicting views? The experimental evidence makes it clear that there are real differences between the cranial and caudal halves of each sclerotome; that sclerotomal cells do indeed migrate medially to surround the notochord and the neural tube; that resegmentation does occur, so that each vertebra receives contributions from two adjacent sclerotomes. In short, the classical view of vertebral development is vindicated in the outcome. It must be said, however, that although Verbout's exquisitely detailed morphological analysis led him to an erroneous conclusion, it is still of value in revealing as crudely mechanistic the classical concept of splitting of each sclerotome and the mass migration of the cells of its caudal half. The processes of resegmentation, migration and recombination of the sclerotomal contributors are evidently executed much more subtly than is implied in textbook schemas.

Even at the stage of the condensed mesenchymal blastema it is already evident that there are important and characteristic regional differences between, e.g., cervical and thoracic vertebrae, even though vertebrae from each region conform to a common plan, of centrum, neural arch and costal elements (see below).

What determines these regional differences, and the timing of that determination, are obviously of interest to the clinician concerned with aberrant vertebral development. The experimental evidence makes it quite clear that regionalization is determined very early: if *unsegmented* paraxial mesoderm from the cervical region is interchanged with that from the thoracic region, vertebrae with cervical characteristics are produced in the thoracic region, and vice-versa (Kieny *et al.*, 1972). However, it should be noted, as a warning against thinking that there is rigid determinism of the fate of a particular somite, that the chick embryo can recover completely from the removal of a single somite and produce a normal vertebral column (Bagnall *et al.*, 1986).

The cartilaginous stage

The process of transformation of the mesenchymal vertebra into a cartilaginous one begins at a number of centres, from which it spreads so that eventually each vertebra is represented by a single cartilage model. Chondrification begins in the centra at Stage 17 (11–14 mm, about six weeks) and in the laminae, articular processes and pedicles by Stage 19 (16–18 mm; about seven weeks).

A transverse section through a cartilaginous thoracic vertebra of a 22 mm human embryo (Stage 21; *c.* 52 days) (Fig. 2.16a) will serve as a model for each region of the column. In a single section, it shows several important features.

1 That the centrum, and the three components of each half of the neural arch (pedicle, lamina, transverse process) form a virtually continuous mass of cartilage; only the rib is demarcated by its developing joints with the vertebra.

2 The two neural processes extend dorsally to about the level of attachment of the dorsal rootlets of the spinal nerve to the spinal cord.

3 The dorsal surface of the spinal cord has no skeletal covering, but is invested by loose vascular mesenchyme (the future pia-arachnoid) and by the membrana reuniens dorsalis, a fibrous membrane which unites the dorsal ends of the neural processes; its inner layer will form dura mater (Fig. 2.16b).

At this stage therefore the embryo shows, as a normal feature, the condition of spina bifida occulta. The spinal cord normally acquires its complete skeletal investment by the progressive extension of the cartilaginous neural processes, as the result of appositional growth of their dorsal tips, which continues until the two processes fuse, in fetuses of about 50 mm (Sensenig, 1949).

4 The ventral end of the dorsal root ganglion already lies in its definitive position, in the intervertebral foramen, where the dorsal and ventral roots of the spinal nerve unite.

Figure 2.17 shows homologous parts of cartilaginous vertebrae from other regions of the column, as determined by O'Rahilly *et al.* (1990a,b). Attention is drawn particularly to the costal elements (i.e. rib-equivalents) in extrathoracic vertebrae. These become of interest to the surgeon when they give rise to cervical, lumbar and (rarely) sacral ribs (see later).

Since the form of the bony vertebra is largely determined by the form and growth of its cartilaginous

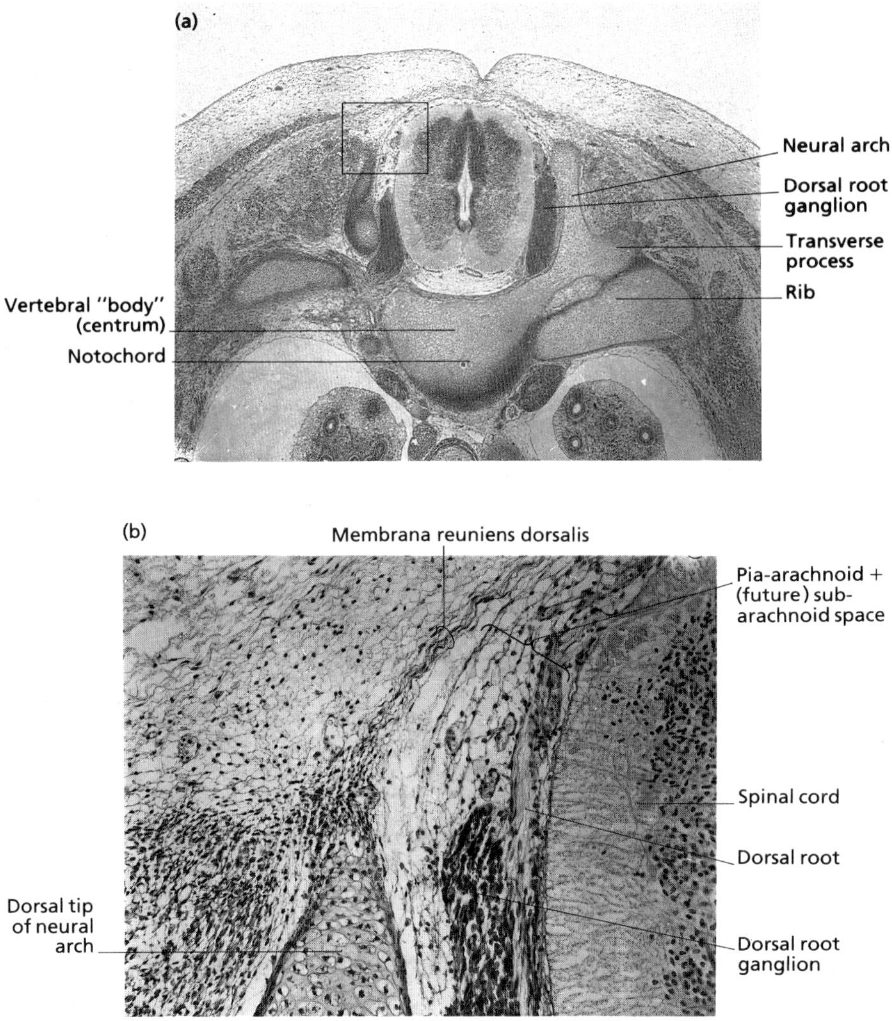

Fig. 2.16 (a) Cartilaginous thoracic vertebra and rib, of 22 mm human embryo (×20). Note: (1) centrum, neural arch and transverse process form continuous cartilaginous model of the vertebra, from which the cartilaginous rib is demarcated by developing costovertebral joints; (2) tip of neural arch extends dorsally to level of dorsal rootlets of spinal nerve. (b) Detail of area corresponding to rectangle marked on (a) but from a 17 mm human embryo (×126). Author's collection.

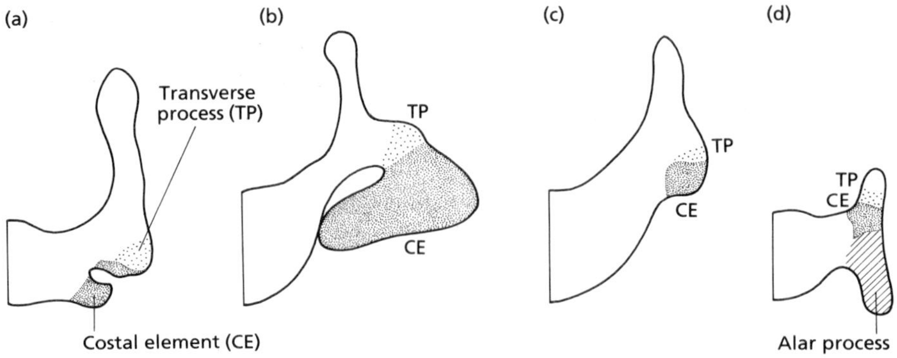

Fig. 2.17 Homologous parts of cervical (a), thoracic (b), lumbar (c) and sacral (d) vertebrae at cartilaginous stage. Note costal element, CE (rib-equivalent) and transverse process, TP. The alar process is thought to be unique to sacral vertebrae. Based on the work of O'Rahilly and Muller (1990a,b).

precursor, the factors which initiate and control the process of chondrification are obviously important. Chondrification depends on inductive interactions between spinal cord and notochord on the one hand, and sclerotomic mesenchyme on the other. Experimental analysis has shown:

1 that the centra do not become cartilaginous if the notochord is extirpated;

2 that neural arch chondrification depends upon the presence of the spinal cord;
3 that the spinal cord and notochord exert their inductive influence only on *sclerotomic* mesenchyme, whose inherent 'chondrogenic bias' is simply accelerated by the inductors (for review, see Nieuwkoop *et al.*, 1985).

DEVELOPMENT OF THE INTERVERTEBRAL DISCS

This account is based largely on the work of Peacock (1951) and Walmsley (1953).

Development of the disc involves a complex series of interactions between the notochord and a surrounding *perichordal disc* of condensed mesenchyme, largely derived, like the vertebral centra between which it lies, from sclerotomic mesenchyme. In longitudinal sections the perichordal discs are seen to lie in a segmental position, alternating with the less densely cellular vertebral centra (Fig. 2.15c).

The cells of the disc show an extensive developmental repertoire.
1 Those at the periphery of the disc begin, in embryos of about 15 mm, to differentiate into fibroblasts, which by the end of the embryonic period (*c.* 30 mm, eight weeks) start to lay down the collagenous lamellae of the outer part of the annulus fibrosus. The complex criss-crossing patterns of fibres in these lamellae seem to be genetically determined, since they develop well in advance of the functional demands which they will be called upon to meet.
2 Where the perichordal disc faces the adjacent vertebral centra, its cells differentiate into chondroblasts, which make a major contribution to the cranial–caudal growth of the cartilaginous vertebral bodies.
3 Within the outer shell of the disc its cells form a flattened sphere, called the inner cell zone, traversed by the notochord, and retaining the developmental potential of mesenchyme. This inner cell zone is of importance for the further development and growth of the disc, since it contributes both to the annulus fibrosus and to the nucleus pulposus.

In embryos of about 20 mm, notochordal cells begin to proliferate at the intervertebral level, to form localized aggregates. At vertebral levels they normally disappear during the cartilaginous stage, leaving behind a 'mucoid streak', or notochordal sheath, which traverses the developing vertebral centrum, and normally disappears in early fetal life as the vertebral bodies ossify. This mucoid streak may persist for some time; if it does so, it appears to inhibit the growth of the cartilage of the vertebral centrum, and Walmsley (1953) suggests that its prolonged persistence may account for disturbances in ossification of the centrum. Taylor (1972) found an associated increase in the heights of affected centra, with a corresponding narrowing of the intervening discs. Notochordal cells persisting in the vertebral body have been regarded as the source of chordomas. That these occur most commonly in the sacrococcygeal region may be related to the persistence of notochordal cells into adulthood in disc remnants in the sacrum.

At the intervertebral level, notochordal cells continue to increase in number and in size during the first six months of fetal life and become surrounded by a 'mucoid' intercellular matrix, produced partly by the notochordal cells, partly by the inner cell zone.

After the sixth month the notochordal cells show progressive signs of senescence and degeneration so that, at birth, the nucleus pulposus, which now forms the main mass of the disc, consists mainly of 'mucoid' matrix. This will be progressively replaced, during childhood, by fibrocartilage, produced centripetally by chondroblasts of the annulus fibrosus and of the cartilage plates on the upper and lower surfaces of the adjacent vertebral bodies.

The discs are avascular at all stages of their development; they are nourished by diffusion of fluid derived from vessels in the adjacent vertebral bodies. Walmsley (1953) points out that the limitation of the epiphysis in humans to a peripheral annulus allows more ready diffusion through most of the upper and lower surfaces of the vertebra into the disc than would be the case if humans were like most pronograde mammals and had complete plate-like epiphyses.

The stage of ossification

Each vertebra ossifies from three primary centres, and five secondary centres.

The primary centres include one for the centrum, and one for each half of the neural arch. Most of them appear in fetuses of about 50–65 mm crown–rump length (10th and 11th weeks), although those in the lower sacral segments do not appear until the 20th to the 30th weeks. The five secondary centres appear at about puberty, and include one for the tip of each spinous process, one for the tip of each transverse process, and an 'annular epiphysis' at the periphery of the upper and lower surface of each vertebral body.

There have been many studies of the timing and sequence of appearance of the primary centres (reviewed by Noback & Robertson, 1951), but the definitive account is that of Bagnall *et al.* (1977b), based on a radiological study of a large number of normal fetuses obtained by hysterotomy. Their findings differ from conventional descriptions for the neural arches, in which centres appear first in a group of lower cervical/upper thoracic vertebrae, followed shortly by centres in the upper cervical region, and then by centres in the lower thoracic/upper lumbar region. The process of ossification spreads from these three areas in cranial and caudal directions. They confirmed the traditional view that centres for the centra always appear first in the lower thoracic/upper lumbar region, from which ossification spreads cranially and, rather more slowly, caudally.

Certain general features are worth comment.

1 In neither the neural arches nor the centra does the sequence of appearance of ossification centres conform to the usual craniocaudal sequence of development, such as occurs in the mesenchymal and cartilaginous stages.

2 Bagnall *et al.* (1977b) found that ossification centres for the neural arches and for the centra develop independently of one another, with no obvious correlation between the patterns in the two components. In seeking to explain the peculiar pattern, they suggested that the onset of ossification 'in these particular regions could provide firm anchorage for the muscles controlling extension of the head and movements of the pectoral girdle and upper limbs', movements which are part of one of the earliest fetal reflexes, the 'gasp' reflex. This ingenious speculation is not supported by experimental evidence that the time of appearance of primary ossification centres is largely determined by genetic factors.

3 Knowledge of the *pattern* of ossification of the vertebral body may be important in understanding some developmental anomalies. Some authors (e.g. Beadle, 1931) have concluded from the study of anomalous vertebrae that each centrum ossifies from two bilateral ossification centres. However, each of the centra studied by Noback (1944) ossified from a single centre. Walmsley (1953) made the important observation that the ossification of the vertebral body is analogous to that of a typical long bone, in that bone first develops in the periosteum. This periosteal collar is restricted initially to the *posterior* surface of the bone. Endochondral ossification of the cartilage model is effected by a large osteogenetic bud which enters the *posterior* surface of the model. It is Walmsley's (1953) view that 'the massive excavation of the cartilage in the interior of the vertebra . . . would appear to be inconsistent with the ossification of a vertebra occurring from one, two or more separate endochondral ossific centres'.

The vertebral column at birth

At birth a typical vertebra is in three parts, ossified from the three primary centres and joined together by cartilage (Fig. 2.18). The centrum is joined to each half of the neural arch by a *neurocentral synchrondrosis*, whose position makes it clear: (a) that the posterolateral parts of the definitive vertebral body are formed from the neural arch and (b) that the rib articulates with the neural arch contribution. The upper and lower surfaces of the body are each covered by a plate of cartilage, which serves as anchorage for the annulus fibrosus of the intervertebral disc and also as a growth plate, providing for the longitudinal growth of the vertebral body (for a quantitative study of longitudinal growth of the column, see Bagnall *et al.*, 1979). The two halves of each neural arch are united by cartilage, so that an X-ray of the spine presents an appearance of spina bifida occulta totalis.

At puberty an annular epiphysis develops on the periphery of each cartilage plate. Growth in diameter of the vertebral body occurs, by subperiosteal deposition of bone, accompanied by internal remodelling. Growth is more rapid on the ventral surface of the vertebral body, resulting in posterior displacement of the nucleus pulposus, which, at birth and during the first postnatal year, is large, soft and gelatinous, and forms a greater proportion of the disc than it does later, when its growth lags, its cells degenerate and it is gradually invaded by the surrounding fibrocartilage of the annulus fibrosus.

Generations of medical students have been taught that the fetal spine shows a uniform kyphotic curve, that the cervical lordosis begins to develop only when the infant starts to raise its head and sit up, and that lumbar lordosis appears only with assumption of the upright stance. This conventional view has been challenged by Bagnall *et al.* (1977a), who found evidence for the appearance, in the early fetal period, of cervical

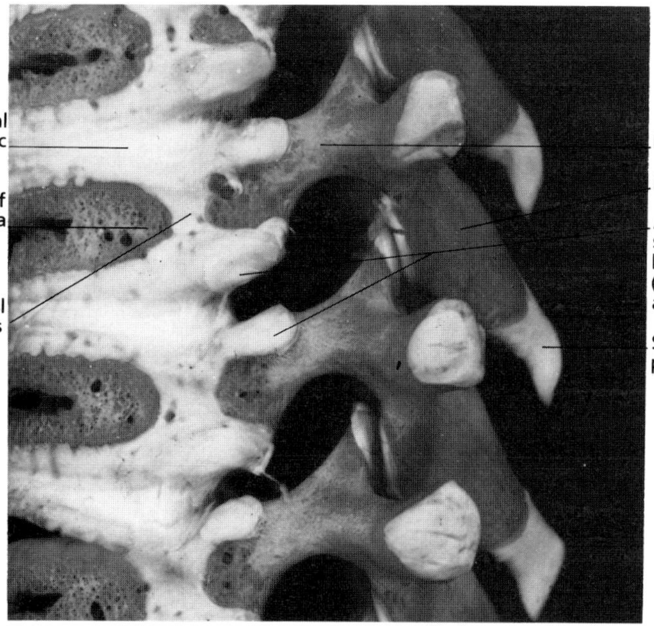

Fig. 2.18 Lateral view of part of thoracic vertebral column of a child 'of about two years'. Note: (1) The neurocentral synchondrosis which unites the centrum to the neural arch; (2) the cartilaginous spinous processes; (3) the articular surfaces on the neural arches for the head of a rib. Photograph of a specimen in the William Hunter Anatomical Museum, University of Glasgow.

lordosis, which they correlated with muscular activity associated with the gasp reflex, and by O'Rahilly *et al.* (1980) who identified a 'slight flattening' in the lumbosacral region, even in the embryonic period (eighth week). It should be said, however, that these secondary curves undoubtedly become *accentuated* at the traditional times, and probably for the traditional reasons. We would do well to remember the wise words of Wood Jones (1946): 'The flexibility of the spine of the infant is notorious, and the general passive mobility of the head is produced . . . by the extreme plasticity of the cervical part of the vertebral column itself. The vertebral column of the infant may be made to assume almost any curvature, but all such curvatures are transient.'

Development of the spinal meninges and subarachnoid space

In an embryo of 18 mm the spinal cord is surrounded by a loose-meshed layer of mesenchyme, thicker ventrally than dorsally. Within this layer the subarachnoid space develops from about seven weeks onwards, splitting it into an inner vascular, pial layer, and an outer layer of arachnoid, in contact with the dura mater (Sensenig, 1951). Attention has already been drawn to the membrana reuniens dorsalis, which is attached to the dorsal tips of the cartilaginous neural processes, and arches over the dorsal surface of the cord. The inner layer of this forms dura mater; the outer layer provides the bed into which the neural arches grow, to meet and fuse in the midline.

It was suggested, in the classic study by Weed (1917) and also by McLone & Bondareff (1975), that the flow of cerebrospinal fluid (CSF) is an important factor in initiating development of the space, but this was not supported by a recent study (Mohamed, 1989) which showed that, in the mouse, the subarachnoid space appears first in areas remote from the roof of the IVth ventricle, before the time of appearance of the lateral foramina (of Luschka) and therefore presumably before the establishment of bulk flow of CSF.

The long-standing controversy over the origin of the mesenchyme from which the spinal meninges develop has been resolved by experimental proof that it arises from somitic mesenchyme (and not from neural crest).

THE EMBRYOLOGY OF NEUROVERTEBRAL DEFECTS: A SPECULATION

For the clinician, this account of normal development of the neurovertebral axis is of value only in so far as it sheds some light on the possible origins of developmental defects.

Neural tube defects

Any interpretation of the embryological origin of spinal cord defects in humans is necessarily speculative, for several reasons: (a) because it is based on a limited number of specimens, each at some unknown point along a pathway of maldevelopment; (b) because malformation seldom arises purely by arrest at some point along the normal developmental route. Development may well continue for some time after the initial aberration, along one of several aberrant pathways; (c) interpretation of the final outcome may be complicated by non-specific secondary changes, e.g. degeneration in an open neural plate, and by compensatory developmental adjustments.

With these cautions in mind we can examine three main hypotheses about the pathogenesis of neural tube defects.

The 'secondary reopening' hypothesis

This maintains that open neural tube defects arise through secondary reopening of a closed tube. It has long been championed by Gardner (1980) who attempted to establish a common pathogenesis for the frequently associated conditions of hydrocephalomyelia, Arnold-Chiari malformation and neural dysraphism. He attributed rupture of the closed roof plate to increased pressure of fluid in the neural canal, due to impermeability of the ependymal roof of the IVth ventricle. This speculation was not supported by the experiments of Warkany and O'Toole (1981) which suggested that these associated conditions were each caused independently by a single teratogenic insult.

Padget (1970) described, in human embryos, defects ('neuroschisis') in the roof plate of the neural tube, which allowed fluid to escape, disrupting the overlying mesenchyme and surface ectoderm, but O'Rahilly & Muller (1988) refute these findings.

There are only a few reports suggesting that reopening can be produced by administration of teratogens *after* the time of closure of the tube (e.g. Padmanabhan, 1984).

Although its bearing on the spontaneous origin of neural tube defects in humans appears to be limited, experimental reopening of the neural tube in chicks by incision of the roof plate provides valuable insights into the possible behaviour of the tube should reopening occur. Fowler (1953) showed that incision led to myeloschisis in some cases, often with overgrowth of the everted neural tube halves, similar to that described in spontaneous myeloschisis in human embryos by Patten (1953), and regarded by him as a cause of 'failure to close'. Rokos & Knowles (1976) showed rapid re-establishment of continuity between neurectoderm and surface ectoderm, to produce a lesion indistinguishable from that usually attributed to failure to close. Clark & Scothorne (1990) have shown that incision of the roof plate in younger embryos is commonly followed by apparently perfect healing, while in older embryos splaying of the margins of the incised tube, and a persistent defect, is the usual outcome (Fig. 2.19). It may be more than coincidence that the neural tube was still occluded at the time of incision in the younger embryos; the forces which produce occlusion may also have resisted splaying open of the incised tube and therefore facilitated healing.

The 'failure-to-close' hypothesis

The newer view, currently more favoured, attributes the defect to failure of the neural tube to close. It is supported by many studies of young human embryos showing such defects (e.g. Patten, 1953; Dekaban and Bartelmez, 1964; Lemire, 1969; Osaka *et al.*, 1978), and by experimental studies in animals, in which defects were produced by teratogens which appeared to act by interfering with one or more of the many mechanisms held to be responsible for closure (see e.g. Warkany *et al.*, 1958; O'Shea & Kaufman, 1980, 1981; Schoenwolf & Fisher, 1983; Lee & Nagele, 1985).

A third view supports the 'failure-to-close' hypothesis but assigns a major causative role either to deficiencies in the adjacent non-neural tissues or to a disturbance in relative growth rates of the (mesodermal) vertebral column and of the (neurectodermal) spinal cord. It is supported by several lines of evidence.

1 In embryos showing early stages in the development of a neural tube defect, there is commonly *overgrowth* of the unfused and everted halves of the neural plate, and Patten (1953) suggested that closure was blocked by its own exuberant overgrowth. (Note that overgrowth may occur secondarily to experimental reopening of chick neural tube: see above.)

2 Barson (1970b) has drawn attention to two associ-

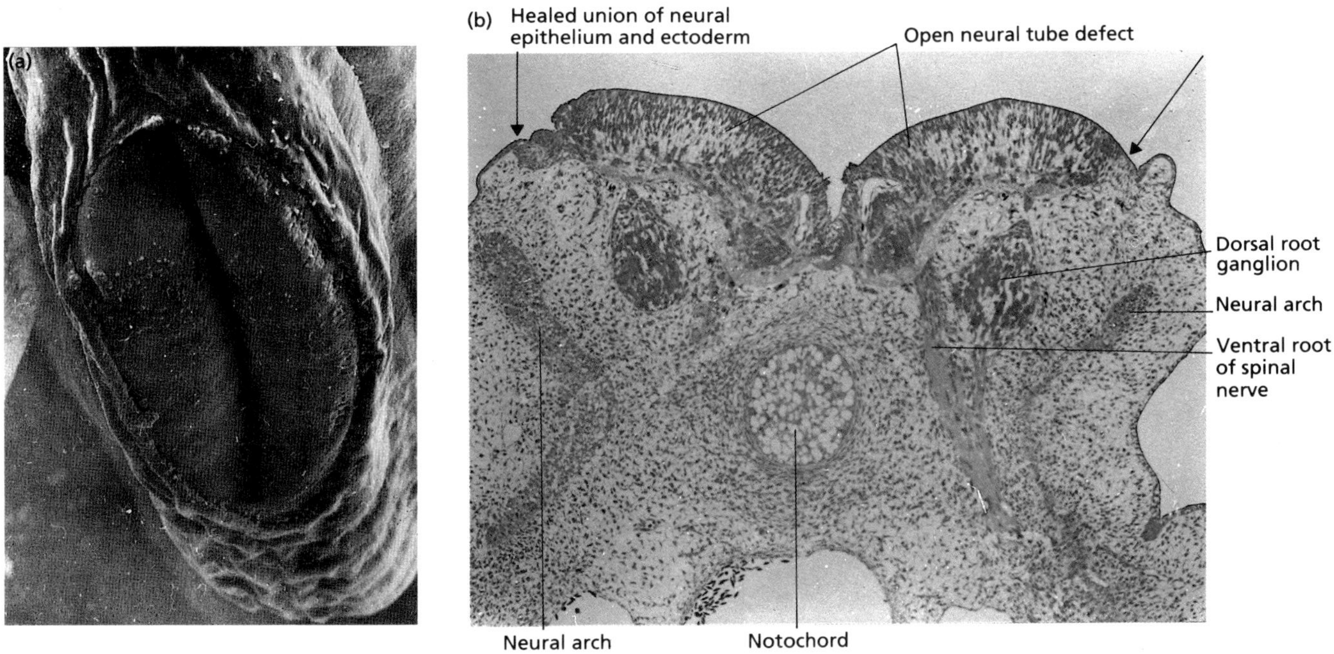

Fig. 2.19 (a) Scanning electron micrograph of open neural tube defect in a chick, produced by incision of roof plate. Note widely splayed walls of neural tube, reminiscent of myeloschisis in human. (b) Transverse section through defect shown in (a) Note: (1) healed union, on each side, of neural epithelium and surface ectoderm (arrows); (2) widely splayed blastemata of neural arches. Specimens prepared by Brian Clark.

ated features in infants with spina bifida and myelocele:

(a) a 25% incidence of lumbar kyphosis, which he suggested might result from an *overgrowth* in length of the neural tube, producing an exaggeration of the normal dorsal convexity of the embryo; and

(b) the abnormally low termination of the cord in many infants with spina bifida and the characteristically altered angulation of the spinal nerve roots, which pass *upwards* in the lumbar region at the level of the myelocele, and downwards below the lesion.

Barson (1970a,b) argued that these associated anomalies point to a derangement of the relative growth of mesodermal and neurectodermal tissues.

3 Strong experimental support has come from the work of Alles & Sulik (1990) on spina bifida in mice, produced by administration of retinoic acid to the pregnant mothers. They found a high incidence of non-closure of the caudal neuropore, with eversion of the neural plate halves, associated with increased cell death in the tissues underlying the caudal end of the neural tube. They attributed the eversion of the neural plate to its continued growth, concomitant with increased cell death and, therefore, delayed growth, in the mesenchymal tissues in the region of the primitive streak and the tail gut, specifically produced by the teratogen. Similar pathogenetic mechanisms have been suggested for other malformations induced by retinoic acid.

4 Caudal neural tube defects in the curly tail mutant mouse have been shown by Copp *et al.* (1988a,b) to be caused by imbalance between growth of ventral and dorsal tissues in the tail.

Defects of vertebrae and ribs

Numerical and regional variation in the vertebral column

In the adult the number of presacral vertebrae is 24 in 90% of the population, 23 or 25 each in 5%, and 24 is the usual number in embryos, although 25 is much more common than 23 (see O'Rahilly *et al.*, 1980). A distinction must be drawn between an absolute increase in number, and an apparent increase, due to variation at the lumbosacral junction and the 'lumbarization' of first sacral vertebra.

In the sacrum there are five vertebrae in about 85%, six in 14%, and four in 1% of the population, although there are significant racial variations. An increase to six may result from sacralization of the last lumbar vertebra (which may be the fifth or sixth lumbar) or of the first coccygeal vertebra. Sacralization of the last lumbar vertebra occurs in about 7–11% of adults. The processes which lead to it are probably already in train early in development: at eight weeks 'the cartilaginous sacral vertebrae are already joined in such a way that the main areas of the definitive bone can be recognised' (O'Rahilly *et al.*, 1990b). Indeed, as indicated above, the characteristics of different regions of the column are already established at the mesenchymal stage of development.

Sacralization of the fifth lumbar vertebra seems to involve development of an alar element normally absent from presacral vertebrae (see Fig. 2.17) and its articulation or fusion, complete or incomplete, on one or both sides, with the alar element of the first sacral vertebra, associated with variable degrees of fusion between the centra and neural processes of the apposed vertebrae.

The junctional region between the skull and the cervical vertebral column is another common site of variation. In the embryo the distinction between these two regions is less clear-cut than it is in the adult. The first four pairs of somites are called occipital, and they bear a relationship to the rootlets of the twelfth cranial (hypoglossal) nerve similar to that of a trunk somite to the ventral rootlets of a spinal nerve. Like trunk somites, occipital somites become divided into myotomes, which (certainly) in birds and (probably) in mammals form the tongue musculature, and sclerotomes, which contribute to the basi- and exoccipital parts of the skull in birds, and probably also in mammals. Occipital sclerotomes resemble those of the trunk in showing subdivision into loose cranial and dense caudal moieties, thereby supporting the idea that the basi- and exoccipitals 'represent' modified cervical vertebrae.

The developmental and evolutionary histories of the first two cervical vertebrae are equally complex. At the end of the embryonic period (Week 8) the body of the axis and its odontoid process are represented by a unitary column of cartilage, subdivided by two shallow horizontal surface grooves into three parts, identified by O'Rahilly *et al.* (1983), in craniocaudal sequence, as X, Y and Z. Of these, Z will form the centrum of the axis, while Y ossifies separately (in fetuses of about 160 mm) to form the basal half of the odontoid process, and represents the centrum of the atlas; the remains of a disc is said to persist throughout life between the two. The most cranial of the three parts (X) also ossifies separately (in the second year after birth); it has been interpreted by Cave (1938) as a separate morphological entity, the proatlas, while Sensenig (1957) regarded it as derived from the cranial half of the first cervical sclerotome.

The 'vertebra-like' developmental history of the basi- and exoccipitals makes less surprising the occurrence of some occipitocervical anomalies, reminiscent of sacralization of the fifth lumbar vertebra (or lumbarization of the first sacral).

VERTEBRAL FUSION ('BLOCKED' VERTEBRAE)

Congenital fusion of cervical and thoracic vertebrae may show various patterns (see e.g. Bustami, 1988, for review, and Chapter 13):

1 fusion of the bodies and laminae, but with independent pedicles and transverse processes;

2 fusion of the bodies, laminae, articular processes and spines;

3 fusion of the bodies, with marked reduction of their height, giving the appearance of hemivertebrae.

Many authors have attributed these defects to nonsegmentation of the sclerotomes, but in the first two groups, at least, anatomical appearances suggested (Bustami, 1988) that fusion had occurred secondarily between essentially normal vertebrae, possibly due to failure of development of the joints between articular processes. In Bustami's (1988) series, fusions were frequently associated with incomplete sacralization of fifth lumbar vertebra and deficient development of sacral neural arches, suggesting interference at the stage of chondrification. A genetic factor is well established for the Klippel–Feil syndrome, but the stage at which the vertebral anomalies are first manifest is not known.

EXTRATHORACIC RIBS

All vertebrae possess a costal element (or 'rib-equivalent') which can be located, even at the cartilaginous stage of development, by its alignment with 'true' (thoracic) ribs, by its shape and by its relationship to the rami of the associated spinal nerve (O'Rahilly *et al.*, 1990a). Exaggerated development of the costal element may produce an extrathoracic rib anywhere in the column, but more commonly at the junctions with the thoracic region. Cervical ribs have been reported in association with each of the cervical vertebrae except the atlas (Sensenig & Hall, 1957), but mostly with the seventh. According to Cave (1975), the costal element comprises most of the lateral part of the anatomical 'transverse process', including the anterior and posterior lamellae and tubercles and the bar of bone between them. The anterior lamella is ossified from a separate centre in about 30% of fetuses (Meyer, 1978), giving rise to some reports of a high incidence of cervical ribs in fetuses, but it usually remains small and fuses with the remainder of the 'transverse process', so that the incidence of cervical rib in adults is less than 1%.

In the lumbar region several authors have reported separate centres of chondrification and of ossification of the costal elements, but these normally fuse rapidly with the transverse process so that, again, the apparent incidence of a first lumbar rib in fetuses is much higher than the real incidence in the adult.

REFERENCES

Alles, A.J. & Sulik, K.K. (1990) Retinoic acid induced spina bifida: evidence for a pathogenetic mechanism. *Development*, **108**, 73–81.

Arey, L.B. (1965) *Developmental Anatomy*, 7th edn. W.B. Saunders, London.

Bagnall, K.M., Harris, P.F. & Jones, P.R.M. (1977a) A radiographic study of the human fetal spine. 1. The development of the secondary cervical curvature. *J. Anat.*, **123**, 777–782.

Bagnall, K.M., Harris, P.F. & Jones, P.R.M. (1977b) A radiographic study of the human fetal spine. 2. The sequence of development of ossification centres in the vertebral column. *J. Anat.*, **124**, 791–802.

Bagnall, K.M., Harris, P.F. & Jones, P.R.M. (1979) A radiographic study of the human fetal spine. 3 Longitudinal growth. *J. Anat.*, **128**, 777–787.

Bagnall, K.M., Higgins, S.J. & Sanders, E.J. (1988) The contribution made by a single somite to the vertebral column: experimental evidence in support of resegmentation using the chick–quail chimaera model. *Development*, **103**, 69–85.

Bagnall, K.M., Higgins, S.J. & Sanders, E.J. (1989) The contribution made by cells from a single somite to tissues within a body segment and assessment of their integration with similar cells from adjacent segments. *Development*, **107**, 931–943.

Bagnall, K.M., Saunders, E.J., Higgins, S.J., Leam, H. & Cheung, E. (1986) The effects on vertebral development of removing a single somite from a 2-day chick embryo. In Bellairs, R., Ede, D.A. & Lash, J.W. (eds) *Somites in Developing Embryos*, pp. 69–78. Plenum Press, New York.

Barry, A. (1956) A quantitative study of the prenatal changes in angulation of the spinal nerves. *Anat. Rec.*, **126**, 97–110.

Barson, A.J. (1970a) The vertebral level of termination of the spinal cord during normal and abnormal development. *J. Anat.*, **106**, 489–497.

Barson, A.J. (1970b) Spina bifida: the significance of the level and extent of the defect to the morphogenesis. *Dev. Med. Child Neurol.*, **12**, 129–144.

Beadle, O.A. (1931) The intervertebral discs; observations on their normal and morbid anatomy in relation to certain spinal deformities. MRC Special Report Series No. 161. HMSO, London.

Burnside, B. (1973) Microtubules and microfilaments in amphibian neurulation. *Am. J. Zool.*, **13**, 989–1006.

Bustami, F. (1988) Some observations on blocked vertebrae. *Jordan Med. J.*, **22**, 63–75.

Campbell, L.R., Dayton, D.H. & Sohal, G.S. (1986) Neural tube defects: a review of human and animal studies on the etiology of neural tube defects. *Teratology*, **34**, 171–187.

Cave, A.J.E. (1938) The morphological constitution of the odontoid process. *J. Anat.*, **72**, 621.

Cave, A.J.E. (1975) The morphology of the mammalian cervical pleurapophysis. *J. Zool.*, **177**, 377–393.

Clark, B.J. & Scothorne, R.J. (1990) Variation in the response of chick embryos to incision of the roof plate of the neural tube at different developmental stages. *J. Anat.*, **168**, 167–184.

Copp, A.J., Brook, F.A. & Roberts, H.J. (1988a) A cell type-specific abnormality of cell proliferation in mutant (curly tail) mouse embryos developing spinal neural tube defects. *Development*, **104**, 285–295.

Copp, A.J., Crolla, J.A. & Brook, F.A. (1988b) Prevention of spinal neural tube defects in the mouse embryo by growth retardation during neurulation. *Development*, **104**, 297–303.

Corner, G.W. (1929) A well preserved human embryo of 10 somites. *Contrib. Embryol. Carnegie Inst.*, **20**, 81–102.

Cowan, W.M. (1982) A synoptic view of the development of the vertebrate nervous system: In Nicholls, J.G. (ed.) *Repair and Regeneration of the Nervous System*, pp. 7–24. Dahlem Konferenzen. Springer-Verlag, Berlin.

Dekaban, A.S. & Bartelmez, G.W. (1964) Complete dysraphism in 14 somite human embryo. A contribution to normal and abnormal morphogenesis. *Am. J. Anat.*, **115**, 27–42.

Desmond, M.E. (1982). A description of occlusion of the lumen of the spinal cord in early human embryos. *Anat. Rec.*, **204**, 89–93.

Desmond, M.E. & Schoenwolf, G.C. (1986) Evaluation of the roles of intrinsic and extrinsic factors in occlusion of the spinal neurocele during rapid brain enlargement in the chick embryo. *J. Embryol. Exp. Morphol.*, **97**, 25–46.

Emery, J.L. & Lendon, R.G. (1973) The local cord lesion in neurospinal dysraphism (meningomyelocele). *J. Pathol.*, **110**, 83–96.

Fowler, I. (1953) Responses of the chick neural tube in mechanically produced spina bifida. *J. Exp. Zool.*, **123**, 115–151.

Gardner, W.J. (1980) Hypothesis: overdistension of the neural tube may cause anomalies of non-neural organs. *Teratology*, **22**, 229–238.

Gasser, R.F. (1979) Evidence that sclerotomal cells do not migrate medially during normal embryonic development of the rat. *Am. J. Anat.*, **154**, 509–523.

Gordon, R. (1985) A review of the theories of vertebrate neurulation and their relationship to the mechanics of neural tube birth defects. *J. Embryol. Exp. Morphol.*, **89** (Suppl.), 229–255.

Heuser, C.H. (1932) A presomite human embryo with a definite chorda canal. *Contrib. Embryol. Carnegie Inst.*, **23**, 251–267.

Hughes, A.F. & Freeman, R.B. (1974) Comparative remarks on the development of the tail cord among higher vertebrates. *J. Embryol. Exp. Morphol.*, **32**, 355–363.

Jacobson, A.G. (1988) Somitomeres: mesodermal segments of vertebrate embryos. *Development*, **104** (Suppl.), 209–220.

Kalcheim, C. & Teillet, M.-A. (1989) Consequences of somite manipulation on the pattern of dorsal root ganglion development. *Development*, **106**, 85–93.

Kernohan, J.W. (1925) The ventriculus terminalis: its growth and development. *J. Comp. Neurol.*, **38**, 107–125.

Keynes, R.J. & Stern, C.D. (1988) The development of neural segmentation in vertebrate embryos. In Parnavelas, J.G., Stern, C.D. & Stirling, R.V. (eds), *The Making of the Nervous System*, pp. 84–100. Oxford University Press, Oxford.

Kieny, M., Mauger, A. & Sengel, P. (1972) Early regionalisation of the somitic mesoderm as studied by development of the axial skeleton of the chick embryo. *Dev. Biol.*, **111**, 243–245.

Kunimoto, K. (1918) The development and reduction of the tail and of the caudal end of the spinal cord. *Contrib. Embryol. Carnegie Inst.*, **8**, 161–198.

Lee, H.Y. & Nagele, R.G. (1985) Neural tube defects caused by local anaesthetics in early chick embryos. *Teratology*, **31**, 119–127.

Lemire, R.J. (1969) Variations in development of the caudal neural tube in human embryos (horizons XIV–XXI). *Teratology*, **2**, 361–370.

Lemire, R.J. (1974) Embryology of the central nervous system. In Davis, J.A. & Dobbing J. (eds) *Scientific Foundations of Paediatrics*, pp. 547–564. Heinemann Medical, London.

Lendon, R.G. & Emery, J.L. (1970) Forking of the central canal in the equinal cord of children. *J. Anat.*, **106**, 499–505.

McClone, D.G. & Bondareff, W. (1975) Developmental morphology of the subarachnoid space and contiguous structures in the mouse. *Am. J. Anat.*, **142**, 273–294.

Meier, S. (1979) Development of the chick mesoblast. Formation of the embryonic axis and establishment of the metameric pattern. *Dev. Biol.*, **73**, 25–45.

Meyer, D.B. (1978) The appearance of 'cervical ribs' during early human fetal development. *Anat. Rec.*, **190**, 481.

Mizoguti, H. (1989) A fifteen somite human embryo. *Adv. Anat. Embryol. Cell Biol.* **116**, 1–102.

Mohamed, A.A. (1989) A correlative developmental study of structures involved in the production, circulation and removal of cerebrospinal fluid. PhD thesis, University of Glasgow.

Muller, F. & O'Rahilly, R. (1986) Somitic-vertebral correlation and vertebral levels in the human embryo. *Am. J. Anat.*, **177**, 3–19.

Muller, F. & O'Rahilly, R. (1987) The development of the human brain, the closure of the caudal neuropore, and the beginning of secondary neurulation at Stage 12. *Anat. Embryol.*, **176**, 413–430.

Nieuwkoop, P.D., Johnen, A.G. & Albers, B. (1985) *The Epigenetic Nature of Early Chordate Development*. Cambridge University Press, Cambridge.

Noback, C.R. (1944) The developmental anatomy of the human osseous skeleton during the embryonic, fetal and circumnatal periods. *Anat. Rec.*, **88**, 91–125.

Noback, C.R. & Robertson, G.G. (1951) Sequences of appearance of ossification centers in the human skeleton during the first five prenatal months. *Am. J. Anat.*, **89**, 1–28.

O'Rahilly, R. & Meyer, D.B. (1979) The timing and sequence of events in the development of the human vertebral column during the embryonic period proper. *Anat. Embryol.*, **157**, 167–176.

O'Rahilly, R. & Muller, F. (1981). The first appearance of the human nervous system at Stage 8. *Anat. Embryol.*, **163**, 1–13.

O'Rahilly, R. & Muller, F. (1987) *Developmental Stages in Human Embryos*. Carnegie Institution of Washington, Publication 637.

O'Rahilly, R. & Muller, F. (1988) 'Neuroschisis' in human embryos. *Teratology*, **38**, 189.

O'Rahilly, R., Muller, F. & Meyer, D.B. (1980) The human vertebral column at the end of the embryonic period proper. 1. The column as a whole. *J. Anat.*, **131**, 565–575.

O'Rahilly, R., Muller, F. & Meyer, D.B. (1983) The human vertebral column at the end of the embryonic period proper. 2. The occipito-cervical region. *J. Anat.*, **136**, 181–195.

O'Rahilly, R., Muller, F. and Meyer, D.B. (1990a) The human vertebral column at the end of the embryonic period proper. 3. The thoracico-lumbar region. *J. Anat.*, **168**, 81–94.

O'Rahilly, R., Muller, F. and Meyer, D.B. (1990b) The human vertebral column at the end of the embryonic period proper. 4. The sacro-coccygeal region. *J. Anat.*, **168**, 95–112.

Osaka, K., Tanimura, T., Hirayama, A. & Matsumoto, S. (1978) Myelomeningocele before birth. *J. Neurosurg.*, **49**, 711–724.

O'Shea, K.S. & Kaufman, M.H. (1980) Neural tube closure defects following in vitro exposure of mouse embryo to xylocaine. *J. Exp. Zool.*, **214**, 235–238.

O'Shea, K.S. & Kaufman, M.H. (1981) Effect of acetaldehyde on the neuroepithelium of early mouse embryos. *J. Anat.*, **132**, 197–218.

Padget, D.H. (1970) Neuroschisis and human embryonic

maldevelopment. *J. Neuropathol. Exp. Neurol.*, **29**, 192–216.

Padmanabhan, R. (1984) Experimental induction of cranioschisis aperta and exencephaly after neural tube closure: a rat model. *J. Neurol. Sci.*, **66**, 235–243.

Patten, B.M. (1953). Embryological stages in the establishing of myeloschisis with spina bifida. *Am. J. Anat.*, **93**, 365–395.

Payne, F. (1925) General description of a 7 somite human embryo. *Contrib. Embryol. Carnegie Inst.*, **16**, 115–124.

Peacock, A. (1951) Observations on the prenatal development of the intervertebral disc in man. *J. Anat.*, **85**, 260–274.

Rokos, J. & Knowles, J. (1976) An experimental contribution to the pathogenesis of spina bifida. *J. Pathol.*, **118**, 21–24.

Schoenwolf, G.C. (1978) An SEM study of posterior spinal cord development in the chick embryo. *Scan. Electron Microsc.*, **II**, 739–746.

Schoenwolf, G.C. (1984) Histological and ultrastructural studies of secondary neurulation in mouse embryos. *Am. J. Anat.*, **169**, 361–376.

Schoenwolf, G.C. & Fisher, M. (1983) Analysis of the effects of *Streptomyces* hyaluronidase on formation of the neural tube. *J. Embryol. Exp. Morphol.*, **73**, 1–15.

Schoenwolf, G.C. & Franks, M.V. (1984) Quantitative analysis of changes in cell shape during bending of the avian neural tube. *Dev. Biol.*, **105**, 257–272.

Sensenig, E.C. (1949) The early development of the human vertebral column. *Contrib. Embryol. Carnegie Inst.*, **33**, 23–41.

Sensenig, E.C. (1951) The early development of the meninges of the spinal cord of human embryos. *Contrib. Embryol. Carnegie Inst.*, **34**, 147–157.

Sensenig, E.C. (1957) The development of the occipital and cervical segments and their associated structures in human embryos. *Contrib. Embryol. Carnegie Inst.*, **36**, 141–152.

Sensenig, E.C. and Hall, V.A. (1957) Cervical ribs: a review with additional embryological and anthropological observations. *Proc. Zool. Soc. Calcutta*, **165**, 165–170.

Stern, C.D. & Keynes, R. (1987) Interactions between somite cells: the formation and maintenance of segment boundaries in the chick embryo. *Development*, **99**, 261–272.

Streeter, G.L. (1919) Factors involved in the formation of the filum terminale. *Am. J. Anat.*, **25**, 1–11.

Taylor, J.R. (1972) Persistence of the notochordal canal in vertebrae. *J. Anat.*, **111**, 211–217.

Tondury, G. (1944) *Entwicklungsgeschichte und Fehlbildungen der Wirbelsaule*. Hippokrates-Verlag, Stuttgart.

Verbout, A.J. (1985) The development of the vertebral column. *Adv. Anat., Embryol. Cell Biol.*, **90**, 1–122.

Walmsley, R. (1953) The development and growth of the intervertebral disc. *Edin. Med. J.*, **60**, 341–364.

Warkany, J. & O'Toole, B. (1981) Experimental spina bifida and associated malformations. *Child's Brain*, **8**, 18–30.

Warkany, J., Wilson, J.G. & Geiger, J.F. (1958) Myeloschisis and myelomeningocele produced experimentally in the rat. *J. Comp. Neurol.*, **109**, 35–64.

Warner, A. (1988) Analysis of induction in the amphibian nervous system. In Parnavelas, J.G., Stern, G.D. & Stirling, R.V. (eds) *The Making of the Nervous System*. Oxford University Press, Oxford.

Weed, L.H. (1917) Development of cerebrospinal fluid spaces in pig and in man. *Contrib. Embryol. Carnegie Inst.*, **5**, 1–116.

Wood Jones, F. (ed.) (1946) *Buchanan's Manual of Anatomy*, 7th edn. Baillière, Tindall & Cox, London.

3 · Anatomy of the Human Spine

By R.E.M. BOWDEN

The main purpose of this contribution is not to abstract readily available textbooks of anatomy, but to collate information which may elucidate the regional vulnerabilities to injury and wear and tear of one of the most complex organs of the body, the normality of which has to be considered in the context of age.

The gross structure and internal architecture of the human vertebrae are influenced by genetic, hormonal, metabolic, environmental and mechanical factors, including posture. The bones, articulations and related soft tissues undergo progressive postnatal changes of development, growth and senescence. These changes affect the ability to resist static and dynamic forces of compression, traction and shear which operate throughout life (Gracovetsky, 1988). Forces vary in magnitude and speed of application, and are also influenced by posture (Nachemson, 1963), occupation, load carrying and locomotion. An extreme example is the rapidly intermittent compressive force equivalent to nine times body weight which is generated during a 100 metre sprint (Cavagna *et al.*, 1971).

There are regional variations in the frequency distribution of fractures associated with differing forms of trauma (Jefferson, 1928; Nicoll, 1949; Saville, 1970; see Figs 3.1 & 3.2). For example the peak incidence of fractures associated with electroconvulsant therapy and chronic epilepsy is between T4 and T7 (Kelly, 1954), in tetanus the peak is between T4 and T9 (Davis & Roland, 1965; Fig. 3.3). The distribution of osteophytes follows neither of these patterns (Boyle, 1954; Fig. 3.4), but the phenomenon is common enough to consider it a normal feature of ageing. This evidence indicates the need for morphometric analysis of gross and internal structure of the bones.

The functions of the spine may be summarized as weight-bearing, movement, protection of the spinal cord and nerve roots, haemopoiesis, articulation with and support of the thoracic cage and provision of attachment for muscles of many functions. The latter include movements of the column itself, the head, upper and lower limb girdles, respiration and protection of abdominal contents. The interdependence of individual vertebrae and discs, and the importance of neuromuscular control are illustrated by the changes induced by traumatic production of an abnormal curve, followed by the development of a compensatory one (Weinmann & Sicher, 1955; Fig. 3.5). Even muscular imbalance alone (e.g. postpoliomyelitis) can lead to gross bony deformity (Mercer, 1950).

STRUCTURAL ANATOMY

Typical vertebrae

Typical vertebrae have a body and neural arch. The latter has a dorsal spinous process and bilateral transverse processes which provide attachments for ligaments and muscles, and levers upon which muscles act. In addition there are costal elements, best developed in the thoracic region. The contributions of these elements to vertebrae of different regions are shown in Fig. 3.6. Reliable distinguishing features for cervical vertebrae are foramina transversaria and for thoracic vertebrae the costal facets. Lumbar vertebrae have neither feature. Other features such as shapes of bodies and lengths and shapes of spinous processes are less reliable, as there are gradual transitional changes between one region and the next.

The articulated adult spine

In the normal column there are no lateral curves but there are well-marked anteroposterior ones. The

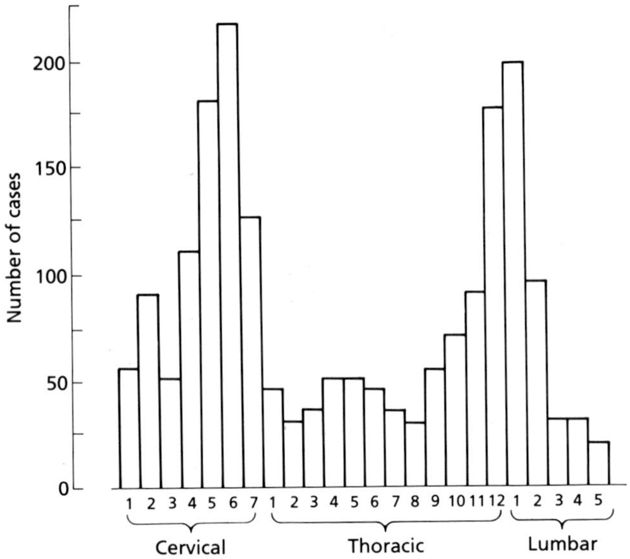

Fig. 3.1 Frequency of vertebral fractures at different levels in 2006 cases (Davis, 1957). Based on Jefferson (1927), by kind permission of Davis (1957).

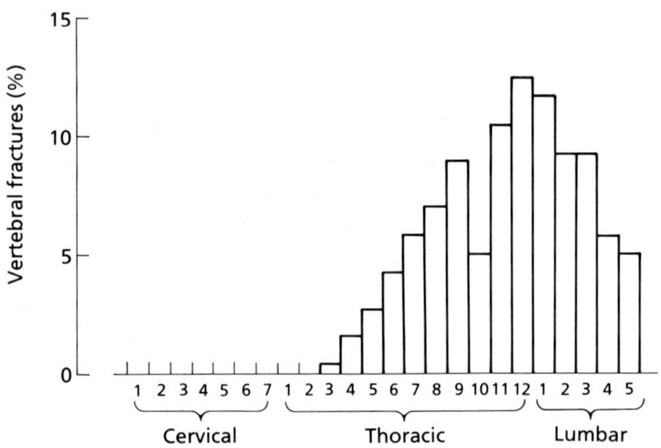

Fig. 3.2 Frequency distribution of 257 vertebral fractures in 80 women at the time of diagnosis of osteoporosis. Based on data of Saville (1970).

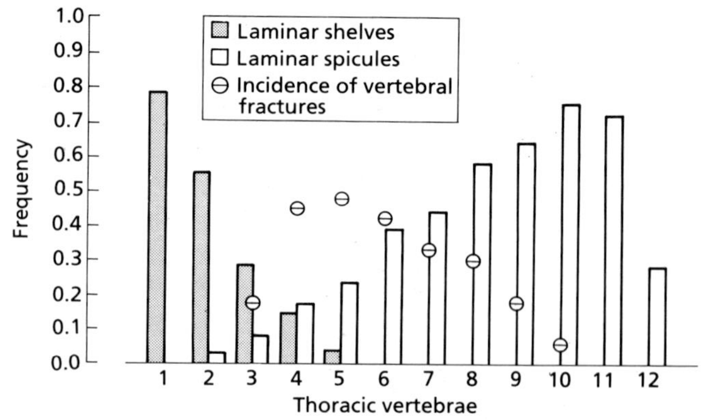

Fig. 3.3 Frequency distribution of fractures in tetanus, the incidence of laminar shelves and spicules on thoracic vertebrae. From Davis & Rowland (1965).

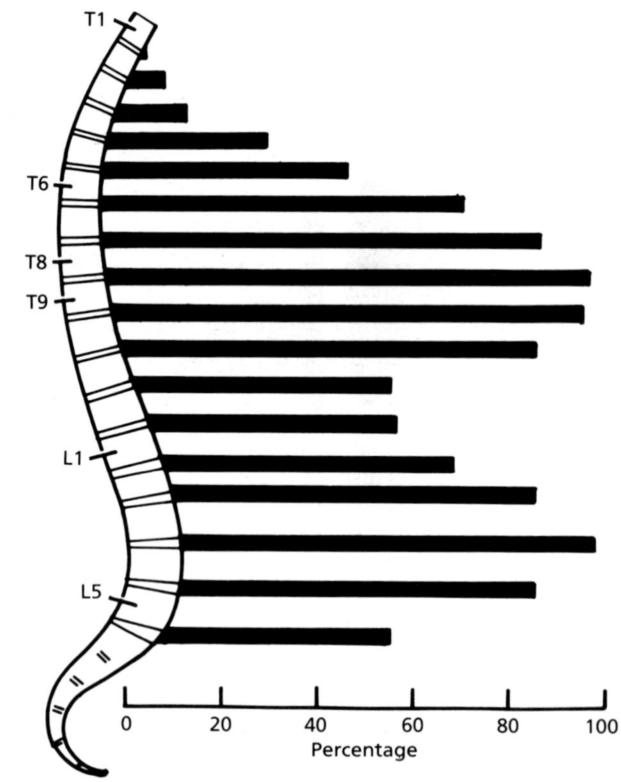

Fig. 3.4 Frequency distribution of osteophytes in 200 patients with no symptoms of spinal disorder. From Boyle (1954). By kind permission of Dr Boyle and Editor of the *Proceedings of the Royal Society of Medicine.*

primary curves are the thoracic and sacral kyphoses which are due to the shapes of the bones. The cervical and lumbar lordoses are largely due to the shapes of intervertebral discs and are maintained by muscular activity. The lumbar lordosis is more marked in females. The transitions between the cervicothoracic and thoracolumbar curves are smooth. The cervical lordosis extends from the upper two thoracic vertebrae, with its apex between the fourth and fifth cervical. The thoracic curve merges into the lumbar lordosis in the region of the eleventh or twelfth thoracic vertebrae. The apices of these curves lie between the sixth and ninth thoracic and at the third lumbar vertebra, respectively.

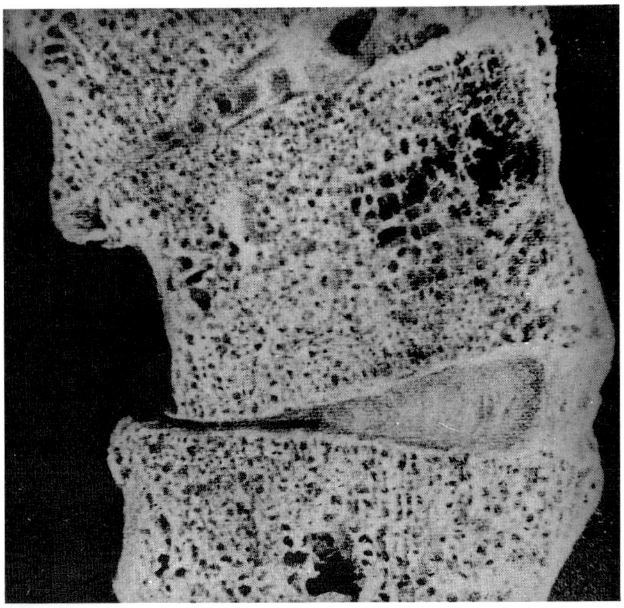

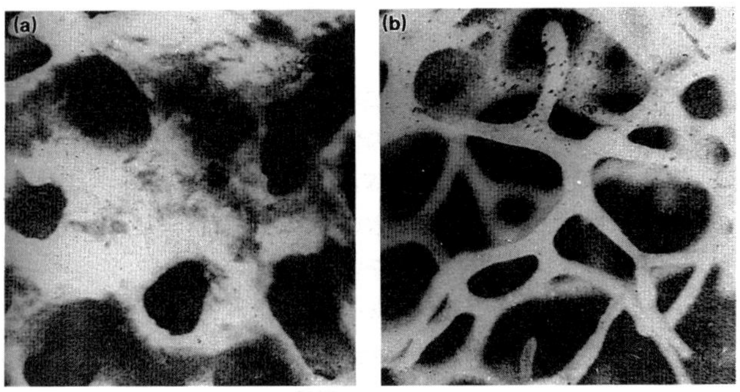

Fig. 3.5 Changes in internal architecture of vertebral bodies in scoliosis due to loss of disc substance. From Weinmann & Sicher (1955). (a) Thickened trabeculae on the concave side. (b) Thinned trabeculae on convex side of abnormal curve. By kind permission of the publishers.

The sharp lumbosacral junction is due to wedging of the fifth lumbar vertebra and the curve and inclination of the sacrum which forms an integral part of the lower limb girdle and the posterior boundary of the lesser pelvis. In the erect posture the plane of the pelvic inlet makes an angle of between 50° and 60° with the horizontal. (For variations at the lumbosacral junction and sexual dimorphism of the sacrum see Chapter 19.)

When standing erect, well-balanced with little or no expenditure of muscle activity (Floyd & Silver, 1955; Klausen, 1965), the line of gravity extends from the level of the external auditory meatus, through the dens of the axis, just anterior to the body of the second thoracic vertebra, through the middle of the

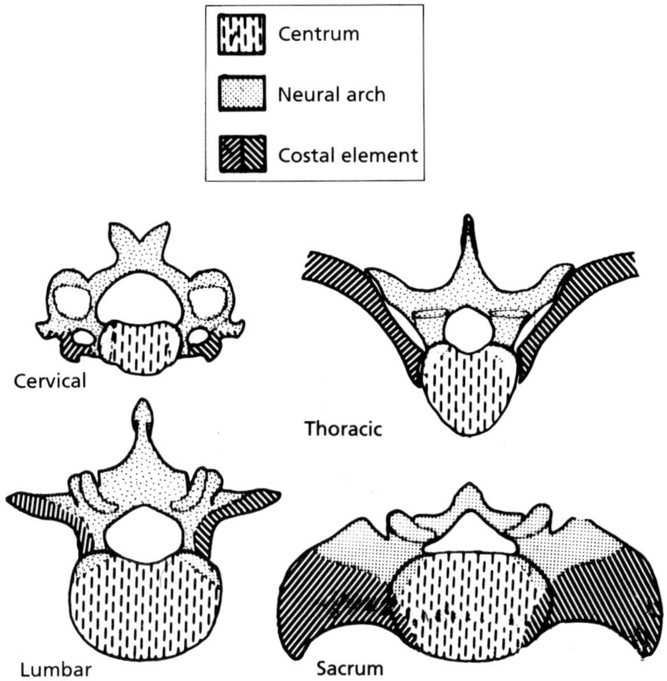

Fig. 3.6 Derivation of parts of vertebrae.

body of the twelfth thoracic and the back of the body of the fifth lumbar vertebra to lie in front of the sacrum (Fig. 3.7). It follows that the bodies and neural arches will play varying roles in transmission of weight. Vertebral bodies and intervertebral discs form a weight-bearing pillar throughout the spine down to the third piece of the sacrum. In this pillar cartilage contributes about 24% of the presacral length. However, this contribution is not evenly distributed either in amount or proportion (Todd & Pyle, 1928a,b; and Fig. 3.8) The ratios of cartilage to bone in the cervical, thoracic and lumbar regions are 1 : 3.4, 1 : 4.6 and 1 : 1.8, respectively.

There is a cephalocaudal increase in the cross-sectional surface area of discs and vertebral bodies. The increase is linear in the neck (Pal & Routal, 1986) but not in the thoracic and lumbar regions (Figs 3.9 & 3.10; Davis, 1955). The rate of increase is slow in the region of ribs articulating with the sternum, and it rises abruptly in relation to the functional thoracolumbar junction with or without mortice joints (Figs 3.9 & 3.10). In females vertebral bodies have a lower ratio of width to depth (Taylor & Twomey, 1984). In some individuals the cross-sectional surface area of the fifth lumbar vertebra is less than the fourth. In such circumstances there are compensatory enlarge-

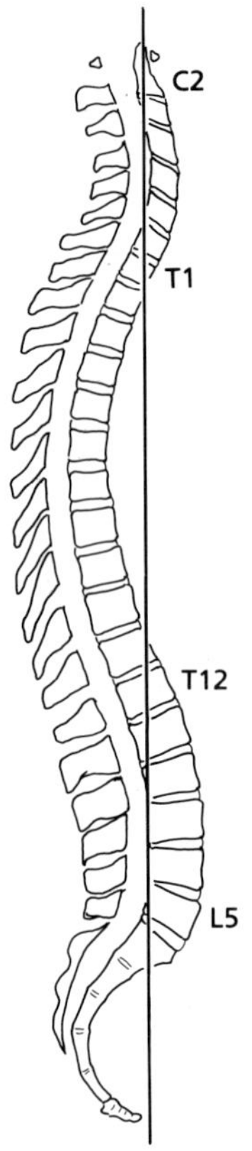

Fig. 3.7 Lateral view of vertebral column with the line of gravity when standing erect.

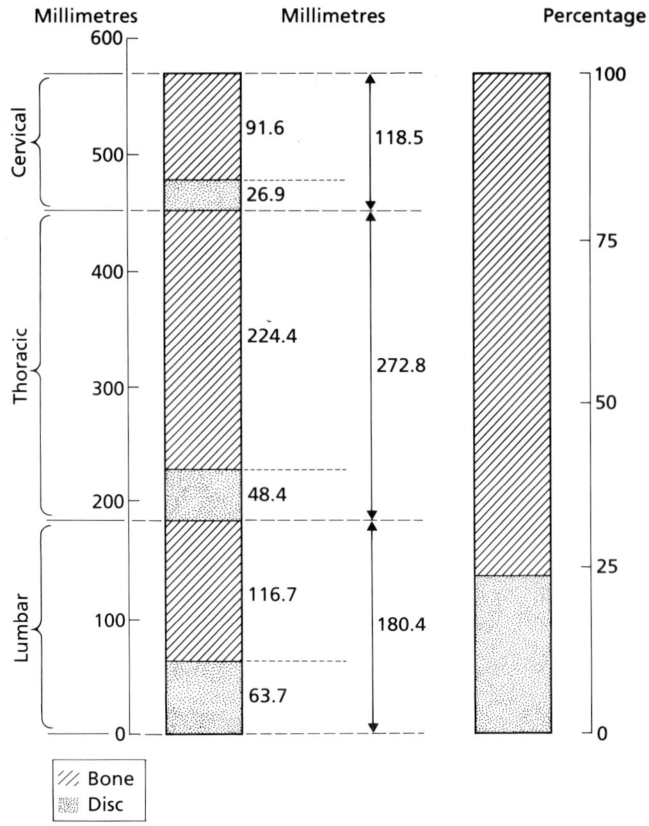

Fig. 3.8 Contribution of vertebral body and intervertebral disc heights to the length of the presacral column. Based on Todd & Pyle (1928b).

ments of pedicles, transverse processes and ligaments (pp. 68 & 72). Below the sacroiliac joints the sacrum diminishes rapidly in all dimensions.

THE CERVICAL SPINE

The cervical spine has three virtually parallel columns for weight-bearing, the bodies and two posterolateral articular pillars (Bowden *et al.*, 1967; Pal & Routal, 1986; Figs 3.11 & 3.12). Pal & Routal showed that the articular weight-bearing area diminished as the surface area of cervical bodies increased. Below the neck, laminae and facet joints play a less obvious role, but the varying stoutness of pedicles indicates transference of forces to the laminae and, in certain postures, to facet joints.

PEDICLES

The cervical pedicles are best seen in a hemisected column. Those of the axis are the most robust in this region; the remainder are more slender but through-

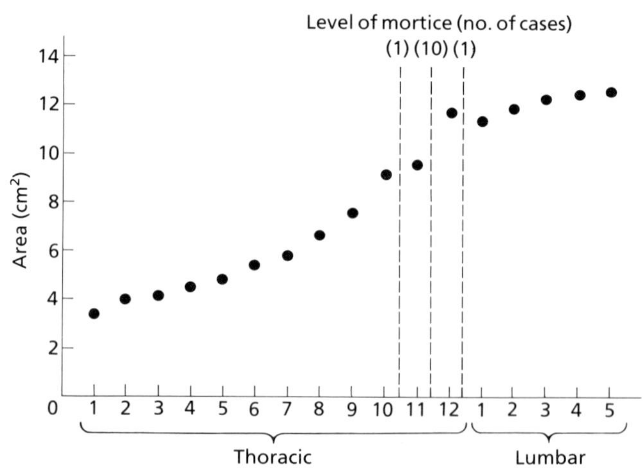

Fig. 3.9 Means of areas of superior surfaces of bodies of thoracic and lumbar vertebrae of 12 columns with mortice joints. After Davis (1957).

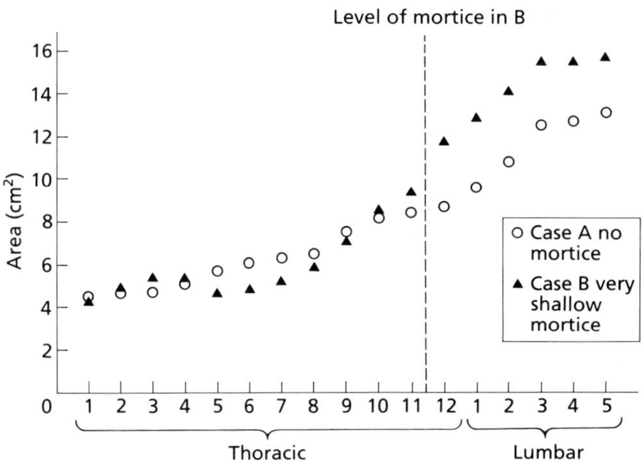

Fig. 3.10 Areas of upper surfaces of thoracic and lumbar vertebrae. After Davis (1957).

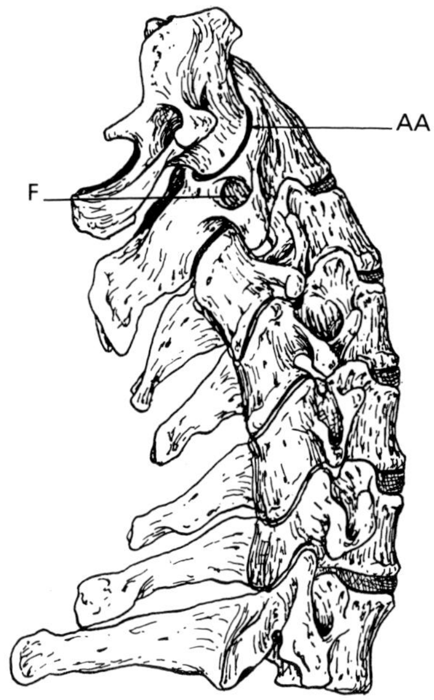

Fig. 3.12 Lateral view of same articulated cervical column. Note: (1) the articular pillar; (2) the atlanto-axial joint (AA) which lies on a plane anterior to the rest of the column; (3) the obliquity of the foramen transversarium of the axis (F). From Bowden *et al.* (1967).

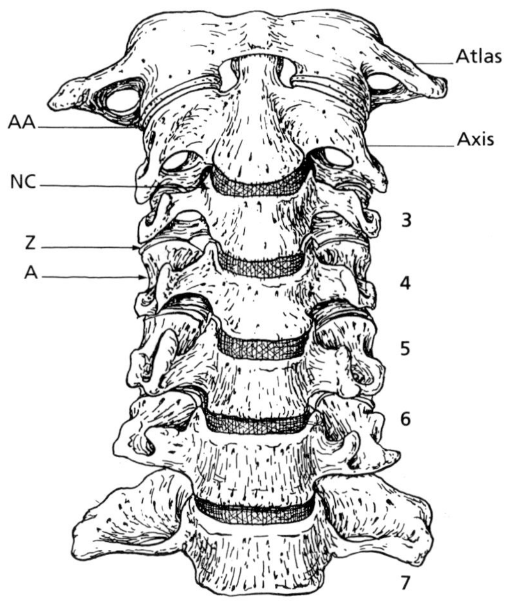

Fig. 3.11 Anterior view of an articulated cervical spine. A, articular pillar; AA, atlanto-axial joint; Z = zygapophyseal joints; NC = neurocentral or uncinate process. From Bowden *et al.* (1967).

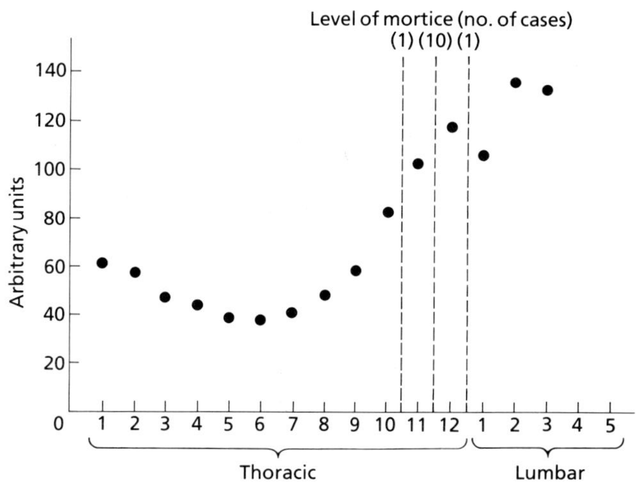

Fig. 3.13 Means of pedicular indices of thoracic and lumbar vertebrae in 12 columns with a mortice joint. After Davis (1957). Pedicular index = breadth × height in millimetres at the most slender part of pedicle.

out the column they increase cephalocaudally in depth; however, the increase is not linear (Figs 3.13 & 3.14). They are directed posterolaterally in the cervical region and anteroposteriorly by the third or fourth thoracic vertebra. The last three lumbar vertebrae have pedicles that slope laterally, especially the fifth, although the triangular cross-section of the lumbar canal is due more to inclination of laminae rather than pedicles. The pedicular elements of the sacrum can be examined only by looking down the canal or, as with cervical vertebrae, in the hemisected column. The pedicles are angulated with respect to the long axis of bodies of the cervical vertebrae (Pal & Routal,

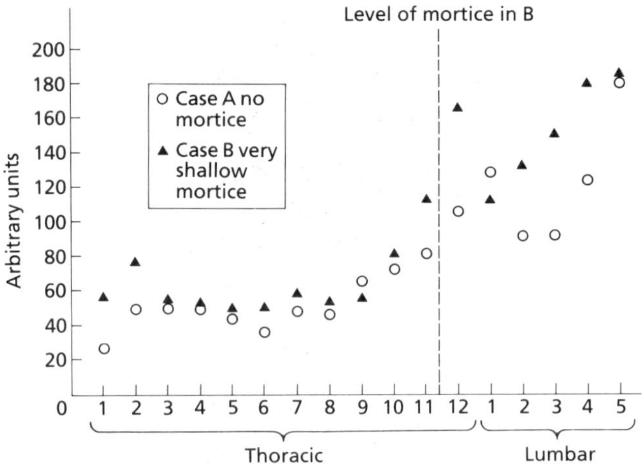

Fig. 3.14 Means of pedicular indices of thoracic and lumbar vertebrae. After Davis (1957).

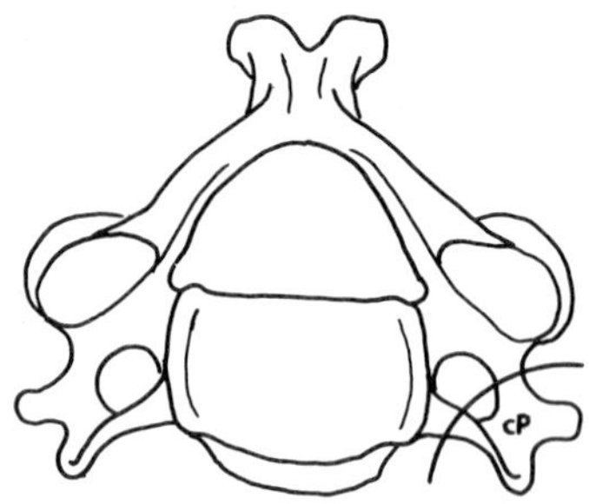

Fig. 3.15 Cervical vertebra showing compound nature of transverse process. CP, Costal process or pleurapophysis. From Cave (1975).

1986). This point has yet to be investigated for other levels. Pedicles are attached to the middle areas of cervical bodies, an appearance due to the upward projection of neurocentral processes (Fig. 3.11). Below the cervical region they are attached to the upper part of the body.

TRANSVERSE PROCESSES

Transverse processes vary in length, robustness and structure. In the neck the longest are those of the atlas, giving better mechanical advantage to the rotator muscles (Fig. 3.16). The compound structures of lower cervical transverse processes (Figs 3.12 & 3.15) provide attachments for many muscles, including the scalenes which suspend and move the upper rib cage (Campbell, 1955). They give support to the vertebral artery and venous plexus and form gutters for the emerging cervical nerves (C3–C8). The artery does not enter the foramen of the seventh vertebra, and this vertebra may have separate unilateral or bilateral cervical ribs (Chapter 13).

THE FIRST THORACIC VERTEBRA

This provides the one osseous, but indirect, connection of the upper limb girdle through the first rib, to the axial skeleton. Its transverse processes are the largest and most robust of the thoracic column and they lie in the coronal plane. Succeeding ones are more posteriorly inclined and become short, stout and rudimentary at the twelfth. The upper ten, sometimes only nine, have facets for the tubercles of ribs. The upper articulations are concave and face downwards, but the shapes change and the lower facets are plane and face medially and upwards, reflecting the orientation of the ribs. The ribs, vertebrocostal joints and ligaments not only have a vital respiratory function, they also effectively elongate the levers by which intrinsic postvertebral and abdominal muscles act upon the column.

The upper four lumbar transverse processes are slender and lie in the coronal plane. The fifth lumbar transverse processes are the most robust. They arise from the body and pedicle and their ligaments are an important element in weight transference (pp. 67, 71, 72). The inclusion of transverse elements in the sacrum is illustrated in Fig. 3.6.

LAMINAE

The broad laminae of the cervical region are continuous laterally with the articular pillars and provide for muscular attachments (Fig. 3.16).

The laminae of the first thoracic vertebra are broad, thereafter they narrow down to the eighth, broaden again, but from the twelfth thoracic to the third lumbar they narrow again. The pars interarticularis and the upper borders of the neural arches are stout in the lower thoracic and the lumbar regions.

SPINOUS PROCESSES

In columns with no lateral curve of vertebral bodies, some individuals have a deflection of spinous processes, said to be related to handedness.

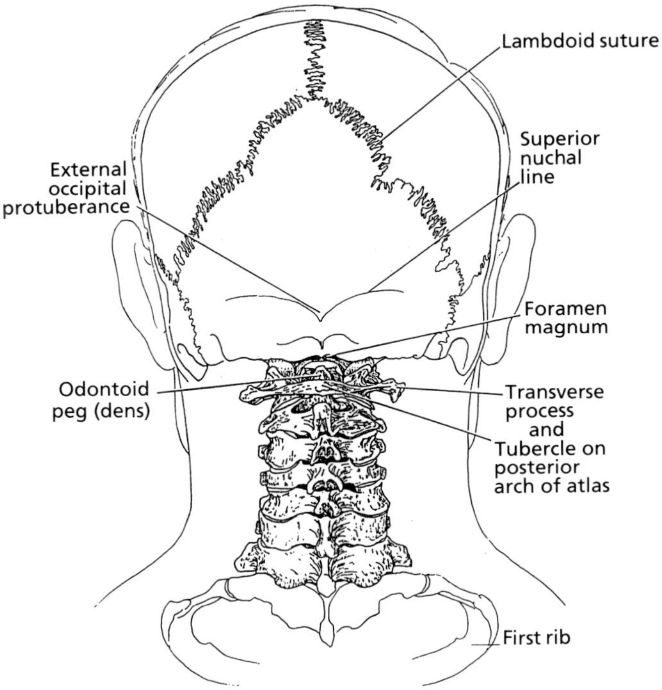

Fig. 3.16 Posterior view of skull, cervical and first thoracic vertebrae and first rib. Note: (1) the massive bifid spine of the axis; (2) the shape of lamina of C7 at the inferior zygapophyseal (facet joint); (3) the transverse processes of atlas and C7. From Bowden *et al.* (1967) by kind permission of the publishers.

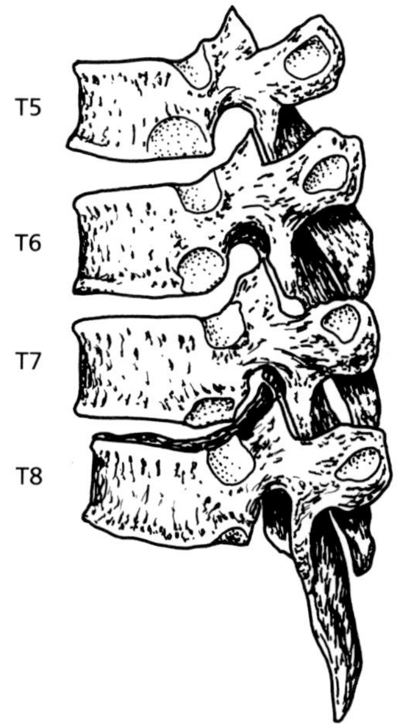

Fig. 3.17 Left lateral view of thoracic vertebrae 5–8. Note: (1) long overlapping spines; (2) changing orientation of costal facets on bodies and transverse processes.

The spinous processes vary considerably. The atlas has a small posterior tubercle which does not interfere with extension of the head, the axis has a massive bifid process for ligamentous and muscular attachments and the seventh is usually the most prominent in the normal; sometimes it is equalled by the first thoracic. In scoliosis there is some variation ranging from the sixth cervical to first thoracic (Stonelake *et al.*, 1988).

Thoracic spines are most variable, the upper four resemble the seventh cervical although they are progressively shorter and inclined inferiorly. The fifth to eighth or ninth are long and overlap each other (Fig. 3.17) and below this they are short and less steeply downward in inclination. The upper four lumbar spines are robust and rectangular, the fifth has a rounded and downturned crest.

INTERVERTEBRAL FORAMINA

The first two cervical segmental nerves appear above the neural arches and behind the synovial joints. Below this level the facet joints are posterior to the emerging spinal nerves. In the cervical spine the articular pillar and the facet joints, the line of which passes obliquely down from lateral to medial, form the posterior boundary of the foramina. The bulk of the pillar thus forms a canal rather than a simple foramen. The superior border is formed by the wide lower margin of the pedicle of the upper vertebra and the lower boundary by the pedicle below. Anteriorly, the neurocentral process of the lower vertebra intervenes between the disc and nerve roots.

In the thoracic and lumbar regions the size of the foramina increases progressively. Facet joints are posterior, the pedicles form upper and lower boundaries and the body of the upper vertebra and the subjacent intervertebral disc are anterior (see Fig. 3.12 & p. 49).

The sacral foramina are illustrated in Figs 3.24 & 3.35 and have no mobile joints related to them.

SPECIAL FEATURES

The atlas. The oval upper articular facets may be partially, or completely, symmetrically or asymmetrically divided (Table 3.1). One out of 30 adult bones had round and completely flat articular surfaces that were medially inclined.

Table 3.1 The shape of upper articular facets of the atlas. RCS (1989)

	Symmetrical	Asymmetrical	
		L	R
Round and flat	1	0	0
Ellipsoid			
Entire, no subdivision	15	2	6
Partial division	3	3	2
Complete division	3	3	0
Total number of bones	22	8	
Total number of facets	44	16	

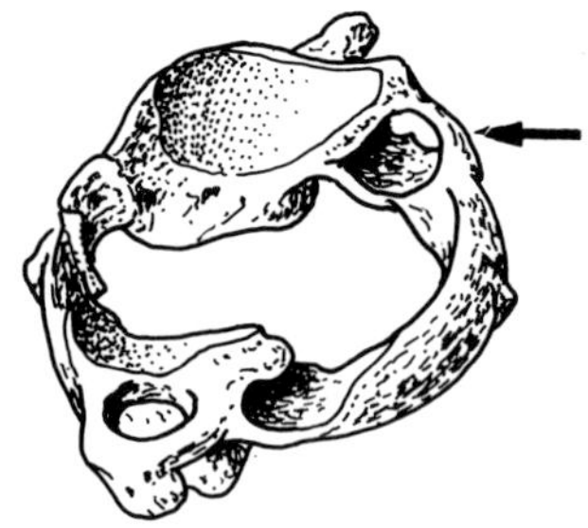

Fig. 3.18 Upper surface of atlas. Note: (1) complete bony ring on right; (2) deep groove and overhang on left.

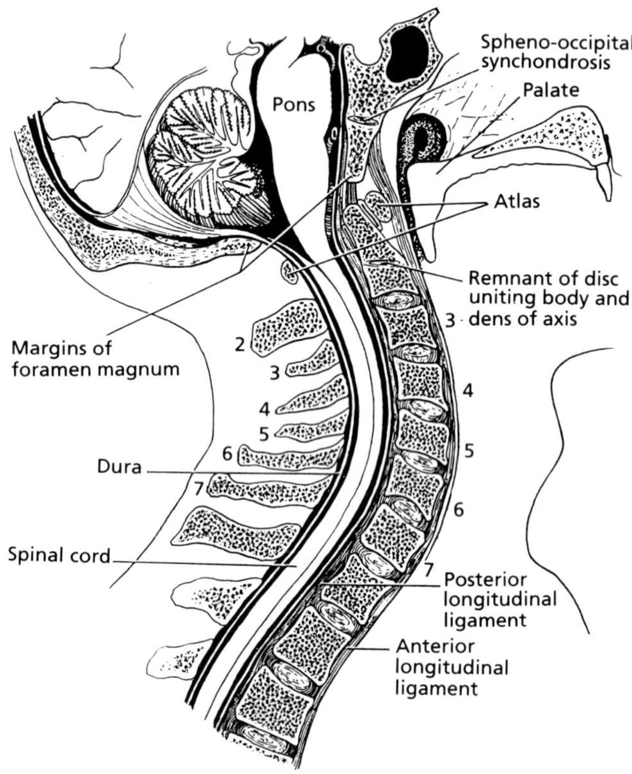

Fig. 3.19 Left side of hemisected head, cervical and upper vertebral column.

There may also be complete or partial rings on the upper surface of the posterior arch; these also may be symmetrical or asymmetrical (Fig. 3.18). They surround the vertebral artery and emerging first cervical nerve (Kendrick & Biggs, 1963). They are not due to degenerative calcification of the opening in the posterior atlanto-occipital membrane as they have been reported in children of two, four and 13 years and are common in other vertebrates. The true incidence is difficult to assess, the figure of 37% has been given from macerated specimens, but in 990 X-rays 7.8% had complete rings and 6.6% incomplete ones (Lamberty & Zinanovic, 1973). Out of 52 specimens (Royal College of Surgeons) one had bilateral rings, three had unilateral rings and in one it was incomplete. These rings have been implicated as possibly being associated with the vertebrobasilar artery syndrome. The depth of the groove and overhang of the lateral mass vary (Fig. 3.18).

The axis. This has oblique vertebro-arterial foramina (Fig. 3.12). The centre for the dens may not fuse completely with the body and a cartilaginous plate may persist with a thin shell of bone (Fig. 3.19).

Thoracic vertebrae. The bodies of the upper thoracic vertebrae resemble those of the cervical region in being wider in the coronal than in the sagittal plane. There may also be neurocentral processes (Table 3.2). Unfortunately these nine out of 32 columns were not taken from wet specimens and the presence or absence of joints of Luschka cannot be assessed. The first vertebra has an entire facet for the head of the first rib, and a demifacet for the head of the second. As the costal articulations are traced downwards they become more posteriorly located, and the single ones for the (tenth), eleventh and twelfth may be mainly on the pedicles. The heart-shaped body, usually considered typical of thoracic vertebrae, is not found throughout the series, considerable variation may exist (Table 3.3). Also the flattening in relation to the descending thoracic aorta is not invariable (Table 3.4). The lower bodies resemble the lumbar series,. and reference has been made to the more slender bodies in females. The facet joints and the mortice joints at the

Table 3.2 Incidence of neurocentral processes of the upper surface of the bodies of thoracic vertebrae. (RCS, 32 columns, 1989)

Level	No. of cases
T1	2
T1–T2	2
T1–T3	2
T1–T4	2
T1–T5	1
Total	9

Table 3.3 Incidence of cordate bodies of thoracic vertebrae. (RCS, 32 columns, 1989)

Level	No. of cases
T3–T6	1
T3–T7	1
T4–T8	2
T4–T9	5
T5–T7	1
T5–T9	2
T6–T8	1
T6–T9	1
Total	14

Table 3.4 Level of asymmetry of bodies of thoracic vertebrae. (RCS, 32 columns, 1989)

Left	Number	Right	Number
T4–T6	1	T5–T8	1
T6–T9	1		
T7–T9	2		

thoracolumbar junction are discussed on pp. 64–67 and mortices are illustrated in Fig. 3.32. When present, laminar shelves of the upper thoracic vertebrae may limit rotation and extension in the erect posture (Table 3.5 & Fig. 3.20). Together with the mortice joint they have been considered as possible aetiological factors in producing fractures associated with the violent and symmetrical muscular contractions of tetanus (Fig 3.3; Davis & Rowland, 1965). Laminar spicules are increasingly frequent as the mortice joint is approached (Table 3.6).

Table 3.5 The incidence of thoracic laminar shelves in 50 columns, RCS (1989)

Level	No. of cases
T1	3
T1–T2	11
T1–T3	10
T1–T4	2
T1–T5	1
Total	27

In articulated skeletons this cannot be assessed.

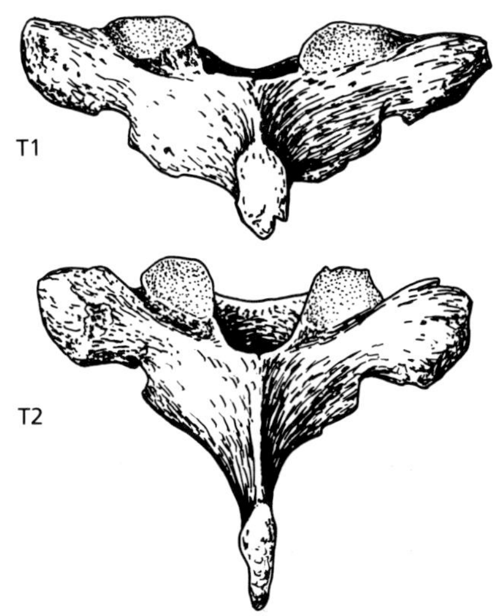

Fig. 3.20 Disarticulated C7, T1 and T2: note laminar shelf.

Lumbar vertebrae. The fifth lumbar vertebra is recognized by the massive transverse processes, and its superior and inferior facet joints are the same distance apart (Fig. 3.21). Wedging of the body appears variable, particularly in elderly spines.

The sacrum is dealt with in detail in Chapter 16. In females the sacrum is relatively broader and shorter than in males, for the lumbosacral disc occupies a third of the upper surface in males and less than a third in females. In females the bone faces more downwards than in males.

The male sacrum is more evenly curved than in the female, whereas in the female the curvature is more marked between the first and second segments and between the third and fifth. The auricular surfaces extend on to the third piece of the sacrum in both male and female, but there are differences in surface

Table 3.6 Incidence of bony lamina spicules in 69 columns (67 with a mortice joint). After Davis (1957)

Vertebral level	Number of columns with spicules		Level related to mortice joint	Number with spicules
T1	2		12	2
T2	4		11	2
T3	2		10	3
T4	6		9	3
T5	22		8	11
T6	30		7	18
T7	45		6	26
T8	58		5	46
T9	61		4	54
T10	64		3	58
T11	59		2	61
T12	22	Above mortice	1	63
L1	1	Below mortice	1	10
L2	2		2	3
L3	1		3	2
L4	0		4	1
L5	0		5	0
			6	0

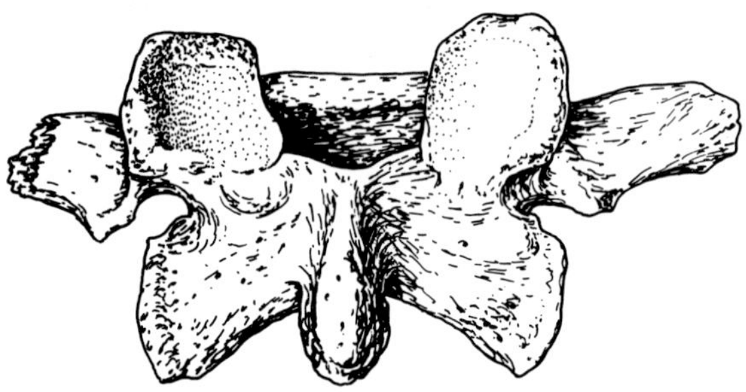

Fig. 3.21 Posterior surface of fifth lumbar vertebra.

area and inclination of the auricular surface which has a more marked concavity on its dorsal border in the female, and this changes with age. In both, the articular surface has conspicuous irregularities in adults; these also increase with age (Weisl, 1954b; Valojerdy & Hogg, 1989).

POSTNATAL DEVELOPMENT OF NORMAL SPINAL CURVATURES, OSSIFICATION AND GROWTH OF THE VERTEBRAL COLUMN

Development of secondary curves

The cervical lordosis, present at birth (Bagnall *et al.*, 1977a), is accentuated when the baby holds up its head and when it sits up. Standing and walking bring the centre of gravity of the trunk over the lower limbs, and lead to the development of the lumbar lordosis with posterior rotation of the pelvis. The primary curves are determined by shapes of the bones, and secondary lordoses are largely due to the shape of intervertebral discs, and are maintained by muscular activity. However, there is usually wedging of the fifth lumbar vertebra as well as the subjacent disc.

The transition between cervical, thoracic and lumbar curves is smooth, unlike the lumbosacral junction. The lumbar lordosis is more marked in females than in males, and in both sexes is more pronounced in the lower three vertebrae. With changes in the height of discs (p. 63) and also compression of osteoporotic bones (p. 61), stature decreases and these curves alter with age. The development of the 'dowager's hump' in the mid and lower thoracic region and/or decrease of lumbar lodosis, result in increasing compensatory cervical lordosis.

Ossification

The atlas, axis, seventh cervical vertebra, sacrum and coccyx will be dealt with separately.

The ossified parts of the vertebral column in a stillborn child are shown in Fig. 3.6.

The two ossific centres for the neural arch unite during the first year, beginning in the lumbar region and extending through the thoracic and cervical regions by the second year (except for the atlas). The neurocentral synchondroses of cervical vertebrae fuse during the third year and the lower lumbar during the sixth (Epstein, 1962).

The fusion of neurocentral joints completes the bony spinal canal and further increase in cross-sectional area occurs by subperiosteal osteoclasis. The ovoid centra seen in X-rays of fetuses (Bagnall *et al.*, 1977b) and infants become more rectangular and their height increases at the expense of the intervening cartilage (Bick & Copel, 1950).

Thoracic and lumbar vertebrae grow at different rates leading to altered body proportions (Taylor, 1975). When measuring vertical heights of the eighth thoracic and fourth lumbar vertebrae and subjacent discs similar growth spurts were seen in subjects ranging from 25 weeks of gestation to 14 years. However, the rates of increase of height of the lumbar vertebrae were greater throughout.

The disc was defined as the total radiolucent area between ossified centres. The thoracic disc showed some slight growth up to six months and then no further increase until after the eighth year when there was slow growth in height. The lumbar disc increased steadily up to two years and more rapidly thereafter. Measuring the components of 'total disc space' in autopsy specimens indicated that up to four years the 'disc proper' increased progressively in height. After birth, and up to two years, the cartilage plates decreased progressively, but after two years lumbar plates increased in thickness, but thoracic ones continued to decrease progressively (Taylor, 1975).

As growth of the vertebral bodies proceeds, radiographs show the development of step-like recesses on the upper and lower borders. The upper and lower surfaces of the bodies have radially arranged grooves which deepen peripherally (Fig. 3.22). Centres of calcification appear in the deep marginal grooves between six and eight years in girls, and seven and nine years in boys (Bick & Copel, 1951; MacEwan & Kirsch, 1971). Later ossification leads to the formation of the annular traction epiphyses at about 12 years. These do not fuse with the bodies until about 25 years of age. Other traction epiphyses appear during puberty at tips of transverse and spinous processes, two appearing when the latter are bifid. Occasionally, secondary centres appear in mamillary processes of lumbar vertebrae and sometimes scale-like centres arise on the costal elements of the fifth.

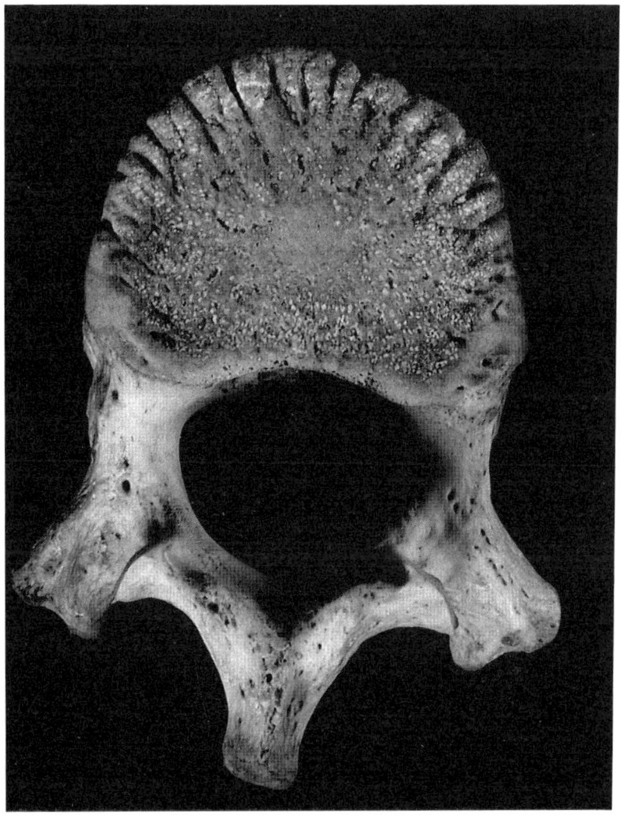

Fig. 3.22 Lower surface of T12 of 15-year-old individual. Note the radial grooves which are deeper peripherally. (Museum of RCS Eng.)

The atlas

Several patterns of ossification occur. At birth there is one for each lateral mass. The anterior arch is fibrocartilaginous. Ossification of the posterior arch is completed by about three to four years. A third centre usually appears in the anterior arch at about one year and fuses with the lateral masses between the sixth and eighth. The line of fusion may cross the upper articular facets and give rise to incomplete or complete subdivision of facets (Table 3.1). Occasionally the two lateral centres fuse together anteriorly. Another variant is the appearance of two centres for each lateral mass.

The axis

Five primary centres are present at birth. The first secondary centre appears at about two years of age at the tip of the dens. The annular epiphysis on the undersurface of the body appears at puberty. The synchondrosis between body and base of dens may fuse or persist with a shell of cortical bone around the cartilage (Fig. 3.19).

Seventh cervical vertebra

The separate centres for costal processes present at birth, fuse with the transverse processes at six years, or remain as cervical ribs. Occasionally separate costal centres also appear in the fourth to sixth vertebrae (Epstein, 1962).

Sacrum

Five primary centres are present at birth for each of the upper three or four sacral segments. Similar centres appear later for the lower segments. The two lateral elements fuse between two and five years, and the conjoined structures fuse with each other dorsally, and with the centra ventrally at about eight years. Hyaline cartilage and a rudimentary intervertebral disc intervene between the bodies. The conjoined costal and transverse processes of successive segments are separated by hyaline cartilage until puberty, at which time they begin to fuse from below upwards. At about 16 years secondary centres develop on upper and lower surfaces of each body (Epstein, 1962), spinous tubercles, transverse tubercles and costal elements. The cortex of the bodies usually unites at about 20 years, leaving remains of discs until the fifth decade or later (Fig. 3.24; McKern & Stewart, 1957).

The coccyx

The four segments each ossify from one primary centre. The first appears between birth and four years, and the cornua may ossify separately. The lower three ossify at widely separated times up to or over 20 years (Epstein, 1962). The second, third and fourth segments unite but the second and first may remain unfused, or fuse as late as 30 years. The coccyx and sacrum may fuse later, this being more common in females.

Growth of the vertebral column

At birth the column is about 24.2 cm in length (Scammon & Calkins, 1929). The lengths of male and female adult columns are 70 cm and 60 cm respectively (Williams *et al.*, 1989). This indicates increases of

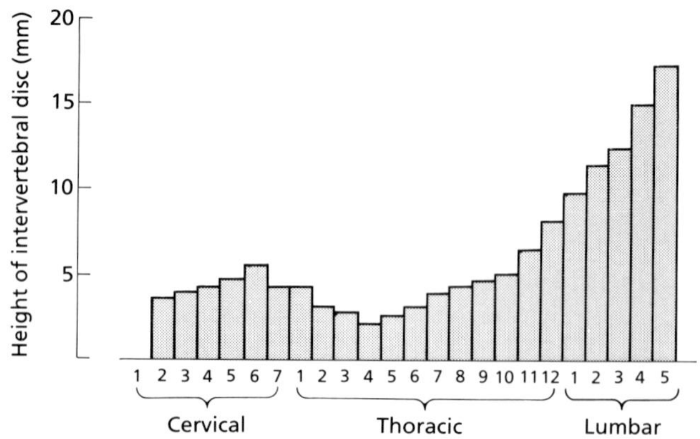

Fig. 3.23 Heights of cervical, thoracic and lumbar intervertebral discs. Based on data of Todd & Pyle (1928b).

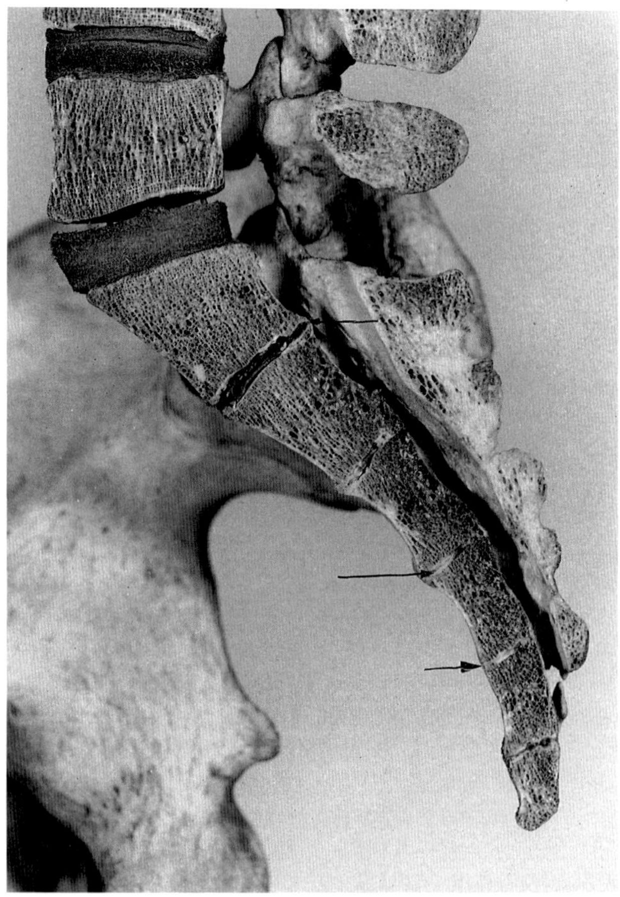

Fig. 3.24 Right side of hemisected adult vertebral column. Note persistent discs within cortical bone of sacrum (↑ ↑). Photograph by J. Fenton, by kind permission of Professor M.H. Day.

Table 3.7 Changes in dimensions of neural arch of a series of lumbar vertebrae. After Roaf (1971)

Age	Width (cm)	A–P (cm)	Height (cm)
Neonate	1.0	1.0	0.8
1 year	1.7	1.5	1.7
1½ years	1.6	1.5	1.8
3 years	1.8	1.5	2.0
5 years	1.8	1.5	3.3
12 years	1.8	1.5	3.5
Adult	2.1	1.7	3.9
Multiple of birth dimension	×2	×1.7	×5

A–P, midsagittal canal.

about three times in males and two and a half in females. However, such generalizations oversimplify the problems associated with prediction of adult height and ignore the many factors other than sexual differences influencing growth and stature (Sinclair, 1973; Falkner & Tanner, 1986).

Absolute and relative size of parts of the body vary with age. Neonatal lumbar and sacral vertebrae are relatively smaller than in the adult, and grow more than the thoracic and cervical ones (Tanner, 1971). Parts of individual vertebrae do not grow to the same extent. The changes in absolute measurements of a lumbar vertebra, from birth to the adult, showed a threefold increase in width of the body and fourfold ones for the height and anteroposterior dimensions of the vertebral body. Increases for the neural arch were twofold for width, fivefold for height and only 1.7 for the anteroposterior diameter of the spinal canal (Table 3.7; Roaf, 1971). Growth patterns of lower lumbar, midthoracic and cervical vertebra in normal and spastic children indicated that growth in height of vertebral bodies might be genetically determined and show sexual dimorphism, whilst intervertebral disc height and anteroposterior growth were more dependent upon activity (Taylor, 1975).

At birth radiological evidence shows that the height of the ossified centra is approximately the same as the translucent intervertebral cartilage; this interval includes the unossified parts of the body, the growth cartilages, as well as the disc itself (Brandner, 1970). The total proportion of cartilage to bone in the adult is approximately 25% and its distribution within regions and between individual vertebrae varies (Figs 3.8 & 3.24, pp. 48 & 56).

The total growth of the column is clearly due to summation of growth in individual vertebrae and discs. The length of the spine is a major component in overall stature (Nicolopoulos *et al.*, 1985). The proliferative processes in the cartilaginous plates become less active after 14–16 years, and after 20 there is little evidence of enchondral growth. The height of discs increases at the expense of the cartilaginous plates (Peacock, 1952). Also as the ossification of the vertebral body proceeds there is diminution in the thickness of the plates. These plates are similar to the epiphyseal cartilages of long bones, and growth in height of the vertebral body takes place at the upper and lower surfaces of the bodies (Bick & Copel, 1950; Peacock, 1952; Siffert & Gilbert, 1969). The annular traction epiphysis is not involved in growth of the body, although its diameter keeps pace with the body. Increase in width of the body is due to subperiosteal deposition of bone which is greater at the upper and lower ends, leaving a waist on lateral and anterior surfaces of the bone. The normally flat or slightly concave posterior surface which forms the anterior wall of the canal is probably maintained by osteoclasis.

Neural arch processes grow from primary centres by extension into cartilage and by subperiosteal deposition. Traction epiphyses appear on the tips of spinous and transverse processes. The facet joints borne on the arches increase in surface area from subarticular growth cartilage (Enneking & Harrington, 1969) and by extension into the extra-articular zone of cartilage (Roaf, 1971). Not only is there growth in extent of the joints, but also with changes of posture and changes in body proportions (Sinclair, 1973) there are alterations in orientation of articular surfaces. The angles of inclination of joints stabilize at different ages (Table 3.8). It is noteworthy that the angle at L2–L3 reached its lowest level of 70° by 14 years, the end of the period of observation, but this does not necessarily indicate that no further change would have taken place (Roaf, 1971). The wide opening angle at L5–S1 is of interest. The orientation of upper sacral facets varies in different individuals (Čihák, 1970; Fig. 3.25). There are correlations between this and the size of transverse processes of the fifth lumbar vertebra which affect transmission of weight from the column to the ilium (p. 68). Figures relating to growth changes in inclination and size of cervical and thoracic facets are not available.

Studies of rates of growth in males and females

Table 3.8 Angles of inclination of planes of facet joints from birth to stabilization. Based on Roaf (1971)

Articulation	Angle at birth	Age of stabilization (years)	Final angle
D12–L1	180°	10	80°
L1–L2	180°	10	75°
L2–L3	180°	14[a]	70°[a]
L3–L4	180°	12	80°
L4–L5	180°	12	110°
L5–S1	180°	12	120°

[a] End of period of observation, but no evidence of stabilization.

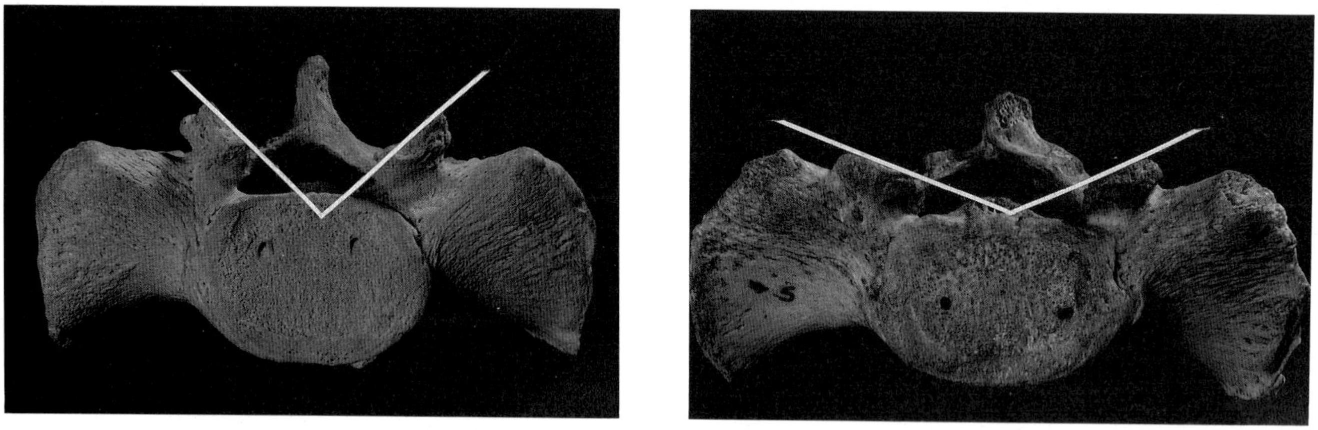

Fig. 3.25 Upper surface of two sacra to show variations in orientation of sacral facets for articulations with L5.

have shown that there is a growth spurt for the spine as for stature, and that there are sexual differences in the time of onset and the end-result. Longitudinal measurements of sitting heights showed an increased and maximum rate of growth in girls between the ages of 11 and 13 years, individual maximum rates ranged from 2.6 to 5.1 cm per annum. The spurt occurred between 13 and 15 years for boys with maximum individual rates of growth ranging from 3.7 to 6.2 cm per annum (Anderson *et al.*, 1965). In a different population and larger sample, longitudinal study of measurements between the first thoracic and fourth lumbar vertebrae made by Taylor & Twomey (1984) showed that between the ages of 5½ and 9½ years there was no significant difference in mean spinal lengths of boys and girls. Between 9½ and 12½ years, growth increments were 61% greater in girls than boys. The spurt began as early as 8½ years in girls in this series, but at 13½ for boys. At 12 and 13 years the mean spinal length was significantly greater in the girls.

In a standardized radiological study of the height/transverse diameter of the vertebral bodies at T6, T9, L1, L3 and L5, no significant differences appeared between males and females in the age range two to eight years. Highly significant differences were found from nine to 25 years for the thoracic vertebrae and from nine to 35 years in the lumbar region. Female vertebrae were significantly more slender (Taylor & Twomey, 1984; Veldhuizen *et al.*, 1986). The latter authors confirmed the relative slenderness of female vertebrae in children between 10 and 17 who had either a single idiopathic thoracic or lumbar scoliosis. They found no significant differences between growth increments of vertebral bodies involved in or outside the abnormal curves.

Growth in standing height of Caucasian girls usually ceases at about 18 years (Tanner *et al.*, 1966) and stabilizes at about 20 years in males, but small increases of 3–4 mm have been reported up to 30 years. The validity of such small measurements is difficult to substantiate unless allowance is made for diurnal variations (p. 63).

In East Africans a significant increase in height of lumbar vertebrae occurred in males between 20 and 45 years, but not in females (Allbrook, 1956). Risser & Ferguson's (1936) estimate that growth ceased at 16 years or less for girls, and about 17 for boys, are now too low. Possibly in 50 years, secular, environmental, dietetic and social factors influencing growth might be operating. Estimations of skeletal maturation based solely on Risser's sign of ossification of the iliac crest are inadequate. Anderson *et al.* (1965) found ossification of the iliac crest occurred between 10 and 16 years in girls (mean 13.26 years) and continued growth of sitting height ranged between 8.4 cm and 0.1 cm, with a mean of 4.05 cm. In boys, ossification of the crest appeared between 11½ and 15½ (mean 14.1 years). Remaining growth of the sitting height ranged from 16.2 to 3.5 cm with a mean of 6.5 cm. The iliac crest and annular epiphyses are traction epiphyses and are not involved in growth. Chronological age is no criterion of skeletal maturity; many factors have to be evaluated including skeletal maturation of hand and wrist bones, dental and sexual maturation; these and other relevant features are reviewed by Roche (1986). Senescent changes are discussed in sections dealing with architecture, the discs, synovial joints and muscles.

THE ARCHITECTURE OF HEALTHY, YOUNG AND AGEING VERTEBRAE

All vertebrae consist of cortical and trabecular bone. The thickness of the cortex and arrangement of trabeculae are related to the forces acting upon them. Trabeculae are visible on the upper and lower surfaces of each vertebral body within the annular epiphysis. Towards the centre of each area porosity is reduced in the area underlying the nucleus pulposus (Fig. 3.26; Beadle, 1931).

In the adult the cortex has small vascular foramina which are plentiful on the bodies and roots of pedicles. In infants large nutrient foramina in the midline of the anterior and posterior surfaces of the body are clearly visible in X-rays. The posterior surfaces of the bodies of mature columns have one, sometimes two,

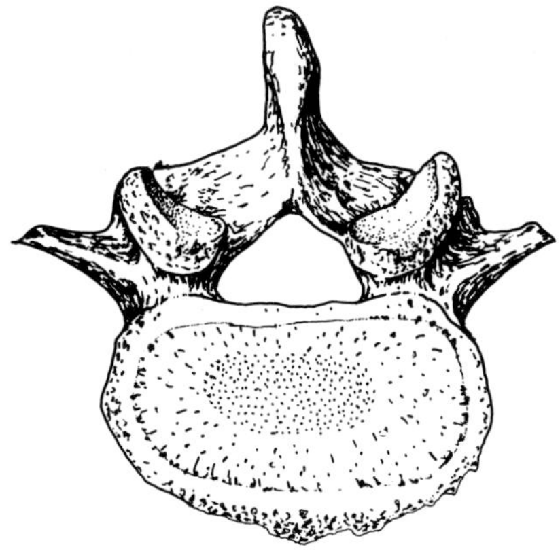

Fig. 3.26 Upper surface of L4; note central area of reduced porosity (openings of trabecular channels of very small diameter).

large openings for basivertebral veins. Small foramina are scattered sparsely over the transverse processes, laminae and spine, but increase in numbers and size in the lower lumbar region in all these areas. At all levels there is a greater concentration of foramina in juxta-articular zones of laminae, presumably in relation to the circulus articuli vasculosus (Barnett *et al.*, 1961).

A sagittal section of the column demonstrates the well-organized pattern of trabeculation in vertical and horizontal strands, the latter being more closely packed towards the upper and lower surfaces of the body (Fig. 2.27). There is no evidence of an epiphyseal scar as seen in long bones. The cortex of the neural arch and its processes are thicker than that of the body, and the trabecular pattern differs. Within a single spinal process there is a change in the density from a loose network at the base to a closer one at the tip.

In non-pathological compact bone of animals, variations in ash mass range from 45% to 85%, and reflect variations in the mechanical properties of Young's modulus of elasticity, bending strength and work of fracture (Currey, 1984). The density of normal human bone also varies, together with the organic and mineral content and the thickness of compact bone. These variables are influenced by race, sex, nutrition and age (Ahuja, 1969). Mechanical factors also operate, as demonstrated by altered deposition of compact and trabecular bone in relation to the convex and concave curves in scoliosis (Weinmann and Sicher, 1955; Fig. 3.5). There is also evidence that

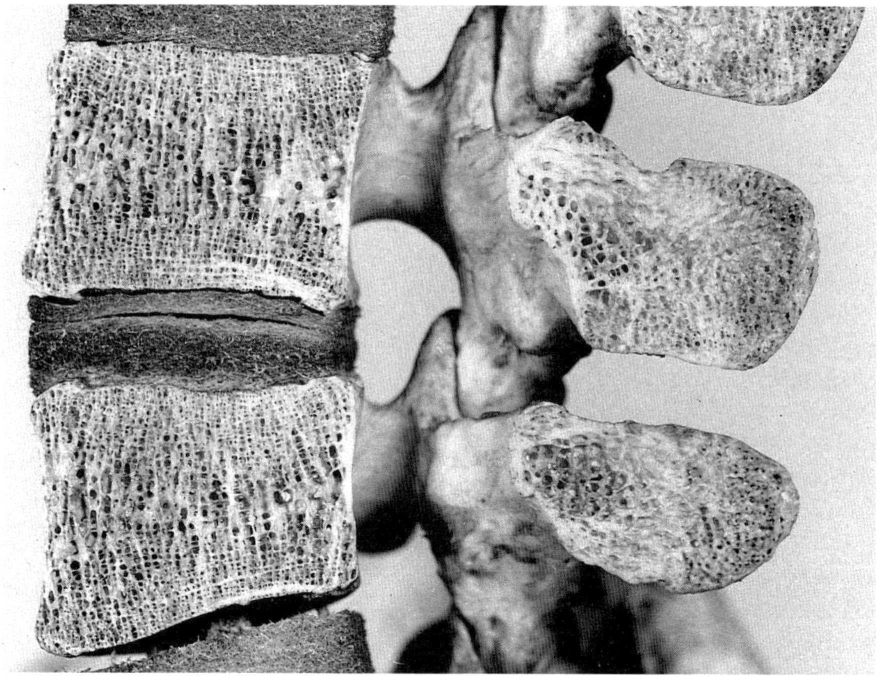

Fig. 3.27 Trabecular patterns in bodies and midline of neural arches of L4 and L5. (Right side of hemisected column shown in Figs 3.24 & 3.28.)

skeletal mass varies in different geographical localities, but this might involve many factors including genetics, diet and economic status (Eddy, 1972).

In healthy human vertebrae the proportions of organic and inorganic mineral matter are respectively about 40% and 60%. The organic matter consists of cells, vessels, collagen and haemopoietic tissue. Both organic and inorganic components undergo non-pathological change with age, and with consequent changes in physical properties. Complete demineralization of a vertebra leaves a tough, spongy collagenous structure displaying every morphological detail of the intact bone. There are four types of cancellous bone. One consists of fine rods built into a meshwork with no well-defined orientation; the second is composed of parallel fenestrated plates linked by fine rods; the third is made up of fenestrated plates forming a meshwork with parallel tubular spaces, and the fourth resembles a honeycomb with small spaces and relatively thick plates. The thickness of plates and rods varies (Singh, 1978).

A reconstruction of the spongiosa of the third lumbar vertebra of a healthy woman of 20 (killed in an accident) showed that it was a complex network of plates with preferential vertical and horizontal orientation, and having many fenestrations of varying sizes (i.e. Type III Singh). The horizontal plates linked the vertical ones at various inclinations, and the amount of horizontal bone was greatest at upper and lower surfaces of the body. Thus there was economy of material with resistance to compressive and shearing forces (Amstutz & Sissons, 1969). Trabeculae in a lumbar articular process are arranged orthogonally and converge towards the apex, an arrangement which coincides with findings in a photoelastic model. This pattern does not extend into the mamillary process (Putz, 1985). These articular processes permit, but also limit, rotation (Putz, 1976). Further information is required for other levels of the column.

In lumbar vertebrae the cortex is very thick where the neural arches join the body (Putz, 1985). This is consistent with the distribution of surface strain found in cadaveric lumbar vertebrae (Shar *et al.*, 1978).

The pars interarticularis of a lower lumbar vertebra has thick cortical bone anterolaterally and posteromedially, the former being the thickest, and in both regions the cortex was thicker at the narrowest part of the bone. The trabeculae found by Krenz & Troup (1973) were stout but sparse (it should be noted that four of their seven subjects were aged 50 years or more). This region of the lumbar neural arch is subject to complex forces, primarily from shearing between the articular processes. The arrangement of cortical bone would tend to resist these forces.

Until the age of 40 the strength of intact vertebral

bodies is directly related to trabecular bone ash content (Rockoff *et al.*, 1969). This is not surprising since 66% of all vertebral bone is cancellous (Twomey *et al.*, 1983). Roaf (1960) attributed some of the capacity to withstand compressive forces to the fluid contents of the trabecular bone which are forced out of the spongiosa into paravertebral vessels, thus acting as an energy dissipating mechanism.

Senescent changes

The thickness of the trabecular plates decreases, and separation between them increases with advancing age (Eder, 1960). This is substantiated by the decrease in percentage volume of cortical and cancellous bone in second lumbar vertebrae of apparently normal subjects (Dunnill *et al.*, 1967). Cortical bone thickness diminishes after the age of 45 (Saville, 1970). After the age of 49 the correlation between strength and trabecular bone is lost (Rockoff *et al.*, 1969). Loss of bone density in lumbar vertebral bodies occurs in men and women, but the rate of loss is greater in women. The primary cause of decline is a significant and selective decrease in transverse trabeculae. This is accompanied by increasing concavity of the vertebral endplates and increases in horizontal dimensions of the bodies, particularly at upper and lower extremities (cf. Figs 3.27 & 3.28; Twomey *et al.*, 1983). This loss of bone affects resistance to trauma, sometimes of a minor degree. The distribution of fractures in osteoporosis demonstrates the vulnerability of the thoracolumbar region (Fig. 3.28; Saville, 1970; Urist *et al.*, 1970).

There is ample evidence of organization of chondrocytes (Poole *et al.*, 1984), fibrils in cartilage (Broom & Marra, 1986) as well as histochemical reactions (Stockwell, 1987) to indicate a close relationship between structure and function in cartilage (see review in Williams *et al.*, 1989). Age-related changes affect all tissues in lumbar facet joints (Taylor & Twomey, 1986; Wang *et al.*, 1989). Articular cartilage thins with age, and degenerative change tends to be more severe in superior than in corresponding inferior facets. Like Engel & Bogduk (1982), Wang *et al.* found little advanced change in the joints up to the age of 37, but the 10-year-old boy in their series was the only one with a complete meniscus. Meniscal damage and other signs of early degenerative change were already present by 19 years. After the age of 40, cartilage showed a variety of changes ranging from complete

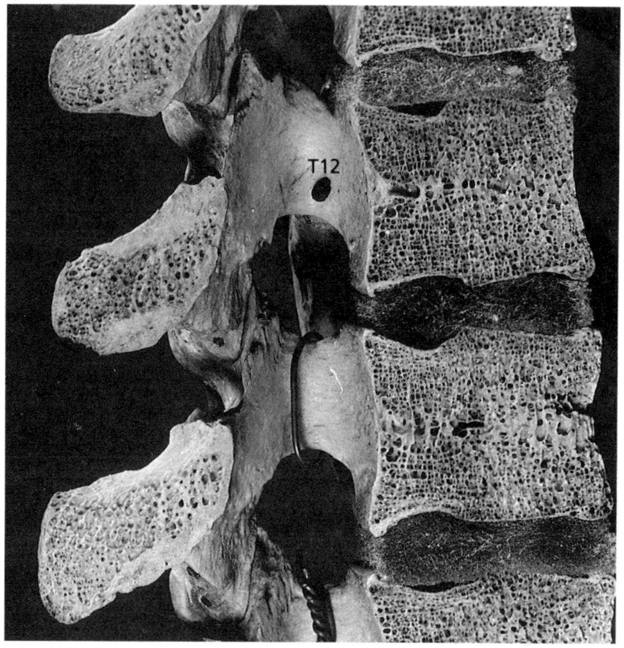

Fig. 3.28 Left hemisection of vertebral column with senescent loss of cortical and trabecular bone. Note irregular concavities on upper and lower surfaces of bodies and loss of concentration of transverse trabeculae seen towards upper and lower surfaces of bodies in Fig. 3.27. (Museum of RCS Eng.)

coverage of the articular bone, despite irregularities and erosions, to either complete absence of, or patchy traces of, cartilage. Meniscal changes ranged from decreased extent, leading to peripheral wedges, to fragmentation and complete absence. Subarticular cortical bone changed from being a smooth evenly thick plate to the final stage of marked irregularity of thickness, erosions and formation of osteophytes.

ARTICULATIONS

The bodies of vertebrae are united by mobile secondary cartilaginous joints (symphyses) from the second cervical vertebra down to the first sacral segment. Below this there are discs but no movements except for the sacrococcygeal joints. Synovial articulations link the atlas and axis and neural arches down to the lumbosacral facet joints.

Fibrocartilaginous discs lie between the hyaline cartilage plates on upper and lower surfaces of vertebral bodies. These symphyses contribute to about 24% of the presacral length of the healthy adult column. However, this contribution is not evenly distributed in amount or proportion (Todd & Pyle, 1928a,b). The axes of movements between vertebrae are largely governed by the shapes of facet joints, whilst the ranges of sagittal movement are related to thickness of discs, bony and ligamentous restraints and neural mechanisms.

Intervertebral discs

Discs conform to the shapes of the bodies of related vertebrae, and vary in thickness in different regions (Fig. 3.24).

The upper four thoracic discs diminish in thickness, and increase slowly to the tenth. Thereafter there is a steady and more rapid rise, the largest, which is also markedly thicker anteriorly, is at the lumbosacral joint.

Discs are attached to vertebral bodies and to the deep layers of anterior and posterior longitudinal ligaments. In the thoracic region they are also attached to the intra-articular ligaments of the heads of the second to ninth or tenth ribs.

Immediately medial to the neurocentral processes in the cervical region cavities develop in the discs. There is no information about the upper thoracic discs where there are neurocentral processes (pp. 52 & 53). These cavities form the joints of Luschka, subjects of controversy (Tondury, 1943). No true synovial membrane was identified by Orofino *et al.* (1960), Hall (1965) found no evidence of a cavity until four years, by 14 it was established. These authors regard it as a regularly occurring degenerate change in discs. Osteophytic changes occur in relation to them and may encroach upon the intervertebral foramina (Cave *et al.*, 1955).

Structure of intervertebral discs

Discs have three components: an outer thin collagenous zone firmly anchored to the annular epiphyses and to the anterior and posterior longitudinal ligaments; an intermediate lamellated fibrocartilaginous annulus fibrosus attached to the cartilage plates and the nucleus pulposus, which is better developed in cervical and lumbar regions. Because of appositional subperiosteal growth in the girth of vertebral bodies the nucleus might tend to be nearer the posterior surface of the body. In a recent study with magnetic resonance and cryomicrotomy, at 10 years the nucleus was more posteriorly placed in the upper lumbar region, and more anteriorly in the lower (Wagner *et al.*, 1988). The nucleus exerts a positive pressure, which increases when loaded, and it is also affected by posture (Nachemson, 1963; Nachemson & Morris, 1964).

The annulus fibrosus is not an homogeneous structure. Within the cartilaginous matrix there are two types of collagen: Type I is found in areas requiring high tensile strength; Type II has a high compressive strength and increases from the periphery inwards. The total amount of collagen decreases as the nucleus is approached. The proportions and distribution of the two types alter with age (Herbert *et al.*, 1975; Brickley-Parsons & Glimcher, 1984). Therefore there are alterations in response to mechanical stress (see Appendix 3 in Gracovetsky, 1988, also p. 63).

The collagen fibres in each lamella are in parallel helices which run with varying degrees of obliquity between the two vertebrae (Inoué, 1973), except posteriorly where they are mainly vertical (Zaki, 1973). In adjacent concentric lamellae the fibres run in opposite directions, thus forming crisscrossed palisades which allow rotation to left and right, but limit it by the length of fibres, which also interconnect adjacent lamellae. Elastic fibres are present in human fetal (Hickey & Hukins, 1981) and adult discs (Johnson *et al.*, 1985). The water content of the annulus at birth is 78%; this declines slowly with age to 70% and affects mechanical properties (Viidik, 1973).

At birth the nucleus pulposus is large, soft, mucoid, gelatinous and round. It contains notochordal cells and others from the surrounding annulus. By 10 years chordal cells have disappeared. Chondrocytes, degenerating necrotic cells and randomly arranged collagen appear within it between four and 18 years. Gradually the nucleus is encroached upon by the inner annulus and upper and lower cartilage plates (Sylven, 1950; Peacock, 1952; Meachim & Cornah, 1970). The water content declines from 88% to 80% by 12 and to 70% at 70 years (Keyes & Compere, 1932; Hendry, 1958). The water-binding capacity and elasticity are due to the mucopolysaccharide and protein content (Sylven *et al.*, 1951; see also Chapter 9). Age-related qualitative changes in proteoglycans lead to increasing interaction with collagen (Adams & Muir, 1976), and limit movement of the nucleus. The nucleus is deformable, but not compressible, and when subjected to compression the annulus bulges (Hirsch & Nachemson, 1954). It exerts a positive pressure which alters with positive load carrying and speed of application of forces (Nachemson & Morris,

1964; Nachemson, 1963). In the young, excessive compression results in fractures of bones before disruption of the discs (Roaf, 1960). However, the changes with age alter biochemical and physical properties (Hendry, 1958; Beard & Stevens, 1980). The more posterior position of the nucleus and the vertical fibres of the annulus predispose to posterior herniation. Fissures appear in cartilaginous plates, probably beginning in the cartilage canals. Dehydration, the presence of these fissures, and persistent notochordal canals (Beadle, 1931) contribute to the small diurnal loss of height which is restored by rest (Taylor & Twomey, 1984). They also contribute to the steady decline in height and narrowed disc spaces in the elderly, in whom there are also bony changes (p. 61).

Nutrition of discs

Cellularity and metabolic demands are highest in the peripheral annulus and the hyaline cartilage nearest the bone. The glucose diffusion coefficient of 2.5 cm per second is comparable with cartilage in other areas (Maroudas *et al.*, 1975). The segmental vessels which supply the outer annulus in infancy do not persist beyond the fourth year (Ehrenhaft, 1942). Nutrition is entirely dependent upon diffusion and flow through the cartilage plates from the underlying trabecular bone, where the porosity is diminished centrally in relation to the nucleus which exerts a positive pressure (Fig. 3.26). The thicker the disc, the greater the risk of central failure of nutrition in both annulus and nucleus.

The outflow of fluid from lumbar discs is larger during flexion than in erect or lordotic postures. This outflow is reversed in the unloaded spine, a finding consistent with the well-authenticated nocturnal restoration of the diurnal loss of height. Adams & Hutton (1983) concluded that fluid exchange within discs was enhanced by flexion. In 1986 they found that flow of large molecules and proteins was assisted by intradiscal pressure changes. Radioactive tracers showed that exchange of smaller molecules was affected by posture. Diffusion into the anterior half of the disc was favoured by the erect posture, and into the posterior half by flexion. Diffusion into the nucleus may be affected by the decreased porosity of bone underlying it. Nuclear resonance demonstrates an early change, in which a dark band bisects the nucleus in the horizontal plane. This was shown to be due to fibrous tissue, and is possibly a reflection of such failure in the depths of the nucleus (Wagner *et al.*, 1988; Fig. 3.26).

Synovial articulations

The atlanto-occipital and atlanto-axial articulations are all synovial and are anterior to those of the succeeding vertebrae. The long axes of the ellipsoid and concave surfaces supported by the lateral masses of the atlas diverge from anterior to posterior. The angle of divergence varies, and in one of 30 bones examined at the Royal College of Surgeons the axes were nearly parallel, and in another they were flat and circular in outline. In infants facets are flat; data regarding the ages at which the concavity develops are lacking. Indentations and varying degrees of subdivision occur and are related to the ossification of the bone (p. 55). The atlanto-occipital joint cavities may communicate with the atlantodental one. There is a bursa between the transverse ligament and the constriction on the neck of the dens (Fig. 3.19).

Macerated specimens show considerable incongruity between articulating facet joints of atlas and axis. The lower facets of the atlas face downwards and medially, and very slightly forwards. The upper axial facets slope slightly posteriorly and more markedly laterally and downwards. The apposed surfaces may be concave, convex or concavoconvex, and lack symmetry. The facets of succeeding joints are circular or slightly ovoid. The surface areas decrease slowly but steadily from C2 down to C7 and the surface area of the bodies increases. Facets account for 46% of the weight-bearing area of the axis, and 39.2% at C7 (Pal & Routal, 1986). Clearly from the line of gravity (Fig. 3.7) these joints contribute to bearing compressive weight, the amount varying with the changes in posture and during movements of the neck and trunk. The joint capsules are somewhat lax, but even with folds, the surface areas of the synovia are small in comparison with the articular cartilages. In healthy spines, branches of the vertebral artery pass perpendicularly into the capsules, but distortion of the artery resulting from degenerative lesions of the spine may obstruct and re-align these branches (Figs 3.29 & 3.30; Abdullah *et al.*, 1967).

THE CERVICOTHORACIC JUNCTION

The inferior facets of the seventh cervical vertebra slope anteriorly and downwards, and may be flat. The

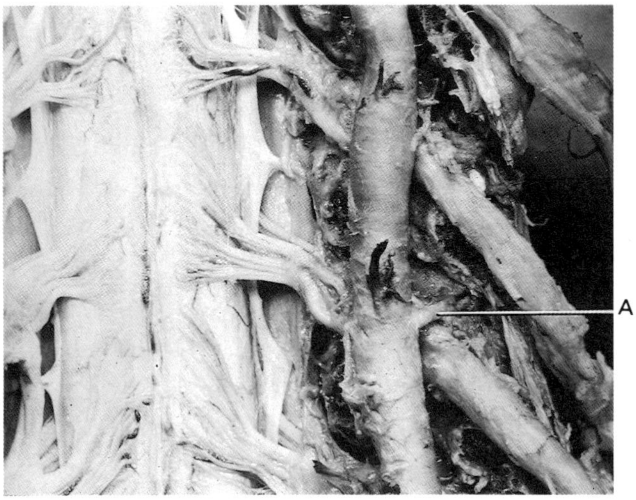

Fig. 3.29 Branch of the vertebral artery entering the fibrous capsule of a zygapophyseal joint A. Dissection by S. Abdullah. From Bowden *et al.* (1967).

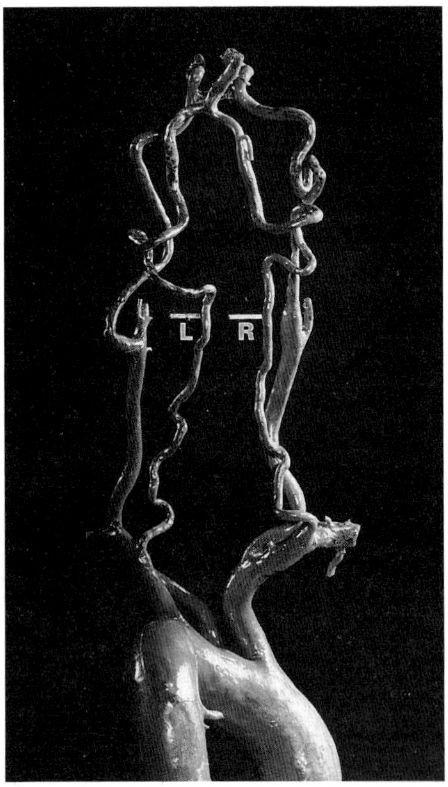

Fig. 3.30 Posterior view of cast of arch of the aorta with branches showing internal carotid and vertebral arteries. L, left; R, right vertebral arteries, which have become tortuous and distorted. Note obliquity of vertebrals in relation to axis and sharp angulation related to upper surface of atlas. (Museum of RCS Eng.)

lower border of the facets is convex and rests against the laminar shelf if present, on the first thoracic vertebra. The latter frequently curves upwards and laterally. In neutral position of the neck or in the erect posture, this limits or obstructs rotation (Figs 3.16 & 3.20).

THORACIC FACET JOINTS

Where the laminar shelf is prominent and occurs in more than one vertebra, the corresponding facets tend to be either flat or on the arcs of circles of larger diameter than those in the middle of the thoracic region. Below shelf level the upper facets are directed laterally and posteriorly, the inferior ones face forwards and medially. The facets form arcs of circles and if perpendiculars to the midpoints of the chords are extended they intersect (Fig. 3.31). To make comparisons between 17 columns, Davis (1959) devised indices for these points with respect to the distance from the midsagittal point of the laminae and the anterior and posterior surfaces of the bodies. When the two points for each vertebra were plotted, in 163/166 joints the intersection points for superior facets were dorsal to the points for inferior ones. There was variation in the position of both in relation to vertebral bodies. In all columns both points lay anterior to the upper one or two thoracic vertebrae. There was considerable variation in the pattern below this, but they never lay behind the middle third of the vertebral body. Conclusions based on this evidence are that:

1 facets are only congruent in the erect posture;
2 centres of rotation vary in individuals, and are anterior to the vertebral canal;
3 in the midthoracic region rotation can take place without a lateral shift of the bodies upon one another;
4 elsewhere lateral shearing of bodies will be associated with rotation unless facets subluxate.

THE THORACOLUMBAR JUNCTION

Theoretically, this lies between the twelfth thoracic and first lumbar vertebrae, but functionally this depends upon the position of the mortice joint when present. Where a single mortice joint exists, invariably the vertebra above has thoracic characteristics, and the one below is a typical lumbar vertebra (Davis, 1955). Where there is more than one mortice joint in a column there are modifications. The mortice is formed by mamillary processes overhanging the

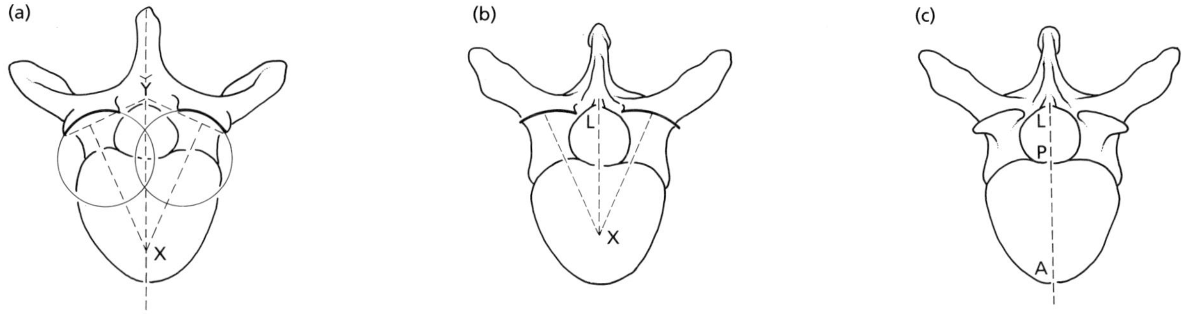

Fig. 3.31 (a): Intersection point X of cords of circles related to inferior facet joints of a typical thoracic vertebra. Note the facetal angle Y; a similar point was determined for superior facets. (b,c) Measurements required for intersection indices: (b), midline distance to intersection point L-X; (c), lamina-body index. Midline distance to posterior surface of body LP. Midline distance to anterior surface of body LA.

$$\text{Intersection Index} = \frac{\text{LX} \times 100}{\text{LA}}. \qquad \text{Lamina-body length index} = \frac{\text{LP} \times 100}{\text{LA}}.$$

From these indices a graph was obtained giving the relationship between intersection points and the vertebral body for each thoracic vertebra.

superior articular facets and enclosing, to varying degrees, the tenon formed by the inferior facets of the vertebra above (Fig. 3.32a–d). The existence of mortices was observed many years ago (Topinard, 1877; Le Double, 1912), but their presence and functional significance are still overlooked (e.g. Gracovetsky, 1988, makes no mention of them). There are three grades of mortice.

Grade I: the mamillary process is attached along the whole length of the lateral border of the upper facet, and therefore encloses the whole tenon in the erect posture.

Grade II: more than half the tenon is enclosed.

Grade III: less than half the tenon is enclosed (Table 3.9).

The frequency distribution of mortices in adults indi-

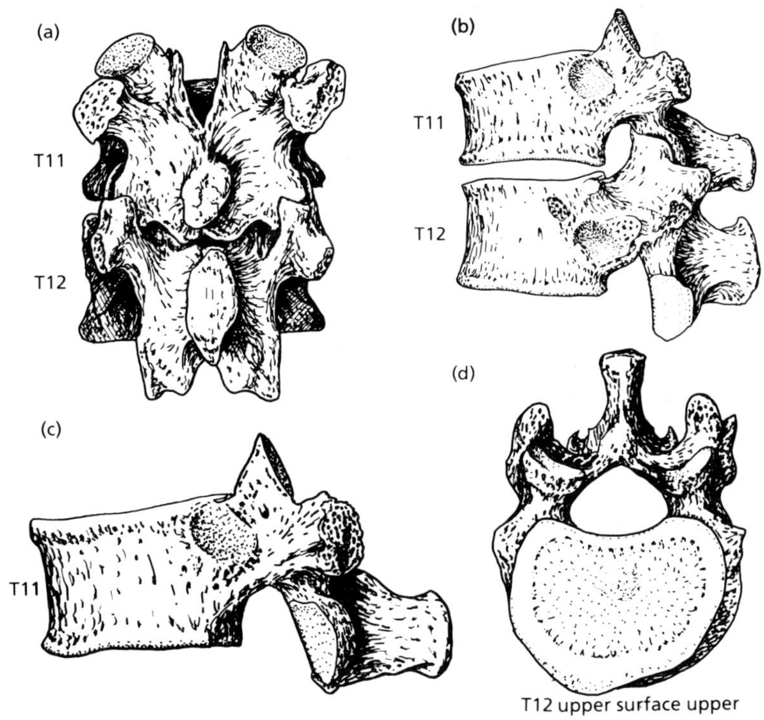

Fig. 3.32 (a) Posterior view of mortice. (b) Lateral view of mortice. (c) Lateral view of T11 with upper facet of thoracic type and lower lumbar type. (d) Upper surface of T12 with typical lumbar facet.

Table 3.9 Depth of mortice and frequency of occurrence in 160 adult and 41 juvenile columns. After Davis (1957)

	Group I	Group II	Group III	Total
Davis (1957)				
Adult	14	50	34	98
Juvenile	2	12	12	26
Davis (1961)[a]				
Adult	6	25	31	62
Juvenile	2	11	2	15
Totals	24	98	79	201
Percentage	11.9	48.8	39.3	100

[a] West African skeletal material.

cates that this should be regarded as a normal feature (Table 3.10). There was no significant difference in incidence in Caucasian and West African adults, or between the juveniles in the two series investigated by Davis (1955, 1961). There was no significant difference in incidence as between male or female, in adults or juveniles in West African skeletons. The levels at which single mortices occur are given in Table 3.10.

In the Caucasian series Davis (1955) found only one double mortice, but there were seven in the West African series (one out of 40 males and six out of 75 females—Davis, 1961). The difference between males and females is significant ($p > 0.02$) and attributable to the fact that women habitually carry heavier head loads than do males. The one male had mortices between T11 and T12, T12 and L1. Five females had them at this level, and the sixth at T10–T11, T11–T12. Eleven out of 50 columns (Royal College of Surgeons) had double mortices, seven were at T10–T11, T11–T12 and four at T11–T12, T12–L1. These were of unknown provenance but probably came from the Indian subcontinent where head-carrying is also practised. No double mortices were found in juvenile columns. The Caucasian specimens ranged in age from birth to 19 years. Of four with no mortices, two were under two years of age. No mortice was found under the age of six years in 53 out of 79 West African columns (Tables 3.11 & 3.12). In view of findings in adults, it is clear that the osseous mortice is a post-natal development. However, it is not possible to exclude the existence of a cartilaginous mortice into which ossification had not yet extended. It is also not possible to determine whether the mortice is genetically determined, or whether it forms as a response to mechanical stress. Its absence before two to six years lends support to the latter view. Head-carrying cannot be invoked for the presence in the Caucasian series. However, in bipedal locomotion there is counter-rotation of pelvis and shoulders (White & Panjabi, 1978) which might produce mechanical stress. This suggestion is supported by pedicular findings in columns with a shallow or no mortice (Fig. 3.14). The presence of a mortice limits extension and, unless very shallow, it also limits rotation. It would add support in resisting compressive forces, and resist any shear or rotational stress. Its possible role in the increased vulnerability of the spine to fractures is of interest (Figs 3.1 & 3.2). There is also a significant relationship between the levels of increased robust-

Table 3.10 Level and frequency of mortice joints in 224 male and female adults

	Level			None	Multiple
	T10–T11	T11–T12	T12–L1		
Davis (1955)	6	72	20	4	1 level not stated, classified by deepest mortice
Davis (1961) West African male and female	2	42	18	6	7
RCS (1989)	6	22	2	5	11
Totals	14	136	40	15	19
Percentage of 224	6.3	60.7	17.9	6.7	8.5

Table 3.11 Age and frequency of mortice joints in 79 juvenile West African columns (43 male, 36 female). After Davis (1961)

Age (years)	Absent		Present		Total	
	Male	Female	Male	Female	Absent	Present
0–2	12	10	—	—	22	—
3–5	16	15	—	—	31	—
6–8	3	2	2	2	5	4
9–11	0	0	2	1	0	3
12–14	1	1	3	2	2	5
15–17	1	1	3	2	2	5
Levels	Males		Females		Total	
T11–T12	7		3		10	
T12–L1	3		2		5	

Table 3.12 Level and frequency of mortice joints in 100 juvenile vertebral columns. After Davis (1957, 1961)

	Absent	T10–T11	T11–T12	T12–L1	Total
1957	8[a]	0	11	2	21
1961	62[b]	—	12	5	79
Totals	70	0	23	7	100

[a] Four under two years of age.
[b] Twenty-two under two years of age; 31 three to five years of age.

ness of pedicles and increase in cross-sectional area of vertebral bodies (Figs 3.9, 3.10 & 3.13).

The laminar spicules which are buried in the lateral borders of the ligamenta flava also increase towards the mortice joints (Fig. 3.3; Table 3.6), also p. 47.

LUMBAR FACET JOINTS

Typically, the superior joints face posteriorly and medially and are concave, the lower ones face antero laterally and are convex. The vertical orientation is suited to flexion and extension. The curvature would allow rotation, but the centre, unlike that of the thoracic region, lies posterior to the vertebral bodies (Fig. 3.2) and the force is countered by the internal architecture (p. 71). The synovial capsule has folds and menisci are present (Engel & Bogduk, 1982; Bogduk & Engle, 1984 and p. 72).

THE LUMBOSACRAL ARTICULATIONS

The wedging of the body of the fifth lumbar vertebra and of the underlying disc, together with the inclination of the sacrum, accounts for the abrupt transition between the two curves.

The compression force to be transmitted to the lower limbs can be resolved into two components at right angles to each other. When standing, one goes obliquely downwards and backwards, and the other inclines forwards and downwards roughly in the plane of the inlet of the lesser pelvis to the acetabulum and femoral head (Fig. 3.33). The tie bar between the two hip bones is formed by the superior ramus and bodies of the pubes and pubic symphysis. There

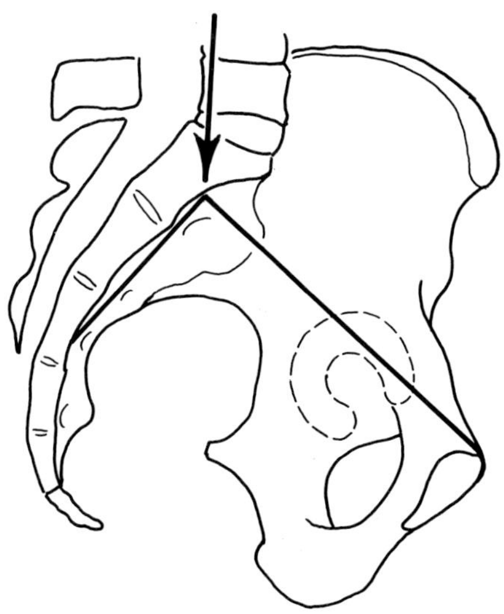

Fig. 3.33 Diagram of resolution of forces acting at L5–S1 in the erect posture.

would be a tendency for the column to slide forwards on the sacrum, and for the sacrum to be rotated still further posteriorly with elevation of the lower end and coccyx. When sitting, weight is transmitted to the ischial tuberosities with the ischiopubic rami, the symphysis and bodies of the pubes being the tie bars in this posture.

As the column is weight-bearing, the cross-sectional area of the body of the fifth lumbar vertebrae might be expected to be the largest in the presacral series. However, this is not invariable (Davis, 1955); therefore, the role of the neural arch requires analysis. The lower articular facets of the fifth lumbar are as wide apart as the superior ones, unlike higher lumbar vertebrae (Fig. 3.34). The angle of inclination to sagittal plane of the facet joints of the sacrum varies (Čihák, 1970), as it does for the lower facet joints of the fifth lumbar, the nearer the inclination of the long axes is to the coronal plane, the greater is the possible contribution to weight-bearing (Fig. 3.25). The stoutness of the pedicles and transverse processes also varies, as demonstrated in two series of adult and juvenile columns (Davis, 1957, 1961). Robustness of lower thoracic pedicles increases at the level of the mortice, decreases in upper lumbar vertebrae and rises sharply in the lower two (Figs 3.13 & 3.14). In a series of adult and juvenile West African columns the area of the lower surface of the body of L4 was slightly larger than L3. In 83% of both adult males and females the area of L4 was larger than L5. In both male and female columns there was an increase in pedicle indices from L3 to L5, but with considerable range of variation between individuals, and no significant differences between the sexes. The greatest range of

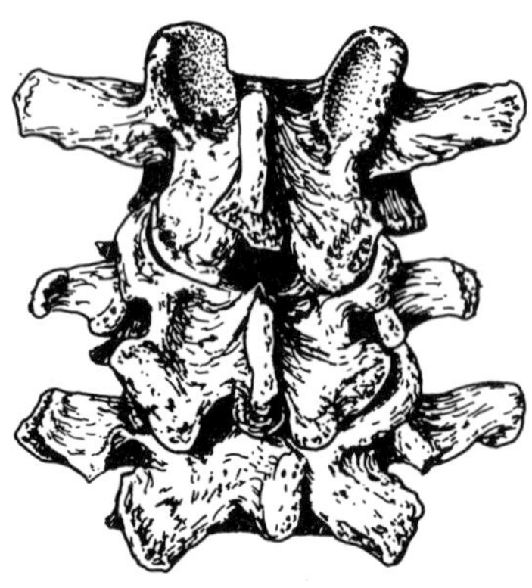

Fig. 3.34 Posterior view of articulated L3, L4 and L5 showing zygapophyseal joints.

variation is in L5. As might be expected, L5 has the stoutest transverse process. In general, the third lumbar transverse process is larger than the fourth. The findings in adults and juveniles were similar. Comparisons between values of pedicle indices and sizes of transverse processes in relation to surface areas of bodies of L4 and L5 showed that the stoutness of pedicles and transverse processes of L5 was greater than in L4 when the body of L4 had the greater surface area. The findings were statistically significant but showed no significant differences between males and females. These findings indicate that, in the upright posture, pressure on the disc at the lumbosacral joint is less than that between L4 and L5, and that the pedicles, transverse and inferior zygapophyseal joints resist some of the compressive forces. Brailsford (1929) found that in 360 out of 3000 subjects (i.e. 12%), the lumbosacral facet joints faced inwards. In such individuals these joints could play little part in resisting the forward component of forces, and the iliolumbar ligaments would be of the greatest importance (pp. 71, 72). The articulating surfaces of the facet joints are reciprocally curved, the lumbar ones facing forwards laterally and downwards, and the sacral ones facing posteromedially and upwards. The degree of curvature, as well as the angle of intersection of the chords, varied, but in none of 55 (Royal College of Surgeons) sacra, was the surface flat. Even one with a persistent synchondrosis between the right transverse process of the fifth lumbar and the transverse element of the sacrum, was slightly curved (Fig. 3.35a,b).

SACROILIAC ARTICULATIONS

The auricular articular surface of the sacrum is irregular. The upper part is confined to the first piece of the sacrum and the lower to the second and third, in both sexes. Although the surface area and length show differences in male and female, Weisl (1954b) considered that the sole difference was a deeper dorsal notch in the female, and greater laxity of the capsule and ligaments, particularly in the puerperium (Weisl, 1954a). However, recently, Valojerdy & Hogg (1989) reported that the articular facets were larger in surface area and longer in the male.

The articular surface on the sacrum is covered with fibrocartilage, and the ilium with hyaline cartilage. In infants both the articular surfaces are virtually flat. Elevations and concavities develop which increase in height and depth with age, and are not exactly recip-

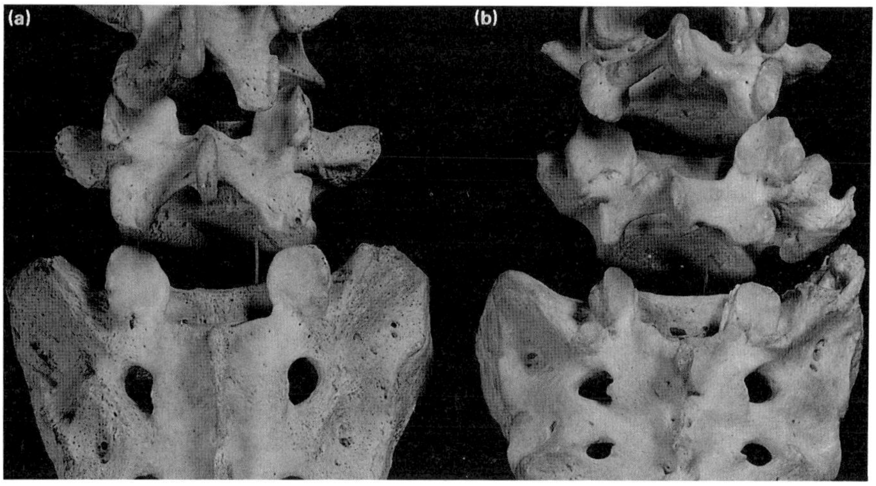

Fig. 3.35 (a) Normal lumbosacral articulation—note the concave sacral zygapophyseal articular surface. (b) Hemisacralization (R) of L5. Bony union had not occurred. Note the orientation of the two sacral zygapophyseal joints is not symmetrical, both surfaces are concave, but only slightly so on the right.

rocal on the two bones (Weisl, 1954b). In the elderly, and especially in males, fibrous, fibrocartilaginous and even osseous adhesions may form. In both sexes the articular surface occupies three pieces of the sacrum and the ventral border follows the slope of the ala and curvature of the bone. According to Weisl the cranial concavity is deeper in females, and the whole surface is proportionately larger and narrower in the male. The differences were recently re-examined in 108 male and 45 female specimens of Indian origin, by Valojerdy & Hogg (1989). They found significantly larger areas and greater lengths of male sacral and iliac articular surfaces, and significant differences in the iliac angle which, on the ilium, was larger in males. The most prominent point on the ventral border of the articular surface was more caudal in females, as was the deepest point on the dorsal border.

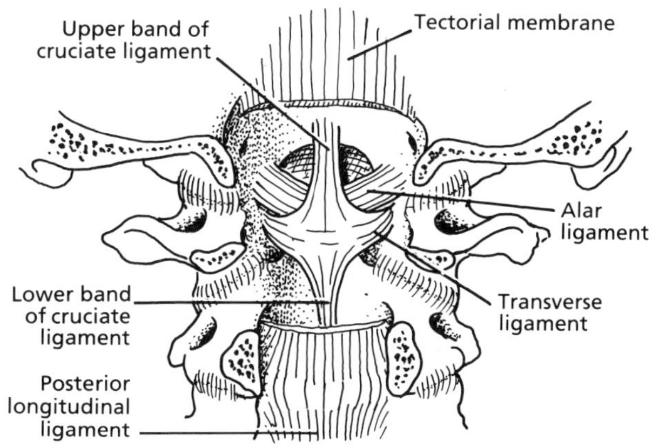

Fig. 3.36 The ligaments of the atlanto-axial and atlanto-occipital joints seen from posteriorly after removal of the neural arches. Note the broad posterior longitudinal ligament which has no free lateral border. It is continuous above with the tectorial membrane, but has been removed to show the cruciate and alar ligaments.

LIGAMENTS

The ligaments of the atlanto-occipital and atlanto-axial joints are illustrated in Figs 3.36 & 3.37.

THE ANTERIOR LONGITUDINAL LIGAMENT

This extends from the basiocciput to the anterior tubercle of the atlas and continues down to the sacrum and coccyx. It broadens as it passes caudally. In the cervical region it envelops the entire ventrolateral surface of the bodies and becomes continuous with the deep layer of the posterior longitudinal ligament (Hayashi *et al.*, 1977). It is thicker and narrower in the thoracic than in the lumbar region.

The ligament is formed of collagen and has three layers. The superficial one crosses three or four vertebrae, the intermediate two or three and the deepest is firmly attached to adjacent vertebrae, the cartilage plates, and also blends with the annulus fibrosus and periosteum. The attachment to the bodies of vertebrae is looser, but the waists are filled out, making a smooth anterior surface.

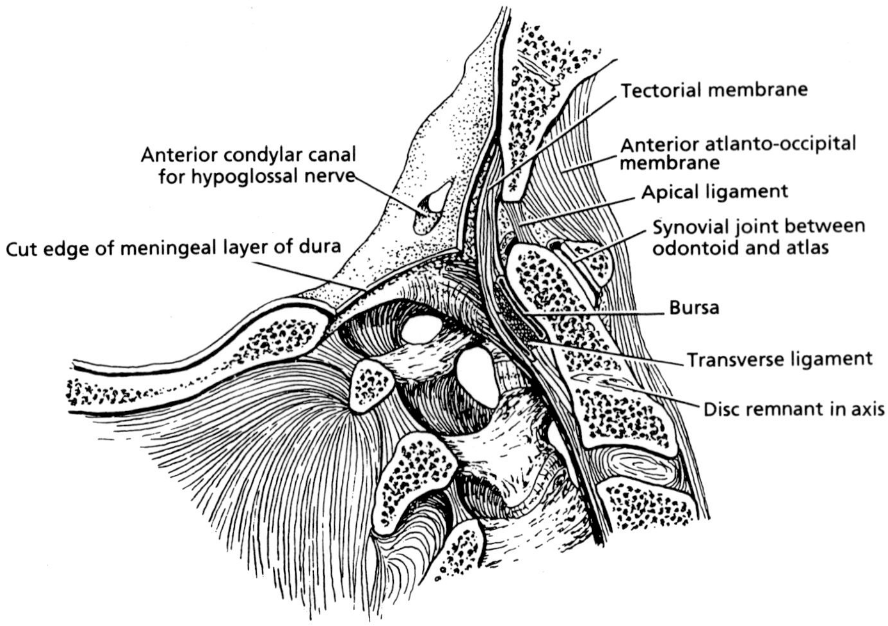

Fig. 3.37 Right hemisection of upper cervical vertebrae and lower posterior cranial fossa.

THE POSTERIOR LONGITUDINAL LIGAMENT

This is continuous above with the tectorial membrane (Fig. 3.36). In the cervical and upper thoracic region it is broad, and in young subjects it has an opaque, glassy appearance, making a smooth lining to the canal. Its attachments to the dura in the cervical region were recognized, but it was not understood until Hayashi *et al.* (1977) demonstrated a loosely adherent posterior superficial layer of the ligament which sends slips to an epidural membrane surrounding the cervical dura, dural root sleeves and the vertebral arteries.

Below the cervical and upper thoracic regions the ligament is denticulate. It is wide and firmly adherent to the annulus, the adjacent cartilage plates and the bones, and narrow and not adherent to the bodies, allowing free passage between basivertebral veins and the anterior vertebral plexus. For ligaments compartmentalizing intervertebral foraminae see p. 81.

Ligaments of vertebral arches

LIGAMENTA FLAVA

These ligaments, composed mainly of perpendicularly arranged yellow elastic fibres, are bilateral and intersegmental. They approach each other in the midline, but fusion is never complete and blood vessels enter and leave the canal. The inclination of the ligaments towards the sagittal plane varies with the shape of the vertebral canal. They are attached to a roughened area on the anterior and inferior aspect of the lamina of the upper vertebra, and the inferior attachment is to the posterior surface and upper margin of the laminae below. Laterally, they extend to the medial aspect of the capsules of the facet joints, where smooth bony spicules of varying size are found (pp. 46, 54, 67; Davis, 1955; Davis & Rowland, 1965). The ligamenta flava permit separation of laminae, and are important in the last phases of flexion of the trunk from the erect posture when there is little or no concentric contraction of erector spinae muscles (Floyd & Silver, 1955).

The facet joint capsules and ligaments

These are attached to the margins of articular facets and are closely related to the lateral margins of the ligamenta flava. They are thin and lax, particularly in the neck.

LIGAMENTUM NUCHAE

This is the homologue of the inter- and supraspinous ligament of the thoracic and lumbar regions. It extends from the external occipital protuberance and the external occipital crest to the posterior tubercle of the atlas, the broad gap in the bifid spine of the axis and successive spinous processes down to the seventh cervical vertebra. Its interspinous portions are thin and short. The supraspinous part provides an additional surface for muscular attachments (see Fig. 3.42, p. 76).

INTERSPINOUS LIGAMENTS

These are thin in the thoracic segments, and very short where spines overlap markedly (Fig. 3.17). They extend from ligamenta flava to the tips of spinous processes. In the lumbar region they are formed of bilateral sheets, with three distinct components. The anterior one contains a few elastic fibres, and possibly may be an extension of the ligamenta flava. The intermediate and largest part, and the dorsal component, are both purely collagenous. The latter is attached to the posterior half of the cranial border of the spinous process of the lower vertebra and the fibres sweep backwards and upwards to enter the supraspinous ligament or to merge with the medial tendons of erector spinae (Heylings, 1978).

THE SUPRASPINOUS LIGAMENT

This extends from the spine of the seventh cervical and links intervening processes down to the spine of the fifth lumbar vertebra, and it links the spines of all intervening ones. It is thin superiorly and broadens as it passes downwards. It is fused with the posterior layer of thoracolumbar fascia. The deepest fibres run between two spines, intermediate ones link two or three, and the most superficial extend over three or four vertebrae. There is no supraspinous ligament between the fifth lumbar spine and the sacrum, but the medial fibres of erector spinae cross over the midline (Heylings, 1978). This arrangement provides strength, and also permits the wide range of sagittal movement at the lumbosacral junction.

INTERTRANSVERSE AND COSTOTRANSVERSE LIGAMENTS OF THE THORACIC REGION

These are illustrated in Figs 3.38 & 3.43.

COSTOVERTEBRAL LIGAMENTS

The articulations and ligamentous attachments between ribs and vertebrae extend the lever arms provided by transverse processes. The joints for the heads of ribs have radiate ligaments attached to adjacent vertebrae and intervening discs. The heads of the first, eleventh, twelfth and sometimes the tenth ribs articulate only with the numerically corresponding vertebral bodies, but the radiate ligaments extend to the vertebra above and intervening discs. The costotransverse articulations have medial and lateral ligaments and, in addition, with the exception of the first rib, superior costotransverse ligaments run between the upper border of the rib to the transverse process of the vertebra above (Fig. 3.38). The accessory ligament, which may be absent, makes a tunnel for the posterior primary ramus of the nerve as it passes into the postvertebral compartment.

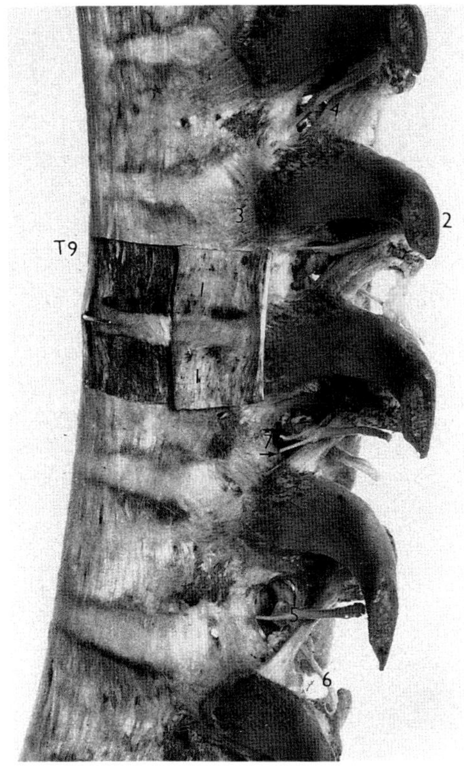

Fig. 3.38 Left side of lower thoracic spine. (1) Flap of cortical bone and anterior longitudinal ligament turned back; (2) ninth rib; (3) radiate ligament; (4) superior costotransverse ligaments; (5) anterior ramus of eleventh thoracic nerve; (6) posterior ramus of eleventh thoracic nerve separating the superior costotransverse ligament from the accessory superior costotransverse ligament; (7) Rami communicantes of tenth thoracic nerve.

Vertebropelvic ligaments

THE ILIOLUMBAR LIGAMENT

This is attached to the ilium, the anterior and lower surfaces of the transverse process of the fifth lumbar

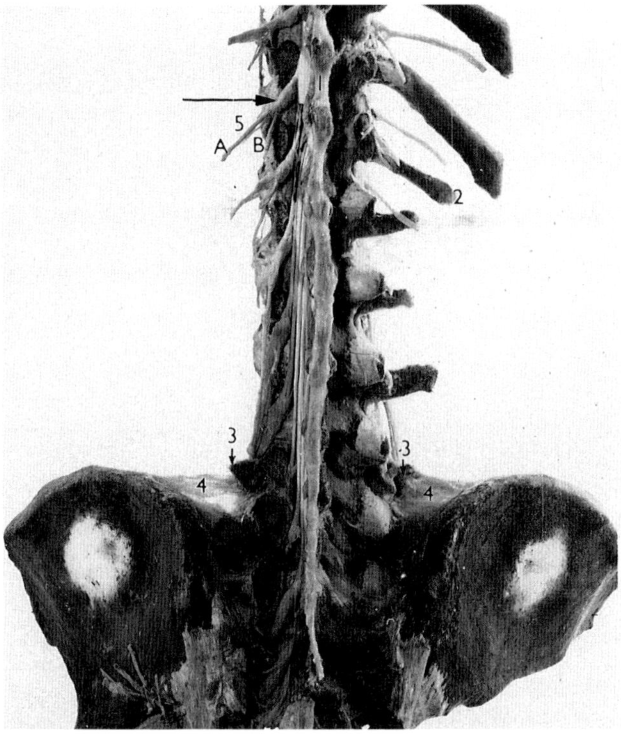

Fig. 3.39 Posterior view of lower thoracic column to sacroiliac region, laminae removed on left. (1) Supraspinous ligament; (2) twelfth rib; (3) transverse process L4; (4) iliolumbar ligament; (5) T11 spinal nerve: (A) intercostal branch, (B) posterior ramus; arrow shows dorsal root ganglion.

vertebra, and sometimes also to the transverse process of the fourth (Fig. 3.39). The fibres fan out in two main bands. The upper band is attached to the iliac crest immediately in front of the sacroiliac joint, is continuous with the anterior layer of the thoracolumbar fasciae and gives origin to some fibres of quadratus lumborum. The lower band consists of fibres running from the lower part of the transverse process of L5 to the anterior and upper part of the ala of the sacrum. It blends with the anterior sacroiliac ligament and is collagenous.

SACROILIAC LIGAMENTS

The ventral fibres from the lateral borders of the ala and anterior margins of the first three sacral vertebrae are inserted close to the anterior and superior borders of the auricular surface of the ilium. The ligament is thin except at the levels of the arcuate line and the posterior inferior iliac spines. These bands are attached respectively to the margin of the preauricular sulcus and third piece of the sacrum.

THE POSTERIOR INTEROSSEUS SACROILIAC LIGAMENTS

This is composed of a well-organized mass of relatively short collagen fibres, running between the rough, pitted area lateral to the transverse tubercles of the sacrum, and the rough, overhanging area of the ilium above and behind the articular surface. The more superficial fibres form a partially divided sheet running laterally, with the upper fibres passing upwards and the lower downwards.

THE DORSAL SACROILIAC LIGAMENT

This is intermediate between the interosseus and the sacrotuberous ligament, which blends superiorly with the long dorsal sacroiliac ligaments.

THE SACROSPINOUS LIGAMENT

This is anterior to the former ligaments and fans out to the lateral margin of the sacrum and coccyx.

The combined effect of these ligaments resists compressive forces tending to drive the sacrum down between the hip bones, and it also resists upward and backward tilting of the sacrum and coccyx (Fig. 3.33 & p. 67). The orientation of fibres in these ligaments appears postnatally (Weisl, 1954a), presumably in response to forces generated by sitting up, standing and walking.

INNERVATION OF VERTEBRAE, INTERVERTEBRAL JOINTS AND LIGAMENTS

Since anterior and posterior rami of every spinal nerve supply the column and/or related ligaments and muscles, the input to the central system is extensive. Skogland (1973) reviewed the role of the four types of articular receptors in control of posture and kinaesthesia.

Type I: slowly adapting Ruffini-type encapsulated endings, supplied by Group II myelinated fibres, are arranged in clusters in superficial layers of articular capsules. They probably signal patterns of stress in the capsules and are important in regulation of posture (Skogland, 1973).

Type II: laminated paciniform receptors, supplied by Group II or III myelinated fibres, are distributed to deeper layers of joint capsules. They respond at low thresholds, are rapidly adapting, and respond to movement, changes in pressure and transient stresses.

Type III: supplied by large fast-conducting myelinated fibres, resemble Golgi tendon organs. They are only found on ligaments, have a high threshold and are slowly adapting and probably prevent excessive articular stress by reflex inhibition of the muscles producing the stress.

Type IV: slowly adapting free endings of fine myelinated and non-myelinated axons ramify in articular capsules, adjacent fat pads and periosteum. These respond to excessive movement, and possibly mediate pain.

Central processes of these neurones are involved in spinal reflex arcs, others synapse with neurones of the spinocerebellar tracts and some run in the posterior columns of the cord. From the latter pathway impulses are relayed to the contralateral thalamus and sensory cerebral cortex (Mountcastle & Powell, 1959; see also Chapter 56).

Branches of segmental and meningeal nerves overlap (Edgar & Nundy, 1966), as do nerve fibres within articular capsules. Those parts liable to stretch in certain movements are supplied by branches of nerves supplying antagonistic muscles. Articular and meningeal nerves contain myelinated afferent fibres up to 10 μm diameter and numerous non-myelinated sensory and postganglionic sympathetic fibres. The meningeal branches supply the dura (mainly anteriorly), periosteum, posterior longitudinal ligaments and outer fibres of lateral parts of the annulus fibrosus. In fetuses and neonates there are many free endings of nerve nets in the anterior and posterior longitudinal ligaments and the outermost parts of the annulus. Perivascular plexuses accompany vessels in cartilage canals. There are numerous encapsulated endings on the anterolateral aspect of the anterior longitudinal ligament (Jackson *et al.*, 1966).

The posterior primary rami of all spinal nerves enter the postvertebral compartment and supply not only the regional facet joints, but also intrinsic vertebral muscles (Badgeley, 1941) which regulate movement and posture of the head and trunk, and have a rich proprioceptive innervation (p. 78). Synovial membrane is devoid of nerve endings, but the perivascular plexus underlying the fibrous capsules of facet joints contains a rich plexus of non-myelinated and small diameter myelinated fibres (2 μm) (Giles *et al.*, 1986). Whilst some of the unmyelinated axons are undoubtedly postganglionic vasomotor fibres, others and the myelinated ones would be afferent fibres. Substance P, one of several pain mediators, has been found in menisci (Giles & Harvey, 1987). Pinching of the synovial folds or menisci and subsequent diffusion of substance P have been postulated as possible causes of pain.

MOVEMENTS OF THE VERTEBRAL COLUMN AS A WHOLE

The cervical and lumbar regions are the most mobile parts of the column, but apart from the atlanto-occipital and atlanto-axial joints, the degrees of movement between adjacent vertebrae are small. However, summation of movements at different levels confers a wide range of mobility. These movements are flexion, extension, lateral flexion to right or left and rotation. Pure circumduction, as defined in strictly anatomical terms, can occur only in the midthoracic region (Davis, 1959). Elsewhere it does not occur because lateral flexion is associated with some rotation. There are regional variations in movements on account of the morphology of the synovial articulations and thickness of intervertebral discs. Flexion and extension are free in cervical and lumbar regions, but restricted in the thoracic.

Movement in the thoracic spine is limited by thin intervertebral discs, the inclinations of the facets and overlapping spinous processes in the midthoracic zone (Fig. 3.17) and by the ribs, in particular the upper seven pairs which articulate with the sternum. Lateral flexion in the cervical and lumbar spine is most free. It is always associated with some rotation that can be compensated by counter-rotation at another level. Rotation is most free at the atlanto-axial joint and occurs in the neck below this, but at the laminar shelf is limited or even prevented (p. 53). It can occur in the thoracic spine, and is least in the lumbar spine. The centres of rotation in the thoracic spine are anterior to the spinal canal and posterior to vertebral bodies in the lumbar region. At the mortice joint rotation is either prevented or limited, or associated with flexion to free the tenon from a low-grade mortice. In osteoligamentous preparations, slight rotation was possible at mortice joints, but decreased with vertical loading.

Analyses of intervertebral movement in the living have been made by fixing external markers to the body, cinematography, chronocyclophotography (Davis *et al.*, 1965) and by radiology (Allbrook, 1957). Isolated autopsy material has been studied in the laboratory.

Movements of the cervical spine

THE ATLANTO-OCCIPITAL JOINTS

The two atlantal surfaces form part of a single ellipsoid. Flexion takes place around a transverse axis, and the absence of an atlantal spine facilitates extension. Approximately half of flexion of the neck occurs at this joint. In the rare case with flat, circular surfaces on the atlas, movement in the sagittal plane would be restricted. The medial inclination of the oval concave surfaces allows a small amount of lateral flexion.

THE ATLANTO-AXIAL JOINTS

Rotation involves movement in all three facet articulations. The lack of congruity and the sloping 'shoulders' of the axis impose a degree of lateral flexion. The long transverse processes of the atlas enhance the mechanical advantages of rotator muscles.

LOWER CERVICAL JOINTS

The shape of discs and the overhanging anterior border of the lower surface of cervical vertebrae 2 to 6, and to a lesser extent C7, leads to forward and backward sliding movements on the lower vertebra during flexion and extension. The movement of each vertebra approximates to an arc of a circle centred in the body of the vertebra below. These centres lie in the coronal plane on a smooth curve. For C6 the centre is midway on the upper surface of C7, and for higher levels they pass posteriorly and inferiorly, the one for the axis lies posteriorly on the inferior surface of C3 (Young, 1967). The ranges of amplitude of flexion and extension in adults (Lysell, 1969) show maximum amplitudes at C5–C6, C4–C5, and minimum at C2–C3 and C7–T1. These ranges are also correlated with the thickness of discs (p. 56). Leysell (1959) found lateral flexion with rotation to be minimal at C7 (mean 2°, SE 0.3, SD ± 1.3), maximal at C4 (5.7°. SE 0.7, SD ± 3.1) followed closely by C2. The centres of motion for rotation and lateral flexion were in the sagittal plane, towards the anterior surface of the vertebrae, and in his series the distribution and severity of degenerative changes varied, being maximal at the C5–C6 articulation, closely followed by C6–C7; and least at C2–C3.

Movements of the thoracic spine

The cumulative effects of mean amplitudes of intervertebral movement for flexion–extension, rotation and lateral bending were respectively 34.4°, 41.4° and 52° (White, 1969). The ranges of flexion–extension were low from T9, but rose at T10–T11 (T12 was not included in any of White's results). Lateral flexion was lowest at T3, T8 and T11 (3.7°) and highest at T1, T4–T6. Axial rotation of T11 was only 2°. A deep mortice joint would preclude rotation, and limit extension, but no comment was made by White with respect to a mortice.

Abdominal and respiratory muscles, including the adductors of vocal cords, are involved in lifting (Davis, 1956, 1963; p. 77, Fig. 3.45). During lifting, electromyographical activity in erector spinae is directly proportional to intratrunkal pressure. Also during coughing and straining, there is increased mechanical and electrical activity in these postvertebral muscles.

Lumbar and lumbosacral movements

The amplitude of sagittal movement is correlated with the thickness of discs and diminishes with age (Figs 3.23, 3.40 & 3.41). Tanz (1953) found the wide range tended to drop during the fourth decade. In none of 62 sacra (Royal College of Surgeons specimens) were the facet joints completely flat, although their inclination to the midline varied. The curvatures would permit some measure of rotation (Fig. 3.35).

Sacroiliac joints

Ranges of movement at this irregular surfaced joint do not differ in healthy males and females between 17 and 23 years of age (Weisl, 1955). The axis of movement lies between 5 and 10 cm vertically below the sacral promontory, but it is a shifting axis, and the movement is not a simple rotation. The posterior margin of the sacral articular surface lies behind the corresponding ilial margin in recumbency. In assuming the erect posture the upper border of the sacral surface rises upon the ilial one, and the ventral one shifts more ventrally. Movement is less consistent

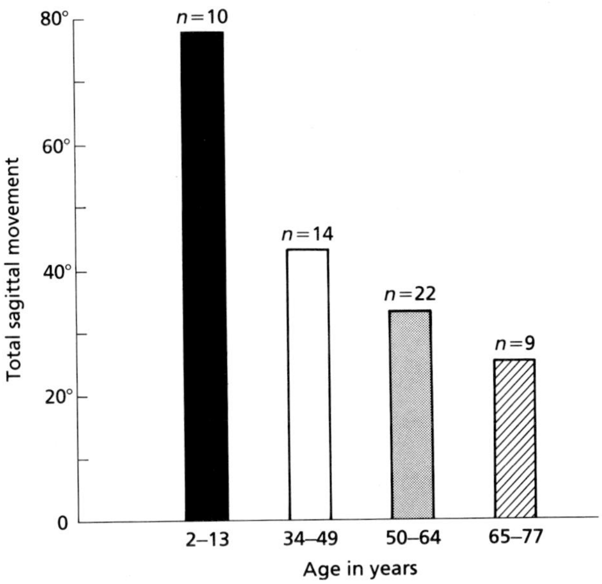

Fig. 3.40 Range of sagittal movement of lumbar spine in relation to age. Based on data of Tanz (1953). After Davis (1957). n = number of individuals examined.

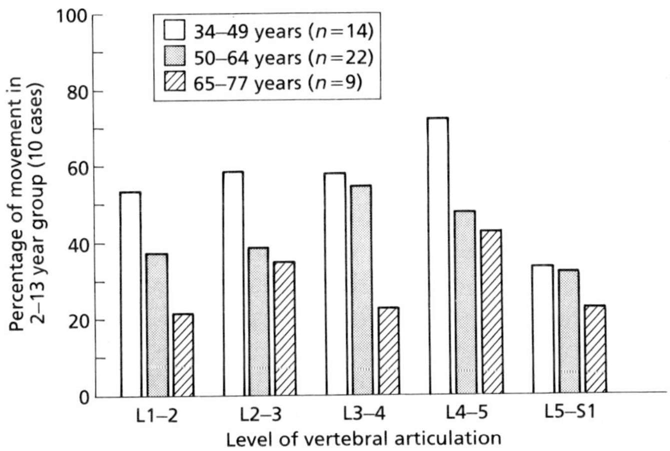

Fig. 3.41 Range of sagittal movements between lumbar vertebrae and L5–S1 in relation to age. Based on data of Tanz (1953). After Davis (1957).

and of short range during flexion and extension of the trunk.

In puerperal subjects the range is increased because of relaxation of ligaments, but decreases later. It is suggested that pain and discomfort ensue if the normal position is not restored before ligaments shorten again. In sitting, the whole pelvis is rotated forwards with reduction of the lumbar lordosis. Change of posture changes pelvic conjugates (Weisl, 1955).

Movements are reduced with adhesions which develop with age. Cohen *et al.* (1967) found radiological changes in the joint in 6% before age 50 and 24% after. Fibrous adhesions may develop into complete bony union, more commonly in males than in females.

THE FASCIAE AND MUSCLES ACTING ON THE VERTEBRAL COLUMN

Arrangements of deep fascia in the neck and trunk differ. In the neck the investing layer is attached to the skull and lower jaw above, to the sternum, clavicle, acromion process and spine of the scapula, and is continued posteriorly to the ligamentum nuchae and the spine of C7. It splits to enclose sternomastoid and trapezius and increases their efficiency of contraction.

The prevertebral fascia extends from the base of the skull to the fourth thoracic vertebra. It encloses the pre-, para- and postvertebral intrinsic muscles of the neck, and fuses with the ligamentum nuchae posteriorly (Fig. 3.42)

The thoracolumbar fascia has three layers between the pelvis and twelfth rib, and one above the rib (Fig. 3.43). The posterior layer extends from the sacrum to the spine of C7. It is attached laterally to the posterior angles of the ribs. Below the thorax it fuses laterally with the other two layers. The middle and anterior layers enclose quadratus lumborum and are attached above to the twelfth rib and below to the crest of the ilium. The middle layer is attached to the tips of the lumbar transverse processes and the anterior to the ridge on the anterior surface of lumber transverse processes (Fig. 3.43). A thickening of the anterior layer gives rise to the lateral arcuate ligament from which fibres of the diaphragm arise. The inferior thickening forms the iliolumbar ligament (p. 72 and Fig. 3.39) from which some fibres of quadratus lumborum arise. The conjoined layers of fascia split into two and provide part of the origins of internal oblique and transversus abdominis. These muscles and the external oblique are attached to the pelvis and to the ribs, and anteriorly their aponeuroses form the rectus sheaths and are inserted into the linea alba, thus forming a fibromuscular cylinder. The fascia, aponeuroses and muscles protect the abdominal contents and act upon the column. The fascia also enhances efficiency of contraction of postvertebral muscles and quadratus lumborum. When tensed by the extensors of the spine the

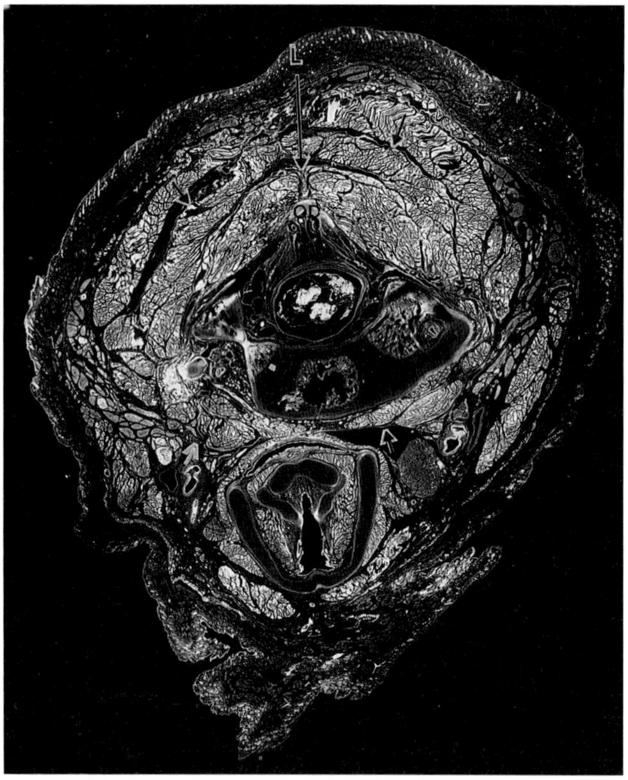

Fig. 3.42 Transverse section through the neck of a seven month human fetus (100 μm thick; × 1.4). The section is slightly oblique and it has been used as the negative in the enlarger. Arrow shows prevertebral fascia; L, ligamentum nuchae.

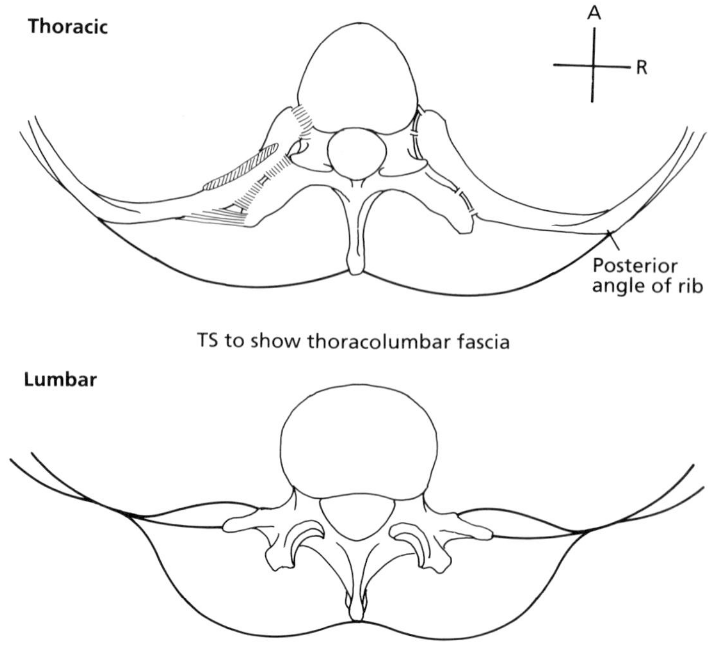

Fig. 3.43 The thoracolumbar fascia in the thoracic and lumbar regions. (1) Superior costotransverse ligament; (2) and (3) medial and lateral costotransverse ligaments

collagen fibres of the fascia also exert an extensile force on the vertebral column (Tesh *et al.*, 1984; Bogduk & Macintosh, 1984).

Postvertebral muscles

There are three layers of muscle superficial to the thoracolumbar fascia; the most superficial consists of trapezius and latissimus dorsi, which overlap from T7 to T12. These upper limb muscles can act on the vertebral column. With sternomastoid the upper fibres of trapezius turn the head (nerve supply spinal accessory nerve C1–C5, and proprioceptor fibres from C2 to C4). With the neck extended, both can continue to extend the head. With a fixed upper limb, latissimus dorsi (long subscapular nerve, C6, C7, C8) elevates one side of the pelvis and laterally flexes the spine, an action exploited in rehabilitation of high thoracic spinal injuries.

Beneath trapezius, levator scapulae (nerve supply C3–C4), and rhomboideus major and minor (nerve supply C5) suspend the scapula from the vertebral column. The third layer consists of the serratus posterior superior and inferior. Both are supplied by intercostal nerves; their action is not yet fully elucidated. All these muscles are innervated by derivatives of anterior primary rami.

THE POSTVERTEBRAL INTRINSIC MUSCLES OF THE SPINE

These are supplied by posterior primary rami of all spinal nerves. The precise arrangements are complex. They are given briefly in anatomical texts (Williams *et al.*, 1989). The following generalizations can be made.

1 The most superficial, but discontinuous, layer extends from sacrum to occiput. The fibres of the different components are mainly vertical, run over many segments, and are extensors.

2 In the intermediate layer the fibres run obliquely and over shorter distances and are capable of rotating and extending the spine.

3 The deepest are intersegmental and particularly well developed in the suboccipital region (Fig. 3.44).

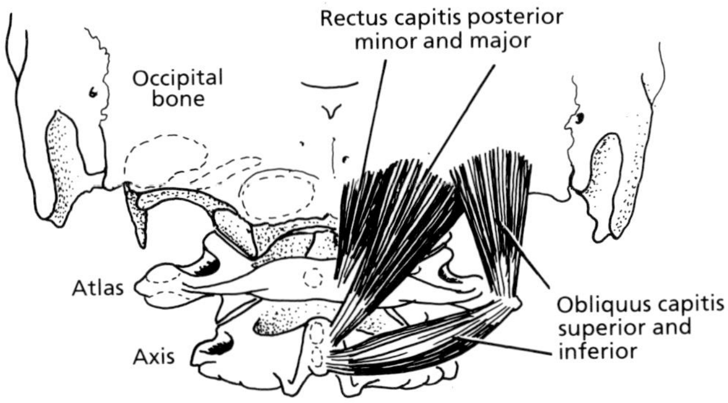

Fig. 3.44 Right suboccipital muscles.

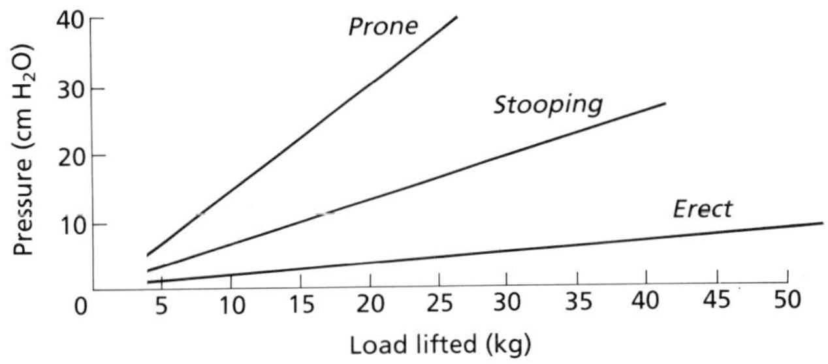

Fig. 3.45 Changes in intra-abdominal pressure during lifting. Based on data of Davis (1957).

This simplistic view is inadequate for a proper understanding of the mechanics of the spine. An holistic approach is necessary and includes appraisal of the combined activities of the post- and paravertebral and abdominal muscles, together with the mechanical effects of the thoracolumbar fascia, the erector spinae, aponeuroses and intermuscular aponeuroses and spinal ligaments (Etemadi, 1974; Bogduk, 1980, Amonoo-Kuofi, 1982b, 1983; Bogduk & Macintosh, 1984, Gracovetsky, 1988). Bogduk (1980) drew attention to the laminated nature of the lumbar fibres of erector spinae which indicated that those to a given vertebra might act independently. A mathematical interpretation of these actions has been given by Gracovetsky (1988). Amongst recent electromyographic studies Vink (1989) demonstrated that all three columns of the intrinsic lumbar back muscles (iliocostalis, longissimus and the medially placed multifidus) are recruited during extension. In submaximal forces the activity of multifidus shows greater activity in relation to the maximal recorded activity of both the other columns. The medial and caudal parts of the combined mass are more active during lateral flexion of lower lumbar vertebrae and the lateral pair are more involved with lateral flexion of upper lumbar vertebrae and the torso.

PARAVERTEBRAL MUSCLES

These are all supplied by anterior primary rami of cervical, brachial and lumbar plexuses. The scalene muscles are active in respiration (Campbell, 1955) and between them support and elevate the upper rib cage. All three act as lateral flexors of the cervical column and scalenus anterior is also a rotator. The only paravertebral muscles in the thoracic region are the intercostals, which have no direct attachment to, or action upon, the spine but have a synergistic action in raising intratrunkal pressure during lifting (Davis, 1957; Fig. 3.45).

QUADRATUS LUMBORUM

The quadratus lumborum (nerve supply T12–L1–L3 (4)) lies between the anterior and middle layers of the thoracolumbar fascia. It fixes the twelfth rib to which the diaphragm is attached. Acting unilaterally, it produces ipsilateral lateral flexion of the vertebral column. When both muscles act, extension of the spine is possibly assisted by the tension produced on and within the fascial sheath.

PSOAS MAJOR

This muscle (nerve supply ventral rami L1, L2 and L3) and the iliacus are powerful flexors of the hip. By acting on the hip joint, both muscles assist in raising the trunk against resistance, e.g. sitting up from recumbency. Electromyography indicates that the psoas major assists the balance of the body when sitting but does not flex the trunk anterolaterally when standing (Keagy *et al.*, 1966).

CRURA OF THE DIAPHRAGM (C3, C4, C5)

The left crus arises from the anterolateral aspect of the upper two lumbar vertebrae and the intervening disc, and the right arises from the upper three lumbar vertebrae and intervening discs. In trunkal support of the column during lifting the diaphragm, glottis, pelvic floor and intercostal muscles are active (Fig. 3.45; Davis, 1961, 1963).

PREVERTEBRAL MUSCLES

Apart from the longus colli, longus capitis, rectus capitus anterior and lateralis, there are no true prevertebral muscles between T3 and the coccyx. However, two powerful pairs of flexors against resistance are the sternomastoid and rectus abdominis. Flexion of the trunk with assistance of gravity takes place at the hip joints and is controlled by concentric contraction of the erector spinae (Floyd & Silver, 1955), the last part of the movement being controlled by the elasticity of the ligamenta flava.

The three pairs of sheet-like abdominal muscles are all attached to the pelvic girdle and the rib cage. The two deepest are attached to the spine through the thoracolumbar fascia. The external oblique, contracting with the contralateral internal oblique, rotate the lumbar and thoracic spine.

All these muscles have postural and dynamic actions upon the vertebral column. Maintenance of the normal curvatures and posture depends upon balanced activity between these groups. Imbalance due to paralysis is capable of producing gross bony deformity (Mercer, 1950).

Imbalance of innervated muscle has been invoked as an aetiological factor in scoliosis (Riddle & Roaf, 1955). Depending upon their function, normal muscles contain varying proportions of fast and slow contracting muscle fibres (Širca & Kostevc, 1985). Disproportion between dynamic and static fibres has been found in scoliosis (Fidler *et al.*, 1974, 1975.) On the convex side the slow fibres predominate. This suggests an attempt to correct the abnormal curve by increasing the tonic fibres. The histochemical nature and physiological properties of muscle are dependent upon the nerve supply, as demonstrated experimentally by cross-reinnervation of fast and slow muscles (Close, 1972), but altered mechanical conditions apparently effect the change and further investigation is required. In ageing muscles there is a loss of the dynamic fast fibres (Jennerken *et al.*, 1971; Fidler *et al.*, 1975).

The large field of afferent and efferent innervation of the intrinsic vertebral muscles, abdominal, respiratory muscles including the larynx, and the pelvic floor, all involved in various patterns of synergistic activity in lifting in different postures, indicates the important role of the nervous system (Morris *et al.*, 1961). Maintenance of posture and 'simple' activities such as walking all involve the muscles acting on the spine.

There is overlap in distribution of posterior primary rami, and a very high density of afferent innervation in the intrinsic muscles, especially the suboccipital muscles (Voss, 1956, 1958; Bowden, 1963; Cooper & Daniel, 1963).

The pattern of segmental muscle mass was demonstrated in fetal and adult postvertebral muscles by Amonoo-Kuofi (1982b, 1983). The intrinsic muscle mass is largest from the lower thoracic to midlumbar region, and although diminishing, down to the first sacral segment, exceeds the bulk found at any other levels. It is fairly bulky in the midcervical region. The number of muscle spindles in fetal muscles (excluding the suboccipital) was remarkably symmetrical, being 1650 on the left and 1634 on the right (Amonoo-Kuofi, 1982b). The smallest numbers were related to the upper two sacral segments, with none below. The largest numbers were found at the cervicothoracic (T1–T2) and thoracolumbar junctions T12, L1 and L2. The largest number in the neck was at C4. Density was lowest in the medial column of muscle. In the intermediate column it was highest at T1, T2, T6, T8 and in the neck at C5. In the lateral column none was found in the sacral and lower two lumbar segments, or above C7. When the three columns were combined, spindles were found from C1 to S2, with the highest densities at T1 and midthoracic regions. The high density in the thoracic region of the lateral column would suggest that they monitor movements of ribs at the costotransverse joints, as well as those of the spinal column.

The very high density in suboccipital muscles, and the presence of spiral endings such as those seen in extrinsic ocular muscles, indicates that these are highly important postural sensors (Daniel, 1946; Voss, 1958; Bowden, 1963; Cooper Daniel, 1963).

THE VERTEBRAL CANAL

The canal curves in conformity with the column (Fig. 3.7) and extends from the foramen magnum to the sacral hiatus where the posterior wall is completed by the superficial dorsal sacrococcygeal ligament. It is widest in the cervical region, narrows below the cervical enlargement of the cord, widens again, but to a lesser extent, in the lumbar region and then narrows progressively. It is triangular in cross-section from the axis down to the upper one or two thoracic vertebrae. Thereafter it is approximately circular, until the thoracolumbar junction where it is once more triangular.

The anterior wall is formed by the tectorial membrane and posterior longitudinal ligaments. These cover the dens and its ligaments, the bodies of succeeding vertebrae and intervertebral discs. The lateral walls are formed of pedicles and intervertebral foramina down to the sacrum. Sacral foramina lead into anterior and posterior channels for the anterior and posterior primary rami of the nerves. The posterior wall is composed of laminae, ligamenta flava and facet joints, the latter form the boundaries of intervertebral foramina. Lateral to the ligaments and medial to the facets there are bony spicules which point downwards, slightly laterally and anteriorly and vary in robustness and length from 1 to 7 mm. The longest may overlap the facets (Table 3.6, p. 54; Davis, 1955; Davis & Rowland, 1965). Soft lobulated fat smooths the contour of this wall where the ligamenta flava lie obliquely to the sagittal plane (Parkin & Harrison, 1985).

Apart from changes in proportion of the trunk with growth, there are variations in dimensions related to age, sex and race. Measurements have been made from skeletal material (Eisenstein, 1977; Porter *et al.*, 1983; Amonoo-Kuofi, 1985). Standardized radiography (Landmesser & Heuberlein, 1953; Verbiest, 1955; Hink *et al.*, 1962, 1966a,b; Epstein, 1962; Epstein & Epstein, 1978; Amonoo-Kuofi, 1982a; Keats, 1988), ultrasound (Porter *et al.*, 1978a,b, 1983) and computerized axial tomography (Harrison, 1986).

Cross-sectional areas of infant and juvenile spinal canals are proportionately greater than in the adult, and differ only slightly in absolute measurement. For precise radiological dimensions reference should be made to the papers already cited. The early fusion of primary centres forming the canal only allows enlargement by subperiosteal osteoclasis (Wolf *et al.*, 1956; Roaf, 1971).

According to Hinck *et al.* (1962) the sagittal diameter in the cervical region in adults is almost the same as, or even slightly less than, in children of three to six years. The same applies to the lumbar region (Hinck *et al.*, 1966b). The dimensions in adult females tended to be less than in males. Torklus & Gehle (1972) give figures for the diameter of the spinal canal, as seen in lateral radiographs of children under 15 and in adults. The values given for the first two vertebrae were larger in children, but the overlap of ranges was such that this may be more apparent than real. Another factor in infants might be incomplete ossification of the cartilaginous atlas and axis. However, an important measurement in radiographs of the upper cervical region in children and adults is the interval between the arch of the atlas and the anterior surface of the dens. In children between three and 15 years this should be less than 4 mm (Locke *et al.*, 1966). Ossification is not complete in early childhood, which explains the difference in the permitted maximum distance of 2.5 mm for adults by the age of 30 years. Conlon *et al.* (1966) gave the adult figures as 2.5 mm for females and 3.0 mm for males.

There is a significant correlation between the sagittal diameters of the cervical and lumbar canals. Porter *et al.* (1983) reported that patients with low back pain are more likely also to suffer pain in the neck than those without low back pain. Gross thickening of laminae (Naylor, 1979) or a trefoil-shaped canal can obstruct emergent nerves (Schatzker & Pennal, 1968; Eisenstein, 1980). Crock (1981) and Porter (1985) stressed the importance of the bell-shaped canal which narrows and lengthens the root canals. Osteophytes around the disc or facet joints would increase the risks of entrapment.

In normal adult Nigerian skeletons the midsagittal diameter of the lumbar canal varied around the means, but all measurements were lower in females. The diameter narrowed from the first to third vertebra in males, and down to the fourth in females. The increase below these levels did not reach the dimensions of the first segment (Amonoo-Kuofi, 1985). Eisenstein (1977) had found a cephalocaudal decline in diameter in Zulus and Sotho. Strict comparison between the two studies was not possible, but it was inferred that the canal was larger in Nigerians than in black South African males, whilst the converse was true for females. Amonoo-Kuofi *et al.* (1991) provide data on adult male and female Saudis. Norms of the canal : body ratio were established. The pattern of segmental variation of the diameters of the lumbar canal in normal adults is similar to that found in other populations.

In 127 autopsies cervical spines from individuals ages 20–99 years showed some degree of disc degeneration in 110 cases. Damage appeared earlier in men. It was estimated that the time course between mild and very severe damage was about 10 years (Holt & Yates, 1966). Wilkinson (1967) and others have shown the severe ridging in the anterior wall of the canal which can produce gross stretching and indentation of the cord and/or nerve roots. In addition, where there has been loss of lumbar lordosis, with or without loss of disc space and bone in the neck, cervical lordosis is exaggerated and the ligamenta flava thicken and bulge forward and produce further narrowing (Stoltmann & Blackwood, 1964; Breig, 1978). A rare but space-occupying calcification of the posterior longitudinal ligament may be another cause of acquired stenosis (Hanai *et al.*, 1977). Congenital stenosis may be due to malformation, and in achondroplasia to short thick pedicles.

NEURO-OSSEOUS RELATIONS

The meningeal layer of dura mater forms the spinal theca, and it and the subarachnoid space extend from the foramen magnum to the junction of the second and third pieces of the sacrum. It is anchored at the foramen magnum, attached to the cervical posterior longitudinal ligament, and to the coccyx by the filum terminale. There are light areolar attachments to the margins of intervertebral foramina. The surrounding epidural space is potential rather than real, containing soft lobulated extradural fat and the venous plexus (Parkin & Harrison, 1985).

With age-related loss of height, the sac ends at a lower level (S3–S4) and it and the lower root sleeves may become adherent to the sacral posterior longitudinal ligament.

The lower medulla, spinal cord, roots of segmental nerves and vessels lie within the spinal meninges (Figs. 3.19 & 3.46). At birth, the cord ends between the second and third lumbar vertebrae, but reaches the adult level between the first and second by two months (Barson, 1970). Levels vary in normal juveniles and young adults from the caudal half of the twelfth thoracic vertebra to the body of the second lumbar vertebra. With loss of height, the cord also drops, and there may be severe angulation of root sleeves and, more seriously, angulation of the nerve rootlets (Fig. 3.47).

The cervical enlargement of the cord extends from the third cervical to the second thoracic vertebra, with its maximum circumference (38 mm) on the body of the sixth cervical. The less bulky lumbar enlargement lies opposite the ninth to twelfth thoracic vertebrae. Relative positions of neurological segments and vertebral spines are as follows:

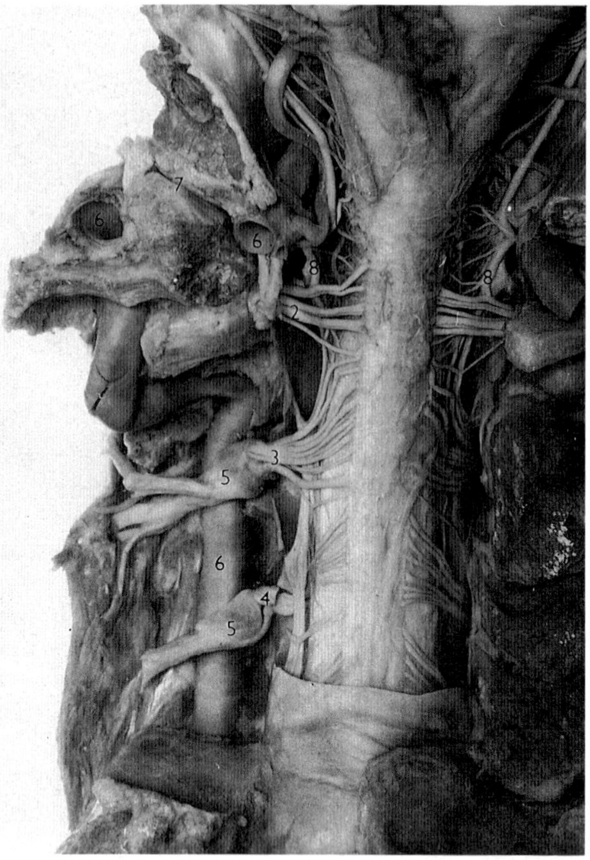

Fig. 3.46 Posterior view of open and closed medulla and upper cervical cord. (1–4) Cervical spinal nerve rootlets; (5) dorsal root ganglia; (6) vertebral artery, note cut ends on left arch of atlas; (7) atlanto-occipital joint; (8) spinal part of accessory nerve. (Museum of the RCS Eng.)

Cord segment	*Vertebral spine*
C3	C2
T6	T4
T9	T6
L1	T9
CX1	L1/2

The relations of dural root sleeves, nerve roots, dorsal root ganglia and the anterior and posterior primary rami of nerves, to the spinal canal, intervertebral foramina, vertebral artery and intertransverse ligaments are shown in Figs 3.46, 3.48, 3.49 & 3.50.

With discrepancy in rates of growth of the spinal cord and vertebral column, root sleeves and nerve roots elongate and become increasingly oblique from above downwards, e.g. the fifth lumbar nerve roots cross five discs before entering the intervertebral fora-

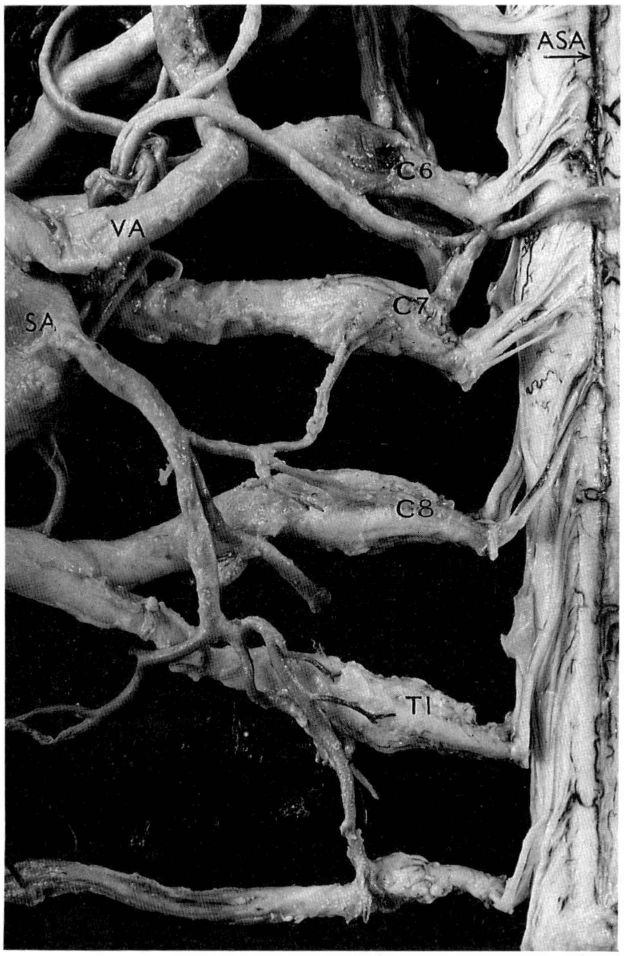

Fig. 3.47 Severe angulation of emergent nerve roots with degenerative changes in the cervical column. From Bowden *et al.* (1967).

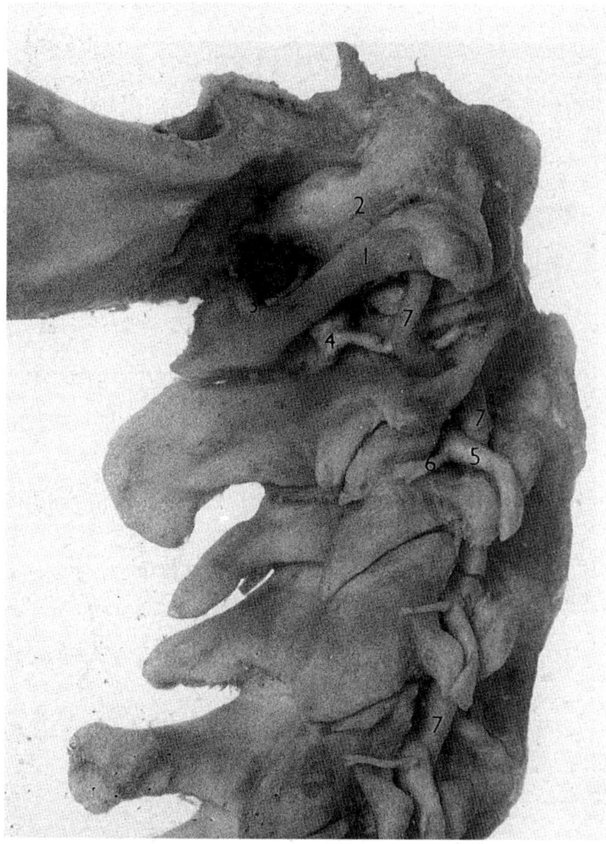

Fig. 3.48 Right lateral view upper cervical vertebrae with part of occipital bone. (1) Atlas; (2) lateral mass of atlas; (3) C1 nerve; (4) C2; (5) C3 anterior ramus; (6) C3 posterior ramus; (7) vertebral artery. Note: the relationship of emerging roots of plexuses to the transverse processes and of the posterior rami to the articular pillar. (Museum of RCS Eng.)

mina. The lateral aspects of lower root sleeves are intimately related to the upper pedicle and the medial aspects are related to the lower one (Fig. 3.50).

The slightly elastic cord and nerve roots move, and may be stretched by flexion of the spine, the shoulder and hip joints, and also by medial rotation at the shoulder and hip. Narrowing of intervertebral foramina and entrapment of nerve roots restricts freedom of movement, and may obstruct blood vessels and damage the nerves. The elastic pia mater forms the intersegmental ligamentum denticulatum. This is attached to the dura and suspends the cord in cerebrospinal fluid, and reduces the effects of stretching upon it (Breig, 1978).

Flexion of the spine reduces angulation of the root sleeves and contained rootlets but stretches the nerves. Extension increases angulation and rotation produces differential traction on nerve roots at the tethering dural ostia. Turning the face to the right stretches the dorsal roots on the right, and the ventral ones on the left, whilst ventral roots are slackened on the right and the dorsal ones on the left (Bowden *et al.*, 1967).

Osseous lumbar intervertebral foramina are large but the exit is reduced and compartmentalized by ligaments (Amonoo-Kuofi *et al.*, 1988a,b). Entrapment may not be confined to the vertebral canal and intervertebral foramina. Other causes of entrapment may involve the roots of the brachial plexus where they lie in the bony troughs of the transverse processes and move with the movement of the shoulder and arm. In addition to a cervical rib, the fibres of scalenus

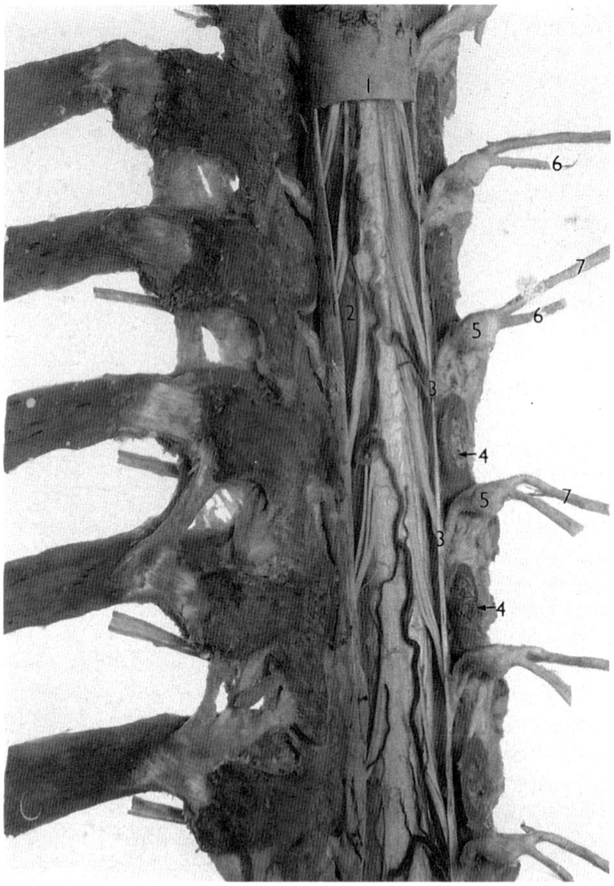

Fig. 3.49 Thoracic spinal cord and nerve roots, seen from behind: (1) dura; (2) ligamentum denticulatum. Note: angulation of nerve roots at: (3) dural ostia; (4) pedicles; (5) dorsal root ganglia; (6) posterior rami and (7) anterior rami of intercostal nerves. (Museum of RCS Eng.)

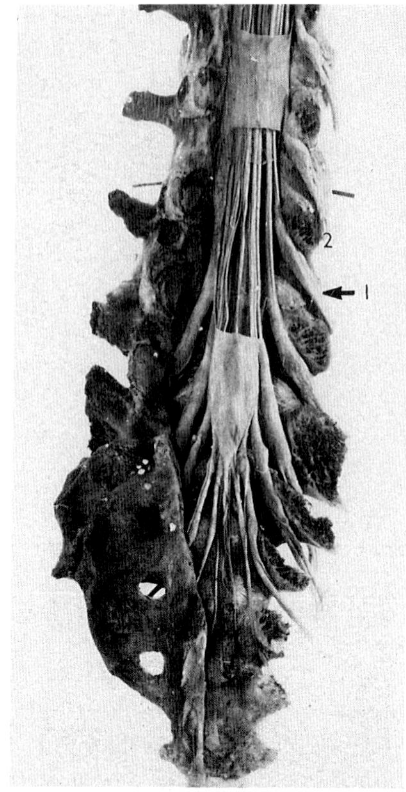

Fig. 3.50 Posterior view of cauda equina, dural sac and root sleeves. (1) Fourth lumbar nerve; (2) pedicle of L4. (Museum of RCS Eng.)

anterior and medius which arise from the perineurium can produce entrapment. The relations of emerging nerves to costotransverse and intertransverse ligaments are shown in Figs 3.38 & 3.49.

Large osteophytes outside the canal may impinge upon the sympathetic chain and splanchnic nerves (Fig. 3.51) and give rise to visceral symptoms (H.V. Crock, 1989, personal communication).

COMMON SENESCENT CHANGES

Some of the changes already discussed are so common that they should be regarded as normal findings in the elderly. These include the changes in architecture of bone, which are more severe in females than males, with loss of height and broadening of the vertbral bodies (Ericksen, 1976), altered collagen content of tissues, the several changes in the discs, synovial articulations and fluid (Jebens & Monk Jones, 1959) and the generalized loss of fast, dynamic muscle fibres which also affects intrinsic vertebral muscles. Tanz (1953) reported steady decline in mobility of the lumbar spine as a whole. The loss between his youngest (two to 13 years) and oldest (65–77 years) subjects, was of the order of 68%. The loss of intersegmental movement between the ages of 34 and 77 years varied; 60% for L1–L2 and L3–L4, approximately 40% for L2–L3 and L4–L5 and 30% for L5–S1 (Fig. 3.41).

The alterations in facet joints due to wear and tear are exacerbated by those secondary to altered alignment following loss of disc substance (Adams & Hutton, 1980; Dunlop *et al.*, 1984; Wilde *et al.*, 1988). The lumbar lordosis is also reduced by loading, which would include increased body weight (Asmussen & Klausen, 1962).

The development of osteophytes is one of the commonest changes. Those appearing in the spinal canal

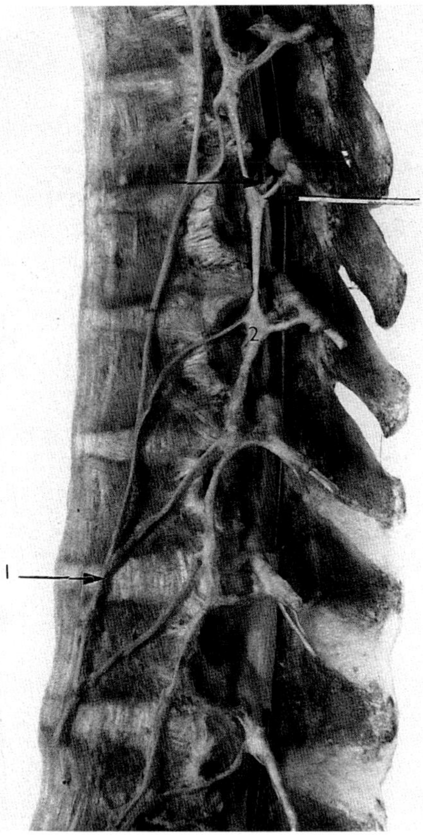

Fig. 3.51 (1) Greater splanchnic nerve intimately related to vertebral bodies and discs; (2) sympathetic chain. Unnumbered arrows show rami communicantes. (Museum of RCS Eng.)

on either side of the disc are usually symmetrical in size, although gross ridging may be formed (Wilkinson, 1967). This would be expected if the precipitating factor was a repetitive posterior bulge of the disc. Extruded disc material may become calcified and ossified, and may be bilateral or median in position. Laminar spicules do not appear to be pathological findings; although Allbrook (1957), classed them amongst osteophytes, they differ in character from the osteophytes on the margins of facet joints.

Spurs on the margins of the anterior and lateral surfaces of bodies arise from compact cortical bone and not from the annular epiphyses. They may range from a millimetre or two to several centimetres in length. In a study of the lumbar spine the incidence in 180 male East Africans was 18.2%, and in females 40% of 28 columns. There was no tribal difference in distribution, and adults of all ages were affected. In wet specimens ossification was proved to be within the anterior longitudinal ligament. Radiological study in the living showed that movement was maximal between the lower lumbar L4–L5, the level of the summit of the lumbar curve in East Africans (Allbrook, 1957). Boyle (1954) analysed 1030 films from 200 patients of all ages. Patients with symptoms referred to the spine were excluded from the study; nevertheless the distribution of osteophytes was widespread (Fig. 3.4). The peak incidences were at T8–T9, T9–T10, followed closely by T7–T8 and T10–T11. In the lumbar region the peak was at L3–L4 (Table 3.13). The thoracic spurs were more plentiful in females than males between the ages of 40 and 45, but the incidence equalized between 60 and 70 years. In the lumbar region spurs were slightly more frequent in men than in women, unlike those in the African series. In East Africa women tend to be responsible for heavy agricultural work as well as carrying heavy head loads. It was noteworthy that none of these subjects reported symptoms. In 346 adult vertebral columns (137 white males and 76 females, 67 black males and 66 females), Nathan (1962) found that over 80% had osteophytes. All groups had some soon after 20 years, and by the early 40s they were present in all, the anterior spurs were much more

Table 3.13 Age and incidence of spondylosis of the lumbar spine. Based on Boyle (1954)

Age (years)	Number of cases			Numbers with spondylosis			Percentage incidence of osteophytes
	Male	Female	Total	Male	Female	Total	
30–39	56	51	107	6	4	10	9.4
40–49	53	52	105	19	17	36	34.3
50–59	52	54	106	30	32	62	58.5
60–69	50	52	102	42	39	81	79.4
70+	50	50	100	47	46	93	93.0
Totals	261	259	520	144	138	282	

common than the posterior, and they were formed invariably of dense bone. The highest incidences in this sample were at the peaks of curves C5, T8, L3–L4, and the lowest incidence was where the line of gravity crosses the spine at T1, T12, L5–S1. The incidence was greater in whites than in blacks, and in both white and black males incidence was higher than in females.

In 127 autopsies Holt & Yates (1966) found evidence of cervical spondylosis in 86.6%.

Osteophytosis was not always associated with symptoms, as demonstrated by Boyle, but in the radiological study in the living Allbrook (1957) found diminished movements. In the Royal College of Surgeons collection of entire columns or regional loops, osteophytic spurs never involved the ring epiphysis, but sprouted from upper or lower borders immediately subjacent to them. In some columns they alternated from left to right, and were larger on the upper border. In others they were central, or found right across the vertebral body. Occasionally complete bony bars formed across the disc space (Nathan, 1962). H.V. Crock (personal communication) has found that spurs may produce visceral symptoms (Fig. 3.51). The massive spurs are attributed to calcification in the anterior longitudinal ligament. Possibly some may arise in tendinous arches of psoas major.

CONCLUSION

Weiss (1975) likened the spine to a tapering curved beam, mass loaded by the head at its narrowest free end, whilst being fixed at the widest end at the sacrum. In such a beam there are nodes where stress is high and deformation low, and antinodes where stress is low and deformation high. He located nodes at the lumbosacral and lower cervical regions. It is suggested that a third node exists at the thoracolumbar junction.

In an epidemiological study of the ageing spine Badley (1987) provided evidence to show that many factors influenced changes, including diet, patterns of activity, economic status, and genetic and hormonal factors (Miall *et al.*, 1976). The complexity of the life cycle of the spine suggests that the concept of the normal spine is as misleading as that of the average individual, and that purely mechanical considerations form only part of the holistic picture.

ACKNOWLEDGEMENTS

Grateful thanks are due to the Royal College of Surgeons of England for permission to photograph specimens in the Wellcome Museum of Anatomy; the dissections are the work of the late Dr David Tompsett. Publishers who have given permission to reproduce illustrations are acknowledged in the captions. Thanks are due to Mrs Audrey Besterman for all line illustrations except Figs 3.2, 3.10, 3.11, 3.15 & 3.16, which were made by Miss Sally Cowley. Photographs of the specimens in the museum were made by Mr Noble. Thanks are also due to Mrs E. de Vaz and Mrs J. Saxton for typing the paper, and to Miss E. Allen for help with processing the reference list.

REFERENCES

Abdullah, S. & Bowden, R.E.M. (1960) The blood supply of the brachial plexus. *Proc. Roy. Soc. Med.*, **53**, 203–205.

Adams, M.A. & Hutton, W.C. (1980) The effect of posture on the role of the apophyseal joints in resisting intervertebral compressive forces. *J. Bone Jt. Surg.*, **62B**, 358–362.

Adams, M.A. & Hutton, W.C. (1983) The effect of posture on the fluid content of lumbar intervertebral discs. *Spine*, **8**, 665–671.

Adams, M.A. & Hutton, W.C. (1986) The effect of posture on diffusion into lumbar intervertebral discs. *J. Anat.*, **147**, 121–134.

Adams, P & Muir, H. (1976) Qualitative changes with age of proteoglycans of human lumbar discs. *Ann. Rheum. Dis.*, **35**, 289–296.

Ahuja, M. (1969) Normal variation in the density of selected human bones in North India. *J. Bone Jt.* Surg., **51B**, 719–735.

Allbrook, D. (1956) Changes in lumbar vertebral body height with age. *Am J. Phys. Anthropol.*, **14**, 35–39.

Allbrook, D.B. (1957) Movements in the lumbar spinal column. *J. Bone Jt. Surg.*, **39B**, 339–345.

Amonoo-Kuofi, H.S. (1982a) Maximum and minimum lumbar interpeduncular distances in normal Nigerians. *J. Anat.*, **135**, 225–233.

Amonoo-Kuofi, H.S. (1982b) The number and distribution of muscle spindles in human intrinsic post-vertebral muscles. *J. Anat.*, **135**, 585–600.

Amonoo-Kuofi, H.S. (1983) The density of muscle spindles in the medial, intermediate and lateral columns of human intrinsic post-vertebral muscles. *J. Anat.*, **136**, 509–519.

Amonoo-Kuofi, H.S. (1985) The sagittal diameter of the lumbar vertebral canal in normal adult Nigerians. *J. Anat.*, **140**, 69–78.

Amonoo-Kuofi, H.S., El-Badawi, M.G. & Fatani, J.A. (1988a) Ligaments associated with lumbar intervertebral foramina 1. L1–4. *J. Anat.*, **156**, 177–183.

Amonoo-Kuofi, H.S., El-Badawi, M.G., Fatani, J.A. & Butt, M.M. (1988b) Ligaments associated with lumbar intervertebral foramina 2. The fifth lumbar level. *J. Anat.*, **159**, 1–10.

Amonoo-Kuofi, H.S., Patel, P.J. & Fatani, J.A. (1991) The sagittal diameters of the lumbar spine canal in normal adult Saudis. *Clin. Anat.*, **4**, 192–199.

Amstutz, H.C. & Sissons, H.A. (1969) The structure of the vertebral spongiosa. *J. Bone Jt. Surg.*, **51B**, 540–550.

Anderson, M, Hwang, S.C. & Green, W.T. (1965) Growth of the normal trunk in boys and girls during the second decade of life. *J. Bone Jt. Surg.*, **47A**, 1554–1564.

Asmussen, E. & Klausen, K. (1962) Form and function of the erect human spine. *Clin. Orthop.*, **25**, 53–63.

Badgeley, C.E. (1941) The articular facets in relation to low back pain and sciatic radiation. *J. Bone Jt. Surg.*, **23**, 481–491.

Badley, E.M. (1987) Epidemiological aspects of the ageing spine. In Hukins, D.W.L. & Nelson, M.A. (eds) *The Ageing Spine*, pp. 1–17. Manchester University Press, Manchester.

Bagnall, K.M., Harris, P.F. & Jones, R.R.M. (1977a) A radiographic study of the human fetal spine. 1. The development of the secondary cervical curvature. *J. Anat.*, **123**, 777–782.

Bagnall, K.M., Harris, P.F. & Jones, R.R.M. (1977b) A radiographic study of the lumbar fetal spine. 2. The sequence of development of ossification in the vertebral column. *J. Anat.*, **124**, 791–802.

Barnett, C.H., Davies, D.V. & MacConaill, M.A. (1961) *Synovial Joints: Their Structure and Mechanisms.* Longman, London.

Barson, A.J. (1970) The vertebral level of termination of the spinal cord during normal and abnormal development. *J. Anat.*, **106**, 489–497.

Beadle, O.A. (1931) The intervertebral discs: observations on their normal and morbid anatomy in relation to certain spinal deformities. Med. Res. Council Spec. Rep. Ser. 161. HMSO, London.

Beard, H.K. & Stevens, R.L. (1980) Biomechanical changes in the intervertebral disc. In Jayson, M.I.V. (ed.) *The Lumbar Spine and Back Pain*, 2nd edn, pp. 407–436. Pitman Medical, Tunbridge Wells.

Bick, E.M. & Copel, J.W. (1950) Longitudinal growth of the human vertebra. *J. Bone Jt. Surg.*, **32A**, 803–814.

Bick, E.M. & Copel, J.W. (1951) The ring apophysis of the human vertebra. *J. Bone Jt. Surg.*, **33A**, 783–787.

Bogduk, N. (1980) A reappraisal of the anatomy of the human lumbar erector spinae. *J. Anat.*, **131**, 525–540.

Bogduk, N. & Engel, R. (1984) The meniscus of lumbar zygapophyseal joints: a review of their anatomy and clinical significance. *Spine*, **9**, 454–460.

Bogduk, N. & Macintosh, J. (1984) Applied anatomy of the thoracolumbar fascia. *J. Anat.*, **139**, 195.

Bowden, R.E.M. (1963) Muscle spindles in the human foetus. *Acta Biol. Szeged.*, **9**, 35–59.

Bowden, R.E.M., Abdullah, S. & Gooding, M.R. (1967) Anatomy of the cervical spine, membranes, spinal cord, nerve roots and brachial plexus. In Lord Brain & Wilkinson M. (eds) *Cervical Spondylosis*, pp. 10–97. William Heinemann Medical Books, London.

Boyle, A.C. (1954) Spondylosis (Discussion), The pathology and incidence of spondylosis. *Proc. Roy. Soc. Med.*, **47**, 49–56.

Brailsford, J. (1929) Deformities of the lumbo-sacral region of the spine. *Br. J. Surg.*, **16**, 64–67.

Brandner, M.E. (1970) Normal values of the vertebral body and intervertebral disc index during growth. *Am. J. Roentgenol.*, **110**, 618–627.

Breig, A. (1978) *Adverse Mechanical Tension in the Central Nervous System.* Wiley, New York.

Brickley-Parsons, D. & Glimcher, M.J. (1984) Is the chemistry of collagen in the intervertebral disc an expression of Wolff's law? A study of the human lumbar spine. *Spine*, **9**, 148–163.

Broom, N.D. & Marra, D.L. (1986) Ultrastructural evidence for fibril-to-fibril associations in articular cartilage and their functional implications. *J. Anat.*, **146**, 185–200.

Campbell, E.J.M. (1955) The role of the scalene muscles, and sternomastoid muscles in breathing in normal subjects. An electromyographical study. *J. Anat.*, **89**, 378–386.

Cavagna, G., Komarek, L. & Mazzoleni, S. (1971) The mechanisms of sprint running. *J. Physiol. (Lond.)*, **217**, 709–721.

Cave, A.J.E. (1975) The morphology of the mammalian cervical pleurapophysis. *J. Zool. Lond.*, **177**, 377–389.

Cave, A.J.E., Griffiths, J.D. & Whiteley, M.M. (1955) Osteo-arthritis deformans of Luschka joints. *Lancet*, **1**, 176–179.

Čihák, R. (1970) Variations in lumbo-sacral joints in their morphogenesis. *Acta Univ. Carol. (Med.) (Praha)*, **16**, 145–165; cited *Gray's Anatomy*, 37th edn; p. 493.

Close, R.I. (1972) Dynamic properties of mammalian skeletal muscles. *Physiol. Rev.*, **52**, 129–197.

Cohen, A.S., McNeill, M., Calkins, E., Sharp, J.T., & Schubart, A. (1967) The 'normal' sacro-iliac joint: analysis of 88 sacroiliac roentgenograms. *Am. J. Roentgenol.*, **100**, 559–563.

Conlon, P.W., Isdale, I.C. & Rose, B.S. (1966) Rheumatoid arthritis of the cervical spine. *Ann. Rheum.* Dis., **25**, 120–126.

Cooper, S. & Daniel, P.M. (1963) Muscle spindles in man; their morphology in the lumbricals and the deep muscles of the neck. *Brain*, **86**, 563–586.

Cornah, M.S., Meachin, G. & Parr, E.W. (1970) Banded structures in the matrix of human and rabbit nucleus pulposus. *J. Anat.*, **107**, 351–362.

Crock, H.V. (1981) Normal and pathological anatomy of the lumbar spinal nerve root canal. *J. Bone Jt. Surg.*, **63B**, 487–490.

Currey, J.D. (1984) Effects of differences in mineralization on the mechanical properties of bone. *Phil. Trans. Roy. Soc. (Biol.)*, **304**, 509–518.

Daniel, P.M. (1946) Spiral endings in the extrinsic ocular muscles of man. *J. Anat.*, **80**, 189–193.

Davis, P.R. (1955) The thoracolumbar mortice joint. *J. Anat.*, **89**, 370–379.

Davis, P.R. (1956) Variations of the human intra-abdominal pressure during weight-lifting in different postures. *J. Anat.*, **90**, 601.

Davis, P.R. (1957) *Functional Anatomy of the Human*

Vertebral Column. Thesis presented for PhD, University of London.

Davis, P.R. (1959) The medial inclination of the human thoracic articular facets. *J. Anat.*, **93**, 68–74.

Davis, P.R. (1961) Human lower lumbar vertebrae: some mechanical and osteological considerations. *J. Anat.*, **95**, 337–344.

Davis, P.R. (1963) Some effects of lifting, pulling and pushing on the human trunk. *Ergonomics*, **6**, 303–304.

Davis, P.R. & Rowland, H.A.K. (1965) Vertebral fractures in West Africans suffering from tetanus. *J. Bone Jt. Surg.*, **47B**, 61–71.

Davis, P.R., Troup, D.G. & Burnard, J.H. (1965) Movements of the thoracic and lumbar spine when lifting: a chrono-cyclophotographic study. *J. Anat.*, **99**, 18–26.

Day, M.H. (1964) The blood supply of the lumbar and sacral plexuses in the human foetus. *J. Anat.*, **98**, 105–116.

Dunlop, R.P., Adam, M.A. & Hutton, W.C. (1984) Disc space narrowing and the lumbar facet joints. *J. Bone Jt. Surg.*, **66B**, 706–710.

Dunnill, M.S., Anderson, J.A. & Whitehead, R. (1967) Quantitative histological studies on age changes in bone. *J. Pathol. Bacteriol.*, **94**, 275.

Eddy, T.P. (1972) Deaths from domestic falls and fractures. *Br. J. Prev. Soc. Med.*, **25**, 173–179.

Eder, M. (1960) Der Strukturumbau der Wirbelspongiosa. *Virchows Arch. Pathol. Anat. Physiol. Klin. Med.*, **333**, 509–522.

Edgar, M.A. & Nundy, S. (1966) Innervation of spinal dura mater. *J. Neurol. Neurosurg. Psychiatry*, **29**, 530–534.

Ehrenhaft, J.L. (1943) Development of the vertebral column as related to certain congenital and pathological changes. *Surg. Gynecol. Obstet.*, **76**, 282–292.

Eisenstein, S. (1977) The morphometry and pathological anatomy of the lumbar spine in South African negroes and caucasoids with special reference to spinal stenosis. *J. Bone Jt. Surg.*, **59B** (Br), 173–180.

Eisenstein, S. (1980) The trefoil configuration of the lumbar vertebral canal. *J. Bone Jt. Surg.*, **62B**, 73–77.

Engel, R. & Bogduk, N. (1982) The menisci of lumbar zygapophysial joints. *J. Anat.*, **135**, 795–809.

Ennerking, W.F. & Harrington, P. (1959) Pathological changes in scoliosis. *J. Bone Jt. Surg.*, **51A**, 165–184.

Epstein, B. (1962) *The Spine Radiological Textbook and Atlas*. Henry Kimpton, London

Epstein, J.A. & Epstein, B. (1978) Stenosis of the lumbar and cervical canal. In Vinken, P.J., Brugh, G.W. & Myrianthopoulos, N.G. (eds) *Handbook of Clinical Neurology, Congenital Malformations of the Spine and Spinal Cord*, vol. 32, pp. 329–345. North-Holland, Amsterdam.

Ericksen, M.F. (1976) Some aspects of aging in the lumbar spine. *Am. J. Phys. Anthropol.*, **45**, 575–560.

Etemadi, A.A. (1974) Extensor power of different parts of the erector spinae musculature in man. *Anat. Anz.*, **135S**, 164–177.

Falkner, F. & Tanner, J.M. (1986) *Human Growth*, vol. 2: *Postnatal Growth Neurobiology*. Plenum Press, New York.

Fidler, M.W., Jowett, R.L. & Troup, J.D.G. (1974) Histological study of multifidus in scoliosis. In Zorab, P.A. (ed.) *Scoliosis and Muscle*. William Heinemann Medical Books, London.

Fidler, M.W., Jowett, R.L. & Troup, J.D.G. (1975) Myosin ATPase activity in multifidus muscle from cases of lumbar spinal derangement. *J. Bone Jt. Surg.*, **57B**, 220–227.

Floyd, W.F. & Silver, P.H.S. (1955) The functions of the erectores spinae muscles in certain movements and postures in man. *J. Physiol. (Lond.)*, **129**, 184–203.

Giles, L.G.F. & Harvey, A.R. (1987) Immunohistochemical demonstration of nociceptors in the capsule and synovial fluid of human zygapophyseal joints. *Br. J. Rheumatol.*, **26**, 362–364.

Giles, L.G.F., Taylor, J.R. & Coxin, A (1986) Human zygapophyseal joint synovial fluids. *Acta Anat. (Basel)*, **126**, 110–114.

Gracovetsky, S. (1988) *The Spinal Engine*, pp. 62–98, 463–476. Springer-Verlag, Vienna.

Hall, D.A. (1987) Structure and function of the ageing intervertebral disc. In Hukins, D.W.L. & Nelson, M.A. (eds) *The Ageing Spine*, pp. 40–60. Manchester University Press, Manchester.

Hall, M.C. (1965) *Luschka's Joint*, p. 127. Charles C. Thomas, Springfield, IL.

Hanai, K., Adachi, H. & Ogasawara, H. (1977) Axial transverse tomography of the cervical spine narrowed by ossification of the posterior longitudinal ligament. *J. Bone Jt. Surg.*, **59B**, 481–484.

Harrison, G.R. (1986) Topographical anatomy of the lumbar epidural region, a study using computerized tomography. *Ann. Roy. Coll. Surg. Eng.*, **68**, 110.

Hayashi, K., Yabuki, T., Kurokawa, T., Seki, H., Hogaki, M. & Minoura, S. (1977) The anterior and posterior longitudinal ligaments of the lower cervical spine. *J. Anat.*, **124**, 633–636.

Hendry, N.G.C. (1958) The hydration of the nucleus pulposus and its relation to intervertebral disc derangement. *J. Bone Jt. Surg.*, **40B**, 132–144.

Herbert, C.M., Lindberg, K.A., Jayson, M.I.V. & Bailey, A.J. (1975) Changes in the collagen of the human intervertebral discs during aging and degenerative disc disease. *J. Mol. Med.*, **1**, 79–91.

Heylings, D.J.A. (1978) Supraspinous and interspinous ligaments of the human lumbar spine. *J. Anat.*, **125**, 127–131.

Hickey, D.S. & Hukins, D.W.L. (1981) Collagen fibril diameters and elastic fibres in the annulus fibrosus of the human fetal intervertebral disc. *J. Anat.*, **133**, 451–457.

Hink, V.C., Clark, W.M. & Hopkins, C.E. (1966a) Normal interpeduncular distances (minimum and maximum) in children and adults. *Am. J. Roentgenol, Radium Ther. Nucl. Med.*, **97**, 141–153.

Hink, V.C., Hopkins, C.E. & Clark, W.M. (1966b) Sagittal diameter of the lumbar spinal canal in children and adults. *Radiology*, **85**, 929–937.

Hink, V.C., Hopkins, C.E. & Savara, B.S. (1962) Sagittal diameter of the cervical spinal canal in children. *Radiology*, **79**, 97–108.

Hirsch, C. & Nachemson, A. (1954) New observations on mechanical behavior of lumbar discs. *Acta Orthop. Scand.*, **23**, 254–283.

Holt, S. & Yates, P.O. (1966) Cervical spondylosis and nerve root lesions. Incidence at routine necropsy. *J. Bone Jt. Surg.*, **48B**, 407–423.

Inoué, S. (1973) Three dimensional observation of the collagen framework of intervertebral discs in rats, dogs and humans. *Arch. Histol. Jpn.*, **136**, 39–56; cited by Williams, Warwick, Dyson, & Bannister in *Gray's Anatomy*, 37th edn, p. 490.

Jackson, H.C., Winkelmann, R.K. & Bickel, H. (1966) Nerve endings in the human lumbar spinal column and related structures. *J. Bone Jt. Surg.*, **48A**, 1272–1281.

Jebens, E.H. & Monk-Jones, M.E. (1959) On the viscosity and pH of synovial fluid and the pH of blood. *J. Bone Jt. Surg.*, **41B**, 388–400.

Jefferson, G. (1928) Discussion on spinal injuries. *Proc. Roy. Soc. Med.*, **21**, 625–637.

Jennerken, F.G.I., Tomlinson, B.E. & Walton, J.N. (1971) Histochemical aspects of five limb muscles in old age: an autopsy study. *J. Neurol. Sci.*, **14**, 259–276.

Johnson, E.F., Berryman, H., Mitchell, R. & Wood, W.B. (1985) Elastic fibres in the annulus fibrosus of the adult human intervertebral disc. A preliminary report. *J. Anat.*, **143**, 57–63.

Keagy, R.D., Brumlik, J. & Bergan, J.L. (1966) Direct electromyography of the psoas muscle in man. *J. Bone Jt. Surg.*, **48A**, 1377–1382.

Keats, T. (1988) *Atlas of Normal Variants that may Simulate Disease*, 4th edn, pp. 167–168. Year Book Medical Publishers, Chicago.

Kelly, J.F. (1954) Fractures complicating electroconvulsive therapy and chronic epilepsy. *J. Bone Jt. Surg.*, **36B**, 70–79.

Kendrick, G.S. & Biggs, N.L. (1963) Incidence of the ponticulus posticus of the first cervical vertebra between the ages of six to seventeen. *Anat. Rec.*, **145**, 449–451.

Keyes, D.C. & Compere, E.L. (1932) The normal and pathological physiology of the nucleus pulposus of the intervertebral disc. *J. Bone Jt. Surg.*, **14A**, 897–938.

Klausen, K. (1965) The form and function of the loaded human spine. *Acta Physiol. Scand.*, **65**, 176–190.

Krenz, J. & Troup, J.D.G. (1973) The structure of the pars interarticularis of the lower lumbar vertebrae and its relation to the etiology of spondylolysis. *J. Bone Jt. Surg.*, **55B**, 735–741.

Kumar, S. & Davis, P.R. (1973) Lumbar vertebral innervation and intra-abdominal pressure. *J. Anat.*, **114**, 47–53.

Lamberty, B.G.N. & Zinanovic, S. (1973) The retro-articular vertebral artery ring of the atlas and its significance. *Acta Anat.*, **85**, 113–122.

Landmesser, W.E. & Heuberlein, G.W. (1953) Measurement of the normal interpeduncular space in the child. *Connecticut Med. J.*, **17**, 310–313.

Le Double, A.F. (1912) *Traité des variations de la colonne vertébrale de L'Homme*, pp. 240–242. Vigot, Paris.

Locke, G.R., Gardner, J.I. & Van Epps, E.K. (1966) Atlanto-dental interval in children and adults. *Am. J. Roentgenol. Radium Ther. Nucl. Med.*, **97**, 135–140.

Lysell, E. (1969) Motion in the cervical spine. An experimental study on autopsy material. *Acta Orthop. Scand.*, **S123**, 5–61.

MacEwen, G.D. & Kirsch, P. (1971) Factors affecting growth of vertebral bodies and intervertebral discs. In Zorab, P.A. (ed.) *Scoliosis and Growth*, pp. 40–46. Churchill Livingstone, Edinburgh.

Maroudas, A., Stockwell, R., Nachemson, A. & Urban, J. (1975) Factors involved in the nutrition of the human lumbar intervertebral disc: cellularity and diffusion of glucose *in vitro*. *J. Anat.*, **120**, 113–130.

McKern, T.W. & Stewart, T.D. (1956) Skeletal age changes in young American males. Tech. Rep. EP 45, Environmental Protection Div. Natick, Mass; cited by Williams, Warwick, Dyson, Bannister in *Gray's Anatomy*, 37th edn, p. 329.

Meachim, G. & Cornah, M.S. (1970) Fine structure of the juvenile human nucleus pulposus. *J. Anat.*, **107**, 337–350.

Mercer, W. (1950) *Orthopaedic Surgery*, 4th edn, p. 678. Williams & Wilkins, Baltimore.

Miall, W.E., Ashcroft, M.T. & Moore, F. (1967) A longitudinal study of decline of adult height with age in two Welsh communities. *Human Biol.*, **39**, 445–454.

Morris, J.M., Lucas, D.B. & Bresler, B. (1961) The role of the trunk in the stability of the spine. *J. Bone Jt. Surg.*, **43A**, 327–351.

Mountcastle, V.B. & Powell, T.P.S. (1959) Central nervous mechanisms subserving position sense and kinesthesis. *Bull. Johns Hopkins Hosp.*, **105**, 173–200.

Nachemson, A. (1963) The influence of spinal movements on the lumbar intradiscal pressure and on the tensile stresses in the annulus fibrosus. *Acta Orthop. Scand.*, **33**, 183–207.

Nachemeson, A. & Morris, J.M. (1944) *In vivo* measurements of intradiscal pressure. *J. Bone Jt. Surg*, **46A**, 1077–1092.

Nathan, H. (1962) Osteophytes of the vertebral column: an anatomical study of their development according to age, race and sex with consideration of their etiology and significance. *J. Bone Jt. Surg.*, **44A**, 243–268.

Naylor, A. (1979) Factors in the development of spinal stenosis syndrome *J. Bone Jt. Surg.*, **61B**, 306–309.

Nicoll, E.A. (1940) Fractures of the dorsolumbar spine. *J. Bone Jt. Surg.*, **31B**, 376–394.

Nicolopoulos, K.S., Burwell, R.G. & Webb, J.K. (1985) Stature in healty children, sexual dimorphism and age related changes. *J. Anat.*, **141**, 105–114.

O'Rahilly, R. & Benson, D.R. (1985) Development of the vertebral column. In Bradford, D.S. & Hensigner, R.M. (eds) *The Pediatric Spine*, pp. 3–17. Thieme, New York.

Orofino, C., Sherman, M.S. & Schechter, D. (1960) Luschka's joint—a degenerative phenomenon. *J. Bone Jt. Surg.*, **42A**, 853–858.

Pal, G.P. & Routal, R.V. (1986) A study of weight transmission through the cervical and upper thoracic regions of the vertebral column in man. *J. Anat.*, **148**, 245–261.

Parkin, I.G. & Harrison, G.R. (1985) The topographical anatomy of the lumbar epidural space. *J. Anat.*, **141**, 211–217.

Peacock, A. (1951) Observations on the prenatal development of the intervertebral disc in man. *J. Anat.*, **85**, 260–274.

Peacock, A. (1952) Observations on the postnatal structure of the intervertebral disc in man. *J. Anat.*, **86**, 162–179.

Pedersen, M.E., Blunck, C.F.J. & Gardner, E. (1956) The anatomy of lumbosacral posterior rami and meningeal branches of spinal nerves. *J. Bone Jt. Surg.*, **38A**, 377–391.

Pennel, G.F. & Schatzkers, J. (1971) Stenosis of the lumbosacral canal. *Clin. Nuerosurg.*, **18**, 86–105.

Poole, C.A., Flint, M.H. & Beaumont, B.W. (1984) Morphological and functional inter-relationships of articular cartilage matrices. *J. Anat.*, **138**, 113–138.

Porter, R.W. (1985) *Management of Back Pain*, pp. 29–39. Churchill Livingstone, Edinburgh.

Porter, R.W., Hibbert, C.S. & Evans, C. (1983) Relationship between the cervical and lumbar canal. *Ann. Roy. Coll. Surg. Eng.*, **63**, 334.

Porter, R.W., Hibbert, C.S. & Wicks, M. (1978a) The spinal canal in symptomatic lumbar disc lesions. *J. Bone Jt. Surg.*, **65B**, 485–487.

Porter, R.W., Wicks, M. & Ottwell, D. (1978b) Measurement of the spinal canal by diagnostic ultrasound. *J. Bone Jt. Surg.*, **48B**, 1–6.

Putz, R. (1976) Zur Morphologie und Rotationsmechanik der kleinen Gelenke der Ledenwirbel. *Z. Orthop.*, **114**, 902–912.

Putz, R. (1985) The functional morphology of the superior articular processes of the lumbar vertebrae. *J. Anat.*, **143**, 181–183.

Riddle, A.F.V. & Roaf, R. (1955) Muscle imbalance in the causation of scoliosis. *Lancet*, **1**, 1245–1247.

Risser, J.C. & Ferguson, A.B. (1936) Scoliosis: its prognosis. *J. Bone Jt. Surg.*, **18**, 667–670.

Roaf, R. (1960) A study of the mechanics of spinal injuries. *J. Bone Jt. Surg.*, **42B**, 810–823.

Roaf, R. (1971) The growth of the spinal articular processes and their clinical significance. In Zorab, P.A. (ed.) *Scoliosis and Growth*, pp. 92–97. Churchill Livingstone, Edinburgh.

Roaf, R. (1977) *Spinal Deformities*, p. 8. Pitman Medical, London.

Roche, A.F. (1986) Bone growth and maturity. In Falkner, F. & Tanner, J.M. (eds) *Postnatal Growth*, vol. 2, pp. 25–60. Plenum Press, New York.

Rockoff, S.D., Sweet, E. & Bleustein, J. (1969) The relative contributions of trabecular and cortical bone to the strength of human lumbar vertebrae. *Calcif. Tiss. Res.*, **3**, 163–175.

Salsabili, N. & Hogg, D.A. (1991) Development of human sacroiliac joint. Clin. Anat., **4**, 99–108.

Saville, P.D. (1970) Observations on 80 women with osteoporotic spine fractures. In Barzel, U.S. (ed.) *Osteoporosis*, pp. 38–46. Grune & Stratton, New York.

Scammon, R.E., & Calkins, L.A. (1929) *The Development and Growth of the External Dimensions of the Human Body in the Fetal Period*. University of Minnesota Press, Minneapolis, MN.

Schatzker, J. & Pennal, G.P. (1968) Spinal stenosis, a cause of cauda equina compression. *J. Bone Jt. Surg.*, **50B**, 606–618.

Schwarz, G.S. (1956) The width of the spinal canal in the growing vertebra, with special reference to the sacrum. Maximum interpeduncular distances in infants and children. *Am. J. Roentgenol.*, **76**, 475–481.

Shar, J.S., Hampson, W.G.J. & Jayson, M.I.V. (1978) The distribution of surface strain in the cadaveric lumbar spine. *J. Bone Jt. Surg.*, **60B**, 246–251.

Siffert, R.S. & Gilbert, M.S. (1969) The anatomy and physiology of the growth plate. In Rang, M. (ed.) *The Growth Plate and its Disorders*, p. 2. Livingstone, Edinburgh.

Sinclair, D. (1973) *Human Growth after Birth*, 2nd edn, pp. 113–118. Oxford Medical Publications, London.

Singh, I. (1978) The architecture of cancellous bone. *J. Anat.*, **127**, 305–310.

Singh, S. (1965) Variations in the superior articular facets of atlas vertebrae. *J. Anat.*, **99**, 565–571.

Širca, A. & Kostevc, V. (1985) The fibre type composition of thoracic and lumbar paravertebral muscles in man. *J. Anat.*, **141**, 131–137.

Skogland, S. (1973) Joint receptors and kinaesthesis. In Iggo, A. (ed.) *Handbook of Sensory Physiology*, vol. 2, pp. 110–136. Springer, Berlin.

Stewart-Brown, S. (1982) *Growth, Child Health and Education Survey*, pp. 132–158. First report to the DHSS on the 10-year follow-up. Department of Child Health, Bristol.

Stockwell, R.A. (1987) Microscopical structure and histochemistry of cervicular cartilage and the marginal transitional zone. *Ann. Roy. Coll. Surg. Eng.*, **69**, 80.

Stoltman, H.F. & Blackwood, W. (1964) The role of ligamenta flava in the pathogenesis of myelopathy. *Brain*, **87**, 45–50.

Stonelake, P.S., Burwell, F.G. & Webb, J.K. (1988) Variations in vertebral levels of the vertebra prominens and sacral dimples in subjects with scoliosis. *J. Anat.*, **159**, 165–172.

Sylven, B. (1950) On the biology of the nucleus pulposus. *Acta Orthop. Scand.*, **20**, 275–279.

Sylven, B., Paulson, S., Hirsch, C. & Snellman, O. (1951) Biophysical and physiological investigations on cartilage and other mesenchymal tissues. 2. *J. Bone Jt. Surg.*, **33A**, 333–340.

Tanner, J.M. (1971) Some main features of growth in normal children. In Zorob, P.A. (ed.) *Scoliosis and Growth*, p. 20. Churchill Livingstone, Edinburgh.

Tanner, J.M., Whitehouse, R.H. & Taraish, I.M. (1966) Standards from birth to maturity for height, weight, height velocity and weight velocity. *Arch. Dis. Childh.*, **4**, 454–471.

Tanz, S.S. (1953) Motion of the lumbar spine: a roentgenologic study. *Am. J. Roentgenol.*, **69**, 399–412.

Taylor, J.R. (1975) Growth of human intervertebral discs and vertebral bodies. *J. Anat.*, **120**, 49–68.

Taylor, J.R. & Twomey, L. (1984) Sexual dimorphism in human vertebral body shape. *J. Anat.*, **138**, 281–286.

Taylor, J.R. & Twomey, L. (1986) Age changes in lumbar

zygapophyseal joints. Observations of structure and function. *Spine*, **11**, 739–745.

Tesh, K.M., Evans, J.H. & Shaw-Dunn, J. (1984) The action of the thoracolumbar fascia in the maintenance of extension of the lumbar spine. *Ann. Roy. Coll. Surg. Eng.*, **66**, 135.

Todd, W.T. & Pyle, S.I. (1982a) Effects of maceration and drying upon the vertebral column. *Am. J. Phys. Anthropol.*, **12**, 303–319.

Todd, W.I. & Pyle, S.I. (1928b) A quantitative study of the vertebral column by direct and roentgenoscopic methods. *Am. J. Phys. Anthropol.*, **12**, 321–337.

Tondury, G. (1943) Zur Anatomiem der Halswirbelsäule, Gibt es Uncovertebral gelenke? *Z. Anat. Entwicklungsgesch.*, **122**, 448–459.

Topinard, P. (1877) Des anomalies de nombre de la colonne vertébrale chez l'homme. *Rev. Anthropol.*, **6**, 577–649.

Torklus, D. von & Gehrle, W. (1972) *Upper Cervical Spine.* (Transl. Michaelis L.S.). Georg Thieme Verlag, Stuttgart; Butterworth, London.

Twomey, L., Taylor, J. & Furniss, B. (1983) Age changes in the bone density and structure of the lumbar vertebral column. *J. Anat.*, **136**, 15–25.

Urist, M.R., Gurvey, M.S. & Fareed, D.O. (1970) Long term observations on aged women with pathologic osteoporosis. In Barzel, U.S. (ed.) *Osteoporosis*, pp. 3–37. Grune & Stratton, New York.

Valojerdy, M.R. & Hogg, D.A. (1989) Sex differences in the morphology of the auricular surfaces of the human sacroiliac joint. *Clin. Anat.*, **2**, 63–68.

Veldhuizen, A.G., Baas, P. & Webb, P.J. (1986) Observations on the growth of the adolescent spine. *J. Bone Jt. Surg.*, **68B**, 724–728.

Verbiest, H. (1955) Further experiences on the pathological influence of a developmental narrowness of the bony lumbar veretebral canal. *J. Bone Jt. Surg.*, **37B**, 576–583.

Viidick, A. (1973) Functional properties of collagenous tissues. *Int. Rev. Connect. Tiss. Res.*, **6**, 127–215.

Vink, P. (1989) Functions of the lumbar back muscles. Thesis for Rijksuniversiteit of Leiden, pp. 1–111 (summary, p. 97).

Voss, H. (1956) Zahl und Anordung der Muskelspindeln in den oberen Zungenbeinmuskel dem M. trapezius und M. latissimus dorsi. *Anat. Anz.*, **103**, 443–446.

Voss, H. (1958) Zahl und Anordung den Muskelspindeln in dem unteren Zungenbeinmuskel dem M sternocleidomastoideus und den Brauch und tiefen Nachenmusleln. *Anat. Anz.*, **105**, 265–275.

Wagner, M., Sether, L.A., Yu, S., Ho, S.P. & Haughton, V.M. (1988) Age changes in the lumbar intervertebral disc studied with magnetic resonance and cryomicrotomy. *Clin. Anat.*, **1**, 93–103.

Wang, Z.L., Yu, S. & Haughton, V.M. (1989) Age related changes in lumbar facet joints. *Clin. Anat.*, **2**, 55–62.

Weinmann, J.P. & Sicher, H. (1955) *Bone and Bones: Fundamentals of Bone Biology*, 2nd edn., p. 135. Kimpton, London.

Weisl, H. (1954a) The ligaments of the sacroiliac joint examined with particular reference to their function. *Acta Anat.*, **20**, 201–213.

Weisl, H. (1954b) The articular surfaces of the sacroiliac joint and their relation to movements of the sacrum. *Acta Anat.*, **22**, 1–14.

Weisl, H. (1955) The movements of the sacroiliac joint. *Acta Anat.*, **23**, 80–91.

Weiss, E.B. (1975) Stresses at the lumbosacral junction. *Orthop. Clin. N. Am.*, **6**, 63–91.

White, A.A. (1969) Analysis of the mechanics of the thoracic spine in man. *Acta Orthop. Scand.*, **S127**, 1–103.

White, A.A. & Panjabi, M.M. (1978) *Clinical Biomechanics of the Spine.* Lippincott, Philadelphia; cited by Gracovetsky (1988), p. 305.

Wilde, G.P., Szypryt, E.P. & Mulholland, R. (1988) Unilateral lumbar facet joint hypertrophy causing nerve root irritation. *Ann. Roy. Coll. Surg. Eng.*, **70**, 307–308.

Wilkinson, M. (1967) Pathology. In Lord Brain & Wilkinson, M. (eds) *Cervical Spondylosis and Other Disorders of the Cervical Spine*, pp. 98–103. William Heinemann Medical Books, London.

Williams, P.L., Warwick, R., Dyson, M. & Bannister, L.H. (1989) *Gray's Anatomy*, 37th edn, p. 329. Churchill Livingstone, Edinburgh.

Wolf, B.S., Khilnani, M. & Malis, L. (1956) Sagittal diameter of the bony cervical spinal canal and its significance. *J. Mt. Sinai Hosp.*, **23**, 283–292.

Young, A.C. (1967) Radiology of cervical spondylosis. In Lord Brain & Wilkinson, M. (eds) *Cervical Spondylosis and Other Disorders of the Cervical Spine*, pp. 142–149. William Heinemann Medical Books, London.

Zaki, W. (1973) Aspect morphologique et fonctionnel de l'annulus fibrosus des disque intervertébral de la colonne dorsale. *Arch. Anat. Pathol.*, **21**, 401–403.

SECTION 3
CLINICAL ASSESSMENT AND INVESTIGATION

4 · Clinical Evaluation of Spinal Disorders

By M.C. LYNCH and L.D. BLUMHARDT

CLINICAL HISTORY

Beyond any doubt the most important factor in the clinical evaluation of a patient presenting with a spinal problem is the clinical history. A careful evaluation of the type of symptom, along with its time scale and the factors which affect it, will produce the foundations of a differential diagnosis. Certain combinations of symptoms, such as the development of radicular pain and foot drop after walking in spinal stenosis, or the association of inadvertent burning of the fingers and a progressive gait disturbance in syringomyelia, may be so typical that they suggest a specific diagnosis from the outset.

Many patients with spinal disorders present with pain and the evaluation of this symptom is of paramount importance. Detailed discussion of the symptomatology of pain as it presents in different conditions is naturally covered in the subsequent chapters of this book. At this stage, however, certain features should be stressed. When a patient complains of spinal pain—whether it be low back pain, neck pain or thoracic or thoracolumbar pain—it is important to attempt to decide whether this indicates serious underlying pathology. Most spinal pains due to degenerative disease tend to fluctuate in severity. Such fluctuation may be on an hourly, daily or weekly basis and may often be affected by position or activity. It is important to recognize, however, that spinal pain which is severely affected by movement may well indicate major structural disease. Pain due to destructive disease such as tumour or infection tends to have a more unremitting time-scale. Whilst it also may be affected by position and movement, such pain tends to become progressively more severe in a relentless fashion. A complaint of spinal pain in a child or teenager should always be taken seriously as degenerative disease or psychological pain is most unusual in these age groups. Pain from intraspinal lesions in such children is frequently more severe at night. Occasionally, patients present with such severe pain and with such gross paraspinal muscle spasm that they may be considered to be showing a hysterical overreaction. Whilst this may be true, it must be remembered that patients with disease such as acute spinal infection (especially, extradural abscess) can show an identical picture.

There are several other types of pain which are common in spinal disease. The differentiation between referred and radicular pain is usually fairly straightforward if a good clinical history is taken, though intercostal radicular pain remains a problem, often being misinterpreted as being due to visceral pathology. Less common is the pain whcih arises from segmental involvement of the central structures of the spinal cord. Such pain has a quality which patients find difficult to describe. It is most often described as burning, and the area affected with such pain is often well below the level of the cord involvement. Pain may have a dysaesthetic quality which, when it involves a limb, may suggest a causalgia. Hypersensitivity is also a common feature of central cord pain.

In addition to the evaluation of pain in the history, many other factors must be elicited. The presence of any instigating factors such as trauma may be of importance. Careful evaluation of sensory symptoms is important. This should not be restricted simply to numbness. Symptoms such as clumsy hands with inability to undo buttons may indicate either a dyspraxia or, more commonly, proprioceptive disturbance in the hands. Evaluation of motor deficit is of obvious importance and a careful analysis of any gait difficulty is essential. Evaluation of sphincteric disturbance is essential, yet sadly often omitted. One of the most frequent errors made in the assessment of disorders such as spinal metastasis is to assume that sphincteric dysfunction in an elderly male has to be due to prostatic disease. It cannot be overstressed that painless urinary retention with or without overflow is a *neurological* rather than a urological emergency.

In addition to obtaining a detailed history of any pain, spinal or neurological symptoms, a full clinical history is obviously necessary. The presence of systemic diseases such as diabetes, malignancy or rheumatoid arthritis may be of great significance. The clinical history should explore the patient's past to the prenatal stage. Hereditary diseases affecting the spine are uncommon and usually obvious, but the family history must be explored. A history of prolonged and difficult birth is of great significance in syringomyelia (see Chapter 54). A surprising number of patients suffering from spinal dysraphism only present in adult life when the significance of a small foot or a hairy patch in the spine may well have been forgotten (Morris & Findlay, 1991). An episode of retrobulbar neuritis or diplopia may have occurred many years before the patient presents with spinal manifestations of multiple sclerosis (MS).

Once a full history has been obtained, the patient should be fully examined. Only then should the spine and the neurological system be examined. Examination of the spine can appear a daunting challenge to those not regularly involved in spinal practice. The correct approach is a systematic one which follows a strict routine. The old orthopaedic maxim of 'look, feel, move' is particularly relevant to examination of the vertebral column.

The techniques of spinal examination are outlined here and detail, in chronological order, the procedures which should be undertaken when a new patient presents. The sequence in which areas of the spine are assessed varies according to the method of examination, i.e. inspection, palpation and movement. For example, the appearance of the thoracic and lumbar spine is examined at the outset of the consultation when the patient is asked to walk; the appearance of the cervical spine is assessed subsequently. By contrast, palpation of the spine should be performed in a craniocaudal direction, and thus the cervical spine is examined before the thoracolumbar area. The description of spinal examination is presented here in the order in which it would be performed in the clinical setting.

INSPECTION

Inspection with the patient walking

Frank abnormalities of gait are unusual in spinal disease without neurological inpairment. There may, of course, be a number of intercurrent orthopaedic abnormalities producing a typical abnormal gait. A short leg produces dipping of the spine and pelvis towards the shortened side, a defective hip abductor mechanism as a consequence of hip disease produces the typical Trendelenburg or lurching type of gait, and a painful joint in the lower limb may result in an antalgic gait in which the patient spends less time on the affected painful limb. General inspection of a patient attired in underclothing only may, however, reveal abnormalities of spinal configuration and abnormal degrees of spinal stiffness which are apparent only on movement. Gross degrees of spondylolisthesis are said to produce tightening of the hamstring muscles and a typical waddling short stride gait.

Inspection from the side

With the patient standing it should be possible to make an assessment of normal spinal postures. There should be a cervical lordosis, a thoracic kyphosis, a lumbar lordosis and a sacral kyphosis. The normal thoracic kyphosis is between 20° and 40° when measured on radiographs, but can be remarkably difficult to assess clinically. A gross increase in the normal thoracic kyphosis or an abnormal flattening of the thoracic spine when marked are usually easy to detect, however. A postural kyphosis will reduce if the patient is asked to stand upright, bracing back the shoulders producing extension. A postural kyphosis increases with forward flexion. A smooth rigid kyphosis is commonly seen in Scheuermann's disease, ankylosing spondylitis and senile kyphosis. When the kyphosis is angular the underlying pathology may be a congenital abnormality of the spine, the result of a previous crush fracture of the thoracic spine or, rarely these days, a result of tuberculous disease of the vertebral bodies.

An abnormally increased lumbar lordosis or hollowing of the back is seen in spondylolisthesis but may, in fact, be a normal finding in females. When the lumbar lordosis is obliterated it is usually an indication of paraspinal muscle spasm set up by an irritative focus in the spine. The most common causes for this are a prolapsed intervertebral disc, ankylosing spondylitis, infections in or round the spine, or a benign tumour of the axial skeleton.

Inspection from the side may show a prominence of the rib cage on one side of the spine giving the false impression of a spinal kyphosis. It is important to distinguish between a rib hump due to the spinal rotation of scoliosis and a true kyphosis of the spine. Most rib prominences associated with scoliosis are, in fact, accompanied by a reduction in the normal thoracic kyphosis.

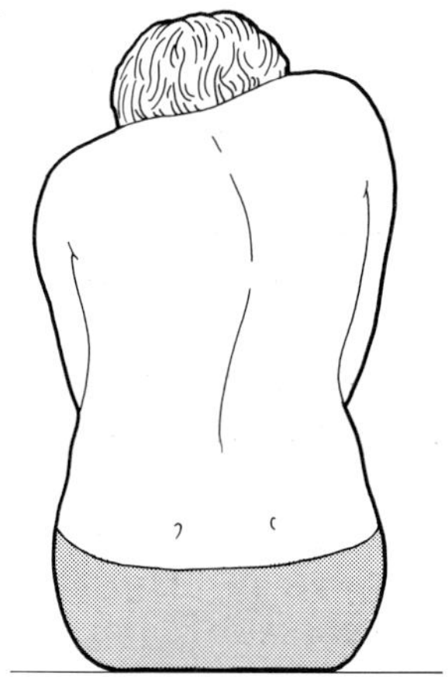

Fig. 4.1 The persistence of scoliosis in the seated position means that it cannot be due to discrepancy in limb length.

Inspection of the spine from the back

A curvature or scoliosis of the spine may be apparent in the coronal plane. Often, however, it is difficult to see minor degrees of curvature, particularly if the spine is in balance, as when the head is directly above the centre of the pelvis. If the patient is asked to bend forwards such that the hands are in contact with the knees, with the legs straight, minor degrees of spinal curvature and rib protrusion become more obvious. In this position of forward flexion the observer can easily look along the length of the spine, which is seen in contour, and quite subtle changes in body shape can be seen. With the patient standing vertically again a plumb-line should be placed from the vertebrae prominens, which is usually T1, and allowed to drop to the region of the natal cleft. If the plumb-line drops to the right or left of the cleft this should be measured in centimetres and referred to as the degree of spinal decompensation. In the standing position the spine should be inspected for the presence of the external features of spinal dysraphism. Such changes as a hairy patch, pigmentation of the skin, the swelling of a lipoma or a pit in the skin may indicate the presence of an underlying developmental abnormality. These changes are more commonly seen in the lumbar region.

If a scoliosis is detected the patient should be asked to sit and the spine observed again for the presence of a lateral curvature (see Fig. 4.1). If the curvature disappears on sitting it would suggest that it was present on standing because of a leg length inequality. This may be confirmed by placing blocks under the shortened limb to again obliterate the curvature when the patient is standing. If the curvature persists on sitting, but disappears on forward flexion, it would suggest that the curvature was postural rather than structural in origin.

If scoliosis is detected in a child who is small enough to be lifted under the arms it is possible to detect whether the curve disappears on suspension. This gives a good test of the mobility of the deformity. In larger children and adults, asking the patient to bend towards and away from the side of the deformity gives a similar indication of curve mobility.

On occasion there may be more than one curvature present in the spine, the common pattern being a curvature of the thoracic spine to one side and in the lumbar spine to the other. Often this is very difficult to detect clinically when of minor degree, and it is often associated with no loss of compensation in the spine. Again, forward flexion tends to accentuate the abnormality.

If a scoliosis is detected in a growing child, a general examination must be carried out for some of the more common causes of the condition. Joint hypermobility needs to be assessed by bending the thumbs onto the forearm in a volar direction and assessing any degree of knee or elbow hyperextension. Abnormal joint laxity is present in conditions such as Marfan's syndrome and other connective tissue abnormalities. A high arched palate and cardiac murmur may also suggest Marfan's syndrome. The skin should be thoroughly assessed for abnormalities of pigmentation which may be present in neurofibromatosis. Freckling in the axillae is almost invariably present in this condition.

Assessment of the size of a rib hump

The size and shape of a rib hump can be measured using a needle template comprising a series of sensing needles mounted between rollers. The tips of the needles can assume the shape of the rib hump and are then locked in position. The shape of the hump can therefore be measured at different levels and transcribed on to a three-dimensional drawing. Moiré fringes have been used to produce a representation of rib prominence. These are produced when a grid of lines is projected optically onto a surface and the illuminated surface is then viewed through a similar grid. Two negatives are produced which, when placed together in the correct alignment on a photograph of the back, can produce a series of lines akin to an Ordnance Survey map representing a hill using height contour lines.

Inspection of the cervical spine

If the patient is viewed from the front, particular attention needs to be directed to the supraclavicular fossa. Occasionally a large tumour at the apex of the lung or a vascular aneurysm may be apparent as a visible swelling. The most common postural derangement of the cervical spine is a torticollis, which results in the head being held in a tilted and slightly rotated attitude due to abnormal tightness in one of the sternomastoid muscles. In infancy this tightness may be due to the so-called 'sternomastoid tumour' which is, in fact, an area of fibrosis within the muscle belly. Some cases of infantile torticollis are not associated with a palpable swelling, and are presumably due to slight contracture of the muscle as a result of an abnormal posture *in utero*. In older child ren and adults a torticollis may be due to a very short-lived spasm in one or other sternomastoid muscle, often attributed to minor trauma, or to sleeping in an abnormal position. When the torticollis lasts for anything longer than two or three days consideration must be given to the diagnoses of pharyngeal infection, vertebral body tumour, vertebral body infection or interposing tumours.

Rarely, a true cervical kyphosis may be present following a widespread upper thoracic or cervical laminectomy in a child, or in cases of advanced ankylosing spondylitis in the adult.

PALPATION

Palpation of the cervical spine

Palpation of the cervical spine should be performed from behind, using both of the examiner's hands. Tenderness should be felt for from the base of the skull to the prominent spinous processes of C7 and T1. Muscle spasm and tenderness may be elicited to one or other sides of the midline in cervical spondylosis and occasionally in infections and tumours of the spine. Tenderness is said to be more easily elicited in the latter two conditions when palpation is performed by striking the spinous processes with the clenched hand. This latter manoeuvre is known as percussion of the spine. No examination of the cervical spine is complete without performing palpation laterally and inferiorly along the sides of the cervical vertebrae to the posterior triangle and supraclavicular region of the neck. Particular attention should be paid towards lymphatic enlargements or swellings of the midline structures of the neck such as the thyroid gland and the position of the trachea. Deep palpation in the region of the scalene muscles occasionally produces pain when underlying nerve root irritation is present in the cervical plexus.

Palpation of the thoracic and lumbar spine

Palpation for spinal tenderness is essentially the same in the thoracic and lumbar spines as in the neck. Both fingertip palpation and percussion should be performed at every spinal level. When a complaint of low back pain has been made the lower lumbar facet joints should be deeply palpated using thumb pressure approximately 2 cm on either side of the spinous processes. Quite marked pressure is required to palpate these joints because of the thickness of the underlying paraspinal musculature at this level. This is best achieved by hooking the remainder of the fingers around the patient's pelvis and applying counterpressure. It must be remembered that there is a two-level nerve supply to the posterior facet joints, and therefore some overlap of sensory supply may give a rather diffuse area of tenderness when only one joint is the source of pain. The sacroiliac joints are close to the facet joints of L4, L5 and L5–S1, and have often been said to be the source of low back pain in the past. With care it should be possible to distinguish tenderness in the posterior facet joints and the sacroiliac joints with careful palpation. Unless disrupted by previous severe trauma, or the appearance of active bacterial infection, it is unlikely that the sacroiliac joints are a common source of low back pain and therefore tenderness. The vast majority of low back pain is generated either in the posterior facet joints or the surrounding ligaments, tendons or muscles. Midline palpation of the lumbosacral region may reveal a step in conditions causing forward slip of one vertebra on another (spondylolisthesis). Minor degrees of forward slip do not give a readily palpable sensation of a step in the spine, and usually quite severe degrees of displacement are required before this clinical sign is easily apparent. In obese or well-muscled individuals even quite marked degrees of spondylolisthesis are not readily apparent on palpation.

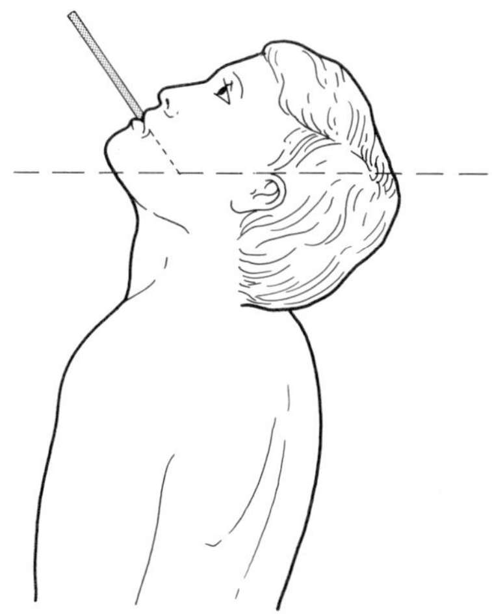

Fig. 4.2 The use of a spatula to assess the range of cervical movement.

MOVEMENT

Because the spine is made up of a number of articulating segments it becomes difficult to measure accurately ranges of motion in most of the directions in which the spine is able to move. In joints such as the elbow or hip there are either one or two long bones which, although covered by a large bulk of soft tissues, are able to act as a pointer on an imaginary protractor. When examining the spine more indirect assessments have to be made of the underlying complex movements contributing to a particular change in position.

Movements of the cervical spine

Flexion of the cervical spine should allow the chin to touch the sternum. This is obviously a highly subjective test because of the quite marked anatomical variation that can occur in the length of the cervical spine and the shape of the upper chest. However, this simple screening test should indicate gross restrictions of movement. Extension should be possible such that it allows the patient's forehead to become parallel with the ceiling when the trunk is held in a vertical position. Again, this is a rather subjective method of assessment but, with practice, it should be possible to make a clinical judgement about the particular range of motion possible. For example if the forehead is only able to angulate such that it measures approximately 45° to the ceiling then a 50% range of cervical extension is recorded. Another method for assessing cervical flexion and extension is to ask the subject to clench an object such as a wooden spatula between the teeth and then describe a full arc of movement from full flexion to full extension (see Fig. 4.2). One should imagine the spatula moving as a pointer across an imaginary protractor scale. The normal range of movement is approximately 120°.

A similar method can be utilized to measure rotation of the cervical spine which occurs largely at the C1–C2 articulation. A normal range of rotation is 0–80° on both sides.

Lateral bending of the cervical spine may be performed by asking the patient to approximate the ear to the shoulder when slightly shrugging. When viewed from the front this test is reasonably reliable as the angle made by the head is usually fairly easy to observe. The normal range is approximately 0–45°. Again, by clenching a spatula sideways in the teeth this movement may become more obvious.

Careful observation should be made of the rhythm of movement. Normally the movements described are made with a smooth, painless progression. Any jerkiness or obvious pain produced is significant.

Movements of the thoracic and lumbar spine

Flexion of the thoracic and lumbar spine is often assessed by asking the patient to touch the toes, with the feet comfortably spread apart and the knees fully extended. The majority of individuals should be able to touch their toes, albeit with some difficulty. The problem with this assessment is that a large proportion of the movement occurs by hip flexion until hamstring tightness prevents further flexion of the hip joints. However, in cases with a rigid lumbar spine it is a common finding that the fingertips usually only reach knee level on attempted full spinal flexion. When these movements of the thoracic and lumbar spines are measured on dynamic radiographs the reported ranges of flexion are approximately 45° and 60°, respectively. Although the gross movement of attempting to touch one's toes is theoretically imprecise it does tend to prove a useful measure when repeated chronological estimations are made of spinal flexion. On each occasion a record should be made of the distance between the fingertips and the floor, in centimetres (see Fig. 4.3).

Extension of the lumbar and thoracic spine is even more difficult to assess. Even an indirect assessment of this movement is very difficult to perform. Clinicians normally express the range of extension in very broad percentage terms based on clinical experience from examining the normal lumbar spine. For example estimates of 25%, 50% and 75% of normal movement are probably as accurate as can be determined by clinical examination alone.

Another method of assessing spinal flexion and extension is to estimate the excursion of the spinous processes at different levels. In conditions such as ankylosing spondylitis, in which the spine may be completely rigid, attempted flexion and extension will show no change between spinous processes even quite far apart when they are measured using a tape measure. Any apparent flexion on extension movements may occur solely at the hip joints. This degree of spinal stiffness may also occur in severe irritative conditions of the spine such as tumours, infections or even prolapsed intervertebral discs when there is marked paraspinal muscle spasm.

Lateral flexion is again a movement of the spine which is difficult to determine accurately. Pure side-bending should allow the fingertips to approximate to knee-level in most normal individuals. This is said to represent a 30° movement to the side, which is obviously a combination of thoracic and lumbar spinal movement.

Similarly, rotation of the spine is a compound movement of the thoracic and lumbar sections. The majority of the movement occurs in the thoracic spine, and it is best estimated viewing the patient from above when the subject is sitting on a flat surface. This position negates pelvic movement and the estimate of rotation is made by viewing the shoulders and estimating the angle made with the fixed pelvis. The normal rotation to either side is from 0° to 45° (see Fig. 4.4).

As in the clinical assessment of the cervical spine the rhythm of spinal movements is as important as the ranges obtained.

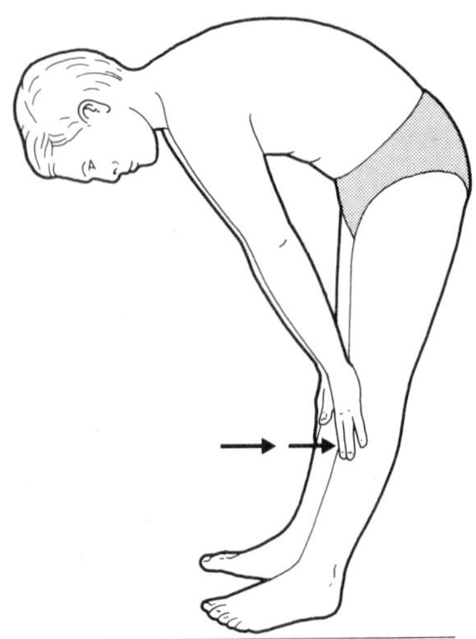

Fig. 4.3 Coarse assessment of lumbar flexion.

REFERRED PAIN IN THE UPPER LIMB FROM THE CERVICAL SPINE

Pain arising in the neck because of cervical disease is often accompanied by pain referred into the upper limb. If pain is present in the upper limb a neurological examination should be performed with emphasis on the diagnosis of nerve root compromise.

Sensation should be assessed by the appreciation of light touch and pinprick. As a guide, C5 supplies the skin on the outer aspect of the shoulder and upper arm. C6 supplies the radial border of the forearm, the thumb and forefinger. C7 supplies the middle finger and C8 the ulnar border of the hand and forearm. T1 supplies the inner border of the upper arm. Sensation should be tested for by the appreciation of light touch and pinprick (see Fig. 4.5).

Muscle power should be graded according to the

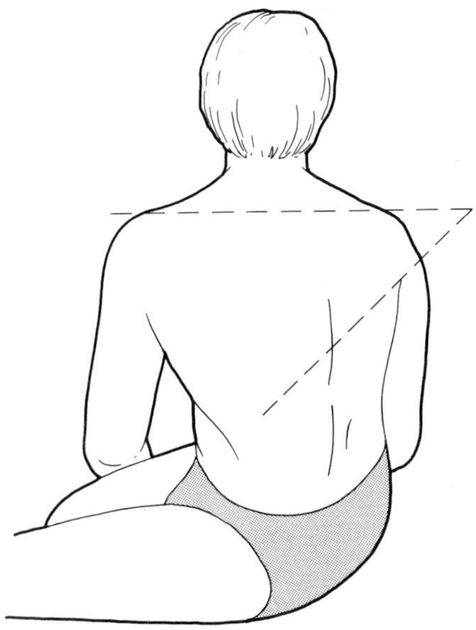

Fig. 4.4 Assessment of combined thoracic and lumbar rotation. The seated position prevents pelvic rotation.

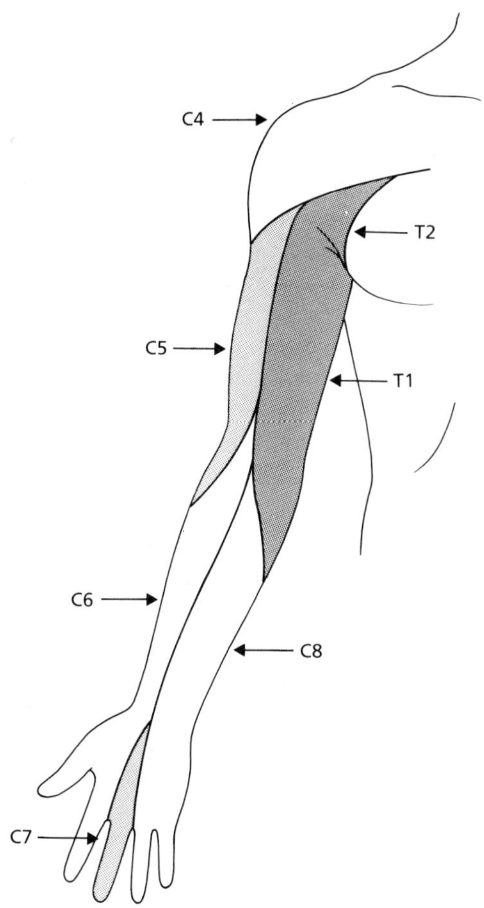

Fig. 4.5 Sensory dermatomes in the upper limb.

MRC classification when the patient attempts full power against resistance. Abduction of the shoulder is a good indication of C5 function. Flexion at the elbow is represented by C5 and C6. Extension at the elbow is an indicator of C7 and C8. Wrist dorsiflexion and palmar flexion is represented by the C6 and C7 nerve roots. The power of grip in the hand is a good test of C7 and C8 function. Tests for intrinsic muscle function in the hand, such as the ability to move the middle finger from side to side in the neutral position, tests for T1 function.

As will be obvious from the description of muscle power the biceps jerk represents C5, C6 and the triceps jerk C7 and C8. These reflexes are best tested with the elbow flexed to 90° and supported across the patient's lap.

PAIN REFERRED TO THE LEG FROM THE LUMBAR SPINE

The commonest cause of pain in the lower limb as a result of back pathology is sciatica as a result of an intervertebral disc prolapse. Disc prolapse is most common at L5–S1 and L4–L5; therefore the two most frequently compromised nerve roots are S1 and L5. In these circumstances pain is usually referred down the posterior aspect of the thigh from the lumbar spine or buttock, terminating in the distribution of the nerve involved. Pain is usually more intense in the upper part of the limb, whereas paraesthesiae—in the form of tingling, numbness or a sensation of trickling in the limb—is usually more common distally. It is important to realize, however, that other nerve roots may be involved by prolapsed disc material such as L3 or L4, resulting in pain in the anterior aspects of the thigh. Frank complaints of weakness are uncommon with an S1 nerve root lesion but are not uncommon when an L5 nerve root is affected. In the latter case a quite profound foot drop may develop before medical advice is sought. It is important to appreciate that pain felt in the back of the thigh but not below the knee is commonly caused by noxious stimuli arising in the lower lumbar facet joints. This pain is not usually caused by direct impingement on the ventral ramus, but is a referred type of pain mediated via the posterior primary ramus. The signs of nerve root irritation to be described later are not apparent in such a case. Nerve root dysfunction in the lumbosacral region is not always caused by a prolapsed disc. Central and lateral canal stenosis of the spine may also lead to nerve root dysfunction by compression. Other more sinister pathologies, such as intra- or extramedullary tumours or spinal infections with collapse, may also mimic the prolapsed disc.

Examination of straight leg raising

The patient's limb should be slowly raised whilst one of the examiner's hands maintains full knee extension (see Fig. 4.6). It should be recorded at which point the patient experiences pain in the leg. The limb should be dropped a few degrees from this position and then the foot slowly dorsiflexed. This manoeuvre again stretches the sciatic nerve and should produce a return of the pain in the same distribution. Also in this position a few degrees below the painful position, firm pressure should be applied to the popliteal fossa over the posterior tibial nerve. Pain in the limb is an indication of nerve root irritation. If pain is appreciated in the affected limb when the normal limb is raised this is a very strong indication of nerve root entrapment. This is because tension is exerted across the dural sac by the nerve root in the normal limb against a relatively fixed root on the painful side which is trapped by extruded disc material. This sign is known as the crossed-leg positive response. If a hysterical response is suspected on performing this straight leg raising test it is useful to ask the patient to sit up from the examination couch with the legs fully extended. Such an individual is often able to do this, and when sitting upright effectively 90° of straight leg raising is produced bilaterally.

Sensation to the anterior aspect of the thighs is mediated by the L3 and L4 nerve roots. The L4 root continues down the inner aspect of the lower leg, stopping short of the ankle joint. L5 nerve root sensation is distributed across the anterior aspect of the shin and on to the dorsomedial aspect of the foot. A highly reliable site for testing the L5 sensation is the skin between the first and second toes dorsally. S1 sensation is appreciated on the lateral side of the shin, the outer border of the foot and the sole of the foot. A most reliable site of testing sensation in the S1 distribution is the skin below and anterior to the lateral malleolus. As in the upper limb, sensation should be tested for both light touch and pinprick (see Fig. 4.7).

As in the upper limb, motor power in the lower limb should be expressed by the MRC grades. In the

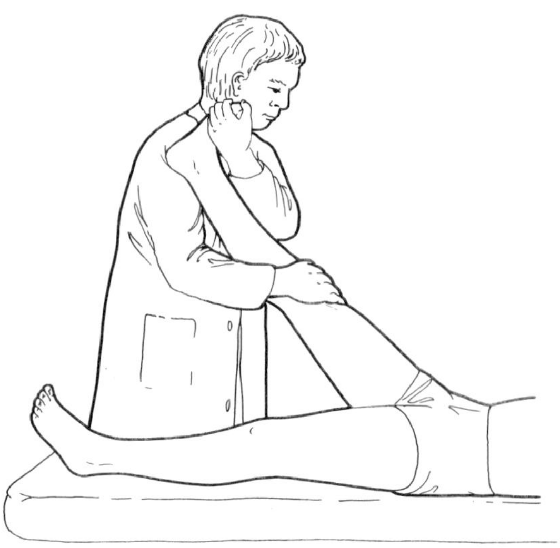

Fig. 4.6 Correct method of examining straight leg raising.

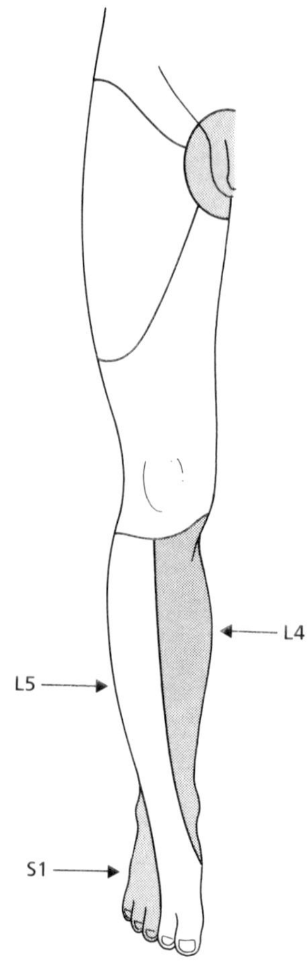

Fig. 4.7 Sensory dermatomes in the lower limb.

presence of sciatica or pain in the femoral nerve distribution testing muscle power around the hip joint is difficult. Extension of the knee represents the L3 and L4 nerve roots and flexion L5. Dorsiflexion of the foot and toes is a mixture of L4 (tibialis anterior) and L5. Plantarflexion is mainly subserved by the S1 nerve root. A profound dysfunction of the L5 nerve root results in a dropped foot. When the S1 nerve root is greatly compromised the patient is unable to stand on tiptoes on the affected side. Wasting of the lower limb may be present in long-standing lesions.

The knee jerk represents the L3, L4 nerve roots. The ankle jerk response is largely subserved by the L5 nerve root but also to a lesser extent by S2. A little-known reflex is the tibialis posterior reflex obtained by tapping the tibialis posterior tendon near to its insertion on the navicular. This response is entirely mediated by the L5 nerve root. Similarly another little-known reflex which is purely for the S1 nerve root is the response produced following scratching the sole of the foot. Normally this stimulation produces a contraction in the tensor fascia lata muscle.

Inappropriate signs

A number of physical signs have been described which are often associated with an hysterical symptom complex (Waddell *et al.*, 1984). If a vertical force is applied to the patient's head by the examiner it is extremely rare for this to reproduce organic back or leg pain. The rare exceptions to this are severe vertebral disease consequent upon infection or tumour. Spinal rotation may indeed induce pain when the pelvis has been anchored. However, the patient may feel that the spine is being rotated if the trunk is turned by holding the pelvis. This movement does not, of course, rotate the spine at all, and should not induce pain in spinal disease. Even in the presence of quite marked spinal tenderness, light pinching of the skin over the tender area should not elicit painful response.

Abdominal and breast examination

No examination of the spine is complete without a routine abdominal examination, and examination of the breasts in a female. Back pain and referred leg pain may be induced by various abdominal malignancies, in particular pancreatic carcinoma. An aortic aneurysm is usually readily palpable and commonly associated with lumbar pain. The breast is a potent site for malignant disease which may produce spinal pain from secondary deposits.

THE EXAMINATION OF NON-DISCOGENIC BACK PAIN

In addition to the syndrome associated with the prolapsed intervertebral disc a number of other syndromes have been described as aetiologies for back and referred pain. The posterior facet syndrome has already been mentioned and is probably the most common cause of acute and chronic low back pain. The cardinal clinical features are local tenderness over the facet joints, pain on hyperextension of the spine and an absence of true neurological signs indicative of nerve root compromise. The sacroiliac syndrome is an ill-understood pain syndrome arising in joints that normally have very little excursion. These joints can be stressed by various manoeuvres usually involving flexion of the ipsilateral hip and rotation. It is hard to imagine how pain can arise in these joints unless they have been disrupted by previous severe trauma. Various other myofascial syndromes are described, such as the gluteus medius syndrome, the gluteus maximus syndrome and the quadratus lumborum syndrome. Specific tests exist to stress all of these muscles. The true nature of these conditions remains poorly documented.

THE ASSESSMENT OF MYELOPATHY

Careful clinical evaluation of the patient as described above, in conjunction with modern radiological assessment, will usually allow an accurate diagnosis to be made. However, in some situations, diagnosis will remain in doubt. This is most frequently encountered in patients presenting with signs and symptoms of spinal cord disease but with normal radiology. Many diseases—some common, some rare—may present in this manner. In fact, virtually any condition which affects the nervous system may present as an apparent spinal cord lesion. The pathological changes may be entirely limited to the spinal cord, its covering meninges, or its blood vessels, or there may be clinical or laboratory evidence providing clues to systemic disease or involvement of extraspinal sites within the nervous system. The surgical causes of spinal cord disease are extensively covered in other chapters of this book. This chapter deals with the differential diagnosis of isolated, non-compressive myelopathies.

Symptoms of spinal cord disease

Whether the pathology is compressive or non-compressive, the initial symptoms in a chronic or insidious cord syndrome are often problems with gait. These can be attributed to involvement of the pyramidal tracts (upper motor neurone). Patients may have difficulty in describing their gait problem, merely noticing that something is wrong with their legs. Complaints of an inability to run may precede difficulty with walking. The legs are felt to be 'heavy', 'stiff' or even 'numb', although no sensory involvement may be obvious on examination. Initial symptoms may only be noted on exercise. Early difficulties may occur while ascending stairs, due to the differential weakness of flexor movements. The patient may complain of cramps, spasms or spontaneous clonus. Relatives or friends may notice the scuffing feet, the stiffness and the unsteadiness. There may be 'unexplained' falls due to tripping over minor obstacles such as paving stones. Formal examination at this stage may reveal no definite signs, but particular care should be taken to observe the patient's gait, which may have a stiff or jerky quality. One limb may move less freely, perhaps with slight circumduction. The toes of the shoes may scuff the ground and show uneven wear. If the upper limbs are involved there may be failure to swing an arm on walking.

Lower motor neurone involvement may cause no symptoms even when clinical signs such as wasting, fasciculation and weakness may be easily detected by a physician. Some patients with motor neurone disease do become aware of thinning of the intrinsic muscles of the hands, particularly if there is clumsiness or loss of dexterity or, occasionally, fasciculation in limb muscles may attract attention. A lower motor neurone foot drop may be a dramatic early symptom of anterior horn cell damage. Pain is frequently an early symptom when there is structural damage to the spine. Pressure effects or erosion of vertebral bone cause pain, which may be related to posture and is non-specifically described as deep, dull or aching. Central pain from cord damage, for example, arising from lesions in the ascending spinothalamic tracts, is usually poorly localized and described as burning or boring sensations below the level of the lesion and without segmental distribution. If the posterior sensory nerve roots are affected by pressure, traction or infiltration, pain may be referred to all or part of the dermatome involved. The pain is usually described as shooting, sharp or tearing. It is characteristically provoked or made worse by coughing or straining and may be worse at night.

Damage to sensory spinal cord pathways results in a wide range of early complaints. Perhaps the most important cause of diagnostic errors in the early stages of a myelopathy are those due to lesions in the spinothalamic tracts. These symptoms are often difficult for the patient to describe and can easily be attributed in error to degenerative skeletal symptoms or to psychiatric problems. The patient may complain of sensations of 'wetness', or of insects moving under the skin (formication), of icy-cold feelings, of warmth or burning, a deep poorly localized aching pain, or peculiar descriptions of pain and dysaesthesiae such as 'razor blades digging into the leg'. Hyperaesthesiae may cause errors in lateralization unless the quality of the stimulus is assessed.

Pathological lesions affecting the posterior columns may give rise to quite different symptoms including tingling paraesthesiae in the limbs and tight, squeezing, band-like sensations around the trunk or joints. The skin may also seem stretched or 'swollen' or covered by a layer of cloth so that any stimulus may seem 'distant'. These paraesthesiae often coexist with segmental pain. They may be present with or without evidence of sensory loss.

Lesions involving the spinal roots or root entry zones may produce sensory symptoms of pain, numbness or paraesthesiae in segmental distribution. Root pains are likely to be exacerbated by coughing or sneezing and by spinal movements. Hyperaesthesiae may precede impairment of light touch or pain in the dermatome. When these symptoms occur on the trunk they may be attributed to intra-abdominal or thoracic pathology, unless the possibility of a root lesion is considered.

Spinal cord lesions which involve the autonomic innervation of the bladder may cause frequency, urgency and urge incontinence. The bladder may be spastic and irritated by quite small volumes. There may be associated loss of potency. It is important to ask for specific details of bladder function as they may not be spontaneously volunteered. In more acute and severe lesions such as transverse myelitis, an automatic bladder may result in reflex emptying. When damage to the motor and sensory control occurs, as with lesions in the cauda equina, there may be lack of sensation of bladder fullness, with resulting high residual volumes and dribbling incontinence.

With high cervical lesions, pain in the occipital region or face may occur with or without pain in the neck and shoulder region. The pain is often exacer bated by coughing, sneezing or movements of the spine. There may be associated complaints of paraesthesiae or numbness of the face due to damage to the descending tract of the trigeminal nerve. Lhermitte's sign, a sudden electric shock-like sensation shooting down the back into the legs, may occur on neck flexion. Either extramedullary or central medullary cord lesions may result in a suspended sensory level, perhaps over the neck, shoulders and upper trunk with normal sensation to pain below, or 'sacral sparing'. In a particularly rapidly evolving cervical cord lesion there may be remarkable discrepancies between the spinothalamic sensory level and the motor level; the sensory level may initially be far below the lesion, later rising perhaps in stepwise fashion to a segment or two below. This phenomenon has been attributed to progressive involvement of the vascular supply to the laminations of the spinothalamic tracts. The ipsilateral arm may be weak with wasting of the small intrinsic muscles of the hand (C8–T1), a finding that has been explained on the basis of involvement of the anterior spinal artery. The highest lesions at foramen magnum level may also produce posterior fossa symptoms, and careful attention should be paid to the lower cranial nerves.

Horner's syndrome, although usually asymptomatic, may be noticed by the patient. It may occur with pathology above the level of the first thoracic segment and may provide localizing clues to a lesion near the cervicothoracic junction if other non-spinal possibilities can be eliminated.

Pain in the thoracic region may be mistaken for gallbladder, intra-abdominal or even hip disease. Lesions of the conus may present with complaints of numbness on the buttocks, often noticed for the first time when sitting on the toilet (saddle analgesia).

Signs of spinal cord disease

It is important that examination of tone, power, reflexes, sensation, coordination, gait and visceral function is careful and complete, to avoid errors of localization of spinal cord lesions. The assessment must include higher function and the cranial nerves, where abnormalities, perhaps subtle, may indicate that the disease process is not confined to, or perhaps not even arising from, the spinal cord.

Although spinal cord anatomy offers only a limited number of possible reactions to disease processes, some common and distinctive patterns allow some syndromes to be described which occur more often with certain pathologies. These include chronic or slowly progressive spastic paraparesis or quadraparesis with or without ataxia and acute partial or complete spinal cord transection

The presentation of a chronic but progressive spastic paraparesis is a common diagnostic problem in both neurological and neurosurgical practice. In young adults, when compression has been excluded, multiple sclerosis (MS) would be the most likely diagnosis, but even in older patients the progressive spinal form of MS is much more commonly encountered than such classical conditions as subacute combined degeneration of the cord, neurosyphilis, syringomyelia or motor neurone disease. If the patient is a child or adolescent with a slowly developing syndrome, then Friedreich's ataxia, hereditary spastic paraparesis or less common forms of spinocerebellar degeneration need to be considered.

In a pure upper motor neurone cord lesion (as in some cases of motor neurone disease and MS) there may be spasticity and clonus in the lower limbs, exaggerated reflexes and extensor plantar responses. To detect a 'spastic catch' in one section of the arc ('clasp-knife' rigidity), the limbs should be rapidly flexed and extended passively through their full range. The ankle should be firmly, rapidly and passively dorsiflexed to demonstrate clonus. Weakness may be apparent in the flexors of the limb, such as the hip and knee flexors and dorsiflexors of the foot. In the early stages, slowness of toe-tapping may be the only sign on the affected side. The abdominal reflexes may all be lost, particularly when the cord lesion is due to MS, but may be retained in the hereditary paraplegias. If the upper limbs become involved (spastic quadraparesis), then a catch on rapid alternating supination and pronation of the forearm ('supinator catch'), may be the earliest sign. Weakness may be apparent in the shoulder abductors, the extensors of elbow, wrist and fingers, and the finger abductors. There may be brisk finger jerks and a Hoffman's reflex. It should be remembered that clumsiness of the hands on rapid alternating movements or on precision movements, as in the 'finger–nose' and 'heel–

shin' tests, is to be expected in the presence of upper motoneurone spasticity and weakness, and should not be attributed to an additional cerebellar problem.

Special attention should be paid to the gait, not only for stiffness, rigidity and balance problems, but for the subtle scuffing of the toes of one foot and the poor swinging of a spastic arm. Can the patient run? Is there instability or hesitation on turning? The limbs and shoulder girdle/scapular area should be inspected for fasciculation or wasting. Absent deep tendon reflexes may also indicate a mixed upper and lower motor neurone syndrome due to additional involvement of nerve roots or anterior horn cell problems.

The sensory examination may reveal loss of vibration and proprioception in the toes or feet of a young adult with suspected MS, or loss of vibration sense below the level of a compressive lesion in the spine. Pain sensation may be lost contralaterally, one or two segments below the level of a lesion in the spinothalamic tract (Brown–Séquard type lesion) or bilaterally, as in transverse myelitis. Light touch is often unhelpful in sorting out a level as it travels in more than one pathway and may be spared until the cord is severely compromised.

Is the pathology in the spinal cord?

Neurological disease in other areas of the nervous system can be confused with pathology in the spinal cord or spine. It is clearly important to make an accurate anatomical diagnosis to avoid potentially dangerous or inappropriate investigations. Possible traps include cerebral disease, particularly diffuse cerebrovascular involvement of both hemispheres, hydrocephalus or a parasagittal meningioma. Rarely, acute peripheral neuropathies (particularly postinfectious polyneuropathy) may be mistaken in the early stages for acute myelitis.

Intracerebral pathology

A tumour of the hemisphere or falx is now, with the aid of the computerized tomography (CT) scan, largely a localization problem of the past. The parasagittal meningioma which results in a symmetric spastic paraparesis is rare. Similarly, posterior fossa tumours causing compression of the lower brain stem or upper cervical cord, will usually give rise to some brain stem signs, for example nystagmus, hearing loss, absent corneal reflex or wasting of the tongue, and should be easily diagnosed in most cases by CT or magnetic resonance imaging (MRI) scans.

A careful history from the patient and the relatives, or the presence on examination of loss of memory or defective cognition, should avoid mistaking the abnormal truncal gait (ataxic heel–toe walking) and bladder symptoms in 'normal-pressure' hydrocephalus with spinal cord pathology, while CT scanning will reveal the diagnosis.

The patient with atherosclerotic cerebral disease may have a shuffling gait and loss of balance associated with extensor plantar responses, but there are usually other clues in the history (e.g. smoking, hypertension, diabetes) or on examination (e.g. emotional incontinence, dysarthria, brisk jaw jerk, personality change, dementia or dysphasia) which indicate that the level is above the foramen magnum.

Peripheral pathology mistaken for spinal cord lesion

Occasionally, patients with a rapid onset of weakness in the lower limbs due to acute radiculopathy or peripheral neuropathy are subjected, unnecessarily, to myelography (particularly when, in the early stages, the weakness appears mainly proximal and when there may be slight difficulty initiating micturition), although the generalized areflexia, lack of upper motor neurone signs or a sensory level on the trunk and the presence perhaps of bulbar signs (such as easily missed mild bilateral facial weakness or sensory symptoms), should all indicate that the pathology is in the peripheral nerves, and the diagnosis to consider is acute postinfectious polyneuropathy (Guillain–Barré syndrome). An electrophysiological examination rather than myelography is indicated.

Similar difficulties occasionally occur when physicians with little experience of spinal cord disease encounter acute muscle or endplate disease such as polymyositis or myasthenia gravis. A careful history and examination will disclose the true nature of these conditions and avoid inappropriate investigations.

Differential diagnosis of non-compressive myelopathies

In many patients, spinal cord signs or symptoms may occur in the context of a known pre-existing systemic illness, for example, neoplasia, polyarteritis or sarcoidosis, so that the diagnosis is usually obvious. In the context of isolated spinal cord disease with no

Table 4.1 Causes of non-compressive myelopathy

Hereditary
Familial spastic paraplegia
Spinocerebellar ataxias
Adrenomyeloleukodystrophy

Congenital/developmental
Arnold–Chiari malformation
Syringomyelia
Diastomyelia

Demyelinating disease
Multiple sclerosis
Acute disseminated encephalomyelitis

Neoplasia
Lymphoma
Ischaemic myelopathy
Acute necrotizing myelopathy
Paraneoplastic myelitis

Infections
Viral myelitis:
  measles, mumps, influenza, poliomyelitis, herpes zoster, herpes simplex, hepatitis, enteroviruses, infectious mononucleosis (Epstein–Barr), varicella, vaccinia, coxsackie, HTLV-I, AIDS, dengue, rabies
Bacterial:
  tuberculous, pyogenic
Spirochaetal:
  syphilis, Lyme disease
Fungal:
  Actinomyces, aspergillosis, *Cryptococcus*
Parasitic:
  schistosomiasis, cysticercosis, malaria, trichinosis

Vascular
Atherosclerotic
Spinal artery thrombosis
Systemic lupus erythematosus
Polyarteritis nodosa
Neoplastic associated (see above)
Polycythaemia
Postcardiac arrest
Heroin addiction
Sarcoidosis
Aortic dissection/coarctation
Vascular malformations

Toxic
Nitrous oxide
Arsenic
Penicillin
Spinal anaesthetics
Lathyrism

Physical agents
Electric shock
Radiation

Allergic or reactive
Postvaccination
Postinfectious (exanthems)
Acute necrotizing haemorrhagic encephalomyelitis

Metabolic and deficiency syndromes
B_{12} deficiency
Folate deficiency
? Hyperparathyroidism
Thyroid disease
Hepatic myelopathy
Leigh's necrotizing encephalomyelitis
Pellagra

known pre-existing condition the diagnostic possibilities are protean, as almost any pathological process that can involve the nervous system may cause selective damage to the spinal cord (Table 4.1). Thus routine tests to exclude treatable conditions are mandatory (Table 4.2) although there are many possible additional tests which could be indicated by specific features of the history or examination. In most cases these tests will be negative and, in the UK, if compression and developmental abnormalities have also been excluded by myelography and there is no family history of spinocerebellar disease, the most likely diagnosis will be MS. The following account will concentrate on the diagnosis of spinal MS and its differentiation from other less commonly encountered conditions.

Multiple sclerosis

It has been estimated that about 45% of patients with MS have symptoms and signs which can be accounted for by a single lesion, and about half of these have only motor weakness (McAlpine, 1972). In one random sample from a large survey, approximately 29% of patients with MS had symptoms and signs limited to the spinal cord (Leibowitz *et al.*, 1967). In that study the authors identified two main spinal cord syndromes, namely a chronic progressive type of spinal MS and a chronic relapsing or remitting form (estimated to be 22% and 7% of the MS population, respectively).

Many of these patients typically present in middle-age, with symptoms or signs resembling a subacute or

Table 4.2 Tests to exclude potentially treatable causes of myelopathy

Condition	Test
In all cases	Myelography/MRI of cord
	CSF, cells, protein, sugar, IgG/albumin, oligoclonal bands
	Routine haematology/biochemistry including ESR, urea, electrolytes blood sugar
	Serum B_{12} Serum/red cell folate
	Syphilis serology, e.g. TPHA etc.
	T4/TSH
Other tests which may be indicated	
Multiple sclerosis	MRI brain (T2-weighted images ± Gadolinium) Visual/auditory evoked potentials
Adrenomyeloleukodsytrophy	Free fatty acids, steroid levels
Viral myelitis	Virology, including HTLV-I if high risk
SLE	Autoantibodies
Sarcoidosis	Ca^{2+}, Kveim, CXR
Malignancy	CSF cytology

chronic cord compression syndrome. The findings are often an asymmetric spastic paraparesis which gives rise to the aphorism, 'symptoms in one leg and signs in both'. Here there may be clues in the past history (perhaps a long-forgotten episode of optic neuritis or vertigo) or on examination (such as optic pallor or nystagmus), but frequently there are no obvious signs or symptoms above the level of the foramen magnum. Nevertheless, careful examination for a paracentral scotoma, testing of colour vision or spatial contrast sensitivity, fundoscopy and visual evoked potentials, may provide evidence of past visual involvement likely to be due to optic neuritis.

MS may also present as an acute or subacute spinal cord syndrome. There may be a transverse myelitis with flaccid paralysis and retention of urine, perhaps with severe pain, or a partial cord lesion (such as Brown–Séquard lesion). In other cases the symptoms may be purely sensory. There may be a rapid onset of numbness or paraesthesiae in the feet, buttocks and perineum, perhaps extending to give symptomatic band-like sensations or numbness on the trunk. There may be little to find on examination; the reflexes may be normal or brisk, the plantar responses flexor or extensor. There may be a clear spinothalamic level to pinprick and/or temperature sensation, or the changes may be more subtle with the patient merely reporting that sensory stimuli seem distant, as though testing is occurring through thick stockings. While the 'syndrome' may be purely sensory, there may be slight motor symptoms such as stiffness or heaviness of the legs and urgency of micturition. Sensory symptoms may be entirely limited to Lhermitte's phenomenon.

In any of these syndromes, myelography or MRI scanning of the cord is essential, as no clinical features appear to reliably separate spinal cord compression from demyelinating disease (Poser *et al.*, 1978). Although segmental wasting, a chronic sensory level on the trunk and radicular pain are more commonly associated with compressive lesions, they may all occur occasionally in MS.

When MS is suspected in patients with syndromes symptomatically and objectively limited to the spinal cord, modern laboratory tests including MRI and evoked potential recordings can provide evidence of multiple lesions elsewhere in the nervous system (Table 4.3). The most sensitive of these is MRI scanning of the brain which can reveal typical (but non-specific) lesions on T2-weighted images in 69–82% of apparently spinal cases. There is less certainty of the relevance of such findings in patients over the age of 50 years, as similar lesions, presumably due to minor asymptomatic vascular changes with age, can be de-

Table 4.3 Prevalence of abnormal tests providing laboratory support for demyelinating disease in patients with 'undiagnosed' myelopathy

		Cerebrospinal fluid			Evoked potentials			
Series	No.	Cells	IgG	OB	VER	AER/BLR	CT	MRI
Paty *et al.* (1978)	72	—	—	44%	44%	56%	4%[a]	—
Paty *et al.* (1988)	52	—	—	62%	54%	—	21%	69%
Miller *et al.* (1987)	94	—	—	33%	28%	15%	—	82%
Blumhardt *et al.* (1991b)	69	36%	41%	38%	20%	19%	4%[a]	74%

[a] Enhancing lesions on double-dose delayed CT.
BLR, blink reflex; IgG, immunoglobulin G/albumin ratio; OB, oligoclonal bands; VER, visual evoked response; AER, auditory evoked response; CT, computerized axial tomography; MRI, magnetic resonance imaging.

monstrated in healthy control subjects (Ormerod *et al.*, 1987). CT scanning, even with the delayed double-dose technique, has a very low sensitivity for the silent demyelinating lesion in such cases, although non-specific cerebral atrophy may be present in a higher proportion.

Other routine investigations which may demonstrate 'clinically silent' extraspinal involvement, or confirm that earlier, perhaps vaguely described or recalled symptoms are relevant to the spinal cord syndrome, include the visual or short-latency brain stem auditory evoked potentials. Here, the sensitivity is lower than that found in clinically definite MS and again the delays are non-specific for demyelinating lesions. Care must be taken to correlate the recordings with the clinical assessment of the visual system to avoid misinterpreting abnormal potentials from unrelated conditions such as glaucoma, amblyopia or high refractive disorder. Other conditions which can cause a combination of spinal cord and optic nerve lesion such as neurosyphilis or sarcoidosis need to be carefully excluded. In acute partial cord syndromes the proportion with abnormalities is even less, perhaps of the order of 5–11% (Blumhardt *et al.*, 1982). In one small series of 12 patients with acute transverse myelitis no EP abnormalities were detected (Ropper *et al.*, 1982).

Further laboratory support may be obtained for the diagnosis of MS by examination of the CSF for abnormal immunoglobulins (elevated IgG/albumin ratio and oligoclonal bands) although again, these are found in a lower proportion of cases than in CDMS (Table 4.3). Although these are non-specific abnormalities, they will allow classification at a higher degree of diagnostic certainty (Poser *et al.*, 1983) providing other inflammatory conditions have been excluded.

Other tests, less often applied as routine investigations, include electro-oculography and electronystagmography (perhaps combined with heating the patient to further impair conduction in demyelinated fibres) which may provide evidence of unsuspected brain stem dysfunction (Jestico & Ellis, 1976) and neuropsychometry or long-latency cognitive evoked potentials, which can reveal defects of memory or impaired intellect impairment (Newton *et al.*, 1990; Blumhardt *et al.*, 1991a). Finally, if a patient with cord disease and negative myelography has no evidence of extraspinal lesions or oligoclonal bands, then he or she should be followed until the symptoms and signs resolve (a course of events which makes MS likely) or the diagnosis becomes clear. Other conditions which mimic MS must be excluded.

The precise proportion of undiagnosed cases in a representative sample of newly presenting myelopathy patients is uncertain. One retrospective survey, carried out prior to the introduction of many of the modern tests, suggested that 6% of patients with paraparesis remained undiagnosed, although a further 2.5% were also undiagnosed but considered to have possible MS on the basis of elevated CSF gammaglobulins (Ungar-Sargon *et al.*, 1980). Other reports have been based on samples of referred cases which may or may not have been representative. An early autopsy study showed that 34% of the chronic undiagnosed cases had MS (Marshall, 1955), but this was before the availability of modern water-soluble contrast agents. Undoubtedly, fewer tumours will now be missed, so that a higher proportion of the patients remaining undiagnosed should turn out to have MS.

Two follow-up studies of undiagnosed chronic progressive spastic paraparesis revealed a similar proportion of patients developing MS (20–25%) some eight to 10 years after presenting (Marshall, 1955; Hubbe & Dam, 1973). By contrast, only 3% of patients with acute transverse myelitis developed MS after a five to 42-year follow-up (Lipton & Teasdale, 1973). No prognostic data are available on the acute, remitting partial spinal cord syndromes which have been considered to be more common.

When a diagnosis of MS is being considered, several other conditions which may have a similar clinical picture must be excluded.

There may be clinically obvious involvement of the nervous system in up to 42% of cases with systemic lupus erythematosus (SLE) (Abel *et al.*, 1980). Although there is often evidence of the systemic nature of the illness, this may be unobtrusive and easily missed. Neurological lesions may cause the initial presentation or may occur in isolation. The symptoms may closely mimic MS; for example, there may be varying combinations of myelopathy with optic nerve lesions. Myelopathy is a rare complication occurring in less than 2% of cases (Ellis & Verity, 1979) when other manifestations of the disease are present, but it may precede the diagnosis (Andreanakos *et al.*, 1975). It may be acute or subacute, suggesting either an infarction or a demyelinating lesion (Kewelramani *et al.*, 1978) or slowly progressive with or without remissions (Penn & Rowan, 1968). Nonspecific findings on laboratory tests may include a raised CSF protein, IgG/albumin ratio, oligoclonal bands, CSF pleocytosis and MRI lesions indistinguishable from MS (Ormerod *et al.*, 1987). Syphilis serology may be positive. More specific tests, such as a search for antinuclear factor or anti-DNA binding antibodies, will provide diagnostic confirmation.

Patients with CNS involvement from polyarteritis nodosa (PAN) are usually systemically ill with other symptoms and signs of the condition, including renal and pulmonary involvement. About 2% of cases with acute necrotizing vasculitis develop an acute or chronic transverse myelopathy (Malamud & Foster, 1942).

The rare granulomatous angiitis may be complicated in 15% of cases by a relapsing and remitting myelopathy (Sigal, 1987) which is often confused with MS (Kolodny *et al.*, 1968; Rawlinson & Braun, 1981). There may be headache, changes in cognition and altered levels of consciousness. The ESR is elevated in 70% of cases.

An estimated 5% of patients with sarcoidosis have CNS involvement (Delaney, 1977) and some have either a progressive or acute spinal cord syndrome indistinguishable from MS. The myelogram may be normal or reveal a granulomatous block (Buge *et al.*, 1975). Most cases have an abnormal CSF with pleocytosis and raised protein, together with other signs of systemic illness such as lymphadenopathy, changes on the chest X-ray, hepatic or dermatological complications.

In the rare Behcet's syndrome, 4–42% may have neurological involvement (Chajek & Fainaru, 1975) including acute or subacute myelopathies, which may mimic MS. Of these, as many as 18% may present as an acute paraplegia (Fadli & Yousef, 1973; Motomura *et al.*, 1980). Coexistent systemic symptoms such as fever, headache, meningeal irritation and perhaps an organic mental syndrome, may be present. The characteristic mucocutaneous ulceration (on history or examination) of the buccal mucosa and the genitalia, provides the necessary evidence for the diagnosis. The relapsing and remitting nature of the symptoms and signs may confuse the condition with MS, although the ESR is often elevated.

The classical syndrome of tabes dorsalis with 'lightning pains', areflexia, ataxia, extensor plantar responses and hypotonia is now rarely seen in the UK. Clues may be found in the loss of deep pain sensation (squeeze the tendoachilles), painless arthopathy ('Charcot joints') and light-near dissociated, small and irregular pupils, perhaps with optic atrophy and delayed visual evoked responses. Meningovascular syphilis may also present as a myelopathy. The diagnosis is often suspected when the CSF reveals a high white cell count and protein, and will be confirmed by serological tests on blood and CSF.

FAMILIAL AND DEGENERATIVE CONDITIONS

Hereditary spastic paraplegia needs to be distinguished from MS. Here there may be a family history or a motor delay in walking. The condition may be dominant or recessive and the age at onset may vary from childhood to as late as the sixth decade (Roe, 1963). Despite the marked spasticity and the severe gait disability, power may be relatively well preserved (Bickerstaff, 1970). The abdominal reflexes are usually preserved (Wilson, 1940) and pes cavus is present in about one-third (Harding, 1981). There may be loss of ankle jerks and vibration sense, but the peripheral sensory conduction is usually intact (Thomas *et al.*, 1981). Progression is slow and bladder involvement is unusual in the early stages. Less common forms occur with associated features such as wasting of the hands, mental retardation, retinal degeneration, optic atrophy, ataxia, skin pigmentation, neuropathy or extrapyramidal signs, and have been reviewed in detail (Harding, 1984).

A rare condition which is not uncommonly mistaken for MS (Elrington *et al.*, 1989) is the adult-onset form of adrenoleukomyelodystrophy. This condition affects adults of both sexes and usually presents as a spastic paraparesis after the second decade along with hypoadrenalism, hypogonadism and polyneuropathy (Hiryama, 1972). The diagnosis rests on the clinical features including hyperpigmentation, the MRI appearances of a leukodystrophy, the accumulation of very long-chain fatty acids in the blood and the demonstration of hypoadrenalism (synacthen test).

In the classic mixed picture of amyotrophic lateral sclerosis, a variety of motor neurone disease, there should be no difficulty with diagnosis. However, some patients who go on eventually to a definite diagnosis of MND, initially present with a 'pure' upper motor neurone syndrome with no sensory loss, their spastic paraparesis then mimicking cord compression. The mistake made most frequently is to proceed to invasive investigation such as myelography when attention paid to the history may reveal emotional change (lability), dysarthria or dysphagia, while careful examination of the relaxed limbs, shoulder girdle and tongue may reveal fasciculation or early wasting of one or both hands. Electrophysiology should be carried out to confirm the presence of chronic denervation in the limb muscles and the absence of a motor neuropathy.

In Friedreich's ataxia there is a positive family history with pes cavus and kyphoscoliosis. The degeneration of the spinocerebellar and pyramidal tracts results in ataxia and extensor plantar responses, while damage to the peripheral nerves causes areflexia.

PHYSICAL AND TOXIC AGENTS

Here the most commonly encountered condition is radiation myelopathy. After irradiation to the chest or pharynx, cervical or mediastinal lymph nodes there is a variable delay of weeks before the symptoms of an early cervical myelopathy occur (Jones, 1964). The early syndrome is characterized by Lhermitte's symptom which usually resolves after some weeks. The prognosis in these cases is good. Chronic syndromes come on usually after a delay of three months, and often after many years. The initial stages of the late form are often characterized by loss of pain sensation and temperature sensation (which may be asymmetric), suggesting that the spinothalamic fibres are unusually susceptible to radiation damage (Jellinger & Sturm, 1971). This may either arrest or progress to a spastic paraparesis. Another form of the delayed myelopathy involves the anterior horn cells with a patchy lower motor neurone syndrome with weakness and loss of reflexes (motor neuronopathy) (Sadowsky *et al.*, 1976).

Rarely, electric shock may result in a permanent neurological abnormality, and this is often a cervical motor myelopathy (Alexander, 1938). There is usually an acute encephalomyelopathy, but eventually the residual myelopathy will become apparent or even develop within days of the shock. There is usually wasting of the upper limbs combined with a spastic paraparesis and little or no sensory involvement. A syndrome similar to motor neurone disease has been described following electric shock or lightning injuries (Paillas & Roger, 1949; Woods, 1952).

Well-recognized spinal toxins which can give rise to a rare toxic myelopathy include arsenic and intrathecal penicillin. Spinal anaesthesiae may also be rarely complicated by myelopathy. This may be acute at the time of the administration of the anaesthetic or delayed by weeks, months or even years and due to adhesive arachnoiditis. An acute transverse myelopathy has been described in heroin addicts, possibly due to a vasculitis (Ell *et al.*, 1981). The myeloneuronopathy which may occur in dentists abusing nitrous oxide has been associated with signs of B_{12} deficiency (Blanco & Peters, 1983). A transient or permanent paraplegia has been associated with the intrathecal use of methotrexate or cytosine arabinoside (Henson & Urich, 1982; Shapiro & Young, 1984).

METABOLIC AND DEFICIENCY DISORDERS

In pernicious anaemia the initial symptoms are usually tingling paraesthesiae progressively worsening and associated with areflexia, both due to peripheral nerve damage. The first evidence of central spinal cord damage (subacute degeneration of the cord) is the development of extensor plantar responses. In an untreated case, further deterioration will result in pyramidal weakness and severe ataxia due to degeneration of the pyramidal tracts and dorsal columns. In rare cases the signs of a neuropathy may be absent with dominant motor symptoms. Vitamin B_{12} estimations should therefore be made in all patients with an acute neuropathy with loss of reflexes and paraesthesiae in order to prevent irreversible central damage and in all undiagnosed myelopathies.

In patients with portocaval shunts (Pant *et al.*, 1968) and severely compromised hepatic function with recurrent encephalopathy, a spastic paraparesis (hepatic myelopathy) may develop insidiously (Bechar *et al.*, 1970). The signs may be misinterpreted as due to a coincident pathology, or confused with those resulting from the encephalopathy. There have been occasional case reports of pyramidal tract signs associated with thyrotoxicosis which have been (sometimes) reversed by treatment (Garcia & Fleming, 1977; Malamed *et al.*, 1975). The rare reports of cases resembling MND, with muscle wasting and extensor plantar responses, may be merely an association of two diseases (Logothetis, 1961; McMenamin & Croxon, 1980).

VIRAL OR POSTVIRAL SYNDROMES

Acute transverse myelitis may be associated with a variety of viruses including measles, mumps, influenza, the Epstein–Barr virus, herpes zoster and simplex and rubella. There may also be evidence of cerebral involvement (acute disseminated encephalomyelopathy). The onset is a variable time after exposure to a virus, although the predisposing agent or event is not always apparent. Usually a child or a young adult several days after the reaction from the infection will develop insidious or sudden weakness and paraplegia (Berman *et al.*, 1981). The condition is usually monophasic. A myelitis may rarely follow inoculation, usually within 10–14 days (postvaccination myelitis). There is usually an encephalomyelitis with the thoracic cord being particularly affected. Influenza immunization has been incriminated by several case reports, although the association may be no more than chance (Beghi *et al.*, 1982). Rabies vaccination with phenol-inactivated preparations containing myelin basic protein may result in myelitis (Hemachudha *et al.*, 1987). Several case reports of young females who have developed transverse myelitis with or without optic neuritis after rubella vaccination (Behan, 1977) may be no more than the onset of MS.

A human retrovirus (HTLV-I) appears to be involved in the pathogenesis of tropical spastic paraparesis (TSP) (HTLV-I myelopathy, HAM/TSP syndrome), a myelopathy formerly of unknown aetiology that was common in tropical areas where this virus is endemic (Osame *et al.*, 1986). Nearly 60% of TSP patients in the French West Indies have been found to have antibodies to this virus, as compared to 4% of controls (Gessain *et al.*, 1985). In a recent French report of cases originating from the West Indies, most had a chronic spastic paraparesis with mean age of onset 45 years (range 30–59 years) and duration of disease from one to 12 years (Gout *et al.*, 1989). Onset is usually insidious with fatiguable asymmetric lower limb weakness or urinary frequency, but the wide variety of features include urgency, incontinence or retention, back pain, paraesthesiae, ataxia, optic atrophy, loss of vibration sense and tinnitus. Laboratory tests show pleocytosis, abnormal IgG/albumin ratios, oligoclonal bands and delayed evoked potentials. MRI scans show appearances similar to MS. Neither steroids nor acyclovir have been shown to modify the disease course in one recent report (Gout *et al.*, 1989).

While a diagnosis of TSP should always be sought in patients from West Indian origins, most patients in the United Kingdom with a non-compressive myelopathy and abnormal signals in the cerebral white matter on MRI, would be assumed to have MS. A recent survey of over 2000 cases, coming to myelo graphy in a regional unit, tested 69 undiagnosed myelopathy cases all of whom were HTLV-I negative (Longson *et al.*, 1991). Nevertheless, occasional cases with an identical clinical and radiological picture, diagnosed as MS and living in non-endemic areas of Europe with no risk factors for infection, have been found to be HTLV-I positive (Annunziata *et al.*, 1987) and the similarities between this condition and MS have led to the recommendation that antibodies should be sought in any patient with an 'unexplained' spastic paraparesis (Tournier-Lasserve *et al.*, 1987).

A paraparesis or quadraparesis with or without mild sensory or bladder symptoms may occur in between 11% and 22% of patients with AIDS (AIDS myelopathy) (Snider *et al.*, 1983). When AIDS dementia is present an associated spinal syndrome (vacuolar myelopathy) in which there are subacute ascending sensory symptoms and multiple tract degeneration, is more commonly seen. This syndrome may resemble subacute combined degeneration (Petito *et al.*, 1985). Other viruses may cause a myelitis in association with the immune deficient state.

OTHER INFECTIONS

Acute bacterial (suppurative) myelitis is uncommon in the antibiotic age but should be considered whenever a septically ill, febrile patient develops an acute or subacute paraparesis. The condition may be partially masked by antibiotics. Paraparesis may evolve slowly over days or weeks but can be sudden. As the infection is often medullary there may be an area of dissociated sensory loss. The method of spread is typically blood-stream-borne from an endocarditis, lung or perhaps direct spread from local vertebral infection. The cord is usually swollen at myelography but the CSF is often normal apart from a raised protein. When a transverse myelopathy occurs as a complication of bacterial or tuberculous meningitis, or epidural abscess, an important clue is the presence of systemic symptoms of infection with fever, rigors and meningeal signs. A special type of acute myelitis which is now very rare is a spinal tuberculoma. This is almost invariably associated with systemic dissemination of tuberculosis.

A variety of rickettsial, fungal and parasitic agents may cause a myelopathy. *Actinomyces*, *Aspergillus* and coccidiomycosis infections may cause chronic spinal abscesses or granulomatous lesions both intra- and extramedullary. Spinal cord involvement in trichinosis is often associated with encephalitic symptoms (headache, fever, photophobia) and muscle pain. Rarely malaria may present with a predominantly spinal cord vascular syndrome. A very variable progressive intrinsic type spinal syndrome with or without low-grade fever and diarrhoea, hepatomegaly and eosinophilia, in a patient with a history of exposure to an endemic area (South East Asia, South America or Africa) should suggest schistosomiasis.

The spirochaete *Borrelia burgdorferi* may cause chronic neurological disease (Lyme disease) in the tertiary stage, including a mostly spinal form which can closely mimic MS. The most frequent neurological signs are spastic paraparesis and tetraparesis occurring in up to 66% of some series (Ackermann *et al.*, 1988). All levels of disability may be seen with or without ataxia, bladder involvement and, less frequently, sensory changes. The spinal signs may occur alone or in association with features of encephalitis including nystagmus, dysarthria, seizures and organic mental disorder. CT and MRI scanning may result in areas of high signal intensity in the white matter indistinguishable from MS. IgG and OB are frequently abnormal in the CSF. The presence of intrathecally synthesized antibodies clinches the diagnosis.

PARANEOPLASTIC SYNDROMES

In some patients before or after presenting with pulmonary carcinoma, lymphoma or leukaemia, a patient may develop back pain and a rapidly ascending myelitis progressing to a flaccid paralysis and eventually within days or weeks to respiratory failure and death. At autopsy a necrotizing myelitis is found. A less fulminant cord lesion associated with neoplastic lesions is usually characterized by asymmetric wasting and weakness, with the accent on the upper limbs. There are often other lesions present in the dorsal root ganglia, posterior columns or autonomic nervous system, sometimes combined with a sensory neuronopathy.

While many cases of lymphoma who present with a myelopathy turn out to have a spinal block and a compressive mass, some cases have an apparently normal myelogram or multiple small nodules which are not compressing but infiltrating the cord. The myelopathy is presumably ischaemic as a result of involvement of the segmental blood supply. The acute necrotizing myelopathy is rarely associated with lymphoma.

REFERENCES

Abel, T., Gladman, D.D. & Urowitz, M.B. (1980) Neuropsychiatric lupus. *J. Rheumatol.*, **7**, 325–333.

Ackerman, R., Rehse-Kupper, B., Gollmer, E. & Schmidt, R. (1988) Chronic neurologic manifestations of erythema migrans borreliosis. *Ann. NY Acad. Sci.*, **539**, 16–23.

Alexander, L. (1938) Clinical and neuropathological aspects of electrical injuries. *J. Indust. Hyg.*, **20**, 191–243.

Andreanakos, A.A., Duffy, J., Suzuki, M. & Sharp, J.T. (1975) Transverse myelopathy in systemic lupus erythematosus: report of three cases and review of the literature. *Ann. Intern. Med.*, **83**, 616–624.

Annunziata, P., Fanetti, G., Giarratana, M. *et al.* (1987). HTLV-I associated spastic paraparesis in an Italian woman. *Lancet*, **2**, 1393–1394.

Bechar, M., Freud, M., Kott, E., Kott, I., Kraavic, H., Stern, J., Sandbank, U. & Bornstein, B. (1970) Hepatic cirrhosis with post-shunt myelopathy. *J. Neurol. Sci.*, **11**, 101–107.

Beghi, E., Kurland, L.T. & Mulder, D.W. (1982) Incidence of acute transverse myelitis in Rochester, Minnesota, 1970–1980, and implications with respect to influenza vaccine. *Neuroepidemiology*, **1**, 176.

Behan, P. (1977) Diffuse myelitis associated with rubella vaccination. *Br. Med. J.*, **2**, 166–167.

Berman, M., Feldman, S., Alter, M., Zilber, N. & Kahana, E. (1981) Acute transverse myelitis, incidence and etiologic considerations. *Neurology*, **31**, 966–972.

Bickerstaff, E.R. (1970) Hereditary spastic paraplegia. *J. Neurol. Neurosurg. Psychiatry*, **13**, 134–145.

Blanco, G. & Peters, H.A. (1983) Myeloneuronopathy and macrocytosis associated with nitrous oxide abuse. *Arch. Neurol.*, **40**, 416–418.

Blumhardt, L.D., Barrett, G. & Halliday, A.M. (1982) The pattern visual evoked potential in the clinical assessment of undiagnosed spinal cord disease. *Adv. Neurol.*, **32**, 463–472.

Blumhardt, L.D., Holly, M., Pelosi, L., Barrett, G., Hayward, M., Ghadiali, E. & Slade, T.J. (1991a) Detection of abnormalities in 'undiagnosed' spinal cord disease using memory-scanning evoked potentials (ERP) *J. Neurol. Neurosurg. Psychiatry* (In press).

Blumbardt, L.D., McDonald, W.I., Sandercock, P.A.G., Moore, P., Brock, L., Dixon, T., Kendall, B., Moseley, I., Woodrow, J. & Findlay, G. (1991b) Isolated non-compressive myelopathy in a regional unit: diagnostic and prognostic value of neuroimaging, evoked potentials and CSF examination. *J. Neurol. Neurosurg. Psychiatry* (In press).

Buge, A., Escarolle, R., Poisson, M., Rancurel, G. & Gray, F. (1975) Sarcoidose medullaire. Observation anatomaclinique. *Ann. Med. Interne*, **126**, 11–16.

Chajek, T. & Fainaru, M. (1975) Behcet's disease. Report of 42 cases and review of literature. *Medicine*, **54**, 179–196.

Delaney, P. (1977) Neurological manifestations of sarcoidosis. *Ann. Intern. Med.*, **87**, 336–345.

Ell, J.J., Uttley, D. & Siver, J.R. (1981) Acute myelopathy in association with heroin addiction. *J. Neurol. Neurosurg. Psychiatry*, **44**, 448–450.

Ellis, S.G. & Verity, M.A. (1979) Central nervous system involvement in systemic lupus erythematosus: a review of neuropathological findings in 57 cases, 1955–1977. *Semin. Arthritis Rheum.*, **8**, 212–221.

Elrington, G.M., Bateman, D.E., Jeffrey, M.J. & Lawton, N.F. (1989) Adrenoleukodystrophy: heterogeneity in two brothers. *J. Neurol. Neurosurg. Psychiatry*, **52**, 310–313.

Fadli, M.E. & Yousef, M.M. (1973) Neuro-Behcet's syndrome in the United Arab Republic. *Eur. Neurol.*, **9**, 76–89.

Garcia, C. & Fleming, H. (1977) Reversible corticospinal tract disease due to hyperthyroidism. *Arch. Neurol.*, **34**, 647–648.

Gessain, A. *et al.* (1985) Antibodies to human T lymphotropic virus type 1 in patients with tropical spastic paraparesis. *Lancet*, **2**, 407–410.

Gout, A., Gessain, A., Boegert, F., Saal, F., Tournier-Lasserre, E., Lasneret, J., Caudie, C., Brunet, P., De-Thé, G., Lhermitte, F. & Lyon-Caen, O. (1989) Chronic myelopathies associated with human T-lymphotrophic virus type I. *Arch. Neurol.*, **46**, 255–260.

Harding, A.E. (1981) Hereditary 'pure' spastic paraplegia: a clinical and genetic study of 22 families. *J. Neurol. Neurosurg. Psychiatry*, **44**, 871–883.

Harding, A.E. (1984) Hereditary 'pure' spastic paraplegia. In Harding, A.E. (ed.) *The Hereditary Ataxias and Related Disorders*, pp. 174–190. Churchill-Livingstone, Edinburgh.

Hemachudha, T., Phanuphak, P., Johnson, R.T., Griffin, D.E., Ratanavongsiri, J., & Siriprasomsup, W. (1987) Neurological complications of semple-type rabies vaccine: clinical and immunologic studies. *Neurology*, **37**, 550–556.

Henson, R.A. & Urich, H. (1982) *Cancer and the Nervous System*. Blackwell Scientific Publications, London.

Hirayama, K. (1972) Juvenile non-progressive muscular atrophy localised in hand and forearm—observation in 38 cases. *Clin. Neurol.*, **12**, 313–324.

Hubbe, P. & Dam, A.M. (1973) Spastic paraplegia of unknown origin. *Acta Neurol. Scand.*, **49**, 536–542.

Jellinger, K. & Sturm, K.W. (1971) Delayed radiation myelopathy in man: report of 12 necropsy cases. *J. Neurol. Sci.*, **14**, 389–408.

Jestico, J. & Ellis, P.D.M. (1976) Changes in nystagmus on raising body temperature in clinically suspected and proven multiple sclerosis. *Br. Med. J.*, **2**, 970–972.

Jones, A. (1964) Transient radiation myelopathy. *Br. J. Radiol.*, **37**, 727–744.

Kewelramani, L.S., Saleem, S. & Bertrand, D. (1978) Myelopathy associated with systemic lupus erythematosus (erythema nodosum). *Paraplegia*, **16**, 282–294.

Kolodny, E.H., Rebeiz, J.J., Caviness, V.S. & Richardson, E.P. (1968) Granulomatous angiitis of the central nervous system. *Arch. Neurol.*, **19**, 510–524.

Leibowitz, U., Halpern, L. & Alter, M. (1967) Clinical studies of multiple sclerosis in Israel. *Neurology*, **17**, 988–992.

Lipton, H.L. & Teasdale, R.D. (1973) Acute transverse myelopathy in adults: a follow up study. *Arch. Neurol.*, **28**, 252–257.

Logothetis, J. (1961) Neurologic and muscular manifestations of hyperthyroidism. *Arch. Neurol.*, **5**, 533–537.

Longson, M., Blumhardt, L.D. & Moore, A.P. (1991) Negative HTLV-I serology in 'undiagnosed myelopathy' in north west England and north Wales. *J. Neurol. Neurosurg. Psychiatry* (In press).

McAlpine, D. (1972) *Multiple Sclerosis: a Reappraisal*, 2nd edn, p. 135. Churchill-Livingstone, Edinburgh.

McMenamin, J. & Croxon, M. (1980) Motoneurone disease and hyperthyroid Graves disease: a chance association? *J. Neurol. Neurosurg. Psychiatry*, **43**, 46–48.

Malamud, N. & Foster, D.B. (1942) Periarteritis nodosa: a clinicopathological report, with special reference to the nervous system. *Arch. Neurol. Psychiatry*, **47**, 828–838.

Malamed, E., Berman, M. & Lavy, S. (1975) Posterolateral myelopathy associated with thyrotoxicosis. *N. Engl. J. Med.*, **293**, 778.

Marshall, J. (1955) Spastic paraplegia of middle age: a clinicopathological study. *Lancet*, **1**, 643–646.

Miller, D., McDonald, W.I., Blumhardt, L.D., Du Boulay, G.H., Halliday, A.M., Johnson, G., Kendall, B.E., Kingsley, D.P.E., Mcmanus, D.G., Mosley, I.F., Rudge, P. & Sandercock, P.A.G. (1987) Magnetic resonance imaging in isolated noncompressive spinal cord syndromes. *Ann. Neurol.*, **22**, 714–723.

Morris, K.M. & Findlay, G. (1991) Spinal dysraphism and the tethered cord syndrome. *Br. J. Neurosurg* (In press).

Motomura, S., Tabira, T. & Kuroiwa, Y. (1980) A clinical comparative study of multiple sclerosis and neuro-Behcet's syndrome. *J. Neurol. Neurosurg. Psychiatry*, **43**, 210–213.

Newton, M.R., Barrett, G., Callanan, M.M. & Towell, A.D. (1990) Cognitive event-related potentials in multiple sclerosis. *Brain*, **112**, 1637–1660.

Ormerod, I.E.C., Miller, D.H., McDonald, W.I., Du Boulay, E.P.G.H., Rudge, P., Kendall, B.E., Moseley, I.F., Johnson, G., Tofts, P.S., Halliday, A.M., Bronstein, A.M., Scaravilli, F., Harding, A.E., Barnes, D. & Zilkha, K.J. (1987) The role of NMR imaging in the assessment of multiple sclerosis and isolated neurological lesions. *Brain*, **110**, 1579–1616.

Osame, M., Usuku, K., Isumu, Z., Ijiche, N., Amifani, W., Igato, A., Matsumoto, M. & Tara, M. (1986) HTLV-I associated myelopathy, a new clinical entity. *Lancet*, **1**, 1031–1032.

Paillas, J. & Roger, J. (1949) Syndrome extenso-progressif a type de sclerose laterale amyotrophique apres electrocution. *Rev. Neurol.*, **81**, 152–154.

Pant, S.S., Rebeiz, J.J. & Richardson, E.P. (1968) Spastic paraparesis following porto-caval shunts. *Neurology*, **18**, 135–141.

Paty, D.W., Blume, W.T., Brown, W.F., Jaatoul, N., Kertesz, A. & McInnes, W. (1978) Chronic progressive myelopathy: Investigation with CSF electrophoresis, evoked potentials and CAT scan. *Trans. Am. Neurol. Assoc.*, **103**, 110–112.

Paty, D.W., Oger, J.J.F., Kastrukoff, L.F., Hashimoto, S.A., Hooge J.P., Eisen, A.A., Eisen, K.A., Purves, S.J., Low, M.D., Brandejs, V., Roberston, W.D. & Li, D.K.B. (1988) MRI in the diagnosis of MS: a prospective study with comparison of clinical evaluation, evoked potentials, oligoclonal banding, and CT. *Neurology*, **30**, 180–185.

Penn, A.S. & Rowan, A.J. (1968) Myelopathy in systemic lupus erythematosus. *Arch. Neurol.*, **18**, 337–349.

Petito, C.K., Navia, B.A., Cho, E., Jordan, B.D., George, D.C. & Price, R.W. (1985) Vacuolar myelopathy pathologically resembling subacute combined degeneration in patients with the acquired immunodeficiency syndrome. *N. Engl. J. Med.*, **312**, 874–879.

Poser, S., Hermann-Gremmels, I., Wikstrom, J. & Poser, W. (1978) Clinical features of the spinal form of multiple sclerosis. *Acta Neurol. Scand.*, **57**, 151–158.

Poser, C.M., Paty, D.W., Scheinberg, L., McDonald, W.I., Davis, F.A., Ebers, G.C., Johnson, K.P., Sibley, W.A., Silberberg, D.H. & Gourtelle, W.W. (1983) New diagnostic criteria for multiple sclerosis: guidelines for research protocols. *Ann. Neurol.*, **13**, 227–231.

Rawlinson, D.G. & Braun, C.W. (1981) Granulomatous angiitis of the nervous system first seen as relapsing myelopathy. *Arch. Neurol.*, **38**, 129–131.

Roe, P.F. (1963) Hereditary spastic paraplegia. *J. Neurol. Neurosurg. Psychiatry*, **26**, 516–519.

Ropper, A.M., Miett, T. & Chiappa, K.H. (1982) Absence of evoked potential abnormalities in acute transverse myelitis. *Neurology*, **32**, 80–82.

Sadowsky, G.H., Sachs, E. & Ochoa, J. (1976) Post-radiation motor neurone syndrome. *Arch. Neurol.*, **33**, 786–787.

Shapiro, W.R. & Young, D.F. (1984) Neurological complications of antineoplastic therapy. *Acta. Neurol. Scand.*, **70**, 125–130.

Sigal, L.H. (1987) The neurological presentation of vasculitic and rheumatological syndromes: a review. *Medicine*, **66**, 157–180.

Snider, W.D., Simpson, D.M., Aronyk, K.E., Nielsen, S., Gold, J.W.M., Metroka, C.E. & Posner, J.B. (1983) Neurological complications of acquired immune deficiency syndrome: analysis of 50 patients. *Ann. Neurol.*, **14**, 403–418.

Thomas, P.K., Jeffreys, J.G.R., Smith, I.S. & Loulakakis, D. (1981) Spinal somatosensory evoked potentials in hereditary spastic paraplegia. *J. Neurol. Neurosurg. Psychiatry*, **44**, 243–246.

Tournier-Lasserve, E., Gout, A., Gessain, A., Iba-Zizen, M.T., Lyon-Caen, O., Lhermitte, F. & De-Thé, G. (1987) HTLV-I, brain abnormalities on magnetic resonance imaging, and relations with multiple sclerosis. *Lancet*, **2**, 49–50.

Ungar-Sargon, J.Y., Lovelace, R.E. & Brust, J.C.M. (1980) Spastic paraplegia–paraparesis, a reappraisal. *J. Neurol. Sci.*, **46**, 1–12.

Waddell, G., Bircher, M., Finlayson, D. & Main, C.J. (1984) Symptoms and signs: physical disease or illness behaviour? *Br. Med. J.*, **289**, 739–741.

Wilson, S.A.K. (1940) In: Bruce, A.N. (ed.) *Neurology*, p. 781. Arnold, London.

Woods, J.D. (1952) Spinal atrophic paralyses following lightning stroke. *S. Afr. Med. J.*, **62**, 92–100.

5 · Radiological Investigation of the Spine in Adults

By E.T.S. SMITH

The radiological investigation of the spine forms only a part of the overall evaluation of the patient. Interpretation of the X-rays alone will lead regularly to incorrect assumptions being made. This is particularly true in spinal radiology as, with increasing age, the finding of a truly normal radiograph becomes unusual. It is only too easy to put undue importance upon the findings of degenerative changes on a plain X-ray which may well have nothing to do with the clinical problem. Equally, apparently alarming radiological appearances may in fact be causing relatively little clinical harm.

To perform adequate radiological assessment of the spine it is necessary that the radiologist should have full access to the relevant clinical information and ideally there should be a close cooperative relationship between radiologist and clinician. Such contact and discussion will lead to appropriate radiological studies being performed. The radiologist not only provides a diagnostic opinion; he or she is trained to assess which of the many and ever-increasing methods of investigation should be utilized, taking into consideration not only diagnostic requirements but also the radiological safety and cost-effectiveness of the investigation. Some investigations will be more appropriate to certain clinical situations and will be further discussed in later chapters. This chapter, however, describes the range of investigations in common usage for spinal investigations with computerized tomography (CT) and magnetic resonance imaging (MRI) being considered in Chapter 7. Such a separation between CT/MRI and other radiology is of course artificial, and in the clinical setting many of the investigations described in this chapter are complementary to CT and MRI.

PLAIN RADIOLOGY OF THE SPINE

Plain films of the spine demonstrate the distribution of crystallized calcium within the region examined. They have the advantages of being inexpensive and readily available. In most situations they are easy to perform with standardized techniques and views being taken, although certain areas of the spine such as the cervicodorsal junction and sacrum can cause difficulties. The main disadvantage of plain films is that they show only bony detail and some less precise detail of the soft tissues which surround the spine. The spinal cord and nerve roots are, of course, not shown. Thus, abnormalities of the intraspinal contents can only be indirectly demonstrated. For example, the presence of an intraspinal tumour may be shown by its effect producing widening of the spinal canal with changes such as increased AP canal diameter, pedicular erosion, scalloping of vertebral bodies or enlargement of an intervertebral foramen.

Plain films show in great detail the presence of any malalignment (Fig. 5.1) or deformity (Fig. 5.2). They also show the presence of any gross congenital anomaly such as abnormal lumbosacral segmentation and thus are normally the initial radiological screening investigation used in studying the spine. Gross abnormalities of bone texture are well shown but it must be recalled that to show a lytic or destructive lesion at least 50% of the normal bone has to be destroyed before any change is visible on plain X-ray.

The exact radiograph required varies with the spinal region being examined. In the cervical spine, AP and lateral projections are standard. In order to completely assess the C1–C2 region an 'open-

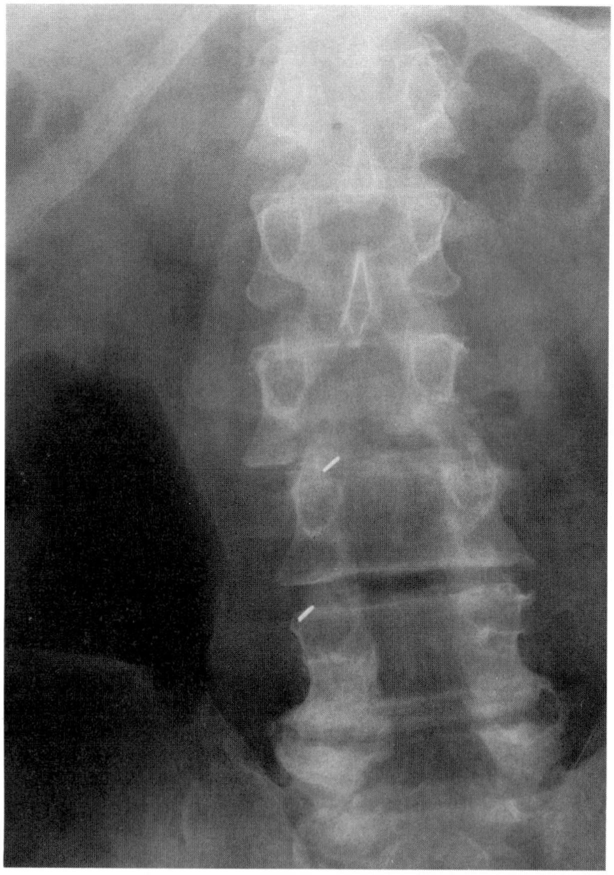

Fig. 5.1 AP radiograph showing obvious malalignment due to postlaminectomy lateral subluxation at L3–L4 with changes of discitis.

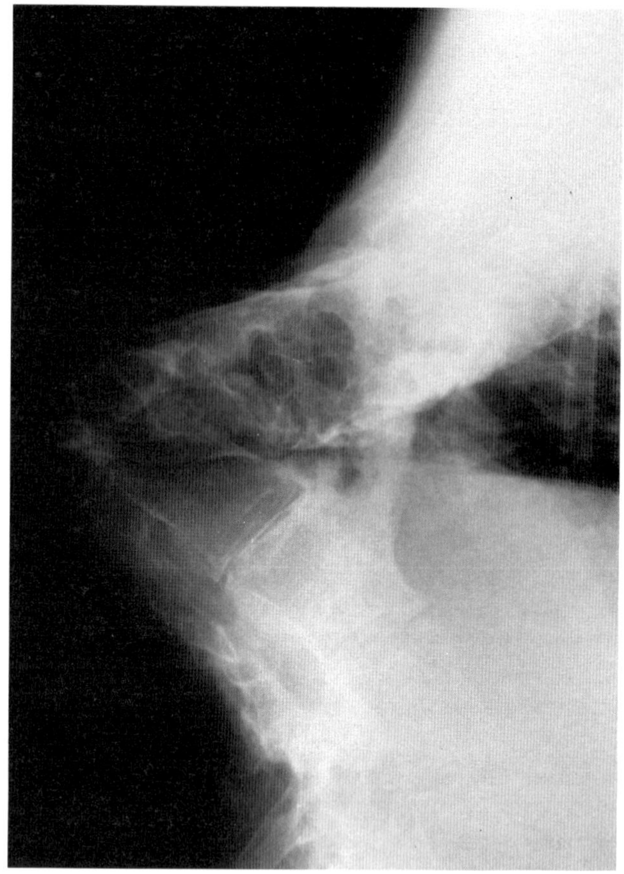

Fig. 5.2 Lateral radiograph showing severe kyphotic deformity in a myelomeningocele patient.

mouth' AP view is necessary to show the odontoid process and atlanto-axial joints fully. Oblique views are used to assess the size of the intervertebral foramina and, in trauma, to show the alignment of individual facets. The routine use of oblique views has been shown to be unhelpful (MacPherson & MacPherson, 1981). In the thoracic region AP and lateral views are standard.

In the lumbar spine, again AP and lateral views are standard, though many units include a coned view of the lumbosacral junction as routine. Oblique projections are useful to reveal defects in the area of the pars interarticularis. Dynamic views are often used in the assessment of low back pain. Simple flexion and extension lateral radiographs will reveal any degree of subluxation which is present. An AP view with the patient in full lateral flexion to each side may reveal abnormal degrees of movement around a disc space, and some authorities will also take radiographs of the lumbar spine in the seated or standing position and also a lateral view with the patient lifting a weight. Whilst it is true that such techniques will often show abnormal movement of one vertebra to another, it is far from certain what relevance this has to the clinical situation. Dynamic views are often used in the cervical spine to assess the presence of atlanto-axial subluxation or hypermobility following trauma. In the acute situation, dynamic cervical radiography should always be supervised by a clinician.

There are few hazards associated with plain film radiography. Excessive manipulation of the patient following trauma either in positioning the patient for the X-ray or in the performance of dynamic views can cause neurological damage. Radiation hazard can be significant if excessive numbers of examinations are performed, especially in the lumbar spine. Following a standard AP and lateral X-ray of the lumbar spine the radiation dose to the testes is approximately 0.05 mGy, and to the ovaries is 2 mGy. The addition of a coned lumbosacral view and obliques increases the doses to 0.12 mGy and 4.7 mGy, respectively. The average dose of radiation to a person from normal background radiation is between 1 and 2 mGy per year; thus it can be seen that the dosage obtained from a single lumbar spine examination is significant.

As with all radiographs, the interpretation of spinal radiographs should be performed systematically. The films should be checked for alignment looking for the presence of abnormal curvatures, scoliosis or spondylolisthesis. The loss of a normal curve may also be significant, usually indicating the presence of paravertebral muscle spasm. The shape of the vertebral bodies should be closely examined, especially in regions such as the cervicodorsal area and at the extremities of the film where abnormalities are often missed. The texture of the skeleton should be assessed, looking for lytic or sclerotic areas. The architecture of the neural arch should be examined closely, looking for pedicular absence or thinning or congenital arch abnormalities. The disc spaces and adjoining endplates require inspection, looking for disc narrowing, osteophytic change or endplate erosion. The alignment and condition of the facet joints should be assessed, as should the condition of paraspinal structures such as the ribs, paravertebral gutter, prevertebral space in the neck, pelvis and sacroiliac joints. Figure 5.3 shows only a few examples of plain spinal radiographs which indicate their diagnostic potential.

Plain radiology represents a most useful screening technique. When applied to large, relatively non-homogeneous, groups such as patients with low back pain, the incidence of clinically important abnormalities is low. Nachemson (1976) estimated that a clinically significant abnormality would be found only once in every 2500 plain film examinations performed for the screening of low back pain patients.

However, where the clinical picture suggests the presence of significant spinal disease, plain radiography represents a moderately sensitive screening investigation. The sensitivity varies with the underlying diagnosis. Plain films are highly sensitive at predicting the presence of degenerative spinal disease but relatively insensitive in the diagnosis of intraspinal tumours. They may also be relatively poor in terms of specificity. For example, it may be impossible to determine whether destructive change in a vertebral body with an adjacent paraspinal mass is due to infection or neoplasm. One further role for plain radiography is that, assuming an abnormality is seen, plain films then serve to localize the region of the spine which needs more detailed examination such as CT or MRI.

CONVENTIONAL TOMOGRAPHY

In certain situations, plain radiology may suggest the presence of an abnormality but sufficient detail is not present to allow an accurate diagnosis. Although in many situations other imaging techniques will resolve this, there remains a place for conventional tomography. This is particularly true when there is a need to show the exact bony detail of the spine in the sagittal plane, as occurs occasionally, for example, in trauma. MRI does not provide the necessary bony detail and sagittal reconstruction of the CT image may be difficult to interpret.

The technique of conventional tomography uses tube and film movements about a fixed point—the fulcrum. The effect of tube movement in one direction and simultaneous film movement in the opposite direction is that only structures sited in one plane of the body—at the level of the fulcrum—are represented by sharp shadows on the developed film. Structures in front of and behind this 'in-focus plane' appear blurred. The movement of the tube may be linear, circular, ellipsoidal or hypocycloidal. By moving the fulcrum the area of the body under scrutiny can be examined in sections. The thickness of each slice or section is controlled by the size of the arc used in the tube movement. The greater the arc of swing, the thinner the slice.

The accumulation of multiple thin tomographic slices in more than one plane allows fine bony detail unencumbered by superimposed tissues to be examined. However, as in plain radiographs, no soft tissue detail of the intraspinal contents can be shown. Other disadvantages are that considerable doses of radiation can be given with this technique and axial views cannot be obtained. Also, as in CT or MR imaging, the presence of metallic implants causes artifacts. The performance of conventional tomography costs approximately twice that of plain spinal radiography.

Tomography is indicated in situations where it is necessary to show the bony anatomy in great detail in the sagittal or coronal plane. The development of CT scanning with sagittal reconstruction has replaced the need for tomography to a large extent, but there remain situations where it may be of use. This is particularly so at the craniocervical junction

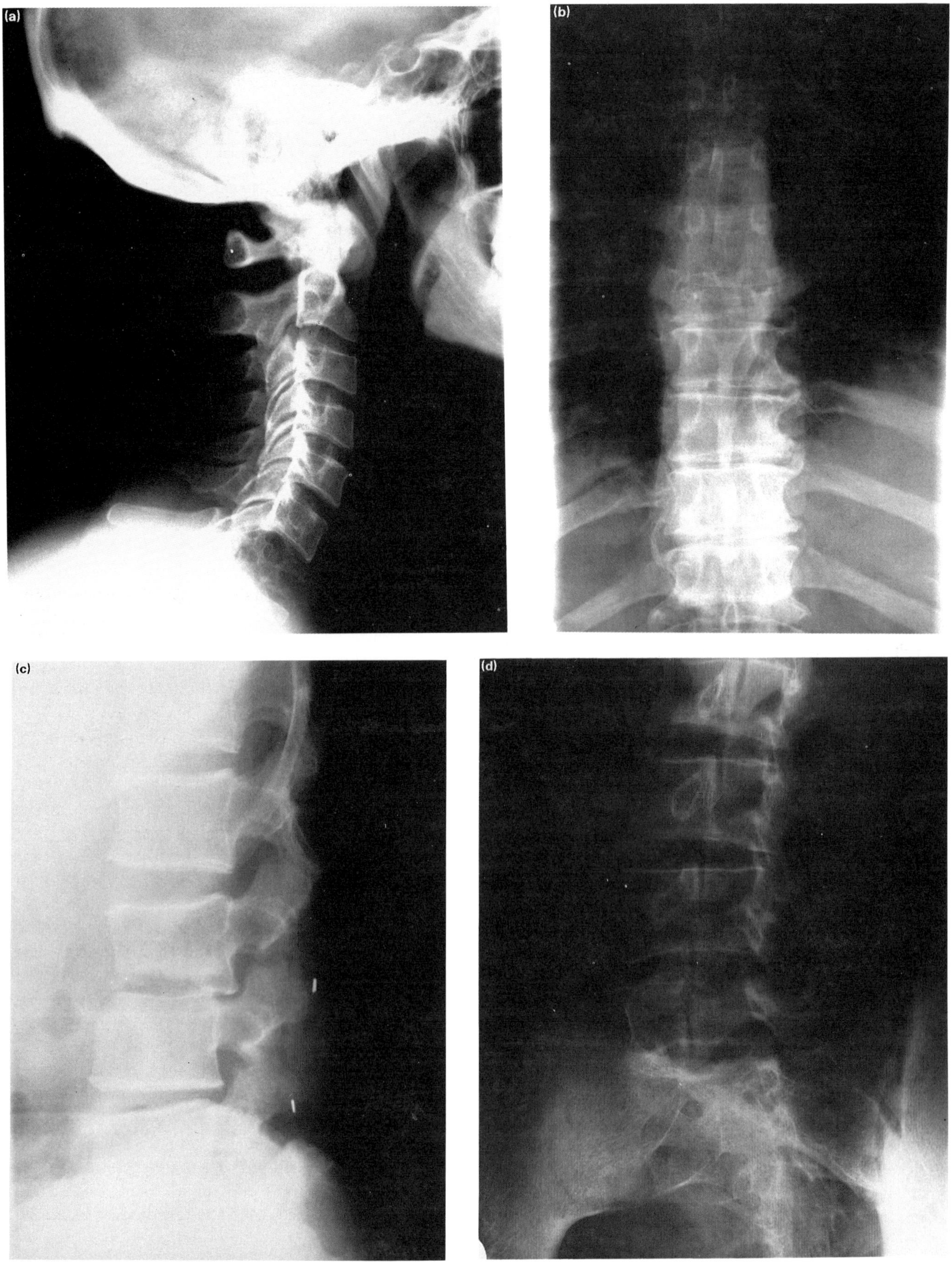

(a)
(b)
(c)
(d)

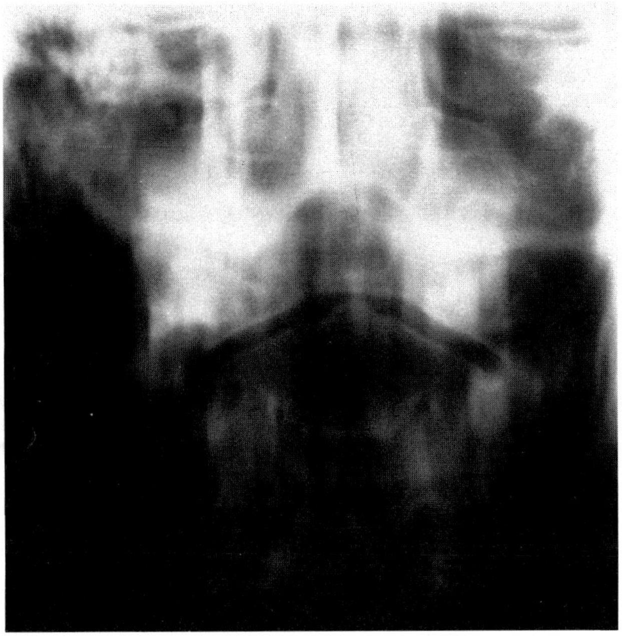

Fig. 5.4 AP tomogram of C2 showing an os odontoideum.

(Fig. 5.4), in certain cases of trauma and in patients with bony diseases which tend to obliterate the normal architecture of the spinal skeleton, such as ankylosing spondylitis or old tuberculosis (Fig. 5.5).

RADIONUCLIDE SCANS

Radionuclide imaging depends on the detection of emitted gamma radiation from radiopharmaceuticals introduced usually by intravenous injection. In order to target the radioactive agent in the appropriate organ the radionuclide is tagged to a biologically active molecule or an organ-specific compound. The most commonly used vehicle in bone scanning is methylene diphosphonate, which localizes technetium (^{99}Tc) in bone. Other radionuclides in usage are indium (^{111}In) and gallium (^{67}Ga). These isotopes differ in their physical half-lives. Technetium has a half-life of six hours whereas ^{111}In is 2.8 days and ^{67}Ga is 78 hours.

The gamma rays emitted by the radionuclide are detected by the measurement of the scintillation which they cause following their absorption in a sodium iodide crystal within the detector. The light produced by the scintillation is photomultiplied and the information computerized to produce a two-dimensional representation of the area being examined. This results in loss of definition due to obscuring of the area of interest by radioactivity existing in front or behind. Thus, the anatomical resolution is far inferior to that of plain radiography. However, radionuclide imaging produces a functional assessment of the metabolic, and to some extent vascular, activity which is actually occurring in the region of bone being examined.

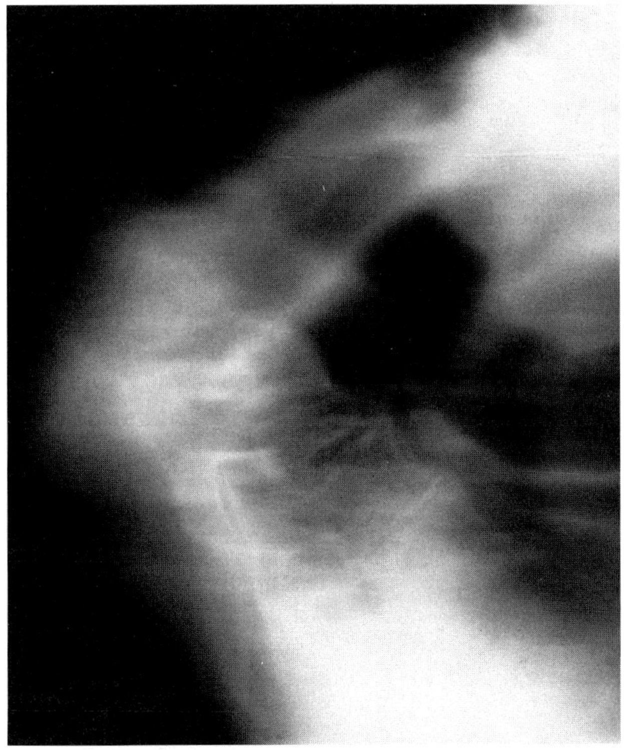

Fig. 5.5 Lateral tomogram showing detail which could not be seen on plain X-ray of an old tuberculous kyphos at T3.

Nuclear medicine techniques are only minimally invasive. However, care must be taken to deal with the resulting radioactive waste such as unused isotope, syringes, etc., and the patient's secretions and excretions. Adverse reactions to the isotope are most uncommon with a reported incidence of one in 100 000. Again, the presence of metallic instrumentation or recent barium will degrade the image quality. Because the isotope must be allowed

Fig. 5.3 (*Opposite*) Examples of diagnostic potential of plain radiographs. (a) Extensive lytic lesion in the body of C7 due to Ewing's sarcoma. (b) Collapse of body and loss of both pedicles of T8 with a small paravertebral mass due to metastatic disease. (c) Postoperative osteomyelitis at L3–L4 (same case as Fig. 5.1). (d) Oblique radiograph showing lytic defect in the pars of L5.

to accumulate within bone, the examination is time-consuming.

The radiation dose resulting from a ^{99}Tc bone scan is greater than that from a lumbar spine X-ray. The dosage varies from 2.7 mGy to the gonads to 14.4 mGy to the bladder. The cost is approximately three times that of plain radiography.

In a standard ^{99}Tc methylene diphosphate bone scan, approximately 50% of the complex is absorbed into the crystalline structures of bone whilst the remainder stays in the body blood pool and contributes to the background activity. With the passage of time this background clears, and the isotope accumulates in areas of increased blood supply and where active bone formation is occurring. This process produces a more sensitive method of detecting bone destruction and reparation than does plain radiography, but it is essentially non-specific. Abnormalities which would result in a positive bone scan range from degenerative disease through infection to neoplasia.

The main indication for a bone scan is in the search for unrecognized metastatic lesions (Fig. 5.6) as part of a diagnostic assessment in order to plan appropriate therapy. Skeletal metastases usually accumulate more activity than adjacent normal bone and so appear 'hot', though such a finding is, of course, non-specific. However, metastases from renal cell carcinoma are frequently negative on bone scan as they tend to be purely destructive lesions. Similarly, myeloma deposits are commonly negative unless a small pathological fracture has occurred resulting in a positive uptake.

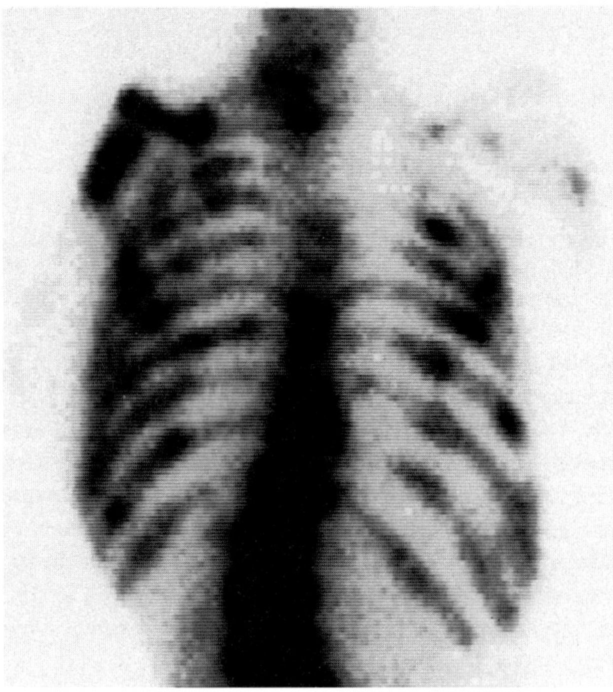

Fig. 5.6 Isotope bone scan showing multiple bony metastases.

Areas of abnormal uptake on the radionuclide scan should be further examined by conventional radiography or CT scanning in an attempt to clarify the cause of the abnormality. It may be seen that there is merely active spondylotic disease. Conventional radiography may, of course, be normal despite the presence of a metastasis. Some 30% of metastases seen on a bone scan will be missed by plain films. On the contrary only 2% of metastases seen on plain films will be negative on a bone scan.

A normal radionuclide scan virtually excludes the presence of osteomyelitis unless performed very soon after the onset of the disease. However, the scan is poor at differentiating between active and inactive infective disease. Where there is strong clinical evidence of infection despite a normal technetium scan, Gallium scanning may be helpful. Gallium-67 citrate has a half-life of 78 hours, much longer than that of technetium. Twenty-four to 78 hours after intravenous injection, gallium accumulates in sites of inflammation. The mechanism of accumulation is ill-understood, but it has been suggested that, in infection, gallium probably penetrates disrupted capillary beds and adheres to pus, perhaps by binding to lactoferrin released by polymorphonuclear neutrophilic leucocytes.

The patient is scanned using the gamma camera at 24, 48 and 72 hours after the intravenous injection of gallium. Gallium accumulates normally in liver, spleen, bone marrow, lungs, adrenals, urinary tract, kidneys, salivary glands, breasts, genitals, and the nasopharynx. It can also accumulate in inflammatory conditions (for example, sarcoidosis, pneumoconiosis, diverticulitis, Crohn's disease) and in a variety of neoplasms (e.g. lung cancer, hepatoma, melanoma, seminoma and Hodgkin's lymphoma). Interpretation of the scan images can be difficult because accumulation of activity in some of these sites can overlie the spine. Colonic excretion is the major route of elimination after the first 24 hours, so thorough bowel preparation is necessary to aid the interpretation of the delayed scans.

The delay of two to three days necessary to obtain the results, and the difficulty in their interpretation, limits the usefulness of this technique. However, a normal gallium scan is strong evidence against an infective process, and gallium scanning can be useful when used to clarify an equivocal technetium scan. It is a very sensitive technique for the detection of osteomyelitis in children but false-negatives can occur in the presence of indolent infections, fungal infections or after prolonged antibiotic therapy.

A further technique for screening for osteomyelitis is the white cell scan. This is performed by harvesting the patient's leucocytes from a sample of venous blood; labelling them with ^{111}In oxime or tropolone and then reinjecting them intravenously.

Oxime and tropolone are lipid-soluble, metal-chelating agents that bind ^{111}In and carry it through the cell membrane. On entering the cell indium binds irreversibly to cytoplasmic protein. Cells labelled in this way have *in vitro* stability; *in vivo* the survival is reduced, but the cells remain sufficiently intact after reintroduction to localize to sites of infection.

This accumulation is less sensitive for bone than for soft tissue infection due to the failure of white cells to accumulate in acute osteomyelitis, which is probably related to increased marrow pressure caused by oedema, preventing entry of labelled cells. However, white cell scanning with indium does have advantages over gallium. Indium is not normally excreted in the gut and so the lumbar spine is not obscured; also, the images are produced only 24 hours following injection and leucocyte penetration of bone is highly specific for osteomyelitis, though haematomas or recent surgery may produce false-positives.

Iodine-131 is a relatively long-lived radionuclide with a half-life of eight days and with a gamma ray emission of 364 keV—too high for optimum imaging—which causes a relatively high radiation dose. It is widely used, nonetheless, because many organic compounds can be readily iodinated and used in scanning procedures.

MIBG is meta-iodo-benzyl-guanidine. This radiopharmaceutical has been used primarily to detect phaeochromocytoma but recently it has been successfully employed to define metastatic neuroblastoma in the skeleton. It is injected intravenously and images are obtained at one, two and three days, using the gamma camera. The thyroid glands must be protected from excessive uptake of free ^{131}I by use of Lugol's iodine or a saturated solution of potassium iodide beginning the day before and continuing for seven days after MIBG administration.

MYELOGRAPHY

Myelography consists of introducing a contrast medium—usually a water-soluble, non-ionic iodine containing contrast medium, into the subarachnoid space by lumbar or cervical puncture for the purpose of outlining the spinal cord and nerve roots. Its value is that the technique allows the assessment of the size, shape and position of the spinal cord and nerve roots. Thus, intrathecal space-occupying lesions are shown as well as compressive lesions, in the extradural space. The technique localizes exactly the level of a cord compression and is usually readily available as an emergency procedure in addition to routine use.

Myelography is, however, an invasive procedure and there are risks associated with the injection of contrast media. The danger of the development of increased neurological deficit due to a lumbar puncture performed caudal to a complete myelographic block is uncommon but well recognized. The contrast agents themselves can be hazardous. The use of oily agents such as myodil is no longer acceptable because of the significant risk of developing arachnoiditis, especially in the presence of blood-stained cerebrospinal fluid. From the point of view of arachnoiditis, ionic and especially non-ionic agents are much safer. Non-ionic agents carry an increased iodine concentration without increased osmolarity, and thus allow lower doses to be used. Non-ionic agents are, however, almost 10 times as expensive as ionic contrast agents.

Myelography is contra-indicated in patients with severe renal insufficiency as the contrast agents are excreted by that route and may themselves be nephrotoxic. It should not be performed on patients with severe coagulation abnormalities since intraspinal haematomas may occur. Certain agents such as metrizamide or iopamidol should not be used in patients taking phenothiazine drugs. Relative contra-indications include a history of a previous severe reaction to intrathecal contrast and a history of epilepsy. Ionic contrast agents are potentially epileptogenic. However, non-ionic agents are much safer. Nevertheless, epileptic patients should continue their normal medication and many radiologists will

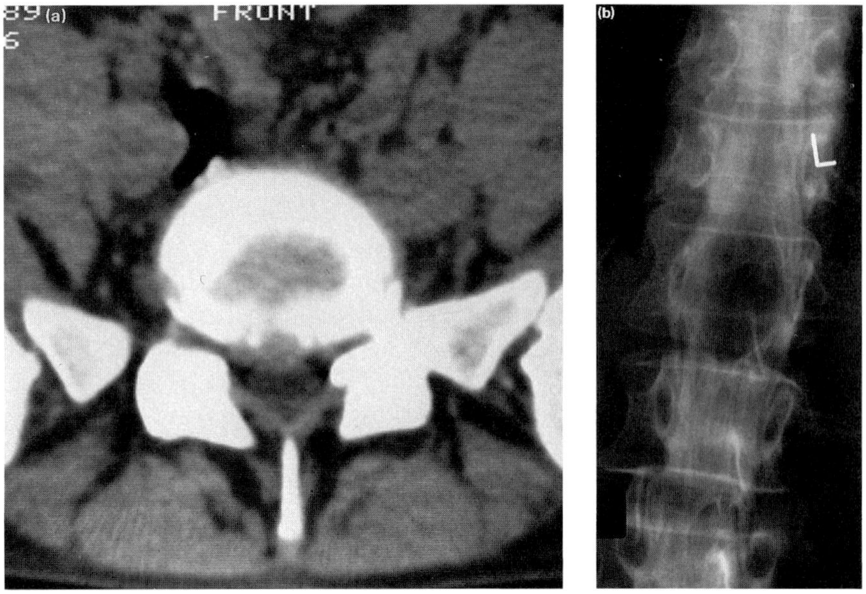

Fig. 5.7 (a) CT scan of a small lumbosacral disc which was removed with no relief of sciatica. (b) When the patient was referred to this unit, a radiculogram was performed which showed an intramedullary conus ependymona. Removal resulted in complete relief of the symptoms.

cover the examination by giving additional anticonvulsants such as clonazepam prior to the procedure.

Postmyelographic complications include headache, nausea and vomiting, as well as increased spinal or radicular pain. Their severity is related to the amount and concentration of the agent used and is much reduced by the use of non-ionic agents. Teasdale & MacPherson (1984) reported the incidence of side-effects following the use of iopamidol, a non-ionic agent. They found a total incidence of symptoms such as headache, nausea and vomiting in 36.5% of patients following lumbar puncture and 29.2% following cervical puncture. Headache was the dominant problem. Local pain on injection was found in 6% following lumbar puncture and in 11.5% after cervical puncture. Only 0.6% of patients had a seizure following myelography. Kendall & Stevens (1984) performed a similar study using another non-ionic agent, iohexol. They reported a lower incidence of problems, but side-effects still occurred in 26.3% following lumbar puncture and 16.3% following cervical puncture. No patients had a fit in their series. Radiation hazard to the gonads is negligible in cervical myelography. Lumbar radiculography produces a dose of 9 mGy (four times that of plain radiography) to the ovaries. The cost of the procedure is also four times greater and to this must be added the cost of the overnight hospital stay customary in most units.

The indications for myelography and radiculography are to localize and delineate a presumed intra-

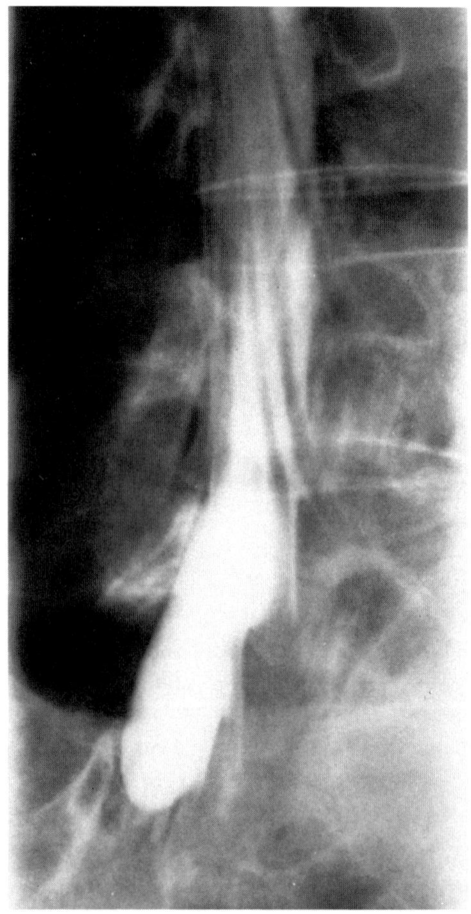

Fig. 5.8 Oblique view of the radiculogram showing root cut-off due to a disc prolapse.

spinal abnormality. It is true that, when available, MRI has largely replaced myelography, as it gives comparable or superior information non-invasively. CT scanning does not, however, produce comparable information. CT inevitably can only examine a restricted area of the spine, and gives poor detail of the intradural structures unless it is combined with myelography. An additional hazard of CT is that it may show evidence of degenerative disease which may be assumed erroneously to be clinically significant whilst the true lesion lies elsewhere (Fig. 5.7).

Myelography shows the presence of an intraspinal abnormality by the displacement or obstruction of the contrast column. If a complete block to the flow of contrast is found, the examination must be completed by the introduction of fresh contrast medium at a higher level in order to exactly delineate the extent of the block and, especially in metastasis, to rule out the possibility of multiple lesions. The information gained from the myelographic study may be greatly enhanced by the performance of a CT scan through the abnormal area while the intrathecal contrast is still present.

Extradural lesions manifest themselves by displacing either a nerve root or the entire dural sac. The most frequent example of the former is the prolapsed lumbar disc (Fig. 5.8) whilst Fig. 5.9 shows the typical 'broken sticks' appearance of a complete block due to an extradural metastasis. Intradural lesions may be manifest in differing ways. A spinal arteriovenous malformation will show evidence of serpiginous filling defects lying on the spinal cord. An extramedullary lesion will show displacement of the cord (Fig. 5.10) while an intramedullary lesion will show cord expansion (Fig. 5.11). In the latter case, myelography will show only the site and sev-

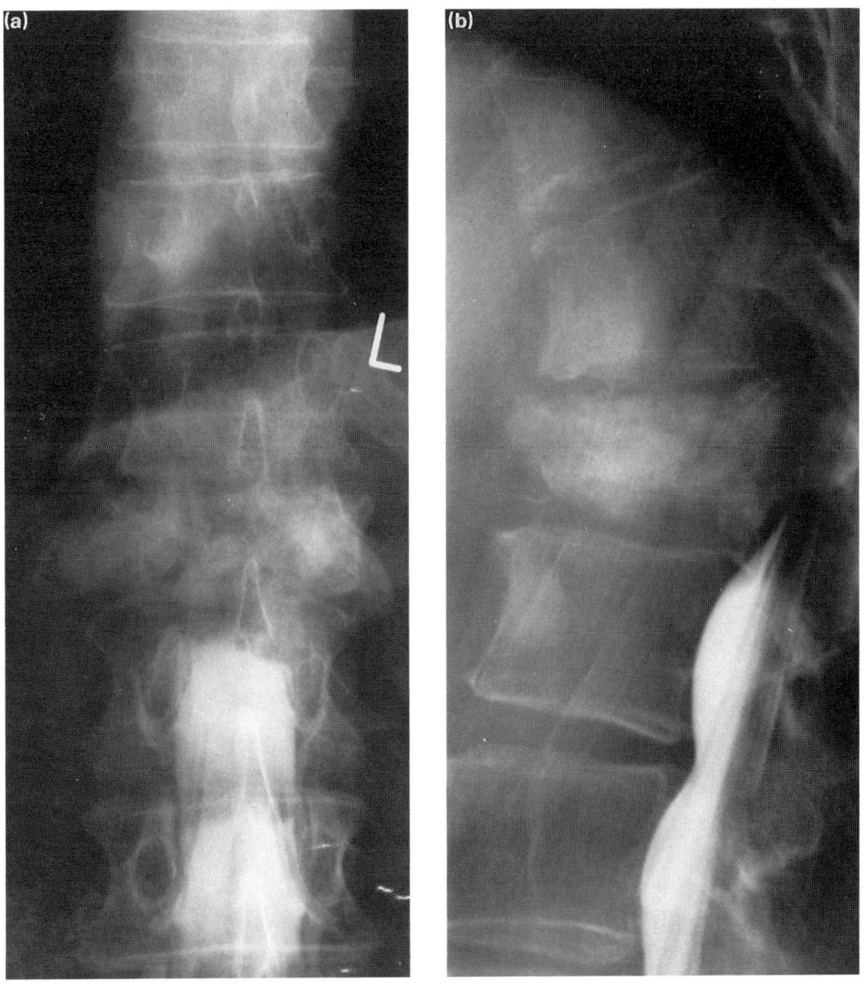

Fig. 5.9 AP (a) and lateral (b) views of a myelogram showing the typical appearance of a complete block due to metastatic disease at the thoracolumbar junction.

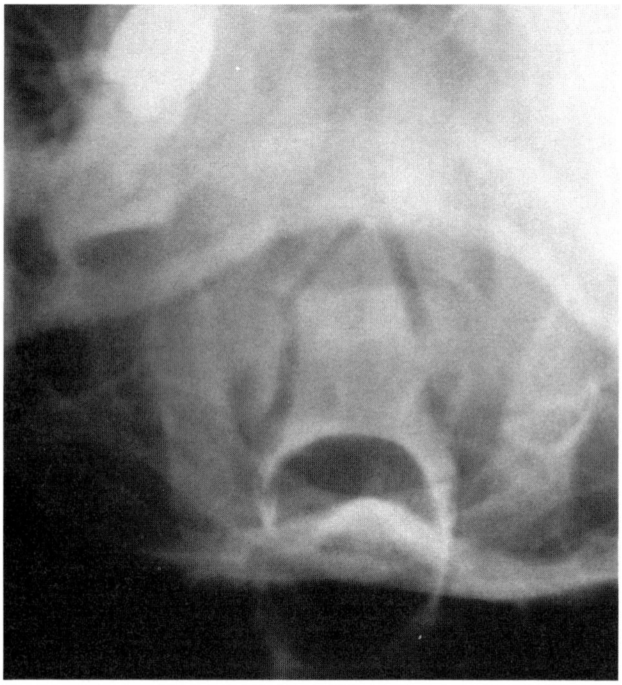

Fig. 5.10 Cervical myelogram showing the appearance of an intradural extramedullary tumour.

erity of cord expansion and will not reveal the cause of such expansion. Further study by MRI is necessary to evaluate intramedullary lesions. Cerebellar ectopia will be seen as a posteriorly sited filling defect at the craniocervical junction when the patient is screened in the supine position.

SPINAL ANGIOGRAPHY

In spinal angiography contrast medium is used to opacify segmental vessels of possible supply to the spinal arteries, thus demonstrating normal and abnormal vasculature. Abnormalities include arteriovenous malformations (AVM) and haemangioblastomas. The normal blood supply of the spinal cord is described in Chapter 49.

Spinal angiomas occur most commonly in the thoracolumbar region and are posterior in position. Most spinal angiomas are supplied by one or more of the radiculomedullary vessels. These feeding vessels usually accompany the posterior nerve roots but they may arise anteriorly, especially in the cer-

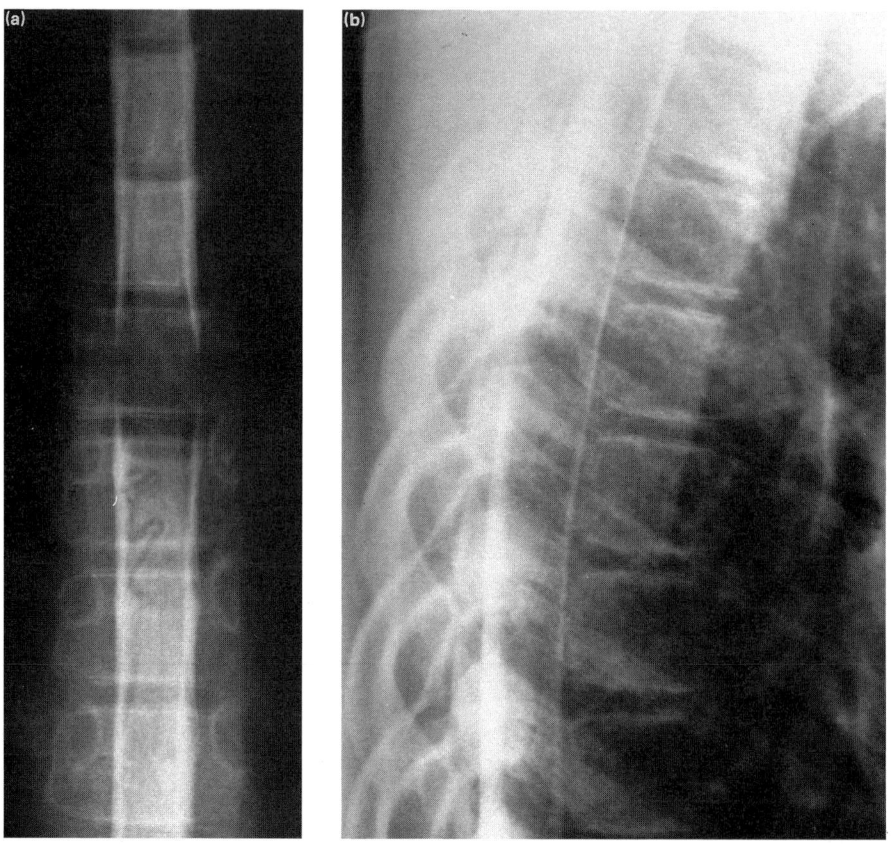

Fig. 5.11 AP (a) and lateral (b) views of a myelogram showing expansion of the spinal cord due to an intramedullary ependymoma. A large draining vein is also seen on the AP.

vical region. Venous drainage is often into longitudinally orientated coronal veins which may be markedly distended.

Neuroradiological investigations are directed at visualizing the angioma and defining its situation, feeding vessels and the local arterial supply to the cord itself. This may necessitate extensive angiographic studies if the malformation is situated in the cervical region, because of the numerous feeding and anastomotic vessels normally found in this area, or if it is in the lumbar region because ascending vessels from the lumbar and lateral sacral arteries may contribute to the circulation there.

In the thoracolumbar region the intramedullary circulation depends predominantly on a single source, the artery of Adamkiewicz, which must always be visualized. The planning of any surgery depends on the information acquired from angiography. The essential feature of a spinal AVM is an arteriovenous shunt. A saccular aneurysm may be present on a feeding artery and this, like the malformation itself, may be a source of haemorrhage. Arteries supplying AVMs are radiculopial or radiculomedullary arteries. The shunt may be fed by a single vessel or by several. In children the arterial supply is more likely to be multiple. There may be drainage by a single coiled vein or by two or more. The existence of more than one shunt is possible though uncommon. Arteries which supply angiomas sited posteriorly in the thoracic region usually arise within two or three segments of the level of the shunt, but feeders to cervical, thoracolumbar and lumbar angiomas frequently have a longer intradural course.

Spinal angiography is an invasive examination and can lead to transient or permanent neurological deterioration. This can arise either from a toxic effect of contrast medium on neurological tissue or, perhaps more likely, from small embolic episodes during the course of the procedure.

Spinal angiography is indicated whenever either myelography or MRI suggest the presence of an arteriovenous malformation. It will allow the exact anatomy and blood supply of the lesion to be identified (Fig. 5.12). Angiography is also indicated in the preoperative assessment of vascular tumours of the spine itself, such as metastasis from renal carcinoma and intramedullary tumours such as haemangioblastoma.

It is essential that the examination is performed methodically to ensure that all vessels which might be supplying a malformation are catheterized and injected. This is particularly true in the upper cervical and lumbosacral regions where the segmental vessel supplying the shunt may lie at a considerable distance from the fistula itself.

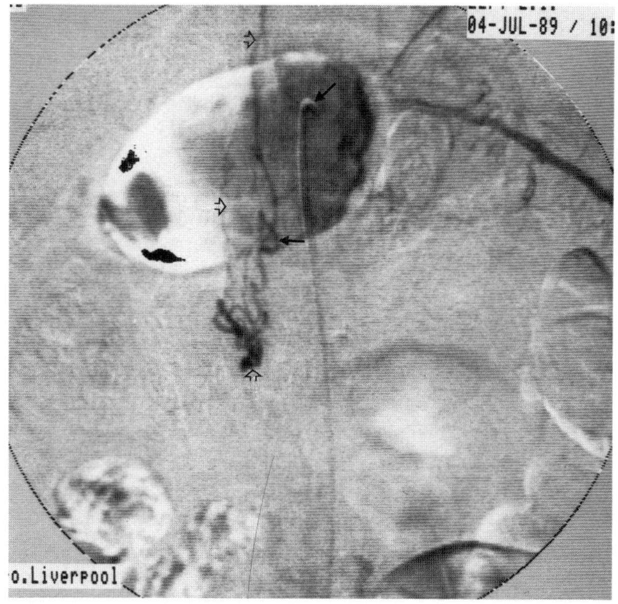

Fig. 5.12 Digital subtraction spinal angiography of a spinal arteriovenous malformation (AVM) seen through a gastric air bubble. Black arrow, catheter in segmental vessel; black arrowhead, feeding artery; open arrow, nidus of the AVM; open arrowheads, draining veins.

DISCOGRAPHY

Discography is most commonly utilized when assessing the integrity of lumbar discs in patients with low back pain. It is less commonly used in the cervical spine. A posterolateral approach is normally utilized (McCulloch & Waddell, 1978) to approach the lumbar disc. A double-needle technique is used to reduce the chance of causing discitis (Fraser *et al.*, 1987). A 21G needle is placed at the posterolateral margin of the disc and the disc is then actually punctured with a 26G needle, which is advanced to the centre of the disc. It is essential that the tip of the needle lies in the centre of the disc to avoid an annular injection.

The interpretation of abnormality is simple in the presence of gross degeneration as when, for example, the contrast passes posteriorly and spreads into the

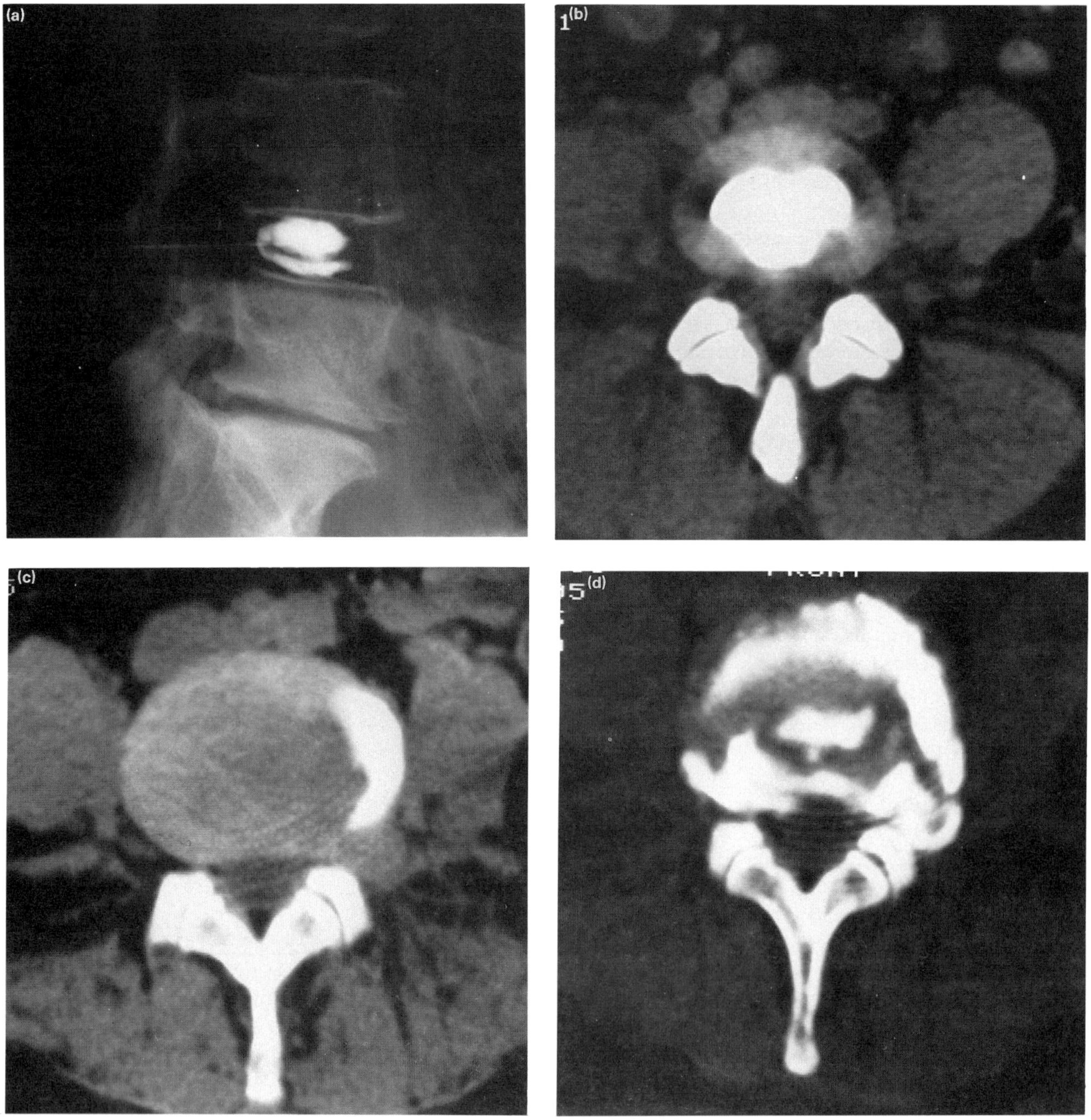

Fig. 5.13 (a) Lateral discogram of L4–L5 which was interpreted as normal. The CT (b) shows early fissuring of the posterior annular fibres. (c) Plain CT showing a mass lying lateral to the root foramen. CT discography (d) shows clearly that this is a far lateral disc herniation and not a neurofibroma.

extradural space. Detecting lesser degrees of abnormality demands knowledge of the normal appearance of the nucleus pulposus. The information gained from the discogram can be enhanced by performing CT following the discogram (Fig. 5.13).

Many authorities place great emphasis on the reproduction of pain during discography. They claim that, should the discographic injection reproduce the identical pain of which the patient complains, and if it is then abolished by the injection, this indicates that the disc is the source of the patient's pain. An equal number of authorities, however, dispute the reliability of pain reproduction. Occasionally, the actual intradiscal pressure is measured. Although this was of enormous potential in experimental studies (Nachemson, 1981), the use of discomanometry has found only a limited place in clinical practice.

MRI allows the assessment of disc degeneration non-invasively. The correlation between MRI and discography has been found to be high, but Heilman & O'Brien (1990) showed that discography can be abnormal, even in the presence of a normal MRI appearance.

REFERENCES

Fraser, R.D., Osti, O.L. & Vernon-Roberts, B. (1987) Discitis after discography. *J. Bone Jt. Surg.*, **69B**, 26–35.

Heilman, A.E. & O'Brien, J.P. (1990) Normal MRI with abnormal discography in patients with disability spinal pain. *J. Bone Jt. Surg.*, **72B**, 1088.

Kendall, B. & Stevens, J. (1984) Cervical myelography with iohexol. *Br. J. Radiol.*, **57**, 785–787.

McCulloch, J.A. & Waddell, G. (1978) Lateral lumbar discography. *Br. J. Radiol.*, **51**, 498–502.

MacPherson, P. & MacPherson, E.L. (1981) Cervical spondylosis—oblique films are unnecessary. *Health Bull. (Edin.)*, **39**, 89–91.

Nachemson, A. (1976) In Jayson, M. (ed.) *The Lumbar Spine and Back Pain*. Sector Publishing, London.

Nachemson, A. (1981) Disc pressure measurements. *Spine*, **6**, 93–97.

Teesdale, E. & MacPherson, P. (1984) Guidelines for cervical myelography; lumbar versus cervical puncture technique. *Br. J. Radiol.*, **57**, 789–793.

6 · Radiological Investigation of the Spine in Children

By H. CARTY

Before any discussion of the radiological assessment of the paediatric spine it is important to emphasize the normal physiological changes that take place with growth. Ossification begins in the vertebral bodies at about three months gestation, first appearing in the lower dorsal and upper lumbar areas. By term, ossification centres for all the bodies and the neural arches are present. The ossification of the arch is complete by 10 years. Secondary ossification centres appear at approximately puberty, at the tips of the bony appendages which arise from the neural arch and fuse with the main mass of bone by about 25 years. Annular ossification centres appear at the upper and lower endplates of the vertebral bodies at about puberty, but may occur as young as seven to eight years. These are also said to be fused by about 25 years at the latest, but for practical purposes are seldom seen on a radiograph beyond the age of 18 years. The importance of all these separate ossification centres is that they may be mistaken for fractures by those not familiar with the paediatric spine.

The spine undergoes a series of changes in its curvature in response to the normal stresses of posture. At birth there is a long single shallow curve concave anteriorly extending from top to bottom. The cervical lordotic curve develops when the child assumes the erect posture. The curve does not become fixed until puberty. At birth the cervical spine constitutes a quarter of the total length, the thoracic spine half and the lumbar spine the remaining quarter. By adulthood the cervical spine forms only one-fifth of truncal length and the lumbar spine one-third (Silverman, 1985).

The longitudinal growth of the vertebral body and the total length of the spine are modified by the stress of weight-bearing. In the absence of weight-bearing due to neuromuscular weakness, there is relative increase in longitudinal growth and decrease in transverse growth. This is maximal in the lumbar vertebrae (Gooding and Neuhauser, 1965).

In the neonate the vertebral bodies tend to be rectangular in the thoracic spine and more ovoid in the lumbar region. The conventional rectangular shape develops in response to weight-bearing as the child begins to sit up and bears weight.

RADIOLOGY OF THE SPINE

The basic examination of the paediatric spine remains the conventional AP and lateral radiographs. The area covered will depend on the clinical indication. In general closely collimated views should be taken when there are good localizing signs, but where symptoms are poorly localized then a wider area should be covered. Localized views can then be taken of any suspicious region. In the young child a single lateral view will adequately display the lumbar spine including the L5–S1 joint, but by the teenage years the lumbar curve may have developed to adult proportions, and a coned lateral view of L5–S1 may be needed to assess this space adequately. This should not be done until the first lateral film is assessed.

Oblique projections are of value only in the cervical and lumbar spine, and are not routinely indicated in children. They should be performed only following review of the AP and lateral projections. They are of most help in evaluating facetal fractures in the cervical spine and the assessment of a suspected or known spondylolisthesis or spondylolysis. Oblique projec-

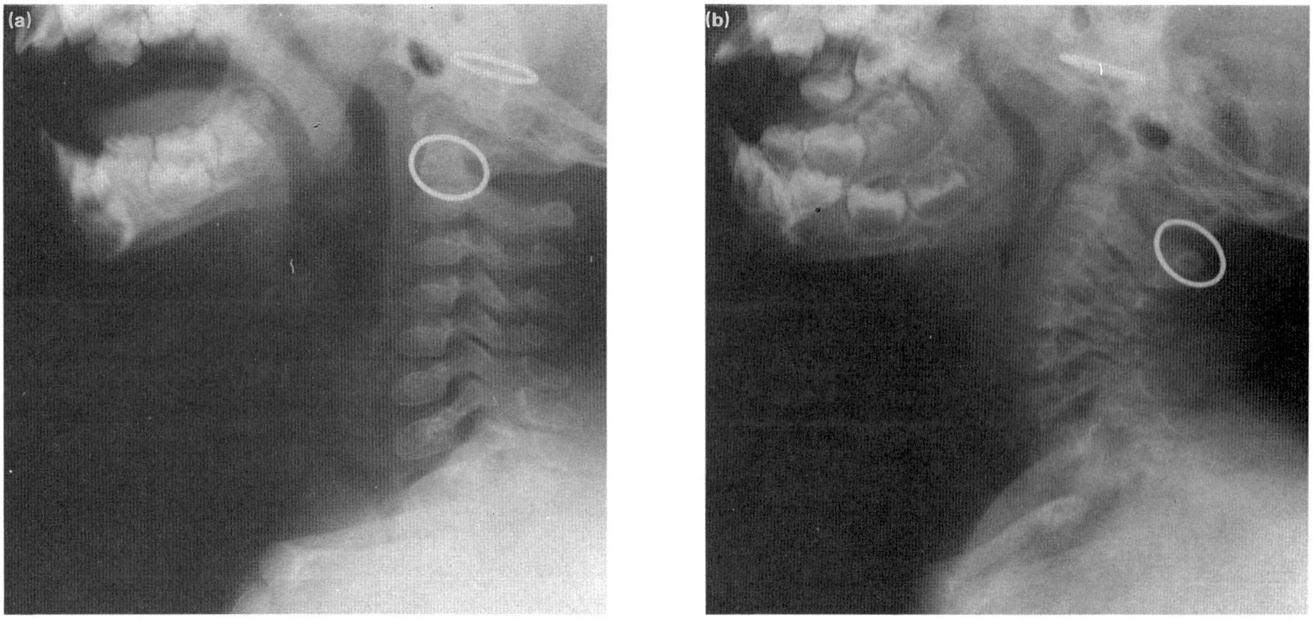

Fig. 6.1 Cervical spine of two-year-old girl. (a) The neck is in slight flexion. There is apparent widening of the retrotracheal soft tissues, which might be mistaken for an abscess. (b) Neck now in extension. The soft tissue is now normal and measures the width of the vertebral body. Note also normal slightly oval vertebral bodies due to non-ossification of the as-yet cartilaginous apophyses.

tions, to be of value, should be centred over the area of interest.

Flexion and extension views are indicated only in the cervical spine in the full assessment of a suspected or expected subluxation, such as might occur in Down's syndrome or the various skeletal dysplasias. They are also indicated in trauma where there is doubtful slip on the straight lateral view, but such flexion and extension views should be supervised by the medical staff. Standing flexion and extension views are very helpful in the assessment of movement in spondylolisthesis. They should not be done as a routine, but requested when there is a specific clinical indication.

There is often pseudosubluxation seen on the cervical spine radiographs of young children, when the X-ray is taken with the neck slightly flexed. This is often coupled with an apparent increase in the retrotracheal soft tissue, which can be alarming and cause great confusion to those not familiar with children's X-rays. If one wishes to confirm normality the X-ray should be repeated with the neck slightly extended. This causes the trachea to straighten, obliterating the apparent soft tissue swelling. With a genuine retropharyngeal abscess or haematoma the child will resist all attempts at neck extension due to the pain. In the normal child during quiet respiration with the neck extended, the retropharyngeal soft tissue should not measure more than the width of the vertebral body (Fig. 6.1).

In children who have severe angular and rotational deformities of the spine it is often impossible to obtain adequate lateral radiographs, important when one is trying to see vertebral foraminal enlargement in suspected neurogenic tumours, or in trying to resolve complex congenital abnormalities, at the apex of a kyphoscoliosis. In these circumstances it is good radiological practice to position the child in the desired projection, using image intensification, and then do the overcouch radiograph once the correct position has been achieved. This will result in far less radiation than would obtain from multiple attempts without screen control.

Conventional tomography has now largely been replaced by computerized tomography (CT) or CT myelography, where these facilities are available. It is occasionally still indicated in the postoperative spine, where metal implants degrade the image, or where there is gross distortion over a long length of the spine which makes CT difficult to interpret, or so many slices are required to resolve the problem that concern might arise from the radiation dose. It is sometimes difficult to appeciate the full extent of a lesion on axial CT images, and for perspective one requires sagittal or coronal reconstruction. Unless the axial slices are taken close together, i.e. no more than 4 mm slices, reconstruction can be very crude and detail obscured. In such a situation conventional linear tomography can sometimes be more useful.

Computerized tomography and magnetic resonance imaging (MRI) of the spine are discussed in detail in Chapter 7. The paediatric applications are very similar to those obtaining in adult practice, i.e. localization of lesions seen on plain X-ray, the assessment of trauma, tumours, vertebral infection and disc lesions. Bony developmental anomalies such as pedicular hypoplasia are best assessed by CT, but thecal and spinal cord anomalies are best investigated by MRI. If MRI is unavailable, then CT is less invasive and a possible alternative to myelography, although for full assessment of a lesion CT myelography is preferred to a non-contrast spinal CT. Lumbar disc lesions are adequately assessed by CT without intrathecal contrast. Intrathecal contrast is essential for assessment of spinal tumours.

The indications for myelography in children largely depend on the local availability of MRI. When this is freely available locally to children of all ages, then it completely replaces myelography. If not available then myelography is still indicated in the full delineation of mass lesions suspected as a result of plain film changes or clinical presentation. It is also necessary to delineate suspected or known congenital lesions such as diastematomyelia or a tethered filum terminale. Myelography is also indicated in the investigation of some children with scoliosis, where there are localizing neurological signs, or an inappropriate clinical course or presentation causing suspicion of an intraspinal tumour or syringomyelia. Facilities should be available to combine the myelogram with CT. The whole spine can be examined by conventional myelography, and CT performed across the area of interest. All myelography in children should be carried out using non-ionic water-soluble contrast medium. The choice of general versus local anaesthetic depends on the age and temperament of the child and the practice of the radiologist. Once intrathecal contrast is introduced for myelography the entire canal including the foramen magnum area should be examined.

Spinal angiography is indicated to fully elucidate vascular anomalies demonstrated by myelography or MRI. It is also possible to embolize many of these anomalies and to effect a cure, but this type of procedure must be carried out only by a radiologist trained in the techniques, and in general should be done only in a specialized centre.

Ultrasound of the spine has received little attention compared with other regions in the body. In intrauterine life it is the means by which neural tube defects are detected. Postpartum, ultrasonic examination of the encephalocele, or meningocele, will very rapidly show the contents of the sac, i.e., whether it contains just cerebrospinal fluid (CSF), or contains theca or brain. It is also possible to define the level of the cord by ultrasonic means in the neonatal spine. All infants with neural tube defects should have cranial ultrasound before closure. Associated Chiari malformations which increase the likelihood of hydrocephalus following closure of the defect are easily identified. Baseline ventricular size is established, making it easier to assess the development of the hydrocephalus. Apart from the Chiari malformation associated with myelomeningocele, other intracranial anomalies such as Dandy Walker cysts and corpus callosum malformations, are also assessable.

Ultrasonic monitoring of the renal tract is the simplest and least invasive means of observing the kidneys in children at risk of neuropathic uropathy.

Bone scintigraphy in children is performed using the radiopharmaceutical technetium-99m (^{99m}Tc) methylene diphosphonate. In cases of suspected infection indium-111-labelled or Tc-labelled HMPAO white cell scanning can be helpful. The major indications in children with spinal symptoms are X-ray negative spinal or sacroiliac pain, painful scoliosis, the further evaluation of a child with pain with doubtful lesions on X-ray, and confirmation of single site pathology in the presence of a known lesion on X-ray and identification of fractures. In practice one of its greatest values is in localizing a lesion in a symptomatic child with vague symptoms. Positive bone scans will be found in infections, trauma and neoplasms. The scan appearance is often non-specific and must be interpreted with other imaging procedures and full clinical biochemical and haematological details.

High-resolution images are essential for interpretation. Sedation may be required to achieve these. Inadequate images will be produced in children with full bladders, and if necessary the bladder must be catheterized to get adequate sacroiliac and pelvic images, if this is the likely site of pathology. Care in interpretation of rotated images and a knowledge of normal scintigraphic appearances in children is essential if mistakes are to be avoided.

Radiation considerations and gonadal protection

The aim of all radiographic technique in children is to obtain the best-quality image with maximum diagnostic information and minimum radiation dose to the patient. Radiology of the spine involves the irradiation of radiosensitive organs, the thyroid, bone marrow, female gonads and the breast. To minimize gonadal exposure, shielding should always be applied in the male. It is probably best omitted on the initial examination in the female, especially if pelvic and hip views are required for initial assessment, but should be applied thereafter.

Good communication between clinical and radiology departments is essential. There should be an agreed protocol as to what films are required; for example, are standing or supine films required? Is a whole spine required on follow-up films or will the region of the curvature suffice? What films are required at initial assessment of a scoliosis and what films are required during follow-up visits? Is a lateral film all that is required in monitoring a kyphos? There is a tendency in busy outpatient departments, for X-ray requests to be filled in by nursing staff, without clear instruction by the consultant as to what information he is seeking, and all too often failure to inform the radiology department when investigation ideas alter. Much unnecessary radiation can be avoided by clear communication.

Breast irradiation is reduced to approximately 10% of the dose received in the AP projection, by simply X-raying PA (Ardran *et al.*, 1980). Further reduction is achieved by the use of an air gap technique and graded or rare earth screens.

Children's radiographs are best taken by technicians trained specifically in paediatric radiography. They should not be left to the mercy of whichever radiographer happens to be rotating through the room on a given day. The technician trained in paediatric technique knows how to communicate with the child, gain his or her confidence and will, therefore, in general produce far higher quality work with a lower incidence of repeats than an 'occasional' paediatric radiographer.

SYSTEMATIC REVIEW OF CHILDREN'S SPINAL X-RAYS

A methodical approach to reviewing the X-rays should be developed. The precise order of review is immaterial. Active consideration of alignment in both frontal and lateral projections is essential, looking for straightness in the frontal view and the presence of the normal cervical and lumbar lordosis, and mild thoracic kyphos in the lateral view. Loss of these is seen most commonly with muscle spasm, but bony abnormalities and intraspinal tumours can also lead to malalignment. Bone texture is best assessed on the lateral view, and any increase or decrease, general or localized, should be noted. The presence of the individual components of each vertebral body—the pedicles, facets, spinous process and body itself—should be individually checked. The interpedicular distance gently widens as it progresses distally. Any sudden deviation from this, or flattening of the normally curved medial border of the pedicles, should lead one to search further for an intrathecal space-occupying lesion. Note should be made of transitional vertebrae in the distal lumbar spine or proximal sacral spine, together with the presence of false articulations. The paravertebral soft tissues should be assessed. These are usually symmetrical. Any unusual prominence or widening over a localized area probably indicates abscess or tumour.

Narrowing of the disc spaces occurs in children both with infection and degeneration, and in the early stages may occur without vertebral endplate abnormality. Disc narrowing is often overlooked in children, especially the young, and this is often the only radiological finding in juvenile discitis. The sacroiliac joints in children are very wide relative to the adult, and they appear irregular in the normal child. Sacroilitis is therefore almost impossible to assess from straight X-rays, and is best assessed by a combination of scintigraphy and CT.

The cranial sutures are usually visible on a cervical spine X-ray and should be actively viewed. The awkward gait, thought to be spinal in origin, may be due to an intracranial tumour. The sutures may be diastased, and the pituitary fossa enlarged.

Normal variants

There are some variants which may cause confusion and lead to unnecessary anxiety and investigation if misinterpreted.

Ossification problems

Ring apophyses appear in the midthoracic and lumbar vertebrae approximately at six years, and fuse with the body by 18 years. These are sometimes mistakenly labelled fractures.

CORONAL CLEFT VERTEBRAE

A lucent cleft at the junction of the anterior two-thirds and posterior one-third of the thoracic or lumbar vertebrae is seen in 2–5% of infants and is found almost exclusively in males. It is due to delay in fusion of the anterior and dorsal vertebral ossification centres. Fusion occurs by the age of one year.

INCOMPLETE FUSION OF NEURAL ARCHES

This is a very common finding at L5 and S1 in children, and is said to occur in up to 60% of children at the age of eight (Sutow & Pryde, 1956). The incidence decreases thereafter as the cartilage ossifies. There is an increased incidence of spondylolisthesis in association with a true spina bifida occulta. Many apparent lesions in the young child have the defects filled with cartilage. In early life the posterior neural arches have commonly a cartilaginous cleft, best seen in the AP projection (Fig. 6.2). This cleft fuses between three and five years, starting in the lumbar region, and finishing with the cervical spine.

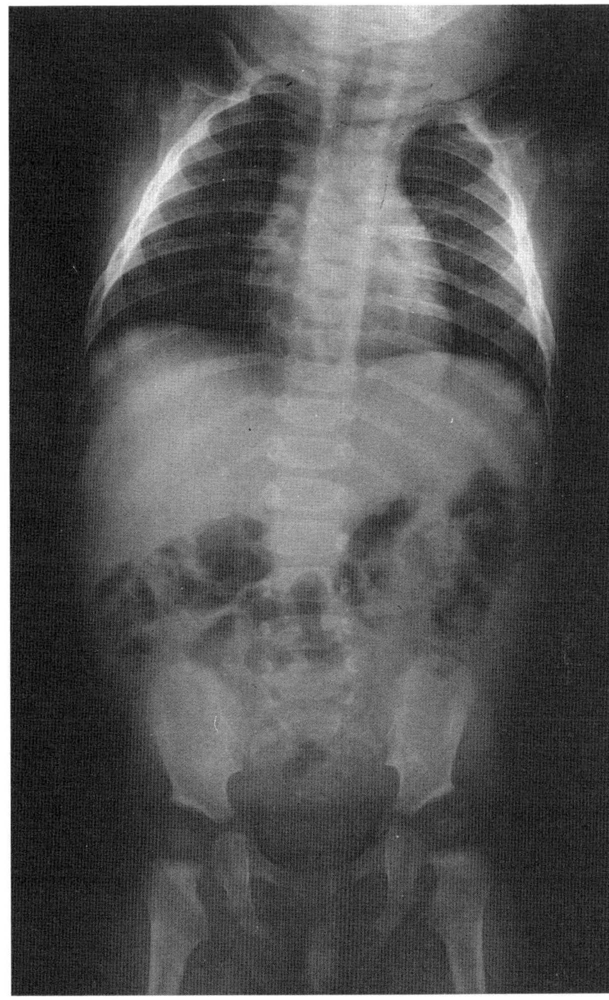

Fig. 6.2 Normal spine of child age nine months. There is incomplete fusion of the neural arches throughout most of the thoracic spine.

OSSIFICATION CENTRE FOR THE DENS

This appears between three and six years and fuses by 12 years. It is known as the os terminale. It must not be confused with the os odontoidonum which is associated with dens hypoplasia (Shapiro & Robinson, 1976).

OSSIFICATION OF THE ATLANTO-OCCIPITAL MEMBRANE

Bony bridging between the occiput and C1 is due to ossification of the lateral edge of the posterior atlanto-occipital membrane behind the superior vertebral notch of C1 (Fig. 6.3). This can be unilateral or bilateral. Congenital absence of part of the vertebral bodies and segmentation defects are abnormal, and not part of the remit of this chapter. These are discussed in the relevant sections elsewhere in this book.

Pseudo-subluxation of the cervical spine

It is common in children to find apparent forward slip of the C1 on C2, or C2 on C3 when the head is slightly flexed. This leads to considerable diagnostic confusion in suspected trauma. A normal atlanto–odontoid measurement in children up to the age of 15 is up to 5 mm (Cattell & Filtzer, 1965). This is partly due to greater normal ligament laxity. Similar appearances occur at C1–C2 where up to 5 mm of movement can be normal (Fig. 6.4). Mistakes can be

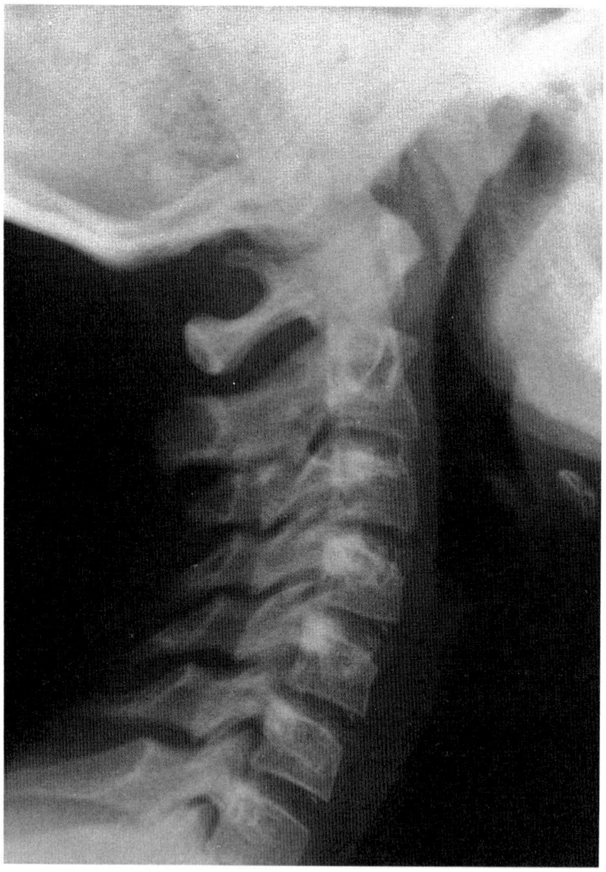

Fig. 6.3 Incomplete ossification of the atlanto-occipital membrane causing incomplete bony bridging between the occiput and C1. Note also unfused ring apophyses of the vertebral endplates. These must not be mistaken for fractures.

avoided by taking lateral neck radiographs in a neutral position or with slight extension, and by observing continuity of the posterior cervical line in which a line connecting the cortices of the post arch of C1 and C3 will pass through, or no more than 1 mm anterior to, the posterior cortex of C2 in physiological subluxation (Swischuk, 1977).

Thickening of the retrotracheal and retropharyngeal space

These tissues can apparently be markedly increased in size in young children when the lateral X-ray is taken in flexion and extension (Fig. 6.1). The tracheal cartilage is not fully developed, allowing the trachea to buckle and giving an appearance suggestive of an abscess. Children who have an abscess will hold their necks stiff with loss of the normal curvatures. The child will also be clinically ill. Extension of the neck will cause all pseudo-mass to disappear.

Pseudo-widening of the interpedicular distance

The normal interpedicular width in the cervical canal in children is relatively wider than in adults (Fig. 6.5). Any obliquity in position of the X-ray will accentuate this. The widening occurs without flattening of the pedicles, and is a gradual appearance. A sudden change in diameter should be viewed with caution and further investigated. As the child matures the relative distance decreases towards adult proportions. The appearance is most pronounced in infancy and has largely disappeared by the age of four to six years, but can persist up to 10 years. Similar appearances are found in relation to the sagittal diameter (Yousefzadeh *et al.*, 1982).

Vertebral height/disc ratio

Normal weight-bearing is necessary to inhibit vertical growth of the vertebral bodies. Absence of normal weight-bearing and neuromuscular tone will lead to a relative increase in height of the vertebral body, with decreased disc space height and poor modelling of the vertebral endplates, which remain normal. An index of normal values and ratios for the vertebral body height versus disc space height has been established (Brandner, 1970).

The infant's lumbar vertebrae are normally oval, while the thoracic vertebrae are rectangular. Normal muscle tone and adoption of the upright posture, together with progressive ossification, gradually effects an alteration in shape, so that the lumbar vertebrae become rectangular when the child is sitting. Some mild apparent anterior wedging of the midthoracic vertebrae is a common finding in children from about the age seven to 14, and must not be mistaken for compression fractures (Fig. 6.6).

Other apparent vertebral anomalies occur. A transitory appearance of a bone within a bone appearance is a normal finding between the ages of one and two months (Brill *et al.*, 1973), disappearing after this. The appearance is prolonged in the premature infant. A mild degree of posterior scalloping in the lumbar spine is a normal appearance in children up to 12–14 years of age and must not be mistaken as evidence of a neurogenic tumour, or skeletal dysplasia.

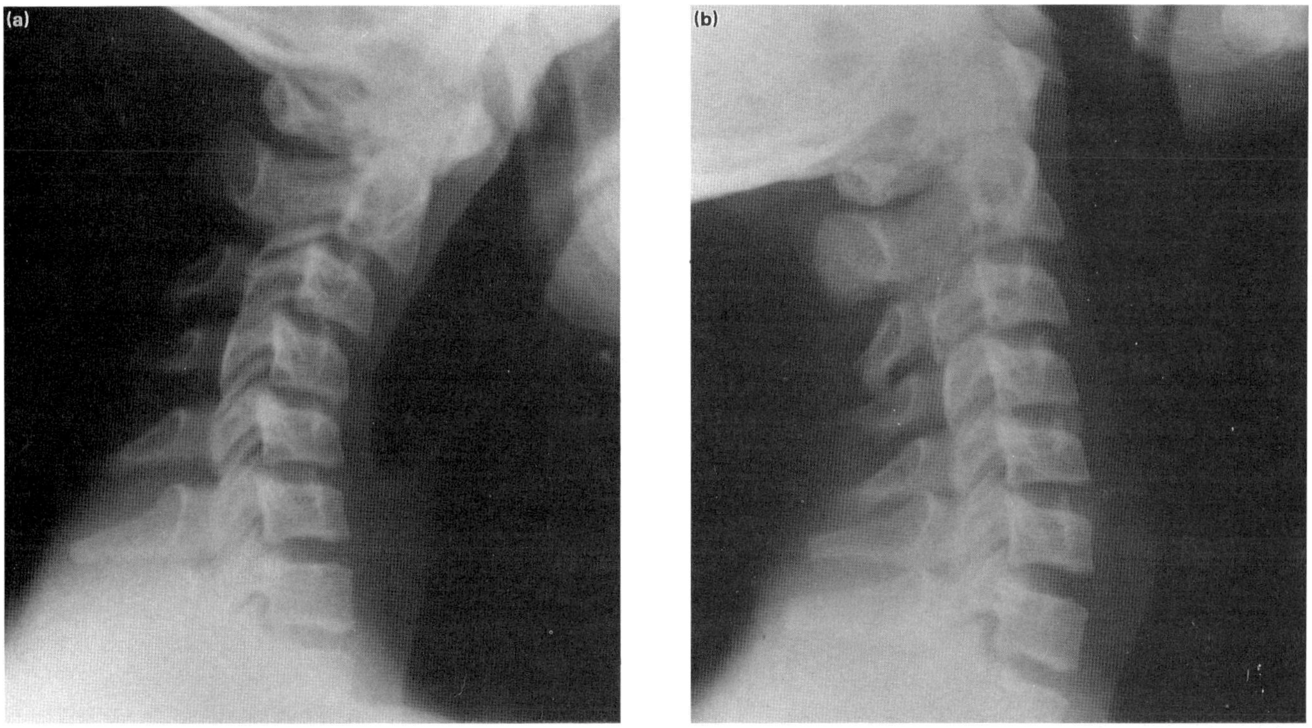

Fig. 6.4 In flexion (a) there is apparent subluxation of the body of C2 on C3. In extension (b) a line drawn through the cortices of the posterior arch of C1 and C3 passes through C2, indicating pseudo-subluxation.

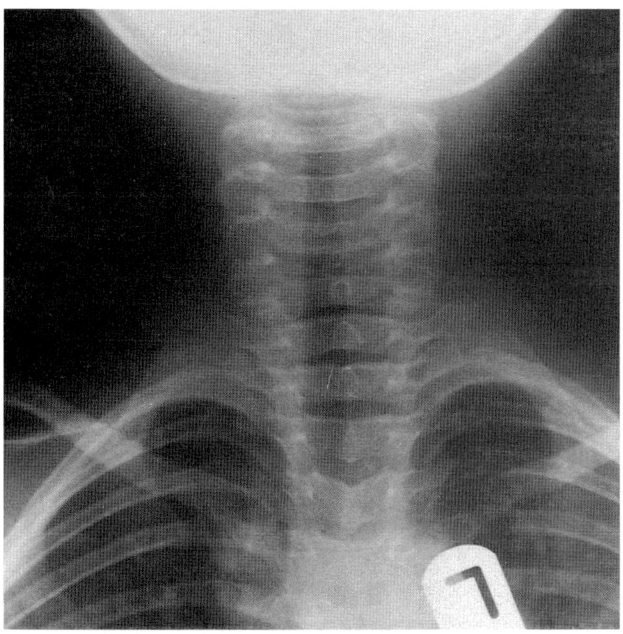

Fig. 6.5 Normal cervical spine AP view in seven-year-old child. The interpedicular distance is apparently widened. Note normal unflattened appearance of the pedicles. This is a normal variant.

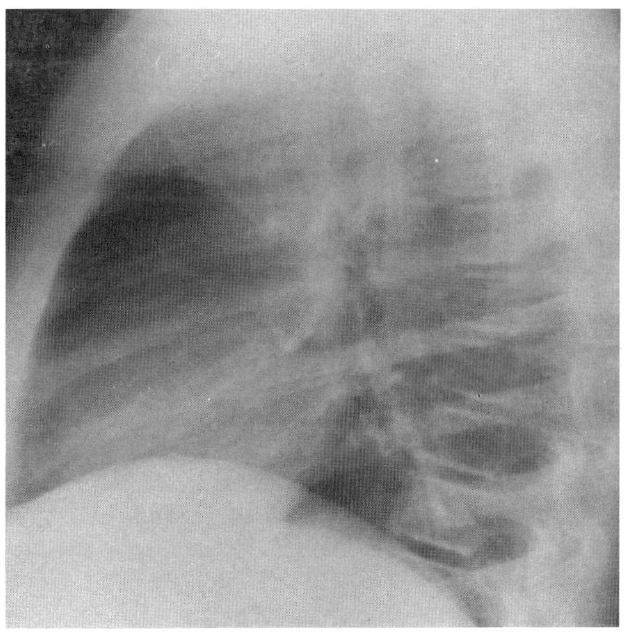

Fig. 6.6 Girl age 12. There is minimal anterior wedging of the bodies of D7–D9, which is normal and due to unossified anterior parts of the vertebral endplates. This spine is normal.

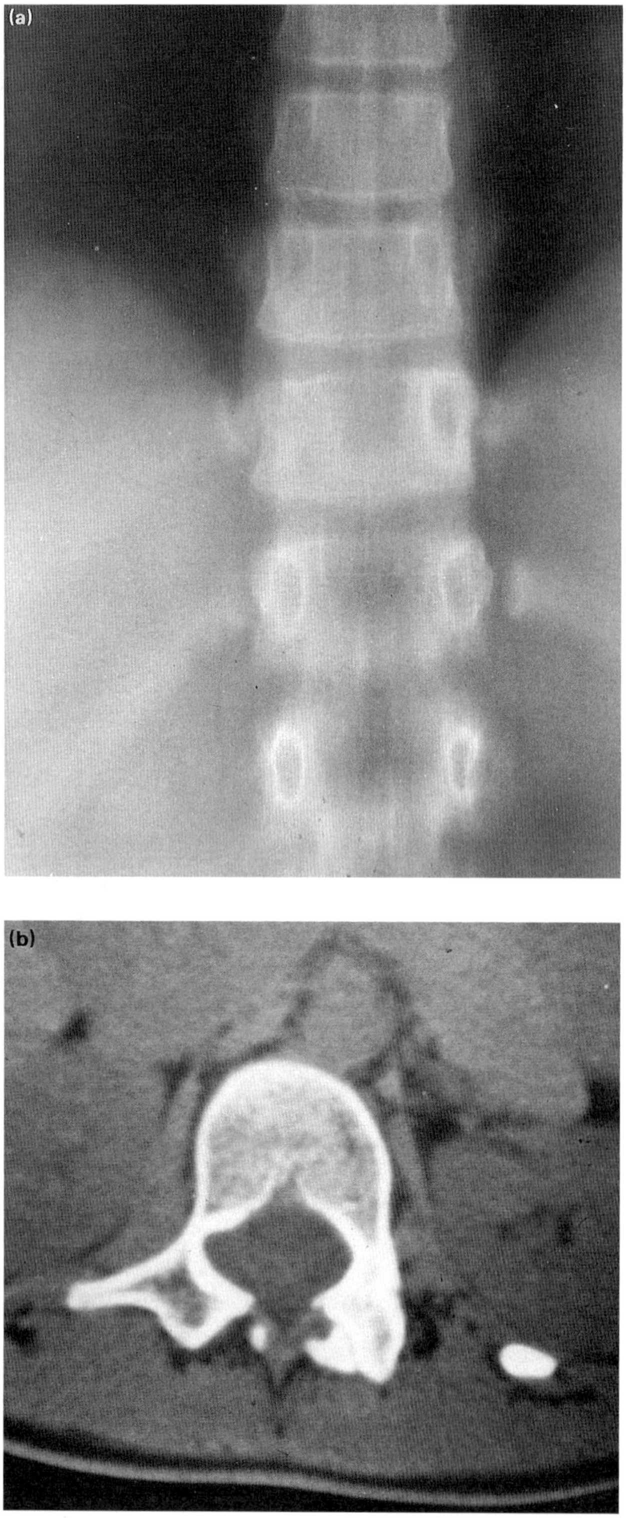

Fig. 6.7 (a) There is absence of the right-hand pedicle of T11, best seen on this tomograph. Girl age 12. (b) CT scan of another patient, girl age 13. There is hypoplasia of the right pedicle with contralateral hypertrophy and sclerosis.

Aplasia or hypoplasia of a pedicle is an uncommon, though well-recognized developmental variant (Fig. 6.7a). Hypoplasia is more frequent than aplasia (Bardsley & Hanelin, 1971; Morin & Palacios, 1974). The lower thoracic and lumbar spine are the most frequent sites. The patients are asymptomatic and the discovery of a lesion is incidental. In adult practice it is common to see contralateral pedicle hypertrophy, but this may not be evident in paediatric practice. There is accompanying abnormality of the ipsilateral transverse process. When an absent pedicle is discovered on an X-ray a CT and isotope bone scan will confirm the nature of the abnormality. The bone scan is normal and the hypoplasia is easy to appreciate on CT (Fig. 6.7b). The lesion must not be mistaken for pedicle destruction secondary to metastatic disease.

Absent or hypoplastic pedicles also occur in the cervical spine. Many of these patients are symptomatic with pain, limb weakness and numbness in the distribution of the nerve roots. Radiological features associated with the absence are a small transverse process and a double vertebral foramen with outpouching of contrast on myelography. The lateral articular mass may also be displaced.

The pedicles in the thoracic spine at the level of the thoracolumbar junction are flat in about 7% of normal children (Benzian *et al.*, 1971). This must not be confused with pedicle erosion. The pedicle is concave laterally and convex medially. The interpedicular distance remains normal, and there is no erosive change. In pathological thinning there is usually some widening of the interpedicular distance.

All movement of a patient with neurological symptoms secondary to tumour, and all movement of a child with spinal trauma, irrespective of neurology, must be carried out by trained staff under medical supervision. Where possible lateral decubitus views should be done in preference to moving the patient for the lateral projection, and collars, etc., removed only if essential. A compromise between moving the patient to the X-ray department to obtain better images and accepting less than optimum portable images, must be agreed between the radiologist and referring clinician.

In the traumatized child the radiologist must be aware of the possibility of trauma other than to the spine, and actively review all X-rays for chest and abdominal complications. These can be overlooked in the anxiety to deal with the spinal trauma. The mechanism of the injury, and the nature of the violence, must be made clear to the radiologist, so that he or she can be alert for the other potential lesions, such as aortic rupture in a decelerating injury in a road traffic accident.

PROBLEM AREAS

Scoliosis

The assessment of spinal curvature deformities is important, and there are frequent indications for referral for X-rays. These children will have repeated radiology to monitor the progress of the curves. It is therefore imperative that there is meticulous attention to the radiographic technique, to avoid unnecessary repeat exposures. The initial assessment should include an AP and lateral erect view of the spine, each on a single film. Iliac crest apophyses must be included to allow assessment of maturity (Wilmot & Sharka, 1987). These are supplemented by coned views of areas of interest such as the cervical spine, or complex congenital anomalies, following review of the initial films. Lateral bending views to differentiate structural and non-structural curves are useful at initial assessment, but should not routinely form part of follow-up. The mobility of the curve can be assessed by traction views, which should be supervised by medical staff. An AP view of the hand and wrist may also be performed for bone age assessment at presentation.

The initial film must be of high quality to allow for assessment of congenital and possible neurogenic lesions. Follow-up films are taken to monitor progress of the curve, and quality is less vital. It is in this situation that the air gap technique (as described by Ardren) is best employed. The techniques of measuring and assessing the deformity are described in Chapter 9.

Following surgical treatment, postoperative X-rays are taken to assess fusion and maintenance of correction of the curves. In general only PA views are taken, but these should be supplemented by lateral views if any loss of correction is observed. Rod fracture and hook dislocation may be appreciated only on the lateral projection. If a child complains of localized pain, possible causes include infection and pseudarthrosis. Oblique views, or linear tomography and scintigraphy, may be required to establish the cause of pain. CT is useless in the spine following instrumentation, as streak artifact from the rod prevents adequate imaging, although computerised subtraction of the CT images may improve this problem.

In the immediate postoperative period, the chest X-rays should be carefully reviewed by a radiologist for complications, such as pleural effusion, pneumothorax, position of drains and lines, and areas of pulmonary collapse or consolidation, all of which may be overlooked by the orthopaedic surgeon whose major concern is the spine. A rare postoperative complication of scoliosis surgery is the development of a persistent CSF pleural effusion. The precise point of leak can be identified by scintigraphy following instillation of intrathecal indium-labelled DTPA.

Neural tube defects

The medical, surgical and orthopaedic details of these lesions are discussed elsewhere. Radiological assessment is fundamental in their management. The extent of the bony defect is assessed on the AP and lateral projection. The contents of the sac are identified by ultrasound. These examinations are supplemented by CT and MRI where indicated. Ultrasound, CT and MRI are used to monitor the intracranial complications, and ultrasound and radionuclides to monitor the renal tract. The cranial and renal progress are cared for by the paediatric surgeon, while the orthopaedic and postural progress are monitored by the orthopaedic surgeons, by a combination of clinical and radiological assessment. The orthopaedic surgeon's assessment of spinal radiographs is excellent, but he may overlook other complications: specifically shunt complications and the development of renal stones, both important to identify and treat prior to spinal surgery. All children with a shunt should have a valve system X-ray prior to spinal surgery. When assessing these films the following points must be actively assessed.

1 The position of the intraventricular catheter. Is it long enough so that the tip is likely to lie within the ventricle?

2 Continuity of the system. Any disruption must be noted and a decision made as to whether the child is shunt-dependent before embarking on surgery.

3 Position of the lower end of the shunt. If this is a ventriculoatrial shunt, is the lower end in a position in which one might reasonably expect it to be, at the right atrium? This can be confirmed by echocardiography. If the system is a ventriculoperitoneal one, is the lower end in the abdomen? A system that has the lower end projected over the liver should be further assessed by a lateral film to ensure that the end is not simply subcutaneous in position.

4 Is there any evidence of a mass effect around the catheter end which suggests an encysted collection of CSF around the lower end and, therefore, impaired function? This can be confirmed by ultrasound.

5 Are renal stones visible on the spinal X-rays? If so a decision about their management should be made prior to surgery.

6 Is there evidence of gross constipation which may lead to faecal impaction and obstruction, during the postoperative period? Appropriate preparation prior to surgery may prevent this complication.

Another complication that occasionally occurs in children with neural tube defects is the development of pressure sores, and ischial or trochanteric abscesses. These are clinically obvious but sinograms with or without CT may be required to assess them fully and allow adequate debridement. Careful and regular monitoring of the renal tract by ultrasound and radionuclide studies, is indicated in all children with sacral anomalies, spinal cord trauma and potential neuropathic uropathy. Annual ultrasound is routinely indicated. Ultrasound is sensitive in the detection of hydronephrosis, ureteral dilatation, assessment of bladder wall thickness and in general in the detection of stones, provided deformity does not preclude a good view. If it does, the ultrasound examination should be supplemented by a plain abdominal X-ray. Renal scarring may be seen on ultrasound but the most sensitive method of detection is by ^{99m}Tc DMSA scintigraphy. This should be done on presentation for baseline assessment, and repeated at three-yearly intervals in the absence of change on ultrasound or clinical infection. Due to the deformity of many of these children, anterior and posterior views should be done, the uptakes calculated for each view independently and then averaged.

Sacral anomalies

In general AP and lateral radiographs are adequate for initial assessment, but if there is severe pelvic rotational deformity associated with the sacral anomaly, CT is invaluable in resolving the anatomy. CT and or MRI are required for the full assessment of anterior meningoceles. The renal tracts are monitored in the usual way.

Segmentation defects

When a segmentation defect which results in a hemivertebra is associated with severe rotational or angular deformity, the full anatomy can be difficult to establish from the plain radiographs and, in particular, the relationship of the spinal cord to the deformity can be difficult to establish. The cord can be visualized with careful MRI but the bony problem is not seen optimally by MRI. As the deformity is usually only over a short segment, axial CT, followed by three-dimensional reconstruction can provide invaluable information, and should be done preoperatively. Simple sagittal or coronal reconstruction of the axial CT images is adequate for demonstration of the extent of the cord splitting associated with diastematomyelia.

Infections and trauma

As in adult practice the primary concern for the radiologist is to demonstrate the extent of the lesion, its bony and intrathecal components, to establish that it is a solitary lesion and not a metastatic one, and where indicated to perform a needle biopsy to provide a specimen for histology or culture. The margins for error in paediatric patients are less than in adult practice, and these procedures should be performed only by a radiologist properly trained or experienced in these techniques. They are best performed under CT control.

REFERENCES

Ardran, L., Coates, R., Dickson, R., Dixon-Brown, A. & Harding, F. (1980) Assessment of scoliosis in children: low dose radiographic technique. *Br. J. Radiol.*, **53**, 146–147.

Bardsley, J.L. & Hanelin, L.G. (1971) The unilateral hypoplastic lumbar pedicle. *Radiology*, **101**, 315–317.

Benzian, S., Mainzer, F. & Gooding, C. (1971) Pedicular thinning: a normal variant at the thoraco lumbar junction. *Br. J. Radiol.*, **44**, 936–939.

Brandner, M.E. (1970) Normal value of the vertebral body and intervertebral disc index during growth. *Am. J. Roentgenol.*, **110**, 618–627

Brill, P., Baker, D. & Ewing, M. (1973) Bone within bone in the neonatal spine: stress change or normal development. *Radiology*, **108**, 363–366.

Cattell, H. & Filtzer, D. (1965) Pseudosubluxation and other normal variations of the cervical spine in children. A study of 160 children. *J. Bone Jt. Surg.* **47A**, 1295–1309.

Gooding, C. & Neuhauser, E. (1965) Growth and development of the normal vertebral body in the presence and the absence of stress. *Am. J. Roentgenol.*, **93**, 388–394.

Morin, M. & Palacios, E. (1974) The aplastic hypoplastic lumbar pedicle. *Am. J. Roentgenol.*, **122**, 639–642.

Shapiro, R. & Robinson, F. (1976) Anomalies of the craniovertebral border. *Am. J. Roentgenol.*, **127**, 281–287.

Silverman, F. (1985) The spine. In Silverman, F. (ed.) *Caffey's Pediatric X-ray Diagnosis*, 8th edn, p. 281. Year Book Medical Publishers, Chicago, IL.

Swischuk, L.E. (1977) Anterior displacement of C_2 in children: physiologic or pathologic? A helpful differentiating line. *Radiology*, **122**, 759–763.

Sutow, W. & Pryde, A. (1956) Incidence of spina bifida occulta in relation to age. *Am. J. Dis. Child.*, **91**, 211–217.

Wilmot, D. & Sharka, G. (1987) Skeletal radiography. In Wilmot, D. & Sharka, G. (eds) *Pediatric Imaging for the Technologist*, Chap. 7, pp. 104–107. Springer, Berlin.

Yousefzadeh, D., El-Khoury, G. & Smith, W. (1982) Normal diameter and variation in the pediatric cervical spine. *Radiology*, **144**, 319–325.

7 · Computerized Tomography and Magnetic Resonance Imaging of the Spine

By K.B. HEITHOFF and R.J. HERZOG

The development of high-resolution computerized tomography (CT) and magnetic resonance imaging (MRI) has greatly enhanced the investigation of patients with spinal disease. High-quality imaging provides essential diagnostic information for the clinician treating spinal pathology. This chapter explores the potential and range which high-resolution CT and MRI provide in a spinal setting. It is impractical to detail the use of those investigations in every region or pathology which affects the spine in one chapter; further information regarding these techniques is given where relevant throughout this book. The subsequent discussion contained in this chapter concentrates on common problem areas—particularly the lumbar spine. It is in the lumbar spine in particular that most experience has been gained, but the mode of application of these technologies may easily be extended to other regions of the spine or to different pathological entities.

CT and MRI have become the mainstays of diagnostic imaging of the lumbar spine for the evaluation of degenerative disease in many practices. Myelography, and to a lesser extent plain radiology, have been relegated to a minor supporting role. The modern spine surgeon, perhaps considering either a microdiscectomy or a percutaneous discectomy for lumbar disc herniation, is no longer satisfied to know there is 'an extradural mass' present that is 'consistent with a disc herniation'. It is necessary to know that it is a definite disc herniation and whether it is contained or non-contained. If it is contained, are outer annular fibres intact, or is it contained by the posterior longitudinal ligament? If it is non-contained, is it a free fragment? Is there definite and demonstrable nerve root compression? Are there other complicating lesions, such as subarticular or lateral stenosis? Is there demonstrated instability, such as lytic or degenerative spondylolisthesis? Is there a conjoined nerve root overlying the disc herniation? Are other soft tissue lesions masquerading as a disc herniation or present in conjunction with it, such as epidural haematoma, hypertrophied ligamentum flavum, or synovial cysts? Is there inflammation of the marrow of the vertebral bodies adjacent to the degenerated, herniated disc?

CT and MRI provide precisely this detailed information, and therefore are the essential diagnostic tools of the spine surgeon. Armed with this knowledge, and excellent surgical judgement and technique, a surgeon can expect a high surgical success rate. It is essential, therefore, that surgeons train themselves in the capabilities of the newer investigative modalities.

Our hope is that just as CT has revolutionized the diagnosis and treatment of lateral stenosis with a concomitant improvement in the care of failed back surgery syndrome patients, MRI will lead to an improvement in our understanding of degenerative disc disease, musculoligamentous pathology, and associated inflammatory responses in the bone marrow, discs, and other soft tissues, and the roles they play in back pain and sciatica. Cooperative studies involving large groups of patients and treatment modalities made possible by telecommunication and computerization of collected data, in conjunction with continued improvements in imaging, will be essential to accomplish this goal in a reasonable time frame.

CT IMAGING PARAMETERS

In the authors' units, CT is the procedure of choice for lumbar spine imaging of non-operated patients presenting with sciatica. In our environment, CT is approximately half the cost of MRI and provides a complete screening examination for degenerative spine disease, including disc herniation (HNP) and stenosis.

High-resolution computerized tomography with multiplanar reformations (CT/MPR) transforms the standard axial CT examination of the spine into a more complete evaluative imaging study (Glenn *et al.*, 1984). The optimal delineation of spinal anatomy and pathology is obtained by studying the spine in complementary orthogonal planes. CT/MPR provides a standardized, integrated approach for evaluating the spine in the axial, sagittal and coronal planes (Glenn *et al.*, 1979; Lancourt *et al.*, 1979).

A high-resolution multiplanar CT examination requires thin contiguous axial sections of the cervical and thoracic spine and overlapping axial sections of the lumbar spine. The quality of the reconstructed images will be no better than the quality of the initial axial CT image data. The reconstructed CT images will have the same contrast resolution as the original axial images, but there will be at least some loss of spatial resolution because of the thickness of the initial axial sections (Ulrich, 1989). To prevent misregistration artifacts on the reconstructed images the patient must remain motionless during the study. Since a complete CT/MPR study can be performed in 25 minutes, it usually is not difficult for the patient to maintain a single position. Rapid scanning techniques have significantly reduced patient X-ray exposure.

In practice, AP and lateral CT scout images should be obtained in every case and may serve as plain films. They are essential for orientation and correlation of the findings noted on axial images. They are adequate for detection of abnormalities of spinal alignment, loss of disc height and gross degenerative changes and/or bony destruction. Additional plain films are only rarely required.

In each case the AP and lateral computerized radiographs are reviewed for disc space narrowing, endplate changes and degenerative spurring. The AP computerized radiograph is used to determine the number of lumbar vertebrae and the presence of any transitional vertebral or other congenital abnormalities.

Disorders of bony alignment, such as lytic or degenerative spondylolisthesis, retrolisthesis, and rotoscoliosis or kyphosis, should be noted. Hyperlordosis, increased lumbosacral angulation, and the

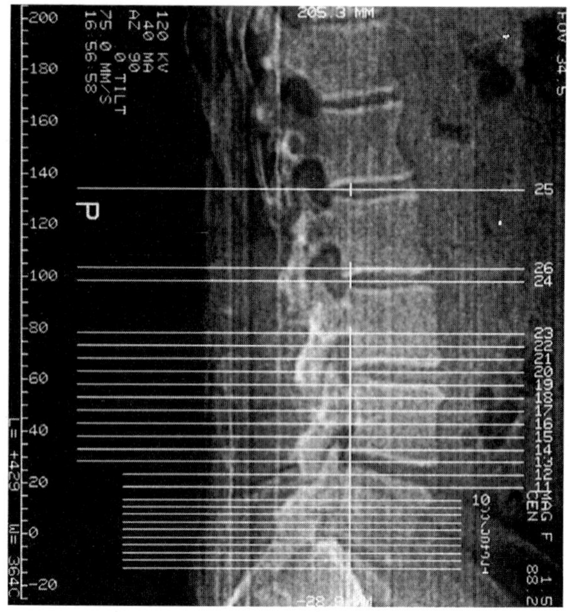

Fig. 7.1 Lateral computed radiograph of the lumbar spine showing the scanning protocol used.

level of the intercristal line are noted on the lateral computerized radiograph. Comment is also made regarding the hip joints and sacroiliac joints, which are routinely included on the AP computerized radiograph.

Detailed clinical information is essential for correct scanning. If full clinical details are not available to the radiologist prior to CT, then patients should be asked to fill out a detailed history of their lumbar spine symptoms, including a pain drawing. Survey images are obtained at L1–L2 and L2–L3 if the lateral computerized radiographs demonstrate abnormalities at those levels or if the patient's pain drawing indicates groin or anterior thigh pain. This routine has been successful in detection of a number of lateral L2–L3 disc herniations and a very occasional L1–L2 herniation. Figure 7.1 shows the protocol used for CT scanning when neither radiculography nor MRI is to be performed, to ensure a complete evaluation of the lumbar spine. Survey images at L1–L2 and L2–L3 are obtained if the lateral topogram shows degenerative change or if the clinical features implicate those levels. Axial adjacent 5 mm images are obtained from the pedicle of L3 to the midpedicle of L5 and, at L5–S1, 3 mm adjacent images are obtained. This sequence of axial images from L3 to S1 shows continuous imaging of the lumbar anatomy and permits sagittal reformatting to allow assessment of lateral spinal stenosis.

Many clinicians have the misconception that the radiation dosage associated with CT of the spine is large because of the large number of images. They incorrectly assume the radiation dose for each slice is additive over the number of slices obtained. However, CT is unlike plain films in that the beam is very tightly collimated and there is very little scatter radiation. Radiation is measured in roentgens per gram radiated, and if one is not overlapping the images the radiation dose for 30 slices is no greater than that for five slices, since each gram of tissue is scanned only once. The usual skin dose is 3–5 rad for a lumbar spine scan, with less exposure of internal structures.

Since the area of the body scanned in lumbar spine imaging is limited and does not extend caudal to the L5–S1 disc, the radiation to the genitals is considerably less than the skin dose of the lower abdomen included within the primary beam. The radiation dose falls off rapidly, and at 10 cm from the caudalmost scan the dose is reduced to 3% of the primary dose. Therefore, radiation of the gonads lying 10 cm or more distal to the inferiormost scan would be in the range 0.15–0.75 rad. In comparison, a full series of spine films with AP, lateral and oblique films has equivalent direct radiation (3–5 rad) and considerably more scatter radiation resulting in greater gonadal radiation than CT. Myelography with use of fluoroscopy has a considerably higher dose of primary and scatter radiation (approximately 8 rad).

When performing a CT/MPR study only a few imaging parameters must be determined at the time of image acquisition. On routine evaluation of the cervical spine, contiguous 1.5 mm thick sections are obtained from the pedicle of C3 to the pedicle of T1. Thin sections are necessary to delineate normal anatomy (Fig. 7.2) and pathological changes in the cervical region. In the thoracic spine, contiguous 3 mm thick sections are obtained in the area of interest. From four to five disc levels can be evaluated on a single thoracic CT/MPR study.

After obtaining the initial axial images, computer-generated contiguous sagittal and coronal images are created with a spacing of 1.5 mm between images in the cervical examination and a spacing of 3 mm in the thoracic and lumbar examination. Approximately 20 sagittal and 20 coronal images are reconstructed from the axial data.

A multiplanar spinal examination must include contiguous sagittal and in some cases coronal reformations to completely evaluate the spine in complementary orthogonal planes. All images are photographed twice to optimally delineate soft tissue and osseous contrast. The strength of the CT/MPR examination resides in its excellent spatial resolution and its superb delineation of calcified or osseous structures. The main limitation of CT/MPR is the radiation exposure, slightly restricted field of view, and poor delineation of intrathecal anatomy and pathology.

Initial axial CT data are reprocessed into additional tomographic projections when performing a CT/MPR examination. With recent advances in software technology, initial axial CT data also can be reconstructed into a three-dimensional (3-D) image. Most 3-D CT images are produced using a surface contour method that permits evaluation of surface anatomy (Ulrich, 1989) (Fig. 7.3). The 3-D CT image adds no new information compared with the multiplanar study. However, with the new 3-D perspective, pathological changes may be more easily appreciated. New 3-D image displays employing non-contour data processing and semitransparent 3-D displays offer potential for new applications for 3-D imaging (Herman, 1988).

CT IN DEGENERATIVE DISC DISEASE OF THE LUMBAR SPINE

In experienced hands CT has been very accurate in the diagnosis of frank disc herniation with nerve root compression as the cause of sciatica. The utility of CT in the evaluation of lumbar herniations has been well described (Hirofuji & Tanaka, 1983; Williams *et al.*, 1983; Firooznia *et al.*, 1984; Wiltse, 1985; Greenough *et al.*, 1986). Criteria must be very specific for a definitive diagnosis of herniation: first, the disc protrusion must be focal and asymmetric, often dorsolateral in position, directly underlying the nerve root traversing that disc. Second, there should be demonstrable nerve root compression and/or displacement. Third, there is often postimpingement swelling of the affected nerve root caudal to the herniation, with enlargement of the nerve and indistinctness of its margin due to oedema, inflammatory exudate, or prominence of adjacent epidural veins (Fig. 7.4a–d). When these findings are present the diagnostic accuracy of CT is very high.

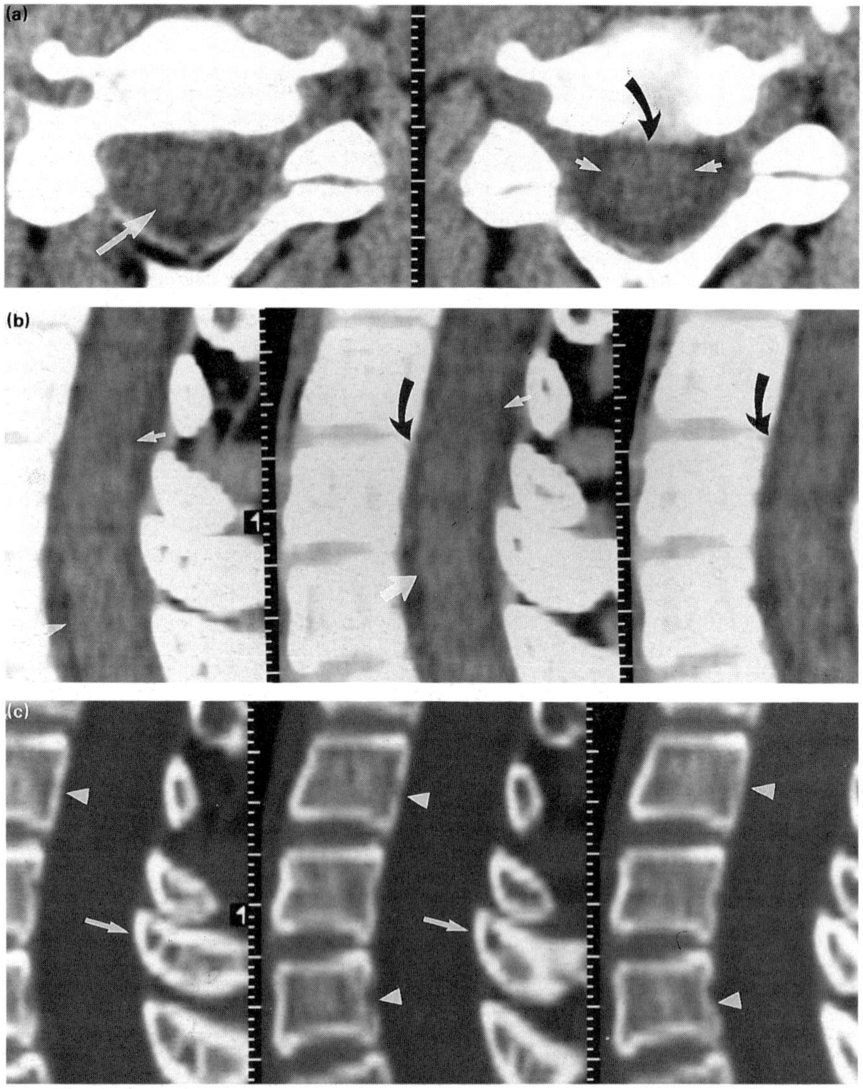

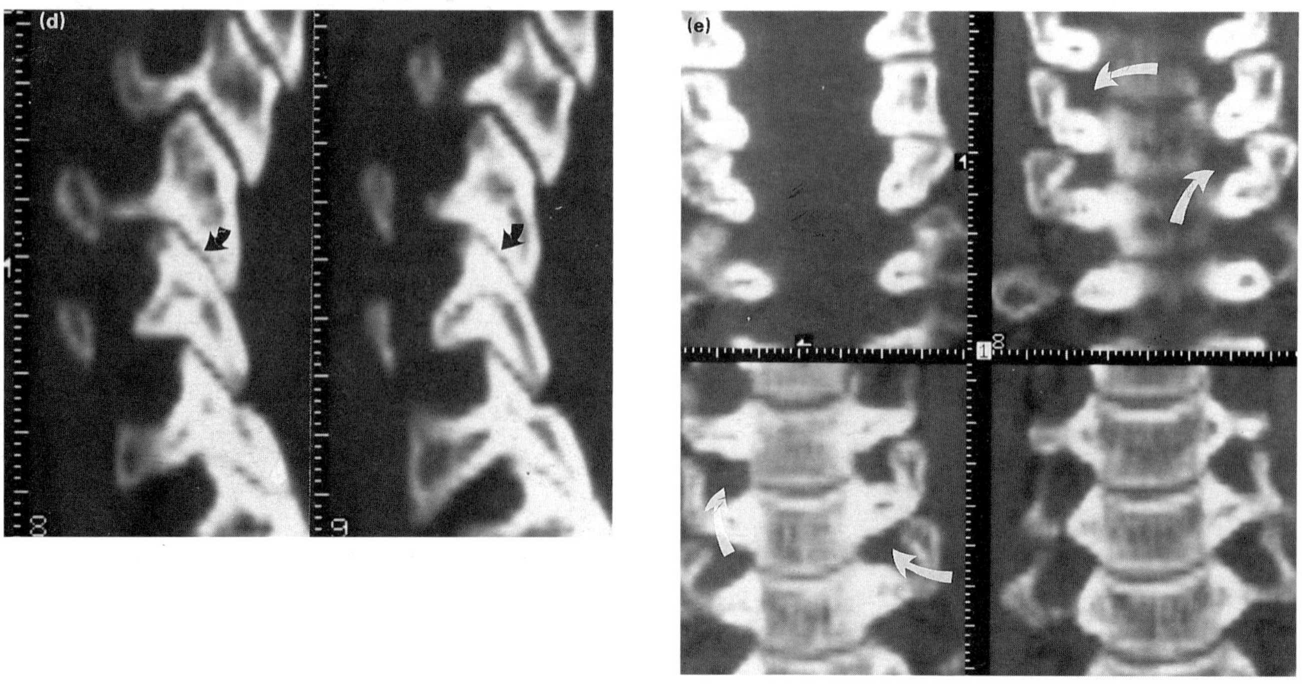

Fig. 7.2 Normal cervical spine anatomy, CT/MPR. On the axial (a) and sagittal (b) images, the spinal cord (white arrows) is delineated along with the posterior margin of the disc (black arrow). The images have been photographed to optimize soft tissue resolution. The sagittal images through the midline (c) and the facet joints (d) and coronal images (e) have been photographed to optimally evaluate the osseous structures. There is excellent delineation of the vertebral bodies (white arrowheads), the laminae (straight white arrows), the facet joints (curved black arrows), and the intervertebral canals (curved white arrows).

Fig. 7.3 (*Right*) Three-dimensional (3-D) image of the lumbar spine looking medially towards the intervertebral nerve root canals. Note the extensive, irregular osteophytic spurring extending into the left L5–S1 intervertebral nerve root canal, which produces severe bony lateral spinal stenosis (arrow). Three-dimensional reconstruction allows the surgeon a better appreciation of the position and extent of bony osteophytes, which produce lateral spinal stenosis and can be helpful in planning surgery, as the osteophytic spur can be viewed with multiple cut-away views. More recent advancements allow 3-D imaging of both bone and soft tissue.

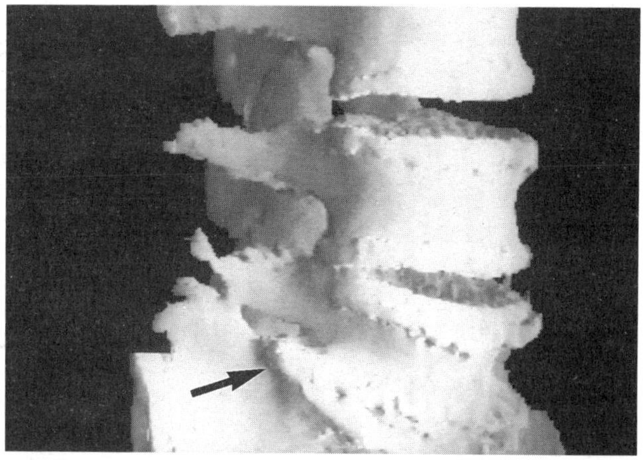

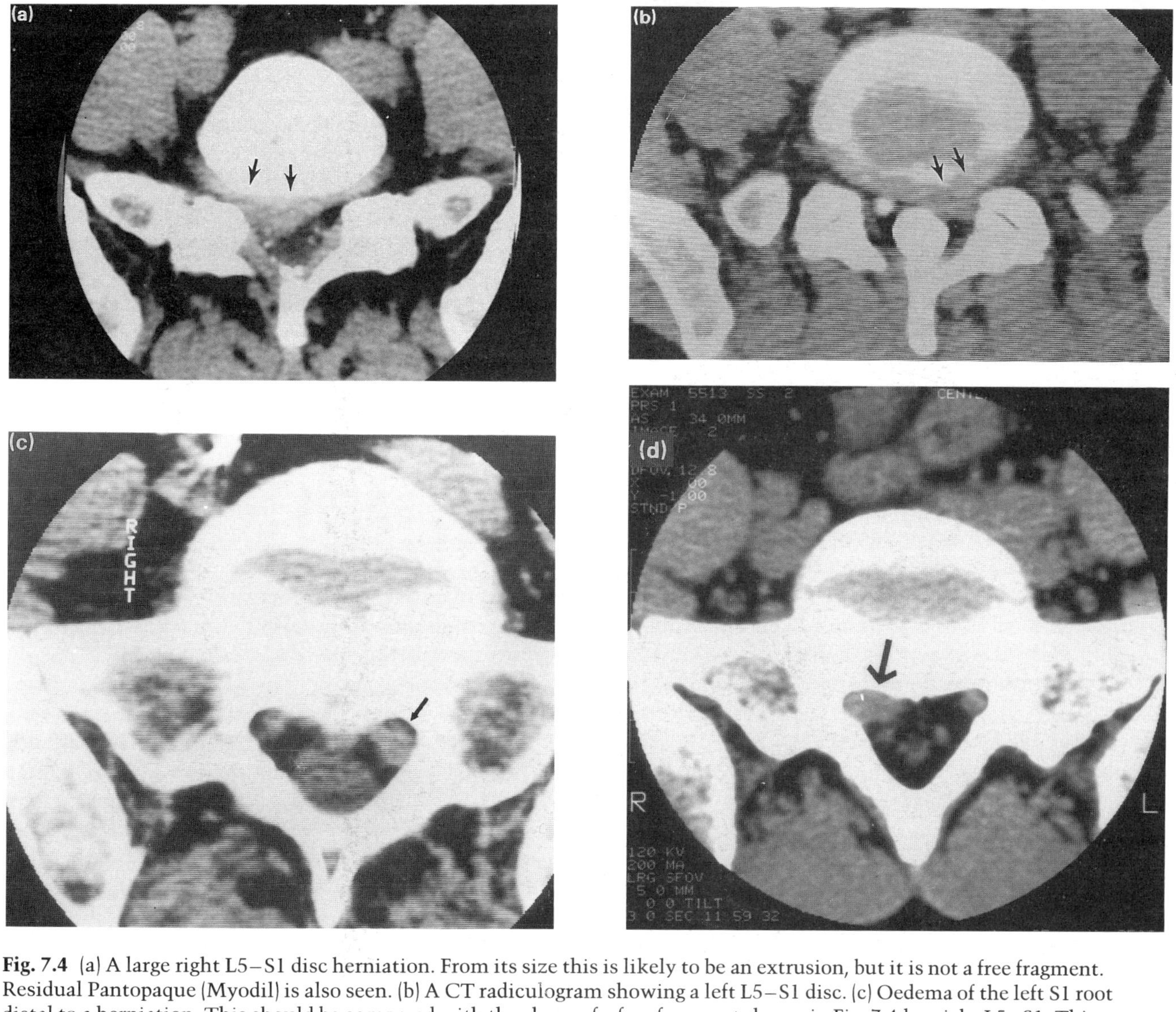

Fig. 7.4 (a) A large right L5–S1 disc herniation. From its size this is likely to be an extrusion, but it is not a free fragment. Residual Pantopaque (Myodil) is also seen. (b) A CT radiculogram showing a left L5–S1 disc. (c) Oedema of the left S1 root distal to a herniation. This should be compared with the shape of a free fragment shown in Fig. 7.4d at right L5–S1. This fragment extends caudal to the disc space and is the hallmark of a free fragment.

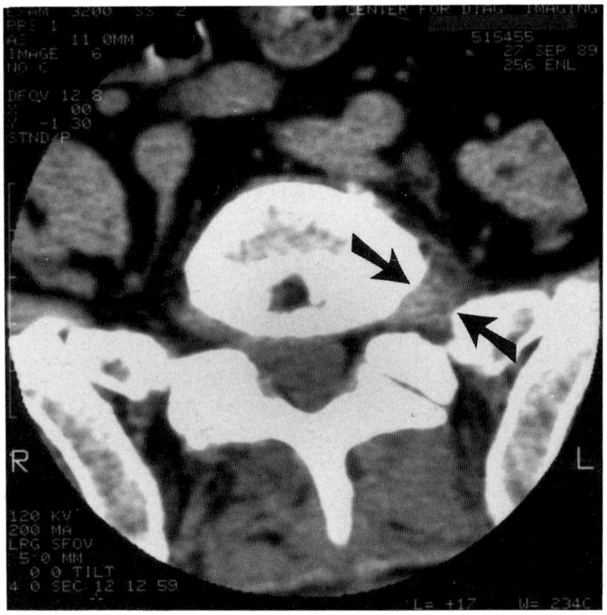

Fig. 7.5 Axial CT showing a far lateral disc herniation at left L5–S1. This is the least common site for such herniations to occur.

Lateral or foraminal disc herniations are not uncommon (Mikhael, 1983; Fries *et al.*, 1984; Godersky *et al.*, 1984), are most common at L4–L5, slightly less common at L3–L4 and relatively rare at L5–S1 (Fig. 7.5). Lateral herniation can also occur at L2–L3 but is very uncommon at L1–L2. Lateral herniations are often extruded and migrate cranially to produce severe compression of the ganglia within the nerve root canal. They are usually very painful, since the ganglia is very sensitive to ischaemia. Paralateral surgical removal has been advocated for the lateral herniations.

Problems arise in the accurate diagnosis of more diffusely bulging or herniated discs, and differentiating these from the normal contours of the L5–S1 disc. The L5–S1 disc 'normally' has a posterior convex configuration on axial CT images because of the normal rounded posterior margin of L5 and the sacrum in most patients and the oblique angle of the L5–S1 disc with the plane of the non-angled axial CT scan. Because of the lumbosacral angulation, the normal L5–S1 disc has an oblique course from its attachment to S1. Therefore, an axial image obtained partially through the inferior margin of L5 and partially through the L5–S1 disc will show an apparent 'bulge'. This is normal. Similarly, minor, symmetrical bulges at L5–S1 are very common and should not be construed as 'herniations'. These disc margins are widely separate from the S1 nerve roots and should never be considered as herniations or a cause of sciatica. Midline sagittal reformatted images are useful in the differentiation between true disc bulges at L5–S1 and CT 'apparent' bulging due to lumbosacral angulation.

More problematic than the classic dorsolateral disc herniation with nerve root impingement is the midline disc herniation. Suffice it to say that the CT scan diagnosis of central disc herniation is the greatest cause of false-positive readings and, perhaps, the cause of the reported high incidence of false-positive diagnosis in some articles in the literature (Wiesel *et al.*, 1984). Since CT (unlike MRI) does not have sufficient soft tissue resolution to differentiate between annulus and nucleus, if the central disc protrusion is symmetrical and small as well as diffuse, one cannot differentiate between a bulging annulus and a symmetrical contained central disc herniation. If there is any asymmetry of the disc protrusion, or any portion of the disc that is focally asymmetric and more prominent, this is strong evidence that one is dealing with a central herniation rather than simple annular bulging (Fig. 7.6).

It is essential to note that a midline central herniation must be shown by either CT or MRI to be responsible for nerve root compression before surgery to relieve sciatica should be contemplated. If the adjacent nerve roots are separated from the disc margin by epidural fat, and no nerve root impingement is identified, the patient is not a discectomy candidate. The reporting radiologist must therefore not only describe the appearance of the disc, but also comment on the presence or absence of nerve root compression to prevent unnecessary surgery resulting from this report of 'herniated disc'.

There is one condition in which a 'bulging disc' or a small, symmetrical contained herniation can cause nerve root entrapment; namely, in patients with trefoil central canals and narrowed bony lateral recesses or pathologically narrowed subarticular recesses due to degenerative facet hypertrophy. In these cases a combination of a widely bulging disc and bony hypertrophy can cause subarticular stenosis and nerve root compression with sciatica (Fig. 7.7).

Since CT cannot differentiate annulus from nucleus as MRI can, it is difficult to differentiate accurately between a contained herniation (intact outer annulus and posterior longitudinal ligament) and a

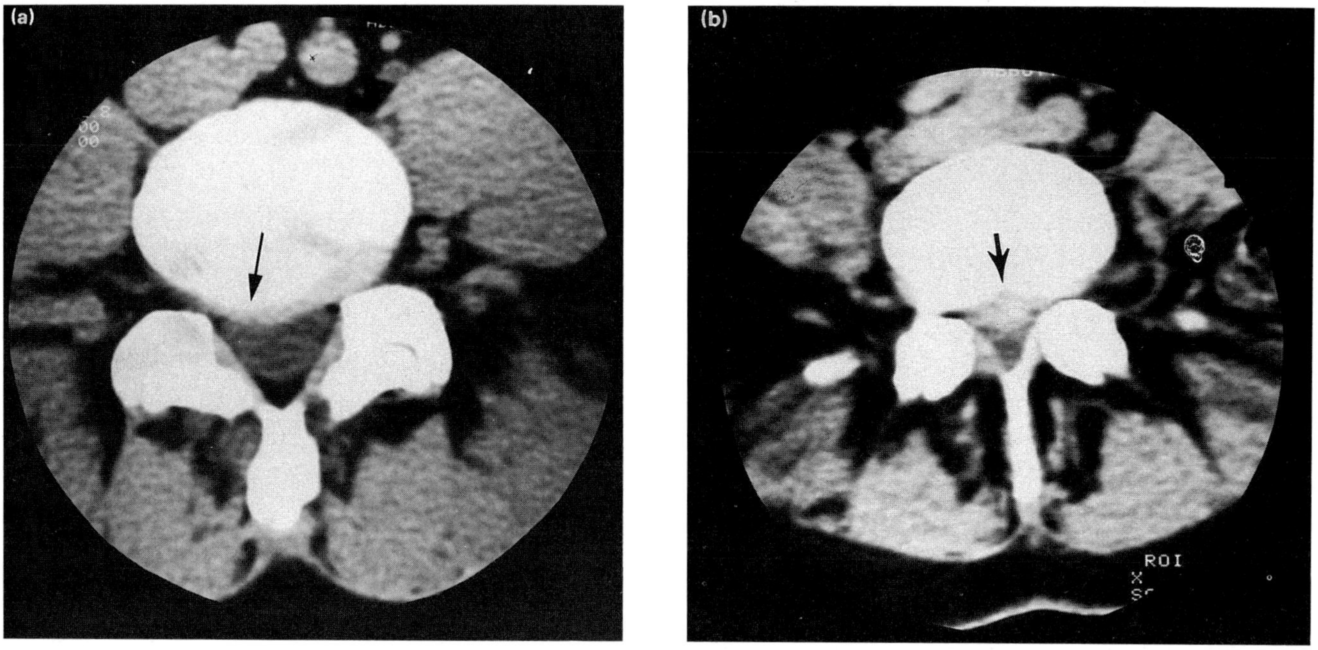

Fig. 7.6 (a) A focal central disc herniation with irregular margination. It is slightly asymmetrical and, on CT, this is probably a contained central disc herniation. (b) A large triangular central disc herniation. From its size it is probably an extrusion but, in both of these cases, the CT diagnosis cannot be certain and would require MRI for differentiation.

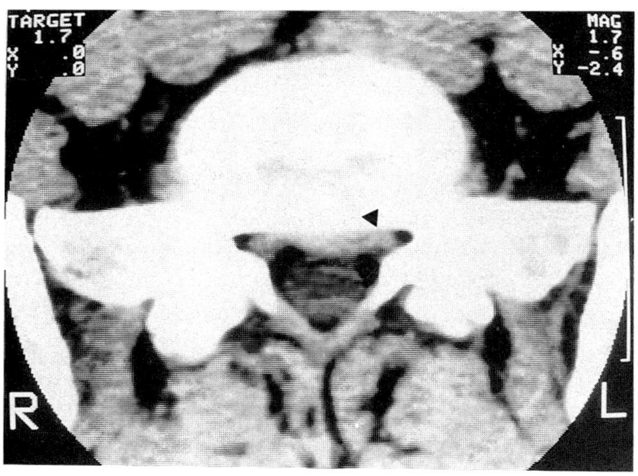

Fig. 7.7 Central disc herniation with subarticular nerve root impingement. Note the asymmetric central and left-sided disc herniation with caudal extension into the subarticular recess. This surgically proven disc herniation is producing moderate subarticular compression of the left S1 nerve root (arrowhead) and mild impingement on the right S1 nerve root.

non-contained herniation. If the disc herniation is large, large and irregular, or extending significantly craniad or caudal to the disc, one can assume it is non-contained, and will most often be correct. However, when the disc is small or moderate in size and smoothly marginated, attempts to differentiate contained from non-contained by means of CT are guesswork. Therefore, if this is necessary, as in the case of percutaneous discectomy where contained herniations are said to have improved results, preoperative MRI evaluation is necessary. MRI has enhanced our understanding of disc pathology and lends itself to a very specific and accurate nomenclature of degenerative disc disease. That is, one can now clearly differentiate thickened, redundant annuli from diffuse contained central disc herniations and visualize complete and incomplete annular tears (both radial and circumferential) and inflammatory fluid within annular tears that may have significance in the prediction of symptomatic disc lesions (Fig. 7.8). Evidence of increased signal within an annular tear on T2-weighted images correlates well with pain reproduction on discography (C. April, personal communication, 1988).

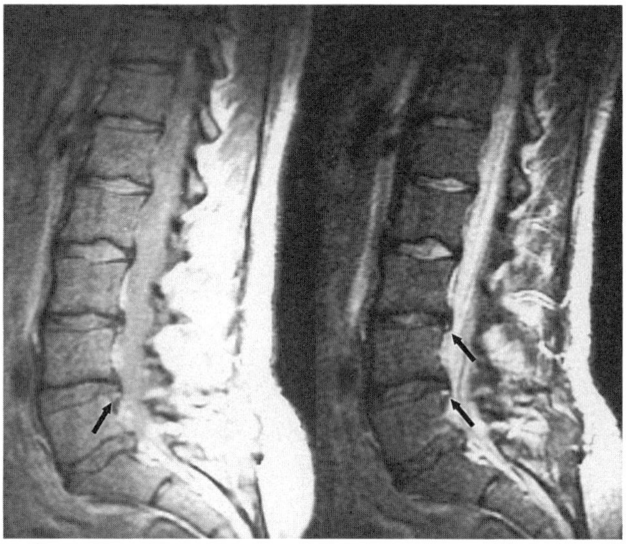

Fig. 7.8 Double-echo, spin-echo sagittal images of the lumbar spine in a patient with degenerative disc disease at L3–L4, L4–L5, and L5–S1 with moderate dehydration of those discs. Note nearly complete annular tears of the L3–L4 and L4–L5 annuli (arrows). There is increased signal intensity in the periphery of the annular tears on the T2-weighted images consistent with inflammation fluid within the annular tear.

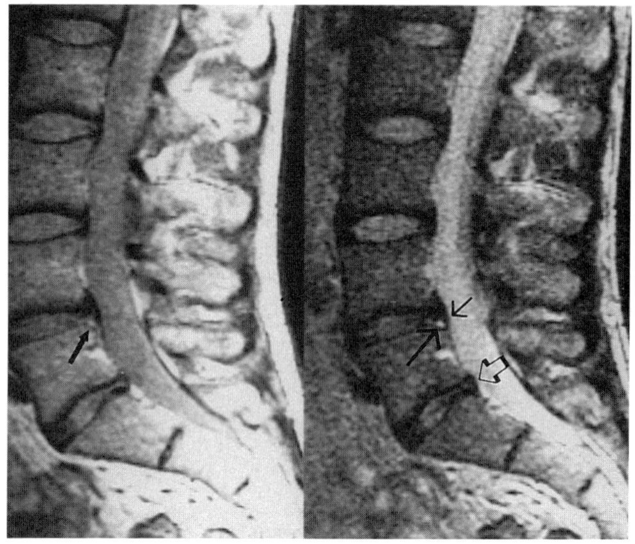

Fig. 7.9 Sagittal spin echo MRI showing a complete annular tear of the L4–L5 disc annulus (arrows). The annulus is torn from its attachment to the posterior superior aspect of L5, and there is increased signal intensity within the annular tear (opposing arrows on the T2-weighted images). The posterior longitudinal ligament is intact. There is no extrusion of nuclear material and this discal abnormality is best described as that of an annular tear and concomitant thickening of the annulus without associated herniation. Note the degenerative dehydration of the L5–S1 disc and thickening of the annulus (open arrow).

MRI has shown that many of the non-specific symmetrical central disc protrusions that, in the past, using CT, were conservatively called 'annular bulges' are in fact contained central herniations with dorsal migration of nuclear material beyond the posterior margin of the vertebral body (Fig. 7.9). Unfortunately, there is no correlative clinical research yet available that indicates there are in fact differing clinical symptoms or responses to treatment between simple degenerative thickening of the annulus, incomplete annular tears, and contained symmetrical central herniations without nerve root impingement. However, now that we can accurately differentiate between them using MRI, clinical research can decide the issue. Hopefully, this added information will lead to more specific treatment modalities and rational compensation schemes.

Normal variations

Several normal variations can lead to nerve root asymmetry, the most common being ectasia of the nerve root sheath. In these cases nerve root asymmetry is the only finding of note, and no pathological impinging lesion, such as a herniated disc or bony stenosis, is identified. The attenuation values of this nerve root enlargement are low and near those of the cerebrospinal fluid (CSF). In cases of nerve root asymmetry and questionable nerve root impingement (such as a narrowed lateral recess), MRI or metrizamide-enhanced CT scanning is definitive.

Tarlov's sacral nerve root cysts also cause enlargement of the imaged nerve root/nerve root sheath complex. These cysts are of CSF density and are often associated with benign expansion of the bony sacral nerve root canals.

The conjoined nerve root is an anatomical variant of considerable interest and importance. It is present in approximately 8% of the population. This most commonly occurs at the L5–S1 level. The conjoined nerve root arises from the thecal sac more caudally than is normal and lies halfway between the nerve roots on the opposite side. The thecal sac is asymmetrical because the opposite, normal, more cephalad nerve root has exited the thecal sac and is surrounded by fat. The conjoined nerve root continues within the sac, producing a local anterolateral expansion of the thecal sac that contains a large, high-density nerve root mass. The attenuation values of the mass are increased (70–80 HU). Because its density is near that of the disc, the conjoined nerve root may be mistakenly diagnosed as an asymmetrical disc protrusion herniation. As reported by Helms *et al.* (1982) the conjoined nerve root is associated with a rounded enlargement of the bony lateral recess of the central canal. This is a useful secondary sign to look for when unsure of the presence of a conjoined nerve root.

At the L5–S1 level the conjoined nerve root divides just medial to the pedicle, the S1 component of the L5–S1 conjoined nerve root mass is more lateral than normal, and no separate origin of the distal nerve root is identifiable. The conjoined nerve root is splayed over the S1 pedicle and the lateral margin of the L5–S1 disc, lying directly dorsal to the disc in the caudal aspect of the L5–S1 nerve root canal (L5), and within the narrowest far lateral portion of the L5–S1 subarticular recess (S1). Thus the conjoined nerve root is fixed in the most restricted and narrowed portion of the L5–S1 nerve root canal and lateral recess.

In this situation very minimal disc bulges/herniations or bony hypertrophy of the superior articular process (SAP) of S1 or hypertrophy of the S1 pedicle can cause stretching or compression of the conjoined nerve root (Fig. 7.10). Identifying an underlying disc herniation may be difficult with CT because the high-density mass of the conjoined nerve root is similar to that of the adjacent disc. MRI, performed with double-echo, spin-echo technique, is the definitive examination for excluding an underlying herniated nucleus pulposus, as it easily distinguishes between the signal intensity of disc and nerve root.

The paired nerve roots are also easily visualized within the thecal sac on T2-weighted axial images. In addition, it is necessary to surgically free up the conjoined nerve root mass prior to removing the herniated fragment that underlies it. This helps to avoid nerve root damage, which otherwise occurs with disturbing frequency (White *et al.*, 1982).

Lumbar epidural haematoma

The characteristic CT features of an epidural hematoma consist of a rounded extradural mass lesion that is largest at the level of the midvertebral body (basivertebral plexus) and has tapering, indistinct margins that extend to the level of the adjacent disc and envelop the involved nerve root. They are ill-defined and nearly isodense with the thecal sac and indistinguishable from the nerve root and ganglia. Most, but not all, extend superiorly from the disc to the basivertebral plexus of the vertebra above (Fig. 7.11a). Review of the first 25 cases of lumbar epidural haematoma seen by the authors revealed a notable absence of a history of trauma. The lesions have been noted in all age groups. Patients present with symptoms indistinguishable from those of a herniated disc. However, the symptoms typically re-

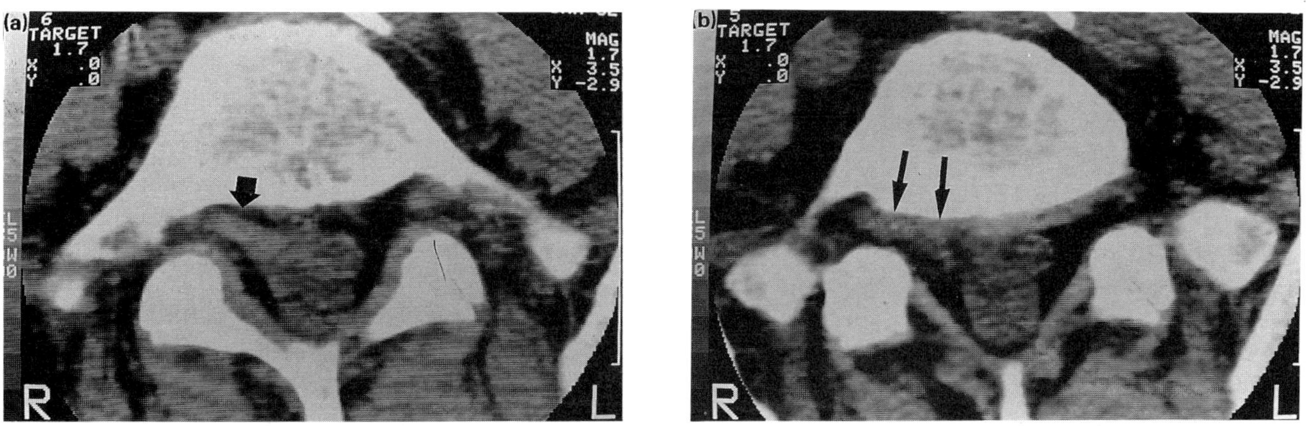

Fig. 7.10 Axial CT showing right-sided conjoint root at L5–S1. In (a) the asymmetrical origin of the conjoint root is seen (arrow); (b) is a more caudal image in the same patient, showing the conjoint root lying adjacent to the annulus and of similar density. On a single image the conjoint root may easily be mistaken for a disc herniation.

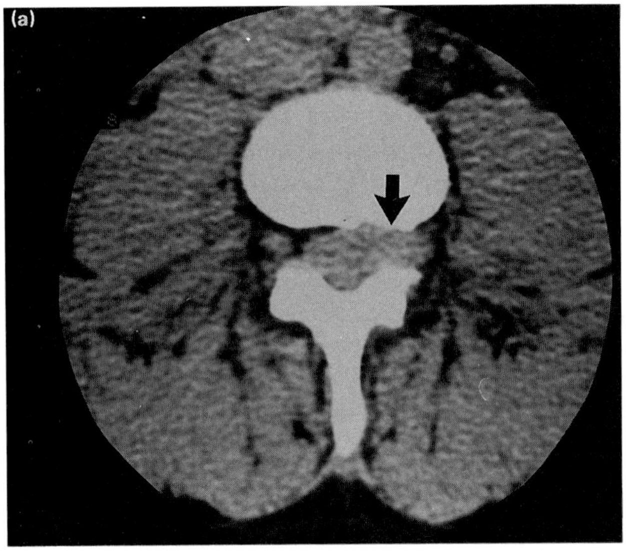

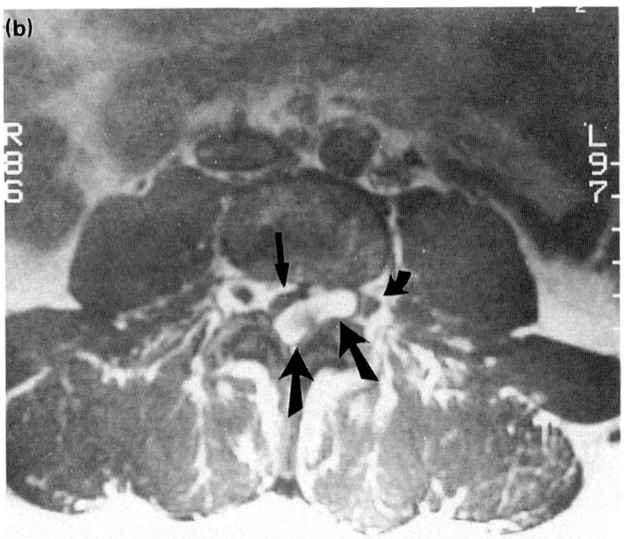

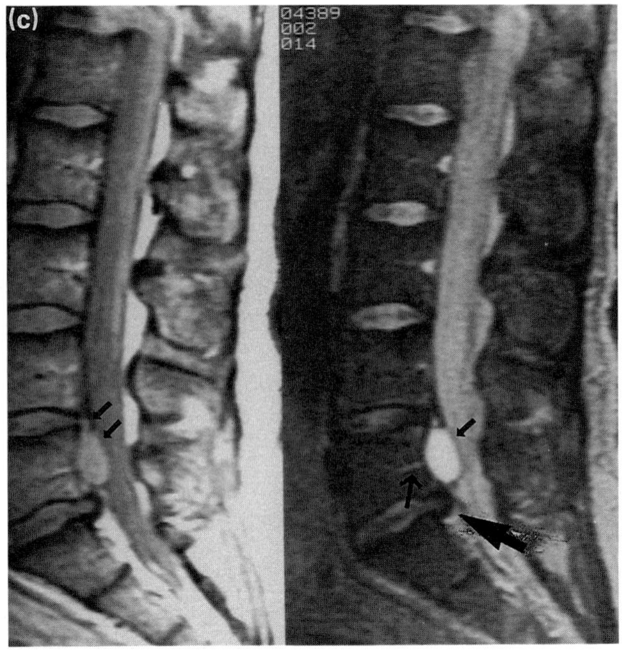

Fig. 7.11 (a) Axial CT at L4–L5 showing large ill-defined soft tissue mass within the left nerve root canal obliterating the epidural fat. (b) The MRI of the same patient. The large arrows indicate the haematoma which has a high though variable signal. The mass displaces the theca forwards and to the right (small arrow) and the left L4 root laterally (curved arrow). (c) A sagittal MRI showing an annular tear (top arrow on T1) with an adjacent haematoma showing very high signal on T2. The basivertebral vein is well shown, as is a central L5–S1 prolapse with an intact thickened annulus (large arrow).

gressed rapidly (three days to weeks) and most commonly (21 of 25 cases) were associated with an underlying small disc herniation or annular tear on follow-up CT examination after the haematoma had regressed.

MRI, performed early, is pathognomonic in most, but not all, cases. The MRI appearance is typical for blood with a high signal intensity of the lesion on T1 proton-density and T2-weighted images (Fig. 7.11b). As the haematoma ages, however, it may become isointense with the disc.

More recently MRI has also shown an underlying annular tear or disc herniation in the vast majority of cases (Fig. 7.11c). Typically the disc herniation comprises a small portion of the mass, whereas most of the mass is haematoma. In all but four patients in our series, the lesions regressed spontaneously, in some cases taking up to four to five months for the mass to resorb entirely. Only one required surgery because of an increase in size and symptoms on follow-up. At surgery this lesion had become encysted and had an open basivertebral vein connecting with it, which bled profusely when the haematoma was removed. All three cases reported by Levitan & Wiens (1983) had become walled off and chronic, and presented with persistent symptoms. Three of the first 20 cases were associated with severe unilateral degenerative facet disease, and the haematoma was based on the medial aspect of the facet joint rather than the disc.

This lesion is remarkably common in our experience, given the paucity of reports of lumbar epidural haematoma in the literature (Post *et al.*, 1982; Levitan & Wiens, 1983; Zilkha *et al.*, 1983; Haykal *et al.*, 1984; Kaiser *et al.*, 1984; Quequet *et al.*, 1987). Because of the almost universal absence of a history of significant trauma, it is likely that the fragile epidural veins adjacent to the disc or facet are torn by relatively minor torsional injury, as a result of instability (facet disease) or by a minor annular disruption. The recognition of epidural haematoma and its distinction from a free fragment is crucial, given the similarity of symptoms and CT appearance of these two lesions but their disparate treatments.

In summary, lumbar epidural haematoma is much more common than is suggested by the few cases reported in the literature. It presents with symptoms indistinguishable from a herniated disc, which, however, regress more rapidly than would be expected with a free fragment disc. It may take months for the haematoma itself to resorb, persisting long after the patient is asymptomatic. It is an important lesion to recognize to avoid unnecessary surgery, since most regress completely and spontaneously. It is probably the lesion responsible for many of the so-called disappearing discs, previously reported in surgical literature, in which large extradural masses noted on myelography are not evident at surgery.

Computerized tomography of lumbar epidural hematoma has a characteristic appearance. However, only a presumptive diagnosis can be made, since a free fragment disc can have an identical appearance. Magnetic resonance imaging is usually diagnostic in the acute or subacute phase when a typical high signal intensity of T1- and T2-weighted images is noted. With age the signal intensity decreases, and may become isointense with the disc.

Synovial cysts

Degenerative spondylolisthesis may be complicated by synovial cyst formation. In fact most patients with synovial cysts have underlying degenerative spondylolisthesis. Contrary to previous reports in the literature, synovial cysts and chondromas are often associated with clinical symptoms resulting from nerve root compression.

Synovial cysts most commonly arise at the medial margin of the degenerated facet joints. The synovial cyst has a characteristic appearance with its flat base paralleling the ligamentum flavum at the medial margin of the zygapophyseal joint. The rounded medial aspect of the cyst projects in an anteromedial direction rather than dorsally as would be expected with disc herniation (Fig 7.12).

MRI can clearly visualize the fluid within the synovial cysts on T2-weighted images and, therefore, differentiates synovial cysts from synovial chondromas. This distinction is important in light of recent clinical research showing that injection of steroids into the zygapophyseal joint, which communicates with the synovial cyst, may dramatically decrease or completely relieve the symptoms related to nerve root compression, and seems to be an alternative to surgery. On the other hand, symptomatic synovial chondromas or non-cystic masses of the ligamentum flavum that produce nerve root compression do not respond to this treatment.

Occasionally, synovial cysts can vary in position and may occur within the lateral aspect of the intervertebral nerve root canal beneath the lateral attachment of the ligamentum flavum to the base of the superior articular facet. The association of these lesions with degenerative spondylolisthesis is so strong that any rounded soft tissue mass projecting into the central spinal canal from the medial margin of the facet joint in a patient with degenerative spondylolisthesis at that segment should be considered to be a synovial cyst and/or chondroma until proven otherwise.

LUMBAR SPONDYLOSIS AND STENOSIS

The pathogenesis of degenerative lumbar spondylosis and stenosis leads to a conglomerate of degenerative changes. Among them are loss of disc height, ligamentous laxity with rotational instability, spondylolisthesis and retrolisthesis, degenerative hypertrophy of the facets, degenerative osteophyte formation, and thickening of the ligamentum flavum. Therefore, a variety of configurations may be present that lead to nerve root entrapment (Osborne *et al.*, 1984).

In contrast with central spinal stenosis, which is usually seen at one or more lumbar spinal levels (typically L4–L5 and above), bony lateral spinal stenosis most often occurs at the lumbosacral level. Several entities occur commonly at this level that do not occur more proximally because of the con-

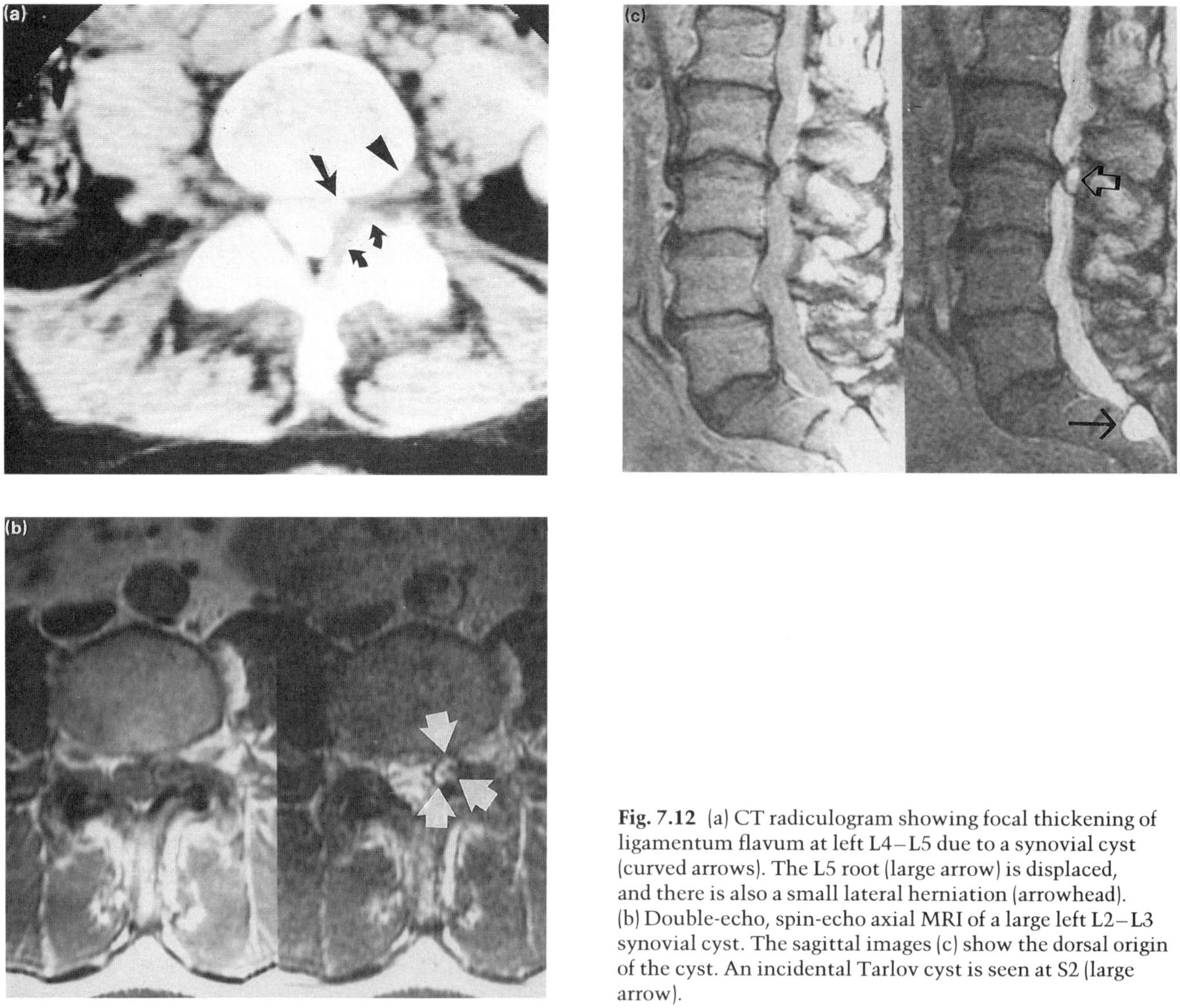

Fig. 7.12 (a) CT radiculogram showing focal thickening of ligamentum flavum at left L4–L5 due to a synovial cyst (curved arrows). The L5 root (large arrow) is displaced, and there is also a small lateral herniation (arrowhead). (b) Double-echo, spin-echo axial MRI of a large left L2–L3 synovial cyst. The sagittal images (c) show the dorsal origin of the cyst. An incidental Tarlov cyst is seen at S2 (large arrow).

figuration of the sacrum and the presence of unique anatomical degenerative (uncinate) spurs arising from L5. However, once the principles of lateral stenosis at L5–S1 are understood, they may be extrapolated to the higher lumbar vertebral spaces.

The margins of the L5–S1 intervertebral nerve root canals are composed of the pedicles of L5 and S1 superiorly and inferiorly, the superior articular processes of S1 dorsally, the L5 vertebral body and L5–S1 intervertebral disc ventrally, and laterally by the iliolumbar and corpotransverse ligaments. Any one of these structures may interface with nerve roots and produce nerve root impingement. Morphologically, this may result in narrowing of the intervertebral nerve root canal in the cephalocaudad and anteroposterior dimensions, as well as in a circumferential narrowing because of a combination of these stenoses. The major classification of lateral spinal stenosis should be divided according to the anatomical narrowing, namely, 'front–back' stenosis and 'up–down' stenosis, since these correspond to specific anatomical pathological entities.

Uncinate spurs

In most cases lateral stenoses are due to a multiplicity of degenerative and proliferative processes that cause the intervertebral nerve root canal to nar-

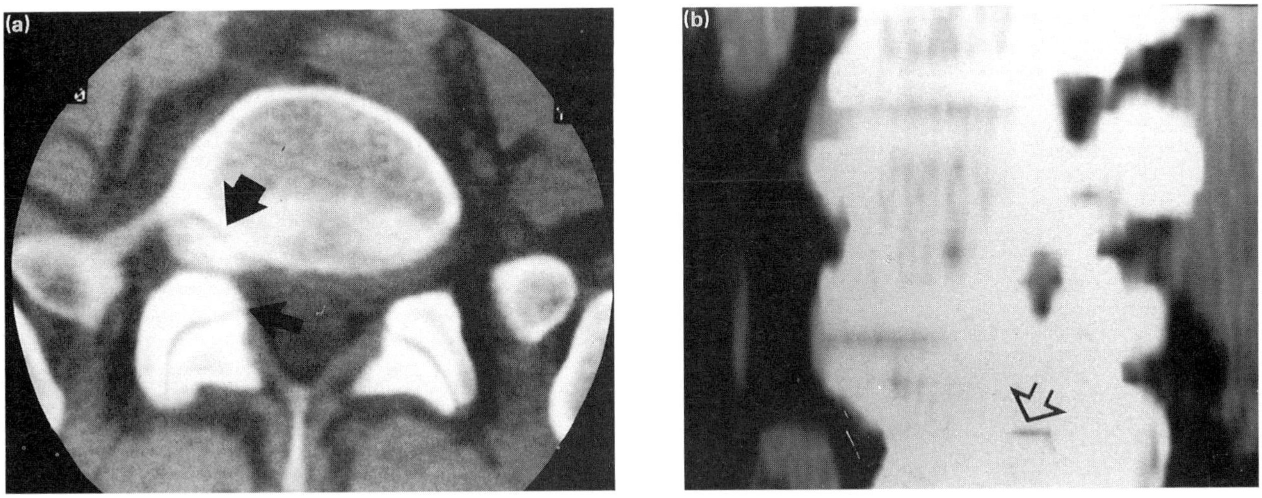

Fig. 7.13 Axial CT (a) showing characteristic uncinate spur at right L5–S1. Sagittal reformatting (b) shows the severity of compromise of the nerve root foramen (arrow) as compared to the normal foramina above.

row in one or more of its several dimensions. Recently, it has become apparent that cephalocaudad stenosis at L5–S1 resulting from spurs (uncinate) arising from the dorsolateral aspect of L5 is the most common cause of lateral spinal stenosis at this level. In most cases degenerative narrowing or collapse of the L5–S1 disc space is found in association with the development of these posterolateral osteophytes.

Uncinate spurs are anatomical correlates of the uncinate spurring found in the cervical spine. The aetiology of uncinate spurs in the adult is believed to be the result of disruption or tearing of the annular and/or Sharpey's fibres from the vertebral endplates and the uncinate process. These osteophytes are visualized on standard CT axial images as dense, rounded bony structures that project dorsally and laterally into the intervertebral nerve root canal from the vertebral body of L5 (Fig. 7.13). The posterolateral location of these spurs correlates anatomically with the uncinate spurs found in the degenerated cervical spine. As they enlarge they project into the intervertebral nerve root canal ventral and lateral to the superior articular process. Because they project into the ventral aspect of the nerve root canal, and the L5 nerve root also lies ventrally tightly opposed to the L5 vertebral body, the spur directly impinges upon the caudal surface of the L5 nerve root or nerve root ganglion. This causes compression of the ganglia against the caudal surface of the pedicle of L5. A surgeon will find these bony processes covered by tough, smooth tissue ligaments or portions of the annulus.

'Up–down' stenosis

As the spinal nerve root emerges from the thecal sac, anatomically and surgically proven small dural ligaments attach the nerve ventrally to the posterior longitudinal ligament, annulus, and fascia covering the posterior and lateral aspect of the vertebral body and intervertebral disc. The emerging neural structure (root, ganglion and spinal nerve) remains relatively fixed in the ventral portion of the canal because of: (a) the close proximity of the root to the inferior aspect of the pedicle as it courses through the canal to exit beyond; (b) the filamentous fibrous extradural ligaments that anchor the nerve root sleeve as it traverses the canal; and (c) a normally slight outward traction of the spinal nerve.

The nerve lies against the vertebral body caudal to the pedicle, almost like a rope passing around a pulley. These natural structures may slide a bit in and out of their foramina, but they have little or no ventral–dorsal mobility. Posterolateral osteophytic (uncinate) spurs that arise from the vertebral body narrow that ventral portion of the canal where the nerve root structures are found, namely the constricted space between the spur caudally and the pedicle cranially. Conversely, the dorsal portion of the nerve root canal may be widely patent in these

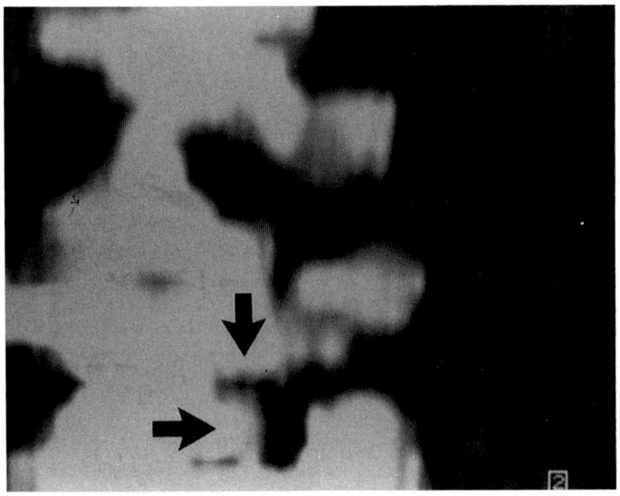

Fig. 7.14 Sagittal reformatted CT image showing severe 'up–down' lateral spinal stenosis. A large osteophyte (horizontal arrow) lies in the ventral half of the root canal. The existing root is severely compressed between the osteophyte and the pedicle (vertical arrow) but the dorsal portion of the root canal remains capacious.

cases and may easily accept a surgical probe (Fig. 7.14). Therefore, surgical probing of a canal does not exclude significant 'up–down' lateral stenosis at L5–S1 due to uncinate spurring. Myelography is negative in these cases because compression of the nerve occurs at or beyond the ganglia distal to the termination of the nerve root sheath. This makes preoperative CT diagnosis and evaluation essential in the prevention of failed lumbar spine surgery that results from unrecognized lateral stenosis.

The anteroposterior dimension of a CT scan image of the craniad portion of the intervertebral nerve root canal that lies cephalad to this spur may appear normal. In many cases the only clue to 'up–down' stenosis compressing the L5 nerve root ganglion by an uncinate spur on axial CT images is an asymmetric enlargement of the L5 ganglion on the affected side resulting from cephalocaudad compression of the ganglion. This 'up–down' compression produces an expansion of the ganglion in the axial plane. Sagittal reformatted images, however, clearly define the severity of the cephalocaudad narrowing and the position and degree of compression of the L5 nerve root ganglion. Similar 'up–down' stenosis may be caused by osteophytes arising from the margin of the L5–S1 disc or by focal, irregular and more laterally located osteophytes.

With advancing age the vertebral bodies frequently reduce in height but widen at the endplate margins. The pedicle, however, increases in diameter and may alter its normally oval configuration into a larger, more rounded shape. The changes are observed best on plain films of the lumbar spine. In effect this represents an apparent relative descent of the pedicle in the vertebral body.

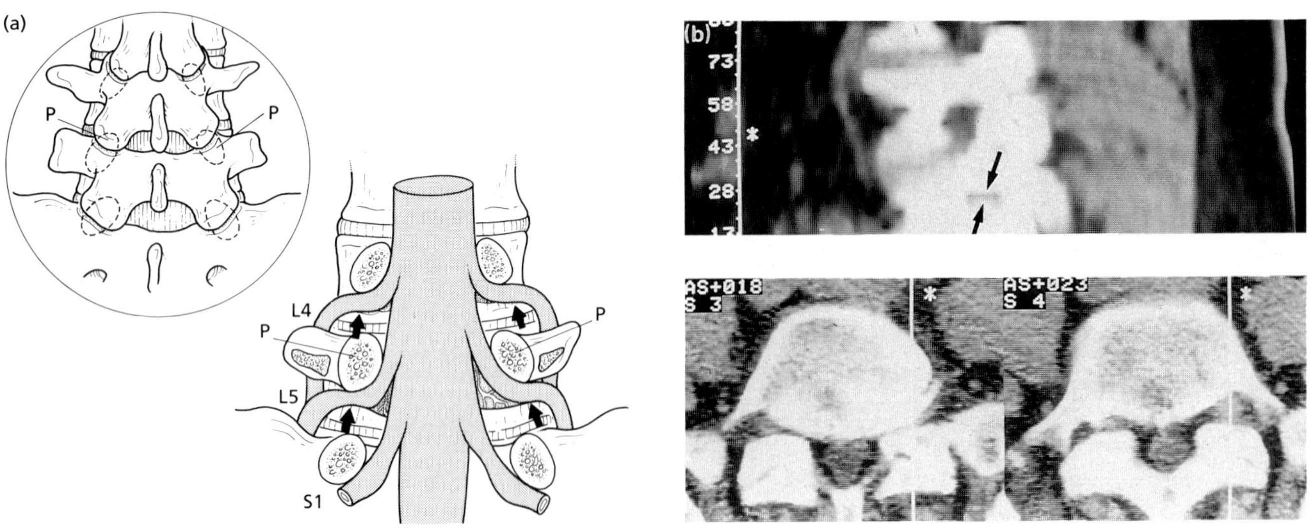

Fig. 7.15 (a) Diagrammatic representation of 'up–down' stenosis at L5–S1. The osteophytic spur arises from the posterior margin of the body of L5 and projects in a cranial direction to produce 'up–down' compression of the existing L5 root (arrow). (b) Axial images of a case of 'up–down' stenosis. Particularly on the left, there is evidence of 'front–back' stenosis, but the sagittal reconstruction reveals the more severe 'up–down' stenosis present.

The pedicles approach each other downward, further restricting the cephalocaudad diameter of the foramen. Disc margins, along which the annulus attaches, become more prominent and often calcified. These bars of the disc margin, especially the uncinate spur, further contribute to 'up–down' narrowing. Thus, loss of disc height combined with osteophytic spurring, produces 'up–down' stenosis; whereas overgrowth of the superior articular facet or osteophyte at the posterior margin of the vertebral body produces 'front–back' stenosis (Fig. 7.15).

'Up–down' stenosis may also occur in the far lateral area of the root canal (Fig. 7.16). Focal osteophytes arising directly beneath the inferior and lateral aspect of the pedicle in association with loss of disc height produce narrowing in the cephalocaudad direction between the pedicle of L5 and the superior aspect of the sacrum. This can result in severe compression of the existing L5 root at the far lateral margin of the nerve root canal.

Lytic spondylolisthesis

Lytic spondylolisthesis at L5–S1 is another entity commonly associated with 'up–down' stenosis. Associated disc space narrowing on plain films is an accurate indicator of the presence of lateral stenosis or far-out stenosis in patients with lytic spondylolisthesis. Lateral spinal stenosis associated with lytic spondylolisthesis L5–S1 is rarely detected in the absence of disc space narrowing. Conversely, lateral spinal stenosis is almost invariably present in patients with both lytic spondylolisthesis and degenerative disc space narrowing. In most patients the forward slip of the vertebral body, pedicle, and pars of L5 is also associated with a caudal settling of the vertebra as the disc space narrows, resulting in entrapment and compression of the L5 nerve root between the pedicle and proximal pars cranially and the L5–S1 disc and body of S1 caudally (McAffee & Yuan, 1982; Teplick *et al.*, 1986).

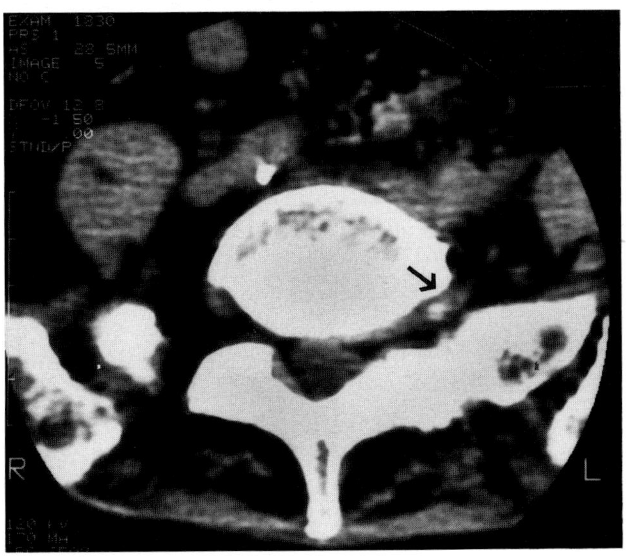

Fig. 7.16 Axial CT showing far lateral 'up–down' stenosis.

Axial images of lytic spondylolisthesis show distortion of the intervertebral nerve root canal with elongation of the anteroposterior dimension of the canals because of the ventral slip of L5. Pre-impingement swelling of the L5 nerve root often occurs. Sagittal reformatted images are the most useful in delineating nerve root compression both within the intervertebral nerve root canal and also laterally between the transverse process of L5 and the sacrum. Coronal and oblique reformatted images are occasionally useful.

Posterolateral bulging of the L5–S1 disc annulus and/or lateral disc herniations at L5–S1 may contribute to the L5 nerve root impingement. Marked narrowing of the cephalocaudad dimension of the intervertebral nerve root canal results in compression and flattening of the L5 nerve root ganglia, which can completely replace the epidural fat within the canal. Distinguishing between the density of the compressed nerve root ganglia and that of a degenerative bulging or laterally herniated L5–S1 disc is often difficult or impossible. Parasagittal reformatted images may be helpful, and when clinically indicated, MRI is definitive. MRI has shown that L5–S1 lateral herniation in patients with L5–S1 spondylolisthesis is not uncommon. Virtually all herniations occurring in these patients are more lateral in position than typical herniations, and because of the more axial orientation of the posterior margin of the L5–S1 disc in patients with lytic spondylolisthesis, a herniation at L5–S1 invariably extends in a cranial direction to compress the L5 nerve root and not S1. We have seen only one such herniation that violated this rule and impinged on S1.

'Front–back' stenosis

For a considerable period of time, hypertrophy of the superior articular facet was considered the major cause of lumbar lateral spinal stenosis. As the disc space collapsed, it seemed plausible that the superior articular facet would rise up in the foramen and compress the nerve cephalad against the pedicle. However, although facet hypertrophy is commonly associated with lateral stenosis, the hypertrophied superior articular process almost always lies dorsal to the nerve. It is unusual for there to be anteroposterior compression of the nerve ganglion against the dorsal aspect of the vertebral body by the enlarged facet unless there is associated uncinate spurring. 'Front–back' stenosis occurred in only 5% of outpatients. A combination of facet hypertrophy and osteophytic spurring may produce severe anteroposterior stenosis. This combination is the most common cause of 'front–back' stenosis (Fig. 7.17).

In the most severe cases all elements of bony hypertrophy (consisting of the dorsolateral osteophyte arising from the vertebral bodies, thickening of the pedicle, overgrowth of the superior articular process, and degenerative narrowing of the disc) are present and lead to severe multidimensional concentric bony stenosis. Sagittal reformatted images show a 'pinhole' intervertebral nerve root canal in these cases.

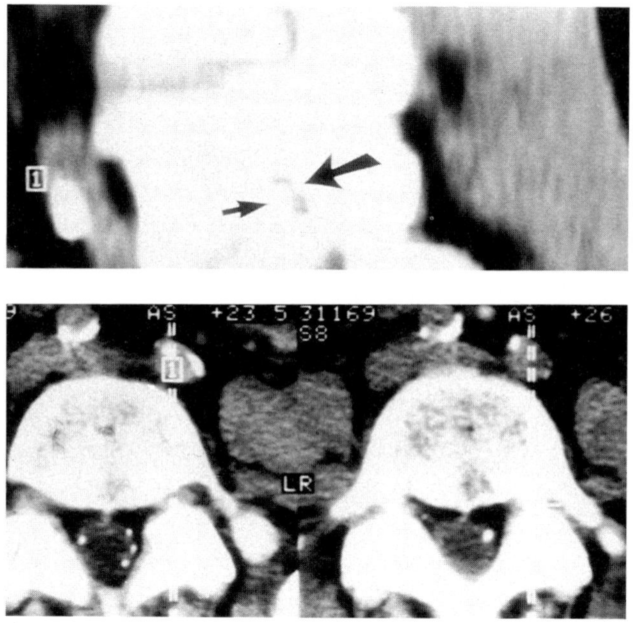

Fig. 7.17 Composite axial and sagittal reformat CT showing severe 'front–back' stenosis due to the combination of hypertrophic overgrowth of the superior articular process (large arrow) and an uncinate spur (small arrow).

Burned-out stenosis

Computerized tomography with sagittal reformatted images accurately depicts the degenerative anatomical processes that lead to lateral spinal stenosis. With CT, degenerative processes that merely involve the facet joints without encroachment on the canal are clearly defined. In most cases CT visualization of bony nerve root compression correlates closely with the clinical symptomatology, particularly if swelling of the affected nerve root is observed. However, there are patients who have definite, and sometimes severe, bony stenosis without the associated clinical symptomatology. Degenerative bony overgrowths and lateral stenosis result from chronic processes occurring over a span of years. Many of these patients, if questioned carefully, reveal a history of sciatica in the distribution of the affected nerve root. This may be followed by slow regression of symptoms, with or without conservative management. While the painful sciatica may disappear, some weakness or other loss of nerve function may remain. In some of these long-standing cases the CT findings are both a severe bony stenosis and a nerve root smaller than its companion on the opposite side. This suggests atrophy of the affected nerve root, which causes symptoms to disappear.

Subarticular stenosis

The subarticular recess is that space within the anterolateral portion of the central spinal canal lying ventral to the base of the superior articular process at its junction with the lamina and dorsal to the intervertebral disc. The subarticular recess is a lateral extension of the central canal and occurs when the canal has a trefoil configuration in conjunction with bulging of the disc or when there is pathological medial hypertrophy of the base of the superior articular process or lamina. Subarticular recess stenosis occurs within the *central* spinal canal, medial to the pedicle (Fig. 7.18) and, therefore, is quite distinct from lateral spinal stenosis which occurs within the *nerve root canal*. Subarticular recess stenosis involves the root traversing the motion segment at that level (S1 root at L5–S1) while lateral spinal stenosis involves the exiting nerve root within its canal. In the more common form of subarticular recess stenosis or entrapment, the nerve is pressed dorsally by a disc bar against the superior ventral edge of the lamina or base of the superior articular process of the segment below.

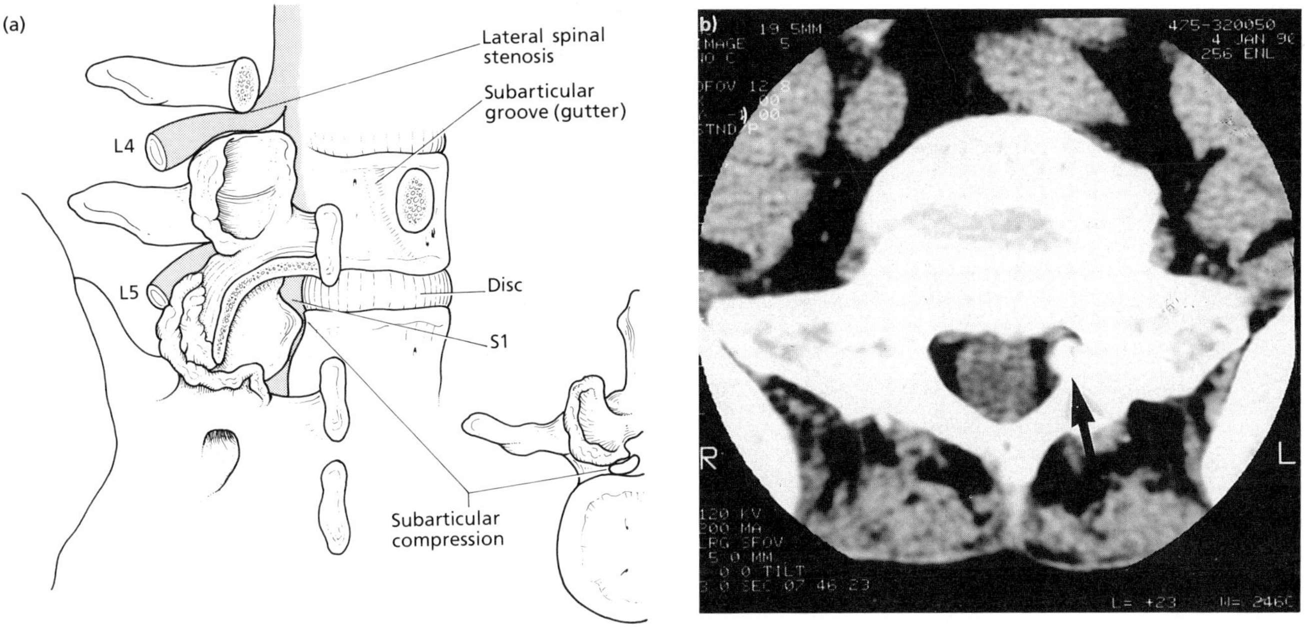

Fig. 7.18 (a) Schematic drawing showing the occurrence of subarticular recess stenosis within the lateral portion of the central spinal canal due to hypertrophy of the superior articular process. (b) An axial CT image showing severe bony subarticular recess stenosis on the left producing 'front–back' stenosis which is compressing the traversing S1 root.

As previously described, the extradural nerve root is tethered ventrally by ligamentous attachments to the posterior longitudinal ligament and disc margin. Therefore, although degenerative processes producing subarticular recess impingement are slowly progressive and chronic, the nerve root becomes entrapped within the subarticular recess because of its immobility. When subarticular recess narrowing becomes severe, the affected nerve root often is not well visualized. Metrizamide-enhanced CT scans confirm the constant position of the affected nerve roots within the far anterolateral aspect of the central canal, and clearly delineate the compression of the nerve roots. Swelling of the affected nerve roots visualized within the nerve root sheath is strong evidence of the pathological significance of the subarticular narrowing and nerve root compression. Myelograms performed in the absence of CT show displacement and broadening of the affected nerve roots and often are misinterpreted as showing disc herniation.

Degenerative spondylolisthesis

Degenerative spondylolisthesis occurs most commonly at the L4–L5 level. Axial CT images clearly show the marked degenerative changes which occur in the zygapophyseal joints producing severe hypertrophic overgrowth and fragmentation of the articular facets. Erosion of the medial portion of the superior articular facet permits the intact lamina of the vertebra above to override the superior facet of the level below, producing the anterior subluxation. The intact lamina arch may cause severe thecal narrowing, and the inferior articular facet causes severe bilateral subarticular impingement of the traversing nerve roots (Fig. 7.19).

In addition to the bony constriction, thickening of the ligamentum flavum and degenerative bulging of the disc annulus occurs. Also, the disc annulus becomes prominent because of the anterior subluxation of the vertebra above. Although the exiting nerve roots are usually indistinct as a result of compression by lateral bulging or contained herniation of the severely degenerated disc into the intervertebral nerve root canals, bony lateral spinal stenosis is unlikely. It appears that bony lateral spinal stenosis is associated with degenerative spondylolisthesis only when there is an associated posterolateral osteophyte projecting into the intervertebral nerve root canal and/or rotational instability with more prominent

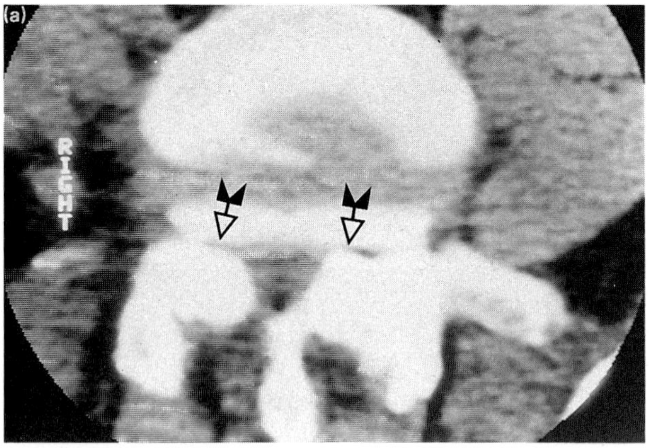

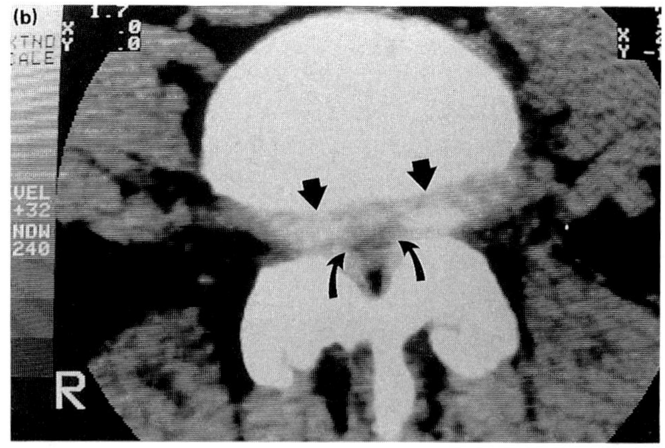

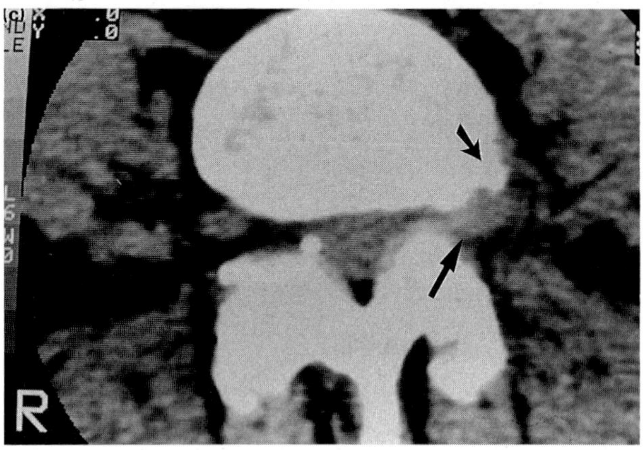

Fig. 7.19 (a) A case of degenerative spondylolisthesis with severe central spinal stenosis due to the intact subluxed neural arch of L4 on L5. The traversing L5 roots are severely compressed by the inferior articular facets. (b) The additional compression effect of the soft tissues. There is marked thickening of the ligamentum flavum (curved arrows) and a broad-based central disc protrusion (broad arrows). (c) The more unusual occurrence of lateral stenosis due to an associated posterolateral osteophyte (small arrow). The existing L4 root is markedly swollen (large arrow).

anterior subluxation of the lamina and inferior facet on one side (Fig. 7.19).

THE ACCURACY OF CT AND MYELOGRAPHY IN THE DIAGNOSIS OF LUMBAR DISC HERNIATION AND STENOSIS

Eighty-four patients were studied from the 20 000 who had undergone CT of the lumbar spine in the authors' unit, and also a myelogram performed elsewhere. All were surgically confirmed. Both the myelograms and the CT scan were evaluated by two spine radiologists without knowledge of the prior interpretations, the clinical information or the surgical findings. All the studies were evaluated for the presence of stenosis (lateral, subarticular and central) as well as disc herniation. Positive correlation between the surgical findings and CT and myelography was accepted only when precise anatomical localization as to level, side and degree of severity was present.

Preoperative CT was 97% accurate in the diagnosis of disc herniation, being truly positive in 92% and truly negative in a further 5%. There was only one false-positive and one false-negative. The diagnostic accuracy for myelography was a true positive rate of 86%. True negatives were found in 3%. False-negatives were found in 6% and false-positives in 5%.

In 19 patients with surgically proven lateral stenosis, CT was 100% accurate in detecting the lateral stenosis but this diagnosis could not be made from any of the myelograms (100% false-negative rate). There were nine cases of central and subarticular stenosis and the diagnosis was made correctly in all cases by both CT and myelography. However, a specific observation of the site and severity of individual nerve root compression could only be made by CT.

A further prospective study was performed in 100 consecutive patients undergoing both the CT examination and the surgical procedure in the authors' department. Surgery confirmed herniated discs in

73% of these patients, lateral stenosis in 62% and a combination of herniation and stenosis in 37%. CT interpretation of these patients resulted in a 96% accuracy of diagnosis. These studies confirm the inability of myelography to delineate lateral entrapment of lumbosacral nerve roots. CT was found to be both more sensitive and specific in the diagnosis of lumbar disc herniation and stenosis. As has already been stated, MRI adds even more detailed information in the assessment of the differing types of disc herniation. The information obtained from high-resolution CT and MRI allows a very precise diagnostic evaluation of lumbar degenerative disease. MRI additionally allows the whole lumbar canal to be imaged. This allows the diagnosis of intradural lesions such as dermoids or neurofibromas which uncommonly, though not rarely (5%), present with a sciatica syndrome. If only CT imaging is used such lesions can easily be missed.

MAGNETIC RESONANCE IMAGING OF THE SPINE

In contrast with CT evaluation, MRI is an operator-intensive imaging study with multiple parameters. Technical considerations to limit various artifacts must be specified for each sequence. With the wide variety of tissue types evaluated in spinal MRI, the standard examination includes T1-weighted, proton-density, and T2-weighted sequences (Berns *et al.*, 1989). In addition, gradient echo sequences are frequently utilized in the evaluation of the cervical spine (Modic *et al.*, 1989).

The MRI examination must be tailored for the unique anatomy of the different parts of the spinal column. It is often tempting to shorten an imaging study when trying to answer a specific clinical question. In the evaluation of spinal disease, clinical symptoms and physical signs of neural dysfunction may not be easily localized to a specific motion segment and they can also be elicited by a variety of pathological processes. For this reason it is critical that, in each spinal region studied, all spinal and paraspinal anatomy must be completely examined and optimally displayed utilizing sagittal, axial and, when appropriate, additional non-orthogonal imaging sequences.

Before undergoing the MRI examination each patient must be carefully questioned to determine if there are any contra-indications to performing the study. Absolute contra-indications include ferromagnetic cerebral aneurysm clips, cardiac pacemakers that may become dysfunctional in high magnetic fields, metallic foreign bodies in the orbit, and ferromagnetic cochlear implants. Pregnancy, recent cardiac or vascular surgery, transcutaneous electrical nerve stimulators, and severe claustrophobia are relative contra-indications that must be handled on an individual basis to determine whether the benefit of a study outweighs the risk. Artifacts can be expected from a variety of metallic instrumentation devices (Shellock, 1988) and from metallic particles in the body from previous trauma or surgery (Heindel *et al.*, 1986). It is difficult to predict the degree of image degradation from metallic devices, and occasionally MRI study will be helpful even in patients with spinal instrumentation.

Cervical spine protocols

Because of the complex geometry and small size of the anatomical components of the cervical spine, imaging with high-resolution surface coils is required. Thin section (3–3.5 mm) with a small interslice gap in both axial and sagittal planes is necessary to delineate the normal neural structures in the spinal central and intervertebral canals (Fig. 7.20).

Sagittal T1-weighted images (Fig. 7.20a) provided excellent anatomical delineation of the vertebral bodies (curved black arrows); intervertebral discs (straight black arrows); and spinal cord (white arrows). A myelographic effect can be created by the utilization of cardiac-gated T2-weighted images (Fig. 7.20b). This produces an excellent interface between the posterior margin of the intervertebral discs and the CSF spaces (curved black arrows). It also produces excellent delineation of the spinal cord (arrowheads).

Axial T1-weighted images (Fig. 7.20c) also provide excellent delineation of the spinal cord (white arrowheads); ventral (short white arrow) and dorsal (long white arrow) nerve roots; and the intervertebral nerve root canals (curved white arrow). The contents of the intervertebral nerve root canals can be shown on oblique T1-weighted images (Fig. 7.20d) where the fat which images as white contrasts the neural (curved arrow) and vascular structures which lie within. The use of gradient echo imaging in the axial phase (Fig. 7.20e) produces a high signal intensity in the CSF which delineates the spinal cord (black

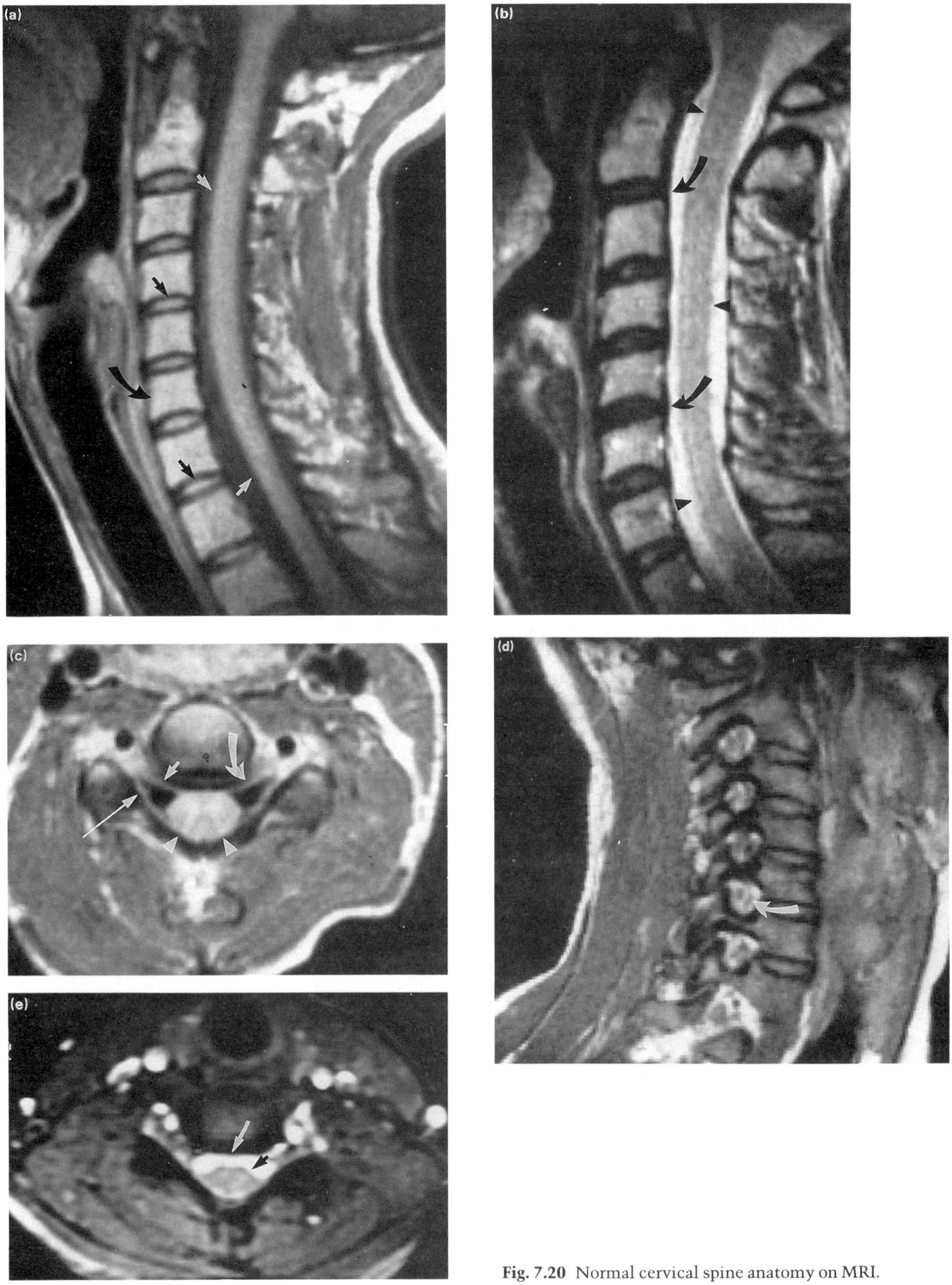

Fig. 7.20 Normal cervical spine anatomy on MRI.

arrow) and the posterior margin of the disc (white arrow).

The routine examination of the cervical spine should include both T1- and T2-weighted sequences to adequately evaluate all spinal and paraspinal anatomy. The sagittal T1-weighted sequence covering from the cervicomedullary junction to the cervicothoracic junction provides an excellent survey of the vertebral bodies, intervertebral discs, spinal cord, thecal sac and posterior elements. Axial T1-weighted images provide an excellent evaluation of spinal cord morphology, intrathecal nerve root anatomy, vertebral bodies, posterior elements, intervertebral canals and paraspinal soft tissues. The main limitation of the T1-weighted sequence is due to the lack of MRI signal from the vertebral body cortex, the posterior annular–posterior longitudinal ligament complex, and the cerebrospinal fluid in the adjacent thecal sac resulting in poor contrast differentiation between these structures. This makes evaluation of small disc herniations, chondro-osseous spurs and hypertrophied or calcified ligaments extremely difficult. To achieve a contrast difference between the posterior margin of the discovertebral joint and the thecal sac, either a cardiac gated or flow compensated T2-weighted sequence or a gradient echo sequence should be performed (Enzmann *et al.*, 1987; Modic *et al.*, 1989). On both of these sequences, CSF will generate high signal intensity, creating a CSF myelographic effect. This provides an excellent CSF–extradural interface and delineates the spinal cord. Gradient echo sequences are helpful in the evaluation of extradural disease, but not as a primary tool in the evaluation of spinal cord pathology or vertebral body marrow disease. Additional pulse sequences helpful in the evaluation of the cervical spine include oblique sequences through the intervertebral canals (Hedberg *et al.*, 1988) and multiple angled sections through the disc spaces (Reicher *et al.*, 1986). Coronal sequences are helpful in the evaluation of spinal cord pathology, extradural masses, paraspinal pathology and vertebral body malalignment or deformation.

Thoracic spine protocols

The initial sequence of a thoracic spine MRI examination should include a sagittal T1-weighted localizer sequence that covers the entire cervical spine and cervicothoracic junction. This sequence provides the best reference for accurately numbering thoracic vertebral bodies, and may also occasionally allow the detection of cervical spine disease presenting as thoracic neural dysfunction. The initial sequence evaluating the thoracic spine should be a sagittal T1-weighted localizer that includes the area from the cervicothoracic junction to the conus medullaris. This is followed by high-resolution sagittal T1 and multiecho T2-weighted sequences (Fig. 7.21).

A surface coil is employed to achieve high spatial resolution, and the field of view of these coils is usually adequate to evaluate the region from T1 or T2 to approximately T10 or T11. After completion of the sagittal sequences the examination should be reviewed by a radiologist to determine whether additional axial sequences are needed. These are obtained when a pathological process is identified, or if the patient's symptomatology suggests a specific location of a disease process, even though this area appears normal on the initial sagittal images. This is particularly true in the evaluation of the intervertebral canals, paravertebral soft tissues, and posterior elements of the vertebrae, which are not adequately evaluated by sagittal sequences alone (Post *et al.*, 1988). In addition to the routine sequences, a coronal T1-weighted sequence is helpful in the evaluation of the spinal cord, extradural or paraspinal masses, scoliosis, and congenital anomalies. In some centres working predominantly with tumour patients, the initial screening study may also include an inversion recovery sequence, which provides excellent delineation of abnormal vertebral body marrow (Cohen *et al.*, 1989).

Lumbar spine protocols

Compared to the cervical and thoracic spine, the greater size of the constituent elements of the lumbar spine, the increased size of the dural sac and the increased amount of epidural fat all combine to directly affect the quality of MRI. To evaluate the lumbar spine optimally, a sagittal T1 and multiecho T2-weighted sequence in conjunction with axial multiecho T2-weighted sequences must be obtained (Fig. 7.22). The sagittal T1-weighted image (Fig. 7.22a) provides optimum imaging of the spinal anatomy with excellent delineation of the vertebral bodies, intervertebral discs, the thecal sac and the conus medullaris (curved white arrow). The cancellous portions of the vertebral bodies are high signal due to the fat content of the marrow. However, the interface between the posterior outer annulus (straight white arrow) and the extradural space is poorly defined on T1-weighted images.

The multiecho T2-weighted sequences provide important information in the assessment of disc degeneration and herniation, marrow oedema, extradural masses and intradural pathology. As part of this sequence, a sagittal proton-density (long TR/short TE) image (Fig. 7.22b) produces increased signal from both the disc and the CSF and is helpful in the assessment of the posterior annular and posterior longitudinal ligamentous areas (arrow). The basivertebral veins are also well shown.

Detailed assessment of nerve root pathology is done by a combination of a sagittal T1-weighted image taken through the invertebral canals (Fig. 7.22c) and by axial T1-weighted image (Fig. 7.22d). Figure 7.22c shows excellent delineation of the dorsal root ganglia (straight arrows) lying subjacent to the pedicles. The posterolateral margins of the discs are also well shown (curved arrows). On the axial image (Fig. 7.22d) the roots of the cauda equina are well shown (white arrow) and the presence of fat within the epidural space provides an excellent soft tissue interface to show individual nerve roots (black arrows).

To produce the highest quality MRI of the lumbar spine high-resolution surface coils must be used. Sagittal images should be 4–5 mm in thickness with a gap of 1 mm between slices. On axial sequences, slices of similar thickness should be obtained contiguously from the L2–L3 or L3–L4 disc level to L5–S1. It is essential that the sagittal images include the conus and the entire sacrum so that additional axial images may be obtained if unsuspected pathology is shown in those areas (Fig. 7.23).

CLINICAL APPLICATIONS

The purpose of an imaging study is to delineate and characterize normal and abnormal tissue. To maximize information obtained from any imaging study

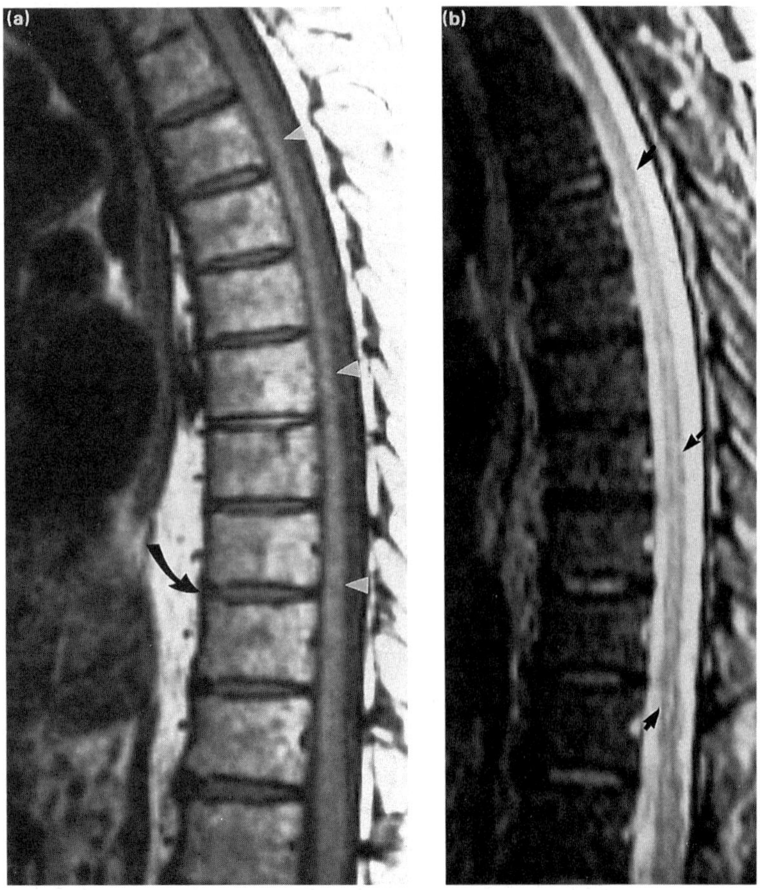

Fig. 7.21 Normal thoracic spine anatomy, MRI. On the sagittal T1-weighted image (a), there is excellent anatomical delineation of the vertebral bodies, intervertebral discs (curved black arrow) and spinal cord (white arrowheads). On the sagittal cardiac gated T2-weighted image (b), as a result of the myelographic effect, there is an excellent CSF–extradural interface along with delineation of the thoracic spinal cord (black arrows).

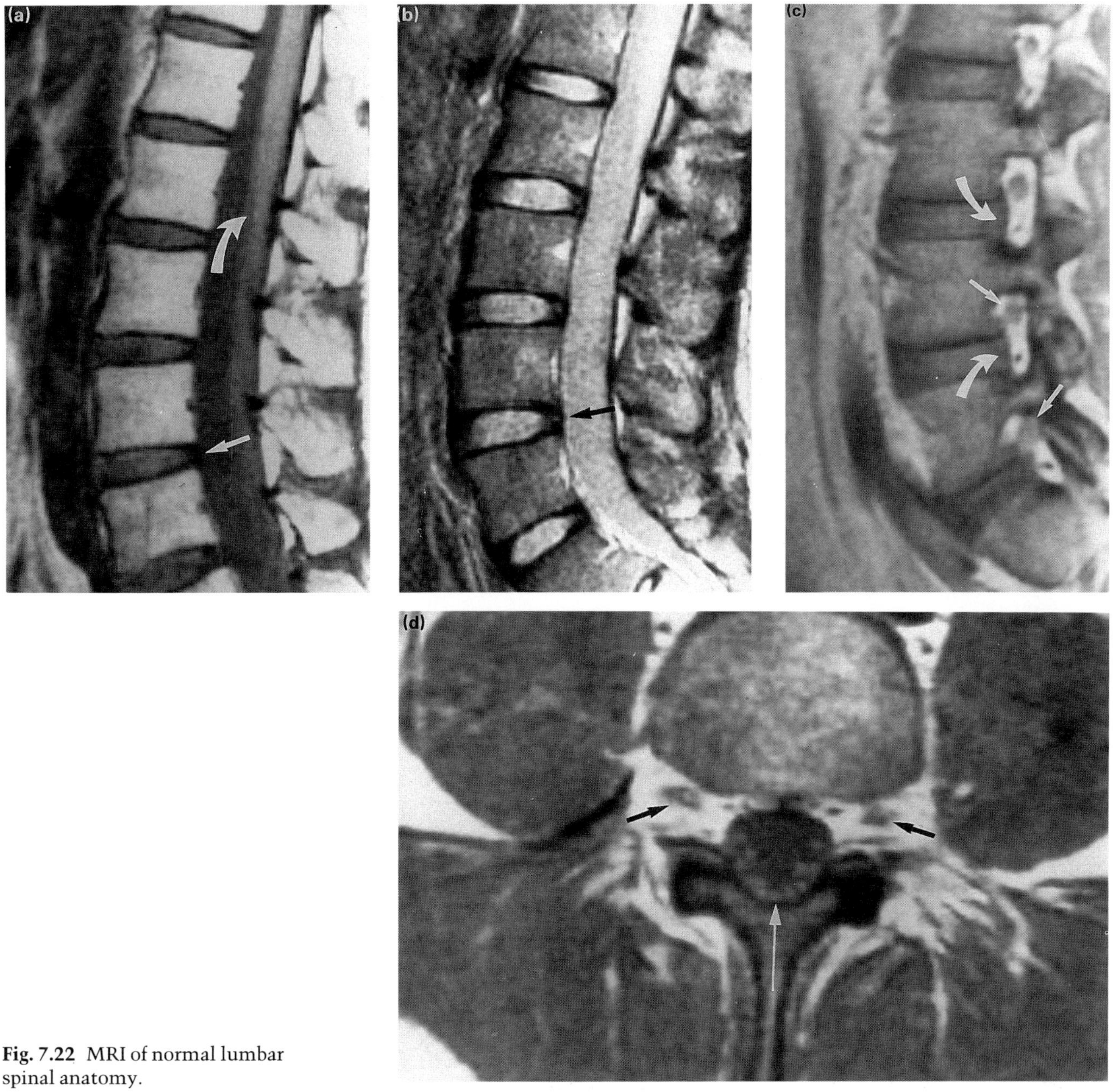

Fig. 7.22 MRI of normal lumbar spinal anatomy.

of the spine, it is first necessary to thoroughly understand normal spinal anatomy and the natural history of spinal diseases. Diagnostic examinations provide information about dynamic disease processes manifesting a spectrum of pathology. The transformation of diagnostic data into useful clinical information is directly dependent on the level of expertise of the clinician interpreting the study.

Degenerative spinal disease

When describing the pathomorphological changes in degenerative spinal disease, it is helpful to consider each disc level as a three-joint complex or motion segment, with the intervertebral disc and facet joints biomechanically linked to form a functional spinal

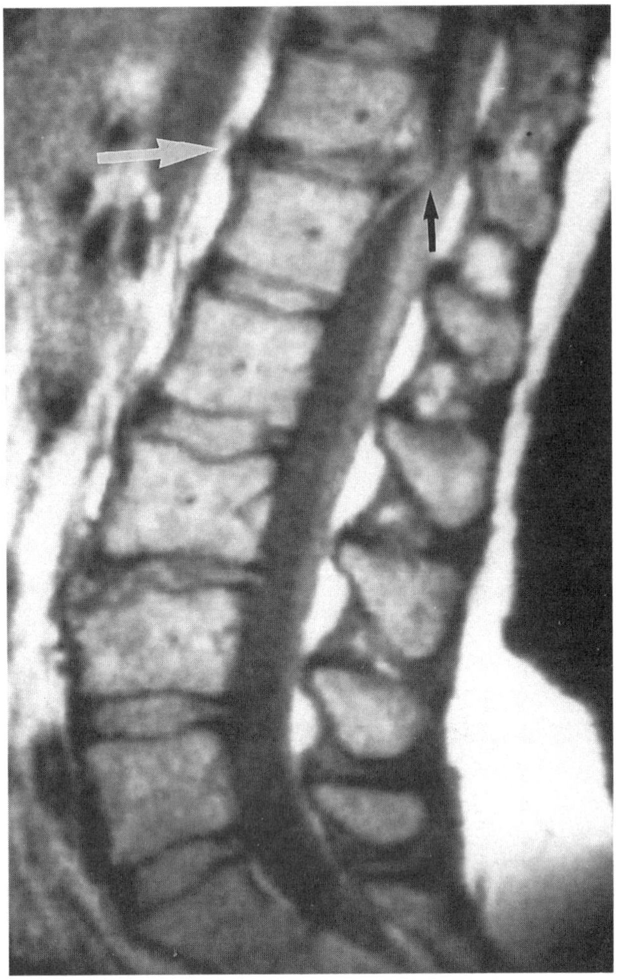

Fig. 7.23 Sagittal T1-weighted image of a patient presenting with a radicular syndrome. Unsuspected cord compression by a posterior disc herniation (black arrow) has been identified at the T12–L1 disc level (white arrow).

unit (Kirkaldy-Willis, 1988). This will promote the critical evaluation of the entire MRI or CT study and not simply focus on one component, such as disc herniation, when evaluating a patient presenting with pain or neural dysfunction.

Degenerative disc disease

Both MRI and high-resolution CT can provide excellent delineation of the morphological changes and effects of a discal herniation. Figure 7.24a shows a sagittal T1-weighted MRI of a patient with a large C5–C6 disc herniation causing cord compression. The axial image (Fig. 7.24b) shows in addition the asymmetrical distribution of the herniation (straight arrow) and the compression of the right-sided nerve root (curved arrow). CT evaluation (Figs 7.24c & d) also demonstrates the herniation, but its effect on the spinal cord is not shown.

MRI, in addition to providing enhanced detail of the effects of disc herniation on intraspinal structures, also permits the assessment of the pathological changes which occur within a disc prior to any disturbance of its contour. Both the nucleus pulposus and the annulus fibrosus consist mainly of water, collagen, and proteoglycans, with the major difference being the relative concentration of the components, level of hydration, and the particular type of collagen that predominates (Ghosh, 1988). On T2-weighted images the high signal intensity in the central portion of the disc originates from both the nucleus pulposus and inner annular fibres (Yu *et al.*, 1988). The signal intensity in the disc is related to its state of hydration and the physicochemical state of discal tissue (Hickey *et al.*, 1986). On T2-weighted images the outer annular fibres demonstrate very low signal intensity, as does the adjacent posterior longitudinal ligament (Pech & Haughton, 1985). With ageing there is a gradual breakdown of proteoglycans in the nucleus, gradual desiccation of the mucoid nuclear material, and loss of anatomical delineation between the nucleus and inner annular fibres (Miller *et al.*, 1988). Over the age of 30, an intranuclear cleft is identified in normal discs on T2-weighted MRI, and this represents normal ingrowth of fibrous tissue (Aguila *et al.*, 1985).

Both experimentally and clinically it appears that the development of a radial annular tear may be the necessary step in the development of disc degeneration or herniation (Lipson & Muir, 1981). Yu *et al.* (1989) were able to delineate small tears in the outer annulus on T2-weighted MRI (Fig. 7.8). Ross *et al.* (1990) also demonstrated such annular tears with gadolinium-DTPA enhancement of T1 images (Fig. 7.25). When the radial tear communicates with the nucleus the disc will begin to degenerate and demonstrate decreased signal intensity on T2-weighted images. With communicating radial tears, displacement of the nuclear material is possible with resultant disc herniation. Displacement of the nuclear material into the region of the outer annular–posterior longitudinal ligament complex will cause altered morphology of the periphery of the disc, resulting in a focal protrusion of the disc beyond the margin of

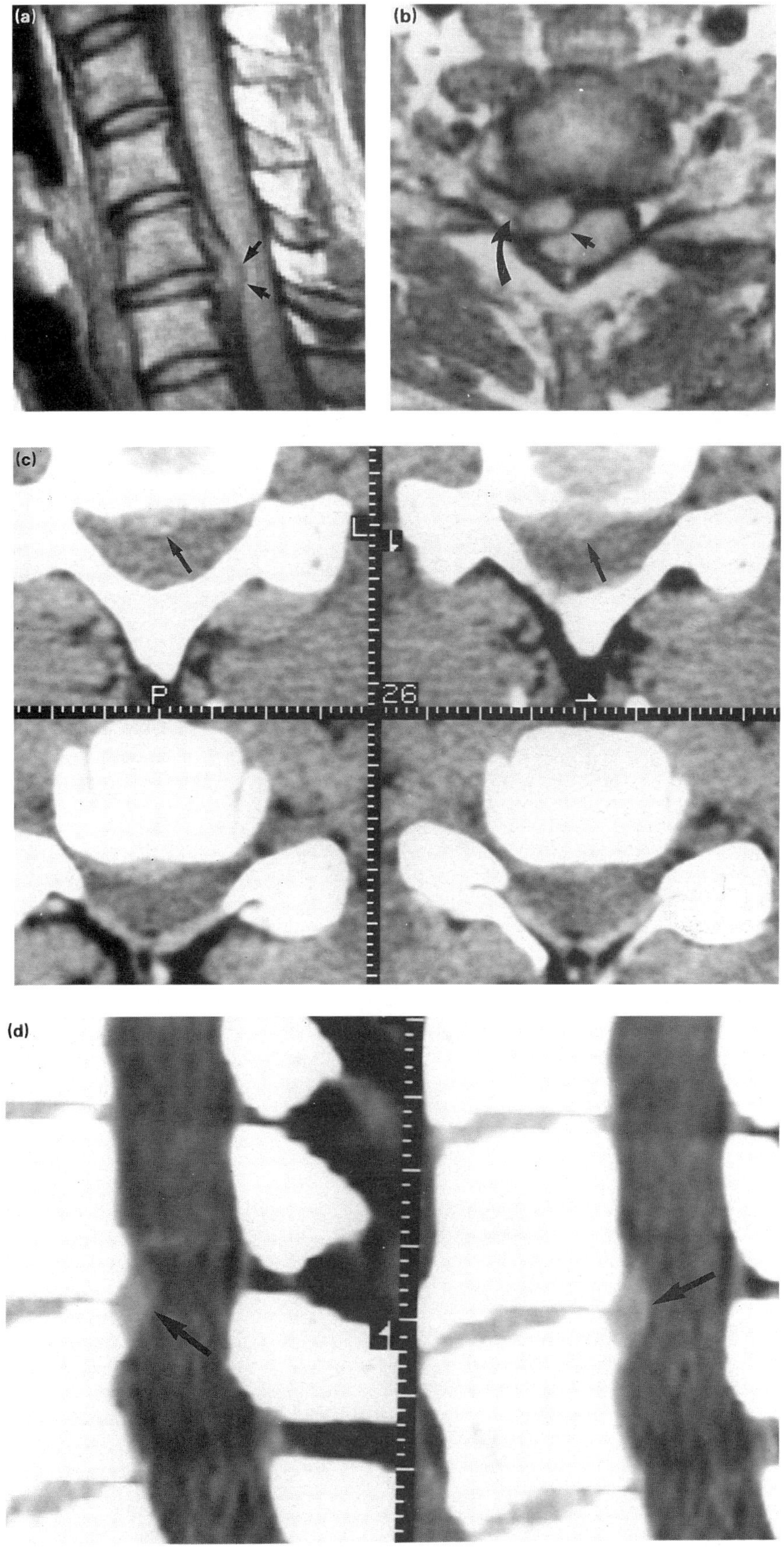

Fig. 7.24 Cervical disc herniation—MRI and high-resolution CT imaging.

the vertebral endplates. Both MRI and CT provide excellent delineation of these contour changes. As long as the disc material is contained by the outer annular fibres or the posterior longitudinal ligament, the herniation is designated a contained herniation. With the superb soft tissue resolution of MRI it is possible to determine whether the disc material is contained by the outer annular–ligamentous complex or has extruded through this complex, becoming an extruded, non-contained, disc herniation (Fig. 7.26) (Grenier *et al.*, 1989).

After disc material has penetrated through the

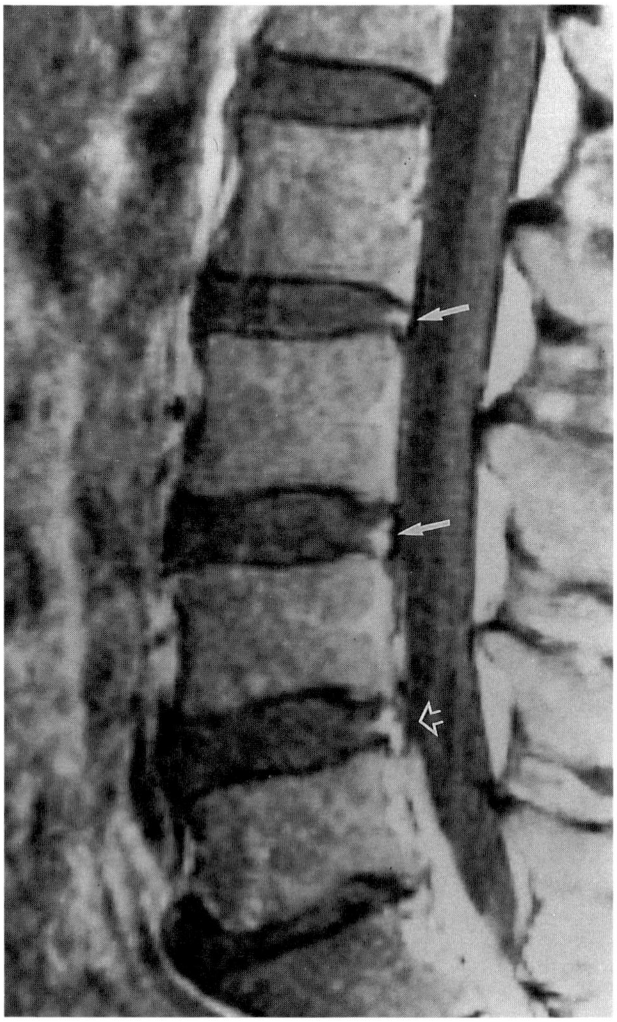

Fig. 7.25 Sagittal T1-weighted MRI following enhancement with gadolinium-DTPA. Posterior annular fissures are seen at the L2–L3 and L3–L4 discs (solid arrows). The small posterior disc herniation at L4–L5 also enhances (open arrow).

posterior longitudinal ligament, it is possible for a portion of the disc material to separate from the disc of origin and become a sequestered fragment. In a prospective MRI study (Masaryk *et al.*, 1988), 80% of sequestered disc fragments demonstrated hyperintensity on T2-weighted images, compared with the degenerated disc of origin. The remaining 20% were isointense. In the same study the accuracy of MRI in differentiating sequestered disc fragments from other forms of lumbar disc herniation was 85% compared with a 65% accuracy for CT–myelography. The differential diagnosis of a sequestered disc fragment includes epidural abscess, extradural tumour, conjoined nerve root, nerve root sheath tumour or cyst, and epidural haematoma.

Following herniation the disc will continue to degenerate and on an MRI study the degenerated disc will demonstrate decreased signal intensity. Disc herniations associated with normal signal intensity from the disc have been reported, and one study demonstrated normal signal intensity in discs that were abnormal morphologically on discography (Zucherman *et al.*, 1988). To date there have been no prospective studies to determine the length of time necessary for a normally hydrated disc to become desiccated after it herniates. Calcification or gas in the disc may be difficult to detect on T2-weighted images due to the decreased signal intensity in the severely degenerated disc and lack of MRI signal from the calcium or gas. T1-weighted or gradient echo images are more useful in delineating a vacuum phenomenon or disc calcification (Modic *et al.*, 1988).

In addition to depicting the degenerative changes of a disc, MRI is sensitive to degenerative changes in the adjacent vertebral body endplates. Modic *et al.* (1988) reported pathological alternations of the vertebral body marrow adjacent to discs undergoing degeneration. With Type I endplate degeneration there was decreased signal intensity in the subchondral cancellous bone on a T1-weighted image and increased signal intensity on a T2-weighted image compared with the normal marrow (Fig. 7.27). The region of altered signal intensity pathologically represents prominent fibrovascular tissue in the marrow adjacent to the vertebral body endplate. Type II endplate degenerative changes, which pathologically represent increased fat in the subchondral bone marrow, demonstrated hyperintensity on T1-weighted images and slight hyperintensity or isointensity on T2-weighted images. Type III endplate degenerative

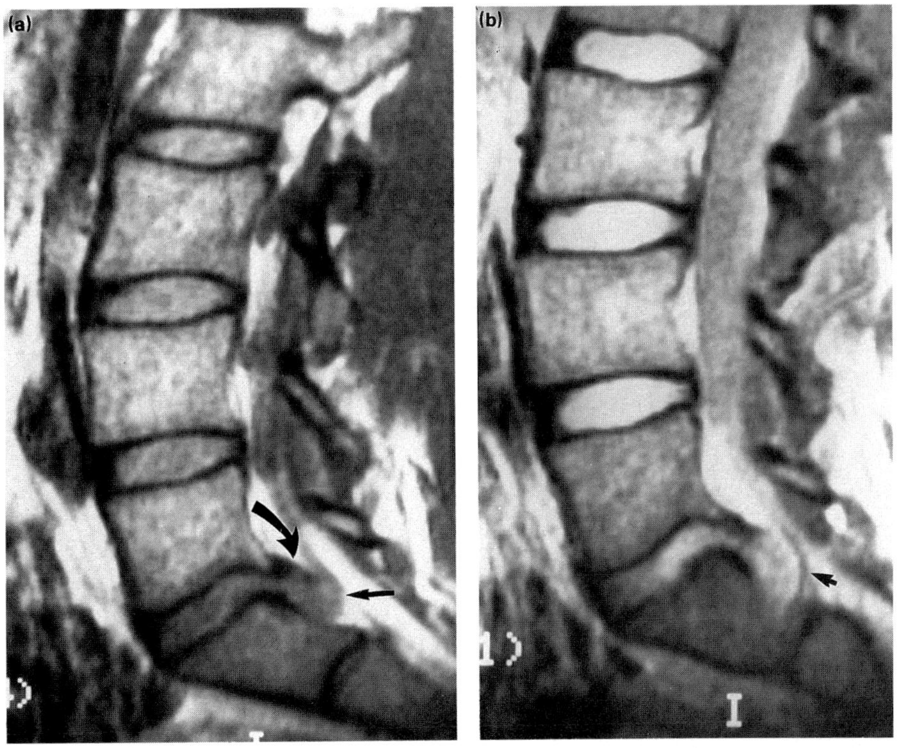

Fig. 7.26 L5–S1 disc extrusion, MRI. On the sagittal proton-density weighted image (a), at the L5–S1 disc level, there is a posterior disc extrusion (straight arrow), which has penetrated through the posterior annular–posterior longitudinal ligament complex (curved arrow). On the T2-weighted image (b), the posterior displacement of the right S1 nerve root (arrow) by the disc extrusion is demonstrated.

changes were represented by coarsening and thickening of the subchondral trabeculae, which was depicted on T1- and T2-weighted images as decreased signal intensity. On a CT evaluation, only endplate sclerosis can be delineated,. and this does not necessarily correlate with Type III changes identified by MRI.

With the excellent characterization of normal and abnormal discs by MRI, it is now possible to non-invasively study the natural history of disc degeneration and herniation. The sensitivity of MRI to early changes of disc degeneration should help in the evaluation of patients with intervertebral disc resorption (Jaffray & O'Brien, 1986) or internal disc disruption (Blumenkopf *et al.*, 1988).

Facet arthrosis

As part of a three-joint complex the facet joints are biomechanically linked to the discovertebral joint. Altered functional status of one component of the complex may induce degeneration of another component of the spinal unit. The size and orientation of the facet joints differ at different levels of the spine and, representing diarthrodial joints, are subject to painful degeneration. In the evaluation of facet orientation and facet arthrosis, CT is unsurpassed (Carerra *et al.*, 1980). Early erosions, cystic changes, hyperostosis and facet capsular calcification are clearly delineated on a CT examination. Degenerative changes of the facet joints resolved by MRI include facet hypertrophy, osteophytic spurring, cartilage narrowing, joint effusions, and capsular hypertrophy (Grenier *et al.*, 1987). Cartilage thickness is difficult to measure accurately because of partial volume averaging and chemical shift artifacts. Gradient echo sequences may prove useful in the evaluation of facet degenerative changes, particularly when evaluating articular cartilage.

Spinal stenosis

Spinal stenosis is defined as local, segmental, or generalized narrowing of the central or intervertebral canals by bony or soft tissue elements that may lead to encroachment on the neural structures. The narrowing may involve the bony canal alone or the dural sac, or both. The degenerative changes most often associated with stenosis include hyperostotic spurring of the vertebral body endplates, uncinate pro-

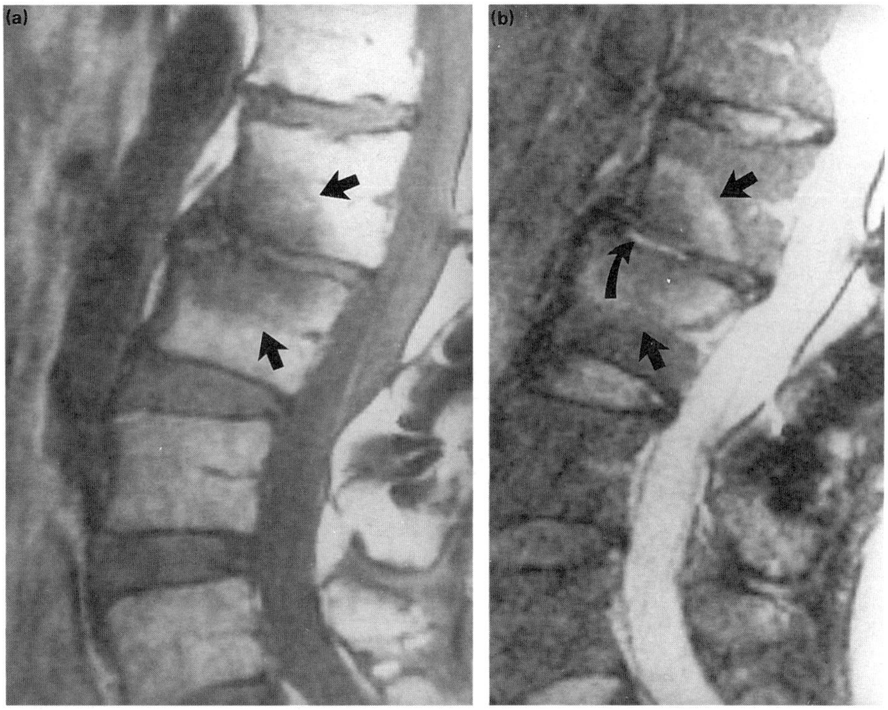

Fig. 7.27 Type I endplate degenerative changes, MRI. On the sagittal T1-weighted image (a), at the L2–L3 disc level, moderately severe decreased disc height is present, along with a minimal retrolisthesis. There is a hemispheric region of decreased signal intensity (straight black arrows) in the cancellous bone adjacent to the degenerative discovertebral joint. On the T2-weighted image (b), there is increased signal intensity (straight black arrows) in the cancellous bone. Increased signal intensity is present in the anterior portion of the disc space (curved black arrow) most likely representing fluid in degenerative fissures.

cesses, and facet joints, along with hypertrophy of the ligamenta flava and anterior facet capsules. The initial size of the central and intervertebral canals is an important factor in determining whether degenerative changes will cause neural impingement or compression. The goal of MRI and CT in the evaluation of the patient presenting with radiculopathy, myeloradiculopathy, or myelopathy is not just to demonstrate that stenosis is present, but to define the relative contributions of each component of the stenotic process.

In the evaluation of patients presenting with cervical myelopathy or radiculopathy, thin-section high-resolution CT has been used as a screening examination for the cervical spine (Miyasaka *et al.*, 1983). However, CT does not directly demonstrate neural impingement or compression, and frequently a contrast study is still needed preoperatively. In the evaluation of cervical spondylosis, CT is excellent in differentiating between disc herniations and spondylotic spurs. This is more difficult with MRI because of the thicker sections and variable signal intensity from degenerative osseous ridges. The strength of MRI is in its clear delineation of the effect of the spondylotic changes on the neural elements in the central and intervertebral canals (Fig. 7.29). In several recent series, excellent results with MRI compared with CT–myelography and myelography alone have been demonstrated when evaluating patients with radiculopathy and myelopathy (Brown *et al.*, 1988; Maravilla & Hartling, 1988).

In addition to the routine sagittal and axial MRI sequences, gradient echo sequences are beneficial in defining the exact aetiology of stenosis. In the cervical spine there is a strong association pathologically

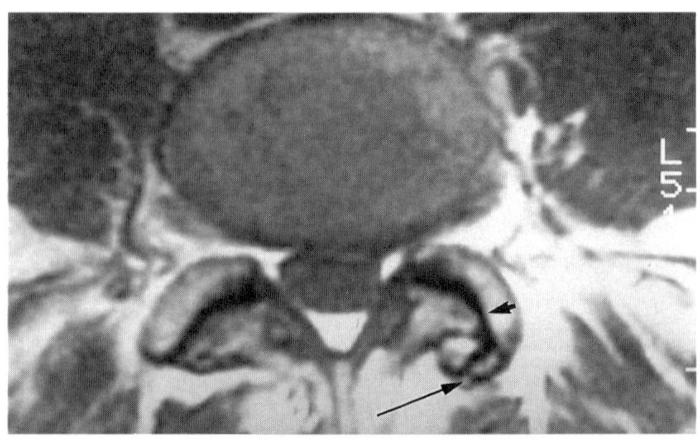

Fig. 7.28 Lumbar facet arthrosis. On the MRI examination, on the axial proton-density weighted image, degeneration of the left facet joint is identified with narrowing of the articular cartilage (short arrow) and osteophytic spurring of the dorsal surface (long arrow) of the left superior articular process.

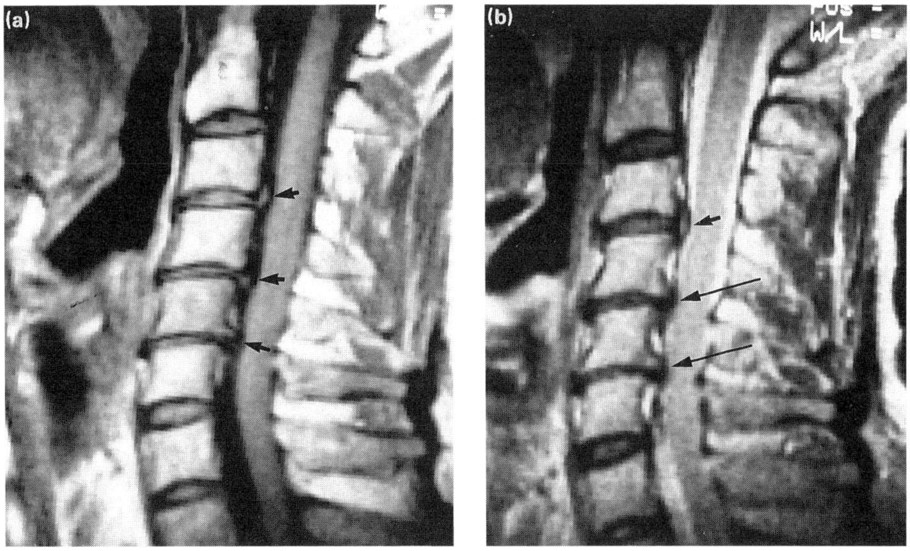

Fig. 7.29 Multilevel cervical spondylosis superimposed on developmental stenosis. Degenerative changes at C3–C4, C4–C5, and C5–C6 are clearly seen on the T1 image (a). The cardiac gated T2 image (b) highlights the CSF producing a myelogram effect. On this image mild cord compression can be seen due to a disc at C3–C4 and spondylotic bars at C4–C5 and C5–C6.

between degenerative changes of the discovertebral joint and uncinate spurs at the same motion segment. Many patients presenting with myelopathy secondary to spondylotic changes will also have an associated radiculopathy. CT with its thin sections is optimal in the evaluation of uncinate spurs projecting into the intervertebral canals. Oblique imaging of the intervertebral canals adds information to a standard MRI scan and should be included if the intervertebral canals cannot be adequately evaluated on standard sequences.

In the evaluation of patients with myelopathy or myeloradiculopathy it is important to determine accurately the size of the central spinal canal. A true osseous diameter can be obtained only from axial images orthogonal to the long axis of the cervical central canal, or by sagittal images. CT, with its excellent osseous delineation, currently provides the most accurate osseous measurements. Osseous stenosis does not necessarily cause cervical myelopathy, and the great advantage of MRI over CT when evaluating stenosis is its demonstration of what effect the degenerative processes and/or a developmentally narrowed central canal have on the neural structures. Patients presenting with myelopathic symptoms frequently have degenerative spondylotic changes superimposed on a developmentally narrowed central canal. In recent studies the best predictor of the clinical course in myelopathic patients, the impact of surgical intervention, and the pathological changes of the spinal cord was the degree of cord compression and measurement of cord volume (Fujiwara *et al.*, 1988, 1989).

Takahashi *et al.* (1989) examined 668 patients with chronic cervical cord compression by MRI and demonstrated high signal intensity within the spinal cord on T2-weighted or proton-density images in 14.8% of the patients. This finding was directly related to increased spinal cord compression and to the severity of clinical myelopathy. Patients with high signal intensity areas responded less favourably to surgical or medical treatment. An exciting future application of MRI will be the dynamic evaluation of the degree of cervical stenosis utilizing flexion and extension sagittal sequences (Condon & Hadley, 1988). MRI is also excellent in the delineation of pathological processes that may mimic spondylotic cervical myelopathy, including spinal cord tumours, intra- and extradural masses, metastatic disease, and demyelinating processes.

In the lumbar spine it has become clear that patients of any age may present with disc degeneration superimposed on a stenotic process, or may present with isolated stenosis as a cause of leg or back pain. The classification of spinal stenosis as congenital, developmental, and acquired is extremely helpful when evaluating a small spinal canal (see Chapter 46). Congenital stenosis is caused by disturbed fetal development and may occur as one element of a congenital malformation of the lumbar spine. Developmental stenosis is a growth disturbance of the posterior elements, involving the pedicles, lamina, and articular processes and resulting in decreased volume of the spinal canal. A true midline osseous sagittal diameter measuring less than 12 mm is considered relative stenosis, and a diameter of less than 10 mm is considered absolute stenosis. This is measured from the middle of the posterior surface of the vertebral body to the point of junction of the base of its spinous process and laminae.

With relative stenosis the reserve capacity of the spinal canal is reduced and a small disc herniation or early degenerative changes may cause symptomatic stenosis in both the young and the older population. Acquired stenosis is the narrowing of the central or intervertebral canals by degenerative changes of the discovertebral joints, facet joints, and ligamenta flava. In a prospective study, Modic *et al.* (1986) examined 60 patients with suspected lumbar disc herniations and/or central stenosis with surface coil MRI, CT and/or myelography, and the results were compared with the findings at surgery. Surgical findings of stenosis agreed with the MRI findings in 77%, CT findings in 79%, and myelographic findings in only 54%. This study did not differentiate between central and intervertebral canal stenosis, and the study also did not include multiplanar reformations, which are helpful in the CT evaluation of central and intervertebral canal stenosis. Bolender *et al.* (1985) found that the cross-sectional area of the thecal sac correlated best to stenotic symptoms. MRI is ideally suited for evaluating the true sagittal dimension and cross-sectional area of the thecal sac, thus obviating the need for CT–myelography.

The role of CT in the evaluation of stenotic disorders and spondylolisthesis has already been stressed in this chapter. However, MRI also provides useful clinical information. Figure 7.30 shows changes of severe multilevel disease with a degree of degenerative spondylolisthesis at L4–L5 but more severe stenosis being produced by the L3–L4 slip (bottom arrow). The other arrows point to further areas of stenosis due to disc bulging at the cranial levels. The delineation of spondylolytic defects is difficult with MRI (Fig. 7.31) but the extent of the associated narrowing of the intervertebral canal is well seen (Heithoff, 1988). MRI is also the ideal medium for assessing the associated disc degeneration which is commonly found at the level of the pars defect (Szypryt *et al.*, 1989) or at the level above (Rothman & Glenn, 1984).

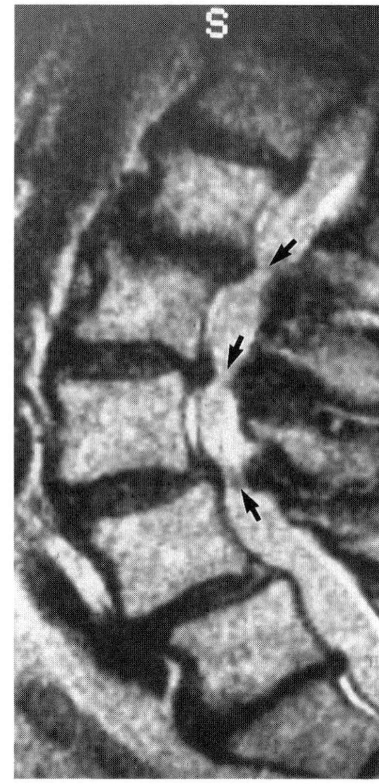

Fig. 7.30 MRI showing multilevel lumbar stenosis.

Spinal trauma

The optimal treatment of cervical cord injury secondary to vertebral fracture and/or dislocation is still in the process of evolution. MRI provides the first non-invasive imaging procedure to directly assess the degree of dural and spinal cord compression and pathological spinal cord changes (Kulkarni *et al.*, 1987; Beers *et al.*, 1988). Injury to posterior ligaments, osseous structures, soft tissues, and discovertebral joints can also be evaluated on the standard MRI examination (Mirvis *et al.*, 1988; Emery *et al.*, 1989; Tracy *et al.*, 1989). The value of MRI in diagnosing spinal cord haemorrhage, oedema, and neural compression has been well documented. Studies have demonstrated that neurological recovery was insignificant in patients with intramedullary spinal cord haemorrhage or extensive contusion, but recovery in neurological function was observed with patients demonstrating only cord oedema (Kulkarni *et al.*, 1987; Schaefer *et al.*, 1989). The sagittal T1-weighted sequence demonstrated altered spinal cord morphology, but the sagittal T2-weighted sequence

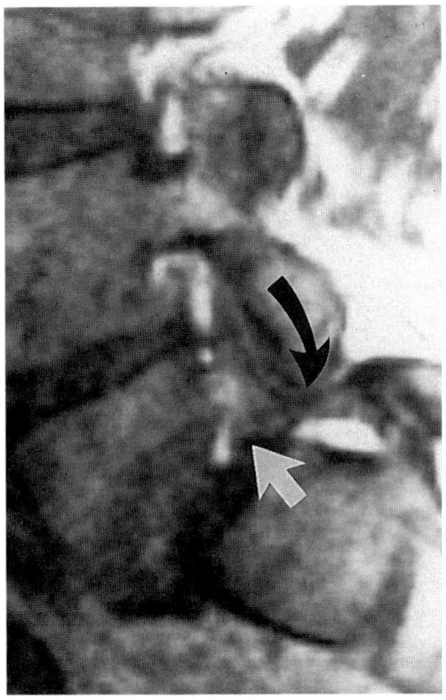

Fig. 7.31 Isthmic spondylolysis. On the sagittal T1-weighted image, the spondylolytic defect (curved arrow) involving the L5 pars interarticularis is difficult to delineate. There is excellent delineation of the cephalocaudal narrowing of the intervertebral canal and compression of the L5 nerve root (straight arrow).

was the most important for delineating abnormal signal intensity from haemorrhage, contusion, or oedema in the spinal cord. The evaluation of the cervico-occipital junction and C1–C2 relationship in patients with an atlantoaxial subluxation can now be easily assessed with MRI (Bundschuch *et al.*, 1988a). In one study comparing MRI with CT–myelography in the evaluation of cervical trauma, MRI was superior in all aspects except in the delineation of cervical spine fractures (Mirvis *et al.*, 1988). Fractures or malalignment of the posterior elements are optimally evaluated utilizing a CT examination (Bergstrom *et al.*, 1983). Figure 7.32 shows a patient with a fracture of the posterior elements of C6 with a partial rotary subluxation at C5–C6. On the axial CT images (Fig. 7.32a), a fracture involving the base of the right lateral mass of C6 (straight arrows) and diastasis of the right facet joint (curved arrow) are shown. It is extremely difficult to assess the degree of malalignment from axial images but the anterior subluxation of the inferior articular process of C5 (straight white arrows) is well seen on the sagittal images (Fig. 7.32b) along with the impacted fracture of the lateral mass of C6 (black arrows). The diastasis of the C5–C6 facet joint is also well seen (curved arrow). Coronal images (Fig. 7.32c) are optimal to delineate the lateral mass fracture. In patients who show late progression of their neurological deficit following spinal trauma, MRI is the optimal study to differentiate myelomalacia from syrinx formation (Quencer *et al.*, 1989).

The role of MRI and CT is complementary in the evaluation of spinal trauma involving the thoracolumbar junction and lumbosacral spine. CT provides excellent delineation of fractures and deformation of the vertebral bodies or posterior elements, while MRI is optimal in evaluating the thecal sac and conus medullaris (Fig. 7.33). Blumenkopf & Huneau (1988) showed that neurological morbidity was related to the level of the conus medullaris and patency of the ventral subarachnoid space demonstrated on the MRI examination.

Spinal tumours

Patients with tumours involving the central spinal canal or vertebrae may present with a rapidly progressive myeloradiculopathy, but most frequently their symptomatology is subacute or chronic in nature. In the evaluation of spinal tumours it is helpful to classify tumour location as either intramedullary, intradural–extramedullary, extradural or osseous. Some tumours may be found in two locations, particularly in the case of metastatic disease that involves the vertebral body and extradural space.

MRI has rapidly become the imaging study of choice in the assessment of intramedullary lesions of the spinal cord (Lee *et al.*, 1985; Sze *et al.*, 1988). In addition to delineating morphological alterations of the spinal cord, MRI is able to characterize the nature of the intramedullary pathology due to the difference in signal intensity of blood, tumour and cyst, compared with the normal spinal cord. The intravenous administration of gadolinium-DTPA is extremely helpful in the delineation of spinal cord tumours and in the differentiation of a benign from a malignant syrinx. In addition to primary and metastatic malignant tumours in the spinal cord, enhancement with gadolinium-DTPA has also been reported with spinal cord infarcts, myelomalacia, myelitis, multiple sclerosis, sarcoidosis and arteriovenous malformations.

Compared with myelography or CT–myelography, MRI has become the method of choice of assessing

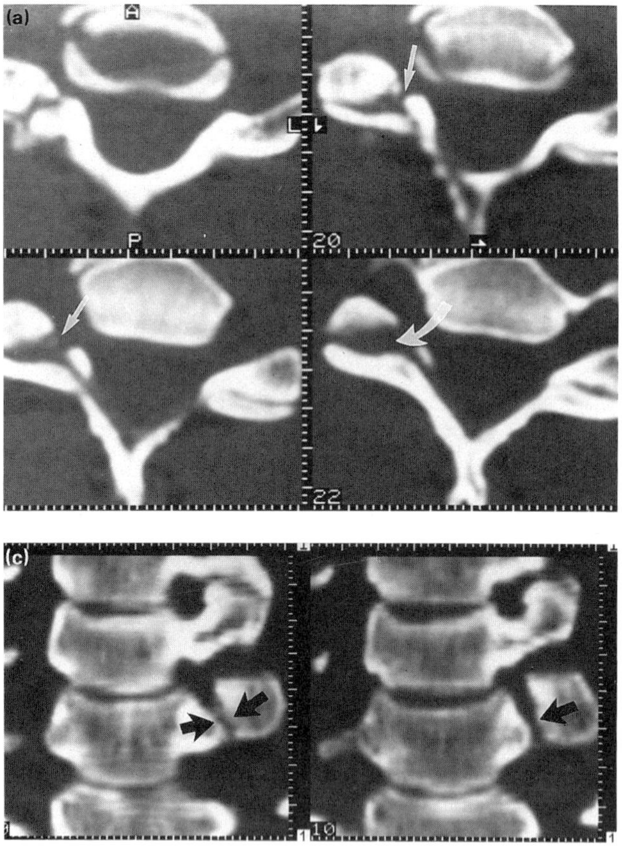

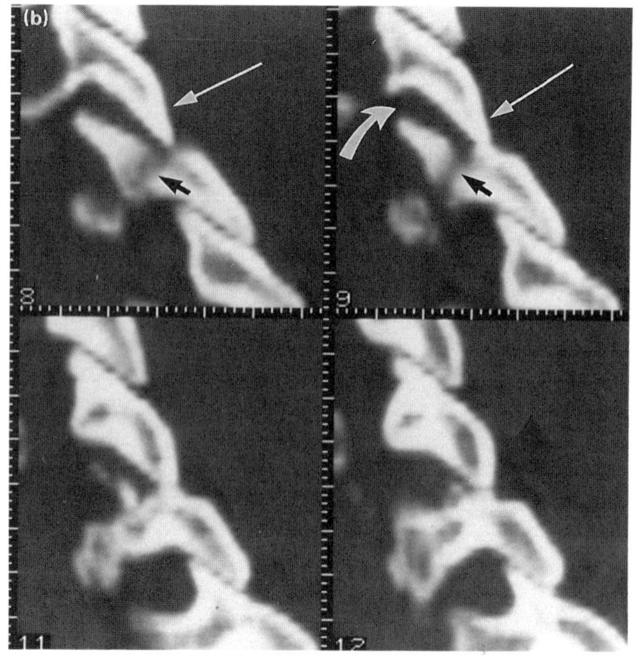

Fig. 7.32 CT in the evaluation of cervical trauma.

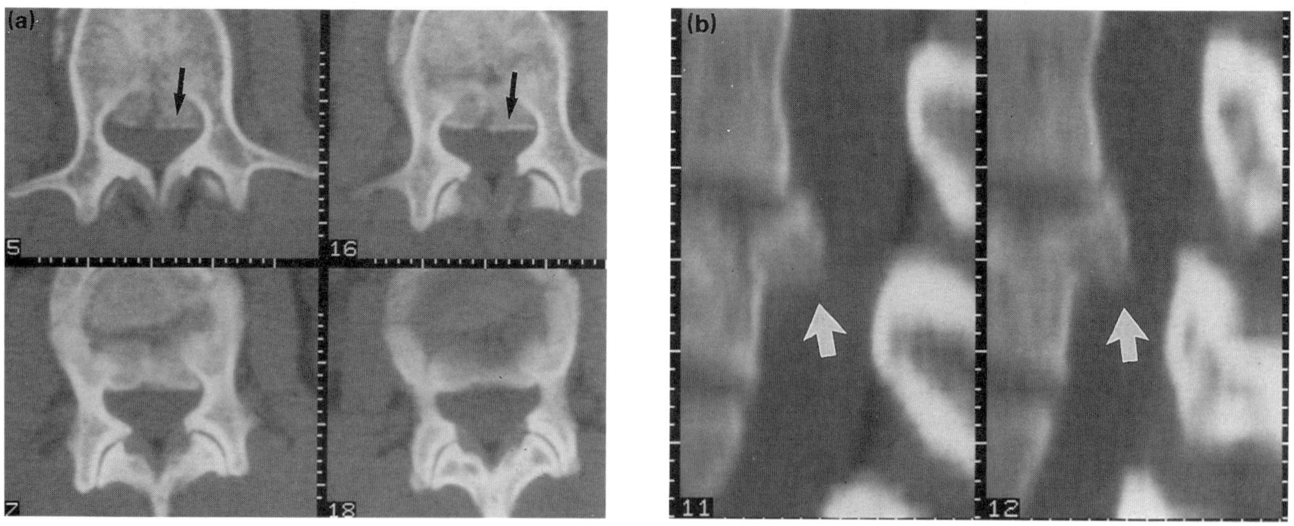

Fig. 7.33 CT of L1 burst fracture showing significant canal compromise due to the retropulsed bone fragment.

other types of spinal tumours (Carmody *et al.*, 1989). Intradural extramedullary tumours are well shown and meningiomas and neurofibromas in particular enhance brightly with gadolinium-DTPA (Fig. 7.34). Metastatic tumours in the vertebral body are normally well shown as areas of decreased signal intensity. Care has to be taken if enhancement with gadolinium-DTPA is used, as this can raise the signal of a vertebral metastasis to a normal level. Krol *et al.* (1988) showed that gadolinium enhancement was very effective at delineating the presence of meningeal carcinomatosis.

Spinal infection

In the adult, infection involving the spinal column usually affects the vertebral bodies and intervening disc. MRI should be the initial screening study in the evaluation of vertebral osteomyelitis. The MRI findings on sagittal images include: (a) confluent decreased signal intensity in the vertebral bodies and intervertebral disc with inability to discern a margin between the disc and the adjacent vertebral bodies on a T1-weighted image; (b) increased signal intensity in the vertebral bodies adjacent to the intervertebral disc on a T2-weighted image; and (c) abnormal configuration and increased signal intensity of the intervertebral disc and absence of the intranuclear cleft on a T2-weighted image (TR 2000–3000 ms, TE 120 ms) (Fig. 7.35). MRI has a reported sensitivity of 96%, specificity of 93%, and accuracy of 94% in diagnosing osteomyelitis, equalling the results of a combined bone scan and gallium study (Modic *et al.*, 1985). The main advantages of MRI over radionuclide studies include acquisition of significant information about the spinal cord, thecal sac and paravertebral soft tissues. The MRI findings of non-pyogenic osteomyelitis may be atypical, suggesting neoplasm rather than infection (Smith *et al.*, 1989). Tuberculous spondylitis occasionally will present with focal involvement of the vertebral body or posterior elements and lack of involvement of the disc and vertebral body endplates (Van Lom *et al.*, 1988). MRI has also rapidly become the screening test for the evaluation of epidural abscesses (Angtuaco *et al.*, 1987).

Postoperative evaluation of the spine

It is not infrequent for patients who have undergone spinal surgery to experience persistent or recurrent back pain. In one series the most frequent findings to explain the patient's symptomatology included stenosis of the central and intervertebral canals, disc herniation, arachnoiditis, epidural fibrosis, and direct nerve injury.

MRI should be the screening evaluation if recurrent or persistent disc herniation is clinically suspected. When performing MRI examinations on the postoperative spine, the interval of time between surgery and an MRI examination is an important factor in the evaluation of MRI findings. Ross *et al.* (1987) found that there was no correlation between the immediate postoperative appearance on an MRI exam and patients' symptomatology, and the authors concluded that the MRI study in the immediate postoperative period was not useful in explaining the aetiology of persistent pain.

Patients with recurrent back pain or failed back surgery syndrome present with a variety of postoperative findings. Epidural fibrosis is frequently present at the operative site and typically demonstrates intermediate signal intensity on T1-weighted images and increased signal intensity on T2-weighted images. Fibrosis is usually poorly marginated and typically generates no mass effect. Recurrent disc herniations are usually contiguous with the disc space, well marginated, and compared with the disc of origin, demonstrate isointensity or hypointensity on T1-weighted images and isointensity or hyperintensity on T2-weighted images. In two studies utilizing the criteria of epidural location, morphological configuration, signal intensity and mass effect, MRI was extremely accurate in differentiating disc herniation from fibrosis (Bundschuch *et al.*, 1988b; Frocain *et al.*, 1989). The intravenous administration of gadolinium-DTPA has also been helpful in differentiating disc material from fibrosis (Hueftle *et al.*, 1988). Disc herniations may enhance with gadolinium-DTPA (Fig. 7.25). Gadolinium does, however, cause intense enhancement of areas of epidural fibrosis. The presence of a non-enhancing mass, particularly if surrounded by a rim of enhanced tissue, in a patient who has undergone previous disc surgery should strongly suggest a recurrence of the discal herniation (Fig. 7.36). In addition to the axial T1-weighted images before and subsequent to enhancement, T2-weighted axial images should be obtained in a previously operated patient as they may show other problems such as epidural abscess, pseudomeningocele or arachnoiditis (Fig. 7.37). One of the

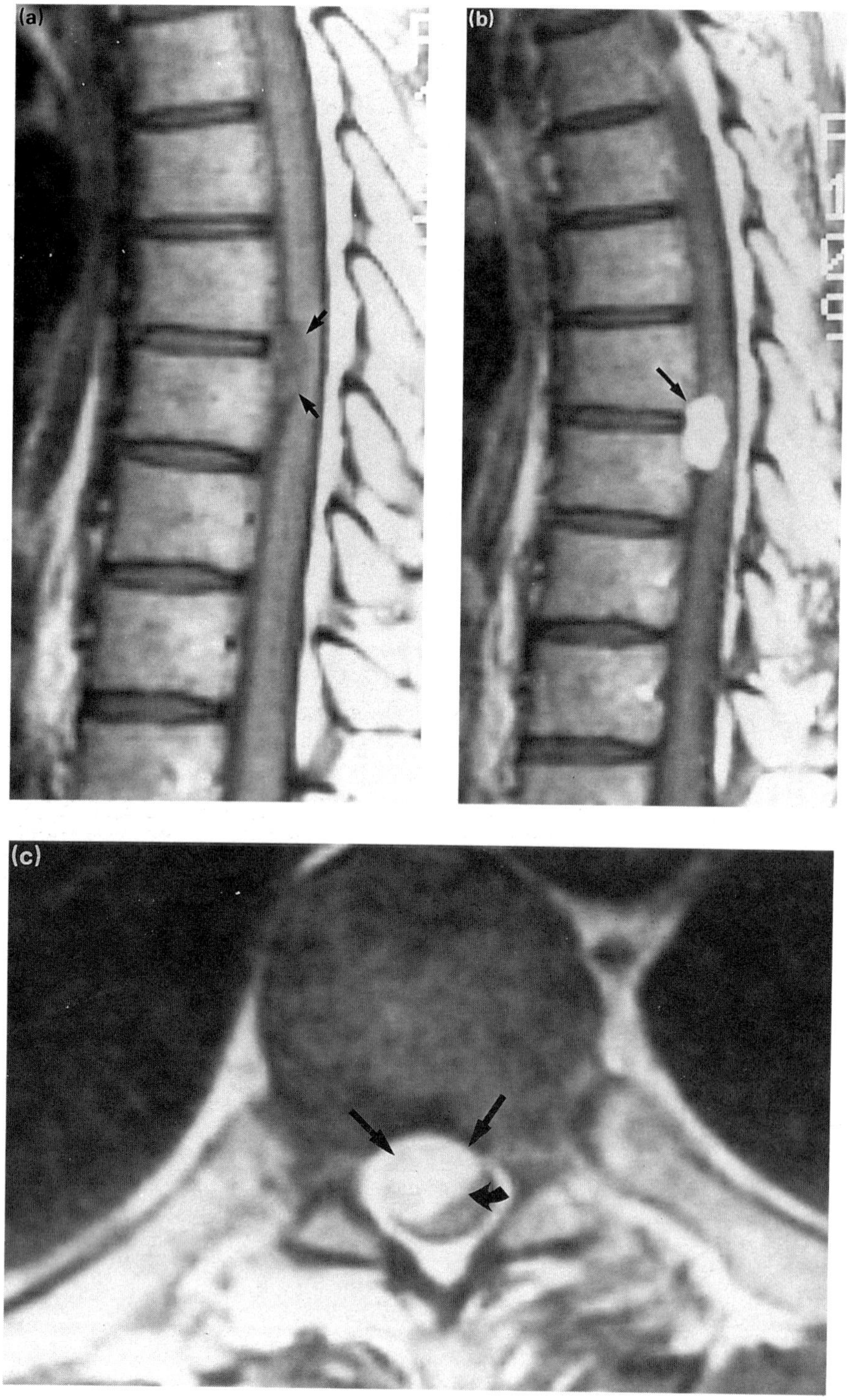

Fig. 7.34 Thoracic meningioma, MRI. On the sagittal T1-weighted image (a), an anterior extradural soft tissue mass (arrows) is identified compressing the thoracic spinal cord. After the administration of gadolinium-DTPA, on the sagittal (b) and the axial (c) T1-weighted images, there is excellent delineation of the enhancing epidural mass (straight arrows). The degree of spinal cord compression (curved arrow) is best delineated on the axial image.

authors routinely utilizes double-echo, spin-echo sagittal and axial images in preference to T1-weighted images with gadolinium-DTPA. Gadolinium-DTPA is only used when this technique does not definitively differentiate between fibrosis and recurrent disc herniation (6%). In a retrospective study of 123 operatively proven cases, surgery agreed with MRI using double-echo, spin-echo technique in 94%. In a pro-

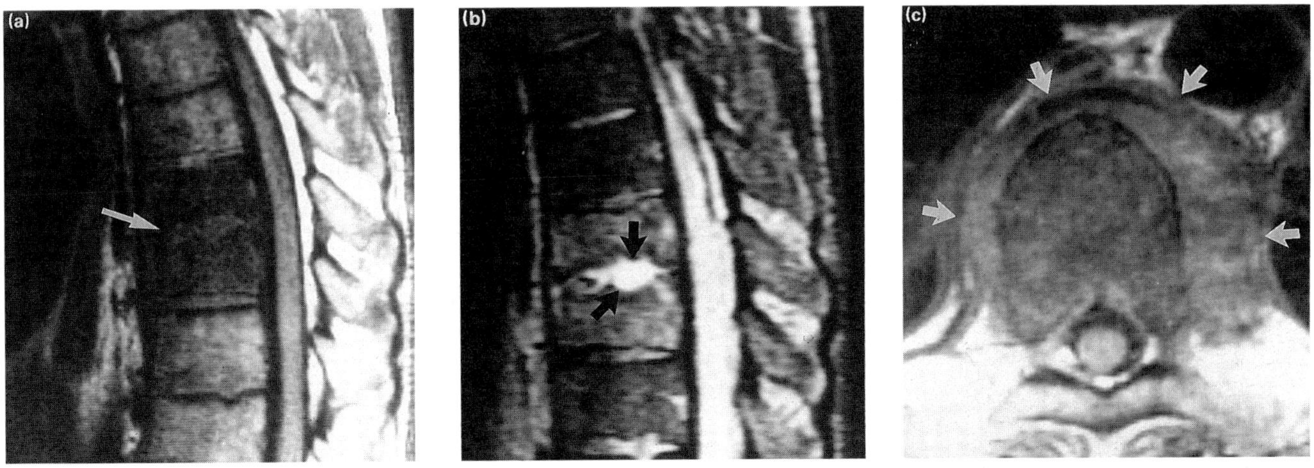

Fig. 7.35 Pyogenic vertebral osteomyelitis, MRI. On the sagittal T1-weighted image (a), there is a confluent area of decreased signal intensity involving the T7 and T8 vertebral bodies and the intervening disc (arrow). On the sagittal T2-weighted image (b), increased signal intensity is identified in the disc space (arrows) along with diffuse increased signal intensity in the adjacent vertebral body marrow. The axial T1-weighted image (c) is needed to determine the degree of extension of the inflammatory process into the paravertebral soft tissue (arrows).

spective comparison of double-echo, spin-echo T2-weighted imaging with gadolinium-DTPA T1-weighted imaging in 35 patients, gadolinium-DTPA was preferred in only two patients.

CT remains the screening modality of choice in the evaluation of postoperative stenosis. With its excellent delineation of osseous structures it is optimal when evaluating encroachment of the central or intervertebral canals secondary to a degenerative process or in the evaluation of postoperative spondylolisthesis. It is also more sensitive than MRI in the evaluation of spinal fusions (Fig. 7.38) and in the delineation of postoperative fractures of the lumbar articular facets.

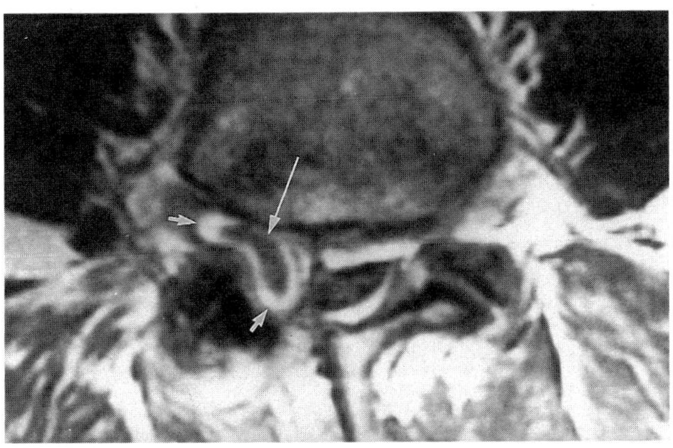

Fig. 7.36 Recurrent right-sided disc protrusion. The neural fragment (large arrow) is surrounded by a rim of epidural fibrosis which has enhanced with gadolinium-DTPA (small arrows).

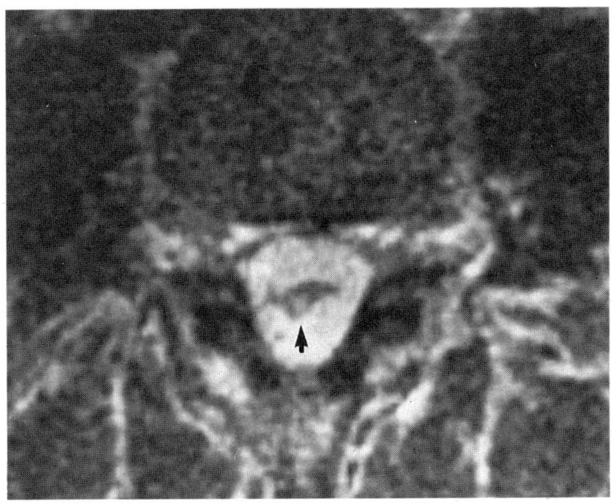

Fig. 7.37 Axial T2-weighted image showing the central clumping of the nerve roots of the cauda equina due to arachnoiditis (arrow).

Spondyloarthropathies

With the spine being a composite of amphiarthroses, diarthroses, and entheses, it may be affected by a

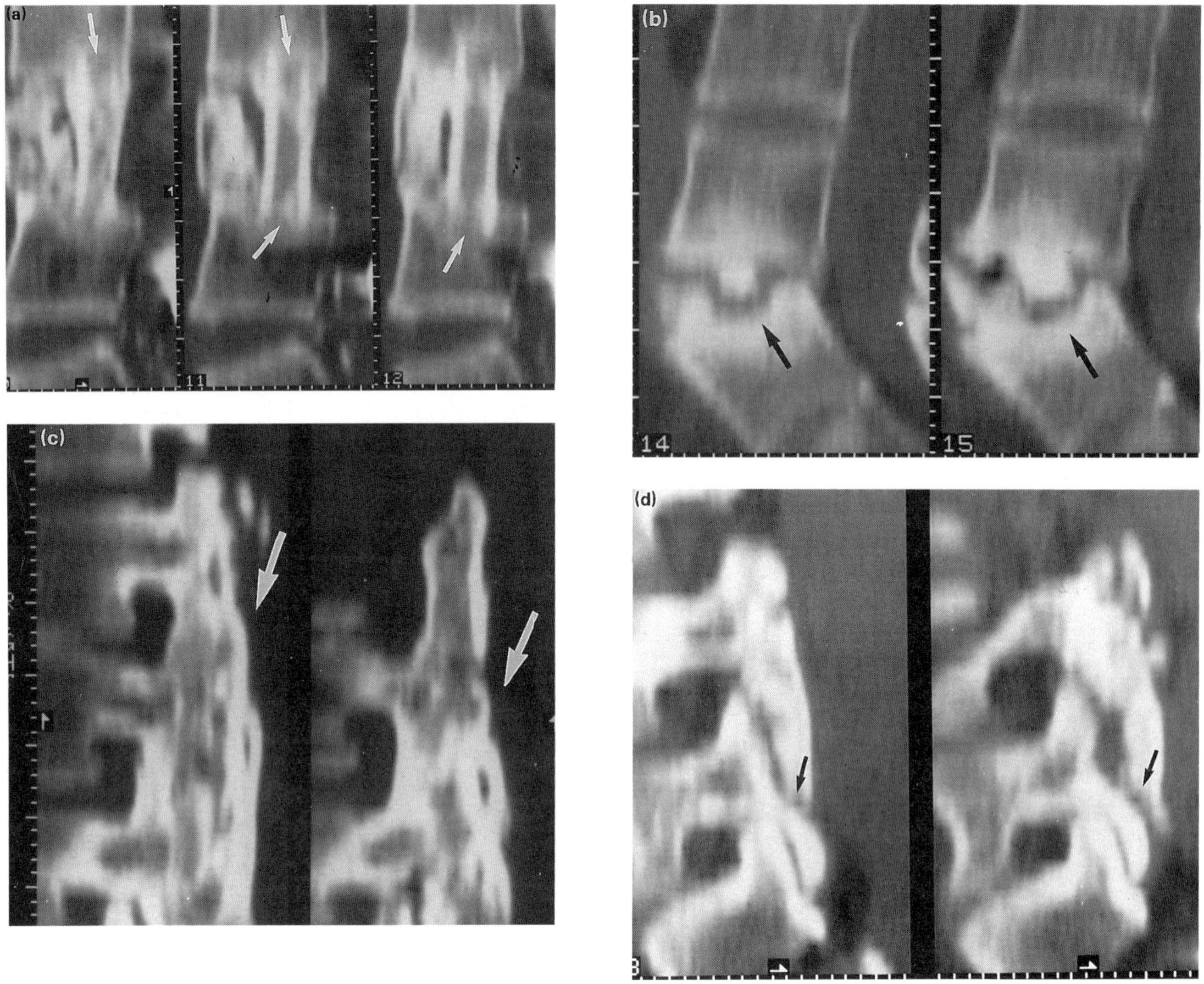

Fig. 7.38 Postoperative evaluation of lumbar fusions, CT/MPR. On the sagittal reconstructed images (a), there is excellent delineation of a solid interbody fusion (arrows). On the examination of another patient the sagittal reconstructed images (b) demonstrate a pseudarthrosis of an interbody fusion (arrows) at the L5–S1 disc level. On the sagittal reconstructed images on two additional patients a solid posterolateral fusion (c) and a pseudarthrosis (d) are demonstrated.

variety of arthritic processes. MRI is particularly useful in evaluating patients with rheumatoid arthritis affecting the cervical spine, who present with symptoms of myelopathy or myeloradiculopathy. Vertical subluxation of the odontoid, atlantoaxial subluxation or subaxial subluxation are frequently identified in patients with long-standing rheumatoid arthritis. MRI can demonstrate the degree of cord impingement on both a static and dynamic examination along with abnormalities of the atlantodental interval and apophyseal joints. In patients with ankylosing spondylitis presenting with spinal pseudarthrosis, or fracture dislocations, CT is the most sensitive study for delineating osseous deformation, but MRI is of benefit for determining whether there is neural compression.

REFERENCES

Aguila, L.A., Piraino, D.W., Modic, M.T., Dudley , A.W. & Duchesneau, P.M. (1985) The intranuclear cleft of the intervertebral disk: magnetic resonance imaging. *Radiology*, **155**, 155–158.

Angtuaco, E.J.C., McConnell, J.R., Chadduck, W.M. &

Flanigan, S. (1987) MR imaging of spinal epidural sepsis. *Am. J. Roentgenol.*, **149**, 1249–1253.

Beers, G.M., Raque, G.H.L., Wagner, G.G., Shields, C.B., Nichols, G.R. II, Johnson, J.R. & Meyer, J.E. (1988) MR imaging in acute cervical spine trauma. *J. Comput. Assist. Tomogr.*, **12**, 755–761.

Bergstrom, K., Nyberg, G., Pech, P., Rausching, W. & Ytterbergh, C. (1983) Multiplanar spinal anatomy: comparison of CT and cryomicrotomy in postmortem specimens. *Am. J. Neuroradiol*, **4**, 590–592.

Berns, D.H., Blaser, S.I. & Modic, M.T. (1989) Magnetic resonance imaging of the spine. *Clin. Orthop. Rel. Res.*, **244**, 78–100.

Blumenkopf, B. & Huneau, P.A. III (1988) Magnetic resonance imaging (MRI) of thoracolumbar fractures. *J. Spinal Disorders*, **1**, 144–150.

Blumenthal, S.L., Baker, J., Cossett, A. & Selby, D.K. (1988) The role of anterior lumbar fusion for internal disc disruption. *Spine*, **13**, 566–569.

Bolender, N.R., Schonstrom, N.S.R. & Spengler, D.M. (1985) Role of computed tomography and myelography in the diagnosis of central spinal stenosis. *J. Bone Jt. Surg.*, **67A**, 240–245.

Brown, B.M., Schwartz, R.H., Frank, E. & Blank, N.K. (1988) Preoperative evaluation of cervical radiculopathy and myelopathy by surface-coil MR imaging. *Am. J. Roentgenol.*, **151**, 1205–1212.

Bundschuh, C., Modic, M.T., Kearney, F., Morris, R. & Deal, C. (1988a) Rheumatoid arthritis of the cervical spine. Surface-coil MR imaging. *Am. J. Roentgenol.*, **151**, 181–187.

Bundschuh, C.V., Modic, M.R., Ross, J.S., Masaryk, T.J. & Bohlman, H. (1988b) Epidural fibrosis and recurrent disk herniation in the lumbar spine: MR imaging assessment. *Am. J. Roentgenol* , **150**, 923–932.

Carmody, R.F., Yang, P.I., Seeley, G.W., Seeger, J.F., Unger, E.C. & Johnson, J.E. (1989) Spinal cord compression due to metastatic disease: diagnosis with MR imaging versus myelography. *Radiology*, **173**, 225–229.

Carrera, G.F., Haughton, V.M., Syvertsen, A. & William, S.L. (1980) Computed tomography of the lumbar facet joints. *Radiology*, **134**, 145–148.

Cohen, W.A., Maravilla, K.R., Shuman, W.P. & Dalley, R.W. (1989) Evaluation of metastatic spinal disease with high-field STIR: comparison of multiple imaging sequences. *Radiology*, **173**(P) (Suppl.), 156.

Condon, B.R. & Hadley, D.M. (1988) Quantification of cord deformation and dynamics during flexion and extension of the cervical spine using MR imaging. *J. Comput. Assist. Tomogr.*, **12**, 947–955.

Emery, S.E., Pathria, M.N., Wilber, R.G., Masaryk, T. & Bohlman, H.N. (1989) Magnetic resonance imaging of posttraumatic spinal ligament injury. *J. Spinal Dis.*, **2**, 229–233.

Enzmann, D.R., Rubin, J.B. & Wright, A. (1987) Cervical spine MR imaging: generating high-signal CSF in sagittal and axial images. *Radiology*, **163**, 233–238.

Firooznia, H., Benjamin, V., Kricheff, I.I., Rafii, M. & Colimbu, C. (1984) CT of lumbar spine disk herniation: correlation with surgical findings. *Am. J. Roentgenol.*, **5**, 91–96.

Fries, J.W., Abodeely, I.D.A., Vijungco, J.G. & Gaffey, W.R. (1984) Lateral L3–4 herniated nucleus pulposus: clinical and imaging considerations. *Comput. Radiol.*, **8**, 341–354.

Frocrain, L., Duvauferrier, R., Husson, J.L., Nuel J., Rammee, A. & Pawlotsky, Y. (1989) Recurrent postoperative sciatica: evaluation with MR imaging and enhanced CT. *Radiology*, **170**, 531–533.

Fujiwara, K., Yonenobu, K., Hiroshima, K., Ebara, S., Yamashita, K. & Ono, K. (1988) Morphometry of the cervical spinal cord and its relation to pathology in cases with compression myelopathy. *Spine*, **13**, 1212–1216.

Fujiwara, K., Yonenobu, K., Ebara, S., Yamashita, K. & Ono, K. (1989) The prognosis of surgery for cervical compression myelopathy. An analysis of the factors involved. *J. Bone Jt. Surg.*, **71B**, 393–398.

Ghosh, P. (ed.) (1988) *The Biology of the Intervertebral Disc*, vol. I. CRC Press, Boca Raton, FL.

Glenn, W.V. Jr, Rhodes, M.L., Altschuler, E.M., Wiltse, L.L., Kostanek, C. & Kuo, Y.M. (1979) Multiplanar display computerized body tomography applications in the lumbar spine. *Spine*, **4**, 282–294.

Glenn, W.V. Jr, Rothman, S.L.G., Rhodes, M.L. & Kerber, C.W. (1984) An overview of lumbar computed tomography/multiplanar reformations: what are its elements and how do they fit together? In Post, M.J.D. (ed.), *Computed Tomography of the Spine*, pp. 135–154. Williams & Wilkins, Baltimore, MD.

Godersky, J.C., Erickson, D.L. & Seljeskog, E.L. (1984) Extreme lateral disc herniation: diagnosis by computed tomographic scanning. *Neurosurgery*, **14**, 549–552.

Greenough, C.G., Dimmock, S., Edwards, D., Ransford, A.O. & Bentley, G. (1986) The role of computerized tomography in intervertebral disc prolapse. *J Bone Jt. Surg.*, **68B**, 729–733.

Grenier, N., Kressel, H.Y., Schiebler, M.L., Grossman, R.I., & Dalinka, M.K. (1987) Normal and degenerative posterior spinal structures: MR imaging. *Radiology*, **165**, 517–525.

Grenier, N., Gresselle, J.F., Vital, J.M., Kien, P., Baulny, D., Broussin, J., Senegas, J. & Caille, J.M. (1989) Normal and disrupted lumbar longitudinal ligaments: correlative MR and anatomic study. *Radiology*, **171**, 197–205.

Haykal, H.A., Wang, A.M., Zamani, A. & Rumbaugh, C.L. (1984) Computed tomography of spontaneous acute cervical epidural hematoma. *J. Comput. Assist. Tomogr.*, **8**, 229–231.

Hedberg, M.C., Drayer, B.P., Flom, R.A., Hodak, J.A. & Bird, C.R. (1988) Gradient echo (GRASS) MR imaging in cervical radiculopathy. *Am. J. Roentgenol.*, **150**, 683–689.

Heindel, W., Friedmann, G., Bunke, J., Thomas, B., Firsching, R. & Ernestus, R.I. (1986) Artifacts in MR imaging after surgical intervention. *J. Comput. Assist. Tomogr.*, **10**, 596–599.

Heithoff, K.B. (1988) Magnetic resonance imaging of the lumbar spine. In Kirkaldy-Willis, W.H. (ed.), *Managing Low Back Pain*, pp. 183–208. Churchill Livingstone, New York.

Helms, C.A., Dorwart, R.H. & Gray, M. (1982) The CT appearance of conjoined nerve roots and differentiation from a herniated nucleus pulposus. *Radiology*, **144**, 803–807.

Herman, G.T. (1988) Three-dimensional imaging on a CT or MR scanner. *J. Comput. Assist. Tomogr.*, **12**, 450–458.

Hickey, D.S., Aspden, R.M., Hukins, D.W.L. *et al.* (1986) Analysis of magnetic resonance images from normal and degenerate lumbar intervertebral discs. *Spine*, **11**, 702–708.

Hirofuji, E. & Tanaka, S. (1983) Computed tomography of lumbar disc herniation. *Spine*, **8**, 300–304.

Hueftle, M.G., Modic, M.T., Ross, J.S., Masaryk, T.J., Carter, J.R., Wilber, R.G., Bohlman, I.I.H., Steinberg, P.M. & Delamarter, R.B. (1988) Lumbar spine: postoperative MR imaging with gadolinium-DTPA. *Radiology*, **167**, 817–824.

Jaffray, D. & O'Brien, J.P. (1986) Isolated intervertebral disc resorption: a source of mechanical and inflammatory back pain? *Spine*, **11**, 397–401.

Kaiser, M.C., Capesius, P., Ohanna, F. & Roilgen, A. (1984) Computed tomography of acute spinal epidural hematoma associated with cervical root avulsion. *J. Comput. Assist. Tomogr.*, **8**, 322–323.

Kirkaldy-Willis, W.H. (1988) The pathology and pathogenesis of low back pain. In Kirkaldy-Willis, W.H. (ed.), *Managing Low Back Pain*, pp. 49–75. Churchill Livingstone, New York.

Krol, G., Sze, G., Malkin, M. & Walker, R. (1988) MR of cranial and spinal meningeal carcinomatosis: comparison with CT and myelography. *Am. J. Roentgenol.*, **151**, 583–588.

Kulkarni, M.W., McArdle, C.B., Kopanicky, D., Miner, M., Cotter, H.B., Lee, K.F. & Harris, J.H. (1987) Acute spinal cord injury: MR imaging at 1.5 T. *Radiology*, **164**, 837–843.

Lancourt, J.E., Glenn, W.V. Jr & Wiltse, L.L. (1979) Multiplanar computerized tomography in the normal spine and in the diagnosis of spinal stenosis: a gross anatomic–computerized tomographic correlation. *Spine*, **4**, 379–390.

Lee, B.C.P., Zimmerman, R.D., Manning, J.J. & Deck, M.D.F. (1985) MR imaging of syringomyelia and hydromyelia. *Am. J. Roentgenol.*, **144**, 1149–1156.

Levitan, L.H. & Wiens, C.W. (1983) Chronic lumbar extradural hematoma: CT findings. *Radiology*, **148**, 707–708.

Lipson, S.J. & Muir, H. (1981) Proteoglycans in experimental intervertebral disc degeneration. *Spine*, **6**, 194–210.

Maravilla, K.R. & Hartling, R.P. (1988) Imaging decisions in degenerative spinal disease: a practical approach. *MRI decisions*, **2**, 2–13.

Masaryk, T.L.J., Ross, J.S., Modic, M.T., Boumphrey, F., Bohlman, H. & Wilber, G. (1988) High resolution MR imaging of sequestered lumbar intervertebral disks. *Am. J. Roentgenol.*, **150**, 1155–1162.

McAffee, P.C. & Yuan, H.A. (1982) Computed tomography in spondylolisthesis. *Clin Orthop.*, **166**, 62–71.

Mikhael, M.A. (1983) High resolution computed tomography in the diagnosis of laterally herniated lumbar discs. *Comput. Radiol.*, **17**, 161–166.

Miller, J.A.A., Schmatz, C. & Schultz, A.B. (1988) Lumbar disc degeneration: correlation with age, sex, and spine level in 600 autopsy specimens. *Spine*, **13**, 173–178.

Mirvis, S.E., Geisler, F.H., Jelinek, J.L., Joslyn, J.N. & Gellnd, F. (1988) Acute cervical spine trauma: evaluation with 1.5-T MR imaging. *Radiology*, **166**, 807–816.

Miyasaka, K., Isu, T., Iwasaki, Y., Abe, S., Takei, H. & Tsuru, M. (1983) High resolution computed tomography in the diagnosis of cervical disc disease. *Neuroradiology*, **24**, 253–257.

Modic, M.T., Feiglin, D.H., Piraino, D.W., Boumphrey, F., Weinstein, M.A., Duchesneau, P.M. & Rehm, S. (1985) Vertebral osteomyelitis: assessment using MR. *Radiology*, **157**, 157–166.

Modic, M.T., Masaryk, T., Boumphrey, F., Goormastic, M. & Bell, G. (1986) Lumbar herniated disk disease and canal stenosis: prospective evaluation by surface coil MR, CT and myelography. *Am. J. Roentgenol.*, **147**, 757–765.

Modic, M.T., Masaryk, T.J., Ross, J.S. & Carter, J.R. (1988a) Imaging of degenerative disk disease. *Radiology*, **168**, 177–186.

Modic, M.T., Steinberg, P.M., Ross, J.S., Masaryk, T.J. & Carter, J.R. (1988b) Degenerative disk disease: assessment of changes in vertebral body marrow with MR imaging. *Radiology*, **166**, 193–199.

Modic, M.T., Ross, J.S. & Masaryk, T.J. (1989) Imaging of degenerative disease of the cervical spine. *Clin. Orthop. Rel. Res.*, **239**, 109–120.

Osborne, D.R., Heinz, E.R., Bullard, D. & Friedman, A. (1984) Role of computed tomography in the radiological evaluation of painful radiculopathy after negative myelography: foraminal neural entrapment. *Neurosurgery*, **14**, 147–153.

Pech, P. & Haughton, V.M. (1985) Lumbar intervertebral disk: correlative MR and anatomic study. *Radiology*, **156**, 699–701.

Post, M.J., Seminer, D.S. & Quencer, R.M. (1982) CT diagnosis of spinal epidural hematoma. *Am. J. Neurol. Res.* **3**, 190–192.

Post, M.J.D., Quencer, R.M., Montalvo, B.M., Katz, B.H., Fismont, F.J. & Green, B.A. (1988) Spinal infection: evaluation with MR imaging and intraoperative US. *Radiology*, **169**, 765–771.

Quequet, P.M., Rosa, A. & Mizon, J.P. (1987) Nontraumatic spinal epidural hematomas (2 cases): contribution of the CT scanner. *Rev. Neurol.*, **143**, 143–146.

Quencer, R.M., Sheldon, J.J., Post, M.J.D., Diaz, R.D., Montalvo, B.M., Green, B.A. & Eismont, F.J. (1989) MRI of the chronically injured cervical spinal cord syndrome. *Am. J. Roentgenol.*, **152**, 843–852.

Reicher, M.A., Lufkin, R.B., Smith, S., Flannigan, B., Olsen, R., Wolf, R., Hertz, D., Winter, J. & Hanafee, W. (1986) Multiple-angle, variable-interval, nonorthogonal MRI. *Am. J. Roentgenol.*, **147**, 363–366.

Ross, J.S., Masaryk, T.J., Modic, M.T., Bohlman, H., Delamater, R. & Wilber, G. (1987) Lumbar spine: postoperative assessment with surface-coil MR imaging. *Radiology*, **164**, 851–860.

Ross, J.S., Modic, M.T. & Masaryk, T.J. (1990) Tears of the anulus fibrosus: assessment with Gd-DTPA-enhanced

MR imaging. *Am. J. Roentgenol.*, **154**, 159–162.

Ross, J.S., Perez-Reyes, N., Masaryk, T.J., Bohlman, H. & Modic, M.T. (1987) Thoracic disk herniation: MR imaging. *Radiology*, **165**, 511–515.

Rothman, S.L.G. & Glenn, W.V. Jr (1984) CT multiplanar reconstruction in 253 cases of lumbar spondylolysis. *Am. J. Neurol. Res.*, **5**, 81–90.

Schaefer, D.M., Flanders, A., Northrup, B.E. & Doan, H.T. (1989) Magnetic resonance imaging of acute cervical spine trauma: correlation with severity of neurologic injury. *Spine*, **14**, 1090–1095.

Shellock, F.G. (1988) MR imaging of metallic implants and materials: A complication of the literature. *Am. J. Roentgenol.*, **151**, 811–814.

Smith, A.S., Weinstein, M.A., Mizushima, A., Coughlin, B., Hayden, S.P., Lakin, M.M. & Lanzieri, O.F. (1989) MR imaging characteristics of tuberculous spondylitis vs vertebral osteomyelitis. *Am. J. Roentgenol.*, **153**, 399–405.

Sze, G., Krol, G., Zimmermann, R.D. & Deck, M.D.F. (1988) Intramedullary disease of the spine: diagnosis using gadolinium-DTPA-enhanced MR imaging. *Am. J. Roentgenol.*, **151**, 1193–1204.

Szypryt, E.P., Twining, P., Mulholland, R.C. & Worthington, B.S. (1989) The prevalence of disc degeneration associated with neural arch defects of the lumbar spine assessed by magnetic resonance imaging. *Spine*, **14**, 977–981.

Takahashi, M., Yamashita, Y., Sakamoto, Y. & Kojima, R. (1989) Chronic cervical cord compression: clinical significance of increased signal intensity on MR images. *Radiology*, **173**, 219–224.

Teplick, J.G., Laffey, P.A., Berman, A. & Haskin, M.E. (1986) Diagnosis and evaluation of spondylolisthesis and/or spondylolysis on axial CT. *Am. J. Neurol. Res.* **7**, 479–491.

Tracy, P.T., Wright, R.M. & Hanigan, W.C. (1989) Magnetic resonance imaging of spinal injury. *Spine*, **14**, 292–301.

Ullrich, C.G. (1989) Three-dimensional CT of the cervical spine: introduction and clinical applications. In: TCSRSE Committee (eds), *The Cervical Spine*, pp. 150–156. Lippincott, Philadelphia, PA.

Van Lom, K.J., Kellerhouse, L.E., Pathria, M.N., Moreland, S.I., Brown, J.J., Zlatkin, M., Sartoris, D.J., Chevrot, A., Resnik, C.S. & Resnick, D. (1988) Infection versus tumor in the spine: criteria for distinction with CT. *Radiology*, **166**, 851–855.

White, III, J.G., Strait, T.A., Binkley, J.R. & Hunter, S.E. (1982) Surgical treatment of 63 cases of conjoined nerve root. *J. Neurosurg.*, **56**, 114–117.

Wiesel, S.W., Tsourmas, N., Feffer, H.L., Citrin, C.M. & Patronas, N. (1984) A study of computer-assisted tomography. I. The incidence of positive CAT scans in an asymptomatic group of patients. *Spine*, **9**, 549–556.

Williams, A.L., Haughton, V.M., Daniels, D.L. & Grogan, J.P. (1983) Differential CT diagnosis of extruded nucleus pulposus. *Radiology*, **148**, 141–148.

Wiltse, L. (1985) "Far-out syndrome". In Rothman, S.L.G. & Glenn, W.V. Jr (eds) *Multiplanar CT of the Spine*, pp. 384–393. University Park Press, Baltimore, MD.

Yu, S., Haughton, V.M., Ho, P.S.P. *et al.* (1988) Progressive and regressive changes in the nucleus pulposus: Part II. The adult. *Radiology*, **169**, 93–97.

Yu, S., Haughton, V.M., Sether, L.A., Ho, K.C. & Wagner, M. (1989) Criteria for classifying normal and degenerated lumbar intervertebral disks. *Radiology*, **170**, 523–526.

Zilkha, A., Irwin, G.A. & Fagelman, D. (1983) Computed tomography of spinal epidural hematoma. *Am. J. Neurol. Res.*, **4**, 1073–1076.

Zucherman, J., Derby, R., Hsu, K., Picetti, G., Kaiser, J., Schofferman, J., Goldthwaite, N. & White, A. (1988) Normal magnetic resonance imaging with abnormal discography. *Spine*, **13**, 1355–1359.

8 · Clinical Assessment Relating to the Urinary Tract

By K.F. PARSONS

Injury to, or disease of, the vertebral column, whether it be congenital or acquired, threatens the integrity of the spinal cord and spinal nerves in their course to the periphery. Any such alteration in innervation of peripheral structures inevitably produces a change in function, which can be subtle if the nerve damage is slight, or may be profound. When considering the clinical manifestation of nerve damage to the genito-urinary tract it is important to have some understanding of its structure, function and innervation. From this standpoint a logical approach can be used in the clinical examination and investigation of patients with neurological lesions producing bladder dysfunction.

It is a truism that the *upper urinary tracts* require no neurological connections to function entirely normally, hence any alteration in upper tract morphology and function which occurs in neurological disease is always a secondary phenomenon, usually to midline neuropathic bladder outflow obstruction. This produces high-pressure fluctuations within a low-compliance bladder which either obstructs and dilates the upper tracts (Lloyd *et al.*, 1987) or provokes vesico-ureteric reflux (Arnold & Cowan, 1988).

The lower urinary tract therefore is the critical end-organ upon which neurological damage has a profound effect, and which has to be analysed in detail.

STRUCTURE AND FUNCTION OF THE LOWER URINARY TRACT

The fundamental requirement of the lower urinary tract is to store urine at low pressure and a suitable volume until such time as micturition is convenient. At this point urine is expelled in a coordinated, convenient and complete manner for the cycle of storage and voiding to be repeated. To fulfil these simple requirements, lower urinary tract function is controlled by the autonomic nervous system, and is governed and modified by higher cerebral influences (Nathan, 1976; Fletcher & Bradley, 1978). The vesico-urethral apparatus must be recognized as a functional single entity with one unit—the bladder, functioning in coordination with the other—the urethra. The bladder must act as a low-pressure storage organ in order that unimpeded transport of urine from the kidneys may occur, thereby preserving normal renal function (Thomas & Clarke, 1979; Webb *et al.*, 1984). During all stages of filling it must remain continent.

The urinary bladder may be considered as a collapsible sphere consisting of a syncytium of elongated smooth muscle fibres and lined by transitional epithelium. The trigone is a specialized triangular muscle plate at the base of the bladder which is formed by an extension of muscle fibres from each ureter, and which condenses as a prolongation into the urethra.

The urethra is formed by an extension of detrusor fibres as a coiled tube in which, in the midzone in females and in the area of the membranous urethra in males, there is a condensation of slow-twitch muscle fibres which constitute the intrinsic urethral mechanism. This complex of muscle is able to sustain prolonged contraction and thus can maintain urethral closure which produces continence (Gosling *et al.*, 1977; Gosling, 1979).

Bladder filling

The ability of the bladder to remain at low pressure during filling is a reflection of both the inherent property of smooth muscle to alter its length without significantly changing its tension, and of the physical properties of the other constituents of the bladder wall, principally elastic tissue and collagen. An elastin fibre, which requires only a small change in tension to produce a relatively large increase in length, may be extended to twice its resting length whilst collagen fibres, which are coiled initially, straighten and contribute to wall tension only when the bladder is considerably distended.

The pressure in the filling bladder is governed by the *Law of Laplace*, which postulates that the pressure within a hollow sphere is equal to twice the wall tension divided by the radius. If the wall tension rises only slightly in proportion to the radius, the pressure within will remain constant. In fact intrinsic bladder pressure rises no more than 10 cmH_2O during filling under normal circumstances.

Continence

In females there is no distinct 'internal sphincter', but in males such a mechanism exists and is an organ of secondary sexual characteristic, for its function is to close tightly at ejaculation to prevent retrograde passage of sperm into the bladder. Bladder neck closure is otherwise a passive phenomenon dependent upon the anatomical arrangement of the smooth muscle fibres and augmented by transmission of abdominal pressure which closes the proximal urethra in a manner which mimics the intra-abdominal oesophagus. It is apparent therefore that the vesico-urethral apparatus must be well supported to facilitate this pressure transmission. The pelvic floor provides this support and normal resting tone in this muscle is necessary for it to function in this way. It comprises the levator ani muscle with additional slings of muscle from the pubis around the tubed structures emerging from the pelvis; the urethra, vagina and rectum, which pass through it. It is somatic, striated muscle and, as such, in common with all striated muscle is not able to maintain sustained contraction for prolonged periods due to fatigue. Thus it does not contribute to active continence, but is able to augment the forces of continence during coughing and sneezing, and is able voluntarily to interrupt the urinary stream temporarily if it is necessary so to do.

Females rely much more heavily than males upon the bladder neck for continence. The bladder neck can be sacrificed in neurologically normal males, as occurs at a prostatectomy with no threat to continence, but in females any destruction of the bladder neck mechanism is likely to produce genuine stress incontinence (Delaere *et al.*, 1983).

Micturition

The mechanism of bladder emptying essentially involves reversal of the forces of continence, and for simplicity may be considered in two phases. Firstly, the 'transition' from the continent to the controlled incontinent state, and secondly the 'period of urination' during which the bladder empties completely.

During the transition phase the bladder neck opens and the urethra relaxes, although experimental studies have shown that the latter precedes the former. Some several seconds before micturition there is active relaxation of the intrinsic urethral mechanism (Torrens, 1978). In order for the urethra to open, the pelvic floor both relaxes and descends, to allow abdominal pressure to be distracted away from the urethra. The descent of the bladder base which this allows also facilitates opening of the bladder neck which is simultaneously achieved by active detrusor contraction and contraction of the urethral prolongation of the trigone. Both are assisted by the secondary phenomenon of the bladder contracting down on the 'bolus' of urine in the fundus, which tends to pull the bladder neck and proximal urethra up into the globular fundus.

Once the bladder pressure has risen, the bladder has descended and the bladder neck and urethra opened, the period of micturition starts. When about two-thirds of the plateau voiding pressure is reached, flow begins. As urine is expelled, the bladder radius is decreased but the pressure within the bladder remains stable. The physical conditions of the Law of Laplace still apply; thus less wall tension is required to sustain voiding. There is also a reduction in the elastic tension because the radius has reduced and active contraction requires a decreasing force because the efficacy of contraction improves with the shorter detrusor muscle fibre length. Once the initial isometric contraction has occurred, therefore, the continuation of voiding requires little further contraction, provided that the urethral resistance remains constant. When full flow is established, and the urethra is widely open, its functional diameter is calculated to be less than 3 mm. Indeed the urinary flow rate is set by the urethral mechanism rather than by the force of detrusor contraction and, theoretically at least, the flow rate cannot be enhanced by abdominal straining.

Towards the end of micturition the detrusor pressure decays to zero and the flow ceases. The contents of the posterior urethra are then returned to the bladder along the gradient of urethral pressure as it is re-established. In the male the distal urethra is emptied by contraction of the bulbospongiosus muscle.

INNERVATION OF THE LOWER URINARY TRACT

The innervation of the urinary tract is complex and still incompletely understood. A practical simplification is necessary to allow a basic understanding of the neurophysiological mechanisms pertaining to micturition and a classification of neuropathic vesico-urethral dysfunction which fits with the dysfunction observed.

The detrusor

The smooth muscle of the detrusor has a rich supply of cholinergic parasympathetic nerves throughout the muscle wall. There is also a presumptive sensory parasympathetic network in the submucosal space (Gosling, 1979). The cell bodies of the motoneurones lie in the pelvic plexus but there are a substantial number of ganglia in the adventitia of the bladder and a few lie within the bladder wall itself. The preganglionic cell bodies to the cholinergic efferent nerves lie in the S2, S3 and S4 segments of the spinal cord in the conus medullaris.

There are few if any adrenergic neurones in the human detrusor muscle.

The bladder neck

There are considerable differences between the innervation of the bladder neck in males and females, and this reflects the difference in function in the two sexes.

Male

In the male the circularly arranged smooth muscle of the bladder neck and preprostatic urethra has a dense supply of nor-adrenergic neurones which have cell bodies in the pelvic plexus. The preganglionic neurones travel in the presacral nerves and the function of this nerve supply would seem to be sexual. The cell bodies of the preganglionic nerves probably lie in the conus (Laruelle, 1948) with ascending fibres in the cord reaching the thoracolumbar sympathetic outflow at the T10–L2 spinal level.

Female

The female bladder neck receives a relatively small supply of nor-adrenergic nerves. There are numerous parasympathetic fibres in the muscle of the bladder neck and proximal urethra in the female.

The urethra

The intrinsic urethral mechanism paradoxically shows functional evidence of an adrenergic innervation without substantive evidence of an abundance of sympathetic nerves. Active urethral relaxation appears to be mediated by a beta-adrenergic response, and midurethral tone can be significantly reduced by sympathetic blockade (Donker *et al.*, 1972).

The peri-urethral striated pelvic floor is supplied by the pudendal nerves with the motor cell bodies in the S2–S4 sacral segments.

Spinal segmental innervation

The spinal innervation to the genito-urinary tract is summarized in Fig. 8.1. Simplistically, there can be considered to be a 'reflex arc' with motor efferents originating in the conus medullaris and travelling in the anterior roots of the S2–S4 segments to the bladder. These nerves branch as the nervi erigentes to travel in the para-rectal plexus to anastomose with the sympathetic neurones which come from the inferior hypogastric plexus. The afferent limb of the 'arc' similarly travels within the plexus to reach the cord through the dorsal roots. The intraspinal connections within the S2–S4 segments constitute the *spinal micturition centre*.

The alpha-adrenergic sympathetic efferents probably have no importance whatever to micturition in the neurologically intact, but may be of critical importance in neuropathic vesico-urethral dysfunction. Sympathetic afferent nerves cannot be morphologically separated. They subserve the sensation of bladder distension and pain and are thought to

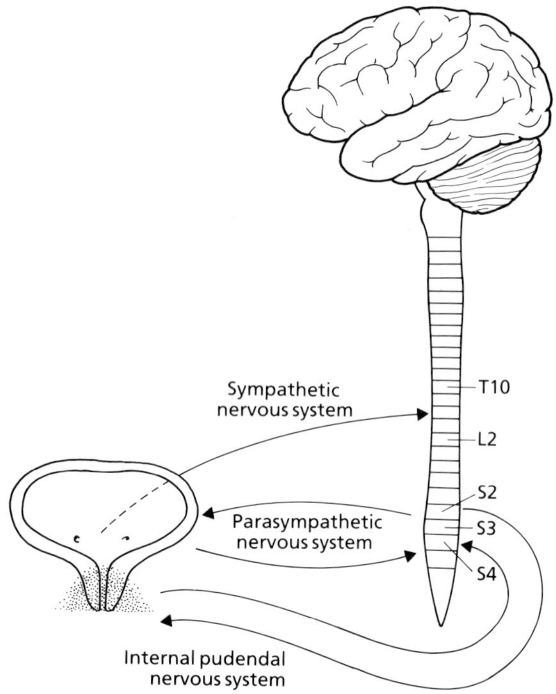

Fig. 8.1 Spinal innervation to the genito-urinary tract.

enter the cord at the thoracolumbar region between T10 and L2. This is important to recognize when local spinal anaesthetic techniques are used when operating on the bladder or urethra, for the anaesthetic level must extend from the sacral segments up to the tenth thoracic segment.

The supraspinal micturition centres are either facilitatory in the paracentral lobule, the anterior cingulate gyrus and the septal area or inhibitory in the cingulate gyrus and the pro-optic nucleus, while the reticular formation and the cerebellum contain both facilitatory and inhibitory centres. From these centres there are descending inhibitory and facilitatory pathways in the cord, which travel in the lateral corticospinal tracts, though the precise position within the cord is difficult to define and may indeed be variable. Ascending pathways to the pons and cerebral cortex can be identified in the spinòthalamic tracts, though some are shown to pass in the medial part of the posterior columns (Kuru, 1965).

It is important to remember the anatomical level of the conus medullaris which is found opposite the lower border of L1. Some expectation of the type of neuropathic vesico-urethral dysfunction can thus be anticipated, depending upon the level of the bony injury in relation to the conus and cauda equina.

CLINICAL EXAMINATION

Any patient in whom it is suspected that there may be a neurological bladder problem should have a complete physical examination, with a careful suprapubic palpation to determine whether the bladder is full or overdistended. In acute spinal transection the onset of spinal shock will guarantee that the detrusor becomes acontractile, and urgent decompression of the bladder by catheterization is mandatory. The longer the bladder is allowed to remain overdistended in this circumstance, the longer is the period of recovery where detrusor acontractility may persist for up to 12 months despite resumption of other reflex activity. If there is any clinical doubt that the bladder is distended an ultrasonographic examination should be performed.

A full and detailed neurological examination should be performed, and perhaps the most pertinent aspect of that examination is the neurological level of the lesion as judged by sensory testing (Fig. 8.2). Some assessment can thus be made as to whether the level is above, at or below the sacral micturition centre. It is important to recognize the areas of skin which are supplied by the sacral segments.

There are specific clinical signs pertinent to vesico-urethral neuropathy which are of crucial importance, and which will help determine the neurological level which relates to bladder function.

The bulbocavernosus reflex

This reflex is used to denote function of the lower sacral segments, and thus by inference to demon-

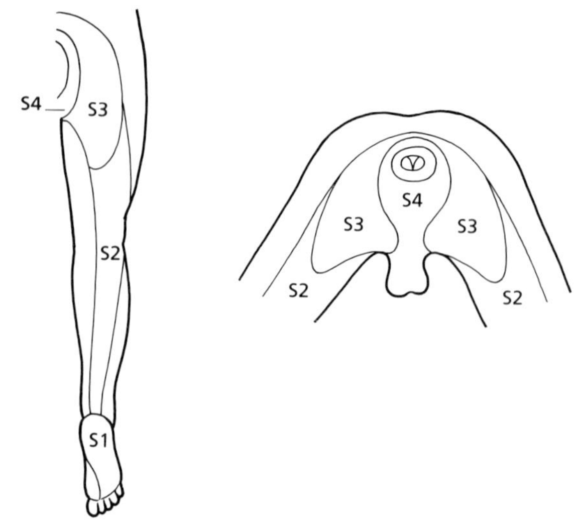

Fig. 8.2 Sensory innervation.

strate that the conus micturition centre is intact. The reflex is elicited by a brisk pinching of the glans penis, which provokes a contraction of the perianal muscles. In females it can be observed by pinching the clitoris, or rather more easily by a single gentle tug on a balloon catheter. The afferent and efferent limbs are in the pudendal nerves and integrity of the conus medullaris, specifically the S2–S4 segments, is required for the reflex to be seen. This reflex is thus absent in conus and cauda equina lesions. In higher lesions the reflex returns within the first 12 hours or so after injury, following the general principle that the more peripheral the reflex, the sooner it is likely to return as spinal shock abates. It is thus important to test this reflex within the first day of injury, for it will help to predict the type of bladder dysfunction which will ensue. The limitation of the bulbocavernosus reflex is that it is absent in 30% of neurologically intact individuals.

The anocutaneous reflex

This reflex can be seen by applying a pinprick to the peri-anal skin. An anal contraction similar to that provoked by the bulbocavernosus reflex will be observed indicating continuity of the S2–S4 reflex arc. The advantage of looking carefully for this reflex is that it can be lateralized depending upon which side of the anal skin evokes the response.

The anal reflex

The third of the three anal responses can be demonstrated by brief finger dilation of the anus at rectal examination. If the conus reflexes are intact this manoeuvre will produce an immediate contraction of the anal ring.

A clear demonstration of the sensory level, and testing of the conus reflexes, will indicate the level of the neurological deficit and allow anticipation of the type of bladder dysfunction which is to be expected. Bors & Comarr (1971) classified neurological lesions as either upper or lower motoneurone lesions in respect of the anatomical relationship of the injury to the sacral cord reflex centres. An upper motoneurone lesion involved disruption of the descending pathways to the bladder and somatic pathways to the lower extremities. Suprasacral spinal cord lesions would thus be expected to result in reflex spasticity of the bladder and the lower extremities. This has been described as a 'reflex' or 'automatic' bladder, but these terms are better abandoned because of the confusion which results from their use, particularly confusion with the 'autonomous' bladder, a term also to be abandoned, used to describe a lower motoneurone lesion involving pre- and postganglionic fibres to the bladder. In these cases the somatic nerves to the lower extremities are involved, and this would be expected to produce vesical and lower extremities flaccidity. A 'mixed lesion' group accounts for the exceptions: lower extremity spasticity with an acontractile bladder, and normal or flaccid lower extremities with a hypercontractile bladder.

The neurological classification can thus be summarized into broadly three groups: *suprasacral*, *sacral* and *mixed* lesions. Unfortunately, neurological examination alone is insufficient to classify bladder behaviour, particularly if the lesion is in the T10–L2 area. The urological presentation may vary depending upon the involvement of the micturition centre or segments immediately above this level. This may lead to a mixed neurological presentation secondary to direct injury to the sacral cord or by descending cord infarction. It is indeed possible to see absence of conus reflexes and acontractility of the bladder with a cord lesion as high as T6, which would normally be associated with a suprasacral type of bladder dysfunction. This is due to vascular injury to the cord below the level of the lesion.

INVESTIGATION

Postmicturitional residual urine

The measurement of postmicturitional residual urine may be used as an additional discriminator if determining the type of bladder dysfunction after cord injury. Voiding efficiency can be expressed as a percentage of the ratio of residual urine to bladder capacity (Bors & Comarr, 1971). This principle was developed to define a 'balanced' bladder and to differentiate from that which was unbalanced. An arbitrary percentage residual urine was used to make the differentiation. Unfortunately this does not separate several significantly different voiding patterns. An elevated residual urine in a suprasacral lesion may imply an acontractile bladder; insufficient reflex bladder contractility, or detrusor sphincter dyssynergia where, despite adequate detrusor contraction, voiding is obstructed by uncoordinated distal sphincteric activity. In an infrasacral lesion the inability to produce significant abdominal straining or the inability to overcome outlet resistance may also produce a residual urine. Of rather more fundamental importance is the inability of the measurement of postmicturitional residual urine to reflect intravesical pressure during voiding or during urinary storage between voiding episodes. Some assessment of detrusor function during filling and emptying is therefore mandatory in the management of neuropathic vesico-urethral dysfunction.

Urodynamic techniques

Perhaps the simplest urodynamic assessment that can be made is a simple test for the presence or absence of detrusor contraction. This can be performed merely by using the catheter tubing as an elementary manometer and observing fluctuations which can be assumed to be detrusor contractions, especially in the paralysed patient. This may provide the barest minimum of information. Most clinicians would, however, find this inadequate, and a full urodynamic assessment of the patient is normally required before treatment can be planned.

It is desirable to obtain as much information as possible about bladder function when undertaking what is, to the patient, an invasive investigation. A full synchronous videocystographic pressure flow study (Thomas, 1979) should thus be used and the components of this will be described in detail.

The crux of the investigation is to determine detrusor function with great accuracy, record it during bladder filling and emptying, relate it to urinary flow rate during micturition, and to watch the cycle by radiographic screening. Where this facility is not available, the bladder neck and proximal urethra can be visualized by transrectal ultrasound scanning, and this provides a reasonably satisfactory alternative imaging (Fellows *et al.*, 1987; Shabsigh *et al.*, 1988).

Detrusor function

The bladder is an intra-abdominal organ, and thus the pressure within it is a summation of extrinsic intraperitoneal pressure and the intrinsic pressure of the muscle within its wall. The latter may be deduced by recording total intravesical pressure and subtracting abdominal pressure from it. This is done in practice reasonably simply. Total bladder pressure is easy to record with a fine pressure line inserted into the bladder. Intra-abdominal pressure can be measured by a similar rectal pressure line passed per anum. Though artifacts of intrinsic rectal activity might be recorded, in practice this is not a problem. The abdominal (intrarectal) pressure is subtracted electronically from the total bladder pressure to allow continuous recording of intrinsic or detrusor pressure. A bladder filled with radiographic contrast via a filling catheter under X-ray screening can thus have the filling limb of the micturitional cycle recorded, during which the detrusor pressure can be measured. Once capacity is reached, micturition can take place, the pressures can be similarly monitored, and the cystogram viewed. Indeed it was in an effort to reduce the screening time at cystography, and to try to identify pertinent episodes during the micturition filling and voiding phases, that the technique of pressure flow video-urodynamics was developed.

Uroflow measurement

It is crucial to know the *rate* at which the bladder empties once the pressure responsible is determined. There are a variety of methods by which this can be done, but all depend upon measurement of mass per unit time of urine passed from the bladder.

The transducers used to measure this value rely on different principles, and each is ingenious, reliable and holds no particular advantage over another. For example, the increasing weight of urine collected in a receptacle can be recorded, and this is plotted as the urinary flow rate. Alternatively, the change in electrical capacitance of a metallic strip vertically hanging in the urine receptacle will also directly relate to the uroflow rate and can be plotted as such; or flow rate can be measured by using a manometer side-arm tube to register on a pressure transducer.

Finally, perhaps the most sophisticated mechanism relies on the principle that uroflow is directly related to the current required to maintain a disc spinning at constant velocity when the urinary stream is directed onto it by a funnel. The forces tending to slow the disc are proportional to mass per unit time of urine passed, hence the current needed can be recorded directly as the uroflow rate.

Any of the uroflowmeters can be incorporated into the schema of urodynamic investigation (Fig. 8.3), so that the relationship between detrusor pressure

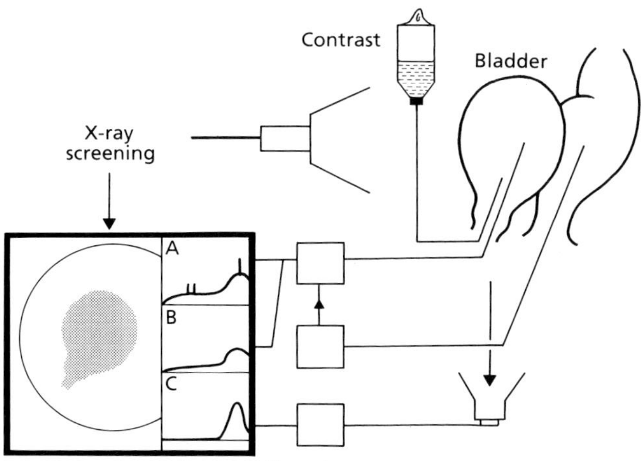

Fig. 8.3 Schema of urodynamic investigation.

and the flow rate that the pressure produces can be analysed. This is the essence of urodynamic investigation and allows the differentiation between the obstructed and the non-obstructed bladder, whilst the radiographic screening identifies the site of obstruction. Furthermore detrusor function can be recognized as normal or abnormal, and the cause of incontinence, if present, accurately identified.

Urodynamic results

The results of urodynamic studies allow objective measurement of a variety of parameters: bladder sensation, capacity, compliance (the ability to accommodate increasing volume), contractility and uroflow may be increased, normal or reduced (Torrens & Abrams, 1979).

Bladder sensation is twofold. Firstly, the sensation when filling is first appreciated, and secondly, the point during filling at which a normal sensation to void is experienced. Each is marked as an absolute value on the filling cystometrogram, but there is no 'normal' value for either. However, the patient who has deficient sensation will be easily recognized, as will one with a hypersensitive bladder.

Maximum cystometric capacity is the point at which the patient feels a normal strong desire to micturate. The bladder should not be overfilled during cystometry because this will influence contractility.

Compliance is the volume increment for a given change in pressure. This is a defined parameter which describes the slope of the filling cystometrogram. Previously this may have been referred to as bladder 'tone', but this confusing concept is best abandoned. Indeed the slope of the filling cystometrogram of the normal bladder should be virtually flat at a low filling rate over the normal range. The normal bladder should not contract under provocation until the patient wishes to void, and the increase in intrinsic detrusor pressure should not exceed 10–15 cmH_2O. Fluctuations in intra-abdominal pressure may be wide and, of course, will alter total bladder pressure, underlining the importance of recording subtracted or detrusor pressure.

Spontaneous bladder contractions during the filling phase have been given many names, of which *detrusor instability* is reserved for those cases in which no identifiable aetiology is recognized, and *uninhibited* or *hyperreflexic* applied to cases with a neuropathic cause. These contractions may lead to involuntary incontinence, and whether or not the patient is aware of this will depend upon sensory integrity.

When compliance is low as recorded by standard cystometric techniques, continuous ambulatory urodynamic monitoring has shown the pressure rise within the bladder generally to be less. Phasic contractions over and above the inexorable bladder pressure increase are recorded, and it is these which seem to correlate with a threat to the upper urinary tracts (Webb *et al.*, 1989).

Contractility is assessed upon the result of an effort to initiate micturition. The pressure required to generate a normal urinary flow rate (see below) should not exceed 50 cmH_2O, and thus outflow obstruction can be diagnosed if the detrusor pressure peaks beyond this point. An acontractile bladder can be recognized easily, though it is one of the failings of urodynamic analysis that the patient who is profoundly inhibited by the circumstance of the test may find it impossible to initiate a detrusor contraction though the bladder may be absolutely normal. Deficient contraction is rather more subjective, and depends upon the uroflow analysis. Decompensation of the detrusor is judged by measurement of postmicturitional residual urine.

Pharmacological tests

Lapides *et al.* (1962) reported a test for peripheral denervation of the bladder based upon Cannon's law that a denervated structure becomes supersensitive to its neurohumoral transmitter. This test is thus useful to determine, in those cases where the bladder is contractile, whether this is due to nerve injury. The Glahn modification of the test (Glahn, 1970) is the simplest to perform. The bladder is filled after cystometry to a volume of 100 ml and the pressure within it monitored continuously. A subcutaneous injection of bethanechol 2.5 mg is given, and if a pressure rise of more than 15 cmH_2O is recorded in the bladder over the subsequent 20 minutes, the test is positive. Others have used prostaglandin as an alternative provocation for this response in neuropathic cases (Kondo *et al.*, 1980).

False-positive results have been attributed to cystitis, emotional stress and rapid diuresis during the monitoring period, and false-negative to myogenic failure, poor absorption of bethanechol, and a delay in conversion of the denervated bladder until some six months after the neurological insult. Accepting these limitations, the test is most useful in differentiating neuropathic from non-neuropathic causes of the non-contractile detrusor.

Uroflowmetry

Uroflowmetry is informative not only for the maximum flow rate produced but also for the characteristics of the flow curves produced. Interrupted flow patterns are common in neuropathic vesico-urethral dysfunction and consideration of the pressure–flow characteristics in conjunction with the radiographic screening allows the distinction between interruption due to an inadequately sustained detrusor contraction, and obstruction due to dyssynergic activity of the urethral mechanism or inadequate opening of the bladder neck.

Urethral pressure profilometry—urostatics

This investigation is used to determine the profile of pressure along the length of the urethra. The technique is based upon the principle that, if a side-holed catheter is perfused at a constant yet slow rate, the pressure required to maintain the fluid flow will vary depending upon the wall pressure of the urethra upon the side-holes. If the catheter is withdrawn slowly from bladder to external meatus a profile pressure can be drawn on an X–Y plotter (Fig. 8.4).

Urethral pressure profiles in isolation can give only the broadest indication of abnormal urethral function, and as such are relatively uninformative. The test can be useful in three circumstances. Firstly, sequential profiles can be drawn over time to identify changes in urethral pressure resistance. This is crucial in cases of vesico-urethral neuropathy where midline neuropathic urethral obstruction may have a devastating effect upon the urinary tract. Secondly, by using pharmacological blocking agents it is possible to determine which element of the urethral sphincteric mechanism behaves abnormally. Specifically, use of an alpha-adrenoreceptor blocker can demonstrate the phenomenon of isolated distal sphincter obstruction. In this condition there is abnormal activity of the intrinsic urethral muscle innervated by the sympathetic nervous system. This phenomenon is found in conus and cauda equina neuropathy. In cases of higher lesions the contribution of the alpha-adrenergically innervated intrinsic urethral muscle within a dyssynergic sphincter can be identified. Finally, using a modified technique of *voiding urethral pressure profilometry* (Desmond & Ramayya, 1988) a baseline profile is drawn to allow accurate

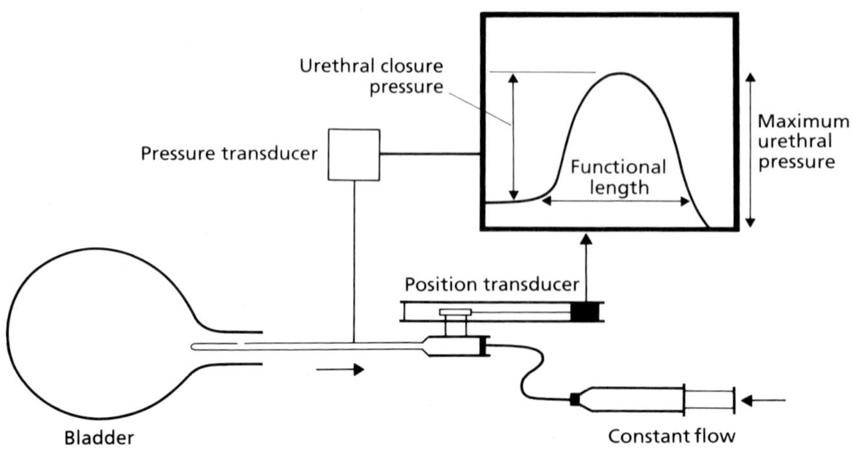

Fig. 8.4 Urethral pressure profilometry.

localization of the bladder neck and the urethral sphincter. These are marked by cursor on a oscilloscope. A second profile is then drawn while the patient is micturating, and this is compared to the pressure constantly recorded in the bladder. Where the two pressure curves separate indicates the site of obstruction within the lower urinary tract. This test can thus distinguish whether obstruction in a neuropathic case is at the bladder neck or at the level of the distal urethral mechanism. This distinction can otherwise prove to be difficult when only videocystography is used.

Urethral pressure has been measured directly by microtransducers mounted on a catheter and placed at the pressure-active area of the urethra (Bary *et al.*, 1982). Urethral activity is thus monitored during voiding and a dynamic assessment of urethral function made.

Electromyography

Direct electromyography (EMG) recording within the urethral mechanism is difficult (Blaivas *et al.*, 1977), but has been reported to be useful. A bipolar needle is inserted directly into the periurethral area and specific patterns of EMG potentials are recognized.

It has been rather more common for electromyograms to be recorded either by anal plug electrodes, skin electrodes or needle electrodes inserted into the levator ani muscle. Patterns of abnormal activity can be seen in those cases with a dyssynergic pelvic floor which produces urethral obstruction. In practical terms EMG recordings have rarely added significantly to urodynamic data, but are a useful adjunct to pressure flow tests.

Sacral evoked potentials

A useful application of EMG technique is direct recording of the conus reflexes (Rockswold & Bradley, 1977; Galloway *et al.*, 1985). The nerve transmission time between the urethral sphincter, the anal sphincter and the dorsal nerve of the penis (or clitoris) is measured. Multiple stimuli are given to ascertain the sensory threshold, and multiple recordings are analysed by an electronic averager. A single evoked potential for each of the reflexes can then be drawn and the reflex latency measured. Normal values are available for comparison with those recorded in neuropathic cases.

The technique is little more than an electrophysiological analysis of the bulbocavernosus (Siroky *et al.*, 1979) and anal reflexes, but its strength is that it allows a degree of objectivity in the assessment of neurological injury. In overt neuropathic cases it adds little to essential data relating to the urinary tract (Lucas & Thomas, 1989) but in cases of subtle or even perhaps disputed neuropathy recording of sacral evoked potentials can be of critical importance. This would certainly apply to cases of vesico-urethral neuropathy, but it can also be of crucial importance in those cases of mild to moderate spinal trauma with little overt evidence of neuropathy who subsequently complain of impotence.

FUNCTIONAL DIAGNOSIS IN THE NEUROPATHIC BLADDER

The aim of diagnosis is to bring together the clinical features and the results of investigations to provide a rational basis for management. The urodynamic patterns in vesico-urethral neuropathy which determine treatment can pragmatically be categorized into relatively simple groups, and they occur whether the neurological lesion is complete or partial, and whether it is congenital or acquired.

The phenomena are: whether the detrusor exhibits contractility; whether that contractility satisfactorily opens the bladder neck; whether urethral resistance to flow, be that by intermittent discoordinated pelvic floor contractions or by a similar unwanted intrinsic urethral muscular contraction, exceeds the contractile force of the detrusor; and finally whether the outflow resistance is incompetent.

In lower motor neurone lesions with a 'sacral' bladder, the expulsive force is provided by abdominal straining and the inappropriate urethral resistance results from contraction of intrinsic urethral muscle, whereas in higher lesions the detrusor will usually, if not always, regain uninhibited contractility while urethral resistance is a combination of striated and intrinsic muscular contraction which is out of synchrony with the detrusor contraction.

Therefore the *neuropathic urethra* is the critical element which merits specific consideration. If the expulsive force is sufficient, the resistance in the urethra is the crucial and fundamental factor (Gibbon *et al.*, 1980; Mundy *et al.*, 1985) in vesico-urethral neuropathy.

REFERENCES

Arnold, E.P. & Cowan, I.M. (1988) Clinical significance of ureteric diameter on intravenous urography after spinal cord injury. *Br. J. Urol.*, **62**, 131–135.

Bary, P.R., Day, G., Lewis, P., Chawla, J., Evans, C. & Stephenson, T.P. (1982) Dynamic urethral function in the assessment of spinal injury patients. *Br. J. Urol.*, **54**, 39–44.

Blaivas, J.G., Labib, K.L., Bauer, S.B. & Retik, A.B. (1977) A new approach to electromyography of the external urethral sphincter. *J. Urol.*, **117**, 773–777.

Bors, E. & Comarr, E. (1971) *Neurologic Urology*. University Park Press, Baltimore.

Delaere, K.P.J., Debruyne, F.M.J. & Moonen, W.A. (1983) Bladder neck incision in the female: a hazardous procedure. *Br. J. Urol.*, **55**, 283–286.

Desmond, A.D. & Ramayya, G.R. (1988) Comparison of pressure flow studies with micturitional urethral pressure profiles in the diagnosis of urinary outflow obstruction. *Br. J. Urol.*, **61**, 224–229.

Donker, P.J., Ivanovici, F. & Noach, E.L. (1972) Analysis of the urethral pressure profile by means of electromyography and the administration of drugs. *Br. J. Urol.*, **44**, 180–193.

Fellows, G.J., Cannell, L.B. & Ravichandran, G. (1987) Transrectal ultrasonography compared with voiding cystourethrography after spinal cord injury. *Br. J. Urol.*, **59**, 218–221.

Fletcher, T.F. & Bradley, W.B. (1978) Neuroanatomy of the bladder/urethra. *J. Urol.*, **119**, 153–160.

Galloway, N.T.M., Chisholm, G.D. & MacInnes, A. (1985) Patterns and significance of sacral evoked response (the urologist's knee jerk). *Br. J. Urol.*, **57**, 145–147.

Gibbon, N.O.K., Parsons, K.F. & Woolfenden, K.A. (1980) The neuropathic urethra. *Paraplegia*, **18**, 221–225.

Glahn, B.E. (1970) Neurogenic bladder diagnosed pharmacologically on the basis of denervation supersensitivity. *Scand. Urol. Nephrol.*, **4**, 13–15.

Gosling, J.A. (1979) The structure of the bladder and urethra in relation to function. *Urol. Clin. N. Am.*, **6**, 31–38.

Gosling, J.A., Dixon, J.S. & Lendon, R.L. (1977) The autonomic innervation of the human male and female bladder neck and proximal urethra. *J. Urol.*, **118**, 302–305.

Kondo, A., Kobayashi, M., Otari, T., Takita, T. & Narita, H. (1980) Supersensitivity to prostaglandin in chronic neurogenic bladders. *Br. J. Urol.*, **52**, 290–294.

Kuru, M. (1965) Nervous control of micturition. *Physiol. Rev.*, **45**, 425–494.

Lapides, J., Friend, C.R., Ajemian, E.P. & Reus, W.S. (1962) Denervation supersensitivity as a test for neurogenic bladder. *Surg. Gynecol. Obstet.*, **114**, 241–244.

Laruelle, L. (1948) Etude d'anatomie microscopique du nevraxe sur coupes longitudinales. *Acta Neurol. Psych. Belg. (Copenhagen)*, **48**, 189–196.

Lloyd, L.K., Kuhlemeier, K.V., Fine, P.R., McEachran, A.B. & Stover, S.C. (1987) Prediction of pyelocaliectsis in follow up of patients with spinal cord injury. *Br. J. Urol.*, **59**, 122–126.

Lucas, M.G. & Thomas, D.G. (1989) Lack of relationship of conus reflexes to bladder function after spinal cord injury. *Br. J. Urol.*, **63**, 24–27.

Mundy, A.R., Shah, P.J.R., Borzyskowski, M. & Saxton, H.M. (1985) Sphincter behaviour in meningomyelocele. *Br. J. Urol.*, **57**, 647–651.

Nathan, P.W. (1976) The central nervous connections of the bladder. In Williams, D.I. & Chisholm, G.D. (eds) *The Scientific Foundations of Urology*, pp. 51–58. Heinemann, London.

Rockswold, G.L. & Bradley, W.E. (1977) The use of evoked electromyographic responses in diagnosing lesions in the cauda equina. *J. Urol.*, **18**, 629–631.

Shabsigh, R., Fiskman, I.J. & Krebs, M. (1988) Combined transrectal sonography and urodynamics in the evaluation of detrusor-sphincter dyssynergia. *Br. J. Urol.*, **62**, 326–330.

Siroky, M.B., Sax, D.S. & Krane, R.J. (1979) Sacral signal tracing: the electrophysiology of the bulbocavernosus reflex. *J. Urol.*, **122**, 661–664.

Thomas, D.G. (1979) Clinical urodynamics in neurogenic bladder dysfunction. *Urol. Clin. N. Am.*, **6**, 227–253.

Thomas, D.G. & Clarke, S.J. (1979) The urological status of 86 females following spinal cord injury. *Br. J. Urol.*, **51**, 515–517.

Torrens, M.J. (1978) Urethral sphincteric responses to stimulation of the sacral nerves in the human female. *Urol. Int.*, **33**, 22–26.

Torrens, M.J. & Abrams, P.H. (1979) Cystometry. *Urol. Clin. N. Am.*, **6**, 79–85.

Webb, D.R., Fitzpatrick, J.M. & O'Flynn, J.D. (1984) A 15 year follow up of 406 consecutive spinal cord injuries. *Br. J. Urol.*, **56**, 614–617.

Webb, R.J., Styles, R.A., Griffiths, C.J., Ramsden, P.D. & Neal, D.E. (1989) Ambulatory monitoring of bladder pressures in patients with low compliance as a result of neurogenic bladder dysfunction. *Br. J. Urol.*, **64**, 150–154.

9 · Anthropometry

By R.G. BURWELL and P.H. DANGERFIELD

Scientists are trained to measure . . .
(The Planets, *Economist*, 1989)

Clinical principles of back-shape appraisal

In examining a child with idiopathic scoliosis the clinician directs his attention to: the patient as a whole; to posture, including shoulder height, the waist and hip asymmetry; to spinal balance, back shape (hump, lateral spinal curvature, kyphosis and lordosis); pelvic tilt and leg-length inequality.

It is customary to record the standing height, sitting height, weight and leg-lengths of the patient at the initial, if not at all visits, to the clinic (see Appendix). Arm-span (or tibial length, Zorab *et al.*, 1964) is used to predict vital capacity. Leg-length inequality is traditionally measured with a tape. The techniques used by most surgeons for measurements made on the surface of the body, with certain exceptions, are inaccurate. Hence X-ray examination is generally used when skeletal measurements are needed—such as of the spinal deformity and of leg-length inequality (scanogram).

Traditionally, the posteroanterior (PA), or anteroposterior (AP) and lateral radiographs provide the principal means for recording and documenting scoliosis. The back hump is rarely evaluated radiologically.

The use of the Cobb (or Ferguson) angle has three major disadvantages (Hierholzer & Lüxmann, 1982):

1 it is a global measure which does not give a description of the degree and distribution of curvature along the spine;

2 it does not take into account the three-dimensional deformity of the scoliotic spine;

3 it depends on the position of the patient relative to the X-ray apparatus.

At present, three-dimensional reconstructions of the radiological deformity of scoliosis are too cumbersome for routine practice.

The Nottingham–Liverpool approach to back-shape appraisal

The system currently being used in our units for trunk asymmetry assessment before and after surgery for scoliosis introduces newer techniques. The methods were built upon previous work on body measurements established since 1972 in Liverpool and Nottingham to evaluate certain orthopaedic deformities of childhood, including scoliosis (Burwell *et al.*, 1980).

To understand the background to such numerical back-shape appraisal it is necessary to discuss some principles of anthropometry and biostereometrics.

Anthropometry and biostereometrics

Anthropometry is the measurement of humans. In orthopaedics, measurements are generally made on the surface of the body, on radiographs, ultrasonographs, computerized tomography (CT) and magnetic resonance imaging (MRI) scans. Some principles of skeletal measurement as applied to orthopaedics are outlined by Burwell *et al.* (1980).

Most readings obtained from instruments applied to the back of patients are simple one- or two-dimensional measurements, such as of a rib hump, a kyphosis angle or a lordosis angle. Occasionally, two readings are obtained, for instance of both thoracic and lumbar humps. A more complete description can be attained by readings procured at several sites on the back, e.g. the 10-level hump measurement (see

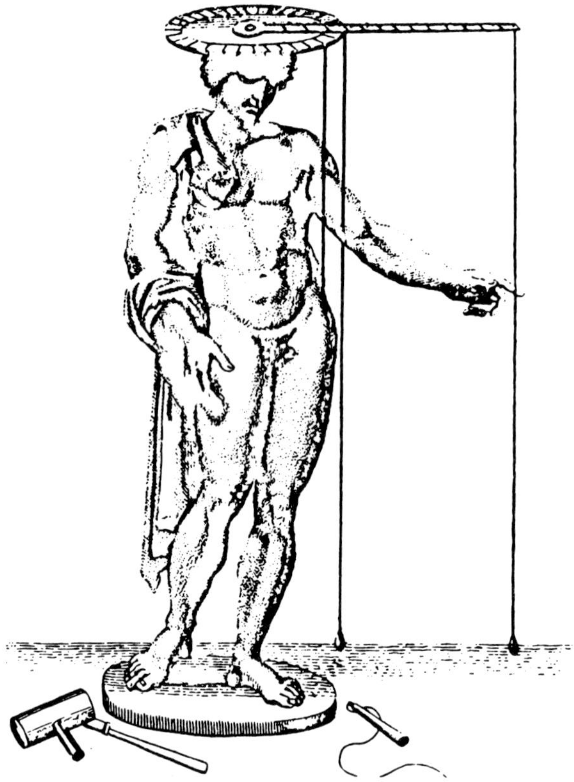

Fig. 9.1 Alberti's 'definer', a modified surveyor's disc which he used to locate points on the body surface in three-dimensional coordinates. Reproduced by kind permission of Dr R. E. Herron and the editor of *Orthopaedic Review*.

below). By taking many readings in different planes at different levels, a three-dimensional description of back shape can be obtained.

CLINICAL APPROACH TO A THREE-DIMENSIONAL DESCRIPTION OF DEFORMITY

Description in words is the principal method of stating and recording orthopaedic data, with the frequent use of images in the form of diagrams and photographs—and to a lesser extent models, drawings and paintings. The mathematics used is both arithmetic and Euclidean geometry. The accurate description in space and time of the body regions as Cartesian coordinates is rarely, if ever, utilized. However, the use of such coordinates in the basic research of orthopaedics is beginning to grow. The method is now being applied, for instance, to manufacture stems for the femoral component of certain non-cemented total hip replacements.

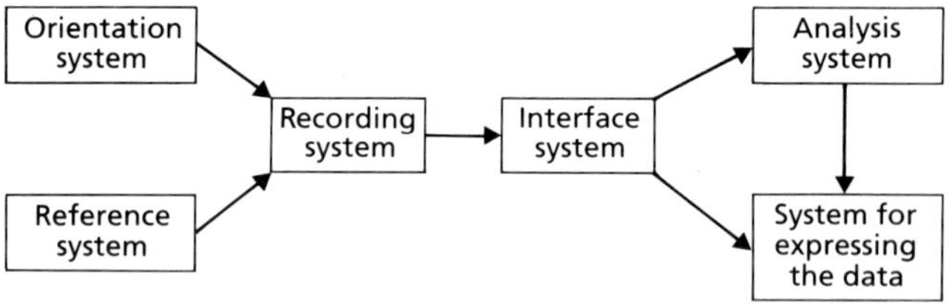

Fig. 9.2 A flow diagram to show the relation of the systems used in biostereometrics.

BIOSTEREOMETRICS

Biostereometrics is the spatial and spatiotemporal analysis of form and function based on principles of analytical geometry (Herron, see Burwell, 1978). The science of biostereometrics deals not only with three-dimensional measurements of biological subjects in space—such as back shape—but also any variation of the measurements with time such as movement and growth. The potential of stereometric measurement of the human body was demonstrated over 500 years ago in Florence by Alberti (Fig. 9.1).

SYSTEMS FOR SPATIAL AND SPATIOTEMPORAL MEASUREMENT

In basic terms, spatial and spatiotemporal measurement of the human body involves using the following systems (Fig. 9.2): orientation, reference, recording, interface, and analysis systems, also systems for expressing the data. The increasing power of digital hardware and software has made it possible to analyse and reconstruct three-dimensional structures. But the problem of how to visualize three dimensions is inherent in all imaging systems, whether they are using coherent or incoherent light, stereo-X-rays, CT and MRI scans or ultrasound. All such systems produce large amounts of data so that even the most powerful computers are not able to do adequate pattern recognition.

Surface anthropometry of the back

The numerical appraisal of back shape is relevant to screening for scoliosis, the natural history of trunk deformity and the evaluation of treatment. Such appraisal is concerned not only with back humps and spinal curvatures, but also shoulder height, hip and waist asymmetry and spinal balance—for which we use the collective term *trunk asymmetry*.

Attempts to measure back shape started in the last century and were concerned with describing the deformity of scoliosis (Schulthess, 1905; see Moe, 1987). After decades in which description of spinal deformity was dominated by radiographs, in recent years engineers and surgeons have been developing and evaluating new methods to quantitate the surface deformity of scoliosis.

The surface deformity of scoliosis is important because it is the disfigurement of which the patient complains. To the surgeon it serves as the reason for X-ray examination of the spine. Because of the hazards of such radiation, attempts are now being made to measure the size of the lateral spinal curvature by automated surface systems (such as ISIS and ultrasound, see below). The relation between the surface deformity and the radiological trunk deformity is then of considerable interest—but it has not yet received the attention it deserves.

Recently the availability of two commercial instruments to record back shape—namely the scoliometer and ISIS—has given considerable impetus to clinical research. It has enabled a few surgeons to describe back shape numerically in patients treated for scoliosis (see p. 217, below). Raster stereography is also contributing to this clinical progress. The findings add to earlier work using the hump-meter, formulator body contour tracer and moiré photography for recording the surface back deformity of scoliosis.

Back shape and the changing attitudes to treatment for adolescent idiopathic scoliosis (AIS)

Such studies on trunk asymmetry before and after surgery for idiopathic scoliosis—as well as evidence from other sources—are currently leading to a re-examination of treatment, including surgery, for AIS. The following points are important:

1 The patient's complaint is of disfigurement, not the radiological appearance.

2 Patients with AIS do not seem to develop life-threatening cardiorespiratory complications secondary to their spinal deformity (Branthwaite, 1986).

3 The need to know whether or not brace treatment is effective for children with AIS (Nachemson, 1991).

4 The cosmetic deformity often progresses despite surgical treatment (Dangerfield & Denton, 1986; Weatherley *et al.*, 1987; Burwell *et al.*, 1992a; Wemyss-Holden *et al.*, 1992).

5 The surgical wiring techniques of segmental spinal instrumentation (SSI) carry neurological hazards (Dove, 1985).

6 The transthoracic surgical approach involved in anterior spinal release, disc excision and bone grafting carries a small risk of the patient developing adult respiratory distress syndrome (ARDS).

7 The cost of new surgical instrumentation (e.g. Cotrel–Dubousset).

8 After school screening, the absence of an agreed policy for early treatment (see Burwell, 1988).

9 The relation of aetiology to the possibility of preventive surgical treatment (Burwell, 1990b).

10 The recent development of a two-stage surgical method for treating progressive infantile idiopathic scoliosis which does not involve spinal fusion (Grivas *et al.*, 1991).

The likelihood that AIS does not threaten life through cardiorespiratory failure implies therefore that any surgical treatment should be of low risk and provide an excellent correction of both the cosmetic and the radiological deformity which is maintained throughout life.

Conventional X-ray examination of the spine (posteroanterior and lateral views) does not reveal the deformity of the rib cage in the transverse plane (rib hump); hence other methods are needed—these include:

1 Surface back shape (see below).

2 Special X-ray methods: skyline views of rib hump (James, 1956); three-dimensional reconstruction of rib cage (Stokes, 1989); CT scans; segmental CT scans (Transfeldt *et al.*, 1990).

3 MRI.

4 Ultrasound methods (see below).

Because of the hazards of X-radiation and the ethical problems involved, attention has been directed by many workers to skin surface anthropometry and more recently to ultrasound anthropometry of the spine and rib cage. MRI has been used to study the nervous system and the discs, but not yet to appraise back shape. Here discussion will be restricted to surface and ultrasound methods.

Papers published on the results of new treatments for idiopathic scoliosis should now include data on back shape. Reports which rely solely on conventional X-ray films are at best incomplete, and at worst misleading.

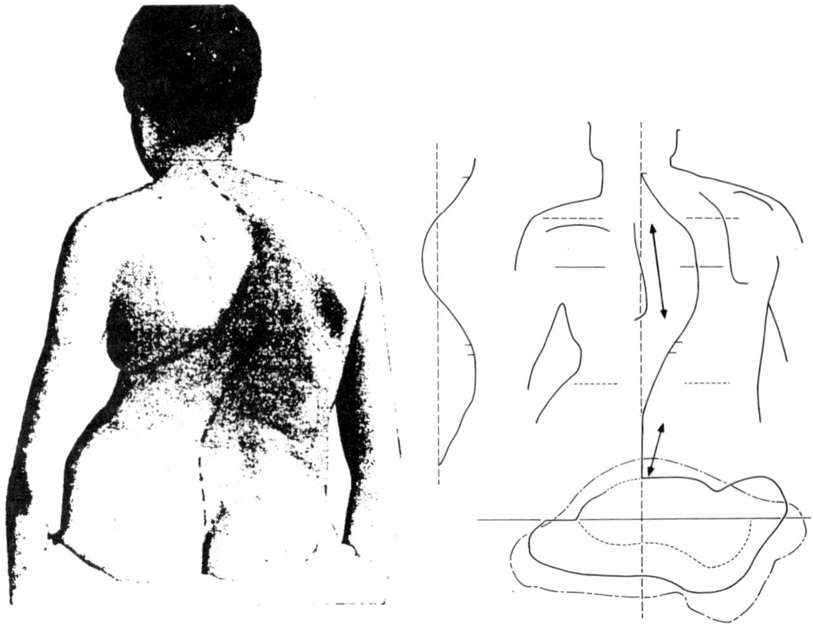

Fig. 9.3 *Left*: clinical photograph of a patient with right thoracic scoliosis. *Right*: tracings of sagittal curves, back and cross-sections made with the Schulthess measuring apparatus. Reproduced from Schulthess (1905).

SOME METHODS USED TO MEASURE SURFACE BACK SHAPE

Back humps

HISTORICAL

Before the discovery of X-rays, plaster casts and photographs were used to record the deformity and demonstrate the effects of treatment. Towards the end of the 19th century a variety of devices were developed to record and measure the deformed back (Schulthess, 1905; Fig. 9.3); and a number of items of such equipment reviewed and demonstrated at a meeting of the Vienna Anthropological Society (1904). Young, in his book *Orthopaedic Surgery*, lists 68 appliances of various forms used to assess scoliosis; and Schulthess mentions 54 different types of apparatus in Joachimstal's *Handbuch für Orthopädische Chirurgie* (see Hovorka, 1904).

SOME MEASURING INSTRUMENTS

Recently a few surgeons and scientists have reported methods for recording the most obvious back deformity, namely the hump (see Horst, 1983). The methods include: hump-meter (Takemitsu, 1981); flexicurve (Pun *et al.*, 1987); formulator body contour tracer (Thulbourne & Gillespie, 1976; Burwell *et al.*, 1983a,b, Dangerfield *et al.*, 1987); inclinometers (e.g. 'scoliometer'—Bunnell, 1984; spirit level—Pruijs, 1989); pantograph (Willner, 1983); vector stereography (Morris & Harris, 1976); moiré photography (Willner, 1979); ISIS (Turner-Smith *et al.*, 1988); stereophotogrammetry (Karara, see Burwell, 1978); raster stereography (Frobin & Hierholzer, 1982, 1990; Stokes *et al.*, 1985); AUSCAN (Assente *et al.*, 1987); optronic torso graph (Dawson *et al.*, 1989); Loughborough anthropometric shadow scanner (Jones *et al.*, 1989).

In some of these methods the child's back is appraised in a standing forward bending position; in others the back is measured with the child standing in a normal relaxed position.

Shoulder, scapular and waist asymmetry were measured by Vercauteren *et al.* (1985) in 160 children aged 11–18 years with 'untreated physiological, postural and idiopathic scoliosis'.

HUMP-METER (Fig. 9.4)

A simple method to measure the size of a rib hump (or lumbar hump) is to ask the child to bend forwards, place a spirit level horizontally across the most prominent part of the back and, using a ruler, measure the distance from the spirit level to the surface of the back on the concavity of the spinal curvature. Instruments have been developed to simplify such measurement of back contour asymmetry (Takemitsu, 1981;

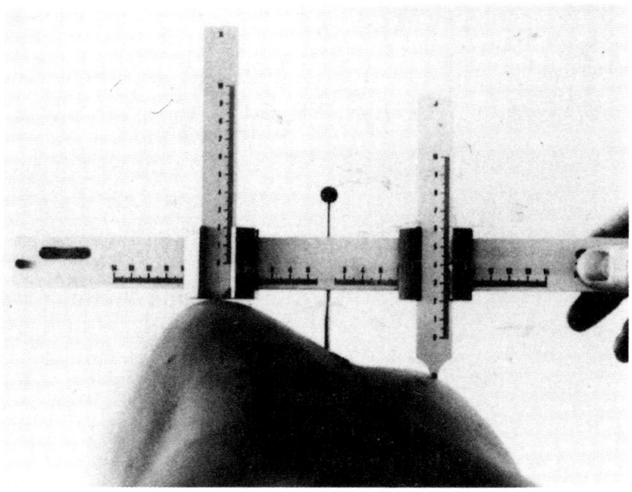

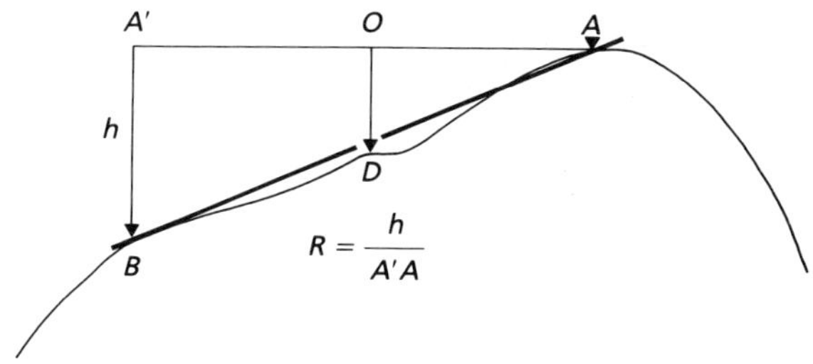

Fig. 9.4 *Left*: rib hump-meter. *Right*: calculation of rotation index. Reproduced from Horst (1983).

Vercauteren *et al.*, 1985). The reading is partly dependent on trunk width; hence it should be corrected for the size of the chest.

FLEXICURVE AND CONTOUR GRAPHS (Figs 9.5 & 9.6)

Another simple method is to prepare a contour graph of the rib hump in scoliosis using a flexicurve (Pun *et al.*, 1987). The tracing can be quantitated as shown in Fig. 9.6.

FORMULATOR BODY CONTOUR TRACER (Figs 9.7–9.9)

This instrument is a rod matrix used to record the back shape in two dimensions with the child in a forward bending position (most usually standing forward bending, but occasionally sitting forward bending) (Thulbourne & Gillespie, 1976). By recording the outline of the back at given spinal levels, calculations of back contour asymmetry can be made and standardized for trunk width (standardized trunk asymmetry scores, TAS, Burwell *et al.*, 1983a,b; Weatherley *et al.*, 1987; Dangerfield *et al.*, 1987). Although the method is useful if applied to several places along the back of a scoliotic child, the instrument is heavy and tedious to use. Nevertheless it provides simple tracings of back shape. We are still using the formulator in the pre- and postoperative appraisal of the scoliosis deformity because the tracings obtained at T4, T8, T12, L3 and S2 provide the surgeon with a ready way of showing the changes in back contours after treatment.

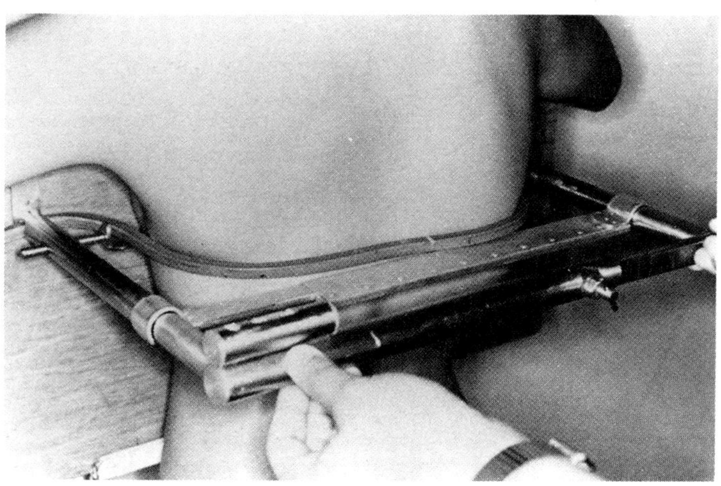

Fig. 9.5 The flexicurve used to obtain the shape of the back. Reproduced by kind permission of Dr W. K. Pun and the editor of *Spine*.

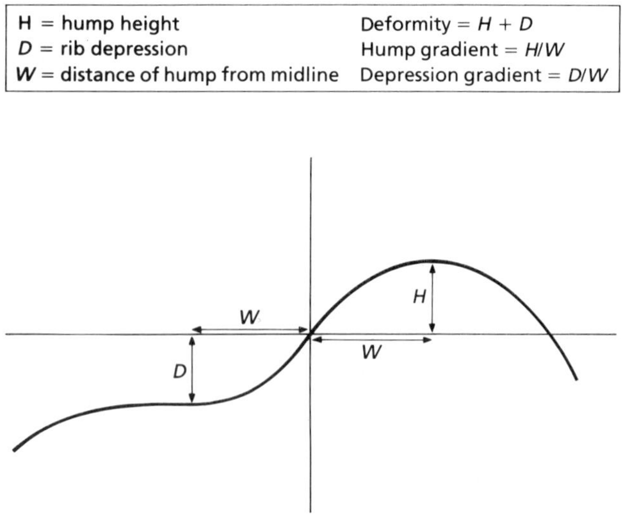

Fig. 9.6 Quantitation of back tracings obtained using the flexicurve. Reproduced by kind permission of Dr W. K. Pun and the editor of *Spine*.

'SCOLIOMETER' (Figs 9.10–9.14)

Schulthess (1905) used a mechanical device ('level indicator') to measure the angle of trunk inclination (ATI) across the back of a child in the standing forward bending position. Recently, Bunnell (1984) introduced a simple inclinometer including a curved spirit level. The reliability of the scoliometer has been evaluated by a few workers. In scoliotic subjects the accuracy of the scoliometer is similar in thoracic and lumbar regions in each of the standing and sitting forward bending positions (±1.28 to ±1.47°, pooled SDs, Upadhyay *et al.*, 1987). We have used the scoliometer in several ways successively to record back shape, namely as: single ATIs (Figs 9.11 & 9.12); ATIs at several spinal levels; compound ATIs (e.g. TLDs, Figs 9.13 & 9.14); multiple ATI system; 10-level ATIs; calculated segmental ATIs (Figs 9.15 & 9.16); segmental ATIs.

Some findings from the use of these methods to record back shape in health, deformity, screening and treatment are considered below (pp. 212, 217).

'SPINAL ROTATION METER' (Fig. 9.17)

The angle of trunk inclination across the back of a child with scoliosis in a standing forward bending position can also be measured using a 'spinal rotation meter' (Pruijs, 1989). It was developed as a simple tool to measure angles on the external surface of the body and on radiographs.

MOIRÉ PHOTOGRAPHY (Fig. 9.18)

This was the first optical method to find widespread use for characterizing deformity patterns of the human back. The method has been used in screening, natural history studies and treatment (Willner, 1979; Suzuki *et al.*, 1981; Daruwalla & Balasubramanian, 1985; Sahlstrand, 1986). Moiré photography uses optical interference to record the three-dimensional image of the shape of a surface. In structural scoliosis, with the child in a relaxed standing position, an asymmetry of the two halves of the back is seen (Fig. 9.18). While moiré photographs are appealing to the eye, their appearance changes with even slight changes of position of the subject so that careful positioning is necessary. Moreover, the interpretation of moiré photographs demands considerable skill and experience, and many different numerical methods have been described which reduce the subjective element in their evaluation (see Turner-Smith *et al.*, 1988).

Reliability and positioning

Bannon & Tredwell (1987) obtained repeated moiré photographs of three normal subjects and one scoliotic subject in three positions: unobstructed free standing (Armstrong); inclined positioning to 10° (Ohtsuka); and a seated forward bending position (Harada). The variability in the normal subjects was insignificant between trial and between method of positioning; but in the scoliotic subject the difference between methods was significant for both rib hump height and rib hump index. They recommended that a study of the variability due to subject positioning be conducted with scoliotic patients.

Transectional contours of the trunk

Suzuki *et al.* (1981) used moiré photography from four directions to obtain transectional contours of the trunk in 21 scoliosis patients. They also examined the effect of respiration upon such contours.

Trunk movements whilst marching on the spot

Asazuma *et al.* (1986) used moiré photography in scoliotic and normal subjects to evaluate pelvic and trunk rotation whilst marching on the spot.

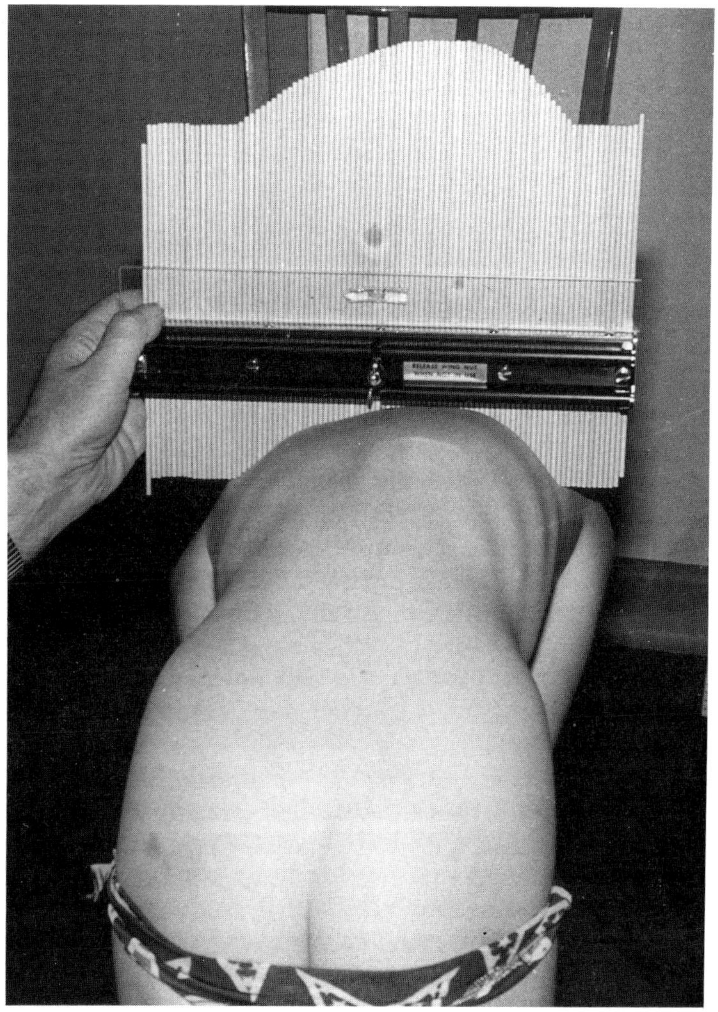

Fig. 9.7 The formulator body contour tracer used to obtain the outline of a child's back in the thoracic region. Note the spirit level supported on the horizontal beam of the apparatus. The rods have dropped to take up the contour of the child's back. Reproduced from Burwell *et al.* (1983a) by kind permission of the editor, *Journal of Bone and Joint Surgery*.

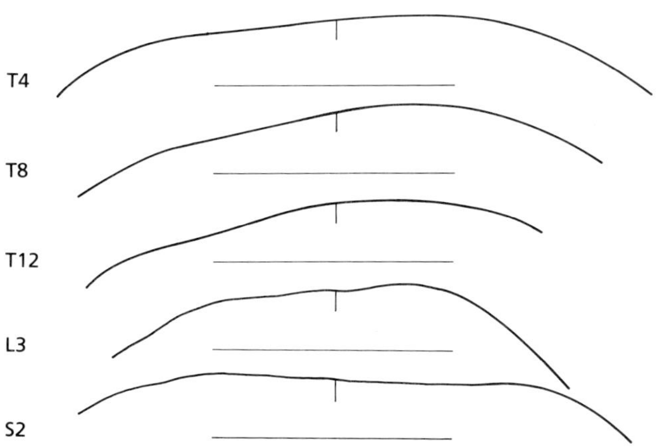

Fig. 9.8 Tracings of the back of a child with a preoperative right thoracic scoliosis (T4, T8, T12, L3 and S2). The spinous process at each level is marked.

INTEGRATED SHAPE INVESTIGATION SYSTEM (ISIS) (Figs 9.19–9.21)

ISIS is a television-scanning method for recording back shape with respect to lateral spinal curve (lateral asymmetry index, LAI), the hump and sagittal spinal curves (Turner-Smith *et al.*, 1988).

The scanning system sweeps a line of light down the back of the child, usually standing in a relaxed position. A television camera records the distortion of the line of light as it moves down the back of the patient. The back shape is displayed graphically (Fig. 9.21). The *lateral asymmetry index* of ISIS is concerned with establishing the line of the spine in the frontal plane, but it does not represent the typical asymmetric hump of a scoliotic back. This asymmetric appearance of the back is best shown on the

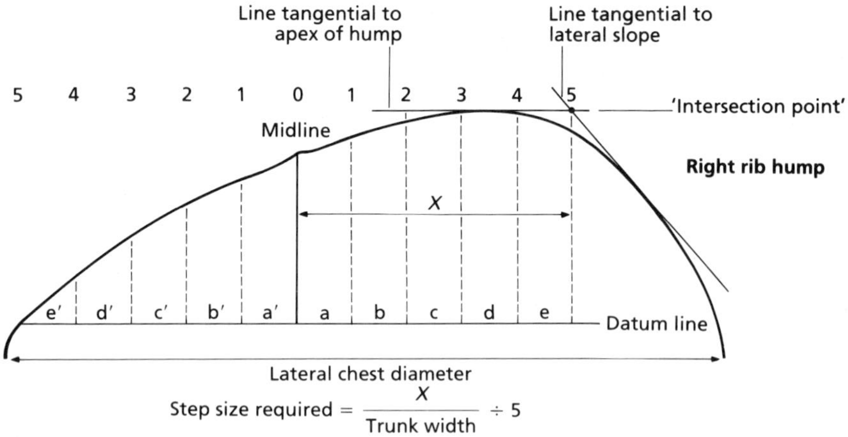

Fig. 9.9 Method of quantitating back contour asymmetry from a formulator tracing at T8. Note the datum line drawn parallel to the horizontal beam of the apparatus. The trunk asymmetry is summated for five positions on each side of the midline to give the crude rib hump score which is then standardized to a 21 cm lateral chest diameter. Reproduced from Burwell (1983b) by kind permission of the editors, *Moiré Fringe Topography and Spinal Deformity*.

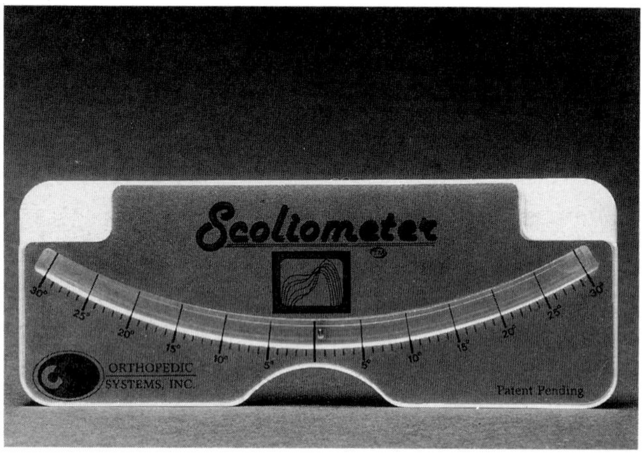

Fig. 9.10 OSI scoliometer. From Bunnell (1984).

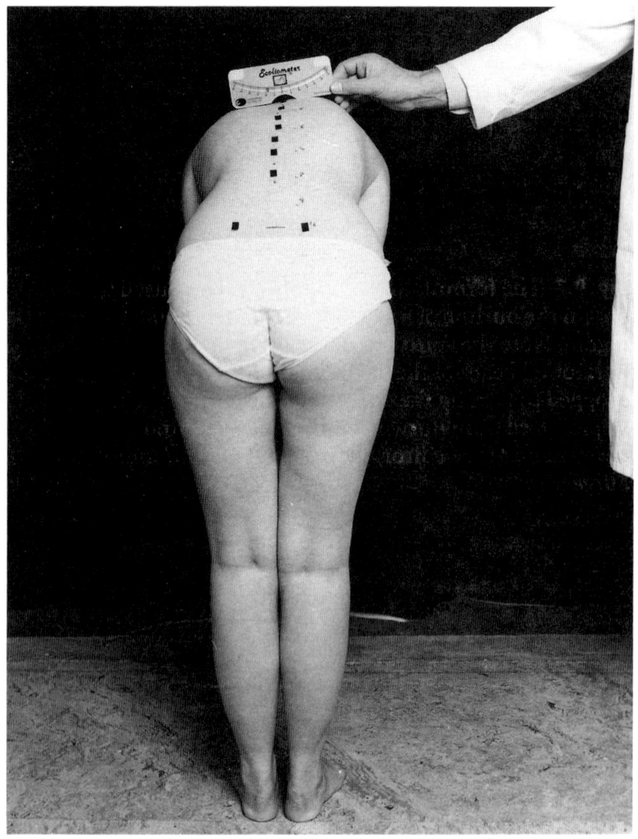

Fig. 9.11 The standard standing forward bending position with a scoliometer being used to measure the thoracic angle of trunk inclination (ATI).

ISIS plot by the 10 'transverse asymmetry' sections. These are horizontal cross-sections of the back and analogous to CT and MRI scan sections. This asymmetry is an important factor to the patient as it is the most obvious manifestation of the disease. It is also an important factor to the surgeon as it clearly shows the improvement in appearance which results from either surgical intervention or conservative treatment (Turner-Smith *et al.*, 1988). Volumetric asymmetries of right and left humps are now calculated.

ISIS has the advantage of being non-contact—especially valuable in sensitive backs after surgery, non-invasive, and simple. Moreover it is observer-independent and produces immediate results as a hard copy—which is an advantage over the use of moiré photography. Disadvantages of ISIS are the relatively low image resolution, its high cost, and the need for a skilled technician.

Comparison with the scoliometer

In preoperative patients with thoracic AIS, ISIS and scoliometer angle and trunk inclination (ATI) data obtained at the maximal hump correlate very highly

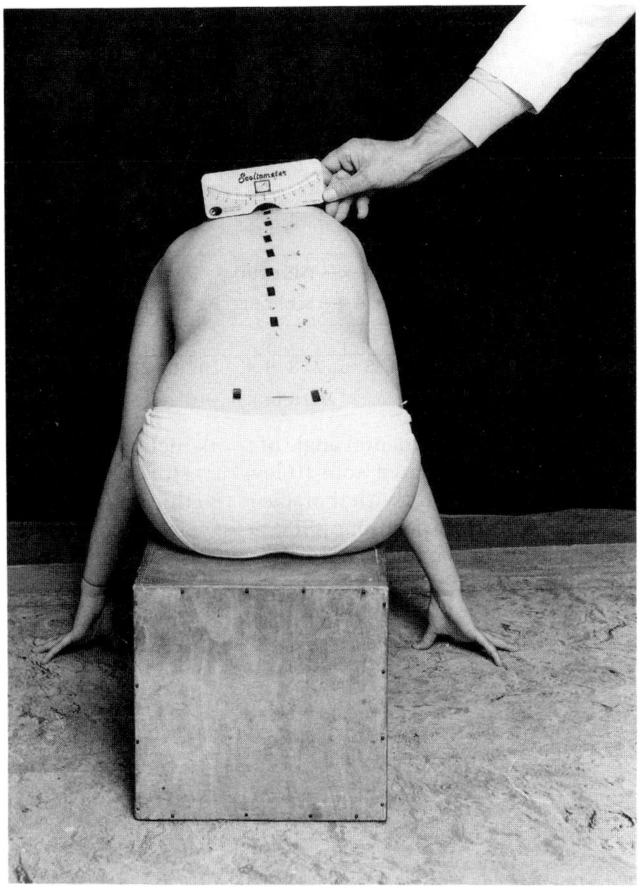

Fig. 9.12 The standard sitting forward bending position with a scoliometer being used to measure the thoracic ATI.

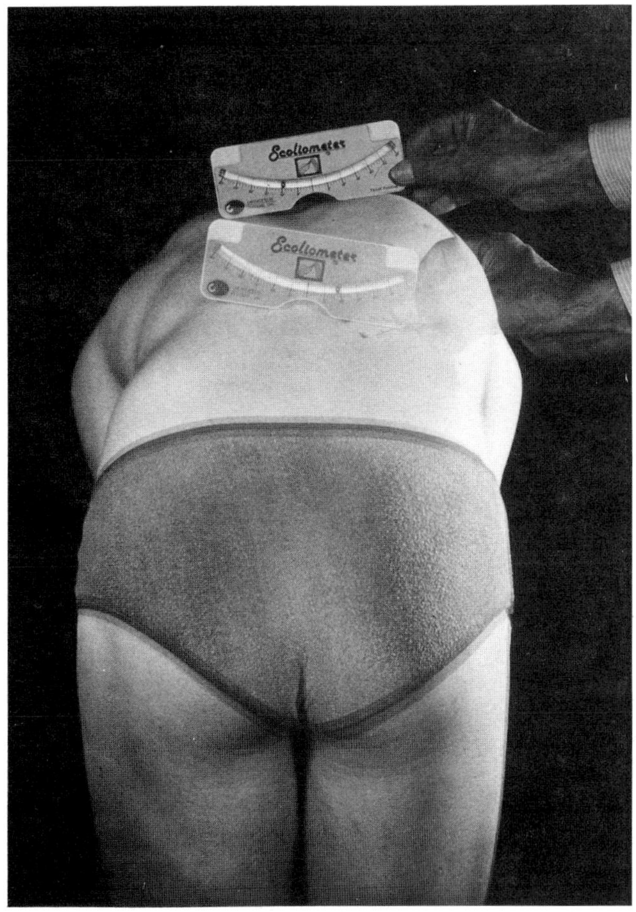

Fig. 9.13 The standing TLD test using the scoliometer (double exposure photograph, for further details, see text).

significantly ($r = 0.73$, $p < 0.001$, $n = 24$, Burwell *et al.*, 1992a, see also Figs 9.15 & 9.16).

STEREOSCOPIC PHOTOGRAPHY WITH MEASUREMENT—STEREOPHOTOGRAMMETRY (Fig. 9.22)

This system was developed for cartography and later applied to medical problems (Karara, see Burwell, 1978). The method of close-range photogrammetry is based on the principle of looking at a subject simultaneously from two points of view, as in stereoscopic vision. In place of the eyes, cameras are used to take overlapping photographs (or stereopairs). When the images comprising a stereopair are suitably orientated in a stereocomparator, or stereoplotter, the observer sees an image in three dimensions. The three-dimensional images can be plotted to produce a contour map and profiles using a stereoplotting instrument. In addition, using a stereocomparator or stereoplotter, the position of chosen points on the body surface can be measured in terms of x, y and z coordinates which are amenable to subsequent computer analysis.

RASTER STEREOGRAPHY (Fig. 9.23)

Grating projection, or raster stereography, uses structured light techniques to generate fringe patterns on the surface of the subject (Frobin & Hierholzer, 1982). Several different systems are being developed using the principle of grating projection. The surface shape of the back outlined by the projected raster can be reconstructed by computer. Although well-suited for scientific research, raster stereography initially was not very appropriate for routine application in the clinic. Since registration was done on photographic

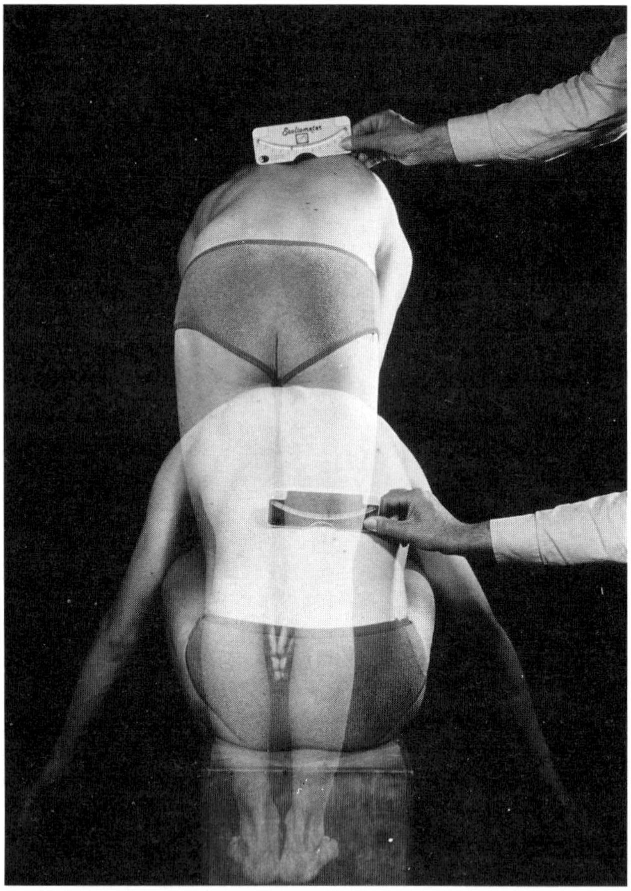

Fig. 9.14 The dynamic TLD test using the scoliometer (double exposure photograph, for further details, see text).

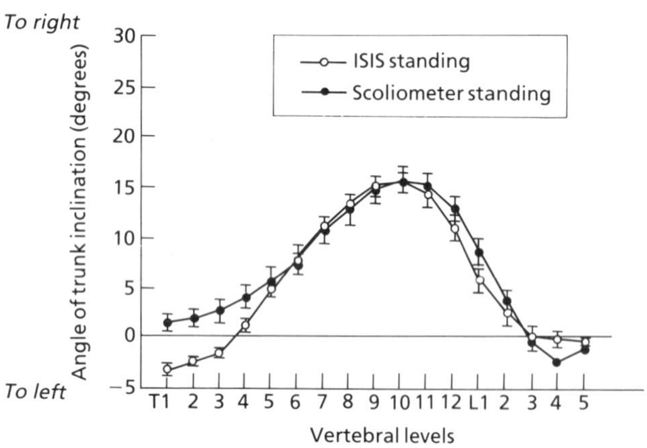

Fig. 9.15 Plot of segmental angle of trunk inclinations (ATIs ± 1 SE) calculated from 10-level data for 30 preoperative patients with thoracic idiopathic scoliosis in each of two *standing* positions (ISIS standing erect; scoliometer standing forward bending). For further details see text. From Wythers *et al.* (1992).

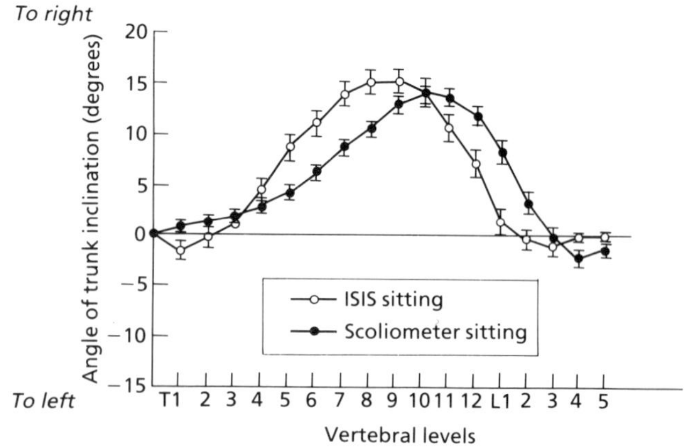

Fig. 9.16 Plot of segmental angle of trunk inclinations (ATIs ± 1 SE) calculated from 10-level data for 30 preoperative patients with thoracic idiopathic scoliosis in each of two *sitting* positions (ISIS, sitting erect; scoliometer, sitting forward bending). For further details see text. From Wythers *et al.* (1992).

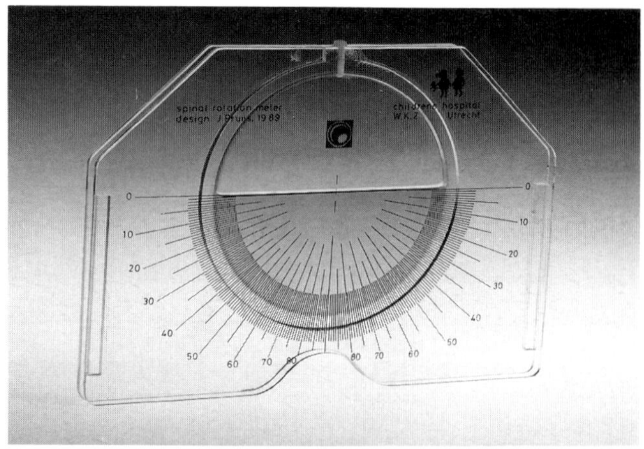

Fig. 9.17 Spinal rotation meter. From Pruijs (1989).

film, a considerable delay was produced by film processing, scanning and image data evaluation. Recently solid state (charge-coupled device, CCD) video cameras with sufficiently high resolution have become available. These cameras contain a rectangular sensor with a large number of pixels. Using such a video camera and a video frame interface connected to a computer allows on-line recording and digitization of raster stereographic images. The subsequent data analysis is performed within a few minutes. Thus, the final data are immediately available for application in the clinic (Frobin & Hierholzer, 1990).

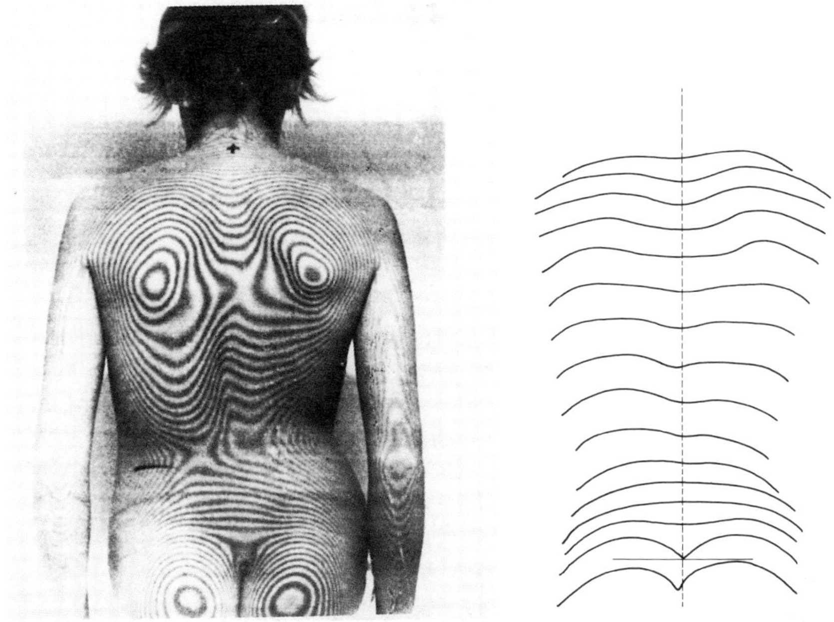

Fig. 9.18 *Left*: moiré photograph of girl with scoliosis. *Right*: transverse sections derived from moiré photograph. Reproduced by kind permission of Jones *et al*. (1987).

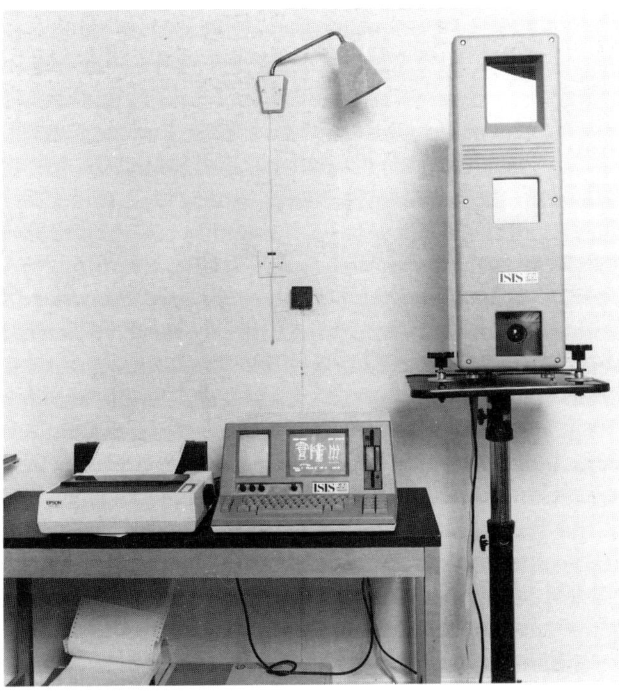

Fig. 9.19 The system configuration of ISIS from right to left: the optical scanner on its stand, the console (showing the display of a patient's back) and the printer. The optical scanner consists essentially of a fixed camera (lower window) and a moving line of light (upper window). Reproduced from Upadhyay *et al*. (1987).

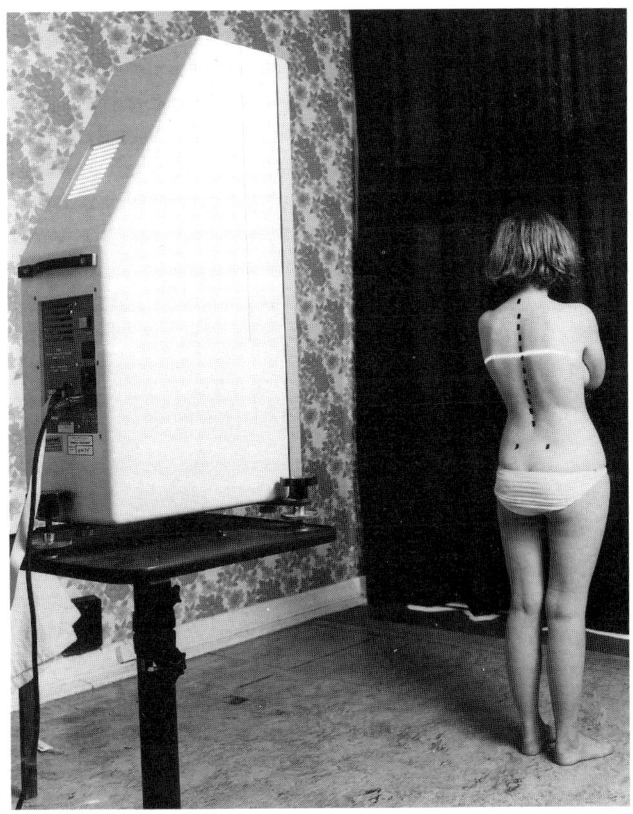

Fig. 9.20 The optical scanner projecting the moving line of light down the back of a patient in the standard standing erect position (see text). Reproduced from Upadhyay *et al*. (1987).

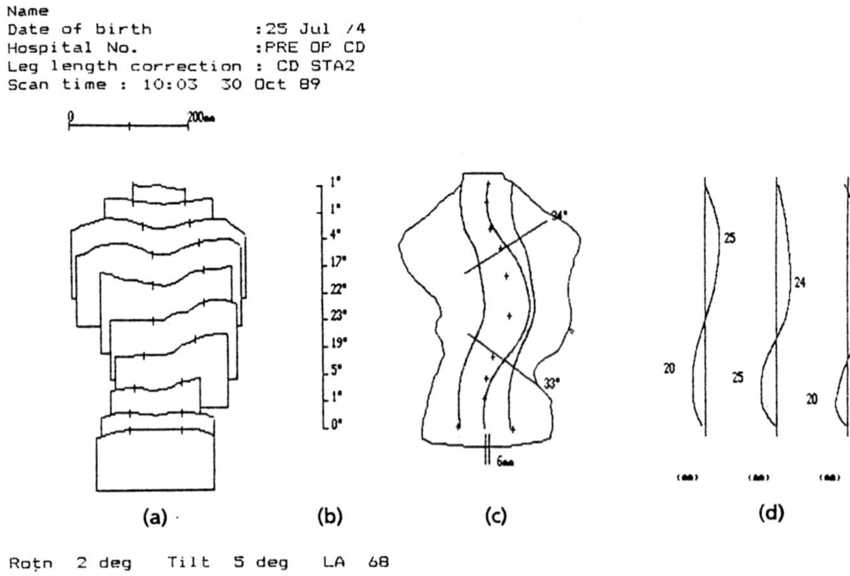

Fig. 9.21 Graphic display of data calculated by ISIS for a patient. (a) Transverse sections (original magnification ×10) across the back from vertebra prominens (above) to the sacrum point below. (b) The vertical line with numbers gives the calculated angle of trunk inclination (ATI) at each of the 10 sections in (a). Right humps are represented by short horizontal lines to the right, and left humps by short horizontal lines to the left. (c) The crosses (+) represent the black patches on spinous processes that have been identified by scanning; the parasagittal lines beside these crosses are separated by one-fifth of the distance between the vertebra prominens and the sacrum point; the angle of trunk inclination (ATI) is calculated for each of the 10 levels using several coordinates about these parasagittal lines; the estimated Cobb angle of 68° is given as lateral asymmetry (LA) index. (d) Sagittal and parasagittal graphic displays of the back showing kyphosis and lordosis, in millimetres, from the plane of the vertical line joining C7 to the sacrum point. 'Rotn' refers to the correction by ISIS of the rotational stance of the patient; 'tilt' refers to the correction by ISIS of the 'flexion' of the patient, which makes the line between the vertebra prominens and the sacrum point vertical (see text).

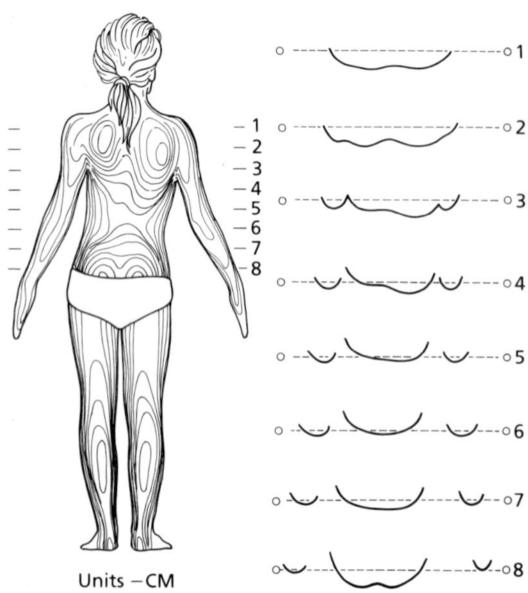

Fig. 9.22 Stereogrammetry. Contour map and profiles of a patient with scoliosis in the standard standing position. Reproduced by kind permission of Mr Hugg and the American Society of Photogrammetry, see Burwell (1978).

A computer imaging system currently under development at Liverpool University and Liverpool Polytechnic uses a structured light technique. A 35 mm slide ruled with a coarse grating is mounted in a conventional 35 mm slide projector. The patient stands in front of a dark screen and the grating is projected onto the surface of the back, upon which a fringe pattern is generated. The back surface is viewed by a CCD video camera mounted horizontally at a predetermined distance from the back surface and a fixed distance below the projector. The camera acquires an image of the back surface in a single frame cycle (1/50 s) using a frame grab/store device and is transferred to a microcomputer for processing. Image processing algorithms are used in the computer program to extract three-dimensional information by comparing the location of fringes on the patient's back with the position of the same fringes projected onto a suitable reference plane. The processing takes 17 s to create reconstructions of the trunk surface (Fig. 9.24, Dangerfield *et al.*, 1990).

Phase measuring profilometry (PMP) is an accurate

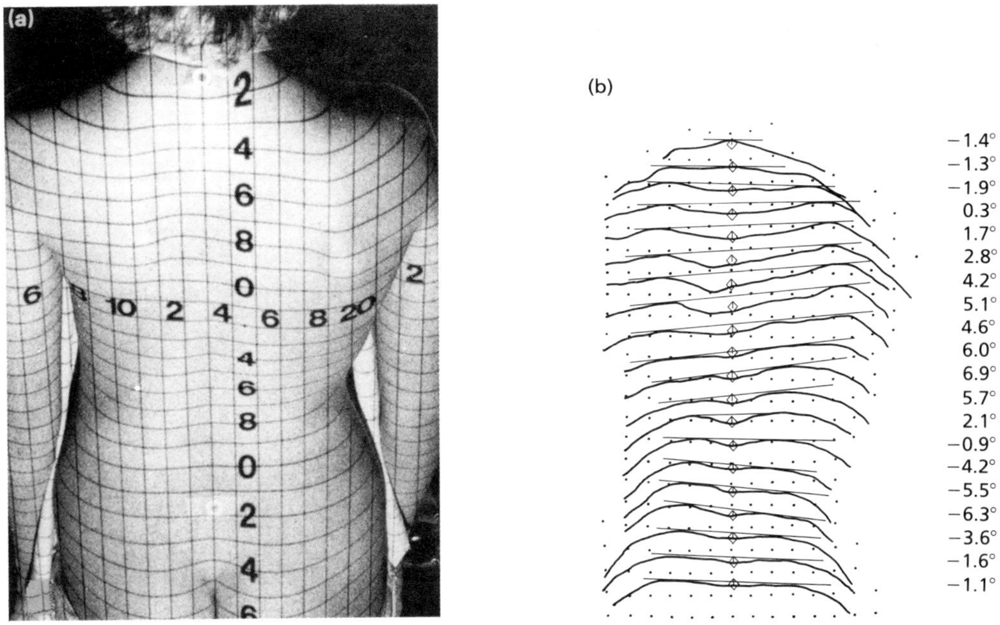

Fig. 9.23 (a) Projected raster photograph of a patient with scoliosis. Projected grid intersections were digitized for computerized analysis to give the three-dimensional coordinates of each point. (b) Subsequently, by interpolation, cross-sections at 20 levels of the back surface were calculated. The angle of the double tangent drawn across the right and left sides of each cross-section was measured as the 'back surface axial rotation'. Reproduced by kind permission of Dr I. A. F. Stokes and Dr M. S. Moreland and the editor of *Spine*.

method for measuring body surface shape using precision optical components and high-speed expensive computer image processing (Halioua *et al.*, 1990).

METHODS USING LIGHT-REFLECTIVE MARKERS

Automatic scoliosis analysis (AUSCAN)

This is a non-invasive system which computes the coordinates in real time of a series of light-reflective markers placed on a subject's back including spinous processes. Developed at the Centre of Bioengineering, Milan, it is considered to be a sensitive and reliable method for assessing the shape of the back and spine (Assente *et al.*, 1987). Further development has enhanced the original system by using four CCD cameras, which allows the computation of three-dimensional information relating to the patient's back. The clinical application has included an investigation of the effects of brace treatment on the progression of scoliosis.

The optronic torso graph (OTG)

This has been used to measure trunk shape in scoliosis patients. It uses 10 light-emitting diodes spaced 10 mm apart on the trunk, and a line sensor camera (Dawson *et al.*, 1989). The light projection system and the camera are rotated about the subject circumferentially in 5 s. Cross-sectional topography at 10 levels is obtained simultaneously and stored in a microcomputer.

Loughborough anthropometric shadow scanner (LASS)

In this method the subject is placed on a turntable and rotated through 360°. Four narrow strips of light are projected from four banks of four special light sources to fall on the body in vertical planes. These planes are arranged to pass through the centre of rotation of the turntable. The whole scene is viewed by banks of seven television cameras interfaced to a computer. The computer is programmed to show the information graphically and a permanent record is obtained by printing out the displayed information. LASS, to date, has been used in computer-aided design (CAD) for textile manufacturing, and in selected medical fields. It has potential application to the deformity of scoliosis.

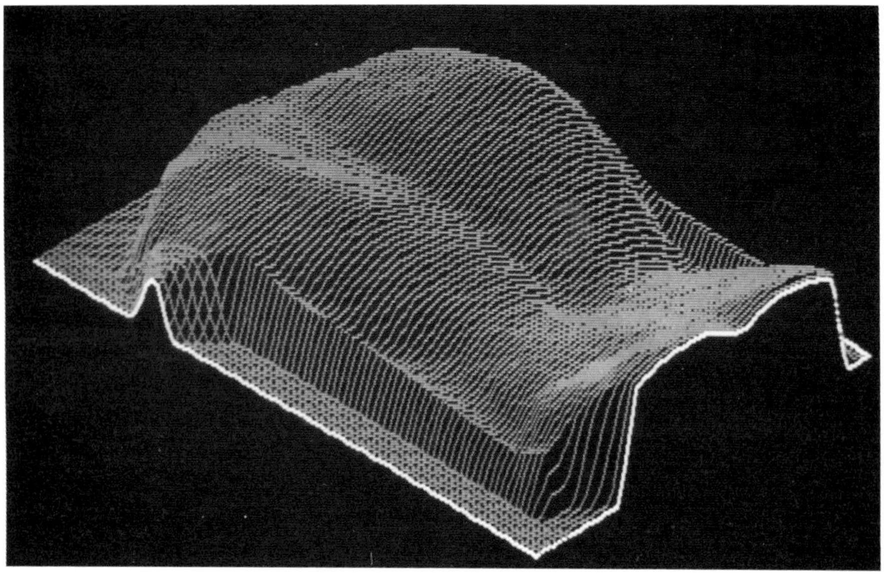

Fig. 9.24 A computer-generated reconstruction of a scoliotic back. From Dangerfield *et al.* (1990).

Lateral spinal curvatures

Schulthess (1905), initially practising before the discovery of X-rays, measured the severity of the lateral spinal curve using a tracing instrument on the body surface (scoliosometer), which also recorded back humps, sagittal curves, and trunk cross-sections (Fig. 9.3).

INTEGRATED SHAPE INVESTIGATION SYSTEM (Figs 9.19–9.21)

ISIS was devised to provide an optical method for recording the lateral spinal curvature. Since a scoliotic vertebra rotates about a posterior axis (at the posterior longitudinal ligament), the lateral spinal curve measured radiologically at the vertebral bodies (Cobb angle) is greater than that measured at the tips of the spinous processes. Hence, the ISIS software corrects the surface spinal curvature (marked by adhesive black patches) by a factor relating to the severity of the back hump; this calculated lateral spinal curvature is termed the 'lateral asymmetry index' (LAI)—so termed because it provides the best correlation with Cobb angle (Turner-Smith *et al.*, 1988).

Turner-Smith & Harris (1986) give the correlation (r) between LAI and Cobb angle to be 0.82 for thoracic idiopathic scoliosis. Johnson *et al.* (1987) scanned the backs four times of 50 patients with idiopathic scoliosis. Cobb angle and vertebral rotation were measured from standing films obtained on the same day. The correlation between LAI and Cobb angle was good for major curves (r = 0.70). Green *et al.* (1987), examining 150 patients with adolescent idiopathic scoliosis, concluded that ISIS is an accurate method for assessing Cobb angles, but not so for curves less than 20°. Harrison & Bettany (1991) have described a footplate to fit into the ISIS position frame to reduce errors caused by variations in the patient's position between scans. It is claimed that both pelvic tilt and rotation are more effectively controlled.

MOIRÉ PHOTOGRAPHY

Benoni *et al.* (1987) compared ISIS with moiré photography for the surface lateral spinal curvature. They write:

> The ISIS method gives a good estimation of the main curve in cases of unoperated scoliosis. Much of the result is expressed in figures which easily can be compared from time to time. However, in some cases the secondary curve is not adequately registered. Unless polaroid photos are used, the Moiré method does not immediately present the results. The information contained in a Moiré picture is more difficult to extract and to reproduce in figures. In this study the correlation between the Moiré

asymmetry and the X-ray findings seems much less than the figures that ISIS gives.

RASTER STEREOGRAPHY

Hierholzer & Drerup (1990) show that their computerized back shape analysis based on raster stereographic surface measurement enables a three-dimensional reconstruction of the spinal midline without the need for manual interaction. In more than 95% of the cases studied the deviation of the results from the corresponding frontal radiographs is in the same order of accuracy as measuring the Cobb angle. Further improvements seem possible by using more sophisticated shape analysis.

OPTRONIC TORSOGRAPH

Dawson *et al.* (1989) have reported a significant correlation between Cobb angle and their 'Torsograph angle'.

Sagittal spinal curvatures

Kyphosis and lordosis angles are usually measured from radiographs obtained in a standing position.

METHODS

In recent years, several workers have described the methods to record the sagittal spinal shape on the surface of the patient (Horst, 1983; Öhlén *et al.*, 1988) which include: profile photography (Towns & Roche, 1968); pegs pushed against the spine (spondylometer, Goff & Rose, 1964); plumb line (Fig. 9.25, Horst, 1983); back-measurer (Das Rückenmessgerät, Neugebauer, 1970); pantograph (Fig. 9.26, Willner, 1983); flexicurve (Milne & Lauder, 1976; Burton & Tillotson, 1988); kyphometer (Fig. 9.27, Debrunner, 1972; Lowden, 1984; Lowden *et al.*, 1986; Dangerfield & Denton, 1986; Dangerfield *et al.*, 1987a,b; Öhlén *et al.*, 1988); moiré photography and profile-measuring device (Suzuki *et al.*, 1981, 1986; Shinoto *et al.*, 1987); ISIS (Figs 9.19–9.21, Nicholson *et al.*, 1987; Carr *et al.*, 1989a, 1991a); raster stereography (Fig. 9.23, Stokes & Moreland, 1987); goniometers (Fig. 9.29, Mellin, 1987); electrogoniometer (Adams *et al.*, 1986).

Vercauteren & Goossens (1986) distinguished three surface *segments* of the sagittal spine profile—upper proclive, declive and lower proclive (Fig. 9.28).

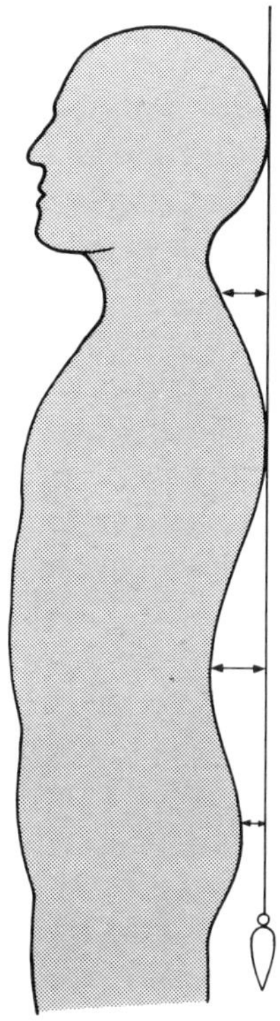

Fig. 9.25 Sagittal spinal curves—plumb line method used by Stagnara. Reproduced by kind permission of Dr M. Horst and the editors, *Moiré Fringe Topography and Spinal Deformity* (1983).

The kyphosis angle is a compound measure of sagittal back shape (declive angle plus upper proclive angle). The latter do not correlate significantly. Likewise, the lordosis angle is a compound measure of sagittal back shape (declive angle plus lower proclive angle) (see Burwell, 1990a; Burwell *et al.*, 1990b).

The surface declive angle at T11–T12 in school screening referrals was flatter in children with the largest spinal curves than in those with the smallest spinal curves (less than 10°) or straight spines (Burwell, 1990a; Burwell *et al.*, 1990b) (Fig. 9.29). The measurement of the surface declive angle with a Myrin goniometer might eliminate referral to hospital of those children with large humps, large declive angles and straight spines.

Finally, Bryant *et al.* (1989) have reported a method by which the location of vertebral bodies can be estimated from the external profile of the spine in the sagittal plane.

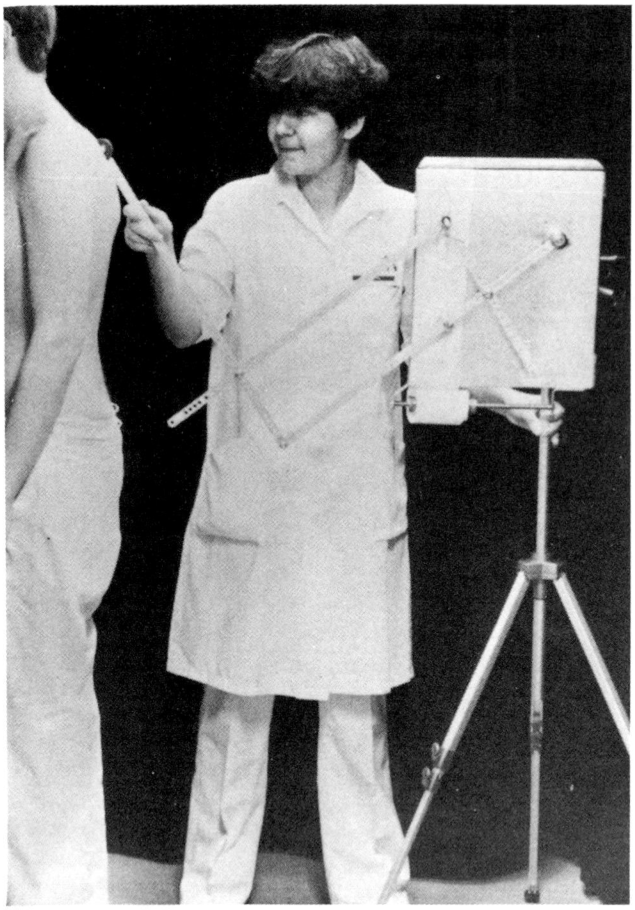

Fig. 9.26 The spinal pantograph. Reproduced by kind permission of Dr S. Willner and the editor of *Acta Paediatrica Scandinavica*.

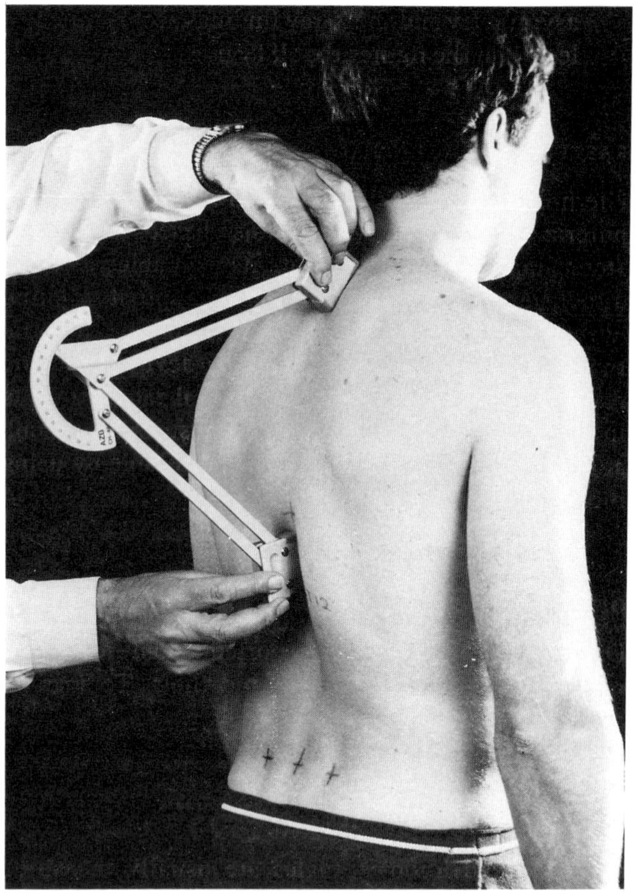

Fig. 9.27 Debrunner's kyphometer being used to measure kyphosis.

Ultrasound examination of the back in spinal deformity

Ultrasound techniques provide X-radiation-free methods for imaging the spine. As a result, ultrasound is currently finding applications in the investigation of spinal problems.

COMPUTERIZED ULTRASONIC MEASUREMENT OF LATERAL SPINAL CURVATURES

Letts *et al.* (1988) developed a simple procedure for identifying and documenting lateral spinal curvature during the performance of the Adams forward bending test, using an ultrasonic sound probe, four sound receivers and a microcomputer. The probe is run along the spinous processes emitting an ultrasonic sound, which is picked up by four receivers mounted

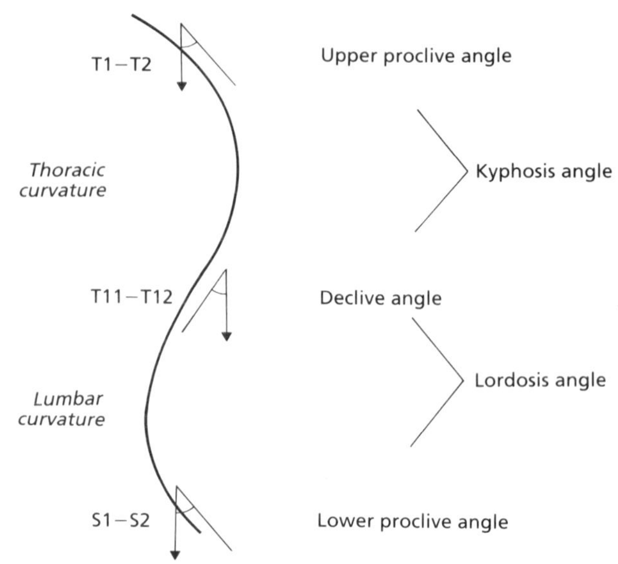

Fig. 9.28 Sagittal back shape angles (see text).

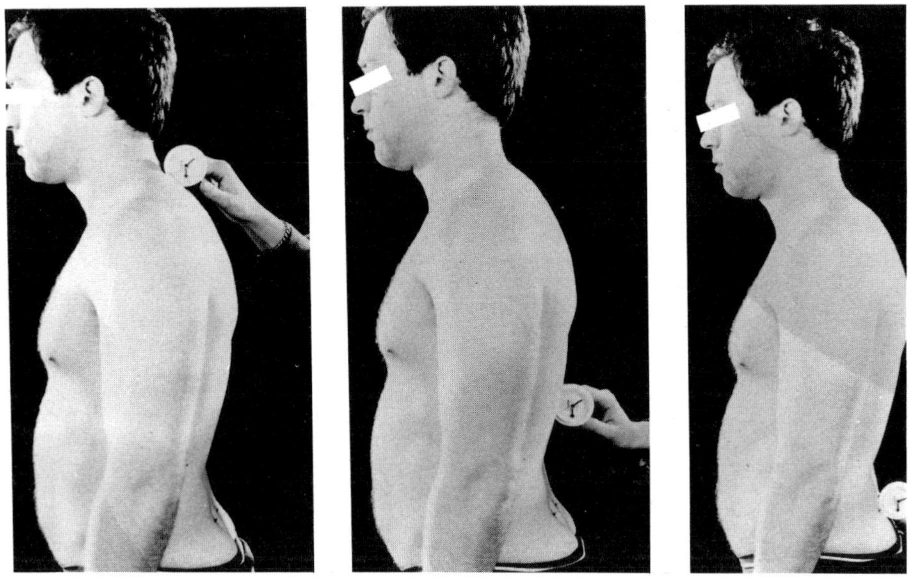

Fig. 9.29 A Myrin goniometer being used to measure: upper proclive angle (left); declive angle at T11–T12 (middle); and lower proclive (sacral tilt) angle (right).

at the corners of a rectangle above the patient. The signal is fed into a microcomputer and the spinal curvature is plotted out. The magnitude of the curve is calculated by the computer, and the actual curve plus the magnitude is printed in hard copy. The reproducibility error and intermeasurer error is less than 5%. Thirty patients with varying magnitudes of scoliosis from 15° to 73° were examined. The results of the ultrasonic digitization were compared with standard scoliosis radiographs of the patient. The average curvature measured from the radiographs was 38°, and from the ultrasonic digitization technique, 30°. The forward bending position contributed to smaller curvature measurement, and measurement in the standing position was thought to be a better technique. Ultrasonic digitization as a method of curve measurement is most accurate in curves over 30°.

THREE-LINEAR ARRAY BACK-SCANNING WITH AIRBORNE ULTRASOUND (ATLAS)

This imaging system uses an airborne ultrasound pulse which is transmitted from an ultrasound transducer directed towards the back of a patient (Mauritzson *et al.*, 1986). The time taken by the sound waves to travel from the transducer to the patient is proportional to the distance. This enables a spinal profile to be obtained if a number of transducers are placed over the back of the patient. The ATLAS system was developed for the screening of schoolchildren for scoliosis; it was considered it could quickly scan the backs of children to detect minor degrees of asymmetry if present.

ULTRASONIC TOPOMETRY

This ultrasound topometric method uses a series of transmitters attached to the back of the patient (Schumpe & Messler, 1987). Four permanently sited receivers are used to measure the transit time of sound waves passing from the transmitters to the receivers. These data have been used to construct cross-sectional profiles of the back and also the dynamic measurement of points on the back while the patient is walking.

B-MODE SCANNING METHODS

Lumbar spinal canal

A B-mode scanner was used by Porter *et al.* (1978) to measure the diameter of the lumbar spinal canal.

Vertebral rotation in scoliosis

Suzuki *et al.* (1989) used a linear B-scanner to measure vertebral rotation in 47 patients with idiopathic scoliosis. There was a strong correlation between the Cobb angle and the rotation of the apical

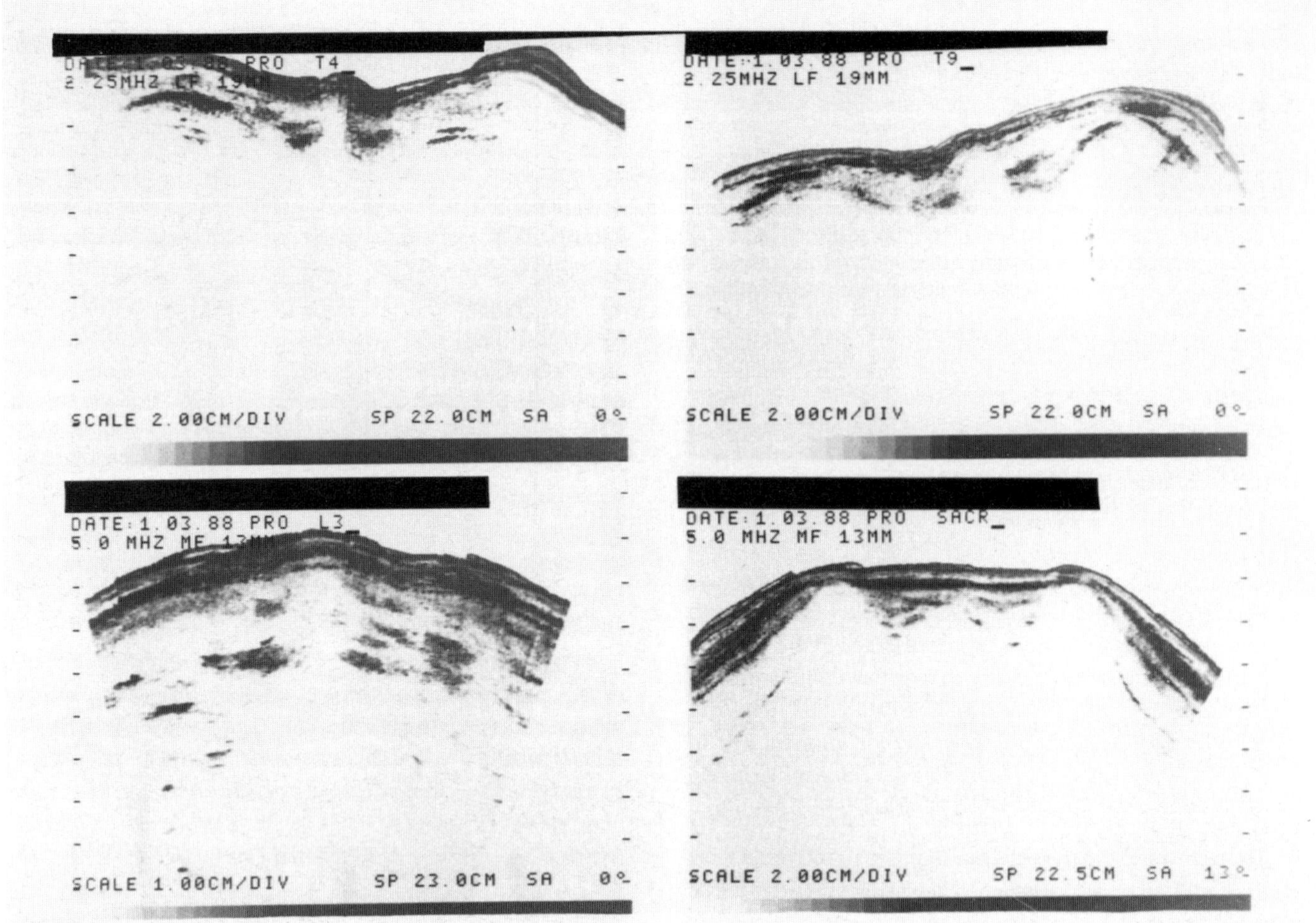

Fig. 9.30 Ultrasonographs of a patient with idiopathic scoliosis (right thoracic curve of 56°) lying prone (T4, T9, L3 and pelvis). Reproduced from Wojcik *et al.* (1990) and by kind permission of the editors of the *Symposium on Surface Topography and Spinal Deformity*.

vertebra in untreated patients; this relationship was lost in patients who had had brace treatment. They concluded that vertebral rotation can easily be measured by ultrasound: it is a harmless and fairly rapid investigation which can be used at the routine follow-up examination of patients with idiopathic scoliosis.

Wojcik *et al.* (1990) reported a new B-mode ultrasound method for measuring the rotational structural deformity of the scoliotic spine using ultrasound (Figs 9.30 & 9.31). The reliability of the method was evaluated on a dissected cadaveric trunk (spine, pelvis and ribs) and on 13 patients with adolescent idiopathic scoliosis. The ultrasound spinal torsion correlated with each of pedicular and spinous process rotation at three spinal levels (33 patients each lying prone). Prone spinal torsion correlated with standing spinal torsion. The ultrasound method of measuring vertebral rotation (spinal torsion) was considered to be of clinical value.

The principle of the ultrasound method of Wojcik *et al.* (1990) for measuring vertebral rotation (spinal torsion) is now being used to measure the rib hump (rib torsion) in patients with scoliosis (Fig. 9.32, Whitwell, 1991).

Kiel *et al.* (1990) used a B-mode scanner to image the sagittal spinal curves and declive angle in healthy children (Fig. 9.33).

REAL-TIME ULTRASOUND METHODS

Real-time linear array ultrasound scanners permit the identification of the laminae of the spinal column as echoes on either side of the shadow cast by the

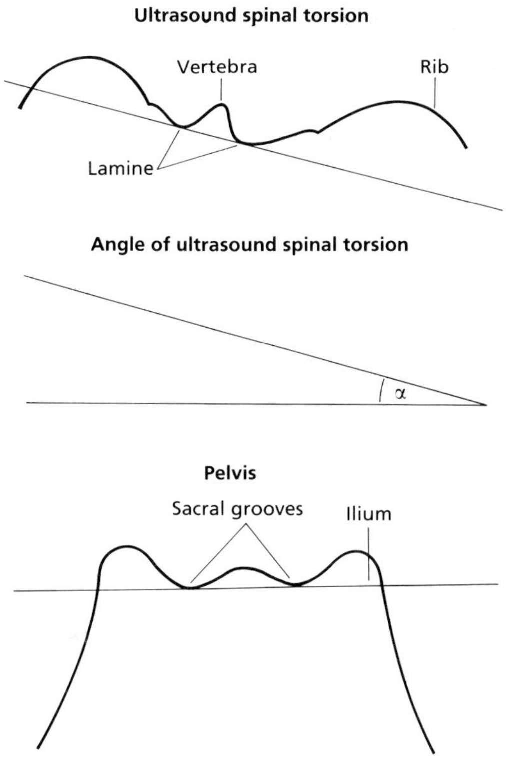

Fig. 9.31 Diagram to show method of calculating angle of ultrasound spinal torsion (see text).

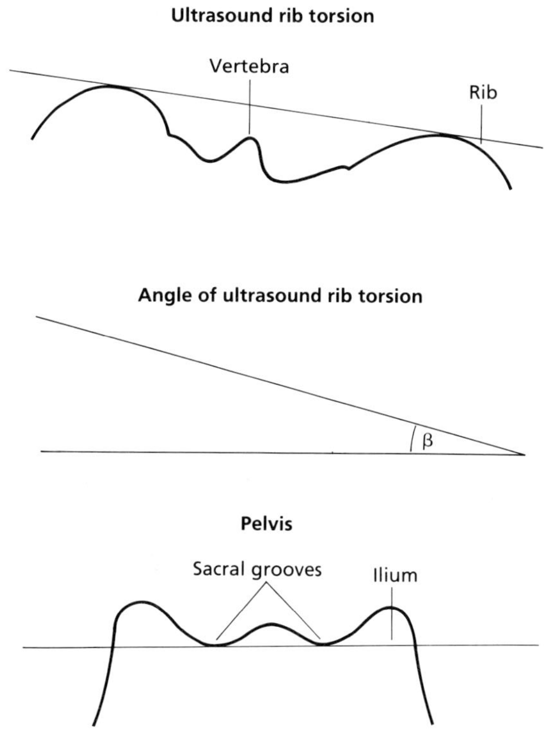

Fig. 9.32 Diagram to show method of calculating angle of ultrasound rib torsion (see text).

spinous process (Oates *et al.*, 1990). The resulting images can then be used to reconstruct a series of images of the spine in the lateral and anteroposterior views.

Real-time ultrasound imaging has also been used to examine spinal movements in fetal and postnatal life (Teot *et al.*, 1989). In adolescent scoliosis caused by syringomyelia, CSF flow dynamics at the foramen magnum of a Chiari I malformation has been demonstrated by colour doppler imaging during posterior fossa decompression, enabling the surgeon to know when sufficient bone has been removed (Jaspan *et al.*, 1991).

SOME FINDINGS ON BACK SHAPE IN HEALTH AND DEFORMITY

Back contour asymmetry in healthy children

School screening for scoliosis continued for many years using the forward bending test without any knowledge of normality with respect to rib and lumbar humps (Burwell *et al.*, 1981). Moreover, the way in which leg-length inequality affects back shape in the forward bending position was not fully understood.

In the early 1980s several papers reported on back contour asymmetry in healthy schoolchildren—in Japan, Belgium, Britain and Sweden (Takemitsu, 1981; Burwell *et al.*, 1983a; Willner, 1984; Vercauteren *et al.*, 1985). The findings are consistent, and show that about 25% of healthy children have a rib or lumbar hump.

CONSTITUTIONAL BACK CONTOUR ASYMMETRY AND CLINICAL LATERAL SPINAL CURVES (Fig. 9.34)

In 636 schoolchildren aged eight to 15 years, Burwell *et al.* (1983a) used the formulator body contour tracer to create standardized trunk asymmetry scores (TAS) at three spinal levels (T8, T12 and L3). Two groups of children were defined: those with clinically straight spines (585 children), and those with clinical evidence of lateral spinal curves (51 children). In the children with clinically straight spines the main findings were: about 1 : 4 had objec-

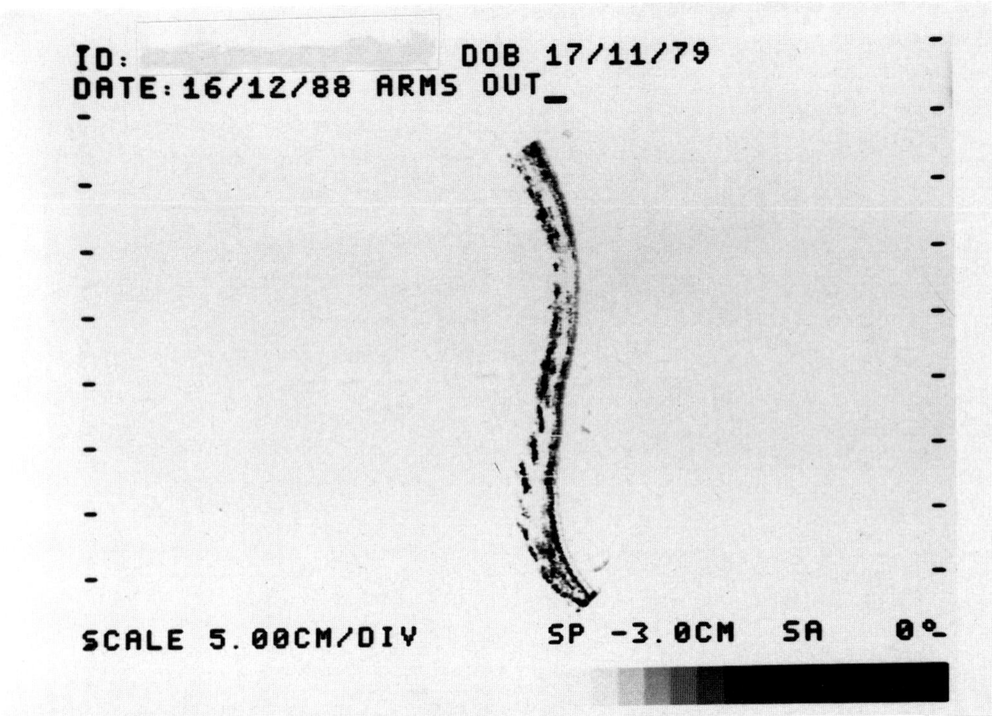

Fig. 9.33 Ultrasonograph of a healthy adolescent child to show sagittal spinal curves. From Kiel *et al.* (1990).

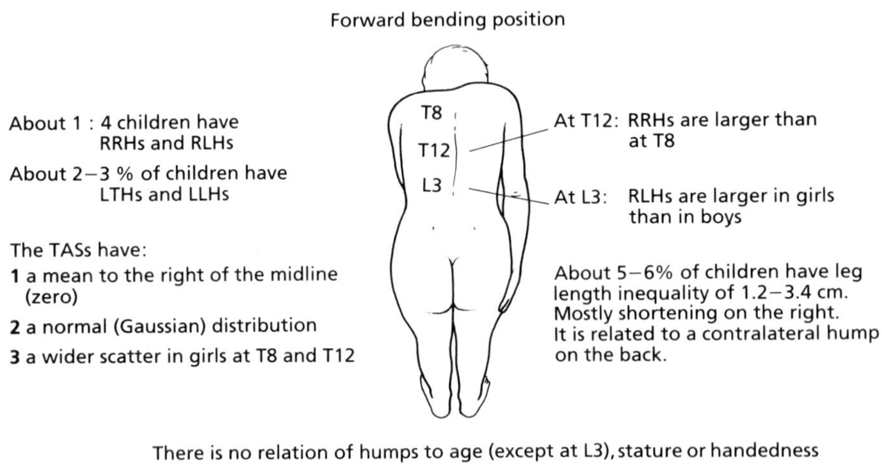

Fig. 9.34 Diagram to summarize the findings for back contour asymmetry in the standard forward bending position for the 585 children with clinically straight spines. TAS, trunk asymmetry score; R, right; L, left; RH, rib hump; LH, lumbar hump. Reproduced from Burwell *et al.* (1983a) and by kind permission of the editor, *Journal of Bone and Joint Surgery*.

tively detectable rib and lumbar humps; female/male ratios were 1.2 : 1 for the thoracic region and 1.4 : 1 for the lumbar region; right humps were about 10 times more common than left; a relationship between shortening of one lower limb and a contralateral hump on the back; and no relation to age (except at L3), stature (corrected for age) or handedness.

The use of the diagnostic label '*constitutional back contour asymmetry*' to describe normal back humps avoids the stigma—social, occupational or economic—which may result from using 'idiopathic scoliosis' as a diagnosis for a healthy schoolchild with a small non-progressive thoracic or lumbar back hump (Dangerfield *et al.*, 1991). Moreover, in constitutional back contour asymmetry, the side ratio of 10 : 1 for right/left thoracic humps is similar to the side ratio of 10 : 1 for idiopathic thoracic spinal curves. This association suggests the hypothesis that the side-pattern of back contour asymmetry in health influences the side-pattern of the idiopathic scoliotic deformity. The hypothesis also accounts for James's (1956) statement for paralytic scoliosis, 'An unexpected and unexplained finding is that, as with idiopathic thoracic curves, there is a predominance of curves to the right'.

SIGNIFICANCE FOR SCOLIOSIS SCREENING

In the light of this new knowledge on back shape in healthy schoolchildren, Burwell *et al.* (1981) wrote to the *Lancet* as follows:

> Our research has led us to conclude that this screening test is unsatisfactory because it has not been based on objective knowledge of the shape of the normal child's back. . . . We support the plea of Warren and his colleagues for a coordinated epidemiological and clinical approach with basic data collection.

Normal back shape data are essential for scientifically based screening programmes (British Scoliosis Society, 1987). More recently, a study of 5350 children aged 11–15 years in five centres in the UK has shown the mean thoracic ATI to be 0.6° for healthy boys and 0.8° for healthy girls as measured by a Scoliometer. There is no significant correlation of thoracic ATIs with age ($r = 0.05$, British Scoliosis Society, 1987). ISIS has been used to examine the backs of healthy schoolchildren and adults (Duff & Draper, 1987; Carr *et al.*, 1991b).

LARGE HUMP STRAIGHT SPINE SYNDROME

Two recent school screening studies have shown that some adolescent children have a large thoracic hump with a radiologically straight spine (British Scoliosis Society, 1987; Burwell *et al.*, 1990b).

Back contour asymmetry of adolescent idiopathic scoliosis

Having obtained data on back contour asymmetry for healthy schoolchildren, the next step was to prepare standard deviation charts of normality (Burwell *et al.*, 1983b; James, 1985). Because trunk asymmetry scores for normal children are site- and sex-specific, charts are needed separately by each level (T4, T8, T12, L3) and sex. Moreover, a method was devised for quantitating formulator contour tracings from the scoliotic back (Fig. 9.9).

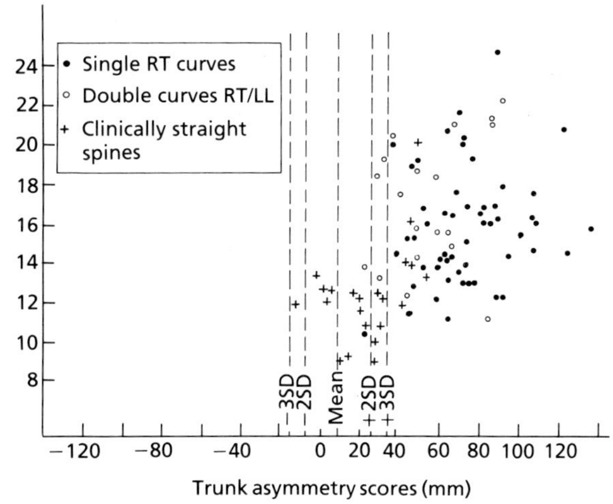

Fig. 9.35 TAS standard deviation chart for T8 prepared from normal girls. The vertical dotted lines represent the mean and standard deviations for the normal population; data are plotted as thoracic TAS for AIS females with single RT curves, and for the RT component of double curves, and also for females with clinically straight spines. TAS, trunk asymmetry score; RT, right thoracic; AIS, adolescent idiopathic scoliosis. From James (1985).

Figure 9.35 shows a TAS standard deviation chart for T8 prepared from normal girls. Data are plotted on this chart for girls with: thoracic AIS, thoracic hump of double-curve AIS, and clinically straight spines. The disadvantage of this method is that plots need to be viewed separately for each vertebral level. Accordingly we developed a chart of *maximum thoracic TAS plotted against maximum lumbar TAS (cruciate plot)*. Figure 9.36 shows such a plot of data from girls with: adolescent idiopathic scoliosis and clinically straight spines (James, 1985). Such a chart prepared from scoliometer ATI data could be valuable in screening for scoliosis by showing instantly where a child's back contour asymmetry lies in relation to normal limits.

The formulator: longitudinal studies of the natural history of infantile idiopathic scoliosis

Dangerfield & Denton (1986) reported longitudinal studies of back shape in 23 boys with infantile idiopathic scoliosis. Seventeen patients had had convex costoplasty and concave release. Six patients received plaster jacket treatment early in the course of the condition.

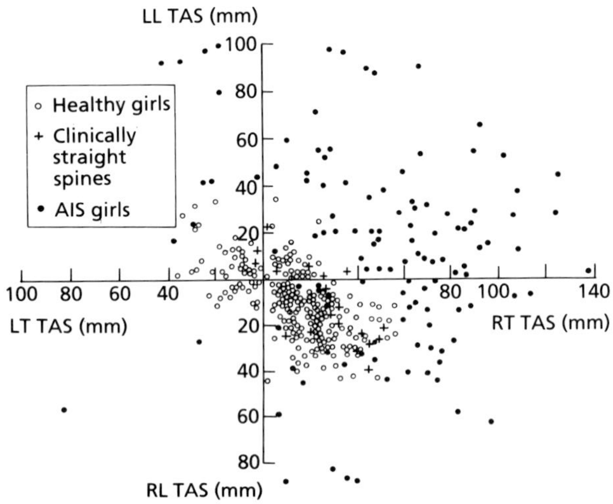

Fig. 9.36 Maximum thoracic TAS plotted against maximum lumbar TAS for normal girls aged 10–15 years, and for female AIS patients and females with clinically straight spines. From James (1985).

The scoliometer: its use in health, deformity and screening

We have used the scoliometer on healthy children in relation to screening, its reliability, in describing the deformity of scoliosis and most recently in treatment evaluation.

SINGLE ATI (Figs 9.11 & 9.12)

Bunnell (1984) recommended that the scoliometer be used to record the maximum ATI across the back of a child in a standing forward bending position; in screening, the ATI threshold for referral to hospital should be 5°. Recent work has shown that this threshold refers to hospital about 7% of the healthy adolescent school population (Burwell *et al.*, 1990b). The 5° ATI threshold is clearly too low; raising it will increase the number of false-negatives. The dilemma seems to have been overcome by using compound ATI recordings (see below).

ATI AT SEVERAL SPINAL LEVELS

The scoliometer (Mark 1) of Bunnell was used to measure the angle of trunk inclination (ATI) of 205 unselected schoolchildren aged 11–14 years as part of a longitudinal study of back contour asymmetry (Burwell *et al.*, 1986). The readings were obtained from each child by one observer. The child first *stood* in a standard forward bending position and recordings were made at each of five vertebral levels (T4, T8, T12, L3 and S2). The child then *sat* on a box (height 30 cm) in a standard forward bending position and the readings were repeated at the same vertebral levels. The sitting position was used in an attempt to eliminate the effect on back contour asymmetry of any leg-length inequality (Burwell *et al.*, 1983a). It was found that only one child in this sample had an ATI of more than 7.5° in the standing position; this was due to a short leg caused by a varus osteotomy on the hip for Perthes' disease. Additionally, in the Scoliosis Clinic, ATI values were measured in the forward bending position on 157 patients with adolescent idiopathic scoliosis (ages 10–24 years; James, 1985). None had had a surgical operation. ATI readings were again made at each of T4, T8, T12, L3 and S2 (and at the maximum ATI if different from these levels). The results showed 87% of the girls with AIS had a single ATI of 7.5° or more.

It was recommended that the scoliometer should be used in both the standing and sitting forward bending positions: two readings should be procured—thoracic and lumbar. This research in the community and clinic formed the basis of the Multicentre Study subsequently undertaken by the British Scoliosis Society (1987) using the OSI scoliometer.

COMPOUND ATI INCLUDING THORACOLUMBAR DIFFERENCE (TLD) TESTS (Figs 9.13 & 9.14)

The simplest compound ATI values are created by adding the ATI readings from two spinal levels (thoracic and lumbar, Burwell *et al.*, 1986; James, 1985).

The Multicentre Study of the British Scoliosis Society (1987) showed first that single ATI readings from a child's back of each of 7.5° and 10° have low predictive values (18–30%) for 20° curves; and secondly, that two new compound ATI measurements of back shape—involving thoracic and lumbar readings, provide better predictive values (56%). These compound ATI measurements are:

1 *The standing thoracolumbar difference test* (standing TLD = standing thoracic ATI plus opposite standing lumbar ATI, Fig. 9.13).

2 *The dynamic thoracolumbar difference test* (dynamic TLD = standing thoracic ATI plus opposite sitting lumbar ATI, Fig. 9.14).

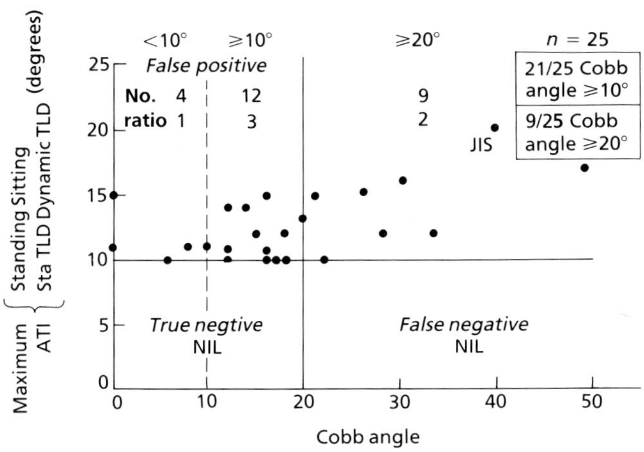

Fig. 9.37 School screening referrals: maximum ATI threshold of 10° more plotted against Cobb angle. Reproduced from Burwell *et al.* (1990b) and by kind permission of the editors of the *Symposium on Surface Topography and Spinal Deformity*.

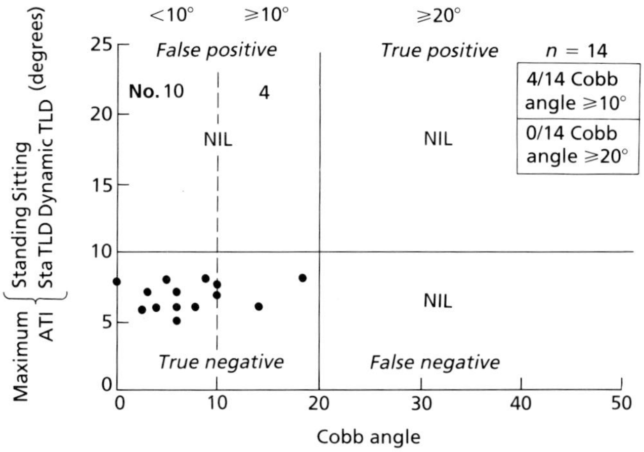

Fig. 9.38 School screening referrals: maximum ATI threshold less than 10° plotted against Cobb angle. From Burwell *et al.* (1990b).

The dynamic TLD test was noted because of previous research on the effect of forward flexion on back contour in patients with scoliosis (hump dynamics, Upadhyay *et al.*, 1987). It was concluded that the TLD tests need further evaluation in screening (British Scoliosis Society, 1987; Burwell, 1988).

MULTIPLE ATI (MATI) SYSTEM (Figs 9.37 & 9.38)

The next step in screening for scoliosis with the scoliometer was to use a combination of single ATIs at high thresholds (8–10°) and the TLD tests (termed the multiple ATI system). These tests were included in six criteria for referral of children to hospital (Burwell, 1990a; Burwell *et al.*, 1990b).

The study population of this School Screening Study in Nottingham was 4890 12-year-old school children. The referral rate was low (0.8%). The prevalence of idiopathic curves of 10° or more was 7.2/1000 girls and 1.7/1000 boys. Using the multiple ATI system at 10° thresholds there is a 60% risk of finding a Cobb angle of 15° or more (for 10° curves, sensitivity = 84%, specificity = 71%, positive predictive value = 84%).

Rationale

The challenge in practical screening for scoliosis is to achieve a low referral rate with a high prevalence of larger curves (20° or more), i.e. the best balance between false-positives and false-negatives. The multiple ATI system, by utilizing several tests, gives the child with back contour asymmetry more chances of being detected than with a single ATI reading. Moreover, the high ATI thresholds will reduce the number of false-positives, including children with minor leg-length inequality causing pelvic tilt scoliosis (Dickson, 1983). The otherwise inevitable increase in the number of false-negatives seems to be offset, at least in part, by using the TLD tests.

TEN-LEVEL ATI

The hump on the back of the child with scoliosis shows variation from above downwards (T1–S1) with considerable variation between individuals. In order to compare scoliometer findings with ISIS data, scoliometer readings were obtained at 10 levels on the back (Upadhyay *et al.*, 1987). When these results are plotted, a fair description is given of the back hump for research purposes (Figs 9.15 & 9.16; Wythers *et al.*, 1992); the 10-level ATI plots for the scoliometer and ISIS data are similar in the standing positions, but differ markedly in the sitting positions.

In appraising back shape after surgery for scoliosis, such back recordings are essential, because deformity often develops below and above the fused segments in hitherto undeformed regions of the back (Burwell *et al.*, 1992a; Wemyss-Holden *et al.*, 1992).

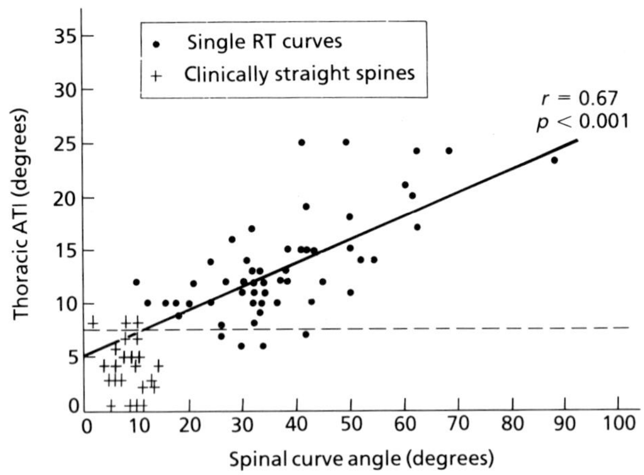

Fig. 9.39 Thoracic ATI plotted against spinal curve angle for single RT curves in female AIS patients and females with clinically straight spines. The horizontal dotted line represents a threshold for referral of 7.5° ATI. From Burwell *et al.* (1986); see James (1985).

CALCULATED SEGMENTAL ATI (Figs 9.15 & 9.16)

In order to establish which radiological features (e.g. vertebral rotation, tilt, displacement and sagittal inclination) are associated with the back contour asymmetry, it is necessary to calculate ATI values for each vertebral segment along the length of the spine. Wythers, who developed this method, studied 30 preoperative patients with adolescent thoracic scoliosis (AIS, apex T8–T9, Wythers *et al.*, 1992).

Using the calculated ATI data, Wythers *et al.* (1991) showed that different radiological features predicted the back deformity at the various vertebral levels. Such analyses are currently being used with other data to evaluate an aetiological concept for adolescent idiopathic scoliosis (Burwell *et al.*, 1992b; Chapter 19).

SEGMENTAL ATI

Most recently, Dangerfield *et al.* (1992) have recorded ATI values at each segmental level from C7 to S1. Radiological segmental data were also obtained and plotted.

Moiré photography: its use in health, deformity and screening

The moiré method has been adopted by some workers for the early detection of scoliosis in schools (Fig. 9.18; Willner, 1979; Suzuki *et al.*, 1981). In such screening, the greatest accuracy in predicting the spinal deformity is obtained at the apex of the curve. A major problem is the high number of false-positives. Sahlstrand (1986), studying children referred to hospital after screening, found no correlation between moiré asymmetry and the Cobb angle. Willner (1984) states that asymmetry of two or more fringes is found in 0.6% of boys and 0.9% of girls. He does not give his referral rate. According to Willner, X-ray examination of a child is indicated if two conditions are fulfilled: (a) asymmetry of two or more fringes on the moiré photograph; and (b) a hump of 1 cm or more. In such children there is a 50% risk of finding a lateral curve of 15° or more (cf. multiple ATI (MATI) system above).

Relation of back humps to radiological deformity in idiopathic scoliosis

FINDINGS FOR UNTREATED PATIENTS

Hump-meter, formulator, moiré and scoliometer findings

Several workers have shown that in idiopathic thoracic scoliosis with severe and moderately severe curves, the thoracic hump correlates with the Cobb angle and apical vertebral rotation (Figs 9.39 & 9.40; see Willner, 1979; Burwell *et al.*, 1983b; Dangerfield *et al.*, 1987b). In double curves the correlation between thoracic hump and radiological deformity is less strong ($r = 0.50$; Burwell *et al.*, 1983b; James, 1985). In children referred after school screening for scoliosis the thoracic (or lumbar) hump severity is a poor predictor of Cobb angle ($r = 0.36$; see Sahlstrand, 1986; British Scoliosis Society, 1987; Stokes, 1989).

Using moiré photographs, Stokes *et al.* (1985) examined a population of 950 patients, attempting to find relationships between measurements of the asymmetry of moiré photographs and the value of the Cobb angle. No good predictive relationships were found. The best correlation was among measurements of 95 patients with midthoracic scolioses where a correlation coefficient (r) of 0.71 was found. A number of characteristic patterns in the moiré photographs were noted which were associated with the level, size and magnitude of each scoliotic curve. A randomized, blind trial involving five observers was devised in order to assess the capability of this

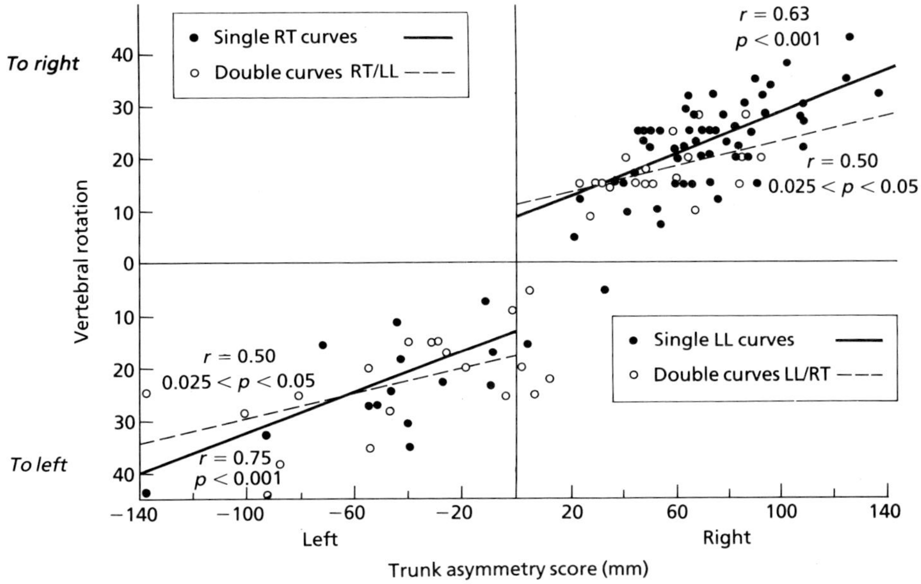

Fig. 9.40 Thoracic or lumbar TAS plotted against vertebral rotation for: single RT curves, RT component of double curves (RT/LL), single LL curves, LL component of double curves (LL/RT) in female AIS patients. From James (1985).

pattern-recognition scheme of diagnosing curve types based on the appearance of the moiré photographs. This study demonstrated that high predictive values could be achieved for assessing the presence, the side and the anatomical region of a scoliotic deformity in a moiré photograph alone, but the ability to assess the magnitude of the deformity was considerably less accurate. These findings highlighted the need for a better measurement of spine shape in three dimensions.

ISIS findings

Using ISIS, it has been found that the maximum skin surface angle has a low correlation with the apical vertebral rotation (Turner-Smith *et al.*, 1988). Recent work on adolescents with thoracic scoliosis has shown that certain preoperative surface and radiological features predict the segmental surface deformity one year after surgery (ISIS and scoliometer data. Wythers *et al.*, 1992; Wemyss-Holden *et al.*, 1992).

Raster stereography

Stokes & Moreland (1989) evaluated the relation of surface hump (moiré and raster stereography) to Cobb angle in 104 patients with mainly single and double idiopathic curves (mean Cobb angle 25°). They concluded that the presence, level, and side of a scoliosis curvature is well demonstrated by back-surface topography in patients with 'standard' rotation; but the magnitude of the scoliosis cannot be determined from topograms sufficiently accurately for most clinical purposes. Stokes (1989) also studied, in 40 patients with idiopathic scoliosis, the relation of surface hump (raster stereography) to skeletal rotations calculated from stereoradiographs of the spine and rib cage. It was found that the rib cage rotation was generally of lesser magnitude than the vertebral rotation; also the back surface rotation was less than both of these skeletal rotations.

Hierholzer & Drerup (1990) used raster stereographs to reconstruct three-dimensionally the spinal midline in patients with scoliosis (Cobb angles up to 52°, $n = 114$). Comparison with radiographs obtained on the same day as the raster stereographs shows that the spinal midline can be reconstructed with an average lateral error of 4.6 mm (the sagittal error could not be determined due to the lack of lateral radiographs). Vertebral rotation was estimated from the surface rotation at the locus of the symmetry line with an average error of 3.1° (compared with vertebral rotation measured by a computer analysis of the corresponding radiographs).

Raso *et al.* (1987) reported a method for combining the internal configuration of the spine obtained from AP and lateral radiographs with surface data from moiré photographs.

Clearly, the relation of the surface deformity (as measured by the hump-meter, formulator, moiré photography, scoliometer, ISIS and raster stereography) to the radiological deformity needs further evaluation.

FINDINGS FOR UNTREATED PATIENTS DURING FOLLOW-UP

Green *et al.* (1987) examined 150 patients with adolescent idiopathic scoliosis followed up for at least six months. They concluded that ISIS is an accurate method for predicting curve change in a known and previously evaluated patient.

In contrast, Stokes *et al.* (1988) examined 35 patients with scoliosis by Cobb radiography and back-surface photogrammetry on each of at least two clinic visits. Each pair of patient visits was classified as showing either a progression, improvement, or no change in the scoliosis using a threshold of 5° change in the Cobb angle. The computer Cobb measurement was the most precise measurement, and the back-surface measurements were the least precise. The Cobb measurement of scoliosis is the most precise for detecting small changes, but can be improved by a computerized analysis of digitized radiographs.

Sagittal spinal curves in idiopathic scoliosis and Scheuermann's disease

Using the spinal pantograph, Willner (1983) showed a diminished kyphosis in idiopathic scoliosis ($n = 15$) and an increased kyphosis in Scheuermann's disease ($n = 16$). The lordosis angle was not significantly different in scoliotics compared with controls; but the lordosis was larger in thoracic Scheuermann's disease than in controls (cf. Carr *et al.*, 1989a).

The kyphometer was used by Lowden (1984) to measure kyphosis and lordosis in 29 girls with adolescent idiopathic scoliosis (AIS). Again the kyphosis, but not the lordosis, was diminished compared with healthy girls. Dangerfield *et al.* (1987a) used the kyphometer to measure kyphosis and lordosis in 170 children with various types of scoliosis. The kyphometer was better at measuring kyphosis ($r = 0.93$) than lordosis ($r = 0.60$). Öhlén *et al.* (1988), using the kyphometer, examined 99 patients with thoracic curves and found the kyphosis and lordosis to be significantly less than that of the controls. Neither the kyphosis nor the lordosis correlated with the Cobb angle. Even patients with small curves had straight spines in the sagittal plane: there was no tendency for the kyphosis and lordosis to decrease when the scoliotic deformity increased. These findings which have aetiological significance for AIS are considered in Chapter 19.

Dangerfield *et al.* (1991) used the kyphometer to measure the kyphosis and lordosis angles (and rib hump) in parents of scoliotic children without finding any familial association. This latter finding does not support Archer & Dickson's (1985) statement that the sagittal shape of the spine is genetically determined, with 'flat-backed' children coming from flat-backed families and 'round-backed' children coming from round-backed families. However, the declive angles (at T11–T12) of school screening referrals and their siblings do correlate significantly (Burwell *et al.*, 1990a; see Carr *et al.*, 1991).

Carr *et al.* (1989a) used ISIS and X-radiation to measure the thoracic kyphosis angles of 16 normal individuals, 10 patients with Scheuermann's disease and 11 with adolescent idiopathic scoliosis. There was a high correlation between the two methods.

EVALUATION OF BACK SHAPE IN TREATMENT

Braces

FORMULATOR BODY CONTOUR TRACER

Thulbourne & Gillespie (1976) examined 37 patients with idiopathic scoliosis treated by Milwaukee brace. The findings showed that, in general, the rib hump on the convexity remained fairly constant; in contrast the rib depression on the concavity gradually became less noticeable until finally it was reversed (Fig. 9.41). This change occurred without change in lateral curvature and with no significant difference in vertebral rotation.

MOIRÉ PHOTOGRAPHY

Benoni & Willner (1986) evaluated 30 patients with idiopathic scoliosis, all treated with braces. The difference between the moiré patterns before and after

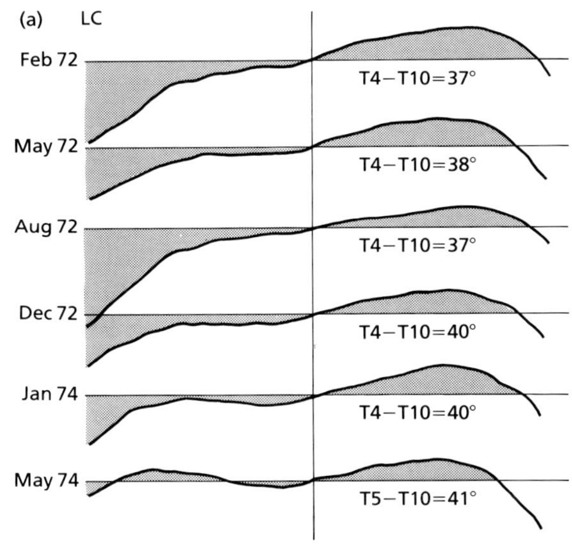

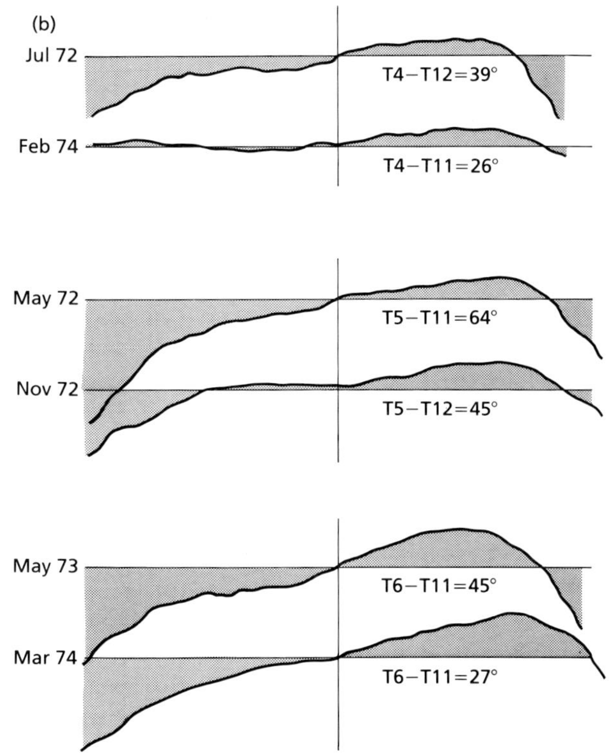

Fig. 9.41 *Left*: formulator body contour tracings in a patient during treatment in a Milwaukee brace. Note the almost unchanged rib hump but marked improvement in rib depression. *Right*: in three patients after Harrington instrumentation. Note the improvement in rib depression but little change in the hump. Reproduced by kind permission of Dr T. Thulbourne, Dr R. Gillespie and editor, *Journal of Bone and Joint Surgery*.

treatment was small. Above the shoulders the asymmetry increased by 3%. The asymmetry lateral to the shoulders decreased by 18% and below the shoulders by 11%. The angle below the shoulders decreased by 10%. None of these differences was statistically significant.

Shinoto *et al.* (1987) used moiré photography to evaluate the back shape of 100 patients treated with a Milwaukee brace (MB), Boston brace (BB) or Boston–Milwaukee brace (BMB) for more than two years. They concluded that correction of surface deformity is affected by brace treatment. After MB and BMB treatment there was a tendency for both the thoracic kyphosis and lumbar lordosis to decrease. After BB, the lumbar lordosis was slightly increased.

ISIS

Jefferson *et al.* (1990) reported 32 AIS patients treated with a Boston brace for at least six months and assessed both radiologically and by ISIS (follow-up 16 months). Surface measurements of lateral curvature improved in 41% of the patients whereas radiological improvement occurred in only 9%. The implication was that the brace, by continuous pressure, affected the surface shape of the back, although the underlying lateral spinal curvature was less affected. Transverse measurements of asymmetry improved in between 16% and 25% of patients depending on the ISIS parameter chosen for assessment. The brace appeared to reduce the rib prominence by dispersing it over a longer length of the back. Over half of the patients showed some reduction in kyphosis after wearing the brace (Carr *et al.*, 1989a); but increase or decrease in kyphosis did not have any bearing on the patients' outcome in terms of curve progression.

Tredwell & Bannon (1988) documented curve progression in 34 adolescent female patients with right thoracic idiopathic scoliosis treated by bracing. They found that a weak positive correlation exists between the change by X-ray examination and the change by ISIS examination. It was concluded that the clinical usefulness of the ISIS method in braced patients has not been proven.

CHANGES IN BACK SHAPE ON REMOVING A BRACE

Fidler & Turner-Smith (1986) used ISIS to record the changes in back shape in a 14-year-old girl with ado-

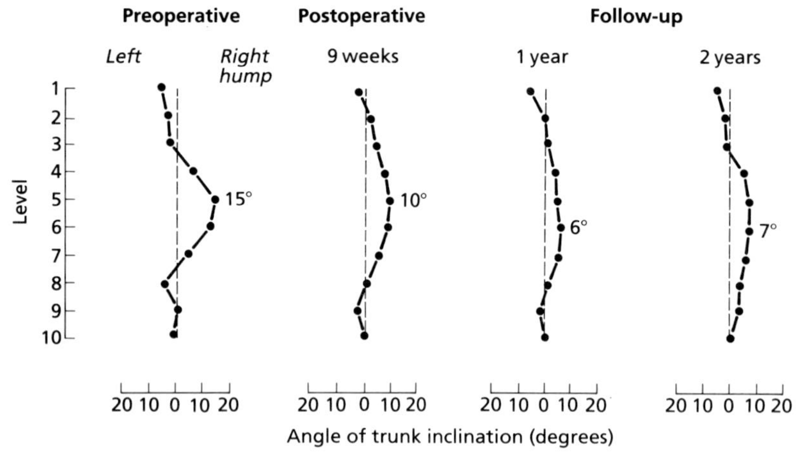

Fig. 9.42 Back shape before and after Cotrel–Dubousset instrumentation. Plots of 10-level ISIS ATI readings procured in the standing erect position. Note the good result. From Burwell *et al.* (1991).

lescent idiopathic scoliosis in the four days after the removal of a Cotrel brace.

Surgery

PREDICTIVE VALUE FOR SURGERY

Weisz *et al.* (1988) reported the value of ISIS scans for assessing progression in 51 patients with adolescent idiopathic scoliosis (mean follow-up more than two years). The mean Cobb angle initially was 35° (range 10° to 55°). ISIS correctly identified curve evolution in 84% of the patients. Eight patients having spinal instrumentation were correctly predicted as candidates for surgery. The writers concluded that ISIS scanning is a reliable and safe method for monitoring scoliosis. Moreover it may be used as a basis for treatment decisions (Fig. 9.42).

HARRINGTON, HARRINGTON–LUQUE (HL), LUQUE AND COTREL–DUBOUSSET (CD) INSTRUMENTATION

In Stockholm, Aaro & Öhlén (1983) examined the effect of Harrington instrumentation on the sagittal spinal curves using a kyphometer and a Myrin goniometer (96 scoliosis patients). After such surgery the mean lordosis angle was reduced to 38° for those fused down to T12; and to 16° for those fused to L5. The thoracic kyphosis angle increases as the top level of the fusion creeps down.

Weatherley *et al.* (1987) used the formulator body contour tracer to investigate changes in the rib hump after operative treatment for 47 patients with AIS by Harrington distraction rod and posterior fusion. Despite operative correction of the lateral curve, there was a progression of the rib deformity in 64% of the cases after four years.

Beaumont *et al.* (1989) reported a preliminary study of five patients who had had CD instrumentation for the correction of idiopathic thoracic scoliosis. Radiological data, ISIS measurement and the range of spinal movements were analysed both pre- and postoperatively with several new techniques. The patients (aged 12–17 years, follow-up maximum six months) showed good maintenance of correction when studied radiologically. However, the surface back shape deteriorated with the re-establishment of thoracic back contour asymmetry. In the lumbar region a hump developed, which has not been evident before operation, on the side of the original curvature. It was concluded that with CD, trunk asymmetry was improved but within three months the rib hump was increasing and a new lumbar asymmetry was forming. Burwell *et al.* (1992a) reported the continuation of this study with the patients examined one year after surgery (by ISIS and scoliometer at 10 levels, CD = 15 patients, HL = nine patients). After one year the mean maximal ATI (scoliometer) with CD was 21% improved and with HL 1% better (Figs 9.43 & 9.44). It was concluded that after CD the correction of the back hump is rarely complete, and may continue with extension distally and proximally in the trunk. Wemyss-Holden *et al.* (1992), continuing this follow-up of 37 patients having CD, concluded that the hump severity before operation is a factor predicting the surface deformity one year after surgery. Scoliometer data may be better predictors than ISIS data. After CD the surface and radiological findings

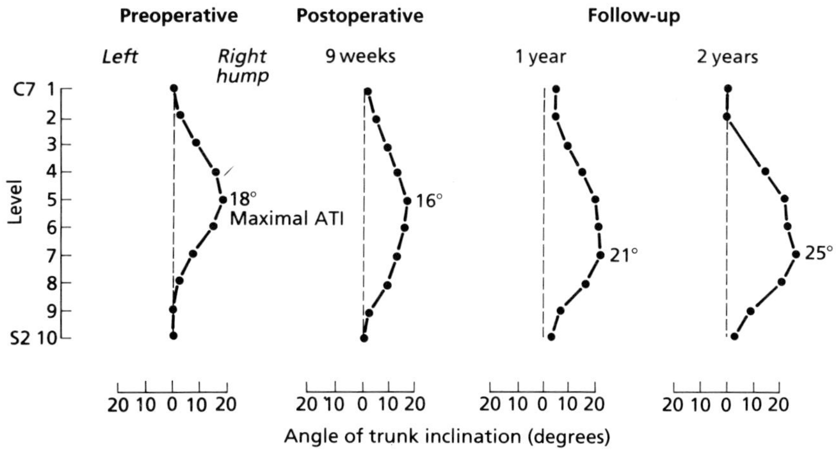

Fig. 9.43 Back shape before and after Cotrel–Dubousset instrumentation. Plots of 10-level scoliometer ATI readings procured in the standing forward bending position (Fig. 9.11). Note the progression of the hump. From Burwell *et al.* (1992a).

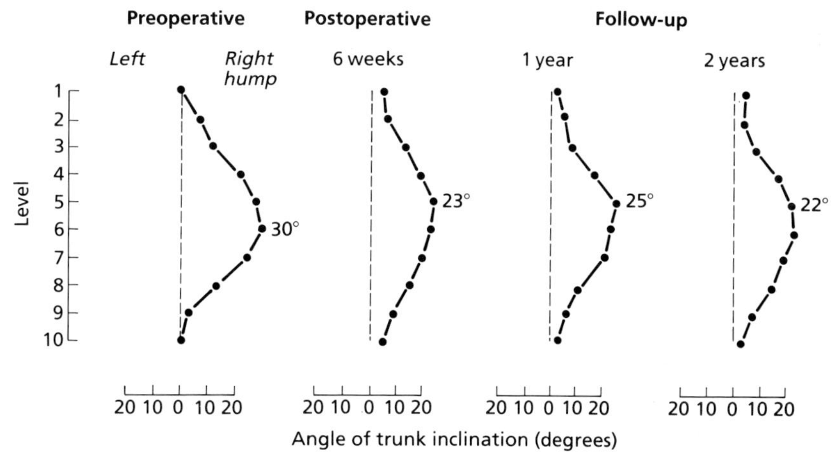

Fig. 9.44 Back shape before and after Harrington–Luque instrumentation. Plots of 10-level scoliometer ATI readings procured in the standing forward bending position (Fig. 9.11). Note that the hump is partly corrected by the operation and shows some distal progression in the trunk. From Burwell *et al.* (1992a).

show that the rib cage continues to deform around the fused spine which is held rigidly by the instrumentation. CD is a good method of treating patients with small scoliotic humps; but for patients with large surface deformities, other forms of treatment including anterior surgery may be more appropriate.

Bannon & Tredwell (1990) used ISIS to study back shape after CD in 37 patients (average follow-up, 122 days). In their Abstract (1988) they concluded that while CD is an effective method for correcting severe spinal curvature, its ability to correct rotation and the cosmetic disfigurement associated with severe spinal curvature has variable results.

Van Ooy and Geukers (1991) studied 38 patients having CD instrumentation and measuring the gibbus (hump) height. They concluded: 'The CD system is a complex system with an important learning curve. Almost all complications occurred in the first half of this series. Loss of correction was minor except in the cases with complications. Derotational effect is good immediately after operation, but worsens with time, with approximately 20% correction at follow-up. With careful handling the system seems safe with respect to neurological problems.'

Hullin *et al.* (1991) studied the change of back shape after Luque instrumentation in 61 patients using ISIS and standard radiological techniques. Luque instrumentation was effective only in improving thoracic curves in the frontal plane; usually it had no effect on the rib hump and only a small effect on the sagittal plane deformity. Of the 40 single thoracic curves, only five had a reduction in the rib hump, 27 were unchanged and seven were made slightly worse.

In contrast, thoracolumbar and lumbar curves could be corrected in all three planes with a significant cosmetic improvement.

Jefferson *et al.* (1988) assessed 34 patients with AIS by radiology and ISIS both before and after spinal surgery. Twenty-seven patients underwent Harrington instrumentation, after which lateral indices of curvature were significantly improved, but changes in the transverse plane were less pronounced. Sublaminar wiring was carried out in two patients whose thoracic lordosis was corrected by the surgery (see Houghton *et al.*, 1987).

Woodland *et al.* (1988) reported a comparison of back shape parameters after Harrington and Harrington–Luque posterior spinal instrumentation for scoliosis in 22 patients. Moiré photographs were used, from which several parameters were calculated at each of 15 levels on the back (a centroid, lateral deviation, rotation effect and shape asymmetry). They found that the most consistent effect of the Harrington–Luque procedure was to lengthen the trunk rotation so that more of the spine is involved in rotation postoperatively. This elongation of the rib prominence tends to reduce the visibility of the deformity; but in five patients the maximum trunk rotation increased postoperatively. For the asymmetry parameter only one patient improved in the Harrington group; in the Harrington–Luque group seven out of 11 improved. The lateral deviation was generally improved in both groups. The average correction of Cobb angle was 31% in the Harrington group and 40% in the Harrington–Luque group.

COSTOPLASTY COMBINED WITH CORRECTIVE SPINAL INSTRUMENTATION

In the above series of Jefferson *et al.* (1988), five patients whose severe deformity had persisted after previous spinal surgery underwent costoplasty, which resulted in a significant improvement in back shape measurements. Jefferson *et al.* concluded that the cosmetic deformity of the back in scoliosis is only partially corrected by operations on the spine itself, whilst costoplasty addresses the problem directly, and improves the surface shape.

Edgar *et al.* (1992a) used ISIS to appraise 17 patients having costoplasty and spinal instrumentation for scoliosis. The maximal skin surface angles and the rib hump were reduced by 50% after costoplasty compared to a 33% reduction of radiological spinal rotation. Edgar *et al.* (1992b), continuing this study in 73 patients with five different operations who had been followed up for one year, reported an increase in rib hump size between the second and twelfth postoperative months. The increase in rib hump is less in the costoplasty group and most marked after Harrington–Luque and CD instrumentation.

ANTERIOR SURGERY FOR LUMBAR AND THORACOLUMBAR CURVES–ZIELKE, WEBB–MORLEY INSTRUMENTATION

Burwell *et al.* (1992a) appraised eight patients having Zielke and Zielke–Harrington instrumentation one year after surgery (Fig. 9.45). The mean maximal ATI was 20° preoperatively and 12° at one year. Bettany *et al.* (1992) used ISIS to evaluate 22 patients with AIS having anterior instrumentation for lumbar and thoracolumbar curves followed up for three months. They observed a large improvement in back shape, which confirmed the place of anterior surgery in the treatment of lumbar scoliosis.

THORACIC KYPHOSIS AFTER HARRINGTON INSTRUMENTATION

Carr *et al.* (1989a) used ISIS to show that after Harrington instrumentation for AIS (30 patients) the thoracic kyphosis was reduced.

SPINAL BALANCE

After Cotrel–Dubousset instrumentation for idiopathic scoliosis, several surgeons have observed loss of spinal balance (decompensation in the frontal plane), particularly of King type II curves. In the series of Richards *et al.* (1989) one-third of all patients developed mild radiological junctional kyphosis at the lower level instrumented, more commonly when instrumentation ended at or above T12. The writers recommend fusing one segment short of the stable vertebra in most Type II curves. Large Type II curves need both curves fused for optimal balance. Type III curves can be fused short of the stable vertebra. Wemyss-Holden *et al.* (1992) find that any spinal imbalance in the frontal plane induced by CD tends to improve spontaneously during follow-up of one to two years.

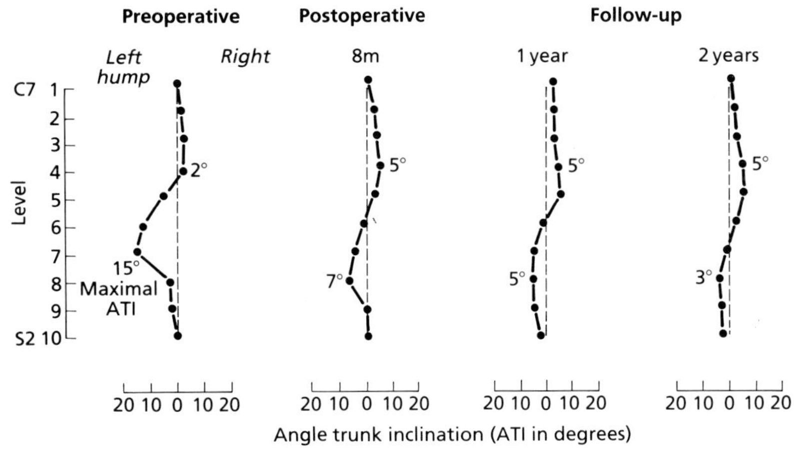

Fig. 9.45 Back shape before and after Zielke instrumentation. Plots of 10-level scoliometer ATI readings procured in the standing forward bending position (Fig. 9.11). Note that the good correction is maintained. From Burwell *et al.* (1992a).

CONCLUSION—THE NEED FOR AN INTEGRATED MULTICENTRE APPROACH

Evidence from several standpoints is leading to a reappraisal of treatment, including surgery for AIS. The patient's complaint is of disfigurement, not the radiological appearance. AIS patients, unlike those with infantile idiopathic scoliosis, do not seem to develop life-threatening cardiorespiratory complications secondary to their spinal deformity. Hence any surgical treatment should be of low risk and provide an excellent correction of both the cosmetic and the radiological deformity which is maintained throughout life.

The recent application of back shape measurement techniques to patients with AIS points to the need for improved surgical methods. A multicentre approach is indicated because of the combination of various types of AIS curves, availability of different types of instrumentation, and use of different methods to appraise back shape quantitatively.

In connection with back shape quantitation, a comparison is needed of methods involving X-radiation, MRI, ultrasound and surface anthropometry. Careful and detailed multicentre studies are likely to add new knowledge to the aetiology of AIS; this is because the various surgical techniques will interfere in different ways with deforming forces in the different types of scoliosis. Hence new therapeutic approaches to scoliosis may emerge.

The immediate need is for an integrated multicentre approach involving clinical, biological and engineering disciplines relating to the spine not only in deformity but also in other disorders and in health. A greater understanding of the factors which lead to the deformity of scoliosis during growth may have relevance to these factors which contribute to the degeneration of lumbar intervertebral discs during adult life.

APPENDIX

Measurement of stature and its correction for spinal curvature

Accurate measurement—even of stature—requires specialist training and careful techniques (Tanner, 1978, cited in Burwell *et al.*, 1980). Anthropometric counter recorder equipment designed for such measurements is also needed.

STATURE AND SCOLIOSIS

The use of the standing height as a measure of the overall size of a child with scoliosis is clearly not ideal—because increasing stature is a function not only of growth but also of the progression (or resolution) of the spinal curvature. Studies of stature in scoliosis must correct for the loss of height due to the lateral spinal curvature. Three methods for attaining such height correction are currently available.

Bjure and Nachemson's method

These writers showed that a height loss of 10 cm corresponded to 110° of curve and resulted also in about 500 ml loss of vital capacity. It should be added that they were unable to measure the height loss due to kyphosis or lordosis (Bjure & Nachemson, 1973).

Hodgett's method

Hodgett reported a study of height loss resulting from idiopathic scoliosis in 50 adolescent and adult patients for whom AP and oblique (Stagnara) radiographs were available (Hodgett *et al.*, 1986). The results show that the measured trunk height loss has a curvilinear relation to Cobb angle. Using $\log_{10}$ trunk height loss the relationship was linear and the two linear regression equations are:

$\log y = 0.014x + 0.626$ ($r = 0.94$) AP radiographs
$\log y = 0.014x + 0.760$ ($r = 0.96$) oblique radiographs

where y = calculated trunk height loss in mm, and x = Cobb angle. The difference (15.3%) for trunk height loss between the AP and oblique radiographs is not statistically significant.

Carr's method

Carr *et al.* (1989b) introduced a new method to correct for changes in height due to spinal deformity in both the frontal and sagittal planes using the ISIS scanner.

REFERENCES

Aaro, S. & Öhlén, G (1983) The effect of Harrington instrumentation on the sagittal configuration and mobility of the spine in scoliosis. *Spine*, **8**, 570–575.

Adams, M.A., Dolan, P., Marx, C. & Hutton, W.C. (1986) An electronic inclinometer technique for measuring lumbar curvature. *Clin. Biomech.*, **1**, 130–134.

Archer, I.A. & Dickson, R.A. (1985) Stature and idiopathic scoliosis: a prospective study. *J. Bone Jt. Surg.*, **67B**, 185–188.

Asazuma, T., Suzuki, N. & Hirabayashi, K. (1986) Analysis of human dynamic posture in normal and scoliotic patients. In Harris, J.D. & Turner-Smith, A.R. (eds) *Surface Topography and Spinal Deformity*, Proceedings of the Third International Symposium, 27–28 September 1984, Oxford, England, pp. 223–233. Gustav Fischer, Stuttgart.

Assente, R., Ferrigno, G., Santambrogio, G.C. & Vigano, R. (1987) Application of AUSCAN system for evaluation of postural changes induced by brace. In Stokes, I.A.F., Pekelsky, J.R. & Moreland, M.S. (eds) *Surface Topography and Spinal Deformity*, Proceedings of the Fourth International Symposium, 29–30 September 1986, Mont Sainte Marie, Quebec, pp. 97–104. Gustav Fischer, Stuttgart.

Bannon, M.A. & Tredwell, S. (1987) Variability due to subject positioning. In Stokes, I.A.F., Pekelsky, J.R. & Moreland, M.S. (eds) *Surface Topography and Spinal Deformity*, Proceedings of the Fourth International Symposium. 29–30 September 1986, Mont Sainte Marie, Quebec, pp. 283–291. Gustav Fischer, Stuttgart.

Bannon, M.A. & Tredwell, S. (1990) Post-operative changes occurring with Cotrel–Dubousset instrumentation. In Neugebauer, H. & Windischbauer, G. (eds) *Proceedings of the Fifth International Symposium*, 29 September–1 October 1988, Vienna, Austria, pp. 73–76. Gustav Fischer, Stuttgart.

Beaumont, S.E., Burwell, R.G. Webb, J.K. & Wojcik A.S. (1989) The effects of the Cotrel–Dubousset operation on back shape: preliminary findings. *J. Bone Jt. Surg.*, **71B**, 153.

Benoni, G. & Willner, S. (1986) A comparison of the moire pattern before and after brace treatment of scoliosis. In Harris, J.D. & Turner-Smith A.R. (eds) *Surface Topography and Spinal Deformity*, Proceedings of the Third International Symposium, 27–28 September 1984, Oxford, England, pp. 161–4. Gustav Fischer, Stuttgart.

Benoni, G., Turner-Smith, A. & Willner, S. (1987) A comparison between ISIS and the moiré method in the assessment of scoliosis. In Stokes, I.A.F., Pekelsky, J.R. & Moreland, M.S. (eds) *Surface Topography and Spinal Deformity*, Proceedings of the Fourth International Symposium, 29–30 September 1986, Mont Sainte Marie, Quebec, pp. 213–221. Gustav Fischer, Stuttgart.

Bettany, J.A., Harrison, D.J., Edgar, M.A., Ransford, A.O., Webb, P.J. & Morley, T.R. (1992) The effect of anterior instrumentation on back shape in adolescent idiopathic scoliosis: preliminary results. In Alberti, A., Drerup, B. & Hierholzer, E. (eds) *Sixth International Symposium on Surface Topography and Spinal Deformity*, pp. 76–82. Gustav Fischer, Stuttgart.

Bjure, J. & Nachemson, A. (1973) Non-treated scoliosis. *Clin. Orthop.*, **93**, 44–52.

Branthwaite, M.A. (1986) Cardiorespiratory consequences of unfused idiopathic scoliosis. *Br. J. Dis. Chest*, **80**, 360–369.

British Scoliosis Society: Natural History Committee (Chairman R.G. Burwell) (1987) A multicentre study of back shape in schoolchildren. A progress report: positional changes in back contour in relation to a new screening test for scoliosis. In Stokes, I.A.F., Pekelsky, J.R. & Moreland, M.S. (eds) *Surface Topography and Spinal Deformity*, Proceedings of the Fourth International Symposium, 29–30 September 1986, Mont Sainte Marie, Quebec, pp. 139–151. Gustav Fischer, Stuttgart.

Bryant, J.T., Reid, J.G., Smith, B.L. & Stevenson, J.M. (1989) Method for determining vertebral body positions in the sagittal plane using skin markers. *Spine*, **14**, 258–265.

Bunnell, W.P. (1984) An objective criterion for scoliosis screening. *J. Bone Jt. Surg.*, **66A**, 1381–1387.

Burton, A.K. & Tillotson, K.M. (1988). Reference values for 'normal' regional lumbar sagittal mobility. *Clin. Biomech.*, **3**, 106–113.

Burwell, R.G. (1978) Biostereometrics, shape replication and orthopaedics. In Harris, J.D. & Copeland, K. (eds) *Conference on Bioengineering*, Nuffield Orthopaedic Centre, 29–30 September 1977, Oxford, England, pp. 51–85. Biological Engineering Society, London.

Burwell, R.G. (1988) Symposium on school screening for scoliosis. The British decision and subsequent events. *Spine*, **13**, 1192–1194.

Burwell, R.G. (1990a) Current status of screening. In Siegler, D., Harrison, D. & Edgar, M. (eds) *Proceedings of the Eighth Phillip Zorab Scoliosis Symposium*, 26–28 October 1988, London, pp. 13–33. Phillip Zorab Scoliosis Research Fund, London.

Burwell, R.G. (1990b). British Scoliosis Society: The 1989 report on school screening for scoliosis: the relation to aetiology. *J. Bone Jt. Surg.*, **72B**, 333–334.

Burwell, R.G., Vernon, C.L. & Dangerfield, P.H. (1980) Skeletal measurement. In Owen, R., Goodfellow, J. & Bullough, P. (eds) *Scientific Foundations of Orthopaedics and Traumatology*, pp. 317–329. Heinemann, London.

Burwell, R.G., Webb, J.K. & More, E.J. (1981) School screening for scoliosis. *Lancet*, **2**, 863.

Burwell, R.G., James, N.J., Johnson, F., Webb, J.K. & Wilson, Y.G. (1983a) Standardised trunk asymmetry scores—a study of back contour in healthy children. *J. Bone Jt. Surg.*, **65B**, 452–462.

Burwell, R.G., James, N.J., Johnson, F., Webb, J.K. & Wilson, Y.G. (1983b). Trunk asymmetry scores: application to subjects with idiopathic scoliosis with particular reference to radiological findings. In Drerup, B., Frobin, W. & Hierholzer, E. (eds) *Moiré Fringe Topography and Spinal Deformity*, Proceedings of the Second International Symposium, 12–15 September 1982, Münster, Germany, pp. 41–50. Gustav Fischer, Stuttgart.

Burwell, R.G., Elwood, J.M., James, N.J. and Webb, J.K. (1986) The use of the Scoliometer in the school and clinic. In *Proceedings of the European Spinal Deformities Society, First Congress*, 16–19 April Rome, p. 101.

Burwell, R.G., Upadhyay, S.S., Wojcik, A.S., Bacon, N.C.M., Moulton, A. and Webb, J.K. (1990a). Ultrasound in evaluating scoliosis. In Siegler, D., Harrison, D. & Edgar, M. (eds) *Proceedings of the Eighth Phillip Zorab Scoliosis Symposium*, 26–28 October, 1988, London, pp. 48–67. London: Phillip Zorab Scoliosis Research Fund.

Burwell, R.G., Patterson, J.F., Webb, J.K. and Wojcik, A.S. (1990b). School screening for scoliosis. In Neugebauer, H. & Windischbauer, G. (eds) *Surface Topography and Body Deformity*. Proceedings of the Fifth International Symposium, 29 September–1 October 1988, Vienna, Austria, pp. 17–23. Gustav Fischer, Stuttgart.

Burwell, R.G., Jacobs, K.J., Polak, F.J., Webb, J.K., Wojcik, A.S. & Wythers, D.J. (1992a) The back hump after Cotrel–Dubousset, Harrington–Luque and Zielke instrumentation: a segmental appraisal of findings at one year, with implications calling for an international multicentre study of new instrumentations. In Alberti, A., Drerup, B. & Hierholzer, E. (eds) *Sixth International Symposium on Surface Topography and Spinal Deformity*, pp. 180–195. Gustav Fischer, Stuttgart.

Burwell, R.G., Cole, A.A., Cook, T.A., Grivas, T.B., Kiel, A.W., Moulton, A., Thirlwall, S.A., Upadhyay, S.S., Webb, J.K., Wemyss-Holden, S.A., Whitwell, D.J., Wojcik, A.S. & Wythers, D.J. (1992b) Pathogenesis of idiopathic scoliosis: the Nottingham concept. In Proceedings of the Combined Meeting of the British Scoliosis Society and the Nordic Scoliosis Society, Newcastle-upon-Tyne, 5–6 June 1991. *J. Bone Jt. Surg. Orthop. Proc.* (In press).

Carr, A.J., Jefferson, R.J., Turner-Smith, A.R., Weisz, I., Thomas, D.C., Stavrakis, T. & Houghton, G.R. (1989a) Surface stereophotogrammetry of thoracic kyphosis. *Acta Orthop. Scand.*, **60**, 177–180.

Carr, A.J., Jefferson, R.J., Weisz, I. & Turner-Smith, A.R. (1989b) Correction of body height in scoliotic patients using ISIS scanning. *Spine*, **14**, 220–222.

Carr, A.J., Jefferson, R.J. & Turner-Smith, A.R. (1991a) Familial back shape in adolescent scoliosis. A photogrammetric population study. *Acta Orthop. Scand.*, **62**, 131–135.

Carr, A.J., Jefferson, R.J., Turner-Smith, A.R. & Beavis, A. (1991b) An analysis of normal back shape measured by ISIS scanning. *Spine*, **16**, 656–659.

Dangerfield, P.H. & Denton, J.S. (1986) A preliminary examination of the relationship between the rib-hump, spinal angle and vertebral rotation in idiopathic scoliosis. In Harris, J.D. & Turner-Smith, A.R. (eds) *Surface Topography and Spinal Deformity*, Proceedings of the Third International Symposium, 27–28 September 1984, Oxford, England, pp. 213–221. Gustav Fischer, Stuttgart.

Dangerfield, P.H., Barnes, S., Owen, R. & Dorgan, J.C. (1987a) Kyphosis and lordosis in scoliosis. *J. Pediatr. Orthop.*, **7**, 350.

Dangerfield, P.H., Denton, J.S., Barnes, S.B. & Drake, N.B. (1987b). The assessment of rib-cage and spinal deformity in scoliosis. In Stokes, I.A.F., Pekelsky, J.R. & Moreland, M.S. (eds) *Surface Topography and Spinal Deformity*, Proceedings of the Fourth International Symposium, 29–30 September 1985, Mont Sainte Marie, Quebec, pp. 53–65. Gustav Fischer, Stuttgart.

Dangerfield, P.H., Groves, D. & Pearson, J. (1990) Advanced computer analysis of moiré contour images and the assessment of ribcage deformity in scoliosis. *J. Bone Jt. Surg.*, **72B**, 338.

Dangerfield, P.H., Drake, N. & Dorgan, J.C. (1991) Rib cage deformity and sagittal plane profile in parents of children with scoliosis. *J. Bone Jt. Surg.* **73B**, *Orthop. Proc.* **I**, 30.

Dangerfield, P.H., Williams, L., Dorgan, J.C. & Rajasekaran, S. (1992) Multiple spinal level measurement of body surface deformity in scoliosis. In Alberti, A., Drerup, B. & Hierholzer, E. (eds) *Sixth International Symposium on Surface Topography and Spinal Deformity*, pp. 212–216. Gustav Fischer, Stuttgart.

Daruwalla, J.S. & Balasubramanian, P. (1985) Moiré topography in scoliosis: its accuracy in detecting the site and size of the curve. *J. Bone Jt. Surg.*, **67B**, 211–213.

Dawson, E.G., Kropf, M.A., Purcell, G.A., Kanim, L.E.A., Kabo, J.M. & Burt, C.M. (1989) Optoelectronic evaluation of trunk deformity in scoliosis. In *Combined Meeting of Scoliosis Research Society and European Spinal*

Deformities Society, Amsterdam, 17–22 September, 1989.

Debrunner, H.U. (1972) Das Kyphometer. *Z. Orthop. Grenzgebiete*, **110**, 389–392.

Dickson, R.A. (1983) Scoliosis in the community. *Br. Med. J.*, **286**, 615–618.

Dove, J. (1985) British Scoliosis Society: Morbidity study. In *Proceedings of Scoliosis Research Society, 20th Annual Meeting*, 17–20 September 1985, Coronado, California, USA.

Duff, E.S. & Draper, E.R.C. (1987) Survey of normal adolescent back shape as measured by ISIS. In Stokes, I.A.F., Pekelsky, J.R. & Moreland, M.S. (eds) *Surface Topography and Spinal Deformity*, Proceedings of the Fourth International Symposium, 29–30 September 1986, Mont Sainte Marie, Quebec, pp. 163–70. Gustav Fischer, Stuttgart.

Edgar, M.A., Bettany, J.A. Ransford, A.O. & Harrison, D.J. (1992a) ISIS assessment of costoplasty: preliminary results. In Alberti, A., Drerup B. & Hierholzer, E. (eds) *Sixth International Symposium on Surface Topography and Spinal Deformity*, pp. 83–88. Gustav Fischer, Stuttgart.

Edgar, M.A., Ransford, A.O., Goldie, B., Irvine, B. & Bettany, J. (1992b). A comparative study of rib hump recurrence following different surgical techniques. In Proceedings of the Combined Meeting of the British Scoliosis Society and the Nordic Scoliosis Society, Newcastle-upon-Tyne, 5–6 June 1991, *J. Bone Jt. Surg. (Br.) Orthop. Proc.* (In press).

Fidler, C. & Turner-Smith, A.R. (1986). Changes in back shape on removing a brace. In Harris, J.D. & Turner-Smith, A.R. (eds) *Surface Topography and Spinal Deformity*, Proceedings of the Third International Symposium, 27–28 September 1984, Oxford, England, pp. 145–150. Gustav Fischer, Stuttgart.

Frobin, W. & Hierholzer, E. (1982) Analysis of human back shape using surface curvatures. *J. Biomech.*, **15**, 379–390.

Frobin, W. & Hierholzer, E. (1990) Video rasterstereography, a method for on-line surface measurement. In Neugebauer, H. & Windischbauer, G. (eds) *Surface Topography and Body Deformity*. Proceedings of the Fifth International Symposium, 29 September–1 October 1988, Vienna, Austria, pp. 155–157. Gustav Fischer, Stuttgart.

Goff, B. & Rose, G.K. (1964) The use of a modified spondylometer in the treatment of ankylosing spondylitis. *Rheumatism*, **20**, 63–66.

Green, N.E., Homra, L., Doll, D. & Szalay, E. (1987) The use of ISIS to determine severity and progression of adolescent idiopathic scoliosis. In: *Proceedings of Scoliosis Research Society, Twenty-second Annual Meeting*, 15–19 September 1987, Vancouver, BC, Canada, p. 90.

Grivas, T.B., Webb, J.K. & Burwell, R.G. (1991). The effects of epiphysiodesis and rodding for early onset scoliosis. *J. Bone Jt. Surg.* **73B**, *Orthop. Proc.*, **I**, 32–33.

Halioua, M., Liu, H-C., Chin, A. & Bowings, T.S. (1990) Automated topography of the human forms by phase-measuring profilometry and model analysis. In Neugebauer, H. & Windischbauer, G. (eds) *Proceedings of the Fifth International Symposium*, 29 September–1 October 1988, Vienna, Austria, pp. 91–100. Gustav Fischer, Stuttgart.

Harrison, D.J. & Bettany, J.A. (1991). The Stanmore footplate: improving ISIS scan reliability. *J. Bone Jt. Surg.*, **73B**, *Orthop. Proc.*, **I**, 35–36.

Hierholzer, E. & Drerup, B. (1990). Three-dimensional reconstruction of the spinal midline from rasterstereographs. In Neugebauer, H. & Windischbauer, G. (eds) *Surface Topography and Body Deformity*, Proceedings of the Fifth International Symposium, 29 September–1 October 1988, Vienna, Austria, pp. 53–55. Gustav Fischer, Stuttgart.

Hierholzer, E. & Lüxmann, G. (1982). Three-dimensional shape analysis of the scoliotic spine using the invariant shape parameters. *J. Biomech.*, **15**, 581–598.

Hodgett, S.G., Burwell, R.G. & Webb, J.K. (1986). Trunk height loss in idiopathic scoliosis in AP and oblique spinal radiographs. In *Proceedings of the European Spinal Deformities Society First Congress*, 16–19 April, Rome, p. 92.

Horst, M. (1983). Skeletal deformities and trunk shape: a survey of diagnostic methods. In Drerup, B., Frobin, W. & Hierholzer, E. (eds) *Surface Topography and Spinal Deformity*, Proceedings of the Second International Symposium, 12–15 September 1982, Münster, Germany, pp. 3–16. Gustav Fischer, Stuttgart.

Houghton, G.R., Jefferson, R.J., Thomas, D.C., Harris, J.D. & Turner-Smith, A.R. (1987) Effects of scoliosis surgery on back shape. In Stokes, I.A.F., Pekelsky, J.R. & Moreland, M.S. (eds) *Surface Topography and Spinal Deformity*, Proceedings of the Fourth International Symposium, 29–30 September 1986, Mont Sainte Marie, Quebec, pp. 24–34. Gustav Fischer, Stuttgart.

Hovorka, O.V. (1904) Über die anthropologisch-orthopädischen Meßmethoden des Rückens. Mittheilungen der anthropologischen *Gesellschaft in Wien*, **34**, 275–315.

Hullin, M.G., McMaster, M.J., Draper, E.R.C. & Duff, E.S. (1991) The effect of Luque segmental sublaminar instrumentation on the rib hump in idiopathic scoliosis. *Spine*, **16**, 402–408.

James, J.I.P. (1956) Paralytic scoliosis. *J. Bone Jt. Surg.*, **38B**, 660–685.

James, N.J. (1985) *A morphological study of the clinical and radiological deformity in patients with idiopathic scoliosis*. M. Phil. thesis, University of Nottingham.

Jaspan, T., Turnbull, A.E., Burwell, R.G. & Firth, J.L. (1991) CSF flow dynamics at the foramen magnum of a Chiari I malformation demonstrated by colour doppler imaging. In: Proceedings of British Association of Clinical Anatomists, 20 December 1990, London. *Clin. Anat.*, **4**, 382.

Jefferson, R.J., Weisz, I., Turner-Smith, A.R., Harris, J.D. & Houghton, G.R. (1988) Scoliosis surgery and its effect on back shape. *J. Bone Jt. Surg.*, **70B**, 261–266.

Jefferson, R.J., Weisz, I., Carr, A.J., Turner-Smith, A.R. & Houghton, G.R. (1990) Back shape in brace treatment of idiopathic scoliosis. *J. Bone Jt. Surg.*, **72B**, 338.

Johnson, M.R., Upadhyay, S.S., Burwell, R.G. & Webb,

J.K. (1987) Integrated Shape Imaging System (ISIS): an evaluation of its capacity to measure lateral spinal curves and appraise hump dynamics on forward flexion. *J. Bone Jt. Surg.*, **69B**, 851–852.

Jones, P.R.M., West, G.M., Harris, D.H. & Read, J.B. (1989) The Loughborough anthropometric shadow scanner (LASS). *Endeavour*, new series, **13**, 162–168.

Jones, T.J., Scull, E.R., Dutton, K.E., White, K.L., Slinger, B.S. & O'Connor, J.C. (1987) Analytical assessment of back symmetry and its reliability in a clinical setting. In Stokes, I.A.F., Pekelsky, J.R. & Moreland, M.S. *Surface Topography and Spinal Deformity, Proceedings of the 4th International Symposium*. September 29–30, 1986, Mont Sainte Marie, Quebec, pp. 301–332. Gustav Fischer, Stuttgart.

Kiel, A.W., Burwell, R.G., Cattle, J., Jacobs, K., Moulton, A., Webb, J.K. & Wojcik, A.S. (1990) A segmental analysis of the lateral profile of the spine revealing changes in the thoracolumbar region of thoracic curves. *J. Bone Jt. Surg.*, **72B**, 333.

Letts, M., Quanbury, A., Gouw, G., Kolsun, W. & Letts, E. (1988) Computerized ultrasonic digitization in the measurement of spinal curvature. *Spine*, **13**, 1106–1110.

Lowden, M.C. (1984) *Sagittal spinal curves and their flexibility during growth in health and scoliosis*. Thesis, University of Nottingham.

Lowden, M.C., Burwell, R.G. & Webb, J.K. (1986) Sagittal spinal curves and their flexibility in healthy children. *Ann. Roy. Coll. Surg. Engl.*, **68**, 110.

Mauritzson, L., Benoni, G., Ilver, J., Lindstrom, K. & Willner, S. (1986) Three linear array back scanning with airborne ultrasound. In Harris, J.D. & Turner-Smith, A.R. (eds) *Surface Topography and Spinal Deformity*, Proceedings of the Third International Symposium, 27–28 September 1984, Oxford, England, pp. 47–51. Gustav Fischer, Stuttgart.

Mellin, G. (1987) Correlations of spinal mobility with degree of chronic low back pain after correction for age and anthropometric factors. *Spine*, **12**, 464–468.

Milne, J.S. & Lauder, I.J. (1976) The relationship of kyphosis to the shape of vertebral bodies. *Ann. Hum. Biol.*, **3**, 173–179.

Moe, J.H. (1987) Historical aspects of scoliosis. In: *Moe's Textbook of Scoliosis and Other Spinal Deformities*, 2nd edn, pp. 1–6. W.B. Saunders, Philadelphia, PA.

Moreland, M.S., Bigalow, L.C. & Stokes, I.A.F. (1986) Concordance of back surface rotation and scoliosis. In Harris, J.D. & Turner-Smith, A.R. (eds) *Surface Topography and Spinal Deformity*, Proceedings of the Third International Symposium, 27–28 September 1984, Oxford, England, pp. 165–179. Gustav Fischer, Stuttgart.

Morris, J.R.W. & Harris, J.D. (1967) Three-dimensional shapes. *Lancet*, **1**, 1189–1190.

Nachemson, A. (1991) Prospective Scoliosis Study Report. In Proceedings of 25th Annual Meeting of Scoliosis Research Society, 23–27 September 1990, Honolulu, Hawaii. *J. Pediatr. Orthop.* (In press).

Neugebauer, von H. (1970). Rückenmeβgerät für Reihenuntersuchungen. *Z. Orthop. Grenzgebiete*, **108**, 395–406.

Nicholson, U.J.L., Burwell, R.G., Upadhyay, S.S. & Webb, J.K. (1987) Kyphosis and lordosis measured by ISIS. An appraisal on a plaster model and the effects of arm position in healthy subjects and patients with low back pain and scoliosis. In Stokes, I.A.F., Pekelsky, J.R. & Moreland, M.S. (eds) *Surface Topography and Spinal Deformity*, Proceedings of the Fourth International Symposium, 29–30 September 1986, Mont Sainte Marie, Quebec, pp. 187–99. Gustav Fischer, Stuttgart.

Oates, C.P., Whittingham, T.A. & Leonard, M.A. (1990) The Newcastle ultrasonic spine image system. In Neugebauer, H. & Windischbauer, G. (eds) *Surface Topography and Body Deformity*. Proceedings of the Fifth International Symposium, 29 September–1 October 1988, Vienna, Austria, pp. 31–33. Gustav Fischer, Stuttgart.

Öhlén, G., Aaro, S. & Bylund, P. (1988) The sagittal configuration, and mobility of the spine in idiopathic scoliosis. *Spine*, **13**, 413–416.

Porter, R.W., Wicks, M.A. & Ottewell, D. (1978) Measurement of the spinal canal by diagnostic ultrasound. *J. Bone Jt. Surg.*, **60B**, 481–484.

Pruijs, J.F.H. (1989) Poster presentation, Combined Meeting of Scoliosis Research Society and European Spinal Deformities Society, 17–22 September 1989, Amsterdam, Netherlands.

Pun, W.K., Luk, K.D.K., Lee, W. & Leong, J.C.Y. (1987) A simple method to estimate the rib hump in scoliosis. *Spine*, **12**, 342–345.

Raso, V.J., Greenhill, B., Moreau, M.J. & Budney, D. (1987). The combined reconstruction of spinal and surface deformity. In Stokes, I.A.F., Pekelsky, J.R. & Moreland, M.S. (eds) *Surface Topography and Spinal Deformity*, Proceedings of the Fourth International Symposium, 29–30 September 1986, Mont Sainte Marie, Quebec, pp. 13–20. Gustav Fischer, Stuttgart.

Richards, B.S., Birch, J.G., Herring, J.A., Johnston, C.E. & Roach, J.W. (1989) Frontal and sagittal plane balance following Cotrel-Dubousset instrumentation for idiopathic scoliosis. *Spine*, **14**, 733–737.

Sahlstrand, T. (1986) The clinical value of Moiré topography in the management of scoliosis. *Spine*, **11**, 409–417.

Schulthess, W. (1905) Die Pathologie der Scoliose. *Z. Orthop. Chirur.*, **14**, 478–524.

Schumpe, G. & Messler, H. (1987) Comparison of parameters used for the measurement of spinal deformity by means of optrimetric, ultrasonic and radiographic technique. In Stokes, I.A.F., Pekelsky, J.R. & Moreland, M.S. (eds) *Surface Topography and Spinal Deformity*, Proceedings of the Fourth International Symposium, 29–30 September 1986, Mont Sainte Marie, Quebec, pp. 203–212. Gustav Fischer, Stuttgart.

Shinoto, A., Ohtsuka, Y. & Inoue, S. (1987) Three dimensional analysis of the effect of brace treatment on idiopathic scoliosis. In Stokes, I.A.F., Pekelsky, J.R. & Moreland, M.S. (eds) *Surface Topography and Spinal Deformity*, Proceedings of the Fourth International

Symposium, 29–30 September 1986, Mont Sainte Marie, Quebec, pp. 113–30. Gustav Fischer, Stuttgart.

Stokes, I.A.F. (1989). Axial rotation component of thoracic scoliosis. *J. Orthop. Res.* **7**, 702–708.

Stokes, I.A.F. and Moreland, M.S. (1987) Measurement of the shape of the surface of the back in patients with scoliosis: the standing and forward-bending positions. *J. Bone Jt. Surg.*, **69A**, 203–211.

Stokes, I.A.F. & Moreland, M.S. (1989) Concordance of back surface asymmetry and spine shape in idiopathic scoliosis. *Spine*, **14**, 73–78.

Stokes, I.A.F., Cobb, L.C., Pope, M.H. & Moreland, M.S. (1985) Back surface shape relationship to spinal deformity. In Whittle, M.W. & Harris, J.D. (eds) *Biomechanical Measurement in Orthopaedic Practice*, pp. 114–24. Clarendon Press, Oxford.

Stokes, I.A.F., Shuma-Harswick, D. & Moreland, M.S. (1988) Spine and back-shape changes in scoliosis. *Acta Orthop. Scand.*, **59**, 128–133.

Suzuki, N., Yamaguchi, Y. & Armstrong, G.W.D. (1981) Measurement of posture using Moire topography. In Moreland, M.S., Pope, M.H. & Armstrong, G.W.D. (eds) *Moiré Fringe Topography and Spinal Deformity*, pp. 122–131. Pergamon Press, New York.

Suzuki, N., Yamashita, Y. & Akamatsu, M. (1986) An analysis of normal range of thoracic kyphosis. *J. Pediatr. Orthop.*, **6**, 367.

Suzuki, S., Yamamuro, T., Shikata, J., Shimizu, K. & Iida, H. (1989) Ultrasound measurement of vertebral rotation in idiopathic scoliosis. *J. Bone Jt. Surg.*, **71B**, 252–255.

Takemitsu, Y. (1981) Scoliosis: screeening methods and the subsequent management. *J. Jpn. Orthop. Assoc.*, **55**, 243–257 (in Japanese).

Teot, L., Deschamps, F., Perdriolle, R. & Vidal, J. (1989) Ultrasonographic imaging of the spine. In *Combined Meeting of Scoliosis Research Society and European Spinal Deformities Society*, Amsterdam, 17–22 September.

Thulbourne, T. & Gillespie, R. (1976). The rib hump in idiopathic scoliosis. Measurement, analysis and response to treatment. *J. Bone Jt. Surg.*, **58B**, 64–71.

Towns, J.W. & Roche, A.F. (1968) Age-associated changes in the shape of the lateral silhouette of the trunk. *Growth*, **32**, 205–210.

Transfeldt, E.E., Heithoff, K.B., Bradford, D.S., Coscia, M., Cohen, M. & Thompson, P. (1990) Changes in segmental coupling and vertebral rotation following Cotrel-Dubousset for idiopathic scoliosis. *J. Bone Jt. Surg.*, **72B**, 334–335.

Tredwell, S.J. & Bannon, M. (1988) The use of the ISIS optical scanner in the management of the braced adolescent idiopathic scoliosis patient. *Spine*, **13**, 1104–1105.

Turner-Smith, A.R. & Harris, J.D. (eds) (1986) ISIS—an automated shape measurement and analysis system. In *Surface Topography and Spinal Deformity*, pp. 31–38. Gustav Fischer, Stuttgart.

Turner-Smith, A.R., Harris, J.D., Houghton, G.R. & Jefferson, R.J. (1988) A method for analysis of backshape in scoliosis. *J. Biomech.*, **21**, 497–509.

Upadhyay, S.S., Burwell, R.G., Nicholson, U.J.L. & Webb, J.K. (1987) The Integrated Shape Imaging System (ISIS) and the Scoliometer for recording back shape in scoliosis. A reliability and comparative study revealing positional changes in back contour (hump dynamics). In Stokes, I.A.F., Pekelsky, J.R. & Moreland, M.S. (eds) *Surface Topography and Spinal Deformity*, Proceedings of the Fourth International Symposium, 29–30 September 1986, Mont Sainte Marie, Quebec; pp. 233–248. Gustav Fischer, Stuttgart.

van Ooy, A. & Geukers, Ch.W.G.M. (1991) Results of CD operation in idiopathic scoliosis. In D. Uyttendaele (ed.) *Symposium on Idiopathic Scoliosis, Orthopaedica Belgica, Gent*, 20–23 March, 1991, *Acta Orthopaedica Belgica* (In press).

Vercauteren, M. & Goossens, M. (1986) Differences in spine profile in boys and girls around puberty with special reference to the etiopathogenesis of idiopathic scoliosis. In: *Proceedings of the European Spinal Deformities Society First Congress*, 16–19 April Rome, p. 4.

Vercauteren, M., Uyttendaele, D. & De Smet, L. (1985) Trunk asymmetries and scoliosis. In Warner, J.O. & Mehta, M.H. (eds) *Scoliosis Prevention*, Proceedings of the Seventh Phillip Zorab Symposium, 1983. Chap. 6, pp. 83–90. Praeger, New York.

Weatherley, C.R., Draycott, V., O'Brien, J.F., Benson, D.R., Gopalakrishnan, K.C., Evans, J.H. & O'Brien, J.P. (1987) The rib deformity in adolescent idiopathic scoliosis. A prospective study to evaluate changes after Harrington distraction and posterior fusion. *J. Bone Jt. Surg.*, **69B**, 179–182.

Weisz, I., Jefferson, R.J., Turner-Smith, A.R., Houghton, G.R. & Harris, J.D. (1988) ISIS scanning: a useful assessment technique in the management of scoliosis. *Spine*, **13**, 405–408.

Wemyss-Holden, S.A., Burwell, R.G., Jacobs, K.J., Polak, F.J., McNeill, S.A., Webb, J.K. & Moulton, A. (1992). Predicting the deformation of the rib-cage around the fused spine after Cotrel–Dubousset instrumentation (CD) for adolescent idiopathic scoliosis (AIS). In: Proceedings of the Combined Meeting of the British Scoliosis Society and the Nordic Scoliosis Society, Newcastle-upon-Tyne, 5–6 June 1991, *J. Bone Jt. Surg. Orthop. Proc.* (In press).

Whitwell, D.J. (1991) *A new segmental ultrasound method to measure rib and spinal torsion: a comparison to the surface and radiological appraisal of adolescent idiopathic scoliosis and school-screening referrals.* Thesis, University of Nottingham.

Willner, S. (1979) Moiré topography for the diagnosis and documentation of scoliosis. *Acta Orthop. Scand.*, **50**, 295–302.

Willner, S. (1983) Spinal pantograph—a non-invasive anthropometric device for describing postures and asymmetries of the trunk. *J. Pediatr. Orthop.*, **3**, 245–249.

Willner, W. (1984) Prevalence study of trunk asymmetries and structural scoliosis in 10-year-old school children. *Spine*, **9**, 644–647.

Wojcik, A.S., Burwell, R.G., Webb, J.K. & Moulton, A.

(1990) A new ultrasound method for measuring spinal torsion in scoliosis. In Neugebauer, H. & Windischbauer, G. (eds) *Surface Topography and Body Deformity*, Proceedings of the Fifth International Symposium, 29 September–1 October 1988, Vienna, Austria, pp. 25–30. Gustav Fischer, Stuttgart.

Woodland, P.R., Jones, T.J., O'Conner, J.C.B & Slinger, B.S. (1988) A comparison of back shape parameters following Harrington and Harrington–Luque posterior spinal instrumentation for scoliosis. In *Fifth International Symposium on Surface Topography and Body Deformity*, Vienna, Austria, 29 September–1 October 1988 (Abstract).

Wythers, D.J., Burwell, R.G., Webb, J.K. & Wojcik, A.S. (1992) The segmental surface and rib deformity of progressive adolescent idiopathic scoliosis: a preoperative segmental appraisal suggesting aetiological factors in the lumbar spine. In Alberti, A., Drerup, B. & Hierholzer, E. (eds) *Sixth International Symposium on Surface Topography and Spinal Deformity*, pp. 119–135. Gustav Fischer, Stuttgart.

Zorab, P.A., Harrison, A. & Harrison, W.J. (1964) Estimation of height from tibial length. *Lancet*, **2**, 1063.

10 · Clinical Neurophysiology

By A.I. WEIR

The techniques evolved by clinical neurophysiologists to investigate peripheral and central nervous system function have many applications in the management of patients with disorders of the bony spine and the spinal cord. The major roles of such investigations are in diagnosis, prognosis and latterly the monitoring of function during and after surgical procedures on the spine.

Neurophysiological investigation must be considered as an extension of the clinical examination. It is designed to demonstrate and categorize disorders of function that may already be clinically evident. Moreover, it may demonstrate disorders of function that are subclinical, providing explanations for clinical symptoms unaccompanied by signs. In many cases the neurophysiological examination is complementary to other techniques of investigation of the spinal cord, particularly imaging, but gives additional and sometimes unique information as to the nature of a lesion.

Information about the location of a lesion within the length of a pathway may be gained. For example, an area of sensory disturbance arising from a lesion lying within the spinal cord may be distinguished from one lying preganglionically at the spinal root or in the peripheral nerve. Secondly, direct evidence of involvement of a number of pathways may allow the inference of an anatomical localization. Thirdly, neurophysiological investigation may detect 'non-surgical' spinal cord diseases or conditions of the peripheral nervous system that may be mimicking a surgical spinal cord lesion. For example the diagnosis of motor neurone disease in a patient with a spastic paraparesis, or of an hereditary sensory and motor neuropathy in a patient suspected of a cauda equina lesion.

Neurophysiological examination gives only indirect evidence of the pathological nature of a lesion but the dynamics of the situation may allow assessment of the age of the lesion. An estimate of the prognosis of any condition depends on the analysis of many aspects of the investigation. The degree of abnormality, evidence of regeneration and the knowledge of the behaviour of individual lesions at particular locations are all important. Even with the most detailed objective neurophysiological data such estimates are at best subjective and can be considered only as guidelines. Repeated neurophysiological testing may be useful in making such analysis as objective as possible, and to demonstrate trends in the recovery from a lesion.

NEUROPHYSIOLOGICAL TECHNIQUES

In order to appreciate the role of neurophysiological examination in clinical practice, some understanding of the techniques involved is necessary. This is particularly true when one comes to interpreting the results. A brief description of the methods and place of the more common investigations will be made, but readers requiring more detailed information are referred to texts such as those by Kimura (1983), Aminoff (1986) or Chu-Andrews & Johnson (1986).

Nerve conduction studies

Motor

Most of the major limb nerves are accessible to stimulation and can be examined. Recording electrodes are placed on the skin surface over a muscle of interest usually deriving its nerve supply from the terminal branch of the motor nerve under investigation (e.g. extensor digitorum brevis for the deep peroneal nerve and abductor pollicis brevis for the median nerve). The electrodes are constructed of silver, often with a coating of silver chloride. One electrode (stigmatic) is placed over the muscle endplate zone (coincident with the motor point) whilst the other is placed at an electrically indifferent point, usually on the tendon of the muscle or a distal digit. The voltage between these electrodes is then measured, amplified and displayed on an oscilloscope or computer screen with respect to time.

Although surface electrode recording is the norm for nerve conduction studies a needle electrode is sometimes used. By comparison with the surface electrode the recording zone (c. 0.5–1 mm) is much smaller, and this technique records only the action potentials from a small sample of the muscle motor units, whereas the surface recording aims, at least in distal muscles, to record the total activity. The advantage of the needle recording is a more abrupt onset of the response on activation of the muscle, making latency measurement easier. Conversely amplitude measurement is less useful, reflecting only a small sample of the total activity. A needle recording may be helpful if the muscle is severely wasted, or when activation of adjacent muscles innervated by another nerve interferes with the surface recording.

The nerve is stimulated with a square-wave voltage or constant-current pulse through two stimulating electrodes placed on the skin over the nerve at a site proximal to the recording point. The cathode is always placed closest to the recording electrodes or in the direction of propagation being studied. The strength of the stimulus is gradually increased (and the duration if necessary) until a voltage change is recorded. This is the compound muscle action potential (CMAP). The stimulus is further increased until the size of the CMAP is at a maximum. At this point, however much the stimulus is increased in voltage, current or duration no further increase in size of this supramaximal CMAP occurs. It is inferred that all axons capable of stimulation are recruited and all muscle fibres in the relevant muscle are activated. Various parameters of the CMAP can be measured (Fig. 10.1). The distal latency (DL) is the time taken from the stimulus onset to the onset of the CMAP. The amplitude may be taken as the amplitude of the major negativity compared with the isoelectric zero, or the peak-to-peak amplitude between the major negativity and the positivity. The area under the CMAP is also a further useful measure.

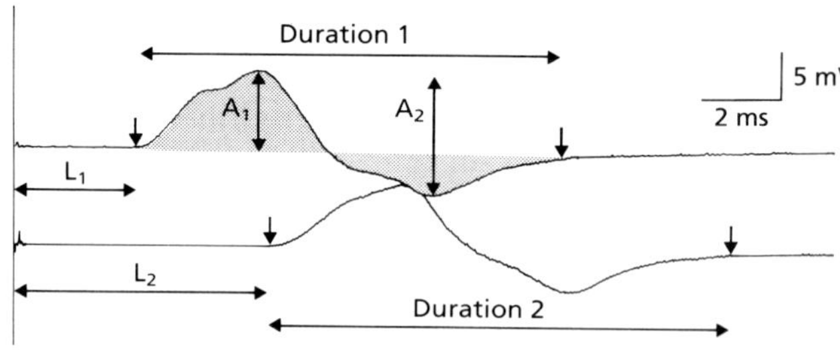

Fig. 10.1 Motor nerve conduction study of the median nerve. Surface recording site over abductor pollicis brevis muscle. Upper trace stimulation at wrist. Lower trace stimulation at elbow. L_1, distal latency (DL); L_2, latency from elbow stimulation; A_1, negative peak amplitude; A_2, peak-to-peak amplitude; total area, hatched area under curve.

The procedure is repeated with a different stimulation point on the same nerve. The distance between the sites in millimetres is then divided by the difference in latency between adjacent stimulation points in milliseconds to give the fastest motor nerve conduction velocity (FMNCV) in metres per second. It should be emphasized that the measurement of the latency to the first deflection of the CMAP means that the velocity quoted is of the fastest axons that respond. Thus if pathology affects a more slowly conducting population of axons then the FMNCV may be entirely normal.

The stimulator locations are chosen to 'straddle' likely sites of nerve entrapment such as at the carpal tunnel, cubital tunnel, pronator fossa, or head of the fibula. However, conduction velocity measurements over segments of less than 10 cm tend to have higher errors. More proximal stimulation of the upper limb nerves at the brachial plexus is possible with a surface stimulator, although the exact spatial location of activation of the deeper structures may be less clear-cut. Surface stimulation of the major lower limb nerves is possible only to the sciatic notch posteriorly and above the inguinal ligament for the femoral nerve. In many cases the stimulation of the sciatic nerve at the sciatic notch is much less painfully achieved by using a monopolar needle electrode inserted equidistant between the ischial tuberosity and the greater trochanter in the gluteal fold as the cathode and a surface anode on the anterior thigh. The more proximal structures of the roots at all levels are available to direct stimulation by a modification of the above technique, where a monopolar stimulating needle is inserted approximately 1 cm lateral to the spinous process until the relevant transverse process is reached (MacLean, 1979). This allows, for example, direct stimulation of the C8–T1 spinal nerves by positioning the needle on the C7 transverse process. A similar technique for the lumbosacral roots is available. It is thought that this technique stimulates the spinal root at the intervertebral foramen; it is thus particularly useful for distinguishing plexus from root lesions.

In addition to the calculation of the FMNCV between points along a peripheral nerve, comparison of the measurements of amplitude and area are important, as they may indicate both temporal dispersion and conduction block at sites of dysfunction.

Sensory nerve conduction

Sensory nerve conduction studies are primarily directed at the detection of sensory neuropathy. In the context of this chapter, however, such studies are particularly useful in locating a lesion causing loss or alteration in sensation either in the pre- or postganglionic afferent sensory pathways.

Stimulation of a sensory nerve can be performed either in the 'physiological' direction (orthodromic), or in the opposite direction (antidromic). Antidromic sensory potentials are larger and stimulation is usually less uncomfortable than orthodromic, but problems can arise when the proximal stimulation excites both motor and sensory fibres. Orthodromic responses are considerably smaller in amplitude but motor responses do not interfere.

In upper limb studies of both types, electrodes are placed round the digits to encompass the digital nerves or in the palm. In the orthodromic technique recording electrodes are surface-pad or near-nerve needle electrodes placed proximal to the wrist crease and separated by 3–4 cm.

In the lower limb, recordings can be made of the sural nerve from a site at the lateral side of the Achilles tendon (orthodromic) or inferior to the lateral malleolus (antidromic).

The nerve is stimulated distally in the upper limb using digital electrodes on the index finger for the median, thumb for the radial and little finger for the ulnar nerve. For the sural nerve the stimulation is applied by a surface bipolar electrode on the skin inferior to the lateral malleolus (orthodromic) or lateral to the Achilles tendon (antidromic).

The sensory action potential (SAP) (Fig. 10.2) is in the order of microvolts amplitude; therefore electronic averaging of a number of responses to the same stimulus is usually required. Measurements are made of the latency of the SAP, and it is conventional to use

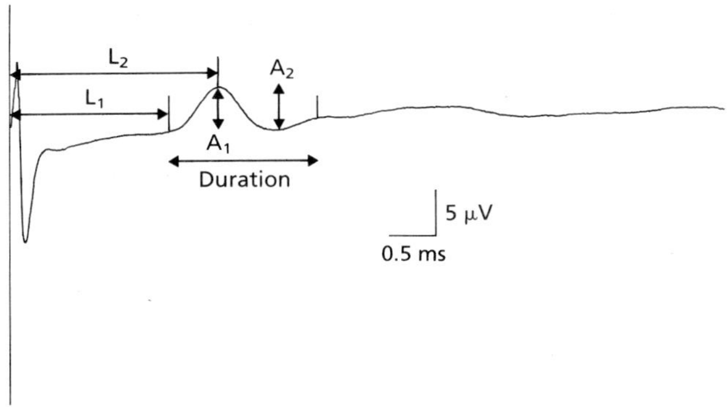

Fig. 10.2 Orthodromic median nerve sensory action potential. L_1, latency to onset; L_2, latency to negative peak; A_1, negative peak amplitude; A_2, peak-to-peak amplitude.

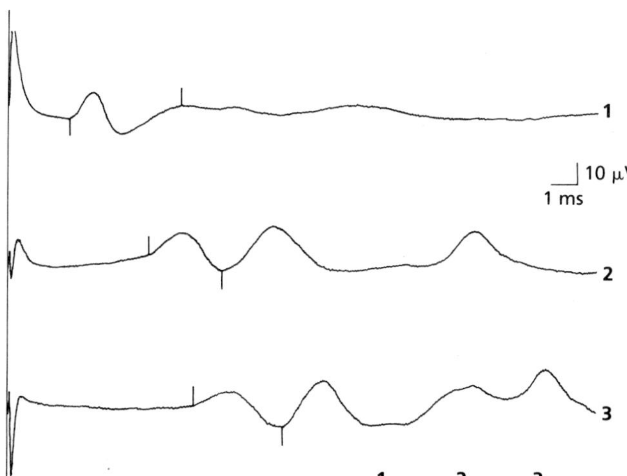

		1	2	3
Latency	(ms)	2.20	4.84	6.32
Distance	(cm)	13.0	17.5	8.20
Peak	(μV)	13.0	17.3	10.7
Peak–peak	(μV)	23.4	20.7	19.0
Area	(μV/ms)	22.1	24.5	21.0
Velocity	(m/s)	59.1	66.3	55.4

Fig. 10.3 Antidromic ulnar nerve sensory action potentials. Recording electrodes over the digital nerves in the little finger. Stimulation sites at the wrist, below elbow and above elbow. Note the fall in amplitude and increased dispersion as the stimulus is moved proximally.

the time from the stimulus to the peak of the response. Whilst this does not represent the fastest conducting sensory axons, and therefore is not strictly correct physiologically, it is a more reliable point of measurement than the onset of the sensory potential, which may be more diffuse. The latency can be related immediately to the recording distance and a sensory conduction velocity (SCV) calculated. The amplitude of the sensory potential is measured either peak-to-peak or the absolute amplitude of the negative peak.

In an antidromic study several proximal stimulation sites are possible (Fig. 10.3). Again, stimulation sites are chosen to straddle sites of possible damage or entrapment. Velocity, amplitude and area measurements are made on the averaged responses from stimulation at each site.

The sensory nerves available for study orthodromically include the median, radial, ulnar, sural, medial and lateral plantar and lateral cutaneous nerves of thigh. Antidromic studies include all the above, as well as the superficial peroneal, saphenous, musculocutaneous and lateral cutaneous of forearm.

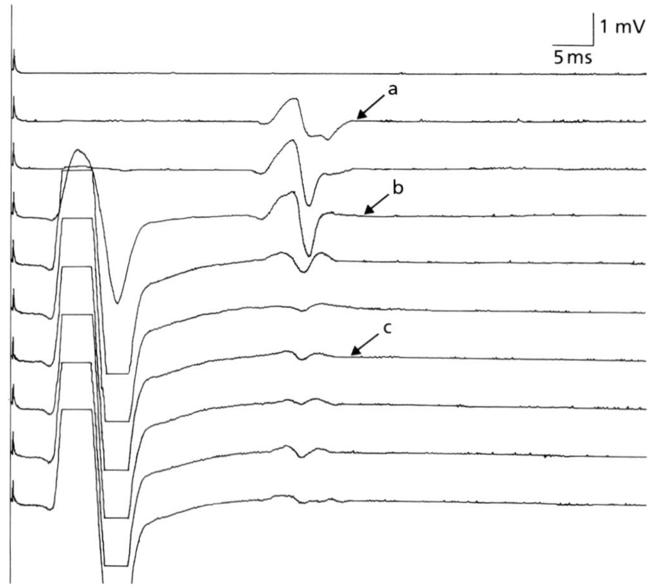

Fig. 10.4 H wave acquisition sequence with surface recording over the soleus muscle. Stimulation of the tibial nerve in the popliteal fossa. Stimulus strength increases with each trace moving from top to bottom. At (a) the H wave is recruited without the direct CMAP (M response); at (b) the H and M are present; at (c) the H wave has been replaced by the F response.

Reflex studies and late responses

Reflex studies and late responses are particularly useful in studying subtle changes in nerve conduction occurring at any point in a peripheral nerve, but specifically abnormalities in direct or reflex pathways at root level or within the spinal cord. In addition, some studies can give indications as to the supraspinal influences acting on the segmental reflex arcs.

In routine clinical use are the Hoffman (H) reflex, the tendon (T) reflex and the F wave. Other reflexes used less frequently are the silent period and the long loop reflexes.

The electrically elicited H reflex attributed to Hoffman (1922) is the electrical equivalent of the 'monosynaptic' deep tendon reflex at the ankle. It has been reliably recorded only from the tibial nerve in the lower limb where it relates to the S1 'monosynaptic' ankle deep tendon reflex and in the upper limb from the radial nerve supply to flexor carpi radialis. For the lower limb study the recording arrangement is the same as a motor nerve conduction study (see above) with recording electrodes applied over the belly of the soleus muscle and stimulation of the tibial nerve in the popliteal fossa. As the stimulus intensity is increased the H reflex appears either at the same threshold as the direct CMAP or at a lower threshold (Fig. 10.4). The H wave is identified by its longer latency compared with the CMAP (M wave), by its reproducible shape, and by its response to the stimulus intensity. As this is increased both the M and H wave increase in amplitude. However, before the M wave is supramaximal the H wave begins to diminish and is replaced by the F wave. The H reflex arises because of the recruitment of the fast-conducting afferent nerve fibres to the spinal cord which then relay monosynaptically with the anterior horn cell motor pool. The resultant impulses travel down the efferent pathway to the muscle, producing a late contraction.

The H reflex and the mechanically elicited tendon jerk (T reflex) may be compared. In the latter the recording arrangement is the same, but the trace is initiated by an inertia switch on the tendon hammer. From a physiological point of view the comparison can give information about the activation state of the γ-motor neurone pool controlling the sensitivity of the muscle spindles. This is because the H reflex effectively bypasses the muscle spindle in the afferent pathway of the reflex arc.

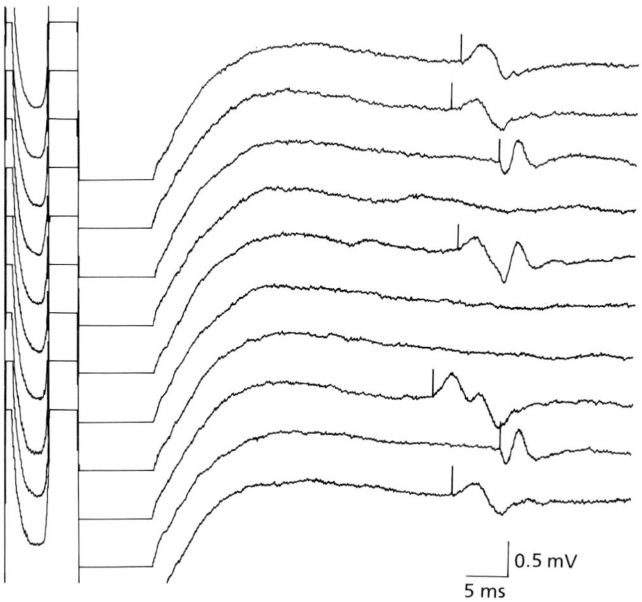

Fig. 10.5 F waves recorded from surface electrodes over the soleus muscle. Stimulation of the tibial nerve in the popliteal fossa. Abnormal chronodispersion and some failures.

The amplitude of the H reflex and its persistence on increasing stimulation strength depends on the excitability of the γ-motor neurone pool. Thus facilitation in a normal subject or pathological loss of inhibition in a suprasegmental or corticospinal tract lesion will give a measurable change in the H reflex.

The F wave is a much more widespread phenomenon, being recordable from most distal limb muscles. The F wave was so named because of its first recording from foot muscles. The recording arrangement is exactly the same as a motor conduction study; therefore this test is a convenient one to follow it. With a supramaximal stimulus and at a longer latency than the M wave (CMAP) a waveform is obtained that varies in latency and shape with each successive stimulus. The majority opinion is that this F wave represents a recurrent discharge arising from the antidromic volley of impulses passing from the stimulation point proximally up the motor axons to the spinal cord, with activation of the anterior horn cells and subsequent passage of impulses orthodromically down to the muscle. There are a number of parameters that are normally measured in an F-wave study which should include 20 successive responses. The minimum latency to the onset of response is the most frequently quoted, but the maximum latency, the variability of latency or 'chronodispersion' and the mean latency are all used as routine values in several centres (Fig. 10.5). In all cases the latency values have to be related both to the age of the subject and to the limb length. This may be done directly using a nomogram of height or limb length/age versus F-wave latency.

An additional parameter that is useful is the F ratio (Kimura, 1978b). A lesion in the pathway studied by the F wave may be very small in length and thus a local prolongation of latency at the lesion may be diluted by the long total pathway tested. To make the F wave effective for detecting localized proximal lesions at root level, for example, a shorter pathway would be useful. Thus the F ratio can be used to compare the above- and below-elbow segments of the median and ulnar nerves by stimulation at the antecubital crease. The conduction distal and proximal to these stimulation points is compared where: F ratio = (F latency − M latency − 1)/2 × M latency. The assumption is that the conducting distance is equal between the proximal and distal segments of the pathway. A normal ratio is close to 1.0, and significant distal slowing is indicated by a ratio significantly less than 1 and a proximal lesion by the converse.

In all the latency measures of the F wave the comparison between the symptomatic and asymptomatic side may be the most useful measurement as well as comparison with normal tables. The amplitude of the F wave does vary with suprasegmental influences, but this is of little practical use in diagnosis. However, the character of the waveform and its variability or lack of variability is another indication of abnormality. The F wave is a variable response from stimulus to stimulus because of the lack of preferential responses from one selective group of neurones. If there is a lesion in the pathway there may be such a group of neurones with a lower threshold to stimulation. This produces the 'repeater' F wave which is characterized by similar morphology from stimulus to stimulus and a much less variable latency.

All measurements of nerve conduction parameters are compared with data from a normal population. In an ideal situation each laboratory creates a normal control group for every study undertaken. In practice this is performed only for the commonly studied nerves, and for unusual studies reference to other laboratories' data is made. In these circumstances care as to the similarity of technique is important.

Comparison of individual nerves from a symptomatic limb compared with the contralateral side is an additional useful technique. In all cases skin temperature should be controlled or compensated for, and allowance made for the age of the subject, and in the late responses a measure of the limb length or height is also needed.

There are certain basic patterns of abnormality in the motor nerve conduction study. Four parameters need to be considered: the DL; the FMNCV; the amplitude and area of the CMAP from stimulation at any site; and the changes in amplitude and area between two sites.

The DL represents nerve conduction velocity in the terminal nerve branches and the time taken for neuromuscular transmission. It may be prolonged in isolation from any other abnormality. The commonest cause of this is low temperature, and this is corrected either by external heating or by a mathematical correction factor introduced into the calculations. Symmetrical long latencies may be an indication of peripheral neuropathy either due to demyelination or axonal damage. In the former process abnormality relates either to pathological loss of myelin or to the shorter internodal length in nerve fibres that are remyelinating. In an axonal neuropathy the distal motor latency may be significantly prolonged with a normal FMNCV proximally. In this circumstance the amplitude of the CMAP is reduced. This pattern is particularly typical of the 'dying-back' neuropathies related to toxic or metabolic insult.

An asymmetrical distal latency prolongation can be the indication of nerve compression such as the carpal tunnel syndrome or a more focal peripheral neuropathy due, for example, to ischaemia.

The FMNCV may also be affected by temperature, but pathologically is most commonly abnormal in a peripheral neuropathy. If this involves significant demyelination the FMNCV may fall by at least 30% of its normal value. Such abnormality may be generalized or quite localized, indicating the necessity of studying many nerve segments and using the late responses to study proximal nerve conduction. However, in the presence of an axonal neuropathy the FMNCV may remain within the normal range despite loss of many or most conducting fibres, although a modest reduction of less that 20% is more usual. This applies to any condition producing axonal loss. Thus in an acute radiculopathy with substantial Wallerian degeneration the FMNCV may fall slightly outwith the normal range, usually with a profound drop in the size of the CMAP and prolongation of the DL. The unwary might think this represented more peripheral pathology, but it merely indicates the degree of axonal damage.

Comparison of the amplitude and area of the CMAP from various sites may indicate the nature of a degenerative process. In addition to the profound slowing of conduction that occurs in a demyelinating neuropathy, the CMAP tends to fall in amplitude and increase in duration as the stimulation site is moved proximally. The waveform also tends to become more complex as the differential conduction slowing of some fibres compared with others is more evident (temporal dispersion). If, in addition, the area of the response reduces, then it can be inferred that conduction block has occurred in some fibres between the stimulus sites. This is again relevant to other conditions closer to the spine. In an acute radicular compression, conduction block, demyelination and axonal loss may coexist, producing abnormalities of proximal nerve conduction.

In the sensory conduction study, the crucial measurements are of sensory latency (SL), SCV, amplitude, area and duration of the SAP. Sensory involvement in a peripheral neuropathy is indicated by a prolonged latency, slowed SCV, reduced amplitude and area with or without evidence of dispersion of the SAP. It must, however, be noted that the SAP is largely generated by activation of the fastest conducting 20% of the total numbers of afferent nerve fibres. Thus if a neuropathy affects only the small-diameter fibres subserving pain, autonomic function and thermal sensation, the SAP may remain within normal limits. In this circumstance modality-specific quantitative sensory testing may need to be used for diagnosis (Jamal *et al.*, 1985). Focal nerve lesions can produce localized changes in SCV and in SAP parameters in the same way as the motor studies. Localized entrapments can differentially affect motor fibres more than sensory or vice-versa, or both together (Kimura, 1978a).

Abnormalities of sensory conduction studies are particularly useful in delineating lesions that lie within the spinal column from those outside. The logic of this is based on the location of the cell bodies of the primary afferent sensory axons in the dorsal root ganglion (DRG) lying within the intervertebral foramina. In the presence of a complaint of cutaneous sensory disturbance and sensory signs on examination, the presence of a normal sensory potential indicates that the sensory pathway *distal* to the DRG remains intact, and that the lesion lies proximal to the ganglion. The lesion could be in the root, or indeed anywhere in the afferent pathway to the somatosensory cortex. While this is a most useful rule, it must be remembered that the normal range for amplitude of a sensory potential within the population is wide, and a fall from 'high normal' to 'low normal' may indicate a postganglionic lesion. This is where comparison between a symptomatic limb and a normal limb is useful, as well as repeated studies over some days or weeks to show trends.

Abnormalities of the H reflex comprise: an increase in minimum latency or dispersion of latencies, a change in the ratio of the amplitude of the CMAP to the H reflex amplitude or the absence of the response. An absent response may be normal after the age of 60 years and therefore mirrors the significance of absent ankle deep tendon reflexes after that age. The response may be absent early in peripheral neuropathy; indeed an increase in minimum latency or its absence may be the first electrophysiological sign of abnormality in diabetes, alcoholic neuropathy or uraemia.

The H reflex indicates conduction in the S1 reflex arc, and is thus useful in the diagnosis of radiculopathy. Taken with electromyographic abnormalities of muscles supplied by the S1 root, an unilateral prolongation of H-reflex latency or its absence is a useful indicator of an S1 root lesion, if a more distal mononeuropathy of the sciatic or tibial nerves has been excluded.

The H to M amplitude ratio is an indicator of the suprasegmental influence on the reflex arc and therefore may be used semiquantitatively to assess spasticity.

F-wave abnormalities can be considered in the same way. Prolongation of the minimum latency indicates slowing of conduction along some part of the nerve proximal to the stimulation point or distal to the recording site. It should be recalled that a small localized entrapment, for example, may give exactly the same or a smaller delay as a more generalized neuropathy. The abnormality related to the small area of entrapment is 'diluted' by the long pathway that is tested. Thus an F-wave abnormality recorded from the abductor pollicis brevis muscle could indicate a carpal tunnel compression of the median nerve or a plexus or root compression syndrome. However, the F-wave study is not performed in isolation, and distal motor and sensory conduction studies should indicate the peripheral entrapment. The nerve fibres contributing to the shortest F latency are the same as those in the FMNCV; thus comparisons between proximal nerve conduction measured with F waves and distal nerve conduction studies are appropriate. If the distal conduction studies are normal and the F ratio is considerably greater than 1.0, this indicates a lesion proximally, perhaps in the plexus or at the spinal root. If the sensory potential is normal, the lesion is preganglionic and lies at the root or cord level. This is a good example of how the neurophysiologist puts together the isolated pieces of evidence to locate the lesion. An increased variability of F-wave latency and/or increased maximal latency can be considered in exactly the same way from a diagnostic point of view as a minimal latency increase.

Electromyography

Electromyography (EMG) is the study of the electrical activity of skeletal muscles both at rest and under voluntary contraction. In EMG the preferred electrode for recording is a concentric needle, and surface recording is used only when mass movements of muscle are being studied, such as in biofeedback. The activity recorded by the needle is amplified and filtered before being presented on the oscilloscope screen of the electromyograph for analysis. There are a variety of needles used in such studies but, in the context of this chapter, two should be mentioned: the concentric needle and the single fibre needle.

The concentric EMG needle consists of an outer sheath insulated from an inner core which is brought to the surface at the bevel of the needle. Once inserted in a muscle the voltage between the core and the outer sheath reflects muscle activity over a cone of height less than 1 mm. This volume contains muscle fibres from some four to six motor units; therefore if the needle is located at eight to 10 different locations within each muscle through the same skin puncture this will provide an acceptable sample of most muscles.

The single fibre EMG needle consists of a shaft insulated from a core, this time of only 25 μm diameter. This core is brought out through the wall of the needle on the side opposite to the bevel. This arrangement facilitates the recording of the single muscle fibre action potentials within a motor unit. The maximum recording distance from the active electrode is approximately 300 μm.

A routine EMG study with a concentric needle involves insertion into the muscle and observation of the electrical activity in four phases: (a) during complete relaxation; (b) during weak contraction; (c) during graded contraction; (d) during maximum voluntary contraction. The choice of muscle studied relates to the clinical problem, so that the pattern of involvement is defined. Thus if a a peripheral neuropathy is suspected distal muscles will be studied first and then more proximal ones. The neurophysiologist will be careful to include muscles subserved by a number of peripheral nerves, to determine whether the neuropathy is a monor neuropathy, mononeuropathy multiplex or generalized. In the same way, in the study of a radiculopathy, muscles will be chosen to represent specific myotomes and exclude others, so that a single root level involvement may be inferred.

The aim of concentric needle electromyography is the detection of the characteristics of a lower motor neurone lesion, an upper motor neurone lesion and a myopathy. This is of course a gross oversimplification, and it needs to be stated that the descriptions below are only guidelines. As before, all the neurophysiological data have to be taken together with the clinical history and examination to give an overall diagnosis.

Insertion of a concentric needle into a muscle at rest should produce only a transient (<0.5 s) disturbance of the oscilloscope tracing termed insertional activity. This comprises both biphasic waves and monophasic positive waves. Increased or prolonged insertional activity is noted when there are runs of the positive sharp waves or other more complex waves termed 'bizarre repetitive discharges' that persist after needle movement has ceased (Fig. 10.6). These can occur acutely and chronically in neuropathy, neuronopathy and myopathy. Once the insertional activity has died down the phase of spontaneous activity is studied. In the normal state no potentials should be seen. Abnormal discharges comprise fibrillations which are biphasic potentials of approximately 100 μV amplitude and positive sharp waves of variable amplitude but characteristic morphology (Fig. 10.7). Both these waveforms occur singly or in groups or bursts, and represent spontaneous activity in single muscle fibres. These may be contrasted with fasciculation potentials, which are much larger (<10 mV) and occur singly. They arise as spontaneous discharges of groups of muscle fibres which represent the whole or part of a motor unit.

Fibrillations and positive sharp waves can be seen in both lower motor neurone disorders, signifying denervation, and primary muscle disease such as myopathy.

Fasciculations are seen commonly in neuronopathies such as motor neurone disease. They are also present in a radicular distribution in chronic radiculopathy, but only relatively rarely in generalized neuropathy.

The search for spontaneous activity in each muscle is carried out through a single skin insertion but with the needle tip placed at eight to 10 separate sites in various directions and depths from the skin insertion. Abnormalities are noted only if they occur at two spatially separated locations within the muscle, and if there is doubt a further skin insertion in another region of the muscle is performed. The degree of spontaneous activity is usually recorded on a scale of 0–4+, but these scales are arbitrary and should not be considered anything more than qualitative information.

The next phase of the study is the analysis of the single motor unit potentials recruited voluntarily. The patient is asked to contract the muscle gently and the needle is moved to a position where a few single motor unit potentials are seen firing at a slow rate, and which can be clearly separated on the screen. The amplitude, duration, numbers of phases (baseline crossings) and variability of the potentials are then

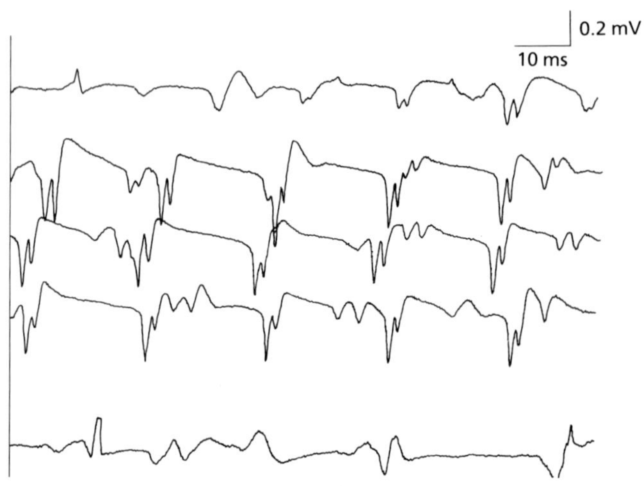

Fig. 10.6 Bizarre repetitive discharges.

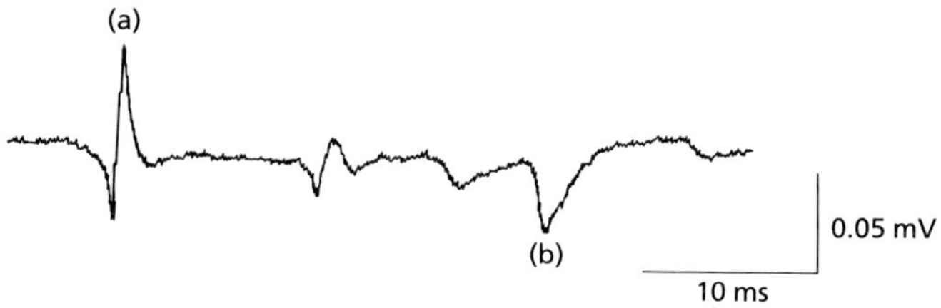

Fig. 10.7 Abnormal spontaneous activity: (a) fibrillation potential; (b) positive sharp wave.

noted and the needle moved to other sites until 10–20 motor unit potentials (MUP) are identified.

There are two approaches to data assessment. On the one hand, detailed analysis of the potentials is made by measurement of printouts or utilizing a computer to analyse the potential. In both situations comparison is made with tables of normal potentials for each muscle and a quantitative answer obtained. In addition computer analysis of the interference pattern during maximal voluntary contraction may be performed. The alternative technique is to adopt a more qualitative approach. The amplitudes, durations and phases of each motor unit potential are assessed by eye and comparison made with normal data and a record of discrepancies made. This is undoubtedly less objective, and is not satisfactory when subtle differences between a mild myopathy or neuropathy are sought. However, in routine studies of a suspected radiculopathy or neuropathy it is entirely satisfactory both for diagnosis and the assessment of the dynamics of the condition.

A normal MUP is triphasic (Fig. 10.8). In myopathy the MUP is of short duration, often small amplitude and polyphasic indicating a reduced number and spatial spread of muscle fibres in that motor unit. Late components may indicate regenerating muscle fibres. Normal or increased amplitude MUP occur in neuropathy with an increase in duration and number of phases. Some components may be unstable with increased 'jitter' on single fibre EMG examination reflecting immature endplate connections. Large-amplitude MUP indicate more sustained reinnervation and these may become less polyphasic as the security of the new connections improves. Giant MUP may appear in any chronic reinnervating condition.

Once the single motor unit potentials are recorded the recruitment can be assessed. The patient is asked to contract the muscle smoothly and the rate of recruitment of new MUP and the frequency of firing of the units assessed. This is again a situation where detailed analysis with some automation may be utilized. Again as an oversimplification certain patterns can be summarized:

1 The upper motor neurone pattern. The numbers of MUP increase moderately but the speed of firing of all the units only increases slightly, if at all.

2 The 'non-organic' pattern. This title implies that the reason for neuromuscular weakness is related not to structural neuromuscular disease but to a failure of volition, whether intentional or subconscious. On the command to contract the muscle the number of MUP recruited may fall, and the rate of firing remains static or reduces, often with accompanying sounds of extreme effort from the patient. In addition the MUP may form into phasic groups which are clinically accompanied by a tremulous contraction of the whole muscle.

3 The lower neurone pattern. There is a modest increase in the numbers of MUP recruited (polyphasic, if reinnervation is active). The firing rate of the MUP

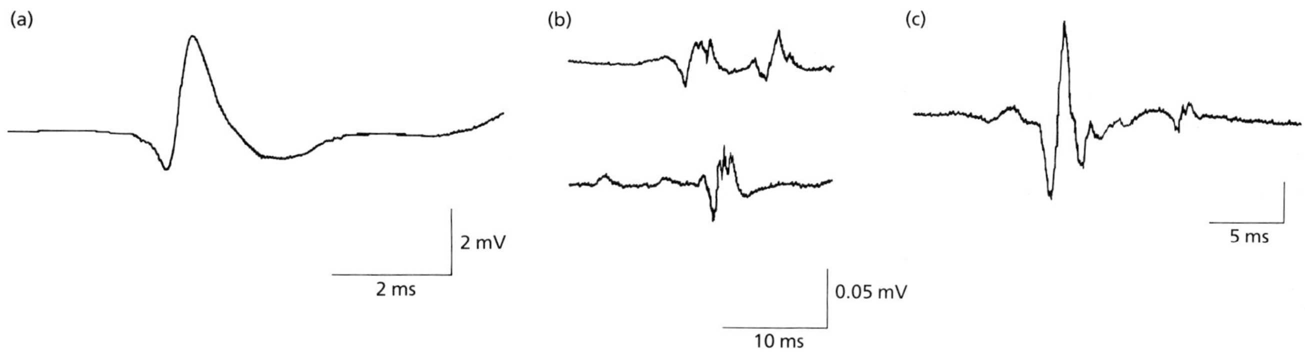

Fig. 10.8 (a) Normal motor unit potential (MUP); (b) small-amplitude, short-duration polyphasic MUP in myopathy; (c) normal-amplitude, long-duration MUP with satellite potential in reinnervating neuropathy.

increases with the muscle power in a gradual fashion but peaks at a rate higher than would normally be expected for that muscle.

4 The myopathic pattern. As soon as the muscle contracts there is an instantaneous recruitment of all MUP available, with a very high overall firing frequency. This rapid recruitment may be in the presence of minimal muscle power.

The final part of the concentric needle EMG examination is the assessment of recruitment with maximal voluntary effort. A normal pattern is defined such that at normal gain and sweep settings on the electromyograph the baseline trace is fully obliterated by the MUP discharges. The interference pattern thus created may be full, reduced in density by varying degrees, or created instantaneously by rapid recruitment. This reflects normality, an upper or lower motor neurone lesion or myopathy, respectively.

A single fibre EMG study usually incorporates the measurement of fibre density and jitter. There are major texts describing this technique in great detail (Stalberg & Trontelj, 1979). Briefly, in the fibre density study the needle is inserted into the muscle under study, and the subject is instructed to contract the muscle gently. The needle is then adjusted until there is a single, well-defined single muscle fibre action potential reproducibly recorded, and the potential is at its maximum amplitude. The numbers of other single fibre action potentials time-locked to the triggering potential (and which derive from the same motor unit) are then counted. This procedure is repeated at 20 locations and the fibre density expressed as the mean number of single fibre potentials present at each recording site.

The single fibre EMG jitter estimation involves the location of the needle at a position to record two or more of the single muscle fibre action potentials from a single motor unit. A timing device is triggered from the first potential and the variance or 'jitter' of the time between the first and second potential is measured for a train of 100 potentials. Mathematical adjustments are made to reduce the influence of changes in muscle fibre conduction velocity, and of trends related to the variable recruitment rate of the firing of the motor unit, and a figure termed the mean consecutive difference (MCD) is derived. This procedure is repeated at up to 20 locations and the individual jitter values for each potential pair are compared with normal data for that muscle. Usually the percentage of abnormal pairs and the mean jitter for the whole study are used in diagnosis.

Spinal cord conduction

Somatosensory evoked potentials (SEP)

Evoked potentials (EP) are electrical potentials recorded from the nervous system in response to an applied peripheral stimulus to the sensory receptors or a point on the afferent sensory pathway. The advent of motor evoked potentials has required this definition to be widened to include stimulation of one or several sites in the motor pathway and recording more caudally in the pathway. Analysis of EP is much more complex than of peripheral nerve conduction.

EP are an order of magnitude smaller in amplitude than the sensory action potential, and are easily lost in the background physiological and electronic noise from a surface voltage recording. Thus for detection, stimuli are applied repetitively and multiple responses are averaged, thus enhancing the signal to noise ratio.

SEP may be recorded by many different protocols. The vast majority use an electrical stimulus to a mixed peripheral nerve in the upper or lower limb with surface recording sites over the proximal limb, spinal column and the contralateral somatosensory cortex. The mixed nerves contain fibres destined for several roots, and workers interested in EP abnormalities in radiculopathies have introduced the use of dermatomal cutaneous stimulation, with the surface stimulus in the signature area for the dermatome under investigation (Katafi & Sedgwick, 1987).

For upper limb SEP studies the median or ulnar nerve at the wrist are commonly stimulated, and the recording sites lie over the brachial plexus at Erb's point, over the cervical spinous process at C7 and/or C2, and on the scalp over the somatosensory cortex (Fig. 10.9). For lower limb studies the posterior tibial nerve at the ankle is the preferred stimulation site, although the common peroneal nerve at the knee is also suitable.

For a routine SEP either 256 or 512 averages are usually required, but a lesser number may be required if only the thoracolumbar potential is of interest. In all EP recordings it is desirable to repeat the test at least once, and make a permanent record of both samples.

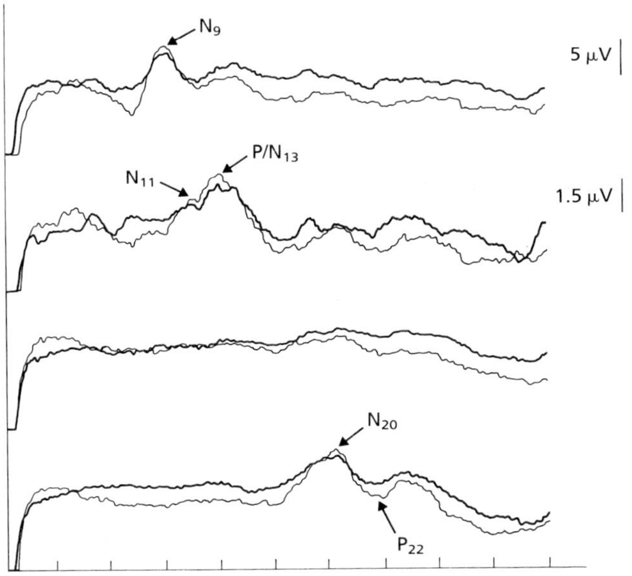

Fig. 10.9 SEP recordings. The upper trace is recorded from the brachial plexus, the lower traces being from C6, ipsilateral scalp and contralateral scalp in descending order. Two trials of 256 averages are superimposed in each trace.

Most of the available data supports the hypothesis that the SEP travels in the large fibre dorsal column/lemniscal afferent pathway. Clinical studies have found normal SEP associated with disorders of the small fibre afferent pathways but abnormalities have been found if touch, vibration or joint position were affected.

There is not universal agreement about the nomenclature of EP waveforms as they have historically been identified by many different techniques in different laboratories. Conventionally EP waveforms are identified by the prefix P or N, denoting that the wave is positive or negative, followed by a number which identifies the normal latency of that component or a number denoting the position of the wave in a sequential sequence, e.g. N75, P100, P1, P2, P3. The amplitude of the component may be expressed as an absolute value or peak-to-peak relative to the following waveform. Thus the N20 cortical response to median nerve stimulation denotes a negative peak occurring 20 ms after the stimulus.

Waveform origins may be summarized using the Fz referential montage. Stimulation of the median nerve produces a diphasic or triphasic potential recorded at Erb's point (N9) reflecting the afferent volley of action potentials in the low-threshold, large-diameter sensory and antidromic activation of the motor nerve fibres. The motor contribution is not substantial as the potential may be largely unchanged in the presence of long-standing lower neurone degeneration following ventral root avulsion. In the cervical spine recording the N11 potential was originally thought to be a fixed generator but is now considered to be a presynaptic travelling wave. The P/N13 is the dominant spinal evoked potential which is positive recording from ventral neck and negative over the dorsal surface. It reflects an anteroposterior generator thought to be the dorsal horn and dorsal column nuclei. At the scalp electrode, N20 reflects a generator either in the thalamocortical radiations or more likely in the posterior bank of the central sulcus.

SEP may be used to measure spinal conduction and can be recorded both invasively and non-invasively either by direct or indirect EP measurements. The direct non-invasive method utilizes the lower limb SEP technique with surface recording electrodes over the thoracolumbar and cervical spinal vertebrae. Thus a conduction time may be measured over a known distance and the conduction velocity of the fastest afferent fibres may then be calculated. The problem with this technique is the difficulty in obtaining reproducible potentials above the thoracolumbar region even in normal subjects. In practical terms these direct non-invasive methods fail to have the necessary reliability in adults, although maturational studies in infants and children have been successful (Cracco & Cracco, 1979).

Direct methods of measuring conduction in the *motor* pathways have been used experimentally in animals for many years. In 1980 Merton & Morton described the use of a rapid, high-voltage condensor discharge to stimulate the cerebral cortex through the scalp. Subsequent studies demonstrated that the stimulating voltage could be reduced by at least 50% if the target muscle was contracted to approximately 10% of its maximal voluntary contraction (Levy *et al.*, 1984). Cervical spinal cord stimulation was also found to be possible; therefore a direct method for measuring the central motor conduction time was developed (Marsden *et al.*, 1982).

A further advance has been the development of painless stimulation of the cortex and spinal cord utilizing a pulsed magnetic field of strength *c.* 1.5 Tesla from a hand-held electromagnet (Barker *et al.*, 1985). The latency of response comparison between magnetic and electrical stimulation demonstrates a consistent increase in latency from magnetic stimulation of approximately 2 ms. A wide variety of clinical applications have been developed for this technique (Chokroverty, 1990) including diagnosis of MS, stroke and peripheral nerve disorders.

Spinal cord monitoring

Monitoring of the spinal cord using somatosensory evoked potentials has become a major new role of the clinical neurophysiologist in the surgical management of spinal cord disease. EP monitoring has two separate roles: first to identify the development of spinal cord dysfunction undetectable by the surgeon at a time when an alteration of technique may restore function, and second to identify in some cases the incompleteness of a decompressive procedure.

SEP monitoring has been utilized during many different types of procedure, but their most frequent use has been in the elective correction of spinal deformity (e.g. Lueders *et al.*, 1982; Tamaki *et al.*, 1984; Whittle *et al.*, 1986; Mostegl *et al.*, 1988; Roy *et al.*, 1988). Their use in other conditions is limited by the delay involved in the averaging process, which means that during resections of , for example, an intramedullary tumour, any alteration to the EP will become evident only after the event. However, a place for their use has been reported in: odontoidectomy (Spetzler *et al.*, 1979); excision or embolization of arteriovenous malformations (Owen *et al.*, 1979; Berenstein *et al.*, 1984); the tethered cord (Roy *et al.*, 1986); spinal stenosis (Herron *et al.*, 1987); and certain neuroablative procedures for the relief of pain or spasticity (Macon *et al.*, 1982; Thomas & Jones, 1984).

It is essential that great attention to technical detail is taken when recording intraoperative EP, as the waveform may be affected by many factors such as electrode movement, hypotension, hypothermia and the effect of anaesthetic agents. The posterior tibial or common peroneal nerves are the most commonly used sites for stimulation, and recording may be non-invasive or invasive. For non-invasive recording surface electrodes over the spine itself may be used, but the most common site is a scalp electrode over the somatosensory cortex. Invasive recordings normally use epidural electrodes or less frequently needles inserted into the spinous processes or interspinous ligaments. In invasive techniques direct root or cauda equina stimulation may be used.

Non-invasive techniques have the advantage of simplicity and safety, but the disadvantage of lower amplitude responses and a long neural pathway leading away from the operation site, resulting in reduced sensitivity. As the non-invasive techniques use a cortical response they are vulnerable to factors affecting cortical and subcortical function such as anaesthetic agents and hypotension. York *et al.* (1987) examined the factors affecting the SEP during scoliosis surgery. Amongst other factors they found that merely saline irrigation of the wound produced the prompt loss of the SEP. Some control of these factors can be obtained in thoracic and lumbar surgery where the use of a control SEP from the upper limb can monitor such factors.

The area of greatest concern in the clinical use of these techniques lies in their sensitivity. The fact that SEP studies by their very nature only monitor ascending pathways raises the spectre of a patient becoming paraplegic during an operation in which the SEP has remained normal. The converse is where the SEP deteriorates in the absence of any clinical disturbance. Assessing the true incidence of such events is difficult as most studies have used differing criteria to decide when a change in SEP is significant. A change of amplitude in excess of 50% is the most widely used, but Roy *et al.* (1988) found a decrease in amplitude greater than 60% in 11% of a series of 63 patients, none of whom had any postoperative deficit.

Reviewing several large scoliosis series (Jones *et al.*, Lueders et al., 1982; Maccabee *et al.*, 1983; Bradshaw *et al.*, 1984; Nuwer & Dawson, 1984; Tamaki *et al.*, 1984; Wilber *et al.*, 1984; Dinner *et al.*, 1986; Ryan & Britt, 1986; Whittle *et al.*, 1986; York *et al.*, 1987; Bieber *et al.*, 1988; Mostegl *et al.*, 1988; Roy *et al.*, 1988) it is seen that the rate for the detection of SEP abnormalities thought to be significant ranged from 0 in 108 operations to 28 in 137. Over the 1582 procedures reported, the mean rate was 4.4%. Of those cases which were abnormal, the SEPs reverted to normal after either altering the surgical technique or removing the instrumentation in 59%. In the remaining cases there were: 13 cases of persisting neurological deficit with persisting SEP abnormality, two had transient deficit where action had resolved a SEP abnormality, five patients had only transient paraesthesiae despite an abnormal SEP and were defined as false-negatives, and there was one case of pure motor paraplegia despite normal intraoperative SEP.

Taking all the cases where significant postoperative

neurological deficit occurred despite intraoperative monitoring produces an incidence of 0.82%. This is very similar to the incidence of 0.72% reported by MacEwan (1975) without monitoring in scoliosis surgery. A more recent review of 1168 cases from London (Forbes *et al.*, 1991) reported a 10.2% detection of SEP abnormality and 0.27% with a significant postoperative neurological deficit. This substantially better result emphasizes the advantage of experience in a centre where monitoring is routine. There still remains doubt in some centres about the efficacy of spinal cord monitoring. This is a question which could only be finally answered by the conduction of a properly controlled trial, including the use of a 'wake-up' test in the non-monitored arm. The well-established 'wake-up' test allows assessment of motor function during the procedure by allowing the patient to become partially conscious and then checking lower limb function.

Levy (1987) has used cortical electrical stimulation during surgery to assess motor function, and studies of magnetic motor stimulation are under way. The value of such assessment of motor tracts has not been established as yet.

The place of monitoring to ensure the completeness of a surgical procedure is in its infacy. Studies such as that by Herron *et al.* (1987), where the completeness of root decompression during spinal stenosis surgery was monitored by the improvement in the dermatomal SEP, suggest that this approach might have a place, but the results are not statistically significant. They can have a place only where the cause of neurological deficit is related to neuropraxia due to the compression. They cannot assess the later improvement which can result from postoperative axonal regeneration and remyelination.

SEP monitoring of the spinal cord is presented as a major advance in the surgery of the spine and spinal cord. It has been demonstrated to have a role in monitoring at least some of the pathways that are at risk from mechanical or vascular interference. The evidence to date does not yet prove the hypothesis that this technique has substantially changed the incidence of intraoperative damage in scoliosis surgery, but in view of the potential catastrophe that postoperative paraplegia presents it is now a permanent part of the neurophysiological armamentarium. It has given insights into the physiological effects of pre-existing trauma and compression on the spinal cord and roots. In the latter area it does seem that the SEP monitor may have a role in demonstrating the adequacy of decompressive procedures.

Electrophysiological assessment along with clinical examination assesses neurological function as opposed to radiological investigation, which merely assesses pathological anatomy. The place of neurophysiology in certain common syndromes is now discussed.

In the clinical syndrome of *myelopathy*, electrophysiological abnormalities correlate with the degree, distribution and progression of the cord lesion but do not indicate the cause. Thus, a single-level cord lesion due to a cervical disc protrusion will produce exactly the same neurophysiological abnormalities as will a neurofibroma at the same site. In cervical spondylotic myelopathy, nerve conduction studies are invariably normal and the presence of normal sensory conduction velocities in a patient with pyramidal signs and distal sensory loss excludes a peripheral neuropathic cause for the sensory loss. Detailed EMG studies may show the effects of radiculopathy affecting the arms in conjunction with myelopathy. The most relevant investigation in patients with compressive myelopathy is that of SEP. This can indicate marked latency differences between the normal brachial plexus/lumbar potential and that arising in the cervical cord and cortex, or loss of all potentials above the level of the lesion.

In the differential diagnosis of cervical spondylotic myelopathy, the most frequent areas of doubt occur with multiple sclerosis and motoneurone disease. The assessment of peripheral and spinal function is the same in cervical spondylotic myelopathy and multiple sclerosis. However, patients with the latter diagnosis will often show changes in the visual evoked and brain stem auditory responses and characteristic MRI imaging. In patients with motoneurone disease, nerve conduction studies may show low-amplitude CMAP, prolonged distal latency and normal motor conduction velocity due to axonal loss. Sensory conduction studies are normal. EMG studies may show evidence of widespread fasciculation which can often be differentiated electrophysiologically from benign fasciculation seen in normal individuals. The cardinal signs of motoneurone disease on needle EMG are evidence of denervation with fibrillation and positive sharp waves with fasciculation in a widespread distribution encompassing the territories of several peripheral nerves and roots in both upper and lower limbs. Giant motor unit potentials may be seen in cases with chronic reinnervation.

In *radiculopathy*, patients with a single root entrapment will show normal distal motor nerve conduction studies with prolonged distal latency and reduced amplitude of the CMAP being exceptional, and only if there is substantial axonal degeneration. Changes in motor conduction velocity suggest the diagnosis of peripheral neuropathy such as in diabetes mellitus where a myotrophy may mimic a lumbosacral radiculopathy. Sensory conduction studies are also normal in the presence of a compressive radiculopathy such as lumbar disc prolapse as the lesion lies distal to the dorsal root ganglion. Analysis of the H and F waves may be of help in assessing the level of radicular compression, but are less reliable in the upper limb due to the presence of contributions from multiple roots to each peripheral limb nerve. EMG is the most fruitful investigation in radiculopathy and may produce evidence not only of the nature of the abnormality of neural function but also of which roots or nerves are affected (Aminoff *et al.*, 1985). EMG evidence of denervation in the paravertebral muscles indicates involvement of the posterior primary rami, indicating spinal rather than peripheral disease, though they are of no significance if there has been previous lumbar surgery.

In the situation of sphincteric dysfunction thought to be due to either a *conus* or a *cauda equina* lesion, electrophysiological studies combined with urodynamics may be very helpful. Apart from EMG studies of sacrally innervated muscles, attention is given to abnormalities of the bulbocavernosus and anal reflex arcs and EMG of the anal sphincters.

Studies of the SEP in patients with *traumatic injury to the spinal cord* indicate that, in general, the more gross the SEP abnormality the more severe is the lesion. Chabot *et al.* (1985) correlated the complete loss of the SEP with a complete lesion. Spielholz *et al.* (1979) found that an early return of the SEP to normal was a good prognostic sign. However, Chabot *et al.* (1985) did not find the use of serial SEP measurement to be of help in assessing outcome. Both nerve conduction and EMG studies may be of considerable help in the assessment of traumatic injury to the brachial and lumbosacral plexuses.

Both the performance and interpretation of neurophysiological testing requires great expertise. However, when combined with sound clinical assessment, it can produce information of great diagnostic and prognostic importance.

REFERENCES

Aminoff, M.J. (1986) *Electrodiagnosis in Clinical Neurology*, 2nd edn. Churchill Livingstone, New York.

Aminoff M.J, Goodin, D.S., Parry, G.J., Barbaro, N.M., Weinstein, P.R. & Rosenblum, M.L. (1985) Electrophysiological evaluation of lumbosacral radiculopathies: electromyography, late responses and somato sensory evoked potential. *Neurology (NY)*, **35**, 1514–1518.

Barker, A.T., Jalinous, R. & Freeston, I.L. (1985) Non-invasive magnetic stimulation of the human motor cortex *Lancet*, **i**, 1106–1107.

Berenstein, A., Young, W., Ransohoff, J., Benjamin, V. & Merkin, H. (1984) Somatosensory evoked potentials during spinal angiography and therapeutic transvascular embolisation. *J. Neurosurg.*, **60**, 777–785.

Bieber, E., Tolo, V. & Uematsu, S. (1988) Spinal cord monitoring during posterior spinal instrumentation and fusion. *Clin. Orthop.*, **229**, 94–98.

Bradshaw, K., Webb, J.K. & Fraser, A.M. (1984) Clinical evaluation of spinal cord monitoring in scoliosis surgery. *Spine*, **9**, 636–643.

Chabot, R., York, D.H., Watts, C. & Waugh, W.A. (1985) Somatosensory evoked potentials evaluated in normal subjects and spinal cord injured patients. *J. Neurosurg.*, **63**, 544–551.

Chokroverty, S. (1990) *Magnetic Stimulation in Clinical Neurophysiology*. Butterworths, London.

Chu-Andrews, J. & Johnson, R.J. (1986) *Electrodiagnosis: an Anatomical and Clinical Approach*. J.B. Lippincott, Philadelphia, PA.

Cracco, J.B., Cracco, R.Q. & Stolove, R. (1979) Spinal evoked potential in man: a maturational study. *Electroencephalogr. Clin. Neurophysiol.*, **46**, 58–64.

Dawson, G.D. (1947) Investigations on a patient subject to seizures after sensory stimulation. *J. Neurol. Neurosurg. Psychiatry*, **10**, 141–162.

Dinner, D.S., Lueders, H., Lesser, R.P., Morris, H.H., Barnett, G. & Klem, G. (1986) Intraoperative spinal somatosensory evoked potential monitoring. *J. Neurosurg.*, **65**, 807–814.

Forbes, H.J., Allen, P.A., Waller, C.S., Jones, S.J., Edgar, M.A., Bentley, G., Webb, P.J., Ransford, A.O. & Morley, T.R. (1991) Spinal cord monitoring: experience with 1168 cases. *J. Bone Jt. Surg.*, **73B**, 487–489.

Herron, L.D., Trippi, A.C. & Gonyeau, H. (1987) Intraoperative use of dermatomal somatosensory evoked potentials in lumbar stenosis surgery. *Spine*, **12**, 379–383.

Hoffman, P. (1922) *Untersuchungen uber die Eigenreflexe (Sehnenreflexe) mensichlicher Muskeln*. Springer, Berlin.

Jamal, G.A., Hansen, S., Weir, A.I. & Ballantyne, J.P. (1989) An improved automated method for the measurement of thermal thresholds. *J. Neurol. Neurosurg. Psychiatry*, **48**, 354–360.

Jones, S.J., Edgar, M.A. & Ransford, A.O. (1982) Sensory nerve conduction in the human spinal cord: epidural recordings made during scoliosis surgery. *J. Neurol. Neurosurg. Psychiatry*, **45**, 446–451.

Katafi, H.A. & Sedgwick, E.M. (1987) Evaluation of the dermatomal somatosensory evoked potential in the diagnosis of lumbosacral root compression. *J. Neurol. Neurosurg. Psychiatry*, **50**, 1204–1210.

Kimura, J. (1983) *Electrodiagnosis in Diseases of Nerve and Muscle: Principles and Practice.* F.A. Davis, Philadelphia, PA.

Kimura, J. (1978a) A method for determining median nerve conduction velocity across the carpal tunnel. *J. Neurol. Sci.*, **38**, 1.

Kimura, J. (1978b) Proximal versus distal slowing of motor nerve conduction velocity in the Guillain–Barré syndrome. *Ann. Neurol.*, **3**, 344.

Levy, W.J. (1987) Clinical experience with motor and cerebellar evoked potential monitoring. *Neurosurgery*, **20**, 169–182.

Levy W.J., York, D.H., McCaffrey, M. & Tanzer, F. (1984) Motor evoked potentials from transcranial stimulation of the motor cortex in humans. *Neurosurgery*, **15**, 287–302.

Lueders, H., Gurd, A., Hahn, J., Andrish, J., Werker, G. & Klem, G. (1982) A new technique for intra-operative monitoring of spinal cord function: Multichannel recording of spinal cord and subcortical evoked potentials. *Spine*, **7**, 100–115.

Maccabee, P.J., Levine, D.B., Pinkhasov, E.I., Cracco, R.Q. & Tsairis, P. (1983) Evoked potentials recorded from scalp and spinous processes during spinal column surgery. *Electroencephalogr. Clin. Neurophysiol.*, **56**, 569–582.

MacEwan, G.D. (1975) Acute neurological complication in the treatment of scoliosis. *J. Bone Jt. Surg.*, **57A**, 404–408.

Maclean, I.C. (1979) Nerve root stimulation to evaluate conduction across the lumbosacral plexus. *Acta Neurol. Scand.*, **60** (Suppl. 73), 270.

Macon, J.B., Poletti, C.E., Sweet, W.H., Ojemann, R.G. & Zervas, N.T. (1982) Conducted somatosensory evoked potentials during spinal surgery. Part 2: Clinical applications. *J. Neurosurg.*, **57**, 354–359.

Marsden, C.D., Merton, P.A. & Morton, H.B. (1982) Percutaneous stimulation of spinal cord and brain: pyramidal tract conduction velocities in man. *J. Physiol.*, **328**, 69.

Merton, P.A. & Morton, H.B. (1980) Stimulation of the cerebral cortex in the intact human subject. *Nature*, **285**, 227.

Mostegl, A., Bauer, R. & Eichenauer, M. (1988) Intraoperative somatosensory evoked potential monitoring. A clinical analysis of 127 surgical procedures. *Spine*, **13**, 396–400.

Nuwer, M.R. & Dawson, E. (1984) Intraoperative evoked potential monitoring of the spinal cord: enhanced stability of cortical recordings. *Electroencephalogr. Clin. Neurophysiol.*, **59**, 318–327.

Owen, M.P., Brown, R.H., Spetzler, R.F., Nash, C.L. Jr, Brodkey, J.S. & Nulsen, F.E. (1979) Excision of intramedullary arteriovenous malformation using intraoperative spinal cord monitoring. *Surg. Neurol.*, **12**, 271–276.

Roy, E.P., Guttmann, L., Riggs, J.E., Jones, E.T., Byrd, J.A. & Ringel, R.A. (1988) Intraoperative somatosensory evoked potential monitoring in scoliosis. *Clin. Orthop.*, **229**, 94–98.

Roy, M.W., Gilmore, R. & Walsh, J.W. (1986) Evaluation of children and young adults with tethered spinal cord syndrome. Utility of spinal and scalp recorded somatosensory evoked potentials. *Surg. Neurol.*, **26**, 241–248.

Ryan, T.P. & Britt, R.H. (1986) Spinal and cortical somatosensory evoked potential monitoring during corrective spinal surgery with 108 patients. *Spine*, **11**, 352–361.

Scarff, T.B., Dallman, D.E., Toleikis, J.R. & Bunch, W.H. (1981) Dermatomal somatosensory evoked potentials in the diagnosis of lumbar root entrapment. *Surg. Forum*, **32**, 489–491.

Spetzler, R.F., Selman, W.R., Nash, C.L. Jr & Brown, R.H. (1979) Transoral microsurgical odontoid resection and spinal cord monitoring. *Spine*, **4**, 506–510.

Spielholz, N.J., Benjamin, M.V. & Engler, G. (1979) Somatosensory evoked potentials and clinical outcome in spinal cord injury. In Popp, A.J. (ed.), *Neural Trauma*, pp. 217–222. Raven Press, New York.

Stalberg, E. & Trontelj, J.V. (1979) *Single Fibre Electromyography.* Miravelle Press, Old Woking, Surrey.

Tamaki, T., Naguchi, T., Takano, H., Tsuji, H., Nakagawa, T., Imai, K. & Inoue, S. (1984) Spinal cord monitoring as a clinical utilisation of the spinal evoked potential. *Clin. Orthop.*, **184**, 58–64.

Thomas, D.G. & Jones, S.J. (1984) dorsal root entry zone lesions (Nasold's procedure) in brachial plexus avulsion. *Neurosurgery*, **15**, 966–968.

Whittle, I.R., Johnston, I.H. & Besser, M. (1986) Recording of spinal somatosensory evoked potentials for intraoperative spinal monitoring. *J. Neurosurg.*, **64**, 601–612.

Wilber, R.G., Thompson, G.H., Shaffer, J.W., Brown, R.H. & Nash, C.L. Jr (1984) Postoperative neurological deficits in segmental spinal instrumentation. A study using spinal cord monitoring. *J. Bone Jt. Surg.*, **66A**, 1178–1187.

York, D.H., Chabot, R.J. & Gaines, R.W. (1987) Response variability of somatosensory evoked potentials during scoliosis surgery. *Spine*, **12**, 864–876.

11 · Examination of Cerebrospinal Fluid

By S.H. BIGNER, M. GLANTZ and S.C. SCHOLD

Sampling of cerebrospinal fluid (CSF) by lumbar puncture is a diagnostic procedure which has been utilized for more than 100 years. Although the earliest applications involved the analysis of the cellular components, the progressive addition of biochemical procedures, radioimmunoassays and immunoelectrophoresis has greatly expanded the breadth of parameters which can be evaluated. Examination of this fluid is among the most direct and effective means of diagnosing conditions which primarily involve the subarachnoid space such as leptomeningitis, subarachnoid haemorrhage, and leptomeningeal neoplasms. In addition, the contact of the subarachnoid space with the entire brain and spinal cord, as well as its continuity with the ventricular system, means that CSF often indirectly reflects disorders located primarily within the parenchyma of the central nervous system.

Correct interpretation of an individual sample of CSF requires that the studies appropriate for that patient be performed, and that these findings be evaluated in the context of the clinical setting. The basic types of analyses which are conducted on CSF will be described, and their application to the diagnoses of conditions which are manifested in CSF will be discussed with emphasis on disorders which occur primarily in the subarachnoid space.

NORMAL CEREBROSPINAL FLUID

The CSF is produced at a rate of 450–500 cm^3 per day in adults, and 30–60 cm^3 per day in newborns. Since the subarachnoid space of the normal adult contains about 150 cm^3 of CSF, the entire CSF volume is replenished three or four times daily. Of this production 60–80% is the result of plasma ultrafiltration and active transport by the intraventricular choroid plexus. The remainder is elaborated by the ventricular ependymal cells and the brain parenchyma. Hydrostatic pressure carries the newly produced CSF out from the ventricles and into the subarachnoid space through the foramina of Luschka and Magendie. The fluid then circulates along the spinal cord and over the convexities of the brain, where it is reabsorbed into the vascular system through multiple arachnoid granulations located within the walls of the dural sinuses and around spinal nerve roots.

The chemical composition of 'normal' CSF varies with age, with site within the neuraxis, and with different study populations. With several specific exceptions, including glucose and the CSF proteins, the chemical content of the CSF is of great physiological importance, but has little clinical relevance. The CSF concentration of most ions differs little from the corresponding plasma level (Table 11.1). Lumbar CSF glucose concentration is related to serum glucose concentration, and in adults is about 60% of the serum level. This ratio decreases as serum glucose increases beyond the normal range (Powers, 1981). Equilibration between these two compartments requires 3–4 h. The cisternal CSF glucose level is slightly higher than the lumbar level, and the ventricular fluid level is still higher. The lumbar CSF glucose level in premature infants ranges from 24 to 63 mg%, and at term is 34–119 (CSF to blood glucose ratios of 0.81 and 0.74, respectively). The protein concentration varies by laboratory and measurement technique, but mean values range from 23 to 38 mg% in the series quoted by Fishman (1980) for lumbar fluid. The ventricular fluid level rarely exceeds 25 mg% in the absence of pathology.

Table 11.1 Normal values for CSF and plasma. After Davson *et al.* (1987)

	CSF	Plasma
Opening pressure (lying)	50–200 mm CSF	
Total protein	25–45 mg%	5000–8000 mg%
Glucose	45–80 mg%	70–110 mg%
Sodium	147 mmol/l	150 mmol/l
Chloride	113 mmol/l	99 mmol/l
Potassium	2.86 mmol/l	4.63 mmol/l
Magnesium	1.61 mmol/l	2.23 mmol/l
Calcium	2.28 mmol/l	4.70 mmol/l
Bicarbonate	23.3 mmol/l	26.8 mmol/l
Osmolarity	295 mosmol/l	295 mosmol/l
pH	7.31	7.40

CSF is seldom obtained from individuals without neurological or spinal symptoms, making opportunities to examine truly 'normal' CSF rare. Based on evaluation of samples from patients in whom no neurological disorder is found, as well as from patients with seizures and those undergoing myelography, one concludes that CSF normally contains only scattered mature lymphocytes and monocytes. In the adult, cell counts considered to be within the normal range are less than five cells per mm^3. Slightly higher cell counts may be seen in neonates, although there are seldom opportunities to examine fluid from neurologically uninvolved individuals in this age group.

The composition of the cellular component and the morphology of the individual cells are equally important as the cell count in determining whether the presence of cells in a sample of CSF is within normal range. Cell types seen in normal CSF are mature lymphocytes of small or intermediate size and monocytes, presumably derived from blood. The presence of polymorphonuclear leucocytes, enlarged, atypical lymphocytes, or monocytes which have become phagocytic, as well as an increase in absolute cell number, are all indications that a pathological condition exists.

Most normal brain and spinal cord elements such as neurones and glia are rarely if ever detected in CSF derived by lumbar puncture. Papillary fragments of cuboidal cells, probably originating in the choroid plexus, are common in ventricular fluids and are occasionally seen in CSF derived by lumbar puncture (Fig. 11.1). These cells are termed 'ependymal–choroidal' by some observers, who correctly point out that cells from the choroid plexus cannot be reliably

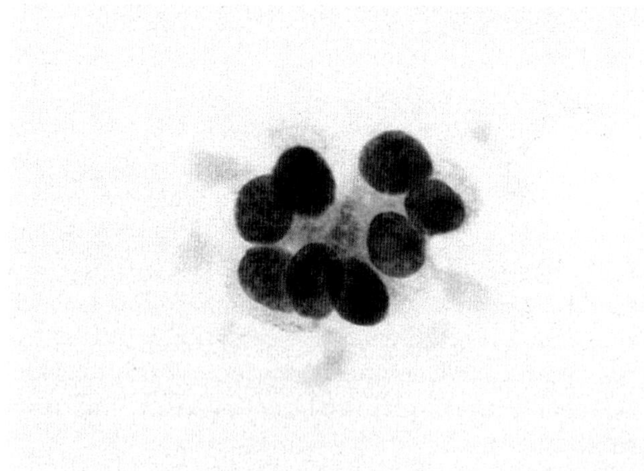

Fig. 11.1 Choroid plexus cells in a sample of cerebrospinal fluid obtained from the ventricle of a three-year-old boy. (Diff-quik stain ×1000.)

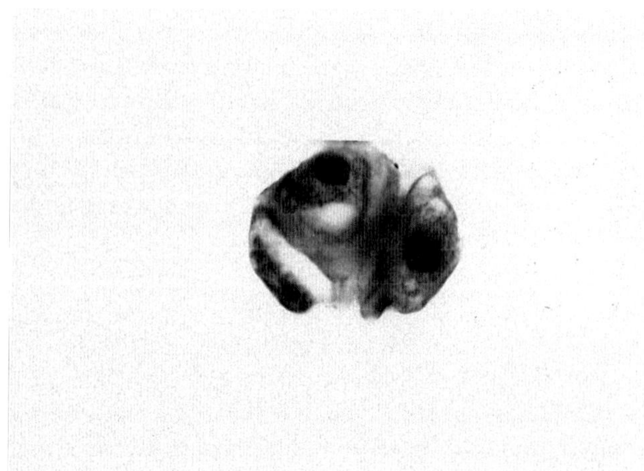

Fig. 11.2 Cartilage cells in a sample of cerebrospinal fluid derived by lumbar puncture. (Papanicolaou stain ×1000.)

distinguished cytologically from ependymal cells. Regardless of the histogenesis of these cells in an individual case, it is important to recognize this normal cellular component to avoid mistaking these fragments for neoplasia. Other normal elements which are sometimes encountered in CSF obtained by lumbar puncture are chondrocytes from the intervertebral disc (Fig. 11.2). The presence of these cells is of no known pathological significance, and is probably a physical phenomenon, related to direct contact of the sampling needle with the disc. Rarely, isolated, benign spindle-shaped cells are encountered. Although some observers have considered them to represent astrocytes, an alternative interpretation is that they are fibroblasts from the loose connective tissue of the subarachnoid space.

INFECTIOUS CONDITIONS

Biochemistry

An elevated CSF protein concentration is the nonspecific hallmark of a pathological process within or adjacent to the subarachnoid space. Infectious conditions are among the most common of these pathological processes, and include diseases within the subarachnoid space itself (meningitis), adjacent to it (subdural empyema, epidural abscess, vertebral discitis, osteomyelitis), within the brain parenchyma (abscess, cerebritis), and within the intracranial venous system (septic sinus thrombosis). The range of protein elevation varies with the site and type of process. A normal protein concentration is seen in approximately 10% of patients with viral meningitis and, with the exception of disease caused by the mumps and lymphocytic choriomeningitis (LCM) viruses, is less than 100 mg% in most of the remainder. Bacterial, tuberculous, and fungal meningitides reliably produce pronounced elevations (>200 mg%), while parasitic and spirochaetal diseases and non-meningitic infections produce intermediate elevations. Human immunodeficiency virus (HIV) infected individuals present a difficult and increasingly common problem of CSF interpretation. Oligoclonal bands and mild-to-moderate increases in protein concentration (45–75 mg%) and IgG index are seen in all stages of infection (asymptomatic seroconverters, patients with lymphadenopathy syndrome, AIDS-related complex, and full-blown AIDS), probably reflecting prompt CNS invasion by the virus (Snider *et al.*, 1983; Elovaara *et al.*, 1987). These CSF abnormalities become more frequent and pronounced as the disease progresses clinically.

A low CSF glucose level is a less common but more specific characteristic of the CSF in the setting of CNS infection. In one very large series, viral meningitis produced CSF glucose levels below 50 mg% in 3% of patients; parameningeal infections in 11%; neurosyphilis in 21%; bacterial meningitis in 64%; tuberculous meningitis in 89%; and fungal infections in 100% (Merritt & Freemont-Smith, 1938). Among the viral agents, mumps, LCM, herpes simplex viruses (HSV) I and II, and (rarely) herpes zoster can also depress the CSF glucose level. Glucose concentration remains unaltered in the absence of superimposed infectious or neoplastic disorders in the CSF of HIV-infected patients.

Several more specific biochemical abnormalities have also been observed in the CSF in the setting of infection. Lactic acid and lactic dehydrogenase (total and isoenzymes 4 and 5) are elevated in bacterial meningitis, and have been used to distinguish between viral and bacterial infections, and to follow the course of bacterial meningitis during treatment (Jordan *et al.*, 1983). Counterimmunoelectrophoresis exploits the reaction between antigens (in infected CSF) and known bacterial antibodies (in standard sera) as these proteins migrate in a polarized agar block to diagnose certain infections (*Haemophilus* influenza B, *Streptococcus, Pneumococcus, Staphylococcus aureus*, group B *Streptococcus* and *Meningococcus*) within 30–60 min (Kaplan, 1983). Commercially available latex agglutination kits provide an even more rapid and sensitive technique for diagnosing these same bacterial infections (Martin, 1983). Radioimmunoassay and enzyme-linked immunoabsorbent assay technology allows measurement of the intrathecal production rate of pathogen-specific IgG or IgM, and permits quick and reliable diagnosis of many infections. Finally, two serological tests, the fluorescent treponemal antibody absorption test (FTA-ABS), and the Venereal Disease Research Laboratory test (VDRL) can be performed on CSF to aid in the diagnosis of neurosyphilis. The specificity of the CSF-VDRL is high, but its sensitivity is low (100% and 27–60%). High sensitivity and low specificity mar the CSF-FTA-ABS. In up to one-quarter of patients with neurosyphilis the CSF is entirely normal.

Cellular composition

The presence of increased numbers of inflammatory cells in a sample of CSF with a component of polymorphonuclear leucocytes, enlarged and atypical lymphocytes, or of monocytes behaving as phagocytes, are indications that a pathological process exists. Although higher cell counts are more likely to be present if the disorder is occurring predominantly in the subarachnoid space, neither cell count nor cellular composition reliably distinguishes meningeal disease from a meningeal infiltrate secondary to primary parenchymal disease of the brain or spinal cord. The nature of the cellular infiltrate may suggest that the process in an individual patient is likely to be infectious rather than a reaction to a non-infectious disorder, and may favour a bacterial, viral, or fungal aetiology. Nevertheless, diagnosis of an infection requires demonstration of the responsible organism either by direct visualization, by culture, or by antibody titre.

The most typical cellular presentation of acute bacterial meningitis is an infiltrate composed predominantly of polymorphonuclear leucocytes. This pattern is not specific for this disorder, however, as an acute inflammatory infiltrate can also be seen in CSF from patients with acute cerebral infarctions, and occasionally in the early stages of viral and fungal infections.

Viral meningoencephalitis most frequently presents in CSF as an infiltrate composed predominantly of lymphocytes. These cells often show atypical features such as clumped chromatin and prominent nucleoli, and care must be taken not to confuse them with lymphoma. The viruses which usually produce this disorder are the enteroviruses, which do not display characteristic cellular inclusions in cells of CSF. Other viruses which involve the parenchyma of the brain and spinal cord, and produce a meningeal infiltrate are cytomegalovirus (CMV), HSV, herpes zoster and Creutzfeld–Jacob virus. Although cells containing the characteristic nuclear inclusions of these viruses can be demonstrated in open biopsies and needle biopsies of the parenchymal lesions, inclusion-bearing cells have only rarely been identified in the CSF.

Patients with AIDS acquire three types of CNS disorders (Katz *et al.*, 1989). First there are lesions resulting directly or indirectly from infection of cells by the AIDS virus within the brain or spinal cord, termed AIDS encephalopathy. Histologically the lesions consist of glial nodules, chronic inflammation, gliosis, and sometimes multinucleated giant cells. The CSF from these patients usually reveals only a non-specific chronic inflammatory infiltrate, although rarely multinucleated giant cells may be encountered. The second group of abnormalities consists of opportunistic infections which are most frequently produced by *Cryptococcus neoformans*, *Toxoplasma gondii*, *Mycobacteria*, *Candida*, and viruses such as CMV and the viruses of PML. These organisms or their characteristic cellular inclusions can frequently be demonstrated by open-brain biopsy or needle aspirates of the cerebral lesions. Among these infections, cryptococcal meningitis is the only process in which examination of CSF yields a specific diagnosis in a high percentage of cases. A non-specific chronic inflammatory response is usually seen in CSF from AIDS patients with these other CNS infections, with the exception of rare cases of CMV inclusion-bearing cells in CSF. The third disorder involving the CNS of AIDS patients is neoplasia, which is most frequently lymphoma. Examination of the CSF often reveals the characteristic malignant cells of lymphoma both in AIDS patients with primary CNS lymphoma involving the subarachnoid space and in patients with systemic lymphoma and CNS metastases. Since the majority of these lymphomas are of B-cell type immunohistochemical markers are useful in helping to establish this diagnosis.

Cryptococcus neoformans is the fungus which most frequently causes meningitis. This organism usually enters the body through the respiratory system and disseminates to the CNS haematogenously (Fetter *et al.*, 1967). Cryptococcal meningitis may be a complication of immunosuppression as is seen in recipients of organ transplants, patients with lymphoma and leukaemia, and in patients with AIDS. This disease occasionally occurs, however, in otherwise healthy individuals. In the immunosuppressed patient, in particular, there may be very little cellular reaction and the CSF may contain multitudes of organisms. In some cases, however, a brisk inflammatory reaction may occur. The cells can be predominantly lymphocytes, although occasionally polymorphonuclear leucocytes or macrophages predominate. The organisms are frequently demonstrable morphologically as round yeast forms of variable diameter which produce thin-necked buds and often possess a thick, mucopolysaccharide capsule (Fig. 11.3). Other

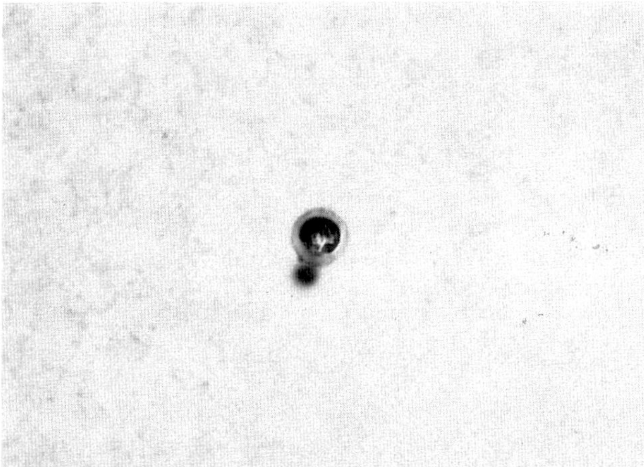

Fig. 11.3 Cryptococcal yeast form in cerebrospinal fluid. (Papanicolaou stain ×1300.)

means of diagnosing cryptococcal meningitis are by growing the organism in culture and by demonstrating cryptococcal antigen by radioimmunoassay.

DEMYELINATING DISEASE

Biochemistry

A variety of demyelinating processes produce biochemical abnormalities in the CSF. In two of these disorders, multiple sclerosis (MS) and the Guillain–Barré syndrome (GBS), the CSF examination constitutes an integral part of the diagnostic evaluation. The glucose level is unaffected in both conditions. The protein concentration is elevated in about 30% of patients with MS, but rarely exceeds 100 mg%. More than 75% of patients with GBS develop CSF protein levels between 40 and 1000 mg%, but a delay of one to six weeks after the onset of symptoms is not uncommon. A preferential increase in the IgG fraction of CSF protein occurs in 75–90% of patients with MS, and calculations correcting for disturbances in the brain–blood barrier ('IgG index') show that this elevation is due to intrathecal immunoglobulin production (Tourtellotte & Ma, 1978; McFarlin & McFarland, 1982). Less than 25% of patients with other neurological disorders (infections, tumours, inflammatory diseases) show similar abnormalities.

Electrophoresis of CSF proteins from patients with MS often shows two or more discrete bands ('oligoclonal bands'). This qualitative abnormality has been reported in 100% of patients with definite MS, and 82% of patients with possible MS (Miller *et al.*, 1983). Again, a variety of nervous system disorders (including GBS) may occasionally show similar abnormalities. Nevertheless, the IgG index and oligoclonal banding are the only laboratory abnormalities recognized in the New Diagnostic Criteria for Multiple Sclerosis (Poser *et al.*, 1982). A variety of other biochemical (mostly protein) CSF abnormalities have been examined, chiefly in MS. Myelin basic protein (MBP) (and antibodies to MBP) may be increased during active phases of MS and other demyelinating processes. The significance of abnormalities in immunoglobulin classes, viral antigens, and lymphocyte subsets remains uncertain. Mild-to-moderate protein elevations are also seen in systemic disorders (diabetes mellitus, pernicious anaemia, postinfectious encephalomyeloradiculopathies, hereditary leucodystrophies, heavy-metal poisoning) which produce some degree of demyelination.

Cellular composition

The cellular components in CSF from patients with demyelinating diseases are variable, depending on the specific diagnosis, and the phase and extent of the disease. In MS, for example, the cell counts and constitution may be normal during quiescent phases of the disease while increased numbers of lymphocytes are often seen during active phases of the disease. Immunophenotyping of the lymphocyte populations generally reveals T-cell predominance with mature T cells expressing either the helper or suppressor phenotype. Some observers have described a decreased suppressor/helper cell ratio in both CSF and peripheral blood of MS patients during exacerbation due to an absolute decrease in the number of suppressor cells. Other studies, however, have failed to demonstrate differences in suppressor/helper cell ratios between CSF from patients with MS and patients with other CNS disorders such as GBS and CNS infections. Rarely, in acute, rapidly progressive cases, other cell types including polymorphonuclear leucocytes and macrophages may be seen.

In most cases of GBS the CSF is acellular, but when inflammatory cells are present a lymphocytic response predominates. The picture is similar to that seen in viral meningoencephalitis with a polyclonal lymphocytic population with T-cell predominance. For the other diseases in which demyelination is a component, the nature and extent of cellular elements in CSF reflects the nature of the infiltrate within the parenchyma of the brain and spinal cord.

OTHER NON-NEOPLASTIC CONDITIONS

Biochemistry

Many miscellaneous neurological and non-neurological disorders alter the chemical composition of the CSF, in particular the glucose and protein concentrations. Among the more common and unexpected causes of an elevated protein level, seizures, migraine headaches, bloody CSF (traumatic as well as truly haemorrhagic), treatment with non-steroidal anti-inflammatory drugs (especially ibuprofen), renal and hepatic failure, and severe degenerative disc disease deserve special mention. Decreased CSF protein levels occur less commonly. High CSF glucose levels always indicate hyperglycaemia. Hypoglycorrhacia occurs in bloody CSF, after metrizamide myelography, and in other more familiar settings (Table 11.2). Angiotensin-converting enzyme may be increased in the CSF of patients with neurosarcoidoses (as well as in cases of neoplastic and bacterial meningitis), and may reflect disease activity in these patients. An almost endless array of biochemical alterations without clear clinical significance has also been reported.

Table 11.2 Causes of a decreased CSF glucose concentration

Meningitis
Bacterial
Tuberculous
Fungal
Viral (mumps, LCM, herpes simplex I and II, herpes zoster)
Amoebic
Chemical (after intrathecal chemotherapy)
Other (syphilitic, leptospiral, cysticercosis, etc.)
Inflammatory
Rheumatoid meningitis
CNS lupus
Sarcoidosis
Leptomeningeal metastases
Subarachnoid haemorrhage
Metrizamide myelography

Cellular composition

A variety of other conditions may produce non-specific elevations in cell counts in CSF. For example, cellular infiltrates are seen in CSF from victims of CNS trauma which are indistinguishable from the cells seen in subarachnoid haemorrhage and destructive lesions of other aetiologies.

NEOPLASIA

Biochemistry

The incidence and magnitude of biochemical abnormalities in the CSF of patients with cancer depends primarily on the extent of nervous system involvement, and on the proximity of the tumour to the ventricular system or subarachnoid space (Table 10.3). Independent of these features, tumour type has some additional bearing, particularly on the presence of various tumour 'markers'. An elevated protein is the most sensitive indicator of malignant CNS disease, and was present in 30% of patients with primary and metastatic brain lesions at the time of their first lumbar puncture in the study of Merritt & Freemont-Smith (1938). This was much more common with tumours invading the ventricular system or growing within the subarachnoid space (acoustic neuromas, for example). Except in these latter two instances the protein concentration was usually less than 100 mg%. With acoustic neuromas, protein concentrations of 200–500 mg% were typical. Earlier diagnosis of brain tumours in the age of magnetic resonance imaging has made the finding of a normal CSF formula at the time of diagnosis more common. The CSF glucose concentration is normal in each of these instances.

Intramedullary, intradural, and epidural spinal cord tumours are more commonly associated with an elevated CSF protein level, usually between 100 and 500 mg%. Extraordinarily elevated protein concentrations (usually greater than 1000 mg%) are seen in cases of complete subarachnoid block. The presence of fibrinogen within the CSF may allow the fluid to clot after removal (Froin's syndrome). Both a markedly elevated protein and formation of a CSF clot are more common with lumbar blocks, and are rare with blocks at the high thoracic or cervical level. Again, unless the CSF is haemorrhagic, the glucose level is normal.

Table 11.3 CSF glucose and protein concentrations in patients with CNS tumours

	Glucose (percentage of patients)	Protein (percentage of patients)	Comment
Brain tumour (first degree of metastatic)	Normal	↑ (30)	Highest in acoustic intraventricular neuromas and tumours
Spinal cord tumour	Normal	↑ (65–84)	Very high protein concentrations with subarachnoid block
Leptomeningeal tumour	↓ (31–76)	↑ (>75)	Tumour markers useful

In patients with leptomeningeal spread of tumour the CSF protein concentration is increased on the initial spinal fluid examination in more than 75%, and is >500 mg% in about 20% and the CSF glucose concentration is depressed. Less than 3% of patients with leptomeningeal tumour have a normal CSF on their first lumbar puncture (Wasserstrom *et al.*, 1982).

Biochemical tumour markers (enzymes, metabolites, oncofetal antigens) represent a final type of abnormality present in the CSF of patients with cancer. Because false-negative results are common for each of these markers, and false-positive values are seen with some markers in a variety of CNS infections and inflammatory conditions, they are usually not as useful in making a definitive diagnosis of cancer as in monitoring response to therapy. CSF markers may also portend a CNS relapse before more conventional signs, symptoms, and CSF abnormalities develop.

Cellular composition

Neoplastic processes which involve the subarachnoid space, and can be detected by examination of CSF, include leukaemia, lymphoma, carcinoma, melanoma, and primary CNS tumours. Since more than 90% of patients with meningeal tumour have a known tumour diagnosis at the time of subarachnoid dissemination, the question is usually whether or not cells similar to those in the original biopsy are present in CSF. In the few cases where a patient without a previous diagnosis of neoplasia presents with neoplastic cells in CSF, knowledge of the age of the patient, location of other tumour masses in the body, and morphology of the cells, including their expression of specific antigens using immunohistochemistry, will usually allow an accurate diagnosis.

Leukaemia

When leukaemia involves the CNS the most frequent pattern is infiltration of the subarachnoid space with little or no parenchymal disease. The types of leukaemia most likely to behave in this manner are composed of primitive cells, with acute lymphocytic leukaemia (ALL) and undifferentiated stem cell leukaemia of childhood being among the most prevalent types. With the advent in the 1960s of chemotherapeutic protocols capable of producing systemic remission, CNS relapse occurred in more than 50% of these patients. This observation led to the routine administration of CNS prophylaxis with radiation or chemotherapy, a practice which has dramatically reduced the likelihood of CNS disease. Nevertheless, this complication still occurs in approximately 10% of cases, making routine examination of CSF in patients with ALL a component of standard protocols.

The cells of ALL are typical blast forms with high nuclear to cytoplasmic ratios and round or convoluted nuclei. All varieties of ALL including null, B, T and pre-B cell types can involve the CSF with a possible tendency for T-cell disorders to behave in this fashion most frequently. When large numbers of blast forms are present they can be readily identified on routine preparations, making immunohistochemical procedures for lymphoid antigens unnecessary. Occasionally, a problem in differential diagnosis arises between recurrent leukaemia and pleocytosis due to infection in a patient with ALL. Here, immunohistochemical demonstration of polyclonality, or of a monoclonal population expressing the same phenotype as was seen in the marrow, may resolve the problem. The most difficult problems in diagnosis arise when only a few abnormal cells are seen, particularly in specimens of normal cell count.

CNS involvement is also seen in patients with acute myelogenous leukaemia, acute monocytic leukaemia and acute myelomonocytic leukaemia, particularly those with inversion of chromosome 16. The absolute incidence of this complication is lower than in ALL due to the shorter survival of these patients, but with improvements in treatment of these disorders the incidence of this complication is increasing. The cells of acute non-lymphocytic leukaemia resemble the cells seen in the marrow and peripheral blood, and can be readily identified on routine preparations. In contrast to the acute leukaemias, CNS involvement is unusual in the chronic phase of chronic myelogenous leukaemia. When patients enter the accelerated phase or blast crisis, however, immature myeloid forms may be seen in the CSF of some patients.

Lymphoma

As with leukaemia, the most common pattern of CNS involvement from systemic lymphoma is subarachnoid dissemination with little or no parenchymal disease. Occasionally, however, multifocal infiltrates will occur within the brain and spinal cord of patients with bulky disease elsewhere. Although primary CNS lymphoma generally presents as a solitary mass lesion, CSF dissemination is common during the course of the disease.

The varieties of lymphoma which tend to seed the subarachnoid space are among the most aggressive histological types, and include large-cell lymphoma and immunoblastic sarcoma in the adult as well as Burkitt's lymphoma, lymphoblastic lymphoma and undifferentiated lymphoma in the child. Cytological features which allow detection of these cells are the presence of a monomorphous population with cellular characteristics of the lymphoma type demonstrated elsewhere in the patient. Since the majority of lymphomas involving the CSF are B-cell type, while reactive lymphocytoses contain mainly T cells, the demonstration of a monoclonal population expressing one type of light chain and one type of heavy chain is a helpful diagnostic adjunct in difficult cases. If the phenotype has previously been demonstrated in nodal tissue, documentation of the same pattern in cells in CSF allows a specific and definitive diagnosis. For T-cell lymphoma, interpretation of lymphoid marker panels may be more difficult due to the mixture of neoplastic and reactive T cells which is frequently encountered.

The better-differentiated forms of lymphoma, including nodular lymphomas and small cell lymphoma of the cleaved and non-cleaved varieties, in contrast, uncommonly produce symptomatic CNS involvement. As with chronic lymphatic leukaemia, infectious processes should be considered in patients with these disorders who develop neurological problems and the immunohistochemical application of lymphoid antibodies is often definitive in distinguishing lymphoma from reactive conditions in samples of CSF from these patients. Hodgkin's disease also rarely involves the CNS directly, and is almost never seen in the subarachnoid space or CSF.

Metastatic carcinoma and meningeal carcinomatosis

The ability to diagnose metastatic carcinoma to the CNS by examination of CSF is directly proportional to the extent to which the process involves the subarachnoid space. In cases where the metastatic lesions are confined to either the brain and spinal cord parenchyma or to the bones and extradural space of the skull or spine, cells have no access to the CSF. In many cases of brain metastases, however, large lesions or small multiple foci impinge upon the surface of the brain and cord and shed diagnostic cells into CSF. The cells may be few in number and are frequently mixed with a dense infiltrate of lymphocytes and macrophages, making multiple samplings and careful study of the fluid necessary to establish the diagnosis. The application of anticytokeratin or anticarcinoma antibodies can be extremely useful in these situations to highlight rare malignant cells within an inflammatory background (Bigner, 1986).

In approximately 5% of cases of brain metastases a

pattern consisting almost entirely of subarachnoid involvement is encountered. This condition, termed meningeal carcinomatosis or carcinomatous meningitis, may be difficult to diagnose clinically, particularly in the patient without previous documentation of cancer. The demonstration of cranial nerve palsies or compression of spinal nerve roots may lead to suspicion of this process, and examination of CSF is the most practical and definitive means of establishing this diagnosis.

Carcinomas of the lung and the breast, with their tendency to disseminate haematogenously, are the tumour types encountered most frequently in CSF, as the result of both multifocal metastases and meningeal carcinomatosis. Although adenocarcinoma of the stomach is considerably less common than it was in the early part of this century, cases of meningeal carcinomatosis from this source are still seen, and this tumour type remains responsible for many cases of meningeal carcinomatosis which present with an occult primary. Other tumour types which are reasonably frequent in the population, including renal cell carcinoma and adenocarcinoma of the colon, are uncommonly seen in CSF as they tend to produce solitary brain metastases rather than multifocal lesions or meningeal carcinomatosis (Fig. 10.4). In addition to these tumour types which involve the subarachnoid space haematogenously, some neoplasms arising in the head and sinuses, such as squamous cell carcinoma in the adult and embryonal rhabdomyosarcoma in the child, enter CSF by direct invasion of bone or travel along cranial nerves. Rarely, a similar process occurs in the pelvis when squamous cell carcinoma of the uterine cervix, or adenocarcinoma of the colon, grows directly into the subarachnoid space of the spinal cord.

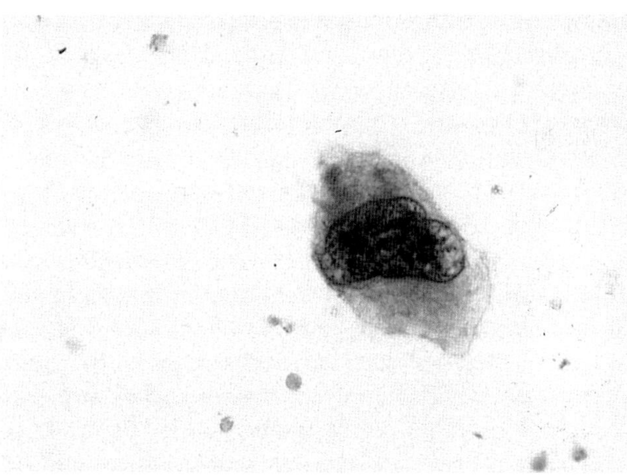

Fig. 11.4 Large malignant tumour cell in cerebrospinal fluid from a patient with disseminated renal cell carcinoma. (Papanicolaou stain ×1000.)

Cutaneous melanoma is among the tumour types with the greatest likelihood of CNS metastasis. The majority of patients dying of disseminated melanoma have nervous system involvement at the time of autopsy. Cells can be identified in CSF from patients with multifocal lesions of the brain and cord if the subarachnoid space is invaded, and tumour spread is readily diagnosed in cases of diffuse subarachnoid melanomatosis. In patients who present with melanoma in CSF in the absence of an identified primary tumour in the skin or mucous membranes, it may be impossible to determine whether or not the process actually began in the meninges as a primary meningeal melanoma. In general, complete autopsy examination with no demonstration of lesions outside the CNS is required to establish this diagnosis.

Cells of malignant melanoma are characteristically large with coarse nuclear chromatin, and prominent macronucleoli. When cytoplasmic melanin pigment is present, a specific diagnosis of melanoma can be made, even in the absence of previous documentation of melanoma elsewhere in the body. In the absence of pigment it may be difficult to distinguish these cells from other large cell malignancies such as large-cell undifferentiated carcinoma of the lung and large-cell lymphoma (Fig. 10.5). Here, positive reactivity with antimelanoma antibodies such as HM-45 or ME1–14 with absence of cytoplasmic cytokeratin, and lack of expression of anticarcinoma antibodies and panleucocyte reagents is useful in helping to establish the diagnosis (Fig. 10.6).

Primary central nervous system tumours

As with metastatic tumours, the only primary CNS tumours which are detectable by examination of CSF are those which involve the ventricles or subarachnoid space by direct extension, and those which disseminate through the spinal fluid pathways. Although any histological type of malignant adult glioma may produce this picture, advanced glioblastoma multiforme is the tumour type which most frequently spreads in this fashion. The morphology of the cells seen in CSF in these cases is as varied as the spectrum seen histologically. Cells may be anaplas-

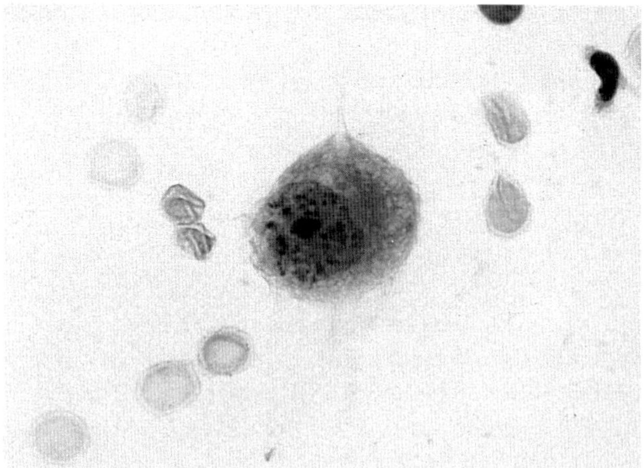

Fig. 11.5 Malignant tumour cell in cerebrospinal fluid from a patient with cutaneous melanoma. (Papanicolaou stain ×1000.)

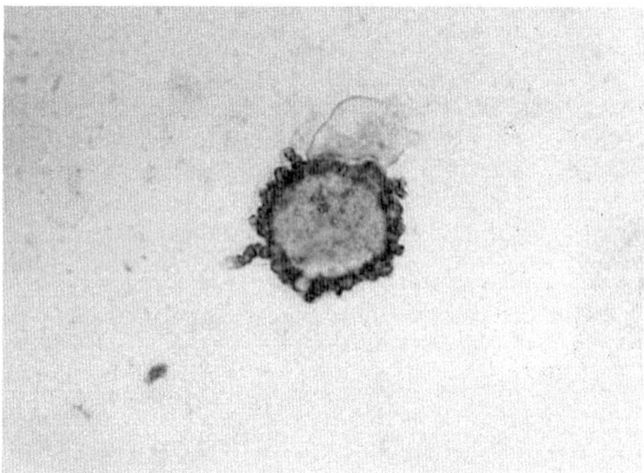

Fig. 11.6 Melanoma cell from the same sample shown in Fig. 11.5, using a polyclonal antiserum against S-100 protein. Monoclonal antibody ME1–14 also stained these tumour cells, but they were negative for cytokeratins, anticarcinoma antibody B72.3, and a panleukocyte reagent. (Immunoperoxidase ×1000.)

tic, ranging from small to large in size, or may retain their resemblance to astrocytes. Fortunately, even the most poorly differentiated tumours usually retain the expression of glial fibrillary acidic protein (GFAP) in at least some cells, allowing for a specific diagnosis using antibodies against GFAP. Another tumour type also exhibiting this type of behaviour is the malignant ependymoma, which also sheds into CSF as morphologically undifferentiated cells. Low-grade gliomas, including astrocytomas, ependymomas, and oli-

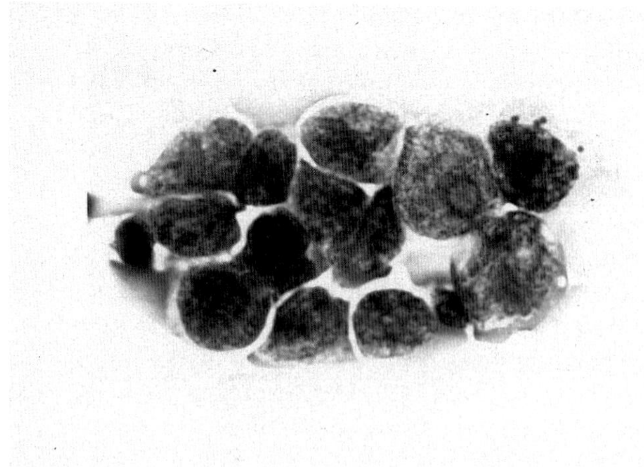

Fig. 11.7 Small malignant tumour cells in cerebrospinal fluid from a boy with a cerebellar medulloblastoma. (Diff-quik stain ×1000.)

godendrogliomas, may also metastasize throughout the ventricular system and subarachnoid space. These tumours are not always demonstrable by cytological examination of CSF, however, since they often produce cohesive implants which exfoliate poorly. In addition, since these cells are cytologically benign, they can be difficult to distinguish from macrophages and monocytes unless specific antibodies are employed.

The most common malignant primary brain tumour of childhood, the medulloblastoma, commonly spreads through the neuroaxis by way of the spinal fluid pathway. This tumour presents as cell clusters and isolated cells with high nuclear to cytoplasmic ratios, hyperchromatic nuclei, and scant cytoplasm (Fig. 11.7). These cells express pan-neuroectodermal antigens such as those detected by monoclonal antibodies UJ13A, are usually negative for GFAP, and sometimes express neurofilament proteins. Gliomas represent another relatively large group of childhood brain tumours. Although most of these neoplasms are low-grade and slow-growing, the most malignant variety of astrocytic glioma, glioblastoma multiforme, is capable of disseminating in the subarachnoid space. This pattern of behaviour is particularly characteristic of malignant brain stem gliomas. These cells are frequently small in size and anaplastic in their cellular characteristics, making them difficult to distinguish from other small-cell neoplasms such as medulloblastoma and ependymoblastoma. Precise localization of the primary tumour in the brain stem as opposed to the fourth ventricle or cerebellum is helpful in making this distinction. In addition, the expression of large amounts of GFAP while characteristic of gliomas is unusual in medulloblastomas.

The examination of the CSF is often neglected as merely a routine adjunct to myelography. With the increasing usage of magnetic resonance imaging, it is even more important to realize the necessity for comprehensive CSF examination. This is especially true in cases where investigation fails to reveal an obvious 'surgical' lesion, and it is in such situations where detailed study of the CSF by biochemical and cellular techniques may be especially helpful.

REFERENCES

Bigner, S.H. (1986) The application of immunocytochemical techniques to specimens derived from the central nervous system (CNS). *Cytopathology*, **14**, 1–5.

Davson, H., Welch, K. & Segal, M.B. (1987) *The Physiology and Pathophysiology of the Cerebrospinal Fluid*. Churchill Livingstone, London, p. 24.

Elovaara, I., Iivanainen, M, Valle, S-L., Suni, J., Tervo, T. & Lahdevirta, J. (1987) CSF protein and cellular profiles in various stages of HIV infection related to neurological manifestations. *J. Neurol. Sci.*, **78**, 331–342.

Fetter, B.F., Klintworth, G.K. & Hendry, W.S. (1967) *Mycoses of the Central Nervous System*. Williams & Williams, Baltimore, MD, p. 131.

Fishman, R.A. (1980) *Cerebrospinal Fluid in Disease of the Nervous System*. W.B. Saunders, Philadelphia, PA.

Jordan, L.G., Shatland, B. & Halsted, C. (1983) CSF lactate in diseases of the CNS. *Arch. Intern. Med.*, **143**, 85–87.

Kaplan, S.L. (1983) Antigen detection in cerebrospinal fluid—pros and cons. *Am. J. Med.*, **75**, 109–118.

Katz, R.L., Alappattu, C., Glass, P.J. & Bruner, J.M. (1989) Cerebrospinal fluid manifestations of the neurologic complications of human immunodeficiency virus infection. *Acta Cytol.*, **33**, 233–244.

Martin, W.J. (1983) Rapid and reliable techniques for the laboratory detection of bacterial meningitis. *Am. J. Med.*, **75**, 119–123.

McFarlin, D.E. & McFarland, H.F. (1982) Multiple sclerosis. *N. Engl. J. Med.*, **307**, 1183–1188.

Merritt, H.H. & Freemont-Smith, F. (1938) *The Cerebrospinal Fluid*, W.B. Saunders, Philadelphia, PA.

Miller, J.R., Burke, A.M. & Bever, C.T. (1983) Occurrence of oligoclonal bands in multiple sclerosis and other CNS diseases. *Ann. Neurol.*, **13**, 53–58.

Poser, C.M., Patv, D.W., Schenberg, L., McDonald, W.I., David, F.A., Ebers, G.C., Johnson, K.P., Siblev, W.A., Silberberg, D.H. & Tourtellotte, W.W. (1982) New diagnostic criteria for multiple sclerosis. Guidelines for Research Protocols. Workshop on the diagnosis of MS. 26–27 April, Washington, DC.

Powers, W.J. (1981) Cerebrospinal fluid to serum glucose ratios in diabetes mellitus and bacterial meningitis. *Am. J. Med.*, **71**, 217–220.

Snider, W.D., Simpson, D.M., Nielsen, S., Gold, J.W.M., Metroka, C.E. & Posner, J.B. (1983) Neurological complications of acquired immune deficiency syndrome: Analysis of 50 patients. *Ann. Neurol.*, **14**, 403–418.

Tourtellotte, W.W. & Ma, B.I. (1978) Multiple sclerosis: the blood–brain barrier in the measurement of de novo central nervous system IgG synthesis. *Neurology (Minneapolis)*, **28**, 76–83.

Wasserstrom, W.R., Glass, J.P. & Posner, J.B. (1982) Diagnosis and treatment of leptomeningeal metastases from solid tumors. Experience with 90 patients. *Cancer*, **49**, 759–772.

12 · Assessment of Neuromuscular Disease

By R.A. SAVAGE, R.D. GRIFFITHS and R.H.T. EDWARDS

This chapter aims to describe the structure and function of normal and diseased skeletal muscle, and provides a brief summary of some of the features of the neuromuscular diseases relevant to surgery of the spine. The chapter includes an account of the quantitative examination of the gross structure of spinal musculature by modern imaging techniques: computerized tomography (CT), magnetic resonance imaging (MRI) and ultrasound.

Spinal muscles are some of the strongest in the body, and are obviously important for erect posture and bipedal locomotion. Spinal muscles are involved in every activity from coughing to giving birth. In any clinical presentation of a spinal problem it is important to consider the possibility of an underlying muscle disease. The stigmas which may suggest this cause include ptosis, bat ears, lack of facial expression or forehead wrinkles, squint (strabismus) or failure to move the eyes normally (such as ophthalmoplegia) and weakness of limb muscles. Referral to a muscle specialist for diagnosis and practical assessments, including respiratory function, can be useful before proceeding to surgical considerations.

Structure and function of human skeletal muscle

The motor unit is the key functional component of the peripheral neuromuscular system, comprising the anterior horn cell, axon, and a varied number of scattered individual muscle fibres. The number of fibres varies depending on the degree of control required; for instance the hand muscles have few (tens) muscle fibres per motor unit, while in the quadriceps each motor unit contains hundreds of fibres (Saltin & Gollnick, 1983). The metabolic characteristics of a muscle fibre depend on the habitual neuronal activity. All the fibres of one motor unit are metabolically identical, and are spread out in a mosaic pattern interdigitating with a number of other motor units. In broad terms there are two major muscle fibre types identified by their different histochemical staining (see Fig. 12.1). Type 1 muscle fibres are more oxidative, with a higher mitochondrial content and less glycolytic activity. The myosin type are slower, and they are analogous to the slow-twitch red muscle of lower animals. These fibres are innervated by motor units which fire at a slower rate and for longer, and as such are more involved in maintenance of posture. Type 2 muscle fibres, in contrast, are predominantly glycolytic, with less oxidative activity. These faster twitch fibres are recruited when sudden rapid movements or high forces are required.

During development, individual nucleated myoblasts fuse longitudinally to form tube-like structures, called myotubes, with multiple centrally situated nuclei. With maturation the nuclei migrate to the periphery of the fibre just beneath the sarcolemma to form a multinucleated cell, the muscle fibre, surrounded by a very thin layer of endomysial connective tissue. Initially fibres are of indeterminate fibre type, probably nearer to Type 2 fibres in character, but with increasing neuronal activity they mature to their definitive fibre type. Several fibres are collected into bundles surrounded by perimysial connective tissue. These fascicles are surrounded by a much thicker epimysial connective tissue sheath. Blood vessels and peripheral nerves course in the connective tissue spaces, then ramify in a fascicle into fine branches to supply each fibre.

A muscle fibre is innervated at the motor endplate or myoneural junction. A nerve impulse releases acetylcholine, which diffuses across the neuromuscu-

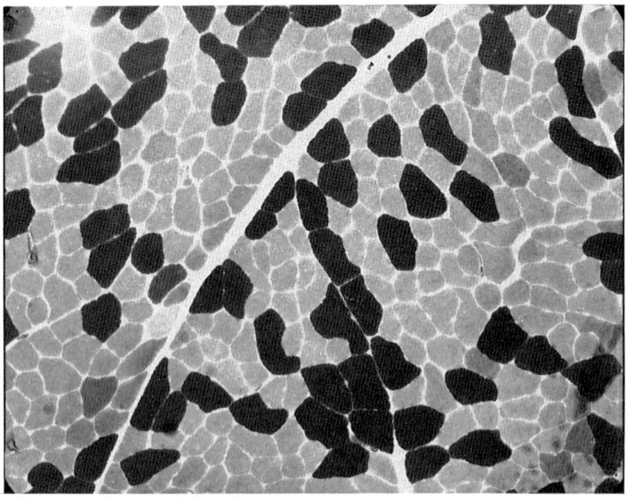

Fig. 12.1 Histochemical properties of human skeletal muscle fibre types.

lar junction to attach to receptors on the muscle. The depolarization of the muscle membrane is propagated through a transverse tubular system deep into the muscle fibre to the sarcoplasmic reticulum. Release of calcium activates the contractile process which involves the interaction between myosin and actin filaments. With energy supplied from the dephosphorylation of adenosine triphosphate (ATP) the filaments slide past one another and the sarcomere shortens.

The arrangement of fibres in a whole muscle is related closely to the range of muscle movement and the forces produced. Attachment of the muscle fibres to connective tissue septa at an angle allows the total length of a fibre to be kept much shorter than the actual length of the muscle, a process called pennation. This reduces the stress per individual fibre and its risk of damage. One of the longest muscles, the longissimus dorsi of the back, has fibres only a few centimetres long attached to a tough collagen sheath both laterally and dorsally.

Clinical assessment

Using a combination of careful clinical assessment and a few physiological investigations (Edwards *et al.*, 1986) it is generally possible to decide whether a neuromuscular problem is the cause of an orthopaedic deformity. The aim is then to differentiate between a primary muscle disease and a neural/neuronal disease. However, superficially there is often a considerable degree of overlap between neurogenic and myopathic disorders, since weakness, manifested as impairment of a particular function, is the common presenting complaint whatever the cause. Table 12.1 lists the major nerve and muscle disorders.

The pattern of muscle weakness or wasting provides the clinical clue to many of the disorders. Some disorders have names derived from early clinical descriptions (e.g. facioscapulohumeral muscular dystrophy). The most common cause of progressive distal weakness is peripheral nerve disease, where sensory findings are present to a variable degree. In motor neurone disease sensory findings are absent, but in this disorder upper motor neurone signs may also be present. Progressive distal weakness is a feature of myotonic dystrophy. A primary muscle disorder (e.g. a muscular dystrophy) is more likely if the features are symmetrical and if there is proximal (pelvic or pectoral) girdle weakness. Reflexes are normal or only moderately depressed in the early stages of the disease, but are lost as the disease progresses. There is an absence of sensory findings or fasciculation. Muscle hypertrophy and pseudo-hypertrophy (replacement by fat and fibrous tissue) are often seen with the muscular dystrophies but the findings are not specific. Calf muscle hypertrophy, a feature of Duchenne and Becker muscular dystrophies, can be seen in proximal spinal muscular atrophy (Kugelberg–Welander disease). Sometimes associated features confirm a diagnosis. In the Emery–Dreyfuss type of scapuloperoneal muscular dystrophy there are characteristically contractures of the elbows and posterior neck muscles and a high incidence of heart block.

A careful history of exercise performance and related symptoms such as pain and fatigue will identify disorders of energy metabolism (e.g. McArdle's disease), and the neuromuscular junction (e.g. myasthenia gravis). These disorders cause their symptoms for reasons which can be largely explained on the basis of disordered physiology (Edwards & Jones, 1983). Pain is not a common complaint of primary muscle disorders, but it may occur in neurogenic disorders such as Guillain–Barré syndrome and motor neurone disease.

In paediatric practice the floppy infant provides a complex diagnostic problem. This can be classified into those conditions where a primary neuromuscular disease exists (i.e. truly weak) and those who are hypotonic for other reasons (see Dubowitz, 1978, for a review).

Table 12.1 Classification of neuromuscular disorders. After Walton & Gardner-Medwin (1988)

Neurogenic disorders	Myopathic disorders
A *Disorders of anterior horn cells*	**A** *Genetically determined myopathies*
1 Spinal muscular atrophies (SMA)	**1** Muscular dystrophies
(a) Severe (infantile) (Werdnig–Hoffmann disease)	(a) Duchenne muscular dystrophy
(b) Intermediate SMA	(b) Becker muscular dystrophy and other X-linked dystrophies (Emery–Dreyfuss)
(c) Mild juvenile SMA (Kugelberg–Welander disease)	(c) Limb-girdle muscular dystrophy
(d) SMA in adults	(d) Ocular myopathy
2 Motor neurone disease	(e) Ocular–pharyngeal syndrome
3 Poliomyelitis and other viral disorders	(f) Ocular–pharyngeal muscular dystrophy
4 Other anterior horn cell disorders	**2** Myotonic syndromes
	(a) Myotonic dystrophy
B *Peripheral neuropathies*	(b) Myotonia congenita
1 Hereditary motor sensory neuropathies	(c) Paramyotonia congenita
(a) Type 1 (peroneal muscular atrophy)	(d) Other myotonic syndromes
(b) Type 2 (neuronal type of peroneal muscular atrophy)	**3** Congenital myopathies of childhood
(c) Type 3 (hypertrophic neuropathy of Dejerine and Sottas)	(a) Central core and multicore disease
(d) Type 4 (hypertrophic neuropathy with phytanic acid storage—Refsum's disease)	(b) Nemaline myopathy
(e) Type 5 (neuropathy with spastic paraplegia)	(c) Myotubular (centronuclear) myopathy
Other genetically determined neuropathies	(d) Congenital fibre-type disproportion
Metachromatic leukodystrophy	(e) Congenital muscular dystrophy
Acute intermittent porphyria	(f) Others
Amyloid neuropathy	**4** Metabolic myopathies
2 Acquired neuropathies	(a) Glycogenoses
(a) Monor neuropathies	(b) Periodic paralysis
(i) Traumatic	(c) Disorders of lipid metabolism, e.g. carnitine deficiency
(ii) Entrapment and compressive	(d) Malignant hyperpyrexia
(iii) Brachial neuritis (neuralgic amyotrophy)	(e) Mitochondrial myopathies
(b) Polyneuropathies	
(i) Inflammatory polyradiculoneuropathy (Guillain–Barré syndrome)	**B** *Endocrine myopathies*
(ii) Metabolic, e.g. diabetes mellitus; renal and hepatic disease; vitamin deficiencies; alcoholic	**1** Thyroid myopathies
(iii) Toxic and drug-induced neuropathies	**2** Osteomalacia
(iv) Associated with malignant disease	**3** Steroid myopathy
(v) Infections, e.g. diphtheria and leprosy	
(vi) Associated with connective tissue disease	**C** *Inflammatory myopathies*
	1 Idiopathic
C *Disorders of neuromuscular transmission (endplate disorders)*	(a) Polymyositis
1 Myasthenia gravis	(b) Dermatomyositis
2 Myasthenic syndrome (Eaton–Lambert syndrome)	(c) Granulomatous polymyositis (sarcoidosis)
3 Botulism, and other toxins	**2** Infections
	(a) Viral (e.g. Coxsackie)
	(b) Bacterial (e.g. staphylococcal)
	(c) Infestations (e.g. trichinosis)
	D *Toxic drug-induced myopathies*

The postural deformities that are recognized in the arthrogryposis syndrome are probably secondary to immobility of the limbs *in utero*. A wide range of disorders, some neurological and others unconnected with a neurological deficit (e.g. oligohydramnios), produce this symptom complex. Muscles disused and kept in a shortened state will atrophy and develop contractures.

After infancy children present with some delay in attaining a motor milestone (Dubowitz, 1978). Duchenne muscular dystrophy, the most common and severe of the progressive muscle wasting disorders, is often only recognized by about three years (Emery, 1986). However, there is often a history of some minor delay in walking which was not picked up. Any child not walking by 18 months should be clinically reviewed. The congenital myopathies can present at any age and are variable in severity and prognosis. While some are non-progressive, a few improve with age and others are rapidly progressive (Dubowitz, 1978). Even within one diagnostic category the clinical features can be variable.

It must be emphasized that delayed motor milestones, difficulty with gait, and progressive scoliosis are not confined to the primary neuromuscular disorders and can occur in connective tissue disorders, e.g. Ehlers–Danlos syndrome. Scoliosis is commonly a feature of the proximal spinal muscular atrophies (presenting earlier as the condition becomes more severe), Duchenne muscular dystrophy (in the second decade), some of the congenital myopathies, and several of the hereditary ataxias (e.g. Friedreich's). Conventional neurological examination of children should be accompanied by careful observation of the child at play. Gowers' sign is the manoeuvre whereby patients with proximal pelvic weakness 'climb up themselves' when rising from the floor.

It is diagnostically helpful to construct a detailed family history to identify the mode of inheritance. The gene for Duchenne dystrophy is on the short arm of the X chromosome, and hence inheritance is via the mother. However, a family history is present only in two-thirds of those with Duchenne dystrophy; the remaining cases are a result of gene mutation. The same gene is responsible for the milder Becker dystrophy, while the gene for Emery–Dreyfuss dystrophy is on the long arm of the X chromosome. Myotonic dystrophy and facioscapulohumeral muscle dystro-

Table 12.2 Neuromuscular diseases with possible orthopaedic consequences to the spine. Modified from Walton & Gardner-Medwin (1988)

Inheritance	Disease	Onset
The spinal muscular atrophies (SMA)		
Autosomal recessive	Type 2 SMA	Childhood
Autosomal recessive	Type 3 SMA (Kugelberg-Welander)	Childhood/teens
The muscular dystrophies		
X-linked Short arm of X chromosome (dystrophin deficiency)	Duchenne dystrophy	Three to five years; scoliosis as severely disabled teenager
	Becker dystrophy	Childhood
Long arm of X chromosome	Emery–Dreyfuss (scapuloperoneal)	Childhood
Autosomal recessive	Scapulohumeral	Early adult life
	Limb girdle	Childhood or early adulthood
	Congenital	Hypotonia at birth
	Chondrodystrophic myotonia (Schwartz–Jampel syndrome)	Muscle stiffness in childhood
Autosomal dominant	Fascioscapulohumeral	Any age
Chromosome 19	Myotonic dystrophy	Childhood or early adulthood

phy are autosomal dominant, as is hereditary motor sensory neuropathy Type 1 (Charcot–Marie–Tooth disease). The inheritance of some of the more common disorders in which scoliosis may be a feature is shown in Table 12.2.

Measurement of muscle strength

The observation of a patient performing a familiar daily task provides useful information about the patient's functional capabilities, and gives a general overview of the distribution of muscle weakness. However, it must be remembered that complex functional activities can be achieved in a number of ways by the use of 'trick' movements that may mask the underlying muscle weakness. Therefore, in addition to a functional assessment it is necessary to assess formally the force-generating capacity of individual muscles or muscle groups.

The Medical Research Council (MRC) scale is the classic method of assessing the force of a muscle contraction. The examiner grades the muscle according to its ability to perform a movement against gravity or an additional resistance. It is a useful test which provides a quick means of assessing the degree and distribution of weakness, and because it does not require any specialized equipment can be performed at the bedside. However, it is not totally objective since it requires the clinician to make a judgement about the appropriate grade, and this may lead to interpretation differences between observers and sequential measurements. Furthermore, discrete changes in muscle force cannot be quantified by this technique since it was developed to assess recovery from nerve injury. As such the gradations describe only broad ranges of muscle force.

A simple hand-held dynamometer (Edwards & McDonnell, 1974) such as the 'Hammersmith myometer' or the electromyometer can be used to measure the contraction force of a muscle objectively (Scott *et al.*, 1982). The myometer records the peak force applied by the examiner in order to just overcome the contraction of a muscle group. Consequently, the technique is limited by the strength of the examiner and can only be used reliably on children or on adults who display a significant degree of muscle weakness. It is not suitable for assessing adults with mild muscle weakness. If the myometer is applied at standard anatomical positions the measurements are reproducible and can be recorded sequentially to follow the course of a disease (Edwards *et al.*, 1987).

A more detailed assessment of muscle strength can be achieved by measuring isometric force with a fixed dynamometer. The quadriceps has been extensively tested by this technique (Edwards *et al.*, 1977), since the quadriceps is frequently affected by muscle disease, and is an important weight-bearing muscle. Whilst seated in a purpose-built testing chair, that ensures correct joint angulation and limb position, the subject is encouraged to make a maximum voluntary contraction (MVC). In a normal population the quadriceps MVC force can be related to body weight, according to the equation $y = 7.91x - 37.7$ (Edwards *et al.*, 1977).

If there is any doubt about a patient's motivation from inconsistency of voluntary efforts, or if a defect of the central motor pathways is suspected for other reasons, the muscle can be stimulated percutaneously to give twitches during voluntary muscle force production. Any increase in force with electrical stimulation implies reduced central neuronal drive (Belanger & McComas, 1981; Chapman *et al.*, 1984a). Electrical stimulation can also provide information about a muscle's susceptibility to fatigue if a programmed stimulation electromyogram is recorded (Edwards, 1984).

Clinical investigations

BLOOD TESTS

The enzyme creatine kinase (CK), previously called creatine phosphokinase, is present in skeletal muscle in high concentrations. It is released into the blood in many neuromuscular disorders, and its concentration is the most useful preliminary investigation. Serum CK activity reaches several thousand international units in the muscular dystrophies, but may be only moderately elevated in the neurogenic atrophies. It rises with strenuous exercise, and in any disorder where muscle is damaged. In some of the congenital myopathies CK activity may be normal; therefore a normal recording cannot exclude a myopathy. Erythrocyte sedimentation rate (ESR) or plasma viscosity is also useful to detect a treatable inflammatory myopathy or underlying malignancy. If either ataxia or peripheral nerve disorder exist more extensive investigations into the aetiology are warranted, outside the scope of this chapter.

ELECTROCARDIOGRAM

The electrocardiogram (ECG) will show evidence of ventricular strain or hypertrophy in the generalized muscular dystrophies, and is characteristic even early in childhood with Duchenne dystrophy. The more mobile the patient the greater the risk of arythmias or heart block (Becker muscular dystrophy, and Emery–Dreyfuss). The ECG in spinal muscular atrophy is normal.

RESPIRATORY FUNCTION

Measurement of respiratory function is essential in any patient suspected of having a neuromuscular disease (Smith *et al.*, 1987). Not only does it aid diagnosis but it also provides an important indicator for prognosis and preoperative assessment (Rideau *et al.*, 1981). In many generalized myopathies the respiratory muscle power follows that of the limb muscles. Measurement of maximal respiratory muscle effort provides a reproducible indicator of muscle disease progress that is clinically relevant to life. Routine measurement of forced vital capacity (FVC) and forced expiratory volume in 1 second (FEV_1) should be performed at each review, and allows the influence of scoliosis and its correction to be assessed (Kurtz *et al.*, 1983). Measurements made when lying and sitting/standing can disclose hidden diaphragmatic weakness. Certain disorders show increased respiratory muscle weakness such as acid-maltase deficiency, the glycogen storage disorder of the lysosome that can affect children and adults. In the presence of significant facial weakness measurement may not always be reliable unless great care is taken to ensure complete sealing of the lips around the mouthpiece.

ELECTROMYOGRAPHY

Needle electromyography is not disease-specific but is particularly useful to differentiate between a primary myopathic and a neurogenic disorder. In myopathic disorders there will be hyper-recruitment of motor units that are of reduced amplitude and duration due to the random loss of muscle fibres across motor units. In contrast in neurogenic atrophies with loss of motor units there will be evidence of denervation (fibrillation) and reinnervation with larger motor units producing giant action potentials. Fasciculation of complete motor units is sometimes seen. Fibrillation potentials and positive sharp waves also occur in myopathic processes with active muscle fibre damage (for example, polymyositis). Electromyography is definitive for confirming myotonia. The technique requires needle sampling of more than one muscle, often in several sites. This can sometimes be quite painful, and requires cooperation from the patient so that records at rest and with different degrees of activity can be recorded. As a result it is of limited use as a screening investigation in children. It is useful to answer specific questions, particularly to confirm myotonia or a neurogenic atrophy (Edwards *et al.*, 1986).

Nerve conduction studies are useful in both children and adults to confirm the existence of a peripheral neuropathy due to demyelination. Nerve conduction may be normal in the early stages of axonopathies and in disorders of the anterior horn cell.

Muscle biopsy

This is required for a definitive diagnosis in the myopathies and in several of the neurogenic disorders. Particularly in children, muscle biopsy is the most important investigation and has replaced EMG studies except for certain indications. The development of percutaneous techniques (Edwards *et al.*, 1983; Dietrichson *et al.*, 1987) over the past 15 years has meant that muscle biopsy is more widely available. Only in exceptional circumstances, where motor endplates or major vessels need be examined, are large open muscle biopsies indicated. The percutaneous techniques performed with local anaesthetic allow biopsy from any patient at any age, even in the neonate. Needle muscle biopsy is most useful for sampling deep inside large muscles, such as the quadriceps or gastrocnemius. In contrast the conchotome forceps generally takes a more superficial sample and is useful for smaller muscles (such as tibialis anterior, deltoid, biceps brachialis, supraspinatus). Once the overlying tissues are anaesthetized there is little pain, and the technique is readily tolerated by children without any other form of sedation. The biopsied limb can be used directly after the procedure, making this an outpatient investigation.

A totally paretic, severely wasted or end-stage muscle is not suitable for biopsy as useful interpretation is impossible. Muscle biopsy in such circumstances is justified only if a moderately affected muscle is accessible. Certain disorders exhibit selective muscle involvement. Ultrasound or magnetic resonance imaging in such circumstances can be useful to identify the involved group.

The muscle biopsy is orientated and frozen so that sections may be taken for histochemical and more recently immunochemical analysis (Dubowitz, 1985). Accurate interpretation depends on a detailed knowledge of the clinical picture, as in many cases the findings are not pathognomonic for a given disease.

Neurogenic disorders are characterized by small angular atrophic fibres in clusters. Enzyme histochemical staining reveals that there is grouping of fibres of the same type, which indicates reinnervation. Myopathic disorders show random variation in fibre size, internalization of nuclei, and increase in endomysial fibrous tissue. In Duchenne muscular dystrophy there is a striking increase in endomysial fibrous tissue, hyperdense opaque fibres, necrotic fibres, and areas of fat. In polymyositis mononuclear inflammatory cells infiltrate muscle fibres, with necrosis, while in dermatomyositis the infiltrate is more epimysial with fibre atrophy being perifascicular.

Glycogen and lipid accumulation can be identified and further investigated either histochemically or by biochemical analysis of a separate muscle sample. Accumulations of abnormal mitochondria which occur in certain mitochondrial myopathies are seen as 'ragged red fibres' or on electron microscopy.

The congenital myopathies are named and characterized by their morphological findings. Type 1 fibres often predominate, or the fibres are all of one indeterminate fibre type. In central core disease there are centrally placed zones of decreased enzyme staining, while in nemaline myopathy there are accumulations of tiny red thread-like structures. In myotubular or central nuclear myopathy the tissue resembles immature undifferentiated muscle, while in fibre-type disproportion there is an overabundance of smaller type 1 fibres.

Muscle imaging techniques

Muscle weakness is often judged in terms of the relationship between a muscle's strength and its bulk (cross-sectional area). Prior to modern imaging techniques assessment of muscle bulk was based on surface measurements and anthropometric calculations. Many of these calculations compensate for subcutaneous fat by subtracting skinfold thickness measurements (Jones & Pearson, 1969) but despite this they only provide estimates of the whole muscle cross-sectional area (CSA) and do not discriminate between contractile and non-contractile elements. For example they are not capable of discriminating between muscle hypertrophy and the pseudohypertrophy which commonly occurs in the calf muscles of Duchenne and Becker muscular dystrophy patients. Since the force that can be generated by a muscle is proportional to the total CSA of the actin–myosin interactions, and not the CSA of the whole muscle, anthropometric estimates of muscle CSA are inadequate in the assessment of the force-generating capacity of muscle. The relationship between the CSA and force-generating capacity of the quadriceps muscle is shown in Fig. 12.2.

Computerized real-time sonography (CRS), CT and MRI are non-invasive techniques that can be used to measure muscle size, position, and composition. They can provide useful supplementary information about the extent and distribution of a number of neuromuscular disorders and can aid in the selection of muscle biopsy sites. All three of these techniques have their advantages and limitations; these are listed in Table 12.3.

Most muscle imaging has been performed on the

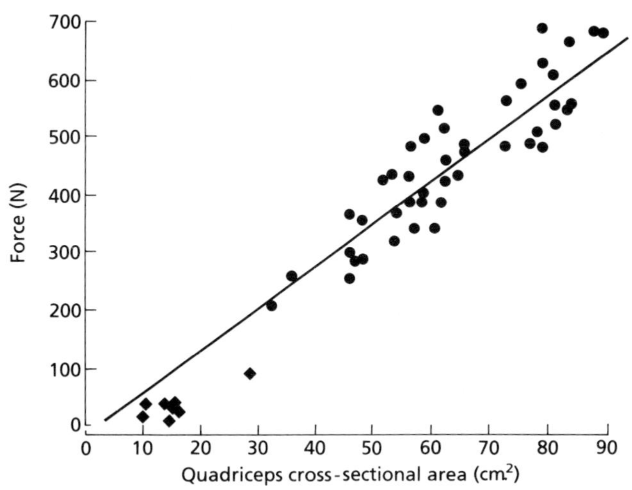

Fig. 12.2 Relationship between quadriceps cross-sectional area and force in normal subjects and Duchenne muscular dystrophy patients (DMD). Normal data (●) obtained from subjects aged 10–34 years, male and female (Chapman *et al.*, 1984b). DMD data (◆) for quadriceps area have been corrected for fat content, but not for connective tissue. Reproduced from Jones and Edwards (1986).

Table 12.3 Comparison of imaging techniques for assessing neuromuscular disorders

	MRI	CT	CRS
Availability	Limited	Readily available	Readily available
Equipment cost	Very expensive	Expensive	Inexpensive
Portability	Fixed	Fixed	Portable
Soft-tissue contrast	Excellent	Good	Fair
Muscle detail	Good	None	Fair
Harmful effects	None	Ionizing radiation	None
Longitudinal assessments	Yes	No	Yes
Infant preparation	Sedation	Sedation	None

extremities, and relatively little attention has been given to the trunk muscles. The paraspinal and abdominal muscles play a vital role in posture and gait. They stabilize the spine and pelvis and in so doing aid balance. One of the main reasons for patients with Duchenne muscular dystrophy becoming unable to walk is inability to balance the upper body in such a way that the knee joint can be locked. Studies have shown that the loss in walking ability does not coincide with the reduction in strength of individual leg muscles (Edwards *et al.*, 1987).

The CSA area of a given muscle or muscle group can be expressed as a ratio of the CSA of another anatomical structure. This provides an index of muscularity that can be compared with a predicted ratio. For example the paraspinal CSA can be expressed as a ratio of the CSA of the appropriate intervertebral disc (Millerchip *et al.*, 1988). Muscle moment arm lengths can also be measured with the scans obtained from modern imaging techniques, and when combined with appropriate muscle CSA measurements the force-generating capacity of individual muscles can be estimated (McGill *et al.*, 1988).

Computerized real-time sonography

Ultrasonography can be used to image the muscle to give an estimation of the CSA, and also to give a

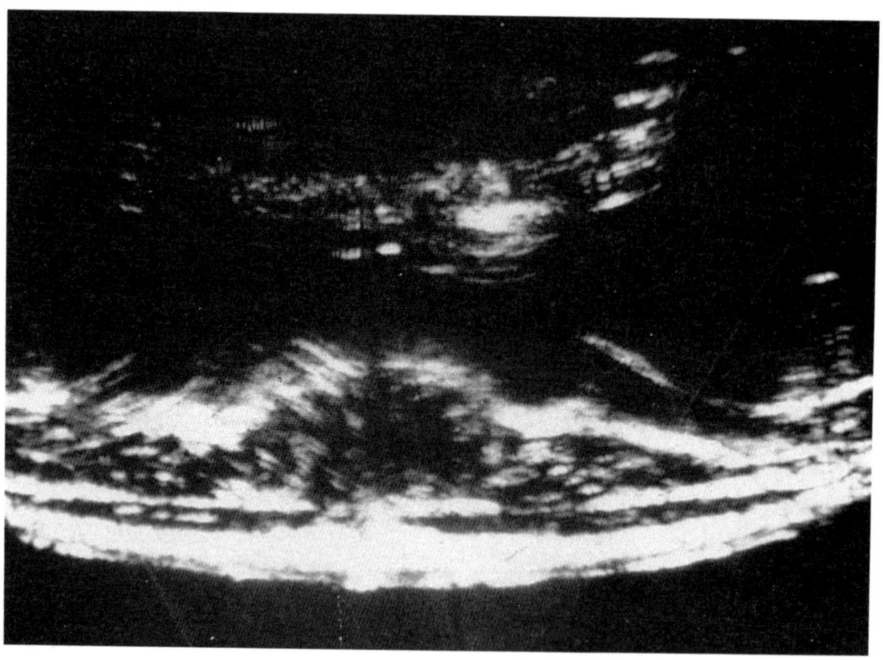

Fig. 12.3 Ultrasound scan of the spinal musculature of a healthy adult.

quantitative measure of the 'texture' of the muscle tissue (Cady *et al.*, 1983). When healthy adult muscle is examined by CRS (Fig. 12.3) the muscle parenchyma appears as a homogeneous echogenic matrix, separated internally by hyperechoic fascial planes, which probably surround muscle fascicles. Each muscle group is enclosed by a hyperechoic intermuscular septum. At the mid-thigh level the bone edge appears as a hyperechoic structure and a clearly defined bone shadow can be observed (Fischer *et al.*, 1988).

In comparison the muscle parenchyma of a normal infant is hypoechoic and has fewer myofascial planes. As the muscle develops the echogenicity and the number of myofascial planes increase up until the age of five years, when the muscle structure resembles that of adult muscle (Fischer & Stephens, 1988).

A number of sonographic abnormalities can be demonstrated in the limb muscles of patients with neuromuscular disorders. Heckmatt *et al.* (1988), and Fischer *et al.* (1988) have shown that CRS can differentiate between dystrophies and neurogenic atrophies, and that floppy infants with central hypotonia can be separated from those with neuromuscular diseases.

In myopathic dystrophies the echogenicity of the muscle parenchyma is severely increased and is homogeneous, producing a brightly speckled or granular appearance. This is probably caused by attenuation of the ultrasound signal as it passes through an increased amount of connective tissue. Also the bone edge cannot be detected, and the bone shadow is absent. The observed abnormalities are dependent on the disease and its extent. Fischer *et al.* (1988) reported that in Duchenne muscular dystrophy the muscle echo is markedly increased, whereas in facioscapulohumeral dystrophy there is only a moderate increase. Neurogenic atrophies are characterized by a moderate increase in echogenicity, which is heterogeneous. The bone edge is usually absent but the bone shadow can often be detected. It has been suggested that the surviving motor units amongst hypoechoic diseased muscle are responsible for the characteristic pattern of punched-out lesions. In addition muscle atrophy is usually associated with neurogenic disorders, whereas muscle thickness is maintained or increased in many myopathies. The degree of atrophy can be expressed in terms of the ratio of muscle to subcutaneous tissue depth, the normal ratio in the thigh being 2 : 1 or more (Heckmatt *et al.*, 1988).

Floppy infants with central nervous system disorders present with normal sonograms. If, however, the hypotonia is peripheral in origin a minimal or moderate increase in echogenicity is observed which may be homogeneous or heterogeneous. The bone echo is diminished but the fascial interfaces appear normal (Fischer *et al.*, 1988).

In terms of patient comfort the CRS examination procedure is more suitable for assessing infants with neuromuscular disorders than CT or MRI. The procedure does not distress the patient in any way, since the equipment is unobtrusive and the child is in constant contact with the examiner. Unlike in CT or MRI, sedation, to prevent 'wriggling' and its associated movement artifacts, is not required. What is more the equipment is portable and can be used in an outpatient clinic to perform sequential assessments.

Computerized tomography

Computerized tomography clearly demonstrates demarcation of diseased and healthy muscle (Fig. 12.4). In the presence of a neurological disorder affecting a particular nerve supply selective muscle involvement can be identified. In myopathies the pattern of muscle involvement may aid diagnosis. Attempts have been made to quantify the degree of fatty infiltration in myopathic disorders (Grindrod *et al.*, 1983). The purpose of this is to provide an objective means of assessing the severity of a disease and following its development. However, the radiation dose that accompanies each CT examination limits the usefulness of this imaging technique in follow-up studies. For the same reason it is recommended that each CT examination of a neuromuscular disorder should be confined to a number of well-selected scan levels (Bulcke & Baert, 1982). The proportion of fat replacement in the quadriceps muscle can be calculated from its average Hounsfield number.

Magnetic resonance imaging

Of the three imaging techniques MRI achieves the best soft-tissue contrast and internal muscle detail. Like CRS it has no known harmful effects and can therefore be used in longitudinal follow-up studies. Images can be obtained in any plane, enabling scans to be made perpendicular to the direction of muscle

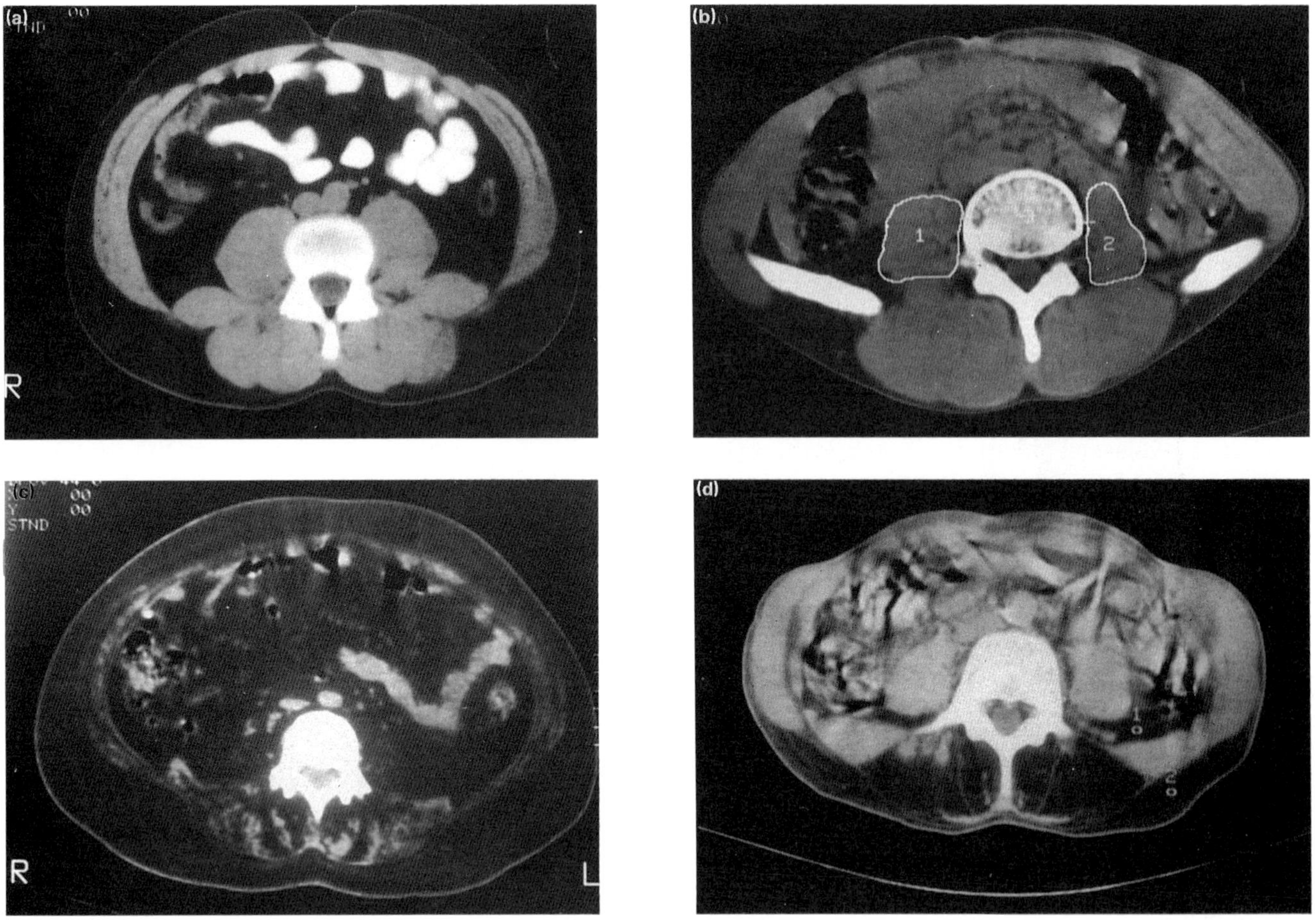

Fig. 12.4 Computerized tomograph of the lumbar spine: (a) normal muscle, (b) scoliosis, (c) Duchenne muscular dystrophy, (d) limb-girdle muscular dystrophy.

fibres. This facility is particularly useful when quantifying the CSA of the paraspinal muscles, which tend to follow the curvature of the spine (Fig. 12.5).

In MRI, tissue signal intensity (SI) depends on the pulse sequence used. However, with the exception of fluid-filled structures which display low signal intensity on T1 weighting and high signal intensity on T2 weighting, the relative brightness of many musculoskeletal tissues remains comparatively constant. Fat has a relatively high SI, muscle has a medium SI and cortical bone, ligaments, tendons and air have very low SI values.

Fat replacement in muscle, typical of many dystrophies, appears as a non-homogeneous increase in SI. Estimates of the degree of fatty infiltration made from magnetic resonance images have been found to correlate well with the clinical stage of the disease (Schreiber *et al.*, 1987). The muscles affected by the disease process can be easily identified and the pattern of muscle involvement used in diagnosis.

Conclusion

It will be appreciated, therefore, that the advances in the field of muscle research, and the advent of new investigative and imaging techniques described in this chapter, have created unique opportunities for clinicians to more accurately assess patients who present with ill-defined spinal and locomotor dysfunction. The diagnostic difficulties of deciding whether a patient is exhibiting early manifestations of the myopathies, neuromuscular diseases, connective tissue anomalies or other entities are much diminished.

Although an accurate history and clinical examination is most essential these added facilities allow

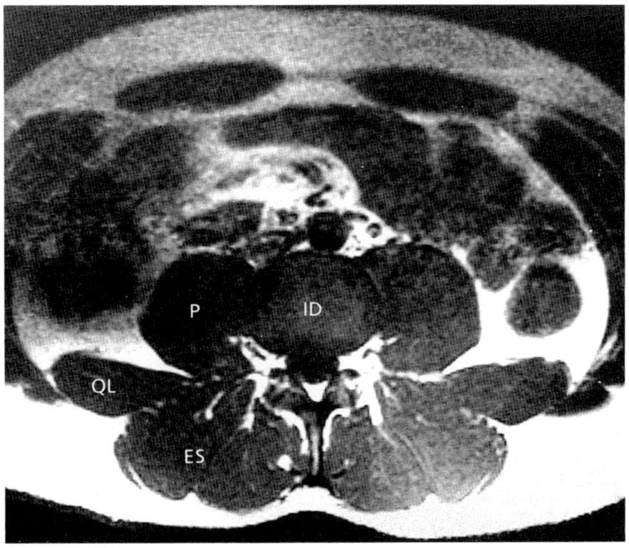

Fig. 12.5 Oblique magnetic resonance scan through L3–L4 intervertebral disc: ID, intervertebral disc: QL, quadratus lumborum; ES, erector spinae; P, psoas.

more realistic evaluation of pathophysiology and long-term prognosis of disease patterns in individual patients, before the surgeon embarks on major spinal surgery. Furthermore anaesthetic and postoperative management, in particular the avoidance of physiological complications such as unforeseen crises from cardiomyopathy or hyperpyrexia, will ensure lesser morbidity and mortality in these high-risk patients.

REFERENCES

Belanger, A.V. & McComas, A.J. (1981) Extent of motor unit activation during effort. *J. Appl. Physiol.*, **51**, 1131–1135.

Bulcke, J.A.L. & Baert, A.L. (1982) *Clinical and Radiological Aspects of Myopathies.* Springer-Verlag, Berlin.

Cady, E.B., Gardner, J.E. & Edwards, R.H.T. (1983) Utrasonic tissue characterisation of skeletal muscle. *Eur. J. Clin. Invest.*, **13**, 469–473.

Chapman, S.J., Edwards, R.H.T., Greig, C. & Rutherford, O. (1984a). Practical application of the twitch interpolation technique for the study of voluntary contraction of the quadriceps muscle in man. *J. Physiol.*, **353**, 19P.

Chapman, S.J., Grindrod, S.R. & Jones, D.A. (1984b) Cross-sectional area and force production of the quadriceps muscle. *J. Physiol.*, **353**, 53P.

Dietrichson, P., Coakley, J., Smith, P.E.M., Griffiths, R.D., Helliwell, T.R. & Edwards, R.H.T. (1987) Conchotome and needle percutaneous biopsy of skeletal muscle. *J. Neurol. Neurosurg. Psychiatry*, **50**, 1461–1467.

Dubowitz, V. (1978) *Muscle Disorders in Childhood.* W.B. Saunders, London, pp. 1–282.

Dubowitz, V. (1985) *Muscle Biopsy: a Practical Approach*, 2nd edn, pp. 3–18. Baillière Tindall, London.

Edwards, R.H.T. (1984) New techniques for studying human muscle function, metabolism, and fatigue. *Muscle and Nerve*, **7**, 599–609.

Edwards, R.H.T. & Jones, D.A. (1983) Diseases of skeletal muscle. In Peachey, L.D. & Adrian, R.D. (eds) *Handbook of Physiology*, Section 10: *Skeletal Muscle*, pp. 633–672. American Physiological Society, Bethesda, MD.

Edwards, R.H.T. & McDonnell, M. (1974) Hand held dynamometer for evaluating voluntary-muscle function. *Lancet*, **ii**, 757–758.

Edwards, R.H.T., Chapman, S.J., Newham, D.J. & Jones, D.A. (1987) Practical analysis of variability of muscle function measurements in Duchenne muscular dystrophy. *Muscle and Nerve*, **10**, 6–14.

Edwards, R.H.T., Griffiths, R.D., Hayward, M., & Helliwell, T.R. (1986) Modern methods of diagnosis of muscle diseases. *J. Roy. Coll. Phys. Lond.*, **20**, 49–55.

Edwards, R.H.T., Round, J.M. & Jones, D.A. (1983) Needle biopsy of skeletal muscle: a review of 10 years experience. *Muscle and Nerve*, **6**, 676–683.

Edwards, R.H.T., Young, A., Hosking, G.P. & Jones, D.A. (1977) Human skeletal muscle function: description of tests and normal values. *Clin. Sci. Mol. Med.*, **52**, 283.

Emery, A. (1986) *Duchenne Muscular Dystrophy.* Oxford University Press, Oxford.

Fischer, A.Q. & Stephens, S. (1988) Computerized real-time sonography: a new application, techniques and methods. *J. Child Neurol.*, **3**, 69–74.

Fischer, A.Q., Carpenter, D.W., Hartlage, P.L., Carroll, J.E. & Stephens, S. (1988) Muscle imaging in neuromuscular disease using computerized real-time sonography. *Muscle and Nerve*, **11**, 270–275.

Grindrod, S., Tofts, P. & Edwards, R. (1983) Investigation of human skeletal muscle structure and composition by X-ray computerised tomography. *Eur. J. Clin. Invest.*, **13**, 465–468.

Heckmatt, J.Z., Pier, N. & Dubowitz, V. (1988) Real-time ultrasound imaging of muscles. *Muscle and Nerve*, **11**, 56–65.

Jones, D.A. & Edwards, R.H.T. (1986) Muscle strength and metabolism. In: Dimitrijevic, M., Kakulas, B. & Vrbova, G. (eds) *Recent Achievements in Restorative Neurology*, vol. 2: *Progressive Neuromuscular Diseases.* Karger, Basel.

Jones, P.R.M. & Pearson, J. (1969) Anthropometric determination of leg fat and muscle plus bone volume in young male and female adults. *J. Physiol.*, **204**, 63P.

Kurtz, L.T., Mubarak, S.J., Schultz, P., Park, S.M. & Leach J. (1983) Correlation of scoliosis and pulmonary function in Duchenne muscular dystrophy. *J. Pediatr. Orthop.*, **3**, 347–353.

McGill, S.M., Patt, N. & Norman, R.W. (1988) Measurement of the trunk musculature of active males using CT scan radiography: implications for force and moment generating capacity about the L4/L5 joint. *J. Biomech.*, **21**, 329–341.

Millerchip, R., Savage, R.A. & Edwards, R.H.T. (1988) Magnetic resonance anthropometry of muscles stabilising the lumbar spine. *Clin. Sci.*, **75**, 39P.

Rideau, Y., Jankowski, L.W. & Grellet, J. (1981) Respiratory function in the muscular dystrophies. *Muscle and Nerve*, **4**, 155–164.

Saltin, B. & Gollinck, P.D. (1983) Skeletal muscle adaptability: significance for metabolism and performance. In *Handbook of Physiology*, Section 10: *Skeletal Muscle*, pp. 555–631. American Physiological Society, Bethesda, MD.

Schrieber, A., Smith W.L., Lonasescu, V., Zellweger, H., Franken, E.A., Dunn, V. & Ehrhardt, J. (1987) Magnetic resonance imaging of children with Duchenne muscular dystrophy. *Pediatr. Radiol.*, **17**, 495–497.

Scott, O.M., Goddard, C. & Dubowitz, V. (1982) Quantitation of muscle function in children: a prospective study in Duchenne muscular dystrophy. *Muscle and Nerve*, **5**, 291–301.

Smith, P.E.M., Calverley, P.M.A., Edwards, R.H.T., Evans, G.A. & Campbell, E.J.M. (1987) Practical problems in the respiratory care of patients with muscular dystrophy. *N. Engl. J. Med.*, **316**, 1197–1205.

Walton, J.N. & Gardner-Medwin, D. (1988) The muscular dystrophies. In Walton, J.N. (ed.) *Disorders of Voluntary Muscle*, Ch. 15. Churchill Livingstone, London.

SECTION 4
CONGENITAL SPINAL ABNORMALITIES

13 · Congenital Deformities of the Spine

By M.J. McMASTER

The term 'congenital deformity of the spine' is misleading because it implies that the spine deformity is present at birth, whereas this is not necessarily so. The developmental vertebral anomalies which cause the deformity are present at birth, hence the term congenital, but the deformity does not usually become apparent until later in childhood when the diagnosis is made radiographically by noting the presence of vertebral malformations lying within the curvature. On occasion there may be an additional failure of development of the posterior spinal elements and an 'open' spinal defect with abnormalities of the spinal cord and overlying tissues, as seen in the myelomeningocoele patient. This, however, is a separate problem usually associated with severe neurological impairment and paralysis of the trunk muscles which contributes to the development of the spinal deformity. This chapter deals only with 'closed' congenital deformities in which the skin overlying the spine is intact.

Congenital deformities of the spine are relatively uncommon and account for less than 5% of patients seen with significant structural deformities at a normal spinal deformity clinic. However, some anomalies cause so little deformity that they remain undetected, and the true prevalence of congenital spine deformity in the general population remains unknown. Wynne-Davies (1975) found that multiple vertebral anomalies were often hereditary in origin and carried a 5–10% risk of occurrence in subsequent siblings, but an isolated single anomaly was usually sporadic and there was no risk to subsequent siblings. In contrast Winter (1983) found that only 1% of patients with a congenital spine deformity had a known relative with the problem.

Patients with a congenital spine deformity present at all ages, but the majority are diagnosed either in the first few years of life or at puberty. All degrees of severity of curvature are seen at all ages. Some patients are first seen in their teenage years with small curves which progress minimally, whereas others present at a younger age with curves which deteriorate rapidly and result in an extreme deformity (see Figs 13.7 & 13.8). Correction of these severe deformities is often difficult and dangerous because of their rigidity. It is therefore important to be able to anticipate when a congenital spine deformity is at risk of rapid deterioration, and to initiate treatment when the curve is small, rather than to attempt the dangerous surgical salvage procedures that are necessary when the curve is severe. Planning such a prophylactic course of treatment requires a thorough knowledge of the natural history of all types of congenital spine deformity and the methods of treatment which are available.

Pathogenesis

In order to understand the great disparity in prognosis for congenital spine deformities it is necessary to correlate the principles of normal growth of the spine with the pathological anatomy of the various types of congenital vertebral anomaly that may cause the deformity (for details see Chapter 2).

The development of the spine is a very rapid process and the complete anatomical pattern is formed in mesenchyme during the first six weeks of intrauterine life. Vertebral anomalies develop during this period, and once the mesenchymal mould is established the cartilaginous and bony stages follow that pattern. The development of the neural axis also occurs at the same time, and it is therefore not surprising that neural and vertebral malformations often coexist. At the beginning of the third week the embryo is basically a three-layered structure and the ectodermal layer invaginates towards the notochord to form the neural tube. Part of the columns of mesoderm on either side of the neural tube then migrate to surround the notochord from either side to form the primitive vertebral body. At this stage there may be a *defect of formation* of a vertebra resulting in wedge-shaped vertebra or a hemivertebra which usually lies laterally or posterolaterally. Each primitive vertebral body then segments longitudinally into two portions. The caudal portion of one unites with the cephalic portion of the other to form the definitive vertebral body. At this stage there may be a *defect of segmentation* resulting in an unsegmented bar joining together one side of a number of vertebrae or a block of vertebrae which are completely fused together.

Normal longitudinal growth of the spine is the sum total of growth occurring at the endplates on the upper and lower surfaces of the vertebral bodies (Bick & Copel, 1950). This growth occurs symmetrically, and as a result the spine grows in a balanced manner and without a pathological curvature. However, in the presence of a congenital vertebral anomaly there is as asymmetrical deficiency in either a number of endplates or their rate of growth on one side of the spine, resulting in a longitudinal growth imbalance and an increasing spinal deformity as the child grows. An early onset of the deformity carries a bad prognosis because it indicates a severe growth imbalance. The final severity of the deformity is proportional to the degree of growth imbalance produced by the vertebral anomalies, and deterioration stops only at skeletal maturity when the growth plates fuse. However, the rate of deterioration is not uniform and accelerates during the adolescent growth spurt which is at its peak in girls around age 12 years and in boys at 14 years.

The pattern of the spinal deformity that develops may be a scoliosis or kyphosis depending on whether the impaired longitudinal growth, due to the vertebral anomaly, lies laterally or anteriorly. However, it is not uncommon for kyphoscoliosis to occur due to an anterolateral growth impairment with either the scoliosis or kyphosis predominating. A lordosis, due to impaired posterior growth of the spine, is uncommon by itself and is usually associated with a scoliosis as the major component.

CONGENITAL SCOLIOSIS

Scoliosis is the commonest type of congenital spine deformity and is a lateral curvature of the spine due to the presence of developmental anomalies which produce a predominantly lateral longitudinal growth imbalance (Winter *et al.*, 1968; McMaster & Ohtsuka, 1982). This type of scoliosis must not be confused with infantile idiopathic scoliosis which can also present with a severe curvature in early childhood, but in these patients the spinal radiograph shows that there is apparently normal vertebral development.

The prognosis for a congenital scoliosis depends on the age of the patient, the type and site of the vertebral anomaly and the degree of growth imbalance it produces (McMaster & Ohtsuka, 1982). There are basically two groups of congenital anomalies which produce a scoliosis, and these are due either to a *defect of formation* or a *defect of segmentation* of one or more vertebrae (Table 13.1; Fig. 13.1). Approximately 80% of vertebral anomalies can usually be classified in this way, but the remaining 20% cannot be classified, either because there is a complex jumble of anomalies or because the severity of the deformity is so great as to obscure the radiographic characteristics of the anomaly. The site of the anomaly also has an effect, and for any given type of vertebral anomaly the rate of deterioration of the resulting scoliosis is most severe in the thoracic and thoracolumbar regions, and is usually less severe in the upper thoracic and lumbar regions (Fig. 13.2). The age of the patient is important because the scoliosis will continue to deteriorate until skeletal maturity.

Defects of formation

A partial failure of formation of a vertebra on one side results in a *wedge vertebra* with retarded longitudinal

Table 13.1 Types of developmental vertebral anomaly causing a congenital scoliosis

Defects of formation
Partial unilateral—wedge vertebra
Complete unilateral—hemivertebra: fully segmented, semisegmented, incarcerated
Defects of segmentation
Bilateral—block vertebra
Unilateral—unilateral unsegmented bar; unilateral unsegmented bar with contralateral hemivertebrae
Mixed or unclassifiable anomalies

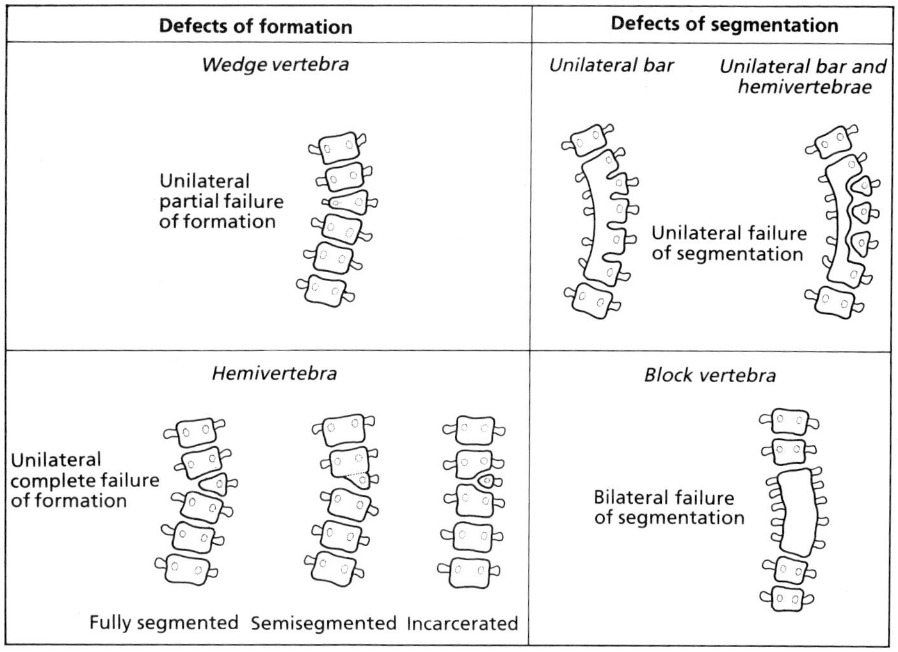

Fig. 13.1 Congenital scoliosis.

Site of curvature	Type of congenital anomaly					
	Block vertebra	Wedged vertebra	Hemivertebra: Single	Hemivertebra: Double	Unilateral unsegmented bar	Unilateral unsegmented bar and contralateral hemivertebrae
Upper thoracic	<1° – 1°	* – 2°	1° – 2°	2° – 2.5°	2° – 4°	5° – 6°
Lower thoracic	<1° – 1°	2° – 2°	2° – 2.5°	2° – 3°	5° – 6.5°	6° – 7°
Thoracolumbar	<1° – 1°	1.5° – 2°	2° – 3.5°	5° – *	6° – 9°	>10° – *
Lumbar	<1° – *	<1° – *	<1° – 1°	*	>5° – *	*
Lumbosacral	*	*	<1°–1.5°	*	*	*

☐ No treatment required
▨ May require spinal fusion
■ Require spinal fusion
* Too few or no curves

Fig. 13.2 Congenital scoliosis: median yearly rate of deterioration (in degrees) without treatment for each type of congenital vertebral anomaly in each region of the spine (before 10 years–after 10 years of age). From McMaster & Ohtsuka (1982).

growth on the hypoplastic side. These curves deteriorate relatively slowly, rarely exceeding 35° at skeletal maturity, and they only very occasionally require treatment.

One of the commonest causes of a congenital scoliosis is complete failure of a vertebra to form on one side, resulting in a *hemivertebra* (McMaster & David, 1986). Longitudinal growth occurs on the upper and lower surfaces of the hemivertebra but there is an absence of two growth plates on the unformed side; as a result the hemivertebra acts as an enlarging wedge on one side of the spine. The hemivertebra may be fully segmented (non-incarcerated), which is most common; semisegmented, which is less common; or incarcerated, which is the least common (Fig. 13.1).

A single fully segmented (non-incarcerated) hemivertebra usually causes a slowly progressive scoliosis (1–2° per year), which can on occasion produce a moderately severe deformity in the lower thoracic and thoracolumbar regions, but this does not usually become significant until after the age of 10 years. However, a hemivertebra at the lumbosacral junction is a particularly pernicious anomaly because it causes the lumbar spine to take off obliquely from the sacrum. This produces a compensatory thoracolumbar scoliosis which is initially mobile but later becomes fixed. This secondary curve, combined with a tendency to list to one side, can produce a very significant cosmetic deformity (Figs 13.3 & 13.4) and requires very early prophylactic treatment.

Two fully segmented unilateral hemivertebrae are less common but cause a much greater growth imbalance because there is an absence of four growth plates on the concavity of the curve. These curves deteriorate more rapidly (approximately 3° per year) than those due to a single hemivertebra and all exceed 50° by 10 years of age (Figs 13.5 & 13.6). These curves all require early prophylactic treatment.

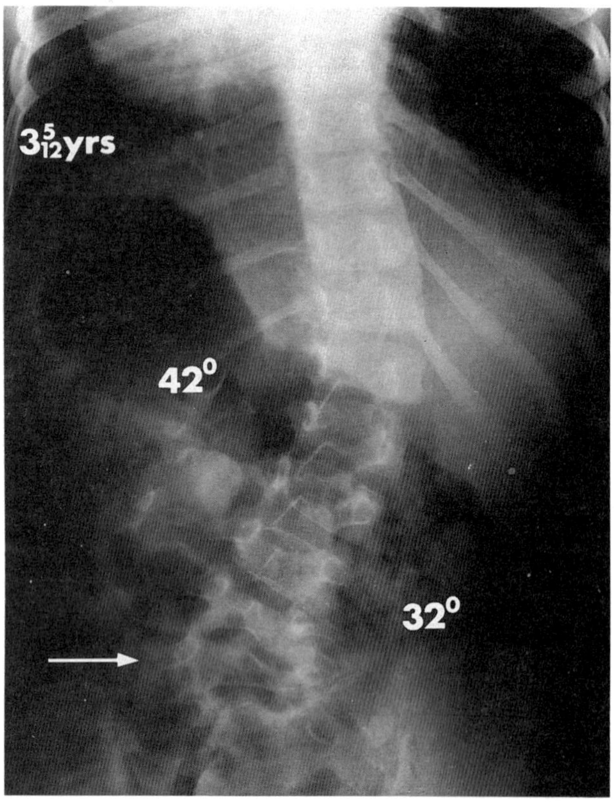

Fig. 13.3 A girl aged three years five months, with a 32° left lumbosacral scoliosis due to a single hemivertebra at the lumbosacral junction. There was also a 42° right thoracolumbar scoliosis in which there are no congenital anomalies. The pelvis was level but the upper body listed to the right.

If there are two opposing hemivertebrae, the prognosis depends on whether the hemivertebrae are close together or in different regions of the spine. If they are close together they tend to balance each other, causing only two small kinks in the spine with minimal cosmetic deformity, and no treatment is required. However, if the hemivertebrae are in different regions the resulting curves are often unbalanced, causing the trunk to list to one side, and prophylactic treatment may be required.

A semisegmented hemivertebra is congenitally synostosed to one of its neighbouring vertebrae and, as a result, two growth plates are obliterated on the convex side and this tends to balance the absence of the two growth plates on the unformed side of the hemivertebra. Although growth of the spine is theoretically balanced, the hemivertebra causes tilting of the vertebral column but the scoliosis never becomes severe or requires treatment.

An incarcerated hemivertebra is a small ovoid piece of bone tucked into the spine and set into a niche scalloped out of the adjacent vertebra. It has a very poor growth potential and as a result there is only a very mild scoliosis which never requires treatment.

Defects of segmentation

A bilateral failure of segmentation of a number of vertebrae results in a *block vertebra*, which is an uncommon cause of scoliosis. This type of anomaly is most commonly found in the thoracic region and usually involves two to five adjacent vertebrae. Longitudinal growth is impaired on both sides of the spine but not always symmetrically, and this may result in a mild degree of curvature which rarely exceeds 20° at skeletal maturity. These curves do not require treatment.

A unilateral failure of segmentation of a number of vertebrae results in a *unilateral unsegmented bar*, and is one of the commonest types of anomaly producing a scoliosis. The unsegmented bar does not contain growth plates and therefore does not grow longitudinally, whereas normal or near-normal growth occurs on the opposite side of the spine. This always produces a severe scoliosis which deteriorates at approximately 5° per year and all exceed 50° by 10 years of age (see Fig. 13.17). This type of congenital scoliosis requires early prophylactic surgical treatment as soon as the diagnosis is made. It is important to appreciate that it is not possible to create growth

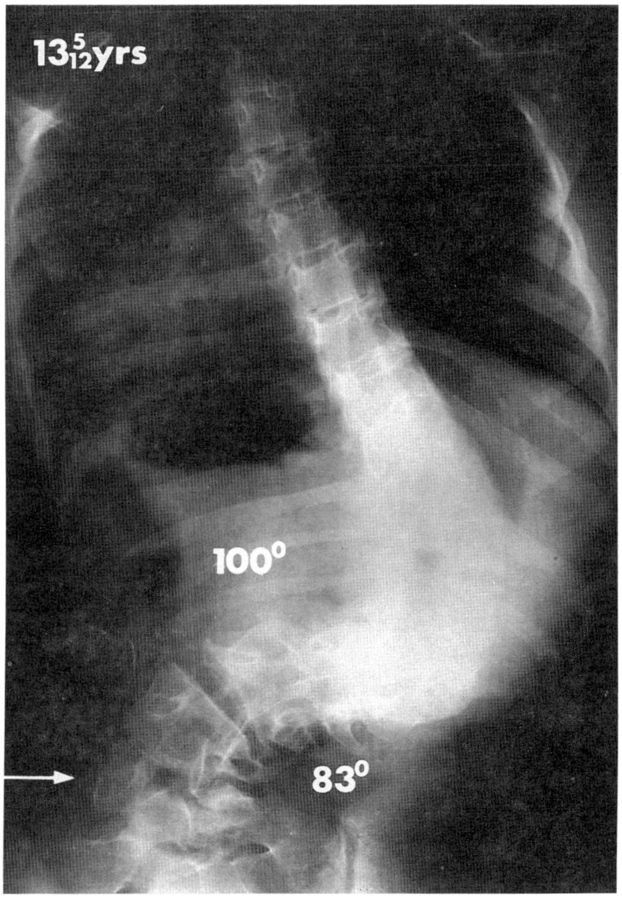

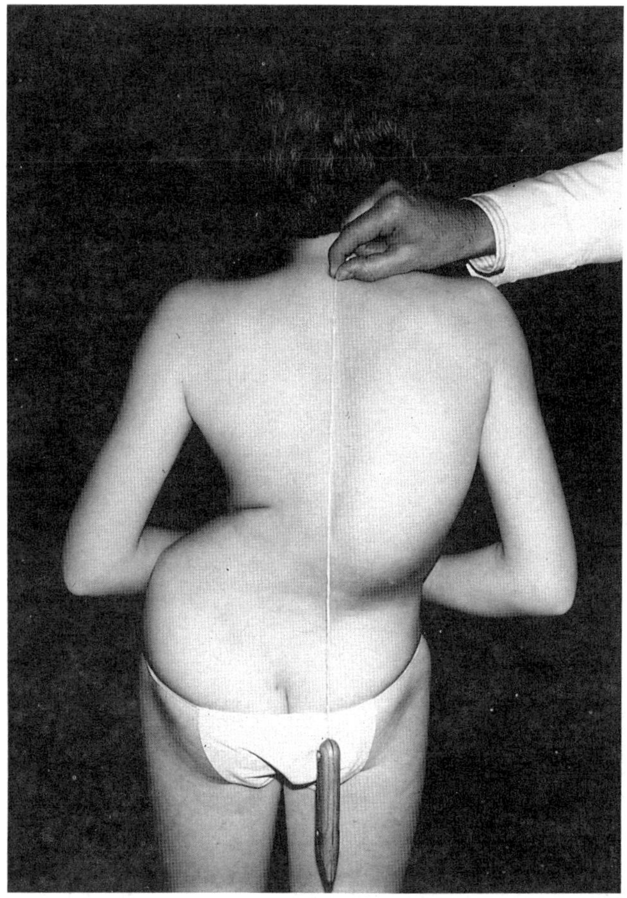

Fig. 13.4 No treatment was given, and by 13 years five months the congenital lumbosacral curve had deteriorated to 83°. The thoracolumbar curve measured 100° and had become structural and severely rotated. The list had increased but the pelvis remained level. The major deformity was due to the severe thoracolumbar scoliosis which, despite its size, failed to compensate for the list to the right.

on the concave side of the spine where none exists, and the aim of treatment is to balance the growth of the spine by preventing further growth on the convex side opposite the anomaly.

It is very important to recognize a *unilateral unsegmented bar with contralateral hemivertebrae* (Nasca *et al.*, 1975) because this produces the most malignant of all types of congenital scoliosis. Although there is no longitudinal growth at the side of the bar, there is a greater growth potential on the convexity than in those patients with an unsegmented bar alone. This causes the most severe growth imbalance of all, and these curves deteriorate at 6° or more per year and usually exceed 50° by four years of age. If left untreated they become extreme at skeletal maturity (Figs 13.7 & 13.8). All require very early surgical treatment as soon as the diagnosis is made, in order to control their progress.

The type of congenital vertebral anomaly which causes the most severe scoliosis, regardless of the area of the spine in which it occurs, is a unilateral unsegmented bar with contralateral hemivertebrae at the same level. Second in severity is a scoliosis due to a unilateral unsegmented bar alone, followed by two unilateral hemivertebrae, a single hemivertebra, and a wedge vertebra. The least severe scoliosis is caused by a block vertebra. A congenital scoliosis caused by a mixture of unclassifiable anomalies can be difficult to predict and requires careful monitoring.

Secondary features

Apart from the severity of the congenital scoliosis there are also a number of important secondary features which contribute to the overall disability and deformity of the patient.

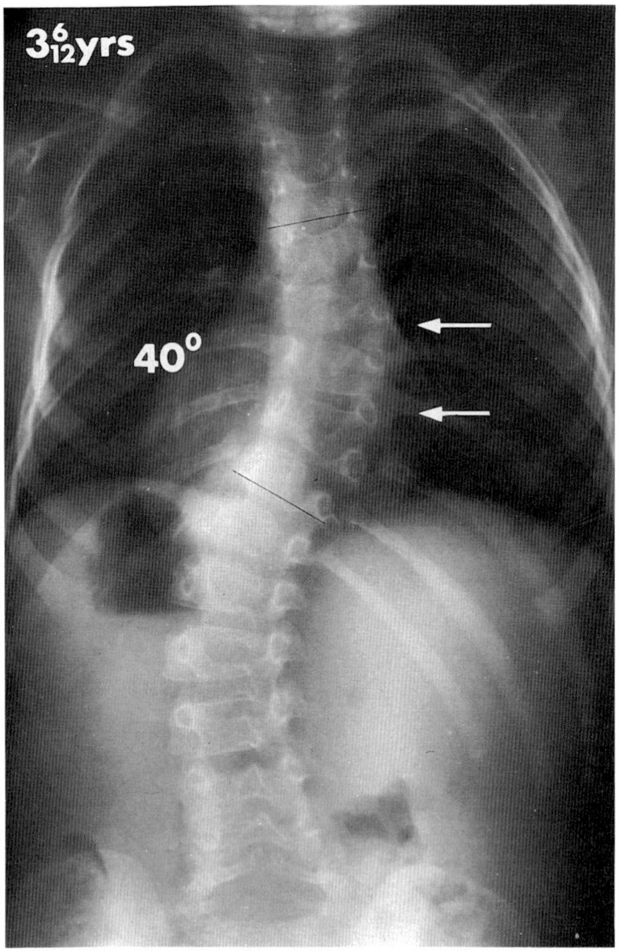

Fig. 13.5 A boy aged three years six months with a 40° right thoracic scoliosis due to two unilateral hemivertebrae on the convexity at the seventh and tenth thoracic levels.

A congenital scoliosis, as distinct from an idiopathic scoliosis, commonly occurs in the upper thoracic region, and although the majority of these curves never become large they can produce a significant cosmetic deformity due to elevation of the shoulder line and occasionally tilting of the head. A 30° curve is probably at the upper limit of acceptance, and anything greater is severely deforming, especially in girls.

An additional problem associated with upper thoracic curves, especially those with their apex at T6 or T7, is the development of a large secondary structural curve below the congenital curve. This curve, which has no congenital anomalies, usually deteriorates even more rapidly than the congenital curve above, and soon becomes the major deformity requiring treatment.

Patients with lower thoracic and thoracolumbar curves, especially those due to a unilateral unsegmented bar with or without a contralateral hemivertebra, often fail to develop compensatory curves, above or below, which are adequate to balance the congenital curve. The reason for this is that there are often too few normal mobile vertebrae between the anomaly and either the upper end of the spine or the sacrum. This results in severe malalignment of the body (see Fig. 13.17), which is very difficult to correct and requires early prophylactic treatment.

CONGENITAL KYPHOSIS

A congenital kyphosis is an abnormal posterior curvature of the spine due to the presence of developmental

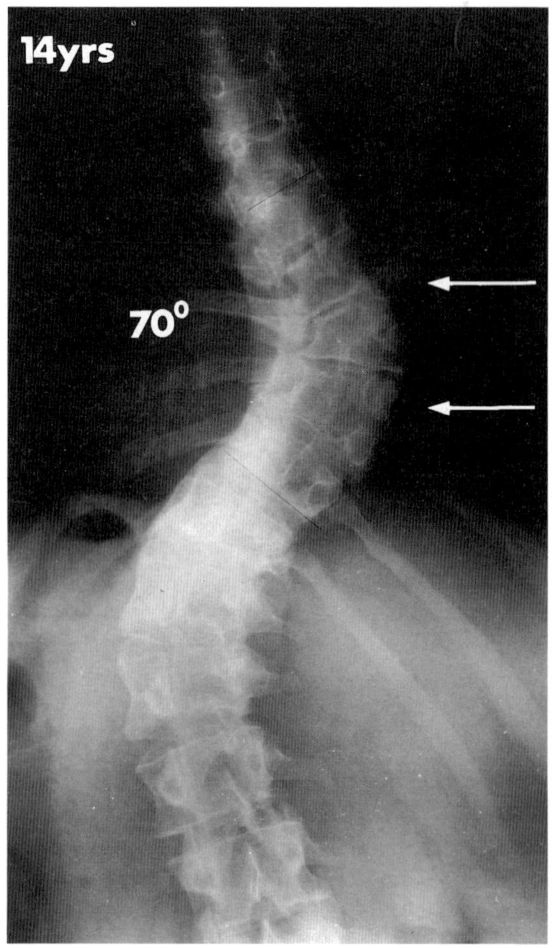

Fig. 13.6 No treatment was given, and by 14 years the curve had deteriorated to 70°.

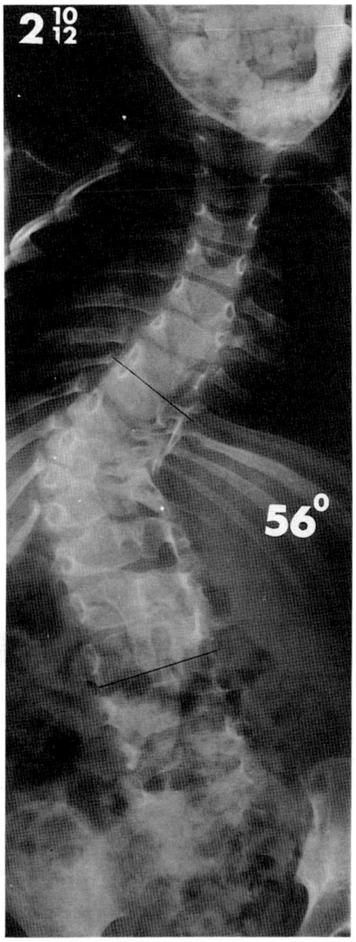

Fig. 13.7 A girl aged two years 10 months, with a 56° left thoracolumbar scoliosis due to a unilateral unsegmented bar on the right extending from the eighth to the twelfth thoracic vertebra with four adjacent contralateral hemivertebrae at the ninth to the twelfth thoracic levels. Note the localized spina bifida occulta associated with widening of the interpedicular distance and narrowing of the disc spaces associated with diastematomyelia which is not obvious.

vertebral anomalies which impair the anterior longitudinal growth of the spine. Although a congenital kyphosis is much less common than a congenital scoliosis, it is even more important to understand and diagnose early, because if left untreated it can, on occasion, lead to spinal cord compression and paraplegia. In contrast, neurological abnormalities occur only in congenital scoliosis as a consequence of an associated intraspinal anomaly, and are not caused by direct compression of the spinal cord by the deformity.

It should be emphasized that early prophylactic treatment of congenital kyphosis is relatively simple, but delayed treatment of a severe deformity or neurological complication is difficult and dangerous.

Table 13.2 Types of developmental vertebral anomaly causing a congenital kyphosis

Anterior failure of formation
Posterior or posterolateral hemivertebra
Anterior failure of segmentation
Anterior unsegmented bar
Mixed or unclassifiable anomalies

The classification of the various types of congenital kyphosis is very similar to that for congenital scoliosis (Table 13.2). A congenital kyphosis may be due to either an anterior failure of formation of a vertebra or a failure of segmentation of one or more vertebrae (Fig. 13.9). A third type can also occur due to a mixture of these anomalies.

Anterior failure of formation

The commonest cause of a congenital kyphosis is an anterior failure of formation of one or more vertebral bodies. The degree of malformation can vary from a mild anterior wedging of the vertebral body to a posterior hemivertebra, or at the extreme there may be a complete absence of the vertebral body with only the posterior elements remaining. Depending on the degree of malformation, there is a varying degree of anterior growth impairment while normal growth continues posteriorly, resulting in an increasing kyphosis. A symmetrically situated posterior hemivertebra will produce a pure kyphosis, but it is more common for the hemivertebra to be situated posterolaterally, resulting in a kyphoscoliosis with the kyphosis being the major deformity (Fig. 13.10).

This type of congenital kyphosis produces a much more angular deformity than that due to an anterior unsegmented bar, and also deteriorates more rapidly at 3–7° per year. The rate of deterioration is proportional to the degree of failure of formation of the vertebrae, and varies from mild progression where there is slight anterior wedging of a vertebra to much more severe progression if there is a complete absence of several vertebral bodies. During the adolescent growth spurt the rate of deterioration increases and stops only at skeletal maturity when the growth plates fuse.

The most major complication associated with this

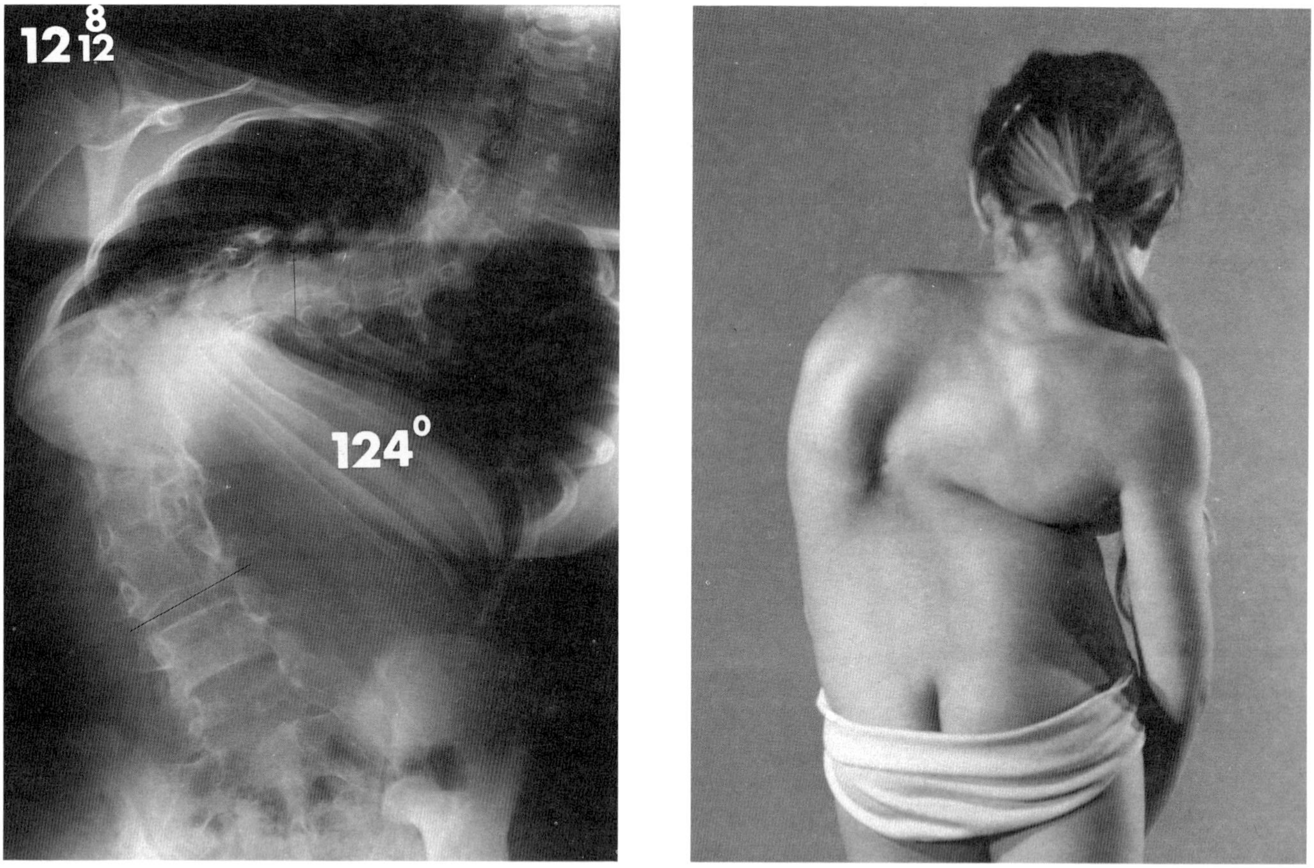

Fig. 13.8 No treatment was given, and by 12 years eight months the scoliosis had increased to 124° and the contralateral hemivertebrae were no longer visible. There was pelvic obliquity, and a severe list of the upper body to the right, producing a very severe cosmetic deformity.

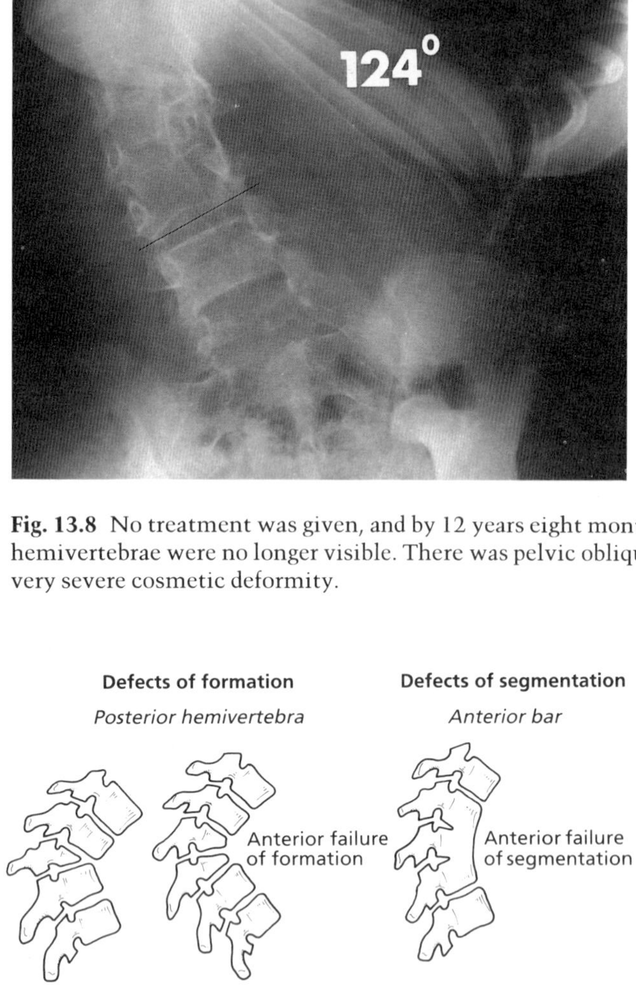

Fig. 13.9 Congenital kyphosis.

type of congenital kyphosis is the development of spinal cord compression progressing to paraplegia as the hemivertebra is extruded backwards into the spinal canal (Figs 13.10 & 13.11). The neurological abnormalities usually develop during the adolescent growth spurt when the deformity is deteriorating most rapidly, and the greatest risk is in high to mid-thoracic curves with their apex between T4 and T9 where the spinal canal is narrowest, the neural structures are least elastic and the blood supply to the cord is least abundant (Winter *et al.*, 1973; Lonstein *et al.*, 1980). If a neurological deficit develops it is always progressive and requires immediate treatment.

A further complication associated with severe angular kyphotic deformities in the thoracic region is distortion and compression of the rib cage leading to respiratory failure and death from cor pulmonale.

Anterior failure of segmentation

Of the two main types of congenital kyphosis this is the least common and relatively more benign (Mayfield *et al.*, 1980). The anterior failure of seg-

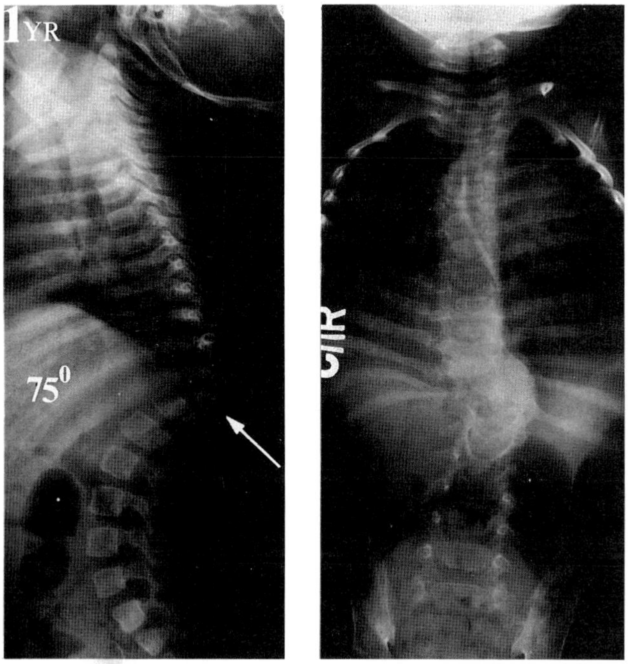

Fig. 13.10 A boy aged one year with a 75° thoracolumbar kyphosis due to a posterolateral hemivertebra at the twelfth thoracic level.

mentation results in a bar of bone extending anteriorly across two or more vertebral bodies (Fig. 13.12). This bar of bone does not contain growth plates, whereas normal growth continues posteriorly resulting in an increasing kyphos. This is usually a smooth pure kyphosis rather than the angular kyphoscoliosis seen with anterior failure of formation of a vertebra. The rate of deterioration of the kyphosis is variable but is more severe if the anterior bar extends over a number of segments. This can result in a severe deformity, but it is never as extreme as that seen with anterior failure of formation. Spinal cord compression does not occur with this type of kyphosis even with severe degrees of deformity, and the respiratory function is seldom significantly impaired. However, low backache can occur in later life as a consequence of secondary degenerative changes developing in the lumbar hyperlordosis below the congenital kyphosis.

ASSOCIATED OCCULT INTRASPINAL ANOMALIES

The development of the spinal cord is closely associated with that of the vertebral column, and it is therefore not surprising that neural and vertebral malformations often coexist. The spinal deformity may be obvious, but the intraspinal anomaly may not be recognized because the associated neural deficit may be mild or absent. It is, however, very important to detect these intraspinal anomalies because they may restrict movement of the spinal cord within the spinal canal, and any attempt to correct the deformity could result in stretching of the spinal cord and serious neurological complications.

The incidence of intraspinal anomalies is more common in a congenital scoliosis than kyphosis. A diastematomyelia is found in 5–20% of patients with congenital scoliosis (Winter *et al.*, 1974; Hood *et al.*, 1980; McMaster, 1984; Goldberg *et al.*, 1984). Other types of congenital intraspinal anomaly are less frequent, and may be found either alone or in association with a diastematomyelia. These anomalies are epidermoid cysts, dermoid cysts, neurenteric cysts, lipomas and teratomas. The spinal cord or cauda equina can also be tethered by fibrous bands, a tight filum terminale, ectopic posterior nerve roots, or arachnoid adhesions to the dura or vertebral column.

Intraspinal anomalies may be associated with all sites and types of congenital deformity, but the most commonly associated deformity is a scoliosis in the lower thoracic or thoracolumbar regions due to a unilateral unsegmented bar with contralateral hemivertebrae (see Fig. 13.7); 50% of these patients have an intraspinal anomaly (McMaster, 1984).

The intraspinal anomaly may not be immediately obvious, but there may be a number of clues to its presence. An abnormality of the skin overlying the spine—such as a dimple, naevus, hairy patch or a lipoma—is present in approximately 50% of patients. Neurological abnormalities may also be present but are often very mild and easily missed. Frequently only one leg is affected, and this is usually slightly short with a small foot which may have a mild cavus deformity and slight clawing of the toes (James & Lassman, 1970). In addition the spinal radiograph may show a localized spina bifida occulta associated with widening of the interpedicular distance and narrowing of the disc spaces (see Fig. 13.7). Occasionally the midline bony spur associated with a diastematomyelia may be visible on the plane spinal radiograph, but a myelogram or MRI is necessary to confirm its presence.

It is widely accepted that an intraspinal anomaly should be treated surgically if there is a progressive neurological deficit, or before attempting to correct a spinal deformity. Excision of the intraspinal anomaly

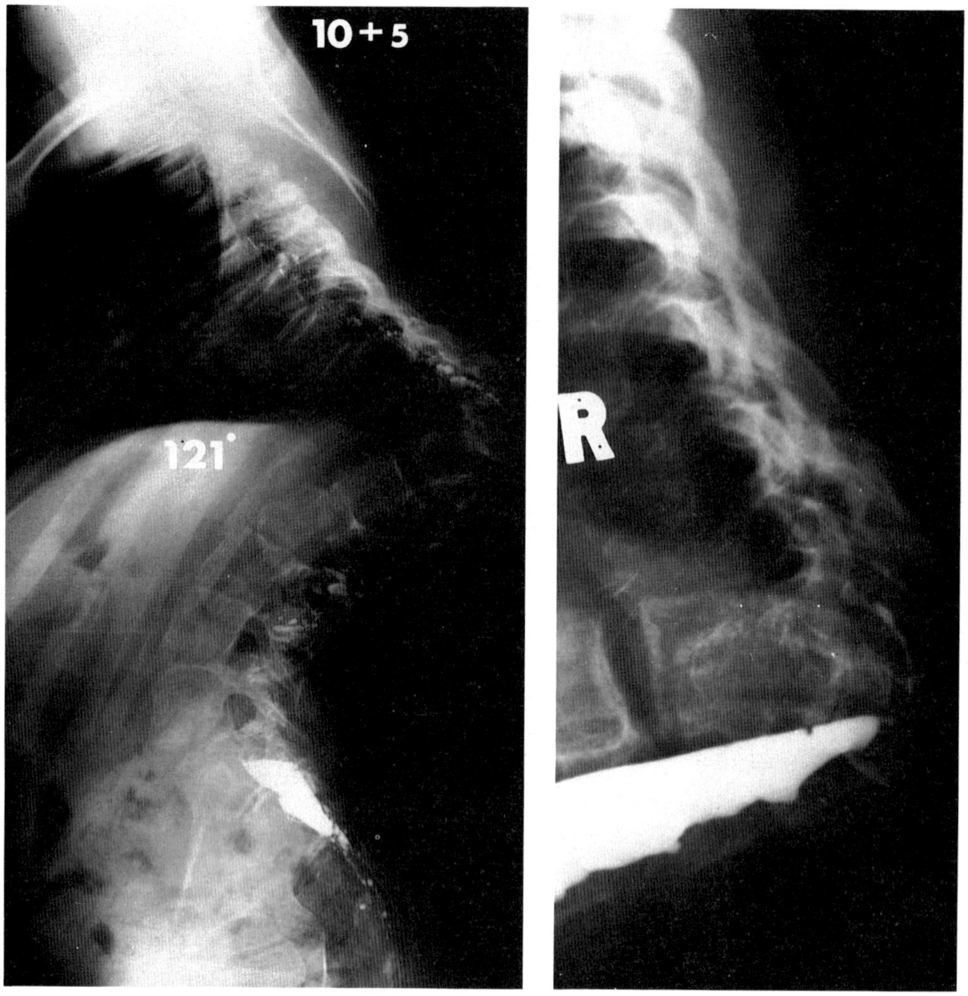

Fig. 13.11 No treatment was given, and by 10 years five months the kyphosis deteriorated to 121°. The patient had developed a spastic paraplegia and the myelogram showed a complete intraspinal block at the apex of the kyphosis.

will not improve the neurological status but should prevent further deterioration and decrease the risk of neurological complications developing following correction of the spinal deformity. However, routine myelography or MRI should not be performed on all patients with congenital spinal deformities, but only on those with clinical or radiological evidence suspicious of an intraspinal anomaly and on those who are about to undergo surgery to correct a spinal deformity. If the intraspinal deformity is diagnosed on the routine assessment it should probably be removed as a prophylactic measure on children who are less than six years of age, to prevent the possible development of neurological abnormalities. However, some authorities may hold the contrasting view in the absence of neurological signs.

Other congenital abnormalities

Congenital deformities of the spine are also frequently associated with congenital abnormalities in other systems (see Chapter 18). The genito-urinary system is most frequently affected (25% of patients) and the most common anomalies are a unilateral kidney, duplication of the kidney or ureteric obstruction (MacEwen *et al.*, 1972). However, these anomalies are usually asymptomatic and renal investigations are necessary to make the diagnosis. Congenital heart disease may also be present in up to 10% of patients (Reckles *et al.*, 1975). Other abnormalities found less frequently are Klippel–Feil anomaly (Hensinger *et al.*, 1974), Sprengel's deformity and deformities of the limbs.

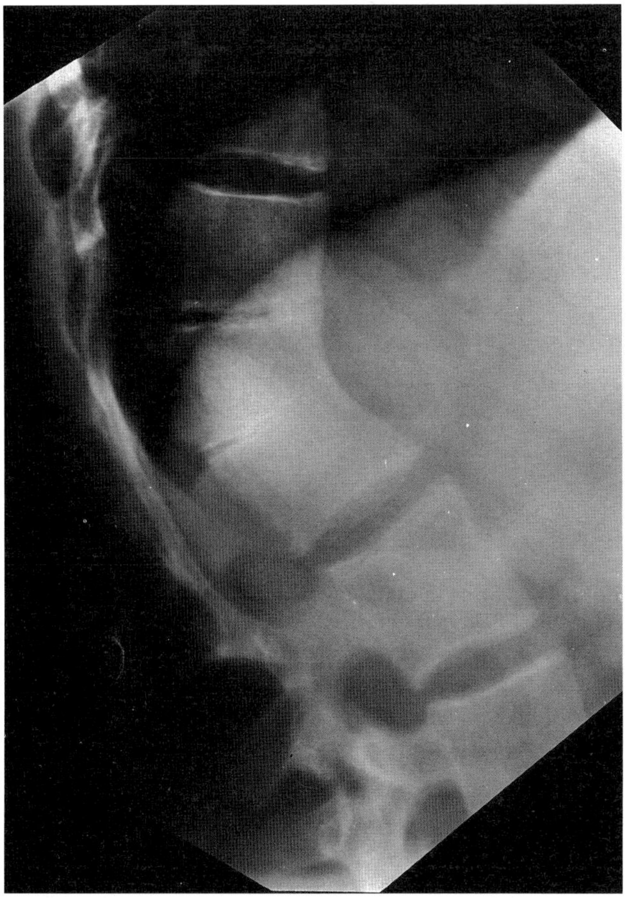

Fig. 13.12 A kyphosis due to an anterior failure of segmentation of three vertebrae at the thoracolumbar junction.

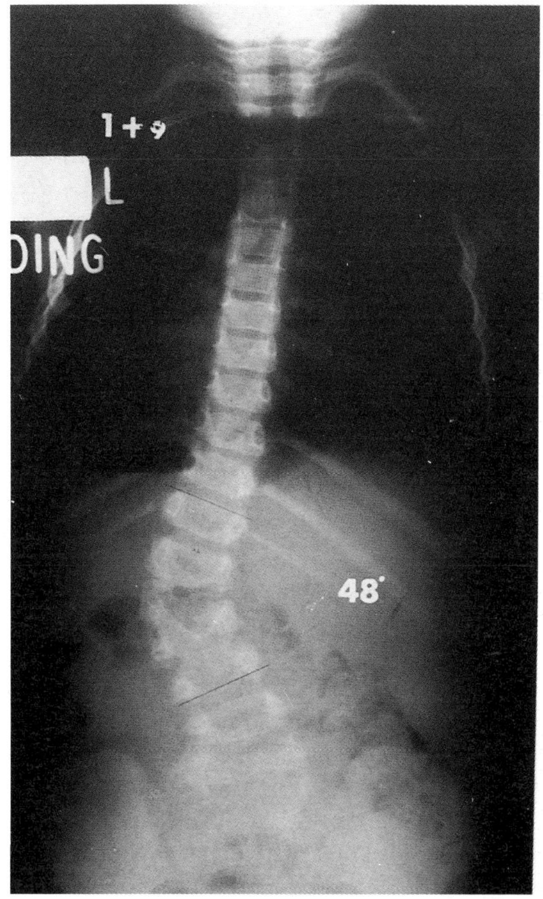

Fig. 13.13 A girl aged one year nine months with 48° lumbar scoliosis due to a single fully segmented hemivertebra on the convexity at the second lumbar level.

TREATMENT

There are three key factors to the successful management of a congenital spine deformity.

1 The diagnosis should be made as early as possible while the curvature is still small.

2 The prognosis should be anticipated based on the amount of spinal growth remaining, taken in conjunction with the type and site of the vertebral anomaly and the degree of growth imbalance it produces. This requires a careful study of good-quality anteroposterior, lateral and oblique spinal radiographs taken with the patient supine. An oblique radiograph often gives a true anteroposterior view of the more severely rotated spine, and may detect hidden vertebral anomalies at the apex of the curve. A misdiagnosis is occasionally possible in very young infants because a short-segment unilateral unsegmented bar may not be apparent radiographically until it becomes fully ossified over the next few years. Tomograms may also help, but a computerized axial tomography (CAT) scan is usually of less value because of the three-dimensional nature of the deformity. Occasionally it is difficult to assess the prognosis in young infants with small curves, due to a jumble of vertebral anomalies, and they require careful radiological follow-up to detect deterioration.

3 Deterioration must be prevented at all costs because it is easier to prevent than to correct a severe deformity. One of the commonest errors is a failure to recognize the slow and relentless deterioration of some curves, and all patients require careful radiological assessment at four-monthly intervals. These follow-up radiographs are taken with the patient standing, and the Cobb angle is measured at exactly the same level with reference to the standing radio-

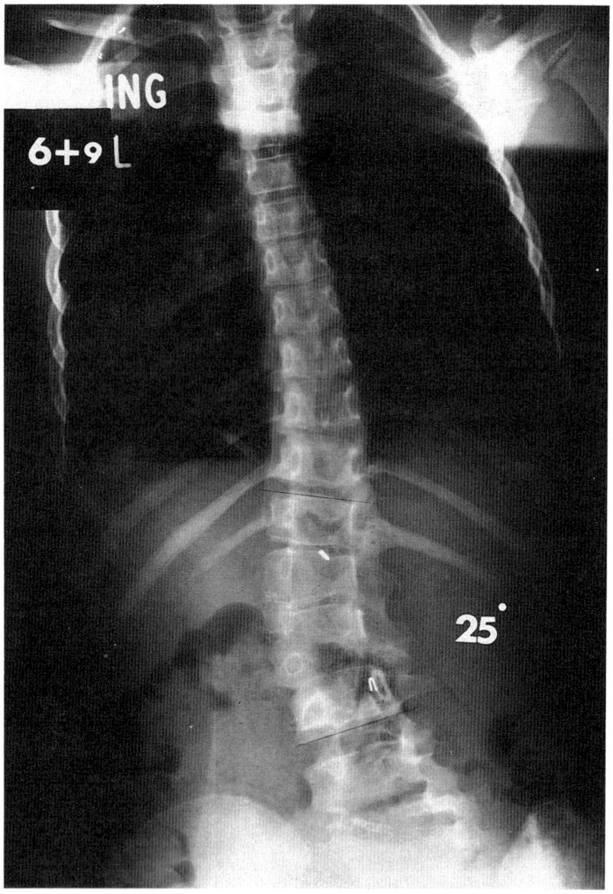

Fig. 13.14 Following a combined anterior and posterior convex epiphyseodesis from the first to the third lumbar vertebrae the scoliosis slowly corrected due to continued growth on the concavity, and by six years nine months the curve measured 25°.

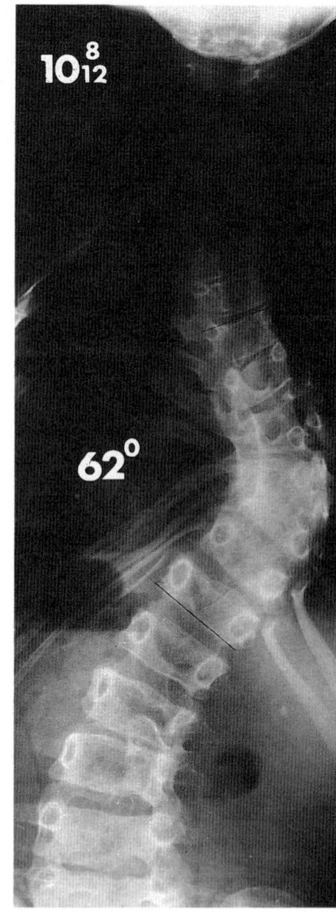

Fig. 13.15 A girl aged 10 years eight months with a 62° right thoracic scoliosis due to a unilateral unsegmentated bar on the concavity extending from the sixth to the tenth thoracic vertebra. The upper body listed to the right.

graph taken when the patient was first seen. Only in this way will deterioration be recognized before it is too late. Once progression is established, immediate treatment is necessary to prevent further deterioration.

In deciding on the method of treatment it is important to appreciate that it is not possible to create growth on the concavity of the deformity where it is retarded or non-existent (Winter *et al.*, 1968). Often the best that can be achieved is to balance the spinal growth by retarding the growth on the convexity, and this may require spinal surgery in the first few years of life. An early simple operation to prevent deformity is much better than a hazardous multistage procedure to correct a severe rigid deformity at a later stage.

Non-operative treatment

A congenital kyphosis cannot be treated by non-operative means and frequently requires surgery at an early age.

Certain types of congenital scoliosis can on occasion be managed by the application of an external support, but this has a very limited application and is never a definitive treatment by itself. It is important to appreciate that the problem being treated is one of spinal growth imbalance and an external support will never be effective in the presence of severe growth imbalance or a large rigid curve. A corrective Risser–Cotrel plaster jacket may be used as a holding device in very young infants with relatively slowly progres-

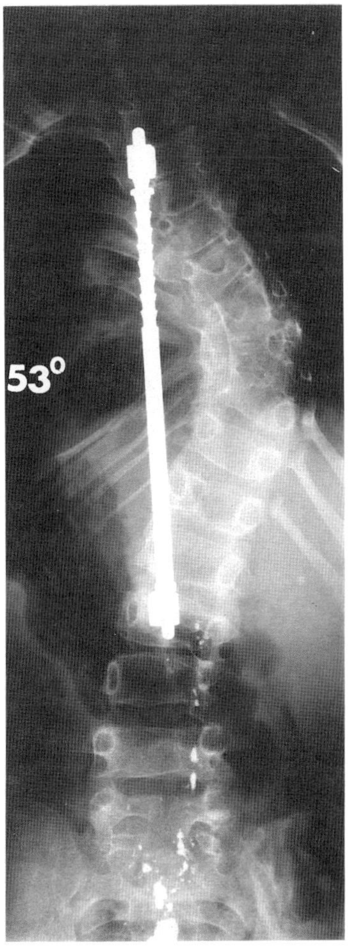

Fig. 13.16 Following posterior spinal fusion with Harrington instrumentation, the curve which was very rigid was only slightly corrected to 53°, but the list was completely corrected.

sive scoliotic curves. A Milwaukee brace may be applied to the older child, and works best in those with long flexible lower thoracic or thoracolumbar curves with a single short anomalous segment such as a hemivertebra at the apex of the curve (Winter *et al.*, 1976). The brace may also be used to improve spinal balance by controlling the development of the secondary compensatory curves which can develop above and below the congenital curve. These secondary structural curves occur in areas of the spine in which there are relatively normal vertebrae, and are therefore much more mobile than the congenital curve itself, which is usually rigid.

If the brace or jacket does not control the congenital deformity it is pointless to continue, and the patient requires immediate surgery.

SURGICAL TREATMENT

Surgical treatment is frequently necessary for congenital spine deformities, and is indicated at any age no matter how young, if the deformity is severe or the curve is increasing and cannot be controlled by any other means. There is no one operative procedure which can be applied to all types of deformity, and the method of surgery is selected depending on the age of the patient, the size of the curvature and the site and type of the vertebral anomalies.

The operative procedures fall into two main groups. Firstly, *prophylactic procedures* which are applied to young patients who have small curves with a bad prognosis. Correction of these curves is unnecessary if they are diagnosed at a sufficiently early stage. The second group of operations are *salvage procedures* because they are applied to patients diagnosed at a later stage when the deformity is greater and correction is necessary. However, the primary objective is to prevent further deterioration, and correction is attempted only if it can be safely achieved.

Congenital scoliosis

Prophylactic convex growth arrest

Prophylactic convex growth arrest (combined anterior and posterior convex hemiepiphyseodesis) is the optimum form of surgical treatment for patients seen at an early stage with small scoliotic curves in which there is some growth potential on the concavity at the site of the vertebral anomaly. This procedure is best applied to patients under the age of five years with progressive short curves of less than 60° due to a hemivertebra on the convexity (Winter, 1981; Andrew & Piggott, 1985). The objective of the surgery is to balance the growth of the spine by stopping the excessive growth on the convexity at the site of the hemivertebra. Theoretically this should allow the scoliosis to correct slowly, due to continuing growth on the concavity, but this does not always occur and the curvature may only be stabilized. To obtain the best results the surgery should be performed as early as possible, even in the first year of life (Figs 13.13 & 13.14).

The surgery consists of two separate procedures which are usually carried out under the same anaesthetic. Firstly, the spine is exposed anteriorly on the convexity of the scoliosis through a thoracotomy, a thoraco-abdominal retroperitoneal exposure or a

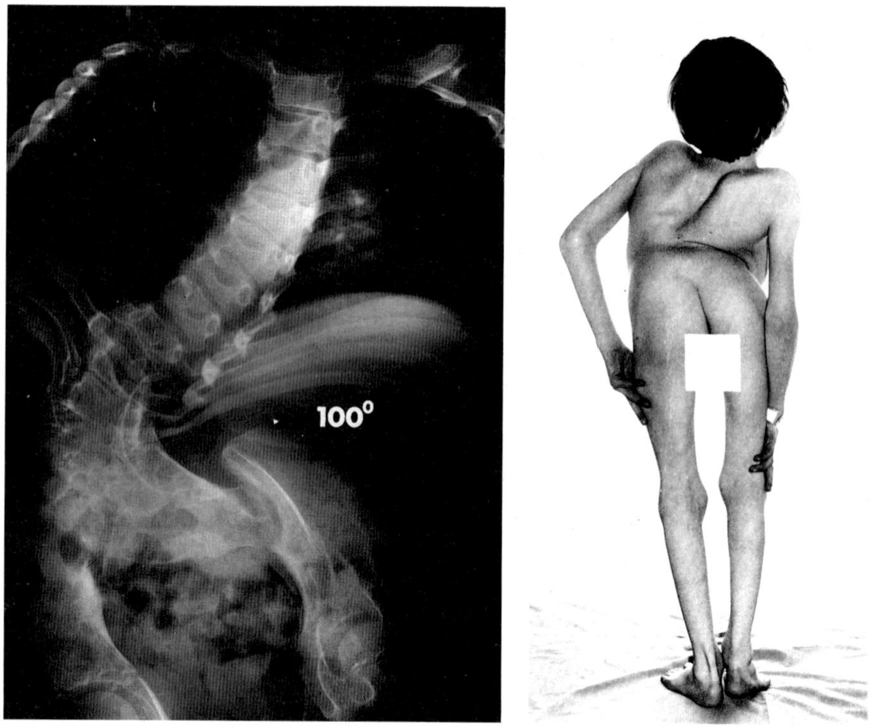

Fig. 13.17 A boy aged nine years six months, with a 100° left lumbar scoliosis due to a unilateral unsegmented bar on the concavity extending from the tenth thoracic vertebra to the sacrum. There was a very severe cosmetic deformity with displacement of the upper body to the right, pelvic obliquity and an apparent shortening of the right leg.

purely retroperitoneal approach beneath the diaphragm, depending on the site of the anomaly. The lateral half of the discs and their associated endplates are removed at the site of the anomalous vertebra and also for one level above and below. An anterior convex fusion is performed by packing the excised disc spaces with homologous bone graft or chips of bone taken from an excised rib. The second procedure is performed through a separate posterior exposure of the convexity of the curve at the site of the anomaly. Care is taken to avoid stripping the paraspinal muscles on the concavity and so possibly interfering with the growth potential on this side. A posterior convex fusion is performed by excising the facet joints and decorticating the posterior elements to one level above and below the anomalous segment. Chips of bone, either from the excised rib or homologous bone, are applied to the fusion area. Correction is attempted several days after the surgery by means of traction and the application of a Risser localizer jacket, which is maintained for six months until the convex growth arrest is soundly healed.

Prophylactic fusion *in situ*

This is the optimum form of surgical treatment for patients with small scoliotic curves due to a unilateral unsegmented bar with or without contralateral hemivertebrae. These anomalies produce very rigid deformities with a known potential for severe progression. There is no growth potential on the concavity at the site of the anomaly, and a convex growth arrest procedure would therefore not produce correction of the deformity as the child grows. In these patients the main objective is to stabilize the deformity by creating a solid spinal fusion which stops the unbalanced growth at the site of the anomaly (Winter & Moe, 1982). It is usual to proceed first with a posterior spinal fusion over the anomalous segment, extending to one vertebra above and below. However, this may not be sufficient by itself, and even a solid posterior fusion may bend in the presence of continued unbalanced anterior growth occurring in the anomalous vertebral bodies. In these circumstances the patient requires a supplementary anterior spinal fusion to prevent further progression. It is often better to perform a primary combined anterior and posterior spinal fusion if there is very severe growth imbalance such as produced by a unilateral unsegmented bar with contralateral hemivertebrae.

A Milwaukee brace may be necessary after either a convex growth arrest or posterior fusion *in situ* if such surgery has been carried out only at the apex of a long curve in which there are normal unfused vertebrae above and below the fused segment. The brace will help to control this unfused part of the curve until the child is old enough to have the posterior fusion extended to the upper and lower limits of the scoliosis and also possibly further corrected by means of instrumentation.

Primary subcutaneous Harrington instrumentation of the whole curve, carried out at the time of either a convex growth arrest or a localized posterior fusion, will also stabilize the whole of the deformity and allow extension of the posterior fusion to be postponed until the child is older (Bradford, 1982). The stunting effect of such an extension of the fusion is much less if it can be postponed until after the age of 10 years.

It has been argued that an early spinal fusion will stunt the growth of the spine, but this is of no relevance in congenital scoliosis because growth in the abnormal segment is not contributing to vertical height and is only causing the spine to curve to the side. There is no perfect treatment for these patients, and often the best that can be achieved is a short relatively straight fused spine rather than an unfused crooked spine which may be even shorter.

Correction of deformity and posterior spinal fusion

This is the usual surgical procedure for an older child with a moderately severe curve which is still relatively flexible. The deformity is corrected either at the time of the posterior spine fusion by spinal instrumentation, or after the surgery by the application of a Risser jacket. The main objective is to achieve trunk balance rather than excessive correction of the curve, which may be dangerous.

A preoperative myelogram is essential in all such patients before attempting correction, especially when using intraoperative instrumentation. This will reveal the presence of any intraspinal anomaly such as a diastematomyelia which may be tethering the cord, and must be removed, otherwise the patient could become paralysed when a distraction force is applied to correct the deformity. It is usually best to remove the intraspinal anomaly at a separate neurosurgical procedure approximately six weeks before the attempted correction of the deformity and posterior spinal fusion.

The posterior fusion is performed not just at the site of the anomalous vertebrae but throughout the length of the deformity from the upper to the lower neutral vertebrae. Care should be taken at the time of surgery to recognize any congenital bony defects in the laminae and so avoid accidental trauma to the spinal cord. In order to obtain a solid stable fusion it is necessary to perform a wide bilateral subperiosteal dissection of the muscles out to the tips of the transverse processes, followed by excision of the facet joints, decortication of all the posterior bony structures and the application of a wide thick layer of iliac crest bone grafts to all the fusion area. Homologous bone from the bone bank is used in those children who do not have sufficient bone in their iliac crests to provide graft material.

The safest method of correcting the deformity is by applying a Risser localizer jacket seven to 10 days after the posterior spine fusion. The patient is awake and the jacket is applied while the spine is distracted on a plaster table. Using this technique there is negligible risk of neurological complications but it has the disadvantage of producing relatively little correction and also the patient having to wear a cumbersome jacket extending from the neck to the pelvis for nine months, until the fusion is solid. This method is usually applied only to young children whose bones are too small or underdeveloped to allow the effective application of internal fixation, and also to patients with cervicothoracic curves where it is hazardous to insert a spine hook above C7 because of the weakness of the laminae and the danger of damaging the vertebral artery.

The intraoperative use of Harrington instrumentation to correct a congenital scoliosis at the time of the posterior spinal fusion is a much more controversial procedure (Figs 13.15 & 13.16). This technique has the advantage of achieving moderately better correction, as well as reducing the incidence of pseudarthrosis when compared with a posterior spinal fusion in a Risser jacket alone (Hall *et al.*, 1981; Winter *et al.*, 1984). However, it has a greater risk of producing neurological complications due to the effect of distraction on the spinal cord while the patient is anaesthetized or soon thereafter. Of all types of scoliosis, the congenital variety carries the highest risk of intraoperative neurological complications, and it has been suggested that, in this type of curvature, Harrington instrumentation should be used only as an internal strut to support the spine and aid the development of a solid fusion (MacEwen *et al.*, 1975). This technique without distraction should certainly be used if there is any suspicion of an intraspinal anomaly, even if it has been removed prior to the surgery. However, despite the risks Harrington instrumentation is frequently used to correct a congenital scoliosis in patients who have no evidence of

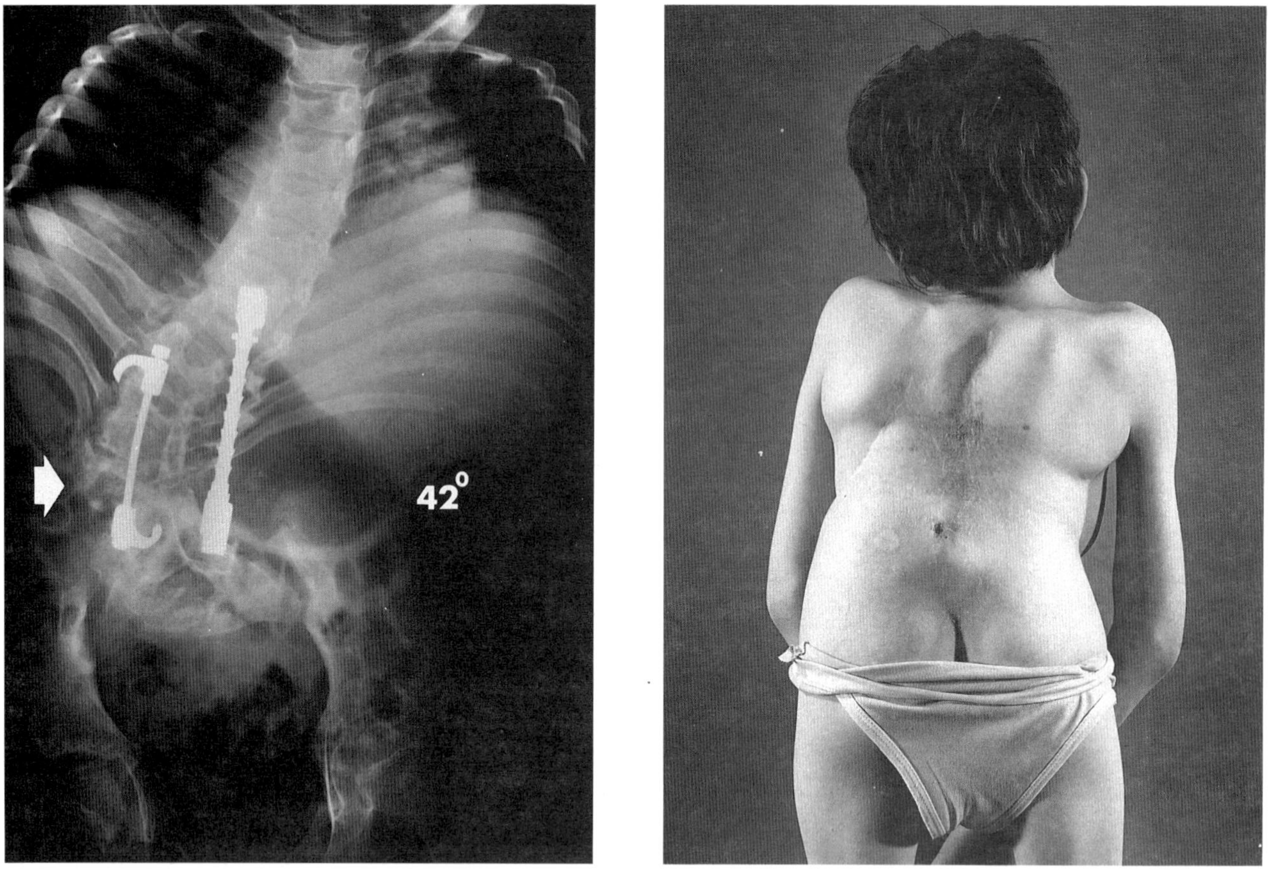

Fig. 13.18 Following an anterior and posterior wedge osteotomy of the spine in the midlumbar region, and correction with Harrington instrumentation, the scoliosis corrected to 42°, the pelvis was level and the upper body displacement was corrected.

an intraspinal anomaly provided specific measures are taken during the surgery to detect the possible development of neurological complications. Unfortunately, these measures are not completely reliable. Spinal cord monitoring using evoked potentials monitors only the function of the posterior spinal columns, and is sometimes difficult to interpret. The 'wake-up test' during surgery can be used immediately following distraction of the spine, but only monitors the neurological status at this time and it is possible for neurological abnormalities to develop later (Letts & Hollenberg, 1977; Hall *et al.*, 1978). If there is any suspicion that a neurological abnormality may have developed during surgery the instrumentation should be removed immediately.

The technique of spinal fusion following Harrington instrumentation is the same as discussed earlier, but postoperatively the patient need only wear an under-arm jacket, which is much more acceptable than a Risser jacket.

Other forms of spinal instrumentation such as the Cotrel–Dubousset system or Luque instrumentation are even more controversial in their application to congenital scoliosis. The anomalous posterior elements at the apex of the curve make it difficult to apply either of these types of instrumentation and the rigidity of the curve prevents significant derotation or correction. It may also be dangerous to pass wires or hooks into the spinal canal at the apex of the curve where it may be congenitally narrowed or contain an abnormal cord.

Anterior and posterior spinal osteotomy, correction and fusion

This is a major salvage procedure which theoretically should never be necessary, and is indicative of a failure to apply the basic principles of early diagnosis, anticipation and prevention. Patients requiring a spinal osteotomy would all have been better treated at a much earlier stage, either by a convex growth arrest or by a posterior spinal fusion with or without instrumentation.

The indication for a spinal osteotomy is a severe rigid deformity with either fixed pelvic obliquity or marked decompensation of the upper trunk relative to the pelvis (Figs 13.17 & 13.18). These deformities are usually caused by a unilateral unsegmented bar with or without hemivertebra, and cannot be satisfactorily corrected by posterior surgery alone.

The object of surgery is to balance the spine so that the head is directly above a level pelvis. The only safe way to correct such a rigid deformity without incurring the danger of neurological complications is to shorten the spinal column and so relax the neural structures as well as straightening the spine (Leatherman & Dickson, 1979). This requires a two-stage procedure in which the spine is osteotomized both anteriorly and posteriorly (Figs 13.17 & 13.18).

The first stage is an anterior approach to the spine via a thoracotomy or a thoraco-abdominal retroperitoneal exposure, depending on the site of the apex of the curve. This allows an anterior excision of the discs and their associated endplates over the whole extent of the curve followed by multiple osteotomies of the unsegmented bar on the concavity. Simply dividing the unsegmented bar will not allow the spine to grow straight, because there is no growth potential on that side of the spine. It may also be necessary to resect the vertebral body at the apex of the curve as a wedge osteotomy with its base on the convexity and tapering towards the concavity. However, it is not possible to close the wedge at this stage because the posterior bony structures are still intact and there is therefore no point in applying corrective Dwyer or Zeilke instrumentation.

The second stage is performed approximately 10–14 days later. The spine is approached posteriorly and the whole of the scoliosis exposed subperiosteally. The area of the anterior wedge resection is identified and the osteotomy completed by removing the posterior elements including the pedicle and transverse process on the convex side. The unsegmented bar may also be osteotomized at a number of levels on the concavity. The wedge osteotomy is then closed by means of a Harrington compression rod, and hooks applied to the convex side of the spine. This shortens the vertebral column and so relaxes the spinal cord, decreasing the risk of neurological complications. The best site for an osteotomy is in the lumbar region, where it is easier to close the wedge because there is no interference from the rib cage and the cauda equina is less vulnerable to damage. Additional stability and correction is usually obtained by inserting a Harrington distraction rod to act as a strut on the concave side of the scoliosis. A posterior fusion is then performed over the entire scoliosis and not just at the site of the osteotomy. Postoperatively the patient is mobilized in an under-arm plaster jacket, which is maintained until the spine is solidly fused at approximately nine months.

Excision of a hemivertebra

This procedure is basically a wedge osteotomy of the spine which, when closed, produces correction of the deformity. Although this is an attractive technique it has a relatively limited application. The majority of hemivertebrae do not unbalance the spine, and are therefore more simply treated by an anterior and posterior convex growth arrest, which is a less risky procedure. The main indication for excising a hemivertebra is when it occurs at the lumbosacral junction, because this unbalances the spine and causes tilting of the trunk which is corrected when the osteotomy is closed (Slabaugh *et al.*, 1980).

The hemivertebra is excised in two stages, which may or may not be carried out under the same anaesthetic. The spine is first approached anteriorly and the body of the hemivertebra is removed along with the adjacent discs and the anterior part of the pedicle. In the second stage the spine is exposed posteriorly and the posterior elements of the hemivertebra are removed along with the transverse process and posterior part of the pedicle. The osteotomy is then closed by applying Harrington compression instrumentation to the convexity of the curve above and below the excised hemivertebra. Care must be taken not to compress the L5 nerve root as the osteotomy is closed. In small children it is difficult to apply instrumentation, and the osteotomy is best closed by applying a hinged body cast incorporating a hip spica.

Congenital kyphosis

The prognosis for an untreated congenital kyphosis is usually poor, and surgery is nearly always indicated. The type of surgery depends on the age of the patient, the size of the curve and the type of congenital anomaly (Winter *et al.*, 1973, 1985; Mayfield *et al.*, 1980).

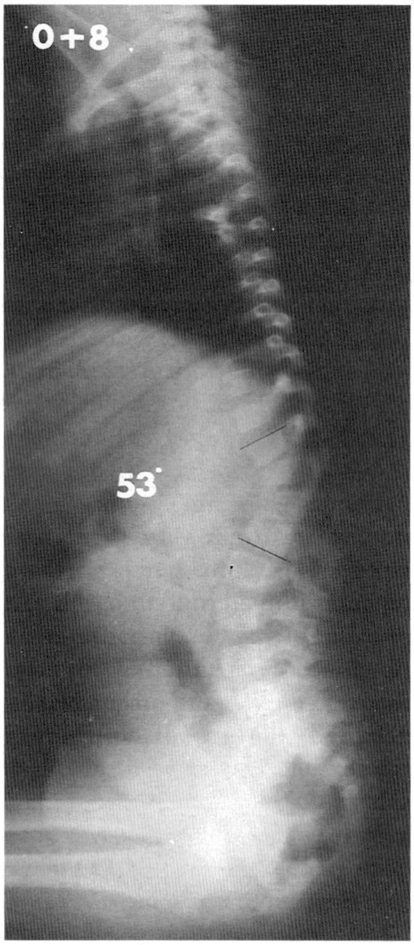

Fig. 13.19 A girl aged eight months with a 53° thoracolumbar kyphosis due to an anterior failure of formation of two vertebrae at the twelfth thoracic and first lumbar levels.

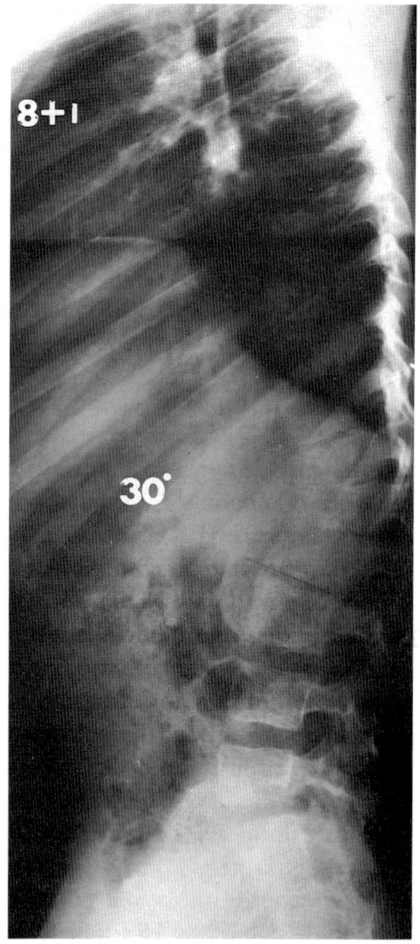

Fig. 13.20 Following a prophylactic localized posterior fusion from the eleventh thoracic vertebra to the second lumbar vertebra the kyphosis gradually corrected due to continued anterior growth, and by eight years one month it measured 30°.

Prophylactic posterior fusion (posterior epiphyseodesis)

This is the optimum treatment for a congenital kyphosis and is indicated in young children under the age of five years with a progressive kyphosis less than 50°. The younger the child, and the smaller the kyphosis, the more successful the result.

A posterior fusion is performed over the anomalous segments at the apex of the curve and extended to one normal vertebra above and below this level. It is important to produce a thick fusion mass which is strong enough to stabilize the spine, and homologous bone grafts are usually necessary as there is insufficient bone graft material in the iliac crests of these small children.

A successful fusion will tether the spinal growth posteriorly, and if the kyphosis is due to a posterior or posterolateral hemivertebra there may be some continuing growth anteriorly, resulting in a gradual correction of the deformity over a number of years (Figs 13.19 & 13.20) (Winter & Moe, 1982). In the presence of an anterior unsegmented bar there is no anterior growth potential, and the posterior fusion will only prevent deterioration of the kyphosis, although further anterior growth in the posteriorly fused normal segments above and below the bar may improve the cosmetic appearance due to the development of small compensatory lordotic curves. After the surgery the child is treated for six months in a Risser jacket for thoracic curves, and in an under-arm jacket for thoracolumbar curves.

The development of a pseudarthrosis is not uncommon because the posterior grafts are under a distraction force, and it has been suggested that the fusion should be explored after six months to repair any defects and strengthen the fusion by the addition of further bone graft material. Following this a brace is worn for six months to allow the fusion mass to mature.

Posterior spinal fusion with instrumentation

This procedure is indicated for the older child or adolescent whose kyphosis is still less than 60°. In these circumstances it is necessary to extend the posterior fusion over the full length of the deformity, and not just over the anomalous vertebrae. It is also usual to attempt to correct the deformity by some form of instrumentation, and this has the additional advantage of lowering the incidence of pseudarthrosis. Harrington compression instrumentation or Luque-type segmental instrumentation is used if the deformity is mainly a kyphosis. However, if there is a kyphoscoliosis the deformity is usually corrected by means of a bent Harrington distraction rod on the concavity combined with compression instrumentation on the convexity of the curve. Postoperatively a spinal jacket is worn for a period of nine months. If a pseudarthrosis should develop it is repaired posteriorly and reinforced by a supplementary anterior spinal fusion.

Anterior and posterior spinal correction and fusion

This is the procedure of choice for patients whose kyphosis is greater than 60°, especially those with a severe rigid unacceptable deformity (Montgomery & Hall, 1982; Winter *et al.*, 1985). In this situation a much greater degree of correction is required, and also a very strong fusion to prevent further deterioration as a result of the large bending force. These objectives can be achieved only by a combination of both anterior and posterior surgery, for several reasons. A posterior fusion alone is very likely to develop a pseudarthrosis because in this severity of curve the bone grafts are under a significant distracting force. With an anterior fusion the bone grafts are under a compression force, and are therefore much more likely to heal. However, an anterior fusion alone would not be sufficient, because it would not prevent increasing deformity due to continued growth in the posterior elements. The most successful results are from a combined anterior and posterior fusion which produces a very strong stable fusion and prevents deterioration. In addition the two-stage procedure allows a release of the spine both anteriorly and posteriorly, and a much greater degree of correction.

The surgery is carried out in two stages. Firstly, the spine is approached anteriorly through either a thoracotomy or a thoraco-abdominal retroperitoneal approach. If there is a kyphoscoliosis it is best to approach it on the convexity of the scoliosis. The spine is released anteriorly by a radical excision of all the intervertebral discs and their associated end-plates, over as wide an area as possible. If there is an anterior unsegmented bar, correction cannot take place until this is osteotomized at two or more levels. The kyphosis is then corrected either manually by pressure over the apex or by the insertion of an anterior distraction device which is usually removed once the bone grafts are *in situ*. The entire length of the kyphos is strutted anteriorly either by a fibular graft or multiple rib grafts. These grafts are placed as far anteriorly as possible, and surrounded by iliac bone grafts extending back to the decorticated vertebral bodies and packed into the excised disc spaces. A free strut graft takes up to two years to incorporate fully, and may fracture during this period of revascularization and healing (Bradford *et al.*, 1982). However, a vascularized rib graft on a pedicle containing the intercostal vessels heals much more rapidly and becomes stronger as it incorporates (Rose *et al.*, 1975; Bradford & Youssef, 1986).

The second stage of the surgery takes place two weeks later, when the correction is improved and maintained by posterior instrumentation and fusion as discussed earlier (Figs 13.21 & 13.22). It is necessary to posteriorly fuse the entire length of the deformity to upper and lower levels which are as close as possible to the line of gravity as seen on the lateral X-ray.

Some surgeons apply halofemoral traction between the two stages of the surgery, but this can be dangerous, especially if the curve is rigid, because the spinal cord is pulled against the apex of the kyphosis and can result in neurological complications.

Postoperatively a spinal jacket is applied and maintained for a period of nine months until the fusion is solid.

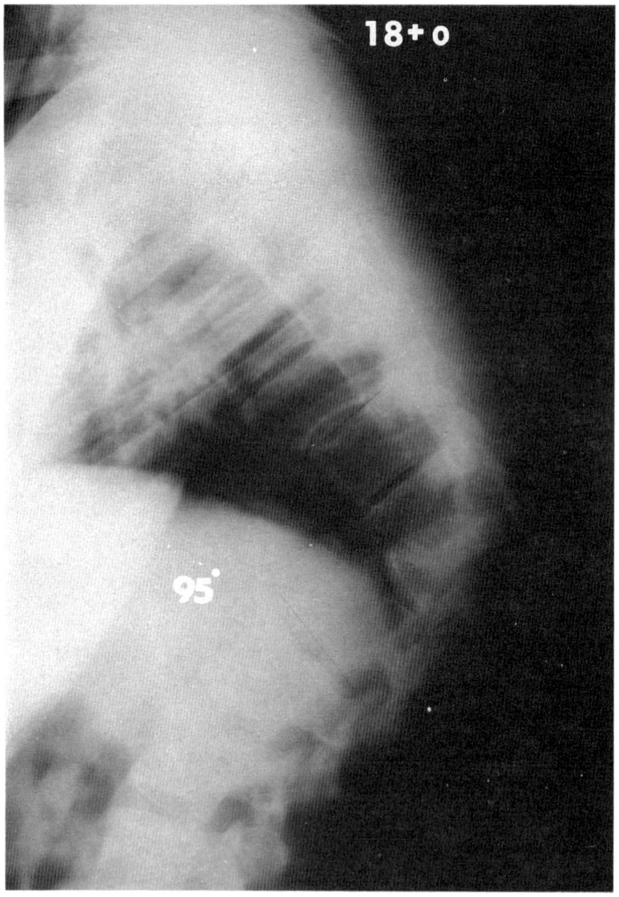

Fig. 13.21 A boy aged 18 years with a 95° rigid thoracolumbar kyphosis due to a posterior hemivertebra at the eleventh and twelfth thoracic levels.

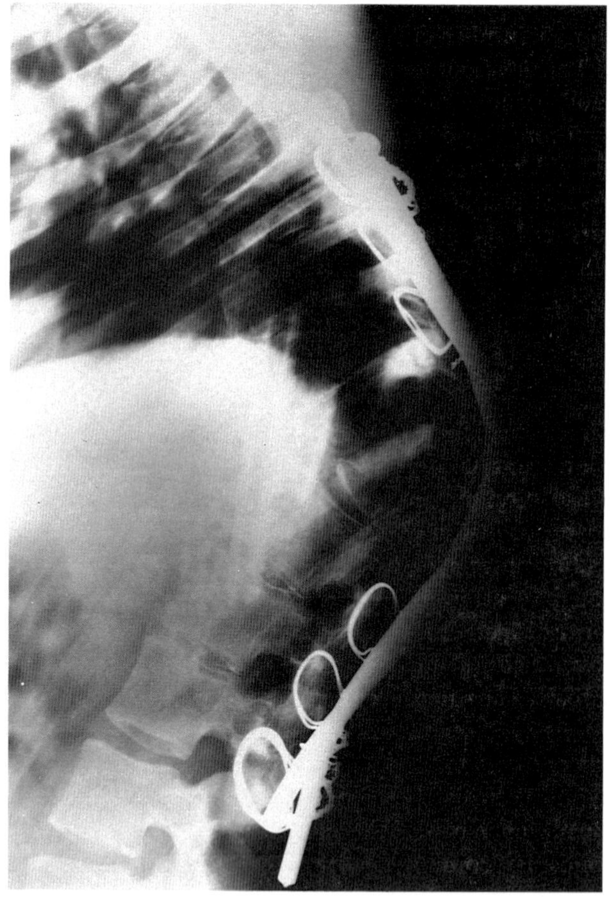

Fig. 13.22 The kyphosis was corrected by a two-stage procedure. The first stage was a transthoracic retroperitoneal spinal release by multiple disc excisions followed by an anterior strut fusion using a combination of fibular and rib strut grafts. The second stage was performed 10 days later and was a posterior spinal fusion from the seventh thoracic vertebra to the fourth lumbar vertebra, with further corrections by means of Luque rods and segmented sublaminar wiring.

Neurological complications

Of all types of spinal deformity, a congenital kyphosis is the most common cause of neurological complication and paralysis (Lonstein *et al.*, 1980). However, this can easily be prevented if the kyphosis is recognized at an early stage and fused to prevent deterioration. Laminectomy is absolutely contra-indicated in these circumstances and is of no value; this is because the neural compression is anterior to the spinal cord at the apex of the kyphosis and this cannot be safely decompressed through a posterior approach. In addition, a laminectomy removes the posterior stabilizing structures and allows the kyphosis to deteriorate even more rapidly, resulting in an increasing neurological deficit. Traction is also dangerous because it lengthens the vertebral column by correcting the relatively mobile compensatory curves above and below the rigid kyphosis, which remains unchanged. This results in the spinal cord being pulled against the apex of the kyphosis and further neurological loss.

A myelogram and, if available, magnetic resonance imaging, is necessary to exclude tethering of the spinal cord, and also to identify the precise site of the neural compression. If the spinal cord compression is mild and of relatively early onset, a period of two to four weeks bed rest may often aid neurological recovery before surgery is performed.

The treatment of neurological complications in a

patient with a congenital kyphosis requires both anterior decompression of the neural structures and stabilization of the kyphosis to prevent further deterioration. The type of surgery depends on the severity of the neurological deficit. If there is very early spinal cord compression resulting in mild spasticity it is possible to decompress the neural structures by correcting the kyphosis by anterior and posterior surgery without exposing the spinal cord. However, if the paralysis is more severe it is necessary to carry out direct anterior decompression by removing the posterior half of the apical vertebrae and allowing the spinal cord to move forward. If there is a kyphoscoliosis it may also be necessary to carry out further decompression posteriorly by removing the pedicle on the concavity at the apex of the curve. Following any of these procedures it is always necessary to perform an extensive posterior spinal fusion with possible further correction by means of instrumentation.

If the neurological loss has been present for more than a year it is very unlikely that any surgery will aid recovery, but it can prevent further neurological deterioration.

CONCLUSION

A congenital spine deformity, whether it be a scoliosis or a kyphosis, is a potentially serious condition. In order to prevent the development of severe deformity and possibly even more serious neurological complications it is necessary to:

1 make an early diagnosis while the curve is still small;

2 anticipate the likely prognosis based on the amount of spinal growth remaining taken in conjunction with the type and site of vertebral anomaly and the degree of growth imbalance it produces;

3 prevent deterioration of the deformity, because it is easier to prevent than to correct a severe rigid deformity. This often necessitates prophylactic surgery at an early age.

REFERENCES

Andrew, T. & Piggott, H. (1985) Growth arrest for progressive scoliosis: combined anterior and posterior fusion of the convexity. *J. Bone Jt. Surg.*, **67B**, 193–197.

Bick, E.M. & Copel, J.W. (1950) Longitudinal growth of the human vertebra: a contribution to human osteogeny. *J. Bone Jt. Surg.*, **32A**, 803–814.

Bradford, D.S. (1982) Partial epiphyseal arrest and supplemental fixation for progressive correction of congenital spine deformity. *J. Bone Jt. Surg.*, **64A**, 610–614.

Bradford, D.S., Ganjavian, S., Antonious, D., Winter, R.B., Longstein, J.C. & Moe, J.H. (1982) Anterior strut grafting for the treatment of kyphosis; review of experience in 48 patients. *J. Bone Jt. Surg.*, **64A**, 680–690.

Bradford, D.S. & Youssef, H.D. (1986) Vascularised rib grafts for stabilisation of kyphosis. *J. Bone Jt. Surg.*, **68B**, 357–361.

Goldberg, C., Fenton, G. & Blacke, N.S. (1984) Diastematomyelia: a critical review of the natural history and treatment. *Spine*, **9**, 367–372.

Hall, J.E., Herndon, W.A. & Levine, C.R. (1981) Surgical treatment of congenital scoliosis with or without Harrington instrumentation. *J. Bone Jt. Surg.*, **63A**, 608–619.

Hall, J.E., Levine, C.R. & Sudhir, K.G. (1978) Intraoperative awakening to monitor spinal cord function during Harrington instrumentation and spine fusion. *J. Bone Jt. Surg.*, **60A**, 533–536.

Hensinger, R., Lang, J.E. & MacEwen, G.D. (1974) Klippel–Feil syndrome; a constellation of associated anomalies. *J. Bone Jt. Surg.*, **56A**, 1246–1253.

Hood, R.W., Riseborough, E., Hehme, A., Micheli, L.J., Stand, R.D. & Neuhauser, E.B.D. (1980) Diastematomyelia and structural spinal deformities. *J. Bone Jt. Surg.*, **62A**, 520–528.

James, C.C.M. & Lassman, L.P. (1970) Diastematomyelia and the tight filum terminale. *J. Neurol. Sci.*, **10**, 193–196.

Leatherman, K.D. & Dickson, R.A. (1979) Two-stage corrective surgery for congenital deformities of the spine. *J. Bone Jt. Surg.*, **61B**, 324–328.

Letts, R.M. & Hollenberg, C. (1977) Delayed paresis following spinal fusion with Harrington instrumentation. *Clin. Orthop.*, **125**, 45–48.

Lonstein, J.E., Winter, R., Moe, J. (1980) Neurologic deficits secondary to spinal deformity: a review of the literature and report of 43 cases. *Spine*, **5**, 331–355.

MacEwen, G.D., Bunnell, W.P. & Sriram, K. (1975) Acute neurological complications in the treatment of scoliosis, a report of the Scoliosis Research Society. *J. Bone Jt. Surg.*, **57A**, 404–408.

MacEwen, G.D., Winter, R.B. & Hardy, J.H. (1972) Evaluation of kidney anomalies in congenital scoliosis. *J. Bone Jt. Surg.*, **54A**, 1341–1454.

Mayfield, J.K., Winter, R.B., Bradford, D.S. & Moe, J.H. (1980) Congenital kyphosis due to defects of anterior segmentation. *J. Bone Jt. Surg.*, **62A**, 1291–1301.

McMaster, M.J. (1984) Occult intraspinal anomalies and congenital scoliosis. *J. Bone Jt. Surg.*, **66A**, 588–601.

McMaster, M.J. & David, C.V. (1986) Hemivertebra as a cause of scoliosis. *J. Bone Jt. Surg.*, **68B**, 588–595.

McMaster, M.J. & Ohtsuka, K. (1982) The natural history of congenital scoliosis: a study of 251 patients. *J. Bone Jt. Surg.*, **64A**, 1128–1147.

Montgomery, S.P. & Hall, J.E. (1982) Congenital kyphosis. *Spine*, **7**, 360–364.

Nasca, R.J., Stelling, F.H. & Steel, H.H. (1975) Progression of congenital scoliosis due to hemivertebrae and hemivertebrae with bars. *J. Bone Jt. Surg.*, **57A**, 456–466.

Reckles, L.H., Peterson, H.A., Bianco, A.J. & Weidman, W.H. (1975) The association of scoliosis and congenital heart defects. *J. Bone Jt. Surg.*, **57A**, 449–455.

Rose, G.K., Owen, R. & Sanderson, J.M. (1975) Transposition of rib with blood supply for stabilisation of a spinal kyphosis. *J. Bone Jt. Surg.*, **57B**, 112.

Slabaugh, P., Winter, R., Lonstein, J. & Moe, J. (1980) Lumbosacral hemivertebrae. A review of 24 patients with resection in eight. *Spine*, **5**, 234–244.

Winter, R.B. (1981) Convex anterior and posterior hemiarthrodesis and epiphyseodesis in young children with progressive congenital scoliosis. *J. Pediatr. Orthop.*, **1**, 361–366.

Winter, R.B. (1983) *Congenital Deformities of the Spine.* Thiéme-Stratton, New York.

Winter, R.B. & Moe, J.H. (1982) The results of spinal arthrodesis for congenital spine deformity in patients younger than 5 years old. *J. Bone Jt. Surg.*, **64A**, 419–432.

Winter, R.B., Haven, J.J., Moe, J.H. & Lagaard, S.M. (1974) Diastematomyelia and congenital spine deformities. *J. Bone Jt. Surg.*, **56A**, 27–39.

Winter, R.B., Moe, J.H., MacEwen, G.D. & Peon-Vidales, H. (1976) The Milwaukee brace in the non-operative treatment of congenital scoliosis. *Spine*, **1**, 85–96.

Winter, R.B., Moe, J.H. & Eilers, V.E. (1968) Congenital scoliosis: a study of 234 patients treated and untreated. *J. Bone Jt. Surg.*, **50A**, 1–47.

Winter, R.B., Moe, J.H. & Lonstein, J.E. (1984) Posterior spinal arthrodesis for congenital scoliosis. *J. Bone Jt. Surg.*, **66A**, 1188–1197.

Winter, R.B., Moe, J.H. & Lonstein, J.E. (1985) The surgical treatment of congenital kyphosis: a review of 94 patients age 5 years or older with 2 years or more followup in 77 patients. *Spine*, **10**, 224–231.

Winter, R.B., Moe, J.H., MacEwen, G.D. & Peon-Vidales, H. (1976) The Milwaukee brace in the non-operative treatment of congenital scoliosis. *Spine*, **1**, 85–96.

Winter, R.B., Moe, J.H. & Wang, J.F. (1973) Congenital kyphosis. *J. Bone Jt.* Surg., **55A**, 223–256.

Wynne-Davies, R. (1975) Congenital vertebral anomalies: etiology and relationship to spina bifida cystica. *J. Med. Genet.*, **12**, 280–288.

14 · Tethered Spinal Cord and Other Intradural Abnormalities

By H.J. HOFFMAN

The condition known as tethered spinal cord consists of a group of malformations and conditions of the caudal neural tube that result in tethering or anchoring of the distal spinal cord in a lower than normal position. The lesions that result in tethering include: the thick, tight filum terminale; the attached spinal cord; diastematomyelia; lipomyelomeningocele; myelocystocele; and tethering at the site of myelomeningocele repair.

EMBRYOLOGY

The neural tube which is the basis of the central nervous system forms through the process of neurulation from Days 18 to 27 of the gestational period and by Day 22 the neural tube is fully formed. Mesoderm interposes itself between the ectoderm and the neural tube to form the skeletal and muscular structures that encase the spinal cord, with neurulation complete by Day 26.

The most distal part of the spinal cord forms through the process of cannulization from Days 28 to 48 of the gestational period. Through this process the caudal cell mass becomes cannulized and forms the terminal neural tube that eventually becomes the conus medullaris. Through a process called regression the most caudal portion of the neural tube atrophies and forms a fibrous band called the filum terminale which is initially identifiable at Day 52. The conus medullaris then ascends within the spinal canal largely through the disproportionate growth of the vertebral column relative to that of the neural tube. At 20 weeks after gestation the termination of the conus medullaris is at the level of the space between the fourth and fifth lumbar vertebrae. By 40 weeks after gestation, or at term, the conus is at L3 level and by two months postnatal age it has reached the adult L1–L2 level (Barson, 1970).

Developmental problems occurring during cannulization are largely responsible for the conditions that lead to tethering of the spinal cord. If dural schisis occurs early in the development of the caudal neural tube it causes the caudal neural tube to adhere to the overlying mesodermal tissue, and thus the formation of lipomyelomeningocele. Such patients will frequently have a terminal syrinx in their spinal cord (Fig. 14.1). Rarely they may have a very distended syrinx in the terminal spinal cord, which is termed a myelocystocele. Such patients have associated anomalies in the region including cloacal extrophy.

In patients in whom the dural closure is complete but regression has failed, the terminal spinal cord remains attached to the terminal dural sac, a condition known as attached spinal cord (Fig. 14.2). In patients with incomplete regression a thickened filum terminale develops, effectively tethering the spinal cord.

The notochord, which actively stimulates the development of the neural tube, occasionally splits over part of its length. In association with this, the spinal cord may also split over several segments. When this occurs within a single dural sac, the split spinal cord may rejoin to form a low-lying conus that remains tethered by a thickened filum to the end of the dural sac. Occasionally the split spinal cord within a single dural tube may remain split with two terminal thickened fila terminale tethering the two conuses to the end of the dural tube (Fig. 14.3).

When the split notochord stimulates the formation of two separate dural tubes encasing the split spinal cord, usually with a bony peg protruding between the two dural tubes, a true diastematomyelia is formed.

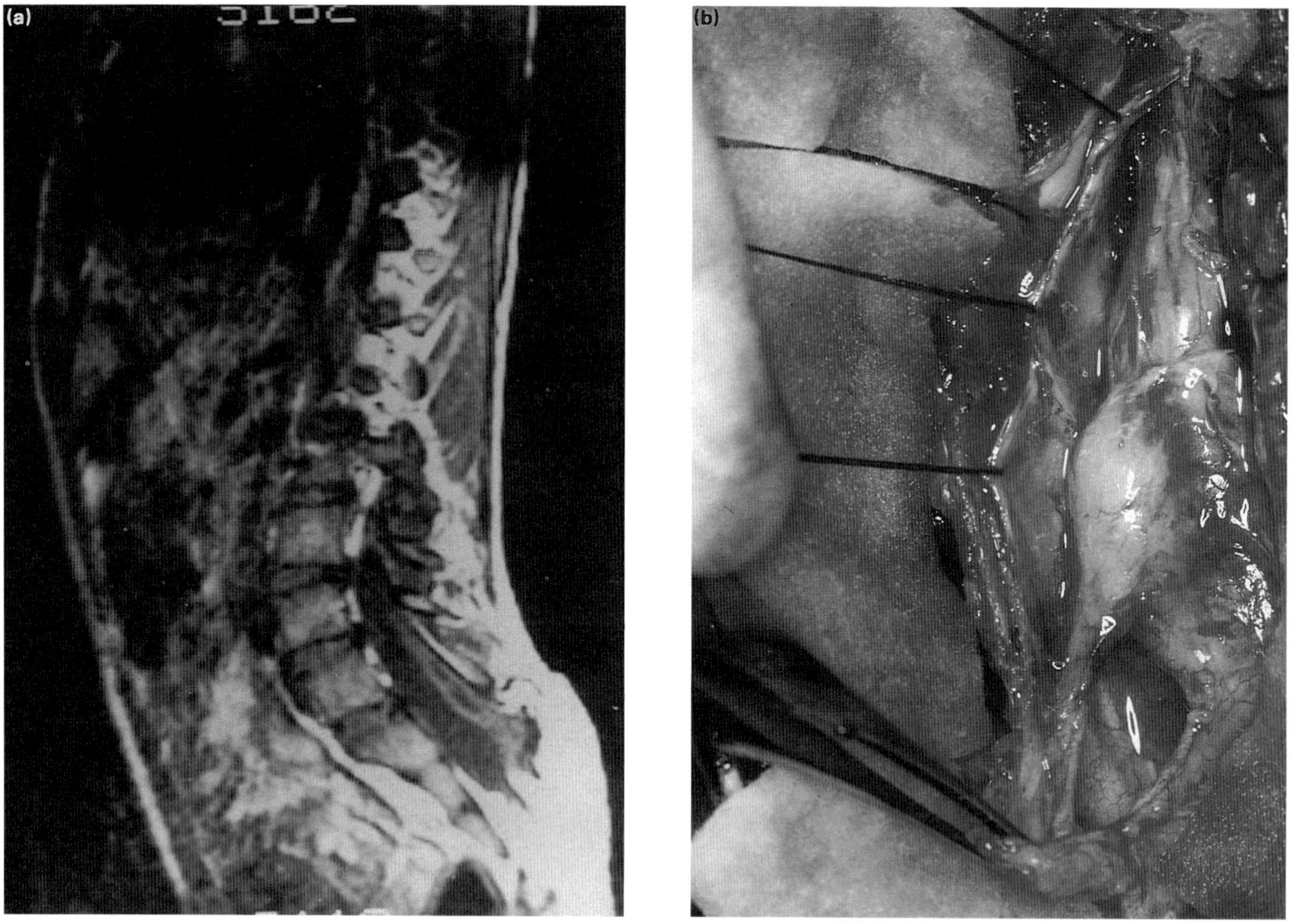

Fig. 14.1 (a) MRI scan of patient with terminal lipomyelomeningocele, showing syrinx (low density) in terminal portion of spinal cord which is adherent to the lipomatous mass (high density). (b) Operative photograph showing terminal syrinx in patient with lipomyelomeningocele.

The two dural tubes remain separate for several segments above the peg and join as a single tube just below the peg; the two spinal cords rejoin at the point where the dural tube becomes single. These patients are thus tethered at the site of the split by the dura and the bony peg, and distally by a thick filum terminale which anchors the conus to the end of the dural tube (Fig. 14.4).

Occasionally, dural schisis may be associated with a split spinal cord. In such cases each spinal cord is tethered to the overlying tissues and shows evidence of a dural defect; thus the patient has a dual lipomye lomeningocele. The split spinal cord may on occasion have dural schisis over only one half of the spinal cord with a lipomyelomeningocele involving one half of the cord, and with the other half of the cord being normally formed.

PATHOPHYSIOLOGY

All patients with a tethered spinal cord have some form of developmental anomaly that affects the caudal spinal cord and spine. They will therefore all have evidence of spina bifida occulta. The patients with an attached spinal cord have a broad attachment of their conus medullaris to the end of the dural sac. In patients with incomplete regression of the caudal neural tube the filum terminale forms, but it is short and thick and frequently infiltrated with lipoma. The conus in these patients is situated below the normal L1–L2 level. In patients with diastematomyelia and with a dorsal lipomyelomeningocele there is similarly incomplete regression producing a thickened filum which anchors the conus to the end of the dural sac. In true diastematomyelia, which James & Lass-

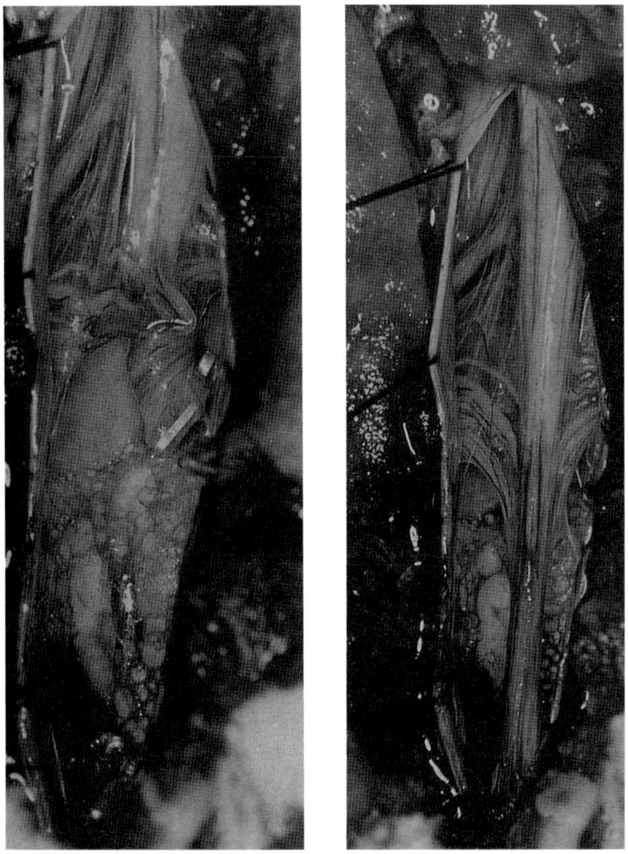

Fig. 14.2 Operative photograph showing spinal cord attached to termination of dural sac with caudal nerve roots running upwards (left). After freeing of spinal cord from end of dural sac, caudal nerve roots take a horizontal course (right). An intradural lipomatous mass is also present.

man (1981) referred to as diastematomyelia with septum, each half of the spinal cord is invested in its own dural tube. The split in the spinal cord ends at the level of the split dura so that the united spinal cord distal to the split is anchored by the split dural tube that usually surrounds the bony spike. The bony spike has a broad base of attachment to the vertebral bodies anteriorly, and broadens out again posteriorly at its attachment to the laminae. Occasionally, the spike may only be anchored anteriorly. The vertebral bodies are abnormal; the disc is usually missing and the two vertebral bodies to which the broad base of the spike is attached are malformed. The spike of bone travels caudally and dorsally and attaches to a proliferative expanse of mesodermal tissue which includes bone, cartilage and fibrous tissue. The split in the dura is relatively short; the dural sac rejoins one or two segments cephalad to the bony spike. The split in the dura and the spinal cord ends immediately caudal to the bony spike. However, the split in the spinal cord may continue for several segments above the level of the bony spike. The two halves of the spinal cord may be unequal in size with a smaller spinal cord going to a smaller leg and smaller foot (Fig. 14.5).

Although James & Lassman (1981) preferred to use the term 'diastematomyelia without septum' for patients who have a split spinal cord within a single sac, it is best to regard such patients as having a split spinal cord, and to reserve the term 'diastematomyelia' for those patients with a split dural sac encasing a split spinal cord. The spinal cords of this latter group of patients are tethered both by the split in the dural sac and by a thick filum. On the other hand, the spinal cords of patients with a single dural sac and

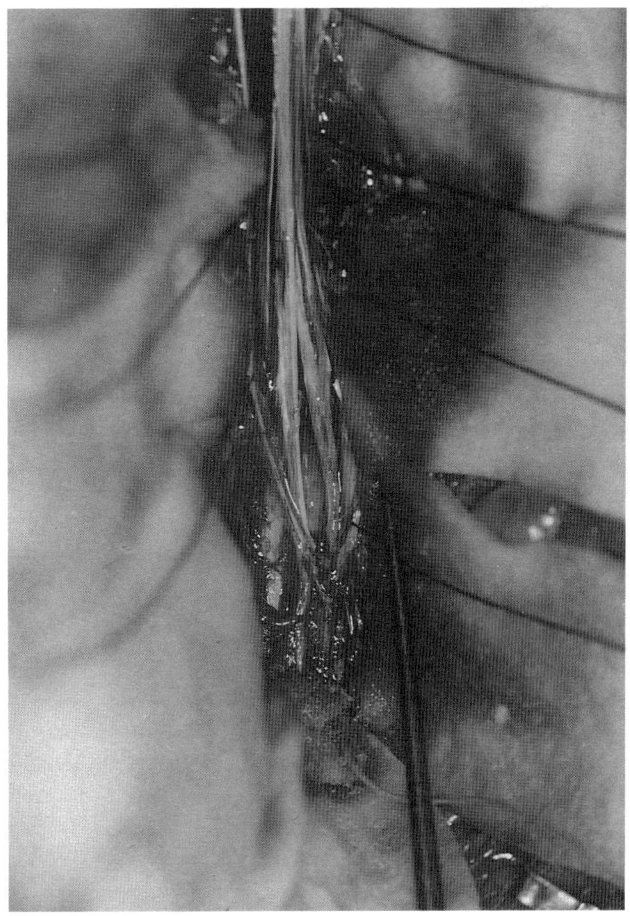

Fig. 14.3 Operative photograph showing split spinal cord ending in two separate fila terminale.

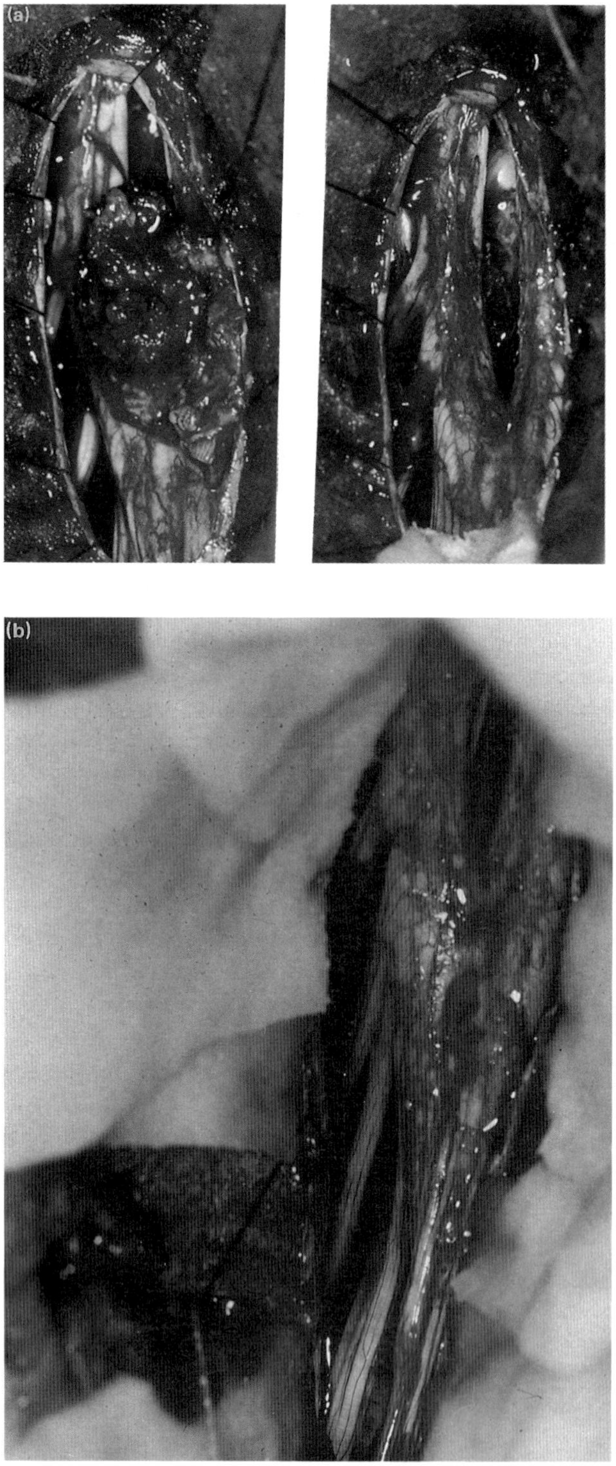

Fig. 14.4 (a) Operative photograph of diastematomyelia showing bony spike encased by dura and fat traversing split in spinal cord (left). After removal of bony spike, the split in spinal cord can be clearly seen (right). (b) Operative photograph below the split in spinal cord in patient in (a) showing thick filum tethering spinal cord.

a split spinal cord are usually tethered only by a thickened filum. This latter group of patients typically have a split in the spinal cord that rejoins to form a low-lying conus from which a single thick filum terminale extends to the bottom of the dural sac.

The lipomatous mass in patients with a lipomyelomeningocele can vary greatly in size and location. It may be small and take the form of a fatty, tail-like appendage, or it may consist of gross amounts of fat occupying most of the lumbosacral region of the back (Figs 14.6 & 14.7). Chapman (1982) divided lipomyelomeningoceles into three anatomical types: dorsal, terminal and transitional (Fig. 14.8). In patients with a dorsal lipomyelomeningocele the fat extends directly from the dorsal aspect of the spinal cord through a dural defect to the overlying skin. The conus continues distal to this lipomatous attachment and ends in a thickened filum attached to the termination of the dural sac. In patients with a terminal lipomyelomeningocele the fat extends from the end of the spinal cord through a dural defect at the end of the dural sac onto the overlying skin. The attachment is frequently asymmetric, spreading into one buttock. In those patients with a transitional lipomyelomeningocele the fat extends from the dorsal aspect and the termination of the spinal cord through a dural defect to the overlying skin.

Those patients who develop tethering after myelomeningocele repair are born with their spinal cord in its primitive neural plate form and attached to skin. In the course of repair the neural plate is freed from the skin and dura and allowed to ride freely in a newly constructed dural tube, where it floats in a bath of cerebrospinal fluid. Nevertheless, some of these children develop adhesions between the neural plate and the dural tube that anchors the spinal cord dorsally. McLone (1980) advocated reconstructing the neural tube during the repair of a myelomeningocele to avoid the possibility of tethering, but Guthkelch *et al.* (1981) felt that reconstitution of the spinal cord offered no advantages over simple replacement of the placode within the dural tube. J. Venes (personal communication) has in the past advocated utilizing silastic sheeting between the neural plate and the dural repair in order to avoid tethering, but has found this to be ineffective. Tamaki *et al.* (1988), amongst others, have reported that magnetic resonance imaging (MRI) studies have shown that all patients show tethering at the site of repair. They associated the development of delayed deficit with the additional occurrence of

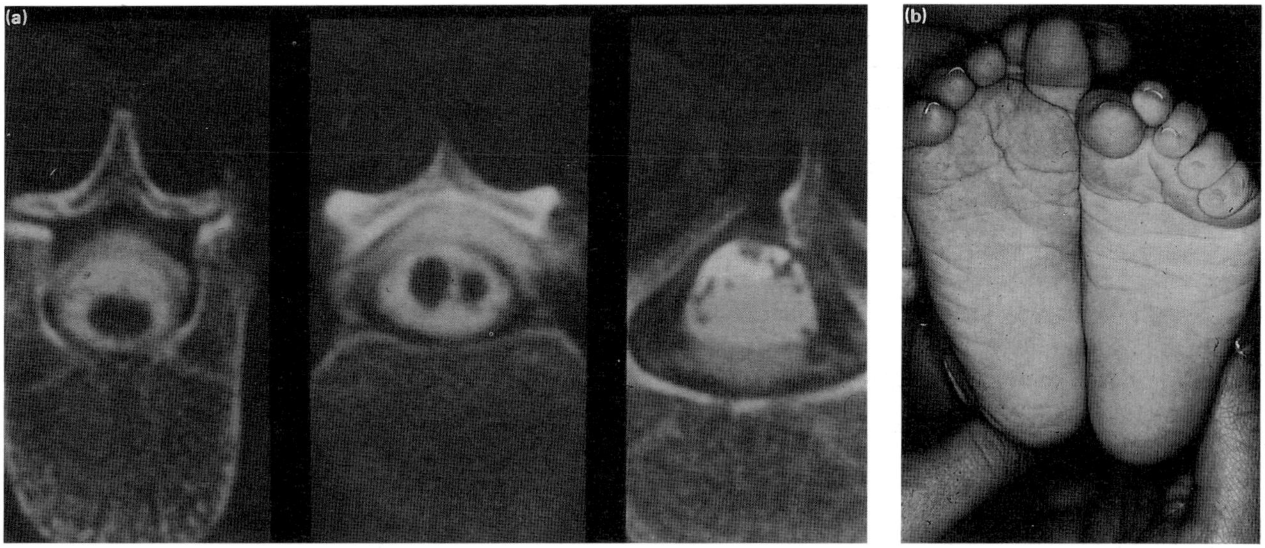

Fig. 14.5 (a) CT metrizamide myelogram of patient with split spinal cord. Note unequal sizes of split cord. (b) Note asymmetry of feet in this patient with the smaller foot being on the side of the smaller cord.

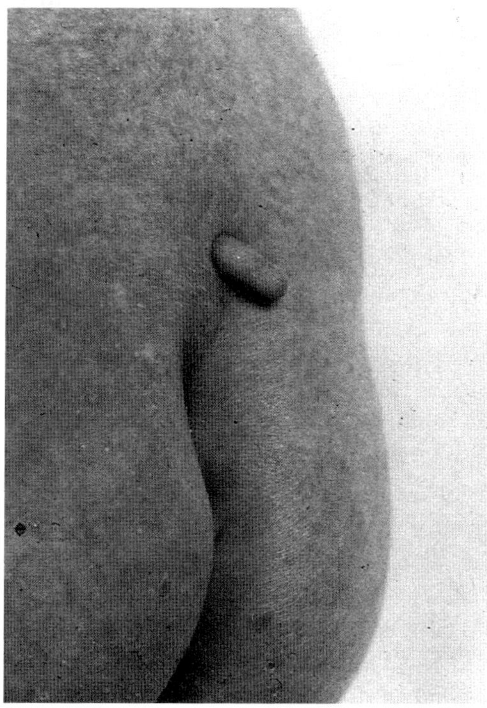

Fig. 14.6 Patient with tail-like appendage emanating from lipomyelomeningocele.

adhesions at the level of the lowest formed lamina, and that laminectomy and division of adhesions was helpful.

Each and all of the processes which have been discussed may be associated with the onset of neurological deficit either in childhood or in later life, but what mechanism actually produces such deficit is not clear.

The anatomical studies by Breig (1970) have shown that, as the normal spine flexes, the spinal cord moves towards the fourth cervical spinal level. This upward movement during flexion is not allowed in a conus medullaris that remains tethered. A sudden flexion movement of the spine in a patient with a tethered cord may produce the onset of neurological deficit but it is more commonly the cumulative effects of repetitive flexion movements in association with trauma which produces the damage. In childhood the effect of repeated flexion is exacerbated by the effects of spinal growth spurts which increase the vulnerability of the tethered cord. It should be recalled that the period of most intense postnatal growth of the spine occurs in the first two years of life when neurological damage may only show itself by the development of foot deformity or unrecognized sphincteric damage.

Yamada *et al.* (1981), using sophisticated intraoperative spectrophotometric techniques, made direct observations on spinal cord metabolism both in cats as an experimental model and in humans with a tethered cord. They showed a relative insensitivity of the intracellular cytochrome system to hypoxia which could be reverted to normal by the release of the tethering. A later study (Yamada *et al.*, 1985) showed a slight reduction in the blood flow in the

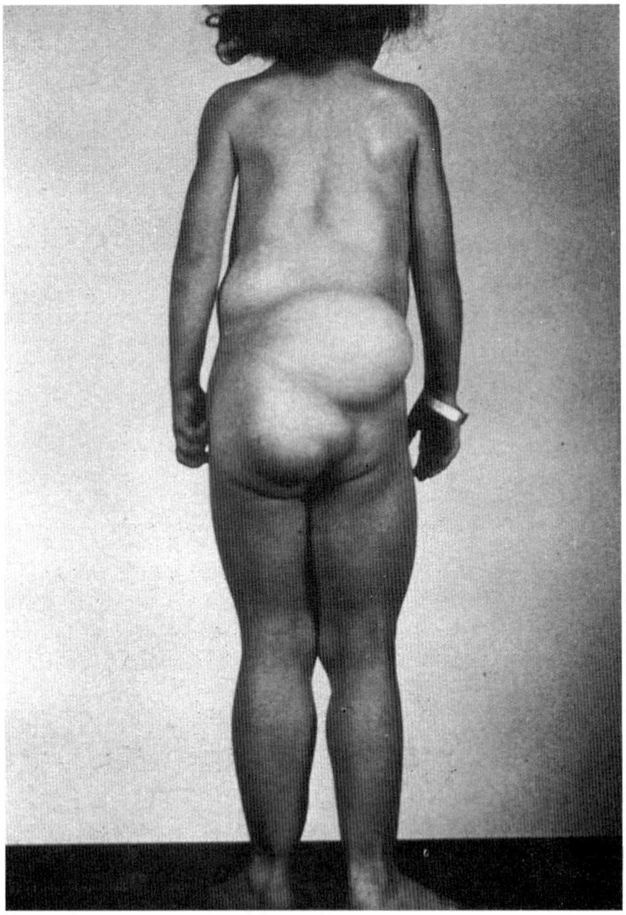

Fig. 14.7 Patient with large fatty mass of lipomyelomeningocele.

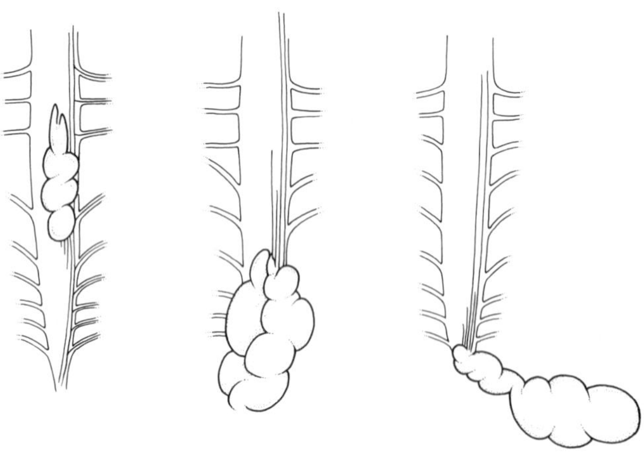

Fig. 14.8 Dorsal lipomyelomeningocele (left), transitional lipomyelomeningocele (middle), and terminal lipomyelomeningocele (right).

tethered cord but, perhaps more significant, evidence of neuronal cell membrane damage. Such damage seemed to be reparable, but they postulated that repetitive flexion might lead to permanent structural damage.

The normal filum terminale is a more elastic structure than the spinal cord (Tani *et al.*, 1987) and therefore cushions the normal cord from flexion stresses. It is likely that the pathologically thickened filum loses its elasticity, and therefore directly transmits stresses to the cord. Additionally, in other tethered states such as lipomyelomeningocele, the cord is vulnerable to direct impulses transmitted through the tethered mass.

CLINICAL FEATURES

Cutaneous manifestations are common in patients with a tethered spinal cord. About 30% of patients without dural schisis but with a thickened filum, an attached spinal cord, or a split spinal cord will have cutaneous manifestations visible in the lumbosacral region. These skin manifestations may consist of: a hairy patch, a dimple, a haemangioma, a lipoma, or an area of thin atrophic skin. Patients with lipomyelomeningoceles will always have a fatty mass visible in the lumbosacral region, which can vary from a very large expansive fatty mass, to a small lipoma, to a caudal tail-like appendage (Figs 14.6 & 14.7). Although the lipomatous mass is typically midline, it can be asymmetric to one side or even off in one buttock. Patients with true diastematomyelia will typically have a large hairy patch overlying the area of the bony spike (Fig. 14.9).

In cases with a spinal cord tethered by a tight filum, or with a spinal cord attached to the end of the dural sac, the presentation is usually that of a progressive motor or sensory deficit in the lower limbs (Hoffman *et al.*, 1976). Many will present to an orthopaedic surgeon with a foot deformity which is often progressive (Fig. 14.10), and trophic ulceration in the foot may occur due to impaired sensation (Fig. 14.11). Scoliosis is a common presenting feature in these patients, and frequently becomes apparent during spurts of growth. Twenty per cent of patients will have evidence of a neurogenic bladder at presentation, and this may be the only evidence of their tethered cord. Back pain frequently associated with sciatic pain can be one of the major presenting features in

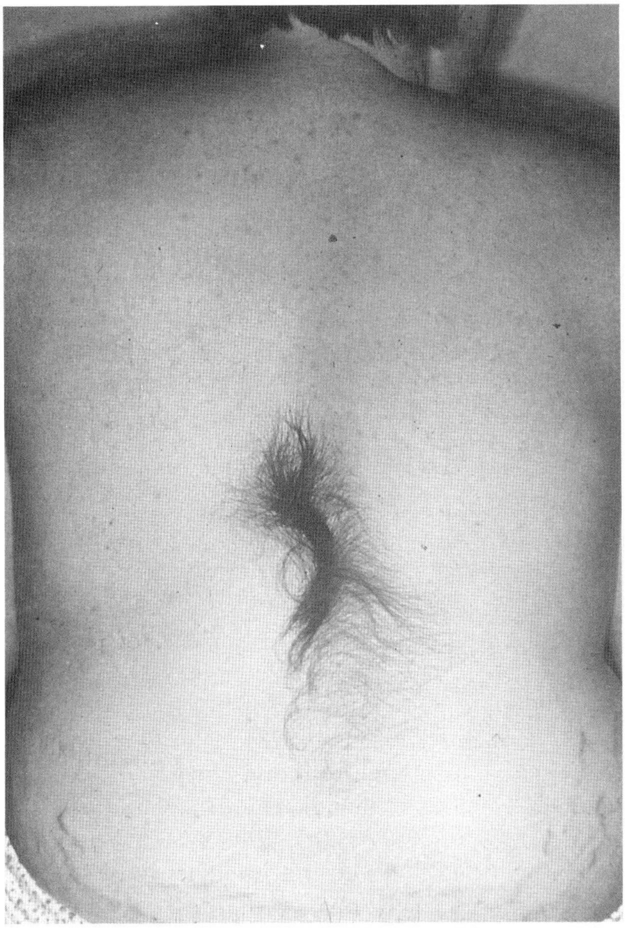

Fig. 14.9 Patient with diastematomyelia showing hairy patch overlying the area of the bone spike.

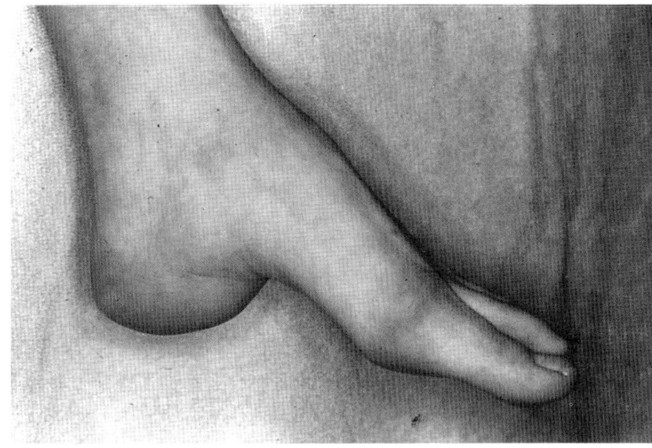

Fig. 14.10 Pes cavus deformity in a patient with tethered spinal cord.

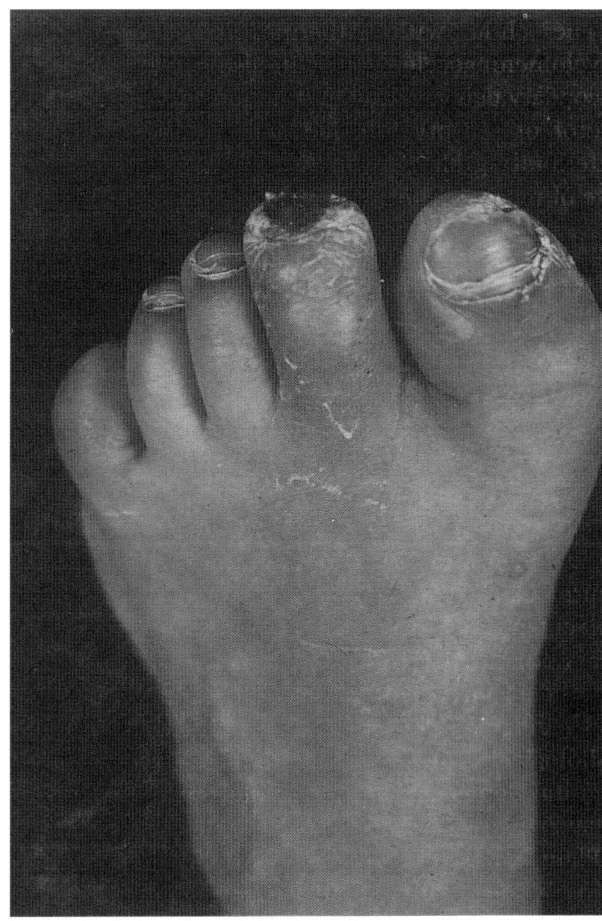

Fig. 14.11 Trophic ulceration of toes in patient with tethered spinal cord.

these children, and again may be the only presenting feature. Patients with diastematomyelia present in a similar manner with motor and/or sensory deficits in their lower limbs or with scoliosis or a neurogenic bladder. If the two halves of the split spinal cord are asymmetric one leg may be more neurologically impaired than the other and the foot or the whole leg on the side of the smaller hemichord may be reduced in size.

The majority of children born with a lipomyelomeningocele are normal neurologically at birth (Hoffman *et al.*, 1985). If these patients are left untreated they all develop progressive deficits consisting of motor and/or sensory loss in their limbs, as well as a neurogenic bladder. The cause of this progressive deterioration in function is due not only to tethering but to local trauma to the fatty mass which transmits the force to the attached conus medullaris in a water-hammer-like effect.

Patients with a myelocystocele are born with a large skin-covered mass over the sacral region which transilluminates brightly. These children usually have cloacal extrophy with the bladder on the abdominal surface, and the gonads are not properly formed. They are born with varying loss of function over the sacral nerve segments. The urologist can correct the bladder and gonadal deformity. However, these patients have a lipomyelomeningocele, with a large terminal syrinx and a dural defect, with the fat tethered to the overlying skin. With appropriate repair they can be left with a relatively minor sacral neurological deficit. If they are not appropriately repaired their deficit progresses and they become severely handicapped neurologically.

The child with tethering at the site of a myelomeningocele repair will also show evidence of secondary deterioration in function that may involve motor or sensory function and may be evident in deteriorating bladder function. Pain localized at the site of repair is common.

INVESTIGATION

All patients who present with evidence of a dysraphic state require careful and repeated documentation of their neurological status. As there is a real risk of further neurological loss, they should all be fully investigated at the time of presentation regardless of their age so that a decision regarding the necessity of prophylactic repair can be made. This is particularly so in the cases of the neonate as progression of the neurological deficit and especially of sphincteric involvement may easily pass unnoticed in the first two years of life. Also, any patient presenting with a pes cavus deformity should have the back both examined and radiographed. Any evidence, either clinically or radiologically, of dysraphism, or merely a spina bifida occulta, demands full neuroradiological assessment in such a case.

Plain X-rays of the spine will show evidence of spina bifida occulta in all patients with a tethered spinal cord, usually involving more than one level. Ultrasound helps delineate the level of the conus in the infant and will show a pulsating conus in the normal individual. MRI scanning is the investigation of choice, and will show changes such as: a low-lying spinal cord (Fig. 14.12); tethering by a lipomyelomeningocele (Fig. 14.13); or a split spinal cord in a patient with diastematomyelia (Fig. 14.14). In some cases of a thickened filum, MRI scanning may not give sufficient detail. In such cases CT metrizamide myelography is still useful in demonstrating a thickened filum terminale with a filum greater than 2 mm in diameter being pathological (Piatt & Hoffman, 1987). In patients with tethering at the site of a myelomeningocoele repair, ultrasound will demonstrate that the spinal cord is immobile and fixed dorsally at the site of repair. This can also be vividly seen with MRI (Fig. 14.15).

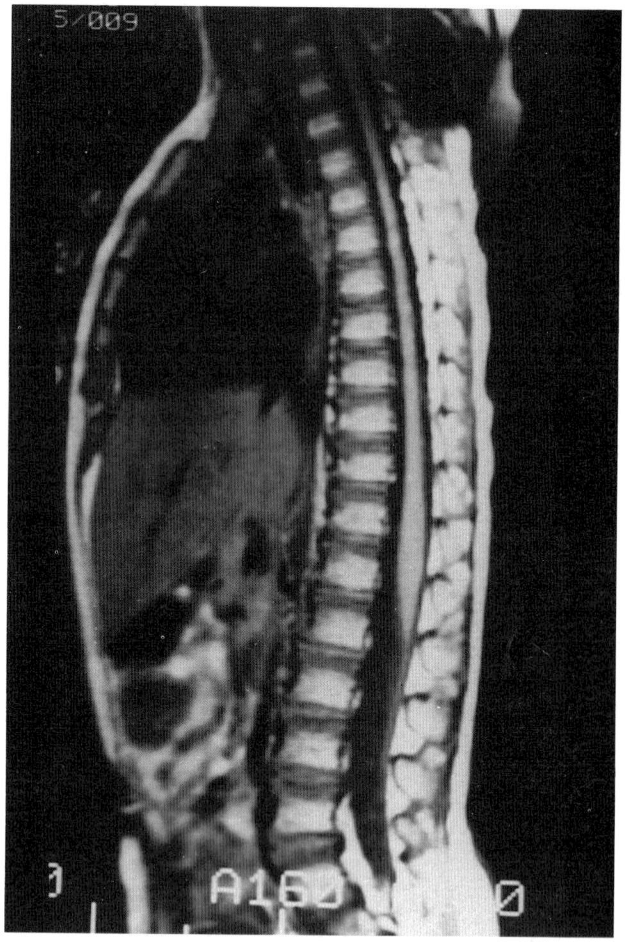

Fig. 14.12 MRI scan showing slightly low-lying spinal cord and thick filum.

Urodynamic testing is an important adjunct to the assessment of these patients both before and after therapy, because it helps identify patients with neurogenic bladders and records objective improvement after untethering.

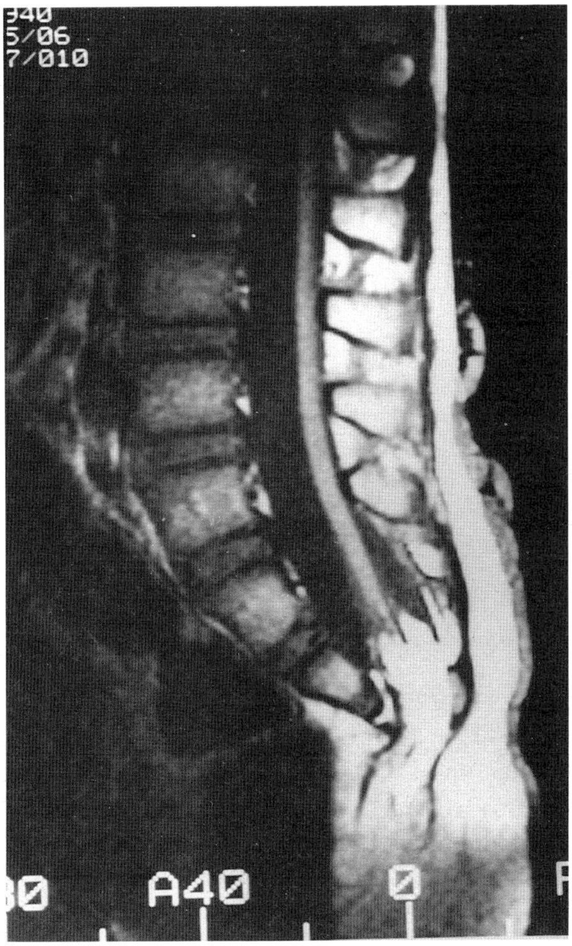

Fig. 14.13 MRI scan of patient with terminal lipomyelomeningocele showing spinal cord tethered to fat.

As in all congenital lesions, it is necessary to carefully exclude the presence of abnormalities in other systems.

TREATMENT

The necessity or otherwise for the operative release of lesions causing spinal cord tethering has been widely debated. There are two possible scenarios where surgery might be considered, namely when there is overt evidence of neurological deterioration or alternatively when the patient presents with either normal neurology or an apparently static lesion. In the case of overt deterioration there is widespread agreement that the cord should be untethered as soon as possible. In static cases, however, there has been less general agreement as to the role of surgery.

Previously, it was felt that surgery was unlikely to result in improvement but studies such as those of Anderson (1975), Hendrick *et al.* (1982), Reigel (1983), Hoffman *et al.* (1985), Pierre-Kann *et al.* (1986) and Tamaki *et al.* (1988) have shown that worthwhile improvement can occur with significant frequency. Moreover, the papers by Hendrick *et al.* and by Reigel reported very satisfactory relief of back pain following release of either a tight filum or of tethering following myelomeningocele closure.

It is now well established that patients with tethered cords carry a high risk of subsequent neurological progression. The risk is perhaps highest in myelomeningocele and least where there is simply a tethered filum. Surgical release, if performed by an experienced surgical team, has a low morbidity, and should therefore be considered in all patients with tethered cord syndrome either as a therapeutic or prophylactic procedure at the time of diagnosis. Experience also suggests that such procedures may often be technically simpler when performed at an early age prior to the development of arachnoiditic changes.

The salient points of each procedure will now be discussed.

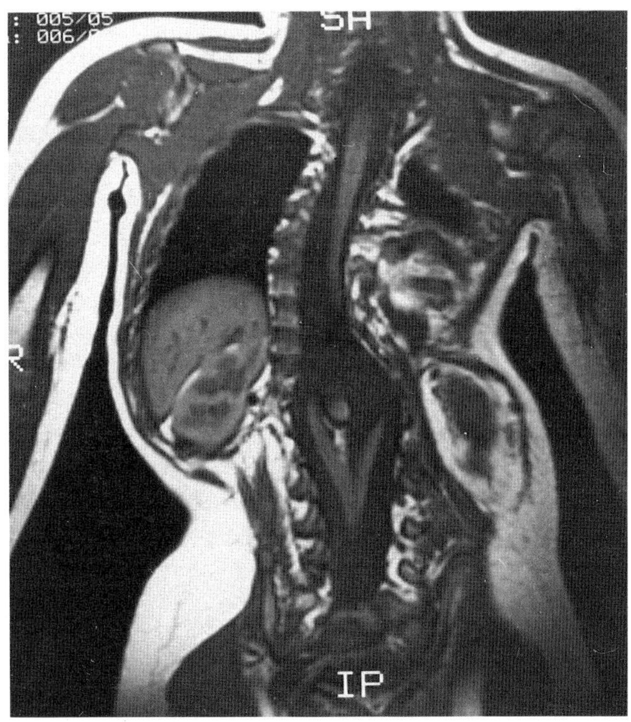

Fig. 14.14 MRI scan of patient with diastematomyelia.

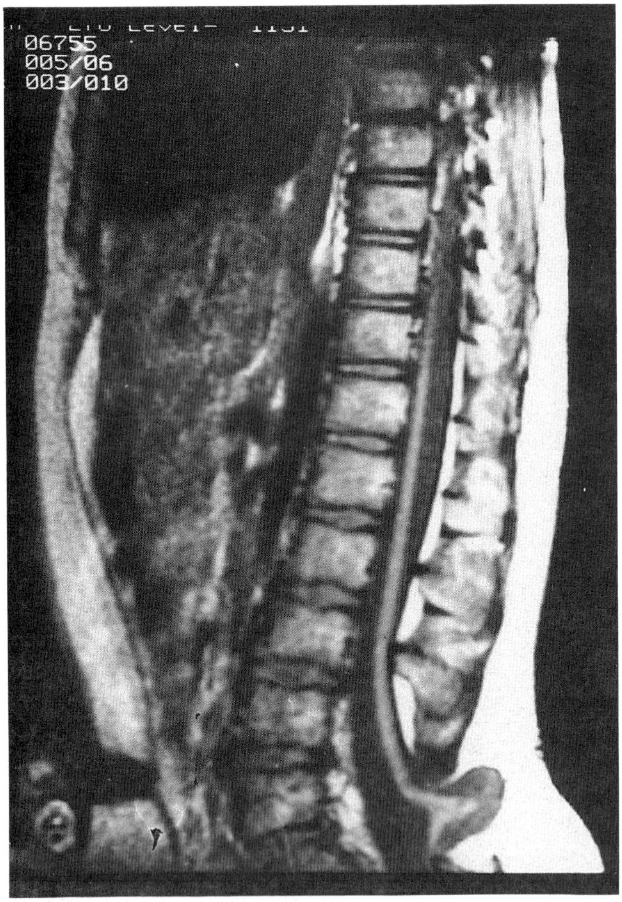

Fig. 14.15 MRI scan showing spinal cord tethered at site of myelomeningocele repair.

Thick filum terminale

Patients with a thickened filum need a single-level laminectomy, usually at the level of the fifth lumbar and first sacral vertebrae. Because the thickened filum is very different from the adjacent nerve roots due to its size, its tautness, and its profusion of blood vessels, it is rarely necessary to stimulate the filum to differentiate it from the surrounding nerve roots (Fig. 14.16). The thickened filum is divided after coagulation but the old practice of placing surgical clips on the cut ends to allow monitoring of cord ascent should be abandoned, as such clips destroy the appearance of postoperative MRI scans due to metallic artifact.

Attached spinal cord

Patients with an attached spinal cord are treated similarly to patients with a thick filum terminale. However, the laminectomy is performed over the mid-to-low sacral region. The cord is detached from the terminal dural sac and allowed to ride free. Frequently, the attached spinal cord is thinned out and stretched because of the tethering, and may mimic a thick filum terminale on neuroimaging. During surgery, however, the nerve roots can readily be seen leaving the spinal cord and ascending to reach their exit foramina (see Fig. 14.2).

Diastematomyelia

To correct diastematomyelia the surgeon makes an incision over the abnormal vertebrae extending downwards to below the level of the diastematomyelia. The laminae are removed over the normal dural sac below the diastematomyelia. The bony removal

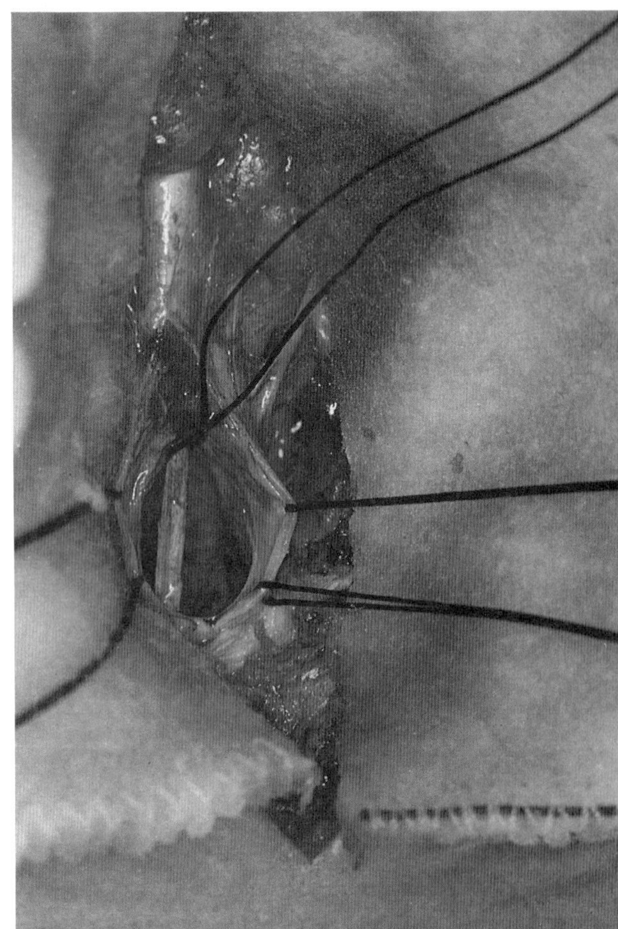

Fig. 14.16 Operative photograph showing thick, taut filum terminale.

then continues in a cephalad direction over the split dural sacs until the normal dural sac is reached. Between the split dural sacs there is usually a massive amount of bone and fat that, as it is removed, leaves a thin spike that travels in a cephalad direction between the split dural tubes and ends in a broad-based attachment to two vertebral bodies at the level of an absent disc space. The dura is now opened over the caudal single dural tube and extended in a cephalad direction over the split dural tube, exposing the split spinal cord (see Fig. 14.4). The spinal cord distal to the split is normally tight against the split in the dural tube and the bony spike. A high-speed drill is used to drill the bony spike down to the vertebra anteriorly. Typically, an arterial blood vessel in the centre of this bony spike bleeds profusely. Waxing the bone will control this bleeding. The anterior dura is then either left open or closed, if possible, with one or two sutures. The posterior dura is reconstituted, either directly or with a dural graft. Since all patients with diastematomyelia have an associated thick filum, the dural opening is continued in a caudal direction to expose the conus and the filum terminale which is then divided (see Fig. 14.4). If the diastematomyelia is not in the lumbosacral area, a separate small laminectomy at L5–S1 is necessary.

Lipomyelomeningocele

To repair a lipomyelomeningocele or a myelocystocele the surgeon makes an incision in the skin in the midline. The dissection is then carried out at the cephalad extent to the last intact lamina which is removed. This exposes the intact dural tube. The dura is then opened at this level, and the dural opening is continued down to the region of the lipomyelomeningocele where the dura is deficient. At the level of the lipomyelomeningocele there are no posterior bony elements. A grooved director is used to divide the dura laterally on either side of the lipomatous mass just at its attachment to the lipoma. If the lipomyelomeningocele is dorsal, the dural tube is intact distally so the dural opening is continued down into the normal distal dural tube. If the lipomyelomeningocele is terminal or transitional the distal dural tube will be abnormal because of dural schisis. The dural incision is then continued to the lowermost portion of the anterior dural tube.

The massive proliferation of dorsal fat can now be identified and separated from the overlying mesodermal tissues (Fig. 14.17). The fat is removed initially with scissors and gradually shaved down. A laser is an effective tool for melting and removing the fat. Complete removal of all the fat, however, may jeopardize normal conus function so that some fat is usually left.

In those patients with a dorsal lipomyelomeningocele the terminal thickened filum must also be divided to untether the spinal cord effectively. In patients with a terminal syrinx, as seen particularly in patients with a myelocystocele, the syrinx is effectively drained as the fat is removed (see Fig. 14.1). Patients with a repaired lipomyelomeningocele are always left with a large dural defect. Cadaver freeze-dried dura provides ideal material for the reconstitu-

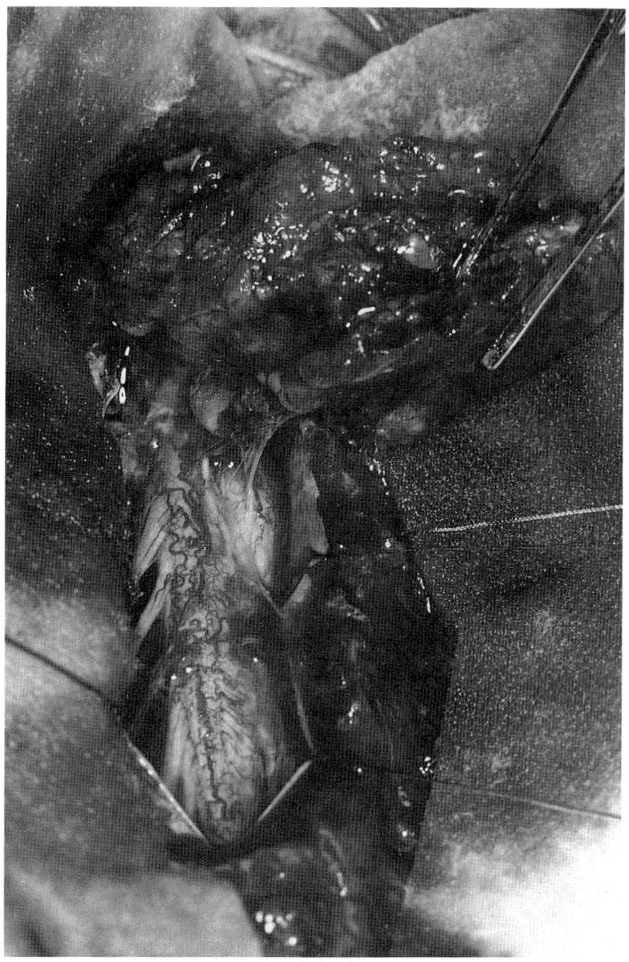

Fig. 14.17 Operative photograph of dorsal lipomyelomeningocele showing spinal cord continuing distally where it eventually ends in thick filum terminale.

tion of the dural tube which is necessary to prevent re-tethering.

Tethering at the site of myelomeningocele repair

Frequently the diagnosis of tethering at the site of repair is a diagnosis of exclusion. The child with a repaired myelomeningocele who shows evidence of secondary deterioration probably has some condition other than tethering: shunt malfunction, Chiari malformation, hydrosyringomyelia, spinal dermoid cysts, diastematomyelia, or intracranial midline cysts. Only when these conditions are excluded should tethering at the site of repair be considered as the cause of the patient's symptoms. This is particularly important since all patients with a repaired myelomeningocele have a low-lying spinal cord. Lack of movement and pulsation of the conus during ultrasound examination may confirm tethering.

The repair of tethering at the site of the myelomeningocele repair must be performed with care under magnification; the cord must be freed from mesodermal tissue. In these cases the dural repair is often inadequate. Fat can frequently be seen extending from subcutaneous tissue into the spinal cord, mimicking the appearance of a lipomyelomeningocele.

Occasionally, in addition to tethering, other conditions such as diastematomyelia or dermoid tumour may be found. These conditions should be dealt with when the cord is untethered. Once the spinal cord is free the dural closure must be secure to prevent neural tissue adhering to mesodermal tissue. The use of cadaver freeze-dried dura helps ensure adequate dural closure.

A further problem arises in the patient with a congenital scoliosis which requires correction. All such patients should be fully investigated either by CT myelography or, preferably, MRI scanning to rule out an associated intraspinal anomaly. Such anomalies are typically those of a thickened filum or a diastematomyelia, though syringomelia or an intramedullary tumour may occasionally occur. If either a bony spur or a tethered filum are present, historically these were released prior to scoliosis surgery. Corrective surgery is often a two-stage procedure and it is now normal practice not to remove the intraspinal anomaly prior to correction if the first stage of the scoliosis surgery is only an anterior release type of procedure involving no lengthening. The diastematomyelia or tethered cord can conveniently be dealt with during the second-stage posterior procedure.

Patients who already show evidence of neurological deficit prior to their scoliosis surgery should all also have their cords released. However, many units do not routinely release a tethered filum in the neurologically intact patient, relying on intraoperative monitoring and a 'wake-up' test to assess cord function during the correction.

THE TETHERED CORD IN ADULTS

It should be appreciated that it is possible for patients to present with a tethered cord syndrome as adults. Such presentation may often be as a deterioration in a patient who has had evidence of a tethered cord as a child but whose clinical picture had been static during maturation. Such a patient may, for example, have had either a hairy patch or a foot deformity as a child but only showed progression in adult life, often after minor trauma.

It is also possible for a completely normal childhood to be followed by the onset of either pain or frank neurological deficit as an adult. Pang & Wilberger (1982) reported 23 cases where a tethered cord syndrome presented as an adult, the oldest being 76 years of age. Ten of those patients had had a pre-existing but static childhood problem, but the remaining 13 had had normal childhoods. Although they found that the mechanism of tethering was similar to that in children, the adults tended to present with a much greater frequency of pain (including perineal pain) and sphincteric disturbance as compared to childhood cases. They found that release produced gratifying results in relation to pain and motor deficits, but sphincteric dysfunction only rarely showed improvement.

The syndrome of the tethered spinal cord can present at any age, from the very old to the very young. The development of neurological deficit in infancy is particularly dangerous as much damage may occur prior to diagnosis. Early, appropriate surgical release of the tethered cord can prevent further neurological damage and may result in neurological improvement more frequently than is commonly appreciated. Full assessment of the patient is mandatory at the time of diagnosis, irrespective of age, and surgical release should be performed at that time in the majority of cases. Finally, it cannot be sufficiently stressed that, in any child presenting with a cavus foot deformity, the back and gluteal cleft should be carefully examined and radiographed to search for any evidence of a dysraphic problem.

REFERENCES

Anderson, F.M. (1975) Occult spinal dysraphism: a series of 73 cases. *Paediatrics*, **55**, 826–835.

Barson, A.J. (1970) The vertebral level of termination of the spinal cord during normal and abnormal development. *J. Anat.*, **106**, 489–497.

Breig, A. (1970) Overstretching of and circumscribed pathological tension in the spinal cord—a basic cause of symptoms in cord disorders. *J. Biochem.*, **3**, 7–9.

Chapman, P.H. (1982) Congenital intraspinal lipomas. Anatomic considerations and surgical treatment. *Child's Brain*, **9**, 37–47.

Guthkelch, A.N., Pang, D. & Vries, J. (1979) Influence of closure technique on results in myelomeningocele. *Child's Brain*, **8**, 350–355.

Hendrick, E.B., Hoffman, H.J. & Humphreys, R.P. (1982) The tethered spinal cord. *Clin. Neurosurg.*, **30**, 457–463.

Hoffman, H.J. Hendrick, E.B. & Humphreys, R.P. (1976) The tethered spinal cord: Its protean manifestations and surgical correction. *Child's Brain*, **2**, 145–155.

Hoffman, H.J., Taecholarn, C., Hendrick, E.B. & Humphreys, R.P. (1985) Management of lipomyelomeningoceles: experience at the Hospital for Sick Children. *J. Neurosurg.*, **62**, 1–8.

James, C.C. & Lassman, L.P. (1981) *Spina Bifida Occulta*. Grune & Stratton, New York, pp. 131–159.

McLone, D.G. (1980) Technique for closure of myelomeningocele. *Child's Brain*, **6**, 65–73.

Pang, D. & Wilberger, J.E. (1982) Tethered cord syndrome in adults. *J. Neurosurg.*, **57**, 32–47.

Piatt, J.H. & Hoffman, H.J. (1987) The tethered spinal cord with focus on the tight filum terminale (Part I). *Neuro-orthopaedics*, **3**, 67–75.

Pierre-Kann, A., Lacombe, J., Pichon, J., Giudicelli, Y., Renier, D., Sainte-Rose, C., Perrigot, M. & Hirsch, J.F. (1986) Intraspinal lipomas with spina bifida. Prognosis and treatment in 73 cases. *J. Neurosurg.*, **65**, 756–761.

Reigel, D.H. (1983) The tethered spinal cord. *Concepts Pediat. Neurosurg.*, **4**, 142–164.

Tamaki, N., Shirataki, K., Kojima, N., Shouse, Y. & Matsumoto, S. (1988) Tethered cord syndrome of delayed onset following repair of myelomeningocele. *J. Neurosurg.*, **69**, 393–398.

Tani, S., Yamada, S. & Knighton, R.M. (1987) Extensibility of the lumbar and sacral cord. Pathophysiology of the tethered spinal cord in cats. *J. Neurosurg.*, **66**, 116–123.

Yamada, S., Schreider, S., Ashwal, S. & Knierim, D. (1985) Pathophysiologic mechanisms in the tethered spinal cord syndrome. In Holtzman, R.N.N. & Stein, B.M. (eds) *The Tethered Spinal Cord*, pp. 29–40. Thieme-Stratton, New York.

Yamada, S., Zinke, D.E. & Sanders, D. (1981) Pathophysiology of tethered cord syndrome. *Neurosurgery*, **54**, 494–503.

15 · Craniocervical Anomalies

By T.E. JEFFREYS

Congenital anomalies or malformations of the cervical spine and the craniovertebral junction are many and varied. They often coexist in a manner which defies tidy classification. They are frequently accompanied by developmental anomalies of the brain stem and spinal cord. An anomaly of the cervical spine may be but one of a number of defects involving skeletal and visceral systems. The bony malformations may be innocuous in themselves, but will become clinically significant if they are responsible for cervical instability. Clinical presentation may be delayed until adult life when degenerative changes reduce the margin of safety in a vulnerable canal. Whenever a cervical anomaly is found the examining surgeon must establish:

1 Is the lesion unstable?

2 Is there a risk of neurological damage from instability?

3 Is there an associated anomaly of the brain stem or cord?

4 Are there other congenital defects lower down in the spine or in other systems?

The malformations are:

1 Anomalies of the craniovertebral junction.
- (a) Basilar coarctation.
- (b) Hypoplasia of the occipital condyles.
- (c) Occipitalization of the atlas.
- (d) Aplasia and hypoplasia of the arch of the atlas.
- (e) Atlanto-axial fusion.

2 Anomalies of the axis.
- (a) Aplasia and hypoplasia of the odontoid.
- (b) Os odontoideum.
- (c) Spondylolisthesis of the axis.
- (d) Fusion of the axis and C3.

3 Anomalies below C2.
- (a) Congenital cervical fusion; the Klippel–Feil syndrome.
- (b) Aplasia and hypoplasia of individual vertebrae.
- (c) Spondylolisthesis.
- (d) Diastometamyelia.

4 Cervical anomalies associated with multisystem defect.
- (a) Dwarfism.
- (b) Spondyloepiphyseal dysplasias.
- (c) Down's syndrome.
- (d) Neurofibromatosis.

The anatomical relations between the base of the skull and the upper two cervical vertebrae are disturbed in a number of congenital and acquired conditions. The terms used to describe these altered relations are often confused, and need to be defined precisely.

Platybasia is an anthropometric term describing flattening of the base of the skull as measured by the angle subtended between the planes of the clivus and the episthion. The word 'platybasia' has no clinical significance. Basilar coarctation is a congenital anomaly where the odontoid is invaginated into the foramen magnum. Basilar impression is an acquired abnormality where the odontoid is invaginated into the foramen magnum. These terms are not synonymous (O'Connell & Turner, 1950) but the convention has arisen to use 'primary basilar impression' for coarctation and 'secondary basilar impression' for impression (Fielding *et al.*, 1978).

It can be difficult to interpret the various relations on standard radiographs, and several diagnostic lines have been described (Figs 15.1 & 15.2). Chamberlain's line runs from the posterior edge of the hard palate to the posterior rim of the foramen magnum, the epis-

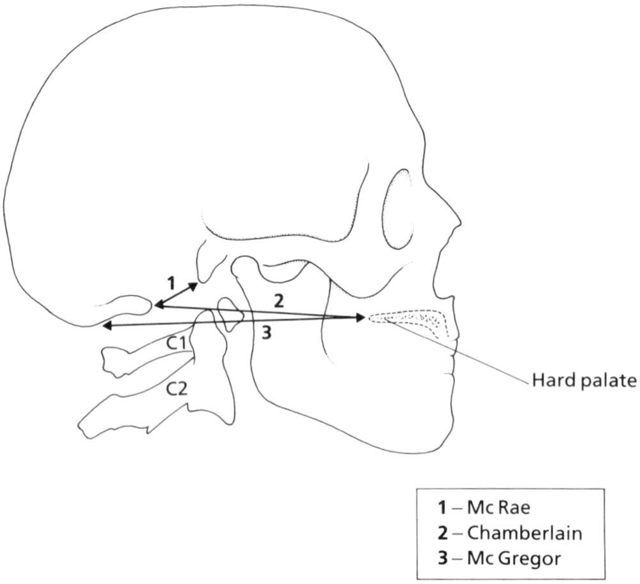

Fig. 15.1 Diagnostic lines at craniovertebral junction—sagittal.

thion; McGregor's line runs from the posterior edge of the hard palate to the most caudal point of the occiput, and McRae's line runs from the anterior to the posterior rims of the foramen magnum (Chamberlain, 1939; McGregor, 1948; McRae, 1953). The margins of the foramen magnum can be deformed, or difficult to define, in congenital anomalies. McGregor's line, by linking bony points remote from the abnormal area, is the most useful in practice as well as being the easiest to draw. Lines can also be drawn in the coronal plane on anteroposterior radiographs (Fig. 15.2). The tip of the odontoid normally lies on a line drawn between the points of the mastoid processes, or below one drawn between the digastric grooves (Fishgold & Metzger, 1952).

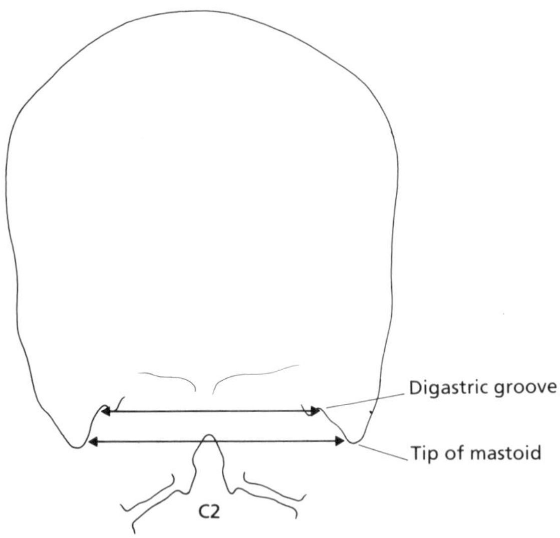

Fig. 15.2 Diagnostic lines at craniovertebral junction—coronal.

It is difficult to define these bony points in standard radiographs of the infantile skull and spine. Fortunately the newer methods of imaging such as computerized tomography (CI) ànd magnetic resonance imaging (MRI) provide pictures of startling clarity.

Basilar coarctation (basilar invagination: primary basilar impression)

Congenital malformation of the occiput around the foramen magnum allows the tip of the axis to be higher than normal, even penetrating the foramen and compromising the brain stem. Other skeletal anomalies—such as the Klippel–Feil syndrome, anomalies of the atlas and axis, and facial asymmetry—may also be present. Congenital anomalies rarely come singly; but the peculiar association of basilar coarctation is with malformations of the hind brain and brain stem, such as the Arnold–Chiari phenomenon, and syringomyelia.

The Arnold–Chiari malformation consists of caudal prolapse of the cerebellar tonsils through the foramen magnum (Fig. 15.3). Degrees of caudal prolapse have been described, from simple prolapse of the tonsils to extension of the IVth ventricle through the foramen (Arnold, 1894; Chiari, 1896). The aqueduct of Sylvius may be blocked, producing hydrocephalus, and there is a high association with lumbosacral myelomeningocoele. The vertebral arteries are often abnormal and, even if morphologically normal, may be compromised by the local congestion. It has been suggested that the resulting ischaemia causes the syringomyelia often found with the other abnormalities (Michie & Clark, 1968).

Basilar coarctation in itself may not be a cause of symptoms, and when symptoms do occur their onset may be delayed until adolescence or adult life. It will be appreciated that the clinical presentation may be varied and complex. The odontoid can impinge on the brain stem, producing motor and sensory problems from long tract pressure. Compression of the prolapsed cerebellar components will result in ataxia, nystagmus and giddiness. The lower cranial nerves

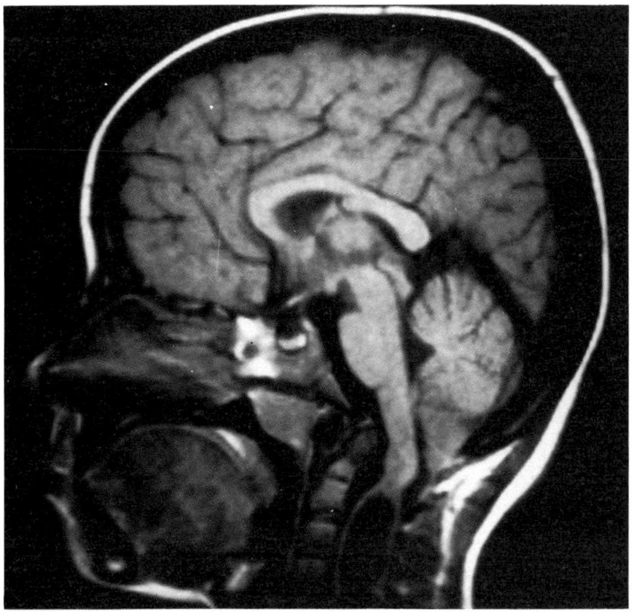

Fig. 15.3 Arnold–Chiari malformation (MRI), associated cervical syringomyelia.

may be affected. Arterial compression can produce a clinical picture ranging from intermittent 'blackouts' to the fully developed lateral medullary, or Wallenburg syndrome (Wallenburg, 1897; Klein *et al.*, 1976).

The delayed onset of symptoms is probably due to progressive instability from ligamentous laxity. Early degenerative changes in the cervical spine will cause restricted movement in segments adjacent to the anomaly, so increasing the vulnerability of the craniovertebral area. When onset of symptoms is delayed into adult life, diagnosis is difficult, and in a review of 68 cases of compressive lesions of the foramen magnum, all amenable to surgical decompression, 53 had originally been diagnosed as suffering from progressive, incurable neurological diseases (McRae, 1953).

With such a protean clinical picture, advice on management can be only in very general terms. The mechanical problems are of foraminal stenosis or craniovertebral instability. The two may be present together, the instability producing intermittent compression. Decompression and stabilization may be necessary together in combined procedures such as those described by Crockard and Ransford (1985). Suboccipital decompression may need to be combined with posterior fusion. The extension of internal fixation devices such as the Hartshill system, the Ransford loop or modified plates, to the skull have allowed more aggressive decompression procedures to be relieved of worries about postoperative instability.

Occipitilization of the atlas (assimilation of the atlas; occipitocervical fusion)

In this anomaly all or part of the atlas is congenitally fused to the occiput by bone or fibrous tissue (MacAlister, 1892) (Figs 15.4a,b). The basiocciput, all the atlas apart from the anterior arch, and the ossiculum terminale of the odontoid develop from a single scler-

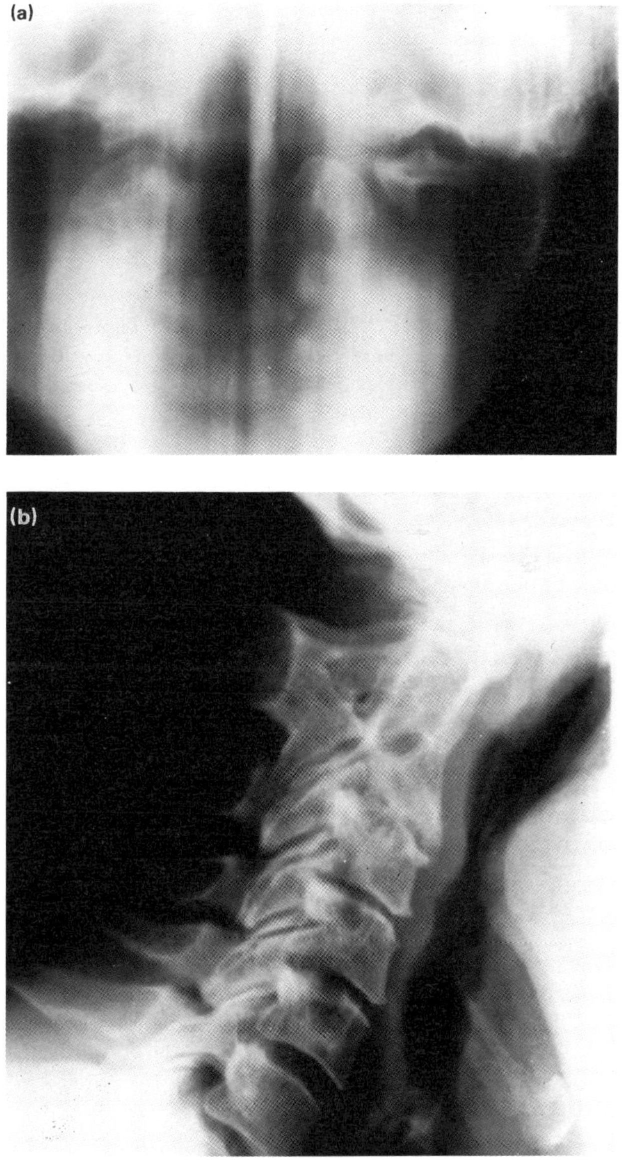

Fig. 15.4 (a) Occipitalization of atlas (AP tomogram); (b) occipitalization of atlas and synostosis of C2–C3.

otome, the pro-atlas. Segmentation occurs during fetal life and precedes ossification. The anomaly of occipitocervical fusion has been described as a failure of segmentation and not a congenital fusion (Hadley, 1956) but this does not explain why the anterior arch of the atlas, which develops from the hypochordal bow, is the element most often fused to the skull. The lateral masses and the superior facets are usually included in the synostosis; the posterior arch less frequently. The latter is often hypoplastic and malaligned, grooving the dura and the cord (Geehr *et al.*, 1978). The transverse processes of the atlas may be dysplastic or fused, the inferior facets asymmetrical and the vertebral artery foramina absent.

The atlas may lie in a relatively posterior position to the occiput. This displaces the odontoid backwards and reduces the capacity of the spinal canal. The odontoid itself can be abnormal in shape, size and direction; sometimes being longer than usual and angled backwards. The assimilation can reduce the height of the atlanto-occipital interval. This can allow the tip of the odontoid to penetrate into the foramen magnum, particularly if it is long, and produce a relative basilar coarctation. The critical distance of the tip of the odontoid above McGregor's line is 4.5 mm. If the tip of the odontoid projects into the foramen magnum, symptoms of basilar coarctation are likely. If the tip lies below the foramen, symptoms are unlikely. The odontoid may be displaced posteriorly by the abnormally located anterior arch, or may be displaced behind the arch by more than the normal 3 mm atlas–dens interval (ADI). If the odontoid rides high such posterior displacement will diminish the depth of the canal between the posterior surface of the odontoid and the posterior lip of the foramen magnum. This depth is least when the neck is flexed, and a measurement of 19 mm or less in this position is critical to the production of a neurological defect (McRae, 1953).

Congenital fusion of C2 and C3 occurs in 70% of patients with occipitalization of the atlas (McRae, 1953). This leaves the atlanto-axial joint the only moving articulation between two rigid segments, and the resulting demand, even without dysplasia or malalignment of the odontoid, will produce instability and the possibility of spinal compromise (Von Torklus & Gehle, 1972). Associated with the anomaly, the dura may be constricted posteriorly by a fibrous band. This occurs independently of a hypoplastic posterior arch. It can be a cause of neural compression and has been observed to occur with tonsillar herniation of the cerebellum (Spillane *et al.*, 1957).

Congenital anomalies of other systems are often found. The spine below may be affected by kyphosis or scoliosis. Facial malformations such as asymmetry, jaw defects and cleft palate; pes cavus and syndactyly, congenital ear defects, hypospadias, and malformations of the genito-urinary tract have been reported (McRae, 1953; Spillane *et al.*, 1957). Unlike patients with other anomalies of the craniovertebral region, patients with occipitalization of the atlas have an appearance remarkably like those afflicted with the Klippel–Feil syndrome; that is to say they have a low hairline, a short stiff neck and, often, torticollis (McRae & Barnum, 1953; Spillane *et al.*, 1957).

As with basilar coarctation, neurological symptoms and signs may not develop until adult life, unless precipitated by injury. The majority of patients present with symptoms produced by anterior compression of the medulla by an abnormally long, angled or hypermobile odontoid. Post-mortem examination has shown indentation of the brain stem (Bharucha & Dastur, 1964). This anterior compression will produce long tract signs of spastic weakness and increased reflexes. The lower cranial nerves may be involved. Less commonly, posterior compression from the lip of the foramen magnum, the hypoplastic posterior arch of the dural groove, will cause loss of proprioception and vibration sense. Nystagmus will indicate cerebellar compression, and vertigo can arise from vertebral artery compromise.

The precipitating mechanical cause of these compressive factors is atlanto-axial instability. This is an intermittent force whose effects accumulate until they become progressive, or may be immediately catastrophic after injury. The delayed onset of symptoms into adult life probably reflects the decreasing tolerance to insult of ageing neural tissue, the loss of elasticity in soft tissue, the increasing rigidity, due to degeneration of adjacent articular segments and, possibly, vascular deterioration.

The operative treatment of this anomaly, once neurological signs have appeared, has a bad reputation. Increased neurological defects and death have been reported. Particularly hazardous is any attempt to reduce atlanto-axial dislocation during operation (Wadia, 1967; Nicholson & Sherk, 1968; Sinto & Pandya, 1968). If symptoms are precipitated by injury, simple immobilization of the neck in a collar may be sufficient to allow remission. Progressive neurological signs, however, dictate an operative approach. The problem is considered fully below, but transoral decompression combined with posterior occipitocervical fusion using internal fixation is probably the safest and most effective procedure (Crockard & Ransford, 1985).

Anomalies of the axis

Anomalies of the odontoid

Congenital malformations of the odontoid, or dens, are clinically significant because they can cause atlanto-axial instability. The variations of anomaly which are described share this tendency, and their separation is of academic importance only.

The development of the odontoid is complex (Fig. 15.5). The apex of the process derives from the pro-atlas. The body derives from the first cervical sclerotome, and is the centrum of the atlas which fuses with the body of the axis. Two ossification centres, lying either side of the midline, appear within the first five intrauterine months, and fuse by birth. At birth the original 'disc space' between the atlas and axis is represented by a cartilaginous plate, the neurocentral synchondrosis. This lies below the level of the superior articular facets of the axis; that is, below the base of the adult dens. A considerable part of the body of the axis is thus formed from the odontoid. Fusion of the odontoid and body occurs in most children by the age of six years. If the synchondrosis persists into adolescence it may be misinterpreted on radiographs as a fracture, but fractures of the odontoid occur at the base of the process, at the level of the articular facets.

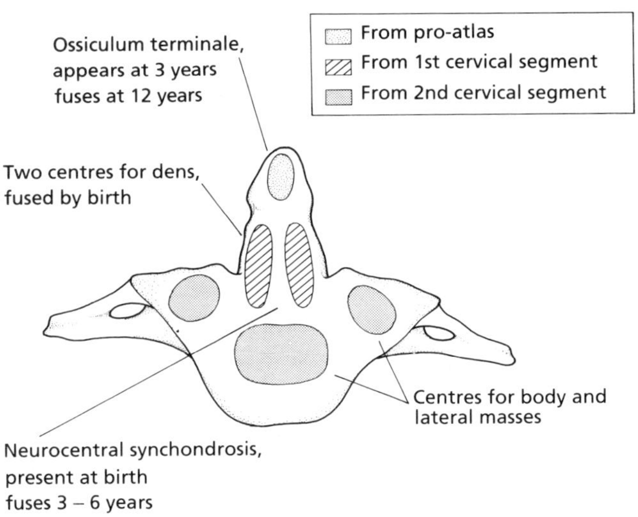

Fig. 15.5 Ossification of the axis.

A separate ossification centre for the apex appears after birth, usually in the second year, and unites with the rest of the odontoid at puberty. It may persist as a separate ossiculum terminale, attached to the body of the dens by cartilage. It is not, as a rule, a cause of atlanto-axial instability; but a case has been reported of fatal atlanto-axial dislocation in a child afflicted with Down's syndrome. At post-mortem examination the transverse ligament of the atlas was found to be interposed between an ossiculum terminale and the body of the odontoid, preventing reduction of the dislocation (Sherk & Nicholson, 1969). A similar case, who survived, was presumed to have the same lesion (Finerman *et al.*, 1976). In radiographs of infants the unossified apex may be falsely interpreted as odontoid hypoplasia, or even atlanto-axial subluxation as the anterior arch of the atlas will appear to lie above the tip of the odontoid.

The blood supply of the dens reflects its ossification pattern. Branches arise from the vertebral arteries at the level of C2 and ascend in front of and behind the dens, to end in a vascular arcade around the apex. This arcade anastomoses with branches of the carotid via the alar ligaments of the atlas (Schiff & Parke, 1972). There is a vascular watershed between the odontoid and the body of the axis, at the level of the neurocentral synchondrosis, which can be a contributory factor in the development of non-union in fractures of the odontoid.

Three variations of odontoid anomaly, other than ossiculum terminale, are recognized. They are agenesis or aplasia, hypoplasia and os odontoideum (Fig. 15.6). It is doubtful whether true agenesis of the odontoid exists. What is often called aplasia is really hypoplasia; that is to say, there is a short stub of odontoid projecting above the level of the articular facets. In true aplasia there would be no bony structure above the level of the neurocentral synchondrosis, and a depression would be visible between the facets.

Os odontoideum is a discrete round or oval ossicle widely separated from a hypoplastic odontoid base. The ossicle is situated in the position of the tip of the odontoid but is considerably larger than an ossiculum terminale. Sometimes the fragment lies near the basi

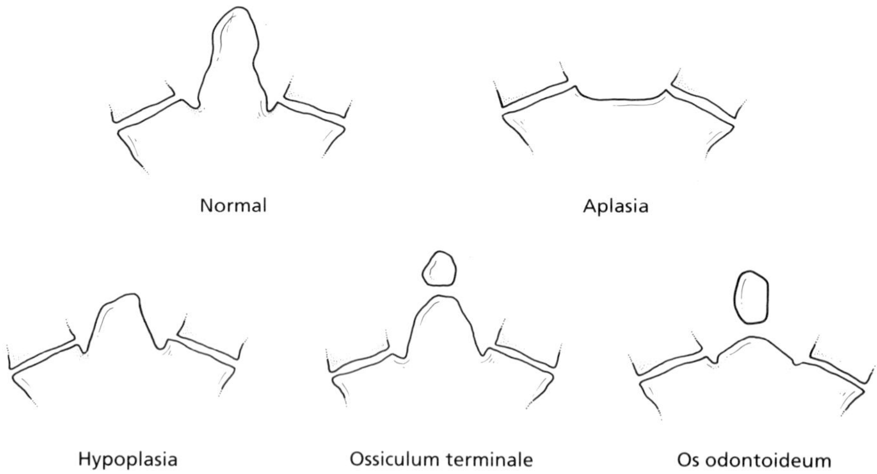

Fig. 15.6 Anomalies of the odontoid.

occiput and may fuse with the clivus. Radiographically the ossicle has a dense rim surrounding a radiolucent centre (Fig. 15.7).

There is controversy whether os odontoideum represents a true congenital anomaly or is an un-united fracture of the base of the odontoid. The congenital theory postulates either a failure of fusion of the ossiculum terminale to the odontoid, or a failure of fusion of the odontoid to the axis. There are cogent

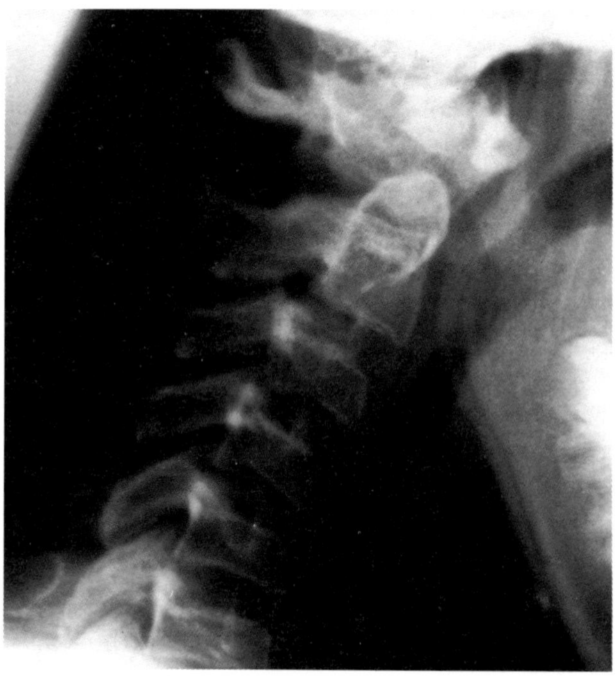

Fig. 15.7 Os odontoideum.

objections to both postulates. As mentioned above, the ossiculum terminale, when present, is much smaller than the os odontoideum. If there were a failure of fusion to the axis one would expect the line of demarcation to lie below the level of the articular facets, at the level of the neurocentral synchondrosis. Os odontoideum always lies above a hypoplastic stub of odontoid base. However, the post-mortem findings in one case claim to support a congenital theory of origin. The patient, a male adult, suffered a fatal atlanto-axial dislocation. The os odontoideum was found to contain three ossified segments surrounded by cartilage. It lay above a bony stub continuous with the body of the axis. There was no remnant of the neurocentral synchondrosis. The junction between the ossicle and the hypoplastic stub was occupied by loose fibrous strands. The short stub arising from the body of the axis was explained as a failed attempt by the early-developing axis to fuse with the separate odontoid (Michaels *et al.*, 1969).

The case for a traumatic origin to os odontoideum has been well put by Fielding and his associates (Fielding, 1965; Fielding & Griffin, 1974, Fielding *et al.*, 1980). Their most recent paper is based on a review of 35 patients. While accepting the increased frequency of odontoid anomalies in patients with Down's syndrome and spondyloepiphyseal dysplasias it observes that if os odontoideum were a true congenital anomaly there would be a higher incidence of association with other craniovertebral malformations.

A significant number of reported cases of os odontoideum have been known to have normal odontoid processes previously. One such case, examined by post mortem, had a normal odontoid process at the age of 10 and os odontoideum at the age of 17. He also had multiple congenital anomalies including hydrocephalus, myelodysplasia and Klippel–Feil syndrome. Seventeen of the 35 reported cases had a history of significant injury to the neck, occurring some time—varying from months to years—before the diagnosis of os odontoideum was made.

Fielding and his associates put forward the following hypothesis to explain these observed facts. An unrecognized fracture of the base of the odontoid occurs. There is, initially, little displacement of the fragments, but eventual contraction of the alar ligaments pulls the body of the odontoid away from the axis. The peculiar arrangement of the blood supply to the dens predisposes to non-union, and the absence of any fracture healing allows wide separation. It is known that avascular necrosis of the odontoid can be caused by the distraction of prolonged halopelvic traction (Tredwell & O'Brien, 1975). A 'fresh' case of odontoid fracture does not look like os odontoideum. The gap between the fragments is narrow and irregular, and the upper fragment looks like a normal odontoid. Fielding explains the wide gap and the smooth round ossicle of the os odontoideum as changes wrought by the passage of time. The associated hypertrophy of the anterior arch of the atlas is also explained as a response to attempts at healing.

The same arguments are used to explain odontoid hypoplasia, although familial hypoplasia has been observed (Shepard, 1966). Hypoplasia and os odontoideum have also been reported after pyogenic osteomyelitis (Ahlback & Collert, 1920; Freiberger *et al.*, 1965).

The clinical presentation of patients with odontoid anomalies varies from local discomfort to progressive myelopathy. Many have no symptoms until they are subjected to injury. The symptoms are due to atlanto-axial instability. When this is slight the symptoms are local, such as neck pain, headache, or torticollis from muscle spasm. Neurological symptoms are due to compression of the cord from atlanto-axial displacement. Involvement of cranial nerves is rare (Minderhoud *et al.*, 1969). Symptoms of vertigo and syncope are uncommon and assumed to be due to vertebral artery compression (McKeever, 1968).

Radiographs will demonstrate the presence of an odontoid anomaly, and more significantly, the degree of atlanto-axial instability. Studies in flexion and extension are needed, and cine-radiography is invaluable. The ossicle of os odontoideum will move with the anterior arch of the atlas, to which is it firmly bound. The relationship of the arch of the atlas to the body of the axis will indicate the extent of displacement, but the sagittal diameter of the spinal canal behind the odontoid must also be measured.

The management of patients with odontoid anomalies can be difficult. Where a neurological defect exists with instability, the segment must be stabilized by posterior atlanto-axial fusion. Management is controversial in those patients whose symptoms are minimal, and in those whose anomaly is found by chance on routine radiography. The case for prophylactic stabilization is that these patients are at considerable risk from minor injury (Shepard, 1966; Fielding *et al.*, 1980).

The case against prophylactic stabilization is that operation is associated with high mortality and morbidity, and that patients with these anomalies are not at risk if they take care to avoid potentially dangerous activities (Gillman, 1959; Garber, 1964; Minderhoud *et al.*, 1969). This author feels that such advice is unrealistic in modern western society, and that prophylactic stabilization should be advised to these patients.

The atlanto-axial displacement should be reduced before operation. This can usually be achieved by positioning of the head or by skull traction. If the displacement is associated with a neurological defect it should be reduced at least seven to 10 days before operation, to allow the irritated cord to settle. When the displacement cannot be reduced before operation a choice must be made between a fusion *in situ*, and a combined anterior and posterior procedure. Where there is no neurological defect, fusion *in situ* is the operation of choice. When there is a defect, and decompression is needed, the combined transoral and posterior approach is suitable (Crockard & Ransford, 1985). The risk of infection following the procedure is not as high as has been suggested (Whitesides & Pendleton, 1975).

In view of the accepted association between injury and the development of os odontoideum, some difficulty may be thought to arise over the management of fractures of the odontoid. There should be none: fresh fractures of the odontoid should be managed conservatively, avoiding distraction. Only if established non-union is diagnosed should operative stabilization be considered.

Spondylolysis and spondylolisthesis of the axis

Failure of fusion between the neural arch and the centrum can occur on one or both sides. The degree of displacement is not great, and the lesion is not usually a source of symptoms. It has been described in association with hypoplasia of the odontoid (Jeffreys, 1980).

Congenital laxity of the transverse ligaments of the atlas

When atlanto-axial instability occurs without any apparent cause, the diagnosis of congenital laxity of the transverse atlantal ligament is made. Congenital anomaly, injury and infection must be excluded as responsible factors.

Cervical anomalies in skeletal dysplasia

Nearly half of patients with skeletal dysplasia (osteochondrodystrophy) have anomalies of the upper cervical spine, and craniovertebral junction. Most of these anomalies are of the odontoid (Wynne Davies *et al.*, 1989). In Morquio's disease the incidence is 100%; in the other dysplasias less (Table 15.1) (see also Chapter 17). The finding of an odontoid anomaly does not in itself imply atlanto-axial instability. The integrity of the articulation depends on the strength of the supporting ligaments. The incidence of neurological damage is less than that of bony anomalies. Flexion and extension lateral radiographs are necessary to demonstrate any instability, and should be included in the routine screening of these children, as soon as they are old enough to cooperate. The ADI and the sagittal diameter of the spinal canal, or space available for the cord (SAC) must be measured as outlined above. These views are obtained by active movement of the head and neck. Passive movement in infants is dangerous.

In Morquio's disease, in addition to the bony anomaly, the soft tissue structures are faulty. Atlanto-axial subluxation is inevitable, and cord compression probable (Fig. 15.8). The assessment of neurological signs is difficult because of the associated lower-limb problems of joint laxity. Deterioration usually begins after the age of four, and is insidious in onset. Fatigue occurs and there may be episodes of tingling in the hands and arms. The child may hold the head and neck extended because it 'feels safe'. Long tract

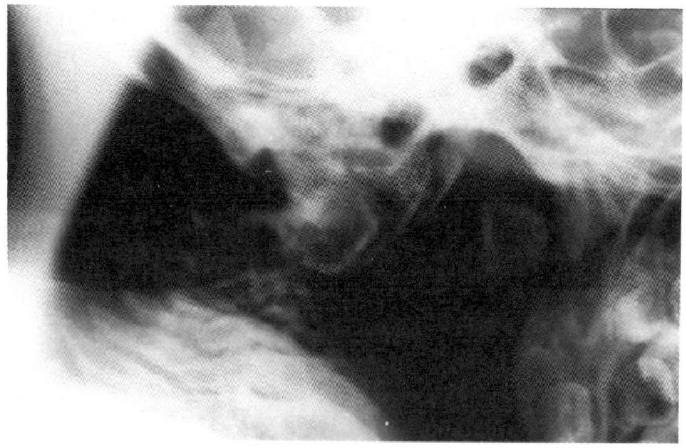

Fig. 15.8 Atlanto-axial instability in Morquio's syndrome.

signs and bladder involvement appear later. Frequent examination, at three-monthly periods, is recommended by the Skeletal Dysplasia Group, and parents should be warned to be alert for changes in the child's physical behaviour.

When neurological signs appear, the atlanto-axial joint must be stabilized by posterior fusion of the arch of the atlas to the spinous process of the axis (Fig. 15.9). There is a strong case for prophylactic fusion but, in the absence of neurological signs, this should be deferred until the child has grown enough to offer an adequate operation field, at eight to 10 years old. The area involved in the posterior operation is less than 2 cm^2. There is an excess of cartilage, and bony fusion is difficult to achieve. Skilled anaesthetic and surgical technique is essential. This expertise is usually available only in specialist spinal centres.

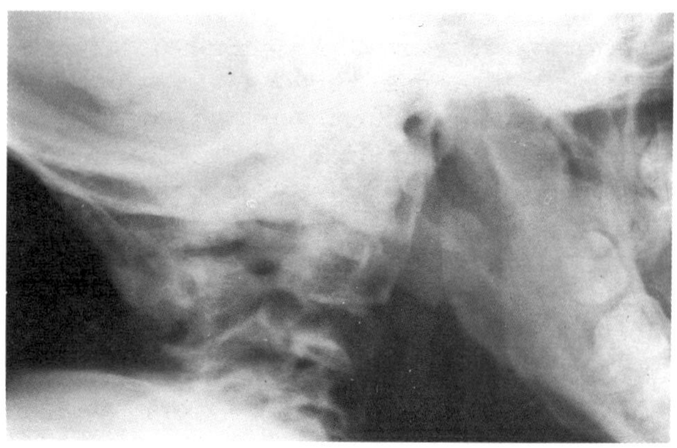

Fig. 15.9 Morquio's syndrome—successful occipitocervical fusion.

Table 15.1 Cervical anomalies in skeletal dysplasia (percentages). After Wynne-Davies *et al.* (1989)

Disease	Odontoid anomaly	Other craniovertebral anomalies	Neurological complications
Morquio's disease	100		30
Other mucopolysaccharide syndromes	75	25	0
Spondyloepiphyseal dysplasia	83	15	4
Other dysplasias	5–50	20	1–2

Atlanto-axial instability in Down's syndrome

It is estimated that 18–20% of patients suffering from Down's syndrome have atlanto-axial instability due to attenuation of the transverse ligaments of the atlas (Burke *et al.*, 1985). The intact alar ligaments provide the restraining support to the odontoid. Despite this alarmingly high incidence of instability, very few have signs of cord compression and a recent review found only 37 published cases of neurological damage (Davidson, 1988). There were five deaths in the reported cases, two of these being sudden with no previous history. Four patients in all had no premonitory symptoms, and these were injured during trampolining or gymnastics. All the others developed symptoms of neck pain, torticollis, weakness of a limb or an abnormality of gait at least one month before neurological signs appeared.

The natural history of atlanto-axial instability in Down's syndrome is not clear. The radiographic demonstration of instability does not mean there is symptomatic atlanto-axial dislocation. Patients who are radiographically stable can become unstable within a period of three years, but others with demonstrable instability can stabilize within a similar time. It is significant that many of the patients reviewed by Davidson had an upper respiratory infection before they developed signs of cord compression. The association between such infections and atlanto-axial instability has been known for some time (Watson Jones, 1932).

Sport enhances the quality of life for Down's syndrome patients, and it would be cruel to restrict them unnecessarily. There is a risk, however, particularly in activities such as gymnastics, trampolining and horse-riding. Previous reports have issued warnings against the dangers of sporting activities (American Academy of Sports Medicine, 1984; Acheson, 1986). Humane wisdom suggests that Down's patients who wish to indulge in athletics should be screened, advised of the risk, and warned to report any premonitory symptoms, but not barred from games. Prophylactic fusion of C1–C2 would not appear to be justified, but obviously the stability or otherwise of the articulation must be assessed before any general anaesthetic is given to these patients.

Congenital atlanto-axial instability

The various individual anomalies described above have in common that their clinical importance lies in the existence of atlanto-axial instability, causing neurological damage from narrowing of the spinal canal.

The atlanto-axial joint is a highly mobile articulation lying between two joints of much more limited movement, the atlanto-occipital joint and the joint between the axis and the third cervical vertebra. If either, or both, of these two is ankylosed by congenital anomaly the stress on the atlanto-axial joint is even greater. The loss of whatever little movement occurs at the neighbouring joints has to be compensated by increased atlanto-axial movement.

The stability of the atlanto-axial joint depends on the integrity of the odontoid process and of the check ligaments which retain it in relation to the atlas. Little, if any, stability derives from the lateral joints between atlas and axis, which are shallow arcs of a large circle (Fig. 15.10).

The intact odontoid is held in close relation to the anterior arch of the atlas by two ligaments, or groups of ligaments. The transverse atlantal ligament passes between the lateral masses of the atlas, and behind the odontoid, holding it against the anterior arch of the atlas while allowing it to rotate. It is strong and is the first line of defence against atlanto-axial subluxation. It is reinforced by the alar ligaments which pass

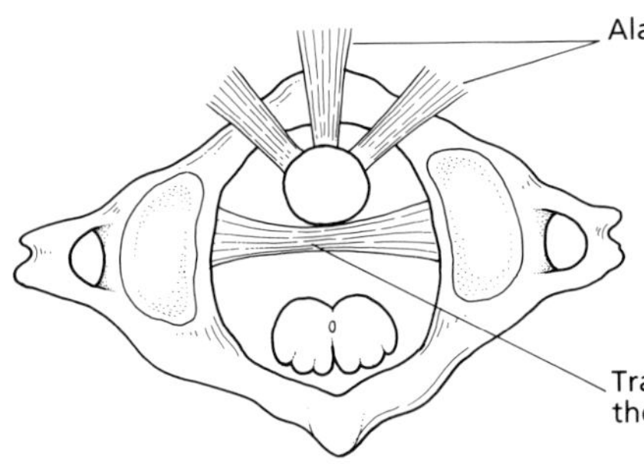

Fig. 15.10 Supporting ligaments of the odontoid.

from the tip of the odontoid to the margins of the foramen magnum. They are check reins, designed to limit rotation, and are inadequate to prevent atlanto-axial displacement if the transverse ligament has been ruptured (Werne, 1957; Fielding, 1973).

Clearly, if atlanto-axial instability exists in the presence of an intact odontoid, the spinal cord is in more danger of compression in flexion than extension. If the odontoid is absent, or if there is an os odontoideum which moves forwards with the anterior arch of the atlas, the cord is compromised in both directions.

The assessment of the degree of atlanto-axial instability is radiographic, and certain spaces and intervals can be identified and measured. The atlas–dens interval (ADI) is the space between the anterior aspect of the odontoid and the posterior aspect of the anterior arch of the atlas. In normal children this distance should not be greater than 4 mm in flexion. In adults it should be less than 3 mm. A measurement greater than this in the healthy adult implies a rupture of the transverse ligament (Fielding, 1973) (Fig. 15.11). These values do not apply where there is chronic

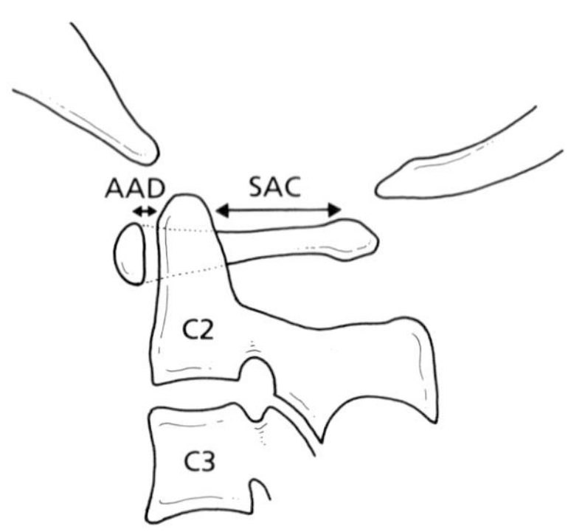

Fig. 15.11 The atlanto-axial distance (AAD) and the space available for the cord (SAC).

atlanto-axial instability due to congenital anomalies or congenital laxity of the transverse ligament in Down's syndrome. In these cases a wider gap than the accepted norm is not necessarily associated with neurological problems.

The other important measurement is the distance between the posterior aspect of the odontoid and the anterior aspect of the posterior arch of the atlas. The spinal cord occupies half of this diameter, and so the measurement shows how much space is available for the cord (SAC). If the odontoid is intact this space is unaffected in extension but reduced in flexion. If the odontoid is fractured or if there is an os odontoideum the space between the posterior arch of the atlas and the anterior edge of the axial canal, is diminished in flexion and the distance between the mobile base of the odontoid peg and the arch of the axis is reduced in extension (Fig. 15.12).

The clinical picture of atlanto-axial instability is of compression of the cervical cord or, if there is basilar coarctation, of the brain stem. The vertebral vessels and the lower cranial nerves may also be compromised. Intermittent compression is more harmful to the cord than is continuous compression (Spillane *et al.*, 1957). The compressive force may be exerted anteriorly by the odontoid, or posteriorly by the posterior arch of the atlas or the posterior rim of the foramen magnum. If an associated Arnold–Chiari malformation is present, cerebellar tissue will also be compressed. The presenting clinical symptoms and signs can therefore be complex and difficult to interpret. Presentation is often delayed into adult life, and may or may not be associated with a history of injury to the neck. Intermittent pressure can give a fluctuating but progressive picture, and it is not surprising that many patients are initially thought to have multiple sclerosis.

Anterior pressure from the odontoid will produce a progressive spastic tetraparesis. Pressure on the posterior columns will cause loss of joint position sense, vibration sense and deep pain. Cerebellar symptoms include ataxia and nystagmus; and vertebral arterial compromise may further complicate the presentation by producing complaints of vertigo, dizziness or episodes of unconsciousness.

The principles of management of atlanto-axial instability can be stated briefly: first reduce the subluxation and then stabilize the articulation. How and when these should be done is not so clear. There are few hard-and-fast rules. Progressive neurological de-

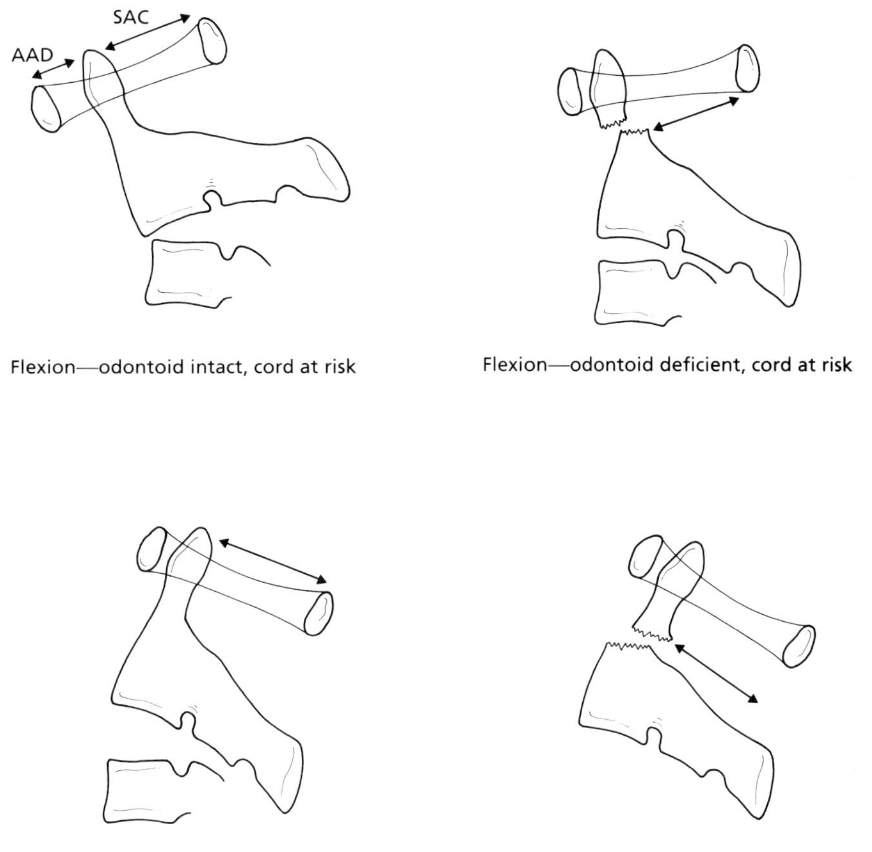

Fig. 15.12 Atlanto-axial instability.

terioration demands interference. The subluxation must be reduced before, never during, operation. The adult patient can be made aware of the risks and the choices. But how can one hold a sensible discussion with a small child who is regarded as being at risk, and whose parents may be too emotionally involved to reach an informed decision? The clinicians responsible for the management of these patients bear a heavy burden.

Congenital cervical fusion: the Klippel–Feil syndrome

Congenital fusion of cervical vertebrae was observed in the 18th and 19th centuries, but in 1912 Klippel and Feil described in detail the syndrome which bears their name. They reported the clinical features and post-mortem findings of a middle-aged man who in life had been known to have a short, stiff neck and a low posterior hairline. He had died of pneumonia and renal failure, although the significance of this was not realized. At post mortem they found all the cervical vertebrae to be fused together, and the base of the skull to approximate to the thoracic cage. They described the case as an 'absence' of cervical vertebrae, but it is only recently that a case of true agenesis of the cervical spine has been reported (Nisan *et al.*, 1988). Feil later collected 13 other cases and appreciated that there could be considerable variation in the extent and pattern of the synostoses. He divided the variants into three types.

Type I, cervical synostosis associated with the clinical triad of a short, stiff neck with a low posterior hairline.

Type II, fusion of two or more cervical vertebrae but without the clinical features of Type I.

Type III, extensive cervical, thoracic and even lumbar synostosis.

This division has little practical significance, and is only of historical interest (Feil, 1919). The term Klippel–Feil syndrome is now used loosely to describe all variations of congenital cervical fusion. The exact incidence is unknown, as many two-segment fusions must remain unrecognized, but the original, classical syndrome accounts for less than half of reported cases.

Formation of the vertebral bodies, combining the caudal and cephalic halves of adjacent protovertebrae, occurs by the fourth intrauterine week. The mature vertebral body is intersegmental. The intervertebral disc is formed from condensed tissue around the sclerotomic fissure which bisects the original protovertebra. Radiographs of congenital fusions in infants show incomplete ossification at the level of the definitive discs, and radiographs of congenital fusions in the adult show the 'ghosts' of disc spaces at the same levels; so the synostosis is not caused by a failure of segmentation. A few cases of hereditary cervical fusions have been reported (Gunderson *et al.*, 1967), but in most the teratogenic effect must occur after embryological segmentation, probably about the eighth week.

The scapula is formed from mesodermal tissue adjacent to the high cervical spine, at the level of the third and fourth vertebrae. It descends to its final position in the eighth week. The frequent association of a congenital high scapula and the Klippel–Feil syndrome is therefore not surprising, and suggests a common teratogenic cause.

The radiographic features of the classical case are unmistakable (Fig. 15.13), but may be difficult to demonstrate in the infant. Vertebral body synostosis is accompanied by bony fusion of the posterior elements (Fig. 15.14) and this will be radiographically apparent in the young patient in whom endplate ossification of the body is incomplete. When ossification is complete the 'ghosts' of the disc spaces will be visible. The less severe degrees of the condition, when

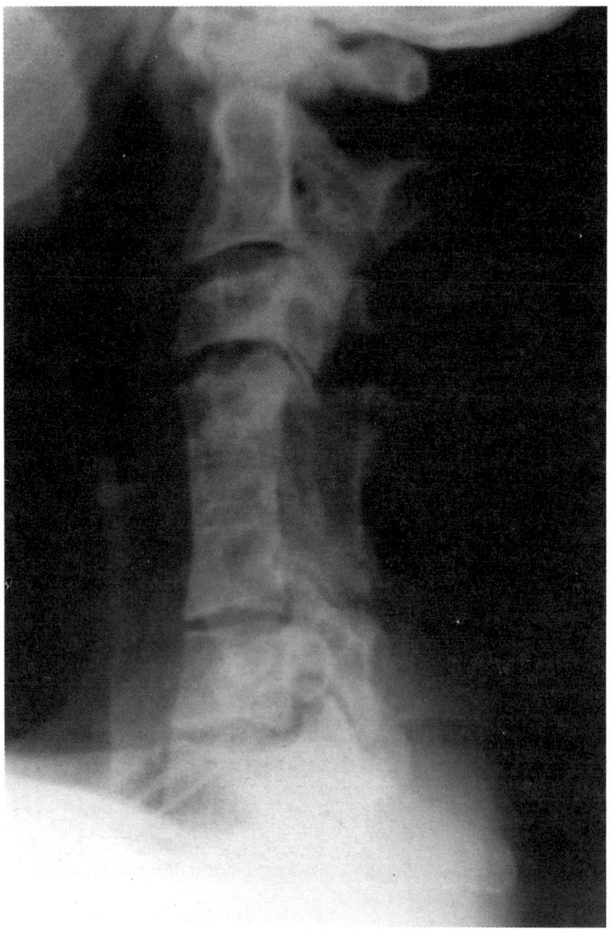

Fig. 15.13 Klippel–Feil syndrome.

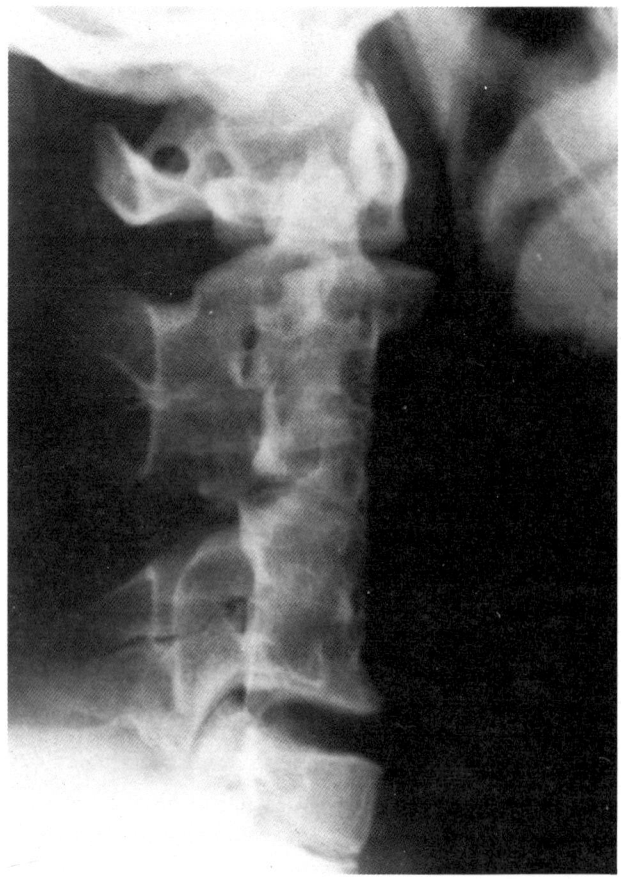

Fig. 15.14 Klippel–Feil syndrome; odontoid hypoplasia; hypertrophy of posterior arch of atlas; fracture through fused segment.

two or three segments are fused, need to be distinguished from fusions caused by injury, surgery or disease. In congenital synostoses the posterior elements are also fused. The sagittal width of the fused mass is smaller at the level of the obliterated disc (Fig. 15.15a). In acquired fusion the sagittal width at the disc level is greater than that of the adjacent bodies (Fig. 15.15b).

The sagittal width of the spinal canal behind the fused segment is usually normal or greater than normal. Cases have been reported of congenital spinal stenosis associated with the Klippel–Feil syndrome, and the stenosis has been held responsible for increasing the susceptibility to cervical myelopathy (Lee & Weiss, 1981; Prusick *et al.*, 1985). The problem of cervical myelopathy is discussed later, but it is arguable whether congenital spinal stenosis is a true entity. The 'normal' minimum sagittal diameter at C5–C6 is 14 mm (Boijsen, 1954). Measurements below this are held to be abnormal and contributory to myelopathy, but are all deviations from the norm to be regarded as congenital defects?

The intervertebral foramina in the fused segments are smaller and rounder than the normal. It has not been thought that this can constrict the nerve root. Indeed, the absence of radiculopathy in the fused segments has been advanced as an argument against trying to achieve distraction of the bodies and decompression of the foramina in anterior fusion for cervical disc disease. A recent report, however, casts doubt on

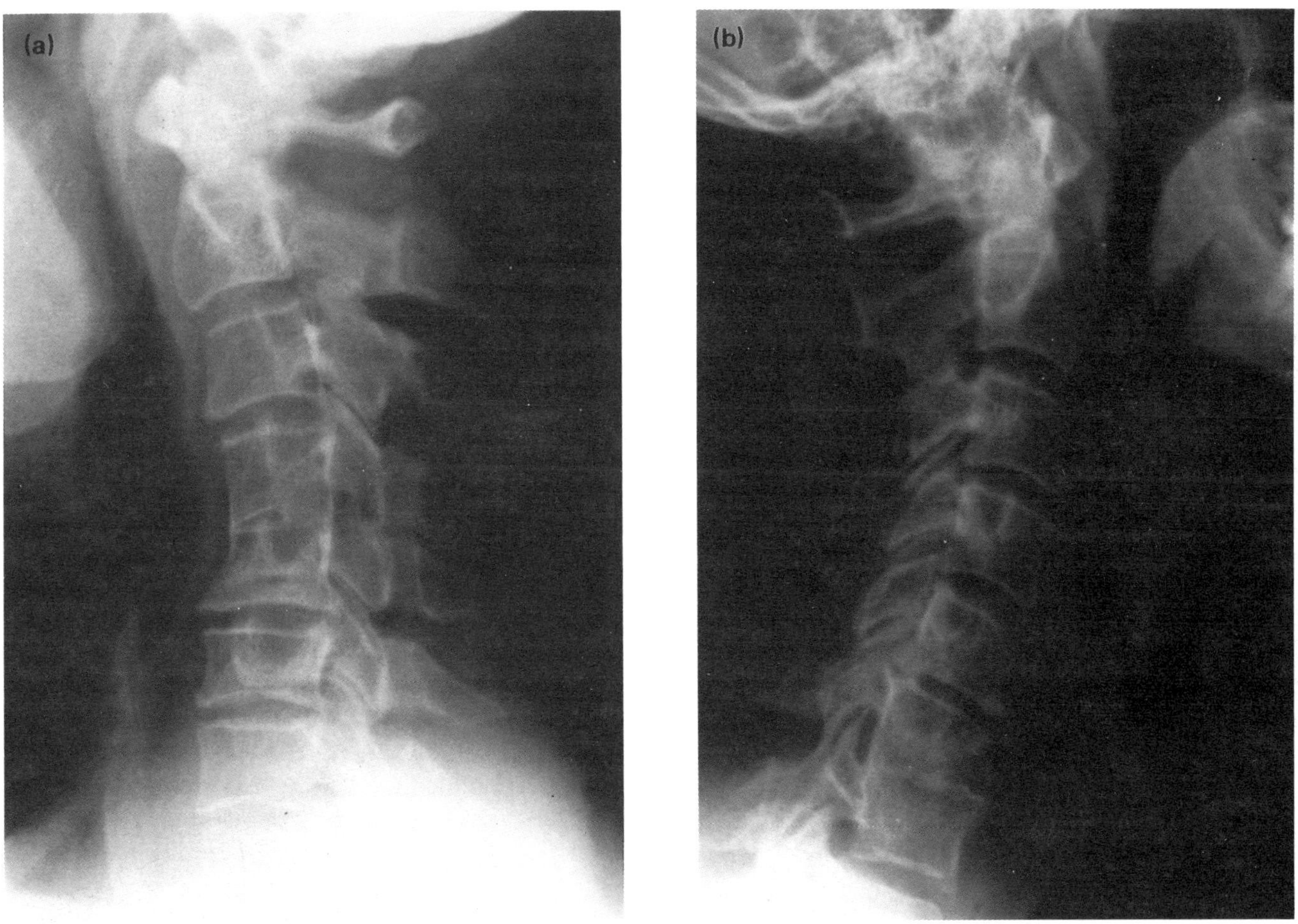

Fig. 15.15 (a) Congenital block vertebrae C4–C5; note 'wasp waist' of fused bodies, and fused posterior elements (b) Acquired fusion of C6–C7 (postinfection); note increased sagittal depth of vertebral bodies at disc space level and separate posterior elements.

this conventional wisdom. A case is described where the sixth cervical root was compromised by a small foramen in a congenitally fused segment (Okada *et al.*, 1988).

When the Klippel–Feil syndrome is recognized it is as well to look for anomalies elsewhere, which are present in the majority of cases. In a memorable phrase the syndrome has been called 'a constellation of associated anomalies' (Hensinger *et al.*, 1974). These other defects can be of other parts of the skeleton, or of other systems. Table 15.2 lists the defects which have been reported. Some of these defects may well be more threatening to the patient's life than the cervical synostosis. In Hensinger's series over half the cases had an associated thoracic scoliosis and over a third had renal abnormality. Every child with a Klippel–Feil syndrome must have radiographs of the whole spine and an intravenous pyelogram.

The scoliosis is usually of the congenital variety and associated with a bony abnormality such as a hemivertebra, but a progressive secondary curve may develop in the apparently normal spine below (Hensinger, 1974). In the treatment of these curves great care must be exercised with distraction methods such as halopelvic traction. Occult neural anomalies of the cervical spine or cranial outlet may be present and traction may produce a neurological defect.

The renal abnormality is most commonly an absent kidney, but other anomalies such as ureteric atresias and reduplications, horseshoe kidneys and hydronephrosis are also found. When one kidney is absent the survivor may be affected by one of these defects, thus making it, and the patient, vulnerable to renal infection.

Most of the other associated anomalies will be obvious on routine clinical examination, or may provide the clinical presentation, when the neck lesion is an incidental finding.

Table 15.2 Reported defects

Skeletal abnormalities	Abnormalities of other systems
Scoliosis	Renal deformities
Congenital high scapula (Sprengel's shoulder)	Cardiovascular anomalies
Webbing of the neck	Enteric cysts
Turner's syndrome (webbing of the neck, gonadal hypoplasia, cubitus valgus)	Deafness
Hemivertebra and spina bifida	Ptosis
Basilar impression	Duane's contracture
Occipitalization of the atlas	Lateral rectus palsy
Hypoplasia of the upper limb	Reduplication of the cord (with synkinesis or mirror movements)
Hypoplasia of the first metacarpal	
Syndactyly	

Management of the Klippel–Feil syndrome

The ugly deformity of the classical clinical triad defies correction. Webbing of skin can be excised, leaving ugly scars, but neck movement will be unchanged. Bilateral upper thoracoplasty has been described, and in the single case so reported, the patient's appearance was improved (Bonola, 1956). It is possible to achieve a 'medical' thoracoplasty. The 'giraffe-necked' women of the Kadang tribe in central Burma obtain their extraordinary appearance by the application of brass rings around the neck, one by one during the years of growth. The effect is produced by depression of the shoulder girdle and upper ribs. The neck itself is, of course, unaffected and remains surprisingly stable when the rings are removed (Roaf, 1961; Jeffreys, 1980).

A Sprengel's shoulder can exaggerate shortness of the neck. The scapula is tethered to the upper cervical spine by a soft tissue band or a bony omovertebral bar. This attachment can be divided and the scapula mobilized downwards, to be held in its new position by fixation to the iliac crest until healing is established (F.G. Allen, personal communication, 1960).

None of these procedures has any effect on neck movement. The fused segment of the spine in itself produces no symptoms other than the rare compression of a nerve root in a small intervertebral foramen. In synostoses short of total, compensatory movement occurs at the junctional segment, and may be of such a degree that the patient is unaware of any stiffness.

Clinical problems can arise at the junctional levels between fixed and mobile segments of the cervical spine. Increased movement at these levels compensates for lack of movement elsewhere, and the changes of disc degeneration may result. Lee and his associates reported a series of radiculopathy and myelopathy following minor trauma or developing without history of injury.

The pathogenesis was thought to be spondylosis

and instability of the junctional segment (Lee & Weiss, 1981). When spinal stenosis coexists with these changes the margin of safety is reduced (Payne & Spillane, 1957; Prusick *et al.*, 1985).

The management of these problems requires fine judgement. It must be remembered that neurological anomalies may coexist with synostosis, and it should not be automatically assumed that the morphological changes seen on radiographs, or with the greater definition of CT are solely responsible for the neurological picture. If it is certain that the spondylotic changes are responsible for the root or cord compression, thorough conservative splinting should be tried. If conservative treatment is unsuccessful, anterior discectomy or decompression followed by anterior fusion is the operation of choice. The neck will be rendered even stiffer as a result, but the alternative of posterior decompression will cause disastrous instability.

Instability at the hypermobile junctional segment can be a greater problem than spondylosis, and Fielding and his associates have drawn particular attention to this (Fielding *et al.*, 1978). They describe three patterns of instability.

Pattern I, fusion of C2 and C3 with occipitalization of the atlas—there is atlanto-axial instability with risk of cord compromise.

Pattern II, extensive subaxial fusion with or without an associated craniovertebral anomaly.

Pattern III, hypermobility at one open junction between two fused segments.

The risk in these patients is that minor trauma can cause neurological lesions of greater severity than would occur if a normal spine were subjected to the same trauma. Elster (1984) reports a case where dislocation with bilateral jumped facets occurred at a mobile segment at C4–C5 between block vertebrae above and below. Permanent tetraplegia followed.

Patients with such identifiable problems of instability are at risk, and as with all patients with potentially hazardous neck lesions, the question of prophylactic stabilization arises. The patient must be made aware of the risks, and should be advised to have the neck fused.

Agenesis of the cervical spine

Hemivertebrae are seen in the cervical spine, usually in association with other anomalies, but true agenesis of five vertebrae has only recently been reported in one case (Nisan *et al.*, 1988). It is interesting to remember that Klippel and Feil described their case as 'absence' of the cervical spine.

Miscellaneous anomalies of the cervical spine

Various anomalies affecting the lower spine are also found in the neck.

SPINA BIFIDA

Spina bifida is a common cervical defect either alone, or in association with other malformation.

SPONDYLOLYSIS OR SPONDYLOLISTHESIS

Failures of fusion between the neural arch and the centrum can be unilateral or bilateral. When the latter exists, forward displacement of the vertebral body can occur, resulting in neurological symptoms from cord compression (Durbin, 1956; Guillane *et al.*, 1976).

CERVICAL DIASTEMATOMYELIA

Diastematomyelia is a condition where the spinal cord is split longitudinally, with a fibrous or bony spur occupying the split. Hemivertebrae and abnormally thickened laminae can be associated. The condition is found predominantly in the lower spine, and very rarely in the cervical spine (James & Lashman, 1972; Okada *et al.*, 1980).

NEUROFIBROMATOSIS

Kyphoscoliosis, vertebral body destruction and enlargement of the intervertebral foramina from 'dumbell' tumours, can all be seen in the cervical spine. The destroyed bone can be replaced by neurofibroma or by undifferentiated fibrous tissue (Heard *et al.*, 1962; Scott, 1965).

MYOSITIS OSSIFICANS PROGRESSIVA

In this condition the longitudinal ligaments, the interspinous ligaments and the ligamentum nuchae are all ossified. There are invariably plaques of ossification elsewhere in the body, and the big toe is small and in valgus (Rosborough, 1967).

REFERENCES

Acheson, E.D. (1986) *Atlantoaxial Instability in People with Down's Syndrome.* DHSS, CMO 86/9.

Ahlback, S. & Collert, S. (1920) Destruction of the odontoid process due to pyogenic osteomyelitis. *Acta Radiol.*, **10**, 394.

American Academy Paediatric Committee On Sports Medicine (1984). Atlantoaxial instability in Down syndrome. *Paediatrics*, **74**, 152.

Arnold, J. (1894) Myelocystele transposition van gewebskeimen und sympodie. *Beitr. Pathol. Anat.*, **16**, 1.

Bharucha, E.P. & Dastur, H.M. (1964) Craniovertebral anomalies. *Brain*, **87**, 469.

Boijsen, E. (1954) The cervical spinal canal in intraspinal expansive processes. *Acta Radiol.*, **42**, 101.

Bonola, A. (1956) Surgical treatment of the Klippel–Feil syndrome. *J. Bone Jt. Surg.*, **38B**, 440.

Burke S.W., French H.G. and Roberts J.M. (1985) Chronic atlantoaxial instability in Down's syndrome. *J. Bone Jt. Surg.*, **67A**, 1356.

Chamberlain, W.E. (1939) Basilar impression (platybasia). *Yale J. Biol. Med.*, **11**, 487.

Chiari, H. (1896) Uber Die Veranderungen Des Kleinhirns Des Und Der Medulla Oblongata. *Denkschr. Akad. Wissench. Wein*, **63**, 71.

Crockard, A. & Ransford, A. (1985) One-stage transoral decompression and posterior stabilisation in cervical myelopathy. *J. Bone Jt. Surg.*, **67B**, 498.

Davidson, R.G. (1988) Atlantoaxial instability in Down's syndrome. *Paediatrics*, **81**, 857.

Durbin, F. (1956) Spondylolisthesis of the cervical spine. *J. Bone Jt. Surg.*, **38B**, 734.

Elster, A.D. (1984) Quadriplegia after minor trauma in the Klippel–Feil syndrome. *J. Bone Jt. Surg.*, **66A**, 1473.

Feil, A.L. (1919) *L'absence et la diminution des vertibres cervicales*. Theses de Paris.

Fielding, J.W. (1965) Disappearance of the central portion of the odontoid process. *J. Bone Jt. Surg.*, **47A**, 1228.

Fielding, J.W. (1973) The cervical spine in the child. *Curr. Pract. Orthop. Surg.*, **5**, 31.

Fielding, J.W. & Griffin, P.P. (1974) Os odontoideum. *J. Bone Jt. Surg.*, **56A**, 187.

Fielding, J.W., Hensinger, R.N. & Hawkins, R.J. (1978) The cervical spine. In Lovell, (ed.) *Paediatric Orthopaedics*, p. 531.

Fielding, J.W., Hensinger, R.N. & Hawkins, R.J. (1980) Os odontoideum. *J. Bone Jt. Surg.*, **62A**, 376.

Finerman, G.A., Sakai, D. & Weingarten, S. (1976) Atlanto-axial dislocation in a Mongoloid child. *J. Bone Jt. Surg.*, **58A**, 408.

Fishgold, H. & Metzger, J. (1952) Etude Radiotomographique De L'Impression Basilaire. *Rev. Rheum.*, **19**, 261.

Freiberger, R.H., Wilson, P.D. & Nicholas, J.A. (1965) Acquired absence of the odontoid process. *J. Bone Jt. Surg.*, **47A**, 1231.

Garber, J.N. (1964) Abnormalities of the atlas and axis. *J. Bone Jt. Surg.*, **46A**, 1782.

Geehr, R.N., Rothman, S.L.G. & Kier, E.L. (1978) The role of C.T. in the evaluation of upper cervical spine pathology. *Comput. Tomogr.*, **2**, 79.

Gillman, C.L. (1959) Congenital absence of the odontoid process. *J. Bone Jt. Surg.*, **41A**, 340.

Guillane, J., Roulleau, J., Fardou, H., Treil, J. & Manelfe, C. (1976) Congenital spondylolysis of cervical vertebrae with spondylolisthesis. *Neuroradiology*, **11**, 159.

Gunderson, C.H., Greensran, R.H., Glaser, G.H. & Lubs, H.A. (1967) Kleippel-Feil syndrome. *Medicine*, **46**, 491

Hadley, L.A. (1956) *The Spine*. Charles C. Thomas, Springfield, IL.

Heard, G., Holt, J.F. & Taylor, B. (1962) Cervical vertebral deformity in von Recklinghausen's disease. *J. Bone Jt. Surg.*, **44B**, 880.

Hensinger, R.N., Lang, J.R. & McEwan, G.D. (1974) The Kleppel–Feil syndrome. *J. Bone Jt. Surg.*, **56A**, 1246.

James, C.C.M. & Lashman, L.P. (1972) *Spinal Dysraphism*. Butterworths, London.

Jeffreys, T.E. (1980) *Disorders of the Cervical Spine*. Butterworths, London, pp. 131, 136.

Klein, R.A., Snyder, R.A. & Schwartz, J.H. (1976) Lateral medullary syndrome in a child. *J. Am. Med. Assoc.*, **253**, 940.

Klippel, M. & Feil, A. (1912) Un cas d'absence des vertibres cervicales avec cage thoracique remontant jusqu'a la Base du Crane. *Nouv. Icon. Salpetriere*, **25**, 223.

Lee, C.K. & Weiss, A.B. (1981) Isolated congenital cervical block vertebrae below the axis with neurological symptoms. *Spine*, **6**, 118.

MacAlister, A. (1892) Notes on the development of the atlas. *J. Anat. Physiol.*, **27**, 519.

McGregor, M. (1948) The significance of certain measurements of the skull. *Br. J. Radiol.*, **21**, 171.

McKeever, F.M. (1968) Atlantoaxial instability. *Surg. Clin. N. Am.*, **48**, 1375.

McRae, D.L. (1953) Bony abnormalities in the region of the foramen magnum. *Acta Radiol.*, **40**, 335.

McRae, D.L. & Barnum, A.S. (1953) Occipitalisation of the atlas. *Am. J. Roentgenol.*, **70**, 23.

Michaels, L., Prevost, M.J. & Crong, D.F. (1969) Pathological changes in a case of os odontoideum. *J. Bone Jt. Surg.*, **51A**, 965.

Michie, I. & Clark, M. (1968) Neurological syndromes associated with cervical and craniocervical anomalies. *Arch. Neurol.*, **18**, 241.

Minderhoud, J.M., Brakman, R. & Penning, L. (1969) Os odontoideum. *J. Neurol. Sci.*, **8**, 521.

Nicholson, J.S. & Sherk, H.H. (1968) Abnormalities of the occipitocervical junction. *J. Bone Jt. Surg.*, **50A**, 295.

Nisan, N., Hiz, M. & Saner, H. (1988) Total agenesis of five cervical vertebrae. *J. Bone Jt. Surg.*, **70B**, 668.

O'Connell, J.E.A. & Turner, J.W.A. (1950) Basilar impression of the skull. *Brain*, **73**, 405.

Okada, K., Hayashi, M., Nitta, M., Owada, T. & Hayashi, H. (1988) Cervical radiculopathy in a congenitally fused segment. *J. Bone Jt. Surg.*, **70**, 1399.

Okada, K., Kagawa, T.F., Yonenobo, K. & Ono, K. (1980) Cervical diastematomyelia with a stable neurological defect. *J. Bone Jt. Surg.*, **68A**, 934.

Payne, E.E. & Spillane, J.D. (1957) The cervical spine: an anatomico-pathological study. *Brain*, **80**, 571.

Prusick, V.R., Samberg, L.C. & Wesolowski, D.P. (1985) Klippel-Feil syndrome associated with spinal stenosis. *J.*

Bone Jt. Surg., **67A**, 161.
Roaf, R. (1961) Giraffe-necked women. *J. Bone Jt. Surg.*, **43B**, 114.
Rosborough, D. (1967) Myositis ossificans progressiva. *J. Bone Jt. Surg.*, **43B**, 485.
Schiff, D.C.M. & Parke, W.W. (1972) Arterial blood supply of the odontoid process. *Anat. Rec.*, **172**, 399.
Scott, J.C. (1965) Scoliosis and neurofibromatosis. *J. Bone Jt. Surg.*, **47B**, 240.
Shepard, C.N. (1966) Familial hypoplasia of the odontoid process. *J. Bone Jt. Surg.*, **48A**, 1224.
Sherk, H.H. & Nicholson, J.T. (1969) Rotatory atlantoaxial dislocation with ossiculum terminale and mongolism. *J. Bone Jt. Surg.*, **51A**, 957.
Sinto, G. & Pandya, S.K. (1968) Treatment of congenital atlantoaxial dislocation. *Proc. Aust. Assoc. Neurol.*, **5**, 507.
Spillane, J.D., Pallis, C. & Jones, A.M. (1957) Developmental abnormalities in the region of the foramen magnum. *Brain*, **80**, 11.
Tredwell, S.S. & O'Brien, J.P. (1975) Avascular necrosis of the proximal end of the dens. *J. Bone Jt. Surg.*, **57A**, 332.
Von Torklus, D. & Gehle, W. (1972) *The Upper Cervical Spine*. Grune & Stratton, New York.
Wadia, N.H. (1967) Myelopathy complicating congenital atlantoaxial dislocation. *Brain*, **90**, 449.
Wallenburg, V.A. (1897) Embolie Der Arterie Cerebellaris Postero-Inferior Sinistra. *Arch. Psychol.*, **27**, 504.
Watson-Jones, R. (1932) Spontaneous hyperaemic dislocation of the atlas. *Proc. R. Soc. Med.*, **25**, 586.
Werne, S. (1957) Studies in spontaneous atlas dislocations. *Acta Orthop. Scand.*, **23**, 1.
Whitesides, T.E. & Pendleton, E.B. (1975) Lateral approach to the upper cervical spine. *J. Bone Jt. Surg.*, **57A**, 1025.
Wynne-Davies, R., Hall, C.M., Howell, C.J., Baker, G.C.E., Crossan, J., Evans, G.A., Fulford, G.E., Smith, M.A. & Witherow, P.J. (1989) *Instability of the Upper Cervical Spine*. Skeletal Dysplasia Group for Teaching and Research, Oxford.

16 · Congenital Sacral Abnormalities

By N.J. TREBLE and R. OWEN

Patients with a congenital abnormality of the sacrum fall into three distinct groups:

1 Those with a quantitative loss of sacral bone which may be transverse, lateral or posterior, and commonly termed 'sacral agenesis'. Often associated with the bony loss are neurological deficit and other congenital abnormalities. As shall be discussed, within this group, recognizable patterns occur.

2 The second group is characterized by a deficiency of the anterior aspect of the sacrum which is generally accompanied by a tumorous mass and abnormalities of the pelvic organs; this is sometimes referred to as the 'Currarino triad'.

3 The most common type consists of minor abnormalities of the shape of the sacrum, for example spina bifida occulta. Whilst these are usually of little or no clinical significance they may be an indicator of significant pathology.

SACRAL AGENESIS

As determination of the lower spine takes place at so fundamental a stage of development any insult leading to a serious congenital abnormality of the sacrum is likely to be incompatible with life; consequently significant congenital abnormalities of the sacrum are rare. Nevertheless, the phenomenon is probably more common than is generally diagnosed as mildly affected cases are often symptom-free while severely afflicted patients may be so extensively handicapped that the sacral anomaly goes unnoticed. The overall incidence of sacral agenesis is reported as being between 0.09 and 0.45% of the general population (Shands & Bundens, 1956; Koontz & Prout, 1968), although in 2707 randomly selected normal individuals Fidas *et al.* (1987) found none.

It is unfortunate that since the first description of major sacral malformation (Hohl, 1852) no generally accepted terminology has been developed. Instead terms such as 'sacral agenesis' and the 'syndrome of caudal regression' have been invoked to describe almost any form of sacral maldevelopment. Those not directly involved in this field may be forgiven for believing that all patients with a deficiency of the sacrum suffer, to a greater or lesser extent, from the same affliction.

As the term sacral agenesis has become entrenched in medical parlance it will be used to describe the situation wherein there is a quantitative lack of sacral bone. It has been shown in large series of patients with sacral agenesis that recognizable patterns of deformity emerge, each with their own particular problems (Stanley *et al.*, 1979; Treble *et al.*, 1988).

Classification

A diagnosis of 'sacral agenesis' without further qualification is little more meaningful than that of 'a broken leg'. The lack of a universally accepted classification of congenital sacral abnormalities results in confusion in the literature and obscures the diversity of what is in fact a range of conditions.

Many classifications of congenital sacral abnormalities have been propounded, some based upon the radiographic appearance of the sacral remnant (Foix & Hillemand, 1924; Durham-Smith, 1959); others on the mechanical consequences of the deformity (Renshaw, 1978). The classification in use at Alder Hey Children's Hospital, Liverpool, is a modification of that of Stanley *et al.* (1979) developed after the analysis of 58 affected patients (Treble *et al.*, 1988). Four types are recognized, based upon the radiographic appearance of the whole spinal column rather than only of the sacrum. While the classification is radiographically based each type demonstrates a discrete clinical picture.

Type Ia, the spinal column terminates abruptly over no more than one level. The vertebrae above this are normal (Fig. 16.1a).

Type Ib, the spinal column terminates abruptly over no more than one level, but there are congenital abnormalities in vertebrae higher in the spine (Fig. 16.1b).

Type II, the terminal segments are deformed, usually represented by hemivertebrae. There will commonly be more proximal abnormalities (Fig. 16.1c).

Type III, the posterior elements of the sacrum are dysraphic (Fig. 16.1d).

This classification is an empirical one, arrived at after the analysis of observed patterns of deformity. It has proved possible to correlate these patterns with events in the early stages of embryogenesis to produce a theory which explains how each type might come about. It is necessary, however, to understand the clinical features associated with each type to fully appreciate the abnormal embryological process.

Characteristic features

A patient with sacral agenesis is liable to suffer as a consequence of one or more of the following:

1 neurological deficiency,

2 congenital abnormalities in other systems,

3 mechanical instability of the spino-pelvic articulation.

The severity of each varies according to the type of sacral agenesis.

While all the above might be confidently predicted in the light of the vertebral malformation, certain unexpected phenomena also occur which deserve special mention.

In most examples of congenital spinal malformation it is usually safe to assume that the level of skeletal abnormality will reflect the level of neurological compromise. In certain types of congenital sacral, or indeed lumbosacral, agenesis a paradox occurs. While the motor deficit correlates with the bony deficit, there may be extensive preservation of sensory function (Franz & Aitken, 1967; Ignelz & Lehman, 1974). So despite being totally paralysed from the waist down skin sensation and proprioception may be retained down to and including the feet.

Urological problems may arise even in the presence of clinically normal sacral outflow. They may result as a primary deformity due to a failure in the differentiation of the somites leading to gross quantitative lesions such as the absence of a kidney, or as a renal dysplasia either primary or secondary to intra-uterine disease. Urological problems also occur secondary to obstruction or some dynamic problem affecting the renal tract (Wilcock & Emery, 1970). Often an extremely damaging combination of these effects is found.

When the usual clinical signs of reduced bladder innervation are not demonstrated, the danger is of delayed diagnosis and treatment of outflow obstruction with the consequent potential for irreversible upper tract damage (Borrelli *et al.*, 1985). Typical is a series reported by Mariani *et al.* (1979); of 11 patients, 10 presented with orthopaedic problems, yet investigation revealed all 11 to require urological attention.

Any patient shown to have one congenital abnormality must be suspected of harbouring further abnormalities elsewhere. Paradoxically, while this is often so in sacral agenesis, in some types the malformation is isolated.

The three phenomena which may be regarded as typical of sacral agenesis are sensory sparing, neurogenic bladder dysfunction and concomitant congenital abnormalities. While these features affect the group as a whole, Table 16.1 shows that different types manifest differing combinations of these features. Apart from these features this group of patients also demonstrate the effects of neurological deficiency often leading to lower limb deformity and problems of chronic constipation, both of which may be compounded by true developmental abnormalities.

It will be appreciated that such patients are often severely handicapped. However, in contrast to spina bifida sufferers, intellectual capacity is rarely impaired.

Aetiology

To explain the various patterns of sacral agenesis the normal process of embryogenesis and how it might be disrupted must be reviewed (see Chapter 2).

The notochord and the primitive knot from which it arises are the *primary organizers*, so called because they are the first tissues to release chemical evocators

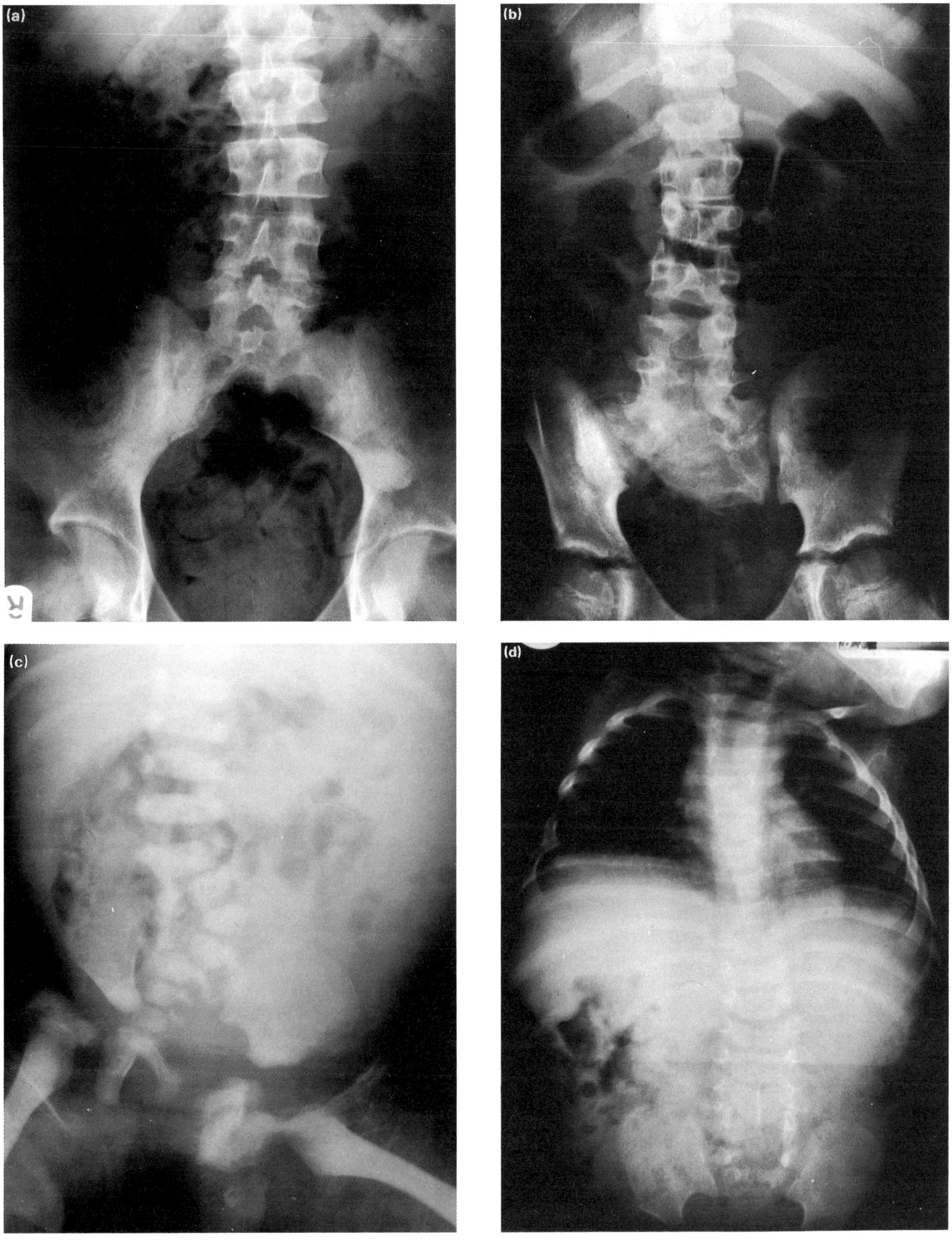

Fig. 16.1 The four types of sacral agenesis: (a) Type Ia; (b) Type Ib; (c) Type II; (d) Type III.

Table 16.1 Liverpool classification of congenital sacral anomalies

Type	Neurological function	Bladder innervation	Other malformations
Type Ia	Motor: corresponds to level of lesion; sensory; often spared	Often impaired despite apparently normal neurology	Very rare
Type Ib	Motor: corresponds to level of lesion; sensory; often spared	Often impaired despite apparently normal neurology	Common
Type II	Corresponds to level of defect	Corresponds to clinical assessment	Common
Type III	Corresponds to level of defect	Corresponds to clinical assessment	Not uncommon

which act on nearby cells inducing them to begin differentiation into their appropriate organs. Having received their organizing influence cells are said to be *determined*, and even if the evocator is withdrawn differentiation will continue. Certain tissues will later adopt the role of secondary organizers, and in turn influence their neighbouring cells.

As the neural groove enfolds to become the neural tube, groups of cells termed the neural crest cells, become separate from the margin of the groove. These cells will develop into the sensory and autonomic systems, while the rest of the spinal cord will arise from the neural tube. It has been shown that the notochord acts as the organizer to the vertebral bodies and the neural tube serves this function for the posterior bony elements (Holzer, 1963). By contrast the neural crest has no organizing capacity.

If a teratogenic insult were to occur soon after the notochord developed from the primitive knot, and to be so mild that it merely interrupted the organizing action of the notochord, the terminal neural crest cells, being already determined, would continue to produce sensory and autonomic elements. However, the failure of the notochordal organizing action would produce failure of the development of the neural tube and vertebral bodies, whilst in turn the absence of the organizing action of the neural tube would lead to failure of development of the posterior bony arches. After a sufficiently brief insult the inductive action of the notochord would resume stimulation of the differentiation of the more cephalad elements, and general organogenesis would continue normally. The effect of such a brief insult would be the loss of entire distal vertebral segments with their corresponding motor elements, but with preservation of sensory function. Moreover, the spinal column above the agenetic segments would develop normally, as would other organs. The resulting fetus would have the characteristics of the Type Ia patient. Cadaveric studies of this type of patient have demonstrated sensory nerve fibres running from the truncated cord to reach their destination often after crossing and recrossing the midline (Durham-Smith, 1959; Anderton & Owen, 1983).

An early insult which abates somewhat more slowly, while having a similar effect on the distal segments, would linger long enough to affect more proximal spinal development as well as the development of other organs which by now has begun, resulting in the picture of the Type Ib patient.

A more severe insult taking place somewhat later in development, after the cartilaginous vertebral anlagen are laid down, might be expected to lead to their disrupted development causing such abnormalities as errors of segmentation and the formation of hemivertebrae. The more severe insult would also upset the developing cord and general organogenesis which is now well under way. The consequence would be the Type II patient.

Type III patients probably arise following an insult later in pregnancy. The effect is on a spinal column which is already largely formed, and the result might be dysraphism and neural damage corresponding to the bony defect. Organogenesis is by now largely complete, so other congenital abnormalities would be relatively uncommon (Fig. 16.2).

This theory is based upon the consideration of the timing of an insult, not of its nature. Yet maternal

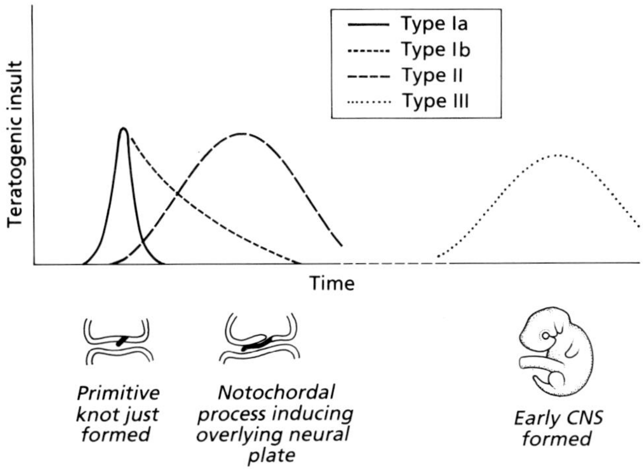

Fig. 16.2 A schematic representation of the temporal relationship between a teratogenic insult and pattern of sacral agenesis.

diabetes, the single most commonly reported aetiological factor in sacral agenesis, may produce the brief insult postulated in Type I cases. The most likely teratogen is an episode of hyperglycaemia, which may be brought about by the detrimental effect of pregnancy on diabetic control perhaps even before the mother is aware of being pregnant.

A multiplicity of agents have been shown in a variety of animal models to be capable of producing anomalies characterized by caudal deficiency or rumplessness; for example trypan blue (Gillman *et al.*, 1948; Beck & Lloyd, 1963; Iwai, 1989), vitamin A (Cohlan, 1954), insulin (Duraiswami, 1950), trauma (Duhamel, 1961) and particularly diabetes (Blumel *et al.*, 1959; Pedersen *et al.*, 1964; Passarge & Lenz, 1966). Moreover, it has been shown that the condition of rumplessness may be inherited as a recessive trait in certain species (Dunn & Landauer, 1934; Chelsey, 1935). More recently it has been concluded that there may be a disturbance of the levels of certain trace elements, primarily zinc (Eriksson & Styrud, 1985).

That particular agents have been shown to produce a given abnormality in laboratory animals must, of course, be viewed very much in the context in which the experiments were conducted, and cannot be directly extrapolated to humans, in whom the majority of cases would appear to arise spontaneously. Nevertheless, the finding that as many as 16% of these children are born to diabetic mothers (Blumel *et al.*, 1959) spawned much research into the identification of those aspects of diabetes which might be responsible for producing fetal malformation. It seems that hyperglycaemia and hyperketonaemia are the most likely teratogens acting either alone or together on a fetus which must already be genetically susceptible (Baker *et al.*, 1981; Welch & Aterman, 1984; Eriksson & Styrud, 1985). The strict control of the diabetic state in the early weeks of pregnancy can do much to reduce the incidence of abnormal offspring.

Congenital sacral abnormality arising as a familial trait has been reported (Cohn & Bay-Nielsen, 1969; Klenerman & Merrick, 1973; Kenefick, 1973; Paris & Laine, 1973; Pierson *et al.*, 1985) but these are isolated cases or small pedigrees and should not be regarded as typical.

As with most human congenital malformations the aetiology of an individual case of sacral agenesis will usually be a matter of conjecture based upon a reflective analysis of events during pregnancy.

Management

Orthopaedic problems

Without motor innervation, embryonic myotubes fail to differentiate into muscle tissue (Rusnak & Driscoll, 1965; Price *et al.*, 1970). Instead, in denervated areas it is common for muscle tissue to be represented by fibrous anlagen. With growth this tissue behaves in a most pernicious way, forming unyielding tethers across joints which result in severe progressive contractures. Soft tissue release of deformed joints is particularly unrewarding as the deformity can be relied upon to recur with further growth.

Lower limb or foot deformity is the usual cause for orthopaedic presentation. In many cases deformity is secondary to neuromuscular deficit, although it is not unusual for there to be true developmental malformations.

Whatever the type of sacral agenesis, before embarking upon treatment it is important that realistic goals are set and discussed. Depending upon the severity of the disability, such goals may vary from the correction of a cosmetically unacceptable toe to the removal of both legs. A radical approach is often called for but, as with all difficult problems in medicine, the management of lower limb deformity enjoys no consensus of opinion. In fact the more proximal the problem, the more the disagreement intensifies.

In Types II and III, lower limb deformity is essentially no different from that encountered in typical spina bifida. The extent of the problem depends upon the neurological deficit, which in these groups is both sensory and motor. Progression of deformity is common in the presence of muscle imbalance and is complicated by reduced sensory perception rendering skin vulnerable to trophic and neuropathic ulceration. Treatment is aimed at retaining normal anatomy by splintage and tendon transfer in younger children, but with recourse where necessary to bony surgery after the age of eight years.

In Type I patients the likelihood that there will be some degree of preservation of sensation must be taken into account when planning a regime of management. Foot deformities are particularly common. When these are due to neuromuscular imbalance, as is usually the case, conservative techniques offer no more than a temporizing measure. Surgery, by soft tissue rebalancing or bony corrections, is usually required. The knee usually adopts an attitude of severe fixed flexion with marked webbing in the popliteal fossa (Fig. 16.3). Some success has been claimed for early posterior release followed by gradual correction to avoid neurovascular compromise (Dal Monte *et al.*, 1979). Unfortunately recurrence is common, which might be overcome only by combined distal femoral and proximal tibial osteotomy. Bone shortening may be required in order to achieve correction.

The hips are also often the site of fixed flexion contracture. Moreover, in a proportion of cases when the level of the neurological defect is such that the flexors are unnopposed, dislocation is not uncommon. The approach to hip problems arouses considerable controversy. On the one hand, in view of the obstinate nature of the contractures in the presence of such dense paralysis, some authorities recommend subtrochanteric amputation (Franz & Aitken, 1967). A pelvithoracic bearing orthosis is then fitted, in which a swing-to or even swing-through gait may be achieved. On the other hand, the phenomenon of sensory sparing excites strong argument against this approach. The consequences of intact sensory perception are threefold. The skin is not liable to break down, proprioception is maintained and body image extends to include the paralysed legs. With this in mind Phillips *et al.* (1982) recommended retention of the femora with through-knee disarticulation. They have found that retained femoral length provides a wider sitting base, allows the use of smaller prostheses and transfer to a chair is easier. Others favour no surgery at all in severe degrees of the condition as the deformed, externally rotated legs act as a stable base for sitting.

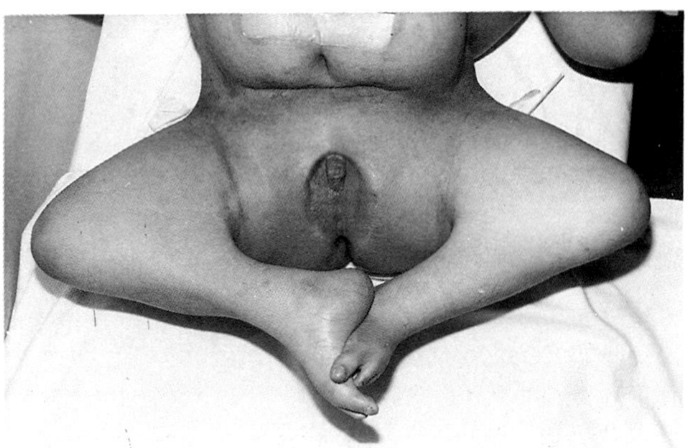

Fig. 16.3 Typical lower limb deformity in sacral agenesis.

The spine itself only rarely requires attention. A proportion of cases will develop a spinal deformity in the thoracic or lumbar regions which may be either of the congenital type with segmental defects or not uncommonly an apparently 'idiopathic' scoliosis.

In most cases the sacral deficit occurs beyond the sacroiliac articulation so that spinopelvic stability is maintained. However, when the agenesis involves the entire sacrum, and even the lower lumbar segments, an unstable situation arises. In that case two opposite views pertain. While some advocate fusion of the lowermost vertebra to the pelvis in order to improve sitting balance, prevent visceral compression and allow the stretching of hip contractures (Perry *et al.*, 1970; Parry *et al.*, 1980; Mayfield *et al.*, 1981), others argue that there is little to be gained by this approach and much to lose (Andrisch *et al.*, 1979; Phillips *et al.*, 1982). Phillips *et al.* report a series of 19 patients with unstable spinopelvic pseudarthroses, of whom 17 were able to sit; they go on to quote three cases in their fourth to seventh decades who were well, and who showed no evidence of visceral compression. As regards the hip flexion contracture, as long as the pelvis remains mobile this presents no problem, but if it is fused to the spine the patient can no longer sit unless the legs are amputated (Fig. 16.4). It is self-evident then that each treatment philosophy carries its own drawbacks. Hence the importance of open discussion with the patient, family and management team.

It must be emphasized that much of the foregoing relates to the severely affected individual, and that

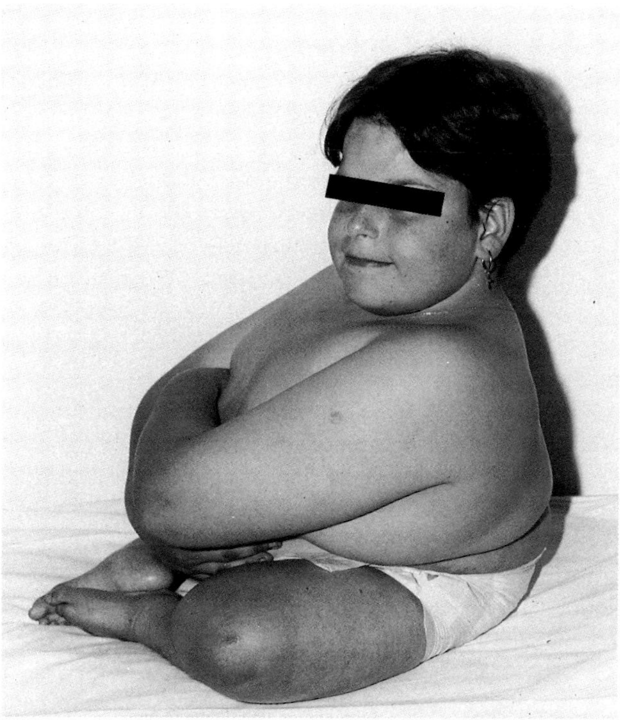

Fig. 16.4 A stable sitting position despite lumbosacral agenesis and hip and knee flexion contractures.

such examples are the exception rather than the rule. The majority of cases requiring orthopaedic attention will have little more than minor deformities and can expect to lead a normal active life.

Urological problems

Although initial presentation of this condition is usually with an orthopaedic complaint considerable morbidity and indeed mortality may arise as a result of urinary problems (Mariani *et al.*, 1979; Borrelli *et al.*, 1985). When there is impairment of sacral outflow from segments S2, S3 and S4, the lower urinary tract is left partially or completely denervated. The pattern and degree of denervation is variable, and upon this depends the resultant malfunction. This may range from normality through slight incontinence to chronic retention with secondary obstructive nephropathy. Today, providing therapy is commenced in good time, modern urological methods can usually be relied upon to render affected sufferers continent and to prevent secondary changes in the upper renal tract (Guzman *et al.*, 1983). Because of this it is of the utmost importance to establish both the presence of urological malfunction and the pattern of denervation.

Both upper and lower motor neurone lesions have been shown to occur in association with sacral agenesis. It must also be realized that the pattern of denervation may change with the passage of time (Koff & Deridder, 1977). Repeated urodynamic analysis of bladder function will reveal such progression and will prompt further investigation.

As previously mentioned, the normal clinical parameters by which sacral outflow is assessed, while helpful in Types II and III, are of poor predictive value when dealing with Type I patients. A high index of suspicion is necessary when dealing with these patients and, if there is the slightest doubt regarding urinary function, specialist attention is mandatory. The literature contains many cases in whom, even at the time of initial urological assessment, irreversible renal damage had already taken place (Thompson *et al.*, 1974; Lebowitz, 1975).

Neurological problems

Whilst sacral agenesis of all types is clearly due to a developmental error, it is a mistake to regard the neurological deficit as being due to a developmental failure, and as such neither amenable to treatment nor progressive. Koff & Deridder (1977) demonstrated neurophysiological findings which changed with time. Pang & Hoffman (1980) reported two cases with progressive neurological findings in whom surgically remediable cauda equina lesions were found. Brooks *et al.* (1981) found that two types of lesion may occur, and that surgery was consistently rewarded by clinical improvement. These were, firstly, a high termination of the subarachnoid space with associated stenosis of the dural tube; and secondly those with features classically associated with spinal dysraphism, e.g. tethered cord, meningocele and congenital tumours.

Investigation of these patients may be with contrast myelography (Brooks *et al.*, 1981), computerized tomography, which is claimed to be as good as or better than myelography (Cerisoli *et al.*, 1983; Shirkhoda *et al.*, 1984) or by magnetic resonance imaging (Brunberg *et al.*, 1988).

The potential for deterioration of neurological function calls for accurate and repeated documentation and further investigation to exclude any remediable condition should there be evidence of progression.

Associated congenital abnormalities

Type Ib, Type II and to a lesser extent Type III patients are particularly liable to exhibit congenital abnormalities in other systems, in particular cardiovascular and gastrointestinal. Many of these will be self-evident but others will only come to light if sought. When managing a patient in one of these categories particular attention must be paid to this.

The most common congenital anomalies involving the gut are imperforate anus and oesophageal atresia, which should be dealt with along accepted lines. As well as suffering true developmental abnormalities all patients, including Type Ia, are prone to functional bowel disturbance with soiling and chronic constipation. While demoralizing, such problems do not have the dire consequences of urinary malfunction; indeed with laxatives and enemas the situation can generally be improved.

It is clear that patients with sacral agenesis are burdened with a wide range of problems. Their management demands the attention of specialists from many disciplines, both medical and paramedical. In order to provide the total care required a team approach must be adopted; comprising orthopaedic surgeon, neurologist/neurosurgeon, urologist, psychologist, nurses, physiotherapists and social worker. The team should be under the overall coordination of one particular practitioner, usually a paediatrician.

By anticipating and treating the conditions suffered by these multiply-handicapped individuals their lot can be made very much more tolerable.

SACRAL MENINGOCELE

In 1969 Cohn & Bay-Nielson reported six related females with sacral defects and anterior sacral meningocele. Kenefick (1973) reported a similar phenomenon which he regarded as hereditary sacral agenesis. While Paris & Laine (1973) were the first to report associated anorectal abnormalities, it is Currarino *et al.* (1981), following their report of three cases and a review of the literature, to whom the honour of eponymous recognition of the triad is accorded by subsequent authors. The 'Currarino triad' comprises:

1 anorectal or urogenital malformation, which may range from minor anal stenosis to rectal atresia;
2 anterior sacral defect, ranging from a minimal 'notch' defect in the sacrum to a major loss leaving what has been termed the 'scimitar' sacrum (Fig. 16.5);
3 a presacral tumour that has been variously reported as meningocele, teratoma or dermoid cyst (Figs 16.6 & 16.7).

Early reports noted a hereditary tendency in this syndrome with some 50% of cases being inherited. Most cases occur in females, a fact which Kofinas *et al.* (1987) felt was explained by the tendency for cases to present during pregnancy. They observed that cases presenting before or after the reproductive years show no such sex predilection.

The embryogenesis of the triad is not beyond doubt, but Currarino postulated adhesions or a fistula between the endoderm of the hindgut and the neurectoderm. Such a connection could displace the notochord or cause it to split, resulting in a failure of anterior closure of the vertebrae. The cells of the fusion are variably resorbed to leave elements which

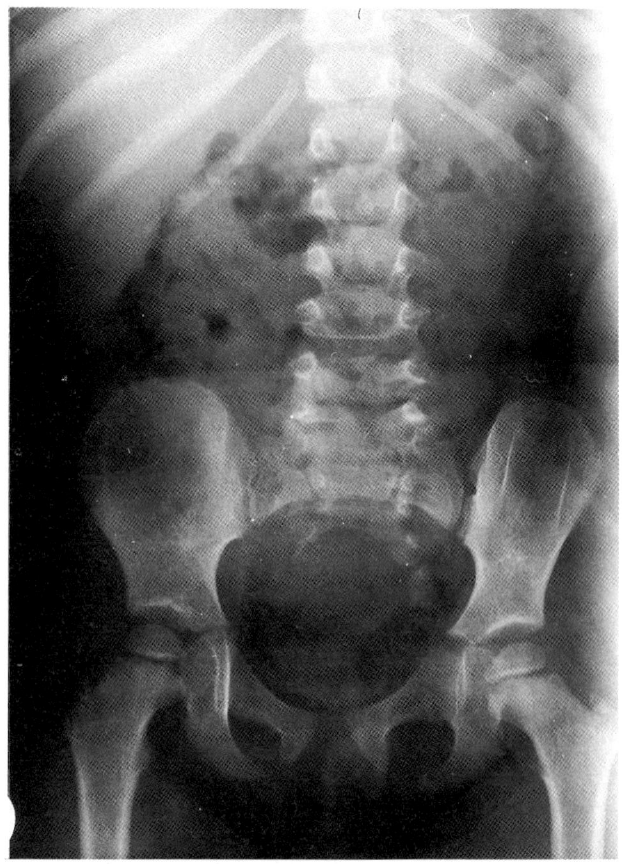

Fig. 16.5 The 'Currarino triad'. Large defect in the anterior wall of sacrum.

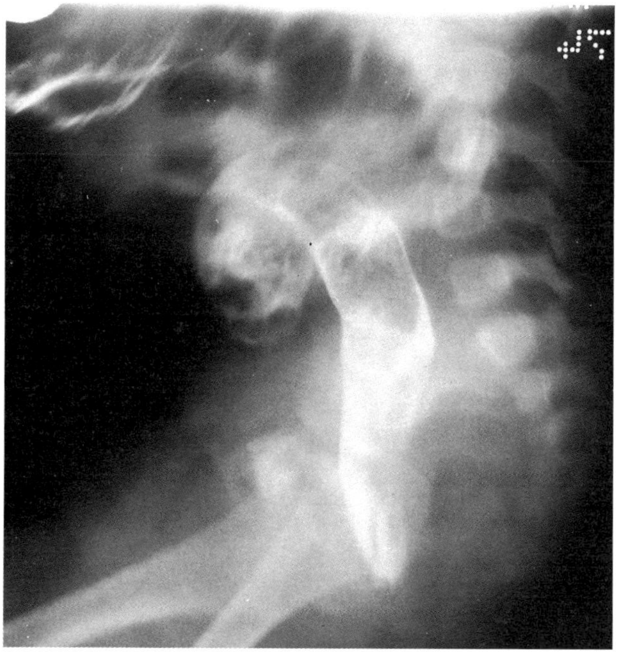

Fig. 16.6 The 'Currarino triad'. Barium enema showing anterior displacement of rectum by presacral mass.

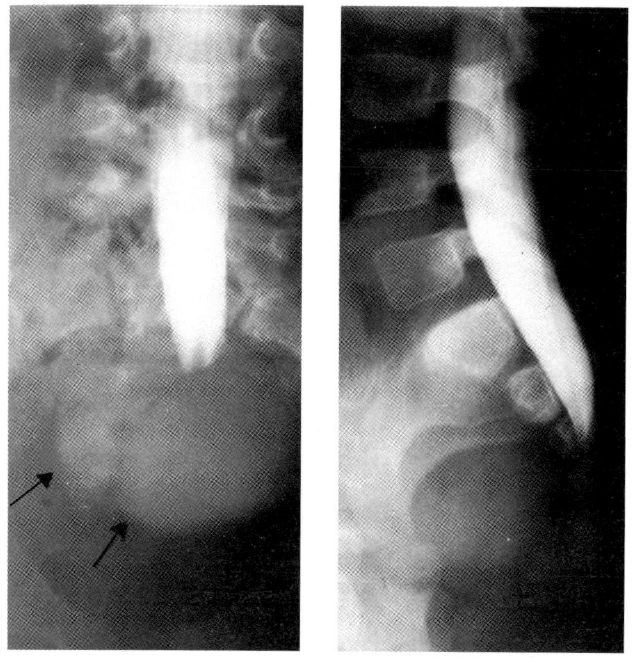

Fig. 16.7 The 'Currarino triad'. Contrast from myelogram fills the presacral mass confirming it to be myelocele.

may form either a meningocele, an enteric cyst or other mass depending upon the tissue remnant.

The syndrome may present in childhood with chronic constipation, or infection of the tumour or meninges. Later diagnosis is usually by the gynaecologist, who notes genital abnormalities, the pelvic tumour or dystocia during delivery. Management depends upon the presenting complaint. The bony sacral defect itself requires no intervention, chronic constipation and anorectal problems present no unique difficulties and should be managed along accepted lines for such conditions.

The optimal treatment of the presacral tumour is not agreed. If left alone, owing to the potential or actual communication between the tumour, the bowel and the meninges, there is a risk of life-threatening infection. This may take the form of a pelvic abscess within the tumour or ascending meningitis. In view of this risk, and because of the small but real possibility of malignant change in a teratoma (Holthusen *et al.*, 1985), most authors recommend surgical resection (Holthusen *et al.*, 1985; Duthel *et al.*, 1988). However, before finally deciding upon surgery a degree of caution is advised because the risks of postoperative infection are high. Furthermore the surgery is difficult, as the intimate embryonic connections between the tumour and adjacent organs obviate any plane of cleavage. Duthel *et al.* (1988) advocated a transsacral approach, which they found easy, and for which they report good results.

When the tumour first presents during pregnancy it should not be interfered with until after delivery. Instead planned Caesarian section should be undertaken (Kofinas *et al.*, 1987) and later resection performed. On no account must a meningocele be aspirated, as out of 11 cases so treated 10 died of meningitis (Amacher *et al.*, 1968).

MINOR QUALITATIVE ABNORMALITIES OF THE SACRUM

The sacrum is often the seat of perhaps less significant, but more common, congenital anomalies. These are usually of no clinical significance but are occasionally what brings the suffering patient to the back clinic.

Failures of segmentation

Of all the intervertebral joints the lumbosacral articulation is the most frequently involved in abnormalities of segmentation. It is not uncommon for there to be complete lumbarization of S1 or complete sacralization of L5. Providing the abnormality is bilaterally symmetrical the finding is generally an asymptomatic chance finding. The main significance of the anomaly lies in the potential difficulties encountered in the identification of the correct level for lumbar spine surgery.

Occasionally there is a unilateral fusion, usually between the transverse process of the lowermost lumbar vertebra and the ala of the sacrum constituting what is termed a transitional vertebra. When symptomatic such a phenomenon is said to cause pain beginning typically at the age of about 20 years. Why a transitional vertebra should cause pain is not clear, but it has been variously attributed to osteoarthritis of the abnormal articulation or to stretching of the nerve roots. The intervertebral discs above the transitional vertebra are particularly prone to degeneration and prolapse (Castellvi *et al.*, 1984; Avrahami *et al.*, 1986).

Spina bifida occulta

Spina bifida occulta (SBO) is so common as to be regarded as a variant of normal development. Fidas *et al.* (1987) found abnormalities of the posterior arches in 23% of a large randomly selected normal population; the incidence in males was twice that in females, and higher in younger than in older adults. The commonest site was S1 alone or S1 and S2 together; it was also noted that where SBO was present the opening of the sacral canal was higher. They identified four radiological patterns of SBO but ascribed no clinical significance to this.

While SBO would seem to be an entirely benign finding this may not always be the case. In 138 patients with urological symptoms attending an incontinence clinic, the prevalence of SBO was significantly higher than in the normal population (Fidas *et al.*, 1989). However, as no correlation could be found between any particular neurophysiological abnormality and sacral SBO they concluded that the relationship is not causal, but rather that there must be a common aetiological factor. Galloway & Tainsch (1985) also reported abnormal neurophysiological findings in patients with SBO and urinary incontinence, concluding that SBO of the upper sacral segments is a useful marker of abnormal sacral neurogenesis in this group of patients.

Facet joint abnormalities

The plane of articulation between the facet joints at the lumbosacral junction is normally both vertical and sagittal. In an anatomical study Brailsford (1929) found that in 57% the fifth lumbar facets faced backwards, in 12% medially and in 31% in different directions on each side. When the two face in different directions the abnormality has been incriminated as a cause of low back pain, possibly due to abnormality of movement.

Spondylolisthesis

Spondylolisthesis is in most cases due to an abnormality of the fifth lumbar vertebra. However in the congenital variety there are undoubted changes in the sacrum itself. More common in females, the sacral facets are hypoplastic and horizontally disposed, while the upper surface of the centrum on lateral projection is seen to be deficient anteriorly. This combination of anomalies allows the lumbar spine to slip forwards on the sacrum. The subject of spondylolisthesis is fully discussed in Chapter 43.

REFERENCES

Square brackets indicate article titles translated to English for ease of reference.

Amacher, A.L., Drake, C.G. & McLachlin, A.D. (1968) Anterior sacral meningocele. *Surg. Gynecol. Obstet.*, **126**, 986–994.

Anderton, J.M. & Owen, R. (1983) Absence of the pituitary gland in a case of congenital sacral agenesis. *J. Bone Jt. Surg.*, **65B**, 182–183.

Andrisch, J., Kalarnchi, A. & MacEwen, G.D. (1979) Sacral agenesis; a clinical evaluation of its management, heredity and associated problems. *Clin. Orthop.*, **139**, 52–57.

Avrahami, E., Cohn, D.F. & Yaron, M. (1986) Computerised tomography, clinical and X-ray correlations in the hemisacralised fifth lumbar vertebra. *Clin. Rheumatol.*, **5**, 332–337.

Baker, L., Egler, J.M., Klein, S.H. & Goldman, A.S. (1981) Meticulous control of diabetes during organogenesis prevents congenital lumbo-sacral defects in rats. *Diabetes*, **11**, 955–999.

Beck, F. & Lloyd, J.B. (1963) An investigation of the relationship between foetal death and foetal malformation. *J. Anat.*, **97**, 555–564.

Blumel, J., Evans, E.B. & Eggars, E.W.N. (1959) Partial and complete agenesis or malformation of the sacrum and associated anomalies. *J. Bone Jt. Surg.*, **41A**, 497–518.

Borrelli, M., Bruschini, H., Nahas, W.C., Figueiredo, J.A., Prado, M.J., Spinola, R., Walligora, M., Freire, G.C. & deGoes, G.M. (1985) Sacral agenesis: why is it so frequently misdiagnosed? *Urology*, **26**, 351–355.

Brailsford, J.F. (1929) *Br. J. Surg.*, **16**, 562.

Brooks, B.S., Gammal, T.E., Hartlage, P. & Beveridge, W. (1981) Myelography of sacral agenesis. *Am. J. Neuroradiol.*, **2**, 319–323.

Brunberg, J.A., Latchaw, R.E., Kanal, E., Burk, D.L. & Albright, L. (1988) Magnetic resonance imaging of spinal dysraphism. *Radiol. Clin. N. Am.*, **26**, 181–205.

Castellvi, A.E., Goldstein, L.A. & Chan, D.P. (1984) Lumbosacral transitional vertebrae and their relationship with lumbar extradural defects. *Spine*, **9**, 493–495.

Cerisoli, M., Davidovits, P. & Giulioni, M. (1983) Sacral agenesis: usefulness of CT study. *J. Neurosurg. Sci.*, **27**, 261–264.

Chelsey, P. (1935) Development of the short-tailed mutant in the house mouse. *J. Exp. Zool.*, **70**, 429–434.

Cohlan, S.Q. (1954) Congenital anomalies in the rat produced by excessive intake of vitamin A during pregnancy. *Pediatrics*, **13**, 556–567.

Cohn, J. & Bay-Nielsen, E. (1969) Hereditary defects of the sacrum and coccyx with anterior sacral meningocele. *Acta Paediatr. Scand.*, **58**, 268–274.

Currarino, G., Coln, D. & Votteler, T. (1981) Triad of anorectal sacral and presacral anomalies. *Am. J. Radiol.*, **137**, 395–398.

Dal Monte, A., Andrisano, A. & Capanna, R. (1979) The treatment of lumbo-sacral coccygeal agenesis. *Ital. J. Orthop. Traumatol.*, **5**, 259–266.

Duhamel, B. (1961) From the mermaid to anal imperforation; the syndrome of caudal regression. *Arch. Dis. Child.*, **36**, 152–155.

Dunn, L.C. & Landauer, W. (1934) The genetics of the rumpless fowl with evidence of a case of changing dominance. *J. Genet.*, **29**, 217–243.

Duraiswami, P.K. (1950) Insulin induced skeletal abnormalities in developing chickens. *Br. Med. J.*, **2**, 384–390.

Durham-Smith, E. (1959) Congenital sacral abnormalities in children. *Aust. N.Z. J. Surg.*, **29**, 165–176.

Duthel, R., Charret, M.C., Huppert, J., Deluzarches, P., Motuo-Fotso, M.J. & Barral, F. (1988) [Anterior sacral meningocele. Apropos of 11 cases]. *Neurochirugie*, **34**, 90–96.

Eriksson, U.J. & Styrud, J. (1985) Congenital malformation in diabetic pregnancy; the clinical relevance of experimental animal studies. *Acta Paediatr. Scand.* (Suppl.), **320**, 72–78.

Fidas, A., Macdonald, H.L., Elton, R.A., Wild, S.R., Chisholm, G.D. & Scott, R. (1987) Prevalence and patterns of spina bifida occulta in 2707 normal adults. *Clin. Radiol.*, **38**, 537–542.

Fidas, A., Macdonald, H.L., Elton, R.A., McInnes, A., Wild, S.R. & Chisholm, G.D. (1989) Prevalence of spina bifida occulta in patients with functional disorders of the lower urinary tract and its relation to urodynamic and neurophysiological measurements. *Br. Med. J.*, **298**, 357–359.

Foix, C. & Hillemand, P. (1924) Dystrophie cruro-vésicofessière par agénésie sacro-coccygienne. *Rev. Neurol.*, **31**, 450–468.

Franz, C.H. & Aitken, G.T. (1967) Complete absence of the lumbar spine and sacrum. *J. Bone Jt. Surg.*, **49A**, 1531–1540.

Galloway, N.T. & Tainsch, J. (1985) Minor defects of the sacrum and neurogenic bladder dysfunction. *Br. J. Urol.*, **57**, 154–155.

Gillman, J., Gilbert, T., Gillman, T. & Spence, I. (1948) A preliminary report on hydrocephalus, spina bifida and other congenital anomalies in the rat produced by trypan blue. *S. Afr. J. Med. Sci.*, **13**, 47–90.

Guzman, L., Bauer, S.B., Hallett, M., Khoshbin, S., Colodny, A.H. & Retik, A.B. (1983) Evaluation and management of children with sacral agenesis. *Urology*, **22**, 506–510.

Hohl, A.F. (1852) *Zur Pathologie des becken.* I: *Das Schräg-oval Becken.* Wilhelm Engelmann, Leipzig, p. 61.

Holthusen, W., Birtel, T., Brinkmann, B., Gunkel, J., Janneck, C. & Richter, E. (1985) [The Currarino triad. An autosomal dominant inherited complex of anorectal malformation, sacrococcygeal defects and presacral tumor. Observation of 9 further cases]. *ROFO*, **143**, 80–83.

Holzer, H. (1963) Comments on induction during cell differentiation. *Unduktion und Morphogenese*, Springer, Berlin.

Ignelz, R.J. & Lehman, R.A.W. (1974) Lumbo-sacral agenesis: management and embryological implications. *J. Neurol. Neurosurg. Psychiatry*, **37**, 1273–1276.

Iwai, K. (1989) [Studies on experimentally induced malformations of the spine and spinal cord; neuropathology of lumbosacral agenesis]. *Nippon Seikeigeka Gakkai Zasshi*, **63**, 116–130.

Kenefick, J.S. (1973) Hereditary sacral agenesis associated with presacral tumours. *Br. J. Surg.*, **60**, 271–274.

Klenermen, L. & Merrick, M.V. (1973) Anterior sacral meningocoele occurring in a family. *J. Bone Jt. Surg.*, **55B**, 331–334.

Koff, S.A. & Deridder, P.D. (1977) Patterns of neurogenic bladder dysfunction in sacral agenesis. *J. Urol.*, **118**, 87–89.

Kofinas, A.D., Hatjis, C.G., Ernest, J.M. & Parker, R.L. Jr. (1987) Anterior sacral meningocele in pregnancy. *Obstet. Gynecol.*, **69**, 441–444.

Koontz, W.W. & Prout, G.R. (1968) Agenesis of the sacrum and the neurogenic bladder. *J. Am. Med. Assoc.*, **203**, 481.

Lebowitz, P. (1975) Sacral agenesis. *Pediatrics*, **55**, 300–301.

Mariani, A.J., Stern, J., Khan, A.U. & Cass, A.S. (1979) Sacral agenesis—an analysis of seven cases and review of literature. *J. Urol.*, **122**, 684–686.

Mayfield, J.K. (1981) Severe spine deformity in myelodysplasia and sacral agenesis; an aggressive surgical approach. *Spine*, **6**, 509–698.

Pang, D. & Hoffman, H.J. (1980) Sacral agenesis with progressive neurological deficit. *Neurosurgery*, **7**, 118–126.

Paris, J. & Laine, E. (1973) Agénésie sacro-coccygienne héréditaire avec perforation anale incomplète. Megarectum dans l'enfance, méningocèle pelvienne a l'âge adulte. *Sem Hôsp (Paris)*, **49**, 1320–1322.

Passarge, E. & Lenz, W. (1966) Syndrome of caudal regression in children of diabetic mothers. Observations of further cases. *Pediatrics*, **37**, 672–675.

Pedersen, L.M., Tygstrup, I. & Pedersen, J. (1964) Congenital malformations in newborn infants of diabetic mothers. The correlation with maternal diabetic vascular complications. *Lancet*, **1**, 1124–1126.

Perry, J., Bonnet, C.A. & Hoffer, M.M. (1970) Vertebral pelvic fusions in the rehabilitation of patients with sacral agenesis. *J. Bone Jt. Surg.*, **52A**, 288–294.

Phillips, W.A., Cooperman, D.R., Lindquist, T.C., Sullivan, R.C. & Millar, E.A., Orthopedic management of lumbosacral agenesis; long-term follow-up. *J. Bone Jt. Surg.*, **64A**, 1282–1294.

Pierson, M., Faulon, M., Vigneron, J. & Leheup B. (1985) [Genetic counselling and the caudal regression syndrome]. *J. Genet. Hum.*, **33**, 405–418.

Price, D.L., Dooling, E.C. & Richardson, E.P. (1970) Caudal dysplasia (caudal regression syndrome). *Arch. Neurol.*, **23**, 212–220.

Renshaw, T.S. (1978) Sacral agenesis: a classification and review of twenty-three cases. *J. Bone Jt. Surg.*, **60A**, 373–383.

Rusnak, S.L. & Driscoll, S.G. (1965) Congenital spinal anomalies in infants of diabetic mothers. *Pediatrics*, **35**, 989–995.

Shands, A.R. & Bundens, W.D. (1956) Congenital deformities of the spine: an analysis of the roentgenograms of 700 children. *Bull. Hosp. Jt. Dis.*, **17**, 110.

Shirkhoda, A., Brashear, H.R., Zelenik, M.E. & Burke, D.C. (1984) Sacral abnormalities—computed tomography versus conventional radiography. *J. Comput. Tomogr.*, **8**, 41–51.

Stanley, J., Owen, R. & Koff, S. (1979) Congenital sacral abnormalities. *J. Bone Jt. Surg.*, **61B**, 401–409.

Thompson, I.M., Kirk, R.M. & Dale, M. (1974) Sacral agenesis. *Pediatrics*, **54**, 236–238.

Treble, N.J. Owen, R. & Rickwood, A.M.K. (1988) Congenital abnormalities of the sacrum; patterns of deformity. *Acta Orthop. Scand.*, **59**, 412–416.

Welch, J.P. & Aterman, K. (1984) The syndrome of caudal dysplasia: a review, including etiologic considerations and evidence of heterogeneity. *Pediatr. Pathol.*, **2**, 313–327.

Wilcock, A.R. & Emery, J.L. (1970) Deformities of the renal tract in children with meningomyelocoele and hydrocephalus compared with those of children showing no such central nervous system deformities. *Br. J. Urol.*, **42**, 152–157.

17 · Skeletal Dysplasias

By P.J. WITHEROW

Spinal problems tend to be most prevalent among those dysplasias which are recognizable at birth, those with ligamentous laxity and those with marked vertebral changes on X-ray. Atlanto-axial instability, cervical and thoracolumbar kyphosis, scoliosis and spinal stenosis all occur.

A knowledge of the natural history of the individual skeletal dysplasias (Bailey, 1973; Maroteaux, 1979; Wynne-Davies *et al.*, 1985; Nicoletti *et al.*, 1988) and of the natural history of the spinal involvement in each dysplasia (Bethem *et al.*, 1981; Tolo, 1985; Winter, 1987; Leatherman & Dickson, 1988) is needed. These cases can be complex and difficult, and there is much to be said for their concentration in centres with a special interest in the problems of short stature. They are also uncommon with prevalences varying between one in 30 000 for achondroplasia and one in a million for diastrophic dysplasia (Wynne-Davies & Gormley, 1985).

Individuals with short stature, in today's society, wish to be treated as such and not as medical or social curiosities. The term 'dwarf' causes distress and should be avoided. Their lack of height tends to generate in others attitudes more appropriate to children than to short adults, and it is important to appreciate this extra dimension when dealing with patients who have both disproportionate short stature and spinal problems.

ACHONDROPLASIA

Achondroplasia is the commonest of the osteochondrodystrophies with a birth incidence of between two and four per 100 000 (Murdoch *et al.*, 1970; Horton *et al.*, 1978). The average height of adults with achondroplasia is 123 cm for women and 131 cm for men, but there is proportionally a greater variation in body measurements between individuals with achondroplasia than there is in the general population.

The facial appearance is characteristic with prominence of the forehead and underdevelopment of the midface. Trunk (and hence sitting) height is on or above the tenth percentile (Ponseti, 1970) but the limbs are notably short and the shortening is rhizomelic, affecting the upper arms and thighs more than the hands and feet (Langer *et al.*, 1967; Bailey, 1973).

Biopsies of iliac and fibular growth cartilage (Ponseti, 1970) show a deficiency in the rate of endochondral ossification. Membrane bones grow normally and periosteal bone growth is relatively increased. Even within the bones ossifying in cartilage there is variation in the severity of their involvement—the changes are more marked in the fibula than the iliac crest, for example—and this accounts for some of the morphological abnormalities.

On X-ray the epiphyses are little affected so that arthritis is not a problem in adult life (Bailey, 1970). The bones tend to be broad and the active periosteal growth produces flaring of the metaphyses and prominent aponeurotic markings.

Mortality in the first year of life is higher than normal, although confusion in the past with thanatophoric dysplasia and with homozygous achondroplasia may have biased the perinatal figures (Murdoch *et al.*, 1970). Middle-ear problems are common and upper airway obstruction may occur due to underdevelopment of the base of the skull (Reid *et al.*, 1988).

The achondroplastic infant shows delayed motor development with head control not well established until six to eight months. Sitting is associated with

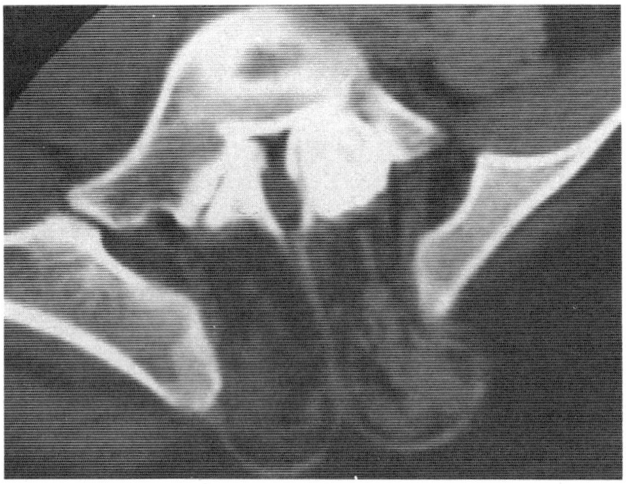

Fig. 17.1 Computerized tomographic scan at the L5–S1 level in achondroplasia, showing marked narrowing of the spinal canal with facet joint intrusion.

a sag thoracolumbar kyphosis. Independent walking starts at an average age of 16 months (Kopits, 1988).

As walking is established there is often a phase of knee laxity and hyperextension before the appearance of the typical bow leg deformity which is associated with fibular overgrowth. At the same time the lumbar lordosis becomes accentuated and hip flexion contractures develop. The elbows also show a flexion contracture of 15–65° with posterior subluxation of the radial heads in some cases, and the arms are relatively short in the young child (Kopits, 1976). Difficulty in opposing the extended fingers (trident hand) is probably due to broadening of the proximal phalangeal bases.

The expectation of life is probably normal. Adults tend to suffer from obesity. Back pain is very common and an estimated 10% will need treatment for potentially serious spinal problems.

The spine in achondroplasia

In the achondroplastic spine growth at the neurocentral growth plate is reduced whereas endochondral growth of the vertebral body is little affected (Ponseti, 1970). The result is a spine of normal length (usually above the 10th percentile) but one in which the pedicles are short and broad. Interpedicular distances tend to narrow between L1 and L5 (Wynne-Davies *et al.*, 1981). The facet joints are both closer to each other in the transverse plane and closer to the vertebral bodies in the sagittal plane. The laminae are probably not thickened. As a result of the underdevelopment of the vertebrae dorsal to the neurocentral joints spinal stenosis develops and the cross-sectional area of the spinal canal may be reduced by more than 50% (Lutter *et al.*, 1977) (Fig. 17.1). The subarachnoid space bears the brunt of this reduction in area (Uematsu *et al.*, 1988) and intraspinal manipulations become very hazardous. This limits the options for internal fixation: pedicular screws may prove to be relatively safe but the passage of segmental wires and the use of distraction or compression hooks should be avoided.

The posterior surfaces of the vertebral bodies are concave in both sagittal and transverse planes and the discs intrude into the spinal canal. Facet joint hypertrophy developing in adult life can result in a further reduction in the limited space available for the normally sized spinal cord and nerve roots. Lumbar extension reduces and flexion increases this space. The sacrum is small and the iliac wings (in contrast to the true pelvis) are of a more normal size. As a result the fifth lumbar vertebra is low-set in the pelvis with half of the L4 vertebra below the level of the iliac crests (Caffey, 1958).

Low back pain is a common complaint from the early teenage years onwards (Hurko *et al.*, 1988). Nelson (1988) surveyed members of the Association for the Study of Restricted Growth in the United Kingdom. Of 67 people with achondroplasia and hypochondroplasia aged over 12 years, 50 had back pain and 17 had none. Kahanovitz *et al.* (1982) found that only 13 of 47 patients with achondroplasia attending a medical genetics clinic were not suffering from backache.

Although spinal canal size is reduced in all achondroplastics only a proportion develop the signs and symptoms of spinal stenosis.

The earliest symptom of stenosis is the development of pain radiating to the legs followed by intermittent paraesthesia in the thighs and lower legs (Hurko *et al.*, 1988). Exercise-related motor weakness affects the foot and ankle dorsiflexors more than the plantarflexors. Objective signs develop relatively late. Ankle reflexes may be absent or increased with clonus and there may be associated mild spasticity. Progressive weakness and objective sensory changes may be followed by paraparesis (or quadriparesis in

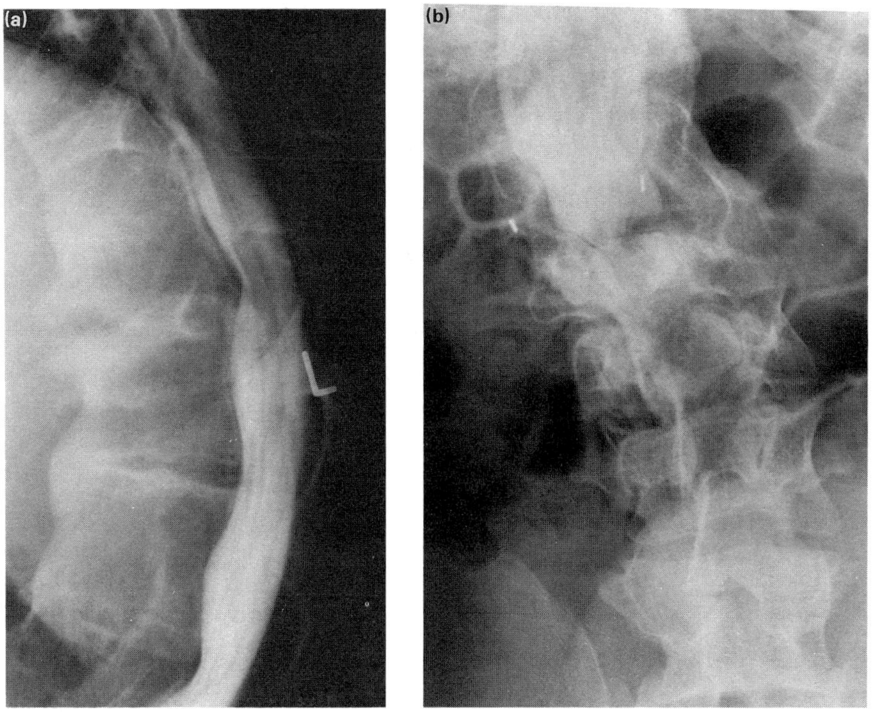

Fig. 17.2 (a) Radiculogram of a 25-year-old patient with achondroplasia and recurrent paraparesis. There is a thoracolumbar kyphosis with intrusion of discs into the spinal canal. A previous thoracic laminectomy has been performed. The cord is narrowed. (b) Stenosis is present at the lower end of the previous laminectomy (marked with clips). There is an apparent scoliosis due to rotation of the thoracolumbar kyphosis.

the case of the uncommon cervical stenosis) in a proportion of patients.

Achondroplastics often tend to accept 'dead legs' as part of their lot and learn to obtain relief by squatting or sitting down. They may not present for treatment until neurological damage has occurred, and once this is the case the prospects of success following surgery are reduced.

Signs of cord and root compression do not develop in all patients with symptoms of spinal claudication. There is a wide range in the age of onset, 14–57 years in Nelson's (1988) series and 10–54 years with a median of 35 in the Johns Hopkins series (Streeten *et al.*, 1988). Once spinal claudication has become disabling surgical decompression should be considered. The selection of levels can be difficult on clinical grounds as superficial sensory objective changes develop late. Computerized tomography (CT) myelography utilizing water-soluble contrast introduced through a lateral C1–C2 puncture has been the standby of investigation (Suss *et al.*, 1983). Lumbar puncture may be impossible due to the minimal subarachnoid space. Magnetic resonance imaging (MRI) scanning may well supplant CT as the resolution of the newer scanners improves. The Johns Hopkins group have emphasized the importance of preoperative studies of bladder function (Streeten *et al.*, 1988). Thirteen out of 15 of their patients had abnormal cystometrograms or postvoiding residues, and knowledge of this helped anticipate problems after extended laminectomy. Preoperative somatosensory evoked potentials are advisable to obtain a baseline, in view of the importance of intraoperative monitoring.

The results of decompressive surgery for spinal stenosis in the past have not been encouraging. This may reflect rather late intervention and possibly the use of too short laminectomies (Fig. 17.2). Bethem *et al.* (1981) treated six patients of whom five needed further surgery and three were made worse. Nelson treated five patients: two were improved and two were rated excellent but there was one death. Recently, good results have been reported by Streeten *et al.* (1988) from long laminectomies. Fourteen of 16 patients were improved and two were unchanged, but the mean follow-up period was only 9.8 months.

A common feature of series with longer follow-ups is the tendency for symptoms to return in association with stenosis at a higher level. Nine of the 20 cases treated by Uematsu (Streeten *et al.*, 1988) had had a previous laminectomy. Surgery for spinal stenosis in achondroplasia is difficult and time-consuming due to the narrow spinal canal and the minimal subarachnoid space. Punches cannot be used to resect the laminae and a high-speed burr is needed to cut a trough through the lamina just medial to the facet joints. The spinous processes and laminae can then be carefully removed without fracturing the facets. In general, provided the facet joints have not been resected or unduly weakened, an anterior fusion is not required; but the situation should be kept under review, for if a kyphosis does develop it may be associated with neurological deterioration and an intersegmental anterior fusion may be required.

Patients with a significant angular kyphosis fall into a separate group with regard to surgery and aftercare, and will be considered further.

With regard to the selection of levels, the spine needs to be decompressed down to S1 and proximally the decompression should be taken four levels above the myelographic stenosis. In exceptional cases the entire spine has been decompressed. In the lower lumbar region muscle flaps can be used to reduce the dead space and minimize the risk of pseudomeningocele (Uematsu *et al.*, 1988).

Kyphosis and hyperlordosis

Donath and Vogl in 1925 first drew attention to the angular kyphosis at the thoracolumbar junction found in a proportion of people with achondroplasia (Vogl & Osborne, 1949).

In early childhood over 90% (Kopits, 1988) of achondroplastic children have a kyphosis which increases to between 60° and 70° between the ages of eight and 18 months. It has been suggested that the large head and narrow thorax, together with hypotonia and delayed motor development, may account for this high incidence.

Independent walking occurs on average at the age of 16 months and with this in most children the kyphosis decreases so that between the ages of two and five years the incidence falls to 39%. In later childhood and adult life between 20% and 35% of achondroplastics have a kyphosis (Kopits, 1988) with a third of these, some 10% overall, developing an angular and progressive deformity (Lonstein, 1988).

The radiological changes in progressive cases (Alexander, 1969; Kopits, 1988) consist of an initial convergence of the anterior part of the L1–L2 disc space as seen on a prone lateral X-ray. The first and second lumbar vertebrae tend to bear the brunt of the changes. Initially there is a failure of the ossific nucleus to grow at the same rate as the adjacent vertebrae followed by notching of the anterosuperior corner and later marked wedging. In severe kyphoses the apical vertebra will be extruded backwards and kyphotic angles of up to 130° can develop (Bethem *et al.*, 1981).

The presence of a kyphosis increases the risk of spinal stenotic symptoms (Duvoisin & Yahr, 1962). Kopits (1988) found that patients with severe spinal stenosis symptoms were twice as likely to have a significant kyphosis as those who were symptom-free. The hyperlordosis found in children and adults with achondroplasia has been shown to further reduce the volume of the lumbar spinal canal (Siebens *et al.*, 1978). It would seem logical to assume that there might be a reciprocal relationship between the degree of lumbar lordosis and the hip flexion contractures on the one hand and the degree of kyphosis on the other. This certainly holds for flexible idiopathic kyphosis in non-achondroplastic children. In angular kyphosis, however, correction of the thoracolumbar curve at operation by an average of 20° had no effect on the lordotic angle (Tolo, 1988).

The soft tissue hip flexion contractures cannot be released sufficiently to correct the lumbar lordosis without dividing the anterior hip joint capsule and this risks anterior dislocation (Kopits, 1988). There may be a place, however, for an extension osteotomy of the upper femur, and certainly as part of a leg elongation programme release of rectus femoris, sartorius and the fascia lata with extension at the femoral elongation site has been claimed to reduce the lordosis in patients without angular kyphosis (Vilarrubias *et al.*, 1988). Orthotic treatment has been tried (Kopits, 1988; Siebens *et al.*, 1988) in the hope of preventing progressive kyphosis. As in scoliosis, assessment of the efficacy of such treatment remains difficult. Kopits failed to control kyphosis in 10 patients (of whom three developed significant curves) out of 76 patients braced at a mean kyphosis angle of 56°.

Physiotherapy aimed at stretching the hip flexors has been tried in an attempt to control sagittal plane deformity but this runs the risk (Kopits, 1988) of producing anterior hip subluxation and is unlikely to affect the development of progressive thoracolumbar kyphosis.

Gravity does seem to play a part in the aetiology of this deformity, and Beighton & Bathfield (1981) have shown that seven of 17 African children with achondroplasia had significant kyphosis (and the majority of these would have been carried on their mothers' backs for long periods), whereas the incidence of kyphosis in white and coloured babies was 5%.

Surgery is probably indicated in kyphosis associated with wedging of the thoracolumbar vertebrae once the kyphosis angle has reached 60° utilizing a one- or two-stage circumferential fusion. In severe cases an anterior strut graft will be required. In mild cases it will usually be possible to carry out a segmental fusion excising the anterior longitudinal ligaments, discs and endplates and inserting grafts into each disc space without necessarily ligating the lumbar segmental vessels.

Posterior instrumentation may well be hazardous. Tolo (1988) reports that three out of four patients who had spinous process (and not sublaminar) segmental wiring developing evoked potential changes necessitating removal of the fixation.

The safest approach is probably to avoid internal fixation and accept that a period of four months recumbent in a plaster cast followed by four months in a brace or cast, until the fusion has consolidated, will be required. In the future it may be possible to obtain secure fixation using pedicle screws and thus obviating a long period of recumbency.

Craniocervical problems

Symptomatic cervical spinal stenosis can occur (Streeten *et al.*, 1988). The age at presentation is similar to that found in thoracolumbar stenosis and the management philosophy follows the same lines.

The question of whether infants with achondroplasia have true hydrocephalus or whether they have megalencephaly has been debated since Dandy's original report (Bergstrom *et al.*, 1971). A degree of ventricular enlargement is present in infants with achondroplasia, but a non-communicating hydrocephalus with loss of the sulcal subarachnoid space is rare. It has been suggested that stenosis of the jugular foramina, part of the general hypoplasia of the base of the skull (Nelson, 1988), may be responsible for a venous outflow obstruction (Yamada *et al.*, 1981). Carson *et al.* (1988) question the need for decompressive surgery in the absence of progressive hydrocephalus and raised intraventricular cerebrospinal fluid pressure.

A more important cause of morbidity, and indeed of mortality, in the first year of life is cervicomedullary cord compression (Hancock & Phillips, 1965; Fremion *et al.*, 1984; Pauli *et al.*, 1984). It may not be easy to separate the effects of high cord compression from those due to the restricted upper airway of the achondroplastic baby. The narrow nasopharynx of the achondroplastic infant predisposes to airway obstruction, particularly if there is adenoid hypertrophy. Sleep apnoea, episodic cyanosis and right ventricular hypertrophy all can occur (Reid *et al.*, 1988). Some achondroplastic infants sleep with the neck extended, to improve airway patency.

The arch of the atlas tends to behave as though it is semioccipitalized and moves with the occiput (Bailey, 1973, p. 74). The basiocciput comes to overlap the posterior arch of the atlas and the relatively large squamous occipital (derived from membrane bone) is associated with elevation of the hind brain and relative angulation of the cervicomedullary junction. Impingement between the posterior rim of the foramen magnum and the upper cord may be worsened by the presence of a large odontoid peg (Yamada *et al.*, 1981).

It may be difficult to determine the exact cause of intermittent respiratory distress in the achondroplastic infant. Reid *et al.* (1988) found that 23% of their patients had primarily a respiratory abnormality and 9% had cervicomedullary compression.

Treatment is by resection of the posterior arch of the atlas, and a painstaking and careful removal of the deeply indenting basiocciput followed by a dural release and patch (Yamada *et al.*, 1981; Carson *et al.*, 1988).

Other aspects of the spine in achondroplasia

Scoliosis is not uncommon, but the curves are rarely of significance. Kopits (1976) reported one case with a double scoliosis of 48° amongst 158 achondroplastic patients. Bailey (1970) found 12 mild curves and one moderate in a group of 41 patients.

DIASTROPHIC DYSPLASIA

Diastrophic dysplasia is a rare condition diagnosable at birth and associated with disproportionate short stature (Hollister & Lachman, 1976). Adult height is very variable, ranging from 80 to 140 cm (Wynne-Davies *et al.*, 1985). It was initially thought that there were two different types of diastrophic dysplasia, a severe and a mild, but it seems more likely that there is in fact a spectrum of severity.

Scoliosis is common and in some cases curves of over 100° develop. Cervical spina bifida occulta may sometimes be associated with severe cervical kyphosis (Langer, 1965).

The clinical features include a characteristic thickening of the ear pinna and proximally placed thumbs ('hitch-hiker thumbs'). A complete or partial cleft palate is common. The fingers are stiff at the interphalangeal joints. Hip dysplasia or dislocation occurs. There are usually knee flexion contractures with varus or more commonly valgus deformity affecting a proportion of patients. A rigid club foot deformity unresponsive to treatment is common. The lumbar lordosis is increased.

Radiological changes in the spine are variable but mild platyspondyly may be present. Interpedicular distances may narrow between L1 and L5, remain the same or widen. Pedicle height may be reduced at L4–L5 level (Langer, 1965). The lumbosacral angle is increased and there may be some wedging of L5 (Tolo, 1985).

Spinal stenosis is not a clinical problem but the cross-sectional area of the spinal canal should be checked prior to any instrumentation involving hook placement.

Scoliosis is common in diastrophic dysplasia (Fig. 17.3). Estimates of the incidence vary. Herring (1978) reported scoliosis in four of five patients over the age of seven; Beighton (1980), in three of six patients; Tolo and Kopits in 71% (Tolo, 1985). Bearing in mind the wide variation in severity of diastrophic dysplasia it seems likely that the incidence of scoliosis may be lower than this. Poussa *et al.* (1990) in Finland found an incidence of 37% with a female to male ratio of approximately two to one. Only 13 patients out of 84 over the age of 11 years had curves in excess of 50°.

This experience parallels that of Tolo and Kopits (Tolo, 1985) who found that 60% of their patients

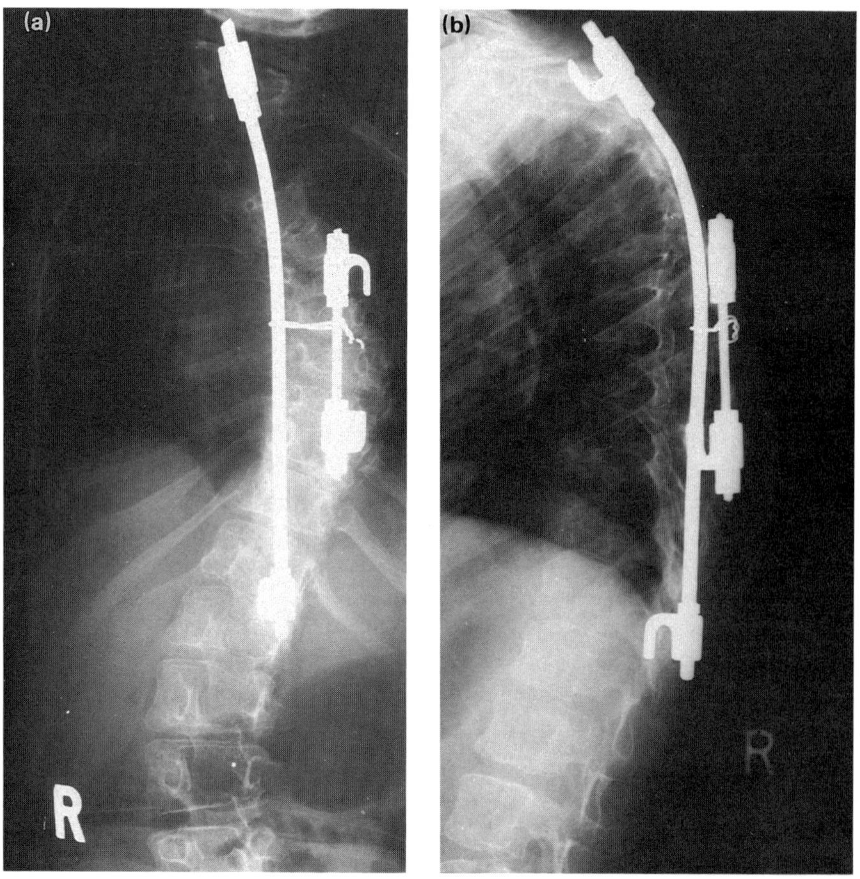

Fig. 17.3 (a) Posterior spinal fusion in a six-year-old patient with diastrophic dysplasia. The preoperative curve measured 95°. The fusion was preceded by anterior discectomies and a period of halo-wheelchair traction. (b) Lateral view showing contouring of the miniature Ulrich distraction rod and hook system.

had curves of under 30°. Scoliosis, however, can appear as early as 10 months (Herring, 1978) and progress to 100° by the age of three years (Poussa *et al.*, 1990). If the child reaches the age of four years without a scoliosis it is likely that the spine will remain straight (Tolo, 1985). The risk of developing a curve of over 100° is probably of the order of 5%. The curve pattern varies, with thoracic, thoracolumbar and double curves represented. Congenital failure of segmentation can occur, producing a true kyphosis in contrast to the more common apparent kyphosis of the rotated lordotic curve.

Treatment should be reserved for the more progressive curve in view of the generally benign natural history of scoliosis in diastrophic dysplasia. Bracing has been advocated (Bethem *et al.*, 1980; Tolo, 1985) but it is doubtful if bracing can control the more difficult curves, and the loss of trunk flexibility associated with bracing poses an additional problem to the young child with disproportionate short stature.

If surgery is required it should probably take the form of a circumferential fusion using small distraction hooks as in the Ulrich system.

Cervical problems

Cervical spina bifida occulta is very common. It usually extends from the second, third or fourth cervical vertebra down to the sixth, seventh or first thoracic vertebrae (Herring, 1978).

Approximately one-third of patients will develop a cervical kyphosis, usually centred on the fourth cervical vertebra, which in a proportion will regress spontaneously. This process, if it is going to occur, will be obvious by the age of 5 years (Poussa *et al.*, 1990). The kyphosis, however, can be rapidly progressive (Amuso, 1968). Kash *et al.* (1974) report the onset of symptoms at the age of 2 years with death at the age of 3½ years from cervical cord compression. The degree of kyphosis can be such that the odontoid process becomes almost horizontal, causing the anterior ring of the atlas to ride up, although atlanto-axial instability is not a problem in general in diastrophic dysplasia (Tolo, 1985).

Treatment should be by circumferential fusion using a strut graft anteriorly once the degree of deformity is such that it is clear that cord cross-sectional shape is being affected. The presence of spina bifida occulta needs to be taken into consideration when making the exposure for the posterior fusion.

MORQUIO–BRAILSFORD MUCOPOLYSACCHARIDOSIS

Cervical myelopathy is a major cause of premature disability and death in the Morquio–Brailsford syndrome (mucopolysaccharidosis IV, MPS IV).

The mucopolysaccharidoses are a group of recessively inherited disorders in which lack of one or other of the enzymes involved in the breakdown of mucopolysaccharide chains leads to the accumulation of these substances in the tissues. In MPS IV the combination of relative longevity and severe bony involvement is seen. A mild and a severe form of the condition exist. At birth affected infants are normal, but by the age of three to four years sternal prominence, a short trunk and facial changes may be apparent. By late childhood the full clinical picture of prominence of the lower face, a high and prominent sternum with horizontal ribs and a relatively rigid chest and lower limb deformities has developed (Brailsford, 1929). Joint laxity is present, and genu valgum may be marked. The corneal clouding seen in other mucopolysaccharidoses occurs, but not to the same extent as in the Hurler and Hunter syndromes.

On X-ray (Caffey, 1952; Langer & Carey, 1966) the skull is relatively normal. The ribs are thick. The metacarpals show a characteristic narrowing of their bases. The pelvis has a wine-glass shape. Coxa valga and marked acetabular dysplasia develop.

The vertebrae have a tongue- or flame-like prolongation of the anterior surface and progressive platyspondyly occurs (Brailsford, 1929; Brandner, 1970). A thoracolumbar kyphus develops, with wedging at the thoracolumbar junction. In some patients this may be progressive.

The most important abnormality is hypoplasia or aplasia of the odontoid associated with instability between the first and second cervical vertebrae (Einhorn *et al.*, 1946; Beighton & Craig, 1973; Lipson, 1977). In most patients this produces a progressive myelopathy. Symptoms usually start around the age of four years, and decreased endurance and pyramidal tract signs may be well established by the age of six (Blaw & Langer, 1969; Tolo, 1985). Motor signs tend to predominate at first, followed by loss of the deep sensory modalities. Superficial sensation is preserved until late and bladder function is lost only terminally (Kopits, 1976). Long tract signs may be asymmetrical. Kopits *et al.* (1972) have shown on gas myelography that the cord may be displaced to one side of the

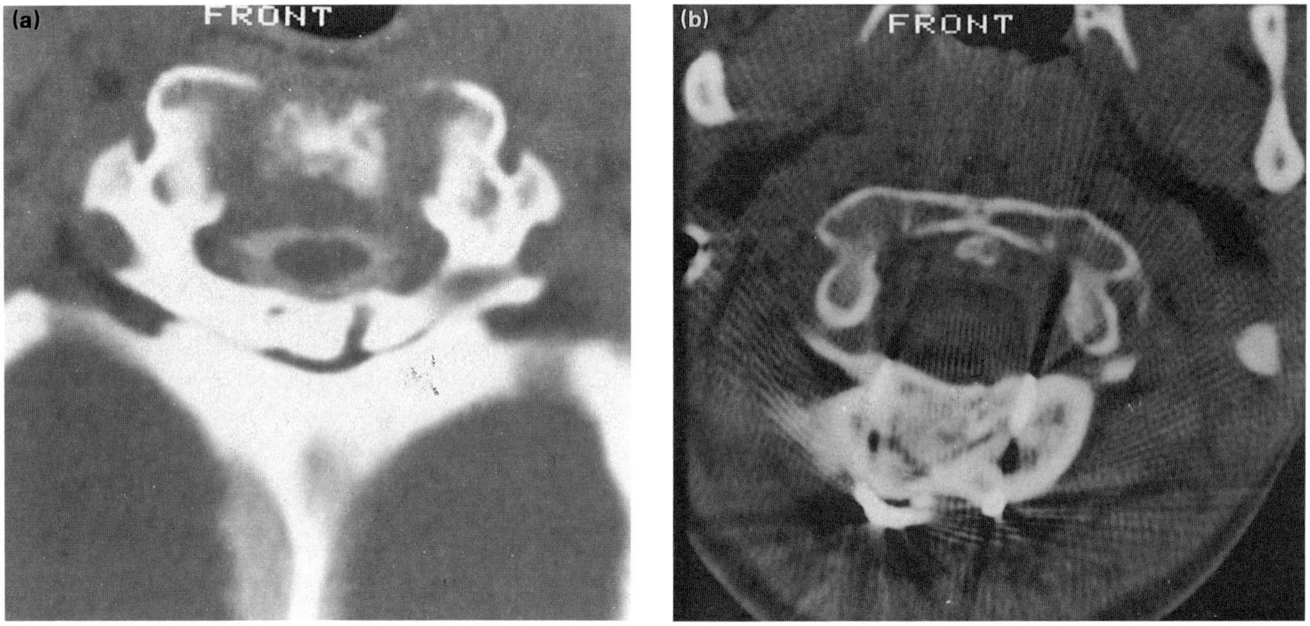

Fig. 17.4 (a) Computerized tomographic scan with cerebrospinal fluid contrast in a patient with Morquio–Brailsford mucopolysaccharidosis and C1–C2 instability. The cord is flattened between the C1 arch and the hypoplastic odontoid. (b) CT scan of the same patient (without contrast) following an occiput to C3 fusion.

midline. The available space in the upper cervical spine may be further compromised by thickening of the transverse odontoid and posterior longitudinal ligaments in association with mucopolysaccharide deposition (Fig. 17.4).

Surgical treatment should be considered between the ages of four and six years in all children with symptoms or signs suggestive of an early myelopathy and confirmed by evidence of cord flattening on MRI or CSF contrast-enhanced CT scans. The surgery is demanding and quite hazardous particularly once long tract signs are established and should probably be carried out in tertiary referral centres.

Because of the very poor quality bone in MPS IV patients (Kopits, 1976) lower femoral or tibial grafts will be required and the surgery should be done with the head immobilized in the optimal position in a halocast. Respiratory failure can occur in the early postoperative period. The legs need to be splinted for six weeks to protect the donor sites and the maintenance of halopin fixation in the thin bone of the skull can be a problem.

METATROPIC DYSPLASIA

At first in metatropic dysplasia the trunk appears relatively normal in contrast to the limbs which are short. The neonate has a narrow chest and sometimes a 1–3 cm sacral tail is present, or there may be an additional skinfold in the upper natal cleft. The major joints tend to be prominent with reduced joint mobility since the epiphyses are affected in this dysplasia. Fixed flexion may develop at the hips in association with a lumbar lordosis, and at the knees there can be either varus or valgus angulation. An increased mortality has been reported during the first year of life (Rimoin *et al.*, 1976; Belik *et al.*, 1985). Adult height is between 110 and 120 cm (Wynne-Davies *et al.*, 1985). During early childhood spinal growth slows and this, together with the development of a progressive double scoliosis, leads to disproportionate short stature of short trunk type. The curves may become rigid early on, or may remain flexible (Bailey, 1973, p. 140). In the transitional zone between the thoracic and lumbar curves a kyphosis may develop (Bethem *et al.*, 1981).

On X-ray the appearance of the spine is dramatic, particularly in early childhood with marked platyspondyly and deep intervertebral spaces (Maroteaux, 1979, p. 49) (Fig. 17.5). The ossified part of the body may be only one-sixth of the total thickness of the vertebra (Rimoin *et al.*, 1976). There may be some reduction in interpedicular distances between L1 and L5, but this is not as marked as in achondroplasia

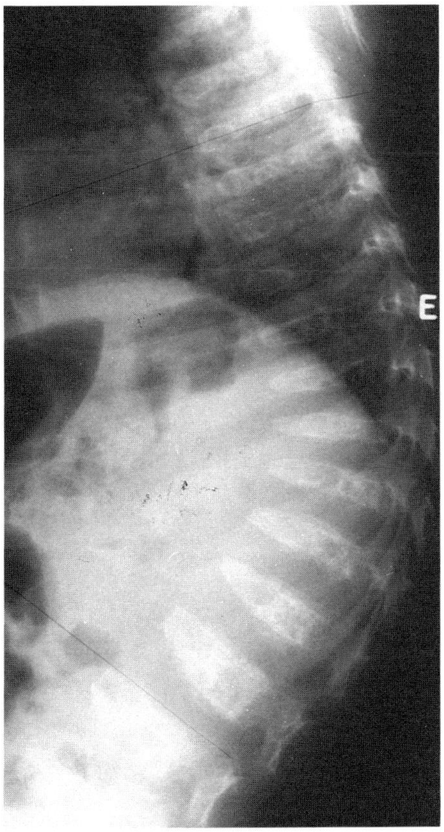

Fig. 17.5 Lateral radiograph of the thoracolumbar spine in metatropic dysplasia. The marked platyspondyly is in part due to delay in endochondral ossification.

(Jenkins *et al.*, 1970; Bailey, 1973). The pedicles may be a little shorter than normal but spinal stenosis is not a problem in practice.

In the cervical spine the odontoid tends to be hypoplastic or aplastic and C1–C2 instability is common (Koop *et al.*, 1984). Congenital vertebral anomalies may be present (Bailey, 1973, p. 140).

In the first year of life, episodes of respiratory obstruction may occur, and there is an increased mortality from sudden unexplained death reminiscent of the problems which sometimes occur in achondroplasia. Belik *et al.* (1985) reported two neonatal deaths associated with intermittent upper airway obstruction: in neither of these was cord compression or atlanto-axial instability present. Odontoid hypoplasia or absence, however, is almost the rule, and many patients have clinically important C1–C2 instability. In the Shohat *et al.* (1989) series three patients were treated for cord compression from this cause; in addition one child died suddenly while waiting to come into hospital for a cervical fusion.

Not all children with metatropic dysplasia develop a severe scoliosis, but the majority do, with a right thoracic and left lumbar pattern being the commonest. There may be a clinically important kyphosis at the transition between the two curves (Bethem *et al.*, 1981) which may be associated with a rotatory vertebral subluxation (Dubousset & Masson, 1988) or a segmentation failure. This transitional kyphosis may need stabilization. If there is associated cord compression a partial vertebrectomy or pedicular resection may also be required. A circumferential fusion should be carried out early in seriously progressive deformity. Curves progressing beyond 60° should be considered for this, even in early childhood. The frequent association of atlanto-axial instability is a complicating factor and an occiput to C2 fusion may be required (Fig. 17.6).

SPONDYLO-EPIPHYSEAL DYSPLASIA CONGENITA

Two forms of this dwarfing dysplasia occur (Wynne-Davies & Hall, 1982); both have a prevalence estimated at between one and two per million. They differ primarily in the severity of hip joint involvement. The form with severe coxa vara tends to have more generalized epiphyseal and some metaphyseal involvement, with a final height between 104 and 127 cm. The type with mild hip involvement has less generalized epiphyseal abnormality and no metaphyseal involvement, with a final height between 130 and 145 cm. Atlanto-axial instability, scoliosis and kyphosis occur. The dysplasia is diagnosable at birth, and initially rhizomelic limb shortening predominates but by the age of three to four years trunk shortening is becoming more obvious, together with pectus carinatum and a lumbar lordosis. The face may be normal or somewhat flat. Some patients have a cleft palate and myopia can be a problem. Walking is often established rather late (around the age of two years) and the children sometimes start to walk with the head in extension. This may be part of an attempt to balance the trunk in the sagittal plane and compensate for hip flexion contractures and lumbar lordosis, but it may also be due to the child adopting this attitude to stabilize the atlanto-axial joint. Coxa vara, a high trochanter and occasionally hip dislocation are all associated with a waddling gait and limited exercise tolerance.

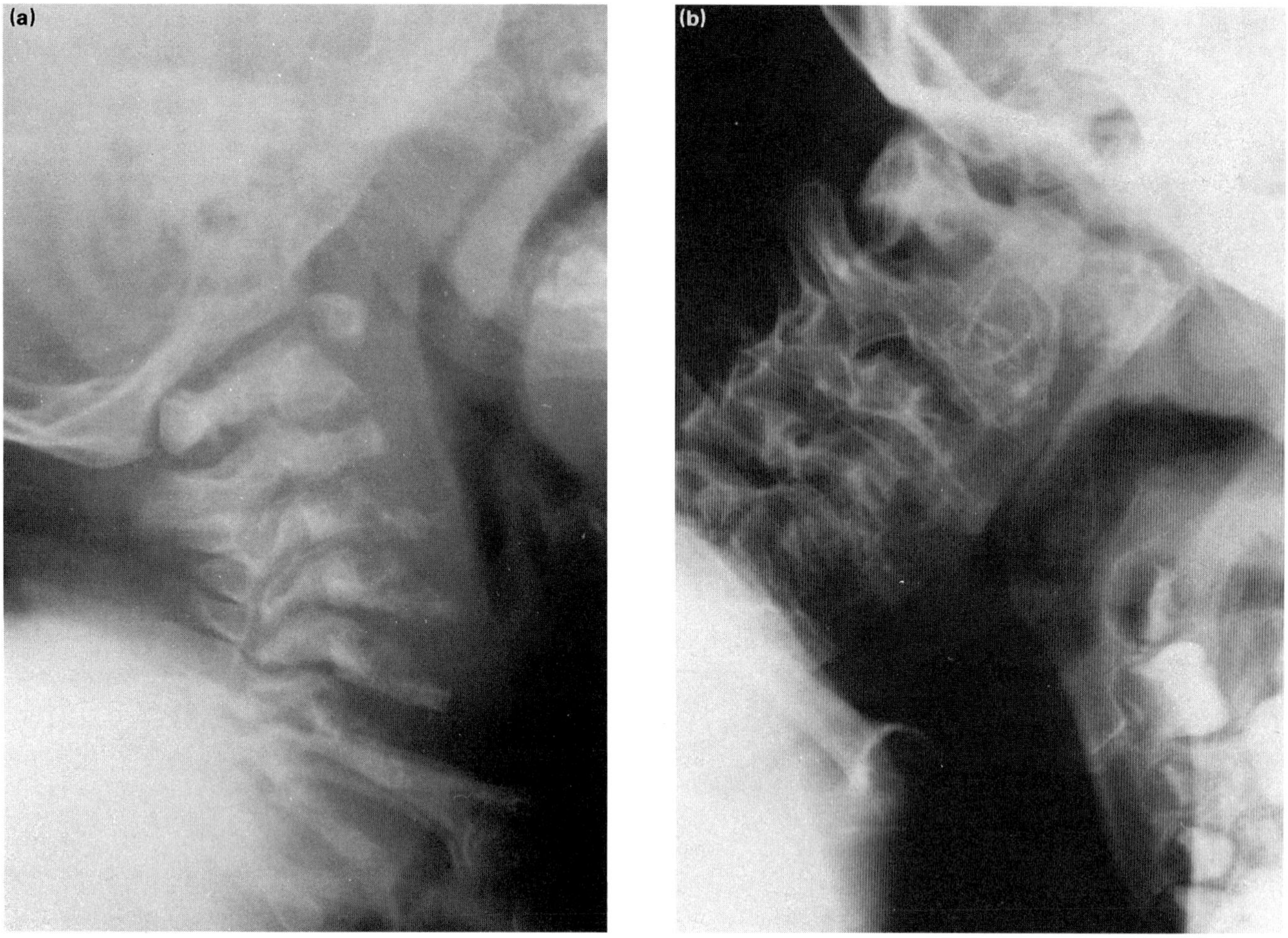

Fig. 17.6 (a) Lateral radiograph of the cervical spine in metatropic dysplasia. Apparent hypoplasia of the odontoid at the age of 10 months. (b) Flexion lateral view of the cervical spine in the same patient, showing development of the odontoid by the age of four years. The instability in this case has not progressed.

Progressive genu valgum may compound the difficulty these children have with walking, and in adult life degenerative joint changes may occur, although these are not always as symptomatic as they are in certain other dysplasias. On X-ray the epiphyses develop late with the capital femoral epiphyses not appearing until the age of four or five years; the pubic rami are also slow to appear.

The vertebral bodies are oval or pear-shaped (Spranger & Langer, 1970) in early childhood. In later childhood the appearances vary from virtually normal to a mild degree of irregular platyspondyly. As is often the case with skeletal dysplasias the characteristic appearances occur in early rather than in late childhood. There may be some wedging of the first lumbar vertebra. There is often delay in the appearance of the odontoid ossific centre and odontoid hypoplasia.

Low back pain can be a problem in childhood. Scoliosis develops commonly. In Wynne-Davies & Hall's series (1982) all but three of 17 patients had a scoliosis by the age of 10 years. The severity varied considerably. In the Bethem *et al.* (1981) series nine patients out of 12 had a scoliosis: five of these had curves of more than 35°. A smooth thoracic kyphosis can occur.

Wynne-Davies & Hall (1982) report two patients developing neurological symptoms. In one case at the age of 10 and in the other at the age of 21. Nelson (1970) reports a paraplegia occurring at the age of 13, responsive to decompression. Bracing has been recommended for the kyphosis but was ineffective in two of the three patients braced in the Bethem *et al.* series (1981). The marked lordosis has been treated by bracing, but Kopits (1976) reported failure of bracing in two patients aged 4 and 5½ because, although the lordosis was corrected in a brace, they were unable to compensate by extending at the hips. Extension osteotomies of the hips could be considered in appropriate cases.

OTHER SKELETAL DYSPLASIAS

Pseudo-achondroplasia

Pseudo-achondroplasia is one of the more common skeletal dysplasias responsible for marked short stature (Cooper *et al.*, 1973). A population frequency of four per million has been estimated (Wynne-Davies *et al.*, 1985). Adult height varies between 82 and 130 cm. At birth the infant is normal. By the age of three to four years disproportionate short stature is evident. In contrast with achondroplasia the epiphyses are involved as well as the metaphyses and the spine. Joint laxity is marked and a proportion of patients develop severe lower limb malalignment with subluxation at the knee. Corrective osteotomies may be necessary at multiple levels. The spine shows a variable degree of platyspondyly with the vertebrae being oval and often cone-shaped anteriorly in the infant. A scoliosis of up to 30 or 40° is quite frequent but troublesome and progressive curves do not, in general, occur. Odontoid hypoplasia is common, but in Kopits' (1976) series only one of 31 patients needed a fusion.

Chondrodysplasia calcificans punctata

There are both mild and severe forms of this condition, with the severe form normally being lethal in infancy. The mild form, Conradi Hunermann disease, has a prevalence estimated at 1.7 per million (Wynne-Davies *et al.*, 1985) although this may be an underestimate in view of the presence of mild and often unrecognized forms. The diagnostic feature is the presence of punctate calcification of the epiphyses with patchy stippling of the vertebral and pelvic ossific nuclei. There may be extracartilaginous ossification. These calcific deposits have largely disappeared by the age of one to four. Cataracts affect 25% of patients and there may be an ichthyoform skin eruption in infancy. The clinical importance of this condition lies in the frequency of congenital vertebral abnormalities and the consequent congenital scoliosis (Herring, 1976). Leg inequality is also common.

The scoliosis should be observed and managed by early hemivertebral anterior and posterior fusion once it is clear that the curve is going to prove seriously progressive (Winter, 1981). The combination of an unscgmented bar and a contralateral hemivertebra should be dealt with early. Adult height in Conradi's disease is above 130 cm and the loss of height consequent on even an early short fusion is likely to be less than that from a seriously progressive congenital curve.

The multiple epiphyseal dysplasias

In general spinal involvement in the various types of multiple epiphyseal dysplasia is minimal and restricted to mild platyspondyly in the thoracolumbar region. Scoliosis can occur (Leatherman & Dickson, 1988, p. 268). Nelson (1970) reported a severe scoliosis in one of his 11 patients.

Spondylo-epiphyseal dysplasia tarda

This dysplasia presents with a short trunk, a stiff back and stiff hips in midchildhood. On a lateral X-ray of the lumbar spine there are characteristic changes with the presence of humps above the upper and below the lower vertebral endplates (Langer, 1964). The pattern of inheritance varies, but is commonly X-linked recessive, in which case only males are affected. Leatherman & Dickson (1988) report two cases with scoliosis. In both there were long tract signs associated with a thoracolumbar kyphosis which recovered after circumferential surgery.

Kniest's disease and Dyggve–Melchior–Clausen disease

These are two extremely rare skeletal dysplasias, both with an incidence of 0.1 per million. The Knicst dysplasia (Rimoin *et al.*, 1976) is diagnosable at birth and in childhood resembles metatropic dysplasia with joint stiffness and prominence, a lordosis, trunk shortening and stiff hips. A scoliosis is usually present but this is not usually progressive. Atlanto-axial instability may occur, and this can be associated with a myelopathy. There is odontoid hypoplasia and platyspondyly.

Dyggve–Melchior–Claussen disease is diagnosable in early childhood rather than at birth. A disproportionately short trunk develops in association with vertebrae which show a characteristic notching of the superior and inferior surfaces on the lateral view. The main diagnostic feature is scalloping of the crest of the ilium. Scoliosis occurs, but in the reported cases does not appear to have been a dominant problem.

REFERENCES

Alexander, E. (1969) Significance of the small lumbar spinal canal: cauda equina compression syndromes due to spondylosis. Part 5: Achondroplasia. *J. Neurosurg.*, **31**, 513–519.

Amuso, S.J. (1968) Diastrophic dwarfism. *J. Bone Jt. Surg.*, **50A**, 113–122.

Bailey, J.A. (1970) Orthopaedic aspects of achondroplasia. *J. Bone Jt. Surg.*, **52A**, 1285–1301.

Bailey, J.A. (1973) *Disproportionate Short Stature.* W.B. Saunders, Philadelphia, PA.

Beighton, P. (1980) Orthopaedic problems in dwarfism. *J. Bone Jt. Surg.*, **62B**, 116.

Beighton, P. & Bathfield, B.A. (1981) Gibbal achondroplasia. *J. Bone Jt. Surg.*, **63B**, 328–329.

Beighton, P. & Craig, J. (1973) Atlanto-axial subluxation in the Morquio syndrome. *J. Bone Jt. Surg.*, **55B**, 478–481.

Belik, J., Anday, E.K., Kaplan, F. & Zakai, E. (1985) Respiratory complications of metatropic dwarfism. *Clin. Pediatr.*, **9**, 504–511.

Bergstrom, K., Laurent, U. & Lundberg, P.O. (1971) Neurological symptoms in achondroplasia. *Acta Neurol. Scand.*, **47**, 59–70.

Bethem, D. (1982) Os odontoideum in chondrodystrophia calcificans congenita, a case report. *J. Bone Jt. Surg.*, **64A**, 1384–1386.

Bethem, D., Winter, R.B. & Lutter, L. (1980) Disorders of the spine in diastrophic dwarfism. A discussion of nine patients and review of the literature. *J. Bone Jt. Surg.*, **62A**, 529–536.

Bethem, D., Winter, R.B. & Lutter, L. (1981) Spinal disorders of dwarfism: review of the literature and report of 80 cases. *J. Bone Jt. Surg.*, **63A**, 1412–1425.

Blaw, M.E. & Langer, L.O. (1969) Spinal cord compression in Morquio–Brailsford's disease. *J. Pediatr.*, **74**, 593–600.

Brailsford, J.F. (1929) Chondro-osteo-dystrophy: roentgenographic and clinical features of a child with dislocation of vertebrae. *Am. J. Surg.*, **7**, 404–410.

Brandner, M.E. (1970) Normal values of the vertebral body and intervertebral disk index during growth. *Am. J. Radiol.*, **110**, 618–627.

Caffey, J. (1952) Gargoylism. Prenatal and neonatal bone lesions and their early postnatal evolution. *Am. J. Roentgenol. Radium Ther. Nucl. Med.*, **67**, 715–731.

Caffey, J. (1958) Achondroplasia of pelvis and lumbosacral spine. *Am. J. Roentgenol. Radium Ther. Nucl. Med.*, **80**, 449–457.

Carson, B., Winfield, J., Wang, H., Reid, C., McPherson, R., Kopits, S. & Uematsu, S. (1988) Surgical management of cervicomedullary compression in achondroplastic patients. In Nicoletti, B., Kopits, S.E., Ascani, E. & McKusick, V.A. (eds) *Human Achondroplasia*, pp. 207–214. Plenum Press, New York.

Cooper, R.R., Ponseti, I.V. & Maynard, J.A. (1973) Pseudoachondroplastic dwarfism: a rough surfaced endoplasmic reticulum storage disorder. *J. Bone Jt. Surg.*, **55A**, 475–484.

Dubousset, J. & Masson, J. Cl. (1988) Spinal disorders: kyphosis and lumbar stenosis. In Nicoletti, B., Kopits, S.E., Ascani, E. & McKusick, V.A. (eds) *Human Achondroplasia*, pp. 299–303. Plenum Press, New York.

Duvoisin, R.C. & Yahr, M.D. (1962) Compressive spinal cord and root syndromes in achondroplastic dwarfs. *Neurology*, **12**, 202–207.

Einhorn, N.H., Moore, J.R. & Rowntree, L.G. (1946) Osteochondrodystrophia deformans (Morquio's disease): observations at autopsy in one case. *Am. J. Dis. Child.*, **72**, 536–544.

Fremion, A.S., Garg, B.P. & Kalsbeck, J. (1984) Apnea as the sole manifestation of cord compression in achondroplasia. *J. Pediatr.*, **104**, 398–401.

Hancock, D.W. & Phillips, D.G. (1965) Spinal compression in achondroplasia. *Paraplegia*, **3**, 23–33.

Herring, J.A. (1976) Rapidly progressive scoliosis in multiple epiphyseal dysplasia. A case report. *J. Bone Jt. Surg.*, **58A**, 703–704.

Herring, J.A. (1978) The spinal disorders in diastrophic dwarfism. *J. Bone Jt. Surg.*, **60A**, 177–182.

Hollister, D.W. & Lachman, R.S. (1976) Diastrophic dwarfism. *Clin. Orthop.*, **114**, 61–69.

Horton, W.A., Rotter, J.I., Rimoin, D.L., Scott, C.I. & Hall, J.G. (1978) Standard growth curves for achondroplasia. *J. Pediatr.*, **93**, 435–438.

Hurko, O., Pyeritz, R. & Uematsu, S. (1988) Neurological considerations in achondroplasia. In Nicoletti, B., Kopits, S.E., Ascani, E. & McKusick, V.A. (eds) *Human Achondroplasia*, pp. 153–62. Plenum Press, New York.

Jenkins, P., Smith, M.B. & McKinnell, J.S. (1970) Metatropic dwarfism. *Br. J. Radiol.*, **43**, 561–565.

Kahanovitz, N., Rimoin, D.L. & Sillence, D.O. (1982) The clinical spectrum of lumbar spine disease in achondroplasia. *Spine*, **7**, 137–170.

Kash, I.J., Sane, S.M., Samaha, F.J. & Briner, J. (1974) Cervical cord compression in diastrophic dwarfism. *J. Pediatr.*, **84**, 862–865.

Koop, S.E., Winter, R.B. & Lonstein, J.E. (1984) The surgical treatment of instability of the upper part of the cervical spine in children and adolescents. *J. Bone Jt. Surg.*, **66A**, 403–411.

Kopits, S.E. (1976) Orthopaedic complications of dwarfism. *Clin. Orthop. Rel. Res.*, **114**, 153–179.

Kopits, S.E. (1988) Thoracolumbar kyphosis and lumbosacral hyperlordosis in achondroplastic children. In Nicoletti, B., Kopits, S.E., Ascani, E. & McKusick, V.A.

(eds) *Human Achondroplasia*, pp. 241–255. Plenum Press, New York.

Kopits, S.E., Perovic, M.N., McKusick, V., Robinson, R.A. & Bailey, J.A. (1972) Congenital atlantoaxial dislocations in various forms of dwarfism. *J. Bone Jt. Surg.*, **54A**, 1349–1350.

Langer, L.O. (1964) Spondyloepiphysial dysplasia tarda. *Radiology*, **82**, 833–839.

Langer, L.O. (1965) Diastrophic dwarfism in early infancy. *Am. J. Roentgenol. Radium Ther. Nucl. Med.*, **93**, 399–404.

Langer, L.O. & Carey, L.S. (1966) The roentgenographic features of the KS mucopolysaccharidosis of Morquio (Morquio-Brailsford's disease). *Am. J. Roentgenol. Radium Ther. Nucl. Med.*, **97**, 1–20.

Langer, L.O., Baumann, P.A. & Gorlin, R.J. (1967) Achondroplasia. *Am. J. Roentgenol. Radium Ther. Nucl. Med.*, **100**, 12–26.

Leatherman, K.D. & Dickson, R.A. (1988) Deformities in association with heritable disorders of connective tissue, mucopolysaccharidoses, skeletal dysplasias and metabolic bone disease. In *The Management of Spinal Deformities*, pp. 253–288. Wright, London.

Lipson, S.J. (1977) Dysplasia of the odontoid process in Morquio's syndrome causing quadriparesis. *J. Bone Jt. Surg.*, **59A**, 340–344.

Lonstein, J.E. (1988) Treatment of kyphosis and lumbar stenosis in achondroplasia. In Nicoletti, B., Kopits, S.E., Ascani, E. & McKusick, V.A. (eds) *Human Achondroplasia*, pp. 283–292. Plenum Press, New York.

Lutter, L.D., Lonstein, J.E., Winter, R.B. & Langer, L.O. (1977) Anatomy of achondroplastic lumbar canal. *Clin. Orthop. Rel. Res.*, **126**, 139–142.

McKusick, V.A. & Scott, C.I. (1971) A nomenclature for constitutional disorders of bone. *J. Bone Jt. Surg.*, **53A**, 978–986.

Maroteaux, P. (1979) *Bone Diseases of Children*. J.B. Lippincott, Philadelphia, PA.

Murdoch, J.L., Walker, B.A., Hall, J.G., Abbey, H., Smith, K.K. & McKusick, V.A. (1970) Achondroplasia: a genetic and statistical study. *Ann. Hum. Genet.*, **33**, 227–244.

Nelson, M.A. (1970) Orthopaedic aspects of the chondrodystrophies. The dwarf and his orthopaedic problems. *Ann. R. Coll. Surg. Engl.*, **47**, 185–210.

Nelson, M.A. (1988) Kyphosis and lumbar stenosis in achondroplasia. In Nicoletti, B., Kopits, S.E., Ascani, E. & McKusick, V.A. (eds) *Human Achondroplasia*, pp. 305–311. Plenum Press, New York.

Nicoletti, B., Kopits, S.E., Ascani, E. & McKusick, V.A. (eds) (1988) *Human Achondroplasia*. Plenum Press, New York.

Pauli, R.M., Scott, C.I., Wassman, E.R., Gilbert, E.F., Leavitt, L.A., Vertloeve, J., Hall, J.G., Partington, J.W., Lyons Jones, K., Sommer, A., Feldman, W., Langer, L.O., Rimoin, D.L., Hecht, J.T. & Lebovitz, R. (1984) Apnea and sudden unexpected death in infants with achondroplasia. *J. Pediatr.*, **104**, 342–348.

Ponseti, I.V. (1970) Skeletal growth in achondroplasia. *J. Bone Jt. Surg.*, **52A**, 701–716.

Poussa, M., Merikanto, J., Ryoppy, S., Martinnen, E. & Kaitila, I. (1990) Spinal deformities in diastrophic dysplasia. Presented to European Paediatric Orthopaedic Society, Athens.

Reid, C.S., Pyeritz, R.E., Kopits, S.E., Maria, B.L., Wang, H., McPherson, R.W., Hurko, O. & Phillips, J.A. (1988) Cervicomedullary cord compression in young children with achondroplasia: value of comprehensive neurologic and respiratory evaluation. In Nicoletti, B., Kopits, S.E., Ascani, E. & McKusick, V.A. (eds) *Human Achondroplasia*, pp. 199–205. Plenum Press, New York.

Rimoin, D.L., Siggers, D.C., Lachman, R.S. & Silberberg, R. (1976) Metatropic dwarfism, the Kneist syndrome and the pseudoachondroplastic dysplasias. *Clin. Orthop. Rel. Res.*, **114**, 70–82.

Shohat, M., Lachman, R. & Rimoin, D.L. (1989) Odontoid hypoplasia with vertebral cervical subluxation and ventriculomegaly in metatropic dysplasia. *J. Pediatr.*, **114**, 239–243.

Siebens, A.A., Hungerford, D.S. & Kirby, N.A. (1978) Curves of achondroplastic spine: a new hypothesis. *Johns Hopkins Med. J.*, **142**, 205–210.

Siebens, A.A., Kirby, N.A. & Hungerford, D.S. (1988) Orthotic correction of sitting abnormality in achondroplastic children. In Nicoletti, B., Kopits, S.E., Ascani, E. & McKusick, V.A. (eds) *Human Achondroplasia*, pp. 313–317. Plenum Press, New York.

Spranger, J.W. & Langer, L.O. (1970) Spondyloepiphyseal dysplasia congenita. *Radiology*, **94**, 313–322.

Stevenson, A.C. (1957) Achondroplasia: an account of the condition in Northern Ireland. *Am. J. Hum. Genet.*, **9**, 81–91.

Streeten, E., Uematsu, S., Hurko, O., Kopits, S., Murphy, E. & Pyeritz, R. (1988) Extended laminectomy for spinal stenosis in achondroplasia. In Nicoletti, B., Kopits, S.E., Ascani, E. & McKusick, V.A. (eds) *Human Achondroplasia*, pp. 261–273. Plenum Press, New York.

Suss, R.A., Uvarhely, G.B., Wang, H., Kumar, A.J., Zinreich, S.J. & Rosenbaum, A.E. (1983) Myelography in achondroplasia: value of a lateral C1–2 puncture and non-ionic water-soluble contrast medium. *Radiology*, **149**, 159–163.

Tolo, V.T. (1985) Spinal deformity in dwarfs. In Bradford, D.S. & Hensinger, R.M. (eds) *The Pediatric Spine*, pp. 338–349. Georg Thième, Stuttgart.

Tolo, V.T. (1988) Surgical treatment of kyphosis in achondroplasia. In Nicoletti, B., Kopits, S.E., Ascani, E. & McKusick, V.A. (eds) *Human Achondroplasia*, pp. 257–259. Plenum Press, New York.

Uematsu, S., Wang, H., Hurko, O. & Kopits, S.E. (1988) The subarachnoid fluid space in achondroplastic spinal stenosis: the surgical implications. In Nicoletti, B., Kopits, S.E., Ascani, E. & McKusick, V.A. (eds) *Human Achondroplasia*, pp. 275–281. Plenum Press, New York.

Vilarrubias, J.M., Cavaliere, P. & Ginebreda, I. (1988) Lengthening of the lower limbs and correction of lumbar hyperlordosis in achondroplasia. In Nicoletti, B., Kopits, S.E., Ascani, E. & McKusick, V.A. (eds) *Human Achondroplasia*, pp. 357–371. Plenum Press, New York.

Vogl, A. & Osborne, R.L. (1949) Lesions of the spinal cord

(transverse myelopathy) in achondroplasia. *Arch. Neurol. Psychiatry*, **61**, 644–662.

Winter, R.B. (1981) Convex anterior and posterior hemiarthrodesis and hemiepiphysiodesis in young children with progressive congenital scoliosis. *J. Pediatr. Orthop.*, **1**, 361–366.

Winter, R.B. (1987) Dwarfs. In Bradford, D.S., Lonstein, J.E., Moe, J.H., Ogilvie, J.W. & Winter, R.B. (eds) *Scoliosis and Other Spinal Deformities*, 2nd edn, pp. 522–540. W.B. Saunders, Philadelphia, PA.

Wynne-Davies, R., Walsh, W.K. & Gormley, J. (1981) Achondroplasia and hypochondroplasia. *J. Bone Jt. Surg.*, **63B**, 508–515.

Wynne-Davies, R. & Hall, C. (1982) Two clinical variants of spondyloepiphyseal dysplasia congenita. *J. Bone Jt. Surg.*, **64B**, 435–441.

Wynne-Davies, R. & Gormley, J. (1985) The prevalence of skeletal dysplasias. *J. Bone Jt. Surg.*, **67B**, 133–137.

Wynne-Davies, R., Hall, C.M. & Apley, A.G. (1985) *Atlas of Skeletal Dysplasias*, 2nd edn. Churchill Livingstone, Edinburgh.

Yamada, H., Nakamura, S., Tajima, M. & Kageyama, N. (1981) Neurological manifestations of pediatric achondroplasia. *J. Neurosurg.*, **54**, 49–57.

18 · Visceral Anomalies Associated with Vertebral Malformations

By R.C.M. COOK

'Sit upright at your work and do not lean or loll, and forbear to carry children in your arms out of a wanton humour; for these, while you are so young, may incline your body to crookedness.' So wrote Mrs Hannah Woolley as part of an exhortation to the schoolgirl in 1675, and human nature both before and since has sought explanation for deformities in outward actions—especially in misuse of the body. We are now more aware of the embryological basis for many conditions which may not manifest themselves until long after birth. Knowledge of embryology, and of the close interaction of the development of different organ systems, may well lead to suspicion that when one anomaly is found others may be present even in apparently unrelated organs. We may be able to provide a slightly clearer picture of the pathogenesis of malformations, but we are often no nearer discovery of the real first cause than was Mrs Woolley.

We are, however, often able to give a comprehensive diagnosis—not just one restricted to a single organ system. This comprehensiveness is essential, not only for the proper management of the presenting lesion, but also for giving the parents an accurate prognosis and appropriate counsel about the need for further treatment later in life. Genetic advice is also often possible and appropriate. Because of their very early close association in formation, the spine and alimentary tract may both be malformed. Later linkage between the development of the gut, the urinary tract, heart, lungs and diaphragm means that a very wide spectrum of visceral defects may be found in association with spinal malformations (see Chapters 13 & 16).

Some grasp of normal, and possible abnormal, routes of embryogenesis is essential to an understanding of the patterns of association of malformations. Some readers may prefer to look at the clinical aspects first and then turn back to the embryology, but the latter is considered first so that the clinical features may seem a logical deduction, backed by observation (see also Chapter 2).

EMBRYOLOGY

In the third week of embryonic life (Day 18 or 19), in the presomitic stage, the notochord begins to form, growing forward from the primitive knot (Hensen's node) between the endoderm and the ectoderm of the embryonic disc. The notochord and the ectoderm are closely attached and form the roof of the archenteron or intraembryonic yolk sac (Bell, 1923). There may be a brief period in the human embryo when there is a dorsal opening in this roof in the region of Hensen's node. This is the neurenteric canal joining the yolk sac to the amniotic cavity (Faris & Crowe, 1975). Hensen's node and the site of the neurenteric canal migrate caudally as axial development continues, and the notochord separates from the roof of the archenteron, and will continue to have endoderm and ectoderm lying ventrally and dorsally, respectively. In this dorsal ectoderm the neural crest differentiates and separates from adjacent ectoderm to form the neural tube. Meanwhile the lateral lying mesodermal masses develop, condense and segment into the sclerotomes that wrap around the notochord and the neural tube to form the vertebral bodies. Errors of segmentation may clearly lead to extra or fewer vertebral bodies than normal.

Abnormal adhesions or growth of the notochord can readily explain intestinal anomalies such as duplication of the gut (Elliot *et al.*, 1970). The notochord and the ectoderm grow faster than the endoderm, so that there is not only folding of the embryo, but also a shearing movement between the layers of tissue. If the endoderm adheres to the notochord, or to the ectoderm, endodermal cells will be dragged upwards or cephalad as a traction diverticulum (Elwood, 1959). If these cells become detached the scene is set for the formation of an isolated cyst; if they remain connected to the gut there will be a long tubular duplication whose caudal end opens into the gut lumen (Fig. 18.1). The earlier in development any abnormal fusion occurs, the longer will be the duplication, and the higher the vertebral level affected.

If the cells remain adherent to the notochord, the mesenchyme destined to form the vertebral bodies cannot fuse ventrally, and hemivertebrae will form. The enteric cyst may be adherent to the dura, grow into the spinal canal and may compress the cord. The term 'neurenteric cyst' is often used for such duplications (Ein *et al.*, 1988). If endoderm and ectoderm remain fused so that the notochord has to split to grow forwards, the mesenchymal condensations that form the vertebrae will be even more disorganized, and more gross vertebral abnormalities will result. Very wide division of the notochord around a persistent neurenteric canal may lead to the most extreme form of the split notochord syndrome, where a dorsal opening of the gut extends through a bifid spine sometimes in association with a myelomeningocele (Bell, 1923; Saunders, 1943; Elwood, 1959; Bentley & Smith, 1960).

Some specific aspects of the embryology of the foregut and hindgut need to be considered, and theories of their normal development need to take into account the known anomalies, and the association of such anomalies with spinal development.

The division of the foregut into a ventral trachea and dorsal oesophagus has traditionally been explained (His, 1887) as a process of septation—lateral ridges appearing in the walls of the foregut which fuse in the midline in a caudocranial direction (Fig. 18.2). This process is analogous to the division of the cloaca into rectum and urogenital sinus by the Tourneux fold and lateral plicae of Rathke (Stephens & Durham Smith, 1971; de Vries & Friedland, 1974) (Fig. 18.3). On the basis of this, a simple mechanical theory of the pathogenesis of anorectal and oesophageal anomalies has been proposed (Piekarski & Stephens, 1976) and this makes the vertebral malformation the primary fault. Excessive folding of the embryo, due either to extra or abnormal vertebrae (Hodson & Shaw, 1973), could lead to malalignment of each fold in both the foregut and the cloaca, so that they are deflected posteriorly. In the foregut this will close off the (posterior) oesophagus and leave the (more anterior) trachea open to the lower oesophagus, and in the hindgut will seal off the rectum. However, in relation to the foregut, the dominant role of the tracheo-oesophageal septum has been called into question in a number of more recent studies (Zwa Tun, 1982; Kluth & Habenich, 1987; Kluth *et al.*, 1987). This work suggests that the trachea and the rest of the respiratory tract develop from a simple 'lung bud' that grows out of the ventral aspect of the common tracheo-oesophageal space, and later faults of organization account for the recognized malformations. The common form of oesophageal atresia

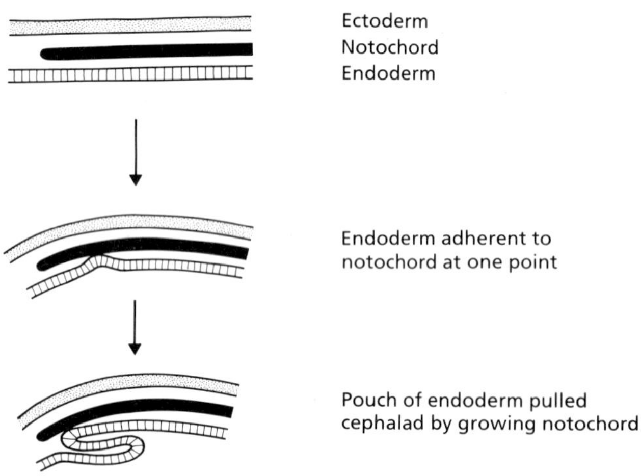

Fig. 18.1 Diagram of the development of intestinal duplication from adherence of endoderm to the lengthening notochord.

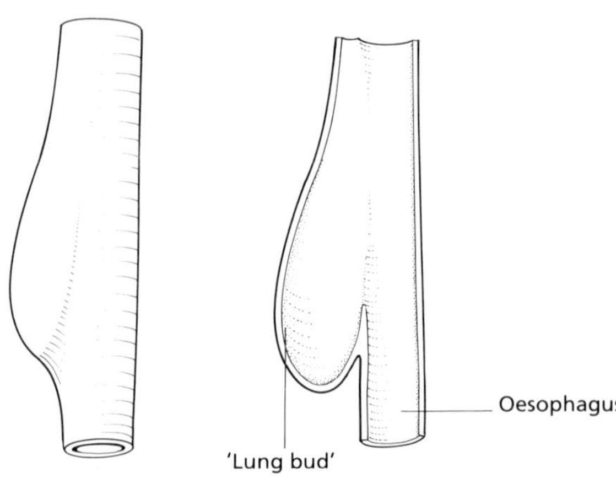

Fig. 18.2 Septation separating the 'lung bud' from the pharynx and oesophagus.

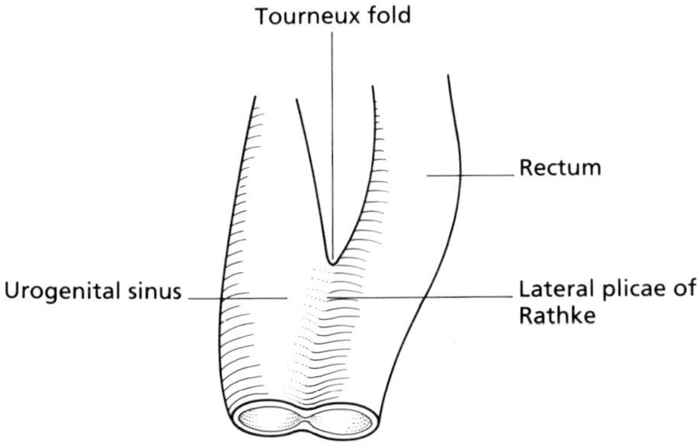

Fig. 18.3 Septation separating the dorsal rectum from the ventral urogenital sinus.

with a tracheo-oesophageal fistula is thought, from electron microscopy studies on chick embryos, to arise because of an excessive ventral displacement of the foregut. Because of its abnormally ventral position it differentiates into trachea, while the pharyngeal pouch above ends blindly, and the lower oesophagus remains attached to the airway (Fig. 18.4).

From studies of the pathological anatomy of infants a high proximal pouch seems to be associated with an especially high incidence of vertebral, rib and sternal anomalies (Touloukian & Keller, 1988). Why derangement of somite formation should particularly be associated with more severe malformation of the foregut is uncertain. The rarer forms of oesophageal anomaly have a less clear association with vertebral malformations, and the 'pure' atresia could develop because of vascular accidents leading to necrosis of an already formed oesophagus, as was suggested some years ago by Lister (1964). Fistulae, without atresia, could be due to breakdown of the two epithelial surfaces if they are in proximity without intervening mesoderm. Such a breakdown is a normal embryological event leading to the disruption of, for instance, the oropharyngeal and cloacal membranes.

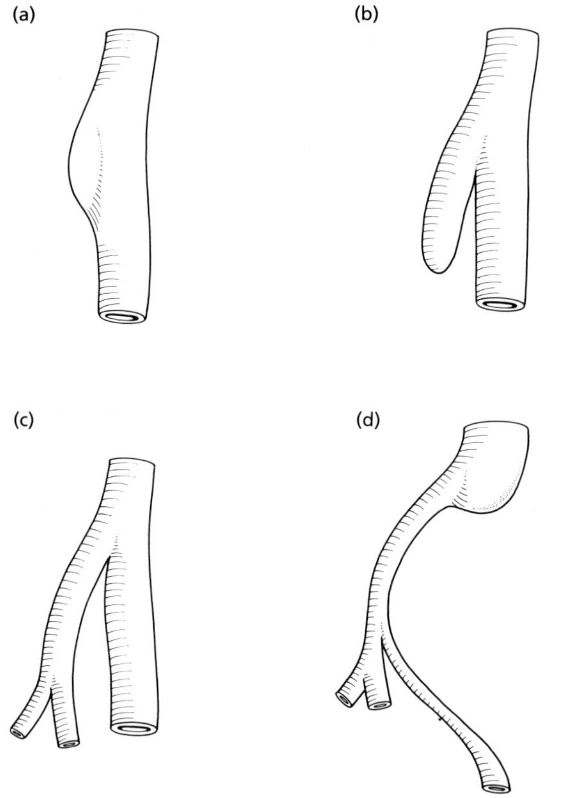

Fig. 18.4 Kluth's theory of separation of the trachea and lungs from the oesophagus. (a)–(c) The lung bud grows out from the ventral aspect of the foregut and the more ventrally sited epithelium differentiates into respiratory type, the more dorsal into oesophageal squamous epithelium; (d) excessive ventral displacement prevents differentiation of a segment of oesophagus.

PATHOGENESIS OF VISCERAL MALFORMATIONS

Folic acid antagonists are known to cause urogenital, skeletal and vertebral anomalies in experimental animals. Other teratogens such as thalidomide and oral contraceptives (Balci *et al.*, 1973; Kaufman, 1973) have been implicated in both oesophageal and anorectal malformations. Genetic factors (Schwoebel *et al.*, 1964; Townes & Brocks, 1972; Boocock & Donnai, 1987) are relevant in some instances, and an autosomal recessive form of inheritance may be responsible for some forms of anorectal anomalies. Uniovular twins have been described (Cozzi & Wilkinson, 1968; Stephens & Durham Smith, 1971) with identical anomalies, but where anorectal malformations occur in twins it is usually only one which is affected. The frequent association of other anomalies, in predictable patterns in any individual, but arising sporadically in the population, fits in with the concept of intrinsic mutagenesis—of random mutations due to errors of DNA replication.

Oesophageal atresia

Oesophageal atresia was a lethal abnormality until 1941 when Cameron Haight achieved a successful end-to-end anastomosis. Earlier, infants had survived with gastrostomies and cervical oesophagostomies, and a fistula without oesophageal atresia had been successfully closed by Imperatori (1939). The incidence of oesophageal anomalies is approximately 1:3500 with an equal number of males and females (Cudmore, 1990).

Classification

Classification by numbered types has been suggested, but it is far more useful to use morphologically accurate names for the different forms of anomaly and to bear in mind that they may have different embryological causes. The common form of oesophageal atresia is associated with a tracheo-oesophageal fistula communicating with the distal oesophagus (Figs 18.5a & 18.7). Oesophageal atresia without a fistula (Fig. 18.5b) is found in 5% or 6% of large series (Myers *et al.*, 1987). Atresia with a fistula to the proximal pouch only is rarer, but found in nearly one-quarter of infants with a gasless abdomen who may easily be assumed to have no fistula at all (Cass & Auldist, 1987). A fistula without oesophageal atresia occurs in about 5% of large series of oesophageal malformations (Fig. 18.5c).

Diagnosis

This condition may be suspected prenatally because of polyhydramnios or from ultrasound. After delivery, drooling of saliva, blowing bubbles and any respiratory difficulty should always raise the possibility of atresia, and the passage of a reasonably firm tube through the mouth should be attempted. If the tube will not pass, a radiograph of the chest is taken. The position of the tip of the tube, the presence or absence of gas in the stomach and intestines will be noted, and the film should also show if the lungs are clear, and demonstrate any gross vertebral anomalies (Figs 18.6 & 18.7). A gasless abdomen is associated with atresia without a fistula, or an isolated fistula to the proximal pouch only.

A fistula without atresia is often difficult to diagnose. It is usually oblique, running caudally from the trachea to the oesophagus. It is therefore more correctly described as an N-type fistula rather than an H-type. Passage of oesophageal (or more hazardously, gastric) contents into the trachea may give acute or recurrent respiratory symptoms. Alternatively the abdomen may become grossly distended because of air passing into the gut. Contrast studies may demonstrate the fistula but tracheoscopy and oesophagoscopy are often more reliable.

Anorectal malformations

Malformations of the anus and rectum are generally said (Stephens & Durham Smith, 1971; Wiener & Kiesewetter, 1973) to occur with an incidence of 1 in 5000, but a figure as high as 1 in 1800 was calculated (Louw *et al.*, 1971) in caucasian and coloured populations in South Africa. The real incidence may be expected to be higher than quoted figures, since although the major 'high' lesions are unlikely to be overlooked, the more minor 'low' lesions may be

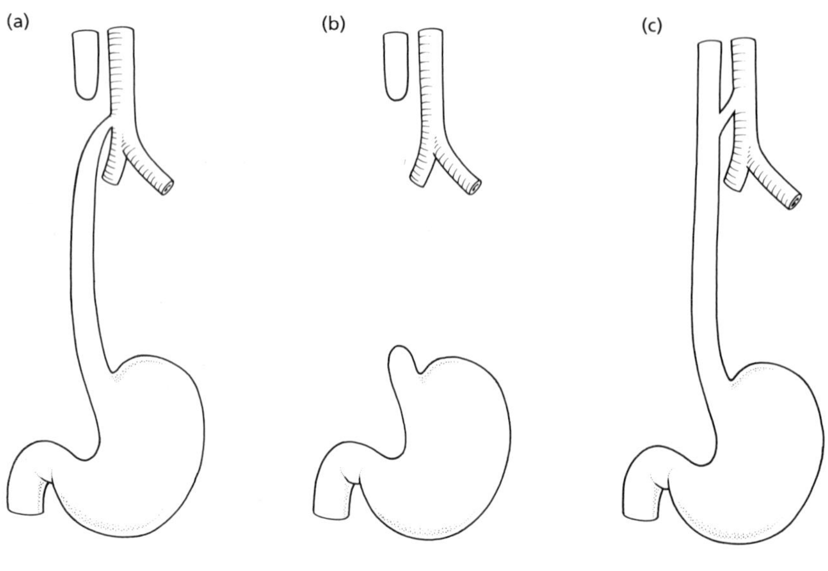

Fig. 18.5 Diagram of the recognized types of oesophageal/tracheal malformations: (a) oesophageal atresia with tracheo-oesophageal fistula; (b) oesophageal atresia without fistula; (c) tracheo-oesophageal fistula (without atresia).

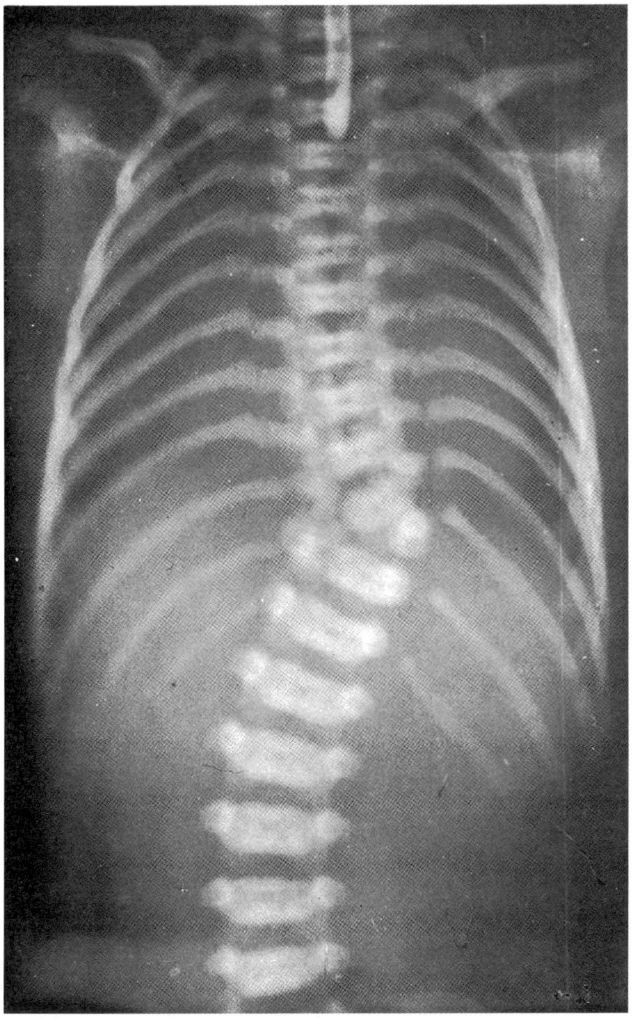

Fig. 18.6 Radiograph of a day-old infant with radio-opaque tube in the upper oesophageal pouch. There is oesophageal atresia without a fistula (no gas in the stomach) and lower thoracic hemivertebrae are evident.

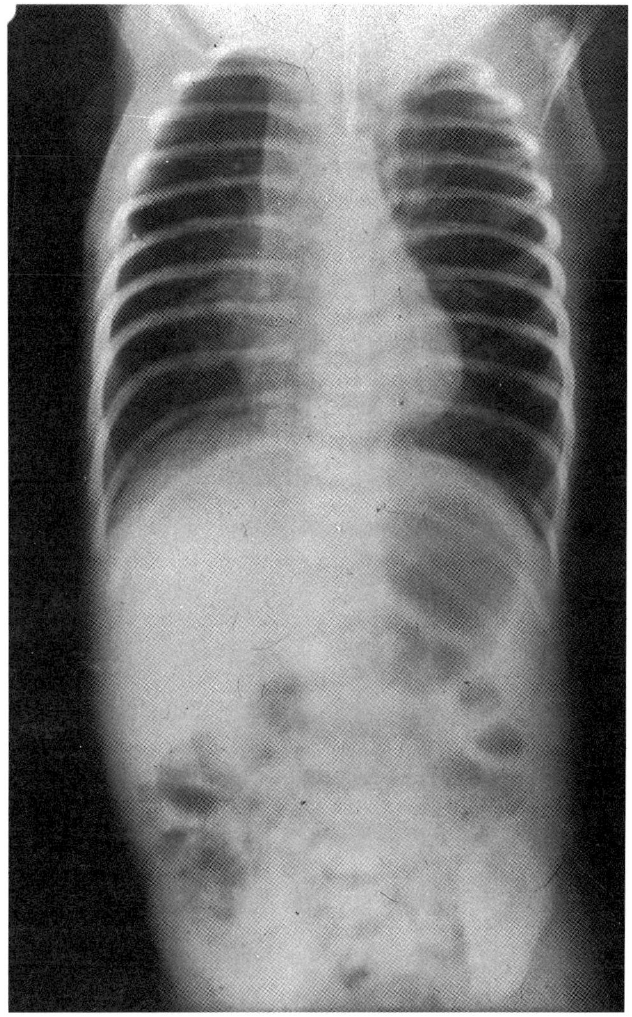

Fig. 18.7 Radiograph of a newborn infant with oesophageal atresia (opaque tube passed as far as possible) and a tracheo-oesophageal fistula (there is gas in the stomach and beyond).

missed in early life and not all appear in statistics of congenital malformations.

The sex incidence shows an overall preponderance of boys, with a greater incidence of high lesions in males and low lesions in females. The incidence of the main types of malformation in recent years in infants admitted to the Regional Neonatal Surgical Centre at Alder Hey is shown in Tables 18.1 & 18.2.

Pathology

The pathological anatomy of anorectal malformations is complex, and attempts to produce an internationally agreed classification have been made to help in comparing methods of treatment. The Melbourne Classification marks an important milestone in the history of paediatric surgery, and its authors bravely grappled with the complexities of the many different forms that are recognized (Stephens & Durham Smith, 1971). Three main groups were distinguished from one another—high, intermediate and low. These were then subdivided to take into account the anatomical configurations, the location of any fistula, and the sex of the infant. Nearly 40 named varieties resulted, and although their names reflected and described the anatomy, the complexity of the classification made it difficult to use with sufficient accuracy to allow comparison to be made between different surgical centres. The Wingspread Conference de-

Table 18.1 Incidence of types of anorectal malformation in male infants in Liverpool

High	
1 Anorectal agenesis	
(a) with rectoprostatic urethral fistula	18
(b) without fistula	8
2 Rectal atresia	3
Intermediate	
1 Rectobulbar–urethral fistula	10
2 Anal agenesis without fistula	2
Low	
1 Anocutaneous fistula	36
2 Anal stenosis	9
'Rare'	
Anorectal agenesis with rectovesical fistula	8
Shared colon in conjoined twins	2
Other	2
Total	98

Table 18.2 Incidence of types of anorectal malformation in female infants in Liverpool

High	
1 Anorectal agenesis	
(a) with rectovaginal fistula	8
(b) without fistula	2
2 Rectal atresia	
Intermediate	
1 Rectovestibular fistula	4
2 Rectovaginal fistula	3
3 Anal agenesis without fistula	
Low	
1 Anovestibular fistula	15
2 Anocutaneous fistula	9
3 Anal stenosis	5
Cloacal anomalies	7
Total	53

veloped a simpler classification in 1984, which omitted many of the rarer anomalies but held firmly to the importance of distinguishing high, intermediate and low lesions in the two sexes (Tables 18.1 & 18.2).

It is the relationship of the termination of the bowel to the pelvic floor and to the sphincter muscle complex which is the central factor in allotting a place in the classification—and, more importantly, in determining the best management, the prognosis and the risk of the presence of associated malformations. Where bowel terminates on the cranial side of the levator muscles, lesions are referred to as 'high' or supralevator; those infants in whom the bowel extends through most of the muscle have 'low' infralevator lesions; whilst in a third 'intermediate' group, even though a fistula is embraced by these muscles, the bowel proper terminates above them (Stephens & Durham Smith, 1971; Pena & de Vries, 1982).

The normal and pathological anatomy of the pelvic floor musculature has been the subject of some study, and even more discussion, in recent years, and the interested reader is referred to recent reviews in the paediatric and adult literature (de Vries and Friedland, 1974; Ayoub, 1979; Pena & de Vries, 1982; Snooks & Swash, 1986; Durham Smith, 1987; Cook, 1990). Suffice it to say here that the pelvic floor and the sphincter muscle complex is of paramount importance, and the correct relationship of the lower bowel to this is essential for continence. It must not be forgotten, however, that the muscles and the lower bowel, and the adjacent skin, must also have their appropriate complement of proprioceptive and other sensory fibres, all linked to centres in the sacral spinal cord segments, and to the brain.

Associated malformations in oesophageal atresia and anorectal malformations

It has long been recognized that the infant born with an anorectal malformation or oesophageal atresia (or both) has a high risk of having other anomalies. An appreciation of particular associations enables appropriate investigations to be carried out, and may well throw light on the embryogenesis of the malformations. With something like anorectal anomalies it is logical to distinguish those conditions that are distinct, even though frequently associated (such as oesophageal atresia and vertebral defects), from those that are an integral part of the primary malformation (such as a recto-urinary fistula) and also from those that are a consequence or complication of it (such as urinary tract infections).

Other anomalies associated with anorectal or oesophageal ones are described in many different organic systems, in varying incidence. Of 132 consecutive recent admissions to Liverpool with anorectal anomalies, who were thoroughly investigated, 85 (64.8%) were found to have other malformations. Stephens & Durham Smith (1971) found that

Table 18.3 Sex and the incidence of anomalies associated with anorectal malformations

	Males with one or more other anomalies	Females with one or more other anomalies
Low	25 out of 45 infants (55.6%)	15 out of 29 infants (51.7%)
Intermediate and high (and cloacal)	40 out of 53 (75.5%)	21 out of 24 (87.5%)
Total	65 out of 98 (66.3%)	36 out of 53 (67.9%)

60.6% (149 out of 246 infants) had one or more associated anomalies. A higher incidence is found in supralevator (high) lesions than in infralevator (low) ones (Obeid & Corkery, 1974). The associated anomalies in the high group are not only more common, but also more severe (Hoekstra *et al.*, 1983). Significant lesions were found in 76.6% of infants with high and intermediate lesions in Liverpool, and in 54.1% of low ones (Table 18.3).

In the Liverpool series of anorectal malformations the incidence of associated lesions was similar in the two sexes in both high and low lesions (Table 18.3). This contrasts with other reports (Stephens & Durham Smith, 1971) in which boys with high lesions have a higher incidence of associated anomalies than girls. Associated anomalies used to be said to be rare in girls with low defects, but recent well-investigated series where large numbers have been studied show, like ours, a significant number of female infants with other anomalies (Wiener & Kiesewetter, 1973; Obeid & Corkery, 1974; Hoekstra *et al.*, 1983) (Table 18.4).

GENITO-URINARY MALFORMATIONS

These form the major group of anomalies associated with 'imperforate anus', which is hardly surprising in view of the closely integrated embryology of the systems. Faulty budding of the ureter from the Wolffian duct seems to be the embryological basis of many of the renal tract anomalies.

Vertebral anomalies

These have long been recognized (Pellerin & Bertin, 1967; Santulli *et al.*, 1971; Thompson & Grossman, 1974; Karrer *et al.*, 1988) as commonly associated with oesophageal and anorectal malformations, but most reported figures of incidence are probably gross underestimates because few infants will have had full spinal radiology. The skeletal malformations in a recent Liverpool series are shown in Table 18.5. Major anomalies causing kyphosis or other spinal deformity will usually be recognized clinically, and lumbosacral vertebral anomalies will usually be apparent in the

Table 18.4 Incidence of anomalies associated with anorectal malformations

	High and intermediate	Low	Total no. of infants	Percentage affected
Urinary tract	38	13	51	33.8
Vertebrae	23	5	28	18.5
Heart and great vessels	14	3	17	11.3
Oesophageal atresia	6	3	9	6.0
Meckel's diverticulum	9	—	9	6.0
Radial aplasia/hypoplasia	7	—	7	4.6
Neural tube defects	2	4	6	4.0
Lip, palate and mandible	2	3	5	3.3
Down's syndrome	4	0	4	2.6
Duodenal atresia	3	0	3	2.0
Malrotation	3	—	3	2.0
Exomphalos	1	1	2	1.3

Table 18.5 Skeletal abnormalies discovered in 339 consecutive cases of oesophageal atresia in Liverpool. After Cudmore (1990)

Malformation	No. of cases	
Anomaly of spine and/or ribs	30	(9%)
Anomaly of fingers	21	(6%)
Absence of radius	9	(3%)
Major anomaly of lower limb	4	(1%)
Phocomelia	2	(<1%)

abdominal and pelvic radiographs taken to elucidate the pathology of the bowel or the urinary tract. Similarly thoracic spinal anomalies will be seen on a chest X-ray taken for oesophageal atresia. Hemivertebrae, absent and extravertebrae, may be found at any level in association with both high and low anorectal malformations. Extra thoracic vertebrae are not uncommon with oesophageal atresia (Stevenson, 1972; Dickens & Myers, 1987). Agenesis or hemiagenesis of vertebrae is of special significance in relation to the ultimate attainment of faecal and urinary continence when the midsacral vertebrae are affected (Louw *et al.*, 1971; Santulli *et al.*, 1971; Carson *et al.*, 1984).

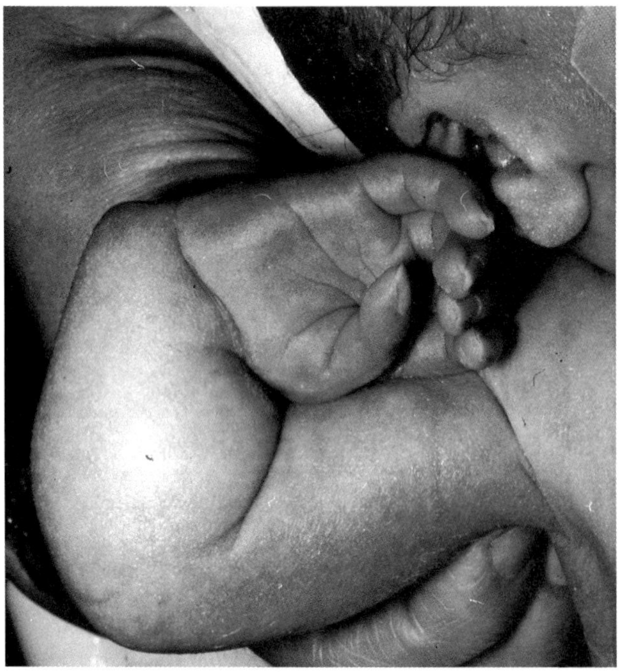

Fig. 18.8 Radial aplasia in an infant with oesophageal atresia.

Fourteen infants in our series of anorectal anomalies are recorded as having agenesis of some or all sacral vertebrae (see Fig. 18.9). Hemivertebrae and wedged vertebrae in the thoracolumbar region may lead to significant scoliosis (Denton, 1982). Eighteen of our infants with anorectal malformations were found to have vertebral anomalies above the sacral zone. Where thoracic vertebrae are abnormal, deformities of the ribs may also be found. The scoliosis associated with oesophageal atresia may also lead to severe neurological problems (Chetcuti *et al.*, 1988).

Half of all infants with oesophageal atresia and tracheo-oesophageal fistula have other significant anomalies, one-fifth of which will be spinal and skeletal (Figs 18.6 & 18.8). In a recent Liverpool series 9% of infants with oesophageal atresia were discovered to have vertebral malformations (Table 18.4). Very high atresias are particularly associated with vertebral (and rib and sternal) malformations

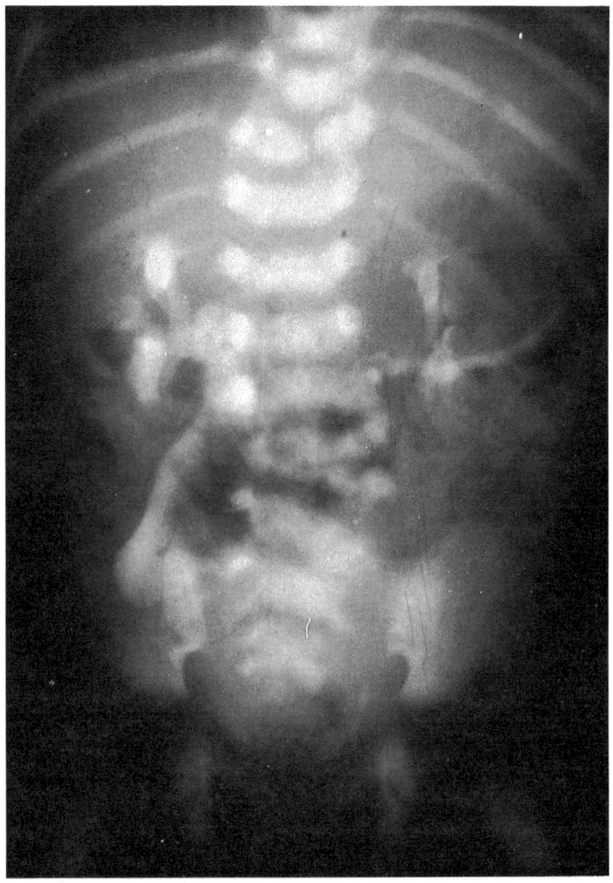

Fig. 18.9 Pyelogram of a child with an anorectal malformation and anomalies of multiple vertebrae.

(Touloukian & Keller, 1988). The rarer forms of oesophageal anomaly show a lower incidence of vertebral malformations, but numbers are necessarily small. In a large and well-investigated series from Melbourne (Myers & Egami, 1987) seven infants with vertebral defects were found in 28 cases of isolated fistula without atresia, but four of 21 infants with atresia but no fistula had spinal abnormalities.

SKELETAL ANOMALIES

Skeletal anomalies other than vertebral ones are also often reported in association with oesophageal and anorectal malformations. Pellerin & Bertin (1967) noted malformations of the lower limbs, and Oberbergerova *et al.* (1975) report a 2% incidence of radial aplasia (Fig. 18.8). This has been found more commonly in a previously reported Liverpool series (Gruchalski *et al.*, 1976) as also having major abnormalities of the lower limbs (hypoplastic leg, absent tibia or fibula, ilial hypoplasia, arthrogryphosis). The extreme form of this association is the mermaid (Duhamel, 1961) (see Chapter 16).

GENITAL, CARDIAC AND OTHER GUT ANOMALIES

These are also found in frequencies higher than expected from simple random association, and this non-random association has been the subject of some interest and study in recent years.

PATTERNS OF MALFORMATION

The idea of a specific syndrome of preaxial polydactyly, imperforate anus and vertebral anomalies was first put forward in 1968 (Fuhrmann, 1968; Say & Gerald, 1968; Say *et al.*, 1971a, b). The association is now well recognized, though preaxial deletion anomalies are as common as, if not more common than, polydactyly (Tunte, 1968, 1969; Kaufman *et al.*, 1970; Say *et al.*, 1971b). There was a very high incidence of skeletal malformations in the Liverpool series of anorectal anomalies, especially where the anorectal anomaly occurred together with oesophageal atresia (Gruchalski *et al.*, 1976). The term VATER association was coined by Quan & Smith (1973) as a mnemonic for '*V*ertebral defects, *A*nal atresia, *T*racheo-*E*sophageal fistula with esophageal atresia, *R*adial and *R*enal dysplasia'. They did not suggest that this was a specific syndrome but rather a non-random association of defects. Cardiac lesions are additional and not infrequent associations, and so the term VACTERL was put forward (Balci *et al.*, 1973) (*V*ertebral, *A*nal, *C*ardiac, *T*racheal, *E*sophageal, *R*enal and *L*imb'), but a simpler expedient was to make the 'V' of VATER stand for vascular as well as vertebral! Children with such patterns of malformation often show significant growth retardation, but usually normal mental development (Temtamy & Miller, 1974).

Apart from some sporadic reports there is little evidence that these groups of anomalies constitute specific syndromes with a single cause. Conversely, it should be borne in mind that the features of the VATER association form part of the list of defects of well-recognized syndromes (such as trisomy 18, and the 13q deletion syndrome). These are specific chromosomal disorders; the affected infant has a very different prognosis, and the parents require accurate counselling both about the prognosis and the genetic implications.

Duplication of the alimentary tract

Duplication of the alimentary tract is a relatively rare anomaly, but may occur at any level from the mouth to the anus. The association of enteric duplications with other anomalies was first clearly described by Gross (1953), and it was Ladd & Gross (1940) who defined the pathological anatomy. Enteric duplications have a smooth muscle wall (usually in two layers), share a common blood supply with the normal gut, have mucosal lining characteristic of any part of the gut, and the lumina may or may not be connected (Forshall, 1961; Lister & Vaos, 1988).

The origin of many enteric duplications can, as we have seen, be traced back to a fault in the separation of the two layers of the embryonic disc and the formation of the notochord. It is often stated (Elwood, 1959; Shepherd, 1965) that duplications below the diaphragm do not commonly have associated vertebral abnormalities. While the spinal abnormalities are more common and more severe in children with foregut duplications, they do occur in a considerable number of those who have duplications of lower levels of the gut (Alrabeeah *et al.*, 1988). The actual vertebral malformations may be of academic and radiological interest only, with no clinical symptoms or signs; or there may be major and significant spinal problems resulting (see Chapters 13 & 16).

The fully expressed split notochord syndrome presents a major malformation for which little corrective surgery is possible. Case reports from around the world suggest that it is not very uncommon (Feller & Sternberg, 1929; Faris & Crowe, 1975; Carachi, 1982; Singh & Singh, 1982; Gupta & Deohar, 1987; Pathak *et al.*, 1988). Useful discussions of the embryology are often included in these reports.

Pharyngeal duplication (to be distinguished from branchial cysts and fistulae) seem rare, but one case is reported in which infection occurred in the duplication and led to osteomyelitis of abnormal cervical vertebrae (and of the femur) (Ein *et al.*, 1988).

Duplications in the thorax, although often referred to as 'oesophageal', may contain mucosa of gastric or lower intestinal type (Wallis, 1967). Seventeen thoracic duplications diagnosed over a period of 28 years were described from Alder Hey Children's Hospital (Baker, 1989). Neonates presented with dyspnoea, cyanosis and feeding difficulty; older infants with stridor, wheeze and cough, or bleeding. Some older children's cysts were found incidentally on chest X-rays. Vertebral anomalies of the upper thoracic and cervical regions were identified in 10 patients. These abnormalities included small irregular vertebral bodies, butterfly and hemivertebrae and segmental defects. Three children had scoliosis that required surgical correction. None of these patients had neurological complications, except one with an extensive thoracolumbar myelomeningocele. Myelography is recommended by Superina *et al.* (1984) because one-quarter of the children in their series who had associated vertebral lesions had intraspinal cysts. Computerized tomographic scanning of the region (or magnetic resonance imaging) would be less invasive an investigation to use if available.

Gastric duplications are among the least frequently reported (Pruksapong *et al.*, 1979) and are often associated with duplications of other parts of the alimentary tract and its derivatives. Their associated vertebral anomalies may affect any part of the spine (Wieczorek *et al.*, 1984).

Jejunal and ileal duplications may be cystic or tubular. The tubular ones may extend for a considerable distance—even the full length of the intestine (Jewett, 1958). Bleeding is the most common presenting symptom, but intestinal obstruction, intussusception, perforation and pseudoascites have all been recorded. Vertebral anomalies are found, if looked for, in at least half the patients (Alrabeeah *et al.*, 1988).

Colonic and rectal duplications are rare, are often associated with some form of 'imperforate anus' and like these are in turn associated with spinal anomalies. The genito-urinary tract may likewise be duplicated.

REFERENCES

Alrabeeah, A., Gillis, D.A., Giacomantonio, P. & Lautt, G. (1988) Neurenteric cysts—a spectrum. *J. Pediatr. Surg.*, **23**, 752–754.

Ayoub, S.F. (1979) Anatomy of the external anal sphincter in man. *Acta Anat.*, **105**, 25–36.

Baker, E.M. (1989) Intrathoracic duplication cyst: a review of 17 patients. *J. Med. Imaging*, **3**, 127–134.

Balci, S., Say, B., Pirnar, T. & Hicsonmez, A. (1973) Birth defects and oral contraceptives. *Lancet*, **ii**, 1098.

Bell, H.H. (1923) Anterior spina bifida and its relation to a persistence of the neurenteric canal. *J. Nerv. Ment. Dis.*, **57**, 445–462.

Bentley, J.F.R. & Smith, J.R. (1960) Developmental posterior enteric remnants and spinal malformation: the split notochord syndrome. *Arch. Dis. Child.*, **35**, 76–86.

Boocock, G.R. & Donnai, D. (1987) Anorectal malformations: familial aspects and associated anomalies. *Arch. Dis. Child.*, **62**, 576–579.

Carachi, R. (1982) The split notochord syndrome: a case report on a mixed spinal enterogenous cyst in a child with spina bifida cystica. *Z. Kinderchir.*, **35**, 32–34.

Carson, J.A., Barnes, P.D., Tunell, W.P., Smith, E.I. & Jolley, S.G. (1984) Imperforate anus: the neurologic implications of sacral abnormalities. *J. Pediatr. Surg.*, **19**, 838–842.

Cass, D. & Auldist, A. (1987) Oesophageal atresia with proximal tracheo-oesophageal fistula. *Pediatr. Surg. Int.*, **2**, 212–215.

Chetcuti, P., Myers, N.A., Phelan, P.D. & Beasley, S.W. (1988) Adults who survived repair of congenital oesophageal atresia and tracheo-oesophageal fistula. *Br. Med. J.*, **297**, 344–346.

Cook, R.C.M. (1990) Anorectal malformations. In Lister, J. & Irving, M. (eds) *Neonatal Surgery*, pp. 547–570. Butterworth, London.

Cozzi, F. & Wilkinson, A.W. (1968) Familial incidence of anorectal anomalies. *Surgery*, **64**, 669.

Cudmore, R.E. (1990) Oesophageal atresia and tracheo-oesophageal fistula. In Listes, J. & Irving, I.M. (eds) *Neonatal Surgery*, pp. 231–258. Butterworth, London.

Denton, J.R. (1982) The association of congenital spinal anomalies with imperforate anus. *Clin. Orthop.*, **162**, 91–98.

Dickens, D.R.V. & Myers, N.A. (1987) Oesophageal atresia and vertebral anomalies. *Pediatr. Surg. Int.*, **2**, 278–281.

Duhamel, B. (1961) From the mermaid to anal imperforation: the syndrome of caudal regression. *Arch. Dis. Child.*, **36**, 152–155.

Durham Smith, E. (1987) The bath water needs changing but don't throw out the baby: an overview of anorectal anomalies. *J. Pediatr. Surg.*, **22**, 335–384.

Ein, S.H., Shandling, B., Humphreys, R. & Krajbich, I. (1988) Osteomyelitis of the cervical spine presenting as a neurenteric cyst. *J. Pediatr. Surg.*, **23**, 779–781.

Elliott, G.B., Tredwell, S.J. & Elliott, K.A. (1970) The notochord as an abnormal organizer in production of congenital intestinal defects. *Am. J. Roentgenol.*, **110**, 628–634.
Elwood, J.S. (1959) Mediastinal duplication of the gut. *Arch. Dis. Child.*, **34**, 474–479.
Faris, J.C. & Crowe, J.E. (1975) The split notochord syndrome. *J. Pediatr. Surg.*, **10**, 467–470.
Feller, A. & Sternberg, H. (1929) Zur Kenntris der Fehlbildungen der Wirbelsaule. I. Die Wirkelkorperspalte und ihre formale Genese. *Virchows Arch. Pathol. Anat.*, **272**, 613–640.
Forshall, I. (1961) Duplication of the intestinal tract. *Postgrad. Med. J.*, **37**, 570.
Fuhrmann, W. (1968) A new polydactyly imperforate anus/vertebral anomalies syndrome? *Lancet*, **ii**, 918.
Gross, R.E. (1953) *The Surgery of Infancy and Childhood*, pp. 221–245. W.B. Saunders, Philadelphia, PA.
Gruchalski, J., Irving, I.M. & Lister, J. (1976) Skeletal anomalies associated with oesophageal, duodenal and anorectal atresias. *Lancet*, **ii**, 517.
Gupta, D.K. & Deohar, M.C. (1987) Split notochord syndrome presenting with meningomyelocele and dorsal enteric fistula. *J. Pediatr. Surg.*, **22**, 382–383.
His, W. (1887) Zur Bildungsgeschichte de Lungen beim menschlichen Embryo. *Arch. Anat.*, **89**, 106.
Hodson, C.J. & Shaw, D.G. (1973) Congenital atresia of the oesophagus and thirteen pairs of ribs. *Pediatr. Radiol.*, **1**, 248–249.
Hoekstra, W.J., Scholtmeijer, R.J., Molenaar, J.C., Schreeve, R.H. & Schroeder, F.H. (1983) Urogenital tract abnormalities associated with congenital anorectal anomalies. *J. Urol.*, **130**, 962–963.
Imperatori, C.J. (1939) Congenital tracheo-oesophageal fistula without atresia of the esophagus. Report of a case with plastic closure and cure. *Arch. Otolaryngol.*, **30**, 352–359.
Jewett, T.C. Jr (1958) Duplication of the entire small intestine with massive melena. *Ann. Surg.*, **147**, 239.
Karrer, F.M., Flannery, A.M., Nelson, M.D., McLowe, D.G. & Raffensperger, J.G. (1988) Anorectal malformations: evaluation of associated spinal dysraphic syndromes. *J. Pediatr. Surg.*, **23**, 45–48.
Kaufman, R.L. (1973) VACTERL associated with oral contraceptives. *Lancet*, **i**, 1396.
Kaufman, R.L., Quinton, B. & Ternber, J.L. (1970) Polydactyly/imperforate anus/vertebral anomalies syndrome. *Lancet*, **i**, 841.
Kluth, D. & Habenich, R. (1987) The embryology of usual and unusual types of esophageal atresia. *Pediatr. Surg. Int.*, **2**, 223–227.
Kluth, D., Steding, G. & Seidl, W. (1987) The embryology of foregut malformations. *J. Pediatr. Surg.*, **22**, 389–393.
Ladd, W.E. & Gross, R.E. (1940) Surgical treatment of duplications of the alimentary tract. *Surg. Gynecol. Obstet.*, **70**, 295.
Lister, J. (1964) The blood supply of the oesophagus in relation to oesophageal atresia. *Arch. Dis. Child.*, **39**, 131–137.
Lister, L. & Vaos, C.G. (1988) Duplication of the alimentary tract. In Spitz, L. & Nixon, H.H. (eds) *Operative Surgery, Paediatric Surgery*, 4th edn, pp. 317–323. Butterworth, London.
Louw, J.H., Cywes, S. & Cremin, B.J. (1971) The management of anorectal agenesis. *S. Afr. J. Surg.*, **9**, 21–26.
Myers, N.A. & Egami, K. (1987) Congenital tracheo-oesophageal fistula. *Pediatr. Surg. Int.*, **2**, 198–211.
Myers, N.A., Beasley, S.W., Auldist, A.W., Kent, M., Wright, V. & Chetcuti, P. (1987) Oesophageal atresia without fistula—anastomosis or replacement. *Pediatr. Surg. Int.*, **2**, 216–222.
Obeid, M.L. & Corkery, J.J. (1974) Importance of the urinary tract in imperforate anus. *Proc. R. Soc. Med.*, **67**, 203.
Oberbergerova, D., Tosousky, V. & Zitkova, M. (1975) Coincidence of atresias of the alimentary tract—in particular of the oesophagus—with skeletal malformations. *Z. Kinderchir.*, **16**, 268.
Pathak, V.B., Singh, S. & Wakhlu, A.K. (1988) Double split of notochord with massive prolapse of the gut. *J. Pediatr. Surg.*, **23**, 1039–1040.
Pellerin, D. & Bertin, P. (1967) Genito-urinary malformations and vertebral anomalies in ano-rectal malformations. *Z. Kinderchir.*, **4**, 375.
Pena, A. & de Vries, P.A. (1982) Posterior sagittal anorectoplasty: important technical considerations and new applications. *J. Pediatr. Surg.*, **17**, 638–643, 796–811.
Piekarski, D. & Stephens, F.D. (1976) The association and embryogenesis of tracheo-oesophageal and anorectal anomalies. *Progr. Pediatr. Surg.*, 63–76.
Pruksapong, C., Donovan, R.G. & Pinit, A. (1979) Gastric duplication. *J. Pediatr. Surg.*, **14**, 83.
Quan, L. & Smith, D.W. (1973) The VATER association. Vertebral defects, anal atresia, TE fistula with oesophageal atresia, radial and renal dysplasia. *J. Pediatr. Surg.*, **82**, 104–106.
Santulli, T.V., Schullinger, J.N., Kiesewetter, W.B. & Bill, A.H. Jr (1971) Imperforate anus: a survey from members of the surgical section of the American Academy of Pediatrics. *J. Pediatr. Surg.*, **6**, 484.
Saunders, R.L. de C.H. (1943) Combined anterior and posterior spina bifida in a living neonatal human female. *Anat. Rec.*, **87**, 255–278.
Say, B. & Gerald, P.S. (1968) A new polydactyly/imperforate anus/vertebral anomalies syndrome? *Lancet*, **ii**, 688.
Say, B., Balci, S., Pirnar, T. & Hiesonmez, A. (1971a) Imperforate anus/polydactyly/vertebral anomalies: a hereditary trait? *J. Pediatr.*, **79**, 1033.
Say, B., Balci, S., Pirnar, T. & Tunebilek, E. (1971b) A new syndrome of dysmorphogenesis: imperforate anus associated with poly-oligodactyly and skeletal (mainly vertebral) anomalies. *Acta Paediatr. Scand*, **60**, 197.
Schwoebel, M.G., Hirsig, J., Schinxel, A. & Stanffer, U.G. (1964) Familial incidence of congenital anorectal anomalies. *J. Pediatr. Surg.*, **19**, 179–182.
Shepherd, M.P. (1965) Thoracic, thoraco-abdominal and abdominal duplication. *Thorax*, **20**, 82–86.
Singh, A. & Singh, R. (1982) Split notochord syndrome with dorsal enteric fistula. *J. Pediatr. Surg.*, **17**, 412–413.
Snooks, S.J. & Swash, M. (1986) The innervation of the muscles of continence. *Ann. R. Coll. Surg. Eng.*, **68**, 45–49.
Stephens, F.D. & Durham Smith, E. (1971) *Anorectal Malformations in Children.* Year Book Medical Publishers, Chicago, IL.
Stephens, F.D. & Durham Smith, E. (1986) Classification, identifications and assessment of surgical treatment of

anorectal anomalies. *Pediatr. Surg. Int.*, **1**, 200–205.

Stevenson, R.E. (1972) Extra vertebrae associated with oesophageal atresia and tracheo-osesophageal fistula. *J. Pediatr. Surg.*, **83**, 1123–1129.

Superina, R.A., Ein, S.H. & Humphreys, R.P. (1984) Cystic duplication of the oesophagus and neurenteric cysts. *J. Pediatr. Surg.*, **19**, 527–530.

Temtamy, S.A. & Miller, J.D. (1974) Extending the scope of the VATER association. Definition of the VATER syndrome. *J. Pediatr. Surg.*, **85**, 345–349.

Thompson, W. & Grossman, H. (1974) The association of spinal and genitourinary abnormalities with low anorectal anomalies (imperforate anus) in female infants. *Radiology*, **113**, 693–698.

Touloukian, R.J. & Keller, M.S. (1988) High proximal pouch oesophageal atresia with vertebral, rib and sternal anomalies. An additional component to the VATER association. *J. Pediatr. Surg.*, **23**, 76–79.

Townes, P.L. & Brocks, E.R. (1972) Hereditary syndrome of imperforate anus with head, foot and ear anomalies. *J. Pediatr.*, **81**, 321.

Tunte, W. (1968) A new polydactyly/imperforate anus/vertebral anomalies syndrome? *Lancet*, **ii**, 1081.

Tunte, W. (1969) Anal atresia bei Zwillingen. *Z. Kinderheilt.*, **105**, 21.

de Vries, P.A. & Friedland, G.W. (1974) The staged sequential development of the anus and rectum in human embryos and fetuses. *J. Pediatr. Surg.*, **9**, 755.

Wallis, P.G. (1967) Enteric duplication cyst in the chest. *Proc. R. Soc. Med.*, **60**, 454.

Wieczorek, R.L., Siedman, I., Ranson, J.H.C. & Ruoff, M. (1984) Congenital duplication of the stomach: case report and review of the English literature. *Ann. J. Gastroenterol.*, **79**, 597.

Wiener, E.S. & Kiesewetter, W.B. (1973) Urologic abnormalities associated with imperforate anus. *J. Pediatr. Surg.*, **6**, 454.

Woolley, Mrs Hannah (1675) Exhortation to the schoolgirl, in *The Gentlewoman's Companion, or a Guide to the Female Sex.*

Zwa Tunn, H.A. (1982) The tracheo-esophageal septum—fact or fantasy? *Acta Anat.*, **114**, 1–21.

SECTION 5
SPINAL DEFORMITY

19 · Pathogenesis and Assessment of Scoliosis

By R.G. BURWELL and P.H. DANGERFIELD

Try to forget the individual deformity of the spinal column, to think of the deformity as one of the shape and efficiency and posture of the trunk as a whole; and to think of the problem as one of restoring the general shape and the coordinate muscular balance of the whole body. (McCrae Aitken, 1928)

No preventive treatment for idiopathic scoliosis (IS) is currently available due to lack of knowledge on aetiology (Figs 19.1 and 19.2). Indeed, there is no generally accepted scientific theory for the causation of IS (Robin, 1990; cf. Burwell, 1971). If there were it might be possible to devise early preventive treatments based on such knowledge.

How may IS develop initially and then progress? Some clarification of concepts about aetiological factors has emerged from school screening for scoliosis. Several abnormal features have been found to be associated with IS, but there is always the problem of interpretation in terms of cause or effect.

Screening for scoliosis

The fact that most children referred to hospital have small scolioses which do not progress led to the suggestion that there are two types of aetiological factors:

1 those which *initiate* a lateral spinal curve;

2 those which lead to curve progression (Tredwell, Yarom).

As we shall explain, this suggestion may be incorrect and, even worse, misleading. With the exception of pelvic tilt scoliosis, research in the 1980s was better at defining factors associated with curve progression than with curve initiation (Lonstein & Carlson, 1984; Bunnell, 1988).

Positive and pseudo-positive findings

Many abnormal features (or anomalies) in the appendicular and axial skeleton, collagen, neuromuscular tissues and hormones are associated with IS (see Byrd, 1988; Robin, 1990). Which of these anomalies are causative ('positive') or consequent to the scoliosis ('pseudo-positive') is unknown (Nachemson). Some resolution of this perennial dilemma has been attempted by also examining:

1 children having scoliosis secondary to a known cause;

2 children without scoliosis who are siblings to the patients;

3 healthy and control children.

Animal research

The complexity of causation of IS suggests that experimental models of the deformity in animals and naturally occurring animal models of scoliosis may not apply to the human state. Many experimentally induced conditions have been shown to produce scoliosis in quadrupeds, usually the rabbit (see Burwell, 1971). The relevance of all such findings for the aetiology of scoliosis in humans at present is obscure. The proper study of humans is humans.

The interaction of aetiological mechanisms?

In the past 5 years we have gained a new insight into the aetiology and pathogenesis of IS by an integrated approach using morphology to interpret function. The

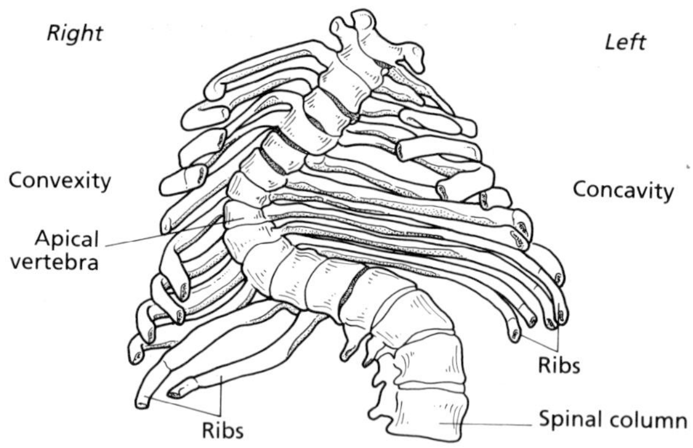

Fig. 19.1 The spine and ribs showing the deformity of structural scoliosis.

evidence suggests that IS results from an abnormality of the physiological mechanisms which interact in the trunk of the immature human to achieve, adapt to and maintain the upright posture and permit bipedal gait.

Our research focuses attention on the rib cage as playing a central and important, but not exclusive, role in scoliosis aetiology. Several other workers are currently attempting to indict the rib cage as the sole cause of IS. This approach cannot accommodate all the evidence, and in our view is too restrictive.

Scoliosis in an evolutionary perspective

As an animal, the human's crucial attributes are: an upright skeleton, manipulative hands, three-dimensional colour vision and a uniquely complex brain. Lambert (1987) writes:

> Our upright skeleton enables us to travel on two legs with a unique heel–toe action, each step a balancing act demanding split-second coordination of muscles in the back, hips, legs and feet. Not only can we walk but run, jump, swim, dive and climb a cliff or tree. Long-distance runners have more endurance than a deer.

A crucial feature in human evolution over the past three million years has been the increase of head and brain size. Evidently, this has been attained by the natural selection of women with large bony pelves and the birth of relatively immature children. The contemporary girl in normal growth and development is then continuously adapting the musculoskeletal framework of her trunk to the changing mechanical demands placed upon it during physical activity and particularly gait by her enlarging pelvis; the latter is detectable at 9 years of age (Nicolopoulos *et al.*, 1985a).

We view scoliosis aetiology in such an evolutionary and developmental perspective.

Previous work

Before we consider our new theory for the aetiology of IS let us examine: (a) the contribution of school screening to our knowledge of pathogenesis, (b) aetiological findings, and (c) some past and present theories of aetiology.

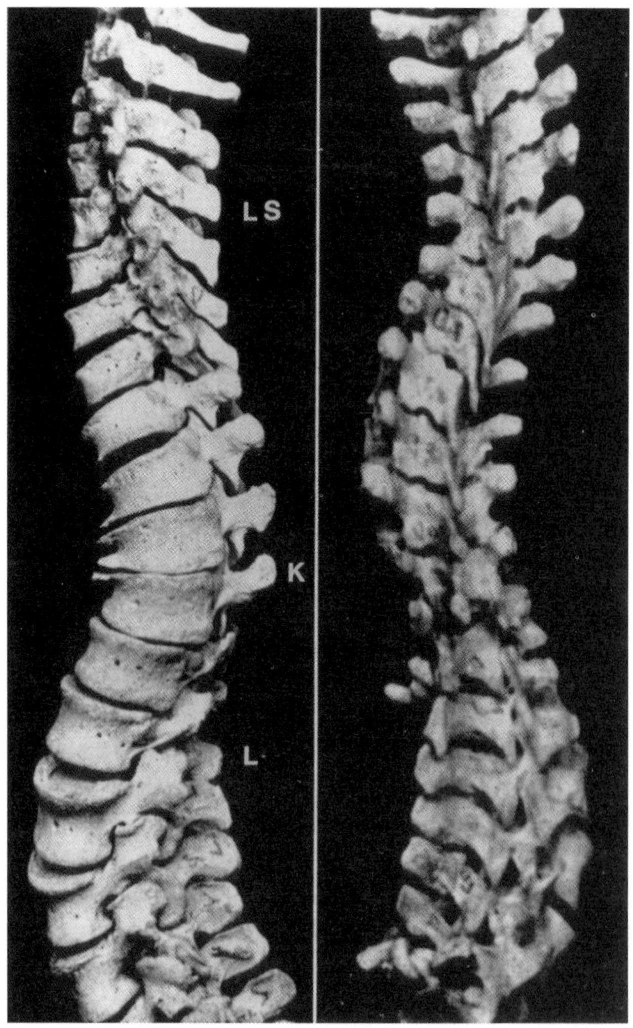

Fig. 19.2 Scoliotic spine. Note: (1) The thoracic kyphosis has disappeared and become lordotic (LS = lordotic segment); (2) the kyphotic angulation at T11–T12 (K): and (3) the lumbar lordosis (L) has increased. From Farkas (1941).

EPIDEMIOLOGY AND NATURAL HISTORY

School screening for adolescent idiopathic scoliosis (AIS) was initially performed to find patients with scoliosis suitable for treatment. Subsequently, the epidemiological approach has provided much new data relating to the prevalence, natural history and factors associated with curve progression. It is now beginning to define aetiological mechanisms of AIS (see Burwell, 1990).

Pelvic tilt scoliosis and spinal scoliosis

The association of leg-length inequality and pelvic asymmetry with static (postural) lumbar scoliosis has been known for many years (Ingelmark & Lindström, 1963). Edelmann (1981) stated that lumbar postural curves may result from: (a) leg-length inequality alone, (b) iliac rotation alone, (c) a combination of leg-length inequality and iliac rotation which summate, and (d) a combination of leg-length inequality and contralateral iliac rotation, with the effect of the latter predominating on the spine.

Dickson and his colleagues, in an epidemiological study of 5303 schoolchildren aged 10–14 years, separated three groups of scoliosis (Dickson, 1983; Walker & Dickson, 1984):

1 pelvic tilt scoliosis (non-progressive)—due to leg-length inequality—40%,
2 spinal scoliosis—minor curves which remain static or resolve—60%,
3 progressive scoliosis—10% of group (2).

Age- and sex-specific prevalence of idiopathic scoliosis

Morais *et al.* (1985) give the age- and sex-specific prevalence for IS at 8–15 years as shown in Table 19.1 (per 1000).

Curve progression

It is customary to define progression of a scoliosis curve as that of 5° or more. This definition is unrelated to curve severity; it therefore has limitations.

Another criterion for progression of a curve is an increase of at least 5°, to 20° curvature or more (Rogala *et al.*, 1978). In Rogala's screening of children aged 12–14 years over a 2-year period, such progression was as shown in Table 19.2.

Perhaps a more meaningful definition of curve progression is that in which the curve reaches a level necessitating brace treatment (Robitaille *et al.*, 1984); but this definition is not in general use.

Prognosis

Lonstein & Carlson (1984) found that the incidence of progression for 20° curves is related to:

1 pattern and magnitude of the curve,
2 patient's age at presentation,
3 Risser sign (iliac apophysis),
4 patient's menarcheal status.

A *progression factor* was calculated:

$$= \frac{\text{Cobb angle} - 3 \times \text{Risser sign}}{\text{Chronological age}}$$

Bunnell (1988), in a retrospective review of 326 female patients with untreated IS, determined what factors might be useful in predicting the risk of curve progression. Predictive indicators included gender, curve pattern and severity, and growth potential. Family history, height–weight ratio, lumbosacral transitional anomalies, kyphosis, lordosis and trunk balance were found not to be significant.

What initiates idiopathic scoliosis?

Once a scoliosis has developed it is difficult, if not impossible, to separate factors which result from,

Table 19.1 Age- and sex-specific prevalence of idiopathic scoliosis

Cobb angle	Boys	Girls
5–14°	29.4	42.0
15–24°	2.2	6.8
25–34°	0.2	2.2
≥35°	0.2	0.9
≥5°	32/1000	51.9/1000

Table 19.2 Progression of scoliosis curve

Curve severity (Cobb angle)	Percentage progression	n
6–10°	2.1	252
≥11°	10.3 (boys 3.8) (girls 15.4)	351

or contribute to, the deformity. Hence aetiological research is difficult. This has led some to express opinions as though they were facts.

SUMMARY OF AETIOLOGICAL FINDINGS

Aetiology

Byrd (1988) summarizes current knowledge on the aetiology of IS as follows:

> [T]he cause of idiopathic scoliosis remains unknown, although research has possibly eliminated some hypothetical causes. Abnormalities of disc, bone, muscle, and collagen do not appear to be etiological factors but, rather, reflect the effects of scoliosis on normal tissues. Although most patients with idiopathic scoliosis are thought of as tall and slender, it has not yet been proven that growth in this condition differs from normal. It is possible that idiopathic scoliosis is caused by multiple factors rather than a single factor. Perhaps there are different factors for curve initiation and curve progression. It appears that a brain stem or equilibrium abnormality does exist in patients with idiopathic scoliosis, although more research is needed to confirm and define the problem. There also may be a genetic basis for idiopathic scoliosis, as it does seem to occur within patients' families more frequently than in the general population. Whether these two factors form the basis for a multifactorial aetiology of idiopathic scoliosis remains to be proven.

Robin (1990), in reviewing the aetiology of IS, concludes: 'The question of aetiology must be answered if logical preventive and therapeutic measures are to be devised.'

Genetics

The fact that IS is often seen in many members of the same family has led researchers to investigate the genetics of this condition in an attempt to uncover its aetiology (see Byrd, 1988). The inheritance is uncertain and suggestions include:

1 familial with a dominant or multiple gene inheritance and raised maternal age;
2 multifactorial inheritance;
3 no simple genetic basis, but maternal influences predominate.

Two problems with this research are the lack of agreed thresholds of lateral spinal curvature (Cobb angle) for the diagnosis of scoliosis, and the use of a rib hump to screen relatives; rib humps are found in about 25% of the population (Burwell *et al.*, 1983).

Multifactorial or unitarian causation?

It is now generally conceded that the *unitarian* approach which makes an observation and then cites the facts that fit the concept of an 'essential lesion' for IS is facile. The *multifactorial* approach is now almost universally accepted. Nachemson, accepting that the aetiology of IS is multifactorial, suggested that it is not one disease, because 'then we go back to those times when "Fever" was a disease'. The view that IS represents a 'final common pathway' to spinal deformity, and which results from more than one possible factor, is supported by other workers (Tredwell, Yarom).

Views, concepts, theories and hypotheses

We shall next examine some past and present theories of aetiology of IS. The early views and even some of the recent work have been put forward didactically. When plausible, ideas became fashionable. When they ceased to satisfy, they were replaced.

Today, the ultimate test of any scientific hypothesis is not can it be proven—no theory ever can; but can it be falsified (Popper)? Most important is whether the concept leads to new and successful treatments for the deformity.

SOME PAST THEORIES OF AETIOLOGY

Starting with the founding fathers, Méry (1706) identified torsion (rotation) in the scoliotic spine of a 16-year-old girl. From the time of Andry (1744) to the discovery of X-rays (1895), many theories of scoliosis causation were adopted. They fall into five main groups: muscular, postural, skeletal, disc and ligamentous (see Rogers, 1933; Brunk, 1951; Valentin, 1991).

Muscular abnormality

Serious attention was at first given to the muscles in producing scoliosis—which had therapeutic implications. Several muscular abnormalities were suggested including: asymmetrical muscle growth (Méry); paralysis of inspiratory muscles (Stromeyer); active muscular contraction (Guérin); a 'primary' muscle affection (Berend); asymmetrical localized weakness, or paralysis of the undernourished child, more pronounced in girls than boys (Carey); and disproportion between growth of muscles and bones in the back (Pravaz).

Bad posture

During the 19th century it became fashionable to view scoliosis as a deformity produced by habitual asymmetric weight-bearing by the spine. As it was commonly seen in children, daily school activities including sitting and writing were impugned but later exonerated (1911). Then, clinicians began to suspect that weight-bearing alone could not produce scoliosis.

Bone abnormality

The next concept to be introduced was that of an abnormal plasticity of vertebrae; it was used to explain why asymmetric weight-bearing could cause habitual scoliosis (Volkmann). Schulthess adopted this view and used the term 'functional osteopathic scoliosis' (1905). Many clinicians changed their opinions and claimed that such 'plasticity' resulted from rickets, endocrine cause or physiological skeletal insufficiency.

A pathomechanical approach to scoliosis causation emerged from the work of Meyer (1866). He considered that the torsion of scoliosis arose from the unequal loading of vertebrae due to variations in the bodies and arches of the vertebrae. Other workers looked for causes in leg-length inequality, pelvic and lumbosacral asymmetry, spinothoracic asymmetry (Hueter) and even cervical ribs.

Discs and ligaments

Delpech proposed that discs, and Lorenz proposed that ligaments, contribute to the cause of scoliosis. In this connection, Harrington wrote:

> It would appear that a relatively minor deficiency in the disk collagen can cause the idiopathic scoliotic development in the spine. A nutritional deficit during the vulnerable growing years (hormonal influence) may initiate the scoliotic process, with the genetic tendency being a recessive factor. Thereafter, given the initial deficit, the spine has no choice—it must react to force, time and direction (mechanics of the spine)—and ultimately produce scoliosis (1977).

The biochemical changes found in scoliotic discs are now generally considered to result from, and not cause, the deformity (T.K.F. Taylor).

These theories provide perspective to our current thoughts about aetiology. The question of whether or not there is 'an essential lesson' for idiopathic progressive scoliosis still remains.

Now let us examine some pathomechanical theories of scoliosis aetiology.

SOME PATHOMECHANICAL THEORIES OF AETIOLOGY

The weight of the head, trunk and upper extremities is largely borne by the flexible column of the vertebral bodies and discs, but it is also supported in a varying degree by the two more rigid posterior columns of the articular processes. Thus the support is tripedal (Adams).

Six types of pathomechanical theories of aetiology will be outlined. These relate to:

1 lateral spinal curves,
2 vertebral rotation,
3 facet joints,
4 sagittal spinal curves,
5 rib cage,
6 trunk muscles.

Lateral spinal curves and aetiology

Sabatier (1791) showed that the great majority of adult spines have a well-defined curve to the right. Bouvier (1858) not only separated rachitic from 'essential' (idiopathic) scoliosis but also suggested that scoliosis was an exaggeration of the normal lateral curvatures of the healthy spine ('état rudimentaire', later termed by others 'Skoliosenkeim').

Farkas (1941) examined 21 normal spines from subjects aged 6–86 years. He concluded that the normal spine becomes asymmetric about the age of 6 years and progresses with advancing age; he termed it 'physiological scoliosis'. The three features which distinguish a physiological from a pathological scoliosis are: the sagittal curves are preserved, there is little vertebral body wedging, and the bony deformity does not involve the whole vertebra. Small lateral spinal curves which do not progress are now confirmed by school screening studies.

Some recent views of aetiology invoke the presence of such 'physiological' scoliosis (White, Dickson, see below).

Vertebral rotation and aetiology

Dods' clinical observation

Adams (1865) wrote:

> The first mention I have met with of rotation of the vertebrae in lateral curvature occurs in a somewhat remarkable book published by the late Dr Dods, of Bath, in the year 1824, entitled 'Pathological Observations on the Rotated or Contorted Spine, commonly called Lateral Curvature'. The author endeavours to prove that the condition generally described as lateral curvature is really one of transverse rotation of the vertebral column. . . . As to the cause and mode of production of this condition of rotation, Dr Dods believed it to be produced by active muscular contraction of the extensor muscles of the spine, acting from the fixed pelvic bones, upon the transverse movable levers, viz.—the ribs and transverse processes of the vertebrae.

Adams' anatomical observations

Adams (1865) then wrote about his own observations and views (p. 110):

> In all the specimens which I have examined, preserved in the museums in London, I have found that the internal is much greater than the external curvature. There can be no doubt that this is the general rule, and so constant does it appear, that I have not yet met with any exception to it. The accompanying diagram [Fig. 19.3] is intended to illustrate the horizontal rotation movement of the bodies of the vertebrae taking place, so that they deviate to the extent of a quarter of a circle, whilst the apices of the spinous processes deviate laterally only to a slight extent.

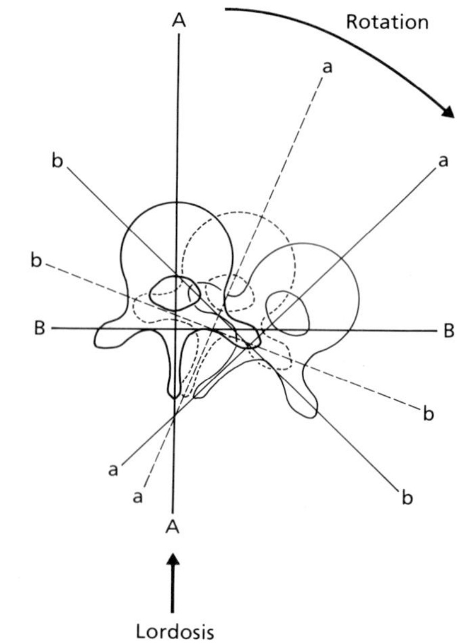

Fig. 19.3 Vertebral rotation in structural scoliosis is about the tip of the spinous process and causes the lordosis and lateral spinal curve. From Adams (1865).

Adams interpreted his findings as follows (p. 116):

> [T]he view I have been led to adopt is, that rotation takes place at the commencement of spinal curvature, and forms an essential part of the series of structural changes which must necessarily exist in slight as well as severe cases, and that the external lateral deviation occurs subsequent, rather than previous to, the rotation movement.

In connection with the flattening of the spine in the sagittal plane, Adams wrote: 'there can be no doubt that it depends upon rotation of the bodies of the vertebrae' (p. 113).

Lovett's clinical and anatomical observations

Lovett (1905) accepted that lateral curvature of the spine, at least in moderate grade, is associated with twisting of the vertebrae in the long axis of the spine. After examining movements of the normal spine in living models and cadavers, Lovett concluded (Fig. 19.4):

1 Torsion and lateral flexion of the spine are parts of

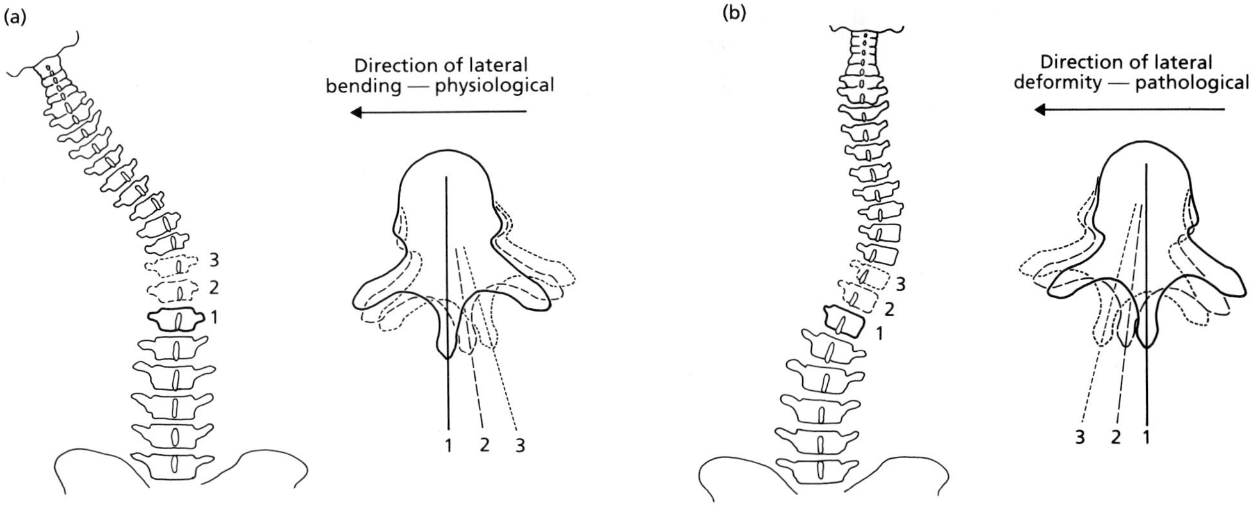

Fig. 19.4 Diagrammatic representation of axial rotation into each of the normal (physiological) lateral curve (a) and the scoliotic curve (b). From White (1971).

one compound movement and neither exists to any extent alone.

2 Lateral flexion in extension of the spine is associated with concave side rotation; and lateral bending in forward flexion with convex side rotation.

Relation to the column theory: the effect of the load

The theory of Euler postulates that under pressure a column will become deformed, as would any other column which is eccentrically loaded, and that the type of the curves of deflection depends upon the manner in which the column is implanted (Steindler, 1955). The spine is not a simple flexible rod. Although many workers from the time of Bigelow have attempted to seek the pathogenesis of scoliosis in Euler's theory, the biological complexity of the spine in the trunk, moved by muscles, makes the comparison difficult, if not impossible.

Vertebral growth asymmetry and rotation

Taylor (1983) reported an

> out of phase appearance of neural arch centres and asymmetrical fusion of neurocentral joints are associated with asymmetry in pedicle length tending to produce vertebral body rotation with thoracic scoliosis which is usually convex to the left in infants and convex to the right in adolescents. Different 'degrees' of asymmetry may be under genetic control.

Facet joints and coupling

Early work

Humphry (1858) pointed out that movements permitted in the spine are mainly due to the shape and position of the facet joints. It is the orientation of these joints that determines their mechanical importance.

Adams (1865) believed that rotation was due to changes in the posterior articular processes. Exception was taken to this a few years later by Judson on the grounds that rotation occurred early in the deformity while changes in the facets were seen only in late cases, and he concluded that such changes were secondary. It seemed highly improbable that the facets could cause rotation in the direction in which it was observed. The lumbar facets allow almost no rotation (see Rogers, 1933).

Coupling of intervertebral motions

In lateral flexion of the normal spine, the connection between it and axial rotation is now termed 'coupling'. It is due to the geometry of the vertebrae, the spinal curvatures and the ligaments and discs (White & Panjabi, 1990).

Roaf's anatomical and radiological studies

Roaf (1958) re-examined the normal movements of the spine, noting in particular whether the spine does, in fact, behave as a tube of unequal flexibilities; whether side-bending and rotation are inevitably linked; and the relationship between movements of the normal spine and the deformity of scoliosis.

Roaf concluded:

> it is possible to explain all the phenomena of severe scoliosis on the basis of a primary rotation deformity alone. The typical rotation type of scoliotic deformity can be reproduced artificially by fitting vertebrae together in an abnormal rotatory relationship without any element of lateral flexion. From this, certain mechanical factors inevitably come into play which must tend to increase the deformity. Above all, the forces responsible for progressive scoliosis are dynamic and not just passive. . . . It is my belief that rotation is usually the dominant factor and that correction and control of severe scoliosis can only be achieved by concentrating on the rotation deformity. I am well aware that this is an old idea but its essential truth has been insufficiently appreciated in recent years and we have not faced its full implications. Failure to correct rotation invites recurrence. Conversely, even a slight reduction in rotation usually produces a marked cosmetic improvement, often out of all proportion to the radiographic appearances.

White's theory of aetiology (Fig. 19.4)

After examining the kinematics of the normal spine in relation to scoliosis, White (1971) proposed a theory of aetiology based on the finding that the spinous processes are occasionally rotated towards the concavity of the lateral curve during lateral flexion in the thoracolumbar region of the spine. White & Panjabi (1990) write:

> The observation that occasional coupling of axial rotations of the vertebrae causes the anterior aspect to point toward the convexity of the lateral curve in normal bending in the middle portion of the thoracic spine must be considered. It is generally acknowledged that scoliosis frequently starts in the mid-thoracic area. There is already a physiologic, slight right thoracic curve in this region. If some precarious balance of the normal thoracic motion should be disturbed, vertebrae in the physiologic, right thoracic curve might somehow rotate too much into the convexity of the curve. Such an occurrence could set off a chain of events leading to asymmetrical loads on the epiphyseal plates and muscle and ligamentous imbalance, with ultimate progression to scoliosis. The precipitating condition may be an abnormal or malaligned facet, a discrete traumatic episode, a chemical hormonal change, extreme handedness of the individual, or any number of other possible embarrassments that upset the delicate balance.

In reappraising White's theory, Stokes (1989) argued that simple coupling of lateral bending and axial rotation on intervertebral joints cannot produce a spinal curvature in which the maximum axial rotation is at the curve apex. Stokes opined that coupling of lateral bending and axial rotation *at each segmental level* would instead produce maximum curvature at the inflection points of the curve. However, the

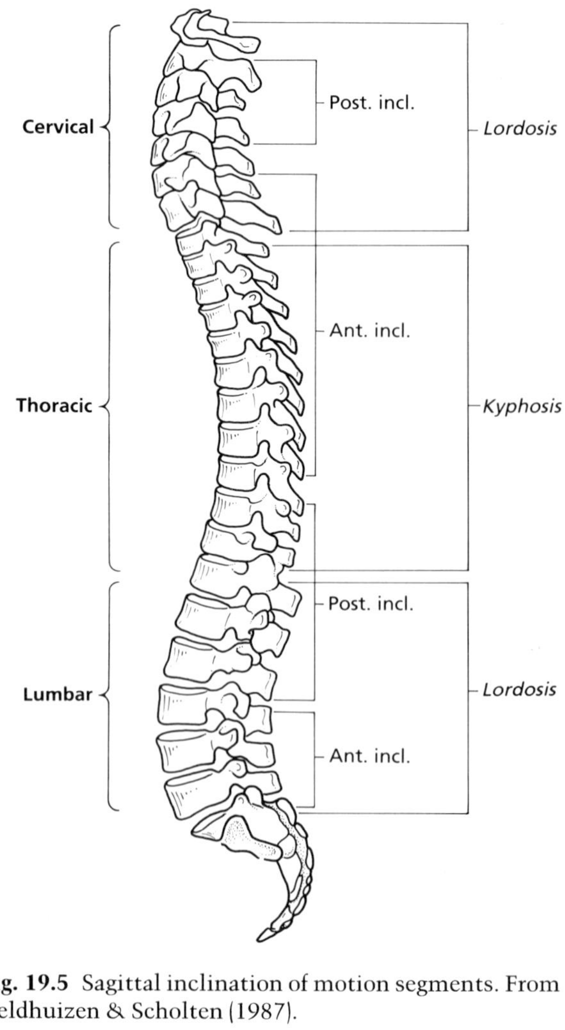

Fig. 19.5 Sagittal inclination of motion segments. From Veldhuizen & Scholten (1987).

findings of Wojcik *et al.* (1992) show that tilt at one level is related to rotation at a *higher* level (and conversely so for the upper half of the curve, Fig. 19.13). These latter findings support the view that in thoracic scoliosis, vertebral tilt and rotation evolve topographically in the development of the lateral spinal curve in order to provide a mechanism for balancing the spine against gravity.

Veldhuizen & Scholten (1987) also take issue with White's theory of aetiology and write:

> This theory considers idiopathic scoliosis as a lateral flexion of a *normal* spine and the axial rotation being due to the normal coupling phenomenon. To suit White's theory, a reverse coupling pattern is required in these areas.

Veldhuizen and Scholten found that the direction of axial rotation during flexion of a *scoliotic* spine does not differ from that of a normal spine. In other words, the posterior (lordotic) inclination and the axially rotated position of the motion segments in the scoliotic spine does not undo the influence of the facet joint orientation on the coupling behaviour between the lateral flexion and axial rotation, although the extent of the axial rotation during lateral flexion may be less. Therefore, the axial rotation in idiopathic scoliosis cannot be explained on the basis of spinal kinematics involving lateral flexion and axial rotation.

Axial vertebral rotation during lateral flexion—influence of facet joints and sagittal spinal shape

Veldhuizen & Scholten (1987) used a biomechanical model of the 'normal' thoracic and lumbar spine to examine the effect of lateral flexion on axial rotation. The direction of such rotation was influenced by: facet joint orientation in the frontal plane; and sagittal plane inclination of the motion segments (Fig. 19.5):

1 if *kyphotic*, lateral flexion rotates the spinous process to the convexity; and

2 if *lordotic*, lateral flexion rotates the spinous process to the concavity.

Sagittal spinal curves and aetiology

Early work

Meyer (1866) based his theory on two findings: firstly the vertebral bodies are compressible, while the laminae are elastic; and secondly strong ligaments exist anteriorly and posteriorly but not lateral to the vertebral bodies. In 1922 MacLennan mentioned unequal growth of the two columns but the principle is the same. Excess length of the column of bodies would cause hyperextension of the spine. Then, in the presence of lateral curvature from habitual position or any other cause, the too-long columnar bodies would tend to deviate from the midline farther than the column of laminae, especially with no lateral ligaments to prevent such deformity (Rogers, 1933).

In 1927 Heuer found that in scoliosis the anterior vertebral components were longer than the posterior elements. He concluded that the primary cause of scoliosis is an isolated growth lengthening of the anterior spinal elements. Schede (1928) could not agree with this interpretation and put forward the view that scoliosis develops as a result of the 'Sitzbuckel' of rachitic children. He claimed that a rachitic child in the sitting position develops a short, slight kyphosis of the thoracolumbar junction and that the vertebra becomes wedge-shaped and fixes the kyphosis, so that when the child stands up, a normal kyphosis is unachievable (Schede, 1928, Fig. 4a), the back straightens out instead, and the child develops a relative lordosis or a flattening of the thoracic spine and in some cases a scoliosis, too, in this region. Farkas (1941) illustrated the kyphotic angulation in a scoliotic spine (Fig. 19.2).

Three aspects need consideration:

1 relative anterior spinal lengthening,

2 lordotic segment,

3 kyphotic angulation.

The findings are not in dispute. The current debate relates to how the facts are interpreted: in particular, which comes first: the vertebral rotation, the lordotic segment or the lateral curvature? On the basis of data obtained from deformed material the question is insoluble; a wider perspective is necessary. Indeed, there is now evidence suggesting that different neuromuscular mechanisms control movements in each of the frontal and transverse planes of the spine.

Relative lengthening of anterior spine in scoliosis

The suggestion that a basic feature of scoliosis is relative lengthening of the anterior spinal components is supported by anatomical studies (Roaf, 1958; Deane & Duthie, 1973; Deacon *et al.*, 1984).

Lordotic segment

Somerville (1952), from radiological studies, concluded that the deformity of thoracic scoliosis consists of lordosis, rotation and lateral flexion. He suggested that the structural lordosis arises from failure of growth of the posterior elements of a segment of the spine. Deacon & Dickson (1987), reporting on 150 patients with thoracic IS, found that in the apical three vertebrae the anterior body height was greater than the posterior body height, an index of which was associated with each of lordosis, apical rotation and Cobb angle. The interpretation they placed upon these findings was that posterior endplate changes cause the short-segment lordosis with the potential to rotate progressively with repeated flexion cycles and growth to produce typical IS. In our view these growth changes are secondary to mechanical factors.

Kyphotic angulation

In recent years the slight kyphosis of the thoracolumbar junction of scoliosis has been studied by several workers (Fig. 19.2). Graf & Dubousset (1980) used frontal and lateral radiographs in an attempt to reconstruct the infantile scoliotic spine in three dimensions ($n = 30$). They found that scoliotic curves usually rotate only one way, and each curve is separated by an acute change in rotation. They write: 'Acute adverse change in vertebral rotation surrounds the kyphosis between two lordo-scoliotic segments' (termed kyphorotatory dislocation). Richards *et al.* (1989) evaluated changes on sagittal spinal profile in right thoracic scoliosis and kyphosis before and after Cotrel–Dubousset instrumentation. If present preoperatively, they found the kyphosis was localized between the two curves in King Type II patterns reflecting the neutral point between the two lordoscoliotic regions. They observed a junctional kyphosis on 19 of 27 patients; the kyphosis was located just above the stable vertebrae, and they state that, with rare exceptions, the junctional kyphosis was very subtle radiographically and, in all, it was not apparent clinically. Cruickshank *et al.* (1989), on the films of seven patients with thoracic curves, used a 'sagittal score' (rotation × wedging) to indicate the presence of kyphosis at the thoracolumbar junction with a normal kyphosis above. They concluded that flexion of the lordosis would be expected to buckle it; the thoracolumbar kyphosis they suggested has a 'centring' effect. No true lateral radiographs were shown to confirm the suggestion of a kyphosis below the thoracic structural rotated lordoscoliosis. Kiel *et al.* (1992) found a kyphotic angulation three or four segments below the apical vertebrae of a thoracic curve (Fig. 19.14); this angulation is in the region of the spinal mortice joint.

Some problems of interpretation (Fig. 19.2)

An important point at issue is: (a) does the kyphosis result from the lordoscoliosis above it (junctional kyphosis); or (b) does the short-segment lordosis result from the kyphotic angulation in the thoracolumbar spine (Schede)?

Then, if the lordoscoliosis precedes the junctional kyphosis, does the short-segment lordosis result from an isolated anterior spinal growth abnormality (Heuer); or from rotation of the apical vertebra (Roaf)? In the latter connection Roaf (1958, 1966) argued that when vertebral rotation is unopposed every muscular contraction pushes the vertebrae further from the midline and increases the lordosis. In turn the secondary lordosis may cause impaired growth of posterior body height about the apex of the curve.

The Leeds view

Dickson *et al.* (1984) suggested that the effect of forward flexion on the lordotic segment of an 'inconsequential' lateral curve causes rotation to the convexity. Their model has four components:

1 a short-segment relatively rigid lordosis (sagittal plane),
2 a small lateral spinal curve (frontal plane),
3 repeated 'flexion cycles',
4 tightening of posterior spinal structures.

The short-segment lordosis is considered to be 'primary' due to the spine growing faster at the front than at the back, i.e. a 'primary' skeletal abnormality (Heuer, 1927, see Somerville, 1952).

The flat back and scoliosis pathogenesis

Staffel (1889) divided human posture into categories including the round, the flat and the lordotic back. The flat back he considered predisposes a child to a scoliosis of the most unfavourable kind (see Bonne, 1969). More recent work using the kyphometer, while confirming that the flat back is commonly a feature of thoracic scoliosis, has failed to find a correlation between the kyphosis angle and the scoliosis (Cobb) angle (Chapter 9).

Dickson and Archer suggested that a flat thoracolumbar profile predisposes an adolescent to IS. But equally the flat thoracolumbar profile could be secondary to the thoracic scoliosis above it. This scientific dilemma should soon be resolved by the current longitudinal studies of the lateral spinal profile in school screening referrals.

In a recent anatomical study of the human vertebral column, Pal and Routal conclude: 'the closer position of the two columns in the lower thoracic region and the high magnitude of load transmission through the anterior column probably make this region more susceptible to scoliosis' (see Pal, 1991).

Spinal mortice joint

Humphry (1858) stated that the lower two thoracic and upper one or two lumbar vertebrae were the weakest part of the spinal column (see Davis, 1955). Davis found that the region of junctional transition between the thoracic and lumbar regions of the human vertebral column is commonly marked by a facet joint comparable with a carpenter's mortice (most commonly at T11–T12, but also at T10–T11 and T12–L1). The anatomy of the mortice joint restricts rotation between the two transitional vertebrae. Davis argued that, with the mortice joint locked in extension, a compression force which is prevented by the lock from forcing the tenon downwards must cause flexion of the joint, by compressing the intervertebral disc. Davis linked the distribution of thoracolumbar fractures to the great increase of pressure that must follow the forced flexion of the locked mortice joint, when such compression forces are applied. He did not mention scoliosis in relation to the mortice joint (see Kiel *et al.*, 1992).

Rib-cage and aetiology

Early work

Stromeyer (1836) suggested that unequal rib pressures cause scoliosis, ascribing the deformity to a disordered action of the muscles of respiration.

Feiss (1907) studied the complex problems of rotation and lateral bending, both by experiments on the living and by a mechanical model of the thorax and a model of a vertebra with its attached ribs. Feiss held that tension on the convex side causes the convex ribs to push the posterior parts of the vertebrae towards the concavity, thereby rotating the anterior part or bodies towards the convexity. Rogers (1933) cast doubt on this theory when it is remembered what a flexible member the rib is in a young child; and more when one reflects how difficult it is to reverse the process, to reduce spinal rotation by pressing on the ribs. Lovett held the opposite view: 'The ribs, of course, follow the rotation of the vertebrae to which they are attached.'

Roaf's work

Roaf (1958, 1968) divided the pressures along the ribs into horizontal and vertical components. On the concave side the pressure is largely horizontal, whereas on the convex side it is largely vertical.

Thoracoplasties and scoliosis

Bisgard (1934) concluded:

> With each successive stage of multistaged thoracoplasties the angle of the curvature is often slightly increased, and usually a more extensive segment of the spine becomes involved. When the stages progress downward from the upper to the lower ribs, the apex of the curve correspondingly moves downward slightly. Lateral deviations of considerable extent are accompanied by rotation of the vertebral bodies and of the thoracic cage. As a result of this mechanical factor, the deformity resembles that of all other rotary scolioses, such as idiopathic and paralytic scoliosis, and differs from that of pleural scoliosis in which there is slight or no rotation of the vertebrae.

Loynes (1972), reviewing the effects of thoracoplasty upon the development of scoliosis in adults, found that scoliosis developed in 99% of cases; and that if the head, neck and tubercle of the rib with the transverse process of the corresponding vertebra were all removed the degree of scoliosis was increased.

Rib resection for infantile idiopathic scoliosis

After experimental work in rabbits, Piggott (1971) reviewed 25-cases of concave posterior rib resection and found that curves progressive before operation showed little progression afterwards; in some cases there was significant retrogression. The best results were produced in children under 5, but he stressed that the average follow-up was only 29 months. In contrast, Barnes (1979) could not find any beneficial effects of concave posterior rib resection for infantile idiopathic scoliosis (IIS).

Rib–vertebra angle difference (RVAD)

In concluding her classical paper on the prognostic value of the apical RVAD in IIS, Mehta (1972) writes:

> The radiological evidence of early rib–vertebra angle difference in scoliosis, thought to be due to a disturbance of the soft tissues in the region of the costo-vertebral joint, supports the experimental and mechanical evidence of the importance of this region in the development of a scoliosis.

Subsequently in 1985, Kristmundsdottir *et al.* found that the apical convex RVA was related to the severity of the Cobb angle (CA), suggesting that common factors determine both the spinal curve and the drooping of the ribs. After a period of relative neglect, several workers are now focusing their attention on the rib cage in an attempt to reveal mechanisms of aetiology in IS. This work will now be outlined.

Rib-length asymmetry

Sevastik and his colleagues (1990) adduced clinical, anatomical and experimental evidence that asymmetric growth of the thorax is possibly an initiating factor in the development of IS. The rib theory of scoliosis is supported by Stokes and his colleagues (1989), who found a tendency for the rib length of patients with scoliosis to be asymmetric. Patients with single right thoracic scoliosis tended to have longer ribs on the right side. Those with single left lumbar curves tended to have longer ribs on the left side.

Stokes & Laible (1990) constructed a biomechanical (finite element) model of the human thorax to investigate how asymmetric growth of the thorax might initiate spinal lateral curvature and axial rotation as seen in scoliosis deformities. They addressed the hypothesis that rib-growth asymmetry produces scoliosis (Fig. 19.6a). The findings demonstrated the feasibility of this mechanism of initiation of thoracic scoliosis. However, the spinal curves which developed were small in all variations of the model tested, so it appears that some other

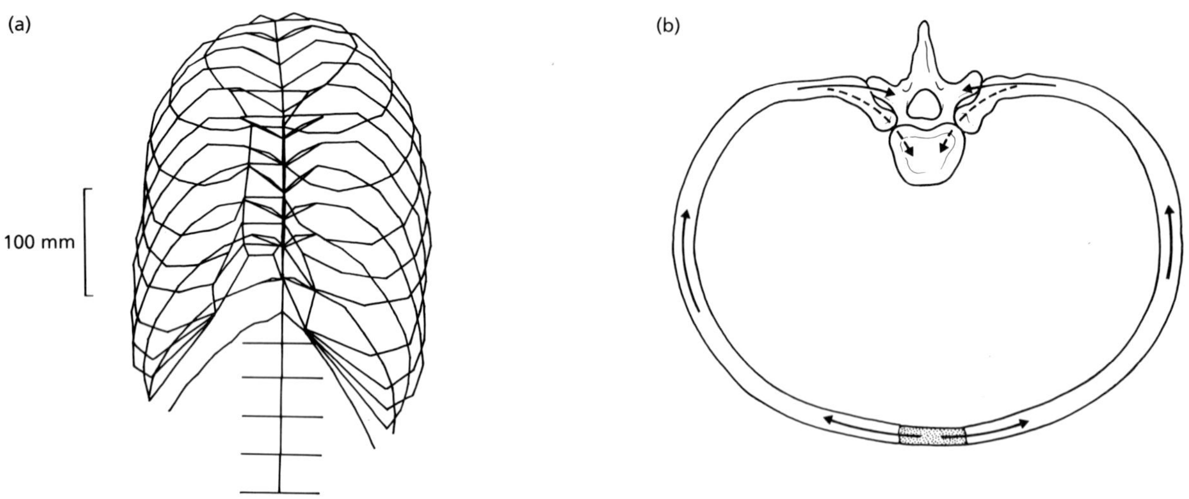

Fig. 19.6 (a) Finite element model of the thorax. Back view of the geometric configuration of the initially symmetric model after deformation resulting from average of 20% growth, but distributed so that the ribs and intercostal ligaments 'grew' four times more at the front than the back, and 1.5 times more on the right side than the left. From Stokes & Laible (1990).
(b) Diagram to show how the ribs balance the thoracic spine. The ribs from each side bring equal load to the spine. The majority of the load passes from the ribs to the laminae through the transverse processes. Compressive forces passing through each vertebra are accentuated at three points—two articular facets and the body. From Pal (1991).

mechanism must participate in the progression of scoliosis to large curvature during growth. It was anticipated that gravity or muscle forces (omitted from their models) might provide that mechanism. A preliminary study of the model with a vertical force applied to the top of the spine, together with asymmetric growth, showed increase in the sagittal spinal curvatures, and not of the scoliosis. Their model ignores the possible contribution of rib–vertebra angle asymmetry to scoliosis aetiology.

Rib-induced imbalance of the thoracic spine

Pal (1991) measured normal vertebral columns and used the morphological data to interpret function. Pal supports the view that vertical stability of the thoracic spine is maintained by equal support through the ribs from both sides due to the equal load brought to the laminae by the ribs through the costotransverse articulations and ligaments (Fig. 19.6b). Any interference in this balancing mechanism disturbs spinal stability which will bend towards the more heavily loaded side. Many factors may act through the ribs to unbalance the spine. In the case of IS, such factors should be investigated on an individual basis.

Trunk muscles and aetiology

Interaction of respiratory and antigravity muscles

McCrae Aitken (1928), writing on scoliosis aetiology, concluded that: 'the static reflex and the respiratory reflex must be taken together when considering those deviations from the normal erect posture of the body commonly called curvature of the spine'. In the *static reflex group* are included all the muscles of the lower limbs, pelvis and trunk which are concerned in keeping the body erect and balanced ('antigravity' muscles). In the *respiratory reflex group* are all the muscles concerned in maintaining respiration.

McCrae Aitken's treatment of scoliosis using plaster-of-Paris was based on Hoke's views that in a deformed thorax the bulging portions of the chest move more freely than the flattened portion; and a rib in moving towards the dorsal bulge exercises a levering action on the vertebrae which rotates the vertebrae. Treatment should aim at reversing this process with two objects in view—that is to increase the mobility of the flattened ribs, and in some measure to achieve a correction of the rotation deformity of the trunk.

Intercostal muscles—postural as well as respiratory functions? 'Autocorrection' and electrical stimulation

Roaf (1974) summarized evidence that intercostal muscles may have a postural as well as a respiratory function. He surmised:

> scoliosis progresses because the body's normal postural and respiratory mechanisms have become deranged. Now, spinal posture is normally maintained by a number of local stretch-reflexes and if the modulating action of the mid-brain on these reflexes is deranged scoliosis can result.

Roaf continued:

> I do not want to give the impression that I believe that the ribs and intercostal muscles are *always* or even *usually* the 'target organs' for the unknown factors which cause the different types of so-called idiopathic scoliosis. On the other hand, I do believe that once a deformity starts the rib-intercostal mechanisms can be an important factor, either in leading to further progression or in stopping it, and that treatment directed to improvement of the function of the ribs as levers can be of benefit. It is hoped, therefore, that further study of the physiological control of rib posture will improve our therapeutic measures.

Later (1980), Roaf wrote:

> For a long time I have used autocorrection, trying to exercise the convex side trunk muscles, as some years ago we found that exercising one's arm increased the electrical activity of the ipsilateral intercostal muscles. I have tried to compare the relative efficacy of different methods of correction; not surprisingly, I found that pre-treatment spinal mobility—if properly assessed—determined the degree of correction far more than the method used.

Schmitt continued the electromyographic work on intercostal muscles and wrote (1981):

> Our investigations showed that in thoracic scoliosis the intercostal muscles on the convex side of the curvature have a significantly higher activity than the muscles on the concave side. This prevailing activity on the convex side

> depends on the degree of the scoliotic angle. It increases with increasing deformity, whereas on the concave side the muscle activity decreases with increasing deformity. These differences of intercostal muscle activity on the two sides of thoracic scoliosis are reduced in prone position and are not seen in Halo extension. With acting or loading one of the upper extremities, the intercostal muscles of the contralateral side show increasing activity. We interpret this prevailing activity on the convex side as natural forces, counteracting against scoliotic deformation. The increased muscle activity that is seen on the contralateral side of the activated upper extremity could produce a thoracic scoliosis and increase an existing one. Therefore, prevailing activities of the right-hand could be one cause of the prevailing of right-sided thoracic scoliosis.

Finally, Schmitt (1986) claimed that with stimulation of convex side muscles, especially of intercostal muscles, the curvature can be corrected. The correction is better in small deformities with a short history.

Deep rotator muscles

Fidler & Jowett (1976) concluded that increased tonic activity of the deep medial paraspinal muscles, such as multifidus, on one side of the spine and a consequent effect on vertebral growth could be of importance in the aetiology of IS. Other workers disagree strongly with this conclusion (Roaf, 1976; Nudelman & Reis, 1990).

Superficial back, chest and abdominal muscles

The function of postvertebral muscles is considered to be primarily postural, maintaining the erect position against gravity (Osmond, 1985). In this connection, Joseph & McColl (1961) studied the activity of the posterior spinal muscles at 12 levels in 20 males standing at ease, and using electromyography. Although there was considerable variation in the detectable activity at any one level, a pattern of activity in a vertical direction was seen. There was little or no activity in the lumbar and cervical regions and moderate or marked activity in the lower thoracic region.

Haderspeck & Schultz (1981) set up a model to study the biomechanics of scoliosis. They investigated muscle action as a cause of curvature of the spine. It was shown that muscles spanning the concavity can cause an increase in the curvature; thus the external oblique and erector spinae muscles can increase the lumbar curvature. Latissimus dorsi, intercostal and erector spinae muscles can increase the thoracic curvature.

More recently, Nudelman & Reis (1990) have proposed that IS results from an imbalance of forces created in a 'triradiate musculoskeletal system' whose points of action are: (a) in the front: the sternum, ribs and clavicle (ventral ray); (b) in the upper back: the cervical and upper thoracic vertebrae (upper thoracic ray); and (c) in the lower back: the lower thoracic and lumbar vertebrae and the iliac crest (lower thoracic ray). No explanation is given as to how such triradiate muscle imbalance may arise.

Muscle tether

The capacity of muscles to tether the spine and create scoliosis is known from the experimental scoliosis in quadrupeds (Langenskiöld). Recent work has suggested that in humans the erector spinae may tether the spine in thoracic scoliosis and after the Zielke operation (see Wojcik *et al.*, 1990; Wythers *et al.*, 1992).

Diaphragmatic balance—a cause of progression in idiopathic scoliosis?

Ransford (1988), from clinical observations, argues that:

> Once a minor lordo-scoliosis has developed the diaphragm begins to lose its mechanical advantage by distortion of its substance. By some subtle mechanism it can distort the ribs in a growing child until the normal shape of the diaphragm has returned. This rib distortion, aided by gravitational forces and spinal flexibility, produces further rotation and deformity of the spine. The direct evidence in support of this hypothesis is that the diaphragm always appears to be 'normal' at surgery, however severe the scoliosis. In double primary curves the forces tending to distort the diaphragm are neutralised and no rib hump develops.

Summary of the forces which may deform and defend the spine

The development of a scoliotic deformity necessitates the movement and displacement of vertebrae. There are only three types of force which can move vertebrae into a deformed position: gravity, growth and muscles.

The contribution of gravity and growth to the deformity of scoliosis is rarely disputed. The role of muscles—despite much research using electromyography and histochemistry—is less certain. In basic terms, muscle actions which could contribute to the deformity of IS are those involved in respiration, posture, bipedal gait and other physical activities.

Equally important in any theoretical interpretation of scoliosis aetiology is a consideration of the structures which can resist such deforming forces; these are bones, joints, ligaments and other muscles. Although the founding fathers identified the need to postulate 'abnormal plasticity of vertebrae' in scoliosis aetiology, this possibility has received but scant attention in recent years. There are only occasional reports associating osteoporosis with AIS (Whitecloud *et al.*, 1987; see Warren *et al.*, 1986).

Conceptual aims

In the present state of knowledge, the aims of any theory of aetiology for IS are to explain many findings, to link previous hypotheses of aetiology, to draw from fields of research other than scoliosis, to make predictions for further work and to devise new treatments based on the understanding of causation.

AN INTEGRATED APPROACH TO SCOLIOSIS AETIOLOGY

During the past 20 years we have developed an integrated approach to scoliosis aetiology using morphological data to interpret function. It has evolved as follows:

1 Reviewing the field and defining problems for aetiological research (Burwell, 1971).

2 Applying and developing anthropometric techniques to children with scoliosis (and other orthopaedic diseases) as well as healthy controls (Chapter 9).

3 Appraising the back shape of normal children (8–15 years) using multisegmental data and applying the results to screening for scoliosis (Chapter 9).

4 Developing an ultrasound method for measuring femoral anteversion and applying it to scoliosis screening referrals, their siblings and healthy children (Burwell *et al.*, 1990; Upadhyay *et al.*, 1990).

5 Defining new ways of appraising sagittal back shape in scoliotic patients (Chapter 9).

6 The introduction of new surgical instrumentation for spinal deformity surgery led us:

(a) To develop new segmental methods for the radiological appraisal of the spine and rib cage (Wojcik *et al.*, 1990; Wythers *et al.*, 1992; Grivas *et al.*, 1991, 1992a,b; Thirlwall, 1991; Austin, 1992; Jones, 1992; Wemyss-Holden *et al.*, 1992b).

(b) To apply new segmental methods of surface back shape appraisal to study and predict the results of surgery (Chapter 9).

7 Extensive data analysis using computers and statistical techniques.

8 New ways of thinking about the aetiology of IS, which include: ceasing to look for 'the essential lesion' of scoliosis, identifying possible mechanisms of aetiology, evaluating how different aetiological mechanisms may interact in life, creating a General Theory of Aetiology, examining publications relating to aetiology in the light of the General Theory of Aetiology, and drawing from other fields of study to help in understanding the cause of IS and other spinal deformities.

9 Anatomical studies of the erector spinae and trunk rotator muscles (Cook *et al.*, 1991; Wemyss-Holden *et al.*, 1991b).

10 Evaluating a mechanical model of the trunk muscles in relation to scoliosis (Wemyss-Holden *et al.*, 1991b).

This integrated morphological approach to solving the idiopathic has helped to create a new theory of aetiology for scoliosis (Burwell *et al.*, 1990, 1991a,b, 1992a,b,c). It will now be described.

THEORY OF AETIOLOGY—GENERAL THEORY

The General Theory of Aetiology (Figs 19.7 & 19.8)

In 1988, findings for both femoral anteversion (ultrasound method) and sagittal spinal shape at T11–T12 of school screening referrals and their siblings suggested a General Theory of Aetiology for AIS. The

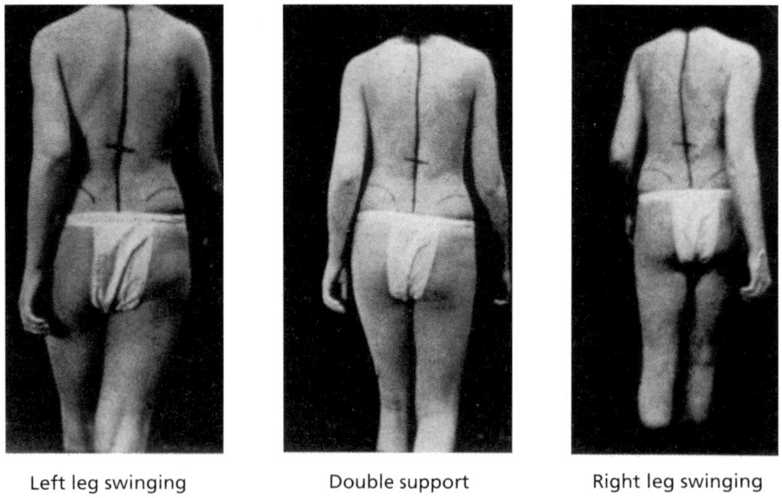

Fig. 19.7 The physiological scoliosis of gait. From Farkas (1941).

General Theory of Aetiology (dinner plate–flagpole concept) states that AIS results from a failure of control of cyclical rotations in the spine during gait due to two mechanisms acting through the spine, namely (Burwell *et al.*, 1990):

1 a pelvic rotation-inducing system involving gait, femoral anteversion and the pelvis ('dinner plate');

2 rotation transmitted to the lumbar and thoracic spine ('flagpole');

3 a spinal rotation-defending system, mainly costal, but also involving discs, ligaments, sagittal spinal shape and neuromuscular mechanisms.

In the light of this theory, some findings of early workers relating to scoliosis, gait and rest were re-examined.

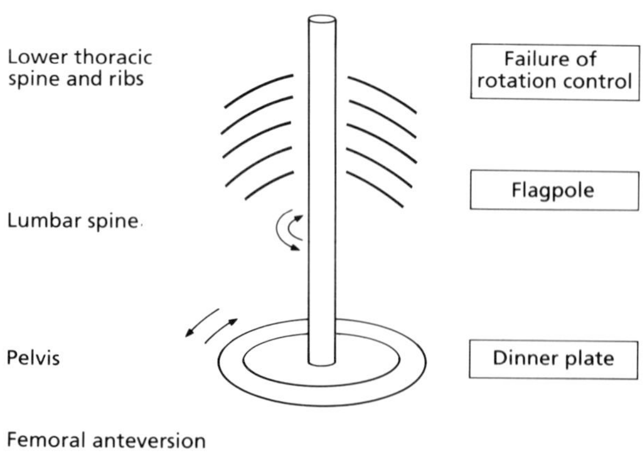

Fig. 19.8 The General Theory of Aetiology (1988) for adolescent idiopathic scoliosis (dinner plate–flagpole concept). From Burwell *et al.* (1990).

Scoliosis, gait and rest

Physiological scoliosis (Fig. 19.7)

Farkas (1941) had concluded that:

> The cause of physiological scoliosis is the human gait, which forces the spine to a threefold curve, alternately changing at every step. However, the

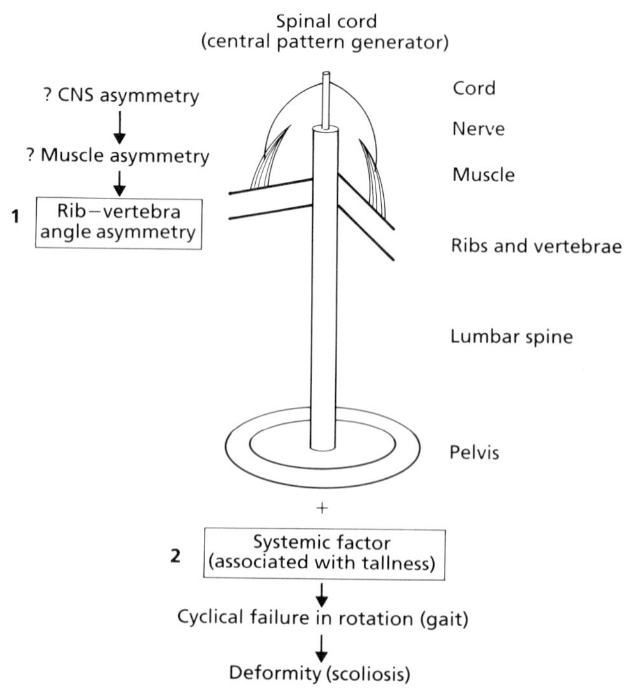

Fig. 19.9 Idiopathic scoliosis: concept of aetiology. From Burwell *et al.* (1992b,c).

innate normal asymmetries of the human body eventually establish permanent lateral curves of the spine, showing marked individual variations within the general law.

Rest in bed and progressive scoliosis

Rogers (1933) noted improvement in the lateral and rotatory elements of scoliosis brought about by prolonged hyperextension in recumbency on a frame. Also, according to Arkin (1949), rest in bed may halt the progress of IS in children. In over 30 cases in which the condition was advancing, Cobb kept the children in bed for 22 hours per day. Except in one case, no progress was noted after 3 months.

Quadrupedal treatment of scoliosis

Klapp's (1873–1948) name is associated with quadrupedal 'crawling exercises' for the treatment of IS in children. In 1956 a book was published on quadrupedal exercises for treating scoliosis (Burger).

Recent data

In the past 4 years we have generated much new data from scoliotic and control subjects. Examination of this evidence in the context of the General Theory (1988) has not rejected it. It has enabled a more detailed theoretical model to be built (Figs 19.9 & 19.10; Burwell *et al.*, 1992a,b,c).

We shall now describe the components of the theory, provide a statement, give a detailed narrative and finally review how the concepts may be used to reinterpret the deformity of IS.

THEORY OF AETIOLOGY—COMPONENTS

The theory of aetiology now has four components:

1 *Mechanical component* (Fig. 19.10a): rotation-

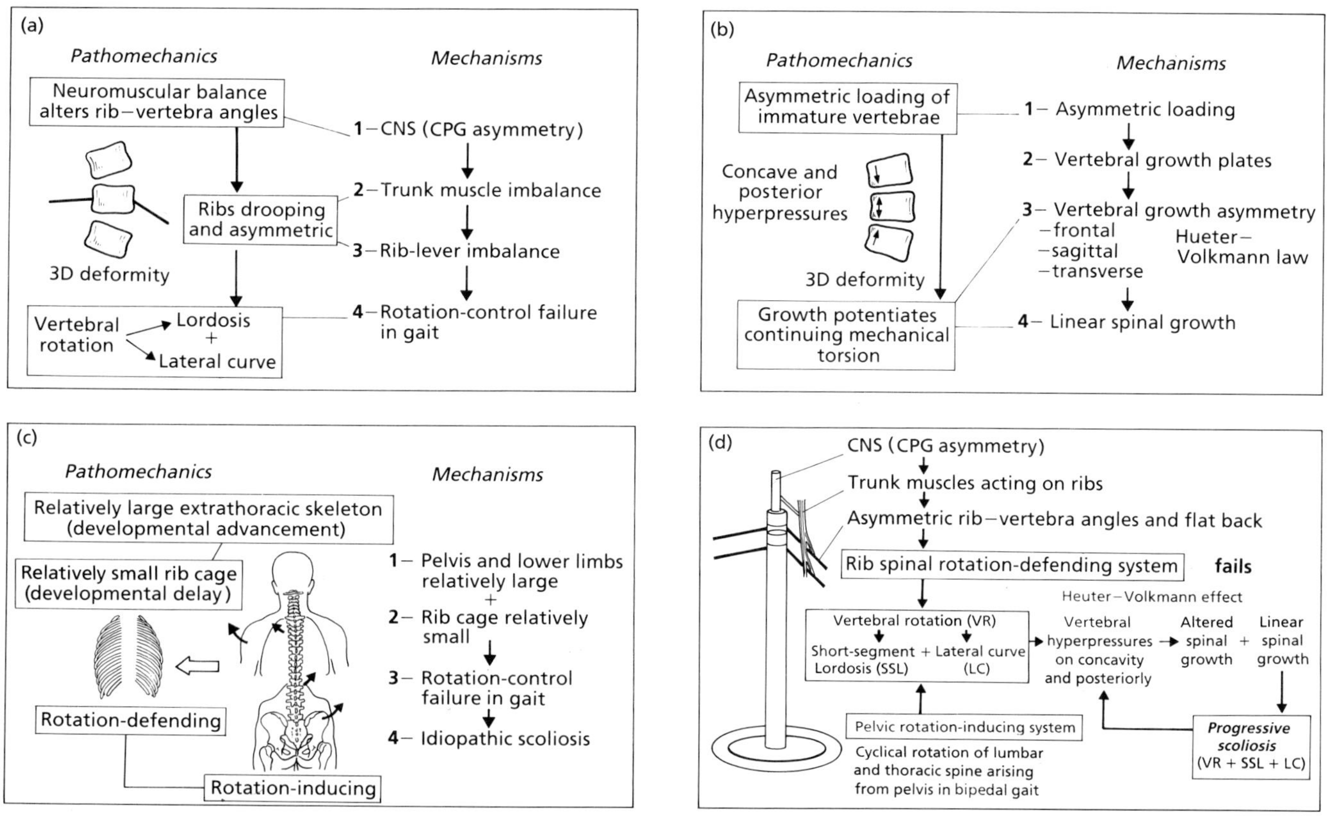

Fig. 19.10 Adolescent idiopathic scoliosis: concept of aetiology: (a) mechanical component (CPG = central pattern generator); (b) growth component; (c) body size disparity (proportion) component; (d) composite drawing. Modified from Burwell *et al.* (1991a).

inducing, mechanisms, rotation-defending mechanisms.
2 *Growth component* (Fig. 19.10b): spinal growth alterations (secondary), rib-cage growth (impaired), growth elsewhere (normal or increased).
3 *Body size disparity (proportion) component* (Fig. 19.10c): relatively small rib cage (local cause), relatively large extrathoracic skeleton (systemic cause).
4 *Nervous component (developmental abnormality)* (Fig. 19.10d): spinal cord development (CPG asymmetry), brain stem and higher centres (sexual dimorphism), peripheral nervous system.

Can extrathoracic growth potentiate scoliosis?

The theory of aetiology predicts that an enlargement of the child's body relative to the thorax, particularly below the waist, by increasing the rotation-inducing forces during gait provides a mechanical mechanism for curve progression (Fig. 19.10c). The findings consistent with this view are:
1 The relatively small rib cage of:
(a) IIS (Grivas *et al.*, 1992a); and
(b) AIS (Thirlwall, 1991; Austin, 1992).
2 The relatively large extrathoracic skeleton of AIS (Nicolopoulos *et al.*, 1985b).
Further research is in hand, including an evaluation of the prognostic value of thoracic shape and body size.

Are respiratory muscles involved in scoliosis aetiology?

It is now generally considered that the intercostal muscles are by no means confined to respiratory functions. They are said to be highly active in postural movements of the chest wall, notably in approximating the ribs during lateral flexion of the trunk (Osmond, 1985). Some workers consider that the intercostal muscles also have a rotatory action on the thoracic spine, rotating the vertebral body towards the convexity (Schmitt, 1981). Whether or not the intercostal muscles also have a function in locomotion, perhaps by contributing to the counter-rotation of the upper thoracic spine during the arm swing of gait, is unknown.

We conclude that the trunk muscles involved in posture and locomotion are the muscles most likely to contribute to scoliosis aetiology. These are mainly the flat rotator muscles, the erector spinae and possibly the intercostal muscles and the diaphragm (Ransford).

THEORY OF AETIOLOGY—A STATEMENT

Trunk movements and posture in gait

In normal gait, spinal movements occur in three dimensions, in the frontal, transverse and sagittal planes (Fig. 19.7). In our concept of aetiology we currently emphasize the role of the transverse plane. In gait, pelvic rotation causes lumbar and lower thoracic spinal rotation with counter-rotation above it (Fig. 19.18).

The pelvispinal rotation we attribute mainly to lower limb movements and particularly to the thrust of toe-off which transmits a force along the straightened limb to initiate pelvic rotation in the transverse plane (Fig. 19.17). The trunk rotator muscles attached to the pelvis may also contribute to this pelvic rotation (a kinetic component of gait, see Fig. 19.27).

The counter-rotation of the upper thoracic spine, we attribute entirely to trunk muscle activity and particularly to the flat rotator muscles and possibly the intercostals.

The erector spinae may act more in the frontal plane to steady the spine when one leg is off the ground during gait (a postural component of gait, see Figs 19.26 & 19.27).

Physiological basis of the theory—trunk rotation equipoise

In the healthy individual there is a dynamic equilibrium in the trunk between the rotation and counter-rotation forces generated during muscular activity and particularly gait. We term this state of balance 'trunk rotation equipoise'. Idiopathic scoliosis and sportsman's scolioses represent a cyclical failure of such trunk equipoise.

By 'rotation equipoise' we mean the capacity of the trunk after activity to return to a neutral position in the transverse plane. The term could also be applied to the frontal and sagittal planes of the trunk. In some idiopathic scolioses the frontal plane component is more evident than the transverse plane component (Agostini).

Pathomechanical concepts (Fig. 19.9)

In essence, when the human rib cage is developmentally unable to control those muscular forces in the spine which are transmitted to it from forces generated elsewhere in the skeleton during physical activity, and particularly gait, a cyclical failure of trunk rotation equipoise occurs which is termed 'idiopathic scoliosis' (IS).

Pelvithoracic size disparity may contribute to this mechanical breakdown of rotation. The latter occurs in association with a lateral spinal curvature and a short-segment lordosis to create the initial three-dimensional deformity of IS.

Biological concepts (Fig. 19.10)

Neuromuscular

The mechanical breakdown of IS is initiated, and then potentiated, by a developmental abnormality in the central nervous system (CNS) involving functional asymmetry of one or more inherited and actively acquired (by movement repetition) spinal cord 'central pattern generators' (CPGs), which control gait (Grillner, 1981). The ensuing neuromuscular asymmetry creates rib–vertebra angle asymmetry which in turn leads to a cyclical failure of mechanisms of rotation control in the trunk; these involve rotation-defending (mainly musculocostal, but also musculospinal, discal and ligamentous) and rotation-inducing (pelvispinal) mechanisms acting mainly in gait.

Resolution of asymmetry in CPGs explains the resolution of infantile and juvenile IS before irreversible changes have occurred in the spine and rib cage (Agadir *et al.*, 1992; Jones, 1992).

Skeletal

The ensuing asymmetrical loading on the immature human spine in the erect position alters spinal growth; this abnormal growth, together with normal linear spinal growth, potentiate the continuing mechanical failure resulting from the opposing rotation-defending and rotation-inducing mechanisms to produce progressive IS. At present there is no evidence to support the concept that progressive scoliosis is determined by 'abnormal vertebral plasticity'.

Discs and ligaments

We envisage that permissive roles are played by discs, ligaments and joint laxity. A strong anterior longitudinal ligament of the spine would be a barrier to progression of the scoliotic deformity.

Functional, developmental and evolutionary perspectives

Our concept views IS in the wider perspective of function in the trunk, development and human evolution, all in relation to bipedalism.

In the last three million years of human evolution the rounding of the thorax and pelvis may have been caused by the CNS and trunk muscles adapting to their new role of oscillating the trunk to give humans their unique bipedal gait; the rounding of the female pelvis seems to have contributed to the rapid evolution of human brain size.

The predisposition of tall adolescent girls to progressive IS is likely to result from several developmental features involving the pelvis, spine, rib cage, trunk muscles, CNS, growth and joint laxity.

THEORY OF AETIOLOGY—DETAILED NARRATIVE

In presenting the conceptual framework of the theory of aetiology, its components need to be defined. These relate to:

1 spinal pathomechanics of scoliosis,
2 femora, hips, pelvis and gait,
3 the spine in gait,
4 rib cage,
5 trunk muscles and gait,
6 central nervous system,
7 growth.

Spinal pathomechanics of scoliosis

The morphology of a primary structural curve—rotation, tilt and lordosis (Figs 19.2, 19.11–19.14)

The three main mechanical components of a primary structural scoliosis curve of the usual rotatory type are rotation, tilt and lordosis (Somerville, 1952; Roaf, 1960). In our view an initial event is a failure of rotation control in the spine. This develops principally during gait due to asymmetrical forces re-

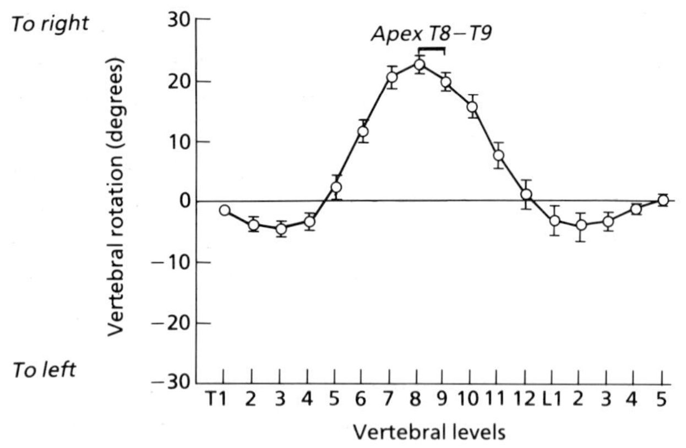

Fig. 19.11 Segmental vertebral rotation (mean ± 1 SE, Perdriolle method). Preoperative thoracic scoliosis apex T8–T9. From Wythers *et al.* (1992).

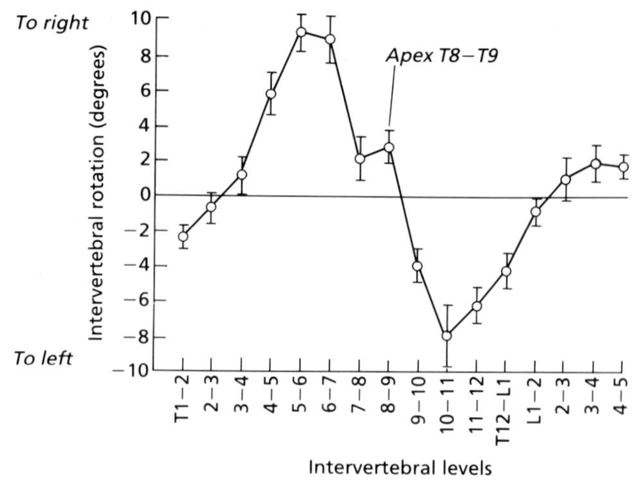

Fig. 19.12 Segmental intervertebral rotation (mean ± 1 SE, calculated from vertebral rotation). Preoperative thoracic scoliosis apex T8–T9. From Wythers *et al.* (1992).

sulting from rib–vertebra angle asymmetry, which in turn is due to a developmental defect in the CNS. The changes of vertebral tilt, in each of the frontal and sagittal planes of the spine, are usually secondary to the vertebral rotation.

VERTEBRAL ROTATION

Figure 19.11 shows vertebral rotation segmentally for preoperative thoracic scoliosis (Wythers *et al.*, 1992). The rotation is maximum at the curve apex (T8–T9).

INTERVERTEBRAL ROTATION

Figure 19.12 shows intervertebral rotation for preoperative thoracic scoliosis (Wythers *et al.*, 1992). The rotation *between* vertebrae is greatest at the ends of the curve (T5–T6 and T10–T11) and least at the curve apex (T8–T9). These findings are consistent with the view that, at the ends of the curve, the thoracic vertebrae are rotating about a normal anterior axis of rotation (Fig. 19.20; Gregersen & Lucas, 1967). In contrast, at the curve apex the thoracic vertebrae are rotating about an abnormal posterior axis of rotation (Fig. 19.3; Adams, 1865), more like a lumbar vertebra.

DISCAL AND INTRAVERTEBRAL TORSION

Axial computerized tomography (CT) scans of scoliotic cadavers confirm the presence and location of the intervertebral rotation. They also reveal the intravertebral torsion which is greater than that in the discs. Both vertebral and discal torsion are present along the length of the spine and are minimal at the curve apex (Wemyss-Holden *et al.*, 1991a).

There are surgical implications for these findings. Posterior instrumentation can derotate the spine only through the discs; it cannot derotate it through the bones. Hence anterior surgery is needed to correct for the torsion within vertebrae. This explains why, after Cotrel–Dubousset instrumentation for scoliosis, there is no consistent derotation of the apical vertebra in relation to the pelvis; the derotation is

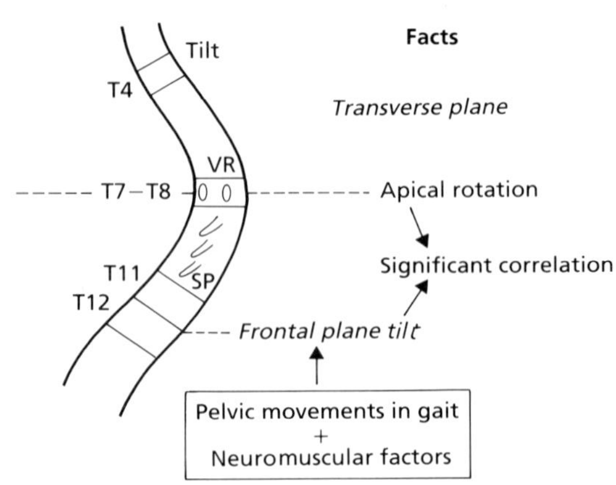

Fig. 19.13 The association between tilt at T11–T12 (frontal plane) and apical vertebral rotation (transverse plane) in radiographs. Preoperative thoracic scoliosis. From Wojcik *et al.* (1992).

merely transmitted down the spine to the pelvis (Fig. 19.8; Wood *et al.*, 1990).

VERTEBRAL TILT AND COBB ANGLE

The Cobb angle is the most obvious radiological feature of a scoliosis. In our view the increased deviation from the midline and vertebral tilt usually occur concomitantly with the rotation; above and below the apical vertebra, the tilts of the end-vertebrae create the Cobb angle (Fig. 19.13; Wojcik *et al.*, 1992). We base this view on findings from preoperative patients with thoracic scoliosis; in these patients the apical rotation correlates with vertebral tilting in the frontal plane at a position three or four segments more distally (and proximally) in the spine.

LORDOTIC SEGMENT—ITS RELATION TO APICAL ROTATION, HUETER–VOLKMANN LAW AND PAUWELS' LAW (Figs 19.2 & 19.14)

In our view the lordotic segment occurs concomitantly with the vertebral rotation; these deformations cannot occur without the anterior longitudinal ligament playing a permissive role (Burwell *et al.*, 1991a). In this connection, Roaf (1958, 1966) has argued that when vertebral rotation is unopposed, every muscular contraction pushes the vertebra further from the midline and increases the lordosis.

In theory, the decreased body height posteriorly at the curve apex results from the effect of altered mechanics on bone growth in two ways:

1 *Posteriorly*, the lordotic segment shifts the mechanical loading of the apical vertebral bodies backwards, which inhibits growth posteriorly (Hueter–Volkmann law).

2 *Anteriorly*, the posterior displacement of the axis of rotation at the apex of a thoracic scoliosis, creates abnormal anterior vertebral shear in the rotationally more mobile vertebrae above T11 (Fig. 19.19) and below the counter-rotations of the upper thoracic spine. In the immature spine under load, repetitive anterior rotational shear arising during gait contributes to the relative anterior spinal overgrowth at the curve apex (Pauwels' law; Burwell, 1990).

LINEAR SPINAL GROWTH AND HUETER–VOLKMANN LAW

Once the spinal pathomechanics of scoliosis have become established, the vertebral wedging (in PA and lateral radiographs) results from altered mechanical loading of vertebral growth-cartilages (Hueter–Volkmann law; see Arkin, 1949; Roaf, 1960). Finally, linear spinal growth and gravity augment the scoliotic deformity.

KYPHOTIC ANGULATION IN SCOLIOSIS (Figs 19.2 & 19.14)

We view the kyphotic angulation as a flexion deformity of the spine resulting from the lordotic segment developing in the primary thoracic curve immediately above it. More specifically, we suggest

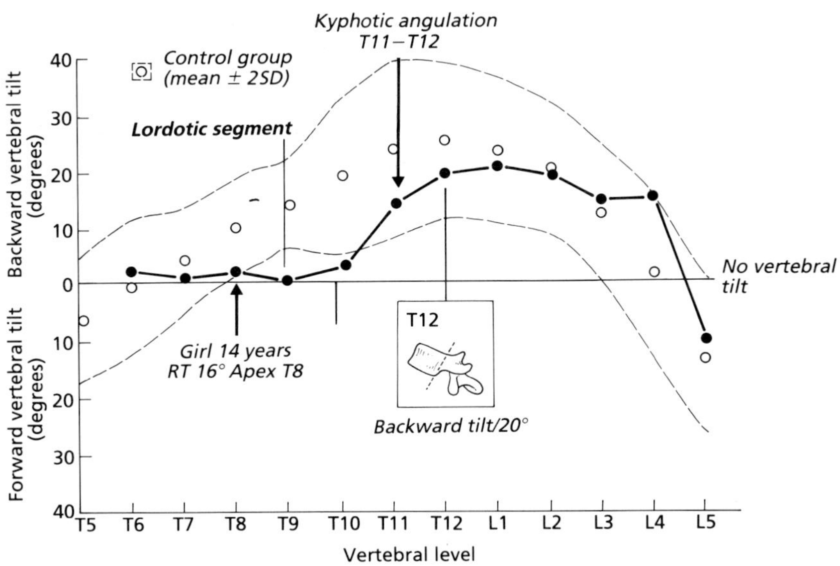

Fig. 19.14 Right thoracic scoliosis in a 14-year-old girl. Segmental sagittal spinal profile showing kyphotic angulation at T11–T12 with the lordotic segment above it. From Kiel *et al.* (1992).

that once a scoliosis starts to develop, the development of a kyphotic angulation in the thoracolumbar or upper lumbar spine is determined by the compressibility of each disc in relation to the length of the articular processes at the corresponding level. Where the combination of disc weakness and facet length is most adverse, forward flexion occurs, as in a spinal fracture, to produce the kyphotic angulation (Kiel *et al.*, 1992).

SAGITTAL SPINAL SHAPE AT T12 AND SCHOOL SCREENING

In the Nottingham School Screening Study the kyphosis and declive angles were significantly flatter for the 10 largest curves compared with the 10 smallest curves (Fig. 19.14; Chapter 9). Our subsequent segmental radiological study of the lateral spinal profile of these children shows an association between a more vertical T12 and each of CA and apical vertebral rotation of thoracic scoliosis curves (Kiel *et al.*, 1992). In preoperative patients, Wythers *et al.* (1992) also showed an association between sagittal back shape and the back hump.

Such flattening at T11–T12 may predispose a child to adolescent idiopathic scoliosis (Burwell, 1990), a view held by Schulthess in the last century (Arkin, 1949); equally the flattening may be secondary to a thoracic structural scoliosis (Wythers *et al.*, 1992).

PELVIC ROTATION, LUMBAR SPINE AND SCOLIOSIS

A segmental surface and radiological evaluation of the spine, rib cage and trunk in 30 preoperative patients with thoracic AIS shows that pathomechanical features in the thoracolumbar spine (in each of the transverse, frontal and sagittal planes) are associated with the surface deformity of AIS; they are possibly linked to the pathomechanical role of rotational forces created in the pelvis during gait (Wythers *et al.*, 1992).

Femora, hips, pelvis and gait

Figure 19.17 gives a plan view of the pelvis and hip rotation in gait. Our data relate to femoral anteversion, hip rotation whilst standing and pelvic movements in gait.

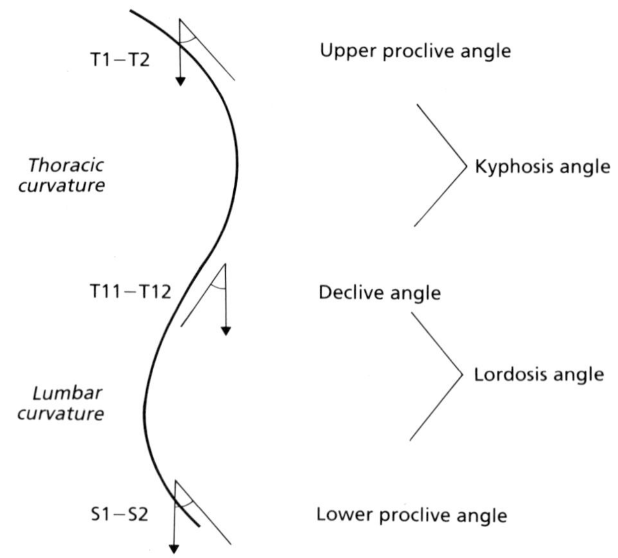

Fig. 19.15 Sagittal spinal curve angles. From Burwell *et al.* (1990).

Femoral anteversion and scoliosis

Prochiantz (1986) studied the femora of eight patients with IS using CT, and concluded that a number of such cases originate in asymmetric femoral anteversion. Burwell *et al.* (1990), using an ultrasound method to measure femoral anteversion, found that anteversion asymmetry is greater in school screening referrals and their siblings than in controls. Moreover, femoral anteversion asymmetry and the flatness of the back at T11–T12 (declive angle, Fig. 19.15) together discriminate as clusters most lumbar curves from thoracic and thoracolumbar curves (Fig. 19.16); this finding suggests that such hip and spinal mechanisms are involved in the aetiology of IS. Finally, a derivative of femoral anteversion and its asymmetry (residual functional anteversion) is related to the CA of the lowest lateral spinal curves of 20° or more. These findings relating to the hips and spine led us to propose the General Theory of Aetiology for IS (Fig. 19.8). There was clearly a need to examine hip rotation in relation to scoliosis curves (Fig. 19.17).

Hip rotation and scoliosis

Cole *et al.* (1990a) used a new instrument to measure the rotation of both hips simultaneously in the standing position in normal and scoliotic subjects. In idiopathic scoliotics, significant correlations are found between hip ratios (external/internal rotation)

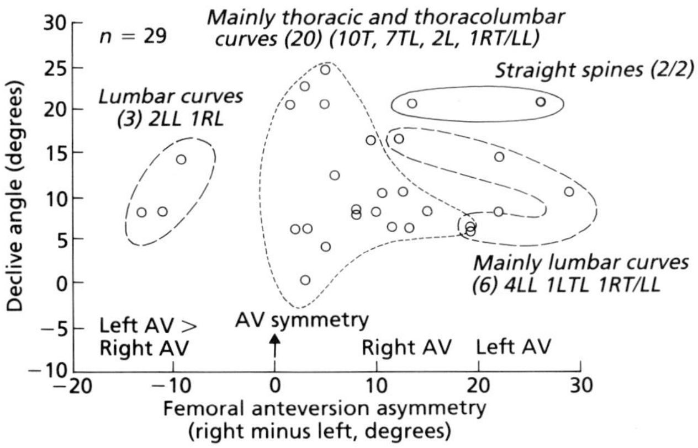

Fig. 19.16 Screening referrals: declive angle plotted against femoral anteversion asymmetry showing discrimination of curve types as clusters. From Burwell *et al.* (1990).

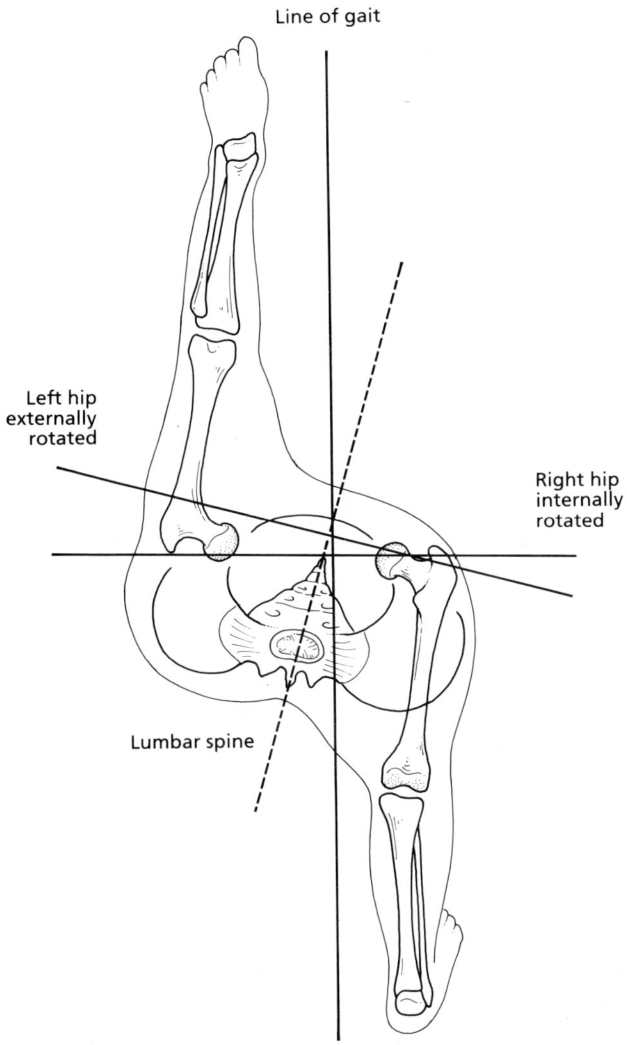

Fig. 19.17 Plan view to show hip rotation in relation to gait at right toe-off. From Wall *et al.* (1981).

and each of CA and vertebral rotation of the lowest lateral spinal curve. The findings are consistent with the hypothesis that the severity of such curves is influenced by the pattern of transverse plane pelvic rotation in gait.

Lower limb torsion

Rotation of the femur at the hip joint in gait is linked to torsion through the knee joint, tibia and subtalar joint.

The spine in gait

There are at least two basic requirements for human bipedal gait to be effective and efficient: (a) the body must be able to balance itself effectively, not only whilst standing but also whilst striding when only one limb is supporting the trunk (Janda, 1983); and (b) the legs must be able to move quickly through a relatively wide arc, which requires the limb can be extended past the vertical to provide propulsion to the stride (Conroy, 1990).

These requirements demand control of the spine in the frontal plane when one leg is off the ground (85% of the gait cycle); in the transverse plane as the pelvis rotates the spine above it, with counter-rotation in the upper thoracic spine; and in the sagittal plane.

When the pelvis rotates, the concurrent and opposite rotation of the thorax probably provides a damping effect. The excursion of the thorax appears most closely related to the arm swing which typically finds the right arm advancing with the left leg and vice-versa (Murray).

Pelvic rotation in gait (Fig. 19.17)

Pelvic movements in gait are complex but can be resolved into each of the transverse, frontal and sagittal planes. Sutherland *et al.* (1980) published pelvic rotation curves during gait for children. It seems likely that both lower limb and trunk muscles contribute to these pelvic movements (the brothers Weber, 1836; Waters and Morris, 1972; Wemyss-Holden *et al.*, 1991b; but see Gracovetsky, 1988).

Spinal rotation in gait (Fig. 19.18)

As the pelvis rotates in the transverse plane, its movements are transmitted directly to the spine.

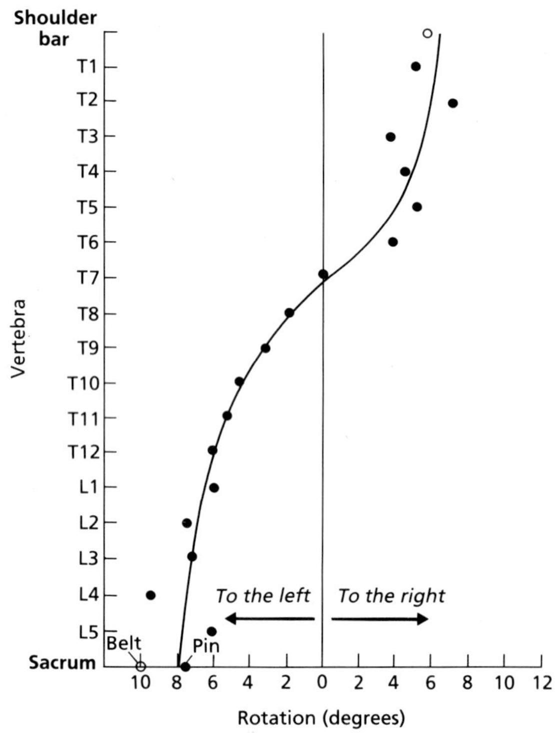

Fig. 19.18 Axial rotation of thoracolumbar spine during gait (left heel strike to right heel strike, 4.38 K/h). From Gregersen & Lucas (1967).

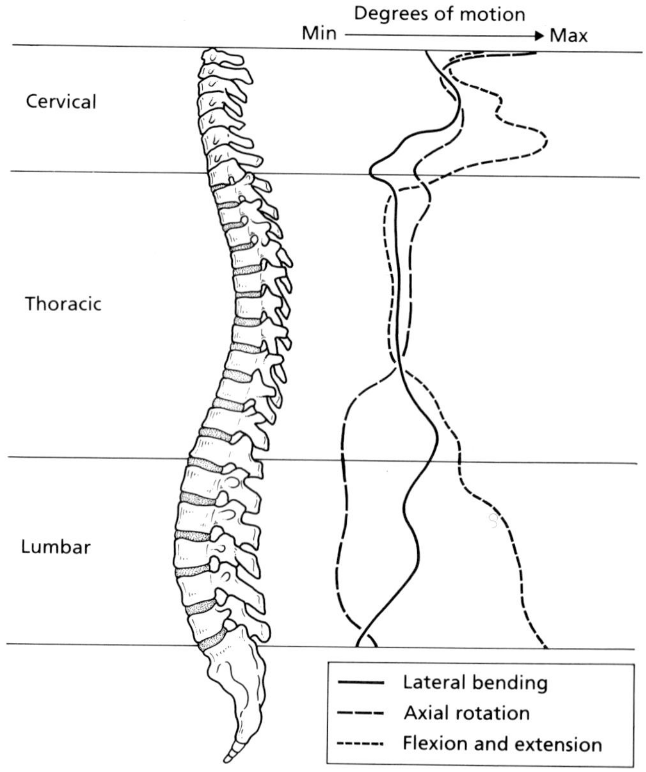

Fig. 19.19 Schematic drawing of spinal mobility at each vertebral level. From Bullough & Boachie-Adjei (1988). See White (1969).

Gregersen & Lucas (1967) described the axial rotation of the thoracic and lumbar spine during locomotion with counter-rotation of the spine above T7. Thurston & Harris (1983) examined the movements of the pelvis and lumbar spine in adult males. Cole *et al.* (1990b) used the Cartesian optoelectronic dynamic anthropometer (CODA) to evaluate pelvic movements in three dimensions during gait in healthy children, and the relation to spinal movement. Hypotheses were developed linking pelvic movements (in both transverse and frontal planes) with spinal movements.

The intervertebral rotation varies along the length of the normal spine; it is least in the lumbar and lower thoracic spine (Figs 19.19 & 19.20; White, 1969). Factors which limit rotation include in the lumbar spine, the discs, and in the thoracic spine, the ribs.

Electrical activity of trunk muscles in gait

Walking requires an upset of the delicate balance of the trunk, which is maintained by minimal muscular activity during standing at rest. During ambulation, the pelvis undergoes significant translational and rotatory motion in the transverse, frontal and sagittal planes. Therefore, the requirements for balancing the trunk by the action of trunk muscles are much more complex than during standing (Waters & Morris, 1972). Some muscles of the trunk, acting through the rib cage, which control trunk rotation during gait, are discussed below.

Rib cage

Functions in respiration, posture, locomotion and other movements

The outstanding function of the thorax is in respiration. In addition, the ribs are the principal agents for the support of the thoracic vertebrae by virtue of their rigidity, not only as bony braces but also because of their service as instruments through which the forces exerted by the attached muscles and ligaments and

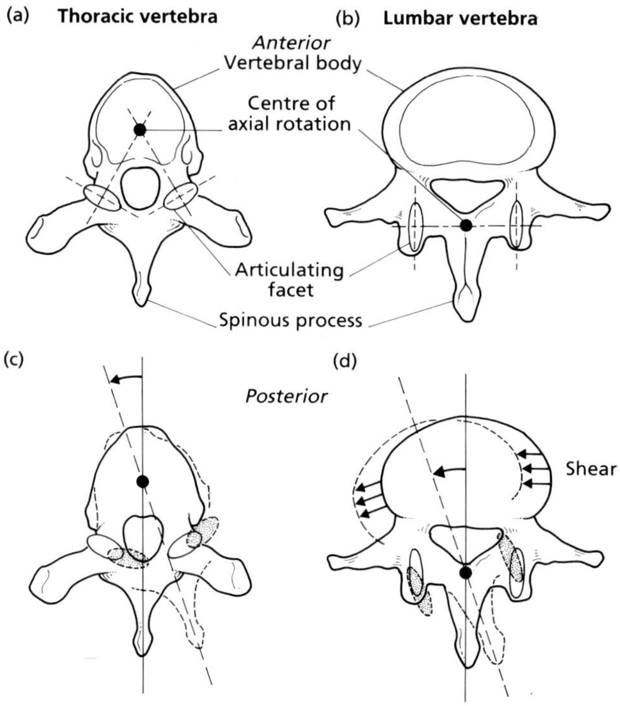

Fig. 19.20 Mechanism of axial rotation in a thoracic and lumbar vertebra. From Gregersen & Lucas (1967).

the forces of intrathoracic pressures and stresses are transmitted to the vertebrae through their costovertebral articulations (Bisgard, 1934; Pal, 1991).

In connection with movements, it is claimed that the contraction of intercostal muscles causes rotational as well as side-bending forces with the vertebral bodies rotating to the convexity (Schmitt, 1981). In standing, sitting and lifting, the trunk must balance on the pelvis, as it must also during walking, as the trunk moves along the vertical and lateral as well as the progressional axis (Waters & Morris, 1972). Finally, in addition to controlling the spine, the ribs are also sites of origin for muscles which run to the scapula and arm, and their firm fixation is important in performing skilled movements of the arms (Roaf, 1974).

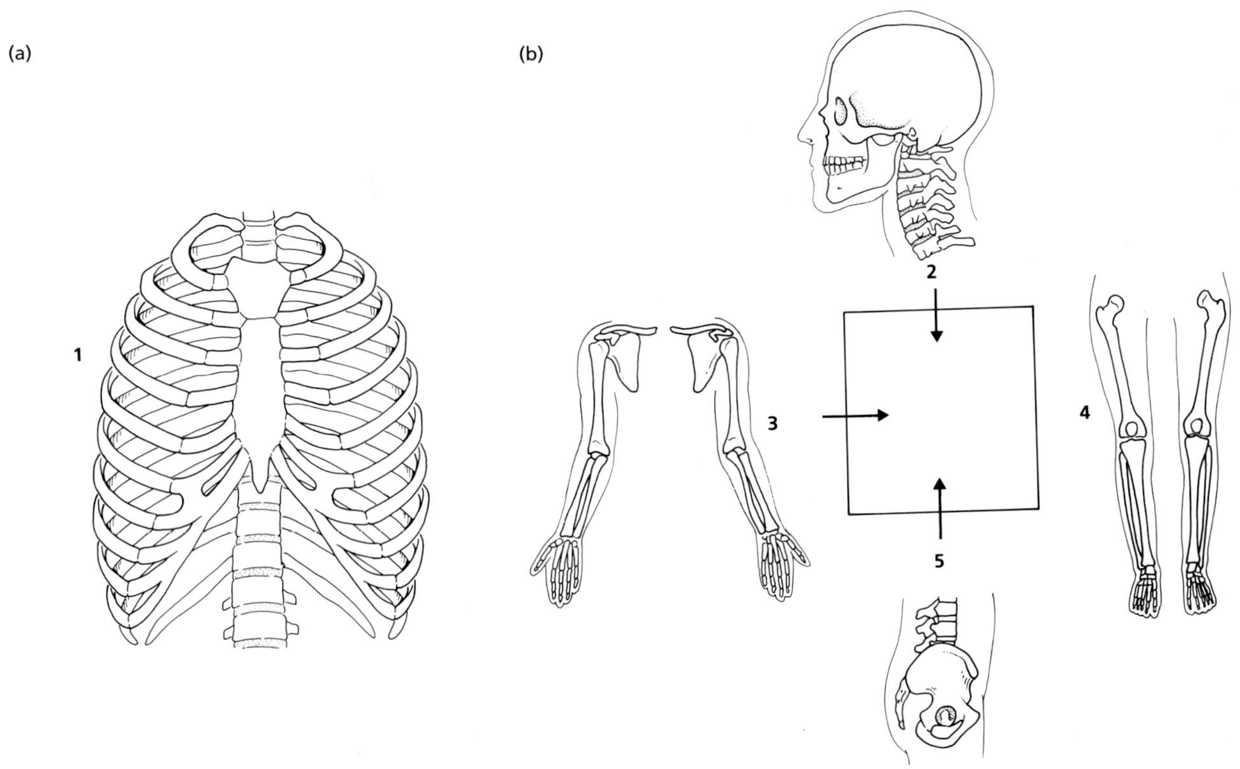

Fig. 19.21 The five functional body segments: left: the body segment thorax (a 'stabile'); right: the four other body segments ('mobiles'). From Klein-Vogelbach (1990).

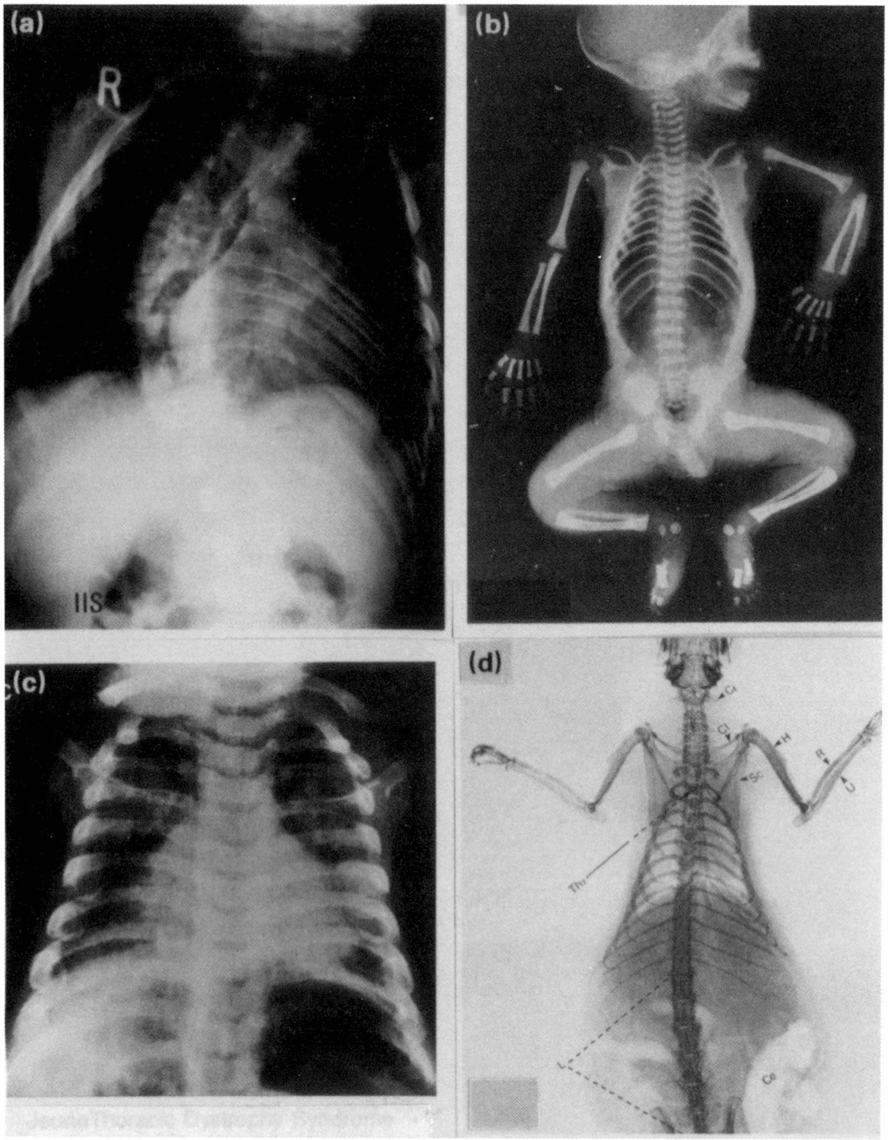

Fig. 19.22 (a) The funnel-shaped upper chest of progressive infantile idiopathic scoliosis (IIS) compared with (b) a normal human foetus, (c) Jeunẹ's thoracic dystrophy syndrome, and (d) adult rabbit. From Grivas *et al.* (1992a).

The thorax as a 'stabilizing centre' for posture and movement

Figure 19.21 shows the concept of the human body as having five functional segments in which the thorax is the stabilizing centre of posture and movement, with impulses coming in from the periphery—from the legs via the pelvis, from the arms via the shoulder girdles, and from the head (Klein-Vogelbach, 1990). The body segment thorax as the *'stabile'* has to withstand the continuous challenges of considerable diversity from the *'mobiles'*. According to this concept, when the stabilizing centre fails to function properly, disruption of normal function occurs.

Segmental RVA asymmetry (RVADs) and scoliosis aetiology

Our segmental RVA findings show that RVA asymmetry is a feature of both progressive infantile and AIS (Grivas *et al.*, 1992a; Wemyss-Holden *et al.*, 1992b). Do these RVA asymmetries result from, or contribute to, the scoliosis? In scoliotic patients the question is difficult to answer; are the observed changes cause or effect?

An apparent escape from this apparent *impasse* emerged from studying the postnatal development of the non-scoliotic thorax (Grivas *et al.*, 1991b, 1992). The findings led to the suggestion that the rib cage contains aetiological mechanisms of IS. Other workers have proposed that rib-length asymmetry causes IS; but their findings are conflicting. Before we summarize the evidence, let us review our findings for the rib cage in IIS.

Infantile idiopathic scoliosis—funnelling of the upper rib cage, RVADs and the predictive value of the upper thoracic spine (Fig. 19.22)

Grivas *et al.* (1992a) showed that the upper rib cage in IIS is abnormal in that: (a) it is funnel-shaped like a foetus, (b) the RVADs increase from T1–T6 above the apical vertebra, (c) the vertebral rotation at T4 predicts apical vertebral rotation at follow-up (compare with the 'specific rotation' of Perdriolle and Vidal, 1985). In the light of these findings, we conclude that progressive IIS is associated with a developmental abnormality of the upper thorax, affecting both the rib cage and the spine. We suggest that the skeletal abnormalities result, in part, from a developmental defect (CPG asymmetry) in the CNS; the abnormalities lead to a cyclical failure of mechanisms of rotation control in the thoracic spine during movements including gait (Burwell *et al.*, 1992a,b,c).

Developmental changes in the normal rib cage between birth and adolescence

Grivas then examined, as controls, the chest radiographs of 412 non-scoliotic children aged 0–17 years divided into three age groups, infancy, childhood and puberty. Attention was directed *segmentally* to:

1 thoracic shape (Fig. 19.23; Grivas *et al.*, 1991);
2 rib–vertebra angles (RVAs, Fig. 19.24, Grivas *et al.*, 1992b);
3 Rib–vertebra angle asymmetries (RVADs, Fig. 19.25, Grivas *et al.*, 1992b).

In summary, the findings show:

1 With increasing age there is narrowing of the chest relative to its height, which is most marked in the lower chest, especially of girls (Fig. 19.23). The relative narrowing of the lower thorax with increasing age may be a mechanism to reduce the rotational inertia created in the thorax by the torque of the rotating pelvis and thoracolumbar spine in gait (Grivas *et al.*, 1991).
2 The upper ribs elevate between birth and adolescence, more marked in boys than girls. The lower ribs droop between infancy and childhood, especially in girls (Fig. 19.24).
3 The RVAD patterns reflect the age, sex and laterality patterns of IS (Fig. 19.25).

Neuromuscular mechanisms as the cause of the age- and sex-related changes in the normal rib cage

Elsewhere we argue that the angle which a rib makes with its vertebra, results in part from the summated muscular forces acting continually in opposite directions along the length of the growing trunk, i.e. RVAs express muscle balance (Grivas *et al.*, 1992b). This

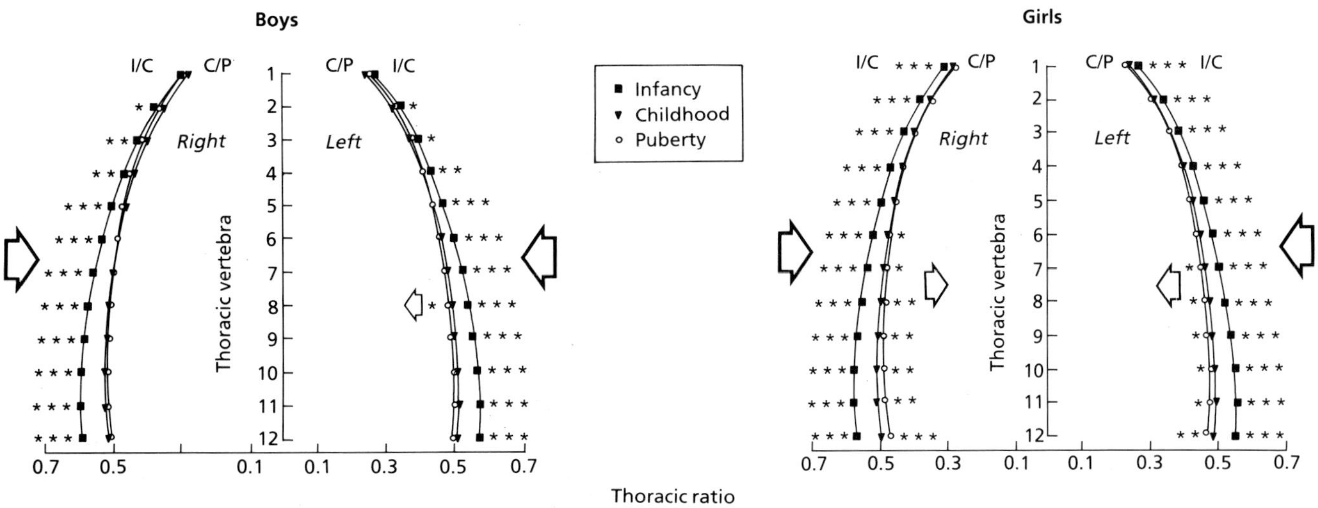

Fig. 19.23 Segmental thoracic ratios (width/height) for control boys and girls plotted by age group, infancy (I), childhood (C) and puberty (P). From Grivas et al. (1991).

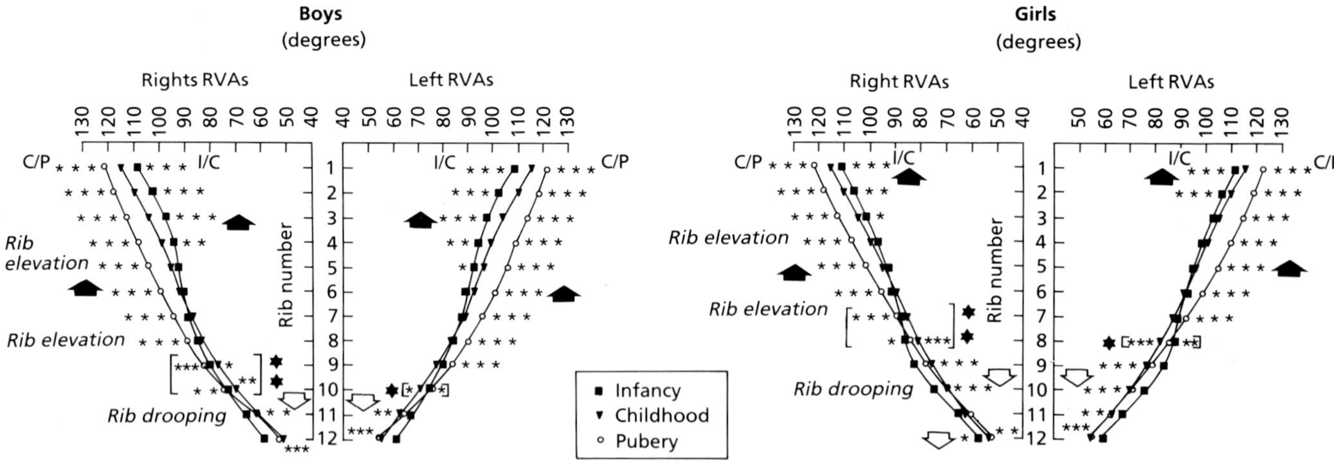

Fig. 19.24 Segmental rib–vertebra angles (RVAs in degrees) in the boys and girls for each of the infancy (I), childhood (C) and puberty (P) age groups by rib level (no. of rib). Note: (1) in infancy at rib 6, RVAs are about 90°; (2) between infancy and childhood (I/C) the RVAs elevate above rib 6 and droop below rib 6; and (3) between childhood and puberty (C/P), RVAs elevate from rib 1 to 10 in boys and from rib 1 to 8 in girls. From Grivas *et al.* (1992a,b).

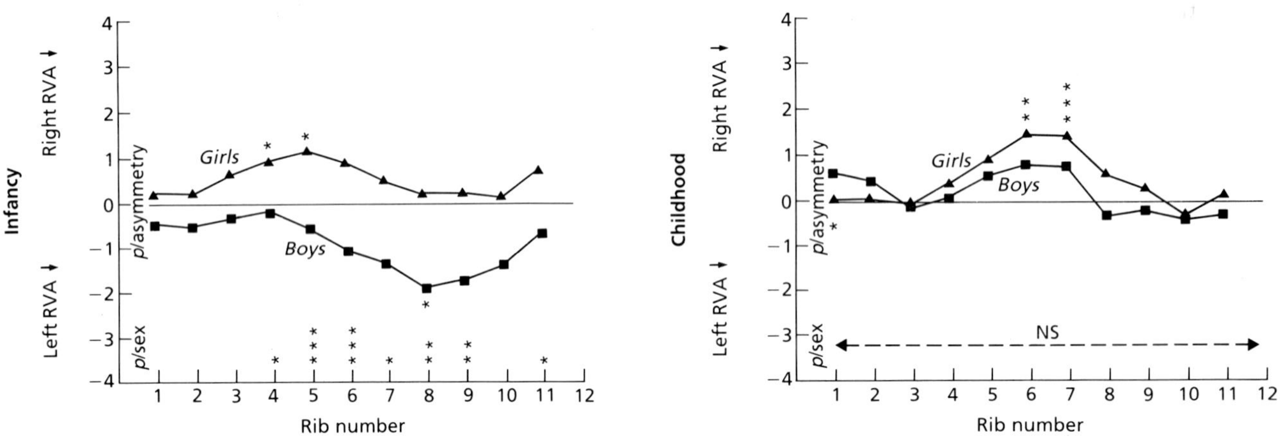

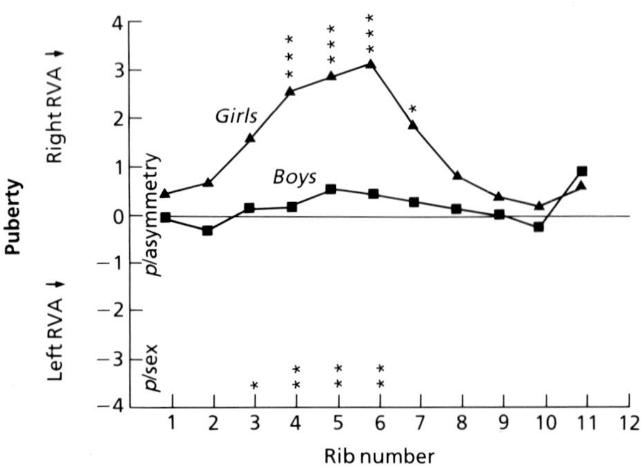

Fig. 19.25 Segmental RVADs (rib–vertebra angle difference = rib vertebral angle asymmetry) for infancy, childhood and puberty age groups. From Grivas *et al.* (1992a,b).

concept implies that there are physiological alterations of the muscle balance acting on ribs during growth; these are likely to be controlled by developmental changes in the CNS, which hitherto were unsuspected.

Adolescent idiopathic scoliosis—preoperative patients

Wemyss-Holden *et al.* (1992b) have recently reported findings relating to segmental RVAs corrected for vertebral tilt in 36 preoperative patients with thoracic AIS, compared with 40 non-scoliotic controls. The findings show a pattern of asymmetrical grouping of the upper concave and lower convex ribs (termed crossed RVA asymmetry); there is little or no abnormality in the ribs contralateral to the drooping.

Pal (1991), studying rib circumference (cross-section) in four scoliotic skeletons, concludes that most load is carried by the upper concave ribs; and also by the apical (and periapical) convex ribs. Pal does not explain his findings. Wemyss-Holden *et al.* suggest that the droop of the upper (and from the work of Pal, ? thicker) concave ribs results from the asymmetrical action of trunk rotator muscles more on the concavity of the scoliotic curve. In addition, by causing a rotational deformity in the trunk, these muscles increase the distance and tension in the abdominal oblique muscles between the lower convex ribs and the contralateral iliac crest (rotational muscle tether). According to this interpretation the drooping of upper concave ribs results directly from 'primary' neuromuscular imbalance; and drooping of the lower convex ribs to mechanical consequences 'secondary' to this neuromuscular imbalance.

Physiological and pathological RVA asymmetry?

Taking our RVA findings in IIS, AIS and control subjects together, the concept is suggested of 'physiological' RVA asymmetry as seen in the controls; and 'pathological' RVA asymmetry as found in the AIS patients.

This concept suggests that if the muscles which control counter-rotation of the upper thoracic spine function asymmetrically but balance pelvispinal rotational forces, the trunk will remain rotationally balanced; but if these muscles function asymmetrically and are unable to balance the pelvispinal rotational forces, a cyclical failure of trunk rotation will occur.

Hence, another factor in scoliosis aetiology may be asymmetrical pelvic rotation in the transverse plane during gait, possibly caused by asymmetry of thrust up the limbs at toe-off. More work is needed.

Trunk muscles, gait and scoliosis

Gravity, inertia and the mechanics of compound pendula are the primary elements of striding gait. Indeed, the great efficiency of this type of locomotion is predicated upon the greatly reduced requirements for muscular contraction (Lovejoy *et al.*, 1973). During normal, relaxed walking, the major function of the skeletal muscles is to accelerate, decelerate and stabilize the body segments in motion. This activity is accomplished not only by contraction with shortening of the muscle but also by elongation occurring during contraction (see Tylkowski, 1990).

Paravertebral muscles cannot control the rib levers of the upper and middle chest

The hypothesis that, in health, the central nervous system, through muscles, elevates the upper ribs to change the RVAs from the funnel-shaped chest at birth to a barrel-shaped thorax in adolescence, led us to examine which trunk muscles may be responsible.

Cook *et al.* (1991) studied the segmental anatomy of the sacrospinalis muscle, with particular reference to iliocostalis in three cadavers (Fig. 19.26). There was a large reduction in the iliocostalis muscle over the lower three ribs, the muscle remaining fairly constant above this region. They suggested that while iliocostalis controlled the movements of the lower thoracic spine, including rotation, it was unlikely to have any rotatory control through the middle and upper ribs. Such control may then involve flat muscles of the trunk including serratus anterior, abdominal muscles and possibly intercostal muscles. If so, aetiological studies on muscles in IS should include the flat rotators of the trunk and intercostal muscles, and not be restricted to paravertebral muscles.

A spiral composite muscle trunk rotator (Fig. 19.27)

Wemyss-Holden *et al.* (1991b) developed the theoretical concept that human trunk rotation in gait is influenced by a spiral composite muscle trunk rotator, comprising on each side: levator scapulae and

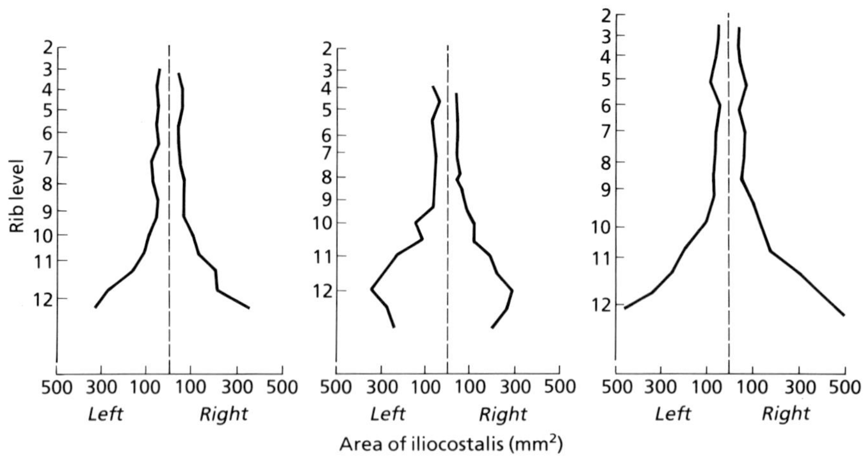

Fig. 19.26 Area of iliocostalis plotted against rib level in three female cadavers. From Cook *et al.* (1991).

rhomboids, serratus anterior, external oblique and the contralateral internal oblique muscle.

A mechanical model of trunk muscles in scoliosis

Wemyss-Holden *et al.* (1991b) then developed a mechanical model of the composite muscle trunk rotator. It was shown, firstly, that asymmetry of one or more of its components creates an axial deformity; and secondly, that the site and type of the induced lateral 'spinal' curve is related to the 'muscle' which is shortened. These findings are consistent with the view that neuromuscular factors are involved in the initiation of IS.

Central nervous system

Many workers have implicated the CNS in the aetiology of IS (see Robin, 1990). Herman *et al.* (1985) concluded that IS may represent a specific impairment of higher cortical function. Moreover, the presence of a visuospatial disorder may be the *common* feature of this clinical entity. Goldberg & Dowling (1990) also found an association between handedness and the side of scoliosis curves; they suggested that cerebral cortical function determines curve laterality.

A normal developmental mechanism in the CNS controlling the shape of the rib cage during growth?

The segmental variation of the RVAs during 'normal' growth suggests that the CNS contains a controlling mechanism, also segmental in the spinal cord, which differs in detail between boys and girls (sexual dimorphism, Grivas *et al.*, 1992b; Burwell *et al.*, 1992a,b,c). The genetic basis of this postnatal developmental process is likely to reflect its evolution (recapitulation concept of ontogeny repeats phylogeny). Such postnatal physiological changes in the spinal cord are likely to be influenced, if not controlled, by higher neural centres.

'Central pattern generators' for locomotion
(Fig. 19.28)

A neurophysiologist writes:

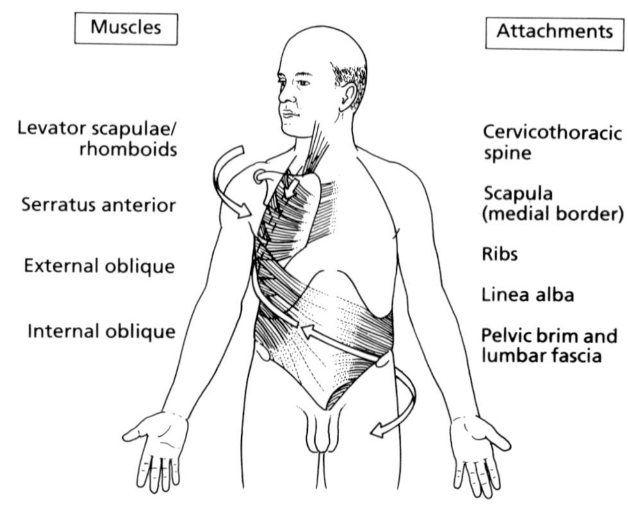

Fig. 19.27 The concept of the spiral 'composite muscle trunk rotator'. From Wemyss-Holden *et al.* (1991b).

(a)

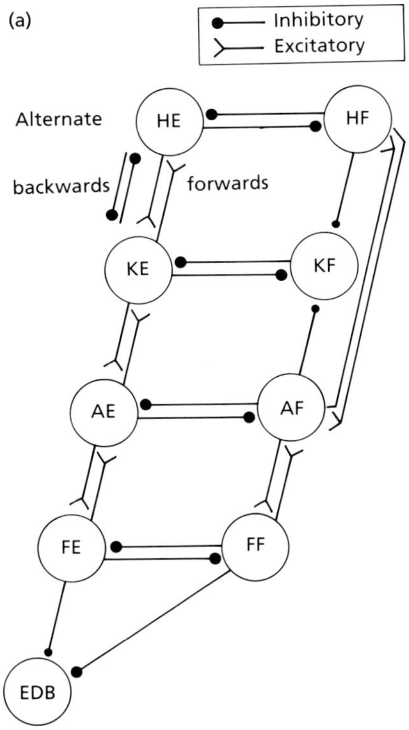

(b)

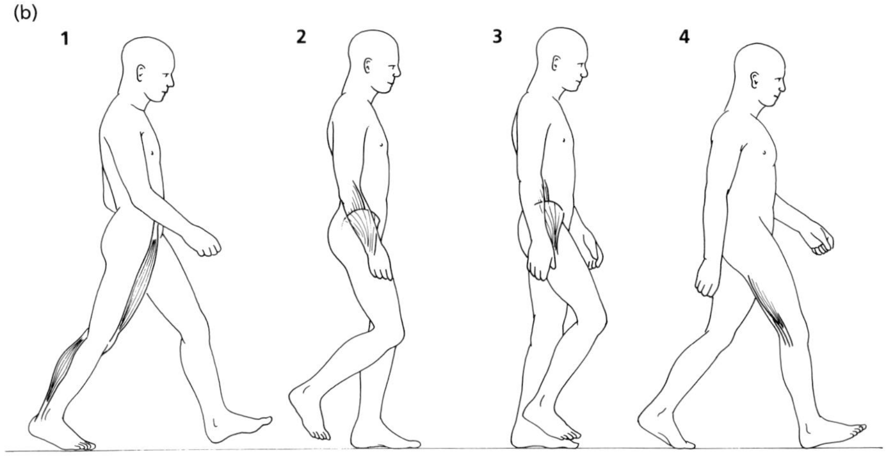

Fig. 19.28 Diagram to show for a limb: (a) central pattern generators (CPGs); (b) muscle activity during human striding. E, extensor; F, flexor; H, hip; K, knee; A, ankle; F, foot; EDB, short toe extensor. From Brooks (1986) and Lovejoy (1988) respectively.

> Locomotion, like many postural reactions, does not require control by the cerebral cortex; it is managed by subcortical and spinal centers, which of course are subject to cortical intervention. . . . Patterns for locomotion are generated in the spinal cord by 'central pattern generators' (CPGs) that operate in a flexible manner under supraspinal control. The most complex controls, emanating from the cerebral cortex, the cerebellum and the brain stem, initiate and maintain patterns of optimal activity by making predictive adjustments based on the circumstances of the moment (Brooks, 1986; see Grillner, 1981).

CPGs are inherited and actively acquired by movement repetition

Studies of newborn babies by Grillner show that a capacity for walking is present at birth—therefore it is inherited. Before birth, a basic walking pattern is imprinted upon the nervous system, a pattern we learn to use when we can walk unassisted for the first time.

The programmes for bipedal gait are acquired gradually during the first year of life. As the nervous system matures and muscles become stronger, the infant pattern is abandoned in favour of 'toddling'. This evolves into a steadier form of walking during the first 4 years, but a child accomplishes a near-normal adult pattern of walking only by about 7 years of age. During a period of 6 years it would have repeated about three million steps to achieve that level of performance. Adult patterns for walking and running are finally acquired during the teens and mature in late adolescence (see Butler & Major, 1992).

Idiopathic scoliosis—an initiating and continuing segmental developmental defect in the CNS?

Our interpretation of the evidence leads us to the following views:

1 There is a physiological mechanism in the CNS for controlling both postnatal changes in RVAs and gait.

2 Extremes of RVA asymmetries result from muscle imbalance.

3 The cause of such muscle imbalance lies in the central nervous system.

4 Aetiological mechanisms for IS include: RVA asymmetry; flat lateral spinal profile at T11–T12; hip rotation and femoral anteversion; growth, normal and abnormal, in the spine; and gait.

Items 1, 2 and 3 suggest that one basic cause of IS is an age-related defect (? CPG asymmetry) affecting certain spinal cord segments. The muscular effects, through asymmetrical trunk muscle action, weaken the spinal rotation-defending system during movements and particularly gait; this leads to a three-dimensional mechanical alteration of the spine, termed scoliosis. The induced mechanical alteration then exposes the spine to other biological factors, including growth which, with mechanical factors, together produce progressive IS (Fig. 19.10d).

The possibility that a mechanism contributing to the aetiology of thoracic IS lies in the CNS, and including lower cervical and upper thoracic spinal cord segments which control some of the muscles moving the upper rib cage, accounts for both the upper arm length asymmetry (Dangerfield *et al.*, 1980; Burwell *et al.*, 1981) and the electromyographic and histochemical abnormalities of deltoid muscles in IS (Yarom).

Syringomyelia and scoliosis

The concepts contained in our theory of aetiology for IS (Fig. 19.10d) explain the association between syringomyelia and scoliosis (Burwell *et al.*, 1991b). In children less than 20 years of age, scoliosis is the initial symptom in 65% of patients with syringomyelia (Isu *et al.*, 1990). Our findings suggest that the CPG asymmetry in the spinal cord interferes with the physiological mechanisms involved in RVA balance; this predisposes the patient to scoliosis, due to impairment of the spinal-rotation defending mechanisms during gait.

Resolution of early-onset scoliosis—reversible changes in the CNS before irreversible changes have occurred in the spine?

In a study of children with resolving IS (infantile 14, juvenile three), Agadir *et al.* (1992) found a group in which the CA started resolving whilst the AVR was still increasing for 2 years before itself starting to resolve. Residual structural rotation in the trunk does not explain such dissociated resolution of CA and AVR. A possible explanation is that biplanar neuromuscular mechanisms involving spinal cord CPGs control the resolution of the spinal asymmetry of scoliosis in each of the frontal plane (CA, postural CPG) and transverse plane (AVR, kinetic CPG). The implication is that resolving IS scoliosis results from reversible asymmetry of those CPGs which control posture (in the frontal plane) and movements (in the transverse plane) of the trunk in gait.

Growth

Spinal growth or extrathoracic growth as aetiological?

When growth is spoken of in relation to scoliosis aetiology it is generally assumed that growth acts through the spine. As already stated, this may be an oversimplification.

Our theory of aetiology suggests that, by enlarging the child's body relative to the thorax, growth may increase the disparity between the rotation-inducing (extrathoracic) and the rotation-defending (largely intrathoracic) mechanisms of the mechanical component of the theory (see Fig. 19.10c). Here we shall restrict discussion to what is generally known about the relation of spinal growth to scoliosis aetiology.

Relative lengthening of the anterior spinal components in scoliosis

We view the relative anterior spinal lengthening as being secondary (adaptive) to the intravertebral torsion along the spinal curvatures of a scoliosis (Wemyss-Holden *et al.*, 1991a).

Is there a cause-and-effect relationship between spinal growth and curve progression?

It is generally considered that growth is an important mechanism in the development of a progressive scoliosis. Indeed, Heuer (1927) concluded that the primary cause of scoliosis is an isolated growth lengthening of the anterior spinal elements, a view supported by Dickson *et al.* (1984). Some French workers take a different view.

There is no simple cause-and-effect relationship

Duval-Beaupère (1971) concluded that there is no 'cause-and-effect' relationship between growth of the vertebral column and scoliosis except as contemporaneous phenomena. According to Perdriolle *et al.* (1989), scoliosis curve progression results from two main factors: (a) a mechanical factor (torsion) which is the three-dimensional rotatory complex movement; and (b) intervertebral localized hyperpressures acting on the concave articular pillar (see Roaf, 1960). Perdriolle minimizes the importance of growth on the progression of a scoliotic curvature. Our findings after Cotrel–Dubousset (CD) instrumentation for AIS accord with, and extend, Perdriolle's conclusion.

CD instrumentation—hump progression without curve progression

In 37 patients having CD, and followed up for 1 year, the back hump reasserted without any detectable change segmentally in the spinal deformity (Wemyss-Holden *et al.*, 1992a). We conclude that the deforming forces of AIS continue to act on the trunk after CD, producing rotatory changes (or deformation) in the rib cage without any detectable progression of the spinal deformity, because the fused spinal segments are held rigidly by the instrumentation. The CD instrumentation seems, then, to have dissociated the pathomechanical relationship between ribs and spine in scoliosis. The interpretation is consistent with our concept of aetiology of AIS; namely that AIS results from a failure of rotation control in the trunk (Fig. 19.9). After CD the surgically fused spinal block may place increasing demands on the muscles controlling the rib cage during trunk movements.

Posterior spinal fusions with less rigidly fixed instrumentation lead to progression of the scoliosis curve as well as the surface hump.

Posterior spinal fusions in young children—hump progression and curve progression

Three groups of workers undertaking extensive posterior spinal fusions on young children with scoliosis have found curve progression with increasing surface deformity ('crankshaft phenomenon', Dubousset *et al.*, 1989; see Hefti & McMaster, 1983). Clearly, a surgically induced tethering at the back of a growing scoliotic spine can aggravate the scoliosis. It does not follow from these observations that untreated progressive IS is caused by posterior 'tethering' and relative anterior spinal overgrowth (see above).

Recently, some insight into the relationship between anterior spinal growth and scoliosis pathogenesis has been obtained from studying a combined surgical procedure for progressive IIS.

Posterior surgery without fusion combined with anterior epiphyseodesis for IIS

Grivas *et al.* (1992a) found that the beneficial effects of such combined surgery compared with posterior rodding alone are: (a) greater derotation postoperatively; (b) maintained correction of the CA; and (c) further derotation during follow-up. The latter derotation is associated with growth in the 'fused' segment which is greater (7%) on the concavity than the convexity. Hence, the epiphyseodesis and rodding do not cause an arrest of growth but a correction of spinal growth.

The mechanism by which the combined procedure, and not posterior rodding alone, improves the rotational deformity of IIS may be as follows: the convex vertebral wedge excisions (epiphyseodesis) help to correct more fully the mechanical alignment of the spine; this reduces the abnormal loading on the vertebral bodies; these are then released from the effect of asymmetric loading on their growth plates (elimination of Hueter–Volkmann effect).

Progression of scoliosis in adults

In our view, growth, both abnormal (secondary to vertebral hyperpressures) and normal (linear spinal growth), with gravity adds to the initiating and continuing neuromuscular mechanisms to augment scoliosis curve progression. There is evidence that muscle tether on the curve concavity may also contribute to progression (Wojcik *et al.*, 1990; Wythers *et al.*, 1992). The continued progression of a scoliosis curve then results from the summation of several mechanisms including spinal pathomechanics (neuromuscular cause), growth, gravity and muscle tether (see Burwell, 1971). The continued rib deformity after CD in adults with AIS in the absence of instrumentation failure we attribute to neuromuscular causes; such causes may also account for the *de novo* development and significant progression of scoliosis in the adult (see Grubb *et al.*, 1988).

Puberty, early maturation, growth spurt and motor performance—the unloading reflex and AIS

The age at adolescence is earlier in girls than boys, and there is some evidence that puberty is earlier in girls with AIS (see Robin, 1990; Ahl *et al.*, 1988; Hägglund *et al.*, 1990). The earlier maturation of

AIS girls may exert its effect not only through the adolescent growth spurt, and extrathoracic growth, but also through neuromuscular mechanisms; for early maturers perform significantly better than late maturers at speed of limb movement, explosive strength and static strength of muscle action (Lefevre *et al.*, 1990). These findings, viewed in the light of our concept of aetiology, call for neuromuscular studies of the flat rotator muscles of the trunk in scoliosis, including the abnormal unloading reflex reported in paraspinal muscles of patients with progressive scoliosis (Dobosiewicz, 1986).

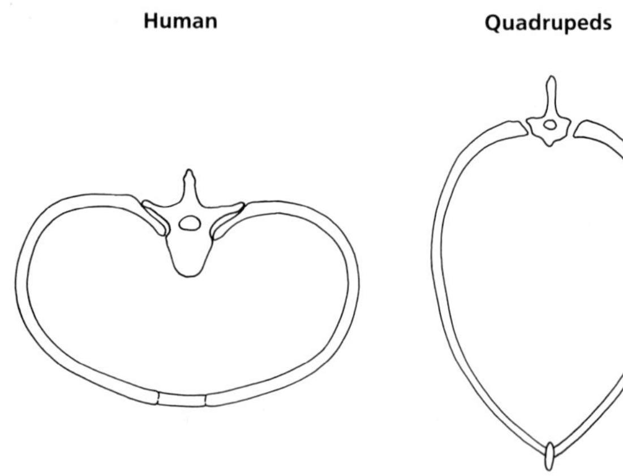

Fig. 19.29 Rib cage of human and quadrupeds. From Schmitt (1981).

Comparative anatomy

The rarity of scoliosis in quadrupeds

Typical 'idiopathic' structural scoliosis occurs rarely in quadrupeds (Arkin, 1949; see Dangerfield *et al.*, 1980). This knowledge is consistent with the view that humans are more vulnerable to scoliosis because of both gait and weight-bearing in the upright position.

The shape of the rib cage in humans, apes and quadrupeds (Figs 19.29 and 19.30)

In both humans and apes the spine has migrated anteriorly towards the centre of gravity in upright posture and lies more within the thorax rather than behind it as it does in other primates. Both the shape of the thorax and the position of the spine develop during infancy in humans and apes. In the foetus the transverse and sagittal diameters of the chest are the same and the spine lies at the back of the thorax. During subsequent growth the transverse diameter of the chest increases much more rapidly than does the sagittal diameter in both humans and apes, but not in monkeys, while the spine migrates to its more central position. Both ontogenetically and phylogenetically these features appear to be related to the development of a more upright position (Aiello & Dean, 1990).

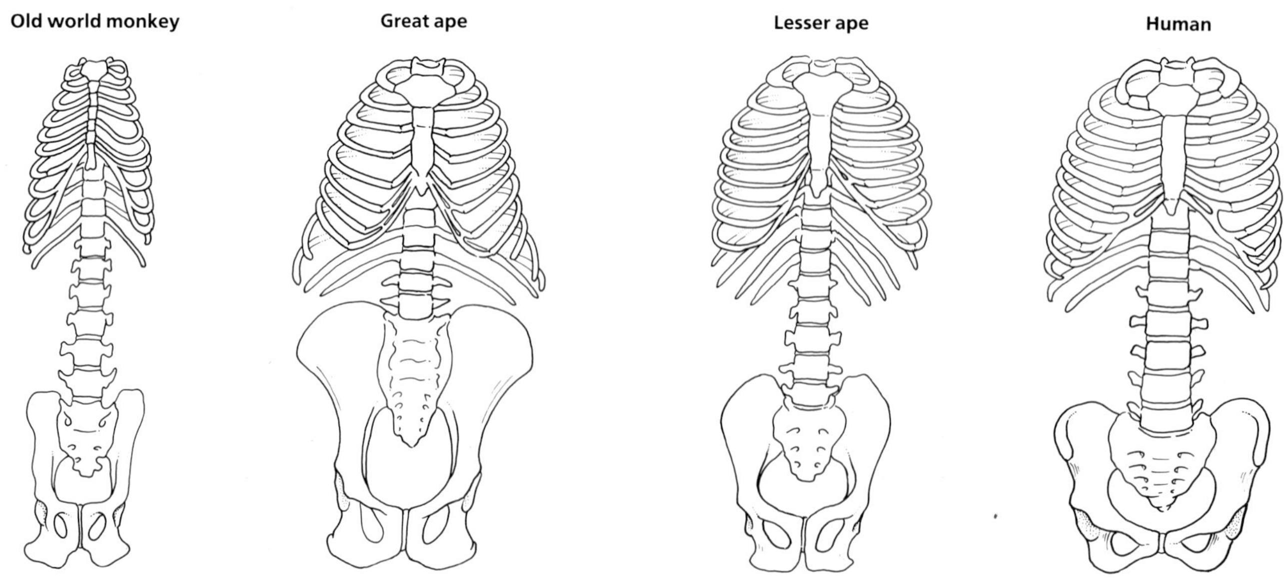

Fig. 19.30 Rib cage, pelvis and spine of primates. From Schultz (1984).

Unique trunk rotation in humans

According to Parry (1966):

> There is one action which man carries out frequently and forcibly, which is not so performed by quadrupeds, and that is rotation of the trunk. A horse that has fallen cannot regain its feet without first rolling, and this is the reason why it is unable to rise when in shafts. Trunk rotation in quadrupeds is limited; thus digging on the part of a dog is mainly a matter of spinal flexion, and in animals built for speed this is achieved by alternate flexion and extension of the spine. No animal other than man carries out such strenuous rotational movements as those involved in digging with a spade, swinging up a sack, or lifting heavy objects with one hand.

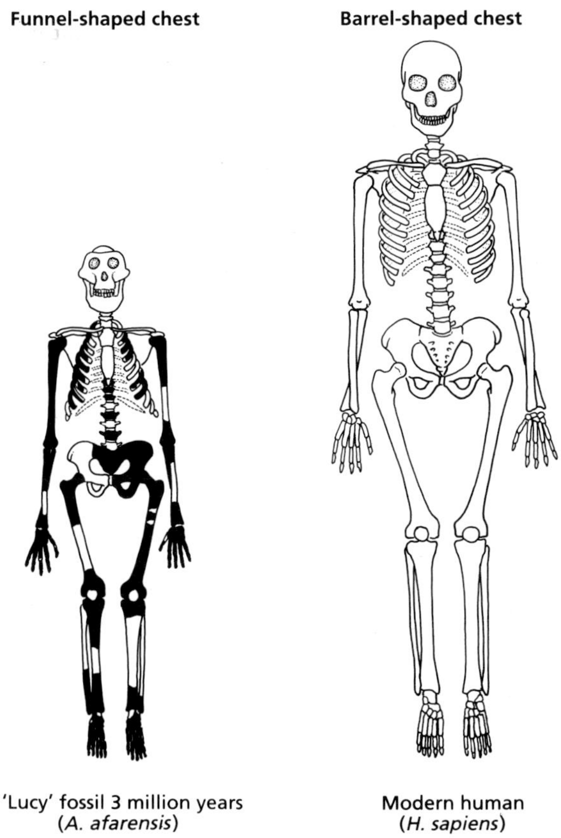

Fig. 19.31 The change in the rib cage from funnel-shaped to barrel-shaped in three million years of bipedalism. Reconstruction of the fossil skeleton of 'Lucy' (*Australopithecus afarensis*) compared with the skeleton of a modern human (*Homo sapiens*). Rearranged from Johanson & Edey (1981). See Aiello & Dean (1990).

Bipedal gait

Lovejoy (1988) writes:

> All other primates are basically quadrupedal, and with good reason: walking on two limbs instead of four has many drawbacks. It deprives us of speed and agility and all but eliminates our capacity to climb trees, which yield many important primate foods, such as fruits and nuts.

The adult human rib cage and pelvis differ in shape from that in the great ape, the lesser ape and the Old World Monkey (Fig. 19.30). We suspect that some of this difference in chest and pelvic shape between humans and non-human primates relates to alterations in skeletal morphology necessary for humans to stand upright with efficient bipedal gait, but also the evolution of human brain size (see below).

Skeletal specializations in humans

In accordance with upright position and bipedal gait, skeletal specializations are found in the human spine, pelvis and his broad thoracic cage, which is boat-shaped in quadrupeds (Parry, 1966).

Evolution and development of the spine, pelvis and rib cage

The evolutionary development of the human from quadrupedalism to bipedalism has involved many adaptive changes in the locomotor system (Aiello & Dean, 1990). Some of the skeletal changes have been observed in fossils; the neuromuscular changes can only be inferred.

Four *skeletal* consequences of humans adopting upright posture are (Fig. 19.31):

1 the creation of a lumbar lordosis (sagittal curves),
2 changes in pelvic shape associated with bipedal gait,
3 changes in rib cage shape,
4 changes in the occipital bone (position of foramen magnum).

Pelvic shape and early bipedal gait (Fig. 19.32)

A pelvic inlet that is wider than it is deep is a uniquely hominid feature. This pelvic configuration is a by-product of a shortening of the distance between sacroiliac and hip joints, which evolved as an adaptation to habitual erect posture and bipedalism in early hominids (Leutenegger, 1982). According to Lovejoy *et al.* (1973):

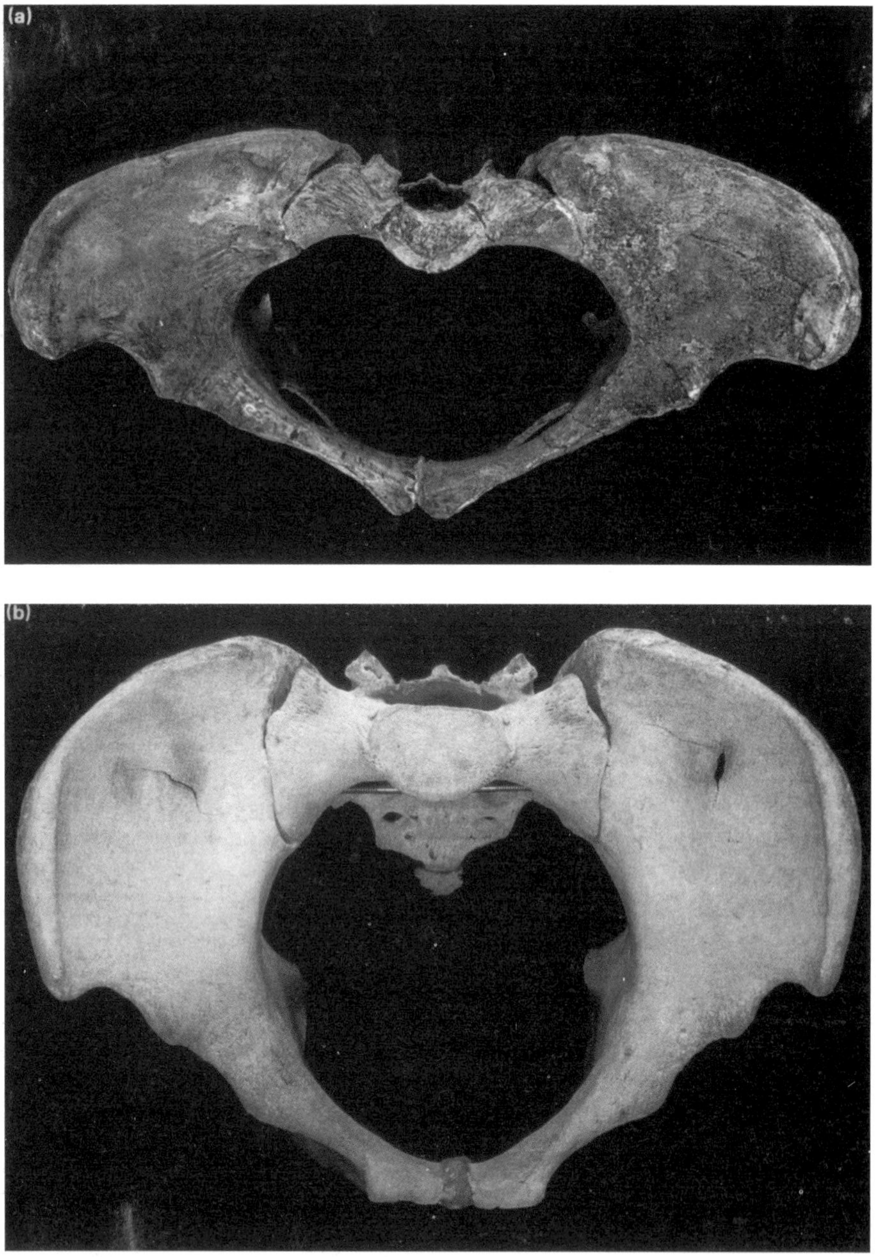

Fig. 19.32 Pelvis of 'Lucy' (a) compared with modern human female (b). The major change visible in this view, namely the more ovoid form of the human pelvis, is accompanied by an expansion of the birth canal. The changes are associated with the increase in brain size since 'Lucy'. From Lovejoy (1988).

> [T]here is a maximum total pelvic breadth which can be efficiently maintained in a biped of any given stature. For example, beyond certain pelvic breadths/stature ratios, rapid locomotion becomes cumbersome and awkward and the efficiency of stride is lost. The pelvic breadth of *Australopithecus* was already great because of the laterally flared ilium and relatively broad interacetabular distance (compared to that of quadrupeds) (Fig. 19.32).

There are strong indications that this and other major modifications in pelvic structure had been established before substantial brain expansion and thus before the emergence of the genus *Homo*. Minor pelvic alterations during the evolution of the genus *Homo*, such as a secondary increase in the sagittal diameter to produce a more cylindrical lesser pelvis, have been interpreted in terms of increased brain size (encephalization, see below).

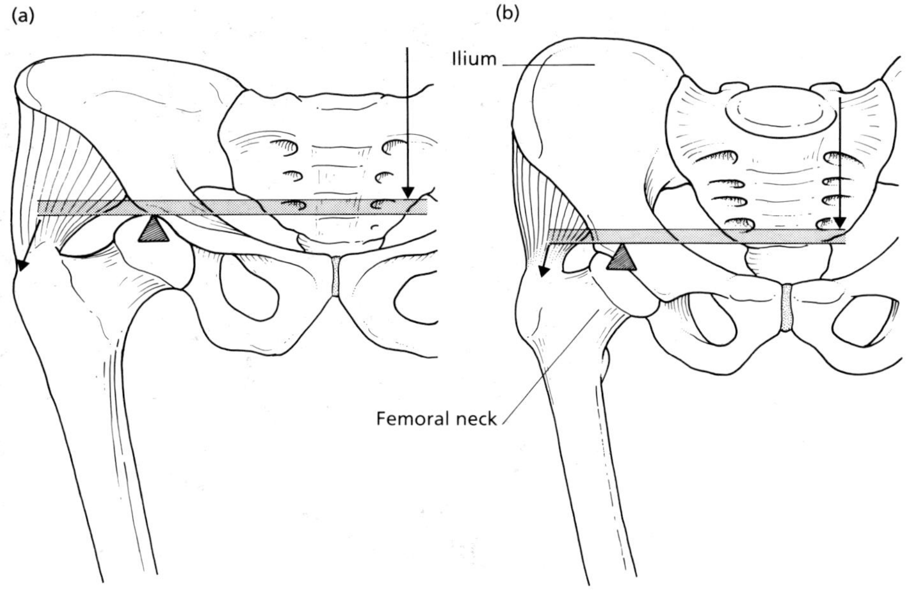

Fig. 19.33 Pelvis of 'Lucy' (a) compared with modern human female (b). In the modern pelvis there is less flare of the ilium and a shorter femoral neck; these changes place the abductors nearer to the hip joint and decrease their mechanical advantage to counterbalance the trunk when one leg is off the ground. Note the fulcrum at the head of the femur and the lengths of the two lever arms (lateral and medial) in each of 'Lucy' and the modern pelvis.

Pelvic shape and later bipedal gait (Fig. 19.33)

Again according to Lovejoy *et al.* (1973):

> In the face of increasing fetal cranial dimensions, adjustments which increased the pelvic ring but which did not increase total pelvic breadth would have been favored. . . . [I]f stature and total pelvic breadth remain unchanged relative to one another, and the dimensions of the parturition canal are to be increased, the only avenue of change is an increase in the medial lever arm length and commensurate reduction in the length of the lateral lever aim [Fig. 19.33]. Such changes would lead to substantially increased femoral head pressures and perhaps the only adaptation available in response to such an increase would be an enlargement of the femoral head. In addition, the resulting increase in the muscle force of the abductor mechanism would require a commensurate increase in the iliac pillar and general robusticity of the ilium.

The inferred *neuromuscular* consequences of the human adopting the upright posture are:

5 changes in trunk muscles for bipedal gait,

6 changes in the CNS associated with bipedal gait.

A neuromuscular cause of the rib cage and pelvic changes?

About three million years ago the adult human rib cage was funnel-shaped (Fig. 19.31). It is now barrel-shaped when viewed from the front. Likewise, the pelvis in the last three million years has dramatically shortened and turned in just the way one might expect if the mechanical requirement were to provide better muscular attachment for erect walking (Johanson & Edey, 1981). These pelvic changes have the effect of both shortening the torso and bringing the centre of pelvic mass much closer to the hip joints (Lovejoy, 1988). The mechanisms for these changes may have involved the trunk musculature acting under the influence of the CNS. Such evolution would select the more efficient individuals.

A CNS role in changing skeletal shape during evolution and development?

We suggest that alterations in the evolving (and developing) CNS provide one mechanism for adapting the femora, pelvis, spine and rib cage to the functional demands placed upon them by bipedalism and, in females, the rounder pelvis; but first, we must examine the evolution of human brain size.

The evolution of human brain size (encephalization)

One of the curious features of the later stages of human evolution was the astonishing rapidity with which the brain became enlarged relative to body size. According to Leakey (1981):

> As the fossils from Africa illustrate, the hominids of about three million years ago had brains that were very ape-like in size. . . . Not until two million years ago is there firm evidence of increasing brain power with the emergence of *Homo habilis*, whose cranial capacity was close to 800 cubic centimetres. . . . With the evolution of *Homo erectus* about one-and-a-half million years ago, there was a further boost to brain power, the cranial capacity increasing over a period of a million years to more than 1000 cubic centimetres. The modern human capacity of 1360 cubic centimetres, on average, was reached within the last 100,000 years.

How could this increasing head size have evolved?

Encephalization and female pelvic morphology (Fig. 19.32)

In *Australopithecus afarensis* ('Lucy', Fig. 19.30), females had much slimmer hips, and therefore narrower birth canals, than modern women and must have given birth to young with relatively far smaller heads and brains than those of modern newborn human babies. In *Homo habilis* the hip bones permit both bipedal walking and giving birth to babies with large heads (Lambert, 1987).

> Encephalization appears to have been fairly rapid during the Pleistocene (2.5 to 3 million years ago), the adult brain apparently tripling in volume. During this period of encephalization, there would have been strong selection upon the female to maintain adequate pelvic dimensions if the size of the fetal cranium were also increasing, and this appears to have been the case. . . . Thus, in the evolution of the hominid hip during the Pleistocene, what appear to have been more significant than changes in gait pattern are selective factors associated with rapid and substantial encephalization (Lovejoy, 1973).

The large brain may have become the survival tool of the species, but it has compromised the earlier asset of bipedal gait; for the hips now work close to the limits of pelvic structural and functional capability (see above). By comparison with the foetal development of other mammals the human infant is born 6 months early, so that the relatively large head may pass through the birth canal.

Now, contemporary growth data show that the human head grows most rapidly in the first 2 years of postnatal life. The postponement of three-quarters of brain growth in humans to postnatal periods should be viewed in terms of obstetric limitations. That is, to pass through the pelvic canal a human neonate must be born at a more immature stage. The most severe constraint is the exceptionally short sagittal diameter of the pelvic inlet. Moreover, the increased encephalization in humans is almost exclusively the result of increased postnatal brain growth. In particular, the remodelling of the human pelvis should be more appropriately viewed as reflecting selection against too low a neonate brain growth advancement and hence too high a degree of immaturity (Leutenegger, 1982).

It seems likely then that the increase in human head size over the last three million years was made possible by the natural selection of females with a rounder pelvis to provide for a larger foetal head at birth (Fig. 19.32). This larger pelvis of females is likely to have secondarily affected the rib-cage development of females differently from that of males; this is because of the need, in gait, to reduce rotational inertia transmitted to the thorax from the larger female pelvis (Fig. 19.8; see Grivas *et al.*, 1991a,c)—a mechanism which explains some of the differences in the rib cage between boys and girls (Figs 19.23–19.25).

Obstetric pelvis in modern humans and apes

Humans, as well as non-human primates that produce infants with a large head relative to the dimensions of the maternal birth canal, are characterized by pelves that are sexually dimorphic (Aiello & Dean, 1990).

The susceptibility of adolescent girls to progressive idiopathic scoliosis

We consider girls to be more susceptible than boys to progressive AIS for several reasons.

1 Larger pelvis and greater torque transmitted to the trunk in gait (Grivas *et al.*, 1991).
2 More slender vertebrae (Schultz *et al.*, 1984).
3 Flatter kyphosis in early adolescence (Archer & Dickson, 1985).
4 Greater joint laxity (Burwell *et al.*, 1981; Binns, 1988).
5 Adolescent growth spurt earlier in neuromuscular development than in boys.

6 Narrower chest width/height ratio (Grivas *et al.*, 1991).
7 Greater drooping of RVAs (Grivas *et al.*, 1992b).
8 Greater RVA symmetry (Grivas *et al.*, 1992b).
9 The physiological balance of muscles attached to ribs which change RVAs during growth may differ in girls and boys (Grivas *et al.*, 1992b).
10 The development of spinal cord CPGs made differ in girls and boys (sexual dimorphism, Burwell 1992a,b,c).

The susceptibility of tall adolescent girls to progressive idiopathic scoliosis

Stature

Several papers have reported cross-sectional data of stature in children with IIS and AIS. The findings are generally consistent and show that, after correcting for loss of height due to lateral spinal curvature, stature at diagnosis is significantly greater in scoliotic patients than in controls (see Nicolopoulos *et al.*, 1985a,b).

Components of stature

Nicolopoulos *et al.* (1985b) examined stature and its components in 143 girls with AIS. Using three components of stature (suprapelvic, pelvic and subischial heights), it was shown that the relatively greater stature of girls with AIS is due to changes in the pelvis and lower limbs but not significantly in the spine. Suprapelvic height is reduced relative to subischial height; this probably represents the growth pattern of predominantly ectomorphic individuals, reflecting the physique of many of these girls. Pelvic height is disproportionately increased, and this is considered to be a true rather than an apparent difference.

Why are tall girls susceptible to progressive AIS?

In the light of the theory of aetiology already outlined, the 'tallness' of an adolescent girl makes her susceptible to progressive AIS during puberty because her rib cage is developmentally unable to control the mechanical forces generated elsewhere in her relatively large growing skeleton during physical activity (Fig. 19.10c). In particular, mention may be made of:

1 Asymmetry of RVAs (local neuromuscular cause, Fig. 19.10a, Wemyss-Holden *et al.*, 1992b).
2 Advanced skeletal development (systemic cause) producing:
(a) Increased stride length from growing legs especially in children who are tall for their age and which is associated with more pelvic rotation.
(b) A wide pelvis increases pelvic torque during gait.
(c) A tall pelvis also increases pelvic torque during gait (Nicolopoulos *et al.*, 1985b).

It is generally considered that physical activity is a contributory factor to scoliosis in some patients. It could act by increasing the frequency and magnitude of pelvic rotations in gait and particularly in fast-walking and running.

Present position and future work

Manning, at the First Zorab Scoliosis Symposium (1965), said:

> Spinal fusion for scoliosis is, I think, as illogical as joint fusion for the elective treatment of joint tuberculosis. Our aim must be to discover the cause and try to apply the appropriate counter-measures so that the patient may retain movement when the deformity has been corrected.

Present position

Idiopathic scoliosis can no longer be regarded as a spinal abnormality in an otherwise normal child. Present knowledge is consistent with the view that the common patterns of spinal pathomechanics in IS result from a wide interaction between neuromuscular activity, the growing skeletal framework of the body (vertebrae, discs, ligaments, ribs, pelvis and lower limbs), gravity and muscle tether.

Research needed

Our theory of aetiology for IS focuses attention on the rib cage and in particular the need for segmental studies of the ribs pre- and postoperatively. We are currently undertaking such research in IIS and AIS.

A basic problem in urgent need of study is how much spinal growth contributes to the progression of scoliosis. The tallness of girls with progressive AIS suggests that growth aggravates a scoliosis by enlarging the child's body relative to the thorax; this could result in increasing disparity between the rotation-inducing (extrathoracic) and rotation-defending (largely intrathoracic) mechanisms of the mechanical component of the theory (Fig. 19.10c). If so, in such children, consideration would need to be given to how the rib-cage function in rotation-control could be strengthened.

Preventive treatment?

It is hoped that greater understanding of the mechanisms which cause IS might lead to that long-desired vantage point where we can base a treatment on some knowledge of causation of the deformity. Preventive treatments, matched to the deformity, may then be attained. The concept of CPG asymmetry suggests the need for a trial of physiotherapy in an attempt to hasten, where possible, symmetrical function of neuromuscular mechanisms involved in gait, and before irreversible changes have occurred in the skeletal and soft tissues of the trunk.

As Harrington said: 'The human spine will develop its inherent form if dynamic balance can be established.'

REFERENCES

Adams, W. (1865) *Lectures on the Pathology and Treatment of Lateral and Other Forms of Curvature of the Spine.* John Churchill & Sons, London.

Agadir, M., Burwell, R.G., Grivas, T.B., Moulton, A., Webb, J.K. & Wemyss-Holden, S.A. (1992) A segmental radiological study of resolving idiopathic scoliosis with aetiological implications. In *Proceedings of the Combined Meeting of the British Scoliosis Society and the Nordic Scoliosis Society*, Newcastle Upon Tyne, 5–6 June 1991.

Ahl, T., Albertsson-Wikland, K. & Kalen, R. (1988) Twenty-four-hour growth hormone profiles in pubertal girls with idiopathic scoliosis. *Spine*, **13**, 139–142.

Aiello, L. & Dean, C. (1990) *An Introduction to Human Evolutionary Anatomy*. Academic Press, London.

Aitken, McCrae D. (1928) Curvature of the spine. In *The Robert Jones Birthday Volume: a collection of surgical essays*, pp. 243–267. Oxford University Press, London.

Archer, I.A. & Dickson, R.A. (1985) Stature and idiopathic scoliosis. A prospective study. *J. Bone Jt. Surg.*, **67B**, 185–188.

Arkin, M. (1949) The mechanism of the structural changes in scoliosis. *J. Bone Jt. Surg.*, **31A**, 519–528.

Austin, J. (1992) Evaluation of segmental thoracic shape, other skeletal factors and certain radiological variables in the prognosis of adolescent idiopathic scoliosis. Thesis, University of Nottingham.

Barnes, J. (1979) Rib resection in infantile idiopathic scoliosis. *J. Bone Jt. Surg.*, **61B**, 31–35.

Binns, M. (1988) Joint laxity in idiopathic adolescent scoliosis. *J. Bone Jt. Surg.*, **70B**, 420–422.

Bisgard, J. (1934) Thoracogenic scoliosis: influence of thoracic disease and thoracic operations on the spine. *Arch. Surg.*, **29**, 417–445.

Bonne, A.J. (1969) On the shape of the human vertebral column. *Acta Orthop. Belg.*, **35**, 567–583.

Brooks, V.B. (1986) Locomotion. In *The Neural Basis of Motor Control*, pp. 181–194. Oxford University Press, New York.

Brunk, M. (1951) The importance of rickets in childhood as a cause of scoliosis in adult age. *Acta Orthop. Scand.* (Suppl.), **9**, 1–114.

Bullough & Boachie-Adjei (1988) In *Atlas of Spinal Diseases*, p. 39. J.B. Lippincott, Philadelphia, PA.

Bunnell, W.P. (1988) The natural history of idiopathic scoliosis. *Clin. Orthop.*, **229**, 20–25.

Burwell, R.G. (1971) The relationship between scoliosis and growth. In Zorab, P.A. (ed.) *Scoliosis and Growth*, pp. 131–150. Proceedings of a Third Symposium. Churchill Livingstone, Edinburgh.

Burwell, R.G. (1990) The 1989 report on school screening for scoliosis: the relation to aetiology. *J. Bone Jt. Surg.*, **72B**, 333–334.

Burwell, R.G., Dangerfield, P.H. & Vernon, C.L. (1981) Bone asymmetry and joint laxity in the upper limbs of children with adolescent idiopathic scoliosis. *Ann. R. Coll. Surg. Engl.*, **63**, 209–210.

Burwell, R.G., James, N.J., Johnson, F., Webb, J.K. & Wilson, Y.G. (1983) Standardised trunk asymmetry scores—a study of back contour in healthy children. *J. Bone Jt. Surg.*, **65B**, 452–462.

Burwell, R.G., Upadhyay, S.S., Wojcik, A.S., Bacon, N.C.M., Moulton, A. & Webb, J.K. (1990) Ultrasound in evaluating scoliosis. In Siegler, D., Harrison, D. & Edgar, M. (eds) *Proceedings of the Eighth Phillip Zorab Scoliosis Symposium*, 26–28 October 1988, London, pp. 48–67. Phillip Zorab Scoliosis Research Fund, London.

Burwell, R.G., Cole, A.A., Grivas, T.B., Kiel, A.W., Moulton, A., Upadhyay, S.S., Webb, J.K., Wojcik, A.S. & Wythers, D.J. (1992a) Screening, aetiology and the Nottingham theory for idiopathic scoliosis. In Alberti, A., Drerup, B. & Hierholzer, E. (ed.) *Sixth International Symposium on Surface Topography and Spinal Deformity*, pp. 136–161. Gustav Fischer, Stuttgart.

Burwell, R.G., Cole, A.A., Cook, T.A., Grivas, T.B., Kiel, A.W., Moulton, A., Thirlwall, A.S., Uphadyay, S.S., Webb, J.K., Wemyss-Holden, S.A., Whitwell, D.J., Wojcik, A.S. & Wythers, D.J. (1992b) Pathogenesis of idiopathic scoliosis: the Nottingham Concept. *Symposium on Idiopathic Scoliosis. Acta Orthop. Belg.* (In press).

Burwell, R.G., Hubbard, M., Wojcik, A.S., Moulton, A., Webb, J.K. (1991a) Some observations on sagittal spinal curvatures and their movements: a relation between lumbar facet length and the anterior longitudinal ligament? *Clin. Anat.*, **3**, 67.

Burwell, R.G., Firth, J.L., Jaspan, T., Thirlwall, A.S., Webb, J.K., Baker, G.C.W. & Wemyss-Holden, S.A. (1991b)

Syringomyelia, scoliosis and the Nottingham theory of aetiology for idiopathic scoliosis. *Clin. Anat.*, **4**, 386.

Burwell, R.G., Cole, A.A., Cook, T.A., Grivas, T.B., Kiel, A.W., Moulton, A., Thirlwall, A.S., Upadhyay, S.S., Webb, J.K., Wemyss-Holden, S.A., Whitwell, D.J., Wojcik, A.S. & Wythers, D.J. (1992) Pathogenesis of idiopathic scoliosis: the Nottingham concept. In *Proceedings of the Combined Meeting of the British Scoliosis Society and the Nordic Scoliosis Society*, 5–6 June 1991. Newcastle Upon Tyne.

Butler, P.B. & Major, R.E. (1992) The learning of motor control: biomechanical considerations. *Physiotherapy*, **78**, 6–11.

Byrd III, J.A. (1988) Current theories on the etiology of idiopathic scoliosis. *Clin. Orthop.*, **229**, 114–119.

Cole, A.A., Burwell, R.G., Jacobs, K.J., Kiel, A.W., Moulton, A., Webb, J.K., Wojcik, A.S., Short, A.H. & Bassey, E.J. (1990a). Hip rotation, knee rotation and femoral anteversion in healthy subjects and children with adolescent idiopathic scoliosis: relation of hip rotation to lateral spinal curves. *Clin. Anat.*, **3**, 65.

Cole, A.A., Barson, R., Burwell, R.G., Jacobs, K.J., Moulton, A., Wallace, W.A., Webb, J.K. & Wojcik, A.S. (1990b) The use of CODA to measure pelvic movements in normal gait: the concept of coupled pelvi-spinal rotation. *Clin. Anat.*, **3**, 65.

Conroy, G.C. (1990) *Primate Evolution*. W.W. Norton, New York.

Cook, T.A., Burwell, R.G., Wemyss-Holden, S.A. & Webb, J.K. (1991) A segmental study of iliocostalis: functional and clinical implications. *Clin. Anat.*, **4**, 387.

Cruickshank, J.L., Koike, M. & Dickson, R.A. (1989) Curve patterns in idiopathic scoliosis. A clinical and radiographic study. *J. Bone Jt. Surg.*, **71B**, 259–263.

Dangerfield, P.H., Burwell, R.G. & Vernon, C.L. (1980) Anthropometry and scoliosis. In Roaf, R. (ed.) *Spinal Deformities*, 2nd edn, pp. 259–280. Pitman Medical, London.

Davis, P.R. (1955) The thoracolumbar mortice joint. *J. Anat. (Lond.)*, **89**, 370–377.

Deacon, P. & Dickson, R.A. (1987) Vertebral shape in the median sagittal plane in idiopathic thoracic scoliosis. A study of true lateral radiographs in 150 patients. *Orthopaedics*, **10**, 893–895.

Deacon, P., Flood, B.M. & Dickson, R.A. (1984) Idiopathic scoliosis in three dimensions: a radiographic and morphometric analysis. *J. Bone Jt. Surg.*, **66B**, 509–512.

Deane, G. & Duthie, R.B. (1973) A new projectional look at articulated scoliotic spines. *Acta Orthop. Scand.*, **44**, 351–365.

Dickson, R.A. (1983) Scoliosis in the community. *Br. Med. J.*, **286**, 615–618.

Dickson, R.A., Lawton, J.O., Archer, I.A. & Butt, W.P. (1984) The pathogenesis of idiopathic scoliosis: biplanar spinal asymmetry. *J. Bone Jt. Surg.*, **66B**, 8–15.

Dobosiewicz, K. (1986) Unloading reflex in the etiology of scoliosis. *Scoliosis: the Last 20 years Experience*, p. 14. Proceedings of the European Spinal Deformities Society First Congress, 16–19 April 1986, Rome.

Dubousset, J., Herring, J.A. & Shufflebarger, H. (1989) The crankshaft phenomenon. *J. Pediatr. Orthop.*, **9**, 541–550.

Duval-Beaupère, G. (1971) Pathogenic relationship between scoliosis and growth. In Zorab, P.A. (ed.) *Scoliosis and Growth*, pp. 58–64. Proceedings of a Third Symposium. Churchill Livingstone, Edinburgh.

Edelmann, P. (1981) Beckengeradstand oder Sakrumgeradstand? *Z. Orthop.*, **119**, 111–114.

Farkas, A. (1941) Physiological scoliosis. *J. Bone Jt. Surg.*, **23**, 607–627.

Feiss, H.O. (1907) Mechanics of lateral curvature. *Am. J. Orthop. Surg.*, **4**, 323–339.

Fidler, M.W. & Jowett, R.L. (1976) Muscle imbalance in the aetiology of scoliosis. *J. Bone Jt. Surg.*, **58B**, 200–201.

Goldberg, C. & Dowling, F.E. (1990) Handedness and scoliosis convexity: a reappraisal. *Spine*, **15**, 61–64.

Gracovetsky, S. (1988) *The Spinal Engine*. Springer-Verlag, New York.

Graf, H. & Dubousset, J. (1980) Tridimensional study of scoliotic spines. Application to infantile scoliosis. In *Proceedings of the 15th Annual Meeting of the Scoliosis Research Society*, p. 46. 17–19 September, Chicago, IL, 1980.

Gregersen, G.G. & Lucas, D.B. (1967) An *in vivo* study of the axial rotation of the human thoracolumbar spine. *J. Bone Jt. Surg.*, **49A**, 247–262.

Grillner, S. (1981) Control of locomotion in bipeds, tetrapods and fish. In Brooks, V.B. (ed.) *Handbook of Physiology*, Section 1, *The Nervous System*, vol. II, *Motor Control*, pp. 1179–1236. American Physiological Society, Bethesda, MD.

Grivas, T.B., Burwell, R.G., Purdue, M., Webb, J.K. & Moulton, A. (1992a) The rib cage deformity in infantile idiopathic scoliosis—the funnel-shaped upper chest in relation to specific rotation as a prognostic factor. An evaluation of thoracic shape in progressive scoliosis and control children during growth. In Alberti, A., Drerup, B. & Hierholzer, E. (ed.) *Sixth International Symposium on Surface Topography and Spinal Deformity*, pp. 93–109. Gustav Fischer, Stuttgart.

Grivas, T.B., Burwell, R.G., Purdue, M., Webb, J.K. & Moulton, A. (1992b) The segmental patterns of rib–vertebra angles in chest radiographs of children. Changes related to rib level, age, sex, side and significance for scoliosis. *Clin. Anat.* (In press).

Grivas, T.B., Burwell, R.G., Purdue, M., Webb, J.K. & Moulton, A. (1991) A segmental analysis of thoracic shape in chest radiographs of children. Changes related to spinal level, age, sex, side and significance for lung growth and scoliosis. *J. Anat. (Lond.)*, **178**, 21–38.

Grubb, S.A., Lipscomb, H.J. & Conrad, R.W. (1988) Degenerative adult onset scoliosis. *Spine*, **13**, 241–245.

Haderspeck, K. & Schultz, A. (1981) Progression of idiopathic scoliosis. *Spine*, **6**, 447–455.

Hägglund, G., Karlberg, J. & Willner, S. (1990) Personal communication from Dr. S. Willner.

Hefti, F.L. & McMaster, M.J. (1983) The effect of the adolescent growth spurt on early posterior spinal fusion in infantile and juvenile idiopathic scoliosis. *J. Bone Jt. Surg.*, **65B**, 247–254.

Herman, R., Mixon, J., Fisher, A., Maulucci, R. & Stuyck, J. (1985) Idiopathic scoliosis and the central nervous system:

a motor control problem. The Harrington Lecture, 1983. Scoliosis Research Society. *Spine*, **10**, 1–14.

Heuer, F. (1927) Ätiologie und Mechanik der Skoliose. *Z. Orthop. Chirur.*, **48**, 157–160.

Ingelmark, B.E. & Lindström, J. (1963) Asymmetries of the lower extremities of pelvis and their relation to lumbar scoliosis. *Acta Morphol. Scand.*, **5**, 221–234.

Isu, T., Iwasaki, Y., Akino, M. & Abe, H. (1990) Hydrosyringomyelia associated with a Chiari I malformation in children and adolescents. *Neurosurgery*, **26**, 591–597.

Janda, V. (1983) On the concept of postural muscles and posture in man. *Austral. J. Physiother.*, **29**, 83–84.

Johanson, D.C. & Edey, M.A. (1981) *Lucy: the Beginnings of Humankind.* Penguin Books, London.

Jones, F.A. (1992) *Ribcage deformity in resolving infantile idiopathic scoliosis—does thoracic shape contribute to expression and resolution of spinal deformity?* Thesis, University of Nottingham.

Joseph, J. & McColl, I. (1961) Electromyography of muscles of posture: posterior vertebral muscles in males. *J. Physiol.*, **157**, 33–37.

Kiel, A.W., Burwell, R.G., Moulton, A., Purdue, M., Webb, J.K. & Wojcik, A.S. (1992) The segmental patterns of sagittal spinal curvatures in children screened for scoliosis. The kyphotic angulation at the thoracolumbar region and the mortice joint. *Clin. Anat.* (In press).

Klein-Vogelbach, S. (1990) Fundamental observation criteria. *Functional Kinetics*, pp. 74–81. Springer-Verlag, Berlin.

Lambert, D. (1987) *The Cambridge Guide to Prehistoric Man.* Cambridge University Press, Cambridge.

Leakey, R.E. (1981) *The Making of Mankind.* Michael Joseph, London.

Lefevre, J., Beunen, G., Steens, G., Claessens, A. & Renson, R. (1990) Motor performance during adolescence and age thirty as related to age at peak height velocity. *Ann. Hum. Biol.*, **17**, 423–435.

Leutenegger, W. (1982) Encephalization and obstetrics in primates with particular reference to human evolution. In Armstrong, E. & Falk, D. (eds) *Primate Brain Evolution: Methods and Concepts*, pp. 85–95. Plenum Press, New York.

Lončar-Dušek, M., Pećina, M. & Prebeg, Ž. (1991) A longitudinal study of growth velocity and development of secondary gender characteristics versus onset of idiopathic scoliosis. *Clin. Orthop.*, **270**, 278–282.

Lonstein, J.E. & Carlson, J.M. (1984) The prediction of curve progression in untreated idiopathic scoliosis during growth. *J. Bone Jt. Surg.*, **66A**, 1061–1071.

Lovejoy, C.O. (1973) The gait of Australopithecines. *Year Book Phys. Anthropol.*, **17**, 147–161.

Lovejoy, C.O. (1988) Evolution of human walking. *Sci. Am.*, **259**, 82–89.

Lovejoy, C.O., Heiple, K.G. & Burstein, A.H. (1973) The gait of *Australopithecus. Am. J. Phys. Anthropol.*, **38**, 757–780.

Lovett, R.W. (1905) The mechanism of the normal spine and its relation to scoliosis. *Boston Med. Surg. J.*, **153**, 349–358.

Loynes, R.D. (1972) Scoliosis after thoracoplasty. *J. Bone Jt. Surg.*, **54B**, 484–498.

Mehta, M. (1972) The rib–vertebra angle in the early diagnosis between resolving and progressive infantile scoliosis. *J. Bone Jt. Surg.*, **54B**, 230–243.

Meyer, H. (1886) Die Mechanik der Skoliose. *Virchows Arch. Path. Anat.*, **35**, 225 and **36**, 144.

Morais, T., Bernier, M. & Turcotte, T. (1985) Age- and sex-specific prevalence of scoliosis and the value of school screening programs. *Am. J. Publ. Health*, **75**, 1377–1380.

Nicolopoulos, K.S., Burwell, R.G. & Webb, J.K. (1985a) Stature and its components in healthy children, sexual dimorphism and age related changes. *J. Anat. (Lond.)*, **141**, 105–114.

Nicolopoulos, K.S., Burwell, R.G. & Webb, J.K. (1985b) Stature and its components in adolescent idiopathic scoliosis. Cephalo-caudal disproportion in the trunk of girls. *J. Bone Jt. Surg.*, **67B**, 594–601.

Nudelman, W. & Reis, N.D. (1990) Anatomy of the extrinsic spinal muscles related to the deformities of scoliosis. *Acta Anat.*, **139**, 220–225.

Osmond, D.G. (1985) Functional anatomy of the chest wall. In Roussos, C. & Macklem, P.T. (eds) *The Thorax*, Part A, pp. 199–233. Marcel Dekker, New York.

Pal, G.P. (1991) Mechanism of production of scoliosis: a hypothesis. *Spine*, **16**, 288–292.

Parry, E. (1966) The influence of rotation of the trunk on the anatomy of the inguinal canal. *Br. J. Surg.*, **53**, 205–210.

Perdriolle, R. & Vidal, J. (1985) Thoracic idiopathic scoliosis curve evolution and prognosis. *Spine*, **10**, 785–791.

Perdriolle, R.J., Vidal, J., Bechetti, S. & Alquier, P. (1989) Torsion: the essential factor for progression in idiopathic scoliosis. In *Combined Meeting of Scoliosis Research Society and European Spinal Deformities Society*, pp. 526–527. Amsterdam, 17–22 September 1989.

Piggott, H. (1971) Posterior rib resection in scoliosis. *J. Bone Jt. Surg.*, **53B**, 663–671.

Prochiantz, A. (1986) Anteversions et scolioses dites essentielles. *Ann. Pediatr. (Paris)*, **33**, 779–787.

Ransford, A.O. (1988) Diaphragmatic balance: a cause of progression in idiopathic scoliosis? *J. Bone Jt. Surg.*, **69B**, 852.

Richards, B.S., Birch, J.G., Herring, J.A., Johnson, C.E. & Roach, J.W. (1989) Frontal plane and sagittal plane balance following Cotrel–Dubousset instrumentation for idiopathic scoliosis. *Spine*, **14**, 733–737.

Roaf, R. (1958) Rotation movements of the spine with special reference to scoliosis. *J. Bone Jt. Surg.*, **40B**, 312–332.

Roaf, R. (1960) Vertebral growth and its mechanical control. *J. Bone Jt. Surg.*, **42B**, 40–59.

Roaf, R. (1966) The basic anatomy of scoliosis. *J. Bone Jt. Surg.*, **48B**, 786–792.

Roaf, R. (1968) Scoliosis. In Zorab, P.A. (ed.) *Proceedings of a Second Symposium on Scoliosis: causation*, pp. 27–30. E.&S. Livingstone, Edinburgh.

Roaf, R. (1974) The postural function of intercostal muscle. In Zorab, P.A. (ed.) *Scoliosis and Muscle*, pp. 46–51. SIMP

Research Monograph No. 4. Heinemann Medical, London.

Roaf, R. (1976) The role of the multifidus muscles and its practical significance. *J. Bone Jt. Surg.*, **58B**, 374.

Robin, G.C. (1990) *The Aetiology of Idiopathic Scoliosis.* CRC Press, Boca Raton, FL.

Robitaille, Y., Villavicencio-Pereda, C. & Gurr, J. (1984) Adolescent idiopathic scoliosis: epidemiology and treatment outcome in a large cohort of children six years after screening. *Int. J. Epidemiol.*, **13**, 319–323.

Rogala, E.J., Drummond, D.S. & Gurr, J. (1978) Scoliosis: incidence and natural history. A prospective epidemiological study. *J. Bone Jt. Surg.*, **60A**, 173–176.

Rogers, S.P. (1933) Mechanics of scoliosis. *Arch. Surg.*, **26**, 962–980.

Schede, Fr. (1928) Der Skoliosenkeim. *Z. Orthop. Chirurg.*, **49**, 74–91.

Schmitt, O. (1981) *Artificial Organs*, **5** (Suppl.), 589–593.

Schmitt, O. (1986) Treatment of idiopathic scoliosis with daily short-term electrostimulation. In Nix, W.A. & Vrbová, G. (eds) *Electrical Stimulation and Neuromuscular Disorders*, pp. 132–143. Springer-Verlag, Heidelberg.

Schultz, A.B. (1984) In Oxnard, C.E. (ed.) *The Order of Man.* Yale University Press, Yale.

Schultz, A.B., Sörensen, S.E. & Anderson, G.B.J. (1984) Measurements of spine morphology in children, ages 10–16. *Spine*, **9**, 70–73.

Sevastik, J.A., Agadir, M. & Sevastik, B. (1990) Effects of the rib elongation on the spine. II. Correction of scoliosis in the rabbit. *Spine*, **15**, 826–829.

Somerville, E.W. (1952) Rotational lordosis: the development of the single curve. *J. Bone Jt. Surg.*, **34B**, 421–427.

Steindler, A. (1955) *Kinesiology of the Human Body under Normal and Pathological Conditions.* C.C. Thomas, Springfield, IL.

Stokes, I.A.F. (1989) Axial rotation component of thoracic scoliosis. *J. Orthop. Res.*, **7**, 702–708.

Stokes, I.A.F. & Laible, J.P. (1990) Three-dimensional osseoligamentous model of the thorax representing initiation of scoliosis by asymmetric growth. *J. Biomech.*, **23**, 589–595.

Stokes, I.A.F., Dansereau, J. & Moreland, M.S. (1989) Rib cage asymmetry in idiopathic scoliosis. In *Proceedings of Combined Meeting of Scoliosis Research Society and European Spinal Deformities Society*, 17–22 September 1989, Amsterdam.

Stromeyer, G.F.L. (1836) Quoted by Keith (1919) *Menders of the Maimed.* Hodder & Stoughton, London.

Sutherland, D.H., Olshen, R., Cooper, L. & Woo, S. (1980) The development of mature gait. *J. Bone Jt. Surg.*, **62**, 336–353.

Taylor, J.R. (1983) Scoliosis and growth: patterns of asymmetry in normal vertebral growth. *Acta Orthop. Scand.*, **54**, 596–602.

Thirlwall, A.S. (1991) *The relation of King curve type to the surface and radiological deformity of preoperative scoliosis.* Thesis, University of Nottingham.

Thurston, A.J. & Harris, J.D. (1983) Normal kinematics of the lumbar spine and pelvis. *Spine*, **8**, 199–205.

Tylkowski, C.M. (1990) Assessment of gait in children and adolescents. In Morrissy, R.T. (ed.) *Lovell and Winter's Pediatric Orthopaedics*, 3rd edn, vol. I, pp. 57–90. J.B. Lippincott, Philadelphia, PA.

Upadhyay, S.S., Burwell, R.G., Moulton, A., Small, P. & Wallace, W.A. (1990) Femoral anteversion in healthy children. Application of a new method using ultrasound. *J. Anat. (Lond.)*, **169**, 49–61.

Valentin, B. (1991) *Geschichte der Orthopädie*, pp. 61–63. Georg Thieme, Stuttgart.

Veldhuizen, A.G. & Scholten, P.J.M. (1987) Kinematics of the scoliotic spine as related to the normal spine. *Spine*, **12**, 852–858.

Walker, A.P. & Dickson, R.A. (1984) School screening and pelvic tilt scoliosis. *Lancet*, 21 July, 152–154.

Wall, J.C., Nottrodt, J.W., Charteris, J. (1981) The effects of uphill and downhill walking on pelvic oscillations in the transverse plane. *Ergonomics*, **24**, 807–816.

Warren, M.P., Brooks-Gunn, J., Hamilton, L.H., Warren, L.F. & Hamilton, W.G. (1986) Scoliosis and fractures in young ballet dancers: relation to delayed menarche and secondary amenorrhea. *N. Engl. J. Med.*, **314**, 1348–1353.

Waters, R.L. & Morris, J.M. (1972) Electrical activity of muscles of the trunk during walking. *J. Anat. (Lond.)*, **111**, 191–199.

Wemyss-Holden, S.A., Butcher, C.A., Burwell, R.G., Webb, J.K. & Moulton, A. (1991a) Segmental evaluation of the rotational (torsional) deformity in scoliosis: clinico-anatomical observations and surgical significance. In *Proceedings of British Association of Clinical Anatomists*, 20 December 1990, London.

Wemyss-Holden, S.A., Burwell, R.G., Cook, T.A., Binch, C., Webb, J.K. & Moulton, A. (1991b) A spiral 'composite muscle trunk rotator' in man? Relevance to gait, idiopathic and sportsman's scolioses and stroke. *Clin. Anat.*, **4**, 386.

Wemyss-Holden, S.A., Burwell, R.G., Jacobs, K.J., Polak, F.J., McNeill, S.A., Webb, J.K. & Moulton, A. (1992a) Predicting the deformation of the rib-cage around the fused spine after Cotrel–Dubousset instrumentation (CD) for adolescent idiopathic scoliosis (AIS). In *Proceedings of the Combined Meeting of the British Scoliosis Society and the Nordic Scoliosis Society*, Newcastle Upon Tyne, 5–6 June 1991.

Wemyss-Holden, S.A., Jacobs, K.J., Burwell, R.G., McNeill, S.A., Polak, F.J., Webb, J.K. & Moulton, A. (1992b) The rib cage in adolescent idiopathic scoliosis (AIS): a segmental analysis of rib-vertebra angles (RVAs) revealing crossed RVA asymmetry with aetiological implications. In *Proceedings of a Joint Meeting of the British Association of Clinical Anatomists and the American Association of Clinical Anatomists*, 8–11 July 1991, Norwich.

White III, A.A. (1969) Analysis of the mechanics of the thoracic spine in man: an experimental study of autopsy specimens. *Acta Orthop. Scand.* (Suppl.), **127**.

White III, A.A. (1971) Kinematics of the normal spine as related to scoliosis. *J. Biomech.*, **4**, 405.

White III, A.A. & Panjabi, M.M. (1990) *Clinical Biomechanics of the Spine*, 2nd edn. J.B. Lippincott, Philadelphia, PA.

Whitecloud, T.S., Cook, S.D., Morgan, E.L., Harding, A.F., Nicholson, R.J. & Thomas, K.A. (1987) An evaluation of trabecular bone mineral density in idiopathic scoliosis. *J. Pediatr. Orthop.*, **7**, 348.

Wojcik, A.S., Webb, J.K. & Burwell, R.G. (1990) Harrington–Luque and Cotrel–Dubousset instrumentation for idiopathic thoracic scoliosis. A postoperative comparison using segmental radiologic analysis. *Spine*, **15**, 424–431.

Wojcik, A.S., Webb, J.K. & Burwell, R.G. (1992) The relation between vertebral rotation and tilt in thoracic idiopathic scoliosis. The concept of rotational load in the spine during gait. In Alberti, A., Drerup, B. & Hierholzer, E. (ed.) *Sixth International Symposium on Surface Topography and Spinal Deformity*, pp. 57–63. Gustav Fischer, Stuttgart.

Wood, K.B., Transfeldt, E.E., Ogilvie, J.W., Bradford, D.S. & Schendel, M.J. (1990) Rotational changes of the vertebral-pelvic axis following Cotrel–Dubousset instrumentation. In *Proceedings of Scoliosis Research Society, 25th Annual Meeting*, 23–27 September 1990, Hilton Hawaiian Village Hotel, Honolulu, Hawaii.

Wythers, D.J., Burwell, R.G., Webb, J.K. & Wojcik, A.S. (1991) The segmental surface and rib deformity of progressive adolescent idiopathic scoliosis: a preoperative segmental appraisal suggesting aetiological factors in the lumbar spine. In Alberti, A., Drerup, B. & Hierholzer, E. (ed.) *Sixth International Symposium on Surface Topography and Spinal Deformity*, pp. 119–135. Gustav Fischer, Stuttgart.

20 · Conservative Management of Spinal Deformities

By M.A. EDGAR

The conservative management of scoliosis and other spinal deformities represents a spectrum starting with the early detection of deformity, with or without the aid of official school screening programmes, through the observation of children who regularly attend spinal deformity clinics and which demands an understanding of the natural history of the condition leading finally to the options for non-surgical treatment in order to reverse or slow down progression. The interface between conservative management and subsequent surgery is also an area that needs consideration.

Early detection and prognosis

The two essential pillars on which conservative management of all spinal deformities rests are (a) the ability to detect early, and (b) a knowledge of the natural history of the various curve patterns. Unfortunately these pillars are far from perfect. Severe spinal deformity still presents at scoliosis clinics having been missed or ignored simply because the clinician at the time was unaware that spinal deformities can deteriorate quite rapidly during childhood or adolescence. On the other hand, the natural histories for many early curves cannot be predicted with accuracy; therefore close observation during childhood and growth is required. Nevertheless with certain types of scoliosis, for example infantile idiopathic curves (see below) and congenital deformities (see also Chapter 13), the predictive factors which denote a good or bad prognosis are known with more reliability.

For early detection to be effective the minimal requirement is that medical, nursing and paramedical personnel involved in assessing or examining children for one reason or another should be made fully aware of the threat of spinal deformity and how it can be diagnosed. The ultimate requirement in early detection is comprehensive screening, the cost-effectiveness of which has been the subject of considerable debate during the past decade as will be discussed further below (Burwell, 1983b; Montgomery, 1989).

The most common presenting scoliosis, namely the adolescent idiopathic type, is usually a mild curve but in 1–5% of cases progression can be rapid, leading to a deformity that will cause considerable morbidity in adult life (Fig. 20.1). Therefore there is no place for blind reassurance by clinicians, as has happened in the past, without the fullest clinical and radiological assessment by an expert in the field. Perhaps one of the distortions that have arisen from those who have looked into the natural history of idiopathic scoliosis, and have reviewed large numbers of minor curves, is that they can lose sight of the occasional deformity that rapidly progresses to cause late problems. In this respect Dickson (1984, 1985), for all his contribution to a better understanding of pathogenesis, tends to regard late-onset idiopathic scoliosis as a self-limiting condition which, even in the face of progression, is of little consequence for morbidity in adult life. This view is not shared by those who have followed idiopathic scoliosis long-term in adult life (Kostuik *et al.*, 1973; Edgar & Mehta, 1988).

Awareness of the factors which denote a potentially severe deformity is therefore all-important, and these factors for the different aetiological types are summarized below.

Infantile idiopathic scoliosis (early-onset)

Idiopathic thoracic curves developing in infancy are usually left-sided, with a slight male preponderance.

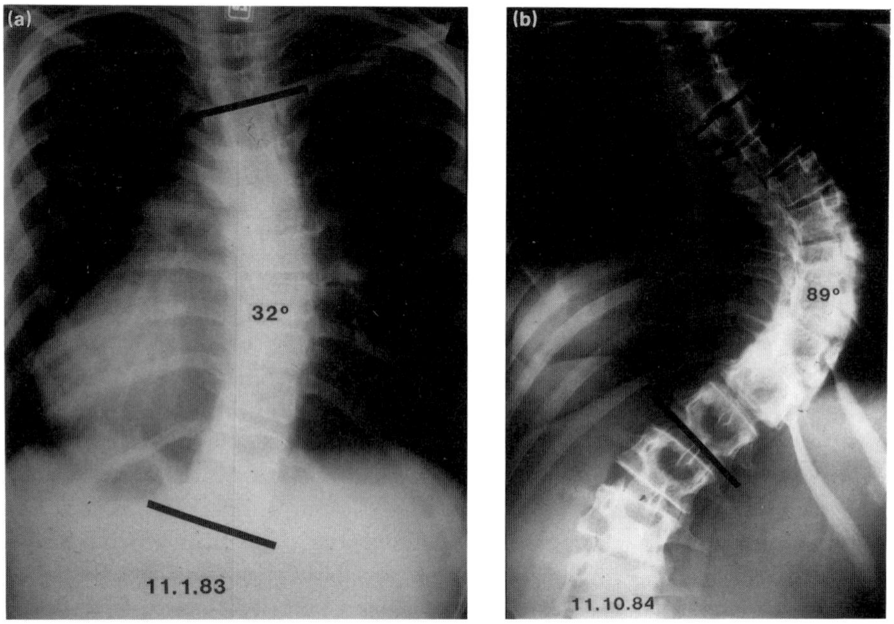

Fig. 20.1 Erect AP X-rays of the spine of a girl aged 12½ with rapidly progressive adolescent idiopathic scoliosis. (a) On first attending in January 1983. (b) She failed to keep her clinic appointments and was next seen in October 1984 with a gross deformity.

Ninety per cent resolve spontaneously (Lloyd Roberts & Pilcher, 1965). However the 10% that progress can result in very severe deformities. It is in this infantile and juvenile phase that an increasing deformity of the chest can lead to long-standing respiratory impairment and premature death. Therefore early detection of the progressive infantile curve is all-important. Mehta (1972) made a brilliant observation in noting that when there is more than a 20° difference between the angles which the apical rib on each side makes with the longitudinal axis of the apical vertebrae then this deformity is likely to progress. This is known as the rib vertebral angle difference, or RVAD (Fig. 20.2). She further identified the malignantly progressive infantile curve which tends to occur in those children of small stature, low body weight, delicate facial features and often a marked plagiocephaly (Mehta, 1977). Double infantile idiopathic curves usually progress, and those with a drooping twelfth rib giving a large RVAD value at T12 also have a bad prognosis. The uncommon infantile thoracolumbar curve also tends to progress rather than resolve.

Adolescent idiopathic scoliosis (late-onset)

Here the pattern of progression in relation to skeletal maturity and curve types is better understood (Lonstein & Carlson, 1984). This is largely because adolescent or late-onset curves are ubiquitous compared with the diminishing number of infantile deformities in western developed countries. Nevertheless, it is still difficult to predict with accuracy the behaviour of individual adolescent idiopathic curves. In addition there is no real equivalent of Mehta's RVAD sign as a criterion on which to judge the curve. As a rule of thumb thoracic or double curves over 30° in premenarcheal females have a 70% chance of significant progression (Lonstein & Carlson, 1984; Bunnell, 1986). A proportion of these curves will progress very rapidly (Fig. 20.1). It has also been our experience that curves which are lordotic and have over 20° of vertebral rotation in the premenarcheal female are set to progress rapidly.

Neuromuscular scoliosis

Here the incidence of progression is a little better defined, but the same criteria apply as in adolescent idiopathic curves (Swank, 1989a). These deformities tend to be long curves and—particularly where there is deficient muscular control, as in poliomyelitis, muscular dystrophy or cerebral palsy—the deformities can collapse and become decompensated with a considerable list that makes balance and mobilization difficult. A higher proportion of curves progress than in idiopathic deformities, and of those that do progress a much higher proportion will progress

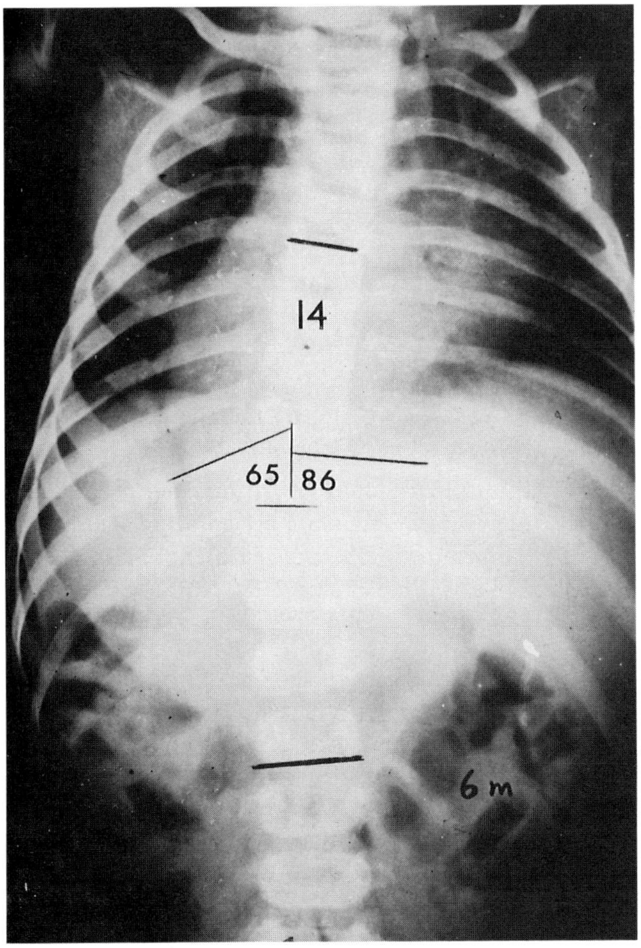

Fig. 20.2 Erect AP X-ray of the spine in a six-month-old, demonstrating a potentially progressive infantile thoracic scoliosis with the rib vertebral angle difference, or Mehta angle, demonstrated. Courtesy of Miss Min Mehta.

rapidly in the adolescent phase. Therefore early detection and intervention is important, even though conservative measures are limited in their effectiveness compared with the idiopathic group (see Chapter 25).

Congenital scoliosis

Factors here are set out in detail in Chapter 13 and further considered in the classic papers by McMaster & Ohtsuka, 1982 and McMaster & David, 1986. Suffice it to say that progression is closely related to the type of osteogenic abnormality and its level in the spine. The worst scenario is seen with an unsegmented unilateral bar with contralateral hemivertebrae over the same levels. A unilateral unsegmented bar with seemingly normal vertebrae on the contralateral side is also likely to progress significantly as, to a lesser extent, are multiple unbalanced hemivertebrae. Single hemivertebrae, if of the incarcerated or semisegmented type, progress minimally, but a fully segmented hemivertebra can cause a severe curvature particularly in the thoracolumbar region. A posteriorly placed hemivertebra producing a kyphos can also progress alarmingly, and through the sharp angulation can become associated with neurological symptoms. This therefore should also be stabilized early. Balance is another important factor with the lumbosacral hemivertebra, which causes pelvic obliquity below and inevitably a compensatory lumbar curve above, which in time can become structural.

It is relevant at this stage to note that active conservative treatment plays no real part in the management of congenital scoliosis except where the compensatory curve threatens (Morley, 1989). Nevertheless, the importance of early detection in congenital scoliosis relates to the ability to stabilize the curve early by fusing the growth plates on the convex side of the curve, thereby halting the asymmetrical growth.

Neurofibromatosis

Prognostic factors relevant to dystrophic curves have been well set out by Calvert and his colleagues (1989). The non-dystrophic curves, which are in the minority, behave very much like adolescent idiopathic deformities. The dystrophic curves are characterized by a short angular scoliosis with scalloping of the vertebral bodies on the AP X-ray so that they are capstan-shaped (Fig. 20.3). In addition there may be pencilling of the ribs, presumably due to pressure erosion from neurofibromata of the intercostal nerves. Lateral X-rays are characterized by an apparent or true kyphosis, and it is the kyphotic component which can progress rapidly during adolescence, leading to neurological complications. Those patients in whom there are several dystrophic changes in the apical vertebrae, and in particular where anterior scalloping is marked, tend to have a poor prognosis. Here early detection relates to the need for early fusion to stabilize the curve anteriorly and posteriorly, rather than to any form of conservative treatment. The appearance of a double-pronged apical

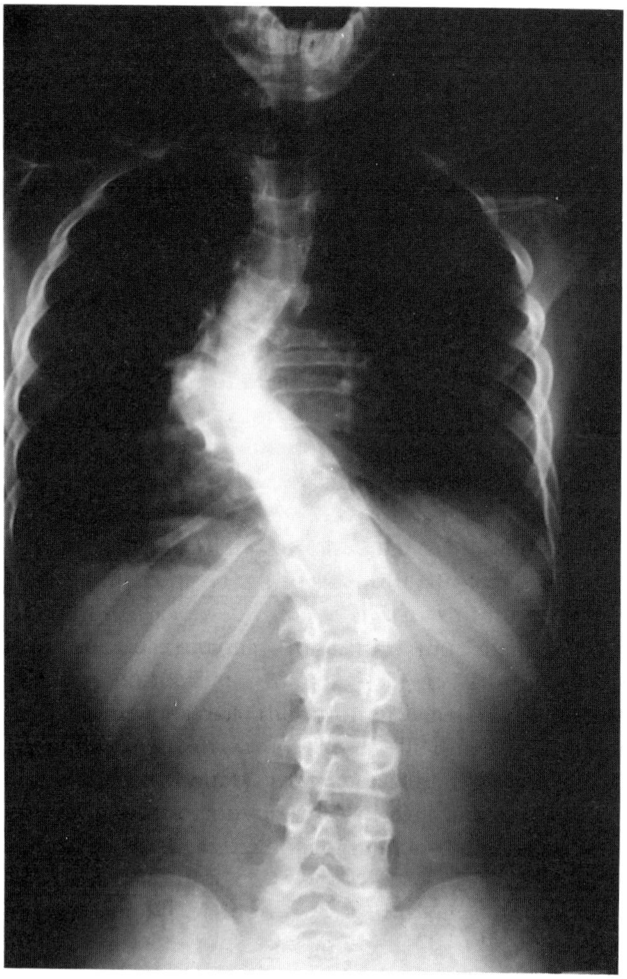

Fig. 20.3 Erect AP X-ray demonstrating typical appearance of a marked dystrophic curve in a girl with neurofibromatosis.

vertebra on the lateral X-ray due to severe anterior scalloping is a particularly bad prognostic sign.

Awareness and school screening

Over the past two decades there has been a growing awareness in the medical and allied professions of the need to diagnose progressive scoliosis and other spinal deformities as early as possible. This is demonstrated in the UK by the overall earlier presentation of children at scoliosis clinics, although there are still worrying exceptions to this. The difference in the presentation pattern of adolescent idiopathic scoliosis to the Scoliosis Unit at the Royal National Orthopaedic Hospital between 1976 and 1985 is shown in Table 20.1. The mean presenting Cobb angle reduced during the period 1976–1985 from 49° to 33°. Although general practitioners referred only a slightly greater proportion of cases by 1985, yet these were significantly smaller deformities. During this period even physical education teachers had become aware of the condition. However, the greatest change was noted in the school medical examinations, the proportion of referrals from which increased threefold (Belstead & Edgar, 1978; Ferris *et al.*, 1988). The increased contribution that school medical examination has made to the diagnostic pattern is also seen in other countries. For example in a study by Torell *et al.* (1981) it was shown that from 1968 to 1978 the proportion of school screening cases which presented in Sweden increased from 45% to 70%. Unlike Britain, school screening became an official Swedish government policy during that period.

Therefore, should the UK institute compulsory school screening for scoliosis? Certainly in Canada, Denmark, Singapore, as well as in Sweden, it is now an authorized routine procedure. In Japan and certain

Table 20.1 A comparison of the pattern of case referral to a scoliosis clinic at the Royal National Orthopaedic Hospital in 1976 and 1985. After Ferris *et al.* (1988)

Diagnosis source	Relative percentage		Mean Cobb angle		Percentage under 40° on presentation	
	1976	1985	1976	1985	1976	1985
Coincidentally by general practitioner	10	14	56	40	12	50
School medical	10	32	49	33	25	72
Family/friends	80	49	56	44	15	37
Physical education teacher	—	5	—	53	—	0

states of the USA screening is mandatory. However, compulsory screening can be justified only if three conditions are fulfilled:

1 that the natural history is known,

2 that early treatment alters the natural history,

3 that the result of screening and early treatment is shown to be cost-effective.

In congenital dislocation of the hip, for instance, screening at birth and during the first year clearly alters the natural history for the vast majority of cases, and the budgetary saving clearly means that it is cost-effective. By contrast in adolescent idiopathic scoliosis, even though the broad trends of the natural history are known, the prediction for an individual case and the best time to screen the patient are not known for certain, and this results in a 'weather forecast' situation. As will be discussed below, there is no established study so far which demonstrates that early treatment can be guaranteed to alter the long-term natural history, even though there are trends which indicate some alteration. In accord with condition 3 above it is not possible, certainly in the UK at present, to justify the expense of screening, and hence this was the conclusion published by the School Screening Committee of the British Scoliosis Society in collaboration with the Council of the British Orthopaedic Association (Burwell *et al.*, 1983b).

However, this report did encourage centres, which at that time were involved in comprehensive screening programmes, to continue on a longitudinal study with the all-important object of further clarifying the natural history, particularly of idiopathic scoliosis. This is clearly one of the advantages of screening, but it need not involve a mandatory policy for the whole country. The report also expressed further reservations. Up to 25% of healthy children had been shown to have some degree of torso asymmetry and therefore screening examinations by school nurses, physiotherapists, doctors or indeed physical education staff, needed to be more specific and better diagnostic tools were required. From statistics there is no doubt that the smaller the curve the less chance it has of progression. This is particularly so for the minor lumbar curves associated with pelvic obliquity (Dickson, 1984). As a result of screening, large numbers of children with trivial or inconsequential curves of the spine had been referred to scoliosis clinics accompanied by parents anxious with the misplaced worry that their child was about to become a hunchback or, worse, paraplegic. The syndrome of a minor non-progressive spinal curvature in a child with overanxious parents referred by screening has been dubbed 'schooliosis'. Apart from the psychological upset, the report was also concerned about the unnecessary number of X-rays that might be carried out on these children with inconsequential curves. This has become all the more important following the recent publication of a report clearly indicating an increased incidence of breast cancer in women who, in their adolescence, attended a scoliosis clinic with routine multiple X-rays (Hoffman *et al.*, 1989).

The British Scoliosis Society report was careful to state in its conclusions that 'it should not be a national policy *at present* to screen children for scoliosis routinely throughout the United Kingdom'. Since 1983 more information has come to light, and in the event of a clearer understanding of the natural history combined with definite evidence that conservative or non-surgical treatment can alter natural history there should be a reconsideration of school screening and whether it will have become cost-effective. This is still not the case in the UK where, as an approximation, 15% of adolescents are usually picked out at the initial screening (Burwell, 1989). This figure is reduced to 2% representing the prevalence of children who on X-ray have a curve measuring 10° or more. Curves of 20° or over, which become eligible for conservative management, represent between 0.2% and 0.6%. Of these only 10–20% have potential for significant progression (Dickson *et al.*, 1980; Dickson 1983). With our current technique only about six children would be effectively helped for every 10 000 screened.

Some form of clinical tool is therefore required to improve the selection process of potentially progressive deformities. In Malmo, the moiré camera technique for a contoured image of the back (Fig. 20.4) is now being used routinely, and a recent study concludes that screening has become cost-effective as a result (Montgomery, 1989). Burwell and his colleagues in Nottingham studied different asymmetry scores of the trunk using a tracing of the transverse contour as different levels (Burwell *et al.*, 1983a). By subtracting the Bunnell inclinometer value at the chest and lumbosacral level (the latter measures leg length inequality), Burwell has been able to derive a formula which more accurately detects the potentially progressive curve (see Chapter 19). Finally the ISIS (Integrated Shape Imaging System) (Jefferson

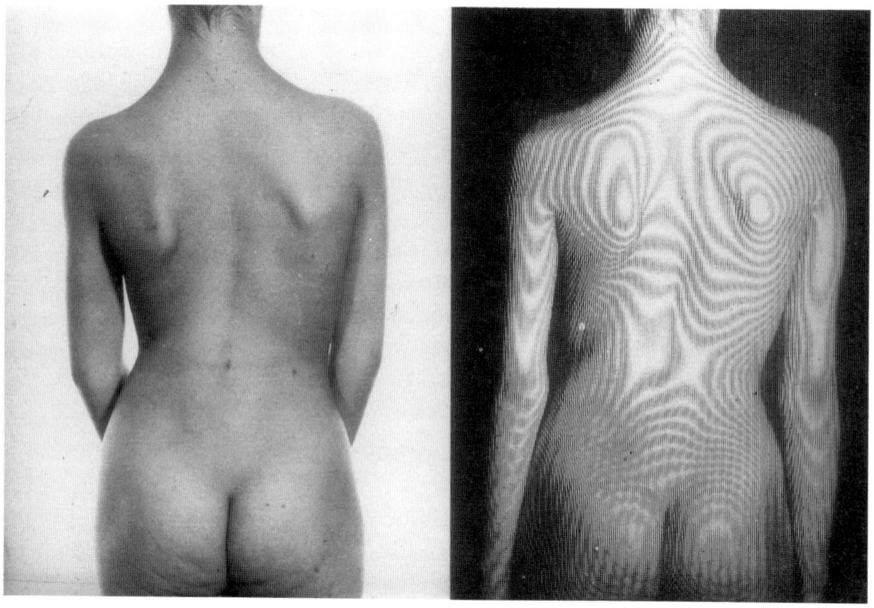

Fig. 20.4 The standard photograph of the back of a girl with adolescent idiopathic scoliosis compared with the moiré fringe photography. The latter demonstrates the asymmetry of contours in relation to the right rib prominence.

et al., 1988) also has potential use in screening evaluation. At present this machine, which is able to provide a more accurate contour map of back shape, is being used experimentally to evaluate progression of scoliosis and the value of certain surgical techniques, yet with more sophistication it could provide a scoring system for use in screening. It has a three-dimensional video camera linked up to a computer system, which is able to numerically record back shape and also print a contour plan of the back with a volumetric difference for each side of the trunk. It also provides an estimation of the Cobb angle (Fig. 20.5).

There is no doubt that, apart from severe congenital deformity, the scoliosis with the greatest potential for progression and morbidity in later life is the infantile idiopathic type. Although there is clear evidence that the incidence of this is reducing in the UK this is still the most important idiopathic curve to pick up early. Treatment can quite definitely alter the natural history (Mehta & Morel, 1980); therefore early childhood is the time when mandatory screening should be put alongside routine examination for other orthopaedic conditions such as club feet and congenital dislocation of the hip. Dickson (1984) also recommends that a child's back should be examined during the first immunization at three to six months, and then later at the routine school medical examination at five years. This all makes such sound sense that it is surprising that one has never seen an official DH document implementing it.

The last word on the effectiveness of school screening in the late-onset type of idiopathic scoliosis must go to Willner (1982) who has no doubts about the efficacy of screening. He reports that in Malmo following 12 years of comprehensive screening surgical intervention has dropped from eight to two cases per 10 000. This is not associated with a decrease in the prevalence of cases being picked up by screening which, using the moiré technique, is 158 per 10 000 children screened (1.58%). Furthermore, the number of children being braced has been increased from 24 to 36 per 10 000, despite stricter criteria for bracing. Finally, Willner does not feel that the natural history of adolescent idiopathic scoliosis is changing. Clearly the debate for screening will go on.

Observation of children in scoliosis clinics

A thorough assessment by a specialist orthopaedic surgeon is essential when a child is first referred to the scoliosis clinic in order to establish the aetiological type of the deformity, its size and radiological features. This is considered in detail in Chapter 19. At this stage it is also important to counsel the child and parents over the likely prognosis, including the possible variables, and to indicate the reasons for observing a child if active treatment is not going to be implemented.

The 'at-risk' factors affecting the curves of different aetiologies have been set out above, and these can be

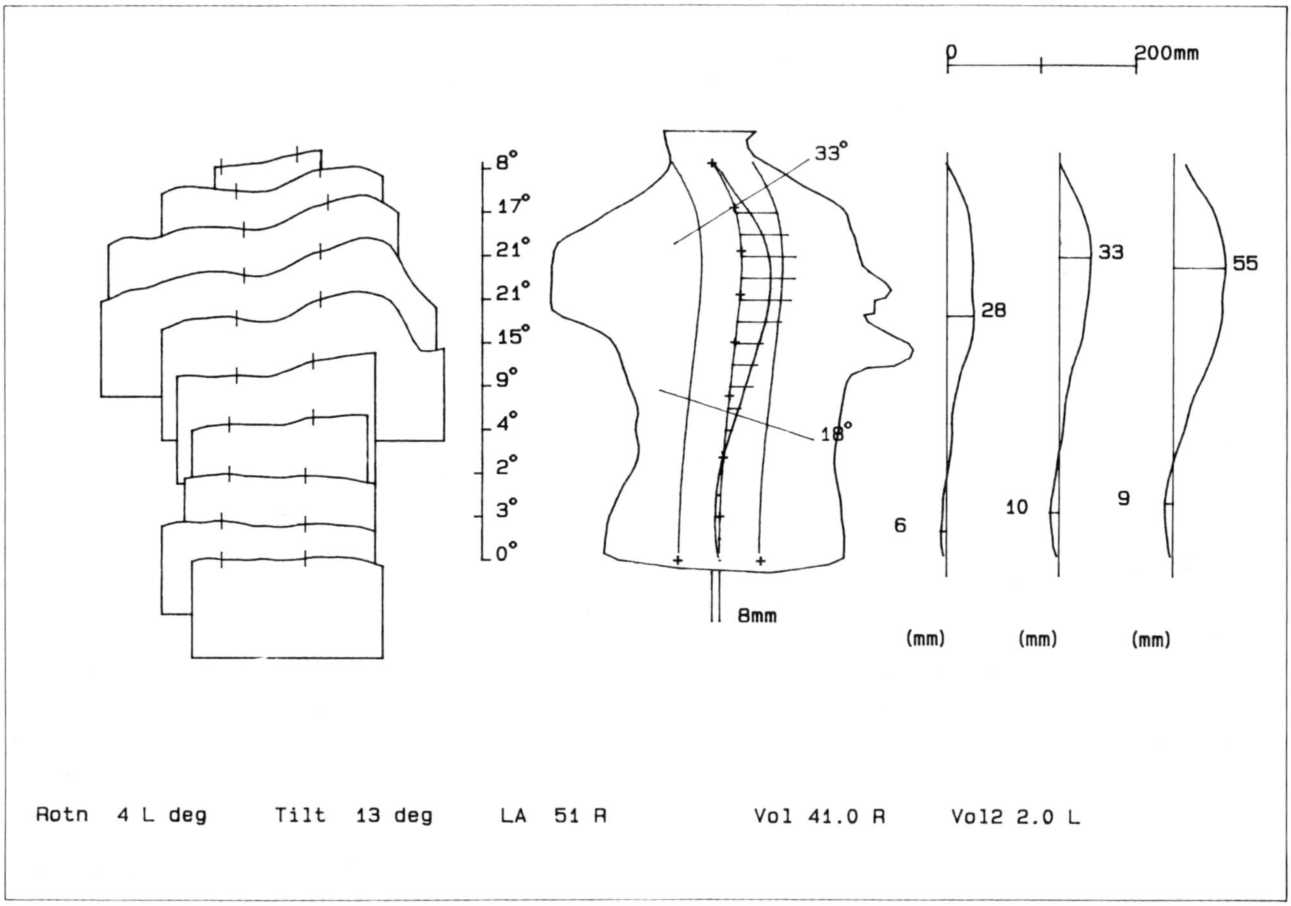

Fig. 20.5 ISIS surface topography printout. From left to right: map of the back contour demonstrated as transverse slices showing the right rib hump; scale according to those slices demonstrating the MSSA (maximal skin surface angle similar to but not identical with the Bunnell angle); lateral asymmetry angle (a computer estimate of the Cobb angle) and the amount of list; sagittal profiles taken to the left of the midline, at the midline and to the right of the midline, respectively. The thoracic difference between D and F is a measure of the size of the rib hump difference at those particular sagittal planes.

used to determine how often a child is followed in the scoliosis clinic. Children with mild curves, who are in the prepubertal stage, that is before 10 years in girls and 12 in boys, can generally be observed six-monthly unless there is evidence from the history that there has been recent noticeable progression. In these cases a four-monthly review is best. Certainly during the adolescent growth phase, if curves are being observed then they should be watched four-monthly in the first instance, and if there is no progression over a period of a year that observation can be extended to six-monthly. Once a girl is postmenarcheal observation can usually be extended to six-monthly reviews, and certainly this applies in all cases where the iliac apophyses are fully developed (Risser Grade IV).

What may be termed the Lonstein rule (Lonstein & Carlson, 1984) states that in postmenarcheal girls, who have idiopathic curves of less than 19°, there will be no significant progression in over 99%, and therefore beyond a final check after the interval of a year they can be discharged. In fact with mild or moderate curves (those less than 40°) patients may be discharged providing the iliac apophyses are fully formed and closing when the girls are over 18 and boys over 20. Previously it was felt that patients could be discharged at an earlier age, but we now know that growth of the vertebral endplates is the last to cease, and may well extend into the early 20s, particularly in boys. In some cases even of mild curvatures this has been associated with progression in adult life, particularly where there is 25° or more vertebral rotation present (Scott & Piggott, 1981).

Therefore young adults with curves of over 30°, and 25° rotation, are best watched yearly until they are 22, particularly if there is some evidence of late progression.

It needs to be emphasized that all curves at risk can deteriorate quite rapidly once the adolescent growth spurt commences. The short sharp dysplastic curve of neurofibromatosis, once it starts to develop a kyphotic element, can deteriorate quite dramatically and, as stated before, these cases must be operated on early. Finally mention must be made of the painful scoliosis, which needs careful investigation particularly if there is night pain or if a short spell of physiotherapy has failed. These are not curves to watch four-monthly. They are discussed further at the end of the chapter.

Options for conservative treatment

Brace management has been the mainstay of non-operative treatment in scoliosis over the last four decades, although indications for this have now become much more selective and rather controversial. Nevertheless, it still has a place in the management of idiopathic scoliosis. It demands a discipline from the adolescent child and the brace requires careful maintenance by the orthotist.

Electrospinal stimulation using surface or deep electrodes to stimulate muscles on the convexity of the curve, either in the paraspinal area or in the mid-axillary line, was originally developed in Toronto by Bobechko (1973), and in Los Angeles by Axelgaard & Brown (1983). It was hoped that mild mobile curves would be controlled by electrospinal stimulation at night only, thereby removing the need for a cumbersome brace with its possible psychological effects. However, the method has been subject to complications, particularly from skin allergy to the skin electrode conduction paste. Although initial success rates of over 80% were reported (Brown *et al.*, 1986), two years later longer-term results showed that it was successful in less than 30% of patients, whose improvement was largely borderline with regard to predicted progression (O'Donnell *et al.*, 1988; Goldberg *et al.*, 1988). Swank (1989b) concludes that with present results the technique is hardly justified, as it only marginally alters the natural history. Similarly a large follow-up study of over 300 patients from Toronto, by Missiuna & Wedge (1989), shows that the pattern of progression in the treated curves again coincided with the expected natural history. Although Bobechko in Toronto maintains enthusiasm for the technique (Herbert & Bobechko, 1989), it has lost much of its credibility as a technique, and is little used at present in the UK. It will not be considered further.

Although it has been established that physiotherapy *per se* does not alter the natural history of major structural scoliosis, nevertheless in mild mobile potentially progressive lumbar and thoracolumbar scoliosis, trunk exercises to correct the scoliosis have met with a certain degree of success and represent a simple and cheap alternative to brace therapy. The technique is still experimental, but the author believes it has a place. It could be particularly valuable for the treatment of children in climates too warm to consider daytime brace-wearing.

Finally, correction of mobile deformities in young children, by moulded plaster of Paris jackets applied with the child on a special frame, has been shown not only to alter the natural history quite significantly, but to reverse a progressive deformity. Serial plaster casts applied in this way are now the mainstay of conservative management to control early-onset idiopathic scoliosis (Dickson, 1985).

Therefore serial plaster jackets, brace therapy and corrective trunk exercises will be considered more fully below.

Serial corrective plaster body jackets in the management of early-onset idiopathic scoliosis

Mehta & Morel (1980), who have the most experience with this technique, have emphasized that this is most useful in the benign progressive thoracic, thoracolumbar and double infantile idiopathic scoliosis. They emphasized that the benign progressive curve, with an RVAD of over 20°, is not intrinsically different from the spontaneously resolving scoliosis which has an RVAD of less than 20°, except that the former suffers from an inability to correct itself spontaneously with growth. By moulding the spine in a plaster jacket which involves elongation, derotation and flexion (EDF technique) the deformity is improved. The technique is undoubtedly encouraging, and benign progressive curves can be made to straighten completely. If these children are straight prior to the onset of the adolescent growth spurt there is every chance that the scoliosis will not reappear. The malignant progressive infantile curve may be

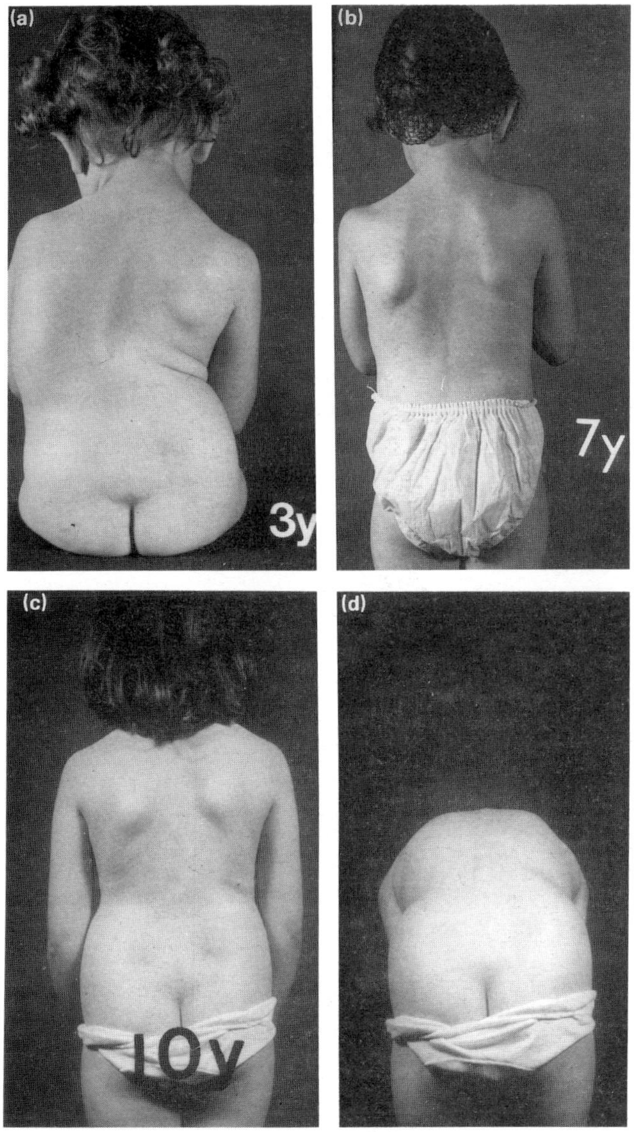

Fig. 20.6 Serial photographs of the spine of a girl with progressive infantile idiopathic scoliosis who was treated with serial localizer casts on a Cotrel plaster frame over a period of six years. The photographs, taken between the ages of 3 and 10, demonstrate the correction achieved.

slowed in its progression by serial plaster casts, but will not usually have its natural history sufficiently altered to prevent surgery at a later date.

Figures 20.6 & 20.7 are photographs of a 65° curvature which was completely straightened through serial corrective casts prior to the adolescent growth spurt. In the Mehta & Morel series, plaster correction was started at a mean age of 3.1 years, ranging from 1.1 to 9 years. There is no doubt that the technique should be started without delay after diagnosis in the young child, and certainly before the RVAD has been allowed to become large. My own technique (following that of Mehta) is to apply the plaster body jacket using the Cotrel table in the small child as described below, and then to repeat the plaster jackets every two months during the autumn, winter and spring periods. For two or three months in the summer the child can be left free in the hot weather, and for holidays. In children over the age of five or six, how-

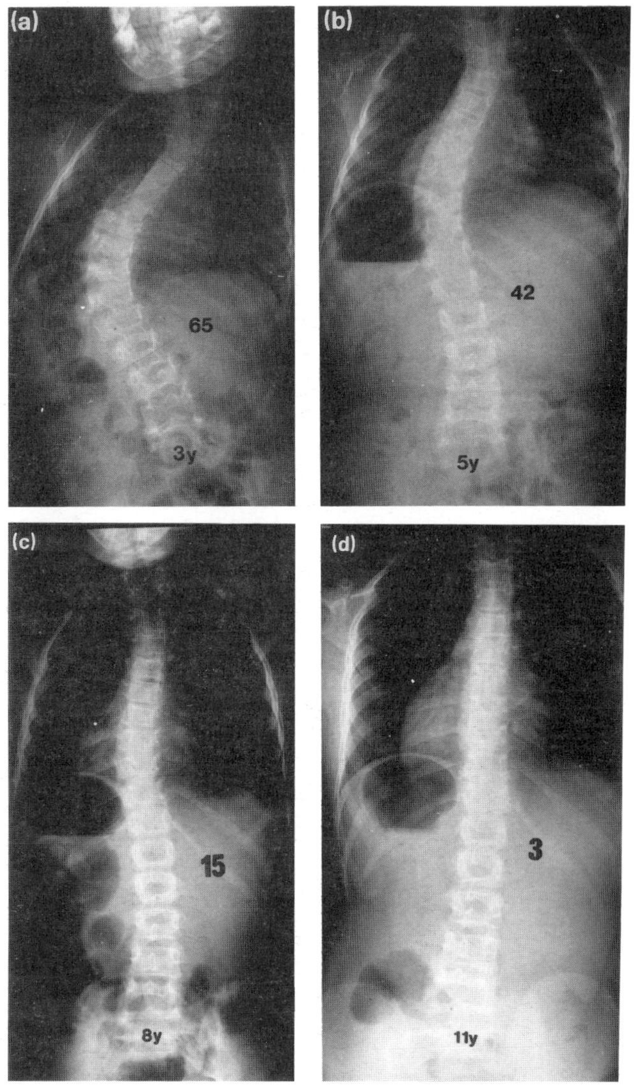

Fig. 20.7 Serial X-rays of the same girl as in Fig. 20.6, demonstrating the improvement in the Cobb angle from 65° to 3° over a similar time scale. She has since passed through her adolescent growth phase without any recurrence of the deformity.

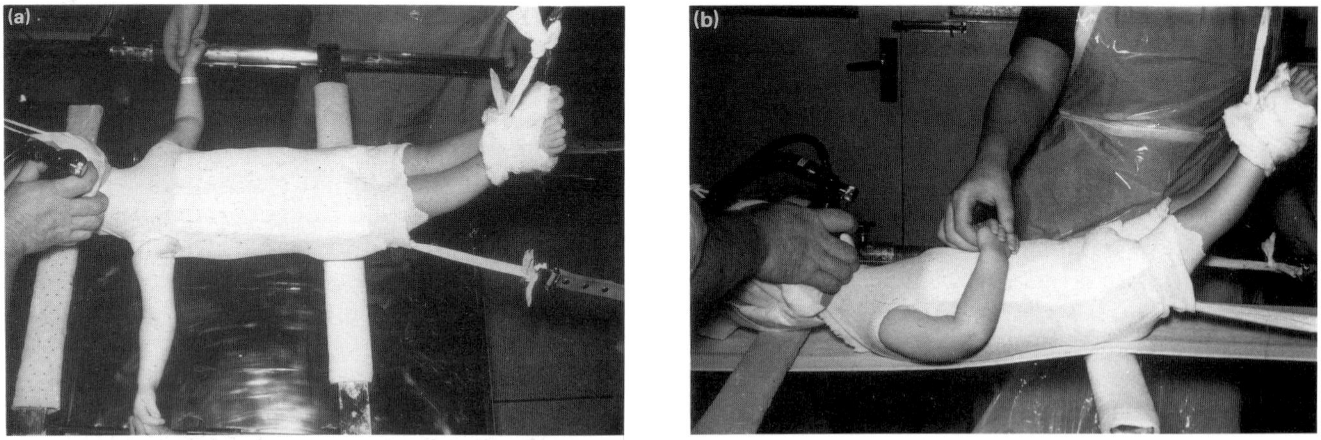

Fig. 20.8 Two views of a child on the Cotrel paediatric spinal plaster frame with neck halter and pelvic traction. The feet are suspended to hold the spine in a slight kyphotic or flexed position as part of the EDF (elongation, derotation, flexion plaster of Cotrel). Courtesy of Miss Min Mehta.

ever, it is best that they do have a TLSO brace fitted during the summer period, which can be taken off for four hours a day to allow for recreation, swimming, etc.

Figure 20.8 shows the Cotrel frame, which is an essential part of applying a corrective plaster cast. For the young child a general anaesthetic is usually required, but in older children sedation is usually sufficient. The child is on the Cotrel frame supported with two transverse straps underneath the pelvis and upper shoulders with woollen flannel traction bandages applied around the pelvis and tied to the crossbars at the lower end of the frame. The neck is supported in a halter with counter-traction again to the crossbar, such that the child hangs banana-wise in flexion. Cross bandages can be placed around the convexity of the curve to correct this and to reduce the rotation, but this is best done with manual moulding of the plaster jacket.

The terminology at the Royal National Orthopaedic Hospital (Fig. 20.9) is that plaster casts that come up to the base of the neck are Type II, and those which have the shoulder straps only are Type III (Fig. 20.10). For thoracic curves and double curves a Type II jacket is advisable, but for the thoracolumbar curve a Type III jacket is sufficient.

A stockinette vest is put on, and felt padding is placed over the rib prominence and bony points of the pelvis, with one layer of orthoband bandages to hold these pads in place and to add to the comfort of the cast. Too much padding can be a hindrance to correction, and can produce a loose uncomfortable jacket a day or two later. Once two or three layers of plaster bandages have been applied, the surgeon

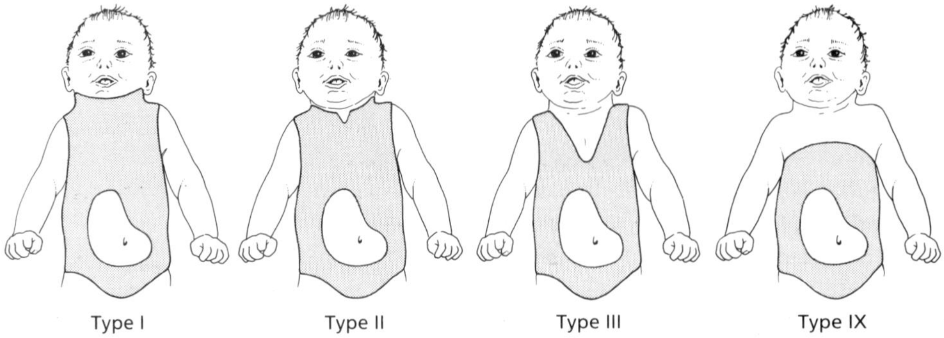

Fig. 20.9 Royal National Orthopaedic Hospital classification of spinal plaster casts according to the extent which they reach upwards over the shoulders and neck. Type I is rarely used these days because of the pressure effect on the developing mandible.

carefully moulds the plaster jacket with both hands, correcting the lateral flexion and also applying one hand under the rib prominence with a counter-derotation effect with the other hand over the contralateral ribs anteriorly. It is important that erect spinal X-rays are to hand so that the level and direction of the moulding can be planned. After the plaster has been further reinforced, and here it is quite useful to put on a surface layer of synthetic plaster bandages such as Scotchcast to keep the jacket light, the cross-straps of the frame are repositioned and the patient transferred after removal of the traction to a trolley for the cutting of an abdominal window and an eccentric posterior window over the concavity of the major curve. The child is then mobilized. It is important that the pressure areas, particularly over the iliac crests, are checked prior to discharge to make sure that there are no impending pressure sores.

Children tolerate this routine surprisingly well from the age of two to 10. Serial plaster cast management is not effective for adolescent curves, and in a sense this is unfortunate as the compliance would clearly be much greater than bracing.

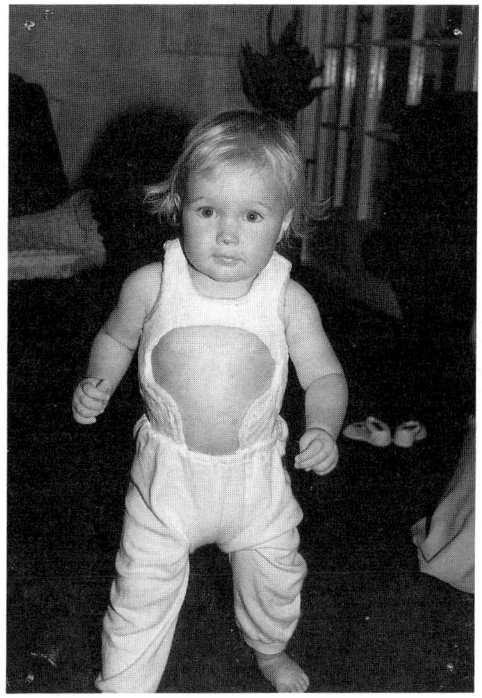

Fig. 20.10 Child with an early-onset idiopathic scoliosis demonstrating a Type corrective plaster body jacket applied with the EDF routine on a Cotrel frame.

TLSO (thoracolumbar sacral orthosis) bracing for adolescent idiopathic scoliosis

Various systems of spinal bracing have been the mainstay of non-operative treatment of scoliosis in the postwar era. The Milwaukee brace, with its neck ring, was developed by Blount in the 1940s in order to hold scoliosis during the preoperative and postoperative phase of spinal fusion in a corrected position, and was applied in adolescents, particularly those with the paralytic type of deformity (Blount *et al.*, 1958). The original action of the brace was essentially one of distraction by means of chin and occipital pads acting against the pelvic support, with some secondary lateral pressure on the rib hump or lumbar prominence (Galante *et al.*, 1970). The chin pads were found to wreak havoc with the development of the child's jaw and teeth, and became an orthodontist's nightmare. Therefore in the 1960s the chin pad was changed to a throat mould, and less emphasis was given to distraction. In fact the neck ring and pelvic support became counter-forces to the pressure pad over the convexity of the scoliosis in a three-point lateral pressure system. Apart from its use as a postoperative support, the modified Milwaukee brace became the standard treatment of mild progressive idiopathic scoliosis in the 1960s. With experience it became evident that it was more effective in controlling deformities under 40° than those over (Carr *et al.*, 1980). This led to great emphasis being placed on the position of the lateral pad, as clearly with mild curves the lateral corrective system is more effective in contrast to the original distraction Milwaukee brace being used for curves of 90° or more.

The unsightly and psychologically upsetting Milwaukee neck ring (Fig. 20.11) was discarded in favour of a 'topless brace' or TLSO (thoracolumbar sacral orthosis) for use in early curves with the three-pressure-pad arrangement built into the structure. A popular modular form of the topless brace became known as the Boston brace system (Fig. 20.12) although equal effectiveness was claimed by those who used custom-built orthoses, such as Wilmington brace (Bassett *et al.*, 1986).

The indications for effective brace treatment were gradually formulated (Nash, 1980) and although dramatic correction was seen in the reports on the

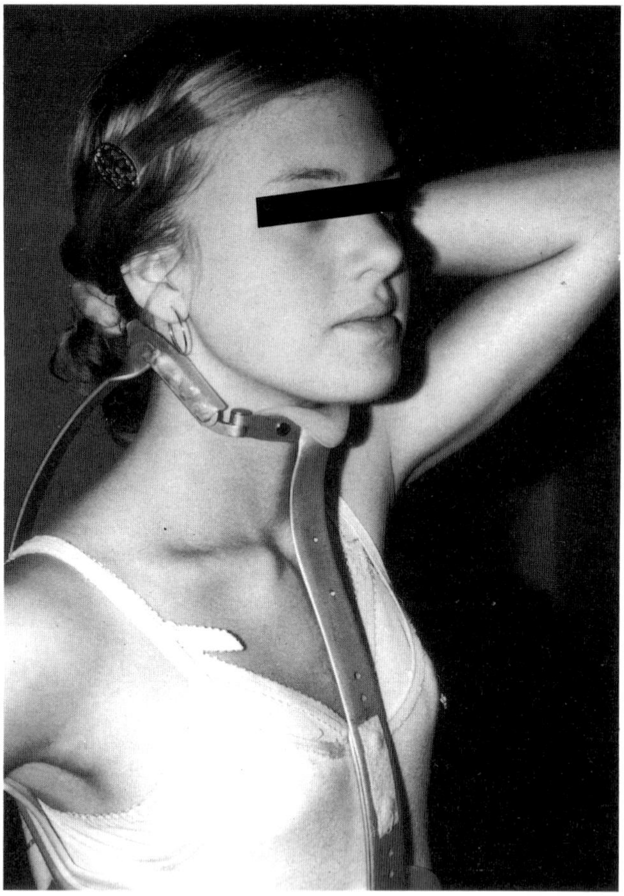

Fig. 20.11 The neck ring and throat mould of the Milwaukee brace.

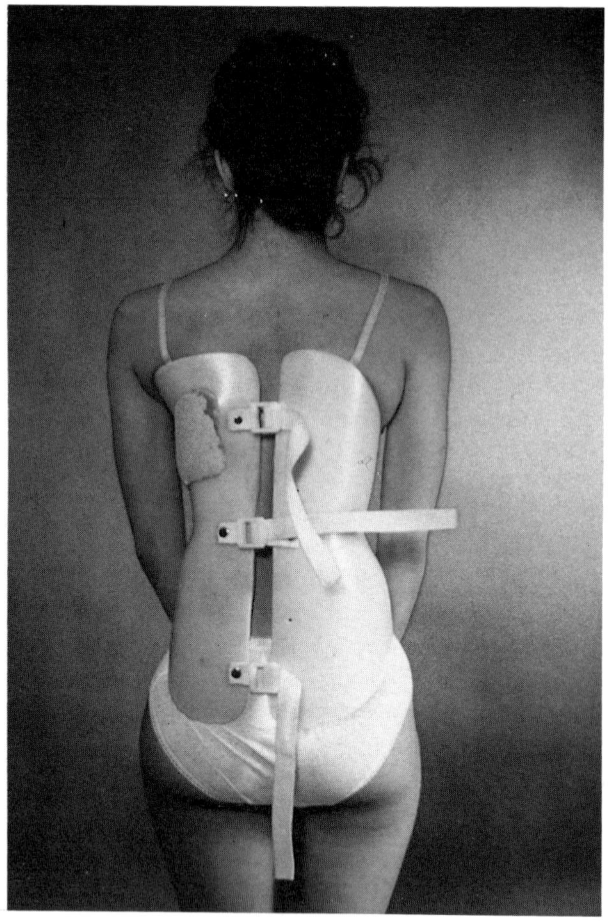

Fig. 20.12 A modular TLSO brace of the Boston type.

early effects, the subsequent long-term results have shown that the mean effect is to produce no more than a curvature at maturity which equals the curve when treatment started. Figure 20.13 shows the typical bar chart of correction against time with bracing. Of course from a knowledge of the natural history this mean final result has to be set against the likelihood that in a fair proportion of cases without treatment the curve will progress, in some cases to the point of surgery.

Perhaps the most effective indicator, that the proposed brace treatment is likely to be successful, is mobility and correctability of the curve with a Cobb angle correction of over 50% shown from X-rays taken in the brace. However, correct brace design, good orthotic care and sufficient period in the brace with adequate patient compliance are all important factors in establishing a successful brace regime. A stiff curve and a large rib hump lead to ineffective

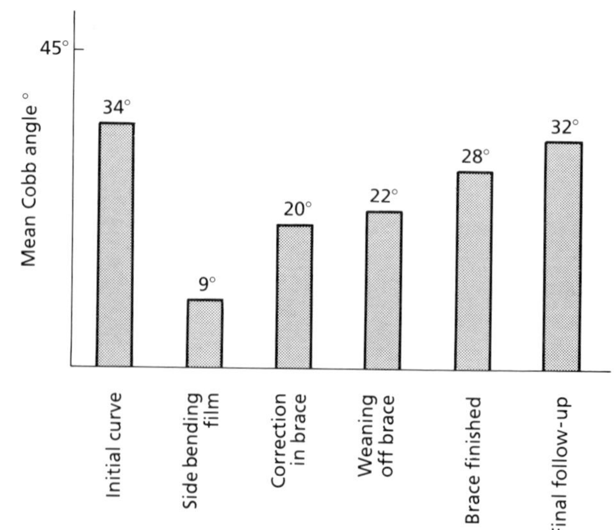

Fig. 20.13 A bar chart to show the mean correction achieved for idiopathic thoracic curves during the adolescent growth period in a series of cases. After Carr *et al.* (1980).

brace correction. An associated thoracic hypokyphosis or marked lordosis is a contra-indication for bracing, which only exaggerates the lordosis and puts respiratory function at risk (Winter *et al.*, 1975).

It is now considered that the brace should be worn by the adolescent child for 20 out of the 24 hours each day. The four hours out of the brace provide opportunity for normal school sport and recreation. Some centres prefer to provide a daily exercise routine to keep the back mobile and muscles active, but clearly it is more natural and less tedious if daily sport of some sort can be encouraged out of the brace. One study (Green, 1986) has shown that 16 hours per day can also be effective.

Conclusions from the latter study, and from studies demonstrating that the brace is more effective in mild curves, which of course have been shown to have less chance of progressing, have raised the question whether bracing *per se* really does alter the natural history of scoliosis. Are curves which achieve the best results those that really have no potential for progression? A number of authorities have challenged the validity of the brace, including Dickson (1985), who felt that, apart from the lack of any evidence of its effectiveness, the brace could not reverse or counter the asymmetrical growth of a rotated lordosis, which he predicted was the primary pathogenetic factor causing the deformity. Of course against this is the fact that a scoliosis is more than just a rotated lordosis. The secondary effect of gravity leads to increase and collapse of the lateral curvature with secondary changes in the disc space ligaments and vertebral body shape. It is the secondary effects of the lateral curvature which can be improved by the brace (Edgar, 1985). Nevertheless, Dickson is right in stating that no controlled long-term prospective study comparing untreated patients with those in a brace has been completed. A number of studies have favourably compared the effects of bracing with the predicted pattern of progression from natural history studies of similar untreated deformities (Bassett *et al.*, 1986). In addition Miller *et al.* (1984) have shown a slight but not statistically confirmed improvement in the progression of a matched controlled study followed over a mean of 1.9 years.

The Scoliosis Research Society has now set up a multicentre trial involving some 10 centres in the USA, Britain and Sweden, in which single curves of between 25° and 35° in idiopathic thoracic scoliosis are allocated in one centre entirely for observation and in another centre entirely for brace management. The early results indicate that the number of curves progressing significantly in the untreated group is four times greater than in the brace group. However, these are unofficial and early findings, and the awaited final result of the long-term effect will be much more important.

In conclusion it is the author's opinion that bracing has a definite place for the mobile 25–35° idiopathic scoliosis in the lower thoracic, thoracolumbar or lumbar region. Braces must be made by well-trained orthotists and there should be a careful follow-up of the patient every four months involving a close check on compliance. Even if the brace slows progression down to the point where surgery can be delayed until the later part of adolescence then considerable benefit can be gained by reducing what would otherwise have been a two-stage surgical procedure to a single-stage operation. A less severe curve will often require a shorter length of fusion also.

Therefore the essential points on brace therapy may be summarized as follows:

1 A child in early adolescence, who has a progressive idiopathic scoliosis in the thoracic, thoracolumbar or lumbar region with the apex of the major curve at or below T8 and with a Cobb angle of between 25° and 35° (or very occasionally 40° if the spine is exceptionally mobile and correctable), should be considered as eligible for bracing.

2 It is important to know that the brace is most effective in the mobile immature curve of the premenarcheal child where the Risser sign is 0. Brace therapy can still be effective when the Risser sign is 3.

3 A scoliosis which corrects well on supine or side-bending films with over 50% correction augurs well for brace treatment. Similarly the initial X-ray in the brace, which shows a 50% or better correction, again is a good prediction.

4 Brace treatment tends to have a poor outcome when there is a rapidly progressive curve with progression of over 20° per year, when there is a marked rib hump and when the major deformity is stiff to side-bending and distraction such that the side-bending X-rays show under 50% correction.

5 Marked lordosis in a thoracic or thoracolumbar deformity is a contra-indication to bracing. In these patients the lateral rib pad will enhance the lordotic posture, producing a decrease in respiratory function.

6 Once a TLSO brace has been applied, the patient will need to be reviewed carefully every four months

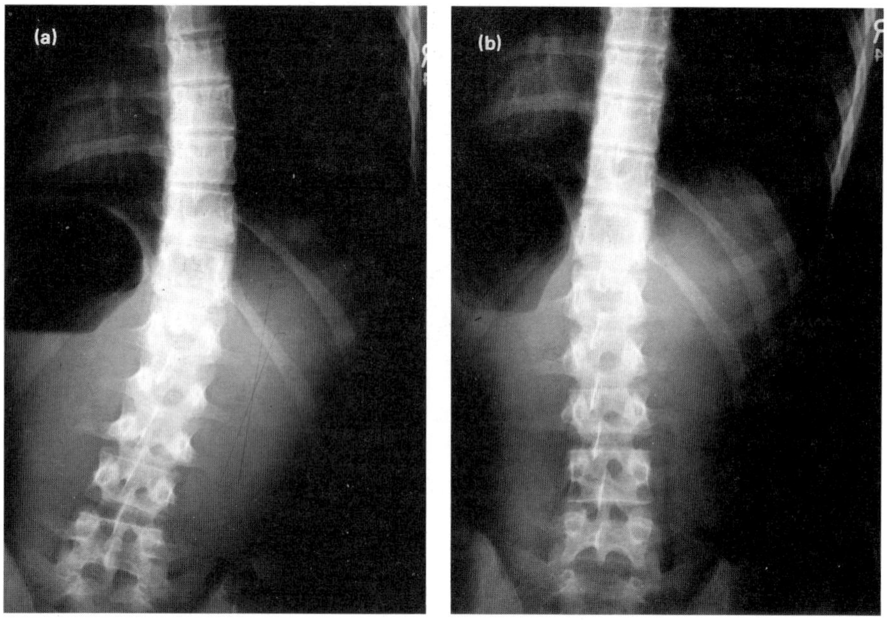

Fig. 20.14 The effect of side-shift exercises on a spinal curve. (a) Before and (b) during side-shift.

with the help of an experienced orthotist. Good brace compliance is often related to a secure and adequately disciplined family scenario. Remember that the poor results of bracing usually reflect the results of poor bracing and poor selection of patients.

Corrective trunk exercises

Some scoliosis surgeons advocate a daily spinal exercise routine for scoliosis children wearing braces, in order to maintain mobility of the spine and strength of the paraspinal and abdominal musculature. Here the physiotherapist's advice and involvement is important. Perhaps of greater importance, particularly where brace-wearing is held at 16–20 hours of the day as opposed to the older regime of 23 hours per day, is the opportunity for the child to take part in normal school sport, gymnastics and recreation. However, there is the occasional child who is not inclined towards sport, and whose place of education does not offer sport and recreation; then the physiotherapist's role is clearly required.

A corrective exercise routine supervised by a physiotherapist was shown in earlier trials to be ineffective, if not harmful, in correcting and preventing deterioration in structural scoliosis (Blount, 1954). Subsequently it was noticed that certain postural exercises, including active pelvic tilt, did correct the curvature, and this led to the development of active correction in combination with a pelvic tilt brace (Jones & Norton, 1956). For some reason this had only limited use, and was probably surpassed by the more comfortable and practical Milwaukee brace at that stage.

However, active postural correction of scoliotic curves has recently been introduced, selecting suitable, very early, progressive idiopathic deformities. This has involved an international multicentre trial (Mehta *et al.*, 1989). Centres in Spain and Malta, where the prevailing weather conditions further reduce compliance of brace-wearing, have been included. Children with mobile idiopathic curves of 15–35° situated in the lower thoracic and thoracolumbar spine have been taught to carry out an active autocorrection procedure, in which the trunk is side-shifted over the pelvis to the concave side of the scoliosis. In lumbar curves with an oblique lower lumbar segment, a pelvic hitch technique is taught, similar to that used by Jones & Norton (1956). These children are instructed to carry out the exercises at regular periods during the day, and many in the trial have become amazingly proficient at them. Side-shifting in lunch queues at school, etc., has started a mini-cult of side-shifting.

So far only early results are available after two years into the trial and these have been presented (Mehta *et al.*, 1989). It is encouraging that overall 80% of curves remained unchanged or actually improved over the study period. This is better than the predicted natural history of such curves in early adolescence. As might be expected, curves of 15–25° magnitude responded better than those over 25°. With the high proportion of non-progressive curves in this range it is not surprising that these results are so far not statistically significant. However, with growing experience, and as the trial extends, there is every evidence that the treatment will have a statistically significant influence on natural history predictions (Mehta, personal communication). Figure 20.14 demonstrates the effect of side-shift in correcting the scoliosis on the initial standing X-ray. The third X-ray shows the position of the curve after two years.

Painful scoliosis in childhood

Back pain in children must be taken seriously because of the relatively high incidence of serious causes (Edgar, 1987). Of particular concern is the painful stiff spinal deformity, when the following conditions must be considered.

SPONDYLOLISTHESIS

As a result of rapid slipping in a Type I congenital dysplastic spondylolisthesis or occasionally a Type II isthmic spondylolytic spondylolisthesis (see the standard classification by Wiltse *et al.*, 1976) an adolescent crisis with a painful rigid lumbar spine associated with a scoliosis can occur (Newman, 1965).

ADOLESCENT DISC HERNIATION

Again a rigid back associated with a marked sciatic scoliosis and very limited straight leg raising can characterize this condition. Pain may be only a minor feature, stiffness being the main disability. As in adult conditions, the lumbosacral or L4–L5 level are the usual sites affected.

NEOPLASMS

Involving either the spinal cord, with an example shown in Fig. 20.15, or the vertebral bodies and pedicles in the form of osteoid osteomas or osteoblastomas, as illustrated in Fig. 20.16. Neoplasms usually present with a stiff painful scoliosis characterized by pain at night.

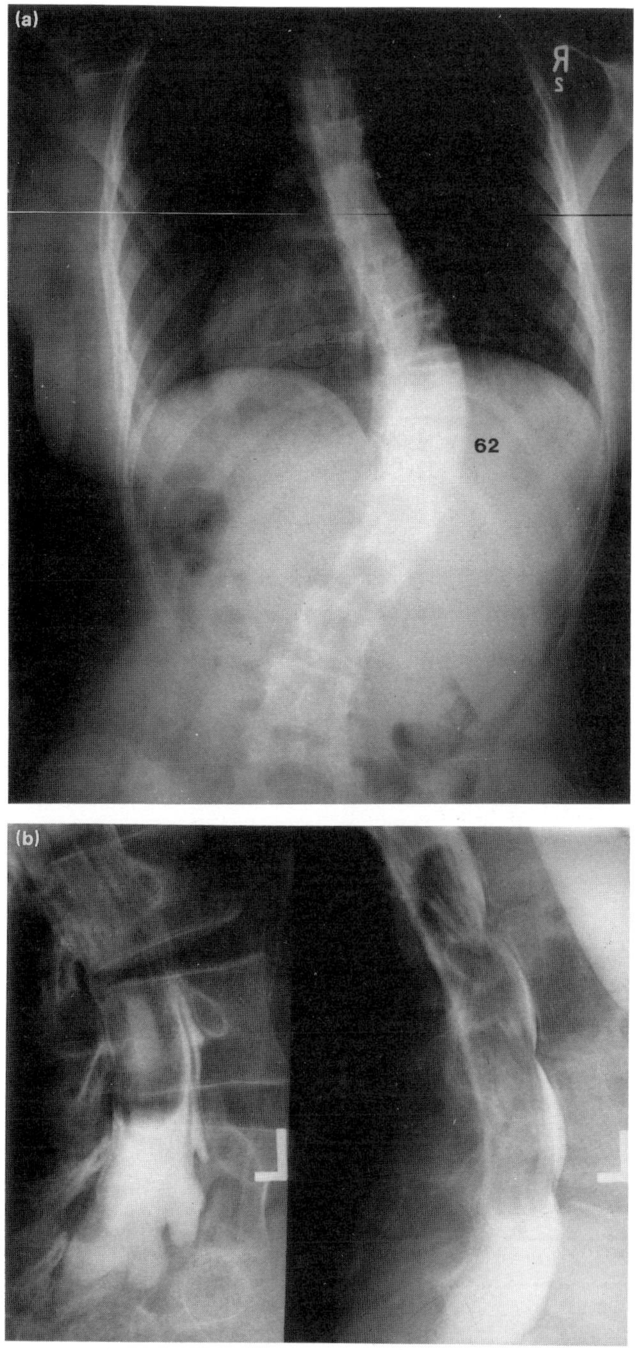

Fig. 20.15 Spinal cord tumour. (a) X-ray of the spine of an adolescent girl with a stiff painful thoracolumbar scoliosis initially thought to be idiopathic. (b) Iohexal myelogram demonstrating tumour mass.

PAINFUL KYPHOSIS

This may be due to osteochondritis of the Scheuermann type affecting usually the thoracic spine, but the lumbar spine may be implicated. Ankylosing spondylitis usually starts in adolescence but rarely it can strike in the juvenile period. Infection may occur at any age and will present with a painful rigid back, and the patient may have developed a kyphos. Occasionally following a spinal burst fracture in adolescence a post-traumatic kyphosis develops with pain due to instability.

Investigations must include a thorough clinical examination, adequate X-rays to be followed by a full blood count, which should raise the suspicion of ankylosing spondylitis or infection. A technetium-99 bone scan will localize an osteoid osteoma, a malignant bone tumour or infection (Fig. 20.16). A computerized tomographic scan of the suspicious area of the spine should define an osteoid osteoma or other bone tumour as well as infection. Finally magnetic resonance imaging or myelography is required for an adolescent disc herniation or spinal cord tumour.

(a)

(b)

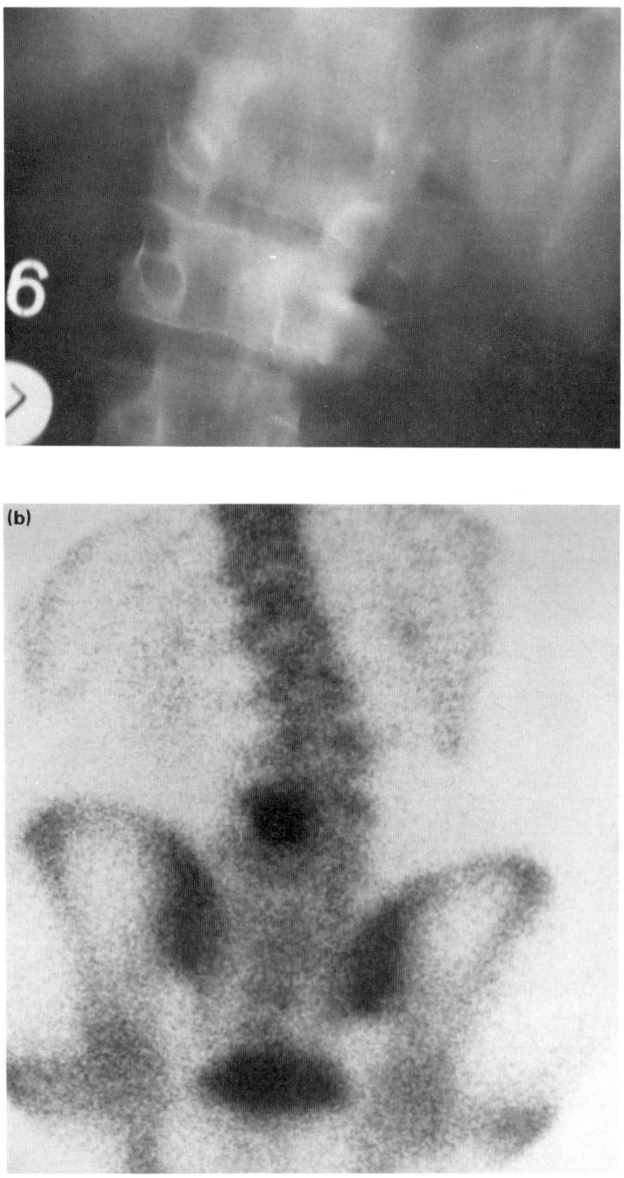

Fig. 20.16 Osteoid osteoma of the lumbar spine. (a) Tomography demonstrating marked thickening of the right pedicle of L4. (b) Technetium-99 bone scan showing the localized hot area. From Kirwan *et al.* (1984).

Clinic attendance

As a postscript to this chapter a protocol has been set out as guidelines to the frequency that children with spinal deformities of different types at different stages should attend the scoliosis clinic.

URGENT REVIEW

1 Children undergoing investigation for painful deformities.
2 Complaint of pain whilst in a corrective localizer cast.
3 Parental complaint of psychological upset as a result of brace or plaster treatment.

FOUR-MONTHLY REVIEW WITH X-RAYS

1 Fast-growing adolescents who are premenarchal with curves over 20°.
2 Any curve in an adolescent where progression is suspected of being over 10° per year or shown to be such as a result of X-rays on previous visits.
3 Curves being actively managed by non-surgical means, i.e. brace or side-shift exercises.
4 Patients in plaster casts generally should not be left longer than four months, and in serial corrective plaster casts changes are best every two months.
5 Scoliosis or spinal deformity awaiting surgery or on a waiting list should not be left longer than four months without reviewing to assess the rate of progression, particularly if they are young adolescents growing fast, or are premenarchal.

SIX-MONTHLY REVIEW WITH X-RAYS

1 Postmenarcheal curves over 20–25° that have been shown to be progressing only slowly.
2 Congenital neuropathic and infantile curves which are changing little during the juvenile period.
3 Adolescents with stable congenital curves.
4 Curves that have been followed up following fusion in adolescence.

TWELVE-MONTH REVIEW

1 All curves that are being followed up if progression is suspected following skeletal maturity (Risser 4–5).
2 Infantile idiopathic curves that are clearly shown to be resolving after several six-monthly visits.

REFERENCES

Axelgaard, J.A. & Brown, J.C. (1983) Lateral electrical surface stimulation for the treatment of progressive idiopathic scoliosis. *Spine*, **8**, 242–260.

Bassett, G.S., Bunnell, W.P. & MacEwen, G.D. (1986) Treatment of idiopathic scoliosis with the Wilmington brace. *J. Bone Jt. Surg.*, **68A**, 602–605.

Belstead, J.S. & Edgar, M.A. (1978) Early detection for scoliosis. *Br. Med. J.*, **2**, 937–938.

Blount, W.P. (1954) Treatment of scoliosis. Report of the sixth SICOT congress, Berne. *J. Bone Jt. Surg.*, **36B**, 686.

Blount, W.P., Schmidt, A.L., Keever, E.D. & Leonard, E.T. (1958) The Milwaukee brace in the operative treatment of scoliosis. *J. Bone Jt. Surg.*, **40A**, 511–525.

Bobenchko, W.P. (1973) Spinal pacemakers in scoliosis. *J. Bone Jt. Surg.*, **55B**, 232.

Brown, J.C., Axelgaard, J.A., Swank, S.M. & Minehart, C. (1986) Multi-centre study of 1221 patients on lateral surface stimulation for idiopathic scoliosis. *Presentation at the 53rd AAOS Meeting*, New Orleans, Louisiana.

Bunnell, W.P. (1986) The natural history of idiopathic scoliosis before skeletal maturity. *Spine*, **II**, 773–776.

Burwell, R.G. (1989) The current status of screening. In Siegler, D., Harrison, D. & Edgar, M.A. (eds) *Proceedings of the Eighth Zorab Scoliosis Symposium: Prognosis in Scoliosis*. Phillip Zorab Scoliosis Research Fund London, pp. 13–33.

Burwell, R.J., James, N.J., Johnson, F., Webb, J.K. & Wilson, Y.G. (1983a) Standardised trunk asymmetry scores. *J. Bone Jt. Surg.*, **65B**, 452–463.

Burwell, R.G., Owen, R. & Mitchell, G.P. (1983b) School screening for scoliosis—Report by the British Orthopaedic Association and the British Scoliosis Society. *Br. Med. J.*, **287**, 963–964.

Calvert, P.T., Edgar, M.A. & Webb, P.J. (1989) Scoliosis in neurofibromatosis—the natural history with or without operation. *J. Bone Jt. Surg.*, **71B**, 246–251.

Carr, W.A., Moe, J.H., Winter, R.B. & Lonstein, J.E. (1980) The treatment of idiopathic scoliosis in the Milwaukee brace. *J. Bone Jt. Surg.*, **62A**, 599–612.

Dickson, R.A., Stamper, P., Sharp, A.M. & Harker, P. (1980) School screening for scoliosis—study of clinical course. *Br. Med. J.*, **281**, 265–267.

Dickson, R.A. (1983) Scoliosis in the community. *Br. Med. J.*, **286**, 615–618.

Dickson, R.A. (1984) Screening for scoliosis. *Br. Med. J.*, **289**, 269–270.

Dickson, R.A. (1985) Conservative treatment for idiopathic scoliosis. *J. Bone Jt. Surg.*, **67B**, 176–181.

Edgar, M.A. (1985) To brace or not to brace (Editorial). *J. Bone Jt. Surg.*, **67B**, 173–174.

Edgar, M.A. (1987) Back pain in childhood and adolescence. *Current Orthopaedics*, vol. I, p. 194. Churchill Livingstone, Edinburgh.

Edgar, M.A. & Mehta, M.H. (1988) Longterm follow-up of fused and unfused scoliosis. *J. Bone Jt. Surg.*, **70B**, 712–716.

Ferris, B., Edgar, M.A. & Leyshon, A. (1988) Screening for scoliosis. *Acta Orthop. Scand.*, **59**, 417–418 (correspondence see **60**, 123–126).

Galante, J., Schults, A., Dewald, R.L. & Ray, R.D. (1970) Forces acting in the Milwaukee brace on patients undergoing treatment for idiopathic scoliosis. *J. Bone Jt. Surg.*, **52A**, 498–506.

Goldberg, C., Dowling, F.E., Fogarty, E.E., Regan, B.F. & Blake, N.S. (1988) Electro-spinal stimulations in children with adolescent and juvenile scoliosis. *Spine*, **13**, 482–484.

Green, N.E. (1986) Part time bracing of adolescent idiopathic scoliosis. *J. Bone Jt. Surg.*, **68A**, 738–742.

Herbert, M.A. & Bobenchko, W.P. (1989) Results of single channel implanted stimulators used to treat idiopathic scoliosis in children. *Abstracts of the Combined Meeting of the Scoliosis Research Society and the European Spinal Deformities Society*, Amsterdam, p. 223.

Hoffman, D.A., Lonstein, J.E., Morim, M.M., Visschu, W., Harris, B.S.H. & Boice, J.D. (1989) Breast cancer in women with scoliosis exposed to multiple diagnostic X-rays. *J. Natl. Cancer Inst.*, **81**, 1307–1312.

Jefferson, R.J., Weisz, I., Turner-Smith, A.R., Harris, J.D. & Houghton, G.R. (1988) Scoliosis surgery and its effect on back shape. *J. Bone Jt. Surg.*, **70B**, 261–266.

Jones, W.N. & Norton, P.L. (1956) A study of the use of pelvic tilt during standing and walking to induce active correction of scoliotic curves. *J. Bone Jt. Surg.*, **38A**, 938.

Kirwan, E., O'G., Hutton, P.A.N., Pozo, J.L. & Ransford, A.R. (1984) Osteoid osteoma and benign osteoblastoma of the spine. *J. Bone Jt. Surg.*, **66B**, 21–26.

Kostuik, J.P., Israel, J. & Hall, J.E. (1973) Scoliosis surgery in adults. *Clin. Orthop.*, **93**, 225–234.

Lloyd-Roberts, G.C. & Pilcher, M.F. (1965) Structural idiopathic scoliosis in infancy: a study of the natural history of 100 patients. *J. Bone Jt. Surg.*, **47B**, 520–523.

Lonstein, J.E. & Carlson, J.M. (1984) The prediction of curve progression in untreated scoliosis during growth. *J. Bone Jt. Surg.*, **66A**, 1061–1071.

McMaster, M.J. & Ohtsuka, K. (1982) The natural history of congenital scoliosis—a study of 251 patients. *J. Bone Jt. Surg.*, **64A**, 1128–1147.

McMaster, M.J. & David, C.V. (1986) Hemivertebra as a cause of scoliosis—a study of 164 patients. *J. Bone Jt. Surg.*, **68B**, 588–595.

Mehta, M.H. (1972) The rib–vertebra angle in the diagnosis between resolving and progressive infantile scoliosis. *J. Bone Jt. Surg.*, **54B**, 230–243.

Mehta, M.H. (1977) The natural history of infantile idiopathic scoliosis. In Zorab, P.A. & Siegler, D. (eds) *Proceedings of a Fifth Symposium: Scoliosis*. Brompton Hospital, London, pp. 103–122.

Mehta, M.H. & Morel, G. (1980) The non-operative treatment of infantile idiopathic scoliosis. In Zorab, P. & Siegler, D. (eds) *Proceedings of the Sixth Zorab Symposium: Scoliosis*, pp. 71–84. Academic Press, New York.

Mehta, M.H., Kurokawa, T., Kojana, T., Pilcher, M., Casaletto, J., Camilleri, D., Bellia, M., Kooijman, M. & Garcia-Alsina, J. (1989) Active auto-correction of scoliosis by side shift: a multi-centre trial. *Abstracts of the Combined Meeting of the Scoliosis Research Society and the European Spinal Deformities Society*, Amsterdam, pp. 368–369.

Miller, J.A.A., Nachemson, A.L. & Schultz, A.B. (1984) Effectiveness of braces in mild idiopathic scoliosis. *Spine*, **9**, 632–635.

Missiuna, P. & Wedge, J.H. (1989) Electrical spinal instrumentation: the longterm results. *Abstracts of the Combined Meeting of the Scoliosis Research Society and the European Spinal Deformities Society*, Amsterdam, p. 385.

Montgomery, F. (1989) *The cost-effectiveness of screening for scoliosis*. Doctoral thesis, Department of Orthopaedics, Lund University, Malmo General Hospital.

Morley, T.R. (1989) Can early decisions affect the outcome of congenital scoliosis? In Siegler, D., Harrison, D.J. & Edgar, M.A. (eds) *Proceedings of the Eighth Zorab Scoliosis Symposium: Prognosis in Scoliosis*. Phillip Zorab Scoliosis Research Fund, London, pp. 104–107.

Nash, C. (1980) Current concepts review: scoliosis bracing. *J. Bone Jt. Surg.*, **62A**, 848–852.

Newman, P.H. (1965) A clinical syndrome associated with severe lumbosacral subluxation. *J. Bone Jt. Surg.*, **47B**, 472–481.

O'Donnell, C.S., Bunnell, W.P., Betz, R.R., Bowen, J.R. & Tipping, C.R. (1988) Electrical stimulation in the treatment of idiopathic scoliosis. *Clin. Orthop.*, **229**, 107–113.

Scott, M.M. & Piggott, H. (1981) A short term follow-up of patients with mild scoliosis. *J. Bone Jt. Surg.*, **63B**, 523–525.

Swank, S.M. (1989a) Prognosis in neuromuscular scoliosis. In Siegler, D., Harrison, D.J. & Edgar, M.A. (eds) *Proceedings of the Eighth Zorab Scoliosis Symposium: Prognosis in Scoliosis*. Phillip Zorab Scoliosis Research Fund, London, pp. 69–73.

Swank, S.M. (1989b) Electro-spinal stimulation; has it worked? In Siegler, D., Harrison, D.J. & Edgar, M.A. (eds) *Proceedings of the Eighth Zorab Scoliosis Symposium: Prognosis in Scoliosis*. Phillip Zorab Scoliosis Research Fund, London, pp. 99–102.

Torell, G., Nordwall, A. & Nachemson, A. (1981) The changing pattern of scoliosis treatment due to effective screening. *J. Bone Jt. Surg.*, **63A**, 337–341.

Willner, S. (1982) A comparative study of the efficiency of different types of school screening for scoliosis. *Acta Orthop. Scand.*, **53**, 769–774.

Wiltse, L.L., Newman, P.H. & McNab, I. (1976) Classification of spondylolysis and spondylolisthesis. *Clin. Orthop.*, **117**, 23–29.

Winter, R.B., Lovell, W.W. & Moe, J.H. (1975) Excessive thoracic lordosis and loss of pulmonary function in patients with idiopathic scoliosis. *J. Bone Jt. Surg.*, **57A**, 972–977.

21 · Anaesthetic Management and Monitoring

By I.M. BOYD

In recent years great advances have been made in the surgical treatment of scoliosis in children. Keim (1972) defined scoliosis as one or more lateral rotatory curvatures of the spine which can be classified according to structural and non-structural characteristics. The most common group of structural scoliosis are classified as 'idiopathic' (65%) and are of unknown aetiology, occurring predominantly in otherwise healthy teenage girls. The rest (35%) can be divided into congenital skeletal abnormalities (15%), neuromuscular disorders (10%), neurofibromatosis (5%), and a miscellaneous group of rareties (5%), e.g. Marfan's syndrome, Morquio's syndrome, spinal tumours, etc. In fact Riseborough (1973) listed 72 possible causes of scoliosis.

The anaesthetist must be aware of these underlying conditions as some of them may pose specific, potentially life-threatening problems intraoperatively and postoperatively, such as difficulty in airway control and intubation in Morquio's syndrome or associated severe cardiothoracic problems in Marfan's syndrome.

Scoliosis may occur at various levels. Cervical scoliosis in children is rare and suggests trauma, destructive disease or congenital deformity. Management here can be technically demanding of both anaesthetist and surgeon.

Thoracic or thoracolumbar curves create maximum physiological effects on respiratory and cardiac function, the degree depending on various factors such as age of onset, aetiology, rate of progression and angle of curvature. Curvature limited to the lumbar spine causes minimal physiological disturbance.

The degree of thoracolumbar curvature is a useful guide to respiratory impairment (Zorab, 1966; Shannon *et al.*, 1971). Children with idiopathic scoliosis and curves less than 65° are unlikely to show any clinical signs of respiratory impairment. This may not be the case where the child has congenital scoliosis, where there may be marked respiratory limitation with lesser degrees of curvature. In general a Cobb angle between 65° and 90° is associated with moderate reduction in lung function. Curves greater than 90° cause a severe impairment of lung function (Riseborough & Davis, 1974).

Evaluation of lung function in small children can be difficult. Exercise tolerance is a good guide, for a child who can walk or run around will have better lung function than a child with similar aetiology who is in a wheelchair or is bed-bound. Dyspnoea and tachypnoea at rest indicate incipient respiratory failure; also, a child who can cough effectively and is able to cooperate with physiotherapy will have a smoother postoperative period than one who lacks these abilities (such as severe cerebral palsy).

Specific tests of pulmonary function, based on armspread rather than height, have practical value if the patient is old enough to cooperate (Relten & Conn 1963; Hardy, 1974; Gibson, 1984). The typical finding is a restrictive defect with a reduction in vital capacity, total lung capacity and functional residual capacity with a normal or proportionately less reduced residual volume. The extent of the restrictive defect is directly related to the degree of angulation (Kafer, 1975).

The simple mechanical explanation for the reduction in lung volumes is increased stiffness (reduced compliance) of the chest wall. This is less marked in young children, where it has been suggested that restriction to expansion is due more to an impaired mechanical advantage of the inspiratory muscles, due to distortion of their normal points of skeletal attachment (Caro & Dubois, 1961).

Localized areas of compression and atelectasis of the underlying lung are likely with such distorted anatomy and a reduction in pulmonary compliance contributes to the volume restriction in some patients. The reduction in lung volumes and poor chest wall compliance cause ventilation/perfusion mismatch and an increase in pulmonary vascular resistance. Blood gases may show hypoxia exaggerated on exercise. With increasing severity of scoliosis tidal volume decreases and hypercapnoea may develop. The hypoxia with or without hypercapnoea is partly responsible for the rise in pulmonary artery pressure. Anatomical factors may also contribute to the high pulmonary vascular resistance and eventually to the development of right heart failure.

Radioisotope studies have shown a more even distribution of regional lung function than normal (Dollery *et al.*, 1965; Littler *et al.*, 1972), sometimes with a reversal of the normal vertical gradients, possibly due to airway closure at the lung bases and to increased pulmonary artery pressure. The volume of the lung on the convex side is larger and contributes greater overall gas exchange than on the concave side of the spinal curve.

In general a reduction of pulmonary function of 70% or more indicates a high probability that a period of postoperative ventilatory support will be required.

Scoliosis that appears late in the growth period may have minimal effects on respiratory and cardiovascular function. In contrast congenital scoliosis where curvature is severe prior to completion of lung development will have a profound effect on respiratory function.

At birth a normal infant's lung contains between 50 000 and 100 000 alveoli which increase to a maximum of 300 000 by two years of age (Reid, 1966). After this the alveoli continue to increase in size until 15 years of age. When curvature appears early in life the compressed lung may reach only one-third the normal size, being defective in both the number and the size of alveoli (Reid, 1966).

In the preoperative assessment the anaesthetist should also assess carefully the cardiovascular system as scoliosis may be associated with congenital heart disease: with a cardiomyopathy, as in Duchenne muscle dystrophy, Friedrich's ataxia, with aneurysmal dilatation of the aorta leading to the possibility of aortic dissection, as in Marfan's syndrome. Thus preparation of patients presenting for spinal surgery requires careful examination and investigation as outlined. Special care should be taken to alleviate apprehension and develop a rapport with both child and parents. Premedication should be carefully prescribed to reduce anxiety without causing undue respiratory depression.

Intraoperatively these patients can pose several particular problems to the anaesthetist. In most centres all patients are intubated and mechanically ventilated throughout the procedure. This can sometimes be technically challenging as some can be very difficult to intubate (such as Klippel-Feil syndrome, Morquio's syndrome). The anaesthetist should remember that a much shorter endotracheal tube than normal may be required, and great care should be taken to avoid endobronchial intubation with the consequent severe ventilation/perfusion mismatch.

Careful positioning of the patient is required especially for posterior spinal surgery. It has been shown that blood normally returning via the inferior vena cava is directed by abdominal pressure to an alternative route via a network of valveless venous plexuses surrounding the spine (Batson, 1940). The patient must therefore be supported either by pads and sandbags or on a special mattress or frame (Relten & Hall, 1967) to ensure the abdomen complete freedom without limiting ventilation. All the various pressure points and areas should be padded, supported and checked as the operation may well proceed for several hours. An indwelling urinary catheter is necessary to monitor urine output intraoperatively and postoperatively.

Adequate ventilation is ensured intraoperatively by mechanical ventilation and continuous monitoring of the end-tidal carbon dioxide and oxygen saturation. In poor-risk patients intermittent blood gas analysis for acid–base control may be necessary. Cardiac stability is maintained throughout by avoidance of light anaesthesia with consequent tachycardia and hypertension, together with avoidance of hypoxia and hypercarbia. Continuous monitoring of heart rate and blood pressure is mandatory. In poor-risk cases, or where hypotensive methods are to be used, continuous monitoring of blood pressure via an indwelling arterial line is essential.

Bleeding is a major problem during spinal surgery. The principal factors contributing to blood loss are related to: (a) the surgical wound and the surgeon's technique of haemostasis, (b) the patient's local vasoconstrictive response and coagulation mechanism, and (c) the additional effects of anaesthetic and ventilatory management.

The surgeon can reduce blood loss by local wound infiltration using adrenaline 1 : 500 000 prior to skin incision, followed by meticulous haemostasis at all stages of the operation.

The anaesthetist can reduce blood loss by using a smooth anaesthetic technique with avoidance of hypoxia, hypercarbia and 'light' anaesthesia with its consequent tachycardia and hypertensive episodes. This, coupled with correct positioning, can do much to control blood loss.

In some adult centres blood loss is further reduced by active hypotension using agents such as sodium nitroglycerine, sodium nitroprusside or trimeprazen infusions, together with β-blockade if necessary. If such methods are used then continuous arterial monitoring via an indwelling arterial cannula is mandatory as is continuous spinal cord monitoring. Monitoring is usually performed using an electrode placed percutaneously into the epidural space by the anaesthetist before profound hypotension is instigated, to ensure that the perfusion pressure is adequate to permit good perfusion of the spinal cord at all times.

Increased stretching of the spinal cord caused by distraction to straighten the curvature introduces the danger of damaging the spinal cord. Figures from the Scoliosis Research Society quote an incidence of between 0.72% and 2% for acute neurological complications after scoliosis correction (MacEwen *et al.*, 1975) without any monitoring. This induced Stagnara and Vauzelle to advocate the 'wake-up' test (Vauzelle *et al.*, 1973). This requires that the patient is woken up, once the spine has been distracted and, commonly with the instrumentation in place, asked to move his or her feet in order to detect any incipient neurological damage. The patient is then re-anaesthetized and the operation is completed.

Most anaesthetic techniques allow for the full and rapid return of cognitive functions and protective reflexes at the end of an operation. It is much more difficult to achieve this for a short period intraoperatively and then return rapidly to anaesthesia of undiminished quality without compromising final awakening, and also ensuring amnesia for this period.

A commonly used method, as described by Abbott & Bentley (1980) is to keep the patient anaesthetized utilizing a muscle relaxant, opiate, nitrous-oxide–oxygen technique until the wake-up test is required. The anaesthetist then gives 100% oxygen, and within a few minutes the patient should be able to obey commands to move feet and/or hands. If the hands are moved but not the feet, or if only one foot is moved, the force on the rod is reduced until both feet move equally. The patient is then rapidly re-anaesthetized with a small dose of thiopentone and diazepam intravenously. On no account should the reversal of the muscle relaxant be attempted, as this could result in sudden violent movements by the patient. This test is unsuitable for small children or the mentally retarded. Increasingly it is being supplanted by continual spinal extradural or cortical recording of somatosensory evoked potentials. For most spinal surgery the stimulating electrodes are placed over the posterior tibial nerve and the recording sites are proximal to the site of surgery. Usually the recording electrode is positioned in the extradural space by the surgeon. However, percutaneous placement by the anaesthetist postinduction but prior to the start of surgery has been advocated (Loughnan & Hall, 1989) to allow continuous spinal cord monitoring during profound hypotension at the start of surgery. Occasionally recording electrodes are placed on the scalp. The increasing use of spinal cord monitoring has reduced the incidence of the 'wake-up' test. However, this occasionally still has to be performed when spinal cord monitoring gives equivocal results.

Spinal surgery may last for several hours, and temperature control in these patients may be a problem. In most instances there is a drop in body temperature, especially when large volumes of blood are transfused rapidly. This heat loss can be minimized by warming the intravenous fluids, humidifying the inspired gases and raising the ambient temperature in the operating room. Heating mattresses are of no value due to the necessity to ensure no abdominal compression.

On the other hand a few cases of malignant hyperpyrexia have been reported related to scoliosis. The incidence has been quoted as 1 : 15 000 anaesthetized children (Britt, 1976). Keaney & Ellis (1971) defined the syndrome in terms of a body temperature rise in excess of 2°C per hour. The disease is manifest as a metabolic crisis and the demonstration, in the presence of fever, of arterial hypercapnia, hyperkalaemia, metabolic acidosis and hypoxia, confirms the diagnosis. The disease is familial and inherited as an autosomal dominant with variable expressivity.

More recently McCarthy *et al.* (1990) have localized the MH gene to chromosome 19, so possibly in the near future susceptible children and adults will be positively identified by locating the abnormal gene. Should malignant hyperpyrexia occur intraoperatively the operation should be aborted, the patient given intravenous dantrolene, arrhythmias treated as necessary, metabolic acidosis corrected and hyperkalaemia controlled with 50% dextrose and soluble insulin as required. The patient should be actively cooled if necessary using cardiopulmonary bypass.

Malignant hyperpyrexia is a rare but exceedingly serious condition although, with the advent of dantrolene, the mortality rate has been greatly reduced. Therefore, all children presenting for scoliosis surgery should have continuous body temperature monitoring and the anaesthetist must be alert for early signs of this condition. It is interesting that the MH gene has been mapped on chromosome 19 and appears to be 25 cM away from the myotonic dystrophy gene—also located on chromosome 19.

Patients with muscle dystrophies may, under anaesthesia, develop a condition akin to malignant hyperpyrexia with hyperkalaemia, metabolic acidosis, myoglobinuria and elevated creatinine kinase. The temperature may or may not be raised. This appears not to be a genetically transmitted trait but due to the underlying disorder of calcium ion flux in the diseased muscle, triggered by anaesthesia. The treatment is identical to that of malignant hyperpyrexia.

At the end of the operation most patients are extubated and immediately encouraged to cough and breathe deeply. Intensive physiotherapy is started on the high-dependency unit. Very poor-risk patients or those with severe muscle disorders may require a period of postoperative ventilation.

Suitable analgesia is prescribed either as a continuous intravenous opiate infusion or epidural opiate via an indwelling epidural catheter. Older children and adults may prefer to use the patient-controlled analgesia system.

Blood loss is constantly monitored and losses are replaced.

Most patients tolerate this major surgery very well. Shannon *et al.* (1971) studied the lung function of adult patients after spinal surgery and found that surgery prevented further deterioration in lung function. In some cases there appeared to be a slight improvement. However, the effects on long-term cardiorespiratory function are as yet to be established.

REFERENCES

Abbott, T.R. & Bentley, G. (1980) Intraoperative awakening during scoliosis surgery. *Anaesthesia*, **35**, 298.

Batson, D.V. (1940) The function of the vertebral veins and their role in the spread of metastases. *Ann. Surg.*, **12**, 129.

Britt, B.A. (1976) *Mod. Med. Can.*, **31**, 511.

Caro, C.G. & Dubois, A.B. (1961) Pulmonary function in kyphoscoliosis. *Thorax*, **16**, 282.

Dollery, C.T., Gillam, P.M.S., Hugh-Jones, P. & Zorab, P.A. (1965) Regional lung function in kyphoscoliosis, *Thorax*, **20**, 175.

Gibson, G.J. (1984) *Clinical Tests of Respiratory Function*, Macmillan, London.

Hardy, J.M. (1974) *Spinal Deformity in Neurological and Muscular Disorders*. C.V. Mosby Co., St Louis, MI.

Kafer, E.R. (1975) Idiopathic scoliosis: mechanical properties of the respiratory system and the ventilatory response to carbon dioxide. *J. Clin. Invest.*, **55**, 1153.

Keaney, N.P. & Ellis, F.R. (1971) *Fr. B. Med. J.*, **4**, 49.

Keim, H.A. (1972) Scoliosis. *Ciba Foundation Symposium*, vol. 24, p. 1. J. Wiley, Chichester.

Littler, W.A., Brown, I.K. & Roaf, R. (1972) Regional lung function in scoliosis. *Thorax*, **27**, 420.

Loughnan, B.A. & Hall, G.M. (1989) Spinal cord monitoring 1989. *Br. J. Anaes.* **63**, 587.

MacEwan, G.D., Bunnell, W.P. & Spiram, K. (1975) Acute neurological complications in the treatment of scoliosis. *J. Bone Jt. Surg.*, **57A**, 404.

McCarthy, T.V., Healy, S.J.M., Heffron, J.J.A., Lehane, M., Duefel, T., Lehmann-Horn, F., Farrall, M. & Johnson, K.J. (1990) Localisation of the malignant hyperthermia susceptibility locus to human chromosome $19_q12-_q13.2$. *Nature (Lond.)*, **343**, 562.

Reid, L. (1966) Autopsy studies of the lung in kyphoscoliosis. In Zorab, P.A. (ed.) *Proceedings of a Symposium on Scoliosis*. Vincent House, London.

Relton, J.E.S. & Conn, A.W. (1963) Anaesthesia for surgical correction of scoliosis by Harrington method in children. *Can. Anaesth. Soc. J.*, **10**, 603.

Relton, J.E.S. & Hall, J.E. (1967) An operating frame for spinal fusion. *J. Bone Jt. Surg.*, **49B**, 327.

Riseborough, E.J. (1973) The anterior approach to the spine for the correction of deformities of the axial skeleton. *Clin. Orthop.*, **93**, 298.

Riseborough, E.J. & Davis, N. (1974) Anaesthesia. In Hardy, J.H. (ed.) *Spinal Deformity in Neurological and Muscular Disorders*, C.V. Mosby Co., St Louis, MI.

Riseborough, E.J. & Herndon, J.H. (1975) *Scoliosis and other Deformities of the Axial Skeleton*, Little, Brown, Boston, MA.

Shannon, D.C., Riseborough, E.J. & Kazemi, H. (1971) Ventilation perfusion relationships following correction of kyphoscoliosis *J. Am. Med. Assoc.*, **217**, 579.

Vauzelle, C., Stagnara, P. & Jouvinroux, P. (1973) Functional monitoring of spinal cord activity during spinal surgery. *Clin. Orthop. Rel. Res.*, **93**, 197.

Zorab, P.A. (ed.) (1966) Assessment of cardiorespiratory function in kyphoscoliosis. In *Proceedings of a Symposium on Scoliosis*, p. 54. Vincent House, London.

22 · Surgical Correction of Scoliosis in the Young

By A.D.H. GARDNER

The development of an idiopathic spinal deformity in a child is the result of an anatomical, physiological and mechanical destabilization of normal spinal posture combined with, and accentuated by, the effects of growth. Once significant destabilization has occurred, then secondary mechanical factors begin to operate such as the effects of gravity and tissue tension on the concave parts of the vertebral epiphyses. These pressures will, in turn, cause differential growth (Hueter–Volkmann principle) with resultant wedging of the vertebral body causing a further deterioration in an increasingly structural deformity.

The net effect of these ill-understood asymmetric forces is to produce a rotated lordosis which appears as a rotated lateral displacement or scoliosis on a frontal X-ray of the spine. For a true scoliosis to be present there must be rotation and deviation of the spine. (For definitions related to spinal deformity see Dickson, 1986.)

Curves without rotation are not true scolioses but are lateral deviations, usually secondary to some definable external cause such as leg-length difference, unilateral muscle spasm secondary to an acute pain source or a compensatory curve adjoining a true scoliosis. Such non-structural curves are correctable by removing their cause, and their importance lies only in their value as a pointer to a possibly significant cause such as an acute disc prolapse, osteoid osteoma, etc.

The development of a scoliosis is accompanied by, and partly caused by, an increasing asymmetry of the individual vertebra. These changes are most marked in the apical vertebrae of a curvature and the change in vertebral shape is best understood by Stagnara's helpful analogy of a man on a delivery tricycle (Fig. 22.1).

Not only is there coronal asymmetry of the apical vertebrae, as illustrated by Stagnara, but there is also a constant sagittal asymmetry. Dickson *et al.* (1984), in particular, have drawn attention to the fact that a true lateral X-ray (a lateral X-ray adjusted for apical vertebral rotation) of the apical vertebrae of an idiopathic curve will invariably show anteroposterior wedging with the front of the vertebral body taller than the back. This is the reverse of Scheuermann's epiphysitis in which a significant rotated scoliosis is very rarely seen. It is a matter of some controversy as to whether this anteroposterior wedging is a primary cause of scoliosis or whether it is a secondary change induced by other factors; it is probably the latter.

Undoubtedly, the causative mechanisms of idiopathic scoliosis are complex and multifactorial and no doubt vary from individual to individual. Simple mechanical explanations of causation are clearly not adequate, as will be discussed in this chapter.

From the patient's point of view, which is of course of the greatest importance, the most obvious outward and visible sign of the scoliosis is the rib hump associated with underlying vertebral rotation (Thulborne & Gillespie, 1976). The rib hump is not wholly a secondary effect as the ribs are themselves asymmetric and rib humps may continue to increase, especially in immature patients even following a secure surgical spinal fusion (Weatherley *et al.*, 1987). Female patients are often concerned that, with their usual right-sided scoliosis, the right breast is less prominent than the left due to rotation of the anterior chest wall as part of the rib deformity. It should be appreciated that of adolescent idiopathic scolioses in

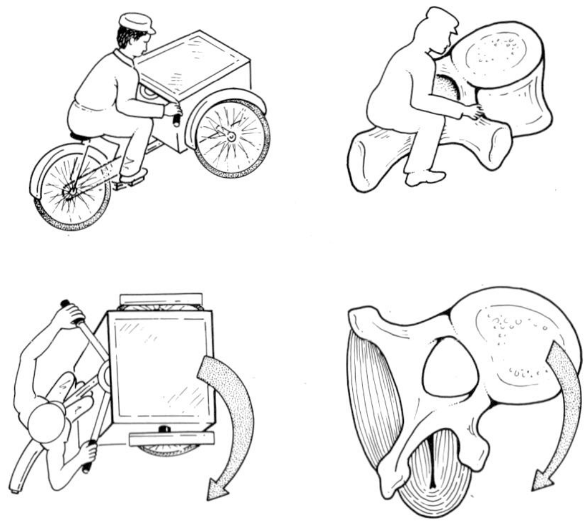

Fig. 22.1 Rotation as preponderant element in progression of scoliosis: tricycle effect. Vertebrae can be compared with delivery tricycle. Load passes through vertebral bodies. Driving force is provided by muscles acting on posterior arches and especially the transverse processes (handlebars). When bend is greater than 30°, driving force is very strongly in rotation and, in addition, muscles on convexity act in same direction. From Stagnara (1988).

excess of 40° Cobb angle, 85% are right-sided and occur in females.

CURVE DEVELOPMENT

The factors leading to the development of idiopathic scoliosis are gradually becoming clear after painstaking research in many centres. There are probably in the region of five to 10 major pieces in the jigsaw puzzle which may have to be present for a scoliosis to develop (see Chapter 19). Probable causative factors are:

1 Genetic: 20–25% of patients with a scoliosis have a close relative with a scoliosis. The mode of inheritance seems to be via a sex-linked autosomal recessive gene of variable penetrance (Wynne-Davies, 1968; Fillio & Thompson, 1971; Cowell *et al.*, 1972; Riseborough & Wynne-Davies, 1973).

2 Neurological abnormalities: evidence of vestibular disturbance has been found in scoliotics and also in their non-scoliotic relatives; these people sway more when blindfolded (Herman *et al.*, 1979; Sahlstrand & Petrusan, 1979; Samberg *et al.*, 1984). Some authors (Leonard, 1981; Dretakis *et al.*, 1988) have reported a higher level of electroencephalograph (EEG) abnormalities in idiopathic scoliotics, but Robb *et al.* (1986) failed to confirm this. Scoliosis is much commoner in children with cerebral palsy. It is likely that some so-called idiopathics have subclinical cortical or subcortical lesions. Unsuspected syrinx formation has been found on MRI scanning in some scoliotics (Isu *et al.*, 1990) and treatment of the syringomyelia by neurosurgical decompression is reported to be beneficial to the scoliosis (see Chapter 54). The absence of abdominal reflexes was reported by Hugus *et al.* (1990) to be the most useful and sometimes the only abnormal neurological sign in patients with syringomyelia and apparently idiopathic scoliosis.

3 Different growth pattern: scoliotic girls are, in general, taller and slimmer than normal, and Nordwall & Willner (1975) found a higher peak growth velocity than normal.

4 Spinal profile: scoliotics have flatter spines than normal, i.e. they are more lordotic in the thoracic region (Willner *et al.*, 1981; Dangerfield *et al.*, 1986). Flexion movements of a lordotic spine will inevitably result in a tendency to lateral rotation, as described by Dickson *et al.* (1984).

5 Kiel *et al.* (1989) have described a fixed and slightly kyphotic segment covering two or three vertebrae below the lordosis, which seems to be a constant factor. Perhaps the rotated lordosis above is secondary to this kyphosis.

6 Burwell and his colleagues (1989) have also identified a correlation between scoliosis and asymmetry of femoral neck anteversion which may result in a torsional moment being applied to the spine via the pelvis with each step.

It is unclear whether some of these factors are primary or secondary to the development of the curvature. No doubt there are other, as yet unidentified, forces at work: why, for instance, when surgery is required for a premenarcheal child, does the rib hump often increase after a solid spinal fusion while the Cobb angle remains the same (Weatherley *et al.*, 1987)? Perhaps the ribs and spine are end-organs responding to subtle neuromuscular forces controlled by the so-called 'central pattern generators' of the central nervous system (Brooks, 1986).

It is probable that one or more of these factors may be predominant in an individual curve, in which case there is less necessity for the other factors to be present.

We have to admit that we are still unable to identify the relevant pieces of the jigsaw in an individual patient to build up a coherent picture which will

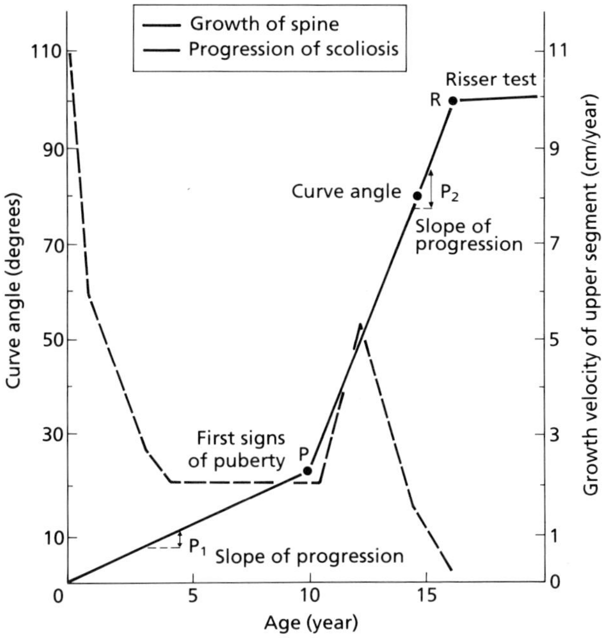

Fig. 22.2 Scheme of progression according to Duval-Beaupère. From Stagnara (1988).

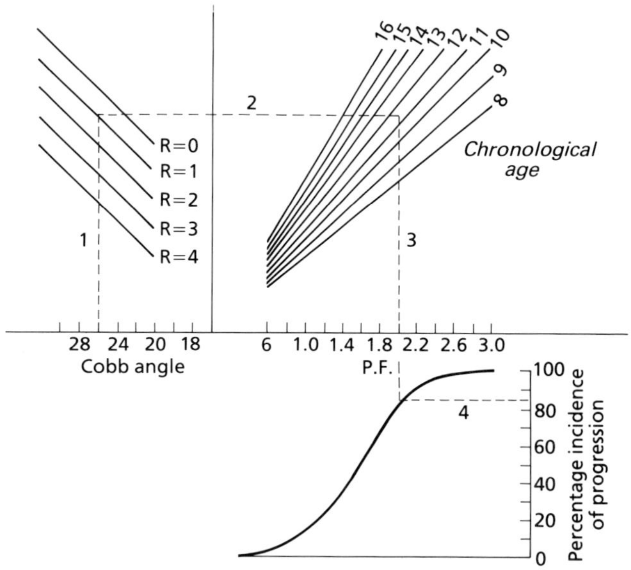

Fig. 22.3 Nomogram constructed for an 11½-year-old child with a 26° curve and a Risser sign of 1. A vertical line (1) is drawn from the Cobb angle to intercept the Risser-sign lines, and a horizontal line (2) is drawn from the intersection of this vertical line and Risser sign 1 (R = 1). Another vertical line (3) is drawn from the intersection of line 2 and the chronological age of 11.5 years, and extended to intersect the progression-factor graph. At the intersection of line 3 and the graph curve, a horizontal line (4) is drawn to the incidence-of-progression axis and the value (85%) is read off. This indicates that there is an 85% chance that the curve will progress. From Lonstein & Carlson (1984).

predict, with certainty, behaviour of an individual curvature. However, there is a general feeling that with continued research it will not be many years before we are able to give an accurate prediction of the natural history of an individual curvature through a full understanding of the causative mechanisms of idiopathic scoliosis.

Duval-Beaupere (1971) reported her studies of scoliosis progression (Fig. 22.2). Her study was carried out using anteroposterior radiographs in the horizontal position. She defined two distinct periods of progression either side of puberty, P1 and P2. Slope P2 indicates the period of rapid growth after puberty. Lonstein & Carlson (1984) (Fig. 22.3), from Minneapolis, have, through a more empirical approach, produced a nomogram combining bone age and Cobb angle to produce a statistically valid prediction of the likely value of the Cobb angle at maturity. Unfortunately, statistical predictions cannot be applied with confidence to the individual, although probabilities are helpful, but they need to be refined so that major decisions can be made with precision, for example the timing of surgery.

We need, in particular, to be able to predict the natural history of a curvature if early, or even prophylactic, surgery is to be considered. If a dominant causative lesion could be identified, such as a kyphotic thoracolumbar segment or marked femoral neck anteversion on one side or pronounced asymmetric rib droop, and we could be sure that a scoliosis would develop as a result, then that lesion could be corrected to prevent the consequences. Clearly, carefully controlled studies would be necessary before such procedures could be recommended.

INDICATIONS FOR SURGERY FOR SPINAL DEFORMITY

The clinical assessment of patients with spinal deformity has been described elsewhere in this book (Chapters 19 & 20). Needless to say, every individual with a significant spinal curvature must be treated as such, and often there will be quite significant differences in the weighting of the various factors which are put in the balance when a decision is being made as to whether or not surgery should be recommended.

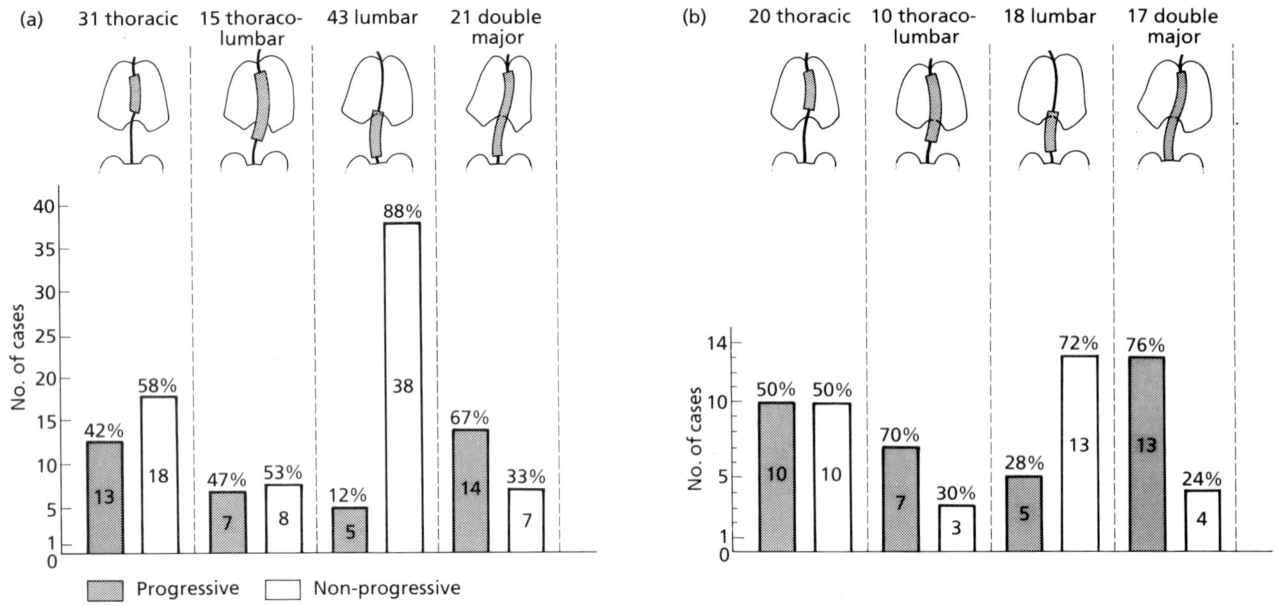

Fig. 22.4 Spontaneous progression of scoliosis from 10° to 29°: stippled columns, having passed 30° at skeletal maturity; clear columns, not having reached 30° at skeletal maturity. (a) Global results; (b) results for juvenile type (Clarisse, 1974). From Stagnara (1988).

A curvature with a Cobb angle of 45° certainly does not always require surgery.

The factors to be considered in approximate order of importance are:

1 curve magnitude,
2 age,
3 flat thoracic spine,
4 pain,
5 external appearance.

These factors will be discussed fully in turn.

Curve magnitude

In general, the threshold for surgery in idiopathic scoliosis is around 40–45° in an adolescent female. In boys, who will often be a year or two older on first presentation, the threshold may be a little higher at 45–50° for two reasons: firstly, cosmetic considerations are not generally as important; and secondly, the curves are often stiffer so that a less satisfactory result is anticipated from surgical correction.

In general, thoracic and thoracolumbar curves are more likely to deteriorate than lumbar curves (Clarisse, 1974) (Fig. 22.4); they also produce a more obvious deformity. The surgical curve threshold for lumbar curves is therefore higher for cosmetic reasons, and also because of a reluctance to fuse below L3 which is more likely to cause long-term pain and stiffness (Edgar & Mehta, 1988).

Double major curves, being well balanced, produce less trunk shift, and they are generally less rotated with a smaller rib hump. Surgery is generally advised for curves in excess of 50°.

Age

The age of the patient when a curvature was first noticed is of considerable importance in determining whether this is an early-onset curve which is likely to produce an ugly and disabling deformity by the end of growth if not treated, or a later-onset curve first becoming noticeable at or after the onset of puberty, which is much less likely to cause pain and disability in later life.

Also of importance is the skeletal age of the patient, which is determined with reference to the atlas of Greulich and Pyle (1959). The left hand and wrist are X-rayed to determine the skeletal age, which gives an indication of the time before skeletal maturity during which the scoliosis may progress relatively rapidly. A less accurate but more practical method of assuming skeletal maturity is that described by Risser (Fig. 22.5). Five stages of excursion of the iliac apophysis are described paralleling development from puberty

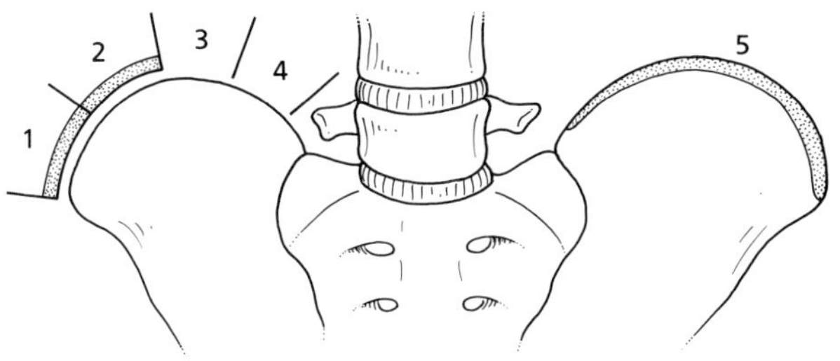

Fig. 22.5 Iliac crest (Risser sign). Skeletal maturity is not precisely definable, but is generally recognized to have occurred when the iliac apophyses have extended to, and fused with, the ilium close to the sacroiliac joint (Risser Stage 5) (Risser, 1958). The ring epiphyses of the vertebral bodies will have disappeared. These changes will generally occur around 4 years after menarche in girls, or puberty in boys.

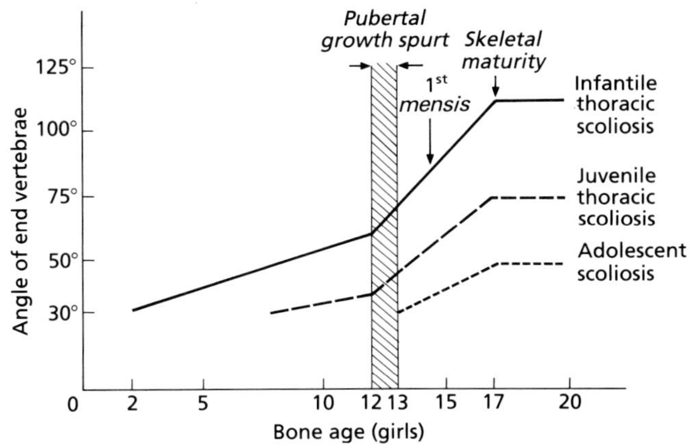

Fig. 22.6 Diagrammatic representation of progression of three types of scoliosis. Skeletal maturity coincides with the end of rapid progression of these curvatures (in fact the most rapid progression occurs just before menarche). From Stagnara (1988).

to skeletal maturity. In general, we can say that the younger the age at presentation of a progressive curve then the more likely it is to progress further and, similarly, the worse the deformity at presentation then the worse it will be at skeletal maturity if the curve is not treated (Fig. 22.6). Curves presenting before menarche or puberty are two or three times more likely to progress than curves presenting afterwards (Lonstein & Carlson, 1984). After skeletal maturity curve progression is much slower: a rule of thumb is that curves tend to progress at a rate of 1° per year through adult life. However, some curves, especially thoracolumbar curves, may go faster and others, especially thoracic curves, may progress less (Collis & Ponseti, 1969).

Patients with spinal curvatures presenting before the age of menarche in girls, and puberty in boys, need to be watched particularly carefully with an erect AP or PA X-ray of the thoracic and lumbar spines being taken every 4–6 months. It has been shown that PA X-rays of the thoracic and lumbar spines result in a significantly smaller radiation dose compared with AP X-rays, although their quality may not be as good (Nash *et al.*, 1979). Unfortunately, since the spine is further from the X-ray plate in a PA X-ray, some detail is lost, which may make it difficult to obtain Cobb angle and other measurements, making repeat X-rays sometimes necessary. Detail of congenital and other lesions may also be obscured. Nash *et al.* (1973) showed that the risk of developing a breast carcinoma was increased from 140 to 290 per million in girls subjected to a three-year Milwaukee brace programme given an average of 22 X-rays. The risk was reduced to 145.3 per million using postero-anterior X-rays. There was no significant risk to other organs and the genetic risk was negligible. Judicious selection and good technical standards were advocated.

A record of the rib hump in the forward-bent position using Bunnel's scoliometer (see Chapter 9), the body contour formulator (Thulborne & Gillespie, 1976) or one of the more elaborate optical methods such as the ISIS scanner, should also be obtained at each consultation (4–6 monthly) during the period of rapid growth prior to skeletal maturity. Less frequent checks (6–12 monthly) are then possible until skeletal maturity is judged to have occurred.

After skeletal maturity, when the curve has been stable on two or three successive visits, it is reasonable to discharge the patient from regular follow-up with the following advice:

1 Your curve is not bad enough to need surgery and you can therefore forget about it and consider your back normal.

2 You may have a little more than your fair share of muscular aching around the shoulders and low back but you would be most unlucky to have major problems. If you are worried in the future seek specialist orthopaedic advice.

3 Curves in excess of 30° Cobb angle may increase slowly over the years, especially thoracolumbar curves. Slowly progressing curves may become symptomatic in late middle age with the onset of spondylotic changes in the tilted vertebrae and discs.

There is some evidence that curvatures may increase more rapidly if pregnancy occurs before the age of 23 years (A. Nachemson, 1983, personal communication).

4 There is a small chance that your children could have a spinal curvature with the daughters much more likely to be affected. Around 20% of people with spinal curvatures have a scoliotic relative. It would be wise to make sure that your daughters are screened at the age of 11 or 12 by bending them forward and looking along the spine for any asymmetry (the Adams test).

Clearly, not all these points will be relevant to every patient, but it is certainly helpful to morale to encourage the patient to lead a normal social, working and sporting life. The girls, and also the boys perhaps to a lesser extent, need to feel that their body image is not seriously compromised and that they are, in fact, normal people with a minor idiosyncrasy which may have to be watched from time to time.

The same positive attitude should, of course, be encouraged in patients who have undergone surgical correction of their curvatures. It is perhaps wise to warn surgically treated patients against the most strenuous and dangerous sports such as horse riding, rugby and American football and other violent body contact sports. Boys should be advised to earn their living with their brains rather than their backs.

We still have no way of predicting the natural history of an individual curve so all must be carefully observed. There are, however, some adverse features which signal the likelihood of a bad prognosis. These are: a noticeably lordotic appearance to the curve, marked rotation with a more prominent rib hump than would be expected for a given Cobb angle, premenarcheal presentation with a curve greater than 30°, rapid growth and joint laxity. The more of these factors that are present, the worse the prognosis. Classification of these curvatures into early-onset and late-onset types is helpful in determining the treatment programme for a particular deformity. This classification was agreed by the British Scoliosis Society in 1986 and is described elsewhere in this book.

Flat thoracic spine

It is generally accepted that patients with noticeably flat thoracic spines (hypokyphosis) have a worse prognosis so far as curve development is concerned. It is reasonable to fuse these curves earlier, but if the patient is prepubertal or premenarcheal it is wise to prevent anterior growth of the apical vertebrae by a transthoracic epiphyseodesis, otherwise a lordosis may develop with growth and the rib hump often increases sharply (Hefti & McMaster, 1983). Unfortunately, anterior fusion does not always prevent increasing rib hump in the immature patient (the crankshaft effect). Patients and their relatives should be warned of this.

Severe thoracic lordosis rarely occurs in idiopathic scoliosis. It can, however, occur in neuromuscular scoliosis and early surgery may be essential to prevent a serious reduction in lung volume.

Pain

It seems remarkable that with such a major structural abnormality as, say, a 30° scoliotic curve, the prevalence of significant pain is variously reported as around 20% (Nachemson *et al.*, 1979), i.e. little above the normal prevalence of back pain in the general population. In general, the older the patient the more likely he or she is to have pain, and on close questioning, most teenagers will admit to some aching at times, particularly after sitting for long periods at school, especially for examinations and particularly towards the end of the day. Aches and pains are generally felt in the region of the rib prominence, usually on the right side of the posterior chest wall, but sometimes in the interscapular and suprascapular regions. A few may complain of upper cervical aching with occipital headaches, usually on the same side as the curvature. Others may complain of low back pain, usually ligamentous in character, usually on the contralateral side to the curve over the posterior iliac crest (Fig. 22.7), often in association with a centimetre or so of pelvic obliquity in the standing position, the left side of the pelvis being palpably lower than the right. (Some shortening, usually left-sided, from the ilium to the foot is common in scoliotics, especially those with lumbar curves, and is presumably part of the growth asymmetry associated with the development of scoliosis.)

All these aches and pains are mechanical in type, and it is certainly very rare to have true nerve root involvement in non-congenital scoliosis before degenerative changes begin in middle age. These symptoms, which are not usually disabling, should be treated initially in the same way as similar symp-

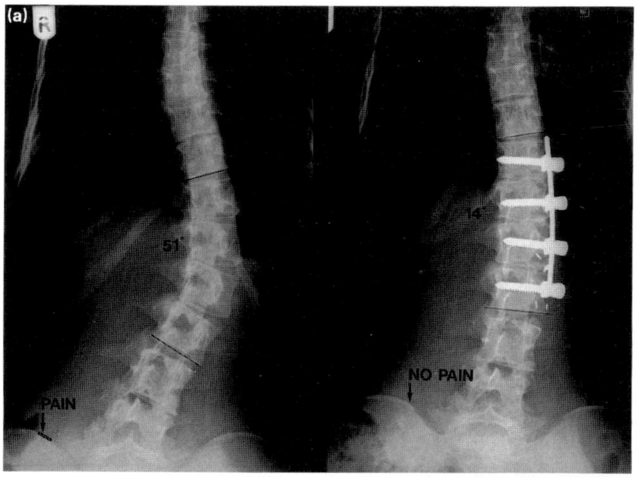

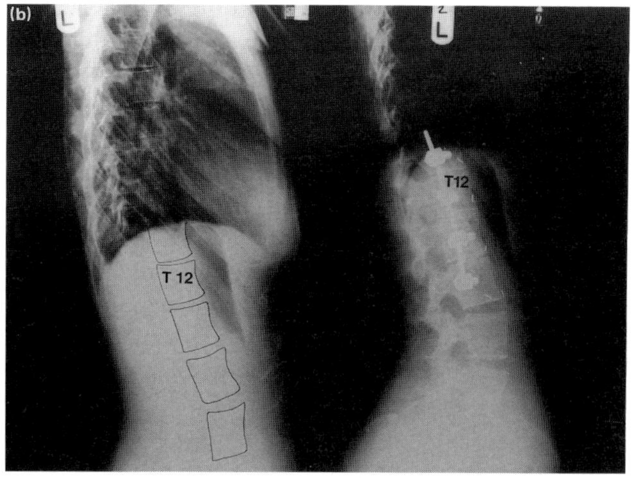

Fig. 22.7 (a) A 32-year-old nursing sister before and one year after surgery with the anterior Webb–Morley technique. Pain is located at the insertion point of the main 'guy ropes' of the spine, namely the iliolumbar ligament, the lumbar fascia and the body wall muscles. One year after surgery she has no pain and for five months has been working normally in a home for the elderly. (b) The lateral view of the same patient. The rod has been slightly contoured to avoid kyphosis.

toms occurring in non-scoliotic patients, that is by physical therapy with manipulation, ultrasound or deep soft tissue massage or by an injection of 5–10 ml of local anaesthetic and a suitable steroid, often combined with physical therapy.

If such treatment is unhelpful, or only temporarily effective, then it may be assumed that the continuing mechanical stresses caused by the scoliosis are at the root of the problem. Some back pains may resolve at skeletal maturity as the tissues mature, but occasionally they become established as a chronic or recurrent problem needing maintenance therapy when necessary.

The presence of significant pain not responding to simple treatment requires further investigation to identify the pain source. If it is eventually decided by a process of elimination and by clinical judgement that the pain is caused by abnormal mechanical stresses as a result of the scoliosis, then this will be a relative indication for surgery. No guarantee can, of course, be given that correction and stabilization of a curve will abolish the pain, but logic dictates that such treatment will probably be beneficial, and this is usually the case in practice.

In general, thoracic pains are much more likely to be improved or eliminated by surgery, but cervical and lumbar pains may persist. The presence of pelvic obliquity in the standing position may be a continuing source of lumbar strain after curve correction. A heel raise can be useful but if a block of more than 2.5–3 cm is required under the foot to level the pelvis then a growth control procedure on the long leg is indicated if the child is young enough; if not, resection of a segment of femur is occasionally necessary and gives good results.

It should be noted that the presence of persistent spinal pain, especially if accompanied by muscle spasm, may indicate intraspinal pathology such as a tumour, juvenile disc prolapse or osteoid osteoma. A significant list or tilt with muscle spasm, with little vertebral rotation, particularly merits further investigation. Isotope scanning will detect an osteoid osteoma, a source of infection and most tumours. Magnetic resonance imaging (MRI) will indicate most pathological lesions and any neural compression, as will thoracic and lumbar myelography. Computerized tomography (CT) scanning may be useful in defining the extent of the lesion once it has been located by these other methods.

The likelihood of future pain is often an important consideration in advising surgery. Unfortunately, without the gift of clairvoyance, there is often little evidence to support a confident prediction. It seems reasonable to assume that if there is pain at present, then there may be pain in the future, but the majority of children with deformities severe enough for surgery have little or no pain.

Nachemson *et al.* (1979) have shown that the

prevalence of pain in scoliotics is no higher than that in the general population. What we do not know is whether scoliotics have the same types of back pain as others, or whether their pain is more severe or resistant to treatment in the presence of the abnormal mechanics created by the spinal deformity. It is even possible that the lordotic deformity of scoliosis, especially in the lumbar spine, protects against some types of spinal pain. There is an impression that acute lumbar disc prolapses are rare in thoracolumbar and lumbar scoliotics.

It is the experience of most established scoliosis surgeons that adult scoliotics with apparent postural and mechanical pain are considerably relieved of symptoms by stabilization and partial correction of their deformity to achieve spinal balance by one of the more modern techniques (see also Chapter 23). It therefore seems reasonable to believe that since reduction of deformity relieves pain, then the deformity must have been a major factor in the development of the pain. The assertion that scoliosis is not an important cause of spinal pain in adults seems difficult to sustain.

Curvatures greater than 30° increase on average by about 1° per year during adult life, but thoracic curves often stabilize at 70–90° in middle age as the ribs on the concave side gradually come together. The lumbar spine is much less stable and thoracolumbar and lumbar curves may become painful as sheering displacements develop in middle age in the midlumbar levels compounded by degenerative changes particularly affecting the concave facet joints. The presence of sheering displacement, often called a 'translation', at one or more midlumbar levels probably carries a bad prognosis and is a relative indication for stabilizing surgery.

External appearance

Although there is a general correlation between Cobb angle and vertebral rotation, there are certainly considerable individual variations. The same applies to the relationship between vertebral rotation and rib hump prominence. This means that a patient with an adolescent idiopathic scoliosis with a Cobb angle of 40° may have quite marked vertebral rotation with a sharp rib hump for which surgery may well be advisable. Another 40° curvature may, on the other hand, have relatively slight rotation with a flat rib hump, and in the absence of other symptoms and approaching skeletal maturity surgery would probably not be advised.

For example, there is, at present, a handsome 18-year-old, with a 59° idiopathic curve who is a prominent fashion model in London. She definitely does not want surgery as she has a fairly rounded rib prominence, but 17° of rotation by scoliometer. She also has a very supple but painless spine and her unusual postural abilities seem to give her an advantage over her straight-spined colleagues! A scar on her back would ruin her career. Similarly, a well-built 17-year-old boy who has had a late growth spurt and is now approaching skeletal maturity, with a 55° curve which is stiff on bending X-rays, with a moderate rib prominence and no significant pain, will also be quite reasonably advised against surgery. That option is still available in future years if the situation changes. The cosmetic appearance is relatively less important to such a patient, although he should be advised to earn his living with his brain rather than his back.

Recommendations for surgery for scoliosis on cosmetic grounds must always be qualified by the understanding that, although traditional surgical techniques are quite good at correcting the Cobb angle on X-ray they are, in general, less good at correcting vertebral rotation, and even where this is achieved, the resulting correction of the rib hump may still be disappointing. We can, however, usually achieve a levelling of the shoulders, some longitudinal spreading of the rib hump and some elevation of the depressed ribs on the concave side.

It seems that the main improvement in trunk shape after surgical correction of scoliosis results from the shift of the apex of the curve and its attached ribs towards the midline, i.e. improvement in the apical vertebral displacement. This is probably a better measure of surgical success than the Cobb angle (Gardner, 1991).

All these factors combine to make for a better external appearance even though objective measurements of rib rotation may be little changed. One can advise patients that there will be about a 50% improvement in the overall appearance of their back, and avoid mentioning specific measurements.

We must remember also that, in idiopathic scoliosis, the usual right-sided posterior rib prominence is accompanied by left-sided posterior rib depression with anterior left-sided rib prominence and right-sided rib depression. In other words, the whole rib

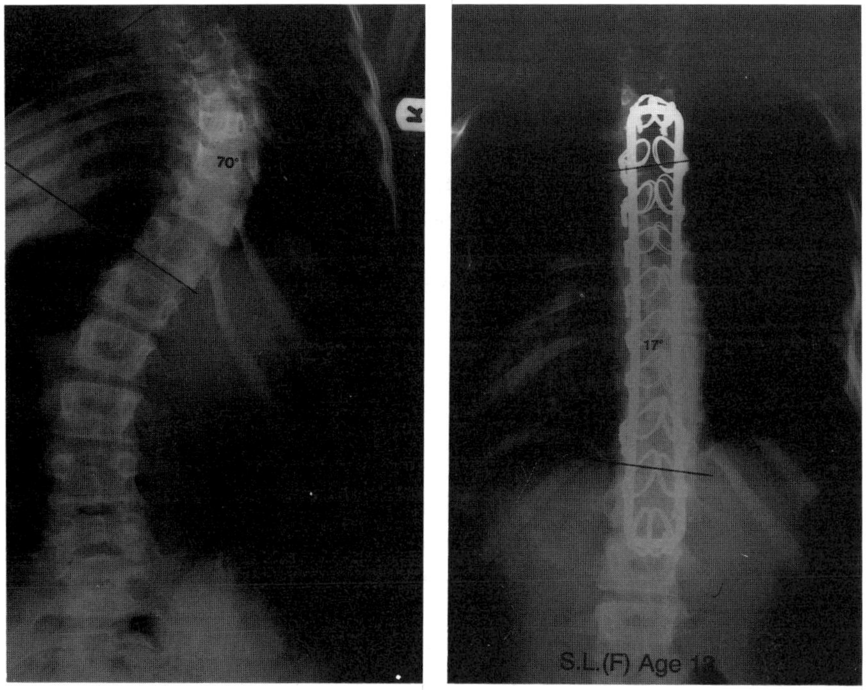

Fig. 22.8 Radiographs showing the powerful corrective ability of Luque segmental sublaminar wiring combined with the Dove–Hartshill rectangle. Spinal cord monitoring is desirable when such major corrections are obtained. In over 10 years experience the author has had no permanent major or minor neurological deficit when using sublaminar wiring techniques for idiopathic scoliosis. It is important to note that other surgeons have reported neurological complications with sublaminar wiring.

cage is rotated, and in girls the left breast will often be much more prominent than the right, which is a component of the deformity often noticed more by the patient herself, who cannot see her back. These patients are often worried that there may be something wrong with their apparently smaller right breast, and are reassured by this explanation. Most patients will increase their height by 2–4 cm after surgery to an idiopathic curve of around 50°. This information is usually well received as an indication that the spine has been considerably straightened.

The above comments certainly apply to the traditional Harrington, Harrington–Luque and early Hartshill–Luque techniques.

In the 1980s, however, powerful new instrumentations became available. These are the complex, technically demanding and expensive Cotrel–Dubousset (CD) system from France (see Fig. 22.13) and the simpler, relatively cheap but also technically demanding Hartshill–Luque system (Fig. 22.8; see also Fig. 22.10) based on the technique of Luque and developed by Dove in the UK. Both these systems rely on multisegmental attachment to the spine of very strong steel rods contoured to the required shape. Such 'overwhelming instrumentation' is capable of correcting substantially, and maintaining correction of, vertebral rotation in the short term. However, follow-up studies of a year or more after surgery show a disappointing tendency for vertebral rotation to recur almost to the preoperative value. Apical vertebral displacement and Cobb angle show only slight loss of correction (Gardner, 1991).

As a result of the very secure fixation achieved with these newer systems it is possible to eliminate, or greatly reduce, the need for postoperative immobilization and bracing. However, in practice many patients feel vulnerable and apprehensive about their backs after such major surgery, and some form of light spinal protection during the first six to eight weeks certainly provides peace of mind for patient and parents, and will also help to prevent slippage of instrumentation with loss of correction, which may occasionally occur.

The CD and Hartshill–Luque techniques are complex, but when correctly performed, these operations, although more prolonged and complicated, produce a pleasing result with simple and relatively quick rehabilitation to a normal life, including sport, within six months. The risk of complications, including paraplegia, is very small, although slightly greater than for a simple Harrington rod (Dove, 1989).

It should be appreciated that the factors listed above constitute the main data on which the surgeon makes up his mind as to whether surgery for a spinal deformity should be advised. However, it goes without saying, but is sometimes forgotten, that the patient and his or her family will also have a point of view which should certainly be expressed. Frequently, the parents feel guilty, either at not having noticed the curvature before, or because they have produced an imperfect offspring. These feelings are particularly strong if one or other parent has a scoliosis, and need to be talked about and put in context so that parents and child are reassured that the situation in which they find themselves is certainly not too unusual, and that they are not alone in facing such problems.

A scoliosis self-help group is often useful in this context, and it is also very helpful for families to be put in touch with other families who have a child with a similar condition who has finished treatment. In the UK there is the Scoliosis Association UK (SAUK), 380–384 Harrow Rd, London W9 2HU.

Some parents may feel angry at any delay, real or apparent, that has occurred in the treatment of their child in the past and, again, it is helpful to explain the natural history of the condition, its relative rarity and the uncertainty as to whether, even if it had been discovered earlier, anything effective could have been done.

Recent studies show that 10–20% of children who come through school screening and then bracing programmes eventually require surgery for their curvatures (Miller *et al.*, 1984). This is, of course, disappointing after 3 or 4 years of perseverance with bracing and the children should have been prepared for this eventuality at the start of their treatment. Once again, time spent in explanation of all the relevant facts and possibilities is always time well spent in alleviating fear and misunderstanding which, if allowed to persist, can affect the relationship with the treatment team and therefore the quality of the treatment. In extreme cases in some communities, litigation may result if discussion time is neglected.

The matter of whether or not bracing or electrical stimulation are worthwhile treatments for adolescent idiopathic scoliosis is, at present, very controversial and will not be covered in this section (see Chapter 20). It can be argued that since modern surgical techniques are so effective and safe, and have a relatively rapid recovery time, this is a more desirable option than several years of bracing during the sensitive years of adolescence with a chance of surgery being eventually necessary anyway.

SELECTION OF SURGICAL TECHNIQUE

The reader will no doubt be aware that there is a confusing number of named surgical techniques available for the treatment of scoliosis and kyphosis, and that the spine can be approached surgically either posteriorly or anteriorly. It is therefore necessary for the individual surgeon who wishes to manage spinal deformity in all its aspects to gain expertise in a sufficient range of techniques to produce the best possible results for his or her patients with a minimum of risk, consistent with any constraints of time or finance within which he or she may have to operate.

In these days of rising expectations from our patients, which we try to satisfy with increasingly complex surgical procedures, there is no doubt that scoliosis surgery should be carried out only in specialized units by experienced surgeons who perform these procedures with sufficient frequency to maintain the highest possible standards. The surgeon, of course, does require the backing of a well-trained team to ensure that he or she has the right equipment, skilled anaesthesia, good postoperative pain relief for the patient, sympathetic and experienced nurses and physiotherapists and good orthotic and outpatient systems. A surgeon working in isolation, however skilful the technique, will quickly become isolated by his poor results.

In selecting a surgical procedure for a deformed spine we must first define our objectives. Our prime aim must be to stabilize the spine and prevent deterioration but, as a bonus, with modern surgical techniques we can also offer the patient substantial correction of the deformity, provided it is flexible. To achieve these aims we must obtain solid bony fusion independent of the instrumentation. If solid fusion is not obtained there is no available implant able to maintain correction without eventually displacing or breaking, with resulting loss of correction and pain developing at the site of the pseudarthrosis.

Stiffer curves do not allow as much correction as flexible curves. Mobilizing procedures such as facetectomy and anterior discectomy may prove disappointing, and closing wedge osteotomy or vertebrectomy may be necessary to obtain flexibility. Such major procedures often require anterior and posterior instrumentation.

Flexibility is assessed in the case of scoliosis by erect lateral bending X-rays to left and right, and for kyphosis, erect and supine views, with traction if necessary, will give the required information. The lateral bending views will also give valuable information on the mobility and movement pattern of the motion segments at either end of the curve, which will help determine the upper and lower levels of instrumentation.

LEVELS OF INSTRUMENTATION

Clearly, the spine must be stabilized over an adequate length to ensure long-term stability, but it is important to save as many thoracic and lumbar discs as possible to preserve function and avoid subsequent postural pain and degenerative change. The length of the stabilized segment will depend on

1 The length of the rotated and relatively fixed deformed segment of the spine.

2 The age of the patient. The immature patient with significant growth to come should always be fused to include one segment above and below the neutral vertebra. The neutral vertebra is that vertebra at either end of a rotated structural scoliosis which, on any erect sagittal X-ray, has its spinous process in the midline, its pedicles symmetrical and has an unwedged, parallel-sided disc adjacent to it.

3 The site of the curvature. With single or double major curves extending into the lumbar region it is very important to preserve the maximum number of mobile lumbar discs consistent with an adequate and long-lasting correction. If possible, instrumentation and fusion should not go below the third lumbar vertebra and the L3–L4 and lower discs should eventually be as horizontal and unwedged as possible. Fusions below L3 result in a considerably raised incidence of long-term low back pain, and the patient is much more aware of stiffness in the spine (Edgar *et al.*, 1983). Badly angulated discs below the fusion are also more likely to cause late low back pain. Another cause of late pain is failure to contour the implant in the sagittal plane, which produces strain on the remaining mobile discs above or below the fusion.

4 Anterior techniques, such as the Dwyer and the Zielke, with their great ability to derotate the lumbar vertebrae, certainly have a place, as it may often be possible to leave mobile an extra lumbar disc. The more recently introduced heavy segmental instrumentation systems of Cotrel and Dubousset (CD), and the Hartshill–Luque system, also derotate to a useful extent, leaving the remaining lumbar discs more horizontal, but it remains to be seen whether they are quite as efficient in this respect as anterior surgery. (For illustrations of these techniques see Figs 22.8–22.15.)

5 Instrumentation above T4 is best avoided, as there is probably a higher incidence of cervicothoracic aching with higher fusions (Nachemson, 1979). Again, it is of great importance to ensure correct sagittal contouring of the instrumentation to avoid postural pain, and also to avoid visible or painful prominence of the upper extremity of the metal, which could as a result require subsequent surgical removal.

In general, fusion is usually carried from neutral vertebra to neutral vertebra, or one vertebra beyond this in the immature patient. Selection of the fusion level is relatively easy in a single idiopathic curve, but more difficult in double curves with a significantly rotated lumbar deformity. The wish to span the two curves to gain maximum correction conflicts with the wish to preserve mobile lumbar discs to ensure good function and freedom from long-term soft tissue pain.

As mentioned above, in double major curves fusion below L3 is undesirable but, on the other hand, a shorter fusion with wedged or non-horizontal discs below it is also likely to result in future low back strain. The CD technique offers a possible solution to this dilemma, with its ability to derotate powerfully a rotated L3 vertebra, but the instrumentation of double curves with this technique is difficult. The Harrington–Luque procedure is also helpful for double major curves in that it has good longitudinal stability and, with skilful contouring, it is possible to derotate the L3 vertebra to some extent. The Hartshill–Luque system is probably less satisfactory in this connection, as its main action is one of correction by transverse traction rather than by longitudinal distraction. It is therefore less stable when considerable lengthening of the spine is required, as when correcting double curves.

A double major curve requires considerable distraction to achieve good alignment. The degrees of rotation of the two components of a double major curve are in opposite directions and are, therefore, usually less than the unidirectional rotation of a single curve; therefore less derotation is required in treating these curves. The Harrington–Luque operation is a relatively simple and satisfactory technique for double major curves (Fig. 22.9). In the author's experience it is rarely necessary to fuse below L3 in double major curves. For further reading on the subject of fusion level the article by King *et al.* (1983) is recommended but the temptation to over-classify should be resisted. Thoracolumbar and lumbar curves are often best corrected anteriorly, and often fusion below L3 can be avoided.

Considerable emphasis has been placed on the importance of leaving the spine mobile below the third lumbar vertebra as this reflects the fact that our patients now demand to be regarded as normal, and that is certainly our objective. It is no good producing a geometrically straight X-ray held by extensive instrumentation into the lower lumbar spine if the patient looks and feels stiff, and develops mechanical low back pain. It is better to accept the persistence of some relatively mild deformity than to precipitate the onset of much more troublesome symptoms of chronic or recurrent low back pain which may prove more disabling than the original scoliosis. Such patients may return to haunt one's consulting room in 10 years' time! (See Fig. 22.10.)

CONSENT FOR SURGERY

If surgery is to be the treatment of choice then the consent of the patient, or of his or her legally competent representatives, must be obtained. Clearly, for this consent to have any ethical meaning, it can only be given against a background of an acceptably full understanding of the main characteristics of the operative procedure, along with its expected risks and benefits. The term 'informed consent' is commonly used to express this concept. What precisely constitutes 'an acceptable level of understanding' of an operation or 'an acceptable level of care and skill' by a surgeon remains debatable and forms a source of income for many members of the legal profession. To summarize: in the UK a doctor's duty of care is judged, among other criteria, by the Bolam test, which states: 'a doctor's duty is fulfilled if the doctor acts in accordance with a practice rightly accepted as proper by a body of skilled and experienced medical men'. In the USA the criteria are more stringent from the surgeon's point of view. The level of informed consent is judged by the so-called 'prudent patient test', which implies that 'all material risks' of which a prudent patient would wish to be aware must be explained by the surgeon. This definition is also open to differences of interpretation but overall, the physician is judged according to the standards of the community in which he practises.

As well as having sufficient information at their disposal on which to base consent for a surgical operation, a patient, or his or her legally competent representatives, must also trust a surgeon and his team to exercise an acceptable level of skill and care, both at the time of operation and subsequently. At the same time, it is also only reasonable that a surgeon advising an operation should expect a patient or his or her legally competent representatives to have given the surgeon a truthful and full account of his or her pathological condition in response to the surgeon's questions, and to provide a satisfactory level of cooperation and obedience to instructions after surgery. In other words, there exists a requirement for knowledge and trust on both sides prior to any major operation. If a significant deficiency in these requirements is detected on either side then, clearly, it is better that surgery does not go ahead until the deficiency has, if possible, been remedied.

In the United Kingdom it has been generally necessary for a patient to prove that he or she has been treated negligently for a damages claim against a doctor or hospital to succeed. There is a proposal that under EEC law that the burden of proof will be reversed so that it will be for the doctor or hospital to prove that negligence has not taken place. This, of course, will take some time to be considered by the EEC and national governments but if ratified its effects will be far reaching.

The prevailing customs with regard to surgical consent do, of course, vary widely in Europe, the USA and elsewhere in the world. It is also an unfortunate fact that in some countries the consent procedures may be inadequate, either in fact or by allegation, so as to form the basis for litigation by patients and their legal advisers who may or may not have a genuine grievance.

One of the major difficulties in this field is, of course, the fact that surgeons and their patients are only human, and they have to communicate with each other. It is well known that, in spite of a full explanation by a surgeon, the patient's perception of, and memory for, what has been said is invariably incomplete and often garbled by pre-existing prejudices derived from so-called friends, popular magazines and other sources. The more technical and complex the surgeon's language, the worse the misunderstanding.

The following phrases, if relevant, have been found

useful in practice: 'One side of your body has been growing a little faster than the other but the rest of you is normal.' 'Some people have bent noses, you have a bend in your back.' 'I can't make your back perfect but it will be a lot better, although not normal.' 'Your spine will be straightened like training a rose up a trellis.' 'The bone graft comes from rearranging the existing bone in the back.' (Many surgeons take additional graft from the pelvis.) 'You should know that all major operations have complications but, fortunately, these are relatively rare in spinal surgery. The main ones are an occasional flaw in the bone graft which may need repairing and result in adjustments to the metalwork a year or so after the operation; also infection occasionally occurs, and I have to mention the rare possibility of paralysis which may be temporary or permanent.'

Patients, of course, come with all levels of intelligence, fortitude and family background. The surgeon will intuitively have to gear his explanation and advice accordingly. The majority of patients and their parents are pleasant and straightforward, but beware of complications such as a pending or recent divorce or other emotional problems.

One intelligent patient may say 'Doctor, you are the expert. I trust you to play your part. I do not wish to know the detail as it scares me/makes me feel ill.' On the other hand, another patient may demand to know the minutest detail of technique and complication, perhaps to satisfy an insecurity. Both extremes must be catered for by the surgeon with patience and understanding.

In legally active societies it must be documented that an adequate explanation of the risks and benefits of the operation has been given, and that this was understood by the patient or his or her legally competent representatives so that they can give adequately informed consent.

In the UK it is now necessary to inform a patient and/or the relatives prior to scoliosis surgery of the possible major complications. These include paralysis, infection and the possibility of future surgery, either for bone graft failure or for removal or adjustment of an implant. There should be some indication of the expected likelihood of such complications. It is also necessary to record in the clinical notes at the time that such information has been given.

The British Scoliosis Society in 1988 produced a special consent form which covers the possibility of neurological complications from spinal cord damage resulting from scoliosis surgery. This form is for use in addition to, and not instead of, the customary full explanation of this and other complications by the surgeon (see Chapter 44).

PREOPERATIVE INVESTIGATION

The assessment of patients with spinal conditions has been covered elsewhere in this book, but it is relevant to describe the essential preoperative work-up for children and adolescents with scoliosis or kyphosis.

A record of the important features of the patient and his or her spinal deformity will have been taken during the outpatient assessment. These will need to be confirmed or re-recorded if the patient was last seen more than, say, three months previously. The objective of the preoperative assessment is to assemble all the necessary facts to ensure a precise diagnosis, record any complicating factors such as drug allergies, asthma or pre-existing neurological deficits which may affect anaesthesia, surgical technique or the recovery from surgery.

It is helpful if, before coming into hospital, both the patient and the parents are supplied with the names and telephone numbers of previous patients and parents who have undergone similar surgery and who are prepared to discuss their experiences. This removes many irrational apprehensions and provides reassurance that there is a future after such surgery. It may be advantageous for the patient and parents to have visited the hospital ward to meet the nursing staff and they may also talk with a liaison officer who can answer individual points of detail concerning schooling, transport, management at home, etc., which may not have been fully covered by the surgeon. Patients for scoliosis surgery are normally admitted to hospital one to three days prior to surgery to allow familiarization with the nursing staff and equipment. As many as possible of the blood and other tests and X-rays are done as an outpatient prior to admission. The preoperative work-up consists of the following tests and procedures:

1 Full radiological examination, including up-to-date erect AP or PA and lateral X-rays with sagittal side bending films to indicate the movement pattern and flexibility of the scoliosis (see Fig. 22.9a,b). For patients with a marked rib hump a tangential longitudinal X-ray with the patient bending forward to skyline the rib hump (see Fig. 22.11d) is useful in showing whether the rib hump contains lung tissue, in which case it can be improved surgically, but if it contains vertebral body and transverse process then little can be done. For kyphosis, erect and supine films, perhaps with a pad beneath the kyphos, or a traction film, will indicate the flexibility of the kyphosis. CT and MRI scanning and myelography are usually not necessary unless there is any indication of a spinal cord or nerve root abnormality, or where there is a sharp angular curve—as for example in dysplastic neurofibromatosis. Any congenital anomaly of the spine, possibly including a spina bifida occulta, or any clinical neurological deficit relating to the spinal cord or nerve roots, needs such further investigation. It is, of course, desirable to keep radiation exposure to sensitive parts such as the developing breast and gonads to a minimum but, on the other hand, excessive screening or poor-quality films which may necessitate repeat exposures, will defeat this objective.

2 All patients should be weighed and their height measured standing and sitting, and the rib hump should be recorded with the Bunnell scoliometer or the body contour formulator (see Chapter 9). These baseline measurements will serve to compare with future measurements after surgery. More sophisticated measurements of surface shape, such as the ISIS scanner, can be used with advantage.

3 It is desirable that the patient should be photographed in standard anteroposterior, posteroanterior, left profile, right profile and forward-bending positions. There is then a clear record of the external deformity for later comparison.

4 Respiratory function tests. The anaesthetist will require the FEV_1 (forced expiratory volume in 1 second) and the FVC (forced vital capacity) values. Blood gas measurements should also be done. These measurements are only likely to be altered significantly in scolioses in excess of 70° Cobb angle.

5 Blood tests. It is usual to cross-match 6 units of blood. This may consist of up to 2 units withdrawn from the patient previously. Recycling of blood withdrawn through the sucker at surgery and through the drains is rarely used in the UK where good blood donor services exist, but is common in the USA. A full blood profile is necessary, along with more specialized investigations if there is any family history of such rare conditions as hyperpyrexia, dysautonomia, bleeding tendencies, etc.

6 A full clinical examination must be made to ensure that the patient has no previously undiscovered heart, lung or neurological abnormality. In other words, the patient must be found to be fit for anaesthesia and surgery.

7 The patient will be seen by a physiotherapist who will teach breathing and bed exercises and give instructions in any specialized apparatus, such as respirators, which may be thought to be necessary.

8 A positive and friendly attitude by all concerned will help to allay anxiety, and provision should be made for a parent to stay with the child for the first few nights after surgery if requested. An experienced member of the nursing staff should talk to the parents and ensure that they know and understand the ward routine, and that they appreciate the necessity for various drips, drains and catheters after surgery. All efforts should be made to allay anxiety so that the child and its parents are as relaxed as is possible under the circumstances.

SURGICAL TECHNIQUES

Introduction

The modern era of spinal surgery can be said to have started with the development by Paul Harrington of the first safe and satisfactory spinal implant. This achieved added correction and provided stability which, along with adequate external support, prevented loss of correction during the first 4–6 months after surgery while the bone graft develops sufficient strength of its own.

Harrington's method, first described in 1960 and initially much criticized, became the standard method of instrumentation in scoliosis surgery around the world (Harrington, 1962, 1972). The Harrington rod does, of course, depend for its success on an adequate spinal fusion, and it remains a matter of regret that we can only correct one structural abnormality, a spinal curvature, by introducing another one, a stiff spinal segment. The stiff straighter spine is, of course, almost always, but certainly not invariably, a more benign deformity than a relatively severe mobile curve.

Perhaps the day will come before too long when the causes of idiopathic scoliosis are sufficiently well understood so that it will be possible to perform relatively minor prophylactic surgery on selected patients at an early stage before the development of a significant deformity. This may then prevent the progressive development of a scoliotic curve which may well be secondary to, and triggered by, one or more initiating abnormalities, themselves amenable to surgical or other treatment.

The 1970s was the decade of certainties in scoliosis treatment. Curvatures in excess of 25° were braced and those that continued to progress or were seen late, and reached a Cobb angle of 40–45°, underwent surgery with a Harrington rod more or less regardless of age and curve type. The only exception to this was the introduction of Dwyer's anterior corrective procedure for thoracolumbar and lumbar curves, first described in 1969.

The Dwyer technique (Dwyer *et al.*, 1969) (see Figs 22.10 & 22.11) was first used for post-polio scoliotics, but it gradually became apparent that superior derotation to that achieved by any posterior procedure resulted in superior corrections and a reduction in the number of discs which had to be fused. Again, the success of the Dwyer technique depended on the development and popularization of anterior approaches to the spine developed by Hodgson and his colleagues in Hong Kong (Hodgson & Stock, 1956; Hodgson *et al.*, 1960) by Leatherman (1969) in the USA and by Cauchoix in France in the 1950s (Cauchoix & Binet, 1956). The author was privileged to assist at some of the early operations carried out by Dwyer in Hong Kong in 1969/70.

Zielke from West Germany described his modification of the Dwyer system in 1976 (Zielke *et al.*, 1976; Moe *et al.*, 1983; see Fig. 22.15) the main difference being the substitution of a solid rod for Dwyer's flexible cable. This gave better stability and, more important, enabled control of the sagittal curve of the spine preventing, to a significant extent, the formation of a relative kyphosis which could occur after Dwyer's procedure (Wojcik *et al.*, 1990).

The next major development was the description by Luque in 1977 (Luque, 1977, 1982) of his method of segmental spinal instrumentation in which sublaminar wires at each level of the curvature were used to attach the spine to stainless-steel rods either side of the spinous processes which could be bent to the required shape. His technique became widely popular in many countries, including the USA and UK, but it became associated with a reported higher incidence of neurological complications, perhaps through inappropriate use, so that it is now much less used and is reserved mainly for patients with neuromuscular disease (Allen, 1984).

In the UK, Dove at Stoke-on-Trent has developed Luque's instrumentation further, and produced the Hartshill rectangle which, in its heavy 6 mm version available since 1988, has, in the author's view, proved to be a very satisfactory and relatively inexpensive implant for the correction of idiopathic scoliosis (Fig. 22.8). A slightly increased incidence of neurological complications with sublaminar wiring has been confirmed in the UK. Dove in 1989 reported a morbidity study conducted among the active surgeons in the British Scoliosis Society. The incidence of significant neurological complications in 130 Harrington–Luque operations was 3 (2.3%). In 339 Luque rod and Luque rectangle operations it was 0.5% compared with 0.32% of 348 Harrington distraction operations. The conclusion is that sublaminar wiring by itself causes little if any extra risk over distraction, but the combination of sublaminar wiring *and* distraction is more dangerous.

Many surgeons have found that a Harrington rod, combined with sublaminar wiring (the Harrington–Luque procedure) was satisfactory for idiopathic scoliosis. It provided superior longitudinal stability by virtue of the hook at each end when compared with a Luque or Hartshill rectangle and, in addition, the added stability of sublaminar wires was superior to a Harrington rod alone, requiring 2–3 months of postoperative bracing compared with 6 months or more for the simple Harrington rod (Fig. 22.9). Most reports have shown no improvement in correction of either the Cobb angle or of vertebral rotation when compared with a Harrington rod alone. This accords with the author's experience and similar results were obtained with the original Luque technique and the earlier 5 mm diameter Hartshill rectangle. However, improved stability with shorter postoperative bracing and a quicker return to normality were significant advantages.

In a series of 18 unselected patients the heavy 6 mm diameter Hartshill rectangle with 18 SWG cold worked semi-annealed Surgicraft wires produced significantly greater improvements in Cobb angle compared with previous techniques 1 year after surgery. Vertebral derotation, as measured by the Perdriolle method, was also improved compared with the Harrington rod, Harrington–Luque and Luque techniques (Targett & Gardner, 1989).

In 1985 Cotrel and Dubousset reported their new (CD) posterior segmental instrumentation of the spine in which multiple hooks are inserted with the bifid distraction hooks engaging the pedicles and with compression hooks in the extradural space. The hooks are then mounted on a pair of heavy-gauge CD rods, one on each side of the midline. These rods are

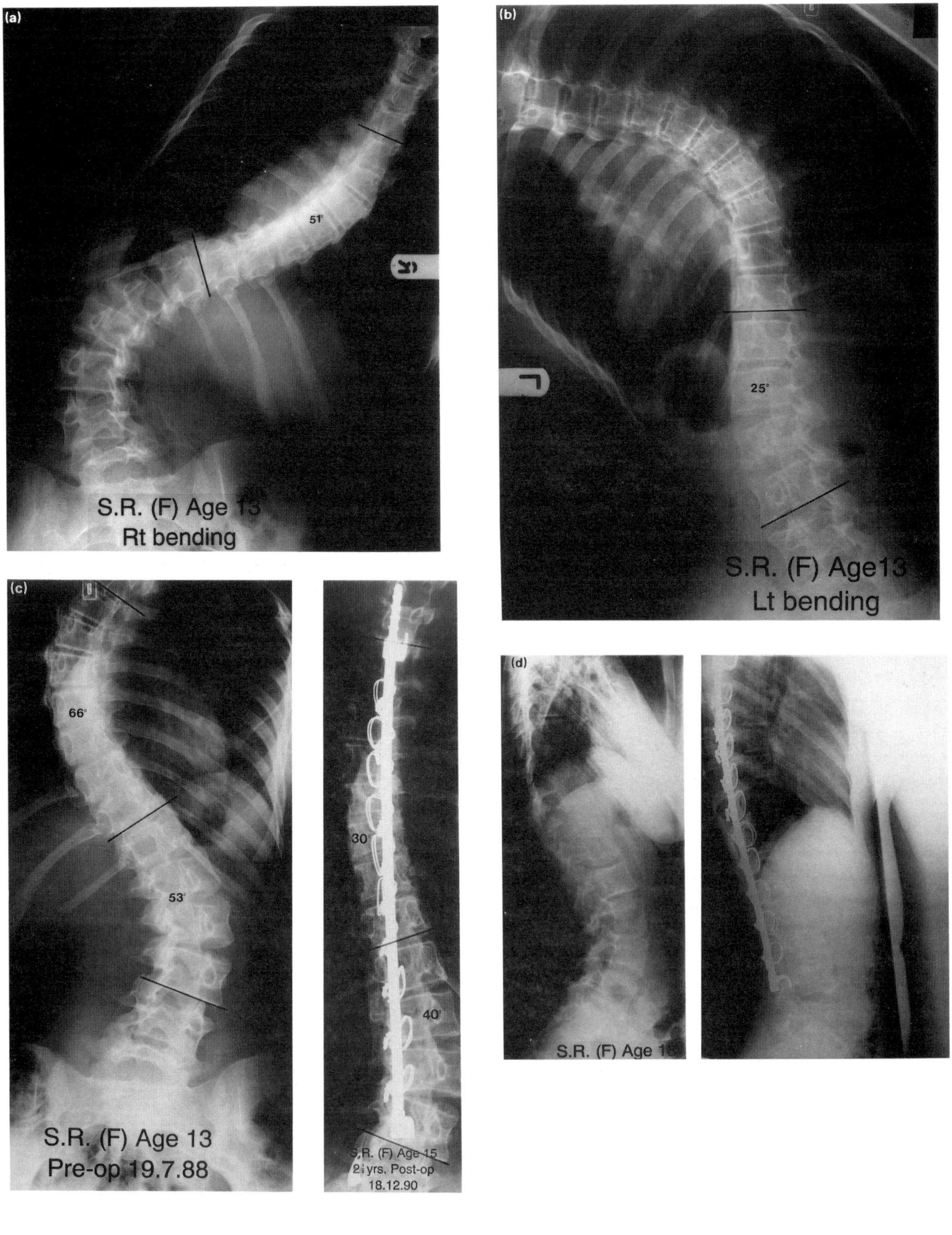
(a)
51°
S.R. (F) Age 13
Rt bending
(b)
25°
S.R. (F) Age13
Lt bending
(c)
66°
53°
S.R. (F) Age 13
Pre-op 19.7.88
30°
40°
S.R. (F) Age 15
2½ yrs. Post-op
18.12.90
(d)

previously contoured to give the correct sagittal angle. When they are inserted the rods lie initially in conformity with the scoliosis. They are then forcibly rotated through 90° so that the scoliosis is powerfully corrected and the curve on the rod dictates the degree of thoracic kyphosis and lumbar lordosis (Fig. 22.13) (Cotrel & Dubousset, 1985).

The CD procedure is expensive and technically demanding, and is now widely used in America and Europe. It is clearly effective not only in correcting the Cobb angle but in derotating the apical vertebrae. This virtue of 'overwhelming instrumentation' is also shared with the heavy Hartshill system, which is also technically demanding, and only time will confirm the relative merits and indications for these types of systems. We must not forget that a solid bony fusion is necessary to guarantee maintenance of our surgically obtained correction in the long term, however strong the instrumentation.

It should be noted that both the CD technique and those requiring sublaminar wiring have considerable learning curves. They should not be attempted unless the surgeon has spent adequate time with an experienced colleague to learn the subtleties of these powerful and potentially dangerous instrumentation systems.

SELECTION OF OPERATIVE TECHNIQUE

The choice of surgical technique will depend to some extent on the surgeon's previous training and the repertoire of techniques with which he or she is comfortable. Today's spinal deformity surgeon should certainly be conversant with the posterior approach to the spine and must have learned a good spinal fusion technique (Cotrel, 1986). In addition, the surgeon should also be able to approach the spine anteriorly or anterolaterally from C2 to the sacrum (Moe, 1972), and should also be able to carry out posterior osteotomies for ankylosing spondylitis and pre-existing spinal fusions, also anterior decompression and grafting techniques for vertebral body disease, deformity or fracture (Hall, 1972).

It is a salutary thought that as recently as 15 years ago many of these techniques would have been available in only a handful of the most major centres. In the later 1980s advances in anaesthetic management and improvements in surgical instrumentation and technique now make these operations fairly commonplace, although they should remain the province of surgeons who perform them relatively frequently, and have advanced training in spinal surgery. Spinal cord monitoring during surgery is an important safety measure now widely in use (see Chapter 9).

It is perhaps easiest to suggest the operative alternatives for different types of curves in different types of patients with idiopathic scoliosis in tabulated form (Table 22.1). Descriptions of the techniques, and some comments on these choices, will follow. No doubt other surgeons will disagree with this selection, which only illustrates the fact that there is no single right answer. The sooner we can understand the aetiology of scoliosis to obviate the need for such major surgery, the better.

SURGICAL TECHNIQUE
(Figs 22.10 and 22.11)

General considerations

Surgery is sometimes considered to be a last resort in scoliosis management and, unfortunately, some parents may be led to believe that its necessity is a near-disaster. In fact there is little justification for

Fig. 22.9 (*Opposite*) (a) The patient is bending to the right. The thoracic curve diminishes from 66° to 51°. This indicates a fairly stiff curve. The upper neutral vertebra is T4. (b) On left bending the lower curve diminishes from 53° to 25°, i.e. by about half—this is a typically mobile lumbar curve. Note the fixed wedging of the L2–L3 disc. Fusion should therefore extend only to L3 even though this is still rotated to some extent. (c) Harrington–Luque fusion has produced a well-balanced and well-corrected curve. A compromise between fusing below L3 in the lumbar spine with a risk of long-term pain and stiffness has had to be made against the risk of similar symptoms from leaving some obliquity and rotation of L4 and L5. The author believes that it is generally more important not to fuse below L3. Note the pedicular slot of the upper hook—an important safety feature preventing medial migration of the hook with sublaminar wiring. (d) Note the contouring of the Harrington rod. Possibly a little more lumbar lordosis would have been desirable, although this was an improvement on the preoperative position which was hyperlordotic. Harrington rods should always be contoured to reproduce the physiological sagittal curves; it is necessary to use rods with square lower ends and square socket hooks otherwise the pull of the sublaminar wires will simply rotate the rods through 90° converting desirable lordotic and kyphotic sagittal curves into undesirable scolioses.

Table 22.1 Operative alternatives in idiopathic scoliosis. (For illustrations of these techniques see Figs 22.7–22.15)

A: Early-onset scoliosis—under the age of five years (old terminology: infantile idiopathic scoliosis)	
1 Rib–vertebral angle difference (Mehta angle) <20°	Observation with expectation of complete resolution within two to three years
2 Mehta angle >20°	Expect progression of curves. If this occurs, serial body casts under anaesthesia repeated two or three times, each for one to two months, followed by custom-made plastic brace until the age of 10–12, then fusion if necessary as in 4
3 Curve in excess of 50°	Luque U rod with sublaminar wiring but no fusion as an internal brace. Anterior hemi-epiphysiodesis has been described but the results are variable. Probable removal of Luque instrumentation and definitive Harrington rod fusion aged 10–12 should be combined with anterior discectomy and fusion at apical four to five levels to prevent anterior growth. Possibility of costoplasty aged 15 or 16 if rib hump increases in spite of solid fusion.
4 Advanced early-onset scoliosis in excess of 70°, aged 5–12	Anterior discectomies and fusion at apical four to five levels combined with posterior Harrington–Luque or, better, 5 mm Hartshill–Luque fusion to derotate. Alternatively, the paediatric CD system may be used. Possibility of costoplasty for rib hump aged 15–16 if the rib hump increases in spite of a solid fusion with instrumentation.
B: Prepubertal late-onset scoliosis aged 5–12 years (old terminology: juvenile idiopathic scoliosis)	
1 Curve <40° shown to be progressing by at least 5° on successive X-rays six months apart.	Probably worth serial body casts with careful moulding to correct curve over six months to one year, followed by removable Boston type brace. Approx. 20% failure rate
2 Curve >50°	Anterior discectomies of apical four to five discs combined with posterior Hartshill–Luque CD or Harrington–Luque fusion. Possibility of costoplasty aged 15–16 if the rib hump increases in spite of a solid fusion.
C: Postpubertal late-onset scoliosis (old terminology: adolescent idiopathic scoliosis)	
1 Curves 20–40°	Observation. Bracing controversial, may improve rib hump in most patients; Cobb angle usually improved by 5° only; 15% failure rate in brace, similar to natural history. Author prefers not to brace.
2 Thoracic curves 40–70°	Generally require surgery. Harrington rod or Harrington–Luque acceptable. Improved derotation and correction with CD or heavy Hartshill technique.
3 Thoracolumbar curves 40–70°	As for thoracic but anterior surgery with Zielke, Webb–Morley or Dwyer will give almost complete correction and derotation. Beware of kyphosis with Dwyer.
4 Lumbar scoliosis 45–70°	Anterior surgery best. Important to prevent kyphosis with anterior placement of bone graft or cement spacers in intervertebral discs. Avoid fusing below L3 if possible.
5 Double or triple major curves >50–55°	Author prefers Harrington–Luque in the so-called 'dollar sign' configuration to maintain spinal balance. The individual curves are less rotated and therefore less prominent than single curves. Fusion usually not below L3. If it is necessary to go to L4, then an anterior technique to the lower curve is probably best. Fusion down to L3 but not below because proximity to great vessels. Will usually obtain good derotation and a near-parallel L4–L5 disc. The upper curve will then usually correct to a satisfactory extent but occasionally needs subsequent posterior surgery. It is rarely necessary to go to L5, which is constrained by the iliolumbar ligaments and therefore not rotated, in idiopathic scolioses. CD system or the Drummond wire and button technique may be used for flexible curves. Remember long fusion equals long surgery and stiff spine for patient and sometimes surgeon.

(Table continued)

6 Severe curves in excess of 70–80° in adolescents:		
	(a) Flexible curves reducing below 40° on bend films:	Two-stage anterior discectomies at apical four to five levels followed 10–14 days later by Harrington, Luque, Luque–Hartshill or CD. Halo-tilting bed traction between stages is occasionally useful. (May be done as one operation.) Costoplasty at second stage often necessary.
	(b) Stiff curves	Two-stage closing wedge vertebrectomy with anterior corpectomy followed 10–14 days later by excision of the posterior element with posterior convex Harrington, Rochester or Wisconsin compression instrumentation inserted first, followed by a concave Harrington rod. Costectomy of five to seven convex ribs is often necessary. Sublaminar and CD techniques may be ineffective or dangerous for stiff deformities. Alternatively, simple Harrington fixation and fusion *in situ* or with limited correction, combined with costectomy, is a safer and less arduous procedure and often gives acceptable results (see Fig. 22.12).

such a negative attitude; indeed the most satisfying results for patient, parents and surgeon are invariably achieved when a constructive and positive attitude, well justified by the facts, is taken from the start.

Scoliosis surgery in the 1990s should be almost complication-free and offers a substantial and permanent improvement in spine and body shape and balance. Although it may take six months or so for the patient to be more or less back to normal, surgery is nothing like the ordeal that it was even 20 years ago. Advances in surgical training, anaesthesia, analgesia, instrumentation, bone grafting techniques and our general understanding of the spine have made a world of difference to the quality and acceptability of surgical treatment. Non-operative treatment may, but only may, inhibit or even prevent the deterioration of a curve, but the only way to achieve substantial correction of a deformity once it has occurred is by surgery.

Clearly, the earlier surgery is performed then the better will be the result, because the curve is likely to be less severe and the spine more flexible and amenable to correction. As our knowledge of the natural history of scoliotic deformity increases, so it should be possible to achieve increasingly early surgery to the point of undertaking prophylactic surgery in carefully selected patients who have either no curve or the most minor curve, but are known to be certain to develop severe curves in the future. Such prophylactic surgery may not, and probably will not, be on the curved segment of the spine itself, but may be directed to a possible primary asymmetry such as a thoracolumbar stiff kyphotic segment, an anteverted femoral neck or pelvic asymmetry. Growth control techniques with the local use of growth hormone also offer interesting possibilities.

We are still some way short of being in a position to carry out prophylactic surgery; indeed, surgery on curves of less than 40° is rare in the absence of significant pain. Our knowledge of the natural history of scoliosis, and therefore our ability to predict spinal shape in an individual, is seriously inadequate, but one can be optimistic that progress is being made (Chapter 19).

The age of modern spinal surgery can be said to have begun with the introduction by Paul Harrington in Texas, USA of the Harrington instrumentation system in the early 1960s (Harrington, 1960, 1962, 1972). As with all revolutionary ideas there was considerable resistance to the concept of placing metalwork in the spine, although others, such as Allen in Birmingham, UK, and Resina and Ferriera-Alves in Portugal, had previously designed metal spinal implants (Resina & Ferriera-Alves, 1977). It was Harrington's total concept of an effective and well-designed implant, combined with a secure spinal fusion, which gradually gained acceptance around the world over the next 10 years.

In the 1970s the Harrington rod reigned more or less supreme, and it remains the basic corrective technique (see Figs 22.9 & 22.12). In the late 1970s and 1980s, however, there was a profusion of further developments in instrumentation, including the Luque segmental spinal instrumentation and its derivatives, Drummond button wiring of the spinous processes (Drummond *et al.*, 1982), and, most im-

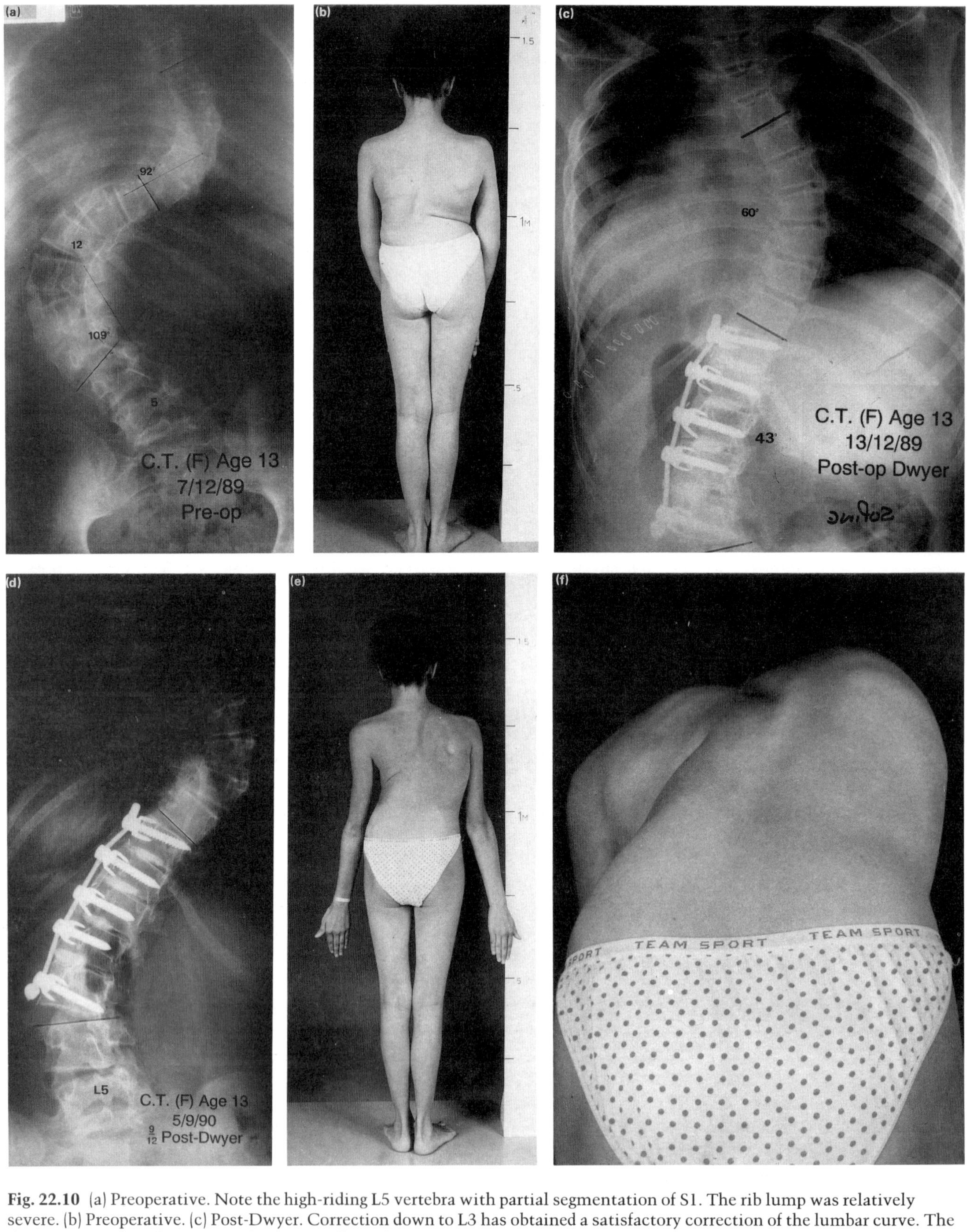

Fig. 22.10 (a) Preoperative. Note the high-riding L5 vertebra with partial segmentation of S1. The rib lump was relatively severe. (b) Preoperative. (c) Post-Dwyer. Correction down to L3 has obtained a satisfactory correction of the lumbar curve. The thoracic curve has also corrected substantially in this supine view giving hope that second-stage posterior surgery to the thoracic curve may not be necessary. (d) Thoracic curve = 94° and is not resolving. Nine months post-Dwyer. Note the anterior bone cement spacers to prevent kyphosis. (e) Nine months post-Dwyer. Marked thoracic deformity still present. (f) Nine months post-Dwyer. Rib rotation on forward bending.

portantly, the Cotrel–Dubousset technique with its complex instrumentation and powerful control of sagittal plane shape (Cotrel & Dubousset, 1985; Cotrel, 1986).

Also of importance are the anterior techniques. Hodgson (1956, 1960) in Hong Kong developed anterior approaches to every level in the spine in the 1950s. Dwyer & Sherwood then produced their anterior instrumentation in Australia in 1968 (Dwyer *et al.*, 1969). This was modified and improved by Zielke in Germany (Zielke *et al.*, 1976) and Morley and Webb in the UK, among others in the 1970s and 1980s.

Anterior approaches to the spine are particularly valuable in the treatment of thoracolumbar and lumbar curves where it is important to fuse a minimum number of motion segments to preserve mobility in as many lumbar discs as possible.

Anaesthesia and positioning of the patient

Needless to say, high-quality anaesthesia and effective postoperative pain control, best monitored by the anaesthetist, are matters of the utmost importance in scoliosis surgery, and advances in these fields are certainly responsible in large measure for our ability to carry out such major procedures safely and without too much discomfort for the patient (see Chapter 21).

Positioning of the patient so that the anaesthetist is happy, and so that the spine is presented to the surgeon in a posture which will allow him to produce the most effective result both physiologically and mechanically, is obviously of great importance. Inevitably, the patient must be face-down for a posterior procedure. This produces some problems for the anaesthetist but, so far as the surgeon is concerned, the most important considerations are to ensure that there is no pressure on the abdomen obstructing the venous return from the lower limbs to the heart, otherwise the venous return will occur through the vertebral venous plexus of Batson and through the sinusoids of the vertebrae provoking increased bleeding. The spine should be in the right posture with the lumbar lordosis preserved, particularly if the lumbar spine is to be operated upon. An over-flattened lumbar lordosis is a well-known pitfall, and is quite disabling to the patient who will have a fatiguing and painful kyphotic posture as a result. To prevent this, the patient's knees should be more or less on a horizontal level with the hips, which will produce pelvic rotation to preserve the lumbar lordosis. A variety of frames, rests, pads and pillows have been developed by various surgeons and anaesthetists to achieve these aims. We prefer to use the Basildon spinal frame, a derivative of the Relton–Hall Toronto frame. It has a headrest and is fully adjustable and portable.

Another important service required of the anaesthetist is the ability to carry out the Stagnara wake-up test (Stagnara, 1988) when instrumentation of the spine is complete, before closure of the wound. Although the use of spinal cord monitoring is the rule in virtually all scoliosis centres, this is not infallible, and a satisfactory trace may not be possible in some patients due to technical failure, obesity or previous neurological deficit. In these circumstances the anaesthetist is asked to raise the level of consciousness sufficiently for the patient to be able to move the hands and feet on command, and thus confirm that at that moment there is no gross compromise of spinal cord function. The wake-up test is a relatively insensitive test of neural conduction, and if this has been impaired no indication as to the moment of impairment is given, as it would be with electronic spinal cord monitoring. If one knows exactly when the trouble occurred then it can often be put right before there is any permanent damage.

When spinal cord monitoring is used, it is generally accepted that the threshold for diagnosing a significant impairment of spinal cord function is a reduction of the amplitude of the signal by 50% or an increase in latency of 1 ms. Lesser changes to the signal complex may be brought about by lengthening the spinal cord by distraction producing some increase in latency, and perhaps conduction may be reduced by cooling of the spinal cord by prolonged exposure and by irrigation with cool fluids during surgery.

If a significant compromise of spinal function is deemed to have occurred, either through an abnormal monitor trace or inability to move one or both feet in the wake-up test, then the following action should be taken:

1 Has any obvious trauma occurred? For example a gouge or periosteal elevator entering the extradural space.

2 With distraction techniques resulting in a net elongation of the vertebral column, take steps to remove the distracting force totally, either by shifting

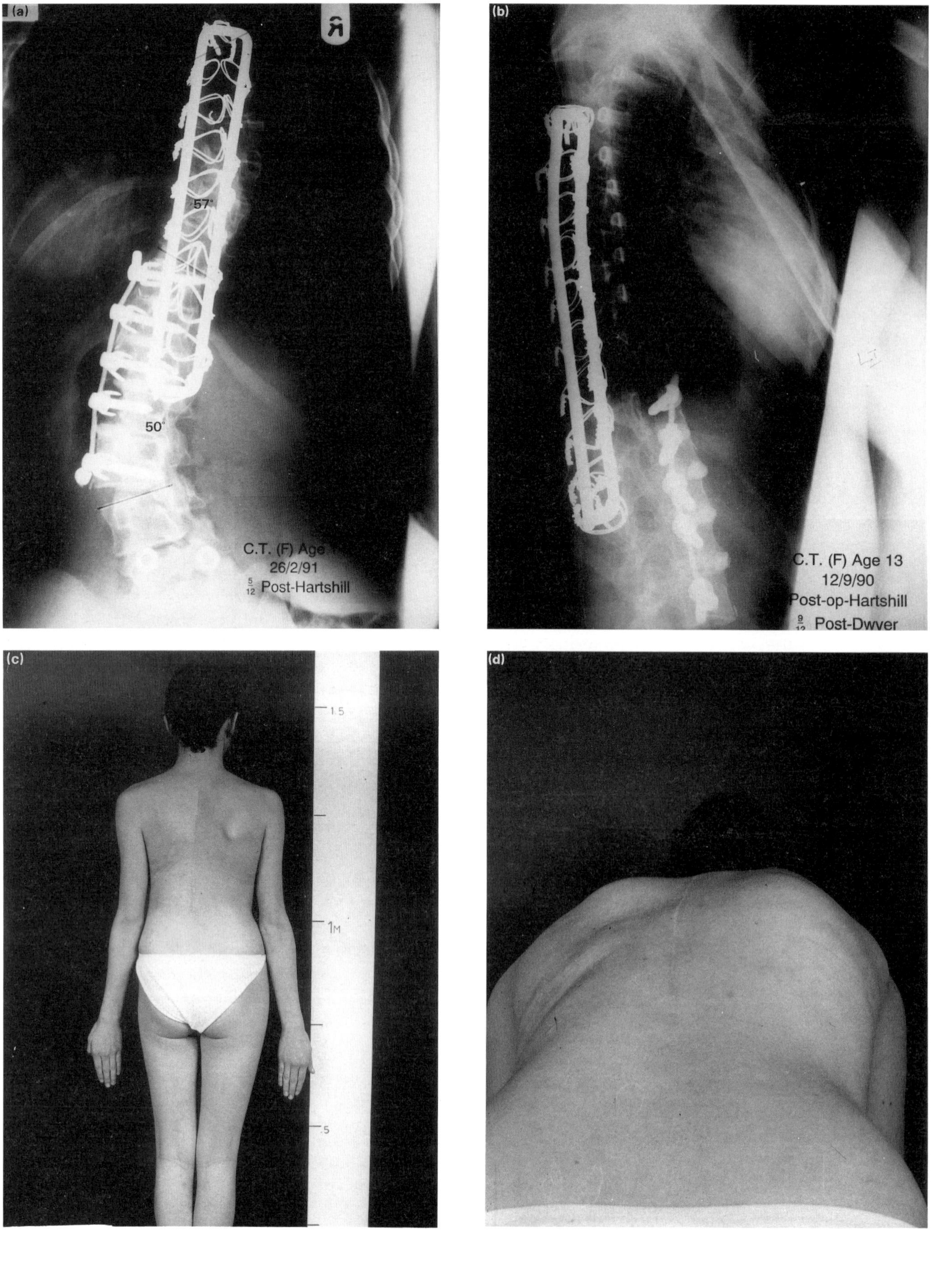

(a)
57°
50°
C.T. (F) Age
26/2/91
5/12 Post-Hartshill
(b)
C.T. (F) Age 13
12/9/90
Post-op-Hartshill
9/12 Post-Dwyer
(c)
1.5
1M
.5
(d)

the upper hook down the ratchet of the Harrington rod, or by cutting the rod. If the trace then gradually returns, cautious distraction may again be tried with a delay of several minutes between each increment of distraction to make sure there is no adverse effect.

3 In techniques employing segmental fixation, either with hooks or wires, each hook or wire must be checked to make sure that it is in the correct position and that there is no possibility of compression on the spinal cord. If a cause is found and rectified then there is no sense in abandoning correction of the deformity, and the management is expectant in the hope that normal function will return.

4 If the surgeon can establish no cause for the deficit in spinal cord function, then he must use his judgement as to whether he thinks the problem is truly in the spine or whether there is a fault in the spinal cord monitor or a fault in the anaesthetic management of the wake-up test. The surgeon may decide that correction of the curvature should be abandoned by cutting the Hartshill or Luque rods, or recontouring the CD rods to reduce correction. In the back of his mind will be the uncomfortable realization that the worst of all worlds is a patient with neurological compromise *and* an unstable spinal deformity little or no better than at the start of surgery. These decisions rarely have to be taken, but when necessary they are among the most difficult and stressful that any surgeon has to make.

Neurological compromise may occur at any stage in the first 24 hours postoperatively, and rarely even after that. Accordingly, all patients must have their vital and neurological functions adequately monitored during this period.

It is generally accepted that, for a neurological deficit of gradual onset, a reasonable chance of a degree of recovery exists if the cause of that deficit is rectified within 6 hours of its onset. Any further delay in the rectification of what is usually thought to be an ischaemic situation is likely to result in permanent damage of the spinal cord. If neurological function is completely lost, including that of the sacral segments, then there is no realistic chance of useful recovery.

Attention to blood volume and restoration of blood gas values are of great importance in ensuring adequate perfusion of the spinal cord. Infusion of dexamethasone probably helps to reduce oedema. By far the best management is prevention, so far as possible, by careful surgical and anaesthetic technique. If there is direct mechanical injury during surgery, however, then recovery will not be aided by removing or slackening the instrumentation; indeed stability and correction of the deformity should be preserved to gain at least some benefit from the operation.

The Harrington rod technique

Paul Harrington of Houston, Texas, USA, was the first to develop an effective internal fixation device which, when combined with an adequate posterior bony fusion, produced consistently successful results in the management of scoliosis (Harrington, 1960, 1962, 1972). When Harrington developed his system in the 1950s, and started using it widely in the early 1960s, there were a large number of children and adults suffering from relatively severe paralytic deformities caused by poliomyelitis. Harrington, in using the principle of distraction, was able to produce dramatic correction and stabilization of these curves (see Figs 22.9 and 22.12).

Over subsequent decades polio has largely faded from the scene and the majority of the curves which now come to surgery are relatively slight idiopathic curves, mostly ranging from 45° to 55° Cobb angle. These curves still respond quite well to distraction in terms of Cobb angle correction where 40–50% improvement can be expected a year after surgery. However, there is no doubt that subsequent tech-

Fig. 22.11 (*Opposite*) (a) After posterior Hartshill–Luque technique. This shows the powerful corrective ability of Luque segmental sublaminar wiring combined with Dove's Hartshill rectangle. Spinal cord monitoring is necessary when such major corrections are obtained. In over 10 years experience the author has had no permanent major or minor neurological deficit when using sublaminar wiring techniques for scoliosis. It is important to note that other surgeons have reported an increased incidence of neurological complications following sublaminar wiring, particularly when distraction is also used. The L3–L4 disc remains wedged and may well cause future problems and require stabilization either by fusion or by a more conservative technique such as the Graf ligament. (b) Postoperative Heavy Hartshill. Note the contouring of the Hartshill rectangle and the cement spacers in front of the Dwyer instrumentation preventing kyphosis. (c) Final result—a well-balanced trunk with relatively inconspicuous rib deformity and posterior midline scar. (d) After posterior surgery. Final result—an acceptable degree of rib rotation.

niques such as the CD and the heavy Hartshill will produce 60–70% correction of the Cobb angle with measurable derotation of the apex of the curve a year after surgery. Although these figures sound advantageous, the actual improvement in the patient's appearance is not quite as impressive. We have still not solved the problem of the increasing rib hump in the presence of solid spinal fusion in patients operated two or three years before skeletal maturity, and we have to remember that the rib hump is one of the most obvious aspects of the deformity so far as the patient is concerned (Weatherley *et al.*, 1987).

It must be said that 30 years after the introduction of the Harrington rod procedure it is still entirely justifiable to treat idiopathic scoliosis by that technique and, indeed, with one or two more modern improvements such as the square-ended rod and the slotted upper hook, the Harrington rod is still competitive in terms of simplicity, speed and economy. It is reasonable that some surgeons judge these advantages to outweigh the disadvantages of more prolonged bracing and a slightly inferior result. However, human nature being what it is, surgeons unceasingly pursue excellence to satisfy their patients and themselves, and provided the results are sufficiently good, the case is made.

The Harrington rod is a ¼ inch (6 mm) stainless-steel rod, notched at one end to form a ratchet proximally, and the distal end is shaped and collared to stand in a stable manner on the distal hook. Correction is achieved by forcing the upper hook up the ratchet to straighten the C-shaped curve of the spine as much as possible. The ability to correct a curve with the Harrington rod is limited only by the strength of the bone in which the hooks are placed at each end. However, overdistraction must certainly be avoided, particularly in fracture work as the spinal cord may be damaged either mechanically or by stretching of its blood supply.

The upper Harrington hook may be inserted beneath the laminar arch into the facet joint or, preferably, with a slotted hook as developed by Cotrel engulfing the pedicle. This latter is the most stable and preferred arrangement. As in all scoliosis techniques with metal implants, a secure spinal fusion of the Moe type is essential: the implant will correct the deformity, the fusion is required to sustain the correction long term (see Figs 22.9 & 22.12).

Detailed description of the Harrington rod technique is beyond the scope of this chapter, and it is recommended that the reader should consult a more specialized text such as Moe *et al.* (1978).

Rib surgery in scoliosis

It is important to emphasize that, so far as the patient is concerned, the rib hump is usually the most major aspect of the deformity in adolescent idiopathic scoliosis. Unfortunately, it is a fact that present surgical techniques are much better at correcting the Cobb angle and the apical vertebral displacement from the midline than they are at correcting the abnormality of surface shape caused by rib rotation.

The more modern techniques such as that of Cotrel–Dubousset and the heavy Hartshill–Luque usually produce gratifying vertebral derotation as measured by the Perdriolle method (Perdriolle *et al.*, 1981), and this certainly reduces rib rotation, but longer-term follow-ups after a year or two show a troublesome tendency for the rib hump to recur, particularly in those patients who undergo surgery well before skeletal maturity (Wojcik *et al.*, 1990) (see Chapter 23). However, others have found this not to be the case, and have found that vertebral rotation and rib hump correction is maintained following Cotrel–Dubousset instrumentation (Cundy *et al.*, 1990).

Before the advent of efficient spinal instrumentation such as the Harrington rod it was customary to obtain as much correction as possible in plaster, then to fuse the spine and combine this either with excision of the prominent border of the scapula or some form of costoplasty. The cosmetic results of such procedures were sometimes quite acceptable in spite of what we would now regard as poor correction of the Cobb angle (Manning *et al.*, 1973). Rib surgery still has an important place in the management of more prominent rib humps, although partial scapulectomy is now rarely performed.

The main indications for rib hump surgery in idiopathic scoliosis are as follows:

1 Early-onset scoliotics who have had to undergo fusion prior to menarche or puberty. These patients, in spite of having had anterior epiphysiodesis of the apical vertebrae combined with a posterior fusion and instrumentation to correct the deformity and arrest growth over the extent of the curvature, will often develop increasing rib humps during the growth spurt, although the spine itself remains well corrected (the crankshaft effect). Rib surgery should

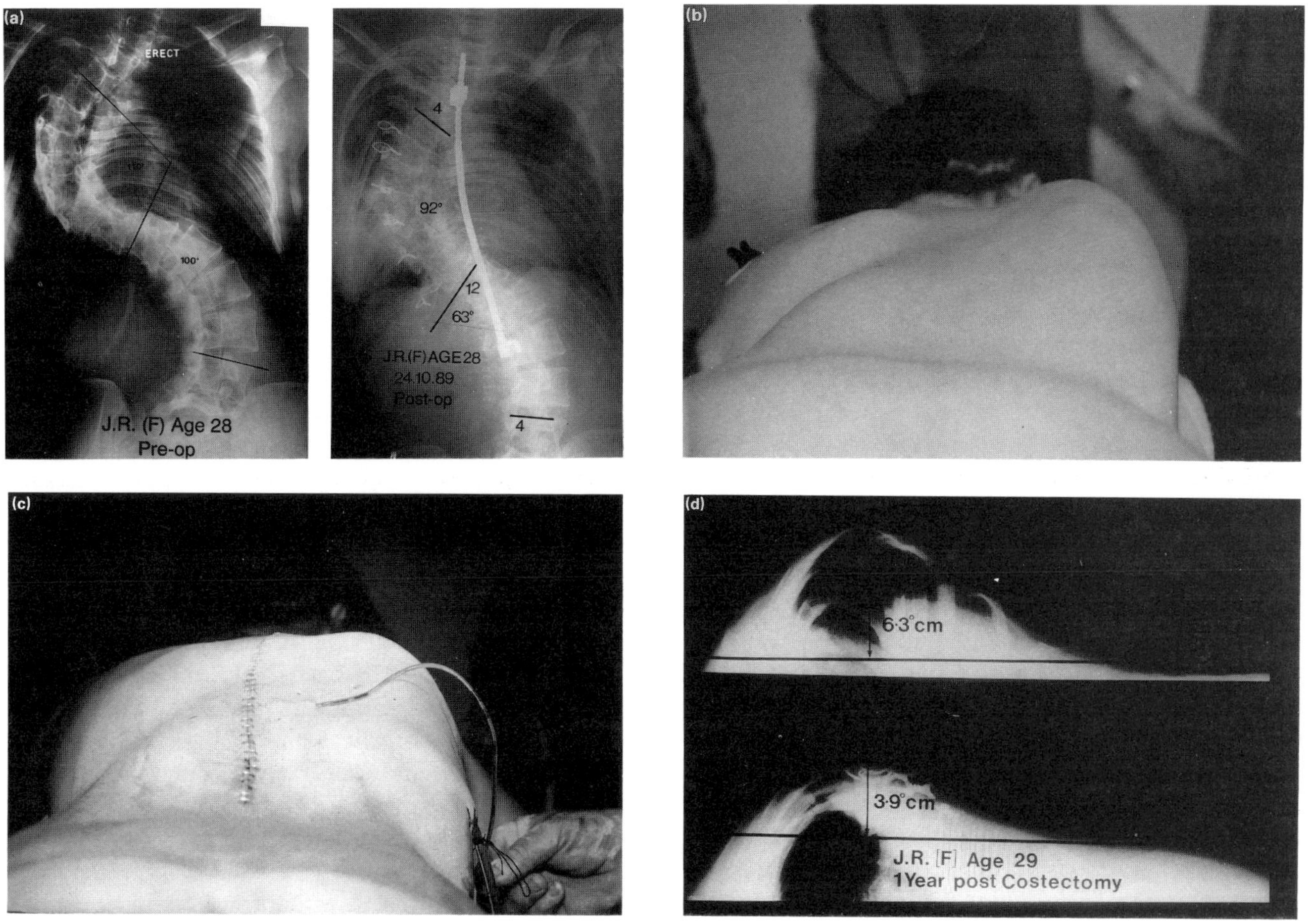

Fig. 22.12 (a) Note the modest correction but important stabilization in this 28-year-old female with a double major adolescent idiopathic scoliosis. She underwent single-stage Harrington rod correction and stabilization with a modified Schollner costoplasty. Note the fourth rib now attached to the stump of the fifth rib. Fusion down to L2 leaves her with a mobile lumbar spine and less likelihood of long-term low back pain than a greater correction with fusion to L3 or below. (b,c) The immediate postoperative surface shape is much improved. These photographs were taken on the operating table. (d) Tangential supero-inferior view. The patient is forward bending with the spine horizontal and the tube shooting along the spine to sky-line the rib hump which is reduced in height by 2.4 cm after surgery.

be delayed, if possible, until the age of 15 or 16 when rapid growth has more or less ceased.

2 It will occasionally be necessary to perform costoplasty on seven or eight year olds with progressive infantile scolioses who have had to undergo early fusion because of severe curve progression. These children often have very major apical vertebral rotation with sharp rib humps, and require reduction of the hump for cosmetic reasons. They should be warned that further rib surgery could be necessary at the age of 15 or 16 years.

3 The more severe adolescent idiopathic scolioses of around 70° or more often have quite prominent rib humps. Although we can obtain good Cobb angle correction and reduction of apical vertebral displacement from the midline with anterior discectomies and posterior instrumentation with today's powerful implants, the rib hump may remain prominent. Costoplasty is often worthwhile at the time of surgical correction.

4 In late adolescence when there is a severe neglected curve of 70° or more, particularly in the male when the curve may be very stiff and the lateral bend films indicate that little correction can be expected, then it may be preferable to provide fairly simple surgery with Harrington rod stabilization and a costoplasty (Fig. 22.12). The alternative would be a one- or two-stage closing wedge vertebrectomy with compression and distraction instrumentation, which is a very major procedure with increased risk of spinal cord damage.

Before advising costoplasty it is often useful to take a supero-inferior X-ray of the spine with the patient bending forward (Fig. 22.12d). This will skyline the rib hump and determine whether it contains lung tissue, in which case correction is relatively straightforward, or whether the rib hump consists of rib tightly wrapping around the severely rotated vertebral body, as in some infantile and early-onset scoliosis. If that is the case little if any correction will be possible.

There are two basic types of costoplasty:

1 Simple costoplasty. This consists of excising the prominent 3–4 cm of the rib hump at each level. This is achieved through the same midline incision used for the scoliosis surgery. The rib segments are excised subperiostially and extrapleurally, usually over five or six levels, and the resulting bone may be a useful supplement to bone grafting the spine if the procedure is being done at the same time as instrumentation and correction of the curvature (Owen *et al.*, 1986).

The patient should be warned that the pleura may be entered, in which case a pleural drain will be necessary for a few days. Some surgeons would use a drain routinely.

It is probably advisable to apply an orthosis to the posterior chest wall for two to three months postoperatively to obtain as much flattening of the rib hump as possible.

2 The modified Schollner costoplasty (Schollner, 1966). In this procedure the approach is similar to simple costoplasty but the major difference is that when the prominent ribs are osteotomized 2 or 3 cm from their ends, they are then reconnected to the stump of the rib below, i.e. the sixth rib is connected to the stump of the seventh rib via holes drilled in the ribs, secured with braided nylon or wire. This has the effect of making the convex ribs more horizontal and nearer to the normal alignment. The concavity of the curvature is then reduced to some extent by transposing the paraspinal muscle mass from the convex side of the midline to the concave side by dividing it at its cephalic end and swinging it across to overlay the concave muscle mass.

If further correction is required, the concave ribs may be divided and excised sections from the convex ribs may be inserted using Judet clips to raise the convex rib depression. This latter manoeuvre may be quite difficult and time-consuming. Broome *et al.* (1990) did not find it worthwhile. Synthetic implants similar to breast prostheses are another possibility under active development. These can be used to fill the rib depression on the concavity of the curve.

Cotrel–Dubousset spinal instrumentation

By A.E. HEILMAN

The Cotrel–Dubousset (CD) technique was developed in France in the early 1980s after extensive computer studies of spinal deformity and mechanical testing (Cotrel, 1986). The CD spinal instrumentation consists of two contourable stainless-steel rods with multiple attachments to the spine via compression and distraction hooks. This system consists of a variation on a theme of previous instrumentation systems. The advantages of this system are that no postoperative cast immobilization is needed, rigid stabilization is obtained, powerful derotation is possible and there is good control of sagittal spinal shape. The hooks are placed at strategic levels, depending on the type of curve, and the two rods are then attached to these hooks and locked to each other by two or more transverse dynamic fixing devices.

By producing compression between hooks lordosis is developed. Distraction between hooks produces kyphosis. This is vital to the understanding of the system. The advantages of the CD system over other fixation systems currently in use are its rigidity and its ability to achieve sagittal derotation of the spine. The procedure is technically demanding and the surgeon has a learning curve which is best shortened by attendance at beginner and advanced training courses for the use of this implant (Cotrel, 1986; Dickson & Erwin, 1989; Berck-Plage, 1990). Furthermore, this technique is only for spinal surgeons who have the time to do extensive preoperative planning (Fig. 22.13). The thought processes concerning CD instrumentation are very different from the Harrington system, inasmuch as three-dimensional correction is planned by hook placement and rod contouring.

The system has a rod that is more flexible than the Luque or Harrington system. Since it is more flexible it can be pre-bent at any part of its length, even after

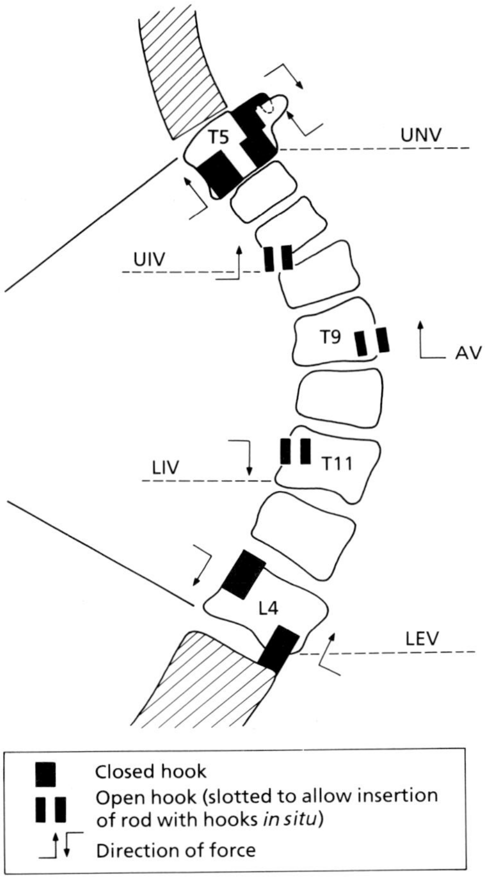

Fig. 22.13 To show a typical planning diagram for a thoracolumbar idiopathic curve. The concave pre-bent rod is inserted with distraction then derotation is performed. The convex rod is then inserted with the hooks in compression and derotated. Note the claw configuration of the hooks on the convex side of the upper neutral vertebra. UNV, upper neutral vertebra; UIV, upper intermediate vertebra; LIV, lower intermediate vertebra; LEV, lower end vertebra.

insertion, but this can be dangerous as, when the rod is bent after engagement with the spinal sockets, forces can be passed through hooks which may either break the hook–bone interface or encroach the hook into the spinal canal.

One of the key points of the system is the placement of hooks so that a double-sided claw is formed. In a routine Harrington rod system the hook is placed free in the canal, and only when a distraction force is placed on the hook is there stability in the construct. With the CD system a claw is formed by placing a hook over the transverse process and under the lamina or pedicle of the same or subsequent vertebrae, which allows immediate fixation of this segment without having to place a distraction force to stabilize the hook. Special low-profile hooks may be necessary in some situations (Fig. 22.14).

Currently, 7 mm rods are used for adult and 6 mm rods for paediatric spines. The specifics of the hooks and the different types of fixation are beyond the scope of this chapter. Each type of curve (right thoracic, thoracolumbar, lumbar double major or double thoracic) requires specific hook placements to allow three-dimensional correction of the spinal deformity. Each curve requires different hook placements to allow correction. It is of extreme importance when planning hook configuration that hooks be avoided in the apical segment of stiff curves in which the rotatory force of the rod would apply the force of the hook towards the spinal canal. There have been reports in the literature of spinal cord injury with these apical hooks.

Hook location is determined by studying standing AP, lateral and right and left side-bending films. If there is significant sagittal plane deformity, lateral views in flexion and extension are necessary. It is of great importance to appreciate junctional kyphosis at the thoracolumbar segment preoperatively. Instrumentation must be extended beyond the level of junctional kyphosis to prevent further worsening of the kyphosis postoperatively (see Fig. 22.14). Traction is not routinely used during instrumentation, but in young children traction views may be necessary.

After careful study of preoperative films a working diagram is a necessity (see Fig. 22.13). This allows the surgeon to plan the appropriate instrumentation during this technically demanding procedure. This planning is done with the aim of obtaining selective correction by the use of compression forces (producing lordosis) and distraction forces (producing kyphosis), as well as the contouring of the rod (producing a sagittal derotation). Closed hooks are used at the end levels and open ones at intermediate sites. Hook blockers and other special instrumentation are required during sagittal rotation of the first rod.

It is of key importance to remember the basic tenet of spinal deformity surgery: that is, that a solid fusion is absolutely essential. It is vital that adequate attention be given to decortication and bone grafting during this procedure. The increased 'fiddle factor' required during instrumentation can lead to inadequate bone grafting unless careful attention is maintained to the grafting part of the surgery. It is

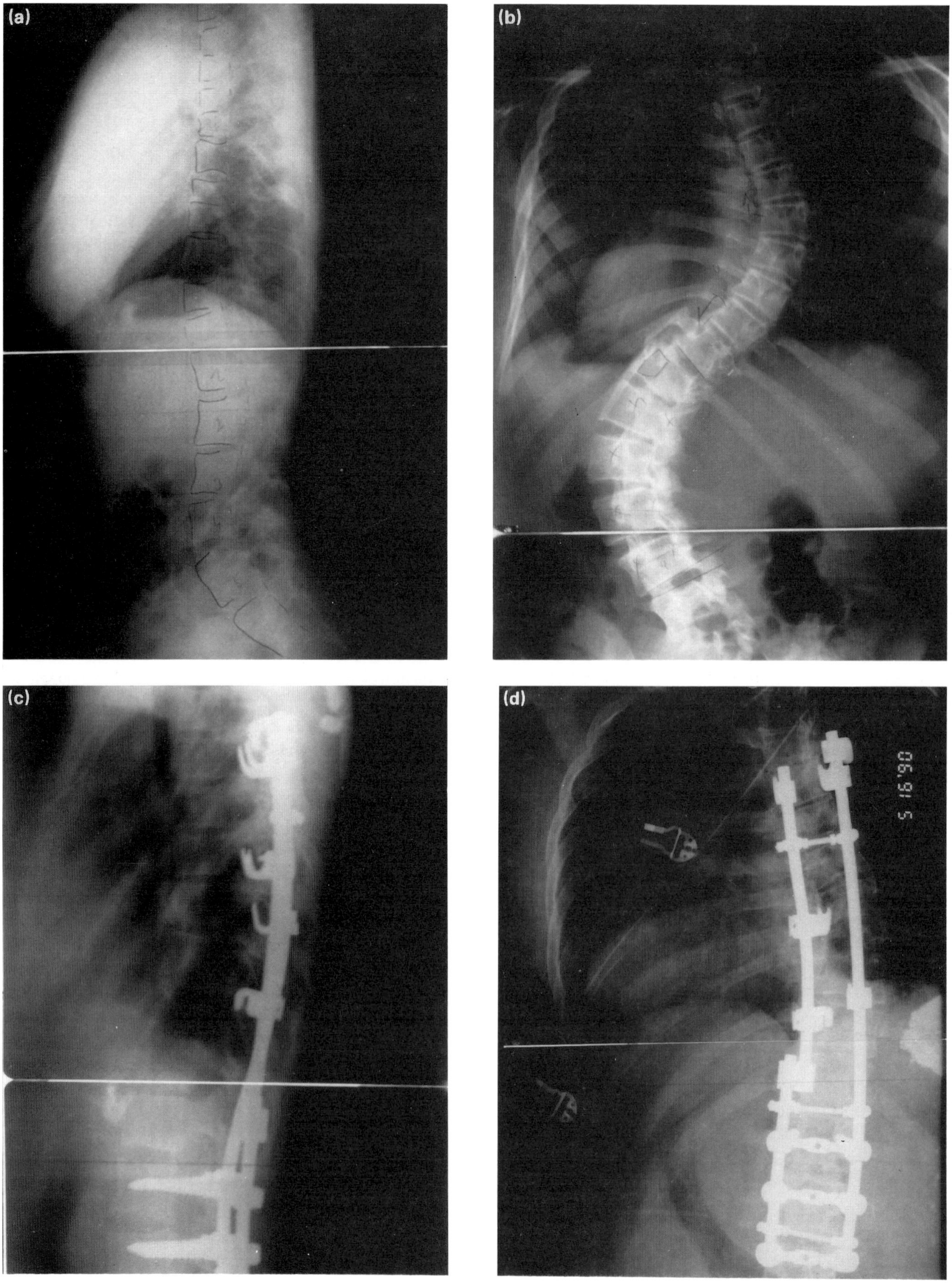
(a)
(b)
(c)
(d)

also important to remember that fixation is extremely rigid mechanically, so that powerful derotation of the spine is possible. There is a definite learning curve as to the extent of safe derotation of the spine so that neurological injury can be avoided; furthermore, intraoperative spinal cord monitoring is important.

This system is ideal for flexible curves. In curves in which there is increased rigidity, especially curves going down into the low lumbar segments, it is technically demanding. Also, this system should not be used for Scheuermann's kyphosis and double thoracic curves unless the surgeon is very experienced. One advantage of this system is that it allows for the interconnection of various-length rods so that segmental fixation of the lumbar spine can be done and then connected to the thoracic correction system. Thus, in some of these more technically demanding procedures, trying to insert one long pre-bent rod is avoided.

Currently it is recommended that fixation in the lumbar spine be primarily with pedicle screws, although claw techniques are acceptable. Sacral fixation with the CD system is currently undergoing new development. The Chopin sacral block shoe (blocker) allows a divergent placement of sacral screws with a very low profile. The widespread use of this sacral system should be discouraged until long-term follow-up is analysed, but early use is promising.

Thus the use of CD instrumentation allows fixed curvatures of the spine to be corrected in three dimensions. The stability achieved makes the use of postoperative external fixation unnecessary, and this may be a strong psychosocial advantage of the system for many adolescent patients.

The Zielke operation

By A.E. HEILMAN

In 1973 Zielke discussed the opportunities, advantages and limitations of the Dwyer method with Dr Dwyer. Subsequently he developed the concept of ventral derotation spondylodesis (VDS) incorporating the basic principles of the Dwyer system (Zielke, 1976; Moe *et al.*, 1983). Besides development of a more sophisticated implant, the basic concept was advanced by the introduction of derotation of the spine. With this concept, unintentional formation of kyphosis by overshortening of the anterior column during correction of scoliosis can usually be avoided (see Chapter 23).

The Zielke system consists of vertebral screws that have a coarse self-cutting thread, angle plates and washers, compression rods and derotational instrumentation. An anterior approach is made to the spine, and after total removal of intervertebral discs back to the posterior longitudinal ligament, a screw is inserted across the vertebral body. In cases where there is posterior ankylosis or a congenital bar, a posterior release operation may need to be done prior to any anterior surgery.

The Zielke instrumentation, as well as other techniques described in this chapter, have a definite learning curve, and it is advised that any surgeon interested in this should spend several sessions with an experienced surgeon and attend appropriate courses describing its use, as well as its complications and pitfalls.

The ideal indications for Zielke instrumentation (Fig. 22.15) are lumbar and thoracolumbar scoliotic deformities. The patient is placed in a lateral flexed position, convex side up. The standard approach is thoraco-abdominal via the rib inserting one level above the highest vertebra to be instrumented. The spine is exposed via a transdiaphragmatic retroperitoneal approach. The intervertebral discs are then removed thoroughly, along with the cartilage endplates, down to cancellous bone using periosteal elevators, osteotomes and curettes. It is of extreme importance that the great vessels be protected from the operative field. Following this dissection the deformity must be flexible when pressure is exerted over its apex. The vertebral screws of correct length, piercing the far cortex, are then inserted along with their washers and with staples for the end vertebrae. The threaded rod, loaded with the required number of hexagonal nuts, is then placed in the slotted heads of the screws. The rod is usually prebent to obtain the correct sagittal curve when rotated through 90° with the derotating instrument.

Fig. 22.14 (*Opposite*) (a) Junctional kyphosis. (b) AP junctional kyphosis. (c) Postoperative lateral X-ray. Note the upper claw hook configuration and the lumbar pedicle screws. (d) Postoperative anteroposterior X-ray. Note the lumbar pedicle screws attached to a two part concave rod for ease of handling.

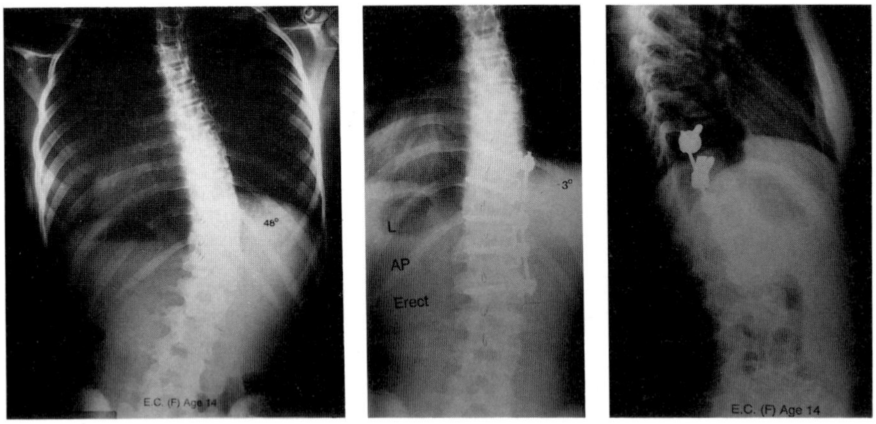

Fig. 22.15 Zielke instrumentation. Note the slight overcorrection which is no problem (−3°). In the lateral view, kyphosis has been avoided. (Courtesy of M.A. Edgar FRCS.)

The implant may be used down to L3, but usually not below, for fear of contact with the great vessels, which may cause erosion and catastrophic haemorrhage. Bone graft derived from the rib removed to allow access is placed in the excised disc spaces prior to curve correction. It is packed especially tightly anteriorly to prevent the development of kyphosis over the instrumented segment.

Postoperatively the patient is carefully monitored for 24–48 hours until neurologically and physiologically stable. A plaster of Paris or synthetic body jacket is applied seven days postoperatively when the patient is able to stand, and is retained for three months, after which a light removable lumbosacral corset is used for a month or two before being gradually discarded. Swimming may be started at four months, and games and physical education at six months. Schooling is resumed three to four months after surgery, depending on the circumstances.

The Dwyer operation

The Dwyer operation was the first successful system to be developed for anterior multilevel scoliosis correction. The system was conceived by Dwyer, and made a practical possibility by his engineer, Sherwood, in Sydney, Australia in the late 1960s (Dwyer *et al.*, 1969; Figs 22.10 & 22.11). The ability to correct and derotate flexible thoracolumbar and lumbar scoliotic curves was, and remains, most impressive. In flexible curves up to around 60° almost complete three-dimensional correction can be obtained by the experienced operator.

The advantage of the Dwyer system is its flexibility. The braided titanium cable is simpler to insert than the rigid rod of the Zielke and its derivative techniques, particularly in patients with rather stiff curves in whom major correction is not possible. These include adult scoliotics and patients with severe meningomyelocele curves (Dwyer *et al.*, 1979).

The main disadvantage of the Dwyer procedure is the tendency of the spine to be pulled into kyphosis following disc excision and tensioning of the cable to correct the deformity. This is because the anterior column of the spine is shortened considerably more than the posterior column. This tendency is minimized by careful annular excision right back to the posterior longitudinal ligament, and by packing bone graft into the anterior part of the intervertebral space prior to tensioning of the cable. The use of bone cement spacers can be recommended, but care must be taken to shape them in a reverse wedge as they can be extruded like an orange pip from the disc space with a possible threat to the great vessels many months after surgery.

The Dwyer procedure is relatively inexpensive and simple to perform, and is probably the preferred technique for relatively stiff or severe thoracolumbar or lumbar curves where near-total correction is not possible. On the other hand, the Zielke technique, having a solid rod, provides greater security of correction.

With these anterior techniques it is usually possible to save an extra lower lumbar disc from fusion with their superior derotation. However, recent developments with posterior pedicle screw fixation can also achieve the same result and it remains to be seen where the balance of advantage lies. Posterior surgery is undoubtedly less severe so far as the patient is concerned.

The Webb–Morley technique

This technique was developed by Webb and Morley at the Royal National Orthopaedic Hospital, London during the mid-1980s. It combines the simplicity and inexpensiveness of the Dwyer system with most of the advantages of the solid rod Zielke system (see Fig. 22.7). The rod can be contoured and rotated using a levered gripping tool such as a Schlein's clamp before finally tightening the locknuts. As in the Zielke procedure, impressive corrections and derotations of flexible scoliotic curves can be obtained. The Webb–Morley technique is being developed further as a pedicle screw system for use in the lumbar spine. For details of the surgical technique see Rob & Smith (1991).

There are a large number of other surgical techniques in clinical use and under development on both sides of the Atlantic for both anterior and posterior scoliosis correction. These are too numerous to describe, and no doubt many of them will fall into disuse as they offer nothing new or are superseded by improved systems. Regrettably, many of the new systems share the disadvantages of technical complexity and high price but no doubt, in the fullness of time, the virtues of effectiveness, safety and economy will prevail.

CONCLUSIONS

Any practitioner aspiring to manage patients with adolescent idiopathic scoliosis must not only be adept at a selection of surgical techniques, both anterior and posterior, but he or she must also have a clear understanding of the natural history of the condition in all its variations. He or she should also be aware of our imperfect but growing knowledge of the pathogenesis of idiopathic scoliosis with its implications for both non-operative and operative treatment. The following points should always be borne in mind:

1 Adolescent idiopathic scoliosis is a basket of conditions, almost certainly with different aetiological factors prevailing in many cases. Subtle genetic, neuromuscular and morphological variations are probably the dominant factors.

2 The spinal deformity—the most obvious abnormality—is quite likely to be a secondary consequence of a combination of other factors. Researchers are struggling to define these factors which, if identified, may open the way to effective prophylactic surgery to correct a primary abnormality, quite possibly in the ribs or femoral necks or another part of the spine.

3 Every patient with a spinal deformity is a frightened and worried individual with a frightened and worried family. Time and effort must be spent in allaying these fears by comprehensive and sensitive explanation at an early stage. This may save much time and anguish later on.

4 Many scolioses do not increase and should not be treated if they are asymptomatic and cosmetically acceptable. Scolioses of between 25° and 35° Cobb angle and progressing may require brace treatment. Scolioses in excess of 40° usually need surgery. However, sometimes a 30° curve with persistent and troublesome thoracic or ligamentous low back pain is best corrected surgically and occasionally a 50° curve, especially in a male, does not need surgery.

The above regimen represents current practice: with improved understanding of the factors influencing individual curves, indications for surgery will no doubt be refined further, with the development of more sophisticated surgical techniques.

5 While modern surgical techniques such as the Cotrel–Dubousset and the 6 mm Hartshill–Luque procedures have been developed for, and are quite good at correcting, the Cobb angle on X-ray, they are not good at correcting the rib hump. The rib hump is the main deformity of which the patient complains. We need to develop much better techniques for preventing and correcting asymmetries of rib shape and position. Successful vertebral derotation, important in the correction of lumbar curves, may have little effect on the shape of the rib deformity, although the concave rib depression is usually elongated and therefore less obvious, and the shoulders become more level.

6 Much more attention needs to be directed towards rib shape and behaviour, both before and after surgery. It seems likely that the upper six ribs, being attached to the sternum, derotate little in spite of successful vertebral derotation, although they become more symmetrical in the vertical plane following Cobb angle correction. The convex ribs become more horizontal and the concave ribs are separated, thus elongating the rib depression but changing the rib hump little. Those patients showing little rib asymmetry will therefore do well cosmetically following surgery compared with those with marked asymmetry. It is vital that patients and their relatives should be warned that their rib hump will be improved to some extent (elevation of the concave depression), but it cannot be eliminated.

The lower six ribs, on the other hand, are often improved in terms of their rib–vertebra angle differences (RVAD) by vertebral derotation, but by a year after surgery they have usually returned to their former obliquity. This is because they have no strong anterior tether, the costal cartilages of ribs 7–9 being quite flexible in adolescents. This suggests that rib obliquity and shape is governed by extravertebral factors rather than being purely secondary to vertebral position.

7 In spite of all these difficulties and imperfections, advances of surgical technology, spinal cord monitoring, pain control and after-care still place surgery in experienced hands as the treatment of choice for adolescent idiopathic curves over a threshold of around 40° Cobb angle.

ACKNOWLEDGMENT

The author would like to thank Alan E. Heilman MD, of Joe W. King Orthopaedic Institute and Bayler College of Medicine Department of Orthopaedic Surgery, Houston, Texas, for his suggestions in the text and help with the references in addition to his sections on Cotrel–Dubousset spinal instrumentation and the Zielke operation. The invaluable help of my secretary Mrs Sylvia Bennett who typed the many drafts of this chapter is also acknowledged.

REFERENCES

Allen, B.L. Jr. (1984) Segmental instrumentation of the spine—indications, results and complications. In Dickson, R. & Bradford, D. (eds) *Management of Spinal Deformities*, pp. 162–192. Butterworths, London.

Benson, D.R., de Wald, R.L. & Schultz, A.B. (1977) Harrington rod distraction and instrumentation: its effect on vertebral rotation and thoracic compensation. *Clin. Orthop*, **125**, 40–44.

Bradford, D.S. (1979) Anterior spinal surgery in the management of scoliosis—indications, techniques, results. *Orthop. Clin. N. Am.*, **10**, 801–812.

Brooks, V.N. (1986) *The Neural Basis of Motor Control.* Oxford University Press, Oxford.

Broome, G., Simpson, A.H. R.W., Catalan, J., Jefferson, R.J. & Houghton, G.R. (1990) The modified Schollner costoplasty. *J. Bone Jt. Surg.*, **72B**, 894–900.

Burwell, R.G., Upadhyay, S.S., Webb, J.K., Patterson, J.F., Wojcik, A.S. & Moulton, A. (1989) Femoral anteversion and sagittal spinal decline angle in adolescents referred after screening for scoliosis. *Clin. Anat.*, **1**, 302 (abstract).

Cauchoix, J. & Binet, J.P. (1956) Anterior approaches to the spine. *Ann. R. Coll. Surg. Eng.*, **21**, 237–243.

Chopin, D. (1990) CD Spinal Instrumentation Course, Berck-Playe.

Clarisse, P. (1974) *Prognostic evolutif des scolioses idiopathiques mineures de 10° a 29° en periode de croissance.* These Med. Lyon.

Collis, D.K. & Ponseti, I.V. (1969) Long term follow-up of patients with idiopathic scoliosis not treated surgically. *J. Bone Jt. Surg.*, **51A**, 425–445.

Cotrel, Y. (1986) *New Instrumentation for Surgery of the Spine.* Freund Publishing House, London. Cotrel, Y. & Dubousset, J. (1985) New segmental posterior instrumentation of the spine. *Orthop. Trans.*, **9**, 118.

Cowell, H.R., Hall, J.N. & MacEwen, G.D. (1972) Genetic aspects of idiopathic scoliosis. *Clin. Orthop. Rel. Res.*, **86**, 121–131.

Cundy, P.J., Paterson, D.C., Hillier, T.M., Sutherland, A.D., Stephen, J.P. & Foster, B.K. (1990) Cotrel–Dubousset instrumentation and vertebral rotation in adolescent idiopathic scoliosis. *J. Bone Jt. Surg.*, **72B**, 670–675.

Dangerfield, P.H., Denton, J.S., Barnes, S.B. & Drake, N.B. (1986) The assessment of ribcage and spinal deformity in scoliosis: surface topography and spinal deformity. In Stokes, I.A.F., Pekelsky, J.R. & Moreland, M.S. (eds) *Proceedings 4th International Symposium*, Quebec, pp. 53–65. Gustav Fischer, Stuttgart.

Dickson, R.A. (1986) Definitions relevant to spinal deformity. Natural History Committee of British Scoliosis Society.

Dickson, J. & Erwin, W. (1989) *Advanced CD Instrumentation Course.* Houston, Texas, June 1989.

Dickson, R.A., Lawton, J.O., Archer, I.A. & Butt, W.T. (1984) The pathogenesis of idiopathic scoliosis. *J. Bone Jt. Surg.*, **66B**, 8–15.

Dove, J. (1989) Segmental wiring for spinal deformity: a morbidity report. Spine, **14**, 229–231.

Dretakis, E.K., Paraskevaidis, C.H., Zarkadoulas, V. & Christodoulou, N. (1988) The electroencephalographic study of schoolchildren with adolescent idiopathic scoliosis. *Spine*, **13**, 143–145.

Drummond, D., Narechania, R., Wenger, D., Corolla, J. & Breed, A.L. (1982) Wisconsin segmental spinal instrumentation. *Orthop. Trans.*, **6**, 22–23.

Duval-Beaupere, G. (1971) Pathogenic relationship between scoliosis and growth: *Proceedings, 3rd Phillip Zorab Symposium*, London.

Dwyer, A.F., Newton, N.C. & Sherwood, A.A. (1969) An anterior approach to scoliosis—a preliminary report. *Clin. Orthop. Rel. Res.*, **62**, 192–202.

Dwyer, A.P., O'Brien, J.P., Seal, V.P., *et al.* (1979) The late complications after the Dwyer anterior spinal instrumentation for scoliosis. *J. Bone Jt. Surg.*, **61A**, 1143–1150.

Edgar, M.A., Mehta, M.A., Michel, C.R., Winter, R., Lonstein, J. & Nachemson, A. (1983) Long term results of operatively treated scoliosis. In Pecina, M. (ed.) *Scoliosis and Kyphosis*, pp. 56–59.

Edgar, M.A. & Mehta, M.H. (1988) Long term follow-up of fused and unfused idiopathic scoliosis. *J. Bone Jt. Surg.*, **70B**, 712–716.

Fillio, N.A. & Thompson, M.W. (1971) Genetic studies in scoliosis. *J. Bone Jt. Surg.*, **53A**, 199.

Gardner, A.D.H. (1991) Correction of adolescent idiopathic scoliosis by the heavy (6 mm) Hartshill rectangle with particular reference to the behaviour of the ribs. Combined meeting, British Scoliosis Society and Scandinavian Scoliosis Societies, Newcastle-on-Tyne, England. *J. Bone Jt. Surg.* (In press).

Greulich, W.W. & Pyle, S.I. (1959) *Radiographic Atlas of Skeletal Development of the Hand and Wrist*, 2nd edn. Stanford University Press, Stanford, CA.

Hall, J.E. (1972) The anterior approach to spinal deformities. *Orthop. Clin. N. Am.*, **3**, 81–98.

Harrington, P.R. (1960) Surgical instrumentation for management of scoliosis. *J. Bone Jt. Surg.*, **42A**, 1448.

Harrington, P.R. (1962) Correction and internal fixation by spine instrumentation. *J. Bone Jt. Surg.*, **44A**, 591.

Harrington, P.R. (1972) Technical details in relation to the successful use of instrumentation in scoliosis. *Orthop. Clin. N. Am.*, **3**, 49.

Hefti, F.L. & McMaster M.J. (1983) The effect of the adolescent growth spurt on early posterior spinal fusion in infantile and juvenile idiopathic scoliosis. *J. Bone Jt. Surg.*, **65B**, 247–254.

Herman, R., Manlucci, R., Stuyck, J. *et al.* (1979) Vestibular functioning in idiopathic scoliosis. *Orthop. Trans.*, **3**, 218.

Hodgson, A.R. & Stock, F.E. (1956) Anterior spine fusion. *Br. J. Surg.*, **44**, 266.

Hodgson, A.R., Stock, F.E., Fang, H.S.Y. & Ong, G.B. (1960) Anterior spine fusion, *Br. J. Surg.*, **48**, 172–178.

Hugus, J.J., Taylor, T.K.F., McGee Collett, M., Besser, M., Gurr, K.R. & Marshfield, W.I. (1990) Syringomyelia and scoliosis: a new view. Presented at Scoliosis Research Society 25th Annual Meeting, Honolulu.

Isu, T., Iwasaki, Y., Akino, M. & Abi, H. (1990) Hydrosyringomyelia associated with a Chiari 1 malformation in children and adolescents. *Neurosurgery*, **26**, 591–597.

Kiel, A.W., Burwell, R.G., Cattle, J., Jacobs, K., Moulton, A., Webb, J.K. & Wozcik, A.S. (1989) A segmental analysis of the lateral profile of the spine revealing changes in the thoraco-lumbar region of thoracic curves: possible relation to the spinal mortice joint. Presented to 14th Annual Meeting of British Scoliosis Society, Basildon, UK.

King, H.A., Moe, J.H., Bradford, D.S. & Winter R.B. (1983) The selection of the fusion levels in thoracic idiopathic scoliosis. *J. Bone Jt. Surg.*, **65A**, 1302–1314.

Leatherman, K.C. (1969) Resection of vertebral bodies. *J. Bone Jt. Surg.*, **51A**, 206.

Leonard, M.A. (1981) Investigation into the electroencephalographic findings in patients with idiopathic scoliosis. *J. Bone Jt. Surg.*, **63B**, 632.

Lonstein, J. & Carlson, J.M. (1984) The prediction of curve progression in untreated idiopathic scoliosis during growth. *J. Bone Jt. Surg.*, **66A**, 1061–1071.

Luque, E.R. (1982) Segmental spinal instrumentation for correction of scoliosis. *Clin. Orthop.*, **163**, 192–198.

Luque, E.R. & Cardoso, A. (1977) Segmental correction of scoliosis with rigid internal fixation. *Orthop. Trans.*, **1**, 136–137.

Manning, C.W., Prince, F.J. & Zorab, P.A. (1973) Partial costectomy as a cosmetic operation in scoliosis. *J. Bone Jt. Surg.*, **55B**, 521–527.

Miller, J.A., Nachemson, A.L. & Schultz, A.B. (1984) The effectiveness of braces in mild idiopathic scoliosis: late results. *Spine*, **9**, 632–635.

Moe, J.H. (1972) Methods of correction and surgical technique in scoliosis. *Orthop. Clin. N. Am.*, **2**, 17.

Moe, J.H., Purcell, G. & Bradford, D.S. (1983) Zielke instrumentation (VDS) for the correction of spinal curvature. Analysis and results of 66 patients. *Clin. Orthop. Rel. Res.*, **180**, 133–154.

Moe, Winter, Bradford & Lonstein (1978) *Scoliosis and other Spinal Deformities*. W.B. Saunders, Philadephia, PA.

Nachemson, A. *et al.* (1979) Symposium on adult scoliosis. *Spine*, **4**, 513–552.

Nash, C.L., Gregg, E.C., Brown, R.H. & Pillai, K. (1979) Risks of exposure to X-rays in patients undergoing long-term treatment for scoliosis. *J. Bone Jt. Surg.*, **61A**, 371–374.

Nordwall, A. & Willner, S. (1975) A study of skeletal age and height in girls with idiopathic scoliosis. *Clin. Orthop. Rel. Res.*, **110**, 6–10.

Owen, R., Turner, A., Bamforth, J.S.G., Taylor, J.F. & Jones R.S. (1986) Costectomy as a first stage of surgery for scoliosis. *J. Bone Jt. Surg.*, **68B**, 91–95.

Perdriolle, R. & Vidal, J. (1981) Édude de la courbure scoliotique. Importance de l'extension et de la rotation vertebrale. Rev. Chir. *Orthop.*, **67**, 25–34.

Resina, J. & Ferriera-Alves, A.F. (1977) A technique of correction and internal fixation for scoliosis *J. Bone Jt. Surg.*, **59B**, 159–165.

Riseborough, E.J. & Wynne-Davies, R. (1973) A genetic survey of idiopathic scoliosis in Boston, Massachusetts. *J. Bone Jt. Surg.*, **55A**, 974–982.

Risser, J.C. (1958) The iliac apophysis, an invaluable sign in the management of scoliosis. *Clin. Orthop.*, **11**, 111.

R. Smith (1991) *Operative Surgery*, 4th edn. Bentley G., (ed) Butterworth and Heinemann, London.

Robb, J. *et al.* (1986) Normal electroencephalography in idiopathic scoliosis. *Acta Orthop. Scand.*, **57**, 220–221.

Sahlstrand, T. & Petrusan, B. (1979) A study of labyrinthine function in patients with adolescent idiopathic scoliosis. *Acta Orthop. Scand.*, **50**, 759–769.

Samberg, L.C., Benitez, J.T., Leisz, M.C. & Mulawka, S.M. (1984) *Study of vestibular function as a prognostic aid in adolescent idiopathic scoliosis.* Presented at 19th Annual Meeting of the Scoliosis Research Society, Orlando, Florida.

Schollner, D. (1966) Steigerung der Vitalkapazitat der Rippenbuckel-resektion mit der Brustkorbdehnungs-tecknik. *Z. Orthop.*, **101**, 323–333.

Stagnara, P. (1988) *Spinal Deformity*, p. 288. Butterworths, London.

Targett, J.P.G. & Gardner, A.D.H. (1989) Comparison of Hartshill/Luque spinal fusions with other sublaminar wiring techniques in idiopathic scoliosis in terms of Cobb angle and Perdriolle rotation. 14th Annual meeting, British Scoliosis Society, Basildon, UK.

Thulborne, T. & Gillespie, R. (1976) The rib hump in idiopathic scoliosis: measurement analysis and response to treatment. *J. Bone Jt. Surg.*, **58B**, 64–71.

Weatherley, C.R., Draycott, V., O'Brien, J.F., Benson, D.R., Gopala Krishnan, K.C., Evans, J.H. & O'Brien, J.P. (1987) The rib deformity in adolescent scoliosis. *J. Bone Jt. Surg.*, **69B**, 179–182.

Willner, S. *et al.* (1981) The spinal pantograph: a non-invasive technique for describing kyphosis and lordosis. *Acta Orthop. Scand.*, **52**, 525–529.

Wojcik, A.S., Webb, J.K. & Burwell, R.G. (1990) An analysis of the effect of the Zielke operation on the rib cage of S-shaped curves in idiopathic scoliosis. *Spine*, **15**, 81–86.

Wojcik, A.S., Webb, J.K. & Burwell, R.G. (1990) Harrington–Luque and Cotrel–Dubousset instrumentation for idiopathic thoracic scoliosis. A post-operative comparison using segmental radiologic analysis. *Spine*, **15**, 424–431.

Wynne-Davies, R. (1968) Familial (idiopathic) scoliosis: a family survey. *J. Bone Jt. Surg.*, **50B**, 24–30.

Zielke, K., Stundat, R. & Beaujean, F. (1976) Ventrale derotations spondylo-disc. Vorlaufiger Ergebuissbericht uber 26 operierte. *Falle. Arch. Orthop. Unfallchir.*, **85**, 257–277.

23 · Management of Adult Spinal Deformity

By J.P. KOSTUIK

Adult scoliosis has been defined as that presenting following skeletal maturity over the age of 20 years.

Thus scolioses in adult life fall into two categories: those curves which were present prior to skeletal maturity, and those deformities which arise '*nouveau*' in adult life because of either osteoporosis, or osteomalacia, or for iatrogenic reasons such as following multiple-level decompression for spinal stenosis and degenerative changes.

In this chapter our concern is primarily with the former category; the principles of management, however, apply to all scoliosis patients regardless of aetiology. Some aspects of acquired kyphosis in the adult will also be addressed.

Prior to the late 1960s it was felt that surgical treatment of scoliotic deformities in the adult, with few exceptions such as of some thoracic curves in people in their third decade, was not considered appropriate. However, the works of Collis (1969), Kostuik (1973), Nilsonne (1968), Ponsetti (1968), Stagnara (1969, 1971), Stagnara *et al.* (1969, 1975) and others (Dawson, 1973; Harrington, 1973; Ponder, 1975; Cummine, 1979; Swank, 1981; Sponseller, 1987; Johnson, 1988; Bradford, 1988; van Dam, 1987, 1988; Winter, 1978, 1988), have shown that curves in the adult may progress, and that frequently these same curves are painful. With the advent of Harrington instrumentation in the late 1950s and the subsequent improvements in Dwyer instrumentation in 1970 (Dwyer, 1973; Winter, 1978; Hall, 1981) Luque instrumentation in 1976 (Luque, 1982a,b), Zielke instrumentation in 1975 (Zielke *et al.*, 1976) and more recently Cotrel–Dubousett instrumentation (CDI) (Cotrel, 1986; Cotrel *et al.*, 1988), together with improvements in preoperative assessment and postoperative care, we have seen marked improvement in the ability to deal with the complex problems of the adult.

Today there is a greater recognition not only by family physicians, but also by paramedical personnel, that the adult scoliotic requiring surgery can safely undergo surgical intervention when necessary.

CURRENT PROBLEMS

Kostuik & Bentivogilio (1981) found an incidence of 3.9% of curves in adults involving the thoracolumbar and lumbar spine. They felt that these curves were truly structural in nature, having commenced in adolescence and progressed in adult life. These were not curves secondary to osteoporosis or to local degenerative changes.

In 1968 James (Vanderpool *et al.*, 1969) stated that in Edinburgh 6% of adults over the age of 50 years showed evidence radiographically of scoliosis, but felt that the majority of these were due to compression fractures associated with osteoporosis and osteomalacia. Dewar in the early 1950s (unpublished data) discovered an incidence of structural thoracic scoliosis of 4% on reviewing 10 000 consecutive chest radiographs taken for routine hospital admission. Since many of these curves are mild to moderate in adolescence, and do not become apparent until the fourth, fifth and sixth decades of life, there will continue to be a group of patients particularly in view of increasing longevity, especially in the industrialized countries in which surgical intervention will be appropriate.

Work by Weinstein & Ponsetti (1983) identified aetiological factors which are responsible for continued progression in adult life. Thoracic curves between 50° and 75° at skeletal maturity increased

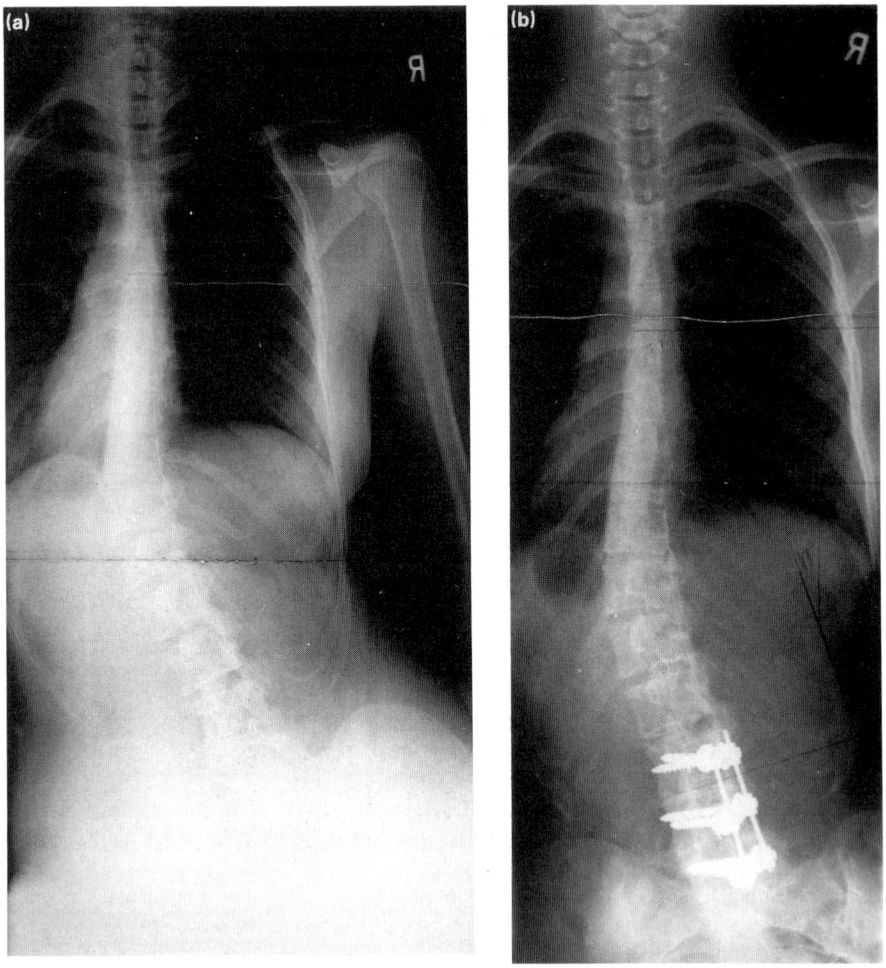

Fig. 23.1 (a) Female age 26 with a painful scoliosis. Note marked imbalance to the left. Pain was reproduced on discography at both L4–L5 and L1–S1 discs. (b) Same case, rebalanced with relief of pain secondary to lateral closing wedges. Note double Zielke rods in order to control rotational forces.

an average of 30° over the follow-up period. Thoracolumbar curves of 50–75° at skeletal maturity increased 22.3° over 40 years. Lumbar spine curves, where the fifth lumbar vertebra was not well seated and where apical rotation was greater than 33%, progressed the most.

In our experience the curve with the worst prognosis in adult life is that of the young person who presents with an unbalanced lumbar or thoracolumbar curve where the fifth lumbar vertebra is not parallel with the sacrum and the curve emanates from the lumbosacral junction (Fig. 23.1a,b). This curve presents the greatest technical difficulties at correction in later life and therefore is best treated at an early age if possible.

Other curves with a poor prognosis include those whose apex fall at the L2–L3 L3–L4 area, who have a significant grade three rotation, are unbalanced and have a secondary compensatory curve which is sharp and angular at the L4–L5 L5–S1 area. These curves in the young adult are best treated and rebalanced by dealing with the compensatory curve at one or two levels, rather than dealing with the entire more proximal curve over five to seven levels.

With the increasing age of our population it is not uncommon for the spinal surgeon to be presented with a complex problem of increasing deformity associated with pain, loss of lumbar lordosis, imbalance, osteoporosis and spinal stenosis. Today, with a better understanding of spinal mechanics, improved instrumentation, improved postoperative care and a better understanding of screw fixation in bone, it is possible to treat these people with relatively little morbidity (Fig. 23.2a–d).

In a review of adult patients with curves in the lumbar and thoracolumbar spine Kostuik & Bentivoglio (1981) found an incidence of back pain in 60%. This was similar in incidence to an un-

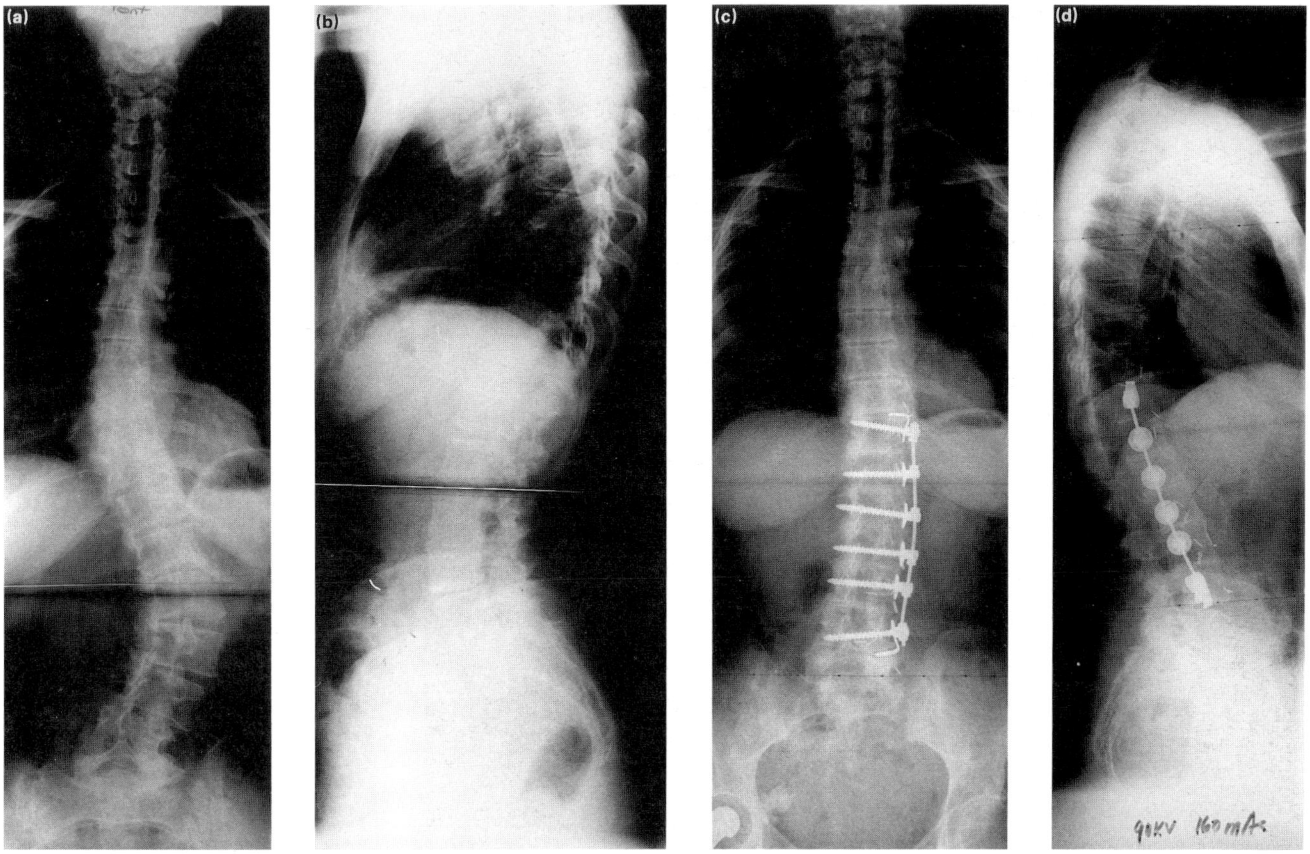

Fig. 23.2 (a) Female age 65 with a documented progressive painful curve of 44°. L4–L5 and L5–S1 discs were not painful on discography; L4–S1 and L5–S1 facet blocks did not relieve pain; note previous total hip. (b) Preoperative lateral 66°. (c) Postoperative Zielke instrumentation 2°. After 6 years follow-up there was no pain. (d) Lordosis has been fully preserved.

selected consecutive series of 100 patients of the same age span without scoliosis. It is recognized that these figures are comparable to population studies in the industrialized world where the incidence of back pain is between 60% and 70% in the general adult population. They also noted that in curves greater than 45% the incidence of pain increased markedly, the pain maximizing between the ages of 40 and 60 years similar to the spondylogenic or discogenic pain patterns in the general population. In 1969 Nachemson (1969, 1983) found a similar incidence of pain amongst scoliotics. However, in contrast the incidence of severe pain seems to be greater in the study of Kostuik & Bentivoglio (1981) than in that of Nachemson (1969, 1983), who noted the pain always to be mild and that it rarely required treatment. It is not the degree of deformity which is so paramount in adults, as compared with adolescents. Most adults should be given a course of non-operative or conservative treatment first. The exception to this is the patient with obvious significant progression, as evidenced either radiologically or by loss of height, who is unbalanced and has a good deal of rotation radiologically with significant disabling pain (Fig. 23.3). In our experience thoracic curves in the adult are rarely painful.

Other major problems in dealing with adult scoliosis (see Doherty, 1973; Grobler *et al.*, 1978; Hasday *et al.*, 1983; Kostuik *et al.*, 1988; Lagrone *et al.*, 1988) are those related to iatrogenic flat back secondary to distraction fusions with Harrington instrumentation extending to the distal lumbar spine, usually L5 or even S1. This problem may also occur as a result of degenerative changes and loss of disc height below a fusion mass ending at the midlumbar level, and indeed may occur above a fusion; for instance from L4 to the sacrum in a female secondary to osteopenia and loss of disc height. A

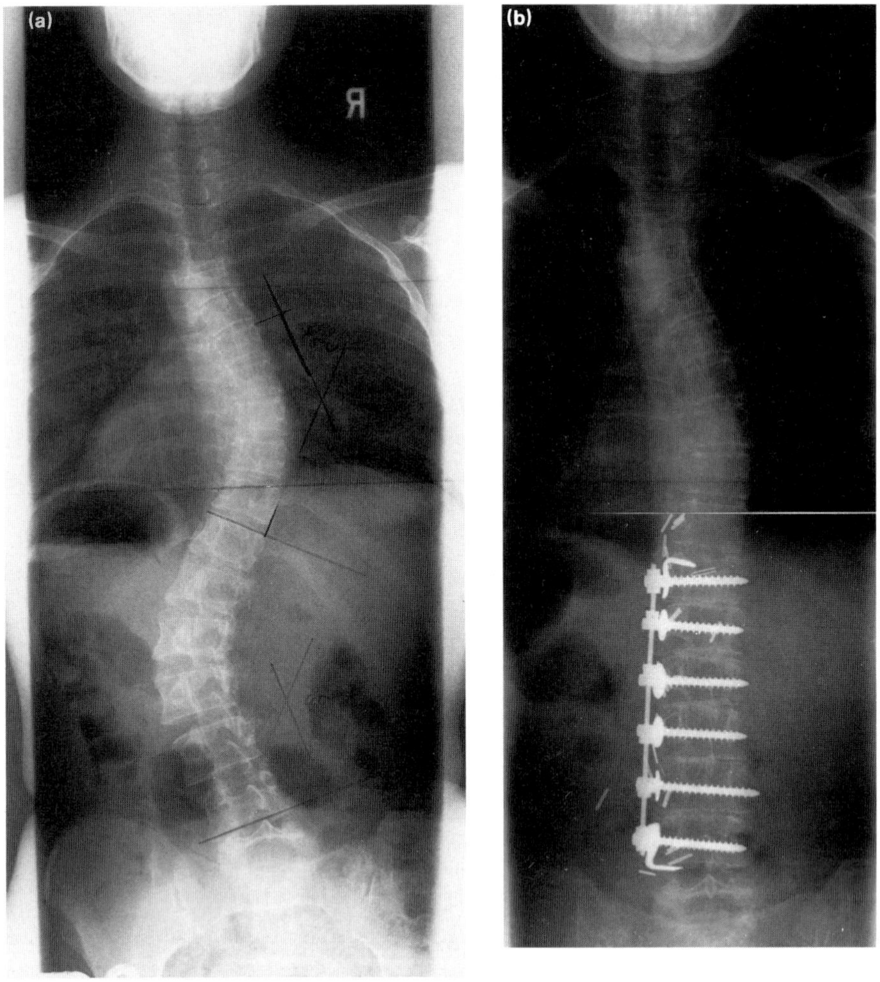

Fig. 23.3 (a) Female age 24. Lumbar curve 60°, thoracic curve 52°. Note obliquity of L5. (b) Postoperative lumbar curve 15°, thoracic curve reduced to 40°. L5 is more parallel to the horizontal.

further problem may result from precocious degenerative changes occurring below a fusion done in adolescence or early adult life.

Cochran *et al.* (1983) in a long-term anatomical and functional review of patients with adolescent idiopathic scoliosis treated by Harrington rod and fusion, have shown a proportionally increased incidence of degenerative changes the more distal the fusion undertaken in adolescence, with an incidence of approximately 20% of degenerative changes with pain below fusions ending at L2; approximately 40% at L3; 60% at L4, and 80% at L5. Edgar (1982) similarly found an increased incidence of degenerative changes associated with pain at levels below a posterior fusion extending to L3 or L4.

When correlating pain with age the pattern seems to follow a bell curve, with the majority of patients with pain falling in the sixth, seventh and eighth decade of life. Pain appears to reach its maximum between 40 and 60 years of age, which corresponds to the maximum incidence of pain from a spondylogenic or discogenic cause in the non-scoliotic population. When correlating occupation and pain there appears to be distinct preference for lighter work by scoliotic patients, although only 21% of patients in the review undertaken by Kostuik & Bentivoglio (1981) were aware that they had a scoliosis. Rogala & Drummond (1978) also suggested a preference for lighter work by scoliotics. The type of occupation was not a predisposing factor regarding pain in this review, although those with heavier-type jobs seemed to be less able to cope, and missed more time from work, or were more likely to be incapacitated. Patients with curves greater than 40° had a statistically greater degree of incapacitating pain than those patients with lesser curves. The increasing incapacity due to pain with greater curves, together with escalating pain with increased age, would suggest that curves 40° or greater at the end of growth will tend to become more clinically significant with time. In both the lumbar and thoracolumbar curves pain was more noticeable the more severe the curve. In attempting to correlate pain with plain radiographic changes, all patients with degenerative changes at the apex of curves also demonstrated similar changes at the lumbosacral junction. Facet sclerosis correlated with a history of pain in 64% of patients.

DEGENERATIVE ADULT SCOLIOSIS

As noted above, considerable controversy has existed in defining 'adult scoliosis'; which curves have progressed from adolescence and which have appeared later in life?

The studies of James (Vanderpool *et al.*, 1969), already referred to, emphasized the importance of osteoporosis and osteomalacia as factors in progression of curves in the adult. However, Kostuik *et al.* (1981), in a review of 5000 myelograms, found an incidence of 3.9% of thoracolumbal lumbar curves; all were considered to have commenced in adolescence.

One difficulty in differentiating between the two groups is that lumbar and thoracolumbar curves are frequently not noticed until the onset of back pain, or until progression occurs as a result of degenerative changes later in life in pre-existing adolescent curves.

Grubb *et al.* (1989) recently analysed two groups of patients: those in which curves commenced in adolescent life and those in which the deformity was felt to occur as a result of degenerative changes. They found significant differences in densitometry measurements between patients with idiopathic adolescent curves and those with adult degenerative curves when compared with age-matched controls.

Pain patterns in both groups were similar, i.e. low back, buttock and leg pains; however, the adult degenerative group had a much higher incidence of stenotic-type symptoms and up to 90% were aggravated by activity compared with 31% in the first group. Activities that provoked stenotic-like symptoms were mainly those involving extension of the lumbar spine. The curve magnitude was significantly different, with the primary adolescent group ranging from 34° to 78° with a mean of 52°. The degenerative group ranged from 15° to 53° with a mean of 28°. Though the curvature in the first group was significantly greater, the mean degree per segment was the same in both groups; 9°. In the first group all were females with a mean age of 42 years, whereas in the degenerative groups male and female numbers were equal, with a mean age of 60 years.

As well as having greater curve magnitude, the primary adolescent cases showed myelographic defects in the compensatory lumbosacral secondary curve, whereas in the degenerative group the myelographic defects were most marked in the main curve; also discography in the latter group revealed gross degenerative disc changes throughout the lumbar spine. Pain was frequently not reproduced on distension of the degenerate disc; indeed the test is of little value in this group, whereas the first group of patients with mechanical back pain discography highlighted the painful discs reproducing symptoms frequently within the curve as Kostuik (1979) has previously noted. Grubb and co-workers (1989) noted that discography at the lower end of the curve in the lumbar spine or in the compensatory lumbosacral curve can reproduce pain. They concluded, as did Kostuik (1979), that although pain can arise in the main structural curve, it can equally arise from the compensatory curve in the lumbosacral area.

With regard to the curves that commence in adolescence the lumbar and thoracolumbar spine lordosis is initially well preserved but with progressive degeneration of the discs in the fifth and sixth decades of life the spine may change from being lordotic in the lumbar area to being kypohotic. The management of such curves is discussed elsewhere in this chapter.

Since the majority of adult-onset curves develop spinal stenosis conventional decompression alone, as also in the adolescent-onset group, should be avoided unless it can be limited to one nerve root with preservation of the facet joints. Any more than this should be accompanied by fusion, either *in situ* or by correcting the deformity (see Fig. 23.17).

Nash *et al.* (1989) have recently analysed fusions done in the lumbar spine to see whether the criteria used for fusion in adolescence was valid for adults. Factors studied were: (a) the stable zone, (b) central sacral line, (c) neutrally rotated vertebra, (d) degenerative arthritis, (e) displaced wedging, (f) rotatory subluxation, (g) vertebral body wedging, (h) lumbosacral take-off, (i) hemi-sacralization. They concluded that many patho-anatomical factors needed to be considered in selecting the number of lumbar vertebrae to be fused in adult scoliosis patients.

The criteria used as listed rarely proved of value in isolation, indeed one factor was only of value in 16 of 53 cases, two factors in 20 of 53 cases, three factors in 11 of 53 cases, four factors in 3 of 53 cases, and five factors in 2 of 53 cases in the series of Nash *et al.* Consideration of the stable zone, although helpful in younger patients in correcting the upper lumbar spine, was of no value in the older patients. Degenerative and deforming factors play a major role in the latter, especially in the lower lumbar spine, necessitating fusions to lower levels as Kostuik (1979) has pointed out. The most important lesson learnt from this review is that degenerative changes must be included in the fusion mass, and that in our estimation are best identified by the use of discography and facet blocks. Despite the limitations identified in the review, Nash *et al.* (1989) concluded that patients undergoing fusion in the lumbar area appeared to have significant relief of pain and were satisfied with their surgery in 89% of cases, provided the selection criteria were applied sensibly.

PATIENT EVALUATION

As with most spinal problems, history is the principal means of evaluation. A relevant family history of deformity may give some indication of prognosis. For example, a close relative who has a progressive severe deformity and is older than the patient may give some indication as to the patient's future. The date of onset of the deformity should be considered, but is not in itself usually important.

Curve progression can be estimated from the history given by the patient or relatives. For example a change in clothes, increasing rib hump, a loss of height and a loss of waistline are relevant. Ideally progression is best determined by serial X-rays, but these are often not available, particularly in the case of thoracolumbar or lumbar curves, where the deformity may not be noticed until adult life. The psychological aspects of the patient's deformity should be considered. Many adults are reluctant to discuss their deformity from an aesthetic point of view, unless directly asked. Many of them have learned to live with their deformity, which does not usually present a problem. Conversely there are a number of patients where deformity continues to play a significant psychological role, and this has occurred in 10% of cases in our series.

A pain questionnaire is important to help determine the location of pain. Pain may be apical or below the apex. Often the patient may indicate with the palm of the hand the source of pain. It is important to know its duration, how it affects activities of daily living, social function, occupation, home and sexual life; also what aggravates and what alleviates the pain. If the pain is suggestive of root irritation it is important to elicit this. Radicular pain may be related to the apex of the curve, and if in the thoracic or thoracolumbar curve area it may be intercostal in nature. It may also arise from the compensatory curve in the case of a thoracolumbar curve, as noted by Jackson *et al.* (1983). The lumbar area pain may be referred into the lower extremities. True sciatica extends below the knee; pain above the knee may simply be referred but can also be of nerve root origin.

A history of bowel and bladder dysfunction is important to elicit. An associated spinal stenosis may present initially with bladder incontinence, particularly in females. Incontinence in the elderly female is often due to spinal stenosis and not, as is commonly assumed, due to the after-effects of childbearing. Thus the recent onset of bladder incontinence is significant.

Respiratory malfunction may be the presenting symptom, but usually only in paralytic or severe congenital curves. The patient may describe respiratory problems such as shortness of breath in climbing stairs or other activities, or simply as tiredness. A review of 200 consecutive adults with idiopathic scoliosis, by the author, revealed no cases of severe dysfunction, even in curves of 100° or more. Ventilation, however, was often decreased, by as much as 25% of predicted normal value, but rarely was of functional significance. Arterial blood gases were generally normal. Severe problems in perfusion or ventilation in the presence of a scoliosis indicate congenital scoliosis or associated congenital cardiac anomalies. There would appear to be a correlation between curve size and pulmonary insufficiency above 60°, but we have not seen, in over 22 years of experience, pulmonary deaths associated with idiopathic scoliosis. All deaths were in congenital or paralytic curves. The only exception to this rule in idiopathic scoliosis is the patient who has a very marked thoracic lordosis, where pulmonary function may be severely affected. Therefore pulmonary function tests are performed only for thoracic curves of greater than 60°, or in cases of paralytic or congenital scoliosis.

Physical examination naturally focuses on the spinal deformity, but a complete examination is necessary, including a full neurological examination as well as cardiopulmonary evaluation. The three-dimensional nature of the curve should be appreciated. A kyphotic or lordotic element should be looked for in the presence of a scoliosis, and its effect on pulmonary function noted.

The degree of decompensation, the flexibility and the size of the rib hump should be measured, as well as the patient's height. Signs of subtle neurological dysfunction should be looked for, particularly in left thoracic 'idiopathic' curves which are sometimes associated with syringomyelia. Mild clawing of the toes may indicate a tethered cord. Muscle fatigue after exercise, in the presence of a history of spinal stenosis associated with scoliosis may be important.

ROENTGENOLOGY

Following clinical assessment initial radiographic analysis should include postero-anterior and lateral radiographs. These will indicate the degree of the deformity; local pathology, if any, and the degree of decompensation. In the presence of pain, localized X-rays are useful to detect such abnormalities as enlarged facets, congenital anomalies, disc narrowing and other relevant pathology.

In our experience, bending X-rays will indicate flexibility of the curve if present, but do not provide any guide as to the degree of correction that might be expected by surgical intervention. In mobile thoracolumbar curves treated by anterior Zielke instrumentation the amount of correction obtained was twice that expected from the bending films.

Traction films are occasionally of value in attempting to show whether distraction will overcome decompensation. A supine postero-anterior film may also help in analysing decompensation. Hyperextension views of the kyphotic area are of value only if the kyphosis is flexible; similarly flexion views are useful in evaluating excessive lordosis. Since scoliosis is a rotational deformity, Stagnara oblique views, particularly in the cases of kyphoscoliosis, demonstrate the deformity well.

Special studies include bone scans, myelography, discography, computerized tomography (CT) and magnetic resonance imaging (MRI). Bone scans are rarely indicated, but are sometimes of value in the young adult with a minor curve in ruling out pathology such as tumour as a cause of the scoliosis. Myelography is indicated in any patient with neuropathology and congenital curves; also in a patient undergoing surgical correction for painful deformity myelography preoperatively is of value to rule out cauda equina or cord compression.

CT has not been of great value in assessing the contents of the dural canal alone; in our experience it is best combined with myelography using non-ionic dyes. The scan is done 3–4 hours following the myelogram. In low back problems of a degenerative nature, myelography or CT scans may yield 30% false-positive results. The combination of myelography and CT scanning, however, has proved to be accurate in more than 90% of cases. The role of MRI is promising; however, it is still somewhat experimental in this field.

The value of discography and the use of facet blocks are discussed under pain evaluation in this chapter.

CONSERVATIVE NON-OPERATIVE CARE

Among those factors which may preclude operative intervention are serious cardiac or respiratory disease or psychological reasons. Conservative care is encouraged in the form of drugs, physical therapeutic modalities and orthotic devices, as well as sympathetic understanding.

Apart from cosmetic deformity, significant progression and/or neurological problems, the major indication for operative intervention is pain. Even then conservative management should be given a trial in the absence of neurological signs.

Non-steroidal anti-inflammatory drugs may be of value; also enteric-coated aspirin, which can be used long term. Muscle relaxants and heavy doses of narcotics should be avoided except for acute phases of severe pain.

Physiotherapy, particularly exercises, is rarely successful in controlling pain in adult scoliotics. Active motion usually aggravates pain; however, flexibility and stretching exercises may be of value in tiding a patient over, for a period, but exercises must be tailored to those motions which avoid pain. Low-thrust aerobics, cycling and swimming exercises may help. Nevertheless, no amount of physiotherapy will prevent the progression of a curve, but it may maintain flexibility to some degree and render subsequent surgical treatment easier.

In patients over 50 years of age, particularly females, the use of orthoses may be of great value. These need to be rigid and modelled to the patient's deformity; they should be worn while the patient is ambulant. These may tide the patient over for many months or even years. However, the majority of patients may eventually come to operative intervention. If an orthosis is provided an attempt should be made to involve the patient in an exercise programme of a general nature to maintain mobility. Diet is also important. Finally, a general understanding of the cause of scoliosis, and prognostic factors involving the patient's individual deformity, is essential.

Since osteoporosis plays a major role in the progression of deformity in the postmenopausal female it is important that those women in particular who are discovered to have a scoliosis before the menopause should exercise. Twenty minutes of general low-impact aerobics four times a week for 10 years before the menopause will prevent subsequent osteoporosis in the majority of women. In the postmenopausal woman exercise combined with hormonal therapy and calcium under the supervision of a physician may also be of benefit, especially in the first 10 years.

SURGICAL INDICATIONS

The indications for surgery are pain, progression of deformity, neurological disability, cosmesis, structural imbalance in paralytic or neuromuscular disease, curve progression associated with pain below previous fusions for spinal deformity and finally iatrogenic flat back.

An adult who presents below the age of 35 years without pain, but who has proven and increasing curvature, whose lumbar or thoracolumbar curve measures approximately 45° and especially if he or she is unbalanced, is best treated surgically, since inevitably the deformity will progress with accompanying low back pain. This is particularly true of female patients in whom a significant lumbar or thoracolumbar curve, because of degenerative changes, may in later life convert from being primarily a scoliosis with lumbar lordosis to a kyphoscoliosis which is rigid, and may be requiring two-stage surgery to correct the problem. The younger adult can be safely treated by anterior surgical correction by Zielke instrumentation with minimal morbidity (Fig. 23.3). There is always concern as to possible degenerative changes occurring below the fusion mass. Edgar & Mehta (1985) and Cochran *et al.* (1983) have stressed, however, that this problem is more related to posterior instrumentation and fusion which has extended to the lower lumbar levels. Following surgery, patients should become involved in athletic endeavours in order to maintain a satisfactory level of physical fitness. This applies to young and old, but in some patients, because of age and often a previous sedentary lifestyle, this is not always practicable.

The younger patient whose major curve may measure 40° or more, extending to L3 or L4, but who has a compensatory curve at L4–L5, L5–S1, and who is unbalanced, may experience improvement in the primary curve by surgically correcting the lower curve; but this should be done only if the lower curve is painful. These patients may run the risk of developing progression of their upper curve at a later date, and it should be explained to them that they may later require extension of their fusion more proximally. The technique has worked satisfactorily in a small number of patients (six), and although the follow-up is short the average correction of the major curve has been more than 40% (Fig. 23.1). Pain patterns must be analysed preoperatively by discography and facet blocks.

Progression is best assessed by a careful history taken from both the patient and relatives, with particular reference to current height, and height at the completion of growth. Radiological documentation, of course, is ideal but rarely available in mature adults. As mentioned previously, Weinstein & Ponselti (1983) showed that curves in the thoracolumbar and lumbar spine may progress, particularly if the fifth lumbar vertebra is not well seated (oblique) and apical rotation is greater than 33°. In our view imbalance seems to play a major role in progression of the curve, together with a significant degree of rotation.

Neurological deficit in our series of more than 1000 adults with scoliosis treated surgically has rarely been an indication for surgical intervention. However, with an increasing ageing population more patients are seen with an associated spinal stenosis (Fig. 23.4a–c). As already stressed, surgical decom-

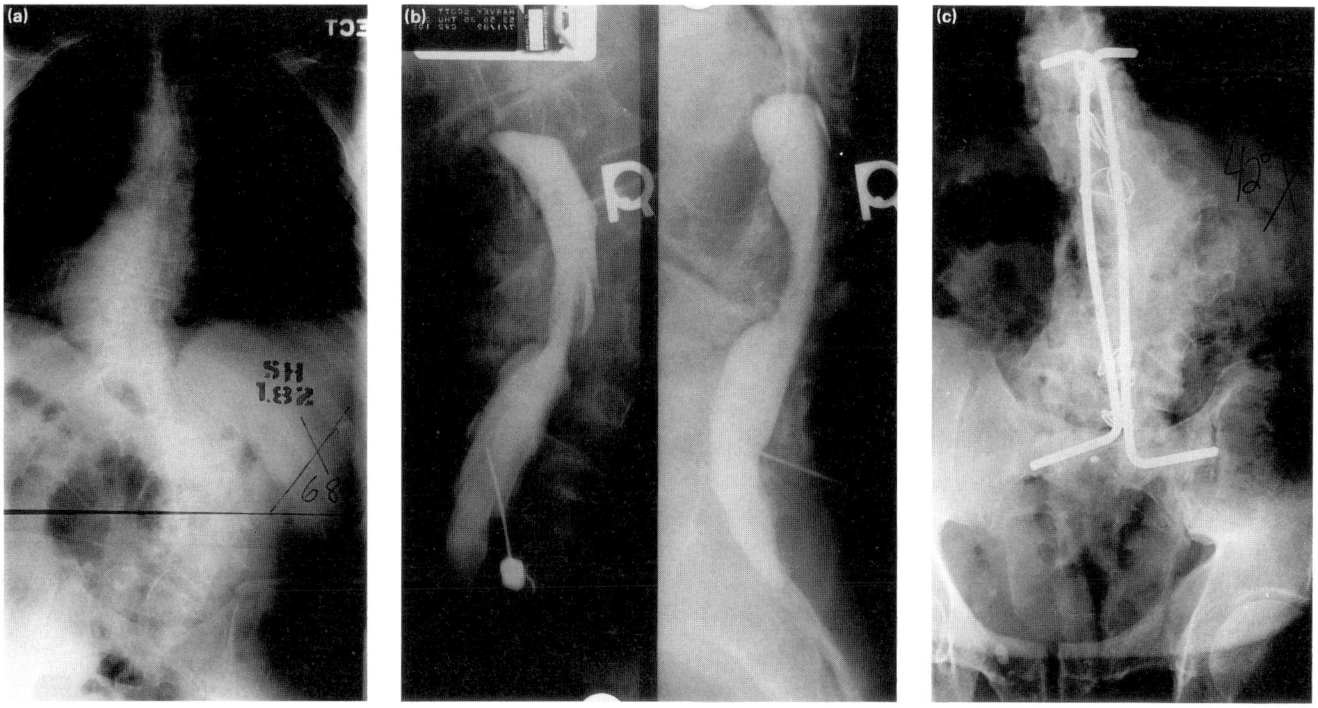

Fig. 23.4 (a) Male age 56 with a curve of 68°. There were marked symptoms, and mild signs of spinal stenosis. (b) Preoperative myelogram indicates severe compromise of canal at the apex of the curve. (c) Postoperative AP curve 42°. Five years later patient is pain-free and working.

pression by laminectomy in our experience is rarely indicated. In a review in 1978 only five patients out of 227 treated surgically for a painful scoliosis required associated decompression (Fig. 23.18).

Jackson *et al.* (1983) showed that frequently patients with radicular symptoms which arise in the compensatory curve may experience marked improvement postoperatively following correction of the major curve by an anterior procedure. In our experience this has been less successful.

We repeat that all patients who complain of significant pain should in our estimation undergo preoperative myelography, to rule out other causes of pain such as intradural or extradural tumours. This also applies to adults with significant lumbar and thoracolumbar curves about 45°, particularly if they have pain, as spinal stenosis may be present, especially in those patients over the age of 60.

The problem of cosmesis in the lumbar and thoracolumbar spine in adults is rare, with the exception of the young adult who is unbalanced. Many adults (10%) with scoliosis, however, present with thoracic curves which are not painful, but require surgical correction for cosmetic reasons. Following a thorough explanation of the complexities of surgery together with the associated risks, should the patient still desire improvement of the deformity, surgical intervention is warrantable, but only after repeated discussion with the patient and close relatives.

With the advent of CDI, especially if the patient is hypokyphotic in the thoracic spine, excellent cosmetic correction can now be obtained in the adult. The use of thoracoplasty will also enhance the postoperative cosmetic appearance.

A recent functional analysis (Kostuik *et al.*, 1990) of 100 patients interviewed more than 10 years postoperatively showed that body image and cosmesis played a much greater role, in the adult, than has hitherto been suspected.

POSTOPERATIVE CARE

Postoperative care of the adult today is much easier. Recumbency is not permitted; patients usually become ambulant by the third or fourth postoperative day. Those with thoracolumbar curves in the postoperative phase are usually fitted with an orthosis either of the modular Boston overlap type or a moulded plastic corset. Thoracic curves require no external support.

PAIN ASSESSMENT

Early attempts by the author (Kostuik *et al.*, 1973) in the late 1960s and 1970s, to treat painful lumbar and thoracolumbar curves, with Harrington instrumentation and fusion, without preoperative pain assessment by discography and facet blocks, left a significant number of patients complaining of pain. Pain relief averaged 65–70%. Subsequent preoperative evaluation of pain using discography and facet blocks has resulted in between 80% and 90% obtaining good pain relief (Kostuik, 1979).

A careful history is most important. Patients may localize their pain to the low back or to the apex of the curvature or to both. Frequently, however, the symptoms may be vague. Macnab (1977) showed that hypertonic saline injection into the supraspinous ligament of the thoracolumbar junction can reproduce pain at the lumbosacral level.

With this in mind the author in the 1970s (Kostuik, 1979) undertook a prospective study using discography to help differentiate sources of pain. The current use of discography is limited to an assessment of the lower levels of the lumbar spine, namely from L3 to the lumbosacral junction. Rarely are discograms now performed at the apex of the curve.

Discography is used to assess whether or not these levels are degenerate and/or painful. Facet blocks are similarly used. Discography is usually done via a posterolateral approach, although occasionally because of deformity it may be necessary to trangress the dura. Facet blocks are done using marcaine with infiltration of the posterior ramus. It is recognized that levels other than the L5–S1 articulation have multiple innervation, and if the L4–L5 level is to be assessed then the L3–L4 level must be infiltrated also. Our current practice in painful lumbar and thoracolumbar curves is to perform discography at the lower levels of the lumbar spine and facet blocks at the L5–S1 level which has a single innervation, and L4–L5 only occasionally.

If facet blocks relieve pain, and discography reproduces pain at the lumbosacral junction, then we feel that fusion should be extended to the sacrum, as previous to discography being available, when fusion was not extended to the sacrum, many patients continued to complain of pain despite correction of the deformity (Kostuik *et al.*, 1973). Such a fusion with preservation of lumbar lordosis has resulted in good results in 90% of such cases.

Conversely, should discograms not reproduce the patient's pain, and facet blocks at the lumbosacral junction not produce relief, then it is assumed that the pain arises in the curve itself. Should L5–S1 not be part of the curve, the curve alone is corrected and the lumbosacral junction left free.

Finally one must be convinced that the pain is mechanical in nature and not clouded by significant psychological difficulties.

SURGICAL TECHNIQUES

Today, Harrington posterior instrumentation is rarely indicated in correcting scoliotic deformity in the adult, especially in the lumbar and thoracolumbar spine. Inevitably, even with the use of sacroalar hooks, broad sleeves or contouring of rods, or the use of square-ended rods, with distraction, loss of lumbar lordosis will occur. In correcting most lumbar and thoracolumbar curves we therefore practise anterior instrumentation of the Zielke type.

The Zielke technique, however, is not suitable in the presence of a true kyphotic deformity as the kyphos may well increase. This can be evaluated only by oblique Stagnara views. In the presence of kyphoscoliosis, a common problem in the lumbar spine of the elderly over the age of 50, to restore balance and relieve pain it is necessary to restore lumbar lordosis. This can be achieved only by a two-stage procedure. Initially via an anterior approach multiple-level discotomies and fusion are undertaken, followed two weeks later by CDI (Figs 23.5a–d & 23.6a–d). If the kyphoscoliosis is mobile, however, correction may be achieved by single-stage posterior CDI. This technique (Cotrel, 1986; Cotrel *et al.*, 1988; Denis, 1988) serves to derotate the spine and restore lordosis, as well as increase spinal rigidity, in comparison with other forms of spinal fixation.

With the advent of Luque instrumentation in 1976 (Luque, 1982a,b; Thompson, 1985) the use of segmental fixation posteriorly gained great popularity. As mentioned above, we do not feel that, for lumbar or thoracolumbar curves, Harrington instrumentation with segmental wiring suffices. The use of

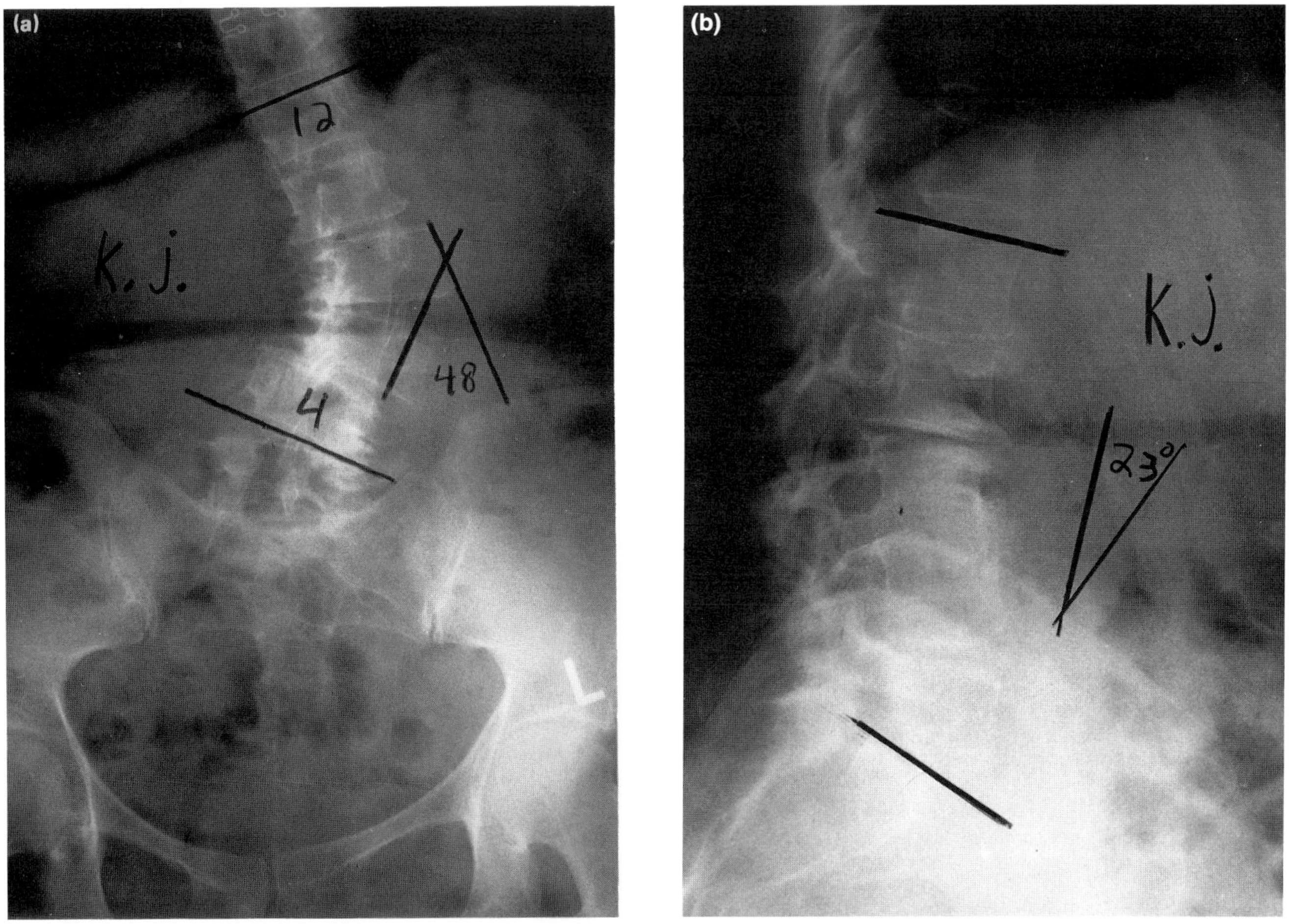

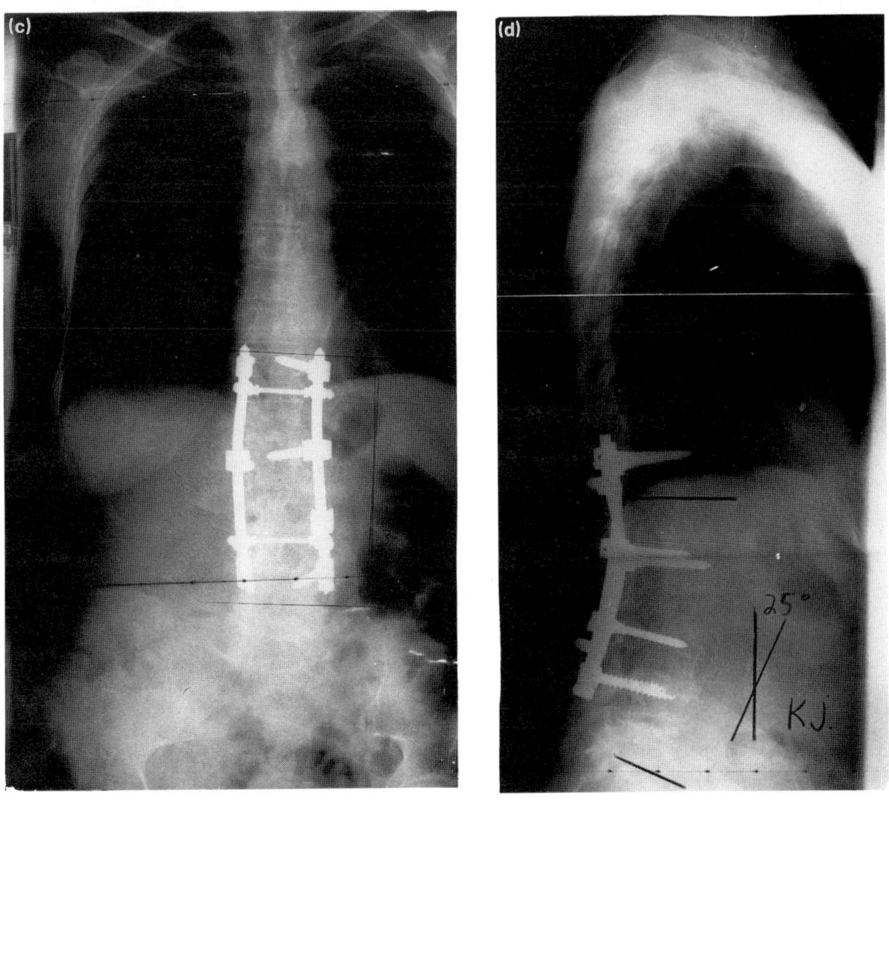

Fig. 23.5 (a) Female age 58 with a progressive painful curve. Stage one, multiple anterior discotomies with morselized bone graft; stage two, Cotrel–Dubousset instrumentation and fusion. (b) Preoperative lateral view; note significant loss of lordosis (−23° L1–S1). (c) Postoperative AP view. (d) Postoperative lateral view. Note significant return of lumbar lordosis due to derotation and anterior release (increase of 48°).

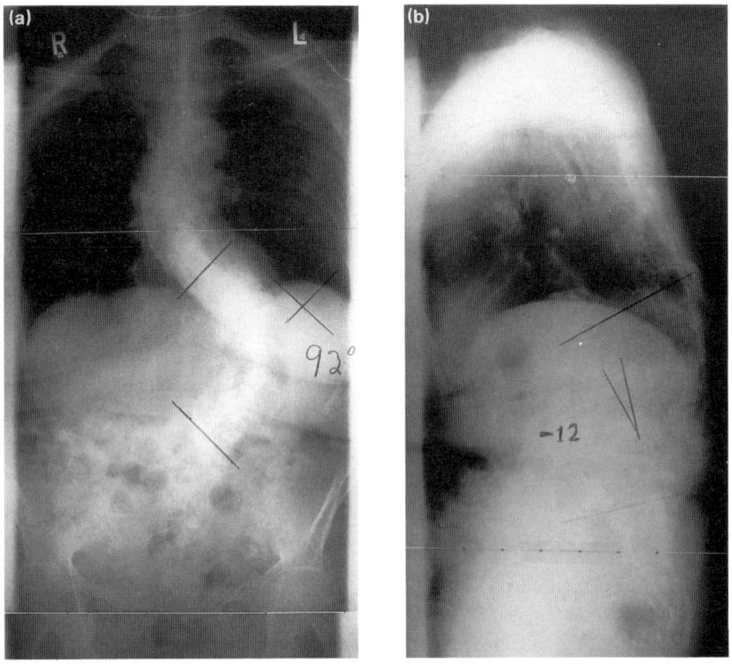

Fig. 23.6 (a) Female age 63 with progressive kyphoscoliosis, curve 92°. Stage one, multiple anterior discotomies morselization of L2–L3. Stage two, Cotrel–Dubousset instrumentation and fusion. (b) Preoperative lateral view; −12° lordosis. (c) Postoperative AP view. Minimal correction. (d) Postoperative lateral view. Marked restoration of lordosis to 42° (gain 54°).

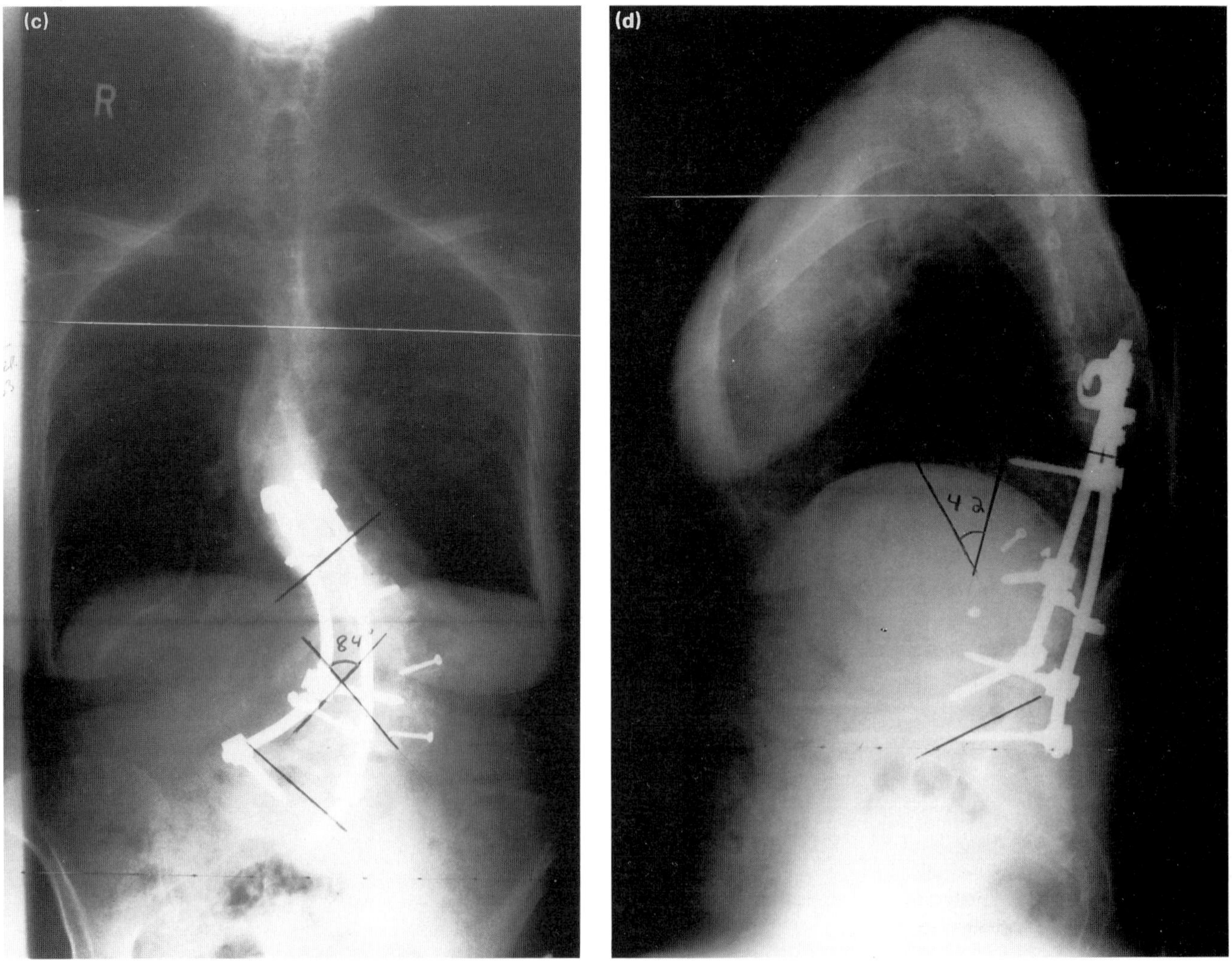

double-L rods or rectangular rods may be indicated (see Fig. 23.10). Initial fixation to the pelvis with Luque rods contoured using the Galveston technique (Allen & Ferguson, 1982; Moe, 1983; Kaneda, 1986; Ogiela, 1986; Herndon, 1987; Kostuik, 1989) showed great promise. Recent reports indicate that many of these patients develop pain related to the sacroiliac joint in the presence of a solid fusion of the lumbar spine. Furthermore, sublaminar wiring has been abandoned in our hands in favour of CDI except in cases of tumour and some cases of paralytic scoliosis (see Chapter 25).

Zielke instrumentation

The prime indication for Zielke instrumentation is a thoracolumbar or lumbar curve which does not require extension of the fusion to the sacrum, is mobile on bending X-rays, and in which lordosis is preserved. In these cases associated with pain, if accurately assessed preoperatively with discography and facet blocks, as indicated previously, correction of the deformity can be achieved using Zielke instrumentation. In the mature adult the entire curve should be incorporated in the procedure. In the less mature a smaller number of segments comparable to that in adolescence will suffice. From a technical viewpoint the major problem in many adults is that of osteoporosis. This can be overcome by injecting methylmethacrylate into predrilled screw-holes in the vertebral bodies. If at all possible the screw should be angled towards the contralateral junction of the pedicle with the vertebral body. This necessitates very careful cleaning of the disc space, including the endplates, back to the posterior longitudinal ligament so that an accurate line can be visualized for insertion of the screws. In order to ensure that the opposite cortex is penetrated a depth gauge is used to measure the line that the screw will follow. Usually 2 mm can be added to the length of the screw, although frequently, if there is lipping of the vertebral body, particularly in cases associated with marked degeneration, this is not necessary. Cooling the methylmethacrylate, or using the low-viscosity variety, will allow increased working time for injection of the material into the enlarged screw-holes (Fig. 23.7a,b). The greatest difficulty encountered technically has been pull-out of the most proximal screw. We do not believe that an extra level should be incorporated across a non-fused space in order

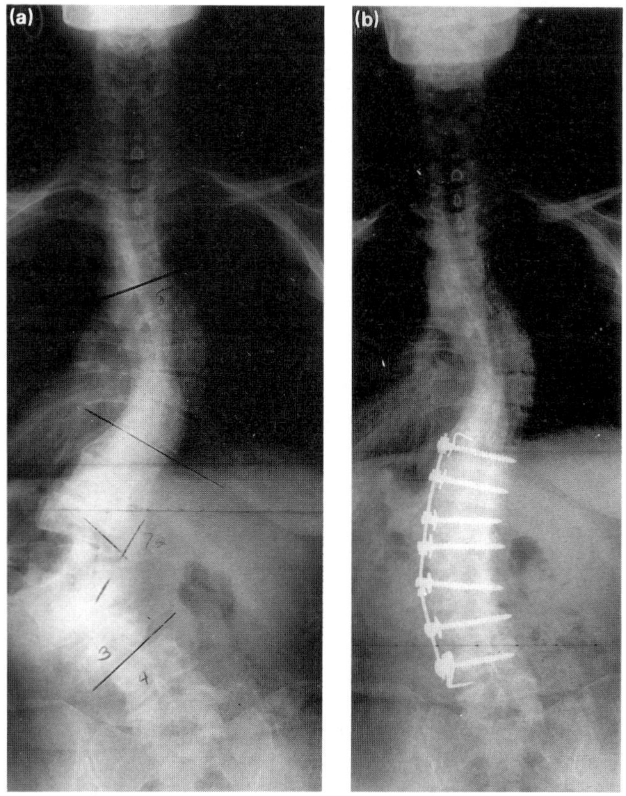

Fig. 23.7 (a) Female age 77 with severe incapacitating painful curve of 75°. (b) Postoperative curve 15°. Methylmethacrylate was used to hold the screws. The patient was pain-free one year postoperatively.

to prevent this problem (Fig. 23.8a–d), but in postmenopausal women we now routinely add cement to the upper level at the time of screw insertion.

There has been no difficulty with fusions extending from L5 proximally, but it is important that the iliolumbar veins at the L5 level are ligated in order to allow mobilization of the common iliac vessels.

Extension of the Zielke implant to the sacrum is practised only in those cases where fusion to the sacrum is based on preoperative assessment, as indicated previously, combined with posterior fusion. Similarly, extension of instrumentation above T9 or T10 is rarely of value, since the disc spaces are so narrow that little correction can be obtained. The use of the derotator is almost routine in order to reproduce lordosis in the lumbar area or reduce kyphosis in the thoracolumbar spine. This offers an advantage over the previously used Dwyer instrumentation, which frequently tended to produce a kyphosis despite accurate screw placement.

In these procedures autogenous bone graft is used,

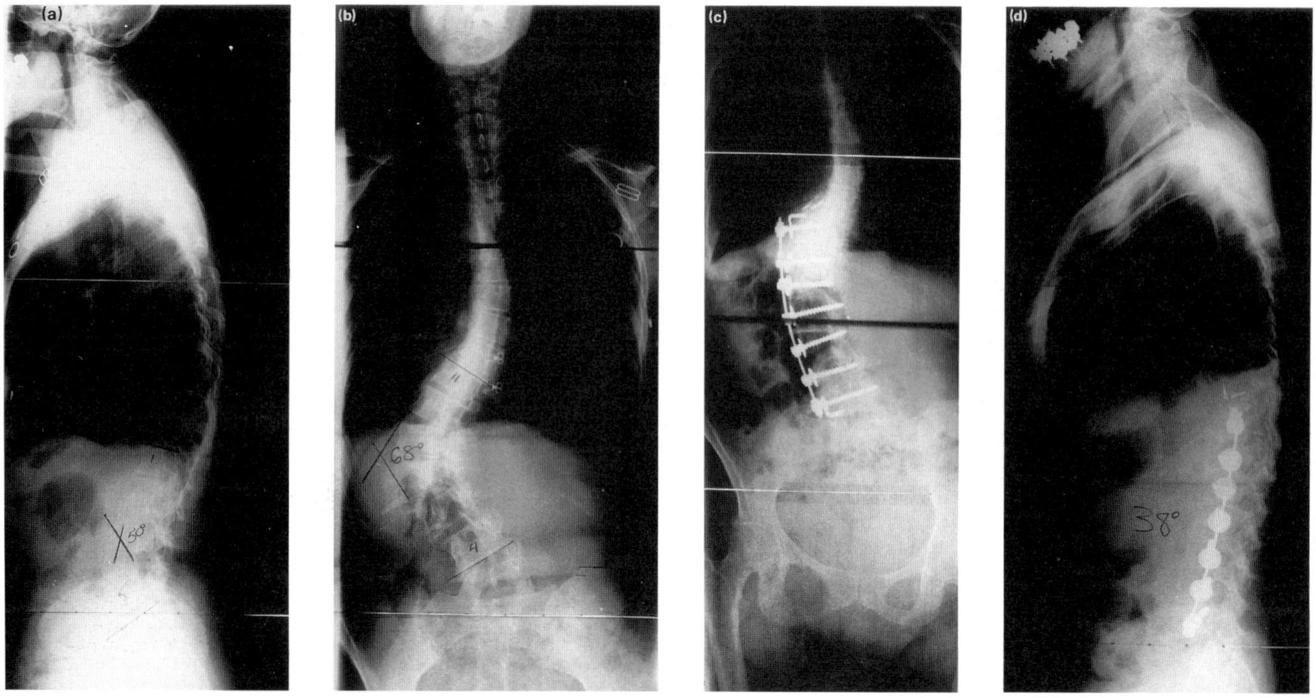

Fig. 23.8 (a,b) Female age 52, curve 68° painful, progressive and rigid. (c) Postoperative curve 34°; note proximal hook pull-out. (d) Postoperative lateral 38°, showing a good long-term result.

consisting usually of the excised rib cut up into small fragments. The use of block and/or minced graft placed more anteriorly in the disc space helps to maintain or increase lordosis. We do not normally use iliac crest bone. By employing hypotensive anaesthesia and cell-savers, average blood loss has been 1750 cm^3. Thus the use of bank blood has been kept to a minimum. However, hypotensive anaesthesia is not advisable in people above the age of 50.

Zielke instrumentation can be used safely into the 70s, although it is usually necessary to incorporate methylmethacrylate with the screws (Fig. 23.7). A recent long-term review of our first 57 patients treated by Zielke instrumentation (Kostuik *et al.*, 1989) showed an average correction of 70% as against 45% with Dwyer instrumentation, with no case of pseudarthrosis.

The use of the derotational device improved correction of the curve both in the sagittal and anteroposterior plane by approximately one grade as assessed by the Nash–Moe (Nash & Moe, 1969) method of rotational classification. Intraoperative complications included five fractured vertebral bodies which were salvaged by injecting methylmethacrylate. Postoperative complications included lateral femoral cutaneous nerve entrapment, temporary post-thoracotomy syndrome, atelectasis and pleural effusions, and instrumentation failure due to proximal staple pull-out at two levels. Nuts backing out of the screw head, and rod disengagement from the screw head, was noted in some cases without loss of correction in the immediate postoperative X-ray. Some patients had partial staple disengagement, including the case noted. At an average follow-up of two years loss of correction was less than one degree.

In double idiopathic curves the average correction at lumbar level was 62%. At 24 months the mean loss was 3.4° (4%). The unoperated proximal thoracic curve improved 38% without deterioration at follow-up. It is of interest that following surgery there was improvement of 50% correction over that anticipated from preoperative bending anterioposterior radiographs.

Reviewing the results of Zielke instrumentation, used posteriorly as pedicle fixation for degenerative disease, has revealed a high incidence of rod breakage. We therefore no longer use the Zielke implant posteriorly; it has been surpassed by the Cotrel–Dubousset system.

Zielke instrumentation has, however, been used

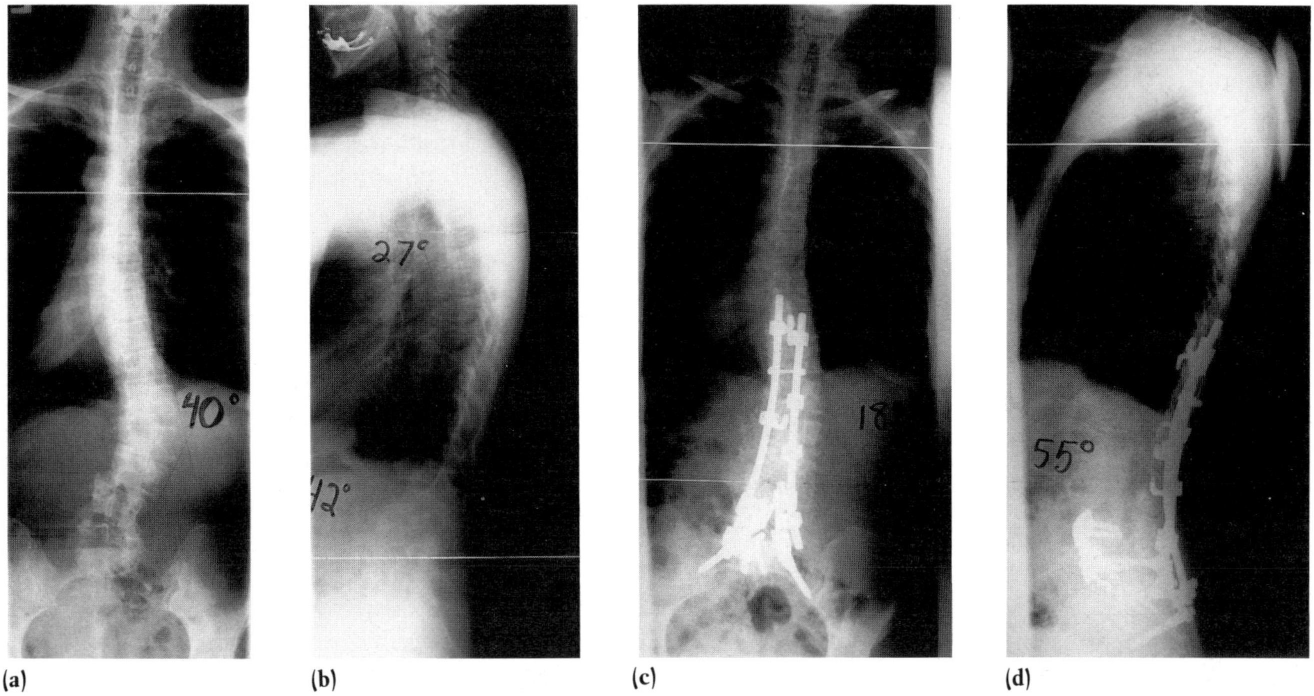

Fig. 23.9 Female age 53 with progressive painful scoliosis of 40°. (b) The curve was flexible. Preoperative discography revealed painful degenerative L4–L5 and L5–S1 discs. (c,d) In order to achieve solid fusion two-stage surgery was performed. The first stage consisted of anterior L4–L5 and L5-S discectomies, interbody iliac crest grafts and internal fixation with an 'I'-beam Yuan plate L4-S and two AO 6.5 mm screws L5–S1. In the second stage Cotrel–Dubousset instrumentation and fusion derotated the spine and increased lordosis. Pain was relieved.

sparingly on the anterior convex aspect of fractional lumbosacral curves where there is imbalance and pain (Fig. 23.1). This has resulted in slightly greater than 40% correction of the proximal major curve. It is recognized, however, that in these patients further treatment of their major curve may be necessary at a later date. The technique therefore should be reserved for those fractional curves in the lower lumbar and lumbosacral spine where there is significant pain confirmed by discography and facet blocks, and the patient is out of balance.

Cotrel–Dubousset instrumentation

This system is designed to ensure rigidity of segmental fixation as well as curve derotation during correction.

Between August 1985 and June 1988, 49 adult patients with deformity secondary to idiopathic scoliosis were operated upon; 43 females and six males. The average age was 43 years, ranging from 21 to 75 years. Curve types were 16 primary thoracic, 15 primary lumbar, 14 double major, and four thoracolumbar. Twelve patients had undergone previous spinal fusions. Curves averaged 60° preoperatively in the frontal plane, ranging from 13° to 115°. The primary thoracic curves averaged 58°, the primary lumbar curves 48°, the thoracolumbar curves 55°, and in the double major curves, the thoracic section 76° and the lumbar section 66°.

The technical details regarding the use of CDI are described elsewhere (Cotrel, 1986; Cotrel *et al.*, 1988) (see Chapter 22). In general, for previously unoperated thoracic curves, the selection of fusion levels as advocated by King *et al.* (1983) and the hook and rod placement as described by Cotrel and Dubousset (Cotrel, 1986; Cotrel *et al.*, 1988) were followed.

For the patient with a severe, rigid thoracic curve greater than 90°, or in the previously fused patient, either an anterior or posterior release as appropriate was performed prior to CDI. In the interval between the two stages, halodependent traction was used in four patients to improve curve flexibility.

Therefore the management of thoracolumbar and lumbar curves often involved staged surgery. This was to reduce the high rate of complications, including pseudarthrosis, poor curve correction, residual truncal imbalance, and loss of or failure to improve lumbar lordosis, associated with single-stage posterior surgery (Figs 23.5 & 23.6). The flexible thoracolumbar or lumbar curve with reasonable preservation of lumbar lordosis not needing fusion to the sacrum was treated with either a single-stage anterior Zielke procedure or a single-stage posterior CDI.

For rigid lumbar kyphoscoliosis, an initial anterior lumbar release with morselized bone grafting of the interspaces, followed by a second stage CDI to derotate the curve and restore lumbar lordosis, was performed (Figs 23.5 & 23.6).

If, in the rigid lumbar kyphoscoliotic curve the fusion had to be extended to the sacrum because of painful disc degeneration, an anterior release extending the length of the curve, including the L4–L5 and L5–S1 interspaces was augmented by wedge-shaped bone blocks to improve lumbosacral lordosis. This was supplemented by anterior internal fixation at these two levels (Fig. 23.9). The remaining higher levels were grafted anteriorly with morselized bone. A second-stage CDI extending posteriorly down to the sacrum was subsequently performed seven to 10 days later (Kostuik, 1987, 1988).

In total, 19 patients had staged or associated surgery including two anterior thoracic releases, two posterior thoracic releases, 10 anterior thoracolumbar or lumbar releases, four nerve root decompressions and one thoracoplasty.

Braces or casts were not routinely used except in the elderly osteoporotic patient in whom fixation was felt to be at risk, in which case a custom-moulded polypropylene thoracolumbar orthosis was provided.

At follow-up (average 28 months) the curves were reduced by an average of 35°, i.e. 42% correction. In previously unoperated patients the curve correction averaged 50%, whilst in those patients previously fused correction averaged 35%.

The amount of correction by curve type revealed significantly greater correction in the primary lumbar and thoracolumbar curves, due to the associated anterior release commonly performed in this group. In the thoracic curves the correction at final follow-up averaged 45% and in the lumbar curves it averaged 58%. In the thoracolumbar curves the correction averaged 60% and in the double major curves both components averaged 41% (see Fig. 23.18).

Apical vertebral rotation as determined by the method of Nash & Moe (1969) improved an average of one-half grade, from 2.5 preoperative to 2.0 postoperative.

Disabling pain present in 44 patients prior to surgery was eliminated in 30, improved in six and was the same or worse in eight.

Complications included pneumothoraces, pancreatitis, urinary tract infections, dural tear closed primarily, superficial wound infection that resolved, haemothorax requiring repeat throacotomy to control bleeding, and chronic post-thoracotomy incisional pain. A few patients complained about prominent rods.

Neurological complications were fortunately transient and consisted of neuropraxias following anterior approaches. The only injury directly attributable to the CDI was a fourth nerve root neurapraxia that resolved. Hook pull-out due to bone failure, and laminar fractures, occurred infrequently. Most failures occurred in the lumbar region at the distal fixation site, mainly occurring in patients over 50 years who had undergone a preliminary anterior lumbar release prior to CDI. It would therefore seem prudent to supplement the distal lumbar fixation with pedicle screws when possible, instead of relying on laminar hooks.

Thus CDI seems to have its greater benefit in the maintenance or improvement of the sagittal plane curves in both the thoracic and lumbar region. In the initial enthusiasm for frontal plane curve correction with Harrington instrumentation the sagittal plane curves were often ignored. Fortunately CDI is able to effect significant improvement in lumbar lordosis and thoracic kyphosis. This improvement in lumbar lordosis is in marked contrast to other instrumentation systems as described above. Furthermore, it would seem that CDI allows the surgeon to take full advantage of preliminary anterior release surgery.

There were numerous complications in the series, but it must be realized that several of these patients had complex deformities, many having undergone previous fusions. A fair proportion underwent staged surgery in the course of their treatment with CDI.

Neurological lesions all amounted to neuropraxias and all resolved. Two of these occurred in multiply operated patients and only one could be attributed to the CDI procedure. The wound infection rate was very low, despite often complex and prolonged operations. Although the incidence of rod irritation was high (16%), due to the bulky implant requiring occasional removal, this is a reasonable trade-off for the initial firm fixation by the somewhat bulkier segmental system of CDI.

In a few patients there was hook dislodgement, due to laminar fracture. This occurred in elderly patients who had undergone staged anterior release. This might be preventable by supplementing the lumbar fixation with pedicle screws, instead of relying on laminar hooks, as already described.

Ultimate satisfaction with the procedure must be judged mainly in terms of pain relief. In 30 patients the preoperative pain was relieved, and in six it was reduced such that they required only occasional analgesics.

Eight patients continued to complain of pain postoperatively because of various identifiable reasons such as pseudarthroses, spinal stenosis and loss of fixation of the implant. Nevertheless, 86% of the patients noted improvement regarding their preoperative pain.

On balance therefore the CDI, although a complex system, provides the surgeon with the versatility necessary to tackle difficult surgical problems. Certainly there is a learning curve involved, and a large 'fiddle factor', but with experience operative time approaches that of other scoliosis procedures.

COSMESIS

In a review of the first 1000 patients with scoliosis treated by the author, approximately 10% were treated essentially for cosmetic reasons. These were primarily thoracic curves with a range from 45° to 75°. The age range was from 20 to 42 years; 90% were females.

Such surgery should not be denied to adults provided the reasons for requesting surgery are carefully assessed, and explanation of the procedure and its postoperative course, also possible complications, is given. The surgeon must be well experienced and supported by full institutional facilities.

The past few years has seen a return to excision of the rib hump. This is particularly valuable in rigid curves in the thoracic spine, especially where there is hypokyphosis. In more mobile curves the advent of CDI, allowing derotation of the spine, helps to decrease the rib hump, although rib excision can be undertaken at the same time.

A review of 20 patients who underwent excision of five or six ribs on the convexity suffering from rigid curves of 90° or greater revealed no untoward morbidity. There were no changes in pre- and postoperative ventilation studies. Thus rib hump excision in the presence of a severe rigid thoracic scoliosis can markedly improve the cosmetic appearance.

But in mobile curves the use of CDI is preferred; indeed because of its enhanced stability it may be used in more rigid curves as well. No postoperative orthoses are necessary.

During these procedures the ribs were all excised subperiosteally and used as graft material. Access is either through an incision created at right angles to the longitudinal spinal incision, whereby two myocutaneous flaps are fashioned; or an intercostal incision is neater. If the spinal curve is not too big, access to the rib hump is feasible from the midline operative field.

THE TREATMENT OF SEVERE RIGID SCOLIOTIC DEFORMITIES

In 1979 the author (Kostuik, 1979) reported on 85 patients with rigid curves of 90° or greater, some due to a primary kyphotic deformity, but the majority scoliotic deformity, either idiopathic or congenital.

Twenty patients had undergone previous fusions and were presenting with progression of their deformity and pain. All patients underwent posterior releases, including where necessary osteotomies of previous fusions or congenitally fused spines. Posterior osteotomies were done at multiple levels, usually averaging four in number. These were accompanied by concave rib releases over three or four levels, also transverse process osteotomies and rib resection of five or six ribs on the convexity. Forty patients had associated anterior osteotomies. The age range of the patients was from 20 to 55 years, with curve magnitude from 75° to 180°.

Second-stage surgery was performed two weeks later. At the time of primary release surgery, traction was usually applied in the form initially of halofemoral traction, but latterly halopelvic traction. The latter form of traction is still favoured in very severe curves, although recently halo-dependent traction, either in the circoelectric bed at 30° of dependency or halo-wheelchair traction was preferred. The second stage procedure consisted of posterior instrumentation, originally with Harrington instrumentation, later by sublaminar wiring techniques and finally by CDI.

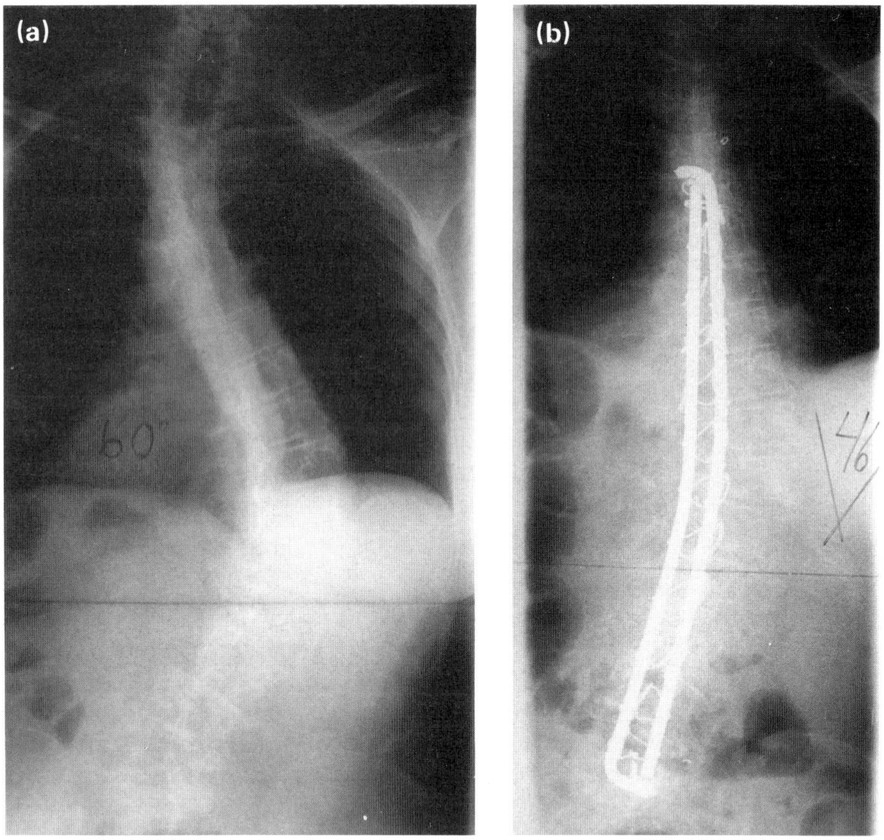

Fig. 23.10 (a) Female age 58 with a progressive painful thoracolumbar kyphoscoliosis. (b) Luque instrumentation; the kyphosis precluded the use of Zielke instrumentation. Today Cotrel–Dubousset instrumentation with derotation would be used.

The degree of correction averaged 40% with halopelvic and 32% with halofemoral distraction. Subsequent Harrington instrumentation added a further 8% to correction. Overall correction in these rigid curves was 40%. This was comparable to a series previously reported in mobile curves. Idiopathic curves corrected an average of 48% and congenital curves 33%.

In cases of significant and rigid kyphoscoliosis CDI has proved to be invaluable in restoring lordosis and relieving pain following anterior multiple discectomies. Instrumentation is carried out some two weeks following anterior surgery, and is suitable even in the presence of extensive laminectomies undertaken for spinal stenosis (Figs 23.5 & 23.6). In our experience there have been no neurological or vascular complications.

STRUCTURAL DISABILITIES

Patients who have a paralytic scoliosis may find sitting at a desk or in a wheelchair difficult because of marked pelvic obliquity or an associated kyphosis with a collapsing spine, or hyperlordosis (Fig. 23.11). The latter is encountered particularly in patients who have had thecoperitoneal shunts in childhood. Patients with paralytic scoliosis are still best treated by a combined anterior and posterior approach, which eliminates the need for postoperative immobilization and allows for early activity in a wheelchair.

Certain patients with paralytic curves of a collapsing nature, where respiratory function is decreased, can be significantly helped by correction of the deformity (Chapter 25). This results in improved diaphragmatic breathing. A preoperative trial of halo-dependent traction may show an improvement in respiratory function and emphasize the advantages of surgical correction of the deformity. The efficacy of CDI has not been sufficiently proven in the treatment of paralytic deformities that extend into the distal lumbar spine; this would suggest an anterior and posterior approach in adults. In children, however, the use of Luque instrumentation extending to the pelvis, or the Galveston or other modification, has been of value.

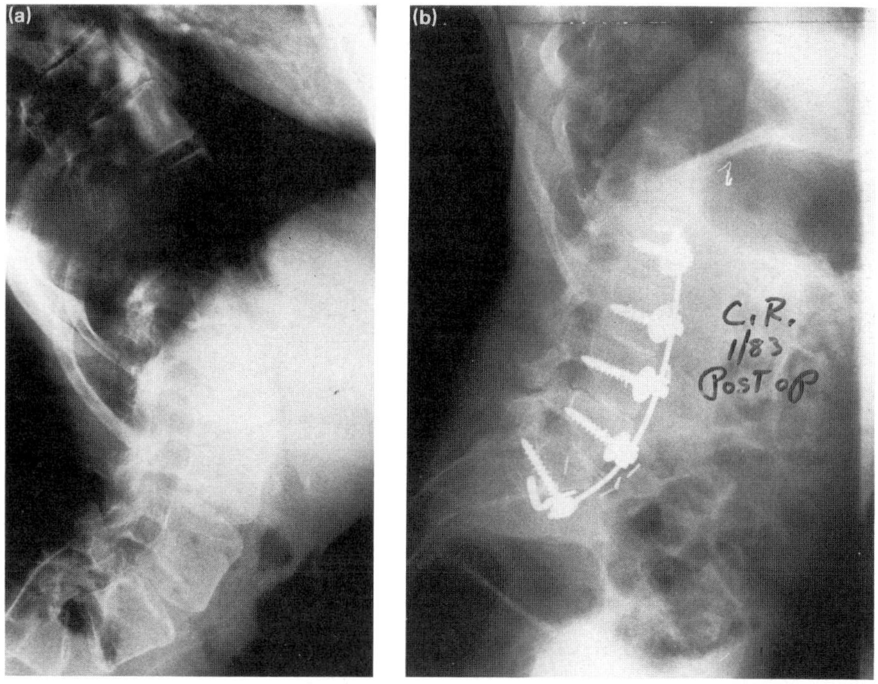

Fig. 23.11 (a) Marked paralytic hyperlordosis. (b) Lordosis has been reduced to 60° L1–S1 by anterior Zielke instrumentation. Note the anterior–posterior orientation of the screws.

SPINAL DEFORMITIES OVER THE AGE OF 50

The adult aged over 50 presents a complex problem; the deformity is often rigid and may be associated with significant imbalance and loss of normal lordosis of the lumbar spine. The bone is frequently osteopenic and there may be associated neurological problems related to spinal stenosis. The major reason for seeking help is pain. The early experience of the author was such that major spinal deformities in patients over the age of 50 could be corrected only at great risk to neurological structures. As a result the majority of such deformities were simply stabilized with Harrington instrumentation, with little attempt at correction. This often resulted in continuing deformity and increasing pain.

With the advent of improved techniques of anterior fixation such as Zielke instrumentation (Zielke *et al.*, 1976) and posterior fixation devices such as CDI (Cotrel, 1986) correction can now be safely achieved. In the presence of a thoracolumbar or lumbar deformity with good preservation of lordosis anterior Zielke instrumentation alone is appropriate. Methylmethacrylate has greatly enhanced the holding power of screws in the vertebral bodies, but it should not be used posteriorly in the pedicles with the exception of the first sacral pedicle, as the cement may exude out of the osteopenic pedicle in elderly adults, resulting in canal compromise. In the presence of a rigid kyphoscoliosis, or where there is minimal lumbar lordosis, a two-stage procedure is preferable, the first stage consisting of multiple disc excisions and interbody grafting followed 10 days later by CDI to correct the curve and restore lumbar lordosis. This has proved to be of much value over the past few years. A recent long-term review of 80 patients over the age of 50 was undertaken by the author. Fifty had idiopathic curves and the remainder either a congenital curve, paralytic curve or a pure kyphotic deformity. Twelve of the idiopathic curves were thoracic, nine thoracolumbar, 17 lumbar and there were 12 double curves. All patients presented with back pain. Eight patients had progressive pulmonary dysfunction, usually related to an increasing kyphosis. Fifty-seven per cent of cases had documented evidence of progression of greater than 10° in three years preoperatively. Sixteen patients had associated root pain. These 80 patients underwent 100 procedures. Twenty had a second stage procedure, either anterior or posterior, for increased stabilization. Twelve patients had concurrent anterior and posterior procedures performed, largely for correction of flat back syndrome through a single-stage combined posterior and anterior osteotomy with anterior and posterior fixation. Although 20 patients underwent a second stage procedure for stabilization, the majority were kyphoscoliotics of a rigid nature. A total of 14 also had a second stage anterior procedure since fusion was carried to the sacrum posteriorly, and in order to ensure a solid fusion anterior fixation and fusion was carried out as described under fusions to the sacrum. In a review of all cases, excellent to good results were achieved in 69%, of which 56.5% were good and 12.5% excellent. Fair and poor results occurred in 6% and 25% respectively. No pain was noted in 27 patients postoperatively (34%); root pain was relieved in all patients.

If, in addition to deformity (mainly kyphosis) there is an element of spinal stenosis or other cause of root pain it may be necessary to perform posterior decompression; in which case a stabilization procedure should also be performed. The author has encountered many patients who have undergone posterior decompression for spinal stenosis in the presence of deformity, only to have the patient present within months or years with significant instability and pain (Fig. 23.9a–d). There is difficulty in obtaining sound fusion of the spine because of lack of bone stock as a result of the decompression and subsequent scarring.

In this group of 80 patients over the age of 50, curve correction was 22% with Harrington instrumentation and 22% with sublaminar wired Harrington rods. A 21% correction was achieved with Harrington rods combined with L rods and 33% in double L rods. Curve correction with Dwyer instrumentation was 42% and 67% with Zielke instrumentation (Figs 23.2 & 23.7). This compares favourably with the 70% of all adults corrected by Zielke instrumentation over the age of 20 (Kostuik *et al.*, 1989). The average correction obtained with CDI was 50% (Figs 23.5 & 23.6). Thirteen of the patients treated with Harrington instrumentation alone developed flat back syndrome. Posterior distraction in the lumbar spine at any age should be avoided at all cost, except for anterior distraction for kyphotic deformities. Pure kyphotic deformities are best treated by anterior instrumentation, as noted in the section on kyphotic deformities. Instrumentation failure in this group of elderly adults occurred in 11 cases, six of which were Harrington rod fractures: dislodgement of rod in one case, two cases of L rod migration, one case of anterior screw breakage and one case of posterior Zielke rod breakage. Infection rate was 1%. Pulmonary complications, including atelectasis and pneumonia and adult respiratory syndrome, occurred in 24%.

Instrumentation failure occurred in 14%. Intraoperative bone fracture of either lamina or vertebral bodies occurred in seven cases and was overcome with the use of methylmethacrylate associated with internal fixation devices. Thirteen patients developed iatrogenic flat back secondary to Harrington distraction. Four of these subsequently underwent restoration of lordosis by single-stage anterior and posterior osteotomies. One patient became paraparetic as a result of surgery with partial improvement. Pseudarthrosis occurred in 21%, primarily in the Harrington series. There was no pseudoarthrosis with the use of Zielke instrumentation or CDI to date; 25% of pseudoarthroses occurred in fusions carried to L5, and 24% when carried to the sacrum. All pseudarthroses to the sacrum occurred prior to the development of two-stage surgery for fusions to the sacrum as described elsewhere in this chapter. Nine patients developed a kyphosis secondary to osteopenic fractures proximal to their instrumentation. Due to improved diagnostic capabilities and improved postoperative care, and the advent of improved fixation such as posterior pedicle fixation, particularly of the Cotrel–Dubousset type and anterior Zielke instrumentation, morbidity has been significantly less in the past five years. The importance of restoration of lordosis cannot be overemphasized, particularly in cases of kyphoscoliosis. The use of multiple-level releases anteriorly, followed by posterior derotation with CDI – and indeed if necessary posterior osteotomy through the pars inter articularis to increase lordosis – markedly improves the quality of life of these senior patients.

FUSIONS TO THE SACRUM

In a review undertaken on behalf of the Scoliosis Research Society in 1978, the author noted that 4% of all scoliosis fusions performed by members resulted in a significant loss of lumbar lordosis (unpublished data). The series included all forms of posterior instrumentation throughout the spine. In a review of fusions to the sacrum, loss of lumbar lordosis was noted to occur in approximately 50% of adult cases (Kostuik & Hall, 1983), and was clinically significant requiring revision surgery in one-half of the patients. Balderson *et al.* (1986) have experienced similar problems. It was not recognized until the late 1970s that posterior distraction of the thoracolumbar and lumbar spine might result in loss of lordosis even with contouring of the Harrington rod as described by Casey *et al.* (1987), and using square-ended Moe rods or sacro-alar hooks. The advent of Luque-L rods (Luque, 1982b) across the sacroiliac joint, and subsequently the refinement of this by the Galveston technique, improved maintenance of lordosis and enhanced the rate of fusion in the lumbosacral area, whereas previously the incidence of pseudoarthrosis using Harrington rods, either with a sacral bar or alar hooks, was 40% (Kostuik & Hall, 1983). The use of CDI has almost eliminated this problem and ensured adequate lordosis.

Since 1981 (Kostuik, 1988), where fusion to the sacrum is indicated, a two-stage procedure had been practised. If the patient has lumbar scoliosis with a reasonable degree of lordosis, initial anterior instrumentation using the Zielke system is undertaken. The use of Zielke instrumentation anterior to the sacrum, although technically demanding, has not resulted in any problems involving the common iliac vessels, either artery or vein, provided one avoids any impingement of screw-heads against the vessels. Rods can safely pass beneath the common iliac vessels as the rods are small and lie close to the vertebral body. Occasionally two rods at the distal two or three levels are used in order to help control rotation at the lumbosacral junction. A second-stage posterior fusion using segmental wiring was initially done, but this has now been superseded by the use of pedicle fixation (CDI or plate instrumentation).

If the patient has a rigid kyphoscoliosis and requires fusion to the sacrum the first stage again is anterior, consisting of multiple discotomies. The interbody spaces are filled with bone chips, except for the fourth to fifth and the fifth lumbar and first sacral interspaces. At those levels bicortical or tricortical grafts are used to heighten the disc spaces and increase lordosis. Internal fixation is performed to enhance stability over these two levels. This is followed about two weeks later by posterior CDI, which serves to derotate the lumbar spine and restore lordosis.

Finally, if the kyphoscoliosis is mobile, it is corrected and lordosis restored by a first-stage posterior CDI, followed by a second stage anterior L4 to sacrum fusion with solid interbody grafts and instrumentation. Over the past two years a rigid contoured I-plate, or two 6.5 mm AO cancellous screws, have been introduced in preference to Zielke instrumentation (Fig. 23.9). During such anterior instrumentation ligation of the segmental vessels, particularly in a left retroperitoneal approach, allows the aorta and common iliac vessels to fall away from the vertebral bodies, ensuring more room for placement of the internal fixation devices. Since the majority of lumbar and thoracolumbar curves are left-sided this approach is most commonly used.

In over 450 cases of anterior instrumentation in both the thoracic and lumbar spine the author has not encountered any late vascular problems.

EXTENSION OF FUSION IN THE LUMBAR SPINE

Recent reports by Edgar & Mehta (1982) and Cochran *et al.* (1983), and a review of our own patients, show that those who have had previous fusion to the mid and lower lumbar level are at increased risk of developing degenerative changes below the fusion mass (Fig. 23.12). These patients require extension of their fusion if non-operative methods fail to control pain and the problem becomes a progressive one, often associated with some degree of spinal stenosis at the level immediately below the fusion. If, following investigative studies – including myelography, CT scanning, discography and facet blocks – a fusion down to the sacrum is not required, then posterior or anterior instrumentation alone will suffice. If, however, extension of the fusion to the sacrum is required, then a combined approach will be necessary (Byrd *et al.*, 1987). This is preferably performed at one sitting, by means of posterior pedicle-screw fixation and anterior instrumentation. In order to improve lordosis a posterior osteotomy through the pars articularis can be done, and compression applied via the pedicles to increase lordosis (Fig. 23.13). Anteriorly interbody grafts are inserted after opening the disc spaces as widely as possible. Anterior instrumentation using Zielke rods or a plate will enhance the fusion.

RESTORATION OF LUMBAR LORDOSIS

As noted previously (Kostuik & Hall, 1983), fusions to the sacrum with posterior instrumentation, particularly that of Harrington, has resulted in a 50%

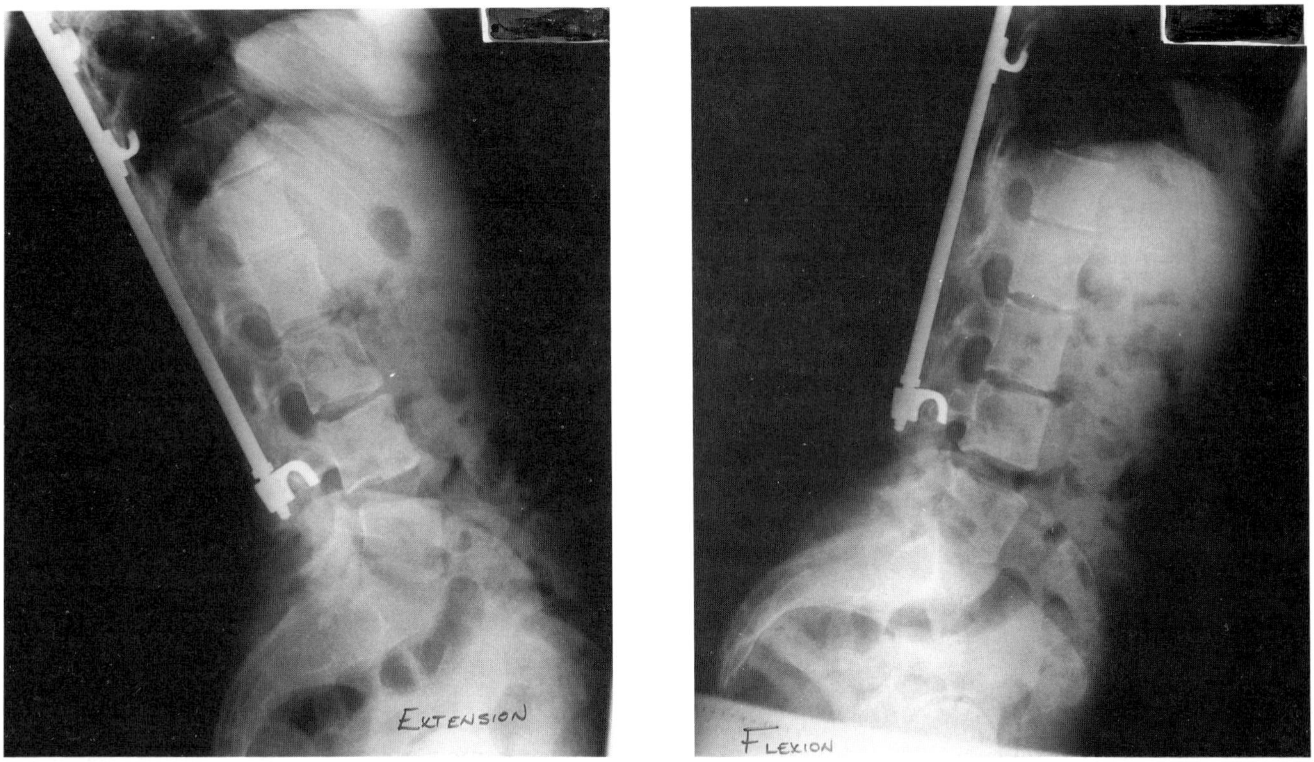

Fig. 23.12 Flexion–extension views demonstrate marked instability at the L4–L5 disc space. The patient had undergone Harrington instrumentation 12 years previously.

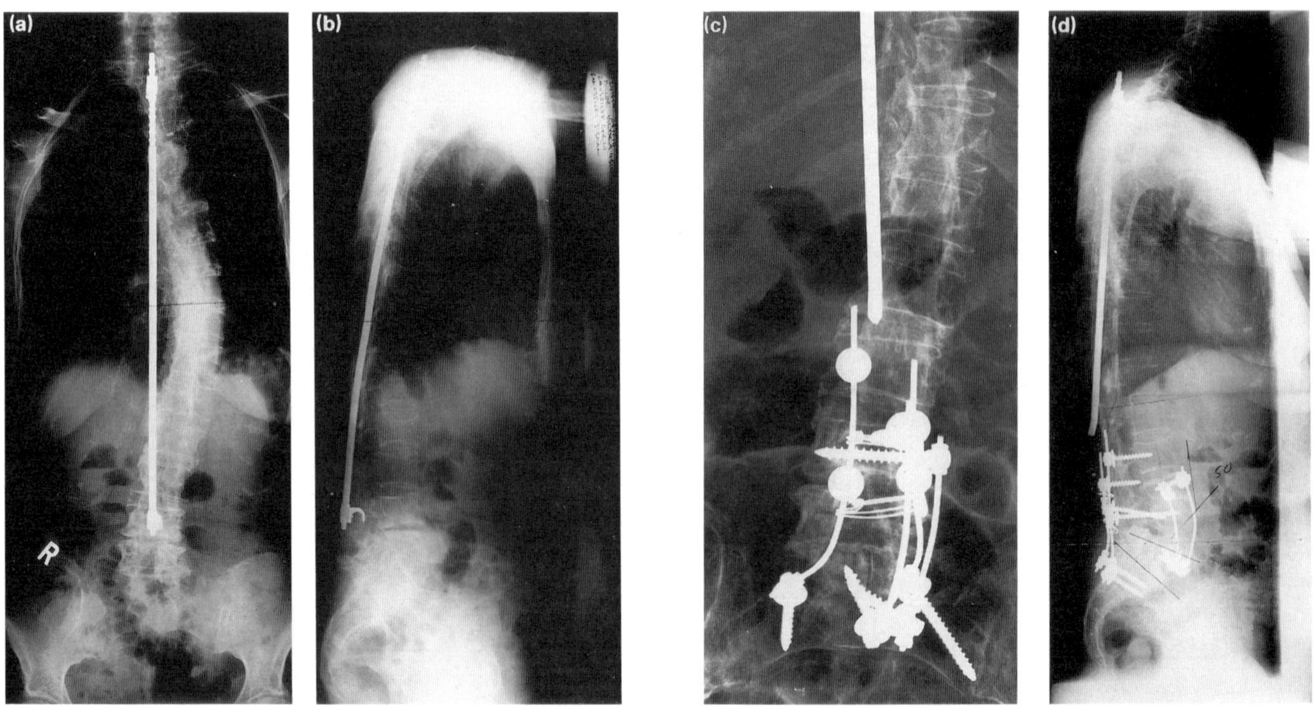

Fig. 23.13 (a) Female age 56 with a previous fusion 25 years ago. (b) AP view demonstrates marked degenerative changes L4–L5, L5–S1 with a flat back (c,d) Postoperative AP-lateral view. Extension of fusion to S1. Note restoration of lordosis; preoperative discography reproduced pain at L4–L5 and L5–S1. Relief was obtained with facet blocks.

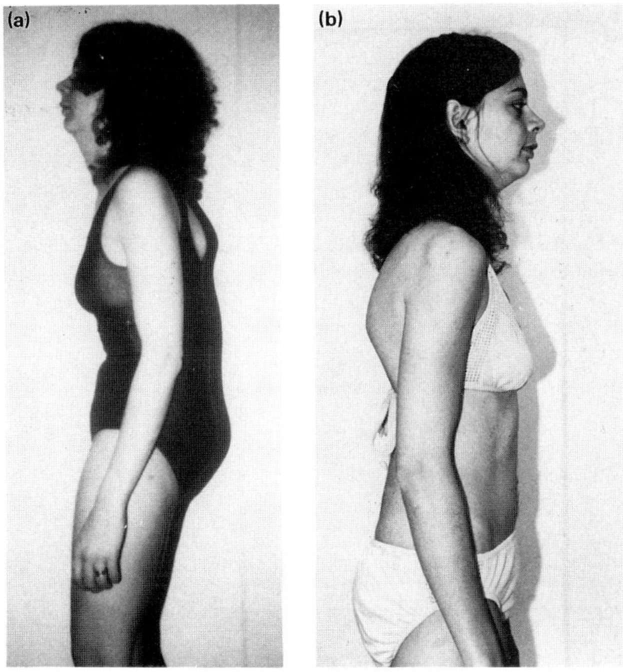

Fig. 23.14 (a) Female age 24 with previous lumbar fusion. Note marked kyphosis (flat back) secondary to distraction. (b) Postoperative result. Note restoration of lordosis.

loss of lumbar lordosis, many patients requiring restorative surgery (Doherty, 1973; Grobler *et al.*, 1978; Kostuik & Hall, 1983; Lagrone *et al.*, 1988). Although adolescents compensate well in early life, by middle age many complain of fatigue and pain in the low back even when there is solid fusion. Pain arising from the sacroiliac joints must be excluded. As the day progresses these patients walk with a forward stoop and with flexed knees and hips; a most unsightly deformity (Fig. 23.14). This problem was not recognized until the late 1970s. To rectify matters a combined anterior and posterior osteotomy approach is superior to a posterior osteotomy of an old fusion mass alone. Greater correction can be obtained, and it is not necessary to immobilize the patient in a hip spica postoperatively. Moreover, the use of posterior osteotomy alone has, in the author's experience, in at least two cases resulted in late recurrence of deformity. The combined approach, supplemented by internal fixation and the use of a simple lumbar orthosis postoperatively, allows early ambulation.

The most important causes of loss of lumbar lordosis are, in descending order of frequency: distraction instrumentation of the lumbar spine extending caudally to the L5 or S1 vertebral level; thoracolumbar junction kyphosis greater than 15°, especially if associated with a hypokyphotic thoracic spine; degenerative changes above and below a previous fusion, associated with loss of disc height occurring more commonly below the previous fusion.

If the loss of lumbar lordosis is associated with a pseudarthrosis, repair of the pseudarthrosis

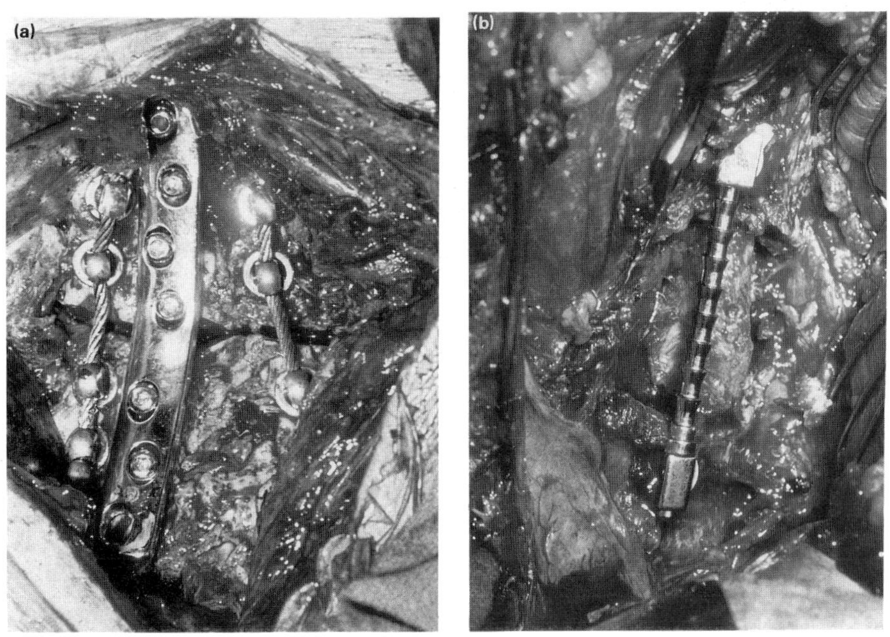

Fig. 23.15 (a) Posterior osteotomy has been closed by the application of Dwyer screws in the lateral fusion mass; an AO plate has been added in the midline to help control rotation. (b) Simultaneous to posterior closure the anterior osteotomy site is opened with Kostuik–Harrington instrumentation. Iliac crest grafts are added and a second Kostuik–Harrington compression rod is added to enhance stability.

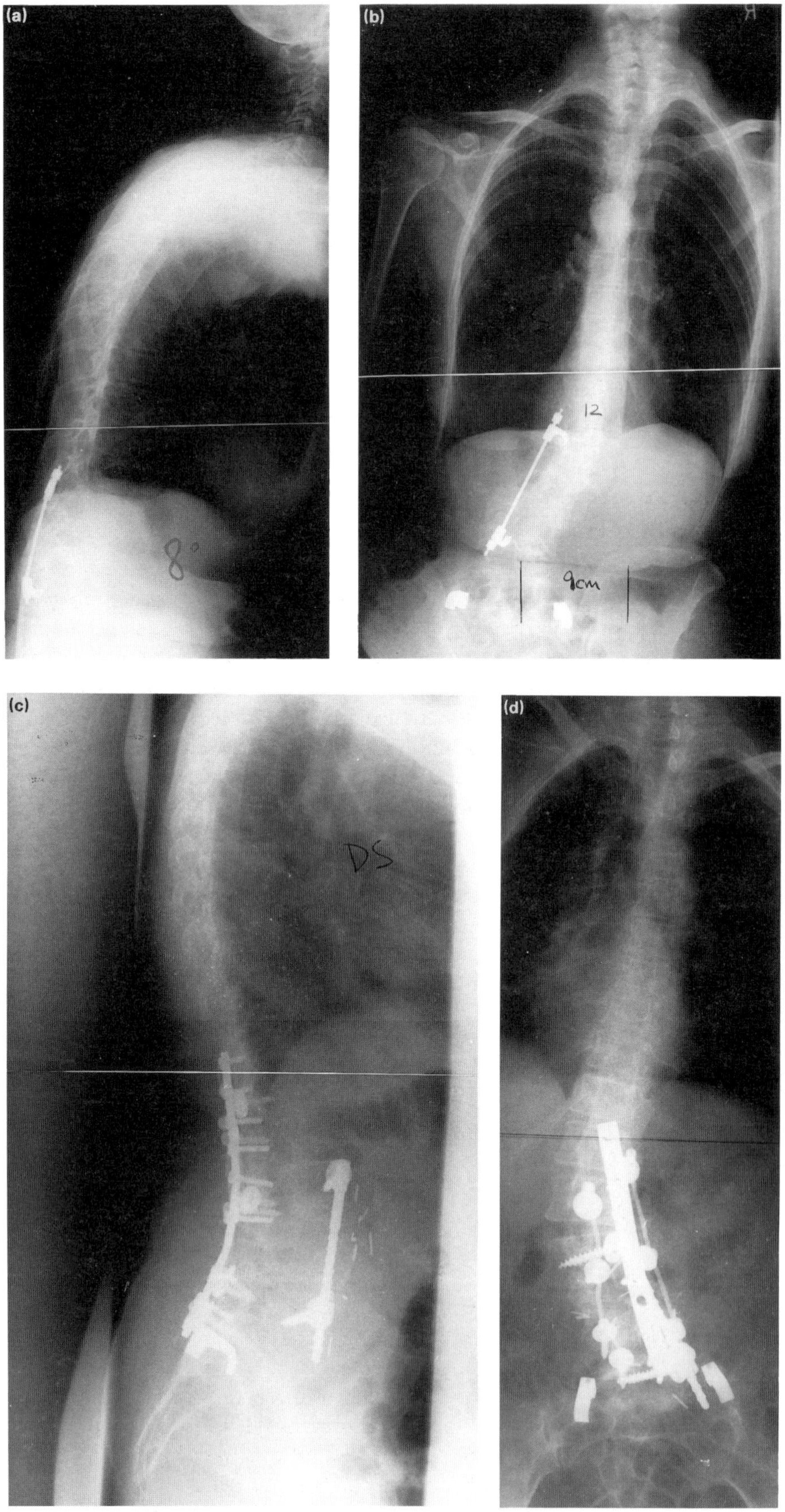

Fig. 23.16 (a) Female age 45. Note loss of lordosis and marked flat back secondary to distraction and fusion of lumbar spine. (b) AP view showing imbalance 9 cm to the right. The Harrington distraction rod has been removed. (c,d) Lordosis and balance has been restored by a single-stage anterior and posterior osteotomy.

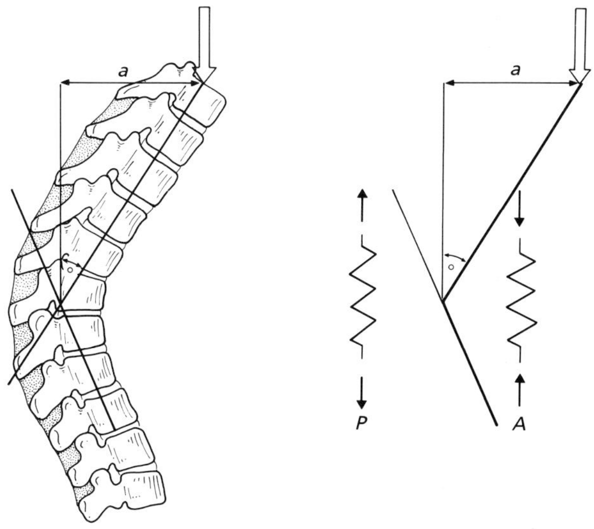

Fig. 23.17 The biomechanics of increasing kyphotic deformity.

alone will not, unfortunately, relieve the patient's symptoms.

If the patient is out of balance, a quadrilateral-type wedge osteotomy done anteriorly and posteriorly will restore balance in the frontal plane as well as restore lumbar lordosis in the sagittal plane. If the fusion is solid the osteotomy is carried out usually at the L3–L4 level or through the posterior pseudarthrosis if present. The nerve roots at the level of the posterior osteotomy must be clearly identified and an osteotomy performed analogous to that described by Smith Peterson. We have found the use of Dwyer screws in the lateral fusion mass posteriorly to be ideal together with the use of posterolateral cables to close the osteotomy site. Eight screws are used for each cable, four screws proximal and four distal to the osteotomy site (Fig. 23.15). A midline contoured AO plate is used to help control rotation, with at least two screws proximal and distal to the osteotomy level. Simultaneous anterior open wedge osteotomy is carried out, preferably at the L3–L4 level, or at the apex of the frontal curve corresponding to the posterior osteotomy utilizing the Kostuik–Harrington system and closing the posterior osteotomy with Dwyer instrumentation. A tricortical or bicortical iliac crest graft is inserted anteriorly (Fig. 23.15). A recent review of 54 patients treated in this fashion (Kostuik *et al.*, 1988) showed excellent results with pain relief in 48 cases (90%) (Fig. 23.16). Non-union occurred in three patients due to anterior graft collapse, and neurological complications occurred in two patients.

ADULT KYPHOTIC DEFORMITIES
(see also Chapter 24)

The posterior elements of the human spine are under tension and the anterior elements under compression. Kyphosis may occur when either of these two components is disrupted. Increased physiological loads, both in magnitude and direction, may result in a kyphotic deformity with a further increase in the moment arm, leading to still further stress on the vertebral bodies (Fig. 23.17).

The treatment of severe kyphosis may involve adequate decompression of the spinal cord anteriorly and correcting the deformity (Fig. 23.18). Posterior fusions are under tension in the kyphotic state, and are usually thin and susceptible to stress fracture; indeed they may bend. The longer the fusion the more stable it is. Nevertheless the pseudarthrosis rate and failure to maintain correction are reported as high as 40% in the treatment of Scheuermann's disease in adults. In contrast, anterior fusions are under compression and stabilize early. Since 1979 the author has used Harrington instrumentation anteriorly for the correction of kyphotic deformities. The system was initially developed for the treatment of burst injuries following decompression anteriorly. Two rods were used: the rachet-ended rod and a heavy Harrington compression rod. These rods were used in rectangular parallelogram fashion, preferably coupled (Fig. 23.19). This led to the subsequent use of the system to correct other kyphotic deformities, and in particularly post-traumatic kyphosis (Fig. 23.20). Scheuermann's kyphosis, as well as a small number of congenital kyphotics and iatrogenic loss of lumbar lordosis, rigid round back, postlaminectomy kyphosis, kyphosis secondary to tumour and secondary to metabolic osteoporosis with fractures were treated in like fashion. Up to October 1988, 304 cases of anterior corrective operations using the system have been carried out. Complications included screw breakage in the earlier cases, distraction rod fractures, and vertebral body fractures in osteoporotic bone salvaged by the use of methylmethacrylate. There have been no early or late vascular or neurological problems.

Previous reports of the surgical treatment of Scheuermann's kyphosis in adults by posterior instrumentation showed a progressive loss of position

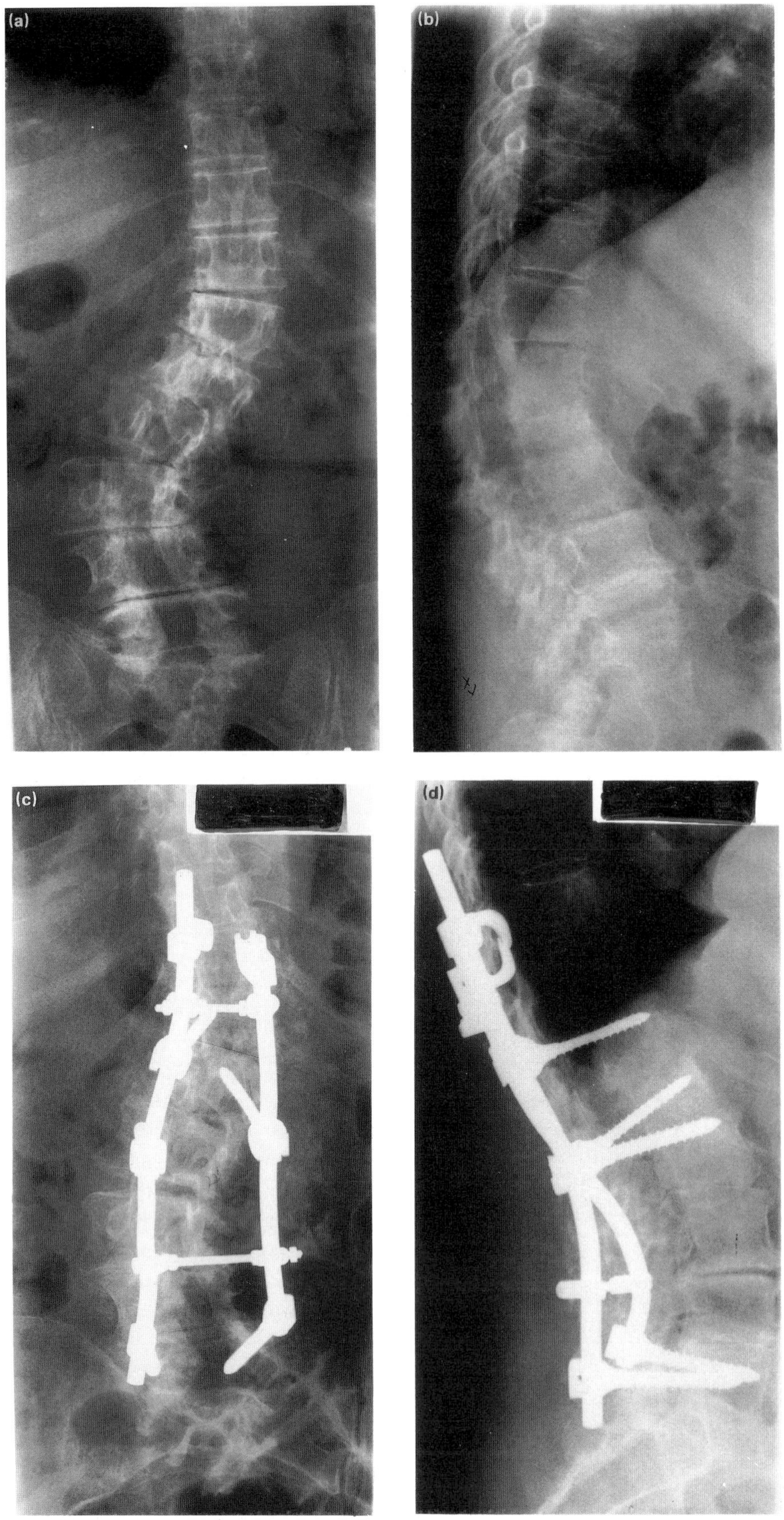

Fig. 23.18 (a,b) Female age 68. Prelaminectomy scoliosis measured 22°. Following decompression the deformity decreased to 32° together with totally disabling back pain, and subsequently to 50°. Note loss of lumbar lordosis post-decompression. (c,d) Two-stage surgery restored lordosis and relieved pain. First stage consisted of multiple anterior discectomies and bone graft. The second stage Cotrel–Dubousset instrumentation and fusion corrected the deformity and restored lordosis.

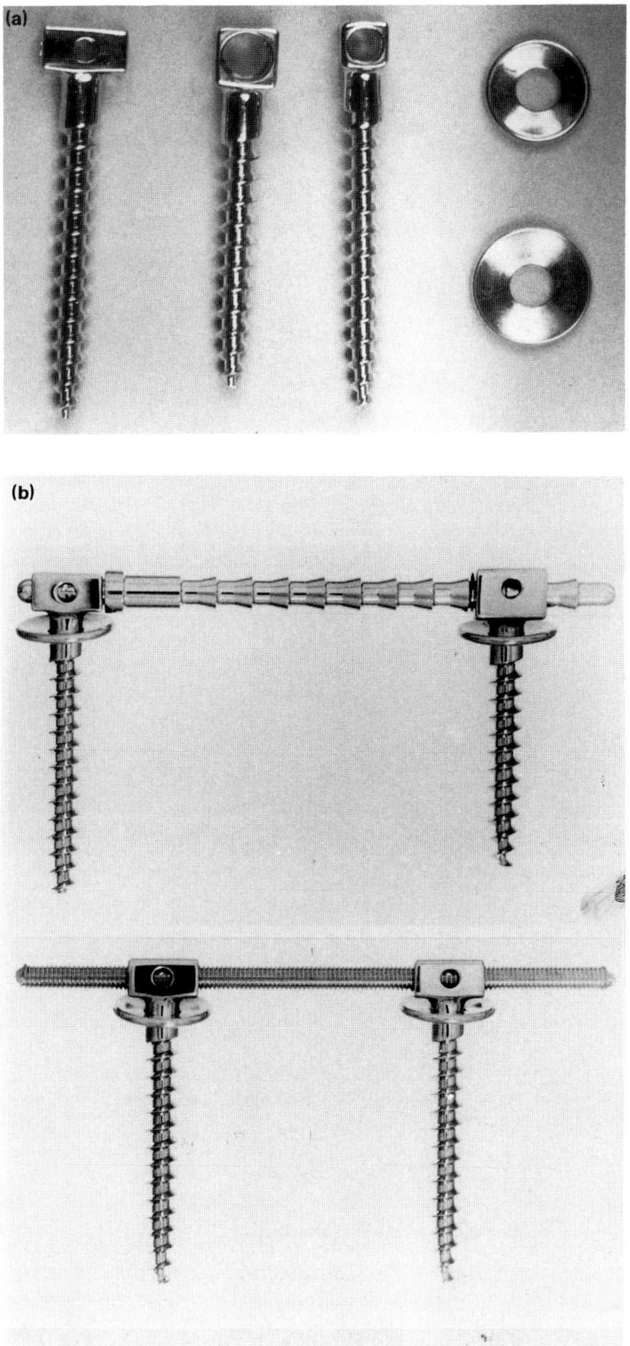

Fig. 23.19 The Kostuik–Harrington system.

of long-term follow-up. Loss of correction was due to the fusion being on the tensile side of the spine resulting in a high pseudarthrosis rate (40%) (Kostuik & Bentivoglio, 1981) and late stress fractures due to repetitive cyclical loading. Previous work showed that anterior interbody fusion alone does not provide adequate correction of the deformity. These factors led to the development of the Kostuik–Harrington system combined with interbody fusion in the correction of Scheuermann's kyphosis (Fig. 23.21).

At surgery the screws must pierce the cortices of both bodies and the holding power in osteopenic bone can be enhanced by the use of methylmethacrylate. Adult patients with Scheuermann's disease with curves of 75° or greater, particularly females with documented evidence of progression, are subjected to surgery. Between 1982 and 1987, 36 patients with an average age of 27.5 years were treated, in this fashion. One pseudarthrosis occurred and four screws fractured with some loss of correction. Postoperatively a plastic orthosis was worn for six months. Anterior instrumentation is therefore important in preventing collapse.

Iliac crest grafts are preferred; these are bicortical in younger patients or tricortical in older osteopenic people. These are preferred to the fibula as iliac crest grafts will revascularize quickly, whereas fibular grafts do not begin to revascularize for 6 months at least. However, anterior instrumentation is necessary if iliac crest grafts are used because these grafts are unable to withstand the loads imposed in the erect position, particularly in the thoracolumbar and lumbar spine.

MORBIDITY AND MORTALITY

The treatment of spinal deformities in the adult is not without risk. Neurological complications in the adolescent have been reported as being approximately 1%, but morbidity reports indicate that neurological complications in the adult lie between 2% and 3%. In the review of the first 1000 patients, by the author, there was an incidence of paraparesis of 0.7% (seven patients). Only two patients remained unable to walk at follow-up. The incidence of nerve root irritatior and of single motor root weakness occurred in 3% The vast majority of these recovered. The secon most dreaded complication is that of pulmonar embolus. Two deaths have occurred as a result of thi complication, but none in the past five years sinc the advent of prophylaxis consisting of intravenou mini-dose heparin 5000 units daily and intravenou persantine 250 mg daily, run as a continuous dri commenced preoperatively and maintained on ave age for 10 days postoperatively. Deep infection rat

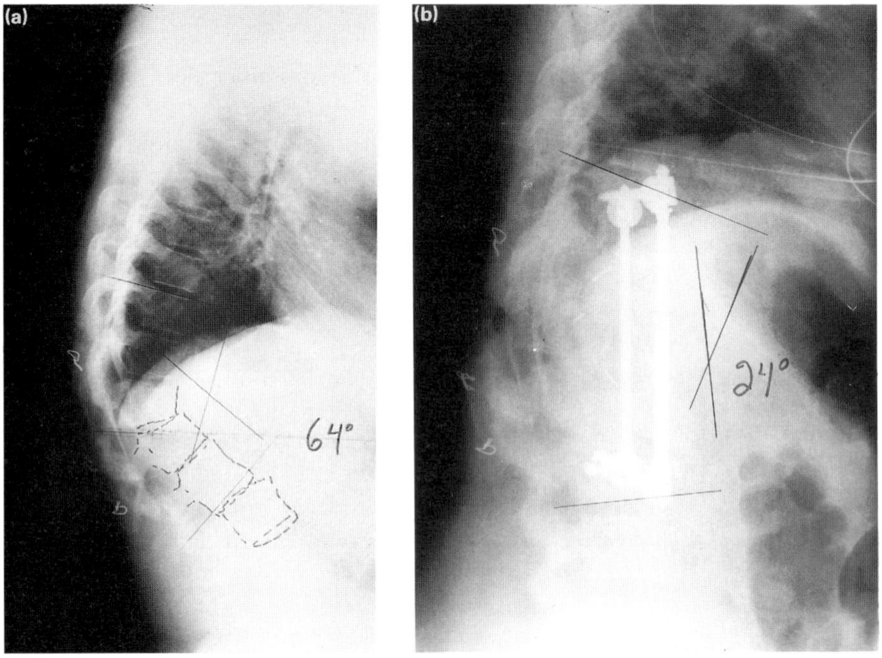

Fig. 23.20 (a) Post-traumatic kyphosis 64° previous posterior fusion (explored), which failed to relieve pain. (b) Pain was relieved following anterior Kostuik–Harrington instrumentation. The thoracolumbar kyphosis is reduced to 24°. No posterior osteotomy was necessary as the fusion was on the tensile side of the spine and thus flexible.

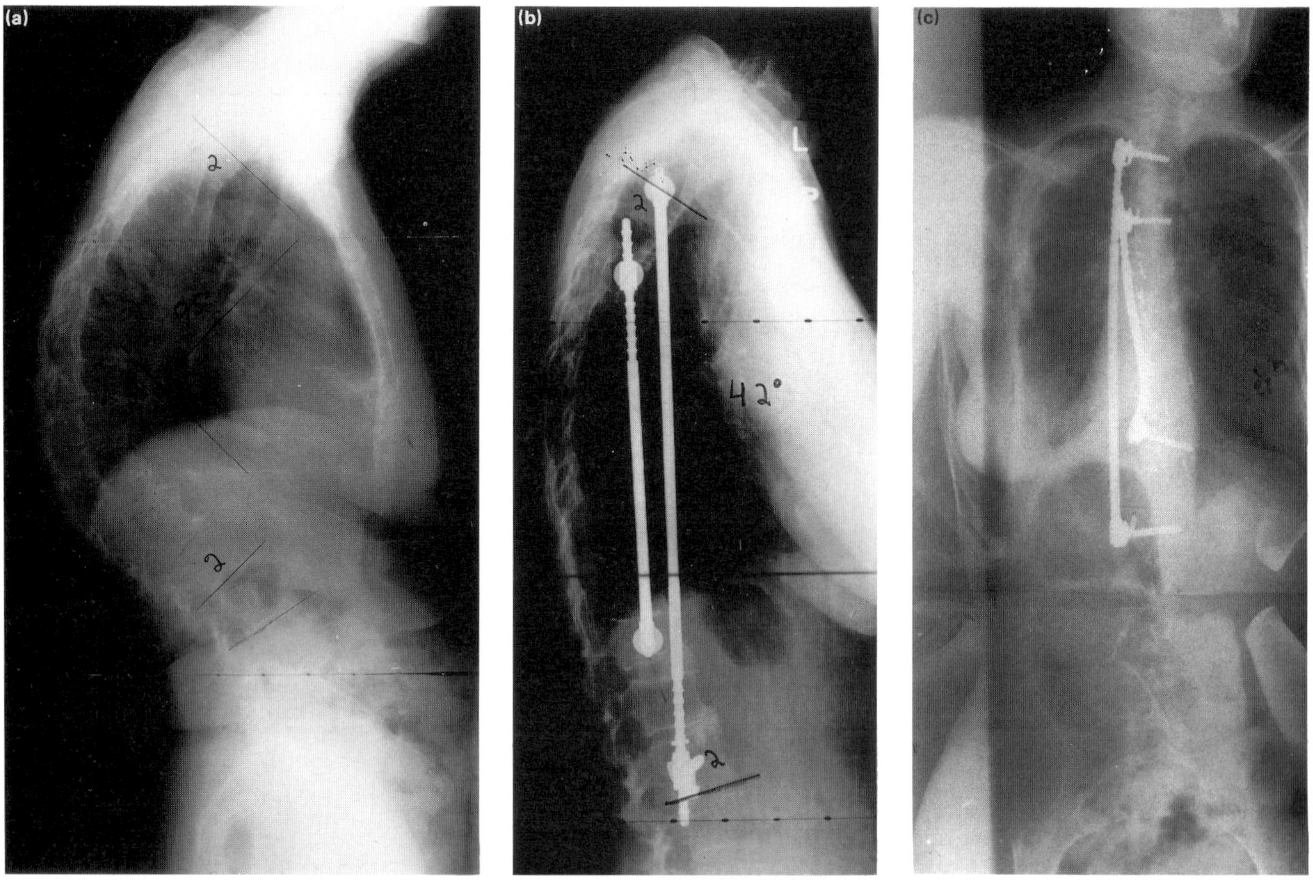

Fig. 23.21 (a) Female age 52 with progressive kyphosis measuring 95°. (b) After surgery the deformity is reduced to 42° by single-stage anterior Kostuik–Harrington instrumentation and fusion. (c) Postoperative AP view demonstrates screw placement.

has been 1% with no major sequelae. Prophylactic antibiotics are used for 48 hours.

There has been a 0.6% mortality rate. Two of these deaths have been from pulmonary embolus, two from adult respiratory distress syndrome and one from a disseminated intravascular coagulopathy.

Other complications, such as instrumentation failure, pseudarthroses and loss of lumbar lordosis, have been discussed in this chapter.

REFERENCES

Allen, B.L. Jr & Ferguson, R.L. (1982) The Galveston technique for L rod instrumentation of the scoliotic spine. *Spine*, **7**, 276–284.

Balderston, R.A., Winter, R.B., Moe, J.H., Bradford, D.S. & Lonstein, J.E. (1986) Fusion to the sacrum for nonparalytic scoliosis in the adult. *Spine*, **11**, 824–829.

Byrd, J.A. III, Scoles, P.V., Winter, R.B., Bradford, D.S., Lonstein, J.E. & Moe, J.H. (1987) Adult idiopathic scoliosis treated by anterior and posterior spinal fusion. *J. Bone Jt. Surg.*, **69A**, 843–850.

Bradford, D.S. (1988) Adult scoliosis: current concepts of treatment. *Clin. Orthop.*, **229**, 70–87.

Cochran, T., Irstam, L. and Nachemson, A. (1983) Long-term anatomic and functional changes in patients with adolescent idiopathic scoliosis treated by Harrington rod fusion. *Spine*, **8**, 576–584.

Collis, D.K. & Ponsetti, I.V. (1969) Long term follow-up of patients with idiopathic scoliosis not treated surgically. *J. Bone Jt. Surg.*, **51A**, 425–445.

Cotrel, Y. (1986) *New Instrumentation for Surgery of the Spine.* Freud Publishing House.

Cotrel, Y., Dubousset, J. & Guillaumat, M. (1988) New universal instrumentation in spinal surgery. *Clin. Orthop.*, **227**, 10–23.

Cummine, J.L., Lonstein, J.E., Moe, J.H., Winter, R.B. & Bradford, D.S. (1979) Reconstructive surgery in the adult for failed scoliosis fusion. *J. Bone Jt. Surg.*, **61A**, 1151–1161.

Dawson, E.G., Caron, A. & Moe, J.H. (1973) Surgical management of scoliosis in the adult. *J. Bone Jt. Surg.*, **55A**, 437.

Denis, F. (1988) Cotrel–Dubousset instrumentation in the treatment of idiopathic scoliosis. *Orthop. Clin. N. Am.*, **19**, 291–311.

Doherty, J.H. (1973) Complications of fusion in lumbar scoliosis. *J. Bone Jt. Surg.*, **55A**, 438.

Dwyer, A.F. (1973) Experience of anterior correction of scoliosis. *Clin. Orthop.*, **93**, 191–206.

Edgar, M.A. & Mehta, M.H. (1982) A longterm review of adults with fused and unfused idiopathic scoliosis. *Orthop. Trans.*, **6**, 462–463.

Grobler, L.J., Moe, J.H., Winter, R.B., Bradford, D.S. & Lonstein, J.E. (1978) Loss of lumbar lordosis following surgical correction of thoracolumbar deformities. *Orthop. Trans.*, **2**, 239.

Grubb, S.A., Lipscomb, H.S. & Conrad, R.W. (1989) Diagnostic findings in painful adult scoliosis. Meeting SRS, Amsterdam, September.

Hall, J.D. (1981) Dwyer Instrumentation in Anterior Fusion of the Spine. *J. Bone Jt. Surg.*, **63A**, 1188.

Harrington, P.R. & Dickson, J.H. (1973) An eleven-year clinical investigation of Harrington instrumentation. A preliminary report on 578 cases. *Clin. Orthop.*, **93**, 113–130.

Hasday, C.A., Passoff, T.L. & Perry, J. (1983) Gait abnormalities arising from iatrogenic loss of lumbar lordosis secondary to Harrington instrumentation in lumbar fractures. *Spine*, **8**, 501–511.

Herndon, W.Q., Sullivan, J.A., Yngve, D.A., Gross, R.H. & Dreher, G. (1987) Segmental spinal instrumentation with sublaminar wires. *J. Bone Jt. Surg.*, **69A**, 851–859.

Herring, J.A. & Wenger, D.R. (1982) Segmental spinal instrumentation. A preliminary report of 40 consecutive cases. *Spine*, **7**, 285–298.

Jackson, R.P., Simmons, E.H. & Stripinus, D. (1983) Incidence and severity of back pain in adult idiopathic scoliosis. *Spine*, **8**, 749–756.

Johnson, J.R. & Holt, R.T. (1988) Combined use of anterior and posterior surgery for adult scoliosis. *Orthop. Clin. N. Am.*, **19**, 361–370.

Kaneda, K., Fujiya, N. & Satoh, S. (1986) Results with Zielke instrumentation for idiopathic thoracolumbar and lumbar scoliosis. *Clin. Orthop.*, **205**, 195–203.

Kostuik, J.P. (1988) Treatment of scoliosis in the adult thoracolumbar spine with special reference to fusion to the sacrum. *Orthop. Clin. N. Am.*, **19**, 371–381.

Kostuik, J.P. (1979) Decision making in adult scoliosis. *Spine*, **4**, 532–525.

Kostuik, J.P. & Bentivoglio, J. (1981) The incidence of low back pain in adult scoliosis. *Spine*, **9**, 268–273.

Kostuik, J.P., Carl, A. & Ferron, S. (1989) Anterior Zielke instrumentation for adult spinal deformity. *J. Bone Jt. Surg.*, **71A**, 898–912.

Kostuik, J.P. & Hall, B.B. (1983) Spinal fusions to the sacrum in adults with scoliosis. *Spine*, **8**, 489–500.

Kostuik, J.P., Israel, J. & Hall, J.E. (1973) Scoliosis surgery in adults. *Clin. Orthop.*, **93**, 225–234.

Kostuik, J.P., Maurais, G.R. & Richardson, W.J. (1989) Primary fusion to the sacrum using Luque instrumentation. *Spine*, **13**, 30.

Kostuik, J.P., Maurais, G.R., Richardson, W.J. & Okajima, Y. (1988) Combined single stage anterior posterior osteotomy for correction of iatrogenic lumbar kyphosis. *Spine*, **13**, 257–266.

Kostuik, J.P., Worden Hawker, R. & Salo, P. (1990) Long-term functional outcome following surgery for adult scoliosis. Presented AOA, Boston, June. SRS Hawadi, September.

Lagrone, M.O., Bradford, D.S., Moe, J.H., Lonstein, J.E., Winter, R.B. & Ogilvie, J.W. (1988) Treatment of symptomatic flatback after spinal fusion. *J. Bone Jt. Surg.*, **70A**, 569–580.

Luque, E.R. (1982a) The anatomic basis and development of segmental spinal instrumentation. *Spine*, **7**, 256–259.

Luque, E.R. (1982b) Segmental spinal instrumentation for correction of scoliosis. *Clin. Orthop.*, **163**, 192–198.

Macnab, I. (1977) *Backache*. Williams & Wilkins, Baltimore, MD.

Moe, J.H., Purcell, G.A. & Bradford, D.S. (1983) Zielke instrumentation (VDS) for the correction of spinal curvature. Analysis of results in the 66 patients. *Clin. Orthop.*, **180**, 133–153.

Nachemson, A. (1969) A longterm follow-up study of non-treated scoliosis. *J. Bone Jt. Surg.*, **50A**, 203.

Nachemson, A. (1983) A longterm follow-up study of non-treated scoliosis. *Acta Orthop. Scand.*, **39**, 489–500.

Nash, C.L. Jr & Moe, J.H. (1969) A study of vertebral rotation. *J. Bone Jt. Surg.*, **51A**, 223–228.

Nash, C.L., Goldstein, J.M. & Wilham, M.R. (1989) Selection of lumbar fusion levels in adult idiopathic scoliosis patients. SRS Meeting, Amsterdam, September.

Nilsonne, U. & Lundgren, D.D. (1968) Longterm prognosis in idiopathic scoliosis. *Acta Orthop. Scand.*, **39**, 455–465.

Nuber, G.W. & Schafer, M.F. (1986) Surgical management of adult scoliosis. *Clin. Orthop.*, **208**, 228–237.

Ogiela, D.M. & Chan, D.P.K. (1986) Ventral derotation spondylodesis. A review of 22 cases. *Spine*, **11**, 18–22.

Ponder, R.C., Dickson, J.H., Harrington, P.R. & Erwin, W.D. (1975) Results of Harrington instrumentation and fusion in the adult idiopathic scoliosis patient. *J. Bone Jt. Surg.*, **57A**, 798–801.

Ponsetti, I.V. (1968) The pathogenesis of adult scoliosis. In Zorab, P.A. (ed.) *Proceedings of Second Symposium on Scoliosis: Causation*. E & S Livingstone, Edinburgh.

Rogala, E.J., Drummond, D.S. & Gurr, J. (1978) Scoliosis: incidence and natural history. A prospective epidemiological study. *J. Bone Jt. Surg.*, **60A**, 173–176.

Sponseller, P.D., Cohen, M.S., Nachemson, A.L., Hall, J.E. & Wohl, M.E.B. (1987) Results of surgical treatment of adults with idiopathic scoliosis. *J. Bone Jt. Surg.*, **69A**, 667–675.

Stagnara, P. (1969) Scoliosis in adults. Surgical treatment of severe forms. *Excerpta Med Found Int. Cong.*, p. 192.

Stagnara, P., Jouvinous, P., Peloux, J. *et al.* (1969) Cyphoscoliosis Essentielles de l'adulte. Formes severe de plus de 100. Redressment partial et arthrodese. Presented at the XI Sicot Congress, Mexico City, Mexico.

Stagnara, P. (1971) Utilization of Harrington's device in the treatment of adult kyphoscoliosis above 100 degrees. *Fourth International Symposium*. George Thieme, Stuttgart.

Stagnara, P., Fleury, D., Faucher, R. *et al.* (1975) Scoliosis majeures de l'adultes supertieures a 100–183 cas traites chirurgicalement. *Rev. Chir. Orthop.*, **61**, 101–122.

Swank, S., Lonstein, J.E., Moe, J.H., Winter, R.B. & Bradford, D.S. (1981) Surgical treatment of adult scoliosis. A review of two hundred and twenty-two cases. *J. Bone Jt. Surg.*, **63A**, 268–287.

Thompson, G.H., Wilber, R.G., Shaffer, J.W., Scoles, P.V. & Nash, C.L. Jr (1985) Segmental spinal instrumentation in idiopathic scoliosis. A preliminary report. *Spine*, **10**, 623–630.

van Dam, B.E. (1988) Nonoperative treatment of adult scoliosis. *Orthop. Clin. N. Am.*, **19**, 347–351.

van Dam, B.E., Bradford, D.S., Lonstein, J.E., Moe, J.H., Ogilvie, J.W. & Winter, R.B. (1987) Adult idiopathic scoliosis treated by posterior spinal fusion and Harrington instrumentation. *Spine*, **12**, 32–36.

Vanderpool, D.W., James, J.I.P. & Wynne-Davies, R. (1969) Scoliosis in the elderly. *J. Bone Jt. Surg.*, **51A**, 446–455.

Weinstein, S.L. & Ponseti, I.V. (1983) Curve progression in idiopathic scoliosis. *J. Bone Jt. Surg.*, **65A**, 447–455.

Winter, R.B., Lonstein, J.E. & Denis, F. (1988) Pain patterns in adult scoliosis. *Orthop. Clin. N. Am.*, **19**, 339–345.

Winter, R.B. (1978) Combined Dwyer and Harrington instrumentation and fusion in the treatment of selected patients with painful adult idiopathic scoliosis. *Spine*, **3**, 135–141.

Zielke, K., Stunkat, R. & Beaujean, F. (1976) Ventrale derotations-spondylodese. *Arch. Orthop. Unfallchir.*, **85**, 257–263.

24 · Acquired Kyphosis

By J.W. OGILVIE

Kyphosis derives from the Greek word 'kyphosos', which means hunchback. In the sagittal plane the normal adult spine has a physiological thoracic kyphosis in the range of 20–40° (Roaf, 1960). When this range is exceeded in the thoracic area the spine is said to be kyphotic. In the lumbar spine, loss of lordosis is called hypolordosis until it exceeds 0°, at which time it is then kyphosis. The term gibbus derives from the Latin word for hump and originally referred to the spinal deformity of Potts' disease. Gibbus infers the presence of a sharp angular sagittal deformity and is measured over the several levels of spine involved. Kyphosis involving the overall sagittal alignment of the thoracic spine is measured from the inferior endplate of T12 to the superior endplate of the highest thoracic vertebra identifiable on the lateral radiograph, usually T3 or higher.

BIOMECHANICS

Kyphosis is important because it may produce pain in the thoracic spine either from chronic strain of the paraspinal musculature or from degenerative changes in the intervertebral discs as they experience excessive anterior weight-bearing. The kyphotic deformity may interfere with pulmonary function by shortening the thoracic cage and decreasing its volume, giving rise to impairment. In the lower thoracic spine, and at the thoracolumbar junction, a sharp angulation forces the contents of the abdominal cavity into the thorax and thus limits respiratory excursion of the diaphragm and subsequently pulmonary expansion. Impingement on the spinal cord and neurological dysfunction may also result from angular deformity of the spinal column. The cosmetic implications of spine deformity vary widely with the individual and the social consequences are often disturbing. Victor Hugo's novel, *Hunchback of Notre Dame*, illustrates the complex interpersonal relationships that may be created around the individual with kyphotic deformity.

Acquired thoracic kyphosis may have many possible aetiologies, and these will be considered separately. While their causes are varied, the pathogenesis has a common mechanical pathway in the adult which can be expressed in Euler's term for short column stability: $P < YA$. When the axial load, P, on a column is less than the term, YA, stability exists. Y is the strength or modulus of the material (disc or vertebral body) and A is the cross-sectional area of the column. In conditions involving disorders of vertebral growth such as the bony dysplasias, mucopolysaccharidoses or Scheuermann's disease, biological factors are most important in addition to purely mechanical considerations.

Therefore, in fractures of the normal vertebral body, an increase in axial load above the fatigue limit of bone is the most important factor. In pathological collapse of the vertebral body due to osteopenia, infection or tumour, a decrease in the strength of bone is responsible for loss of stability. Loss of the hydrophilic glycosaminoglycans in the intervertebral disc, a phenomenon which occurs with the natural ageing process, also leads to collapse of the anterior portion of the vertebral column. These processes are usually manifest in the vertebral body and intervertebral disc and not so much in the neural arch and facet joints. With shortening of the anterior spinal column and maintenance of height in the posterior column, rotation of the spine in the sagittal plane occurs and kyphosis develops.

Fracture

While shear stress and torsional loads occur, flexion–compression and flexion–distraction forces are the most common mechanisms of spinal fracture. When they result in fractures of the low lumbar spine, L4 and L5, which is already in lordosis, the axial load frequently causes a symmetrical compression fracture without increasing the kyphosis. In the thoracic and upper lumbar spine these forces result in an increase of sagittal plane rotation and a kyphotic deformity may result.

Spinal fractures may result in neurological impairment, but in addition to neurological considerations there are three issues concerning the mechanical stability of the spine which must be considered; they are: (1) stability during the initial and early healing stages, (2) late instability with kyphotic progression and possible neural canal compromise after the fracture has healed, (3) late pain in the fracture site.

Sir Frank Holdsworth (1963) introduced the concept of a two-column spine. The anterior column consists of the vertebral body, intervertebral disc and the associated anterior and posterior longitudinal ligaments. The posterior column is the neural arch and the 'posterior ligamentous complex' which he defined as the interspinous ligament, ligamentum flavum and facet capsules. In the thoracic spine the spinal column is greatly stabilized by the presence of the thorax. When there is widening of the interspinous process distance with facet dislocation, mechanical instability is likely to be present. While others have attempted to explain this concept Holdsworth remains the most popular reference for this theory. More recently the three-column concept of Denis has gained general acceptance. Shear fractures and fractures associated with a flail chest or sternal dislocation also have a higher probability of instability. These injuries require prolonged bed rest or surgical stabilization. When traumatic, as opposed to pathological fractures of the thoracic spine are considered, fracture–dislocations and compression fractures compromise more than 90% of all injuries (Hanley & Eskay, 1989).

Late fracture instability manifest as a progressive kyphosis is frequently associated with ligamentous disruption at the intervertebral joint, e.g. dislocation (Fig. 24.1). Bony injuries usually heal satisfactorily, thus providing long-term stability. Leidholt and others (1969) were unable to correlate the degree of residual kyphosis and the presence of pain in paraplegics. Malcolm and others (1981), however, recommend both anterior and posterior fusion for if the post-traumatic kyphosis is greater than 50°; if there is deficient vertebral body bone stock, or if there is deficient posterior bone because of previous laminectomy. After surgery, most of their patients experienced an improvement in the pain associated with their injuries.

The combination of kyphosis and pathological bone may result in a progressive deformity and deteriorating neurological function (see Fig. 24.9).

Tumour

Benign tumours of the spine such as aneurysmal bone cyst, osteoblastoma and osteoid osteoma usually occur in the neural arch and are therefore seldom the cause of kyphosis. When benign lesions involve the vertebral body they usually involve a single level, and if they destroy the integrity of the bone a gibbus may develop. The source of pain may be muscular in origin because of the kyphos or from the deranged intervertebral joints anteriorly or posteriorly. Anterior single-level interbody arthrodesis with correction of the deformity is appropriate treatment for both the deformity and the pain at the intervertebral joints (Fig. 24.3a,b).

When compromise of the spinal canal results from tumour infiltration or kyphosis, decompression should be accomplished through the costotransversectomy or anterior approaches. Anterior and posterior surgery with internal fixation is usually required to achieve both correction of the deformity and long-term stability if a multilevel anterior defect is present (Fig. 24.3c). If the prognosis of the underlying disease is poor, with short survival anticipated, anterior spinal support may be provided with a buttress of polymethylmethacrylate. If survival is anticipated longer than 18–24 months, a biological material should be used that will incorporate and provide long-term stability.

Osteopenia

Loss of bone stock may be due to osteoporosis or osteomalacia. In the elderly there are usually elements of both present. Pathological vertebral body compression fractures may occur with seemingly minor trauma. There is a progressive age-related increase in

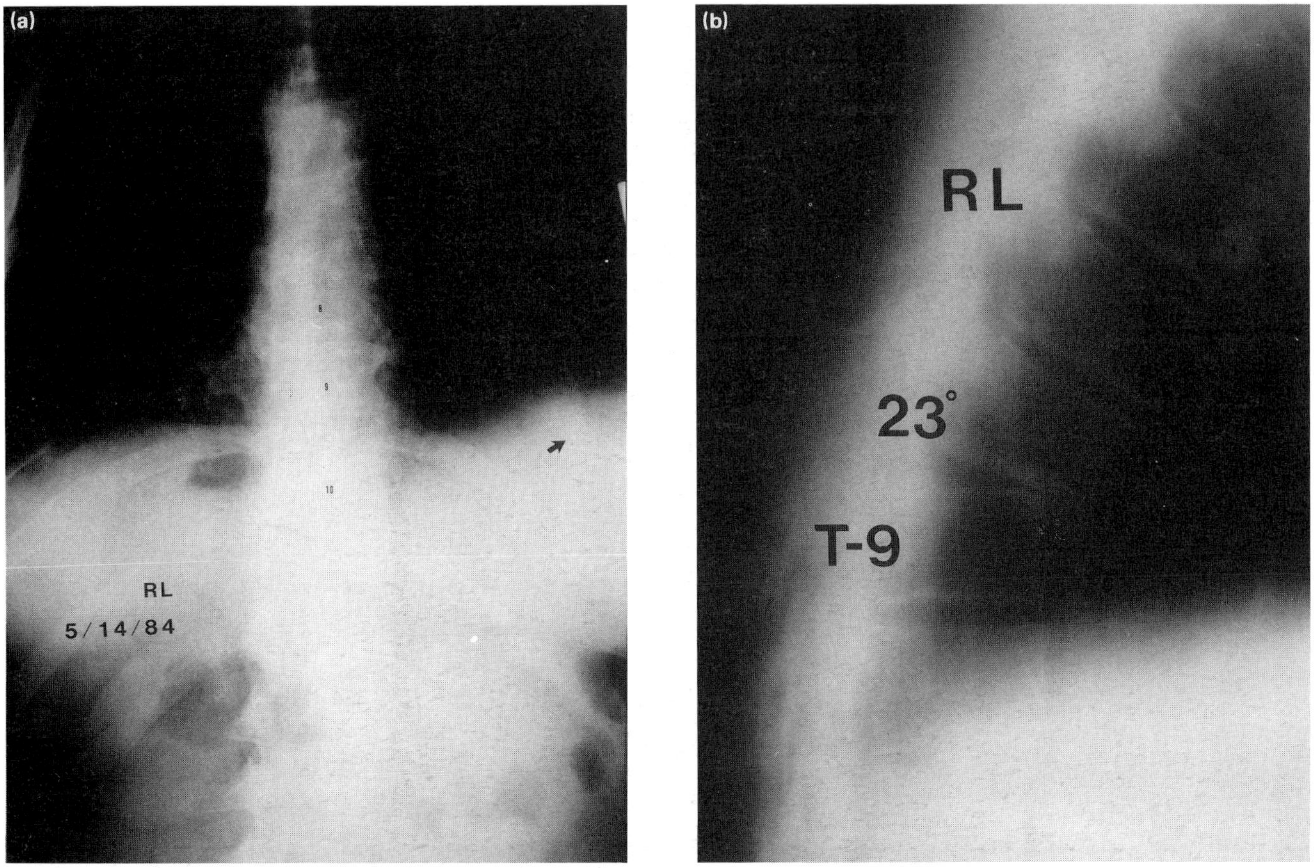

Fig. 24.1 (a) A 37-year-old male was involved in an automobile accident and received penetrating injury to his thorax. One month following injury, his pulmonary status returned to normal. However he noted a progressive painful kyphotic deformity in the lower thoracic spine. Lateral X-rays (b) revealed a subluxation at T8–T9, with disruption of the posterior ligamentous complex. Posterior instrumentation and fusion restored his normal thoracic contour with relief of symptoms.

the wedging of the thoracic vertebrae in both men and women in similar fashion. Additional age-related soft tissue changes occur in women, and this may explain the greater overall kyphosis noted in females (Milne & Lauder, 1976).

In a prospective study of osteoporotic women, anterior wedge fractures were noted most commonly in the midthoracic area, and midbody compression fractures in the lumbar spine (Fig. 24.2a–d). Isolated compression fractures were uncommon above the seventh thoracic level. Even in women without compression fractures, 19% were found to have hyperkyphosis indicating a non-osseous factor contributing to the deformity (Gordan, 1985).

When an additional reason for osteopenia is present, such as the use of corticosteroids or malnutrition from poor diet or malabsorption, the pathological process is accelerated (Fig. 24.4). Treatment is initially directed at identifying a treatable cause of osteopenia. Direct treatment of osteopenia may include the use of vitamin D and calcium supplements. Whether the menopause occurs naturally or surgically, postmenopausal women should be considered for hormone replacement therapy. Fluoride treatment of osteoporosis requires close monitoring for toxic side-effects, and may require long-term treatment before beneficial effects are realized. The use of spinal orthosis may alleviate pain in the acute stage, but is usually unacceptable to the patient in the long term.

Infection

Infection, either granulomatous or pyogenic, can result in destruction of the intervertebral disc and vertebral body by the action of lytic enzymes or by compromise of the blood supply. *Staphylococcus*

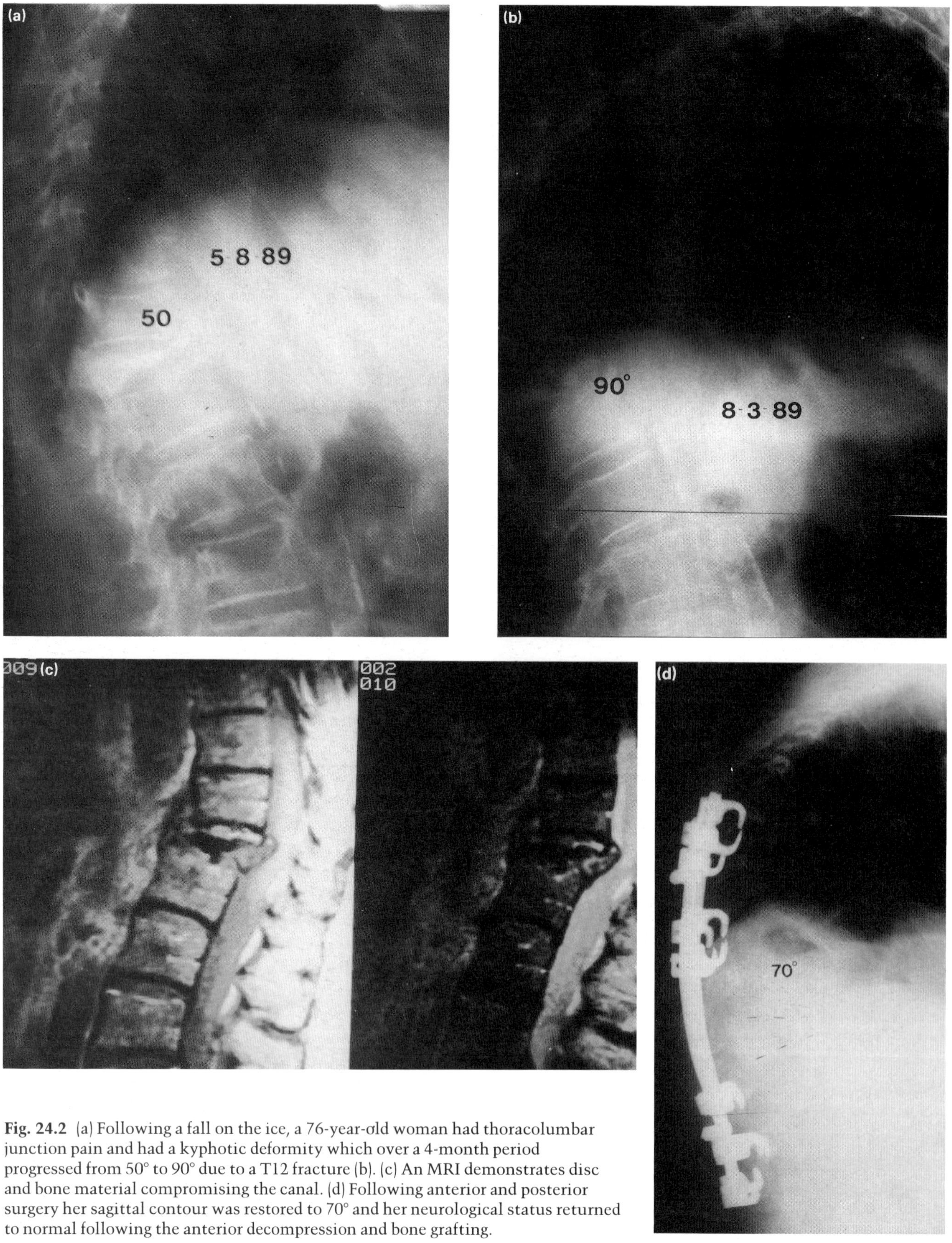

Fig. 24.2 (a) Following a fall on the ice, a 76-year-old woman had thoracolumbar junction pain and had a kyphotic deformity which over a 4-month period progressed from 50° to 90° due to a T12 fracture (b). (c) An MRI demonstrates disc and bone material compromising the canal. (d) Following anterior and posterior surgery her sagittal contour was restored to 70° and her neurological status returned to normal following the anterior decompression and bone grafting.

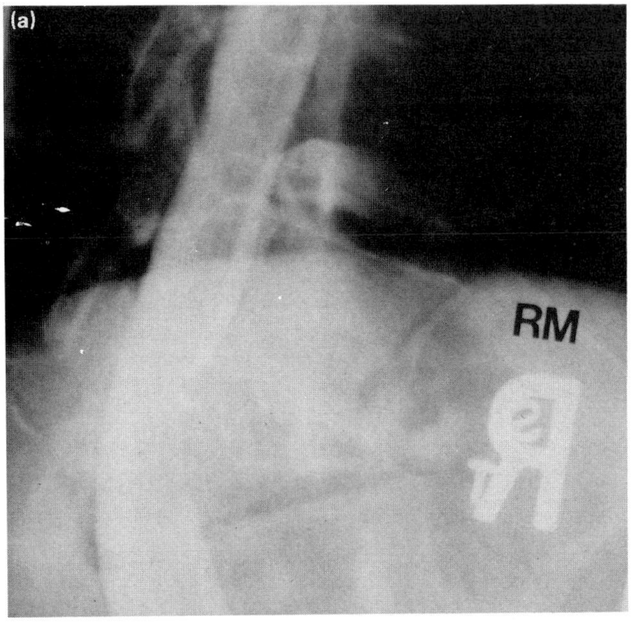

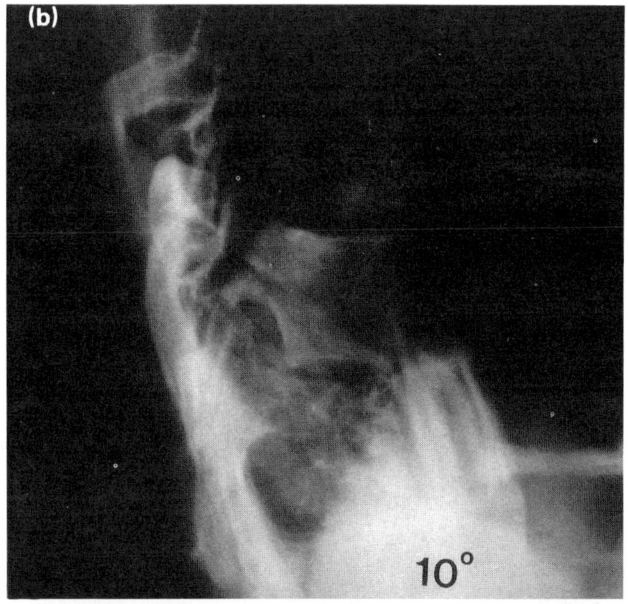

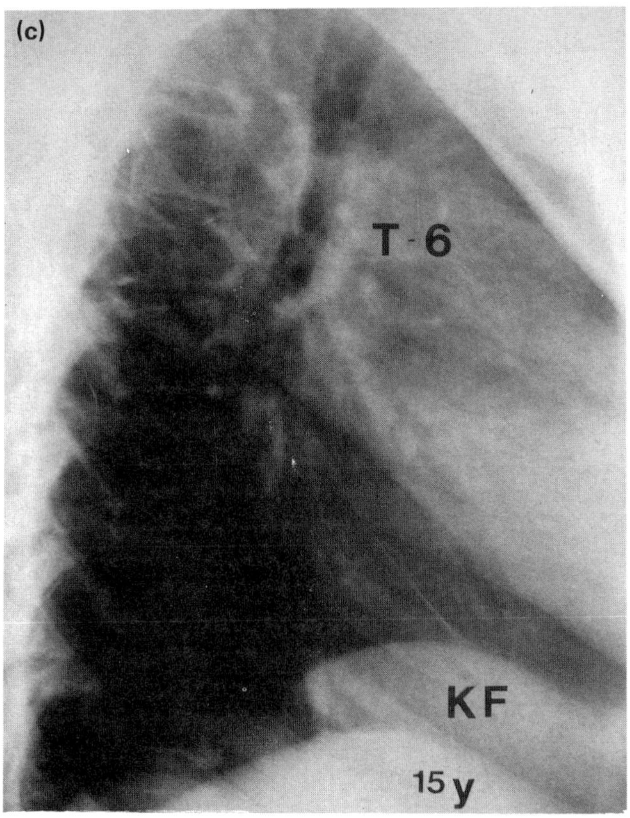

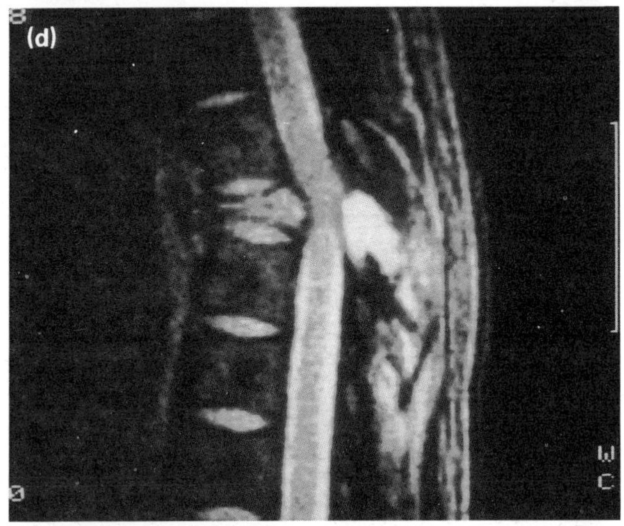

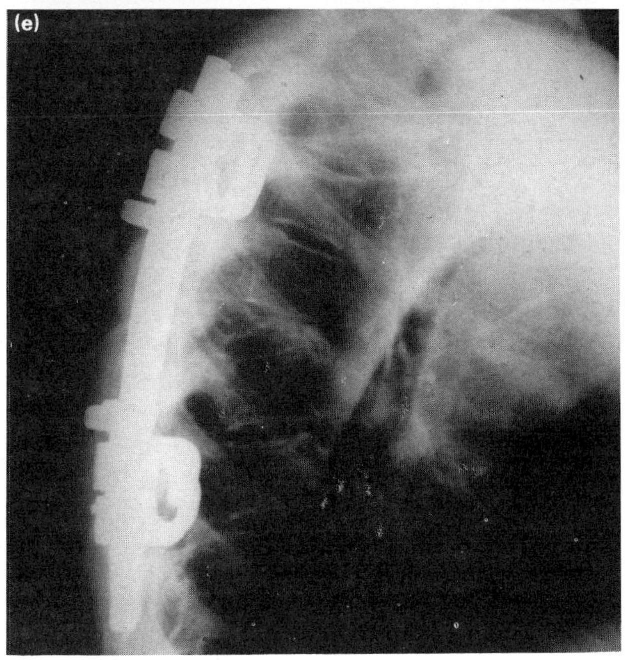

Fig. 24.3 (a) A 20-year-old woman had a painful kyphos with normal neurological examination. Complete collapsı of T12 is noted. Following anterior removal of her aneurysmal bone cyst, solid variant (b) rib strut graft she hı restoration of her normal sagittal contour and relief of pain as noted at three years postsurgery. (c,d) A 15-year-old chilı had back pain and paraparesis due to a T5 aneurysmal bone cyst. (e) Anterior decompression followed by posterior instrumentation was required to relieve the neural compression, correct her deformity, and stabilize the involved segments by fusion.

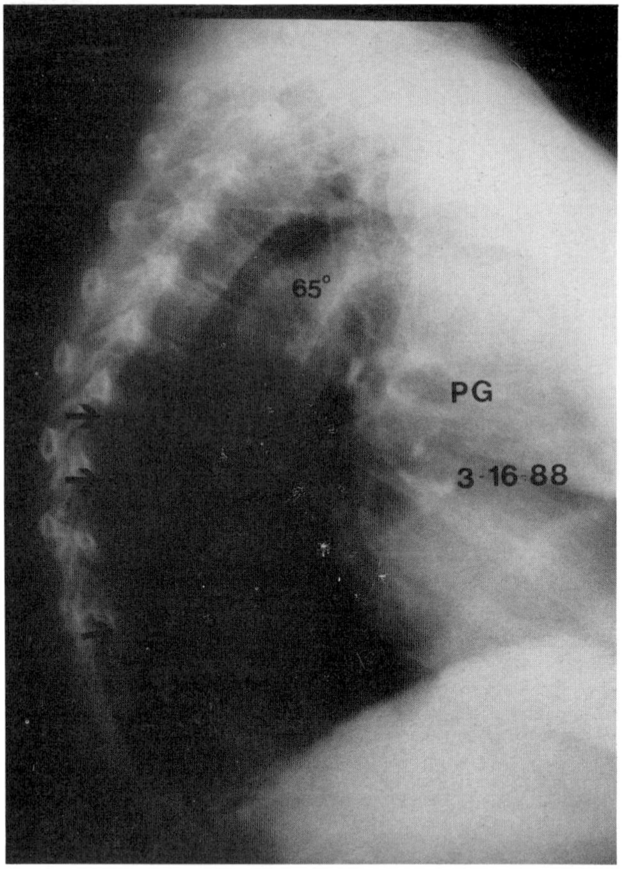

Fig. 24.4 Lateral radiograph of the thoracic spine demonstrates a traumatic compression fracture of the thoracic spine in a 50-year-old woman who was post-cardiac transplant and on high doses of corticosteroids.

aureus is the most common pyogenic organism affecting the vertebral column (Griffiths & Jones, 1971). In tuberculous spondylitis the disc is preserved for a longer period of time than in pyogenic spondylitis, where the disc is destroyed relatively early in the process. When vertebral body and intervertebral disc destruction occurs in the thoracic spine, the resulting kyphotic deformity may impair respiratory function or cause compression of the spinal cord. Direct extension of the infectious process into the spinal canal may cause cord compression, paraplegia, meningitis and death.

Initial treatment is directed towards identifying the infectious agent and antimicrobial-drug administration. When dealing with acute pyogenic spondylitis, blood cultures may be helpful in the identification process. If the patient does not respond by fever defervescence within 72 hours of antibiotic administration, a specimen of the abscess should be obtained for culture, either by needle aspiration or open biopsy.

Pyogenic spondylitis more frequently involves the lumbar spine due to haematogenous spread from Batson's plexus (Hodgson *et al.*, 1969). In the lumbar spine, where physiological lordosis is present, progressive or significant kyphotic deformity usually does not develop.

Tuberculous spondylitis affects more than 58% of those with tuberculosis (Hodgson *et al.*, 1969). The thoracic spine is frequently involved by direct extension from the pulmonary infection. In the skeletally immature patient there is arrested growth in the anterior column and a progressive kyphosis develops as the posterior elements continue their growth (see Fig. 24.5a,b). There is no correlation between the degree of kyphosis and the presence of neurological dysfunction (Rajasekaran & Shanmugasundaram, 1987). If multiple vertebrae are involved, if a progressive neurological deficit is present or when the infection is resistant to antibiotic therapy, surgical debridement and stabilization is usually required (Fig. 24.6a,b). First-stage anterior surgery is performed to remove all infected material and place fresh autogenous cancellous bone graft in the void left by removal of infected or necrotic vertebral body and disc. Second-stage posterior surgery with rigid internal fixation may then be required to correct deformity and to provide additional mechanical stability (Bailey *et al.*, 1972).

Scheuermann's disease

Juvenile kyphosis was first described by the Danish radiologist Holger Scheuermann (1920). Although the precise aetiology is unknown, its pathogenesis is related to juvenile osteoporosis of the vertebral bodies in the thoracic spine. Subsequent wedging of the vertebrae and vertebral growth plate disturbances perpetuate the deformity. When this entity presents in the skeletally immature patient it may be amenable to orthotic treatment. When it presents in the adult it is frequently with the complaint of thoracic and/or lumbar back pain and progression of the kyphosis. Acute neurological dysfunction due to spinal cord compression is rare but has been reported (Ryan & Taylor, 1982). Progression of the deformity is also possible, and when either documented pro-

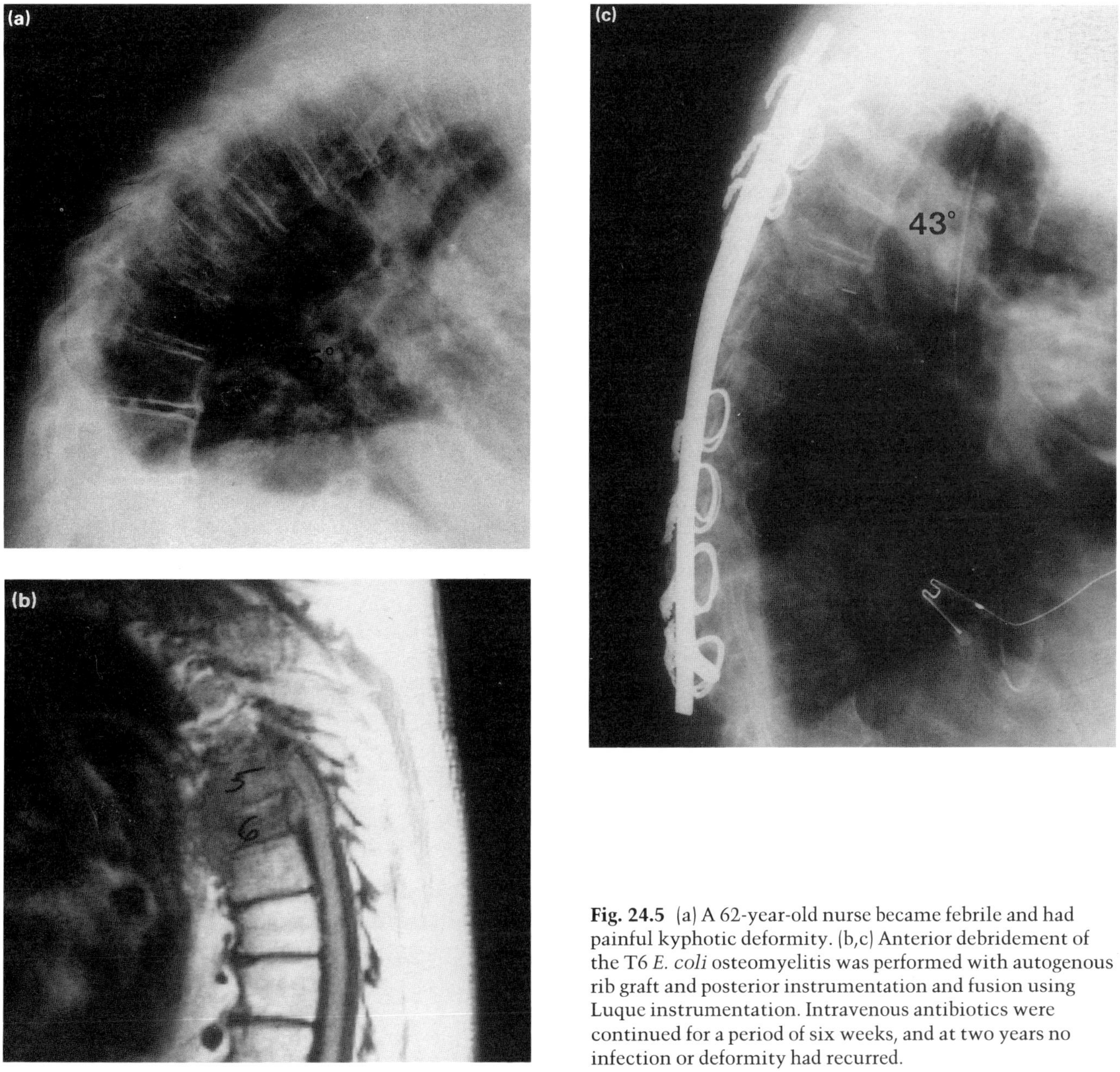

Fig. 24.5 (a) A 62-year-old nurse became febrile and had painful kyphotic deformity. (b,c) Anterior debridement of the T6 *E. coli* osteomyelitis was performed with autogenous rib graft and posterior instrumentation and fusion using Luque instrumentation. Intravenous antibiotics were continued for a period of six weeks, and at two years no infection or deformity had recurred.

gression past 70° or intractable thoracic pain is present, surgical treatment may be considered. Non-operative modalities are first tried in an effort to relieve the chronic fatigue of the thoracic musculature and the symptoms of degenerative disc pain. This may relieve pain but cannot prevent progression of the kyphotic deformity.

If the kyphosis is flexible, that is if it can be corrected to 60° with hyperextension, one-stage posterior fusion with internal fixation is usually sufficient to correct the deformity and achieve spinal arthrodesis, although one must accept that pseudarthrosis may occur. While successful treatment with single-stage Harrington compression instrumentation is usually adequate for flexible kyphoses, if the deformity is rigid, anterior release and fusion of the six apical segments followed by posterior instrumentation and fusion is indicated (Bradford *et al.*, 1980). Instrument-related complications in the form of a proximal junctional kyphosis occur at a high rate when Luque

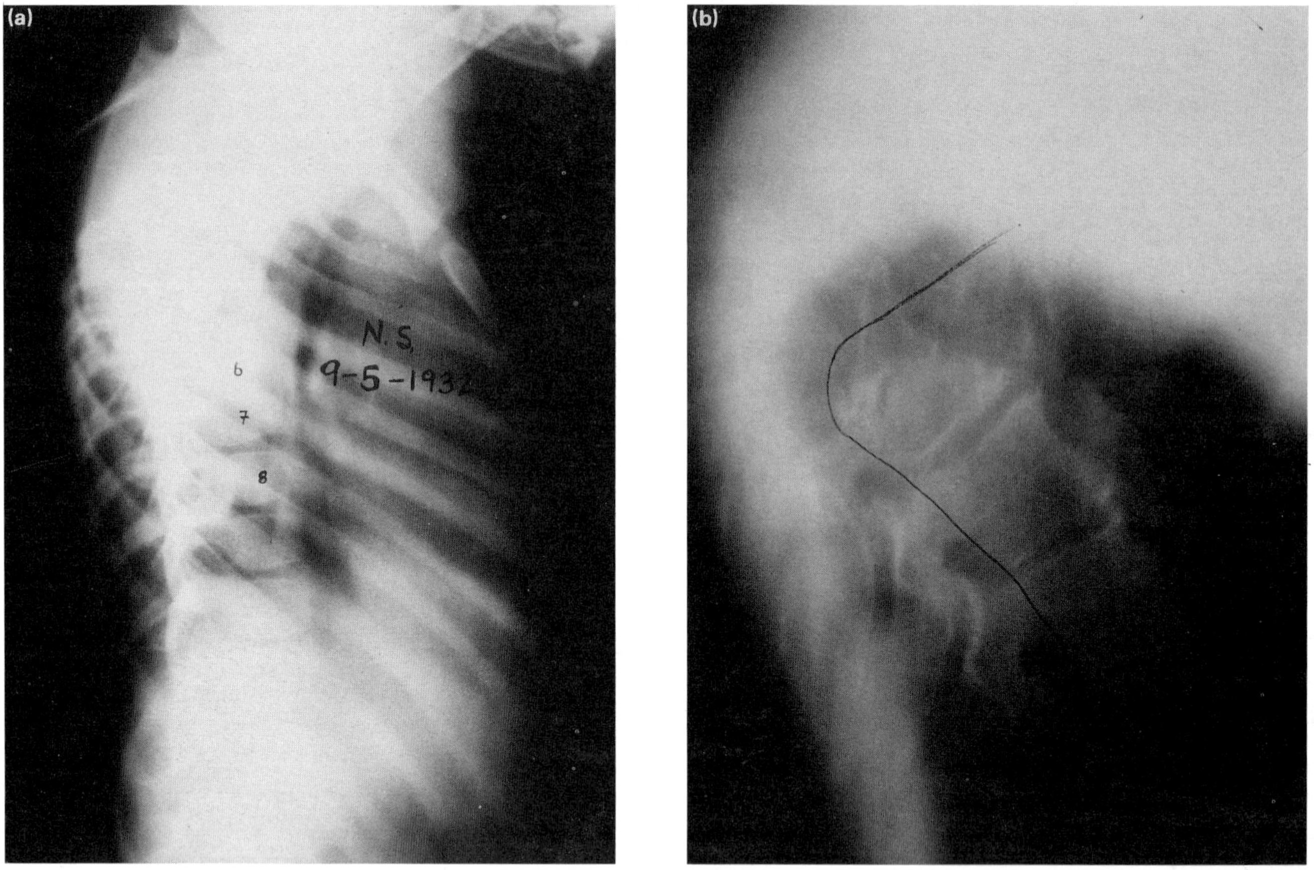

Fig. 24.6 (a) Pulmonary tuberculosis with osteomyelitis was diagnosed in this child at the age of 3 years in 1932. (b) Forty-two years later this man was seen because of respiratory difficulty and recurrent tuberculous osteomyelitis which required anterior surgical debridement and kyphectomy.

instrumentation is used, and this construct is less favoured for kyphotic deformity.

Ankylosing spondylitis

A rigid yet progressive kyphotic deformity is the frequent consequence of this inflammatory disease which affects predominantly young white males who carry the HLA-B27 antigen. While appendicular joints may be affected, the inflammatory process primarily involves the sacroiliac and the intervertebral joints. Ossification of the anterior longitudinal ligament is present initially with progressive involvement of the disc and ultimately the facet joints and ligamentum flavum. Psoriatic arthritis can also produce kyphotic deformity (see Chapter 53).

The kyphotic deformity of ankylosing spondylitis is most prominent in the lumbar spine; however, the thoracic spine is also involved. When the overall kyphotic deformity does not allow the patient to look forward, spinal osteotomy is indicated (Smith-Peterson *et al.*, 1945). This is done in the upper lumbar spine by removing a chevron-shaped wedge through the facet joint area and applying compression instrumentation. By closing the wedge, disruption of the anterior longitudinal ligament results and thus an improvement of the sagittal alignment. Although the thoracic component of the deformity is unchanged, a satisfactory overall posture is achieved. The added safety of osteotomizing the spine in an area occupied by the cauda equina rather than the spinal cord is obvious. If correction of the lumbar kyphosis does not restore the sagittal alignment with T1 vertically oriented over S1, it may be necessary to proceed with an osteotomy through the thoracic portion of the deformity. This is done in staged transthoracic anterior and subsequent posterior osteotomies. Intercurrent traction has not always proved to be effective. (Bradford *et al.*, 1980).

When a cervicothoracic kyphosis is present, a posterior closing wedge osteotomy is performed through the lower cervical laminae. This is done under local anaesthetic so that any loss of neurological function can be determined immediately and the osteotomy correction reversed (Simmons, 1972). (For operative details see Chapter 53.)

Iatrogenic kyphosis

Treatment of the growing spine with radiation therapy for such conditions as Wilm's tumour or neuroblastoma can result in progressive kyphotic deformity. This is most common if the radiation dosage is high and is administered before the child is two years of age (Murphy & Blount, 1962). Therapeutic radiation given after the age of 4 years does not result in significant spinal deformity. Unilateral radiation more commonly leads to scoliosis or kyphoscoliosis while mildline or symmetrical radiation ports predispose to kyphosis.

Multiple-level laminectomy, particularly in the skeletally immature patient, may also lead to kyphosis (Lonstein, 1977). When laminectomy and radiation are combined in the diagnosis and treatment of a condition in the paediatric patient, kyphosis is often rapidly progressive.

Any skeletally immature patient receiving either of these two therapeutic modalities must be observed at regular intervals for spinal deformity. When the thoracic kyphosis exceeds 55–60°, or if a gibbus devel-

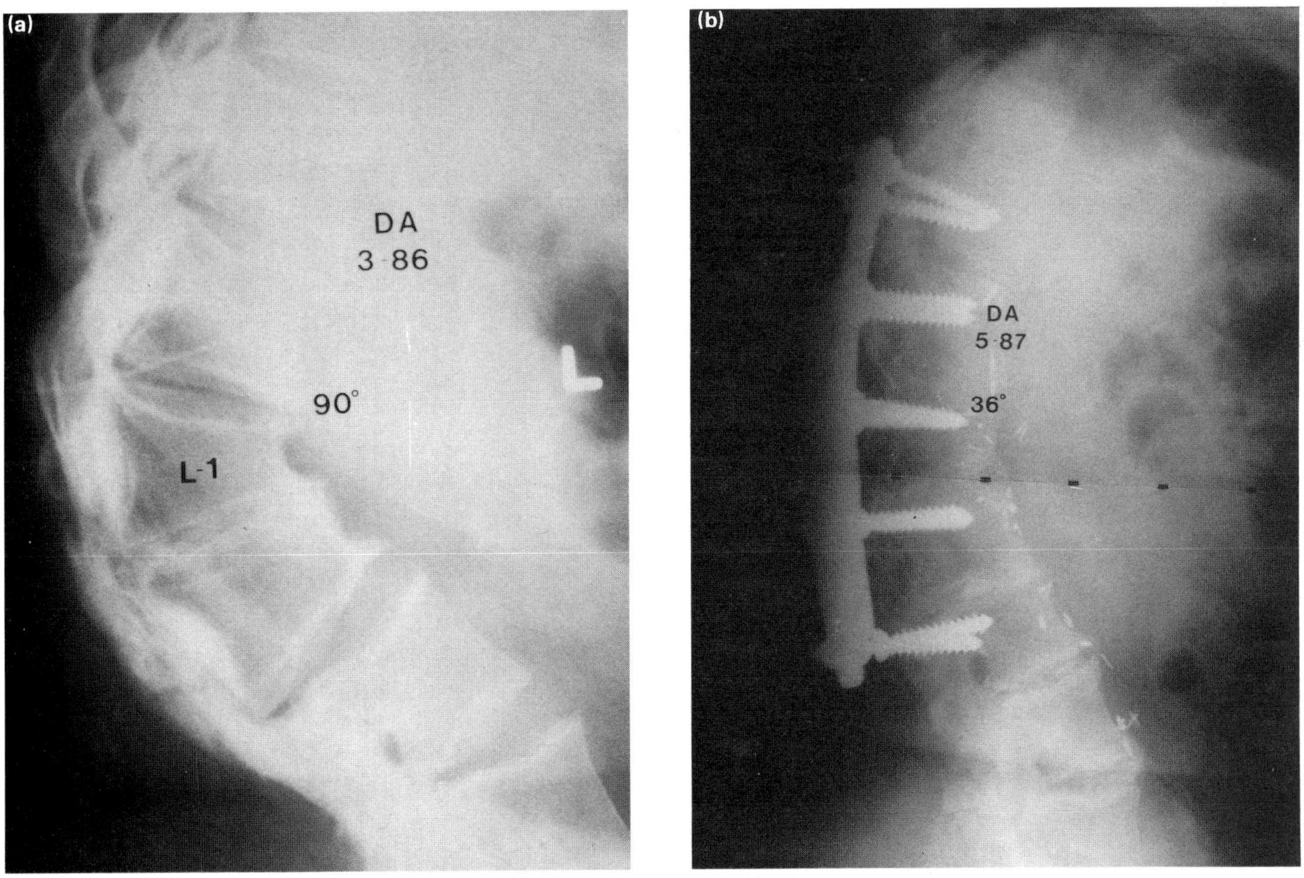

Fig. 24.7 Lateral radiograph of a 42-year-old man with achondroplasia is shown. He had progressive kyphosis and paraparesis following two laminectomies. (b) Anterior interbody fusion with bone grafts and posterior instrumentation with transpedicular screw plate fixation reduced his lumbar kyphos to 36° and improved his paraparesis. Although ambulatory, he did not regain normal bowel and bladder control.

ops, orthotic support is the initial form of treatment. The Milwaukee brace (cervicothoracolumbosacral orthosis CTLSO), is preferred for control of the deformity. If the deformity is uncontrolled by the orthosis, or if the patient has reached early adolescence, surgical correction and stabilization is indicated. In the case of radiation-induced kyphosis there is usually a deficient anterior spinal column, while in kyphosis secondary to laminectomy the posterior spinal column is deficient. For these reasons it is usually necessary to proceed with anterior and posterior spinal fusion when undertaking definitive treatment.

Mucopolysaccharidoses and dysplasias

Developmental kyphosis and spondylolisthesis affects a significant number of patients with disorders such as Morquio–Brailsford's disease, Hurler's syndrome, achondroplasia, metatrophic and diastrophic dwarfism, spondyloepiphyseal dysplasia congenita, and to a lesser extent Maroteaux–Lamy syndrome (Smith-Peterson *et al.*, 1945; Holdsworth, 1963; Blaw & Langer, 1969; Bailey, 1970). With the advent of bone marrow transplantation in Hurler's disease, and other aggressive medical treatment of previously fatal inherited syndromes, many children are living into early adult life. Skeletal deformities which were previously ignored because of the overall poor prognosis may assume greater relative importance. The sagittal plane deformities, in addition to the spinal stenosis which frequently accompanies these conditions, may result in progressive kyphosis and neurological impairment. When surgery is indicated for progressive deformity or neurological deficit, timid procedures such as limited laminectomy may inadequately decompress neurological structures and yet produce mechanical instability which can contribute to a more rapid progression of the kyphotic or spondylolisthetic deformity. Surgical treatment is directed at wide dural and nerve root decompression, improvement of the deformity and arthrodesis. The use of transpedicular segmental fixation allows these goals to be accomplished (Fig. 24.7a,b). If the kyphosis

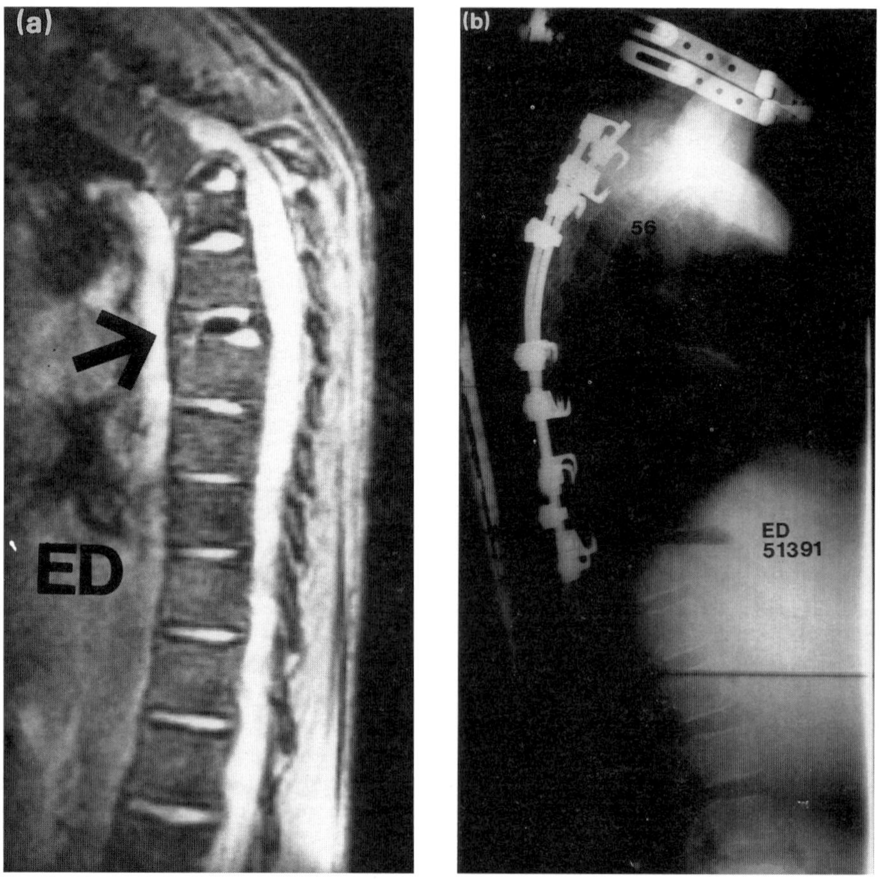

Fig. 24.8 A 15-year-old male, with progressive kyphosis due to T4–T5 collapse from Gauchier's disease. Anterior and posterior surgery was required to decompress the spinal cord and stabilize the spine.

is rigid, preliminary anterior intervertebral disc release and bone grafting may be appropriate.

NON-SURGICAL TREATMENT OF KYPHOSIS

Orthotic treatment of certain acquired kyphotic conditions such as Scheuermann's disease is directed at controlling the deformity rather than correction. In the elderly, an orthosis may relieve the pain associated with senile compression fractures, but it does not correct the deformity.

Such modalities as postural exercises and traction may be effective in mitigating pain, but again are of no value in correcting a kyphotic deformity.

SURGICAL CORRECTION OF KYPHOSIS

Several important principles of biomechanics must be observed in the surgical treatment of kyphosis. These apply to the deformity itself and not necessarily to the disease process which has produced the kyphosis.

Firstly, when kyphosis results in compression of the spinal canal contents, the compression is located anteriorly. Decompression of the spinal cord must then be done through the anterior approach (Fig. 24.8). Laminectomy does not improve anterior cord impingement and is contraindicated.

Secondly, a column under bending moment is analogous to an axial load on the kyphotic spine. The 60% of a column on the concave side is under compression, and the convex 40% of the column is in tension. An isolated posterior fusion mass, therefore, tends to be under tension and does not heal or remodel according to Wolff's law. Posterior fusion alone, for a kyphosis deformity greater then approximately 50° in the thorax and 15° in the lumbar spine, has a high rate of failure. Anterior fusion with the fusion mass as close to the axis of compression as possible is desirable. In a rigid gibbus deformity this may require struts of rib, iliac crest or fibula to span the anterior gap. The use of vascularized rib graft for anterior fusion in kyphosis allows early healing and avoids the extended time required for consolidation of avascular grafts (Rose *et al.*, 1973).

Internal fixation of the thoracic spine should include at least three levels above and below the apex of the kyphosis. Instrumentation should never terminate at the apex of a pre-existing kyphosis. When this occurs a junctional kyphosis frequently results.

SUMMARY

Kyphotic deformity of the thoracic and lumbar spine may result from a wide spectrum of developmental and acquired conditions. This excessive sagittal curvature may cause pain, pulmonary compromise, impingement on the spinal canal contents with accompanying neurological dysfunction and unsightly cosmetic deformity. An understanding of the disease process and its prognosis is necessary before initiating treatment.

The biomechanical implications of kyphosis are important. When surgical correction is attempted, release of the anterior tethering annulus fibrosis and anterior longitudinal ligament plus anterior fusion is needed if the kyphosis exceeds 60°. If there is a gibbus, anterior bridging struts may be required to obtain fusion of the spine. Rigid internal fixation of the spine improves the rate of arthrodesis and allows early postoperative mobilization of the patient. Spinal instrumentation should be extended from the neutral vertebra above to the neutral vertebra below the deformity, and should never terminate at the apex of a pre-existing frontal or sagittal plane deformity.

REFERENCES

Bailey, H.L., Gabriel, M., Hodgson, A.R. & Shin, J.S. (1972) Tuberculosis of the spine in children. Operative findings and results in one hundred consecutive patients treated by removal of the lesion and anterior grafting. *J. Bone Jt. Surg.*, **54A**, 1633–1657.

Bailey, J.A. (1970) Orthopaedic management of dwarfisms recognizable at birth. *Bull. Hosp. Jt. Dis.*, **31**, 27–30.

Blaw, M.E. & Langer, L.O. (1969) Spinal cord compression in Morquio–Brailsford's disease. *J. Pediatr.*, **74**, 593–600.

Bradford, D.S. & Daher, Y.H. (19) Vascularized rib grafts for the stabilization of kyphosis. *J. Bone Jt. Surg.*, **68B**, 357–361.

Bradford, D.S., Khalid, B.A., Moe, J.H. *et al.* (1980) The surgical management of patients with Scheuermann's disease. A review of 24 cases managed by combined anterior and posterior spine fusion. *J. Bone Jt. Surg.*, **62A**, 705.

Bradford, D.S., Schumacher, W., Lonstein, J.E. & Winter, R.B. (1987) Ankylosing spondylitis: experience in the surgical management of 21 patients. *Spine*, **12**, 238–243.

Erickson, R.P., Sandman, R. & Langer, L.O. Jr (1975) A lysosomal storage disease with severe dwarfism, severe joint contractures, mild-moderate mental retardation, corneal opacities and retinal abnormalities. *Birth Defects*, **11**, 317–324.

Gordan, G.S. (1985) Estrogen and bone: Marshall R. Urist's contributions. *Clin. Orthop. Rel. Res.*, **200**, 174–180.

Griffiths, H.E. & Jones, D.M. (1971) Pyogenic infection of the spine. A review of 28 cases. *J. Bone Jt. Surg.*, **53B**, 383–391.

Hanley, E.N. Jr & Eskay, M.L. (1989) Thoracic spine fractures. *Orthopaedics*, **12**, 689–696.

Hodgson, A.R., Wong, Y. & Yau, A. (1969) *X-ray Appearance of Tuberculosis of the Spine*. Charles C. Thomas, Springfield, IL.

Holdsworth, F.W. (1963) Fractures, dislocations and fracture-dislocations of the spine. *J. Bone Jt. Surg.*, **45B**, 6–20.

Kopitis, S.E. (1976) Orthopaedic complications of dwarfism. *Clin. Orthop.*, **114**, 152–179.

Leidholt, J.D., Young, J.J., Hahn, H.R. *et al.* (1969) Evaluation of late spinal deformities with fracture-dislocations of the dorsal and lumbar spine in paraplegias. *Paraplegia*, **7**, 16–28.

Lonstein, J.E. (1977) Post laminectomy kyphosis. *Clin. Orthop.*, **128**, 93–100.

Malcom, B.W., Bradford, D.S., Winter, R.B. *et al.* (1981) Post traumatic kyphosis. A review of forty eight surgically treated patients. *J. Bone Jt. Surg.*, **63A**, 891–899.

Milne, J.S. & Lauder, I.J. (1976) The relationship of kyphosis to the shape of vertebral bodies. *Ann. Hum. Biol.*, **3**, 173–179.

Murphy, F.D. & Blount, W.P. (1962) Cartilagenous exostoses following irradiation. *J. Bone Jt. Surg.*, **44A**, 662.

Rajasekaran, S. & Shanmugasundaram, T.K. (1987) Prediction of the angle of the gibbus deformity in tuberculosis of the spine. *J. Bone Jt. Surg.*, **4**, 503–509.

Roaf, R. (1960) Vertebral growth and its mechanical control. *J. Bone Jt. Surg.*, **42B**, 40.

Rose, Owen & Saunderson (1973)

Ryan, M.D. & Taylor, T.K.F. (1982) Acute spinal cord compression in Scheuermann's disease. *J. Bone Jt. Surg.*, **64B**, 409.

Sachs, B.L., Bradford, D.S., Winter, R.B. *et al.* (1985) Scheuermann's kyphosis: Long term results of Milwaukee brace treatment. *Orthop. Trans.*, **9**, 108.

Scheuermann, H.W. (1920) Kyfosis dorsalis juvenilis. *Ugeskr Laeger.*, **82**, 385.

Simmons, E. (1972) The surgical correction of flexion deformity of the cervical spine of ankylosing spondylitis. *Clin. Orthop.*, **86**, 132.

Smith-Peterson, M.N., Larson, C.B. & Aufranc, O.E. (1945) Osteotomy of the spine for correction of flexion deformity in rheumatoid arthritis. *J. Bone Jt. Surg.*, **27**, 1.

Spranger, J.W. & Langer, L.O. (1970) Spondyloepiphyseal dysplasia congenita. *Radiology*, **94**, 313.

25 · Management of Neuromuscular Deformity

By C.S.B. GALASKO

Neuromuscular deformity is very different from idiopathic or congenital scoliosis. It is a more severe disorder, associated with specific complications, and frequently the patient also suffers from a number of other serious conditions as a result of the underlying neuromuscular disorder, such as respiratory insufficiency, cardiac myopathy or sensory disturbance.

PATTERN OF CURVE

There are three patterns of neuromuscular spinal deformity.

The commonest and most characteristic is a long 'C' curve which involves the dorsal and lumbar spine, extends to the pelvis and is associated with increasing pelvic obliquity. It is probably due to weakness of the trunk muscles and, as a result, the spine 'collapses' under the influence of gravity. Initially the curve may be limited to one part of the spine but gradually extends to involve the dorsal spine, lumbar spine and pelvis. In its early stages the curve is mobile but, with time, gradually becomes rigid.

As a result of the increasing pelvic obliquity the patient can no longer sit squarely, and weight is increasingly taken on one buttock and eventually the lumbar spine (Fig. 25.1). Sitting becomes uncomfortable and the patient is confined to bed, not because of the underlying neuromuscular disorder, but as a result of the progressive scoliosis. Hsu (1983) reported that in Duchenne muscular dystrophy progression of a curve beyond 40° was associated with diminished sitting tolerance, and use of the arms and hands to prop the body up when seated. Progressive pelvic obliquity may also predispose to dislocation of the hip, especially in cerebral palsy and spinal muscle atrophy.

Progressive scoliosis is also associated with diminished lung function. Kurz *et al.* (1983) showed that in Duchenne muscular dystrophy the vital capacity peaked at approximately the age when standing ceased, and then declined rapidly. It deteriorated approximately 4% for each year of life after the patient became wheelchair-bound, and for every 10° of thoracic scoliosis there was an additional 4% loss of vital capacity.

The scoliosis continues to deteriorate after growth has ceased, probably due to the effect of gravity.

The second pattern shows in patients with neuromuscular disease, who may develop a curve which is similar to an idiopathic scoliosis in that only one part of the spine is affected. This may be due to an idiopathic curve in a patient with neuromuscular disease, or may be due to asymmetric weakness of the spinal musculature. This type of curve is uncommon, but probably occurs in Friedreich's ataxia more frequently than in any other neuromuscular disorder. The curve may remain localized to one part of the spine, or may subsequently extend to involve the rest of the spine and deteriorate into a classical neuromuscular collapsing scoliosis.

The third pattern is in myelomeningocele, where an angular kyphotic deformity can occur. Patients have a total paraplegia and the defect in the lumbar region is wider than in the majority of patients with myelomeningocele (Hoppenfeld, 1967). As a result the paraspinal muscles, which normally extend the spine, are carried forward and act at a mechanical disadvantage (Drennan, 1970).

PREVENTION

The incidence of scoliosis varies in the different neuromuscular disorders and, in our experience,

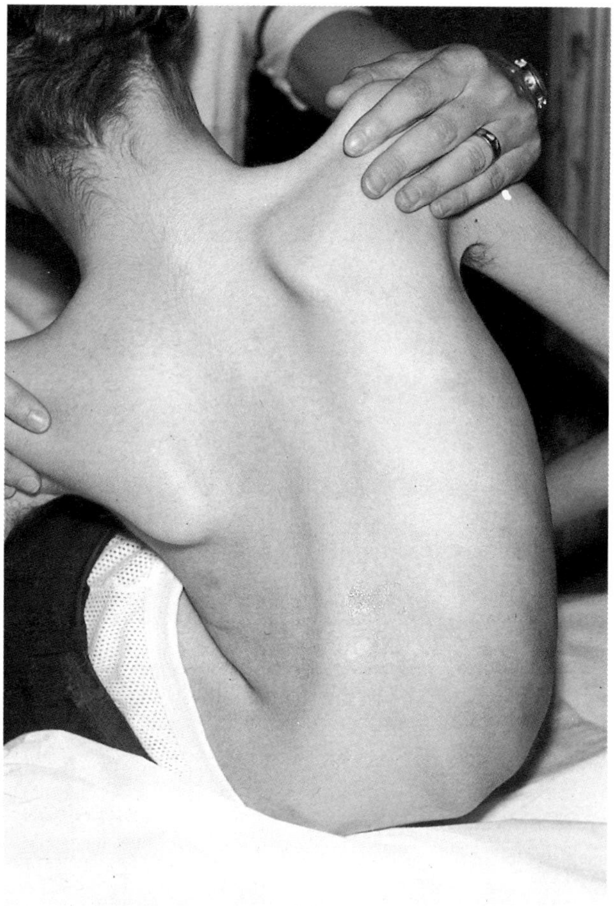

Fig. 25.1 Patient with Duchenne muscular dystrophy demonstrating the typical neuromuscular scoliosis. He has an extensive curve involving his dorsal and lumbar spine, associated with gross pelvic obliquity. He is unable to sit unsupported and when he does sit much of his weight is taken on the lumbar spine. There is some rotation associated with his curve.

occurs most commonly in patients with Duchenne muscular dystrophy. This condition is associated with progressive and rapid increase in weakness, most of the boys losing their ability to walk independently between the ages of eight and 11 years. Most die in their late teens from respiratory infection or cardiomyopathy. Under the age of eight years scoliosis is uncommon. This is thought to be due to the lordotic posture adopted by patients who are still mobile.

Once patients are confined to a wheelchair they lose the lordosis and develop a rapidly deteriorating scoliosis. Rarely, they may develop fibrotic extension contractures of the spine, with fixed lordosis and a mild scoliosis (Gibson & Wilkins, 1975). Two of our 138 patients with Duchenne dystrophy have developed such a contracture (Fig. 25.2). Provision of calipers not only maintains mobility, but also maintains the lordotic posture and slows the development of scoliosis. At the age of 13 years the mean curve in our chair-bound patients was $62 \pm 12°$ compared with $14 \pm 3°$ in patients who were still mobile in their orthoses (Galasko, 1987). Standing, even when the patient is no longer mobile, may also protect the spine and maintain lung function (Galasko & Delaney, 1990).

Several centres have tried to modify the wheelchair to maintain a lordotic posture. However, this design of chair has major disadvantages. Because the patient is reclining he or she is further away from work surfaces, both at school and at home. In practice it has proved extremely difficult to raise work surfaces to the patient's level, so that the patient has to lean forward, adopting a kyphotic posture and putting the spine at risk. These modified chairs have not prevented the development or deterioration of scoliosis, and have been largely abandoned (Galasko, 1987).

The arms of the wheelchair are sometimes removed to allow the child easier access to the wheels. This results in further lack of support to the trunk, the patient leaning to one side and thus perhaps initiating the scoliotic process. It is essential that arm rests are fitted to the wheelchair to allow maximum support. Ideally, the patient should be provided with a powered chair with a central control to obviate the necessity of leaning to one side.

A variety of spinal orthoses have been tried, of which the best is a total contact underarm thoracolumbar orthosis. The spinal orthoses may slow the progression of scoliosis, but there are inherent difficulties. Because patients are sedentary the orthoses are more difficult to fit, and tend to ride up even if carefully moulded; they often are uncomfortable and, if they are too well-fitting, may interfere with respiration. Many patients will not use them regularly. Our results (Galasko, 1987) showed that orthoses slowed the progression of the curve but did not prevent it; this may partly be due to lack of patient cooperation.

Moulded inserts or matrix chairs are extremely useful in patients with cerebral palsy who are grossly affected, mentally retarded and do not have independent sitting balance. However, most patients with Duchenne muscular dystrophy and many other forms

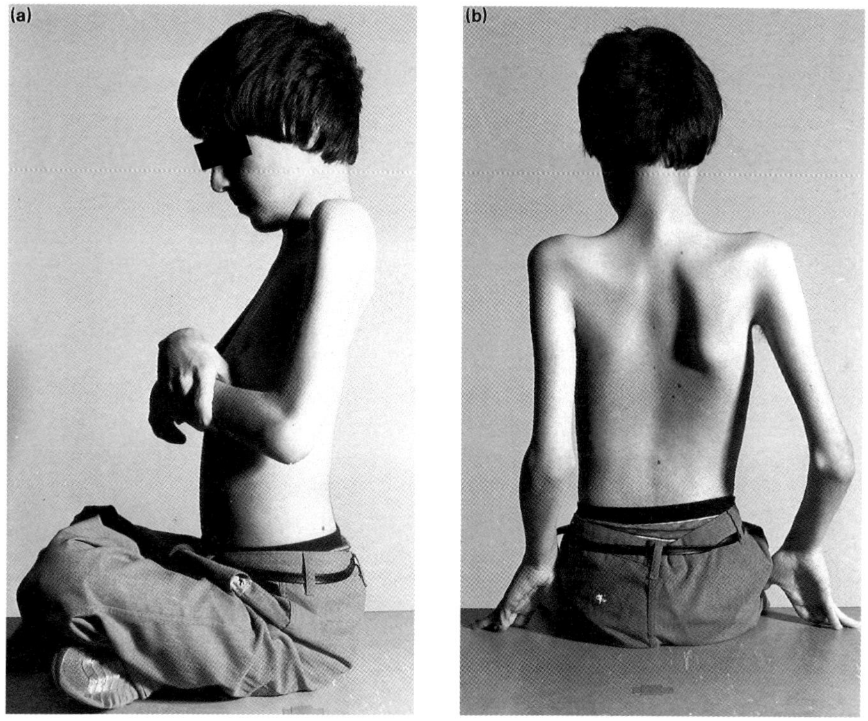

Fig. 25.2 patient with Duchenne muscular dystrophy who has developed an extension contracture of his dorsal and lumbar spine and minimal scoliosis. The development of a lordotic spine tends to protect against scoliosis.

of neuromuscular disorders find them uncomfortable.

TREATMENT

Once scoliosis has developed, the use of a modified chair or orthosis may slow the progression of the curve but will not prevent it. Seeger *et al.* (1984) reported that modular seats, spinal jackets and custom-moulded seats had no effect on the rate of progression of the curve in patients with Duchenne muscular dystrophy of 14 years of age and over. Furthermore, once the curve has reached 50–60° it deteriorates rapidly.

The optimum treatment for a progressive neuromuscular curve is surgical stabilization of the spine. However, in Duchenne muscular dystrophy the patient may no longer be fit for surgery because of rapid and progressive deterioration in pulmonary function by the time he or she has developed a major curve. The concept of 'prophylactic' spinal stabilization has therefore been developed, i.e. stabilization of the spine when the patient is still fit for major surgery, even though the curve is relatively small (Fig. 25.3). The optimum time at which to stabilize the spine in a patient with Duchenne muscular dystrophy is soon after he or she loses the ability to walk independently, when lung function is adequate for major spinal surgery, before the patient has developed cor pulmonale or severe cardiomyopathy, and when the curve is still mobile and preferably less than 30°. Despite the risk of major surgery in these patients, such prophylactic surgery is extremely worthwhile in avoiding the seating problems associated with a late, severe scoliosis, maintains lung function (Table 25.1) and significantly improves life expectancy (Galasko & Delaney, 1990).

In many of the other neuromuscular disorders the patient does not deteriorate as rapidly, and early surgery is not as essential. Nevertheless, it is still preferable to stabilize the spine when the curve is mobile and small, rather than waiting until the patient has developed a severe, extensive rigid curve. Ideally, surgery should not be carried out until the patient is 10–12 years of age, but occasionally early surgery may be required, especially in spinal muscle atrophy. These patients may develop a progressive curve in their first few years.

Patients with Duchenne muscular dystrophy, and many other neuromuscular disorders, may require a six-monthly erect X-ray of the spine, and six-monthly lung function tests. Rapid deterioration in lung func-

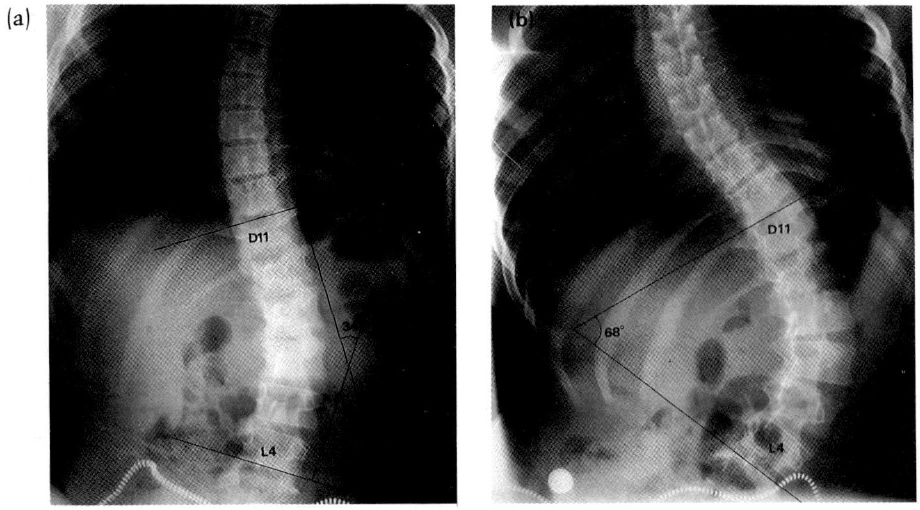

Fig. 25.3 (a) Patient with Duchenne muscular dystrophy with a scoliosis of 34°. Spinal stabilization was recommended, but the family refused surgery. (b) Nine months later the family requested surgery. He had developed pelvic obliquity. His curve had progressed to 68°, but he was no longer fit for major spinal surgery. His vital capacity had fallen to 19%.

tion or progression of a curve suggests early stabilization of the spine. We are also concerned about the cardiac status, and electrocardiography and echocardiography are required before surgery. Many of the neuromuscular conditions are associated with cardiomyopathy, including Duchenne muscular dystrophy, Friedreich's ataxia and many of the congenital myopathies. Provided the cardiac status is reasonable, we have operated on patients with Duchenne muscular dystrophy whose vital capacity was only 23% of the expected normal for age and arm span, although Swank *et al.* (1982) did not recommend surgery if the vital capacity was less than 40%, or the patient had a non-functional cough, symptoms due to cardiomyopathy, or rapidly progressive deterioration in muscle strength.

SURGICAL TREATMENT

Several techniques of spinal fusion are available, and the choice of treatment depends on the extent of the curve, underlying diagnosis, general fitness of the patient, age of the patient, and associated vertebral anomalies.

In the majority of patients we used a modified technique of segmental spinal stabilization. This is particularly the case in patients with Duchenne muscular dystrophy and other neuromuscular disorders associated with respiratory insufficiency or cardiac abnormalities. A square-ended, 'U'-shaped rod is used (Fig. 25.4). It is fixed to the spine from D3 or D4 to the sacrum, by sublaminal wires at every level, after the facet joints have been excised and grafted at each level. The use of a single U-shaped rod fixed to the sacrum obviates the risk of migration if double rods are used. Segmental spinal stabilization also obviates the need for a postoperative plaster of Paris cast, which many patients with severe neuromuscular disorders will not be able to tolerate.

Although these patients have muscle weakness, and may be confined to a wheelchair, their sensation is intact and they have normal bladder and bowel

Table 25.1 Effect of spinal stabilization on pulmonary function as indicated by vital capacity (litres) in Duchenne muscular dystrophy

Group	Preoperative	Postoperative			
		6 months	12 months	24 months	36 months
Underwent spinal stabilization	1.41 ± 0.09	1.38 ± 0.10	1.39 ± 0.13	1.31 ± 0.12	1.39 ± 0.15
Refused surgery	1.43 ± 0.12	1.29 ± 0.16	1.25 ± 0.17	1.14 ± 0.15	0.89 ± 0.16

Figures are mean ± SE.

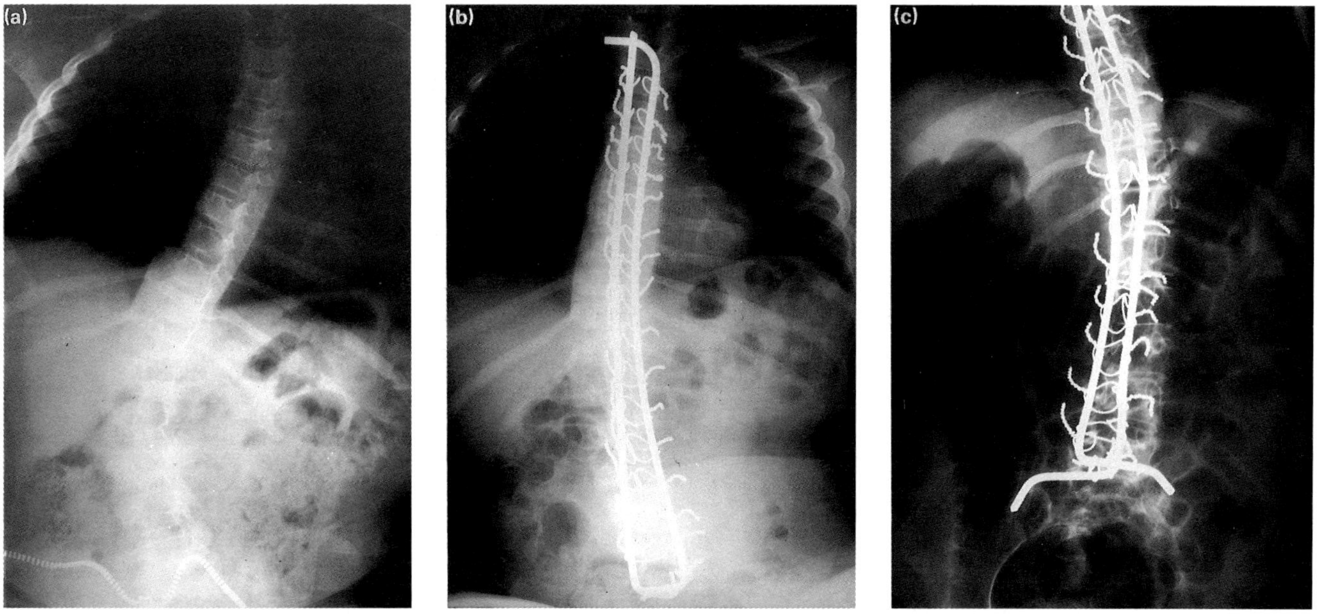

Fig. 25.4 (a) Patient with Duchenne muscular dystrophy with a 50° curve. (b) Postoperative radiograph. The curve has been corrected and held with a 'U'-shaped rod. The rod has been fixed from D3 to the sacrum with sublaminal wires at each level. The top of the rod has been trimmed to the size of the patient, and one end bent over to complete the rectangle. In addition to the spinal stabilization a facet joint fusion was carried out at every level from D3 to the sacrum. (c) Alternative method of stabilizing the spine where two 'L' rods are used, the lower end of the rod being inserted into the pelvis. However, these rods occasionally migrate and, therefore, we prefer the use of a single 'U'-shaped rod. This postoperative radiograph was taken 48 hours following surgery. Note the dilated large bowel. This is typical in patients with Duchenne muscular dystrophy following spinal stabilization.

function. Therefore, it is important to protect the spinal cord, and the operation should be carried out with spinal cord monitoring. However, there may be difficulties with the latter. In a series of 29 patients no responses could be recorded (prior to instrumentation) from one patient with spina bifida, one patient with Friedreich's ataxia, and one patient with peripheral neuropathy (Arafa *et al.*, 1987).

The operation is a major one, and patients must undergo careful preoperative assessment to ensure that they are fit for such surgery (see above).

The postoperative regimen is critical. Patients require nursing in an intensive care unit for at least 24 hours, and they may require intubation for the first 12–24 hours. Analgesia is provided by an intravenous morphine drip, the drip rate being increased or decreased as required. Patients are given prophylactic antibiotics. Virtually all those with Duchenne dystrophy develop a profound ileus and require nasogastric suction and intravenous feeding for three to four days. The degree of correction depends on the mobility of the curve and varies from 25% to 100%. Patients with cerebral palsy tolerate correction of their curve least.

In some circumstances the extent of the fixation should be modified. In the vast majority of patients, irrespective of the extent of the curve, the spine should be stabilized from the upper dorsal region to the sacrum. However, some patients with Friedreich's ataxia may have a curve localized to their thoracic spine. Their ability to walk often depends on the use of the trunk, and if the spine is stabilized to the sacrum they may lose their independent mobility. Under these circumstances it is reasonable to stabilize and fuse the scoliotic segment. If the curve subsequently progresses, as is often the case if the patient becomes wheelchair-bound because of increasing ataxia, the fusion and stabilization can be extended to the sacrum (Fig. 25.5).

The most common error in the surgical treatment of neuromuscular scoliosis is to fuse too short a segment of the spine. The rods must be contoured to provide a lumbar lordosis (Fig. 25.6) and accommodate the kyphosis. A 'flat-back' is to be avoided as this will interfere with sitting balance. Harrington instru-

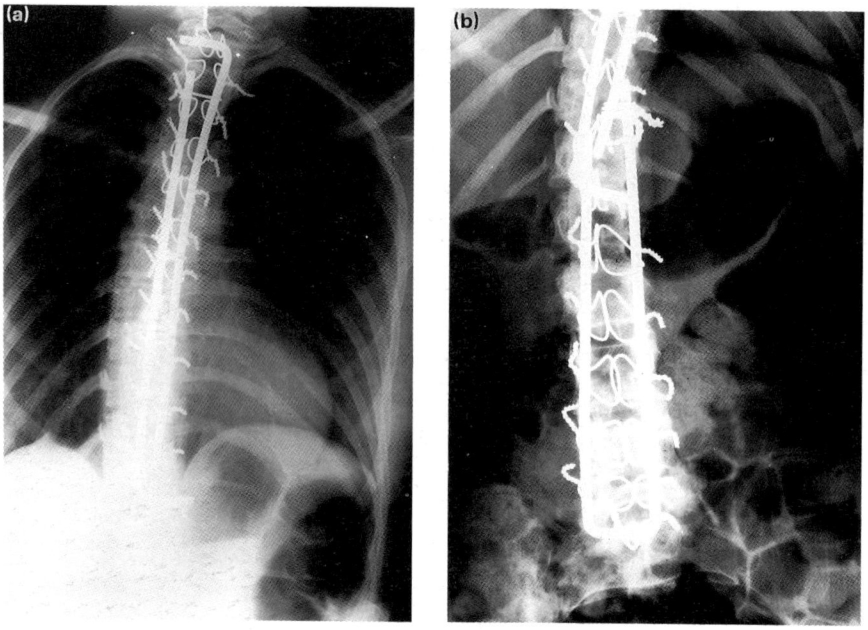

Fig. 25.5 (a) Patient with Friedreich's ataxia. This patient initially presented with a thoracic scoliosis, whilst she was still mobile. A limited fusion was carried out from D1 to D12 with segmental spinal stabilization of the entire dorsal spine. (b) Because of increasing ataxia the patient gradually went off her feet, and two years later was confined to a wheelchair. At this stage she started to develop a progressive lumbar scoliosis below the level of the previous fusion, and three years after the initial operation underwent segmental stabilization of her lumbar curve using a 'U' rod wired to each lumbar vertebra, the sacrum and the distal end of the dorsal rods. An interfacetal fusion was carried out at each level.

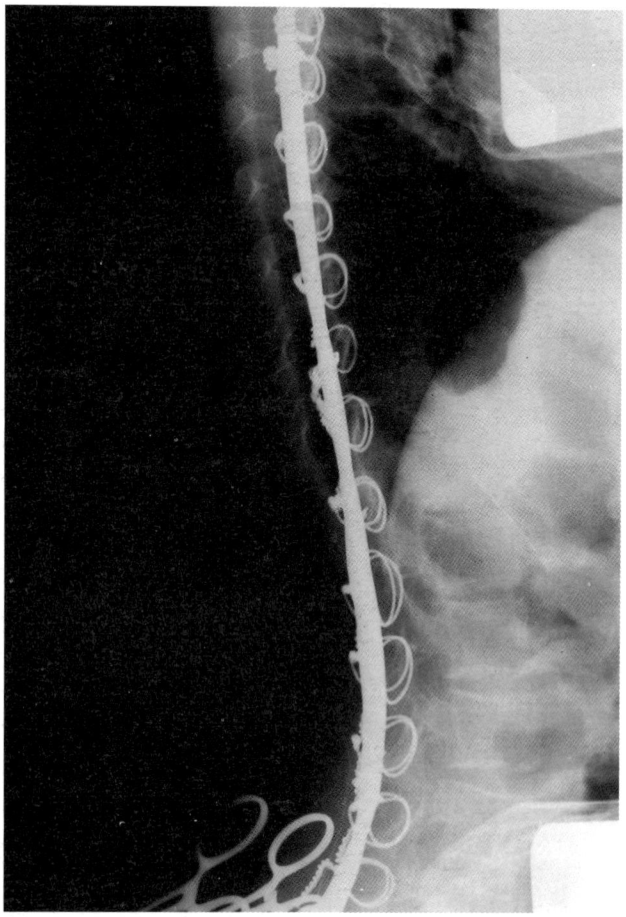

Fig. 25.6 The rods must be contoured to provide a lumbar scoliosis.

mentation can be used as an alternative. However, the Harrington distraction rod must be pre-bent to accommodate both the lumbar lordosis and any kyphosis; therefore a square-ended rod must be used. If the patient has a long collapsing curve, two rods are often used: a long distraction rod extending from the upper thoracic region to the ala of the sacrum with a second distraction rod in the apex of the curve. The patient will require a postoperative spinal support—either a plaster of Paris jacket or a total-body contact orthosis. A fusion is carried out simultaneously, but the incidence of pseudarthrosis is higher than in idiopathic scoliosis, Bonnett *et al.* (1975) reporting an incidence of 27% with Harrington instrumentation and spinal fusion, compared with less than 1% in patients with idiopathic scoliosis (Erwin *et al.*, 1976).

Patients with spina bifida are probably best treated by an anterior correction and fusion with Dwyer, Zielke or similar instrumentation, followed two or three weeks later by posterior correction and fusion with Harrington instrumentation. Great care must be taken in dissecting the skin from the dura, and some surgeons prefer two parallel incisions over the facet joints, stripping the tissues laterally, and leaving intact the scarred and potentially infected tissue overlying the spinal defect (Mayfield, 1981). An interfacetal intertransverse fusion (Moe, 1972) is carried out, followed by a deep and thorough decortication of all the posterior bony structures. Because of the high risk of pseudarthrosis, large amounts of bone graft are laid bilaterally in the paraspinal gutters, on the sides of the defective laminae and on top of the vestigial transverse processes. The fusion is taken down to the sacrum (McMaster, 1987b).

Anterior correction is indicated in spina bifida and in rigid curves in patients who are sufficiently fit for a thoraco-abdominal operation with splitting of the diaphragm. Patients with Duchenne muscular dystrophy, and many of the other neuromuscular diseases, will not tolerate an anterior fusion.

Anterior correction is sometimes indicated in cerebral palsy, and must be used in combination with a posterior fusion. Bonnett *et al.* (1976) reported that, in cerebral palsy, the incidence of pseudarthrosis with Dwyer instrumentation alone was 72%, compared with 40% with Harrington instrumentation alone. The combination of an anterior spinal fusion with Dwyer instrumentation and a posterior fusion with Harrington instrumentation produced an excellent degree of correction, with a very low incidence of pseudarthrosis in a stable spine (McMaster, 1987a), although Brown *et al.* (1982) reported a pseudarthrosis rate of 18%. Lonstein & Akbarnia (1983) reported that, in cerebral palsy, the degree of correction was improved from 55% with Harrington instrumentation alone to 70% by the combined procedure, and the incidence of pseudarthrosis decreased from 22% to 5.9%. Staged anterior and posterior procedures were also recommended for postpoliomyelitic scoliosis (Mayer *et al.*, 1981).

The combined procedure does not provide adequate stability until the graft matures, and a plaster of Paris jacket or brace must be worn for at least nine to 12 months to allow the fusion to mature. Such a support may further restrict an already impaired respiratory function, and produce pressure sores in a patient with anaesthetic skin. It is for this reason that segmental spinal stabilization is the preferred method of treatment. Segmental stabilization alone is associated with a high incidence of instrument failure (Luque, 1982) and an interfacetal fusion must be carried out simultaneously. In myelomeningocele patients there is difficulty in obtaining satisfactory fixation, because of the laminar defects, and Harrington instrumentation may be preferable.

Patients with Duchenne muscular dystrophy, in particular, and neuromuscular diseases in general, do not tolerate prolonged bed rest. They tend to weaken rapidly when confined to bed, and should be rapidly mobilized following surgery.

Angular kyphotic curves in myelomeningocele are rigid. The spine is osteotomized and sufficient vertebrae are resected at the apex of the deformity to correct it. The spine is instrumented and a long posterior fusion carried out. Lindseth & Stelzer (1979) recommended that the fusion extend from the thoracic spine to the sacrum to obviate recurrence of the deformity.

Complications

Spinal surgery in patients with neuromuscular disease is associated with more bleeding during surgery, partly because venous canals in the osteoporotic bone are larger than normal and bleed more freely, and partly because the muscles are weak and fibrotic and do not contract. Muscle contraction aids vasoconstriction.

The incidence of postoperative complications is greater than for other types of scoliosis (Galasko, 1987). The complications in 90 operations for neuromuscular scoliosis are shown in Table 25.2.

There have been no peroperative deaths, although one patient with Friedreich's ataxia died three weeks postoperatively from cardiac failure, as a result of her cardiomyopathy. One patient with nemaline myopathy died whilst on the waiting list for surgery. She had nocturnal apnoea and was on a nocturnal respirator. One further patient with Friedreich's ataxia collapsed under induction of anaesthetic. She was resuscitated, but the operation was abandoned. No patients have required permanent tracheostomy or intubation. Our policy is to avoid tracheostomy, but to intubate the patient for several hours postoperatively, as required. There are no instances of malignant hyperpyrexia in this series.

Two patients with cerebral palsy developed intraoperative spinal cord dysfunction. In one the spinal cord trace returned to normal after the stabilization was slightly loosened. Postoperatively she had temporary unilateral paraesthesia which settled rapidly. In the second patient the trace did not return until the instrumentation was removed. Instrumentation was abandoned and a posterior fusion *in situ* was carried out. One patient with Duchenne muscular dystrophy developed a temporary neuritic pain localized to one buttock and thigh. This was probably due to an isolated nerve root dysfunction caused either when the

Table 25.2 Complications of scoliosis surgery in 90 operations for neuromuscular scoliosis

Complication	No.	Diagnosis
Cardiac and respiratory		
Peroperative deaths	0	
Cardiac arrest (resuscitated)	1	Minicore disease
Postoperative death	1	Freidreich's ataxia; died of cardiac failure three weeks postoperatively
Atrial flutter with 2 : 1 heart block	1	Duchenne muscular dystrophy
Required serial postoperative bronchoscopies	1	Spinal muscle atrophy
Required single postoperative bronchoscopy	1	Duchenne muscular dystrophy
Required temporary tracheostomy	1	Duchenne muscular dystrophy
Malignant hyperpyrexia	0	
Neurological complications		
Intraoperative spinal cord dysfunction	2	Cerebral palsy[a]
Temporary neuritic pain	1	Duchenne muscular dystrophy
Local complications		
Broken 'L' rod	1	Spinal muscle atrophy
Trimming 'L' rod	2	Spinal muscle atrophy; Duchenne muscular dystrophy
Other failure fixation	0	
Pseudarthrosis	2	Friedreich's ataxia; telangiectatic ataxia
Deep infection	0	
Superficial infection	3	Spina bifida; Duchenne muscular dystrophy; cerebral palsy

[a] See text.

sublaminal wire was being passed, by an epidural haematoma, or due to movement of a wire segment against a nerve root in the first few postoperative days.

CONCLUSIONS

Scoliosis is a common and severe complication of neuromuscular disease. It is frequently associated with respiratory insufficiency and pelvic obliquity. The latter may make sitting uncomfortable and may predispose to hip dislocation. Once a scoliosis has developed it is progressive. The progression will not be stopped by modifying the wheelchair, nor by the use of orthoses, although they may slow the progression of the curve.

Prolonged standing may prevent the development of a progressive scoliosis. Once a curve has developed it is best treated by spinal fusion and stabilization. At the moment, for the majority of patients, the optimum form of stabilization is segmental spinal fixation, as it obviates the need for a postoperative plaster of Paris jacket or orthosis. This type of surgery is complex; the patient requires careful preoperative evaluation and postoperative management. Such surgery should be carried out only in specialized units, where the facilities for the preoperative evaluation, operative skills, and postoperative care are available.

The surgery and care of these patients are more complex than for other forms of scoliosis, and the risk of major complications much higher.

REFERENCES

Arafa, M., Morris, P. & Galasko, C.S.B. (1987) Spinal cord monitoring during surgery for scoliosis. In Noble, J. & Galasko, C.S.B. (eds) *Recent Developments in Orthopaedic Surgery*, pp. 143–149. Manchester University Press, Manchester.

Bonnett, C., Brown, J., Perry J., Nickel, V., Walinksi, T., Brooks, L., Hoffer, M., Stiles, C. & Brooks, R. (1975) Evolution of treatment of paralytic scoliosis at Rancho Los Amigos Hospital. *J. Bone Jt. Surg.*, **57A**, 206–215.

Bonnett, C., Brown, J.C. & Grow, T. (1976) Thoracolumbar scoliosis in cerebral palsy. Results of surgical treatment. *J. Bone Jt. Surg.*, **58A**, 328–336.

Brown, J.C., Swank, S. & Specht, L. (1982) Combined anterior and posterior spinal fusion in cerebral palsy. *Spine*, **7**, 570–573.

Drennan, J.C. (1970) The role of muscles in the development of human lumbar kyphosis. *Dev. Med. Child Neurol.* Suppl. 22, 33–38.

Erwin, W.D., Dickson, J.H. & Harrington, P.R. (1976). The post-operative management of scoliosis patients treated with Harrington instrumentation and fusion. *J. Bone Jt. Surg.*, **58A**, 479–482.

Galasko, C.S.B. (1987) The orthopaedic management of the dystrophies, myopathies, atrophies, neuropathies and ataxias. In Galasko, C.S.B. (ed.) *Neuromuscular Problems in Orthopaedics*, pp. 83–105. Blackwell Scientific Publications, Oxford.

Galasko, C.S.B. & Delaney, C. (1990) Scoliosis and lung function in Duchenne muscular dystrophy. *J. Bone Jt. Surg.*, **72B**, 399.

Gibson, D.A. & Wilkins, K.E. (1975) The management of spinal deformities in Duchenne muscular dystrophy: a new concept of spinal bracing. *Clin. Orthop. Rel. Res.*, **108**, 41–51.

Hoppenfield, S. (1967) Congenital kyphosis in myelomeningocele. *J. Bone Jt. Surg.*, **49B**, 276–280.

Hsu, J.D. (1983) The natural history of spine curvature progression in the non-ambulatory Duchenne muscular dystrophy patient. *Spine*, **8**, 771–775.

Kurz, L.T., Mubarak, S.J., Schultz, P., Park, S.M. & Leach, J. (1983) Correlation of scoliosis and pulmonary function in Duchenne muscular dystrophy. *J. Pediatr. Orthop.*, **3**, 347–353.

Lindseth, R.E. & Stelzer, L. (1979) Vertebral excision for kyphosis in children with myelomeningocele. *J. Bone Jt. Surg.*, **61A**, 699–704.

Lonstein, J.E. & Akbarnia, B.A. (1983) Operative treatment of spinal deformities in patients with cerebral palsy or mental retardation; an analysis of 107 cases. *J. Bone Jt. Surg.*, **65A**, 43–55.

Luque, E.R. (1982) Paralytic scoliosis in growing children. *Clin. Orthop. Rel. Res.*, **163**, 202–209.

McMaster, M.J. (1987a) Anterior and posterior spinal instrumentation and fusion of severe paralytic thoracolumbar scoliosis due to myelomeningocele. *J. Bone Jt. Surg.*, **69B**, 20–25.

McMaster, M.J. (1987b) The management of spinal deformity in neuromuscular disease. In Galasko, C.S.B. (ed.) *Neuromuscular Problems in Orthopaedics*, pp. 106–127. Blackwell Scientific Publications, Oxford.

Mayer, P.J., Dore, J., Ditmanson, M. & Shon, Y-S (1981) Post-poliomyelitis paralytic scoliosis. *Spine*, **6**, 573–582.

Mayfield, J.K. (1981) Severe spine deformity in myelodysplasia and sacral agenesis: an aggressive surgical approach. *Spine*, **6**, 498–509.

Miller, G. & Dunn, N. (1982) An outline of the management and prognosis of Duchenne muscular dystrophy in Western Australia. *Austral. Paediatr. J.*, **18**, 277–282.

Moe, J.H. (1972) Methods of correction and surgical techniques in scoliosis. *Orthop. Clin. N. Am.*, **3**, 17–48.

Seeger, B.R., Sutherland, A. D'A. & Clark, M.S. (1984) Orthotic management of scoliosis in Duchenne muscular dystrophy. *Arch. Phys. Med. Rehabil.*, **65**, 83–86.

Swank, S.M., Brown, J.C. & Perry, R.E. (1982) Spinal fusion in Duchenne muscular dystrophy. *Spine*, **7**, 484–491.

SECTION 6
SPINAL NEOPLASIA

26 · Pathology of Spinal Tumours

By R. REID and D.I. GRAHAM

Neurological symptoms and signs due to tumours affecting the spinal cord result from direct pressure on the cord or from interference with its blood supply. The exact clinical picture depends upon the site and rate of progress of the lesion. For the purposes of this chapter the tumours that occur in the spinal column and those which occur within the spinal canal are considered separately.

TUMOURS OF THE SPINAL COLUMN

While there are cases, particularly of metastatic carcinoma and myeloma, where histology alone allows a definite diagnosis to be made, it must be emphasized that the pathologist should not interpret a biopsy without knowledge of the patient's clinical and radiological features. This is particularly important in the field of primary tumours of bone.

The choice of needle or open biopsy is, of course, a clinical decision. Tissue from needle biopsy often shows considerable traumatic artifact; cellular tissue may be crushed beyond recognition. Because of this, it is wise to process not only bony needle cores but also any accompanying blood clot, as this may contain small clumps of tumour cells which often show less cytological distortion. In urgent cases smears/imprints or frozen sections of blood clot or soft tissue may be attempted. In general, the use of such rapid histological techniques in patients with a presumptive diagnosis of tumour will confirm the diagnosis in about 70% of cases. On the other hand, biopsy material from non-tumorous disease is much more difficult to diagnose. If rapid techniques fail to give a diagnosis in an urgent case, the tissue can be processed rapidly and paraffin-embedded sections may be prepared within four hours. The increasing use of microwave irradiation to accelerate fixation and decalcification will allow more rapid tissue processing.

In addition to conventional light microscopy, immunohistochemistry and electron microscopy improve diagnostic accuracy. Immunostaining can often be performed on paraffin-embedded sections, and allows classification of poorly differentiated tumours.

Optimum electron microscopy necessitates immediate fixation of a small representative tissue sample in glutaraldehyde. This is obviously more practical with tissue removed at open surgery than a bony needle core. Valuable diagnostic information, however, may be gained from examination of formalin-fixed tissue, and on occasion material retrieved from a paraffin block, or even a single histological section.

Primary bone tumours are uncommon and only about 12% affect the spine (Dahlin & Unni, 1986). They are far outnumbered by metastatic tumours, even when solitary lesions are considered (Cohen *et al.*, 1964). All segments may be involved; the cervical spine being the least common. In general benign tumours tend to occur in children and young adults, and usually involve the posterior vertebral elements, while lesions in the vertebral body and in older patients are likely to be malignant (Bohlman *et al.*, 1986; Weinstein & McLain, 1987). The relative frequency of the more common tumours in two series is listed in Table 26.1.

Benign tumours

Aneurysmal bone cyst

This non-neoplastic lesion of childhood and young adults may grow rapidly and mimic malignancy. About 15% occur within the spine (Tillman *et al.*,

Table 26.1 Major primary tumours of spine[a]

	Weinstein & McLain (1987)	Dahlin & Unni (1986)
Benign tumours		
Osteoblastoma	7	25
Osteochondroma	7	20
Giant-cell tumour	5	51
Aneurysmal bone cyst	4	40
Haemangioma	3	20
Osteoid osteoma	2	28
Eosinophilic granuloma	2	—
Malignant tumours		
Plasma-cell tumour	15[b]	205[c]
Chordoma	14	165
Chondrosarcoma	6	59
Lymphoma	5	67
Ewing's sarcoma	4	31
Osteosarcoma	3	37
Fibrosarcoma	2	19

[a] Other tumours occasionally arise in the spine, but will not be discussed in this chapter. These are absolute numbers of cases seen from 1935 to 1985 (Weinstein & McLain) and up to 1984 (Dahlin & Unni).
[b] Solitary plasmacytoma.
[c] Myeloma diagnosed on bone biopsy—including solitary and multiple lesions.

1968), especially in the lumbar vertebrae (Hay *et al.*, 1978; Capanna *et al.*, 1985). Almost all involve the vertebral arch, and although extension into the body is common, lesions of the body alone are extremely rare. Aneurysmal bone cysts are expansile osteolytic lesions, often with a thin peripheral shell of bone. They consist of large blood-filled spaces and a network of fibrous tissue containing immature bone, giant cells and macrophages (Fig. 26.1). Extension into adjacent vertebrae or ribs may occur (MacCarty *et al.*, 1961; Stillwell & Fielding, 1984), and cord compression is not uncommon. Recurrence may follow incomplete excision. Since other tumours such as osteoblastoma sometimes contain areas resembling aneurysmal bone cyst, all available tissue should be examined histologically.

Osteoid osteoma

Five per cent of cases of this benign bone-forming tumour occur in the spine, mostly within the vertebral arch and rarely within the bodies (MacLellan & Wilson, 1967; Pettine & Klassen, 1986). Patients typically complain of gnawing pain, sometimes relieved by aspirin. There is often scoliosis and back stiffness (Keim & Reina, 1975; Kirwan *et al.*, 1984). Osteoid osteomas consist of a small (usually less than 1.5 cm) central nidus of irregular trabeculae of woven bone formed by active osteoblasts; this is usually highly vascular and may be radiolucent or opaque. There is often a peripheral zone of reactive sclerosis, but this is less marked than that associated with cortical lesions of long bones. Although entirely benign, local recurrence with return of symptoms may follow incomplete removal.

Benign osteoblastoma

Although histologically similar to osteoid osteomas, osteoblastomas are larger, and may be up to 10 cm in diameter (McLeod *et al.*, 1976). About 30% occur in the spine, usually in the posterior elements (Myles & MacRae, 1988). Stiffness and scoliosis are common but pain is less prominent than with osteoid osteomas. Osteoblastomas (Fig. 26.2) are often sclerotic, but surrounding reactive new bone is rarely marked (Marsh *et al.*, 1975). Most osteoblastomas are cured by conservative surgery, although multifocal lesions may lead to incomplete excision. Rarely osteoblastomas showing atypical histological appearances are

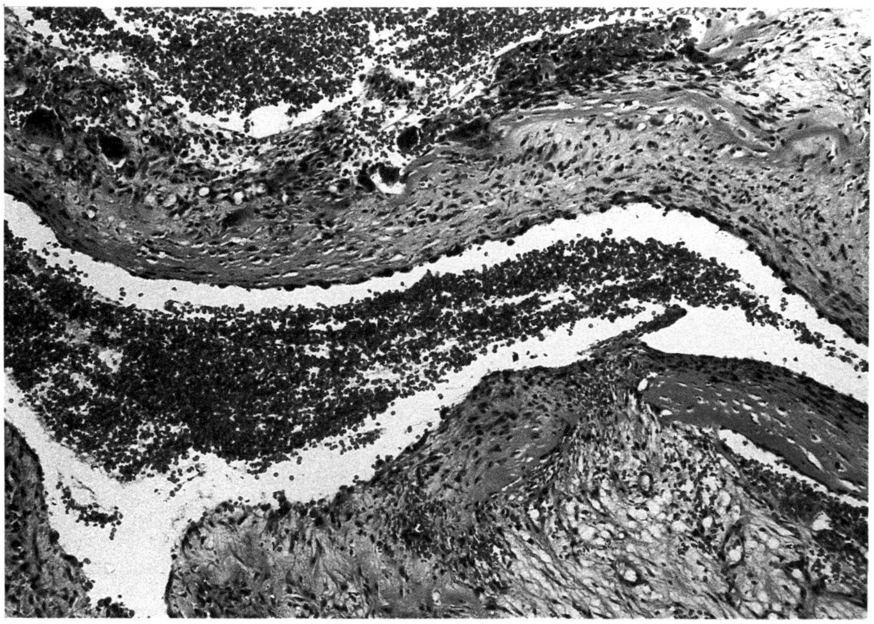

Fig. 26.1 Aneurysmal bone cyst of T2. Blood-filled spaces are separated by trabeculae of fibrous tissue containing giant cells and woven bone. (Haematoxylin and eosin.)

associated with an increased risk of local recurrence. Distinction of these 'aggressive osteoblastomas' from low-grade osteosarcoma may be extremely difficult (Dorfman & Weiss, 1984; Bertoni *et al.*, 1985).

Giant-cell tumour (osteoclastoma)

About 10% of giant-cell tumours are located in the spine, half of these within the sacrum. Most patients are between 20 and 50 years old, and usually present with neurological symptoms. Thoracic and lumbar tumours usually involve the vertebral body, which may collapse. There is often extension into the pedicle or vertebral arch (Dahlin, 1977) and into soft tissue. Giant-cell tumours of the posterior elements are less common except in the cervical spine (Enneking, 1983). The sacrum is often extensively destroyed at presentation.

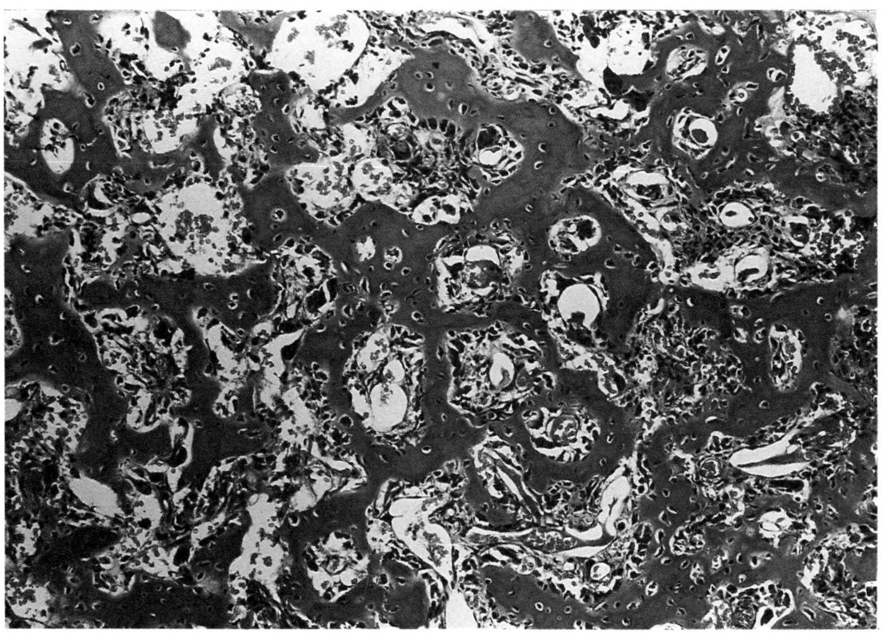

Fig. 26.2 Osteoblastoma. Irregular trabeculae of woven bone are separated by vascular fibrous tissue. Osteoblasts and osteoclasts are present on the bone surface. (Haematoxylin and eosin.)

Giant-cell tumours consist of ovoid mononuclear cells interspersed with large osteoclastic giant cells. Local recurrence after surgery may be less common in the spine than in long bones (Larsson *et al.*, 1975; Savini *et al.*, 1983). Metastatic spread occurs in about 10% of patients, most commonly as high-grade sarcoma often following radiotherapy. Other than tumours showing frank sarcomatous change, histological grading is of little value (Dahlin & Unni, 1986).

Osteochondroma

An osteochondroma is a cartilage-capped bony protuberance found chiefly in young people. Less than 3% arise in the spine, mainly in the posterior elements. Many are symptomless or form a palpable lump (Inglis *et al.*, 1977), but cord compression may occur both with solitary lesions (Julien *et al.*, 1978) and in patients with diaphyseal aclasis (Roman, 1978; O'Connor & Roberts, 1984). Malignant transformation of solitary lesions is rare, and is uncommon in diaphyseal aclasis. Evidence of continued growth, pain and a greatly thickened cartilage cap in adulthood are highly suggestive of chondrosarcoma.

Haemangioma

Asymptomatic vertebral haemangiomas may be found in 10% of adults at necropsy (Schmorl, 1927, quoted by Huvos, 1979). Much less commonly, cord compression may occur due to vertebral expansion or extradural extension (McAllister *et al.*, 1975; Baker, 1986). Vertebral collapse due to a haemangioma is rare. Most haemangiomas involve the vertebral body with a radiological appearance of vertical striations or a honeycomb pattern. Microscopically the lesion is composed of cavernous or capillary vascular channels. Multiple haemangiomas may simulate metastases, and on rare occasions may be sclerotic (Bullough & Boachie-Adjei, 1988).

Eosinophil granuloma

This, the mildest form of histiocytosis X, involves the spine in about 8% of cases (Schajowicz, 1981). One or multiple bones may be affected (Ferris *et al.*, 1974), and less commonly visceral lesions are present. The vertebral body is usually affected, with partial or complete collapse giving a 'vertebra plana' on X-ray, although focal lysis or sclerosis without collapse may be seen (Bullough & Boachie-Adjei, 1988). In about 15% of cases the posterior arch is affected (Robert *et al.*, 1987). Histological examination shows clusters of histiocytic cells (Langerhans' cells) whose cytoplasm contains characteristic organelles (Birbeck granules) seen by electron microscopy. A mixture of eosinophils and giant cells is also present. Eosinophil granuloma usually causes pain and stiffness, but sometimes neurological deficit (Green *et al.*, 1980). Lesions often heal spontaneously in children usually with considerable recovery of vertebral height (Ippolito *et al.*, 1984; Canadell *et al.*, 1986).

Malignant tumours

Myeloma

Myeloma is the commonest primary tumour of bone which rarely occurs in patients under 50 years (Dahlin & Unni, 1986). In most cases multiple lesions are found at the time of presentation with vertebrae almost always involved. Radiographs may show diffuse osteoporosis, a lytic lesion, often with collapse, or rarely sclerosis (Driedger & Pruzanski, 1979). Microscopic examination shows sheets of plasma cells of varying degrees of differentiation (Fig. 26.3).

Rarely solitary lesions (solitary plasmacytomas) are seen. These patients are on average 10 years younger than those with multiple myeloma (Delauche-Cavallier *et al.*, 1988) and more commonly present with cord compression (Valderrama & Bullough, 1968). A third to a half will develop multiple deposits within a few years (Meis *et al.*, 1987; Delauche-Cavallier *et al.*, 1988).

Chordoma

This tumour is thought to arise from notochordal remnants. Half arise in the sacrum (Dahlin & Unni, 1986), usually causing extensive destruction and a palpable presacral mass. About 15% are located in the vertebrae, particularly in the cervical region. These often present early with cord compression, although large retropharyngeal and neck masses may occur.

Involvement of adjacent vertebral bodies is typical (Sundaresan, 1986). Chordomas are gelatinous tumours infiltrating through bone, but often with a well-defined pseudo-capsule in soft tissue. Histologically cords of vacuolated (physaliferous) cells lie

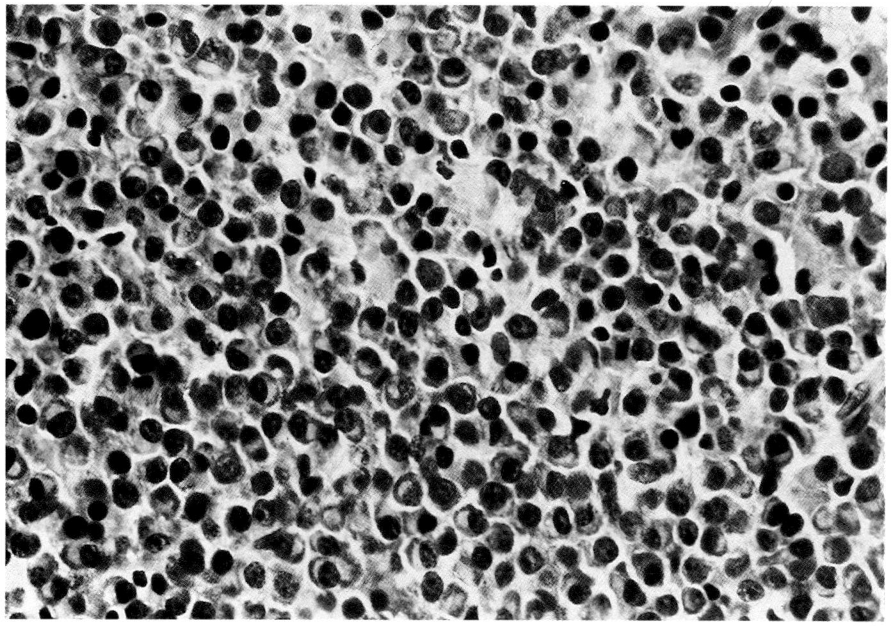

Fig. 26.3 Myeloma. The tumour consists of sheets of abnormal plasma cells. Prominent perinuclear vacuoles representing the Golgi apparatus are seen. (Haematoxylin and eosin.)

within a mucoid matrix (Fig. 26.4). Immunocytochemistry (Salisbury & Isaacson, 1985) and electron microscopy (Pena *et al.*, 1970) allow distinction from metastatic carcinoma and chondrosarcoma. Chordomas grow slowly but with a marked tendency to local extension and recurrence. Although metastases may occur in 30% of cases (Chambers & Schwinn, 1979), death usually results from local disease.

Chondrosarcoma

Less than 8% of chondrosarcomas arise in the spine (Dahlin & Unni, 1986). A tumour mainly of adults, chondrosarcoma can arise within the medullary cavity of the vertebra (central) or from an exostosis (peripheral). Central tumours of the vertebral body or arch cause bone destruction with extension into soft

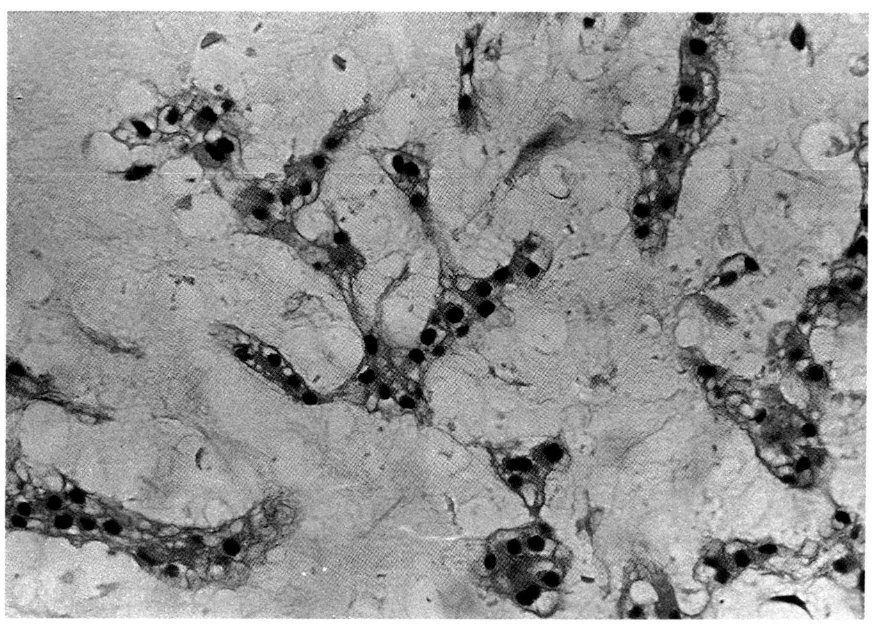

Fig. 26.4 Chordoma of T8. Cords of vacuolated cells lie in myxoid matrix. The patient, a woman of 69 years, died with local recurrence 28 months after surgical decompression and radiotherapy.

tissue or spinal canal (Wronski *et al.*, 1964; Blaylock & Kempe, 1976). Peripheral tumours in particular may present as large masses (Camins *et al.*, 1978), which are usually focally calcified on X-ray. The behaviour of chondrosarcoma depends on the histological grade. Most chondrosarcomas are low-grade tumours which rarely metastasize but, unless completely excised, grow slowly and relentlessly; many prove fatal. Spillage of tumour cells at surgery often results in implantation and local recurrence. About 10% of low-grade chondrosarcomas are associated with a high-grade sarcoma, often an osteosarcoma. These 'dedifferentiated' chondrosarcomas have an extremely poor prognosis (Frassica *et al.*, 1986).

High-grade chondrosarcomas (Fig. 26.5) are highly malignant tumours which spread early to the lungs.

Osteosarcoma

Approximately 3% of osteosarcomas arise within the spine, representing 5% of all malignant primary spinal tumours (Shives *et al.*, 1986). The sacrum is most often affected, while vertebral tumours more often involve the body than vertebral arch. Patients are in general older than those with limb osteosarcoma (Barwick *et al.*, 1980). Spinal osteosarcomas sometimes complicate previous radiation therapy (Dowdle *et al.*, 1977; Shives *et al.*, 1986) or Paget's disease, although the incidence of Paget's sarcoma of the spine is much lower than of long bones (Schajowicz *et al.*, 1983). The histological appearances of osteosarcoma vary greatly, but all show malignant cells directly forming bone or osteoid. The prognosis of spinal osteosarcoma is poor with only occasional exceptions (Ogihara *et al.*, 1984). Occasional cases have been misdiagnosed radiologically and pathologically as osteoblastoma (Marsh & Choi, 1970).

Lymphoma

Primary lymphoma of bone is rare and must be distinguished from bony involvement in a patient with disseminated lymphoma.

About 14% of primary lymphomas occur within the vertebral column (Mirra, 1989). The vertebral body is usually involved, often with lysis but sometimes with considerable sclerosis. Vertebral collapse with extension into the paravertebral soft tissue and spinal canal are common. Histologically, most cases are non-Hodgkin's lymphoma, often of B-cell type (Falini *et al.*, 1988), although Hodgkin's disease may also be seen (Horan, 1969; Newcomer *et al.*, 1982). The prognosis of primary lymphoma of bone is relatively favourable with a five-year survival of 40–50% reported (Dahlin & Unni, 1986).

Ewing's sarcoma

About 8% of Ewing's tumours occur primarily within the spine, particularly the sacrum (Dahlin & Unni,

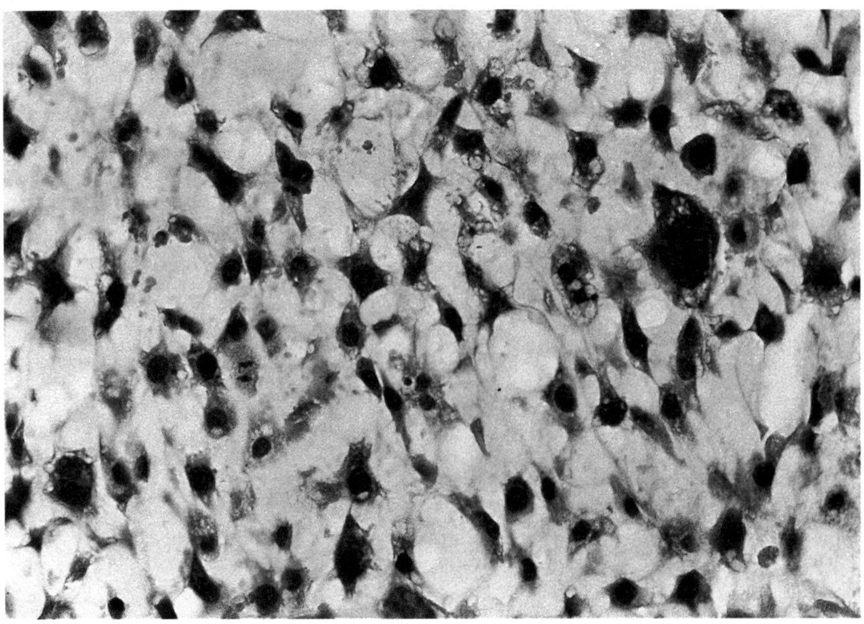

Fig. 26.5 High-grade chondrosarcoma of L1. The tumour is highly cellular with marked nuclear pleomorphism and mitotic activity. The patient, a woman of 63 years, died with extensive local disease one year after surgery and radiotherapy.

1986). In addition, spinal metastases from Ewing's sarcoma elsewhere are fairly common. Most patients are children or adolescents, often presenting with low-grade fever, and elevated white blood count and erythrocyte sedimentation rate, suggesting infection. Typically there is bone destruction with a paravertebral soft tissue mass (Weinstein *et al.*, 1984), and cord compression. Histologically, Ewing's sarcoma consists of sheets of uniform small cells containing glycogen and with very little intercellular reticulin. These features, together with electron microscopy and immunocytochemistry (Triche & Cavazzana, 1988), allow distinction from lymphoma and metastatic neuroblastoma.

Metastatic bone tumours

The spine is the commonest site of skeletal metastases, about three-quarters originating from carcinoma of breast, bronchus, prostate, kidney (Fig. 26.6) and thyroid, and from lymphoma (Fornasier & Horne, 1975; Harrington, 1986). Metastases of neuroblastoma and sarcomas such as Ewing's tumour and osteosarcoma are also seen. Although vertebral metastases are very commonly found in patients dying of cancer at necropsy, most are asymptomatic. Cord compression occurs in 5% of cases, mainly due to vertebral collapse or extradural spread (Boland *et al.*, 1982; Constans *et al.*, 1983; Onimus *et al.*, 1986), this being particularly common in the thoracic spine (Kleinman *et al.*, 1978). The vertebral body is almost always involved. Spread to the vertebrae is blood-borne, either by arterial dissemination or through the valveless vessels of Batson's paravertebral venous plexus. Carcinomas of breast and lung commonly spread to the thoracic spine, while prostatic cancer usually affects the sacrum and lumbar vertebrae. Most metastases are lytic; a minority, mainly of prostate, breast and gastrointestinal origin, induce reactive new bone formation and appear sclerotic on X-ray. Metastases confined to the intradural and extradural spaces, without bone involvement, were found in only 1% and 5% of cases, respectively, in a series of 600 patients with spinal metastases causing neurological complications (Constans *et al.*, 1983).

TUMOURS OF SPINAL CANAL

Tumours of the spinal canal are uncommon, comprising only 10–15% of all tumours of the central nervous system. They occur with equal frequency in men and women, and are most common between the ages of 20 and 60 years (Kurland, 1958; Slooff *et al.*, 1964; Alter, 1975). True prevalence is difficult to establish, but by far the most common tumour affecting the spinal cord is metastatic carcinoma. Of the primary intraspinal tumours about 30% are neurilemmoma, 26% meningioma and 22% glioma (Slooff *et*

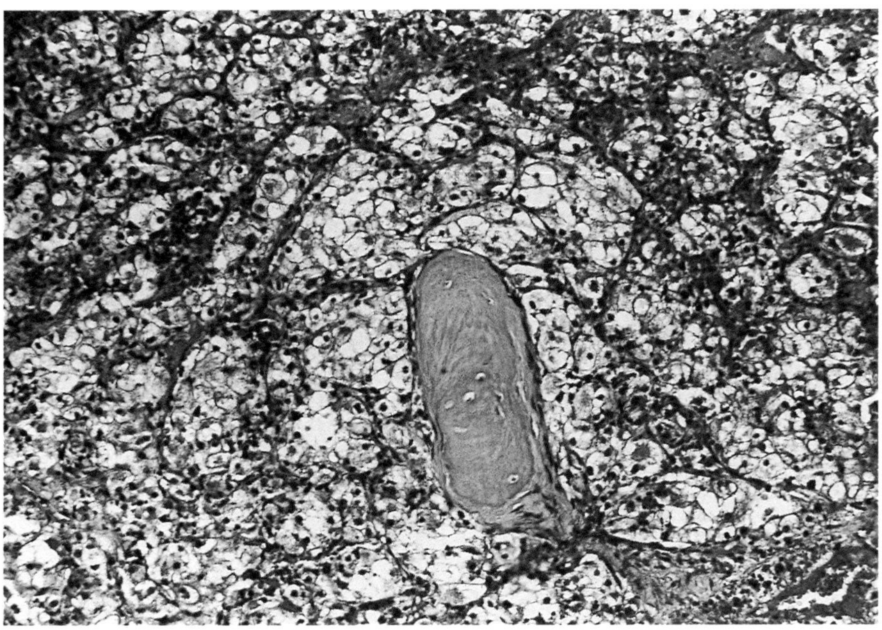

Fig. 26.6 Metastatic renal carcinoma. Packets of cells with clear cytoplasm surround a trabecula of woven bone.

al., 1964). Gliomas occur most commonly in adulthood, although there is a higher proportion of gliomas in childhood because of the low incidence of meningiomas and neurilemmomas in early life (Slooff *et al.*, 1964; Alter, 1975). Table 26.2 shows the types of spinal tumours presenting over a 15-year period to the Institute of Neurological Sciences in Glasgow, which provides a neurosurgical service to a population of some 2.7 million people. Although these figures exclude autopsy findings, the figures should give some idea of the incidence, at least of neuroepithelial tumours.

The examination of a small biopsy from spinal tumours is an important and sometimes difficult task, a particular problem being the distinction between intense reactive changes and a low-grade astrocytoma. The logic of the diagnostic process rests on an understanding of the likely nature of the tumour, this being based predominantly on the site of the biopsy and the age of the patient (Table 26.2). If the immediate diagnosis on smears (Adams *et al.*, 1981) or on cryostat sections is not readily apparent, the pathologist has to bear in mind the possibility that the biopsy has been taken from a rare tumour when some material must be preserved for special diagnostic techniques such as immunohistochemistry or electron microscopy (Russell & Rubinstein, 1989).

The terminology used for tumours of the nervous system is a continuing problem. In the following account a modification of the World Health Organization (1979) classification is used (see Table 26.3), although traditionally tumours of the spinal canal have been classified by their location, viz. extradural, intradural–extramedullary, and intramedullary (Hughes, 1978; Langford *et al.*, 1987).

Tumours of neuroepithelial tissue

Astrocytic tumours

Some 3% of all astrocytomas affect the spinal cord, but of the primary neuroepithelial tumours arising in the spinal cord they comprise some 25% (Sloof *et al.*, 1964). Occurring with equal frequency in men and women in the third and fourth decades, they are found most commonly in the cervical segments where they may develop as a result of downward extension of tumours in the brain stem (Webb *et al.*, 1953). Occasionally they start in the cauda equina. While predominance in the cervical segments may also be true in children and adolescents (Reimer &

Table 26.2 An analysis of the 615 spinal tumours among the 6149 neurosurgically referred biopsies examined in the Department of Neuropathology, Institute of Neurological Sciences, Glasgow, in a 15-year period (1974–88)

	n	Children (up to 15 years)		*n*	Adults (16–64 years)		*n*	Elderly (65 years and over)	
Extradural	15	Neuroblastoma	9	269	Carcinoma	184	129	Carcinoma	99
		Ganglioneuroma	2		Myeloma	22		Lymphoma	17
		Ganglioneuroblastoma	1		Neurofibroma/ neurilemmoma	21		Myeloma	11
		Lymphoma	1		Lymphoma	17		Sarcoma	1
		Neurofibroma	1		Sarcoma	11		Benign bone tumours	1
		Sarcoma	1		Benign bone tumour	11			
					Vascular	2			
					Teratoma	1			
Intradural extramedullary	18	Dermoid/epidermoid	12	87	Neurofibroma/ neurilemmoma	38	45	Meningioma	28
		Other developmental	5		Meningioma	33		Neurofibroma/ neurilemmoma	15
		Meningioma	1		Other developmental	14		Carcinoma	2
					Paraganglioma	2			
Intramedullary	10	Astrocytoma	8	40	Astrocytoma	21	2	Ependymoma	1
		Ependymoma	2		Ependymoma	13		Astrocytoma	1
					Anaplastic astrocytoma	6			

Table 26.3 Classification of tumours of the central nervous system with particular reference to the spinal cord. Modified from WHO (1979)

Tumours of neuroepithelial tissue
Astrocytoma
Oligodendroglioma
Ependymoma
Neuronal tumours
Poorly differentiated and embryonal tumours
Tumours of nerve sheath cells
Neurilemmoma (Schwannoma)
Neurofibroma
Tumours of meningeal and related tissues
Meningioma
Primary melanotic tumours
Primary malignant lymphoma
Tumours of blood vessel origin
Haemangioblastoma
Germ-cell tumours
Other malformative tumours and tumour-like lesions
Epidermoid cyst
Dermoid cyst
Enterogenous cyst
Local extension
Chordomas
Sarcoma
Benign bone tumours
Metastatic tumours

Onofrio, 1985), they commonly extend throughout the whole length of the spinal cord, although the actual solid moiety may be surprisingly small and associated with rostral and caudal cysts (Matson & Tachdjian, 1963; Epstein & Epstein, 1982).

Astrocytomas appear as localized fusiform enlargements of the spinal cord. Usually they are wholly intramedullary but may infiltrate the subarachnoid space. On section the affected segments are diffusely expanded by greyish-white firm tissue: cystic degeneration is common, the cyst containing yellowish-brown proteinaceous fluid.

The histological appearances vary with the grade of tumour. Most, however, resemble the low-grade, diffuse fibrillary astrocytomas of the cerebrum in which there are large numbers of intertwining astrocytic fibrils arising from characteristically stellate cells. The infiltrated tissues are usually well preserved (Fig. 26.7). In tumours of intermediate grade (II and III) there is greater cellularity, an increased number of mitotic figures and some endothelial proliferation. The anaplastic astrocytomas (grade IV), on the other hand, are highly cellular, pleomorphic tumours in which there is a high mitotic figure rate and proliferation of small vessels.

The relatively poor cellularity of the low-grade fibrillary astrocytomas and the frequency of cystic degeneration make the differentiation between astrocytoma and other intrinsic cystic conditions such as syringomyelia very difficult, particularly when only a limited biopsy is available. This is particularly so in the latter instance, for intramedullary cysts accompany a wide variety of intramedullary tumours and the cavitation is not always in anatomical continuity with the tumour (Poser, 1956). However, with the increasing use of open spinal surgery in specialized units, and multiple sampling from the margins of lesions and at the limits of resection, many of the earlier diagnostic difficulties have been overcome. In those cases where the initial biopsy is small and has been used in the preparation of smears or cryostat sections, it should be recalled that diagnostic information may be obtained from material removed with the ultrasonic surgical aspirator (Blackie & Gordon, 1984; Silverman *et al.*, 1989).

Oligodendroglioma

These uncommon, slowly growing tumours occur equally in males and females in the second decade, and occur most frequently in the thoracic segments of the cord (Earnest *et al.*, 1950; Fortuna *et al.*, 1980). Described as firm reddish tumours that are inseparable from the surrounding tissue, or soft, white gelatinous and infiltrating, both types are frequently cystic and have multiple foci of haemorrhage. The tumours consist of enlarged, uniform, closely packed cells with round to oval nuclei, clear cytoplasm and well-defined cell boundaries, giving the appearance of perinuclear haloes in a honeycomb pattern.

Ependymoma

The majority of spinal ependymomas occur between the second and sixth decades with a peak incidence in the fourth: they are slightly more common in males than females.

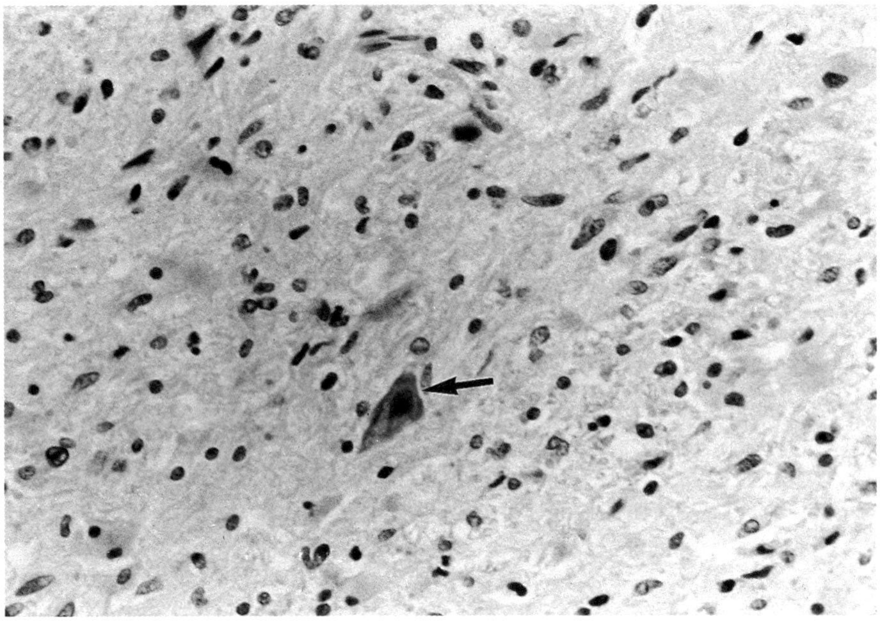

Fig. 26.7 Low-grade astrocytoma. There is increased cellularity by elongated tumour cells that have well-defined processes. Note surviving ventral horn cell (arrow). (Haematoxylin and eosin.)

They are the most common type of glioma of the spinal cord and filum terminale, over two-thirds occurring in the region of the conus medullaris, the filum terminale and the cauda equina: the remainder may be found at any level of the cord (Mork & Loken, 1977). Multiple spinal ependymomas are associated with von Recklinghausen's disease when they may be associated with syringomyelia (Poser, 1956).

Intramedullary ependymomas cause localized fusiform expansions which on section appear as masses of focally cystic homogeneous grey tumour, which often appears well demarcated from surrounding cord. True encapsulation, however, is uncommon, although the tumour can often be enucleated. In contrast, tumours of the filum terminale appear as ovoid nodules expanding, or attached to, the filum, lying free within the cauda equina. Occasionally there is infiltration of the meninges and in those that arise in the region of the cauda equina there may be extension through the dura and even remote metastases (Sonneland *et al.*, 1985).

Histologically the cells in ependymomas frequently have a distinctly epithelial appearance, but the most characteristic feature is the pseudo-rosette which takes the form of a perivascular fibrillary eosinophilic cuff between blood vessels and tumour cells (Fig. 26.8a). In myxopapillary ependymomas, tumour cells are arranged in a papillary fashion around blood vessels, and the distinctive histological feature is due to the mucinous change undergone by the collagenous stroma of the papillae and mucin secretion (Fig. 26.8b). As with astrocytomas, four grades of malignancy in ependymomas have been described: anaplastic (grade IV) features consisting of cellular pleomorphism, mitotic figures, capillary endothelial hyperplasia, necrosis and haemorrhage (Dohrman *et al.*, 1976).

Neuronal tumours

This category includes neuroblastoma, ganglioneuroma and ganglioglioma, all of which are uncommon.

Neuroblastoma may arise either within the cord, or in relation to the cauda equina (Kepes *et al.*, 1985). It consists of densely cellular fields of small round or oval cells with darkly staining nuclei and in which Homer Wright rosettes are often found (Fig. 26.9a). Mitotic figures are numerous.

There are reports of intramedullary ganglioneuroma but more commonly they present as extradural tumours arising from the sympathetic chain. Intramedullary ganglioglioma have also been reported (Bevilacqua & Sarnelli, 1979). Histologically there may be a large number of mature ganglion cells in ganglioneuroma, but the finding of more primitive foci of neuroblastic nature (ganglioneuroblastoma)

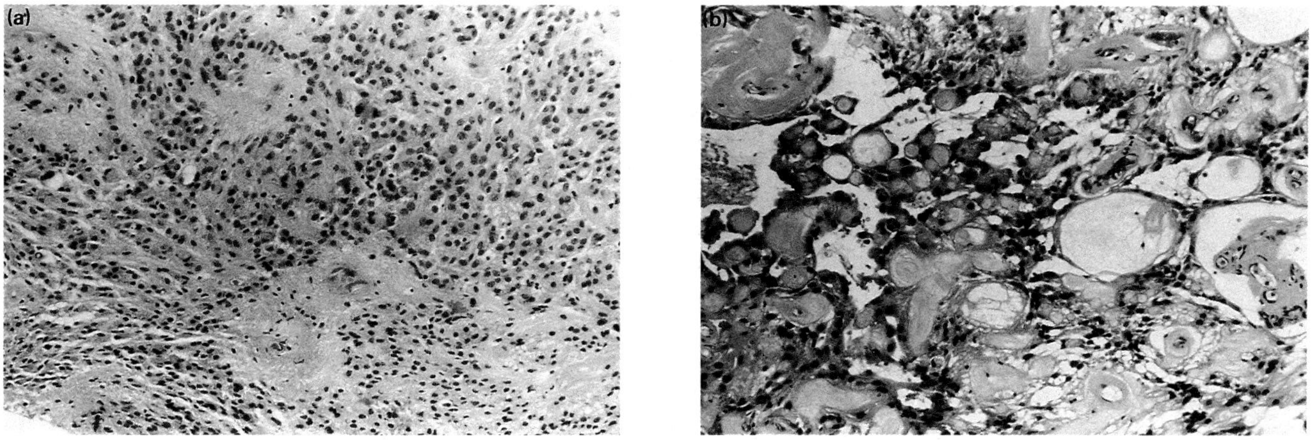

Fig. 26.8 (a) Ependymoma. Note the perivascular fibrillary halo that is highly characteristic of ependymoma. (Haematoxylin and eosin.) (b) Myxopapillary ependymoma of cauda equina. The tumour cells are arranged around myxomatous fibrovascular trabeculae. (Haematoxylin and eosin.)

is of considerable adverse prognostic significance. Ganglioglioma is more common and its microscopic appearances are similar to astrocytoma. Histologically there is a mixture of bizarre cells of ganglionic type in addition to tumour astrocytes. Many of the ganglion cells are binucleate, and throughout the tumour there are groups of small dark cells that are usually interpreted as being neuroblasts (Fig. 26.9b). The bizarre and atypical features of the ganglion cells usually allow this type of tumour to be distinguished quite easily from astrocytoma invading grey matter in which there are residual neurones. Most behave more as hamartomas than true tumours, and mitotic figures are rarely seen. Occasionally, however, anaplastic change occurs within a ganglioglioma and it is usually in the astrocytic element.

A further form of presentation, particularly in children, is that of cord compression by spread of neuroblastoma through extradural tissue. This may occur as direct extension from tumours arising in the mediastinum or retroperitoneal tissues, or as a result of metastases.

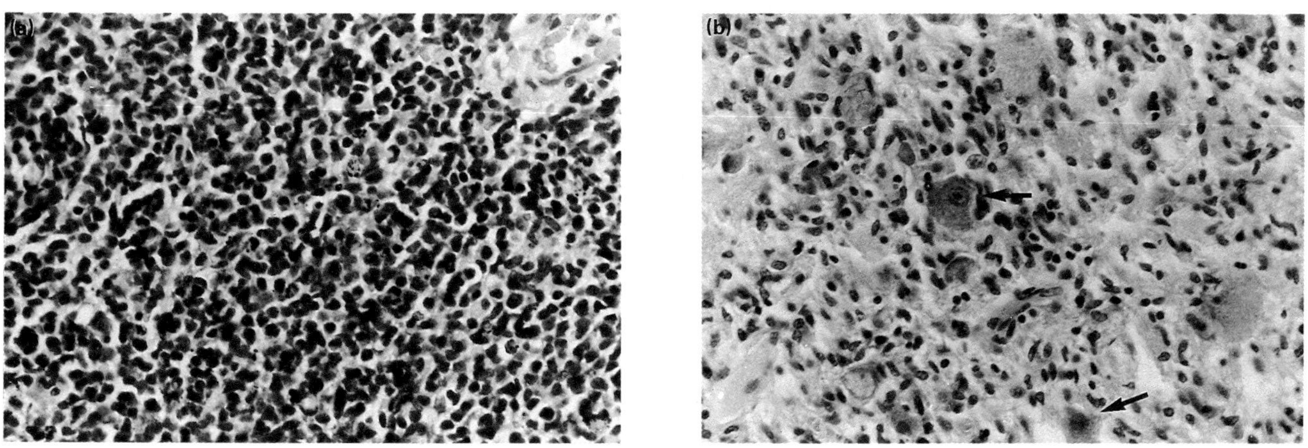

Fig. 26.9 (a) Neuroblastoma. The nuclei of this densely cellular tumour are small, round and hyperchromatic. Cytoplasm is scanty and rosette formation is poor. (Haematoxylin and eosin.) (b) Ganglioglioma. In this part of the tumour there are a few cells that are clearly of ganglionic type (arrows) and others with small hyperchromatic nuclei and scanty cytoplasm. (Haematoxylin and eosin.)

Poorly differentiated and embryonal tumours

There are two main types of tumour in this category. The term 'glioblastoma multiforme' is used for a pleomorphic and anaplastic tumour within which there are no recognizable features by conventional microscopy of astrocytic, oligodendroglial or ependymal origin. The spinal cord is an uncommon site (Sloof *et al.*, 1964). The tumour may occupy and expand several cervical or thoracic segments: the incidence in males and females is roughly equal, occurring usually in patients less than 30 years. Histologically, there is great variety in cell size, from small undifferentiated cells through cells of intermediate size to bizarre giant cells, many of which are multinucleated. There are frequently mitotic figures: haemorrhage, necrosis and vascular proliferation are the rule. Glioblastomas may break through the pia into the subarachnoid space and metastasize widely in the cerebrospinal pathways.

Medulloblastoma is a tumour of the cerebellum that probably arises from nests of cells originating in the external granular layer. It is seen most commonly in children but also in adolescence and occasionally in early adult life. Medulloblastoma has a particular propensity to spread within the subarachnoid space: there are often small nodules of tumour on spinal nerve roots. Occasionally, such deposits may be responsible for neurological signs and symptoms and erroneously interpreted as the primary growth when the cerebellar focus is relatively small and inconspicuous. Histologically, it consists of sheets of closely packed, often slightly elongated cells that have scant cytoplasm. The classical feature is the presence of neuroblastic rosettes but they are not present in every medulloblastoma.

Primary neuroepithelial tumours at unusual sites

Intraspinal extramedullary spread of various types of glioma may be found in between 10% and 15% of cases. There are, however, reports attributing the origin of gliomas to heterotopia of the meninges. Occurring particularly in the lumbosacral region, they have often been associated with congenital abnormality such as spina bifida (Cooper *et al.*, 1951). In spite of its rarity, cases of primary leptomeningeal gliomatosis have been described (Kitahara *et al.*, 1985).

Primary extraspinal sacral gliomas have also been described: they are more often ependymomas than astrocytomas (Russell & Rubinstein, 1989) and are believed to arise from embryological cord remnants.

Tumours of nerve sheath cells

Neurilemmoma/Schwannoma

Probably of Schwann cell origin, the neurilemmoma appears as a well-defined, encapsulated, ovoid mass arising predominantly from sensory roots: they are uncommon in children, and males are more commonly affected than females. The majority are solitary, and intramedullary cases have been reported (Ross *et al.*, 1986): they occur most commonly in the lumbar region. They are also found in the cervical and thoracic regions where they may extend through an intervertebral foramen or even the foramen magnum, resulting in a 'dumb-bell' or 'hourglass' tumour (Webb *et al.*, 1953).

They are benign and slow-growing. On section they are frequently cystic and there may also be distinctly yellow areas. Histologically, the tumour is of variegated appearance, two features being particularly common (Fig. 26.10), *viz.* the occurrence of interlacing bundles of greatly elongated cells, the nuclei of which often show palisading (Antoni A) alternating with tissue of a much looser texture containing large, often pleomorphic, polygonal cells (Antoni B). Small cysts and evidence of previous haemorrhage are common.

An important group affects the intercostal nerves and posterior mediastinum where the tumour may extend into and enlarge the adjacent intervertebral foramina. Another reported site is in the vertebral bodies (Polkey, 1975).

Neurofibroma

These tumours are composed of Schwann cells and fibroblasts and cause fusiform enlargement of the affected segments of nerve: they are frequently in continuity with a paravertebral mass. Several adjacent nerves are often affected, the ensuing condition being known as plexiform neurofibroma. They occur most commonly in adults in relation to the thoracic segments or the cauda equina, and may attain a very large size. On section the tissue has a pale, rather mucoid appearance but may be pigmented. Histologically, the affected nerve is expanded and because of

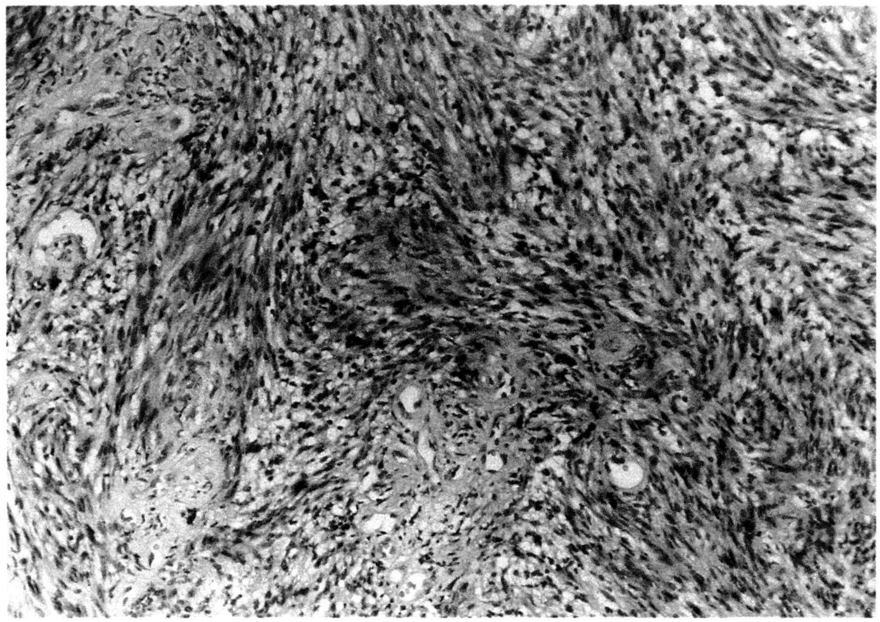

Fig. 26.10 Schwannoma. There is 'palisading' of nuclei in Antoni A areas and cellular pleomorphism of lipid containing cells with clear or foamy cytoplasm in Antoni B areas. (Haematoxylin and eosin.)

the presence of a considerable amount of pale intercellular matrix, often appears of low cellularity. Residual axons can usually be identified (Lassmann *et al.*, 1977). Malignant transformation is most likely to occur in association with von Recklinghausen's disease (Lott & Richardson, 1981; Rubinstein, 1986).

Tumours of meningeal and related tissue

Meningiomas

These are among the most common intraspinal tumours in middle life and in women (Kepes, 1982), taking origin from cells of arachnoidal granulations. Although predominantly intradural in adults, extradural meningioma has also been described, especially in children (Calogero & Moossy, 1972).

Meningiomas may attain a quite remarkable size before giving rise to symptoms. They are solid lobulated tumours, often attached by a broad base to the dura. As they enlarge they excavate a cavity in adjacent cord from which they are usually easily separated. They vary greatly in appearance, some being soft and fleshy while others are hard and gritty. There are several named types of meningioma based on their histological appearances (Fig. 26.11), but there is little correlation between these and the sites of the tumour or its gross appearances (WHO, 1979).

Primary melanotic tumour

Most commonly this takes the form of diffuse meningeal melanomatosis with an origin from pial melanocytes. Rarely, the tumours appear as solid, greyish haemorrhagic masses. Meningeal melanomatosis is particularly common in patients who have one or more benign hairy pigmented naevi on the skin. This syndrome is known as neurocutaneous melanosis (Faillace *et al.*, 1984). In addition, there are well-documented examples of primary meningeal melanoma in which an origin from pial melanocytes is postulated (Bamborschke *et al.*, 1985).

Primary malignant lymphomas

Non-Hodgkin's lymphoma

Lymphomas may affect the central nervous system in several ways, the commonest being compression of the spinal cord by an extradural deposit (Grant *et al.*, 1986). It also occurs intrinsically within the spinal cord (Hautzer *et al.*, 1983), and in the past was often referred to as microgliomatosis. There may be no evidence of systemic lymphoma. The origin, classification and nomenclature of these tumours have been the subject of a great deal of recent study (Jellinger *et al.*, 1975; Simon *et al.*, 1987; Hochberg & Miller, 1988). There is a strong association between

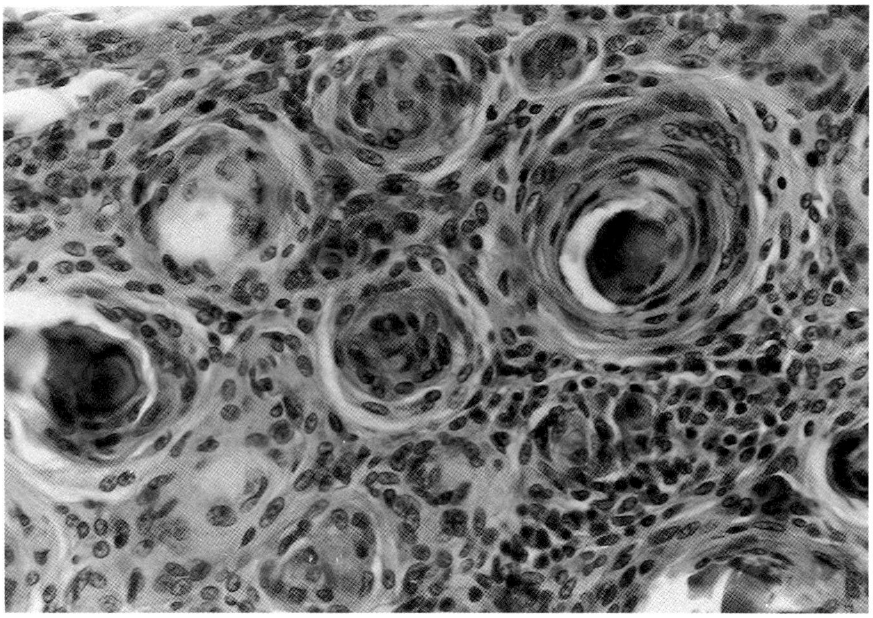

Fig. 26.11 Meningioma. Cell whorls and psammoma bodies are easily recognized. (Haematoxylin and eosin.)

primary central nervous system (CNS) lymphoma and immunodeficiency disorders, either congenital e.g. the Wiskott–Aldrich syndrome, or acquired such as following organ transplantation or during the course of infection by the human immunodeficiency virus (HIV). It has been estimated that primary lymphoma of the nervous system is seen in about 6% of all cases of neurological complications of the acquired immunodeficiency syndrome (AIDS), and by the end of this century may well become the most common intracranial tumour (So *et al.*, 1986; Hochberg & Miller, 1988).

Intrinsic lymphomas vary greatly in appearance. Some are fairly well-defined, rather fleshy masses, whilst others are ill-defined, sometimes rather granular lesions with appearances that can be very similar to those of astrocytoma, including cyst formation. Multicentric deposits are not uncommon. Deposits of lymphoma often seem to replace cord tissue rather than to act as expanding lesions. Histologically, the tumour is composed of round or oval cells with a distinctly lymphoid appearance and usually containing oval or slightly twisted nuclei. Mitotic figures and varying degrees of pleomorphism may be present, and there are sometimes foci of necrosis. Extension into the subarachnoid space is common. In the past, considerable emphasis was placed on the fact that a proportion of the tumour cells in an intrinsic cerebral lymphoma would with silver impregnation show the staining properties of microglia (hence the term 'microgliomatosis'). It now seems likely, however, that these cells are reactive and not an intrinsic component of the tumour. This has been established by immunocytochemical studies which have indicated that nearly all intrinsic cerebral lymphomas are diffuse, non-Hodgkin's lymphomas composed of B cells (Grant *et al.*, 1986; So *et al.*, 1986; Simon *et al.*, 1987).

Hodgkin's disease

Intraspinal involvement by Hodgkin's disease is rarely seen, but may occur as extradural infiltration which is the most common manifestation, and even more rarely as direct extension into the spinal cord (Henson & Urich, 1982).

Leukaemias

The meninges may be affected in acute leukaemia, particularly in acute lymphatic leukaemia in children. There is diffuse infiltration of the meninges by leukaemic cells that are readily identifiable in CSF cytospin preparations. There may also be invasion of the cranial and spinal nerve roots, and rarely there may be large extradural masses of tumour (Wilhyde *et al.*, 1963).

Tumours of blood vessel origin

The most important tumour of the spinal cord in this category is the capillary haemangioblastoma (Wyburn-Mason, 1944; Sloof *et al.*, 1964; Yasargil *et al.*, 1976; Fox et al., 1985): often in the upper cervical cord–medullary region with a multiple arterial supply. They may exist as solitary lesions but also as a component of Lindau's syndrome, when there may be multiple haemangioblastomas, similar tumours occurring in the retinas, congenital cysts of pancreas and kidney, and clear-cell tumours of kidney (Horton *et al.*, 1976; Ismail and Cole, 1984). Syringomyelia or cyst formation is present in many cases, and there is an association with vascular malformations, particularly of the spinal cord (Russell & Rubinstein, 1989). Histologically, the tumour consists of a closely packed network of vascular channels of varying size and a stroma composed of large polygonal cells that are usually distended with lipid. There is a dense reticulin network through the tumour. A good plane of cleavage from cord is often present.

Germ-cell tumours

Teratoma

Teratoma contains tissue from all three germ layers and is a true tumour composed of multiple tissues of kinds foreign to the part in which it arises, the most common components being skin, teeth, CNS tissue, alimentary and respiratory mucosae. Intraspinal teratomas are rare, and may occur at any level. Associated developmental abnormalities are common and spina bifida is present in many cases (Furtado & Marques, 1951; Slooff *et al.*, 1964; Garrison & Kasdon, 1980). Most are cystic and lack a capsule. Histologically, appearances vary considerably depending upon the type of tissue present and the degree to which it forms organized structures. The prognosis depends on the identification of immature elements comprising primitive cells derived from (usually one of) the three principal germinal layers.

Other malformative tumours and tumour-like lesions

Epidermoid and dermoid cysts

These are the same type of developmental cysts that occur elsewhere in the body. Traditionally they are distinguished from teratomas, but whether such a distinction is appropriate is doubtful. Certainly these cysts are more common than teratomas, and they have been described as being either extradural, intradural but extramedullary or intramedullary (Manno *et al.*, 1962), occurring at all levels of the spinal canal but more commonly in the lower portion. Epidermoid cysts are more common than dermoid, occurring between the ages of 20 and 50 years and more commonly in males than females. They are encapsulated lesions, sharply defined from adjacent tissue which they compress. The contents of epidermoid cysts are usually white and rich in keratin and cholesterol, being sometimes referred to as 'pearly tumours', whereas dermoid cysts usually contain an oily or cheesy substance which is a mixture of sebaceous material and desquamated epithelium with hair and more rarely teeth. Histologically both cysts are lined by stratified squamous epithelium; in dermoid cysts skin appendages are also present.

They are commonly associated with evidence of spinal dysraphism. Both epidermoid and dermoid cysts are thought to arise from a developmental abnormality due to inclusion of ectodermal elements at the time of neural groove closure in the third to fifth weeks of embryonic life. Acquired cysts may be found in children who have been subjected to numerous lumbar punctures for tuberculous meningitis (Choremis *et al.*, 1956; Boyd, 1966).

Lipomas

Intraspinal lipomatous masses are commonly associated with congenital abnormalities such as spina bifida. Most occur in the thoracic region but may be present along the length of the cord. They occur with equal frequency in both sexes, and are found most commonly in the first five years or between the second and fifth decades. They are lobulated and surrounded by dense collagen which extends as fibrous septae into the cord. For this reason and although benign, they are difficult to treat.

Enterogenous cyst

Of developmental foregut origin, these intradural cysts, which occur most commonly in the cervical and cervicothoracic segments, are usually extramedullary and are lined by columnar epithelium of intestinal type (Agnoli *el al.*, 1984). They may be associated with mediastinal enterogenous cysts which may connect with the spinal cyst through an anteriorly placed defect in the vertebrae.

There are a number of lesions that occur in relation to the spinal meninges and nerve roots (Burger *et al.* 1991). Some, such as epidermoid, dermoid and enterogenous cysts, have already been described. However, other lesions do occur.

The meningeal cyst is a posteriorly placed extradural pedunculated diverticulum that develops either in the midline or laterally close to a dorsal nerve root. Usually connected to the subarachnoid space, it is made up histologically of a thick collagenous outer wall which resembles dura, and an inner membrane similar to arachnoid. Spinal extradural and subdural arachnoidal cysts also occur as thin-walled structures containing clear colourless fluid. Histologically, the cyst wall is made up of flattened arachnoidal cells. Their origin is not known, but has been attributed to trauma or inflammation. The intradural ependymal cyst develops most often anteriorly to the cervical cord of children. It is lined by cuboidal or columnar ciliated epithelium. Even though benign histologically, it may recur if excised incompletely.

Metastatic tumours

The true incidence of metastatic carcinoma in the central nervous system is difficult to establish. It is, however, a common tumour and may be as frequent as, or even more common than, tumours of neuroepithelial tissue. The lesions are often multiple and often occur in the extradural space of the thoracic spine (Stark *et al.*, 1982): both intradural and intramedullary lesions also occur (Perrin *et al.*, 1982; Costigan & Winkelman, 1985). In many patients there are widespread deposits of tumour. The primary tumours giving rise to extradural metastases are most commonly of bronchus, breast, prostate and kidney, in that order.

Tumours of neuroepithelium, particularly medulloblastoma and lymphoma, may spread throughout the subarachnoid space but meningeal carcinomatosis is the most common type of diffuse meningeal tumour. In many cases there is no other evidence of metastatic carcinoma in the brain. It is often possible to identify some thickening and opalescence of the pia arachnoid, and small nodules of tumour on the nerve roots of the cauda equina, which tend also to be rather matted together and difficult to separate, are also seen (Henson & Urich, 1982). The majority of tumours that cause meningeal carcinomatosis are adenocarcinomas. Histologically, carcinoma cells are seen diffusely throughout the subarachnoid space, and it is not uncommon to see a monolayer of cells growing on the pia. Tumour cells can usually be identified in the CSF, although several specimens may have to be examined (Boyle *et al.*, 1980).

REFERENCES

Adams, J.H., Graham, D.I. & Doyle, D. (1981) *Brain Biopsy: The Smear Technique for Neurosurgical Biopsies.* Chapman & Hall, London.

Agnoli, A.L., Laun, A. & Schonmayr, R. (1984) Enterogenous intraspinal cysts. *J. Neurosurg.*, **61**, 834–840.

Alter, M. (1975) Statistical aspects of spinal cord tumors. In Vinken, P.J. & Bruyn, G.W. (eds) *Handbook of Clinical Neurology*, vol. 19, pp. 1–22. North-Holland, Amsterdam.

Baker, N.D. (1986) Symptomatic vertebral haemangiomas: a report of 4 cases. *Skeletal Radiol.*, **15**, 458–463.

Bamborschke, S., Ebhardt, G., Szelies-Stock, B., Dreesbach, H.A. & Heiss, W.D. (1985) Review and case report: primary melanoblastosis of the leptomeninges. *Clin. Neuropathol.*, **4**, 47–55.

Barwick, K.W., Huvos, A.G. & Smith, J. (1980) Primary osteogenic sarcoma of the vertebral column. A clinicopathologic correlation of ten patients. *Cancer*, **46**, 595–604.

Bertoni, F., Unni, K.K., McLeod, R.A. & Dahlin, D.C. (1985) Osteosarcoma resembling osteoblastoma. *Cancer*, **55**, 416–426.

Bevilacqua, G. & Sarnelli, R. (1979) Ganglioglioma of the spinal cord. A case with a long survival. *Acta Neuropathol.*, **48**, 239–242.

Blackie, R.A.S. & Gordon, A. (1984) Histological appearances of intracranial biopsies obtained using the Cavitron ultrasonic surgical aspirator. *J. Clin. Pathol.*, **37**, 1101–1104.

Blaylock, R.L. & Kempe, L.G. (1976) Chondrosarcoma of the cervical spine. *J. Neurosurg.*, **44**, 500–503.

Bohlman, H.H., Sachs, B.L., Carter, J.R., Riley, L. & Robinson, R.A. (1986) Primary neoplasms of the cervical spine. *J. Bone Jt. Surg.*, **68A**, 483–494.

Boland, P.J., Lane, J.M. & Sundaresan, N. (1982) Metastatic disease of the spine. *Clin. Orthop.*, **169**, 95–102.

Boyd, H.R. (1966) Iatrogenic intraspinal epidermoid. *J. Neurosurg.*, **24**, 105–107.

Boyle, R., Thomas, M. & Adams, J.H. (1980) Diffuse involvement of the leptomeninges by tumour—a clinical and pathological study of 63 cases. *Postgrad. Med. J.*, **56**, 149–158.

Bullough, P.G. & Boachie-Adjei, O. (1988) *Atlas of Spinal Diseases.* Gower, New York.

Burger, P.C., Scheithaver, B.W. & Vogel, F.S. (1991) *Surgical Pathology of the Nervous System and its Coverings*, 3rd edn., pp. 605–660. Churchill Livingstone, New York.

Calogero, J.A. & Moossy, J. (1972) Extradural spinal meningiomas. Report of four cases. *J. Neurosurg.*, **37**, 442–447.

Camins, M.B., Duncan, A.W., Smith, J. & Marcove, R.C. (1978) Chondrosarcoma of the spine. *Spine*, **3**, 202–209.

Canadell, J., Villas, C., Martinez-Densgri, J., Azcarate, J. & Imizcoz, A. (1986) Vertebral eosinophilic granuloma. Long term evolution of a case. *Spine*, **11**, 767–769.

Capanna, R., Albisinni, U., Picci, P., Calderoni, P., Campanacci, M. & Springfield, D.S. (1985) Aneurysmal bone cyst of the spine. *J. Bone Jt. Surg.*, **67A**, 527–531.

Chambers, P.W. & Schwinn, C.P. (1979) Chordoma. A clinicopathologic study of metastases. *Am. J. Clin. Pathol.*, **72**, 765–776.

Choremis, C., Economos, D., Papodatos, C. & Gargoulas, A. (1956) Intraspinal epidermoid tumours (cholesteatomas) in patients treated for tuberculous meningitis. *Lancet*, **ii**, 437–439.

Cohen, D.M., Dahlin, D.C. & MacCarty, C.S. (1964) Apparently solitary tumors of the vertebral column. *Mayo Clin. Proc.*, **39**, 509–528.

Constans, J.P., de Divitiis, E., Donzelli, R., Spaziante, R., Meder, J.F. & Haye, C. (1983) Spinal metastases with neurological manifestations. *J. Neurosurg.*, **59**, 111–118.

Cooper, I.S., Craig, W.McK. & Kernohan, J.W. (1951) Tumors of the spinal cord: primary extramedullary gliomas. *Surg. Gynecol. Obstet.*, **92**, 183–190.

Costigan, D.A. & Winkelman, M.D. (1985) Intramedullary spinal cord metastasis. A clinicopathological study of 13 cases. *J. Neurosurg.*, **62**, 227–233.

Dahlin, D.C. (1977) Giant cell tumor of vertebrae above the sacrum. A review of 31 cases. *Cancer*, **39**, 1350–1356.

Dahlin, D.C. & Unni, K.K. (1986) *Bone Tumors: General Aspects and Data on 8,542 Cases.* Thomas, Springfield.

Delauche-Cavallier, M.C., Laredo, J.D., Wybier, M., Bard, M., Mazabraud, A., Darne, J.L.L., Kuntz, D. & Ryckewaert, A. (1988) Solitary plasmacytoma of the spine. Long term clinical course. *Cancer*, **62**, 1707–1714.

Dohrman, G.J., Farwell, J.R. & Flannery, J.T. (1976) Ependymomas and ependymoblastoma in children. *J. Neurosurg.*, **45**, 273–283.

Dorfman, H.D. & Weiss, S.W. (1984) Borderline osteoblastic tumors: problems in the differential diagnosis of aggressive osteoblastoma and low-grade osteosarcoma. *Semin. Diag. Pathol.*, **1**, 215–234.

Dowdle, J.A. Jr, Winter, R.B. & Dehner, L.P. (1977) Postradiation osteosarcoma of the cervical spine in childhood. A case report. *J Bone Jt. Surg.*, **59A**, 969–971.

Driedger, H. & Pruzanski, W. (1979) Plasma cell neoplasia with osteosclerotic lesions. A study of five cases and a review of the literature. *Arch. Intern. Med.*, **139**, 892–896.

Earnest, F., Kernohan, J.W. & Craig, W.M. (1950) Oligodendrogliomas. A review of two hundred cases. *Arch. Neurol. Psychiatry*, **63**, 964–976.

Enneking, W.F. (1983) *Musculoskeletal Tumor Surgery.* Churchill Livingstone, New York.

Epstein, F. & Epstein, N. (1982) Surgical treatment of spinal cord astrocytoma of childhood. A series of 19 patients. *J. Neurosurg.*, **57**, 685–689.

Faillace, W.J., Okaware, S.-H. & McDonald, J.V. (1984) Neurocutaneous melanomas with extensive intracerebral and spinal involvement. *J. Neurosurg.*, **61**, 782–785.

Falini, B., Binazzi, R., Pileri, S., Mori, A., Bertoni, S., Canino, M., Fagiolo, M., Minelli, O., Ciani, C. & Pellicioli, P. (1988) Large cell lymphoma of bone. A report of three cases of B-cell origin. *Histopathology*, **12**, 177–190.

Ferris, R.A., Pettrone, F.A., McKelvie, A.M., Twigg, H.L. & Chun, B.K. (1974) Eosinophilic granuloma of the spine: an unusual radiographic presentation. *Clin. Orthop.*, **99**, 57–63.

Fornasier, V.L. & Horne, J.G. (1975) Metastases to the vertebral column. *Cancer*, **36**, 590–594.

Fortuna, A., Celli, P. & Palma, L. (1980) Oligodendrogliomas of the spinal cord. *Acta Neurochir.*, **52**, 305–329.

Fox, J.L., Bashir, R., Jinkins, J.R. & Al-Mefty, O. (1985) Syrinx of the conus medullaris and filum terminale in association with multiple hemangioblastomas. *Surg. Neurol.*, **24**, 265–271.

Frassica, F.J., Unni, K.K., Beabout, J.W. & Sim, F.H. (1986) Dedifferentiated chondrosarcoma. A report of the clinicopathological features and treatment of seventy-eight cases. *J. Bone Jt. Surg.*, **68A**, 1197–1205.

Furtado, D. & Marques, V. (1951) Spinal teratoma. *J. Neuropathol. Exp. Neurol.*, **10**, 384–393.

Garrison, J.E. & Kasdon, D.L. (1980) Intramedullary spinal teratoma. Case report and review of the literature. *Neurosurgery*, **7**, 509–512.

Grant, J.W., Kaech, D. & Jones, D.B. (1986) Spinal cord compression as the first presentation of lymphoma—a review of 15 cases. *Histopathology*, **10**, 1191–1202.

Green, N.E., Robertson, W.W. & Kilroy, A.W. (1980) Eosinophilic granuloma of the spine with associated neural deficit. Report of three cases. *J. Bone Jt. Surg.*, **62A**, 1198–1202.

Harrington, K.D. (1986) Metastatic disease of the spine. *J. Bone Jt. Surg.*, **68A**, 1110–1115.

Hay, M.C., Paterson, D. & Taylor, T.K.F. (1978) Aneurysmal bone cysts of the spine. *J. Bone Jt. Surg.*, **60B**, 406–411.

Hautzer, N.W., Aiyesimoju, A. & Robitaille, Y. (1983) 'Primary' spinal intramedullary lymphomas: a review. *Ann. Neurol.*, **14**, 62–66.

Henson, R.A. & Urich, H. (1982) *Cancer and the Nervous System. The Neurological Manifestations of Systemic Malignant Disease.* Blackwell Scientific Publications, Oxford.

Hochberg, F.H. & Miller, D.C. (1988) Primary central nervous system lymphoma. *J. Neurosurg.*, **68**, 835–853.

Horan, F.T. (1969) Bone involvement in Hodgkin's disease. *Br. J. Surg.*, **56**, 277–281.

Horton, W.A., Wong, V. & Eldridge, R. (1976) Von Hippel-Lindau disease. Clinical and pathological manifestations in nine families with 50 affected members. *Arch. Intern. Med.*, **136**, 769–777.

Hughes, J.T. (1978) *Pathology of the Spinal Cord*, pp. 218–241. Lloyd Luke, London.

Huvos, A.G. (1979) *Bone Tumors, Diagnosis, Treatment and Prognosis.* W.B. Saunders, Philadelphia.

Inglis, A.E., Rubin, R.M., Lewis, R.J. & Villacin, A. (1977) Osteochondroma of the cervical spine. *Clin. Orthop.*, **126**, 127–129.

Ippolito, E., Farsetti, P. & Tudisco, C. (1984) Vertebra plana.

Long term follow up in five patients. *J. Bone Jt. Surg.*, **66A**, 1364–1368.

Ismail, S.M. & Cole, G. (1984) Von Hippel–Lindau syndrome with microscopic hemangioblastomas of the spinal nerve roots. *J. Neurosurg.*, **60**, 1279–1281.

Jellinger, K., Radaszkiewicz, T. & Slowik, F. (1975) Primary malignant lymphomas of the central nervous system in man. *Acta Neuropathol. (Berl).*, Suppl VI, 95–102.

Julien, J., Riemens, V., Vital, C., Lagueny, A. & Miet, G. (1978) Cervical cord compression by solitary osteochondroma of the atlas. *J. Neurol. Neurosurg. Psychiatry*, **41**, 479–481.

Keim, H.A. & Reina, E.G. (1975) Osteoid osteoma as a cause of scoliosis. *J. Bone Jt. Surg.*, **57A**, 159–163.

Kepes, J.J. (1982) *Meningiomas. Biology, Pathology and Differential Diagnosis.* Masson, New York.

Kepes, J.J., Belton, K., Roessmann, U. & Ketcherside, W.J. (1985) Primitive neuroectodermal tumours of the cauda equina in adults with no detectable primary intracranial neoplasm—three case studies. *Clin. Neuropathol.*, **4**, 1–11.

Kirwan, E.O'G., Hutton, P.A.N., Pozo, J.L. & Ransford, A.O. (1984) Osteoid osteoma and benign osteoblastoma of the spine. Clinical presentation and treatment. *J. Bone Jt. Surg.*, **66B**, 21–26.

Kitahara, M., Katakura, R., Wada, T., Namiki, T. & Suzuki, J. (1985) Diffuse form of primary leptomeningeal gliomatosis. *J. Neurosurg.*, **63**, 283–287.

Kleinman, W.B., Kiernan, H.A. & Michelsen, W.J. (1978) Metastatic cancer of the spinal column. *Clin. Orthop.*, **136**, 166–172.

Kurland, L.T. (1958) The frequency of intracranial and intraspinal neoplasms in the resident population of Rochester, Minnesota. *J. Neurosurg.*, **15**, 627–641.

Langford, L.A., Cartreras, F.L. & McCormick, W.F. (1987) Tumors of the spinal canal. In Davidoff, R.A. (ed.) *Handbook of the Spinal Cord*, vols 4 and 5, pp. 371–409. Marcel Dekker, New York.

Larsson, S.E., Lorentzon, R. & Boquist, L. (1975) Giant cell tumors of the spine and sacrum causing neurological symptoms. *Clin. Orthop.*, **111**, 201–211.

Lassmann, H., Jurecka, W., Lassmann, G., Gebhart, W., Matras, H. & Watzek, G. (1977) Different types of benign nerve sheath tumours. Light microscopy, electron microscopy and autoradiograpy. *Virch. Arch. (Pathol. Anat).*, **375**, 157–210.

Lott, I.T. & Richardson, E.P. (1981) Neuropathological findings and the biology of neurofibromatosis. In Riccardi, V.M. & Mulvihill, J.J. (eds) *Neurofibromatosis (von Recklinghausen's Disease); Advances in Neurology*, vol. 29, pp. 23–32. Raven Press, New York.

Manno, M.J., Uihlein, A. & Kernohan, J.W. (1962) Intraspinal epidermoid. *J. Neurosurg.*, **19**, 754–765.

Marsh, B.W., Bonfiglio, M., Brady, L.P. & Enneking, W.F. (1975) Benign osteoblastoma: range of manifestations. *J. Bone Jt. Surg.*, **57A**, 1–9.

Marsh, H.O. & Choi, C.-B. (1970) Primary osteogenic sarcoma of the cervical spine originally mistaken for benign osteoblastoma. *J. Bone Jt. Surg.*, **52A**, 1467–1471.

Matson, D.D. & Tachdjian, M.O. (1963) Intraspinal tumours in infants and children. Review of 115 cases. *Postgrad. Med. J.*, **34**, 279–285.

Meis, J.M., Butler, J.J., Osborne, B.M. & Ordonez, N.G. (1987) Solitary plasmacytomas of bone and extramedullary plasmacytomas. *Cancer*, **59**, 1475–1485.

Mirra, J.M. (1989) *Bone Tumors.* Lea & Febiger, Philadelphia.

Mork, S.J. & Loken, A.C. (1977) Ependymoma. A follow-up study of 101 cases. *Cancer*, **40**, 907–915.

Myles, S.T. & MacRae, M.E. (1988) Benign osteoblastoma of the spine in childhood. *J. Neurosurg.*, **68**, 884–888.

McAllister, V.L., Kendall, B.E. & Bull, J.W.D. (1975) Symptomatic vertebral haemangiomas. *Brain*, **98**, 71–80.

MacCarty, C.S., Dahlin, D.C., Doyle, J.B. Jr, Lipscomb, P.R. & Pugh, D.G. (1961) Aneurysmal bone cysts of the neural axis. *J. Neurosurg.*, **18**, 671–677.

MacLellan, D.I. & Wilson, F.C. (1967) Osteoid osteoma of the spine. A review of the literature and report of six new cases. *J. Bone Jt. Surg.*, **49A**, 111–121.

McLeod, R.A., Dahlin, D.C. & Beabout, J.W. (1976) The spectrum of osteoblastoma. *Am. J. Roentgenol.*, **126**, 321–335.

Newcomer, L.N., Silverstein, M.B., Cadman, E.C., Farber, L.R., Bertino, J.R. & Prosnitz, L.R. (1982) Bone involvement in Hodgkin's disease. *Cancer*, **49**, 338–342.

O'Connor, G.A. & Roberts, T.S. (1984) Spinal cord compression by an osteochondroma in a patient with multiple osteochondromatosis. *J. Neurosurg.*, **60**, 420–423.

Ogihara, Y., Sekiguchi, K. & Tsuruta, T. (1984) Osteogenic sarcoma of the fourth thoracic vertebra. Long term survival by chemotherapy only. *Cancer*, **53**, 2615–2618.

Onimus, M., Schraub, S., Bertin, D., Bosset, J.F. & Guidet, M. (1986) Surgical treatment of vertebral metastasis. *Spine*, **11**, 883–891.

Pena, C.E., Horvat, B.L. & Fisher, E.R. (1970) The ultrastructure of chordoma. *Am. J. Clin. Pathol.*, **53**, 544–551.

Perrin, R.G., Livingston, K.E. & Aarbi, B. (1982) Intradural extramedullary spinal metastasis. A report of 10 cases. *J. Neurosurg.*, **56**, 835–837.

Pettine, K.A. & Klassen, R.A. (1986) Osteoid-osteoma and osteoblastoma of the spine. *J. Bone Jt. Surg.*, **68A**, 354–361.

Polkey, C.E. (1975) Intraosseous neurilemmoma of the cervical spine causing paraparesis and treated by resection and grafting. *J. Neurol. Neurosurg. Psychiatry*, **38**, 776–781.

Poser, C.M. (1956) *The Relationship Between Syringomyelia and Neoplasm.* Thomas, Springfield.

Reimer, R. & Onofrio, B.M. (1985) Astrocytomas of the spinal cord in children and adolescents. *J. Neurosurg.*, **63**, 669–675.

Robert, H., Dubousset, J. & Miladi, L. (1987) Histiocytosis X in the juvenile spine. *Spine*, **12**, 167–172.

Roman, G. (1978) Hereditary multiple exostoses. A rare cause of spinal cord compression. *Spine*, **3**, 230–233.

Ross, D.A., Edwards, M.S.B. & Wilson, C.B. (1986) Intramedullary neurilemmoma of the spinal cord: report of two cases and review of the literature. *Neurosurgery*, **19**,

458–464.

Rubinstein, L.J. (1986) The malformative central nervous system lesions in the central and peripheral forms of neurofibromatosis. A neuropathological study of 22 cases. *Ann. NY Acad. Sci.*, **486**, 14–29.

Russell, D.S. & Rubinstein, L.J. (1989) *Pathology of Tumours of the Nervous System*, 5th edn. Edward Arnold, London.

Salisbury, J. & Isaacson, P. (1985) Demonstration of cytokeratins and an epithelial membrane antigen in chordomas and human foetal notochord. *Am. J. Surg. Pathol.*, **9**, 791–797.

Savini, R., Gherlinzoni, F., Morandi, M., Neff, J.R. & Picci, P. (1983) Surgical treatment of giant-cell tumor of the spine. *J. Bone Jt. Surg*, **65A**, 1283–1289.

Schajowicz, F. (1981) *Tumors and Tumorlike Lesions of Bone and Joints*. Springer Verlag, New York.

Schajowicz, F., Araujo, E.S. & Berenstein, M. (1983) Sarcoma complicating Paget's disease of bone. *J. Bone Jt. Surg.*, **65B**, 299–307.

Shives, T.C., Dahlan, D.C., Sim, F.H., Pritchard, D.J. & Earle, J.D. (1986) Osteosarcoma of the spine. *J. Bone Jt. Surg.*, **68A**, 660–668.

Silverman, J.F., Jones, F.D., Unverferth, M. & Berns, L. (1989) Cytopathology of neoplasms of the central nervous system in specimens obtained by the Cavitron ultrasonic surgical aspirator. *Acta Cytol.*, **33**, 576–582.

Simon, J., Jones, E.L., Trumper, M.M. & Salmon, M.V. (1987) Malignant lymphomas involving the central nervous system—a morphological and immunohistochemical study of 32 cases. *Histopathology*, **11**, 335–349.

Slooff, J.L., Kernohan, J.W. & MacCarty, C.S. (1964) *Primary Intramedullary Tumors of the Spinal Cord and Filum Terminale*. Saunders, Philadelphia.

So, Y.T., Beckstead, J.H. & Davis, R.L. (1986) Primary central nervous system lymphoma in acquired immune deficiency syndrome: a clinical and pathological study. *Ann. Neurol.*, **20**, 566–572.

Sonneland, P.R.L., Scheithauer, B.W. & Onofrio, P.M. (1985) Myxopapillary ependymoma. A clinicopathologic and immunocytochemical study of 77 cases. *Cancer*, **56**, 883–893.

Stark, R.J., Henson, R.A. & Evans, S.J.W. (1982) Spinal metastasis. A retrospective survey from a general hospital. *Brain*, **105**, 189–213.

Stillwell, W.T. & Fielding, J.W. (1984) Aneurysmal bone cyst of the cervicodorsal spine. *Clin. Orthop.*, **187**, 144–146.

Sundaresan, N. (1986) Chordomas. *Clin. Orthop.*, **204**, 135–142.

Tillman, B.P., Dahlin, D.C., Lipscomb, P.R. & Stewart, J.R. (1968) Aneurysmal bone cyst; an analysis of 95 cases. *Mayo Clin. Proc.*, **43**, 478–495.

Triche, T. & Cavazzana, A. (1988) Round cell tumors of bone. In Unni, K.K. (ed.) *Contemporary Issues in Surgical Pathology*, vol. 11, pp. 199–223. Churchill Livingstone, New York.

Valderrama, J.A.F. & Bullough, P.G. (1968) Solitary myeloma of the spine. *J. Bone Jt. Surg.*, **50B**, 82–90.

Webb, J.H., Craig, W.M. & Kernohan, J.W. (1953) Intraspinal neoplasms in the cervical region. *J. Neurosurg.*, **10**, 360–366.

Weinstein, J.N. & McLain, R.F. (1987) Primary tumors of the spine. *Spine*, **12**, 843–851.

Weinstein, J.B., Siegel, M.J. & Griffith, R.C. (1984) Spinal Ewing sarcoma: misleading appearances. *Skeletal Radiol.*, **11**, 262–265.

WHO (1979) Histological classification of tumours of the central nervous system. *International Histological Classification of Tumours*, No. 21, WHO, Geneva.

Wilhyde, D.E., Jane, J.A. & Mullan, S. (1963) Spinal epidural leukemia. *Am. J. Med.*, **34**, 281–287.

Wronski, J., Bryc, S., Kaminski, J. & Chibowski, D. (1964) Chondrosarcoma of cervical spine causing compression of the cord. *J. Neurosurg.*, **21**, 419–421.

Wyburn-Mason, R. (1944) *The Vascular Abnormalities and Tumours of the Spinal Cord and its Membrane*. C.V. Mosby, St Louis, MI.

Yasargil, M.G., Antic, J., Laciga, R., de Preux, J., Fideler, R.W. & Brone, S.C. (1976) The microsurgical removal of intramedullary spinal hemangioblastomas. Report of twelve cases and a review of the literature. *Surg. Neurol.*, **6**, 141–148.

27 · Primary Tumours of the Spine

By R.M. MORAN and J.K. WEBB

Primary tumours of the spine can be benign or malignant. Benign tumours are exceedingly rare; it has been estimated that they account for about 1–2% of primary skeletal tumours (Dahlin, 1978). They also account for a minority of primary vertebral tumours, with the estimated incidence varying from about 10% to almost 40% (Paillas *et al.*, 1975; Weinstein & McLain, 1987), the majority being malignant. Clinically, benign tumours are difficult to diagnose, as the lesions are rare, seldom suspected, and lack specific symptoms and signs. The most common presenting symptom is back pain, more commonly presenting in adolescents and young adults. Patients may complain of radiating pain, although specific neurological deficits due to benign tumours are rare. Such deficits will occur only if a benign tumour is strategically located within the spinal canal or the foramina, resulting in spinal cord or nerve root compression. Back pain, with or without radiation, is also the most common presenting feature of primary malignant tumours of the spine (Weinstein & McLain, 1987). The pain pattern is often similar in both benign and malignant lesions. Typically, the pain is constant and unresponsive to conservative measures. It often occurs at night and increases when the patient lies supine (Sim *et al.*, 1977; Friedlander & Southwick, 1982; Delamarter *et al.*, 1990). The severity of the pain increases more rapidly in patients with malignant lesions. Weinstein & McLain found that the mean interval from onset of symptoms to diagnosis was 10.4 months in patients with malignant lesions, and 19.3 months in those with benign lesions. Spinal deformity, particularly scoliosis, can occasionally be a presenting sign of both benign and malignant spinal tumours, particularly in adolescents (Thommesen & Poulsen, 1976).

Age and location can help distinguish benign from malignant primary spinal tumours. In Weinstein & McLain's series the mean age of diagnosis of benign lesions was 21 years, compared with 49 years for malignant lesions. In primary malignant spinal lesions the tumour was located in the vertebral body in 80% of cases, compared with just over 40% of patients with benign lesions. Neurological deficit was a more common finding in patients with primary malignant disease. Fifty-five per cent of patients presenting with primary malignant spinal tumours had neurological involvement, compared with 35% of those with benign spinal lesions.

Patients with spinal cord compression usually present with upper motoneurone lesion signs, including weakness, spasticity, hyperreflexia, upgoing plantar reflexes and sensory loss. Bowel and bladder function may be affected. Patients with extensive involvement may have severe paraparesis, while patients with less significant involvement may present with patchy asymmetric signs. Primary spinal tumours causing such symptoms are usually malignant, as such lesions are usually located in the vertebral bodies from where cord compression due to tumour extension or vertebral body collapse is more likely. Signs of lower motoneurone lesions, such as muscle weakness, fasciculation, diminished reflexes and loss of sensation, are more likely to occur due to nerve root involvement, and are more common with benign lesions.

It is usually not possible to make an accurate diagnosis of a primary spinal tumour from plain radiographs. Only certain primary tumours, such as osteochondroma and haemangioma, have characteristic features on the plain radiograph suggestive of the correct diagnosis. Usually, further radiological investigation, such as bone scan, computerized tomography (CT) with or without contrast, or magnetic resonance imaging (MRI), are necessary. Certain features regarding the location of the tumour may increase the likelihood of it being benign. Osteoid osteoma and osteoblastoma characteristically arise in the posterior elements (Sabanas *et al.*, 1956), while aneurysmal bone cysts and giant-cell tumours often involve both the posterior elements and the vertebral body. Tumours located primarily in the vertebral body are usually malignant, most commonly due to metastatic disease. The incidence of primary tumours is greatest in the proximal spine. Most cervical primary tumours are benign, while the majority of sacrococcygeal tumours are malignant (Weinstein & McLain, 1987).

Benign tumours distinguish themselves by remaining within their tissue of origin. Even within bone they are contained within their own capsule, and grow along lines of least resistance, which is between the trabeculae or along the Haversian systems. These finger-like extensions are a major reason why certain benign tumours, such as giant-cell tumours and osteoblastomas, have a significant recurrence rate following surgery (Askin & Webb, 1991). Recurrence rates of up to 20% have been reported following surgical excision of benign tumours (Weinstein & McLain, 1987).

Malignant lesions, on the other hand, have the capacity to penetrate the capsule. The host reaction is to form a reactive zone around the advancing lesion. The more aggressive the lesion, the more tumour tends to outgrow this reactive zone. Growth occurs by tumour causing compression and stimulated resorption of normal tissue, and also by direct tissue destruction. New bone formation is a frequent feature of such malignant growth. However, in the majority of cases this is as a result of reactive new bone formation. Only osteosarcomas characteristically form primary osteoid and new bone within the tumour.

Primary malignant tumours to the vertebral column are extremely difficult to differentiate from the more common metastatic lesions. Features of vertebral body involvement with bone destruction and collapse and reactive bone formation are common to both. Most primary malignant tumours, however, are solitary, whereas metastatic lesions are frequently multiple. A bone scan revealing either single or multiple lesions is a useful investigation in distinguishing these lesions.

When evaluating either benign or malignant tumours it is necessary to be able to stage the tumours accurately so that appropriate treatment can be recommended, and the risk of local recurrence reasonably evaluated. Most published reports on primary tumours of the spine do not attempt to stage them, as there are usually such small numbers involved in each category. The application of a staging system to these tumours should allow for adequate comparison of tumour types between various centres to be performed, thus enabling evaluation of various treatment modalities. The most appropriate system for staging primary tumours of the spine is to use the staging system for musculoskeletal neoplasms, as proposed by Enneking (1986).

The simplest form of this staging system is shown in Table 27.1. Latent, benign lesions are usually asymptomatic lesions that are discovered incidentally. They can grow to various sizes but are usually limited by contact inhibition. Examples include eosinophilic granuloma and non-ossified fibroma. When excision is undertaken, for example to establish a diagnosis, recurrence is virtually unknown. Active benign lesions can be mildly symptomatic, usually grow larger than latent lesions, and may expand the containing bone. Osteoblastomas are typical of such lesions. There is a significant recurrence rate if the capsule is breached in removing such tumours, although there is very low recurrence rate if extracapsular excision is possible. Enneking (1983) has suggested the use of thermal and/or cryosurgery in addition to surgical excision in questionable cases,

Table 27.1 Staging of musculoskeletal neoplasms

Benign	
1	Latent
2	Active
3	Aggressive
Malignant	
I	Low-grade without metastases
Ia	Intracompartmental
Ib	Extracompartmental
II	High-grade without metastases
IIa	Intracompartmental
IIb	Extracompartmental
III	Low/high-grade with metastases
IIIa	Intracompartmental
IIIb	Extracompartmental

to decrease the likelihood of recurrence. Aggressive benign tumours include the aggressive form of giant-cell tumour. Wide surgical margins are necessary to prevent recurrence of such lesions following excision, and this is particularly difficult to produce in the spine. Fortunately, most giant-cell tumours that do affect the spine are not of the aggressive type, and this reduces the incidence of recurrence.

There are three grades of malignant lesion which are each subdivided into intra- or extracompartmental. In reference to the spine an intracompartmental tumour is one which is completely intra-osseous without any soft tissue extension. This grading system is easy to apply, and has obvious prognostic value, as, for example, a patient with a Type IIIb lesion will have a poor prognosis, irrespective of the tumour type.

A useful classification for benign and malignant tumours is given in Table 27.2, which is based upon the tissue type from which the tumour derives. Benign, tumour-like lesions, such as aneurysmal bone cyst and eosinophilic granuloma, are also included in this chapter, as they should be considered in the differential diagnosis of benign spinal lesions.

TUMOUR TYPES

Benign tumours

Osteoblastoma

This tumour was first described as a distinct entity by Jaffe in 1956. It is a rare tumour, still occasionally reported in the medical literature in the form of case

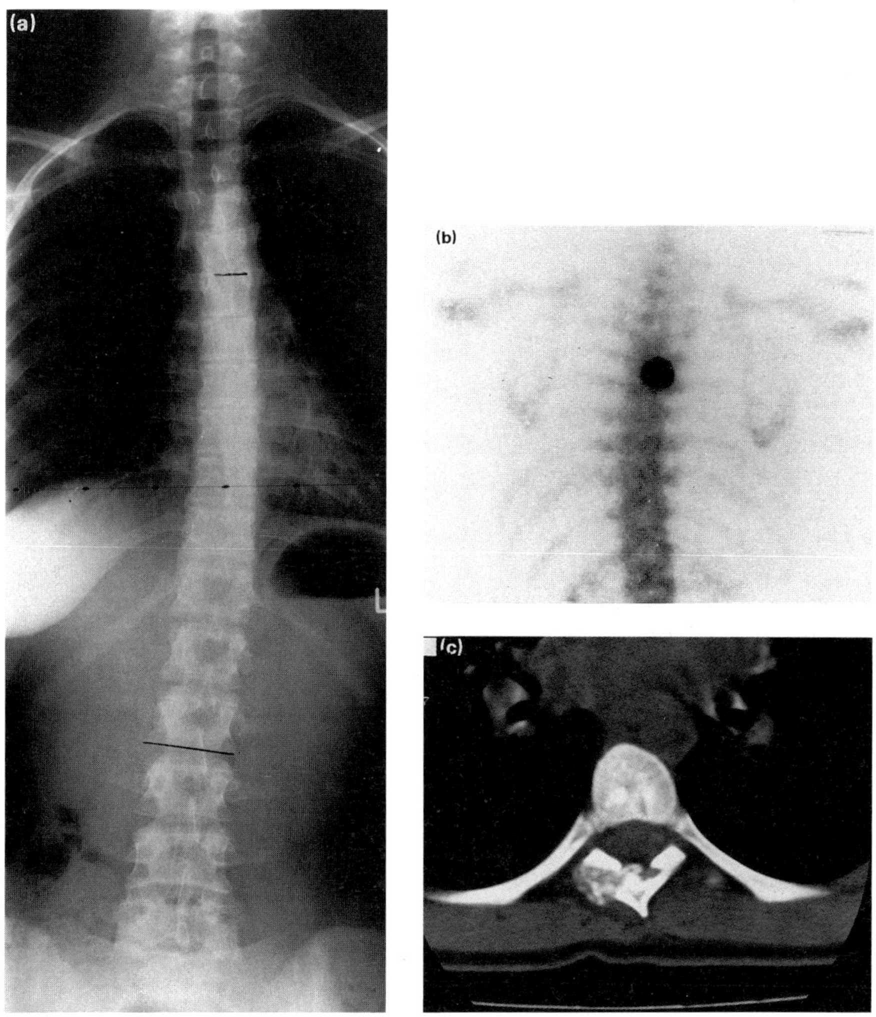

Fig. 27.1 Osteoblastoma. A 14-year-old girl presented with a four-year history of intermittent intrascapular back pain. (a) Plain X-ray shows a mild scoliosis but no specific anomaly in the midthoracic region. (b) Technetium bone scan shows an area of intense increased uptake to the right of the midline at T6. (c) CT scan reveals the typical features of an osteoblastoma with an expansile destructive mass of the lamina, with a finger-like extension into the extradural space. Patient had complete relief of symptoms following surgical excision, combined with a single-level fusion.

Table 27.2 Classification of primary bone tumours according to their tissue of origin

Derivation or type of tumour	Benign	Malignant
Fibrous tissue	Non-ossifying fibroma; desmoplastic fibroma	Fibrosarcoma
Cartilage	Osteocartilaginous exostosis; enchondroma Benign chondroblastoma Chondromyxoid fibroma	Secondary chondrosarcoma Primary chondrosarcoma Mesenchymal chondrosarcoma
Bone	Osteoma; osteoid osteoma Benign osteoblastoma	Osteosarcoma (including some Paget's and postirradiation sarcomas) Parosteal osteosarcoma
Unknown	Giant-cell tumour	Giant-cell tumour; Ewing's tumour; 'adamantinoma' of long bones
Vascular tissue	Haemangioma Glomus tumour	Haemangioendothelioma Haemangiopericytoma
Fat cells	Lipoma	Liposarcoma
Haematopoietic	Solitary plasmacytoma	Myelomatosis; malignant lymphoma
Neural tissue	Schwannoma; neurofibroma	Malignant schwannoma
Notochordal tissue		Chordoma
Histiocytes		Malignant fibrous histiocytoma

reports (Akbarnia & Rooholamini, 1981; Shikata *et al.*, 1987). It occurs twice as commonly in males as in females, usually presenting in the second decade (Huvos, 1979a). It is usually located in the posterior elements (Nemoto *et al.*, 1990) (Fig. 27.1). Once diagnosed, it can grow rapidly in size over a short period of time (Pochaczevsky *et al.*, 1960).

Histological differentiation between osteoblastoma and osteoid osteoma can be difficult. In many cases this is arbitrarily resolved on the basis of size, with lesions greater than 1.5 cm in diameter being considered as osteoblastoma. Occasionally, difficulty has been encountered histologically in differentiating osteoblastoma from osteogenic sarcoma. This difficulty can be compounded by the fact that there is a definite recurrence rate following surgical excision of osteoblastoma. Radiologically, osteoblastoma can appear either as a radiolucent area alone or as a radiolucent area surrounded by an area of sclerosis (McLeod *et al.*, 1976). In the absence of sclerosis there can be some difficulty differentiating it from an aneurysmal bone cyst. Osteoblastomas without surrounding sclerosis may not be visible on plain radiographs.

Patients with osteoblastoma may present with back pain, either diffuse or localized. Patients may also present with radiating pain. Patients presenting with neurological deficits due to direct pressure of osteoblastoma on either the spinal cord or nerve root are well recognized (Myles & MacRae, 1988). Patients who present with a painful scoliosis usually have the osteoblastoma located at the apex of the curve (Dahlin, 1978; Akbarnia & Rooholamini, 1981).

Isotope bone scan is invariably positive, showing a marked increase in uptake at the tumour site. Once the lesion is accurately localized by isotope bone scan, a CT scan of the involved region invariably gives good detail of the lesion. Characteristically, this is an expansile area surrounded by an area of sclerosis.

Treatment is surgical, involving complete excision of the lesion. Lesions that are completely confined to the posterior elements are usually readily accessible by a posterior approach. Larger lesions, and particularly those located in the cervical spine, may demand a combined anterior and posterior approach, increasing the technical difficulty of the operation and therefore the risk of incomplete removal (Shikata *et al.*, 1987). Although recurrence following surgery is well recognized it is unusual, and significant recurrence of the tumour may not occur even following incomplete removal of the tumour (Marsh *et al.*, 1975). If a significant amount of bony resection is necessary to remove the lesion, bone grafting of the defect, usually involving fusion of the involved segment, is often necessary. Postoperative irradiation has often been performed, particularly in cases of incomplete removal, but there is no evidence that this decreases the rate of recurrence, and some evidence to suggest that it may lead to an increase in the incidence of sarcomatous change (Dahlin, 1978; Myles & MacRae, 1988).

Osteoid osteoma

Osteoid osteoma is a rare, benign lesion of bone that was also initially described by Jaffe in 1935. Osteoid osteomas most commonly occur in the thoracic and lumbar regions, although there are several case reports of occurrence in the cervical spine (Janin *et al.*, 1981; Polivy *et al.*, 1986). It is differentiated from osteoblastoma by its size, osteoid osteoma being less than 1.5 cm diameter. The characteristic finding with osteoid osteoma is a radiolucent nidus. This nidus may be difficult to detect, particularly in the vertebral column. It does, however, usually provoke an intense bony reaction with surrounding sclerosis, which is often the only radiographic sign of the lesion.

The differentiation between osteoid osteoma and osteoblastoma is, however, important, as the latter is more likely to be expansile in nature, and so is often associated with a narrowing of the spinal canal or neural foramina, resulting in some neurological deficit. This is not a feature of osteoid osteomas, which are not associated with neurological signs.

Osteoid osteoma usually presents in patients in the second and third decades. The male/female ratio for this lesion in the spine is 6 : 1 (MacLellan & Wilson, 1967; Caldicott, 1969). In common with most other benign tumours it rarely occurs in the vertebral column. Only nine out of 158 osteoid osteomas, reported by Dahlin, occurred in the vertebral column.

Back pain, which is often localized, is invariably the presenting feature of this lesion. Radiating pain can be a feature, due to referred dermatomal pain, but characteristically there is rarely any evidence of neurological deficit (Zwimpfer *et al.*, 1982). Pain is often more pronounced at night-time. Patients may report that the use of aspirin often relieves the symptoms. This feature is peculiar to osteoid osteoma. It has been postulated that osteoid osteoma can produce arachidonic acid, which in the presence of cyclo-oxygenase is metabolized, forming products that create and promote pain and bone resorption. Aspirin, which is a cyclo-oxygenase inhibitor, can prevent the formation of such products (Saville, 1980). Painful scoliosis is an occasional presenting sign, the osteoid osteoma, when present, being found at the apex of the curve.

Plain radiographs seldom reveal a nidus but may show simply an area of sclerosis (Fig. 27.2). A ^{99}Tc bone scan is a very useful investigation, and characteristically shows an area of intense, localized increased uptake. CT scan is the best investigation for demonstrating the nidus. It is important to alert the radiologist of the likely diagnosis, as thin slices are necessary to avoid missing the nidus.

Treatment is by the surgical removal of the lesion. Once the localization of the tumour has been accomplished with bone scan and CT scan, which is usually of the posterior elements, removal of the involved bone by, for example, hemilaminectomy, is performed. As sufficient bone removal is necessary to be sure that the lesion has been completely removed, it is often necessary to stabilize and fuse the involved segment. Removal of the lesion results in a dramatic resolution of the pain. In adolescents with painful scoliosis the curvature usually resolves gradually during the subsequent months following surgery. However, in late adolescence and in patients in their second decade, if the pain has persisted for a significant length of time before diagnosis has been made, structural changes may have occurred in this scoliosis, and full resolution may not occur.

Osteochondroma

While multiple osteochondromatosis is the most common of the bone dysplasias, the presence of these lesions in the vertebral column is found in less than 5% of cases (Larson *et al.*, 1957). These lesions are usually seen in the long bones of the body, with a predilection for the ends of the diaphysis. Characteristically, they consist of a bony exostosis with a cartilaginous cap. Increase in the size of the lesion is often seen during the adolescent growth spurt (Palmer & Blum, 1980). These tumours are usually found in the posterior elements of the vertebrae, particularly the spinous or transverse processes. They have also been reported to occur in the pedicles (Spaziante *et al.*, 1988).

There are no specific symptoms or signs associated with this lesion in the spine. Patients may present

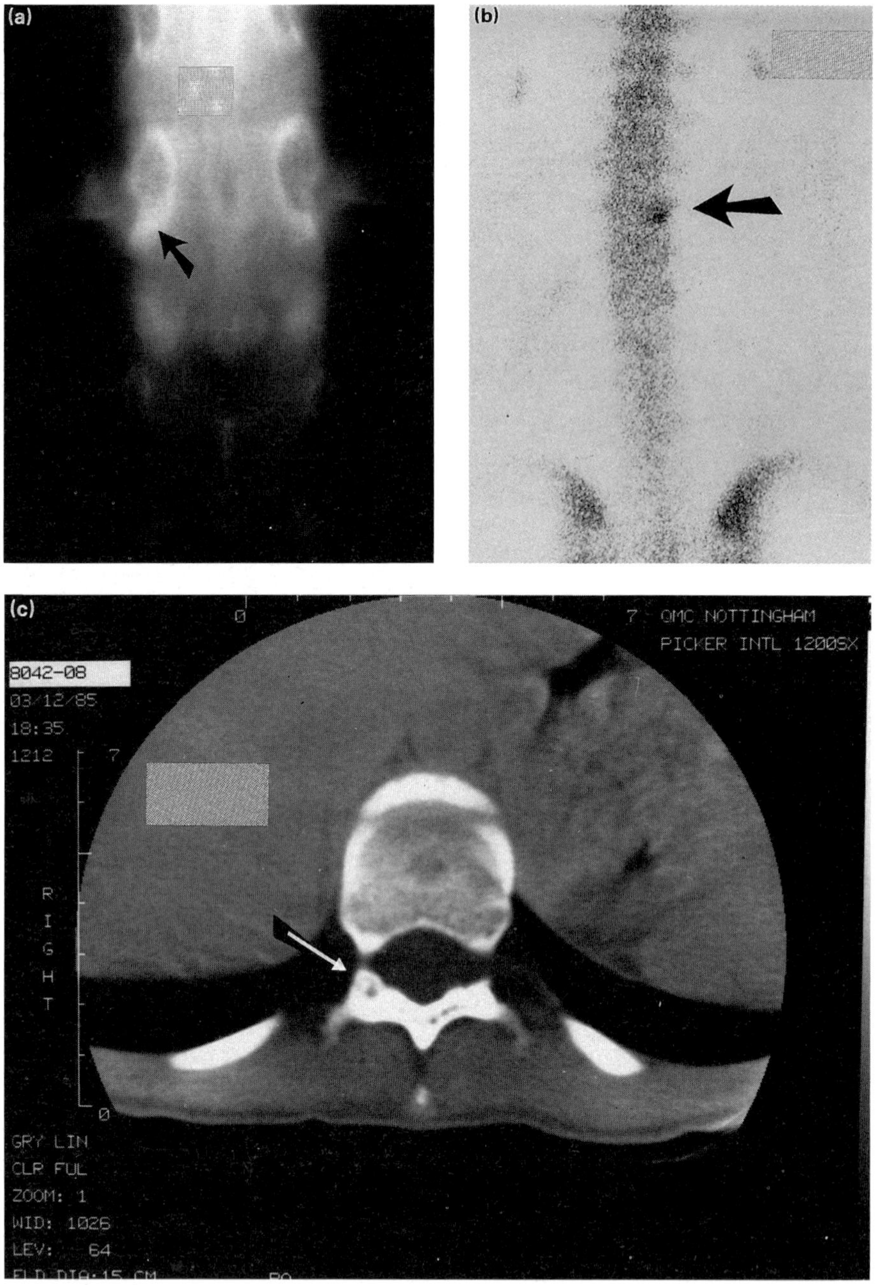

Fig. 27.2 A 15-year-old girl presenting with persistent back pain in the thoracolumbar region. Plain radiographs appear normal. (a) AP tomogram shows an area of sclerosis of the inferior aspect of the right pedicle of T11. (b) Technetium bone scan shows a well-defined area of increased uptake at T11. (c) On CT there is a lytic lesion of the inferior aspect of the right pedicle (arrowed), with a dense sclerotic nidus in its centre typical of an osteoid osteoma.

with pain which can be localized, diffuse or radiating, scoliosis, or progressive neurological signs (Palmer & Blum, 1980; O'Connor & Roberts, 1984; Buckler *et al.*, 1987). It may also present as a palpable mass in the neck (Inglis *et al.*, 1977) Osteochondroma rarely results in spinal cord compression. Such compression usually results from tumours located in the posterior elements, particularly the laminae or pedicles, although anterior spinal cord compression has been reported (Bradford, 1954). The extent of neurological involvement is dependent on the size of the lesion, its rate of growth and its position. Sudden death in an infant, due to an osteochondroma situated on the odontoid, was reported by Rose & Fekete (1964).

A technetium bone scan may show some increase in uptake of the isotope, but lacks the intense uptake occurring with osteoid osteoma. The best investigation for demonstrating the lesion is CT, with or without myelography, depending on the presence of neurological involvement (Loftus *et al.*, 1980).

The presence of osteochondromas within the vertebral column is not an indication for their removal. Normally, these lesions cause a minimum of symptoms and signs, and do not warrant treatment. Osteochondroma resulting in neurological compromise is an absolute indication for removal. Slow but progressive increase in the size of these lesions can occur well after skeletal maturity, as patients often present initially with neurological defects in the third and fourth decades. Removal of most of these lesions is usually accomplished through a posterior approach, utilizing either a hemi- or complete laminectomy, with or without surgical stabilization and fusion, depending on the amount of bone removed.

Giant-cell tumour

True giant-cell tumours frequently present in the long bones, but are much less common in the vertebral column (Cohen *et al.*, 1964; Fors & Stenkvist, 1966). They account for less than 3% of all vertebral tumours (Schajowicz, 1961). Within the vertebral column the most common location is the sacrum. In Dahlin's series (1978), 23 out of 32 spinal giant-cell tumours were located in the sacrum, with an age range from two to 66 years. They are usually located within the vertebral body. However, with larger lesions, both body and posterior elements are frequently involved (Fig. 27.3).

The presenting symptom is usually pain, which can be either localized or radiating. Neurological

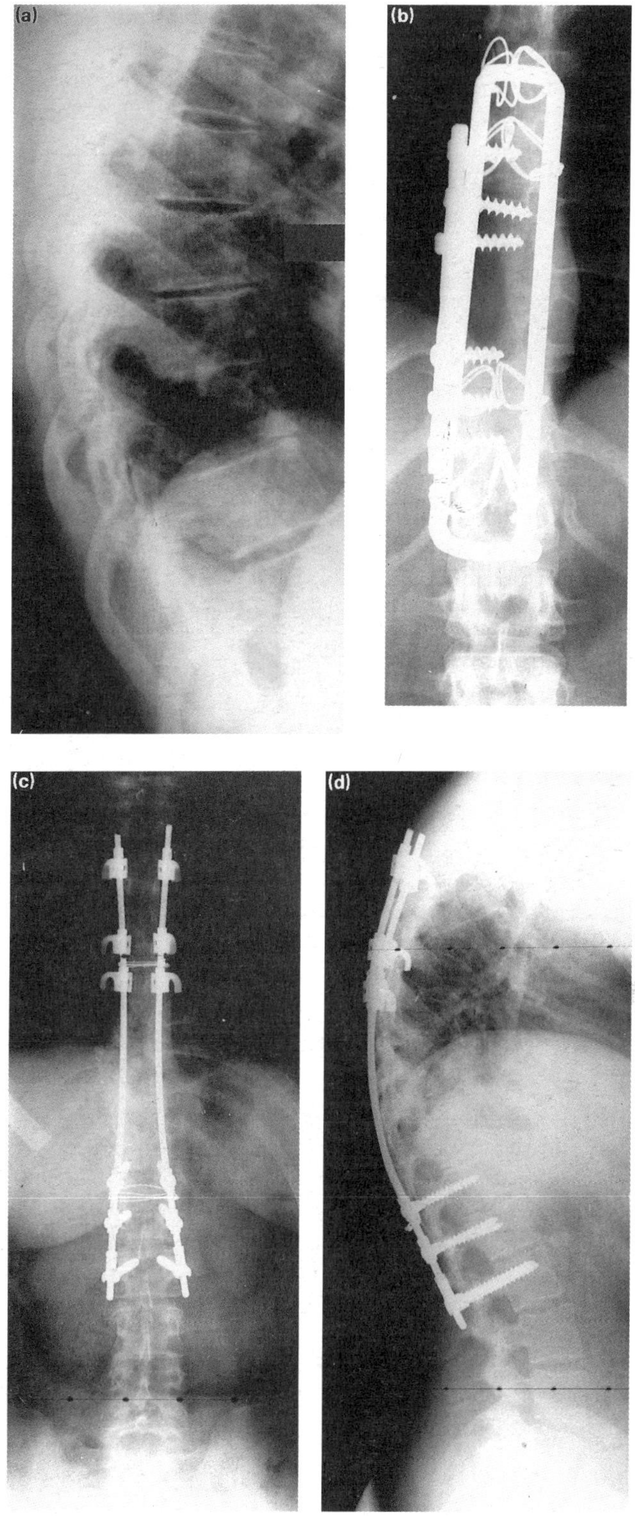

Fig. 27.3 (*Right*) Giant-cell tumour. A 21-year old female presented with back pain and increasing spastic paraparesis. (a) Plain radiographs demonstrate lytic lesion of the body of T9 with loss of outline of the posterior wall due to tumour invasion of the spinal canal. (b) Initial surgical management involved anterior and posterior resection of the tumour with anterior iliac crest graft, anterior stabilization with a plate, and posterior stabilization with a Luque rectangle. Patient developed recurrence three years following initial surgery. (c), (d) Recurrent tumour was again excised and previous metalwork removed. Patient was stabilized using Zilke rods posteriorly, utilizing hooks proximally and pedicle screws distally. Two years following this procedure there is no evidence of recurrence, and the patient is fully ambulant.

involvement is largely dependent on the size and location of the tumour. Patients can present with a small area of numbness or extensive cord and nerve root involvement (Di Lorenzo *et al.*, 1980).

Radiologically the diagnosis can be difficult. Typically, bone rarefaction, cortical expansion, multiloculated cysts, paravertebral invasion, vertebral collapse and osteoblastic activity can be present. The size of the lesion can vary from discrete lesions within the vertebral body to massive expansile lesions occupying a significant amount of the abdominal cavity (Biagiwi *et al.*, 1990). They can be quite difficult to distinguish from aneurysmal bone cysts. Typically, giant-cell tumours are confined to single vertebrae, while aneurysmal bone cysts may involve multiple levels. This distinction is not absolute, however, as giant-cell tumours have also been reported over multiple levels. CT scan is most useful for documenting the extent of the lesion. They usually appear as radiolucent lesions which are well defined and lack a surrounding area of sclerosis. Other lesions to be considered in the differential diagnosis include haemangioma, brown tumour of hyperparathyroidism, fibrous dysplasia and osteoblastoma. Within the sacrum the differential includes aneurysmal bone cyst, chordoma, myeloma and metastases.

Although giant-cell tumours are benign, they do have a marked tendency towards recurrence. Radical removal of these tumours gives the best hope of preventing recurrence. To date this has rarely been possible, when dealing with these tumours located in the vertebral column. This is because of the proximity of major surrounding structures, such as the spinal cord and major vessels, as well as the risk of leaving spinal instability following the procedure. Standard treatment has been partial removal of the tumours, often followed by irradiation. There is, however, no clear evidence to suggest that partial removal with radiation gives rise to a decrease in the recurrence rate (Goldenberg *et al.*, 1970). Malignant transformation in giant-cell tumours is well recognized following high-dose irradiation, and has been reported in up to 10–15% of cases (Murphy & Ackerman, 1956; Johnson & Dahlin, 1959).

Currently, the most accepted treatment approach is as radical a removal of as much tumour as possible. Fears about spinal instability have been decreased because of the improved fixation techniques that are now available. Postoperative, low-dose irradiation is still often used if complete removal of the tumour is not possible. Selective arterial embolization can have a definite role to play in the management of these tumours, particularly when they are large. Biagini *et al.* (1990) reported a massive giant-cell tumour of L3 which showed dramatic reduction in size following the embolization of several lumbar arteries. Two embolizations resulted in a reduction of the mass of the tumour by 80%, which was then satisfactorily removed surgically. Such selective embolization should be reserved for these larger giant-cell tumours, as it is less effective at reducing the mass of smaller ones.

Although recurrence following surgical removal of giant-cell tumours is well recognized, this does not occur as commonly in the axial skeleton as it does when these tumours have been removed from the long bones. It is unknown why giant-cell tumours in the spine act in a less aggressive fashion than they do elsewhere in the body. A management regime that involves subtotal resection with adjuvant postoperative therapy and satisfactory surgical stabilization will lead to a satisfactory outcome in the majority of cases, and a recurrence rate of less than 5%.

Aneurysmal bone cyst

This lesion was originally described by Jaffe & Lichtenstein in 1942. The lesion, although rare, occurs throughout the skeleton and is relatively common in the spine. In the Mayo Clinic series reported by Beaubout *et al.* (1979), 27 (20%) of 134 aneurysmal bone cysts were located in the spine. While most studies have not found a predilection for any particular part of the spine, there has been an increased incidence reported in the lumbar spine (Hay *et al.*, 1978). Clinical symptoms and signs are usually non-specific, with pain, stiffness and occasional swelling. The spectrum of neurological involvement varies from minor numbness to significant neurological deficit. Significant neurological deficit has been reported in up to 30% of cases.

The classical lesion is a lytic expansile lesion, often confined to the posterior elements, but usually involving both the body and posterior elements (Beaubout *et al.*, 1979). On X-ray this expansile lytic lesion is often noted to have fine strands of bone within it, and to be surrounded by an eggshell of the blown-out cortex. The thinned cortex is often difficult to visualize on plain radiographs; therefore the lesion often has a malignant appearance about it. The presence of similar changes on adjacent vertebrae is strongly suggestive of aneurysmal bone cyst. Aneurysmal bone cysts can expand in size at a rapid rate, which can further confuse the diagnosis with that of a malignant lesion. CT scan is perhaps the best radiological investigation for outlining the extent of the lesion, and also for demonstrating the thinned cortical rim. Biopsy is necessary to confirm the diagnosis. Treatment remains somewhat controversial. The ideal treatment is surgical excision, but this is often difficult to achieve in view of the size of the lesions and their inaccessibility on occasions. Hay *et al.* (1978) reviewed the world literature for these lesions in the spine, and the techniques used for treatment. Incomplete excision with radiotherapy had a recurrence rate of 6%; biopsy curettage with incomplete excision had a recurrence rate of 25%; radiotherapy alone had a recurrence rate of 11%, and there was no recorded recurrence following complete excision. Complete or subtotal surgical excision, combined with adequate stabilization, would appear to give the best results.

Haemangioma

The frequency of haemangiomas in the vertebral column is difficult to establish, as it is a bony finding which is often noted in patients who are asymptomatic. Many cases reported radiologically as haemangiomas cannot be verified, as there is no indication to undertake biopsy in patients who are asymptomatic. Post-mortem examination of such lesions has demonstrated many of them to be simple varicosities in the osseous veins, rather than true haemangiomas (Jaffe, 1958). Occasionally they can result in cord compression, and indeed are the most common vascular bone tumour that causes cord compression (Unni *et al.*, 1971). This can result from expansion of the bony neural arch into the epidural space, or can result from pathological compression fractures secondary to the lesion. While haemangiomas most commonly occur as a single lesion they are often found at multiple sites. In 66% they are solitary; there are two to five lesions in 33%, and more than five lesions in less than 1% (Junghanns, 1932). It is important to distinguish multiple bony haemangiomas from diffuse cystic angiomatosis, a condition which is characterized by widespread cystic bone destruction, visceral angiomas and a poor prognosis (Boyle, 1972).

The typical radiographic appearance of a haemangioma is of vertical striations in the vertebral body. The lower thoracic and upper lumbar vertebrae are the most common locations.

It is unusual for patients to present with persistent symptoms due to haemangioma. However, patients with persistent symptoms often benefit by treatment with low-dose radiation therapy. Protection with a spinal orthosis may be necessary to prevent vertebral collapse. There is little in the literature regarding treatment of haemangiomas that are causing neurological compromise. Selective arterial embolization has been used, either alone or as a pre-resection procedure, with some success (Esparza *et al.*, 1978). Often the diagnosis has not been confirmed, as decompression may be undertaken as an emergency procedure, in view of persistent neurological symptoms. Decompression with resection, with or without surgical stabilization depending on the degree of instability, usually yields a satisfactory outcome (Zito & Kadis, 1980).

Eosinophilic granulomas

These are correctly described as tumour-like lesions, as they arise due to defects in lipid metabolism in the reticuloendothelial system of bone rather than being true neoplasms. Eosinophilic granulomas are aggregates of phagocytic histiocytes that normally cause bone resorption. They may be solitary or multiple. Although they can arise anywhere in the reticuloendothelial system they are most commonly found in bone rather than soft tissues. They are most commonly found in the skull (Enneking, 1983).

Pain is the most common presenting symptom. This pain is often constant, unrelated to activity and difficult to gain relief from with aspirin or non-steroidal anti-inflammatory. It usually presents in children and adolescents but may present in adults. Patients may also present with some degree of neurological deficit, which can vary from mild sensory loss to complete paraplegia.

The vertebral body is the site in the spine most commonly involved. The classical lesion presents as a vertebra plana, which is due to the total collapse of the vertebral body due to the histiocytic infiltration of it. The lesion may also present as a lytic lesion, with minimal reaction in the vertebral body but without collapse. The lesion may be present at more than one site (Fig. 27.4).

Technetium-99 isotopic bone scan shows intense increase in uptake at the lesion. It is particularly useful in demonstrating other occult lesions that may not be obvious on the initial radiographs. CT is useful in outlining the bony extent of the lesion in the spine.

Treatment guidelines for this condition are controversial, as there is a proven tendency for the lesion to resolve spontaneously. Some believe that active treatment of these lesions in the spinal column is never indicated. It has also been shown that there is a tendency towards spontaneous restoration of vertebral height in long-term follow-ups on vertebra plana (Nesbit *et al.*, 1969). Patients with neurological compromise often have spinal instability due to this lesion, and in these less common cases decompression, combined with spinal stabilization, may be required. The use of radiation is often advocated, although in the absence of spinal instability it is probably unnecessary.

Fibrous histiocytomas

These lesions, also commonly known as fibrous cortical defects or non-ossified fibromas, occur very rarely in the vertebral column. They commonly occur in the metaphysis of the long bones of children, particularly that of the femur (Compere & Coleman, 1957). These lesions have been reported in the cervical spine and the sacrum (Dahlin, 1978; Destouet

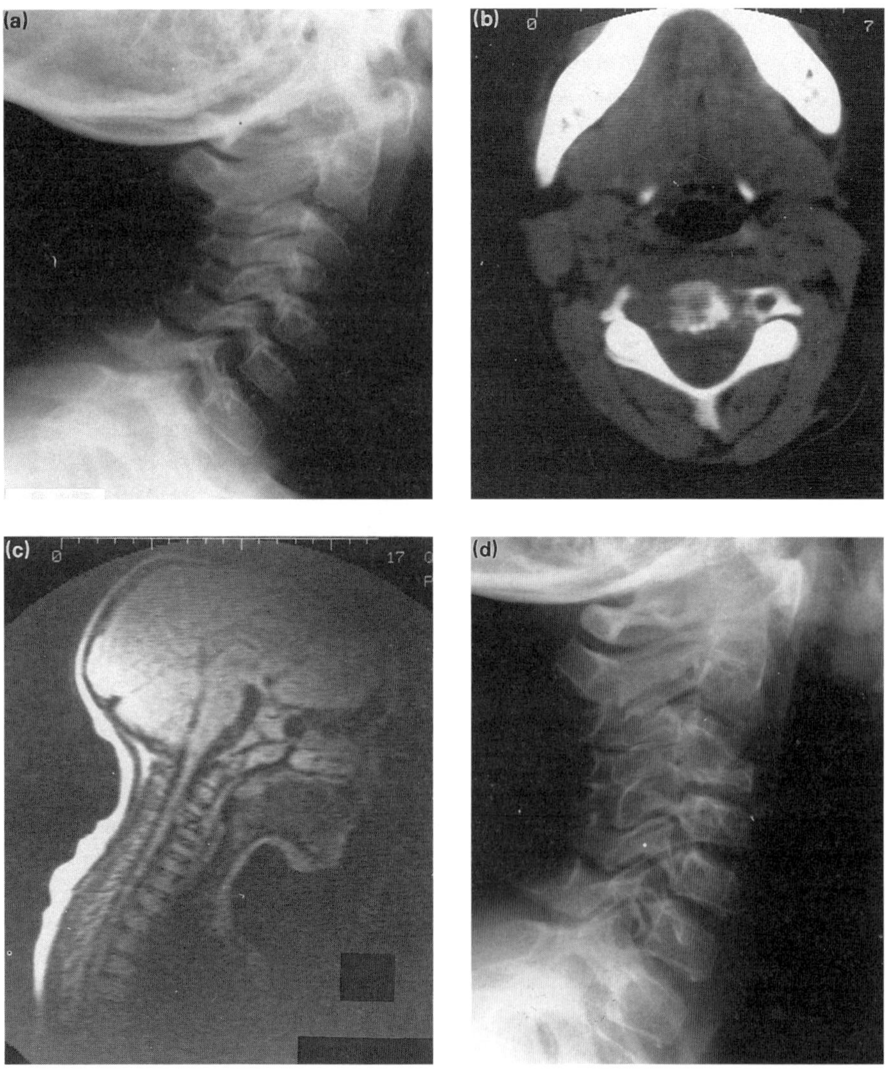

Fig. 27.4 Eosinophilic granuloma. A six-year-old boy who presented with neck pain. (a) X-ray on presentation shows destructive lesion of the body of C4 with partial involvement of the body of C3. (b) CT scan confirms extensive vertebral body involvement with lesion at C4, without involvement of the posterior elements. (c) MRI scan shows some posterior retropulsion of the body of C4 with mild cord compression. Patient had no neurological symptoms or signs. Biopsy confirmed the diagnosis of eosinophilic granuloma. (d) Lateral radiograph at three years follow-up. There is a solid fusion of the bodies of C3 and C4 with a localized kyphosis. The patient is totally asymptomatic and fully active.

et al., 1980). They appear as areas of increased radiolucency, with well-demarcated borders and minimal expansion of the bone. They occur too infrequently to determine the most common anatomical locations within the vertebral body. The case reported by Destouet *et al.* (1980) was of a lesion in the cervical spine, and was noted to involve the spinous process, both laminae, the right pedicle and the right facet joint of the second cervical vertebra. Such lesions would be difficult to differentiate from osteoblastoma, aneurysmal bone cyst and giant-cell tumour. The tumour is sufficiently rare that accurate diagnosis can be established only by histology. Once the histology has been confirmed no further treatment is necessary, unless there is instability as a result of the extent of the lesion or its location. In such cases stabilization may be necessary.

Desmoplastic fibroma

This tumour very rarely affects the spine. It is characterized by cortical expansion, with some trabeculation and marginal sclerosis (Fuji *et al.*, 1988). A review of 50 of these cases in the literature revealed only two that affected the vertebral column (Sugiura, 1976). Patients may present with pain, a palpable lump or increasing neurological defect due to the location of the tumour. Radiologically it is difficult to differentiate from aneurysmal bone cyst, giant-cell tumour and osteoblastoma. Biopsy is necessary to confirm the diagnosis. Once the diagnosis has been established, complete resection is advised, as recurrence occurs in 20% of cases (Huvos, 1979b).

Malignant tumours

Osteosarcoma of the spine

Although osteosarcoma is the most common primary malignant tumour of bone, it rarely affects the spine. Between 1909 and 1980, 1122 patients with osteosarcoma attended the Mayo Clinic, and only 30 of them had the tumour located primarily in the spine (Shives *et al.*, 1986). Primary osteosarcoma of the spine most commonly presents in the second decade (Marcove *et al.*, 1970). A second peak in the incidence of osteosarcoma of the spine occurs later in life, in the sixth and seventh decades. This is due to secondary osteosarcoma occurring in patients with underlying conditions such as Paget's disease, or those who have had previous radiation therapy (Huvos, 1986). Both of these peaks correspond with periods of increased bone turnover. In the second decade the peak corresponds with the adolescent growth spurt, while Paget's disease is also associated with increased turnover of bone.

The majority of patients present either with pain at the site of the tumour or with referred pain due to neurological involvement. The duration of symptoms at the time of presentation is usually between six months and one year. The majority of patients will present with some evidence of neurological involvement which can vary from subtle sensory changes to frank paraplegia (Shives *et al.*, 1986). A minority of patients will also present with a palpable soft tissue mass adjacent to the vertebral lesion.

Osteosarcoma affecting the spine exhibits the typical features of osteosarcoma elsewhere, being either mainly lytic, mainly sclerotic, or mixed. Significant soft tissue extension is common. Although the vertebral body is predominantly affected, the osteosarcoma can arise also in the posterior elements. The radiological features are usually strongly suggestive of malignancy, although it is usually not possible to confidently diagnose the lesion on the plain radiographs, as metastatic lesions and other primary malignant lesions may exhibit similar features. Osteoblastoma is a benign lesion which occasionally presents similar radiological features, and may cause difficulty in diagnosis, particularly if an osteosarcoma is located in the posterior vertebral elements (Mnaymneh *et al.*, 1979). Osteosarcoma and osteoblastoma can be misdiagnosed histologically, as there is close similarity between the two lesions. Giant-cell tumours can be radiologically similar to the lytic type of osteosarcoma.

Bone scanning is a useful investigation to determine if there are other hot spots in the skeleton which would suggest that the lesion is metastatic rather than a primary malignant tumour. Following diagnosis of osteosarcoma, bone scanning can also be useful as a follow-up investigation, to determine if regression of the tumour is occurring with adjuvant therapy, or if recurrence of tumour has occurred following surgical excision. CT and particularly MRI are very useful in accurately assessing the bony and soft tissue extent of such tumours.

Histologically, osteosarcoma can be osteoblastic, chondroblastic, or fibroblastic, depending on the predominant tumour cell type present. The chondroblastic and fibroblastic types of osteosarcoma are often histologically similar to chondrosarcoma and fibrosarcoma, but will always show some small amount of osteoid tissue produced directly by the malignant cells. Shives *et al.* (1986) applied the Enneking classification for surgical staging to his series, and found that the majority were IIb (high-grade; extracompartmental).

Several factors combine to ensure that the prognosis for osteosarcoma of the spine is poor. The preferred method of treatment for this tumour in the long bones is complete surgical removal, either by amputation or limb-sparing resection, combined with adjuvant chemotherapy. In the spine, complete surgical removal is usually impossible, both because there is usually evidence of extracompartmental spread at the time of presentation, and also because of the limitations of resection, due to the surrounding vital structures. Preoperative chemotherapy, as proposed by Rosen *et al.* (1983), is particularly appropriate in the management of osteosarcoma of the spine. Chemotherapeutic agents frequently used in the treatment of osteosarcoma include high-dose methotrexate, doxorubicin, and adriamycin. The combination of complete surgical resection of osteosarcoma and chemotherapy has led to significant improvement in the outlook for these tumours. Prior to the use of chemotherapy, five-year survival rates for osteosarcoma were less than 20%, and these have now improved to around 50% with chemotherapy regimes (Sundaresan *et al.*, 1990). No significant clinical series combining chemotherapy and surgical resection of spinal osteosarcoma have been reported, although the five-year survival is likely to be significantly less than with peripheral osteosarcoma, as complete surgical resection is seldom possible in spinal cases. The object of surgery is resection of the involved portion of the vertebral body with appropriate reconstruction. With tumours that are primarily confined to the vertebral body this usually involves an anterior approach resecting the tumour with reconstruction of the defect using methyl methacrylate or bone graft either from the iliac crest or from the bone bank. If the posterior elements of the vertebra are also involved a two-stage procedure may be necessary for complete removal.

Chondrosarcoma

Chondrosarcoma is the third most frequent primary malignant tumour of bone after multiple myeloma and osteosarcoma. While chondrosarcomas classically are located in the axial skeleton or proximal limb bones, spinal involvement in fact is unusual. Of the 634 cases of chondrosarcoma reported in the Mayo Clinic series (Sunderasan *et al.*, 1990), only 55 affected the vertebral column; nine involved the cervical spine, 18 the thoracic spine, 12 the lumbar spine and 16 the sacrum. Clinical symptoms and signs are similar to those with other malignant spinal tumours. Pain is a predominant symptom; this may be localized or referred. Neurological involvement is a frequent feature. These lessions may arise in new bone or in pre-existing benign cartilaginous lesions such as multiple exostosis or Ollier's disease (Sim, 1984).

Mottled calcification of the tumour mass is a characteristic finding in chondrosarcoma. The diagnosis can often be suspected where such mottled calcification exists in chondrosarcoma that has significant extra-osseous extension. The minority of chondrosarcomas may present as lytic lesions in the vertebra, with minimal calcification, features which are non-specific. Contrast, CT and MRI can be useful in defining the intra- and extra-osseous extent of the tumour.

Surgical excision is the principal method of treatment for chondrosarcoma (Camins *et al.*, 1978; Healy & Lane, 1986). Radical excision is generally advised in the treatment of chondrosarcoma, as the prognosis with this tumour is related to the incidence of local recurrence. However, radical excision is seldom possible with tumours located in the vertebral column, on account of the close proximity of vital structures such as the aorta, vena cava and spinal cord. The surgical aim has to be to remove as much tumour as possible. Patients who have intralesional resection, that is debulking of the tumour, almost invariably will have recurrence. Patients in whom a marginal or wide excision is performed have a lesser incidence of recurrence. It is possible to achieve a radical excision with no recurrence in patients who are detected early with intracompartmental lesions, although this is unusual. Although chondrosarcoma is radioresistant, there is evidence to suggest that some benefit may be derived from treating patients with radiotherapy who have unresectable tumours or following inadequate surgical excision (Suit & Goitein, 1982).

Chordomas

Chordomas are malignant tumours thought to arise from the remnants of the embryonic notochord. Over

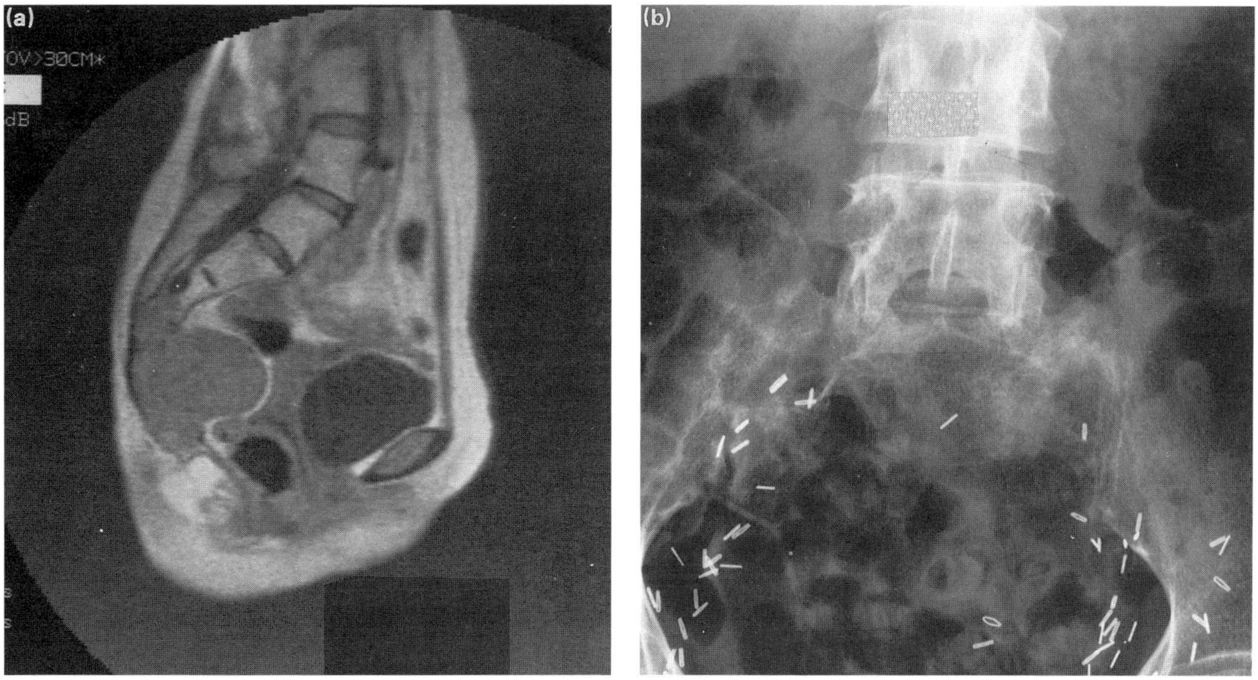

Fig. 27.5 Chordoma (sacral). A 65-year-old female with low back pain. (a) Sagittal T1 weighted spin echo MRI scan demonstrates a large mass over the anterior aspect of the sacrum extending into the body of S2. The margins of the mass are well defined. These are the typical features of a sacral chordoma. (b) Surgery involved initial mobilization of the adjacent structures through an anterior approach, followed by posterior resection, as advocated by Stener & Gunterberg (1978). At two years postresection there has been no clinical or radiological evidence of recurrence, and the patient remains well.

80% occur either in the sacral or in the basiocciput region, other vertebrae rarely being affected. They are twice as common in males, most commonly presenting in the fifth and sixth decades. They can, however, occur at any age, and have been reported in children (Wold & Laws, 1983). Chordomas represent about 4% of primary bone tumours (Dahlin & MacCarty, 1952).

The usual presenting symptom is pain, either localized at the site of the tumour or radiating in a particular dermatome. Patients can also present with a midline palpable mass which is much more common with this lesion than with other malignant lesions. In its early stages the tumour can be difficult to distinguish on plain radiographs, so that these patients often attend clinics for some time and are treated for back pain, due to disc disease, before correct diagnosis is finally made. Motor or sensory neurological deficits can occur, but are less frequent than with other malignant spinal lesions. Local pressure of the sacral chordoma on the rectum may result in patients presenting with altered bowel habit, particularly constipation and occasionally rectal bleeding (Utne & Pugh, 1955).

Radiologically, sacral chordomas usually demonstrate some anterior bony erosion with an anterior soft tissue mass which may be demonstrable due to speckled calcification in its periphery. Enlarged sacral, neural foramina may also be seen on plain radiographs (Hudson & Galcerran, 1983). Evidence of bony erosion can be difficult to detect unless specifically looked for, and in many of these patients the diagnosis is initially missed. CT gives excellent demonstration of both the bony changes and soft tissue mass. MRI gives excellent demonstration of the soft tissue extent of the tumour (Fig. 27.5).

Radiographs of cranial chordomas may demonstrate bony destruction in the spheno-occipital or hypophyseal region, with CT or MRI necessary to adequately demonstrate the soft tissue mass (Mindell, 1981) (Fig. 27.6).

Vertebral chordomas often demonstrate lytic lesions in the vertebral bodies, although osteoblastic changes may be seen. Two or more adjacent vertebrae

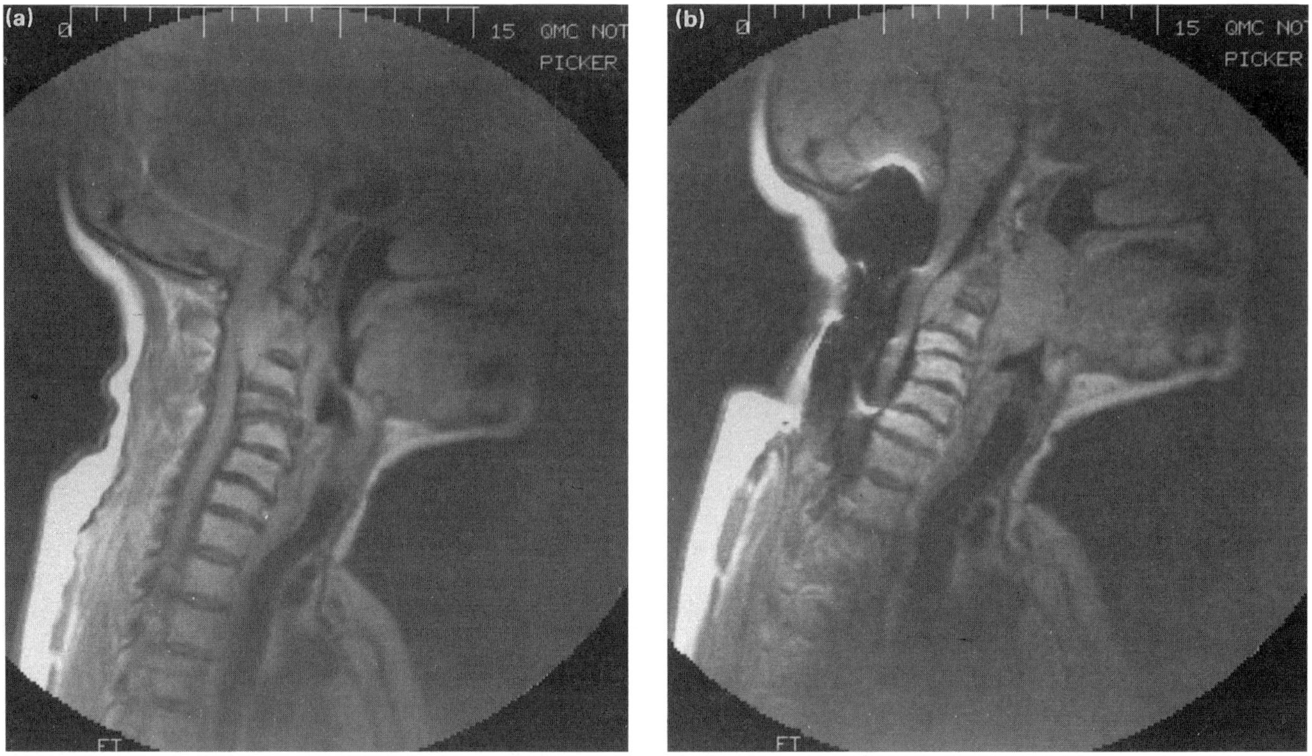

Fig. 27.6 Chordoma (upper cervical). A 66-year-old lady presenting with upper cervical pain and myelopathy. (a) Sagittal T1 weighted spin echo MRI scan reveals chordoma predominantly posterior to the body of C2 and C3 causing cord compression. Patient had transoral resection followed by posterior stabilization. (b) Two years later the patient developed recurrent symptoms. MRI scan revealed a recurrent tumour with less cord compression but significant increase in mass, anterior to vertebral body. Patient underwent multiple debulking procedures over a five-year period prior to finally succumbing to her disease.

may be affected. The radiological features are difficult to distinguish from other vertebral body tumours.

Surgical removal is the standard treatment for these tumours. Complete removal is, however, often difficult to achieve, due to the size of the tumour presentation and its close proximity to vital structures. Complete resection of sacral chordomas can be achieved by a combined anterior and posterior surgical approach, as advocated by Stener & Gunterberg (1978). A large, lower abdominal, semicircular incision is utilized to achieve a bilateral retroperitoneal approach to the tumour. The internal iliac vessels are ligated and divided, as well as the middle sacral artery and veins. The rectum can be mobilized off the tumour. Through a posterior incision, laminectomy is performed, usually at L5 to identify the theca and the S1 nerve roots. For tumours involving up to the S2 segment an osteotomy is used to amputate through the S1 segment. The sacrum is then mobilized by division of the sacrotuberous, sacrospinous ligaments and removed. The gluteal musculature can be turned into the wound to decrease the dead-space.

Results following resection of chordomas at the base of the skull are less favourable, as complete resection here is more difficult. Approaching these tumours through a transoral approach will give a limited exposure, and a transmandibular median glossotomy is preferred.

For sacral chordomas the median survival is about five years, with 20–40% survival at 10 years post-treatment stage (Sundaresan *et al.*, 1990). The median survival for patients with lesions in the basiocciput and vertebral regions is less than five years, and rarely do such patients survive for 10 years. Although the tumour is not very radiosensitive, high-dose radiation therapy may give some pain relief and decrease the progression of neurological involvement. Although the overall results of treatment have not been very satisfactory to date, it is hoped that, with increasing use of radical resection of these tumours, the prognosis will improve.

Myeloma

Myelomas occur as a result of a malignancy arising in B cell lymphocytes, that is those that produce immunoglobulins. They can be either single (plasmacytoma) or multiple. Plasmacytomas are tumours of malignant plasma cells not affecting the bone marrow, while multiple myeloma does affect the bone marrow. Most follow-ups on plasmacytoma affecting the spine, however, eventually show that the condition progresses into multiple myeloma so that plasmacytoma affecting the spine should not be considered an isolated lesion (Bataille & Sany, 1981).

When there is spinal involvement with either lesion, patients usually present with back pain which is often radiating, and frequently have evidence of neurological deficit. In addition, patients with multiple myeloma often exhibit signs of systemic illness, for example weight loss, anaemia and raised erythrocyte sedimentation rate. The typical myeloma

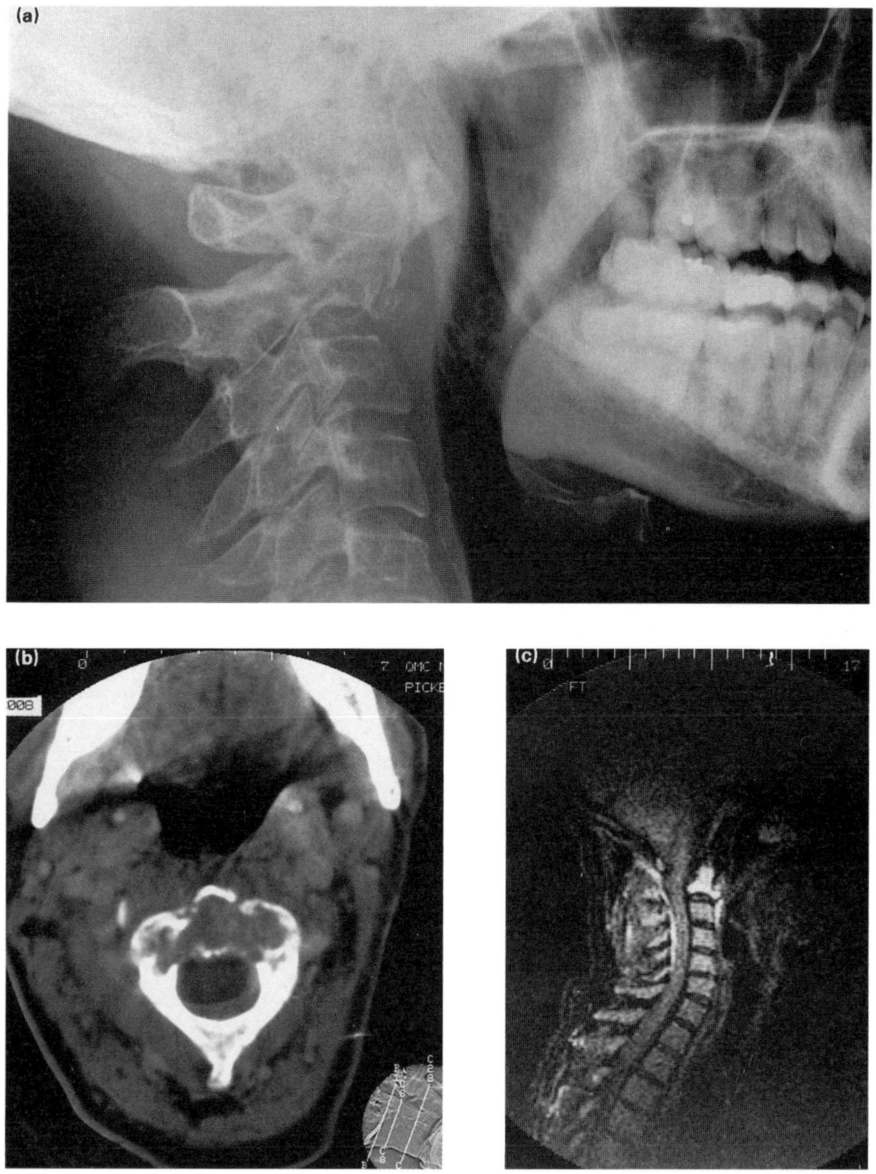

Fig. 27.7 Multiple myeloma. (a) A 47-year-old male presented with severe neck pain and acute torticollis. A lateral cervical radiograph reveals destructive lesion of C2, confirmed on CT (b). (c) MRI sagittal image confirms extensive involvement of odontoid and body of C2. The base of the body of C2 is widened due to collapse of vertebral height because of tumour involvement. Histology confirmed multiple myeloma.

lesion has been described as having a 'soap-bubble' appearance, although in the spine they are often featureless, non-specific, lytic lesions (Fig. 27.7). Bone scans are generally unhelpful, usually being either normal or showing areas of decreased uptake. CT and MRI can detail the bony changes as well as evidence of extra-bony involvement, a feature which has a significantly worse prognosis. Both plasmacytoma and multiple myeloma most frequently occur from the fifth decade onwards. Males and females are about equally affected by multiple myeloma, while plasmacytoma has a higher incidence in males.

As the radiographic features in the spine are quite non-specific a biopsy is necessary for diagnosis. A skeletal survey is necessary to determine if the condition is single or multiple. Serum and urinary paraprotein levels are routinely measured as part of the work-up of these patients, and can be useful indicators of response to treatment at a later stage.

Solitary spinal plasmacytoma responds well to radiation treatment if there is no associated instability or neurological deficit (Mill & Griffith, 1980). Patients with solitary spinal plasmacytoma and instability or extradural involvement with the tumour are best treated with surgical resection and stabilization. Patients with multiple spinal myeloma invariably have systemic marrow involvement elsewhere, and systemic chemotherapy is necessary to adequately treat these patients. Steroids are effective in treating the frequently associated hypocalcaemia and protein urea, as well as affecting the tumour bulk (Alexanian *et al.*, 1972). Radiation is useful as a palliative measure in multiple myeloma for treatment of painful bony lesions.

Ewing's sarcoma

Ewing's sarcoma can be defined as a highly anaplastic, small, round-cell sarcoma with the clinical and X-ray features of a primary osseous lesion. It is thought to arise from undifferentiated mesenchymal tissue. It affects younger patients than most primary malignant tumours of bone, usually occurring before the end of the second decade. It most commonly affects the lower extremities and the pelvic girdle. Dahlin (1978) found 22 cases involving the spinal column out of a total of 299, an incidence of 7%. The sacrum is most frequently involved. Pain, either localized or radiating, is the commonest presenting feature, and there is a high incidence of patients presenting with neurological involvement. Radiological features are non-specific, usually presenting as a lytic area, occasionally with a surrounding area of sclerosis. Soft tissue and extradural involvement are best demonstrated with CT or MRI.

In recent years surgical resection of Ewing's tumours elsewhere in the body has become increasingly advocated as part of a combined treatment, including radiation and chemotherapy (Wilkins *et al.*, 1986). At best, surgical resection for spinal Ewing's will achieve subtotal resection, and adjuvant chemotherapy will always be necessary, as well as localized radiotherapy. Bradway & Pritchard (1990) reviewed 19 patients with spinal Ewing's sarcoma who were treated by this combination. Thirteen patients had died within 33 months, and only one patient had survived more than five years. This indicates the very poor prognosis associated with this tumour, particularly when it presents with spinal involvement.

REFERENCES

Akbarnia, B. & Rooholamini, S. (1981) Scoliosis caused by benign osteoblastoma of the thoracic or lumbar spine. *J. Bone Jt. Surg.*, **63A**, 1146–1155.

Alexanian, R., Bonnet, J. & Gehan, E. (1972) Combination chemotherapy for multiple myeloma. *Cancer*, **30**, 382–389.

Askin, G. & Webb, J. (1991) The management of spinal neoplasia. *Operative Spinal Surgery*, vol. 20, pp. 241–269. Churchill Livingstone, Edinburgh.

Bataille, R. & Sany, J. (1981) Solitary myeloma: clinical and prognostic features of a review of 114 cases. *Cancer*, **48**, 843–851.

Beaubout, J., McLeod, R. & Dahlin, D. (1979) Benign tumours. *Sem. Roentgenol.*, **XIV**, 33–43.

Biagini, R., De Cristogaro, R., Ruggieri, P. & Boriani, S. (1990) Giant cell tumor of the spine. *J. Bone Jt. Surg.*, **72A**, 1102–1107.

Boyle, W. (1972) Cystic angiomatosis of bone. *J. Bone Jt. Surg.*, **54B**, 626–636.

Bradford, F. (1954) Intraspinal tumors. *Dis. Nerv. Syst.*, **15**, 55–60.

Bradway, J. & Pritchard, D. (1990) Ewing's tumor of the spine: diagnosis and clinical management. In Sundaresan, N. *et al.* (eds) W.B. Saunders, Philadelphia.

Buckler, R., Chad, D. *et al.* (1987) Sciatica: an early manifestation of thoracic vertebral osteochondroma. *Neurosurgery*, **21**, 98–100.

Caldicott, W. (1969) Diagnosis of spinal osteoid osteoma. *Radiology*, **92**, 1192–1195.

Camins, M., Duncan, A. *et al.* (1978) Chondrosarcoma of the spine. *Spine*, **3**, 202–209.

Cohen, D., Dahlin, D. & MacCarty, C. (1964) Vertebral giant cell tumor and variants. *Cancer*, **17**, 461–472.

Compere, C. & Coleman, S. (1957) Nonosteogenic fibroma of bone. *Surg. Gynaecol. Obstet.*, **104**, 329.

Dahlin, D. (1978) *Bone Tumors. General Aspects and Data on 6221 Cases*, 3rd edn. Charles C. Thomas, Springfield, IL.

Dahlin, D. & MacCarty, C. (1952) Chordoma: a study of fifty-nine cases. *Cancer*, **5**, 1170–1178.

Delamarter, R., Sachs, B. *et al.* (1990) Primary neoplasms of the thoracic and lumbar spine. *Clin. Orthop. Rel. Res.*, **256**, 87–100.

Destouet, J., Kyriakos, M. & Gilula, L. (1980) Fibrous histiocytoma (fibroxanthoma) of a cervical vertebra. *Skeletal Radiol.*, **5**, 241–246.

Di Lorenzo, N., Spallone, A., Nolletti, A. & Nardi, P. (1980) Giant cell tumors of the spine: a clinical study of six cases, with emphasis on the radiological features, treatment, and follow-up. *Neurosurgery*, **6**, 29–34.

Enneking, W. (1983) *Musculoskeletal Tumour Surgery*, p. 1331. Churchill Livingstone, Edinburgh.

Enneking, W. (1986) A system of staging musculoskeletal neoplasms. *Clin. Orthop.*, **204**, 9–24.

Esparza, J., Castro, S. & Portillo, J. (1978) Vertebral hemangioma: spinal angiography and preoperative embolisation. *Surg. Neurol.*, **10**, 171–173.

Fors, B. & Stenkvist, B. (1966) Giant cell tumor of thoracic vertebra. *Acta Orthop. Scand.*, **37**, 191–196.

Friedlander, F. & Southwick, W. Tumors of the spine. In Rothman, R. & Simeone, F. (eds) *The Spine*, pp. 1022–1054. W.B. Saunders, Philadelphia, PA.

Fuji, T., Hamada, H. *et al.* (1988) Desmoplastic fibroma of the axis. *Clin. Orthop. Rel. Res.*, **234**, 16–20.

Goldenberg, R., Campbell, C. & Bonfiglio, M. (1970) Giant-cell tumor of bone: an analysis of 218 cases. *J. Bone Jt. Surg.*, **52A**, 619–663.

Hay, M., Paterson, D. *et al.* (1978) Aneurysmal bone cysts of the spine. *J. Bone Jt. Surg.*, **60B**, 406–411.

Healy, J. & Lane, J. (1986) Chondrosarcoma. *Clin. Orthop.*, **204**, 119–129.

Hudson, T. & Galcerran, M. (1983) Radiology of sacrocyccygeal chordoma difficulties in detecting soft tissue extension. *Clin. Orthop.*, **175**, 237–242.

Huvos, A. (1979a) *Bone Tumors*, pp. 33–46. W.B. Saunders, Philadelphia, PA.

Huvos, A. (1979b) *Desmoplastic Fibroma and Periosteal 'Desmoid'. Bone Tumors, Diagnosis, Treatment and Prognosis*, p. 243. W.B. Saunders, Philadelphia, PA.

Huvos, A. (1986) Osteogenic sarcoma of bones and soft tissues in older patients: a clinico-pathologic analysis of 117 patients older than 60 years. *Cancer*, **57**, 1442–1449.

Inglis, A., Rubin, R. *et al.* (1977) Osteochondroma of the cervical spine. *Clin. Orthop. Rel. Res.*, **126**, 127–129.

Jaffe, H. (1956) Benign osteoblastoma. *Bull. Hosp. Jt. Dis.*, **17**, 141–151.

Jaffe, H. (1935) Osteoid osteoma. *Arch. Surg.*, **31**, 709.

Jaffe, H. & Lichtenstein, L. (1942) Solitary unicameral bone cyst with emphasis on the Roentgen picture, the pathological appearance and the pathogenesis. *Arch. Surg.*, **44**, 1004–1025.

Jaffe, H. (1958) *Tumors and Tumorous Conditions of the Bones and Joints*, pp. 224–225. Lea & Febiger, Philadelphia, PA.

Janin, Y., Epstein, J. *et al.* (1981) Osteoid osteomas and osteoblastomas of the spine. *Neurosurgery*, **8**, 31–38.

Johnson, E. & Dahlin, D. (1959) Treatment of giant-cell tumor of bone. *J. Bone Jt. Surg.*, **41A**, 895–904.

Junghanns, H. (1932) Uber die Haufigkeit gutartiger Geschwalste in der Wirbelkorpern (angiome, lipome, osteome). *Arch. Klin. Chir.*, **169**, 204–212.

Larson, N., Dodge, H. *et al.* (1957) Hereditary multiple exostoses with compression of the spinal cord. *Proc. Staff Meet. Mayo Clin.*, **32**, 728–734.

Loftus, C., Rozario, *et al.* (1980) Solitary osteochondroma of T4 with thoracic cord compression. *Surg. Neurol.*, **13**, 355–357.

MacLellan, D. & Wilson, F. (1967) Osteoid osteoma of the spine. A review of the literature and report of six new cases. *J. Bone Jt. Surg.*, **49A**, 111–121.

Marcove, R., Mike, V., Hajek, J. *et al.* (1970) Osteogenic sarcoma under the age of 21 years. A review of 145 operative cases. *J. Bone Jt. Surg.*, **52A**, 411–423.

Marsh, B., Bonfiglio, M. *et al.* (1975) Benign osteoblastoma: range of manifestations. *J. Bone Jt. Surg.*, **57A**, 1–9.

McLeod, R., Dahlin, D. *et al.* (1976) The spectrum of osteoblastoma. *Ann. J. Roentgenol.*, **126**, 321–335.

Mill, W. & Griffith, R. (1980) The role of radiation therapy in the management of plasma cell tumours. *Cancer*, **45**, 647–652.

Mindell, E. (1981) Chordoma—current concepts review. *J. Bone Jt. Surg.*, **63A**, 501–505.

Mnaymneh, W., Brown, M. *et al.* (1979) Primary osteogenic sarcoma of the second cervical vertebra. *J. Bone Jt. Surg.*, **61A**, 460–462.

Murphy, W. & Ackerman, L. (1956) Benign and malignant giant-cell tumors of bone. A clinical–pathological evaluation of 31 cases. *Cancer*, **9**, 317–339.

Myles, S. & MacRae, M. (1988) Benign osteoblastoma of the spine in childhood. *J. Neurosurg.*, **68**, 884–888.

Nemoto, O., Moser, R. *et al.* (1990) Osteoblastoma of the spine. A review of 75 cases. *Spine*, **15**, 1272–1280.

Nesbit, M. *et al.* (1969) Reconstitution of vertebral height of histiocytosis. A long term follow up. *J. Bone Jt. Surg.*, **51A**, 1360–1368.

O'Connor, G. & Roberts, T. (1984) Spinal cord compression by an osteochondroma in a patient with multiple osteochondromatosis. *J. Neurosurg.*, **60**, 420–423.

Palmer, F. & Blum, P. (1980) Osteochondroma with spinal cord compression. *J. Neurosurg.*, **52**, 842–845.

Paillas, J., Alliez, B. *et al.* (1975) Primary and secondary tumours of the spine. In Vinken, P. & Bruyn, G. (eds) *Handbook of Clinical Neurology*, vol. 20, pp. 19–54. North-Holland, Amsterdam.

Pochaczevsky, R., Yen, Y. & Sherman, R. (1960) The Roentgen appearance of benign osteoblastoma. *Radiology*, **75**, 429–437.

Polivy, K., Scott, R. & Zimbler, S. (1986) Osteoid osteoma of the cervical spine. *Orthopaedics*, **9**, 1101–1103.

Rose, E. & Fekete, A. (1964) Odontoid osteochondroma causing sudden death. Report of a case and review of the literature. *Ann. J. Clin. Pathol.*, **42**, 606–609.
Rosen, G., Marcove, R. *et al.* (1983) Primary osteogenic sarcoma: eight years experience with adjuvant chemotherapy. *J. Cancer Res. Clin. Oncol.*, **106**, 55–67.
Sabanas, A., Bickel, W. *et al.* (1956) Natural history of osteoid osteoma of the spine. Review of the literature and report of three cases. *Ann. J. Surg.*, **91**, 880–889.
Saville, P. (1980) A medical option for the treatment of osteoid osteoma. *Arthritis Rheum.*, **23**, 1409–1411.
Schajowicz, F. (1961) Giant cell tumors of bone (osteoclastoma). A pathological and histochemical study. *J. Bone Jt. Surg.*, **43A**, 1–29.
Shikata, J., Yamamuro, T. *et al.* (1987) Benign osteoblastoma of the cervical vertebra. *Surg. Neurol.*, **27**, 381–385.
Shives, T., Dahlin, D. *et al.* (1986) Osteosarcoma of the spine. *J. Bone Jt. Surg.*, **68A**, 660–668.
Sim, F., Dahlin, D. *et al.* (1977) Primary bone tumors simulating lumbar disc syndrome. *Spine*, **2**, 65.
Sim, F. (1984) Chondrosarcoma. In Uhthoff, H. (ed.) *Current Concepts of Diagnosis and Treatment of Bone and Soft Tissue Tumors*. Springer-Verlag, Berlin.
Spaziante, R., Irace, C., Gambardella, A. *et al.* (1988) Solitary osteochondroma of the pedicle of L4 causing root compression. *J. Neuro. Sci.*, **32**, 141–145.
Stener, B. & Gunterberg, B. (1978) High amputation of the sacrum for extirpation of tumors: principles and technique. *Spine*, **3**, 351–366.
Sugiura, I. (1976) Desmoplastic fibroma. Case report and review of the literature. *J. Bone Jt. Surg.*, **58A**, 126.
Suit, H. & Goitein, M. (1982) Definitive radiation therapy for chordoma and chondrosarcoma of base of skull and cervical spine. *J. Neurosurg.*, **56**, 377–385.
Sundaresan, N., Schmidek, H. *et al.* (1990) *Tumours of the Spine. Diagnosis and Clinical Management.* W.B. Saunders, Philadelphia, PA.
Thommesen, P. & Poulsen, J. (1976) Primary tumours in the spine and pelvis in adolescents. Clinical and radiological features. *Acta Orthop. Scand.*, **47**, 170–174.
Unni, K., Ivins, J. & Beabout, J. (1971) Hemangioma, hemangiopericytoma, and hemangioendothelioma (angiosarcoma) of bone. *Cancer*, **27**, 1043–1414.
Utne, J. & Pugh, D. (1955) The roentgenologic aspects of chordoma. *Am. J. Roentgenol.*, **74**, 593–608.
Weinstein, J. & McLain, R. (1987) Primary tumors of the spine. *Spine*, **12**, 843–851.
Wilkins, R., Pritchard, D. *et al.* (1986) Ewing's sarcoma of bone. Experience with 140 patients. *Cancer*, **58**, 2551–2555.
Wold, L. & Laws, E. (1983) Cranial chordomas in children and young adults. *J. Neurosurg.*, **59**, 1043–1047.
Zito, G. & Kadis, G. (1980) Multiple vertebral haemangiomas resembling metastases with spinal cord compression. *Arch. Neurol.*, **37**, 247–248.
Zwimpfer, T., Tucker, W. & Faulkner, J. (1982) Osteoid osteoma of the cervical spine; case reports and literature review. *Canad. J. Surg.*, **25**, 637–641.

28 · Metastatic Spinal Disease

By G.F.G. FINDLAY

The commonest neoplastic disease affecting the spine is undoubtedly the problem of metastatic spinal involvement. For far too long the problem of metastatic spinal disease has been neglected. It is only in recent years that scientific attention has turned to this subject, and critical appraisal has led to rationalization and improvement in the overall management of this distressing disease.

It seems probable that it was LeCat, in 1751, who was the first to report the use of laminectomy in the partial removal of a spinal metastasis (Markham, 1951). The use of laminectomy subsequently became the standard therapeutic approach to all such patients. In a paper published in 1963, Bucy stated that all patients with paraplegia due to a spinal metastasis in reasonable general condition should undergo laminectomy. Such an attitude accurately reflected the majority view which continued through to the late 1970s and early 1980s. However, such views were not universal and, as early as 1941, Elsberg wrote that 'in proved metastatic disease, there is very rarely, if ever, any justification for the attempted removal of the malignancy'.

The enthusiasm typified by Bucy's remarks for laminectomy has, however, persisted though the emergence of papers, such as that of Gilbert *et al.* (1978) regarding the role of radiotherapy, and that of Siegal and Siegal (1985) concerning the role of anterior surgery, which have led to a long overdue reappraisal of the overall management. Bucy, in his 1963 paper, did in fact comment on the inadequacies of laminectomy in the presence of anterior structural disease, and Brice & McKissock in 1965 observed that 'no patient with severe neurological deficit and vertebral collapse improved' with laminectomy and radiotherapy. Along with the development of anterior surgical approaches for the management of malignant vertebral collapse came a realization that laminectomy carried a very significant incidence of adverse effects (Findlay, 1984, 1987). It has now become accepted practice that laminectomy as the sole surgical procedure in the management of malignant spinal disease has very little place.

The incidence of metastatic spinal disease has been widely reported. Sundaresan *et al.* (1986a,b) reported that autopsy data suggested that 5% of patients with a primary malignancy develop spinal secondaries. Other papers assess the risk as being as high as 20% (Schaberg & Gainor, 1985). Wong *et al.* (1990) examined the spines of 832 patients who had died from a malignant neoplasm. They found obvious metastatic lesions by either inspection or radiography in 222 cases, but discovered occult metastases in a further 78 cases following sagittal sectioning of the spinal column. This gave an overall incidence of 36.1%. However, they also suspected the presence of a metastasis due to vertebral collapse in a further 34 patients which were subsequently found to be not due to metastatic disease. This stresses the importance of not assuming that vertebral collapse in a patient known to have malignant disease is due to a metastasis. McNeil (1984) found that the isotope bone scan was positive in 39% of the cancer patients he studied, but this is a relatively non-specific investigation. It is clear that not all patients who harbour spinal secondaries develop neurological deficit. Cobb *et al.* (1977) followed over 12 000 patients with primary breast cancer and found that 2467 (19.7%) developed radiological evidence of secondary spinal involvement. In 1735 of them treatment was by radiotherapy and none developed neurological deficit. Signs of spinal cord compression developed in only 2.4% of the whole population.

PATHOPHYSIOLOGY

The most frequent mechanism by which a primary tumour seeds to the spine is by haematogenous spread to the vertebra, settling mainly in either the marrow of the body or the pedicle. Other modes of spread do occur, including: extension of a paravertebral lesion such as a renal neoplasm to involve the spine; perineural spread along spinal nerves; lymphatic permeation through the nerve root foramen; and, possibly, by direct spread through paraspinal venous networks as described by Batson (1940).

Any primary tumour may spread in a manner which causes spinal involvement, but neoplasms of the bronchus and the breast account for the vast majority (Constans *et al.*, 1983). Sundaresan *et al.* (1985) stated that two-thirds of spinal metastases arose from primary tumours of either the breast, lung, prostate, or the haematopoietic system. Other neoplasms such as renal neoplasms, or those of the thyroid, have a high incidence of spinal involvement but usually represent only small percentages of most series.

Although it is often well established that a patient has a primary neoplasm, the clinical presentation of metastatic spinal cord compression is not infrequently the first sign of the presence of a primary neoplasm. It is obvious that the absence of a known primary should not preclude a diagnosis of metastatic spinal compression whilst, on the other hand, spinal disease in a patient with a known primary could well be due to other diseases such as infection.

The reported frequency of metastatic spinal disease presenting as the first sign of an occult distant primary neoplasm varies according to the referral pattern of the patients. Many series where the primary treatment has been radiotherapy report low incidences for occult primaries. Gilbert *et al.* (1978) had only four patients out of 235 where the primary site remained occult, and in only 8% was the spinal metastasis the presenting feature of the neoplasm. Such low incidence in radiotherapy series are explained by two factors: firstly, many of the patients are already under review by radiotherapists who have treated the primary neoplasm; and secondly, because patients without a known primary were often subjected to laminectomy in order to confirm the diagnosis. Shaw *et al.* (1980), however, reported a consecutive unselected series of patients presenting to a neurosurgical unit with cord compression. At the time of presentation, and following initial assessment, the primary neoplasm was occult in 52%. Histological examination subsequent to surgery only reduced that figure to 28%, and in those patients the primary source remained obscure.

Table 28.1 shows the site of spinal involvement as reported by Constans *et al.* (1983). It is evident that extradural involvement accounts for the vast majority of cases. That paper reports a high incidence of 86% for involvement of greater than one level either distant or contiguous to the main lesion as compared to that of 17% found by Gilbert *et al.* (1978). Van der Sande *et al.* (1990) examined the entire thoracic and lumbar canal by myelography in 106 patients who were suspected of having an epidural metastasis. Fifty-four of the patients were found to have a spinal metastasis, and of those, 16 (30%) were found to have at least one additional metastasis remote from the lesion which was causing the neurological deficit. In all of the patients with multiple lesions at least one was asymptomatic. There is much greater agreement about regional involvement with some 50–60% of cases involving the thoracic spine. The lumbosacral spine is next most frequently involved, with the cervical region least common, accounting for some 15%. Most series find that vertebral body involvement is more common than posterior, and that about 20% will have circumferential involvement by the time they present. Siegal & Siegal (1989), however, felt that 85% of cases had anterior disease. Overall, individual tumours seem to have little preference for involving any particular site or region. However, it is well recognized that renal neoplasms often involve the upper lumbar spine by direct extension, and it has been reported that colonic tumours tend to favour the lumbar spine. Intramedullary secondaries

Table 28.1 Site of spinal involvement by metastasis. Data from Constans *et al.* (1983)

Location of metastasis	Percentage of cases
Purely intradural	1.2
Purely extradural	5.0
Purely bony lesion	10.3
Bone and extradural	83.5

are very likely to be metastatic from the bronchus, and Sundaresan *et al.* (1981) state that lesions at C1–C2 are almost always from breast or lymphatic sources.

The effects which a spinal metastasis exerts upon the spinal cord are complex. Neural compression and distortion play a fundamental role either from the extending extradural mass itself or from bony compression subsequent to the development of spinal deformity due to vertebral collapse. Experimental studies such as that of Ushio *et al.* (1977) showed that the compression results in the development of vasogenic oedema within the cord parenchyma. This finding was supported by Ikeda *et al.* (1980) and also by Siegal *et al.* (1988a,b). Siegal and his co-workers also found that the development of oedema was preceded by an increased production of prostanoids, and that there was an associated increase in water content and specific gravity. In addition to the effects of compression, there is little doubt that vascular changes are of importance. Epidural venous compression leading to stasis, as described by Ikeda *et al.* (1980) and Ushio *et al.* (1977), showed that eventually arterial compression occurred within the cord leading ultimately to infarction. Angiographic studies by Doppman & Girton (1976) in the presence of an expanding anterior extradural mass also showed impaired cord blood flow which was not reversed by laminectomy. Shapiro & Posner (1983) also showed that laminectomy was ineffective in the experimental model.

The pathophysiology of metastatic spinal cord compression is therefore a highly complex entity. Despite this it does produce a remarkably uniform clinical picture.

CLINICAL FEATURES

Metastatic spinal cord compression may present as either an acute or a chronic condition. Shapiro & Posner (1983) found the length of history to vary from as little as one day to two years, with a median of seven weeks. Occasionally the occurrence of a true pathological fracture of the spine will produce an even more dramatic presentation. In the series described by Constans *et al.* (1983), 28% of their cases presented with a history of less than two days duration. They felt that lesions at the thoracolumbar junction were particularly likely to present with rapidly evolving deficit, whereas cervical lesions tended to have a more protracted course. With regard to the interval between the onset of the primary neoplasm and the development of a spinal secondary, Gilbert *et al.* (1978) described one case where the interval was as much as 19 years.

Pain is the most common initial symptom, and by the time of presentation almost all patients have pain. The majority of patients experience midline pain local to the level of spinal involvement. The pain is usually present at all times, though it may be either exacerbated or relieved by activity or rest, especially if there is an element of structural instability. The occurrence of continual pain which becomes progressively more severe as time passes should alert suspicion to the presence of serious spinal pathology rather than some musculoskeletal cause for the pain. Obviously pathological processes causing this type of pain are not necessarily neoplastic, but could be due to other serious disease such as infection. Root pain is unusual in the thoracic region but occurs more commonly in the cervical and lumbosacral spine. It is usually possible to differentiate such root pain from that of spondylotic disease by its severity and continual nature, and the higher incidence of sensorimotor root deficit in the neoplastic cases. The more diffuse, regionally distributed, burning pain due to central cord involvement is unusual in extradural lesions but can occur in intramedullary metastases.

Although pain was the presenting symptom in 96% of the Gilbert *et al.* (1978) series it is not uncommon for the patient to present only when neurological deficit develops. Thus, in Constans *et al.* (1983) pain was the actual presenting feature in only 61%. Diagnostic delay is regrettably all too frequent, as shown by series such as that of Shaw *et al.* (1980), where 75% of the patients were non-ambulant at the time of admission to the neurosurgical department and 68% had developed urinary retention. Sundaresan *et al.* (1985) found that 45% were non-ambulant on admission and, in a large review paper, Findlay (1984) showed that 66% of over 1800 patients had lost the ability to walk prior to presentation.

The onset of neurological deficit results usually in a short period where only sensory symptoms are present, rapidly followed by the development of motor and then sphincteric dysfunction. The sensory symptoms are usually of cord type with ascending numbness and paraesthesiae below the level of the lesion. A sense of heaviness in the legs, or of walking on cotton wool, are often described in the initial stages and, as the sensory deficit progresses, loss of balance occurs due to spinal ataxia. A dermatomal distribution of sensory changes is found only in cases with root involvement. Motor deficit produces the expected weakness and functional loss in the affected limbs. Sphincteric involvement results in painless urinary retention leading ultimately to overflow incontinence and loss of anal control.

Examination of the spine may be very revealing and should never be omitted. Localized tenderness on percussion is a useful rough localizing sign to the level involved, as is the finding of a sensory level to pinprick or light touch. In some cases with structural deformity an obvious gibbus may be present, though it must be remembered that such deformity may equally result from non-neoplastic disease such as trauma or infection. Neurological examination will reveal a sensory level usually also with impairment of proprioception. The legs will be spastic with increased reflexes, clonus and extensor plantar responses. If the history of increasing deficit is very rapid, the legs may be flaccid as it does take time for the classical upper motoneurone signs of spasticity to develop. Obviously, if the level of spinal involvement is below the conus, such patients will exhibit flaccidity as cauda equina compression produces lower motoneurone signs. Whilst sensory changes are often fairly symmetrical, the motor deficit is frequently asymmetrical. Particularly in laterally placed lesions, a true Brown–Sequard picture may be evident. Sphincteric involvement produces a distended bladder and a lax anus.

The above clinical picture is common to all pathological processes producing spinal cord compression, but a rapidly evolving picture in a patient beyond middle age who also has pain in the spine should strongly raise suspicion of metastatic spinal disease. Charting of individual muscle strengths does not give a good functional picture, and it is best to assess the patient's disability in terms of his ability to walk. Thus a classification of: normal gait, ambulant with walking aids, paraparetic but non-ambulant, and paraplegic provides an easily understandable functional assessment. The term paraplegic is frequently misused, causing great confusion when assessing reported results (Findlay, 1984). In some papers the term paraplegia is used to include those with sensory preservation but no movement (Shaw *et al.*, 1980) and other papers include people with retained movement but no antigravity function (Siegal & Siegal, 1985). Such patients may have very severe paraparesis but they have incomplete lesions and therefore may have a very different prognosis as opposed to those truly paraplegic.

Having come to a clinical diagnosis of spinal cord compression, consideration must then be paid to differential diagnosis. The differential diagnosis of spinal cord compression conveniently falls into two differing groups depending upon the presence or absence of a mass lesion. With regard to mass lesions, other neoplastic diseases may cause cord compression but are less common than metastases. They comprise the primary neoplasia of bone and cartilage of the spinal column described in Chapter 27 and the intradural tumours described in Chapters 29 and 30. Other mass lesions of importance are those of infection causing compression either from spinal osteomyelitis or from extradural and intradural abscess formation. Thoracic disc protrusion causing cord compression can present in a very similar manner to metastatic disease, as can compression of the cervical cord or cauda equina by a herniated cervical or lumbar disc respectively. It is of vital importance to recognize that benign mass lesions can, of course, occur in a patient known to have a primary systemic neoplasm, and not merely to assume that the episode of cord compression is due to a metastasis.

The list of non-mass lesions which can simulate cord compression is very long. The commonest, however, include diseases such as acute demyelination, transverse myelitis, Guillain–Barré syndrome, acute vascular disease of the cord and carcinomatous meningitis. Many of these conditions can be suspected from the clinical findings, but it is on only very rare occasions that a mass lesion can be confidently excluded purely on clinical grounds. As the presence of a mass lesion causing acute cord compression requires urgent therapy it is advisable without delay to investigate all patients presenting with the syndrome of acute spinal cord compression to exclude the presence of a mass lesion, even if the presumptive clinical diagnosis is that of neurological disease. Such a policy can uncover an unexpectedly high incidence of diseases such as thoracic disc protrusion causing paraparesis (Findlay, 1991).

INVESTIGATION

When a presumptive diagnosis of metastatic spinal cord compression is made, it is imperative that investigation and assessment are carried out without

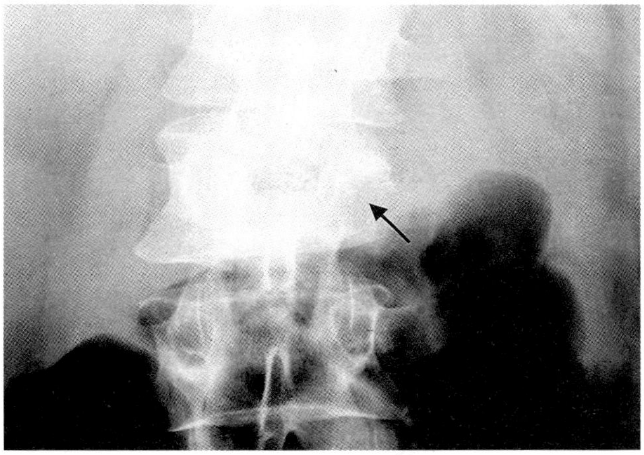

Fig. 28.1 AP radiograph showing partial erosion of the left L2 pedicle (arrow) and some erosion of the vertebral body due to metastasis.

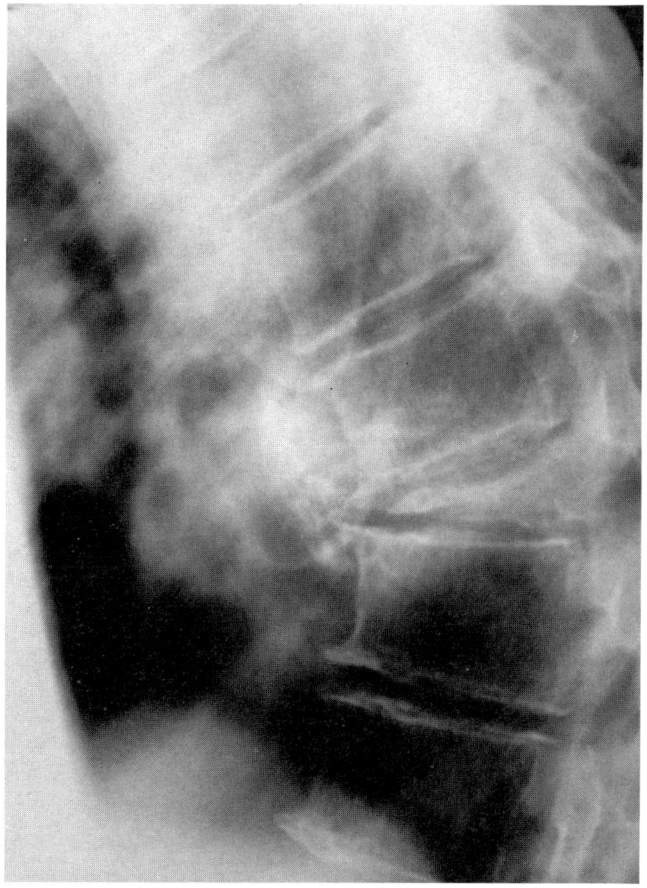

Fig. 28.2 Severe vertebral body collapse due to metastatic involvement.

delay thus allowing appropriate treatment of the spinal lesion before further neurological deterioration ensues. There is no place for the practice of attempting to discover the presumed underlying primary lesion unless this is made obvious by clinical examination or chest X-ray. However, it is appropriate to undertake simple investigations such as full blood count, plasma electrophoresis, liver function tests and acid phosphatase if clinically relevant. The results of such tests should not be awaited prior to undertaking assessment of the spinal problem, though they may prove subsequently to be indicators of the primary source.

Chest X-ray is mandatory as it may reveal evidence of multiple metastases either in the lung parenchyma or in the skeleton. It is also important in that it may show an unexpected primary bronchogenic carcinoma. Such a finding is of great relevance as patients who present with cord compression as the first sign of the presence of such a primary have an extremely poor prognosis with only 50% surviving more than eight weeks (Turner *et al.*, 1988). Only gross lesions in the upper thoracic spine can be seen on the chest X-ray, and formal plain films of the spine are always necessary.

Plain radiology of the spine shows evidence of metastatic disease in approximately 60% of patients with cord or root compression (Black, 1979). Plain X-ray changes usually arise in either the pedicle or the vertebral body, producing either pedicular loss (Fig. 28.1) or vertebral collapse (Fig. 28.2). On occasions the only sign may be a radiolucent area or sclerotic change within the body. Constans *et al.* (1983) found sclerotic metastases in only 8% of their series, but such lesions are usually from primary sources such as lymphoma, breast or prostate. Some patients may show evidence of a paravertebral mass, but it must be remembered that infection also causes such a mass. The differentiation of metastasis from spinal osteomyelitis is obviously of the greatest importance and, although there are no totally diagnostic features on plain X-ray, the presence of an indistinct margin between the affected body and its adjacent disc is highly suggestive of infection (Fig. 28.3). Plain films of the whole spine should be taken rather than merely of the affected region, as multiple spinal deposits occur in up to 17% of cases (Gilbert *et al.*, 1978).

Isotope bone scanning can be useful in assessment, but it is not routinely available on an emergency basis and is itself time-consuming. It is a non-specific test

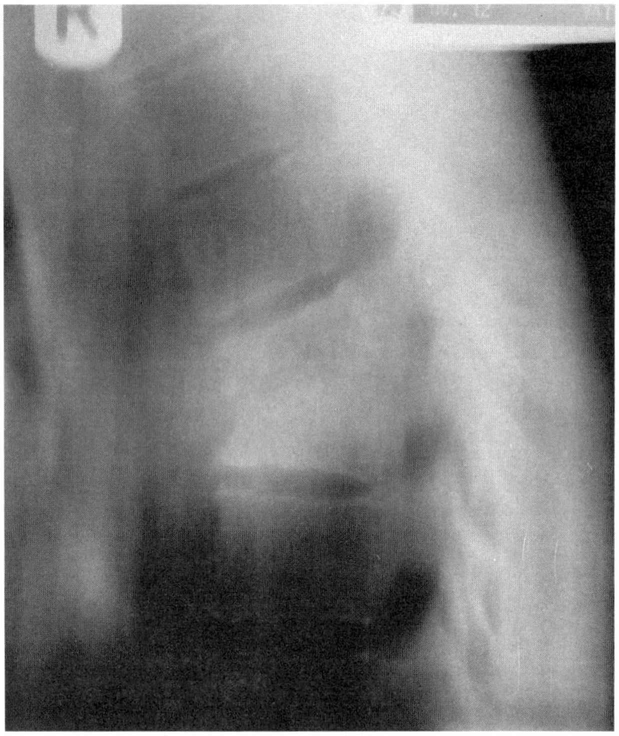

Fig. 28.3 Tomogram showing characteristic changes of osteomyelitis with obliteration of the disc space (compare with Fig. 28.2).

merely indicating either increased blood flow or osteoblastic activity, and therefore may be positive in benign disease such as infection or simple degenerative disease. It is, however, more sensitive than plain radiology and allows assessment of skeletal disease outwith the spine. McNeil (1984) found that 39% of patients with metastatic disease had spinal involvement. One point of great importance is that myeloma deposits are frequently negative on bone scanning (Ell, 1983) and thus both false-positive and false-negative results are not uncommon in isotope bone scanning.

Water-soluble contrast myelography remains the most widely used method of assessing the degree and level of spinal cord compression. It is possible to image the whole spine with this technique though, if a complete block is found during examination by the lumbar route, a cervical puncture is necessary to delineate the upward extent of the block. The myelographic picture of extradural compression is well recognized (Fig. 28.4), but it also is not specific for metastasis. However, the presence of a typical block

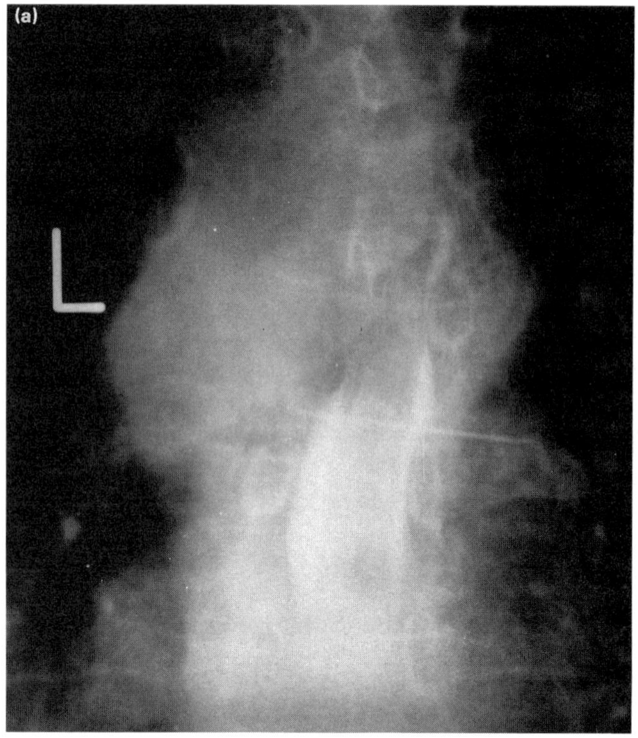

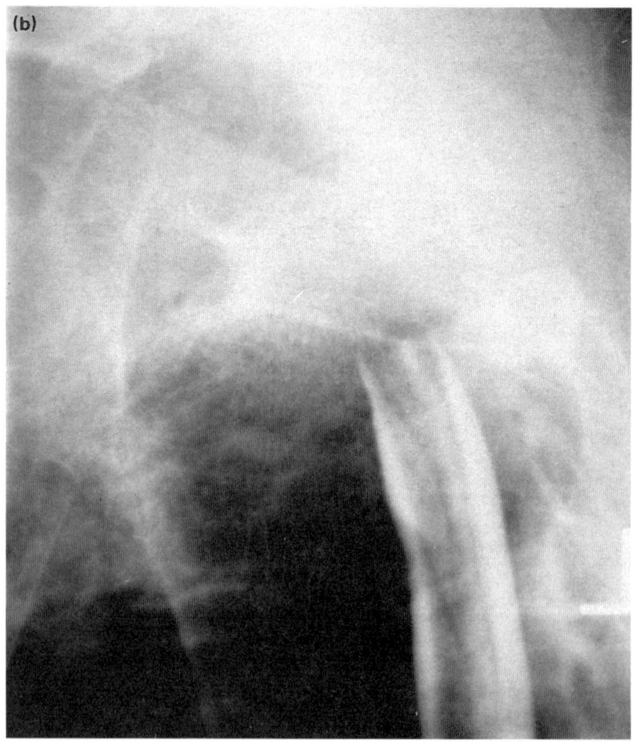

Fig. 28.4 Complete myelographic block due to extradural lesion. Note the paravertebral mass and erosion of pedicle on the left (a). The needle is a skin marker. (b) Typical appearance of an extradural lesion in the lateral view.

in the presence of characteristic plain film changes makes the diagnosis of a metastatic cause highly likely. It is often possible to assess from the myelogram whether the main site of cord compression lies either anteriorly or posteriorly, or is circumferential. This information is of the greatest importance when planning a surgical approach, and even greater detail emerges when a computerized tomography (CT) scan is performed following the myelogram (Fig. 28.5). Weissman *et al.* (1985) discovered extradural extension beyond the limits of the affected bony level in 11% of their patients examined with this technique.

CT scanning alone as the primary investigation is not recommended, as assessment of the whole spine is impossible. If the correct level is imaged it will show the extent of bony disease and the presence of cortical disruption strongly suggests a malignant process (Fig. 28.6). Involvement of the adjacent paravertebral tissues is well seen, and this may be of importance in the rare event of total extirpation of the tumour being under consideration.

Myelography either with or without CT also allows examination of the cerebrospinal fluid (CSF). Usually the CSF changes are relatively non-specific, such as a rise in the CSF protein, but cytological examination can sometimes reveal malignant cells. The nature of such cells can sometimes be discovered by immunological staining methods (Coakham *et al.*, 1984). Acute neurological deterioration can occasionally occur following myelography by the lumbar route in the presence of a complete extradural block (Greenwood, 1973). It is therefore advisable that

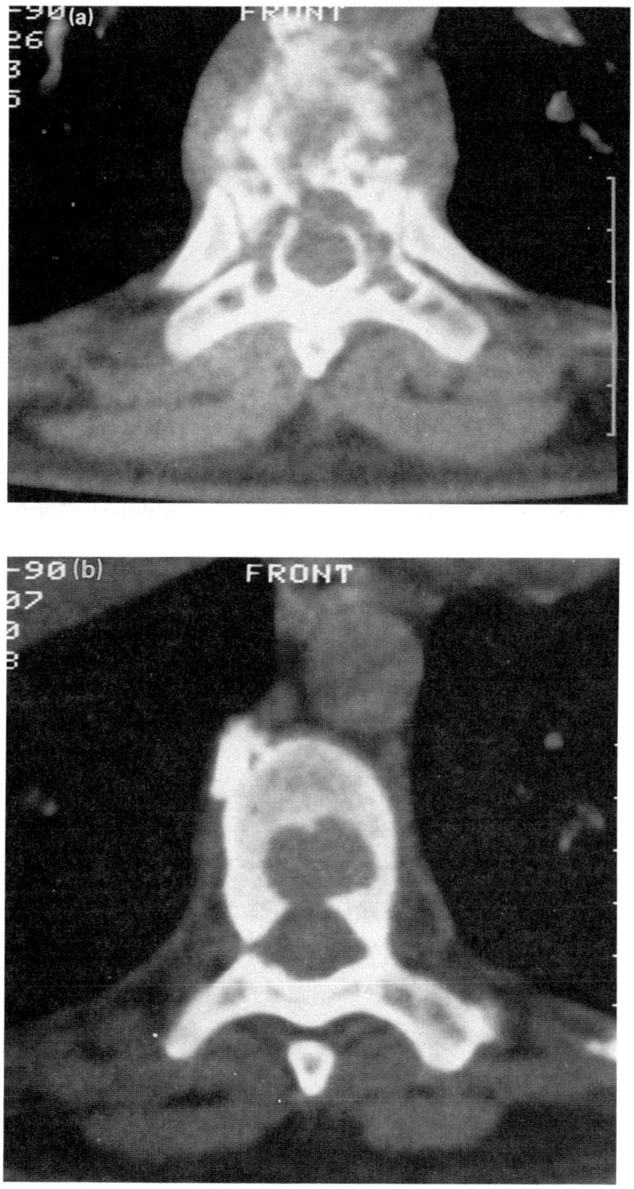

Fig. 28.5 Axial CT scan (a) following myelography showing extensive metastatic involvement of a thoracic vertebral body with extradural tumour surrounding the thecal sac anteriorly and on both sides. (b) Axial CT scan of the vertebral body immediately above that shown in (a). Plain radiographs and the myelogram were normal at this level but the CT clearly shows involvement of the adjacent body. The histology was myeloma.

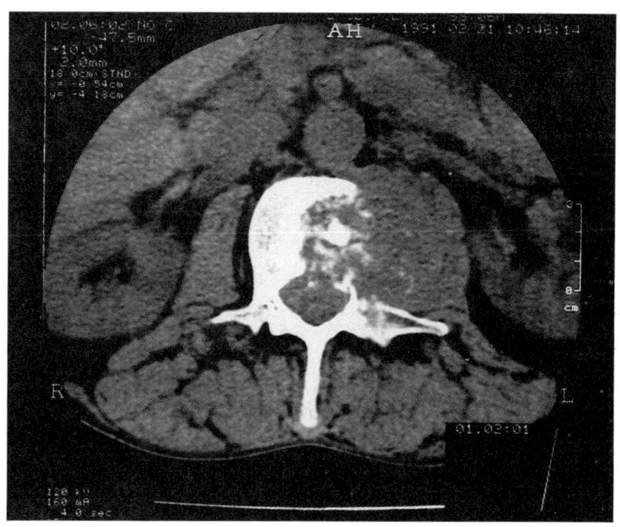

Fig. 28.6 Plain CT scan showing extensive involvement of the body, pedicle and transverse process of a lumbar vertebral body due to metastatic involvement. The large paravertebral mass can easily be biopsied by a CT-guided technique.

myelography is performed only in a unit where emergency surgery is readily available.

The role of magnetic resonance imaging (MRI) in metastatic spinal compression has not been clearly defined (Fig. 28.7). Clearly, the examination allows non-invasive assessment of the whole spinal column. However, although pathological changes in the marrow of the vertebral bodies can be readily seen in some cases (Godersky *et al.*, 1987), cortical bony changes are not well seen. Sarpel *et al.* (1987) compared MRI against myelography in 16 cases and found that MRI showed cord compression in three patients where the myelogram was normal. On the other hand, Hagenau *et al.* (1987) found that, in the presence of an incomplete block, myelography was superior to MRI. Both investigations were comparable in the presence of a complete block. Sze *et al.* (1988) showed that enhancing MRI images with gadolinium could obliterate the plain MRI evidence of the presence of tumour. However, the use of enhanced and unenhanced MRI images improved the delineation and also the characterization of extradural lesions.

In some situations where the existence of a primary neoplasm is certain, it may be possible from clinical and radiological evidence to conclude that an extradural lesion is a metastasis. However, it is advisable that formal histological confirmation is sought in all cases, and it is mandatory if there is no known primary. Obviously histological confirmation is obtained whenever a surgical approach to therapy is chosen, but an alternative means of diagnosis is needed if non-surgical therapy is selected. Percutaneous needle biopsy allows such a diagnosis to be achieved.

In 1955, Ottolenghi published his results of the technique of percutaneous needle aspiration of vertebral body lesions based on a technique described by Robertson & Ball (1935). Ottolenghi was able to achieve a diagnostic aspirate in 73% of his very large series. Fyfe *et al.* (1983) showed that the diagnostic yield could be increased to 90% by the use of a 3 mm trephine needle allowing a core of vertebral tissue to be obtained, thus allowing structural as well as cytological histological methods. The technique was originally confined to lesions in the lumbar spine, but Fyfe *et al.*, and the author's experience, confirm that all vertebrae distal to T3 can be biopsied. It is also possible to biopsy midcervical lesions and even certain sacral tumours. Thus only lesions at the cervicothoracic junction are inaccessible as the body

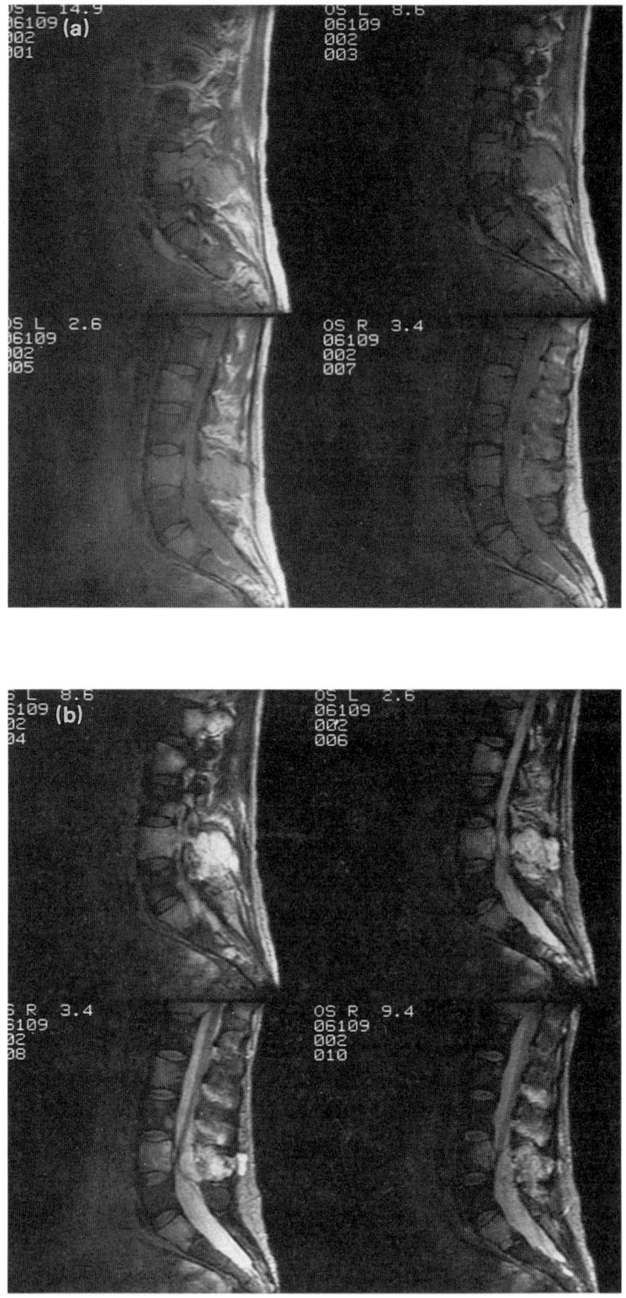

Fig. 28.7 T1 (a) and T2 (b) MRI sagittal images showing extensive involvement of L4 with compression of the cauda equina. Further metastases are present at L1, L2, L3 and S1.

of C2 can be biopsied via a transoral route. Trephine needle biopsy is necessary only when the metastasis remains contained within the confines of the vertebral body. Where CT shows extension of the tumour into the paravertebral tissues, a diagnosis can normally be achieved by a CT-guided Tru-Cut biopsy, as the histological interpretation of tumour within soft tissues is much simpler than the interpretation of bony lesions.

Fyfe *et al.* used conventional histological methods in their series. Although this could allow rapid diagnosis of some lesions such as infection, many specimens have to undergo decalcification prior to histological examination, and the delay which this involves proves unacceptable in patients who present with evolving neurological deficit. In 1988, Findlay *et al.* reported the results of using immediate smear histology routinely on the needle cores. It proved possible to find sufficient soft tissue or marrow to allow an immediate smear in all cases, and the histological correlation between the immediate smear and the final definitive histology was extremely high (97%). Certain information was lacking in the smear results as it was usually not possible to say what type of primary lesion was likely to be involved, but the differentiation of metastatic secondaries, myeloma, lymphoma and infection was easily achieved from the smear. Thus the combination of percutaneous biopsy and smear histology allows an accurate working diagnosis to be made within half an hour of the biopsy being taken.

Some epidural metastases are extremely vascular lesions and spinal angiography may be an appropriate preoperative investigation in certain situations, in particular renal metastases (Sundaresan *et al.*, 1986c). The main advantage of angiography is that it may allow superselective arterial embolization of the main feeding vessels of the tumour prior to surgery. Both Sundaresan *et al.* (1986c) and Broaddus *et al.* (1990) felt that this technique significantly reduced the resulting blood loss at surgery. Embolization is, however, contra-indicated if the vessels feeding the tumour arise from arterial branches which also are seen to supply the spinal cord.

PREDICTION OF OUTCOME

From reviewing the many papers on the subject of metastatic spinal disease it becomes evident that certain factors are of clear importance when predicting the outcome of these unfortunate patients. Equally, there are other factors where their significance in outcome prediction is less certain.

All papers agree that the factors of prime significance are the histological nature of the underlying primary and the severity of the neurological deficit at the time of presentation. It is generally agreed that metastases from primary lesions such as breast, myeloma, lymphoma and prostate have a more favourable prognosis, whereas secondaries from bronchogenic lesions have a poor prognosis. Obviously such a statement can be only a generalization, but Gilbert *et al.* (1978) felt that the biological activity of the primary was of greater importance in determining the outcome than was the nature of the treatment given.

Again there is general agreement that, the more severe the pretreatment neurological deficit is, the worse is the outcome. Findlay (1984) found that there was no significant difference between treatment either by laminectomy with postoperative radiotherapy or by radiotherapy alone. Of those patients who were still able to walk even with aids at the onset of treatment, 71% were still able to walk after the completion of therapy. However, when those patients who had deteriorated further, such that they could no longer stand but were still not paraplegic, were considered, the success in regaining ambulation fell to 37%. Patients who are truly paraplegic only rarely regain the ability to walk after therapy, but occasional cases have been reported. However, careful review of some of those cases reveals that they were not truly paraplegic but had retained some sensory sparing. There is general agreement that, in the presence of true paraplegia of greater than 24 hours duration, functional recovery is of extreme rarity. The severity of the neurological deficit is therefore a powerful predictor of functional recovery, and represents one area where a significant improvement in outcome could be achieved. There is no doubt that continued education of the medical profession to increase the awareness of the diagnosis of metastatic spinal cord compression would lead to an improved outcome following on from early diagnosis.

Several other factors which may affect the outcome of treatment exist. Amongst these are: the location of the tumour within the spinal canal (Barcena *et al.*, 1984); the presence of vertebral collapse (Brice & McKissock, 1965; Findlay, 1987); the radiosensitivity of the tumour (Gilbert *et al.*, 1978; Barcena *et al.*, 1984); the segmental level of spinal involvement (Smith, 1965; White *et al.*, 1971); and the completeness of the myelographic block (Young *et al.*, 1980). Whilst conflicting views exist regarding the importance or otherwise of such factors, there is one further area where its significance is even more debated. That is the role of the rapidity of onset of the neurological deficit. There is a strong feeling that the more rapidly the deficit progresses the worse the outcome becomes. This is supported by many papers, the principal ones being: Tarlov, 1954; Mullan & Evans, 1957; Wild & Porter, 1963; Smith, 1965; and Chade, 1976. Against this, more recent papers tend to suggest the opposite: that the rate of progression of the deficit has no bearing upon surgical outcome (Hall & Mackay, 1973; Shaw *et al.*, 1980; Stark *et al.*, 1982; Barcena *et al.*, 1984). The true importance of this factor is therefore unclear.

The general condition of the patient has an obvious effect on outcome. In normal practice, patients with widespread and terminal disease are often treated symptomatically and not surgically unless surgery is required to abolish otherwise untreatable instability pain. In an attempt to assess the advisability of surgery in a more rational manner, Tokuhashi *et al.* (1990) devised a scoring system based on six variables: Karnofsky performance status; number of extraspinal bony metastases; number of metastases in the vertebral body; metastases to major organs; primary site of the cancer; and the neurological status. They found that patients scoring five or less points did not survive for more than three months after surgery, while patients scoring nine or more had a high chance of surviving for longer than 12 months.

MANAGEMENT

Siegal & Siegal (1985) defined the criteria of successful therapy in metastatic spinal cord compression as: 'preservation or restoration of neurological function—ambulation and control of bowel and bladder'. For years the only therapy used to try to achieve that goal was that of urgent laminectomy followed, if thought appropriate, by radiotherapy. Through the central part of this century many papers were published giving the results of such an approach, but there was little critical evaluation of just what was being achieved. During the 1970s some papers—especially that of Gilbert *et al.* (1978)—appeared, suggesting that primary radiotherapy might be as effective as laminectomy. This was followed in the 1980s by an increased appreciation of the role of spinal stability and the development of more aggressive surgical procedures designed to allow tumour removal whilst maintaining spinal stability. This latter attitude has resulted at last in improvement in outcome, and has gone some way to achieve success as defined above.

The argument as to whether laminectomy or radiotherapy was the best therapy has not been helped by the rarity of any attempts at a controlled trial to evaluate the problem properly. Even the excellent paper by Gilbert *et al.* (1978) compared their radiotherapeutic results against a surgical group who were preselected in that they had either had previous radiotherapy, a more rapid onset, or did not have a proven primary. Gilbert *et al.* concluded that primary radiotherapy was as effective as laminectomy, but the scientific foundation of that conclusion was suspect. Other studies lent support to that conclusion but the absence of a definitive trial still left the question open. Findlay (1984) approached the question by reviewing all the publications on the topic over the previous 25 years. Only papers which clearly showed the extent of any neurological change were included—those using imprecise terms such as 'improvement' were excluded. Ultimately, there were accurate data concerning over 1800 cases available. No significant difference in outcome between patients treated either by primary radiotherapy or by laminectomy and subsequent radiotherapy was found. Overall, only 71% of those who were still ambulant at the time of therapy retained the ability to walk. Of those who were paraparetic and non-ambulant, only 37% regained the ability to walk. These figures led to an appreciation that many of the patients so treated were in fact not only failing to achieve success, but were actually deteriorating despite therapy. Overall, 20% of the patients in that review actually deteriorated either from ambulant to paraparetic but non-ambulant, or to become paraplegic despite apparent optimum therapy.

It had often been thought that laminectomy was the only acceptable therapy in a patient who was deteriorating rapidly. This was based on the feeling that the effects of radiotherapy would initially cause cord swelling, and that any clinical benefit would be delayed. The fear of cord swelling from radiotherapy came from a paper by Lawes & Ham (1953). However, it was found that more modern high-dose radiotherapeutic regimes actually did cause acute shrinkage of the tumour without significant cord oedema (Rubin, 1969; Ushio *et al.*, 1977). Further, Gilbert *et al.* (1978) actually looked at their cases who presented with rapid deterioration and found that radiotherapy was markedly superior to laminectomy in outcome.

Little attention had been paid to the significance of the presence of vertebral body collapse on outcome with either therapy. Brice & McKissock (1965) did observe that no patients with severe neurological deficit with collapse improved following laminectomy. Hall & Mackay (1973) found that only 9% of their patients with collapse improved after laminectomy. Findlay (1987) examined the role of vertebral collapse in a series of patients undergoing laminectomy. He found that those with collapse had a much worse outcome, with only 15% remaining ambulant and over 50% becoming paraplegic. In addition 22% of those undergoing laminectomy in the presence of vertebral body collapse developed spinal instability. Little information exists in the radiotherapy literature about the effect of collapse on outcome, but Tomita *et al.* (1983) certainly showed a much poorer outcome from radiotherapy in this situation, even in the presence of apparently radiosensitive lesions.

With the greater appreciation of the role of spinal instability in producing morbidity, several reports of the use of posterior spinal stabilization at the time of laminectomy have appeared. All such reports depend on spinal instrumentation at the time of laminectomy, as simple bone grafting techniques do not allow immediate stability. The techniques available are those of: Harrington distraction rods with or without segmental wiring (Sundaresan *et al.*, 1984); laminar bar fixation (Miles *et al.*, 1984); the Luque/Hartshill system (Manabe *et al.*, 1989); pedicle screw fixation and the Cotrel–Dubousset instrumentation (Aprin, 1988). Each of these techniques requires considerable surgical experience and expertise as they all carry the potential of causing cord damage. In experienced hands, however, they certainly limit the adverse effects found when laminectomy alone is performed, and prevent spinal instability. There is regrettably little evidence that they actually increase the number of patients successfully regaining the ability to walk. In patients who have undergone previous radiotherapy, posterior spinal instrumentation significantly increases the incidence of wound infection and dehiscence.

The reason for the apparent failure of posterior techniques to improve outcome lies with the fact that the majority of patients have an anterior extradural mass as either the sole cause or part of their spinal cord compression (Siegal & Siegal, 1985). Laminectomy even with instrumentation fails to decompress the cord adequately when severely compressed from in front. The evidence for this is seen in the poor outcome in patients with marked neurological deficit and vertebral collapse who undergo laminectomy. There is also experimental evidence showing that laminectomy fails to decompress an anterior mass and is also unsuccessful in restoring normal cord blood flow (Doppman & Girton, 1976; Bennett & McCallum, 1977). Some papers have advocated a costotransversectomy approach in addition to laminectomy, to allow adequate anterior decompression of the tumour mass. Encouraging results have been reported with this technique. Overby & Rothman (1985) reported 12 patients on whom they used this approach, of whom only one was ambulant preoperatively. Following surgery eight regained the ability to walk. Overby & Rothman did not routinely use spinal instrumentation at the time of surgery, though many would consider it advisable following such a wide decompression.

The increasing realization of the inadequacy of posterior surgical approaches in patients with anteriorly sited metastases leads naturally to the use of anterior approaches to the spine. The anterior approach to the cervical spine is well established, and the transthoracic or thoracoabdominal approaches to the spine were already widely used for non-metastatic conditions such as osteomyelitis. Bailey & Badgley (1960) were the first to report the use of an anterior approach to a tumour in the cervical spine with subsequent bone grafting, and Scoville *et al.* (1967) reported the resection of a cervical vertebral body followed by acrylic stabilization. In 1962, Senning *et al.* reported a prototype vertebral body prosthesis. Gradually, papers reporting the results of small numbers of patients with metastases treated by an anterior approach appeared (Gunn *et al.*, 1974; Jelsma & Kirsch, 1979; Harrington, 1981). More recently, several larger studies have been reported (Sundaresan *et al.*, 1985; Siegal *et al.*, 1985; Siegal & Siegal, 1985; Sundaresan *et al.*, 1986a,b; Perrin & McBroom, 1987; Turner *et al.*, 1988). They all show remarkably consistent results with between 76% and 83% of the patients being able to walk following anterior operation. This is a most striking improvement upon the results of the other techniques already discussed, as the anterior series comprised a very similar mix of patients with regard to histology and neurological deficit. In the anterior surgical series referred to the proportion of patients ambulant prior to treatment ranged from 26% to 38%, with the exception of one with 55% ambulant preoperatively. This compares favourably with the majority of the papers discussing either radiotherapy or laminectomy, where the percentage of patients overall ambulant after treatment was only in the order of 40%.

There is thus a striking improvement in outcome achieved by anterior surgical techniques in the presence of vertebral collapse. Certain series (Siegal & Siegal, 1985; O'Neil *et al.*, 1988; Manabe *et al.*, 1989) have determined their surgical approach upon the topography of the tumour utilizing either a posterior, anterior or combined approach. These series again report overall success in achieving ambulation in between 70% and 82% of their patients, whereas prior to surgery only between 22% and 27% were able to walk. Furthermore, these studies have shown that, in the hands of an experienced surgical team, the morbidity and mortality of anterior or combined procedures is no greater than that of laminectomy alone.

There is considerable variation in the techniques used to replace the excised or partially excised vertebral body following anterior excision. No clear method of choice has emerged. The ideal is to replace the vertebral body with an autologous bone graft which will ultimately become incorporated in the spine. The author's experience is that replacement of a thoracic vertebral body with a carefully fitted tricortical strut graft taken from the iliac crest and inserted under distraction will give adequate stability. Early mobilization with an external brace is feasible and late loss of correction is uncommon. Tumour invasion of such grafts is a concern but, provided that it is delayed for three weeks, radiotherapy does not affect the ultimate incorporation of the graft (Schwartz *et al.*, 1986), and loss of the graft due to tumour invasion has been extremely rare in the author's experience. Whilst the rib cage and an external brace give sufficient stability to allow early mobilization after the replacement of a thoracic body by bone graft alone, additional instrumentation is necessary at the thoracolumbar junction. This may take the form of either anterior fixation or a posterior instrumentation.

Many other techniques for maintaining spinal stability following vertebral body resection have been described. They all either use bone graft as described above or inert devices as spacers to fill the gap in the spine from the decompression. Most authors supplement the bone graft with instrumentation to enhance spinal stability. There are many methods with which to stabilize the spine during an anterior vertebrectomy and these were well discussed by Cybulski (1989). Stability can also be achieved by supplementing the anterior bone graft by posterior instrumentation or pedicle screw fixation. True vertebral body replacements include blocks constructed from various metals or hydroxyapatite-coated ceramics but many surgeons use acrylic cement alone to fashion a vertebral body replacement. This technique also works well but it must be keyed into the spine by inserting Steinmann pins into the adjacent bodies to improve the fixation between the bone–acrylic interface.

The use of the anterior approach allows maximum tumour removal and greatly enhances dural decompression but it does demand great surgical skill as, in the presence of decompressions extending beyond the confines of one vertebral body or at the thoracolumbar junction, spinal reconstruction as discussed above is necessary. At the cervicothoracic junction an anterior approach is more difficult, but is possible in the majority of patients (Sundaresan *et al.*, 1984). Should there be involvement of more than one level at the cervicothoracic junction, then posterior instrumentation is also required to support an anterior fusion.

Thus it is seen that a wide range of therapy is available in the modern management of metastatic spinal disease, ranging from symptomatic treatment to aggressive surgery. No single approach will accommodate all patients, and the therapeutic choice must be tailored to the individual situation. Figure 28.8 shows a flowchart to aid decision-making in the management of metastatic spinal cord compression.

Whilst the majority of patients presenting with cord compression will also have pain, it must be appreciated that some patients will present with pain in the absence of neurological deficit. Such patients should not be denied treatment of their pain. Obviously some can be controlled by pharmacological means, but if the pain is severe the dosage necessary for control may have unwanted side-effects. Radiotherapy itself affords pain relief in many cases, but it is not universally effective, especially if there is structural instability. In those cases it is often possible to achieve a most rewarding

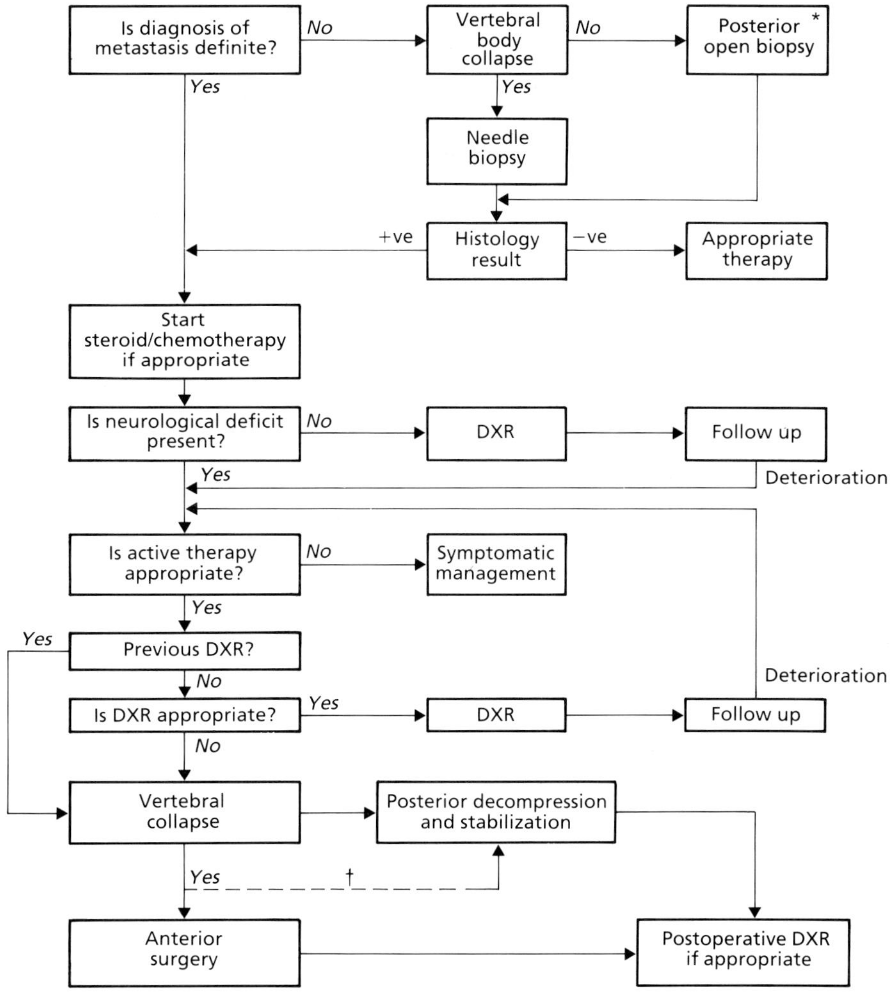

Fig. 28.8 Algorithm for decision-making involved in the management of malignant spinal compression. * May be combined with posterior surgery if that option is selected. † If anterior surgery deemed inappropriate. From Findlay *et al.* (1988).

result by the judicious usage of the techniques of spinal stabilization discussed above, allowing major improvement in the quality of life.

The previous discussion has dealt with therapy directly related to relieving the effects of cord compression. In addition, however, it is important to consider the patient as a whole and to provide adjuvant therapy directed either towards control of the primary neoplasm or towards enhancing the effects of therapy on the compressed cord. Many primary neoplasia are amenable to therapy such as hormonal manipulation, and chemotherapy may be appropriate in both solid tumours as well as those of haematogenous origin. In rare instances such treatment alone may be effective in reversing a trend towards cord compression.

The most widely used adjunct used in the control of the cord compression is steroid therapy. There is little evidence supporting the usage of high-dose regimens, but there is general agreement that conventional doses of steroid do affect the syndrome of metastatic cord compression. Such an effect is, however, only temporary, but it can significantly slow down the evolution of the neurological deficit, and in many cases allow for some improvement. This permits time for more detailed planning of the therapeutic strategy. Marshall & Langfitt (1977) showed that 62% of their patients improved for a period of 24 hours with steroid therapy.

Siegal *et al.* (1988a,b) have examined the role of vasogenic oedema in the early stages of experimental metastastic cord compression. They found that dexamethasone commenced at the onset of neurological deficit in rats with extradural tumours reduced the increase in cord water content, but did not affect the specific gravity changes. The anti-inflammatory agent indomethacin, however, returned both factors back to normal levels. The usage of dexamethasone significantly delayed the progression of neurological deficit by 29% but indomethacin proved more effective, delaying progression in 66%. Siegel *et al.* also examined the effect on the increased prostanoid production which occurs in the compressed cord, an effect which precedes the increase in water content. Dexamethasone had no effect on this, whereas indomethacin inhibited prostanoid formation and returned water content to normal. It remains to be seen whether anti-inflammatory agents will be clinically useful.

There is a much greater role for adjuvant therapy in children with spinal metastatic disease. Klein *et al.* (1991) reported an incidence of spinal cord compression in only 5% of paediatric patients with solid malignant tumours. Patients with Ewing's sarcoma had the greatest incidence of spinal involvement (18%) with spinal involvement occurring in neuroblastoma in 8%. Spinal involvement from metastatic osteosarcoma carried a very poor prognosis.

Klein *et al.* found that, in patients with a sarcomatous primary, chemotherapy and irradiation had a significantly poorer outcome than did appropriate surgical decompression. However, in patients with primary small-cell tumours such as neuroblastoma, Hodgkin's or germ-cell tumours, they found that medical treatment was as effective as surgical therapy except for cases with a rapid onset of neurological deficit or where complete paraplegia was present. They also observed that, unlike the adult patient, complete paraplegia was not a contra-indication to aggressive therapy as 50% became ambulatory following decompression and medical therapy. The authors stress, as have many others, that laminectomy in children is associated with significant risk of progressive kyphotic deformity and the surgical procedure must be planned so as to avoid or prevent postlaminectomy deformity.

INTRAMEDULLARY METASTASES

The occurrence of metastases within the spinal cord itself is much less frequent than in the extradural space. Chason *et al.* (1963) examined the cords of 1066 patients with disseminated cancer at autopsy. They found an intramedullary metastasis in only 10 cases, all of whom had other central nervous system involvement. Nugent *et al.* (1979) found an incidence of 6% for intramedullary metastasis in cases of small-cell carcinoma of the lung. Findlay *et al.* (1987) reported two cases diagnosed in life, and reviewed 144 further reported cases. They estimated the incidence to lie between 0.9% and 2.1% of autopsied cancer cases. The lung was the primary source in 64%. Those cases reported usually present with a rapidly progressive and severe neurological deficit, and surprisingly the finding of malignant cells in the CSF is rare. Initial myelography was often normal, and survival was found to be very poor. Grem *et al.* (1985) found a 55% mortality rate within four weeks of the diagnosis being made, rising to 83% at 12 weeks.

Reports of attempted treatment are uncommon, but the general experience is that attempts at surgical extirpation carry a very high risk of worsening deficit and a high mortality. Most authors advise either no treatment or radiotherapy. This perhaps is dangerous advice, as the finding of an intramedullary mass does not necessarily mean that it is due to a metastasis and surgical exploration should be carried out to achieve at least histological confirmation. The two patients presented by Findlay *et al.* (1987) both had a more gradual presentation and regained the ability to walk after microsurgical removal.

REFERENCES

Aprin, H. (1988) Metastatic tumours of the spine. In Akbarnia, B. (ed.) *Spinal Tumours*, pp. 301–313. Hanley & Belfus, Philadelphia.

Bailey, R. & Badgley, C. (1960) Stabilisation of the cervical spine by anterior fusion. *J. Bone Jt. Surg.*, **42A**, 565–594.

Barcena, A., Lobato, R., Rivas, J., Cordobes, F., de Castro S., Cabrera, A. & Lamas, E. (1984) Spinal metastatic disease: analysis of factors determining functional prognosis and the choice of treatment. *Neurosurgery*, **15**, 820–827.

Batson, O. (1940) The function of the vertebral veins and their role in the spread of metastases. *Ann. Surg.*, **112**, 138–149.

Bennett, M. & McCallum, J. (1977) Experimental decompression of the spinal cord. *Surg. Neurol.*, **8**, 63–67.

Black, P. (1979) Spinal metastasis: current status and recommended guidelines for management. *Neurosurgery*, **5**, 726–746.

Brice, J. & McKissock, W. (1965). Surgical treatment of malignant extradural tumours. *Br. Med. J.*, **1**, 1341–1344.

Broaddus, W., Grady, M., Delashaw, J., Ferguson, R. & Jane, J. (1990) Preoperative superselective arteriolar embolization: a new approach to enhance resectability of spinal tumours. *Neurosurgery*, **27**, 755–759.

Bucy, P. (1963). The treatment of malignant tumours of the spine: a review. *Neurology*, **13**, 938–944.

Chade, H. (1976). Metastatic tumours of the spine and

spinal cord. In Vinken, P. & Bruyn, G. (eds) *Handbook of Clinical Neurology*, vol. 20, pp. 415–433. North-Holland, Amsterdam.

Chason, J., Walker, F. & Landers, J. (1963) Metastatic carcinoma in the central nervous system and dorsal root ganglia: A prospective autopsy study. *Cancer*, **16**, 781–787.

Coakham, H., Garson, J., Brownell, B., Allan, P., Harper, E., Lane, E. & Kemshead, J. (1984) Use of monoclonal antibody panel to identify malignant cells in cerebrospinal fluid. *Lancet*, **2**, 1095–1098.

Cobb, C., Leavens, M. & Eckles, N. (1977). Indications for non-operative treatment of spinal cord compression due to breast cancer. *J. Neurosurg.*, **47**, 653–658.

Constans, J., de Divitiis, E., Donzelli, R., Spazianti, R., Meder, J. & Haye, C. (1983) Spinal metastases with neurological manifestations: review of 600 cases. *J. Neurosurg.*, **59**, 111–118.

Cybulski, G. (1989) Methods of surgical stabilization for metastatic disease of the spine. *Neurosurgery*, **25**, 240–252.

Doppman, J. & Girton, M. (1976) Angiographic study of the effect of laminectomy in the presence of acute anterior epidural masses. *J. Neurosurg.*, **45**, 195–202.

Ell, P. (1983) Bones and joints. In Maisey, M., Britton, K. & Gilday, D. (eds) *Clinical Nuclear Imaging*. Chapman & Hall, London.

Elsberg, C. (1941) *Surgical Diseases of the Spinal Cord, Membranes and Nerve Roots: Symptoms, Diagnosis and Treatment*. Hoeber, New York.

Findlay, G. (1984) Adverse effects of the management of malignant spinal cord compression. *J. Neurol. Neurosurg. Psychiatry*, **47**, 761–768.

Findlay, G. (1987) The role of vertebral body collapse in the management of malignant spinal cord compression. *J. Neurol. Neurosurg. Psychiatry*, **50**, 151–154.

Findlay, G., Sandeman, D. & Buxton, P. (1988) The role of needle biopsy in the management of malignant spinal compression. *Br. J. Neurosurg.*, **2**, 479–484.

Findlay, G. (1991) Transthoracic approach for thoracic disc and kyphectomy. In Torrens, M. & Dickson, R. (eds) *Operative Spinal Surgery*. Churchill Livingstone, London.

Findlay, J., Bernstein, M., Vanderlinden, R. & Resch, L. (1987) Microsurgical resection of solitary intramedullary spinal cord metastases. *Neurosurgery*, **21**, 911–915.

Fyfe, I., Henry, A. & Mulholland, R. (1983) Closed vertebral biopsy. *J. Bone Jt. Surg*, **65B**, 140–143.

Gilbert, R., Kim, J. & Posner, J. (1978) Epidural spinal cord compression from metastatic tumour: diagnosis and treatment. *Ann. Neurol.*, **3**, 40–51.

Godersky, J., Smoker, W. & Knutzon, R. (1987) Use of magnetic resonance imaging in the evaluation of metastatic spinal disease. *Neurosurgery*, **21**, 676–680.

Greenwood, J. (1973) Spinal cord tumours. In Youmans, J. (ed.) *Neurological Surgery*, pp. 1514–1534. W.B. Saunders, Philadelphia, PA.

Grem, J., Burgess, J. & Trump, D. (1985) Clinical features and natural history of intramedullary spinal cord metastasis. *Cancer*, **56**, 2305–2314.

Gunn, D., Tupper, J. & Mullen, M. (1974) Decompression and immediate stabilisation of the spine in patients suffering from malignant disease. *J. Bone Jt. Surg.*, **56A**, 1767–1770.

Hagenau, C., Grosh, W., Currie, M. & Wiley, R. (1987) Comparison of spinal magnetic resonance imaging and myelography in cancer patients. *J. Clin. Oncol.*, **5**, 1663–1669.

Hall, A. & Mackay, N. (1973) The results of laminectomy for compression of the cord and cauda equina by extradural malignant tumour. *J. Bone Jt. Surg.*, **55B**, 497–505.

Harrington, K. (1981) The use of methylmethacrylate for vertebral-body replacement and anterior stabilisation of pathological fracture-dislocations of the spine due to metastatic malignant disease. *J. Bone Jt. Surg.*, **63A**, 36–46.

Ikeda, H., Ushio, Y., Hayakawa, B., Mogami, H. & Hayakawa, T. (1980) Edema and circulatory disturbances in the spinal cord compressed by epidural neoplasms in rabbits. *J. Neurosurg.*, **52**, 203–209.

Jelsma, R. & Kirsch, P. (1979) The treatment of malignancy of a vertebral body. *Surg. Neurol.*, **13**, 189–195.

Klein, S., Sanford, R. & Muhlbauer, M. (1991) Pediatric spinal epidural metastases. *J. Neurosurg.*, **74**, 70–75.

Lawes, F. & Ham, H. (1953) A case of Hodgkins disease with spinal cord involvement treated by nitrogen mustard. *Med. J. Aust.*, **1**, 104–106.

Manabe, S., Tateishi, A., Abe, M. & Ohno, T. (1989) Surgical treatment of metastatic tumours of the spine. *Spine*, **14**, 41–47.

Markham, J. (1951) Surgery in the spinal cord and vertebral column. In Walker, A. (ed.) *A History of Neurological Surgery*, p. 383. Williams & Wilkins, Baltimore, MD.

Marshall, L. & Langfitt, T. (1977) Combined therapy for metastatic extradural tumours of the spine. *Cancer*, **40**, 2067–2070.

McNeil, B. (1984) Value of bone scanning in neoplastic disease. *Semin. Nucl. Med.*, **14**, 277–286.

Miles, J., Banks, A., Dervin, E. & Noori, Z. (1984) Stabilization of the spine affected by malignancy. *J. Neurol. Neurosurg. Psychiatry*, **47**, 897–904.

Mullan, J. & Evans, J. (1957) Neoplastic disease of the spinal extradural space: a review of fifty cases. *Arch. Surg.*, **74**, 900–907.

Nugent, J., Bunn, P., Matthews, M., Ihde, D., Cohen, M., Garzdar, A. & Minna, J. (1979) CNS metastasis in small cell bronchogenic carcinoma. *Cancer*, **44**, 1885–1893.

O'Neil, J., Gardner, V. & Armstrong, G. (1988) Treatment of tumors of the thoracic and lumbar spinal column. *Clin. Orthop.*, **227**, 103–112.

Ottolenghi, C. (1955) Diagnosis of orthopaedic lesions by aspiration biopsy: result of 1061 punctures. *J. Bone Jt. Surg.*, **37A**, 443–464.

Overby, M. & Rothman, S. (1985) Anterolateral decompression for metastatic epidural spinal cord tumors. *J. Neurosurg.*, **62**, 344–348.

Perrin, R. & McBroom, R. (1988) Spinal fixation after anterior decompression for symptomatic spinal metastasis.

Neurosurgery, **22**, 324–327.
Robertson, R. & Ball, R. (1935) Destructive spine lesions: diagnosis by needle biopsy. *J. Bone Jt. Surg.*, **17**, 749–758.
Rubin, P. (1969) Extradural spinal cord compression by tumour: Part 1. Experimental production and treatment trial. *Radiology*, **93**, 1243–1260.
van der Sande, J., Kröger, R. & Boogerd, W. (1990) Multiple spinal epidural metastases; an unexpectedly frequent finding. *J. Neurol. Neurosurg. Psychiatry*, **53**, 1001–1003.
Sarpel, S., Sarpel, G., Yu, E., Hyder, S., Kaufman, B. & Hindo, W. (1987) Early diagnosis of spinal–epidural metastasis by magnetic resonance imaging. *Cancer*, **59**, 1112–1116.
Schaberg, J. & Gainor, B. (1985) A profile of metastatic carcinoma of the spine. *Spine*, **10**, 19–20.
Schwartz, H., Leake, D., Kagan, R., Snow, H. & Pizzoperrato, A. (1985) Postoperative irradiation of fresh autogenic cancellous bone grafts. *Plast. Reconstr. Surg.*, **77**, 122–126.
Scoville, W., Palmer, A., Samra, K. & Chong, G. (1967) The use of acrylic plastic for vertebral replacement of fixation in metastatic disease of the spine. *J. Neurosurg.*, **27**, 274–279.
Senning, A., Weber, G. & Yasargil, M. (1962) Zur operativen Behandlung von Tumoren der Wirbelsaule. *Scheiwz. Med. Wochenschr.*, **92**, 1574–1576.
Shapiro, W. & Posner, J. (1983) Medical versus surgical treatment of metastatic spinal cord tumours. In Thompson, R. & Green, J. (eds) *Controversies in Neurology*, pp. 57–65. Raven Press, New York.
Shaw, M., Rose, J. & Paterson, A. (1980) Metastatic extradural malignancy of the spine. *Acta Neurochir.*, **52**, 113–120.
Siegal, T. & Siegal, T. (1985) Surgical decompression of anterior and posterior malignant epidural tumours compressing the spinal cord: a prospective study. *Neurosurgery*, **17**, 424–432.
Siegal, T. & Siegal, T. (1989) Current considerations in the management of neoplastic spinal cord compression. *Spine*, **14**, 223–228.
Siegal, T., Tiqva, P. & Siegal, T. (1985) Vertebral body resection for epidural compression by malignant tumours. *J. Bone Jt. Surg.*, **67A**, 375–382.
Siegal, T., Siegal, T., Shapira, Y., Sandbank, U. & Catane, R. (1988a) Indomethacin and dexamethasone treatment in experimental neoplastic spinal cord compression: Part 1. *Neurosurgery*, **22**, 328–333.
Siegal, T., Shohami, E., Shapira, Y. & Siegal, T. (1988b) Indomethacin and dexamethasone treatment in experimental neoplastic spinal cord compression: Part 2. *Neurosurgery*, **22**, 334–339.
Smith, R. (1965) An evaluation of surgical treatment for spinal cord compression due to metastatic carcinoma. *J. Neurol. Neurosurg. Psychiatry*, **28**, 152–158.
Stark, R., Henson, R. & Evans, S. (1982) Spinal metastases—a retrospective survey from a general hospital. *Brain*, **105**, 189–213.
Sundaresan, N., Galicich, J. & Lane, J. (1981) Treatment of odontoid fractures in cancer patients. *J. Neurosurg.*, **52**, 187–191.
Sundaresan, N., Galicich, J. & Lane, J. (1984) Harrington rod stabilisation for pathological fractures of the spine. *J. Neurosurg.*, **60**, 282–286.
Sundaresan, N., Galicich, J., Lane, J., Bavis, M. & McCormack, P. (1985) Treatment of neoplastic epidural cord compression by vertebral body resection and stabilisation. *J. Neurosurg.*, **63**, 676–684.
Sundaresan, N., Galicich, J., Lane, J. & Scher, H. (1986a) Stabilisation of the spine involved by cancer. In Dunsker, S. (ed.) *The Unstable Spine*. Grune & Stratton, New York.
Sundaresan, N., DiGiacinto, G. & Hughes, J. (1986b) Surgical treatment of spinal metastases. *Clin. Neurosurg.*, **33**, 503–522.
Sundaresan, N., Scher, H., DiGiacinto, G., Yagoda, A., Whitmore, W. & Choi, I. (1986c) Surgical treatment of spinal cord compression in kidney cancer. *J. Clin. Oncol.*, **4**, 1851–1856.
Sze, G., Krol, G., Zimmerman, R. & Deck, M. (1988) Malignant extradural spinal tumours: MR imaging with Gd-DTPA. *Radiology*, **167**, 217–223.
Tarlov, I. (1954) Spinal cord compression studies: III. Time limits for recovery after gradual compression in dogs. *Arch. Neurol. Psychiatry*, **71**, 588–597.
Tokuhashi, Y., Matsuzaki, H., Toriyama, S., Kawano, H. & Ohsaka, S. (1990) Scoring system for the preoperative evaluation of metastatic spine tumour prognosis. *Spine*, **15**, 1110–1113.
Tomita, T., Galicich, J. & Sundaresan, N. (1983) Radiation therapy for spinal epidural metastases with complete block. *Acta Radiol. Oncol.*, **22**, 135–143.
Turner, P., Prince, H., Webb, J. & Sokal, M. (1988) Surgery for malignant extradural tumours of the spine. *J. Bone Jt. Surg.*, **70B**, 451–456.
Ushio, Y., Posner, R., Posner, J. & Shapiro, W. (1977) Experimental spinal cord compression by epidural neoplasms. *Neurology*, **27**, 422–429.
Weissman, D., Gilbert, M., Wang, H. & Grossman, S. (1985) The use of computed tomography of the spine to identify patients at high risk for epidural metastases. *J. Clin. Oncol.*, **3**, 1541–1544.
White, W., Patterson, R. & Bergland, R. (1971) The role of surgery in the treatment of spinal cord compression by metastatic neoplasm. *Cancer*, **27**, 558–561.
Wild, W. & Porter, R. (1963) Metastatic epidural tumour of the spine: study of 45 cases. *Arch. Surg.*, **87**, 825–830.
Wong, D., Fornasier, V. & MacNab, I. (1990) Spinal metastases: the obvious, the occult, and the imposters. *Spine*, **15**, 1–4.
Young, R., Post, E. & King, G. (1980) Treatment of spinal epidural metastases. Randomised prospective comparison of laminectomy and radiotherapy. *J. Neurosurg.*, **53**, 741–748.

29 · Intradural Extramedullary Tumours

By P.M. FOY

Spinal tumours are classified by histological type and by their anatomical relationship to the dura mater and spinal cord. The dura provides a natural barrier to the spread of malignant tumours and this is of practical surgical importance. Extradural tumours invade the spinal column from surrounding structures and are mostly metastatic. Intradural tumours can be extrinsic to the spinal cord, i.e. extramedullary, or can be intramedullary, arising within the substance of the cord. About 70% of intradural tumours are extramedullary. They are nearly always benign and the majority are either meningiomas or schwannomas. The remainder are accounted for by dermoid and epidermoid tumours, cysts, lipomas and other rare miscellaneous lesions.

INCIDENCE

Primary intraspinal neoplasms are rare and the statistical data on the incidence and frequency of different lesions tend to come from specialist referral centres rather than defined populations. Helseth & Mørk (1989) reported a large population-based survey of primary intraspinal neoplasms from the Norwegian Cancer Registry and quoted an annual incidence of five per million for females and three per million for males. In their 467 patients the incidence of meningiomas was 46.7% but only 10.8% were schwannomas. However, most of the series of spinal tumours from specialist centres show a slight predominance of schwannomas. Nittner (1976) gave a summary from the literature of 4885 cases of spinal cord tumours and other space-occupying lesions, according to their histological classification. Meningiomas accounted for 22.4% of the cases, schwannomas for 23.1% and ependymomas for only 2.5%. The range of incidence from the series surveyed was 13–30% for meningiomas and 11–38% for schwannomas. In the largest series of Sloof *et al.* (1964), who reported 1322 tumours, the incidence of meningiomas was 25.5% and of schwannoma 29%.

CLINICAL FEATURES

Progressive expansion of the tumour, in the limited capacity of the spinal canal, will be initially at the expense of extradural fat, venous blood volume and cerebrospinal fluid (CSF), but later at the expense of the spinal cord. Generally speaking a fast rate of compression produces more neurological damage and carries a worse prognosis for neurological recovery.

The clinical manifestations of an intradural extramedullary tumour are brought about by compression and displacement of the spinal cord and involvement of adjacent nerve roots. In contradistinction from malignant extradural compression, intradural tumours show a chronic compressive syndrome. Chronic compression over months or years allows the cord to be slowly displaced and deformed, producing flattened 'wasted' tissue which still allows for a remarkable degree of neurological function. It would seem that the blood vessels in the compressed area of cord can also accommodate the deformation.

Pain is the commonest initial symptom and frequently precedes by months or years the signs of spinal cord compression. Pain of spinal root origin is described as shooting, stabbing or burning, and by its distribution may help to localize the affected nerve. Movement and straining may aggravate the pain and curiously in some patients the pain is present only at night. Pain due to spinal cord compression may be quite different and is often described as dull, aching and continuous with a wide distribution and not influenced by straining and movement. Extremes of neck flexion and extension in the presence of a tumour in the cervical spine may evoke tingling, pins and needles and electric shock sensations radiating down the spine and perhaps into the limbs (L'Hermitte's sign). Pain in the occipital region and in the neck is a common initial symptom of foramen magnum tumours and is often aggravated by change in posture and by movement of the neck; the head and neck may be held stiffly awry, and this is particularly common in children.

The tumour may produce any combination of neurological signs, depending on the spinal segment involved and the specific site of compression and pattern of deformation of the spinal cord.

Motor disturbances are often the second symptom to be noticed; with cord compression the legs are affected first, the patient complaining of stiffness of muscles, gradually followed by weakness. The neurological findings are those of an upper motor neurone lesion with spasticity and increased reflexes. There may be evidence of a lower motor neurone disorder with flaccid atrophy and fasciculation arising from the cord segment or nerve root which has been directly compressed. Sensory deficits nearly always appear after the motor disturbances. The abnormal signs that develop will depend upon the tracts affected. Posterior column involvement will give loss of joint position and vibration sense. Compression of the anterolateral columns will give impaired pain and temperature sensation. A definite sensory level develops late and gives a valuable guide to the site of cord compression. Sphincter disturbances almost always occur at a late stage after motor and sensory disturbances have developed. It is only in tumours that compress the conus and cauda equina that sphincter disturbances may be the first complaint.

Foramen magnum tumours, sometimes described as spinocranial if the tumour started in the spinal canal, produce a clinical picture which is shared with a variety of malformations and deformations which occur at this level; they may simulate tumours at a distance and certain intrinsic diseases of the brain stem and spinal cord. Love *et al.* (1954) analysed 74 cases of tumour at this level; amongst them were 26 meningiomas, 16 astrocytomas, 14 ependymomas, four medulloblastomas, three schwannomas, two oligodendrogliomas, an intramedullary glioma and an aneurysm of the vertebral artery.

Depending upon the precise situation and extent of the tumour above the foramen magnum there may be involvement of the lower cranial nerves. Dysphagia and respiratory obstruction may occur, and nystagmus occurs in about half the cases (Dodge *et al.*, 1956). Signs of interference with the cervical sympathetic supply (Horner's syndrome) and disturbance of trigeminal sensation due to compression of the descending sensory root may also be present.

Intraspinal tumours may present in unusual ways, posing pitfalls in diagnosis. Hydrocephalus or intracranial hypertension due to intraspinal tumour is rare; this association was found in three of the 289 tumours of the cauda equina reported by Arseni & Maretsis (1967), and eight of the 61 paediatric tumours in the series of Oi & Raimondi (1981). Kudo *et al.* (1987) reported three cases bringing the total in the literature at that time to 67. In cases with headache and dementia the intraspinal tumour is often not diagnosed, and a CSF shunting procedure may be performed without the spinal tumour being recognized. Particularly in patients over 40 years, symptoms of 'normal pressure hydrocephalus'—dementia, gait disturbance and urinary incontinence—may appear, and it is suggested that a lumbar puncture should be carried out prior to any shunting operation to ensure that the CSF is normal.

The pathophysiology of the hydrocephalus is complex and is not completely understood. A raised protein level in the CSF will increase its viscosity and decrease absorption; the protein may also cause blockage of absorption at the arachnoid villi where CSF water and protein are absorbed into the venous system. Compression of the spinal venous plexus may lead to raised venous intracranial pressure and decreased absorption of CSF. Subarachnoid haemorrhage may rarely be the prevailing symptom of a spinal tumour (Scotti *et al.*, 1987; Chalif *et al.*, 1990) and blood in the CSF can contribute to the development of hydrocephalus.

Meningiomas

Cushing & Eisenhardt (1938) gave an account of the earliest descriptions of these tumours and of the controversies which have arisen over their nomenclature and histogenesis. Schmidt (1902) drew attention to the similarity between the microscopical appearances of the cells of the tumour and those of the arachnoidal villi, and it is now accepted that meningiomas arise from the endothelium which lines the leptomeningeal spaces. Some meningiomas are so firmly attached to the dura that they appear to be arising from it, but it is thought that they are derived from sequestered clumps of arachnoidal cells which occur within normal dura mater. In the spinal canal there are nests of arachnoidal cells at the junction of the arachnoid and dura where they encase the nerve roots on their passage towards the intervertebral foramina (Hassin, 1930). The term 'meningioma' was introduced by Cushing in his 1922 Cavendish Lecture as a simple and non-committal designation, and is now universally employed, although many alternatives have been proposed.

The microscopic appearances of meningiomas fall into a variety of different patterns which have led to a multiplicity of classifications and confused terminology. A widely accepted scheme is that of Courville (1945), who classified meningiomas into five basic types: syncytial, transitional, fibrous, angioblastic and malignant. A variety of secondary changes may occur in any of these types, and Kepes (1986) has pointed out their protean microscopic appearances which may mimic other tumours.

Russell & Rubinstein (1989) proposed a regrouping of the meningiomas under three principal headings based on distinctive electron microscopic and immunohistochemical features. The first group comprised the three main types of 'classic meningiomas': syncytial (meningothelial), transitional and fibroblastic. The second group consists of the 'angioblastic meningiomas' which are themselves divided into two distinct variants, the haemangioblastic and the haemangiopericytic. The third group is formed by the 'malignant meningiomas', which include the papillary type as a characteristic variant.

In its simplest form the tumour is seen as a pinkish round or oval mass whose surface may be quite smooth, finely granular or coarsely lobulated. Its texture is usually firm and fibrous but sometimes friable and sufficiently soft to respond to suction. At times the tumour is gritty from calcareous deposits (psammoma bodies) and rarely there is cystic degeneration, haemorrhage or butter-like areas due to lipoid changes.

The tumour is attached to the dura mater and arachnoid and consequently does not have the mobility of an intradural schwannoma. The meningeal attachment may be broad, rendering the tumour sessile, or much narrower than the diameter of the tumour mass. It is through its attachment that the tumour receives its major blood supply; hence the dura mater in this area is often thickened and vascular. The extradural vessels are increased and there may be a particularly rich venous plexus. Although the dura mater is firmly involved, extradural spread is uncommon and primary extradural meningioma is rare. In the series of Tönnis (Becker, 1965) 85% of meningiomas were intradural, 7% were extradural and intradural, and 8% were entirely extradural. Spinal as opposed to intracranial meningiomas do not involve bone, and this is probably due to the space between dura and bone which is filled with fat, venous plexuses and nerve roots.

Meningiomas may develop in any part of the spinal canal but arise most frequently in the thoracic region. Nittner (1976) analysed 705 cases of meningioma reported in various series between 1925 and 1965, and found that 80.9% were in the thoracic spine, 16.8% arose in the cervical area and 2.3% lay near the conus or cauda equina. The capacity of the lumbosacral canal may allow a slow-growing tumour to reach a large size, and there are rare reports of giant lumbosacral meningiomas (Feldenzer *et al.*, 1990). There is no clear explanation for the predilection of meningiomas for the thoracic canal and for their rarity in the lumbosacral region; the rarity of the lumbar site has been attributed to the arrangement of the denticulate ligaments there. The majority of spinal meningiomas present between the ages of 40 and 70 years with a peak in the sixth decade; they are rare in children and young adults.

Very long clinical histories are unusual, with about a half of all patients with spinal meningiomas coming to surgery within a year and over three-quarters within two years. Of the 174 spinal meningiomas reported by Solero *et al.* (1989) 117 patients had a clinical history ranging from six months to three years, the duration being longer than three years in 28 cases and shorter than six months in 29 cases.

There is no difference between the sexes in the incidence of spinal tumours as a whole, but meningiomas predominantly affect females. In most series over 80% of the patients are female (Nittner, 1976; Solero *et al.*, 1989). Meningiomas have been associated with pregnancy and menstruation (Bickerstaff *et al.*, 1958), obesity (Bellur *et al.*, 1983) and breast cancer (Schoenberg *et al.*, 1975), raising the possibility that these tumours are hormonally reactive and may respond to hormonal manipulation.

Several studies have shown that progesterone receptors are present in a high percentage of meningiomas and are more common than oestrogen receptors. Grunberg *et al.* (1987) found that a significant number of meningiomas in tissue culture had their growth suppressed by progesterone and that progesterone receptor positivity was predictive of such an effect in approximately 40% of cases. Benzel & Gelder (1988) suggested that progesterone receptors may play a role in the production of oedema around meningiomas and the use of progesterone antagonists preoperatively may make surgery safer. Olson *et al.* (1986) showed that a progesterone antagonist (RU486) inhibited meningioma growth in culture, raising the possibility that these drugs may be useful clinically in treating aggressive, recurrent or incompletely excised meningiomas. Low levels of oestrogen and progesterone receptors have also been found in spinal schwannomas (Markwalder *et al.*, 1986) but the significance of this is not clear.

It is well recognized that meningiomas, usually multiple, are associated with central neurofibromatosis. Indeed it has been suggested (List, 1943; Delleman *et al.*, 1978) that multiple meningiomas represent a form of neurofibromatosis. Hereditary factors have been demonstrated by the occurrence of multiple meningiomas in families (Sedzimir *et al.*, 1973; Patronas *et al.*, 1980). True multiple meningiomas, with no family history or evidence of neurofibromatosis, are rare, and occurred in 2.4% of the 288 meningiomas reported by Eljamel & Foy (1989).

Schwannoma and neurofibroma

Benign encapsulated tumours arise on cranial, spinal and peripheral nerves and may be solitary or multiple; in the latter case they constitute the chief feature of neurofibromatosis or Von Recklinghausen's disease. A great variety of names has been applied to these tumours; neurofibroma, neurinoma, perineural fibroblastoma, neurolemmoma, peripheral glioma. This diversity of nomenclature has depended upon the interpretations placed upon the histology of the tumours, the identity of their cells and upon opinions regarding their embryological origin, whether mesodermal or ectodermal. However, electron microscopy, immunohistochemistry and tissue culture studies have led to a wide acceptance that in both varieties of tumour the essential neoplastic cell is derived from the sheath of Schwann (Russell & Rubinstein, 1989).

There are macroscopical and microscopical differences between the solitary tumour and those of neurofibromatosis. The solitary tumour is circumscribed, rounded, its nerve of origin incorporated in its capsule and applied to one aspect of the tumour. In Von Recklinghausen's disease the affected portion of nerve is commonly diffusely swollen in spindle fashion, with irregular nodular enlargements; the nerve fibres are incorporated in the tumour. Microscopical examination of schwannomas show that they consist of Schwann cells which may be arranged in two entirely different patterns (Antoni, 1920). Type A tissue consists of strands, shoals and whorls of closely packed spindle cells with elongated, darkly staining nuclei which show a tendency to grouping and even to striking palisading. Type B tissue consists of loosely arranged stellate cells the processes of which form a fine meshwork. The two types of tissue are usually intermingled, although clearly demarcated from each other, one or the other pattern predominating. The stroma of the tumour usually consists of fine reticulin fibres, collagen being scanty. In some long-standing tumours, however, strands of collagen fibres, sometimes hyalinized, may be abundant. Other degenerative changes include intracellular deposition of lipid leading to the formation of xanthomatous areas and frequent aggregations of iron pigment, a residue of old haemorrhages. Both malignant schwannomas and neurofibromas can develop as solitary tumours but are predominantly found in the context of von Recklinghausen's disease. They occur almost exclusively on peripheral nerves, the common spinal root tumour very rarely undergoing malignant change.

Multiple schwannomas are a prominent feature of von Recklinghausen's neurofibromatosis and two forms of the disease, central and peripheral, are well described. The central form is characterized by tumours arising almost exclusively on the cranial and spinal nerve roots, and in the peripheral form the peripheral nerves are predominantly affected, the principal lesions being neurofibromas with schwannomas restricted to the larger nerve trunks.

Spinal schwannomas arise indiscriminately from any of the spinal nerves and almost invariably from the sensory roots (Russell & Rubinstein, 1989) which may account for the high incidence of radicular pain as a first symptom. Intramedullary schwannomas, deeply embedded in the substance of the spinal cord, are very rare—Ross *et al.* (1986) described two cases and reviewed the literature.

To the naked eye at operation a schwannoma is usually a round or oval shape and the surface is smooth and glistening. It lies relatively mobile under the arachnoid but is attached firmly to the relevant nerve root which is incorporated in its capsule. In consistency the tumour is usually slightly elastic but may contain cystic areas and occasionally recent and old haemorrhage. A common size for a thoracic tumour is about 2 cm, although it is often larger in the upper cervical region. Because of the large capacity of the lumbosacral spinal canal tumours here may reach a very large size, practically filling the canal and extending 5 cm or more in length.

Occasionally a schwannoma extends through the intervertebral foramen to form a further mass on the peripheral segment of the nerve. These hourglass or dumbbell tumours occur mostly in the cervical or thoracic regions, and occasional examples are also found behind the peritoneum and in the pelvis. Cervical tumours may produce a palpable mass in the neck, and thoracic tumours may present to the thoracic surgeon before its intraspinal portion has given rise to neurological symptoms.

INVESTIGATION

Generally speaking the initial radiological investigation of a spinal neoplasm should include radiographs of the whole spine; there may be multiple lesions and diffuse changes may be present. A considerable proportion of intradural extramedullary tumours betray their presence by pressure erosion of adjacent bone. Localized radiological changes are found much more frequently in schwannomas than meningiomas, 45% and 10% respectively in the series reported by Bull (1953).

Erosion may cause enlargement of the margins of an intervertebral foramen and this is typical of a schwannoma (Fig. 29.1); the large extraspinal extension of a thoracic schwannoma may also erode adjacent ribs. The medial aspect of corresponding pedicles may be eroded, causing a widening of the spinal canal. At the level of increased interpedicular distance it is often possible to identify a change in shape of the pedicle, the inner margin being flat or concave. The posterior surface of the vertebral body may be hollowed out by chronic pressure from

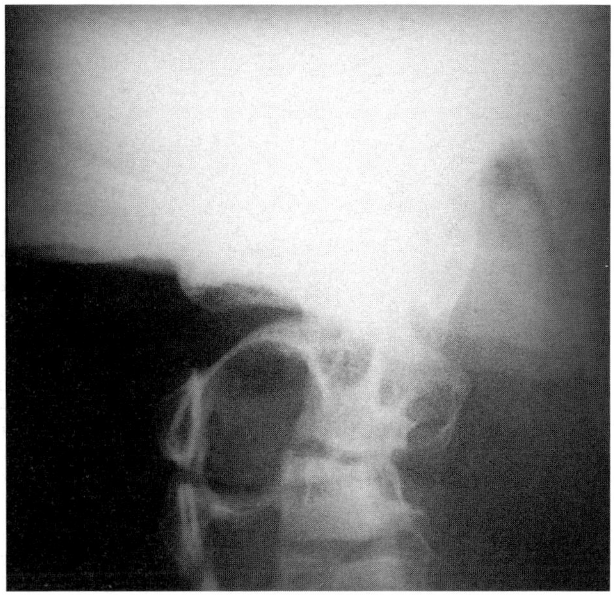

Fig. 29.1 Enlargement of intervertebral foramina at C2–C3 and C3–C4 in a case of neurofibromatosis.

a benign tumour. The intervertebral discs resist this pressure erosion and on lateral radiographs the posterior surfaces of the vertebral bodies cast a series of concavities, described as 'scalloping' (Fig. 29.2). This usually occurs in the lower thoracic, lumbar and sacral regions. The tumour is generally massive and chronic with minimal symptoms; schwannomas and ependymonas of the cauda equina are the commonest tumours to produce scalloping but it very occasionally occurs with massive meningiomas. Scalloping may occur without evidence of spinal neoplasia and has been reported in cases of communicating hydrocephalus (Shealy *et al.*, 1964) and dural ectasia (Heard & Payne, 1962). Calcification may occasionally be seen in meningiomas but rarely in schwannomas (Fig. 29.3).

Myelography is still the diagnostic workhorse in spinal neoplasia. Its introduction by Sicard & Forestier (1922) as a method of radiological examination of the spinal subarachnoid space by the instillation of a radio-opaque medium was a milestone in the history of the surgery of the spinal cord. Modern water-soluble contrast media have considerably reduced the complications, particularly arachnoiditis associated with the older media such as myodil. The general practice is to introduce the dye by lumbar puncture, and from the deformity produced in the

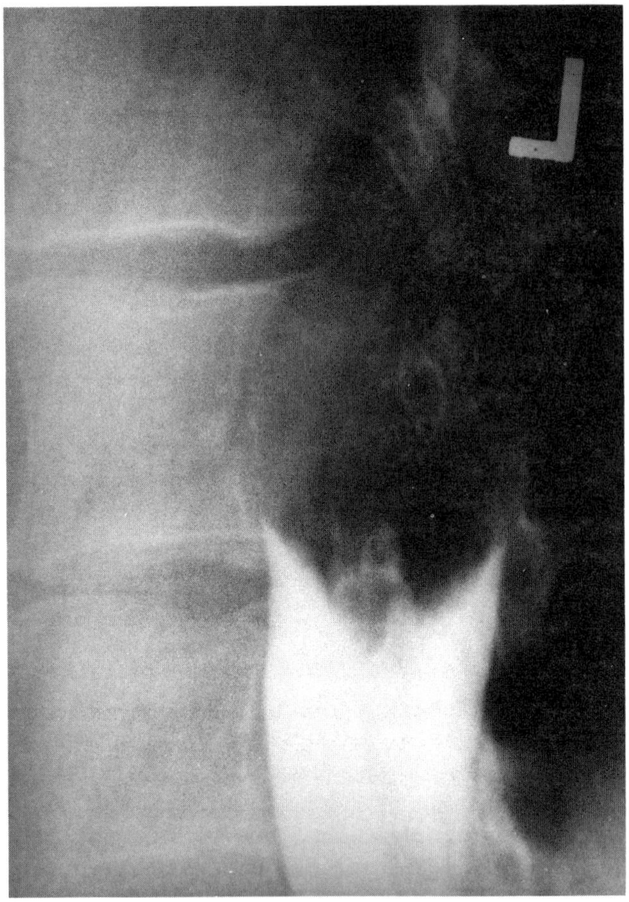

Fig. 29.2 Myelogram of a giant lumbar ependymoma with scalloping of the vertebral bodies.

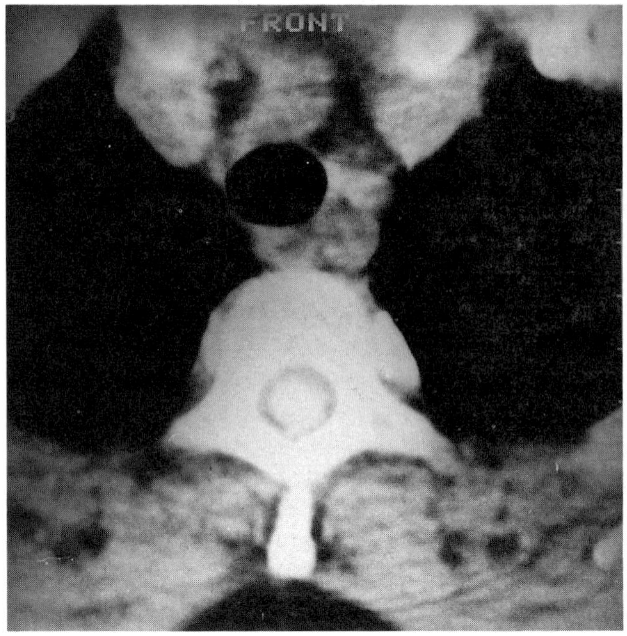

Fig. 29.3 CT scan of calcified thoracic meningioma occupying most of the spinal canal. No intravenous or intrathecal contrast.

contrast column it is usually possible to deduce whether the lesion is extradural, intradural or intramedullary. If there is a complete spinal block to the passage of dye and it is thought necessary to define the upper limit of the lesion then a small amount of dye may be introduced by a lateral cervical puncture. An intradural extramedullary tumour produces a rounded filling defect and in the anteroposterior and lateral films it should be possible to define displacement of the relatively translucent spinal cord (Fig. 29.4). Computerized tomographic (CT) scanning in intraspinal neoplasms has been limited by problems of resolution in distinguishing the subarachnoid space from the spinal cord and tumours. However, this has been improved considerably by combining water-soluble contrast myelography with CT (Di Chiro & Schellinger, 1976) (Fig. 29.5). Magnetic reasonance imaging (MRI) with

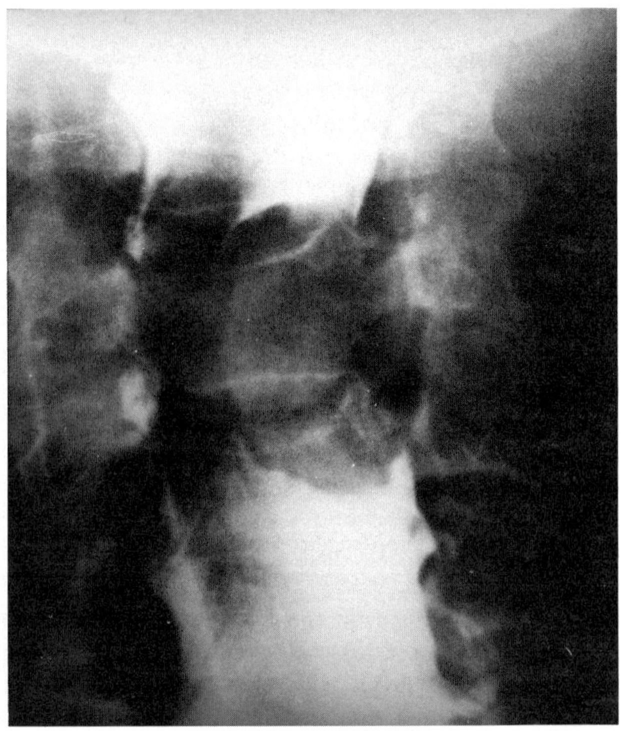

Fig. 29.4 Cervical myelogram, anteroposterior projection, showing large intradural schwannoma displacing the spinal cord laterally.

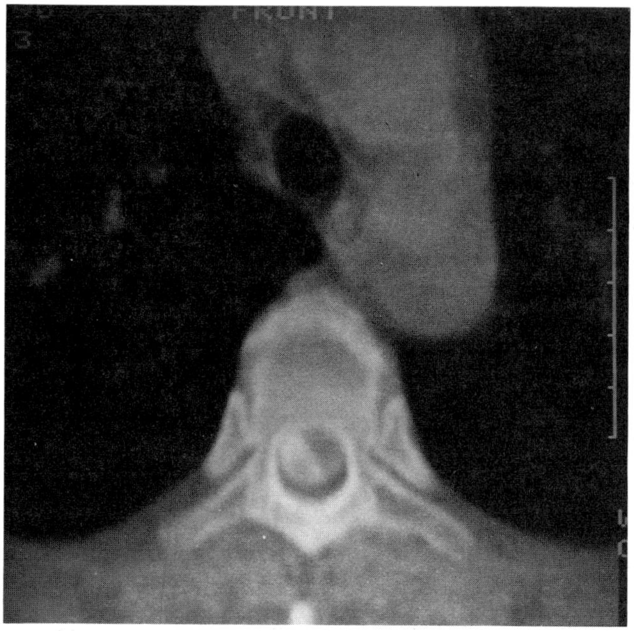

Fig. 29.5 CT myelogram showing displacement of the contrast column by an anterolateral meningioma.

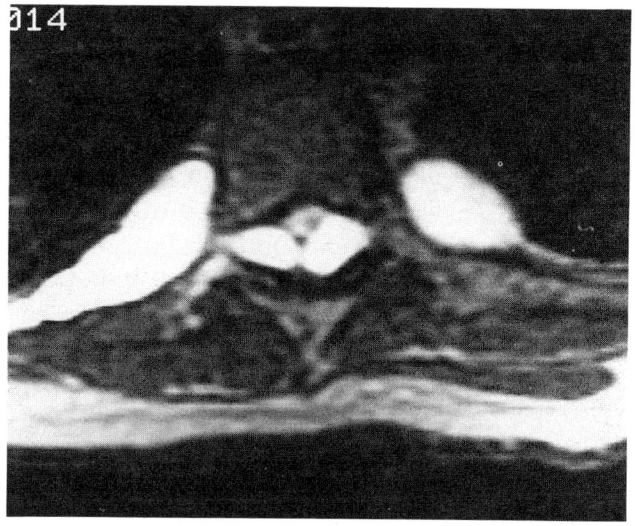

Fig. 29.6 MRI sequence with a TR of 2000 and TE of 80. Neurofibromatosis with intradural tumour and bilateral dumbbell extensions.

paramagnetic contrast enhancement has the potential to replace myelography in the investigation of spinal neoplasms including meningiomas and schwannomas (Fig. 29.6). Schroth *et al.* (1987) reported greater, faster and more consistent tumour enhancement on MRI in meningiomas compared with the more variable enhancement of schwannomas; however, it was not possible to differentiate reliably between the two tumours. MRI seems to be particularly valuable in investigating tumours around the foramen magnum (Wagle *et al.*, 1987).

Lumbar puncture and examination of the CSF should be restricted to the myelographic examination because of the risk of neurological deterioration. This 'spinal coning' is attributed to movement of the tumour as a result of withdrawing CSF from below a block, partial or complete, with subsequent impaction of the tumour against the cord. According to Hollis *et al.* (1986) myelography in the presence of a subarachnoid block carries a 14–20% risk of acute neurological deterioration. The deterioration may be merely an increase in pain or worsening of sensory loss, but total paraplegia can develop rapidly. Other mechanisms which may affect the integrity of the cord are a sudden increase in the size of the tumour as a result of haemorrhage into its substance, and ischaemia of the cord consequent upon compression of an entering arterial radicle or of adjacent veins. If deterioration does occur after myelography then the information is available to allow immediate surgical exploration. It follows that the Queckenstedt test used to assess the presence or absence of a spinal block is potentially dangerous and should no longer be performed.

Loculation of fluid below a total spinal subarachnoid block leads to an increase in its protein constituents derived partly from the transudation of plasma from congested veins and partly from the tumour. The amount of protein in the CSF varies considerably according to the completeness of the block, its proximity to the level of puncture and its duration. In the majority of cases of spinal tumour there is no increase in the number of cells in the CSF; the combination of a high CSF protein and a normal cell count is commonly referred to as Froin's syndrome.

TREATMENT

The treatment of spinal meningiomas and schwannomas is surgical excision. The detailed account of the clinical features and operative findings make it likely that the spinal tumour removed by Horsley (Gowers & Horsley, 1988), the first ever to be removed, was a schwannoma. A laminectomy and removal of a small accessible tumour can be one of the simplest and most rewarding of neurosurgical operations. On the other hand those tumours which lie at the craniovertebral junction or anterior to the cord, or which pass through the intervertebral foramen or occupy the whole of the lumbar canal, can tax the most skilful and experienced surgeon. The overriding consideration is the need to avoid damage to the spinal cord, whose nourishment has already been jeopardized by the tumour. In general terms it is best to debulk the tumour by piecemeal intracapsular removal, thus allowing withdrawal of the capsule and remaining fragments without disturbing the spinal cord. Modern techniques and surgical tools—for example microsurgery, lasers and ultrasonic aspiration—have all contributed to the goal of tumour removal without cord damage.

Large schwannomas with intervertebral extension can cause difficulty on account of haemorrhage from extradural veins and the fixity of the tumour by its extradural extension along the course of the issuing nerve root. Unroofing the intervertebral foramen allows the removal of the foraminal component and if the extraspinal portion of a dumbbell tumour is large it may be judicious to defer its removal to a second operation through an extraspinal approach.

The operative mortality for a spinal schwannoma is low, most series reporting a mortality of less than 2% (Elsberg, 1925; Horrax *et al.*, 1949) although Broager (1953) reported a 7% postoperative mortality. In the majority of cases of schwannoma a high degree of postoperative neurological recovery can be anticipated even in cases of established paraplegia. Nittner (1976) reviewed the literature and concluded that two-thirds of cases of schwannoma have a good postoperative result. Levy *et al.* (1986) reported a series of 66 cases of whom 60% had a full functional recovery following surgery and 85% of those who had pain preoperatively reported complete relief. However, 10% experienced worsening of their motor deficits following surgery and 33% of patients with preoperative bladder or bowel disturbance did not improve. About 10% had persistent pain and this may be the result of abnormal impulses arising in the stump of the affected sensory root, or in the compressed cord. However, functional recovery may be disappointing in large lumbosacral schwannomas because a number of roots may be involved, and removing tumour from them may increase the neurological deficit.

In operations on a spinal nerve schwannoma an attempt should be made to preserve the anatomical continuity and function of the involved root. This may be possible with small tumours, but to obtain complete excision of large tumours the nerve root may have to be sacrificed. A conservative approach has been formerly advocated with partial excision of the tumour in order to preserve the root, particularly if the nerves involved are important for limb function (Stein, 1985). Experience, however, shows that patients with tumours in the lower cervical or lumbar regions can recover without neurological deficit even after resection of the involved nerve root with the tumour. Kim *et al.* (1989) analysed in detail 31 cases of spinal schwannoma, arising from the segments C5–T1 or L3–S1, where the relevant nerve root was sacrificed in order to achieve total tumour removal. Only seven patients (23%) developed detectable motor or sensory deficits postoperatively and none of these deficits was functionally debilitating. They concluded that resection of the nerve root, if necessary to achieve total removal of the schwannoma, was justified. They also found that preoperative electromyography (EMG) had a value in predicting the outcome of surgery; if the EMG showed no evidence of denervation then the risk of a postoperative deficit was extremely low. However, every effort must be made to preserve adherent blood vessels that may be supplying the spinal cord (Iraci *et al.*, 1971).

Recurrence of a schwannoma is likely only where it is difficult to be certain that a total removal has been achieved. This can be the case in tumours with extradural extensions or in large cauda equina tumours.

Multiple spinal neurofibromas are almost always related to von Recklinghausen's disease, and it is usually impossible to remove all of them. The clinical symptoms and signs may identify the symptomatic tumour, which should then be excised. If the culpable lesion cannot be identified on clinical grounds then the largest lesion that could be symptomatic is chosen. Malignant change is most common on peripheral nerves in the presence of multiple tumours (Russell & Rubinstein, 1989).

The removal of a meningioma differs from that of a schwannoma in some respects. A meningioma is fixed by its dural attachment and even a small tumour is not mobile like a schwannoma. It may be possible to remove small posterior tumours in one piece with its dural attachment, but in general terms it is preferable to exenterate the tumour before removing the capsule from the cord and excising the dural origin. Gradual tumour exenteration is an essential step in the surgery of anteriorly based tumours but in such cases dural excision may be impractical. Unlike a schwannoma, a meningioma tends to engulf structures which lie in the direction of its growth and so it may surround a nerve root or important artery. If a watertight dural closure is thought desirable after excising the dural origin then a dural graft will be necessary.

The results of surgical removal of spinal meningiomas are very similar to those for schwannomas apart from the higher incidence of recurrence. Solero *et al.* (1989) reported an operative mortality of 1% in a series of 174 spinal meningiomas. Other large series have reported surgical mortalities ranging from 2% to 5.3% (Kunicki & Maciejak, 1965; Iraci *et al.*, 1971; Levy *et al.*, 1982). There are few long-term follow-up studies concerning the recurrence rate of spinal meningiomas. Levy *et al.* (1982) reported 79 cases of meningiomas with three (4%) symptomatic recurrences at eight, 13 and 16 years following surgery. Phillipon *et al.* (1986) had a similar experience with recurrences from five to 16 years after complete tumour removal. The most reliable estimate is probably that of Mirimanoff *et al.* (1985), who used statistical and life-table analysis to compute a risk of recurrence after total tumour removal of nil within the first five years and 13% at 10 years.

As with schwannomas the prospects of postoperative neurological recovery are good even in those patients who had severe preoperative neurological deficits. Of the cases reported by Levy *et al.* (1982) 85% were said to have had a good neurological recovery six months after surgery, and on long-term follow-up 91% had a good functional result. This is very similar to the series reported by Solero *et al.* (1989)—92% of their patients had a good functional recovery on prolonged follow-up. Again Solero *et al.* observed that 31 of their 37 patients with severe preoperative neurological disability showed significant improvement at long-term follow-up, and only six patients were left severely disabled. Eighty-nine of their cases had mild preoperative neurological dysfunction and four (4.5%) showed significant neurological deterioration after surgery.

It has been advocated that an attempt should be made, whenever possible, radically to excise the dural attachment of spinal meningiomas, and that intraoperative histological examination may be helpful in defining the resection margins (Levy *et al.* 1982). However, in the series reported by Solero *et al.* (1989) there was an 8% recurrence rate when the dura was radically excised, and only 5.6% recurrence if the dural attachment was coagulated. Levy *et al.* (1982) reported no recurrences in their anteriorly located meningiomas where the dural origin was coagulated but there was a 4% recurrence rate when the dural attachment was excised. It would therefore seem that it is not necessary to attempt radical dural excision if this exposes the patient to additional risks, as simple coagulation of the dural attachment still gives very low recurrence rates.

Comparison of schwannomas with meningiomas

Levy *et al.* (1986) reported 66 cases of spinal schwannomas and compared them with a similar series of meningiomas from the same institution over the same time period. They found a one to one male to female ratio with schwannomas as opposed to a one to four ratio with meningiomas. In males both schwannomas and meningiomas were evenly distributed along the spinal axis. In women, however, although the schwannomas were evenly distributed the meningiomas were heavily concentrated in the thoracic region. The duration of symptoms in the two tumour groups was similar, 23 months for meningiomas and 19 months for schwannomas. Neurological deficits including bladder dysfunction were twice as common in the meningioma patients. On the other hand, plain radiographs of the spine were abnormal in 50% of the schwannoma group but in only 20% of the meningiomas. The CSF protein was elevated in both groups, modestly in the case of meningiomas at about 100 mg/100 ml, and four times higher in schwannomas. The incidence of increased postoperative deficits was at the same low level of about 5% in both groups.

Ventral tumours of the foramen magnum and cervical spine

A laminectomy with removal of the pedicle and adopting a lateral approach where necessary will allow removal of the great majority of tumours even when they are anterior or anterolateral to the spinal cord. However, there are a small number of ventral tumours which cannot be removed totally and safely by a posterior approach. These tumours are mainly of the foramen magnum and cervical spine, where the tumour is straddled by the vertebral arteries and lower cranial nerves and the brain stem and spinal cord are displaced posteriorly. Broad-based meningiomas and recurrent tumours in this region pose particular difficulties. Meyer *et al.* (1984) reported 102 benign intradural extramedullary tumours of the foramen magnum with a 5% operative mortality due entirely to ventrally located tumours; another 5% died within three years of surgery because of recurrent disease, and 13% were left severely disabled. Stein *et al.* (1963) reported 25 ventrolateral foramen magnum meningiomas approached posteriorly; 20% died from recurrent disease and 16% were severely disabled following surgery. To overcome these problems a variety of anterior and lateral approaches have been developed.

Anterior approaches using a transoral or transcervical route involve removal of the vertebral bodies to allow direct access to the tumour without retraction of the spinal cord. However, exposure of the lateral margins of the tumour may be inadequate and a spinal fusion may be necessary. A major problem of the transoral approach is the risk of a CSF fistula and meningitis, and several strategies to prevent this have been put forward (Bonkowski *et al.*, 1990; Crockard & Sen, 1991).

Various lateral approaches to the cervical spine have been used. The transuncodiscal approach (Hakuba *et al.*, 1984) and the arterolateral approach (Verbiest, 1968) (see Chapter 46) involve exposure of the vertebral body by dissecting posterior to the carotid sheath. The anterolateral part of the vertebral body is drilled away and the vertebral artery is displaced. The rostral limit to this approach is C2 and an interbody fusion is necessary. Shucart & Kleriga (1980) used an extreme lateral approach to a ventrally located meningioma at C2–C3 and restricted bony removal to the lamina. Sen & Sekhar (1990) have extended this extreme lateral approach to allow access to intradural lesions of the lower clivus, foramen magnum, and the cervical spine down to C5. Depending on the extent of the tumour, bony resection may include a retromastoid craniectomy, partial mastoidectomy, the occipital condyle and part of the lateral mass of C1.

DERMOID AND EPIDERMOID CYSTS

Dermoid and epidermoid cysts are congenital tumours arising from the anomalous inclusion of ectodermal elements at the time of closure of the neural groove, between the third and fifth weeks of embryonic life (Russell & Rubinstein, 1989). The congenital origin of these tumours is confirmed by their association with spina bifida, dermal sinus, myelomeningocele, diastematomyelia and syringomyelic cavities. However, it has been reported that repeated lumbar puncture in the treatment of meningitis in children may lead to the development of lumbar epidermoid cysts many years later (Choremis *et al.*, 1956). Some of these cases had multiple cysts (Blockey & Schorstein, 1961) and it was thought that fragments of skin had been implanted on the end of a lumbar puncture needle used without a stylet. This complication of lumbar puncture has virtually disappeared since the introduction of disposable needles with properly fitting stylets.

Dermoid and epidermoid cysts have been grouped together as 'pearly tumours' (Tytus & Pennybacker, 1956) although it is now generally accepted that the demonstration of hair and other skin appendages separates the dermoid from the epidermoid. They are uncommon tumours accounting for 2.2% of the 680 primary spinal tumours reported by Lunardi *et al.* (1989), and Sloof *et al.* (1964) reported an incidence of 1.4% for combined dermoid and epidermoid tumours and teratomas from a series of 1322 spinal tumours. They are more frequent in children and spinal dermoid cysts account for 17% of primary spinal tumours during the first year of life (Takeuchi *et al.*, 1978).

These tumours are equally distributed between the sexes; they occur at all ages, and the most frequent sites are in the cauda equina or conus medullaris. They may be extramedullary or lie within the substance of the cord—10 of the 16 tumours reported by Lunardi *et al.* (1989) were extramedullary. The presence of a dermal sinus may allow penetration of infection and meningitis, and rarely the cyst may rupture into the subarachnoid space to cause a sterile chemical meningitis. The most irritant content of the cyst is thought to be the cholesterol derived from the breakdown of keratin, and this excites a granulomatous meningitis with a foreign-body giant-cell reaction.

The symptoms, signs and investigations do not differ from other spinal tumours. The diagnosis may be suspected by the presence of associated congenital anomalies. Magnetic resonance imaging permits characterization of the cyst contents, but Awwad *et al.* (1982) suggest that the diagnosis can best be established by correlating MRI and CT images.

The treatment of spinal dermoid and epidermoid tumours is surgery; a radical removal is desirable but not always possible or essential. It may be helpful to evacuate the contents of the cyst, taking care not to spill the contents into the subarachnoid space, before excising the remainder of the cyst wall. If the capsule is very adherent to the spinal cord or nerve roots it is wiser to leave fragments rather than risk neurological damage. In cases where there is an associated dermal sinus it is probably best to isolate or excise the sinus before opening the dura. When operating on these tumours the surgeon should also be prepared to deal with associated malformations such as diastematomyelia and spondylolisthesis.

Lunardi *et al.* (1989) reported total cyst removal in seven of their 16 patients. Their follow-up ranged from five to 30 years and only one patient in whom the capsule removal was incomplete required a second operation. It is concluded that a subtotal excision of the capsule may still allow marked and prolonged improvement in neurological function.

TERATOMAS

Spinal teratomas, excluding the sacrococcygeal variety, are very rare, for only two examples were found in the 1322 intraspinal tumours reported by Sloof *et al.* (1964), and again two cases were quoted by Lunardi *et al.* (1989) from their 680 primary spinal tumours. The tumour may be cystic or solid, and is usually extramedullary although it may be attached to the cord by a pedicle. The lesions are generally dorsal to the cord and various levels in the spinal canal are affected: of the six cases described by Ingraham & Bailey (1946) three were in the lumbar, two in the cervical and one in the thoracic regions. Teratomas may be malignant and subarachnoid and remote metasases have been described (Rand & Rand 1960). The treatment of spinal teratomas is surgical, and the prognosis is good provided there has been no histological evidence of malignancy.

ENTEROGENOUS CYSTS (NEURENTERIC CYST, GASTROCYTOMA)

Enterogenous cysts are lined by columnar epithelium of intestinal character and the contents of the cyst are often said to have a mucoid or stringy consistency. Occasionally areas of focal squamous metaplasma have been noted (Holmes *et al.*, 1978). These cysts occur most frequently in the cervical or cervicothoracic segments and of the six cases reported by Rubinstein (1972), three were in the cervical region, two in the upper thoracic and one in the lumbar regions. High cervical examples are very rare (Fabinyi & Adams, 1979) and Koksel *et al.* (1990) have reported a craniospinal case located anterior to the brain stem and upper cervical spine.

Enterogenous cysts are derived from the embryonic endodermal layer (Rhaney & Barclay, 1959) and are associated with developmental defects of the vertebrae. This, it is claimed, permits the formation of a fistula in the early embryo between the neuroectoderm and the yolk sac. However, vertebral malformation is seen in a minority of cases and occurred in only nine of the 33 cases reviewed by Agnoli *et al.* (1984). In the absence of vertebral anomalies, therefore, the mechanism of development of these cysts remains conjectural.

The majority of enterogenous cysts are extramedullary—29 of the 33 cases reported by Agnoli *et al.* (1984)—and they may lie dorsal or ventral to the spinal cord. Surgical excision of these cysts can be difficult as the wall may be adherent to the spinal cord and nerve roots. If complete excision of the cyst is not feasible, drainage and wide opening of the cyst can produce dramatic and long-lasting recovery of neurological function. However, recurrence is not uncommon and may require reoperation or percutaneous aspiration with the aid of ultrasonic or CT guidance.

ARACHNOIDAL CYSTS

Arachnoidal or leptomeningeal cysts are round or sausage-shaped collections of CSF sequestered within a compartment of arachnoid. There is debate about their origin and a variety of causes have been proposed. They are probably due to a developmental error in the distribution of the arachnoidal trabeculae and their enlargement has been attributed to hydrostatic factors. Despite their apparent developmental origin, intraspinal arachnoidal diverticula and cysts are seldom associated with spinal dysraphism or other spinal anomalies. Arachnoidal cysts may also be caused by arachnoidal adhesions following meningitis, the instillation of drugs, or spinal trauma.

The leptomeninges forming the cyst may appear transparent and entirely normal, or may be opaque from fibrosis. The cysts are found most frequently in the thoracic region dorsal to the spinal cord but ventral examples have been reported (Chan *et al.*, 1985). They may be single or multiple, and Burger & Vogel (1982) claim that multiple cysts are common.

Asymptomatic cysts are common incidental findings during radiological investigations and at operation or post-mortem. On the other hand the rare symptomatic cyst causes compression of the spinal cord or nerve roots (Palmer, 1974; Galzio *et al.*, 1982). Andrews *et al.* (1988) have pointed out that intradural arachnoid cysts and intramedullary cysts may occur together as a late complication of spinal surgery or spinal cord trauma, and either or both lesions may cause delayed neurological deterioration.

The surgical treatment of spinal arachnoidal cysts includes the complete excision of dorsal or lateral cysts, fenestration into the normal subarachnoid space or a shunting procedure to the peritoneum or right atrium.

INTRADURAL SPINAL LIPOMAS

Intradural spinal lipomas are uncommon tumours accounting for only 0.45% of the 1322 primary spinal tumours reported by Sloof *et al.* (1964). The aetiology of these lesions is obscure and there is debate as to whether they are neoplastic or hamartomatous. They have a characteristic appearance at operation, being yellowish in colour, of rubbery consistency and standing out clearly from the spinal cord. They lie within the arachnoid, attached loosely or, more commonly, firmly to the spinal cord, and may be embedded within it; emerging nerve roots may pass through the lipomatous tissue (Ammelman *et al.*, 1976).

Giuffré (1976) reviewed 154 cases of intradural spinal lipoma collected from the literature. Significant clinical features were the early onset and long duration of symptoms. Sixty-eight per cent of patients reported that their symptoms began in the first 30 years of life, but only 46% presented clinically in their first three decades. The duration of symptoms exceeded three years in 56% of cases and 20 years in 10%. The tumours usually extended over at least four or five segments of the cord; 34% were located in the cervical or cervicothoracic areas and a further 33% were in the thoracic region. Characteristically they arise from the posterior aspect of the spinal cord, with the majority being found in the midline and a small number situated laterally. One third of the spinal intradural lipoma patients had associated lesions, most of which were malformations of the vertebrae and the soft tissues around the spine.

According to Giuffré (1976) the lipomas always lie both within and outside the spinal cord, and there is rarely a plane of cleavage between the tumour and the cord. Thomas & Miller (1973) reported a series of 60 patients with spinal lipomas and suggested that, for lipomas that cannot be completely removed, the surgery should be limited to a decompressive laminectomy and biopsy. However, this approach may not prevent neurological deterioration in the long term, and two of the 13 patients with lipomas in the cervicothoracic region required further surgery. An alternative approach is to debulk the tumour, with great care being taken not to transgress the interface between tumour and spinal cord (McGillicuddy *et al.*, 1987). Ultrasonic aspirators and the laser (McClone & Naidick, 1986) are particularly useful tools in achieving this surgical objective. It is claimed that removal of up to 50% of the tumour mass is probably sufficient to allow long-lasting neurological stability or even improvement in many cases. Giuffré (1976) reviewed the surgical results in 132 intradural spinal lipomas—27% of the patients improved after decompression and biopsy whereas 58% improved when the tumour was debulked.

REFERENCES

Agnoli, A.L., Laun, A. & Schönmayr, R. (1984) Enterogenous intraspinal cysts. *J. Neurosurg.*, **61**, 834–840.

Ammelman, B.J., Henry, J.M., De Girolami, U. & Earle, K.M. (1976) Intradural lipomas of the spinal cord. *J. Neurosurg.*, **44**, 331–336.

Andrews, B.T., Weinstein, P.R., Rosenblum, M.L. & Barbaro, N.M. (1988) Intradural arachnoid cysts of the spinal canal associated with intramedullary cysts. *J. Neurosurg.*, **68**, 544–549.

Antoni, N. (1920) *Ueber Rückenmarkstumoren und Neurofibrome.* Bergmann, Munich.

Arseni, C. & Maretsis, M. (1967) Tumors of the low spinal cord associated with increased intracranial pressure and papilledema. *J. Neurosurg.*, **27**, 105–110.

Awwad, E.E., Backer, R. & Archer, C.R. (1987) The imaging of an intraspinal cervical dermoid tumor by MR, CT and sonography. *Comput. Radiol.*, **11**, 169–173.

Becker, J. (1965) *Die Meningiome des Rückenmarks. Klinik und Differentialdiagnose.* Inaugural dissertation, Cologne.

Bellur, S.N., Chandra, V. & Anderson, R.J. (1983) Association of meningiomas with obesity. *Ann. Neurol.*, **13**, 346–347.

Benzel, E.C. & Gelder, F.B. (1988) Correlation between sex hormone binding and peritumoral edema in intracranial meningiomas. *Neurosurgery*, **23**, 169–174.

Bickerstaff, E.R., Small, J.M. & Guest, I.A. (1958) The relapsing course of certain meningiomas in relation to pregnancy and menstruation. *J. Neurol. Neurosurg. Psychiatry*, **21**, 89–91.

Blockey, N.J. & Schorstein, J. (1961) Intraspinal epidermoid tumours in the lumbar region of children. *J. Bone Jt. Surg.*, **43B**, 556–562.

Bonkowski, J.A., Gibson, R.D. & Snape, L. (1990) Foramen magnum meningioma: transoral resection with a bone baffle to prevent CSF leakage. *J. Neurosurg.*, **72**, 493–496.

Broager, B. (1953) Spinal neurinoma. A clinical study comprising 44 cases. *Acta Psychiat. Scand.* Suppl. 85(1).

Bull, J.W.D. (1953) Spinal meningiomas and neurofibromas. *Acta Radiol.*, **40**, 283–300.

Burger, P.C. & Vogel, F.S. (1982) *Surgical Pathology of the Nervous System and its Coverings*, 2nd edn. John Wiley, New York.

Chalif, D.J., Black, K. & Rosenstein, D. (1990) Intradural spinal cord tumor presenting as a subarachnoid hemorrhage: magnetic resonance imaging diagnosis. *Neurosurgery*, **27**, 631–634.

Chan, R.C., Thompson, G.B. & Bratty, P.J.A. (1985). Symptomatic anterior spinal arachnoid diverticulum. *Neurosurgery*, **16**, 663–665.

Choremis, C., Economos, D., Papadotos, C. & Gargoulas, A. (1956) Intraspinal epidermoid tumours (cholesteatomas) in patients treated for tuberculous meningitis. *Lancet*, **2**, 437–439.

Courville, C.B. (1945) *Pathology of the Central Nervous System*, 2nd edn. Pacific Press, Mountain View, CA.

Crockard, H.A. & Sen, C.N. (1991) The transoral approach for the management of intradural lesions at the craniovertebral junction: review of 7 cases. *Neurosurgery*, **28**, 88–98.

Cushing, H. & Eisenhardt, L. (1938). *The Meningiomas.* Charles C. Thomas, Springfield, IL.

Delleman, J.W., De Jong, J.G.Y. & Bleeker, G.M. (1978) Meningiomas in five members of a family over two generations, in one member simultaneously with acoustic neuromas. *Neurology*, **28**, 567–570.

Di Chiro, G. & Schellinger, D. (1976) Computerized tomography of spinal cord after lumbar intrathecal introduction of metrizamide (computer-assisted myelography). *Radiology*, **120**, 101–104.

Dodge, H.W. Jr, Love, J.G. & Gottlieb, C.M. (1956) Benign tumors at the foramen magnum. Surgical considerations. *J. Neurosurg.*, **13**, 603–617.

Eljamel, M.S.M. & Foy, P.M. (1989) Multiple meningiomas and their relation to neurofibromatosis. Review of the literature and report of seven cases. *Surg. Neurol.*, **32**, 131–136.

Elsberg, C.A. (1925) Some aspects of the diagnosis and surgical treatment of tumors of the spinal cord. *Ann. Surg.*, **81**, 1057.

Fabinyi, G.C.A. & Adams, J.E. (1979) High cervical spinal cord compression by an enterogenous cyst. Case report. *J. Neurosurg.*, **51**, 556–559.

Feldenzer, J.A., McGillicuddy, J.E. & Hopkins, J.W. (1990) Giant sacrolumbar meningioma. Case report. *J. Neurosurg.*, **72**, 951–954.

Galzio, R.J., Zenobii, M. & Lucantoni, D. (1982) Spinal intradural arachnoid cyst. *Surg. Neurol.*, **17**, 388–391.

Giuffré, R. (1976) In Vinken, P.J. & Bruyn, G.W. (eds) *Handbook of Clinical Neurology*, Vol. 20, Part II: *Tumours of the Spine and Spinal Cord*, pp. 389–412. North-Holland, Amsterdam.

Gowers, W.R. & Horsley, V. (1988) A case of tumour of the spinal cord: removal: recovery. *Br. Med. J.*, **1**, 1273 (reprinted: *J. Neurosurg.*, 1963; **9**, 815–824).

Grunberg, S.M., Daniels, A.M., Muensch, H., Daniels, J.R., Bernstein, L., Kortes, V. & Weiss, M.H. (1987) Correlation of meningioma hormone receptor status with hormone sensitivity in a tumor stem-cell assay. *J. Neurosurg.*, **66**, 405–408.

Hakuba, A., Komiyama, M., Tsujimoto, T., Ahn, M.S., Nishimura, S., Ohta, T. & Kitano, H. (1984) Transuncodiscal approach to dumbbell tumors of the cervîcal spinal canal. *J. Neurosurg.*, **61**, 1100–1106.

Hassin, G.B. (1930) Villi (Pacchionian bodies) of the spinal arachnoid. *Arch. Neurol. Psychiatry*, **23**, 65.

Heard, C. & Payne, E.E. (1962) *J. Neurosurg. Psychiatry*, **25**, 345.

Helseth, A. & Mørk, S.J. (1989) Primary intraspinal neoplasms in Norway 1955 to 1986. A population-based survey of 467 patients. *J. Neurosurg.*, **71**, 842–845.

Hollis, P.H., Malis, L.I. & Zappulla, R.A. (1986) Neurological deterioration after lumbar puncture below complete spinal subarachnoid block. *J. Neurosurg.*, **64**, 253–256.

Holmes, G.L., Trader, S. & Ignatiadis, P. (1978) Intraspinal enterogenous cysts. *Am. J. Dis. Child.*, **132**, 906.

Horrax, G., Poppen, J.L., Wu, W.Q. & Weadon, P.R. (1949) Meningiomas and neurofibromas of the spinal cord. Certain clinical features and end results. *Surg. Clin. N. Am.*, **29**, 659.

Ingraham, F.D. & Bailey, O.T. (1946) Cystic teratomas and teratoid tumors of the central nervous system in infancy and childhood. *J. Neurosurg.*, **3**, 511.

Iraci, G., Peserico, L. & Salar, G. (1971) Intraspinal neuromas and meningiomas: a clinical survey of 172 cases. *Int. Surg.*, **56**, 289–303.

Kepes, J.J. (1986) The histopathology of meningiomas. A reflection of origins and expected behavior? *J. Neuropathol. Exp. Neurol.*, **45**, 95.

Kim, P., Ebersuld, M.J., Onofrio, B.M. & Quast, L.M. (1989) Surgery of spinal nerve schwannoma. Risk of neurological deficit after resection of involved root. *J. Neurosurg.*, **71**, 810–814.

Koksel, T., Revesz, T. & Crockard, H.A. (1990) Craniospinal neurenteric cyst. *Br. J. Neurosurg.*, **4**, 425–428.

Kudo, H., Tamaki, N., Kim, S., Shirataki, K. & Matsumoto, S. (1987) Intraspinal tumours associated with hydrocephalus. *Neurosurgery*, **21**, 726–731.

Kunicki, A. & Maciejak, A. (1965) Results of operative treatment in 154 cases of extramedullary meningiomas and neurinomas. *Acta Med. Pol.*, **3**, 397–404.

Levy, W., Bay, J. & Dohn, D. (1982). Spinal cord meningioma.

J. Neurosurg., **57**, 804–812.

Levy, W.J., Latchaw, J., Hahn, J.F., Sawhny, B., Bay, J. & Dohn, D.F. (1986) Spinal neurofibromas: a report of 66 cases and a comparison with meningiomas. *Neurosurgery*, **18**, 331–334.

List, C.F. (1943) Multiple meningiomas; removal of four tumours from region of the foramen magnum and upper cervical region of the cord. *Arch. Neurol. Psychiatry*, **50**, 335–341.

Love, J.G., Thelen, E.P. & Dodge, H.W. Jr (1954) Tumors of the foramen magnum. *J. Int. Coll. Surg.*, **22**, 1–17.

Lunardi, P., Missori, P., Gagliardi, F.M. & Fortuna, A. (1989) Long-term results of the surgical treatment of spinal dermoid and epidermoid tumours. *Neurosurgery*, **25**, 860–864.

McClone, D.G. & Naidich, T.P. (1986) Laser resection of fifty spinal lipomas. *Neurosurgery*, **18**, 611–615.

McGillicuddy, G.T., Shucart, W. & Kwan, E.S.K. (1987) Intradural spinal lipomas. *Neurosurgery*, **21**, 343–346.

Markwalder, T.M., Waelti, E. & Markwalder, R.V. (1986) Estrogen and progestin receptors in acoustic and spinal neurilemmomas. Clinicopathologic correlations. *Surg. Neurol.*, **26**, 142.

Meyer, F.B., Ebersold, M.J. & Reese, D.F. (1984) Benign tumors of the foramen magnum. *J. Neurosurg.*, **61**, 136–142.

Mirimanoff, R.V., Dosretz, D.E., Lingood, R.M., Ojemann, R.G. & Martuza, R.L. (1985) Meningiomas: analysis of recurrence and progression following neurosurgical resection. *J. Neurosurg.*, **62**, 18–24.

Nittner, K. (1976). Spinal meningiomas, neurinomas and neurofibromas, and hourglass tumours. In Vinken, P.J. & Bruyn, G.W. (eds) *Handbook of Clinical Neurology*, vol. 20, Part II: *Tumours of the Spine and Spinal Cord*, pp. 177–322. North-Holland, Amsterdam.

Oi, S. & Raimondi, A.J. (1981) Hydrocephalus associated with intraspinal neoplasms in childhood. *Am. J. Dis. Child.*, **135**, 1122–1124.

Olson, J.J., Beck, D.W., Schlechte, J. & Loh, P.M. (1986) Hormonal manipulation of meningiomas *in vitro*. *J. Neurosurg.*, **65**, 99–107.

Palmer, J.J. (1974) Spinal arachnoid cysts. Report of six cases. *J. Neurosurg.*, **41**, 728–735.

Patronas, N.J., Brown, F. & Duda, E.E. (1980) Multiple meningiomas in the spinal canal. *Surg. Neurol.*, **13**, 78–80.

Philippon, J., Cornu, P.R., Grob, R. & Rivierez, M. (1986) Les meningiomes récidivantes. *Neurochirurgie*, **32** (Suppl. 1), 54–62.

Rand, R.W. & Rand, C.W. (1960) *Intraspinal Tumours of Childhood.* Thomas, Springfield, IL.

Rhaney, K. & Barclay, G.P.T. (1959) Enterogenous cysts and congenital diverticula of the alimentary canal with abnormalities of the vertebral column and spinal cord. *J. Pathol. Bacteriol.*, **77**, 457–471.

Ross, D.A., Edwards, M.S.B. & Wilson, C.B. (1986). Intramedullary neurilemmomas of the spinal cord: report of two cases and review of the literature. *Neurosurgery*, **19**, 458.

Rubinstein, L.J. (1972). Tumors of the central nervous system. *Atlas of Tumor Pathology*, second series, fascicle 6. Armed Forces Institute of Pathology, Washington, DC.

Russell, D.S. & Rubinstein, L.J. (1989) *Pathology of Tumours of the Nervous System*, 5th edn. Edward Arnold, London.

Schmidt, M.B. (1902) Ueber die Pacchionischen Granulationen und Ihr Verhaltniss zu den Sarcomen und Psammomen der Dura Mater. *Virchows Arch.*, **170**, 429.

Schoenberg, B.S., Christine, B.W. & Whisnant, J.P. (1975) Nervous system neoplasms and primary malignancies of other sites. The unique association between meningiomas and breast cancer. *Neurology*, **25**, 705–712.

Schroth, G., Thron, A., Guhl, L., Voigt, K., Niendorf, H-P. & Garces, L. R-N. (1987) Magnetic resonance imaging of spinal meningiomas and neurinomas. Improvement of imaging by paramagnetic contrast enhancement. *J. Neurosurg.*, **66**, 695–700.

Scotti, G., Filizzolo, F., Scialfa, G., Tampieri, D. & Versari, P. (1987) Repeated subarachnoid hemorrhage from a cervical meningioma. *J. Neurosurg.*, **66**, 779–781.

Sedzimir, C.B., Frazer, A.K. & Roberts, J.R. (1973). Cranial and spinal meningiomas in a pair of identical twin boys. *J. Neurol. Neurosurg. Psychiatry*, **36**, 368–376.

Sen, C.N. & Sekhar, L.N. (1990) An extreme lateral approach to intradural lesions of the cervical spine and foramen magnum. *Neurosurgery*, **27**, 197–204.

Shealy, C.N., Lemay, M. & Haddad, F.S. (1964) Posterior scalloping of vertebral bodies in uncontrolled hydrocephalus. *J. Neurol. Neurosurg. Psychiatry*, **27**, 567–573.

Shucart, W.A. & Kleriga, E. (1980) Lateral approach to the upper cervical spine. *Neurosurgery*, **6**, 278–281.

Sicard, J.A. & Forestier, A. (1922) Methode generale d'exploration radiologique par l'huile iodée (lipiodol). *Bull. Mem. Soc. Med. Hôp. Paris*, **46**, 463–469.

Sloof, J.L., Kernohan, J.W. & MacCarty, C.S. (1964) *Primary Intramedullary Tumors of the Spinal Cord and Filum Terminale.* W.B. Saunders, Philadelphia, PA.

Solero, C.L., Fornari, M., Giombini, S., Lasio, G., Oliveri, G., Cimino, C. & Pluchino, F. (1989) Spinal meningiomas: review of 174 operated cases. *Neurosurgery*, **25**, 153–160.

Stein, B.M. (1985) Spinal intradural tumours. In Wilkins, R.H. & Rengachary, S.S. (eds) *Neurosurgery*, vol. 1, pp. 1048–1061. McGraw-Hill, New York.

Stein, B.M., Leeds, N.E., Taveras, J.M. & Pool, J.L. (1963) Meningiomas of the foramen magnum. *J. Neurosurg.*, **20**, 740–751.

Takeuchi, J., Ohta, T. & Kajikawa, H. (1978). Congenital tumors of the spinal cord. In Uinken, P.J. & Bruyn, G.W. (eds) *Handbook of Clinical Neurology*, vol. 32, pp. 355–392. North-Holland, Amsterdam.

Thomas, J.E. & Miller, R.H. (1973) Lipomatous tumors of the spinal cord. *Mayo Clin. Proc.*, **48**, 393–400.

Tytus, J.S. & Pennybacker, J. (1956) Pearly tumours in relation to the central nervous system. *J. Neurol. Neurosurg. Psychiatry*, **19**, 241.

Verbiest, J.H. (1968) A lateral approach to the cervical spine: technique and indications. *J. Neurosurg.*, **28**, 191–203.

Wagle, V.G., Villemure, J.G., Melanson, D., Ethier, R., Bertrand, G. & Feindel, W. (1987) Diagnostic potential of magnetic resonance in cases of foramen magnum meningiomas. *Neurosurgery*, **21**, 622–626.

30 · Intramedullary Tumours

By P.R. COOPER and F.J. EPSTEIN

Intramedullary spinal cord tumours are relatively uncommon. Many earlier reports were based on anecdotal experience or small series of patients prior to the advent of surgical adjuncts such as the operating microscope, ultrasonic aspirator, surgical laser and intraoperative ultrasonography. Whilst ependymomas of the spinal cord and cauda equina have been totally excised in the past, the surgical treatment of intramedullary astrocytomas was usually confined to biopsy, dural decompression and radiotherapy (Kopelson *et al.*, 1980) despite the recognition that, after a relatively short remission, serious disability or death ensued. This has been unfortunate as, especially in children, most astrocytomas are low grade and histologically identical to cerebellar astrocytomas, and are potentially curable by surgery. Furthermore, biopsy alone exposes the patient to many of the hazards of operation without the potential benefits of tumour excision. Limited biopsy produces only tiny fragments of tumour for the histopathologist, and may result in misdiagnosis. Cooper (1989) reported that a high percentage of patients referred to him after previous surgery had indeed been misdiagnosed in this fashion.

With the development of technology which enables resection of intramedullary tumours a more aggressive approach to surgery has been adopted, and this chapter reports the combined experience gained by the authors in 266 cases.

PATHOLOGY

Approximately 15% of all primary intradural tumours are intramedullary in location, the most common pathologies being astrocytoma and ependymoma. However, intramedullary tumours constitute only 4% of the central nervous system tumours which occur in childhood (Anderson & Carson, 1953; Arseni *et al.*, 1967). In children astrocytomas predominate (Reimer & Onofrio, 1985). In fact, an intramedullary spinal cord tumour above the conus in children under the age of 15 years has a 90% chance of being an astrocytoma as compared with adults where the ratio is approximately equal. The presence of a local expansion of the cord over only one or two segments makes a diagnosis of ependymoma more likely; while the presence of large rostral and caudal intramedullary cysts favours a diagnosis of astrocytoma. Other lesions such as oligodendroglioma, haemangioblastoma, lipoma, dermoid, epidermoid and metastasis do occur, but are much less common. The problem of intramedullary metastases is discussed in Chapter 28.

The astrocytomas which occur in childhood are usually histologically benign but the incidence of malignant forms increases with increasing age. Intramedullary tumours other than metastasis occur only rarely beyond the age of 60. There is a roughly equal incidence between males and females and intramedullary tumours can occur anywhere within the spinal cord. However, Cooper & Epstein (1985) and Cooper (1989) found that over 50% were located in the cervical or cervicodorsal regions. There appear to be no major predisposing factors in causation, and a familial link occurs only in patients with Von Hippel–Lindau syndrome and in neurofibromatosis where the risk of intramedullary astrocytomas is increased.

Haemangioblastomas and lipomas are normally evident on the surface of the cord once the dura is opened, but ependymomas and astrocytomas usually remain buried within the cord surface. Ependymomas presumably arise from nests of ependymal cells which remain in the centre of the cord once the central canal has closed during development. They are distinct from the surrounding spinal cord, are firm in consistency and are reddish-grey or yellow. Whilst there is usually a clear separation between the cord and the tumour, they may blend imperceptibly at the point of origin of the tumour, making total resection impractical (Woods & Pimenta, 1944). They are frequently associated with cystic cavitation adjacent to the poles of the tumour but such cysts are normally small.

Astrocytomas, however, are infiltrating tumours and, although they can be distinguished from the surrounding cord by their glassy and grey appearance, they blend imperceptibly with the spinal cord at their margins. As has been stated, they are normally of low grade histologically in children and in some two-thirds of adults. However, their continuing slow growth and expansion does not have a benign effect on the surrounding spinal cord, which becomes progressively damaged. Occasionally, even apparently benign tumours may spread through the subarachnoid space (Hardison *et al.*, 1987). Malignant astrocytomas behave in a similar manner to their intracranial counterparts. Complete resection is impossible, and they rapidly recur, inevitably resulting in the patient's demise (Guidetti *et al.*, 1981; Kopelson and Linggood, 1982).

Astrocytomas are frequently associated with extensive rostral and caudal cysts. In such a situation the solid portion of the tumour can occupy a variable length of the cord but the cysts may become huge and extend to the conus or even into the hindbrain. This produces the so-called 'holocord' widening seen at myelography with expansion of the cord over its entire length. Epstein & Epstein (1981) found holocord widening in 60% of their paediatric patients. It is vital to realize that the cysts are non-tumorous. They are lined merely by glia, and the fluid which they contain is produced by the tumour itself. It is therefore possible to limit exposure merely to the solid portion of tumour. Once the poles of the tumour have been reached, the cysts will drain and not recollect. Indeed, reaccumulation of the fluid indicates either incomplete removal or recurrence of the tumour.

CLINICAL PRESENTATION

The clinical manifestations of intramedullary tumours are not pathognomonic, and may be confused with other conditions which cause dysfunction of the spinal cord or nerve roots. The clinical course is variable. Cooper & Epstein (1985) noted that there was less than a 10-month interval from the time of the first clinical manifestations until operation in patients with malignant spinal cord tumours. However, the symptoms of non-malignant intramedullary tumours are more usually subtle and slow in onset, and develop over a period of years (Woods & Pimenta, 1944; Chigasaki & Pennybacker, 1968; Reimer & Onofrio, 1985), suggesting a more benign process. The onset of symptoms will commonly date back several years, with patients able to recall pain, mild clumsiness, weakness or sensory symptoms for lengthy periods prior to diagnosis. A number of patients will be noted to have had a scoliosis at the time of presentation, which may have been present for 10–15 years.

The most common initial symptom is spinal pain. This is particularly the case in children where 80% experience spinal pain. The pain is most acute in the segment occupied by the solid tumour and is due to dural distension. It is aggravated by recumbency due to the epidural venous distension which occurs when lying down, and which then aggravates the dural distension. Thus, it is common for the pain to be worse at night and to be somewhat eased by activity.

Progression will eventually produce the onset of neurological dysfunction. Sensory symptoms with paraesthesiae and dysaesthesiae may occur. A suspended sensory loss involving the arm and trunk may be seen in cervical lesions closely simulating that seen with syringomyelia. Damage to sensory pathways within the cord may produce either distal numbness or burning, and dysaesthetic pain in the lower limbs or trunk. Joint position sense may be relatively little affected in the lower limbs, but deficit of joint position not uncommonly compromises hand function.

Patients with tumours involving the cervical spinal cord will frequently present with upper extremity weakness prior to the onset of symptoms in the legs consistent with the central location of the tumour resulting in invasion or compression of anterior horn cells. Physical examination of the arms will frequently reveal motor deficit of a lower motor neurone variety, with wasting and weakness and decreased deep tendon reflexes. Involvement of the more peripherally located corticospinal tracts occurs later, and will produce spasticity and weakness in the lower extremities and a combination of upper and lower motor signs in the upper extremities.

Thoracic spinal cord lesions will produce a spastic paraparesis and bladder dysfunction consistent with corticospinal tract dysfunction. Lesions of the conus medullaris will characteristically result in a hypotonic bladder, faecal incontinence and impotence. Lower extremity motor weakness is uncommon with lesions at this level, but rostral extension to involve the spinal cord at the level of the L5 or S1 nerve root may produce foot weakness.

Cranial nerve dysfunction is generally absent unless tumours of the upper cervical spinal cord involve the lower medulla. In this situation signs and symptoms may also include hoarseness, dysphagia, a depressed gag reflex, palatal asymmetry, weakness of the muscles innervated by the spinal accessory nerve and atrophy or fasciculation of the tongue.

Hydrocephalus occurs in 1–12.5% of patients with spinal cord tumours (Ammerman & Smith, 1975; Neau *et al.*, 1987). In some patients dissemination of tumour cells from malignant astrocytomas or ependymomas into the subarachnoid space or ventricular system will cause obstruction of the cerebrospinal fluid pathways with ventriculomegaly and signs of elevated intracranial pressure. In other patients hydrocephalus will occur in the absence of tumour dissemination. In the latter instance it is likely that a markedly elevated cerebrospinal fluid protein produced by the tumour results in impaired absorption of cerebrospinal fluid.

In children the clinical course is similar except for the greater incidence of severe pain. In young children the diagnosis may be suspected only if the significance of, for example, a torticollis, or the fact that they have changed 'handedness', is recognized. A subtle deterioration of the ability to run, followed by change in the gait pattern, may be reported by the parents. In children who are too young to have walked, delay in walking or motor regression (starting to crawl again rather than trying to stand or walk) may be the only apparent sign.

The other important sign in children is the development of skeletal deformity, usually scoliosis. Any factor which appears unusual in a child who is developing an apparent idiopathic scoliosis should demand full investigation. Such factors are: the presence of pain, onset at an unusual age, scoliosis developing in a boy, and an unusual side or region for the apex of the curve. Reviewing our own series, 80% of children less than 12 years old already had a progressive scoliosis at the time of clinical presentation.

INVESTIGATION

Magnetic resonance imaging (MRI) is the preferred imaging modality for the diagnosis of intramedullary tumours. With rare exceptions it is the only modality necessary for the diagnosis of this entity. Unlike computerized tomography/myelography, which visualizes the external configuration of the spinal cord, MRI is capable of imaging the pathological anatomy of the interior of the spinal cord as well as the relationship of the spinal cord to surrounding bone and soft tissue structures.

The T1 image is the most informative, disclosing the presence or absence of polar cysts, intratumoral cysts and defining the extent of the solid tumour (Fig. 30.1). Intravenous gadolinium–DPTA allows tumour

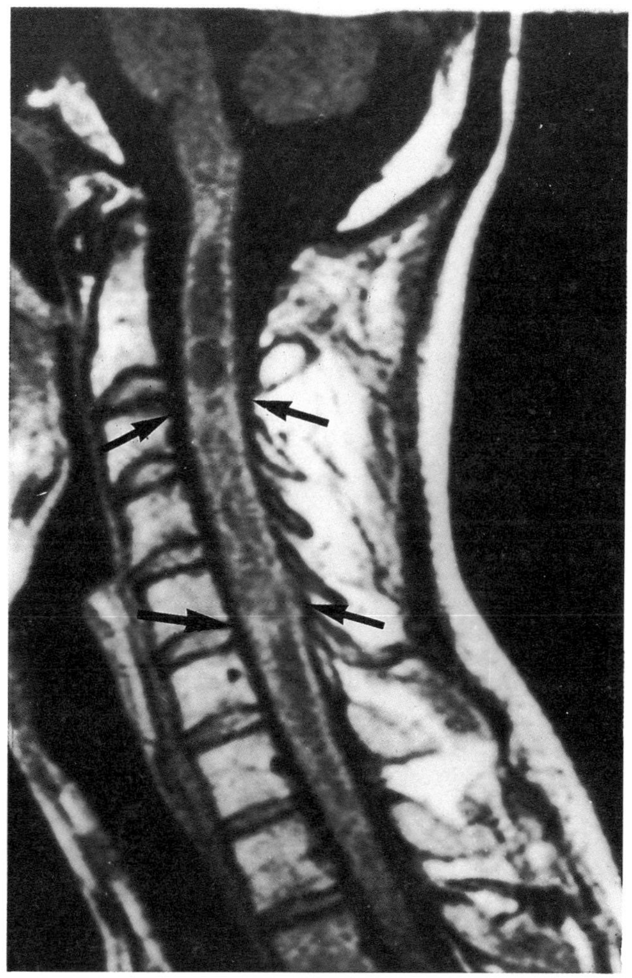

Fig. 30.1 T1-unenhanced MRI scan showing a solid astrocytoma from C3 to C5. At the poles of the tumour (arrows) large cysts extend rostrally and caudally.

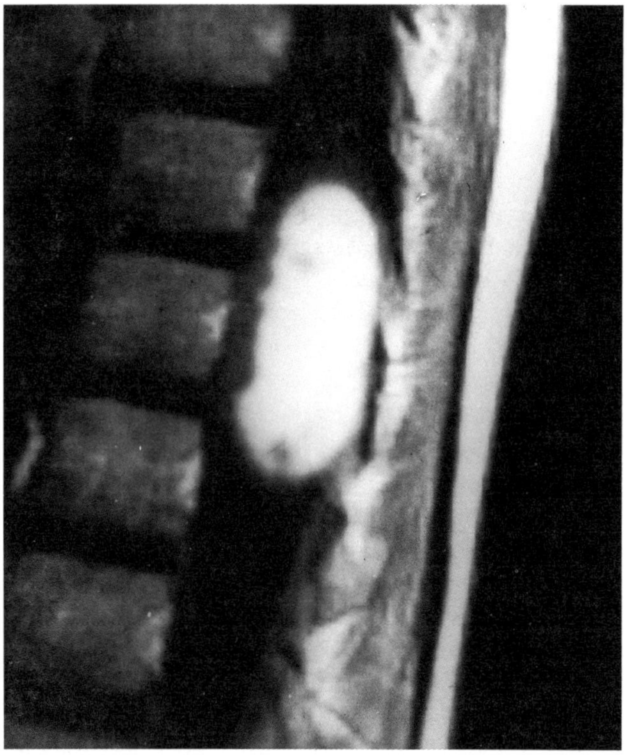

Fig. 30.2 MRI with gadolinium showing a brightly enhancing ependymoma.

enhancement and further defines the solid tumour. Ependymomas usually enhance intensely and homogeneously, producing sharply defined limits to the tumour (Fig. 30.2). Most astrocytomas manifest some degree of enhancement, but this is variable in degree and not homogeneous. The axial gadolinium-enhanced MRI scan can also help in the differentiation of astrocytomas and ependymomas. Ependymomas, arising as they do, tend to produce a symmetric expansion of the cord. These features are only suggestive factors in the diagnosis, and it is often impossible to separate astrocytomas from ependymomas purely by MRI.

Other intramedullary lesions have recognizable MRI features. Lipomas have a characteristic signal intensity on T2 imaging which should suggest the diagnosis (Fig. 30.3). Intense enhancement with gadolinium and areas of flow void around the perimeter of a sharply demarcated lesion should suggest the presence of a haemangioblastoma (Fig. 30.4).

MRI scanning does have some pitfalls. It can be very difficult to completely image the whole cord in patients with a major scoliosis. Small lesions may be missed in this situation and myelography should be used. Tumours with very extensive cystic formation can be difficult to separate from syringomyelia. The presence of an Arnold–Chiari malformation, and the absence of enhancement with gadolinium, suggest a diagnosis of syringomyelia. Some tumour cysts may have the same signal intensity as the adjacent

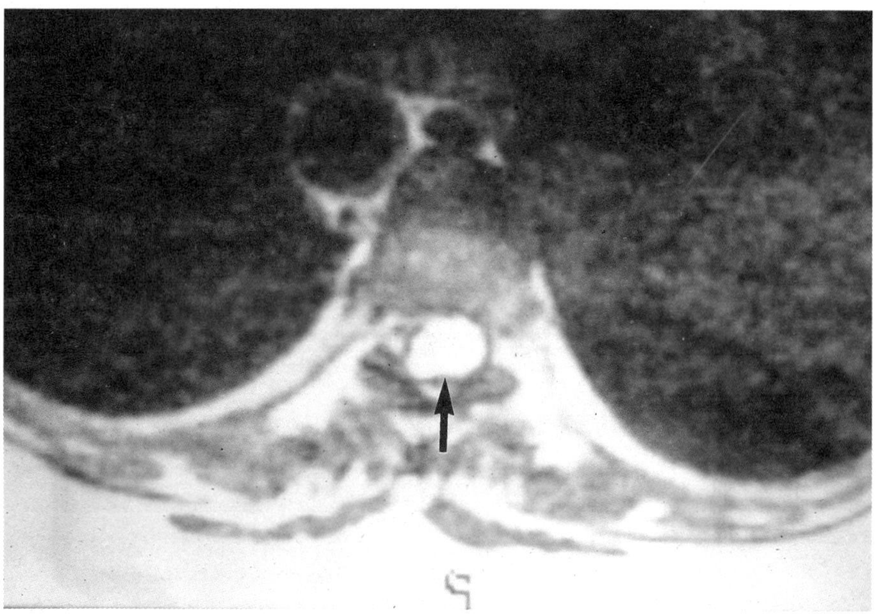

Fig. 30.3 Axial T2 MRI scan showing a hyperintense lesion with the same signal as the subcutaneous fat. This was an intramedullary lipoma.

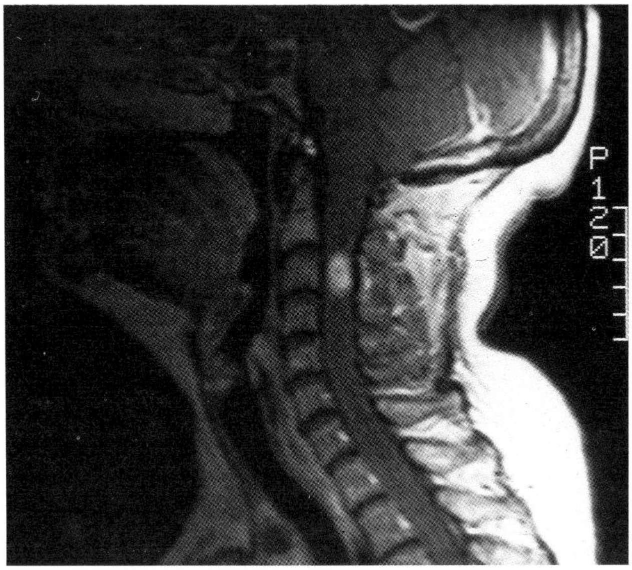

Fig. 30.4 MRI scan with gadolinium showing the typical appearance of a haemangioblastoma.

tumour, giving the misleading appearance of a long solid tumour (Goy *et al.*, 1986).

Prior to the advent of computerized tomography (CT) and MRI, myelography was the only means of diagnosing intraspinal pathology. Roentgenograms obtained following the subarachnoid introduction of the oil-soluble contrast medium, pantopaque, could distinguish gross widening of the spinal cord and intramedullary from extramedullary lesions. The advent of water-soluble contrast agents such as metrizamide and iopamidol, with subsequent imaging using CT, represented an important step forward. For the first time the spinal cord and its relationship to the spine could be viewed in the axial projection. Subtle enlargement of the spinal cord could be more easily appreciated than was the case using routine myelography, and the nature of lesions such as lipomas or epidermoids which differed significantly in radiodensity from the spinal cord could be ascertained. Some cystic lesions of the spinal cord could be identified by their tendency to take up the contrast material after a delay of several hours, but it was frequently difficult to distinguish tumour-associated cysts from non-neoplastic cystic lesions with absolute certainty.

Plain films of the spine still have a certain usefulness as a screening examination in the patient who presents with pain or myelopathy. Widening of the pedicles on the frontal projection will suggest an intraspinal mass, but the compartment that the mass occupies, and the nature of the mass itself, cannot be determined. Overall less than 20% of patients with intramedullary tumours will have abnormal plain films (Woods & Pimenta, 1944).

Angiography of the spinal cord is usually not indicated in the evaluation of these lesions. However, if there is suspicion from the clinical history, or MRI appearance that a lesion may represent an arteriovenous malformation rather than a tumour, spinal angiography will clarify the diagnosis and define the anatomy of the lesion. The presence of an intramedullary lesion on MRI, along with an extensive vascular supply, should suggest the diagnosis of a haemangioblastoma. Here too spinal cord angiography is indicated to aid in the operative removal of the lesion and also to identify additional lesions that may have escaped notice on the MRI.

The advent of MRI scanning has greatly simplified the differential diagnosis of intramedullary tumours. Nevertheless the clinical appearance of two entities may cause confusion. Because the MRI may also be misinterpreted in those conditions, they deserve special mention.

When multiple sclerosis involves the spinal cord the signs and symptoms may resemble those seen with intramedullary tumours. In general, however, the onset of neurological deficit is more rapid in onset in patients with multiple sclerosis, and remissions and exacerbations are a common part of the clinical picture. Although the rapidity of the clinical course in patients with spinal cord tumours may vary from patient to patient and even in the same patient, relentless progression is the rule and remissions are unusual except in the rare instance of intratumoral haemorrhage.

In multiple sclerosis (MS), ancillary tests such as cerebrospinal fluid oligoclonal bands and abnormal visual evoked responses may help to confirm the diagnosis. Cerebral MRI may often be positive but to the inexperienced observer of MRI scans lesions of the spinal cord caused by the demyelination of multiple sclerosis may resemble intramedullary tumours. The spinal cord lesions of MS will almost always be limited to one or two spinal segments in their rostral–caudal extent. Although the signal intensity of the acute lesions of MS may be similar to that seen with intramedullary tumours, and may enhance following the administration of gadolinium, the spinal cord is only minimally widened in cases of MS (Fig. 30.5).

The clinical course of syringomyelia tends to be more indolent than intramedullary tumours, but in all other respects the manifestations of the two conditions may be indistinguishable. The salient features of the MRI scan in syringomyelia have already been mentioned, but it is important to reiterate that the administration of gadolinium is absolutely essential to rule out enhancement from a small tumour. Visualization of the cervicomedullary junction in the sagittal plane is also important to identify tonsillar herniation.

MANAGEMENT

The diagnosis of an intramedullary tumour does not necessarily mandate operative removal. The decision to operate on patients with far-advanced neurological deficit must be made with realistic expectations. These include a desire to preserve residual sensory function in bed-ridden patients who are likely to suffer skin breakdown in anaesthetic areas or preservation of residual sphincter function. However, patients who are unable to stand are unlikely to regain enough motor function to ambulate as a result of tumour resection. Nevertheless, operation may maintain the quality of a patient's life by preserving the ability to transfer or to turn in bed. Patients with complete motor and sensory deficit will not regain function with surgery, and are not operative candidates.

Patients with progressive neurological deficit who are still able to walk represent the ideal candidates. In most, operation provides an opportunity to arrest the progression of neurological deterioration and improve motor and sensory function. Although the risks of an increase in neurological deficit as a result of operation are real, once motor deficit begins its progression is relentless. Although the rate of progression may vary, untreated patients will almost always develop complete neurological deficit. Thus the risks of operation are more than outweighed by the natural history of the disease process.

If the patient presents with already-established total paraplegia, removal of the tumour will not result in neurological recovery. However, there is a fear that the tumour will grow rostrally and ultimately result in quadriplegia and death. Reviewing the authors' cases has shown that benign non-cystic astrocytomas caudal to T4 do not usually extend rostrally. A similar tumour above T4 is more likely to threaten upper limb function. Therefore, tumours close to the cervicodorsal junction should be removed in an attempt to prevent future neurological dysfunction in the upper limb. Thoracic tumours with a rostral cyst must also be removed, as expansion of the cyst will lead to involvement of the cervical canal.

Decision-making in the patient who presents with neck or back pain and mild sensory symptoms, and a

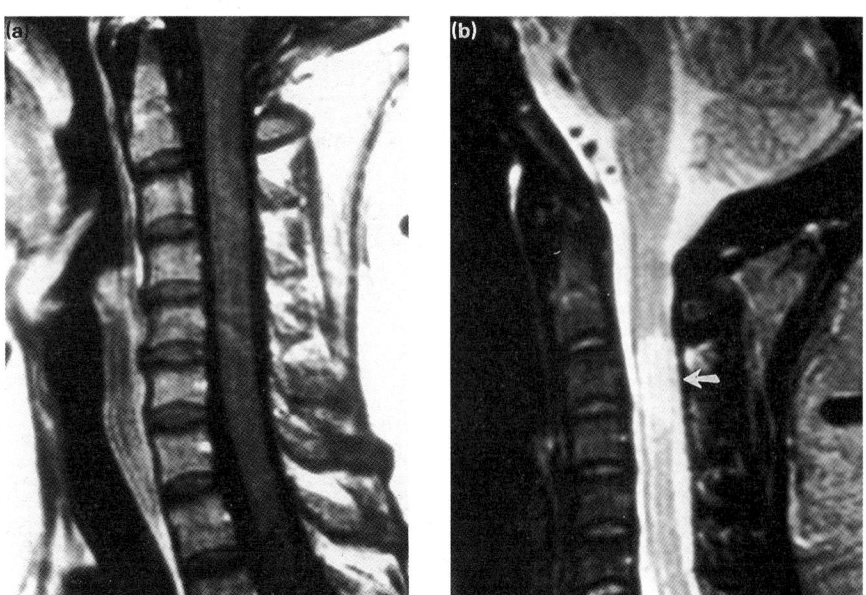

Fig. 30.5 (a) T1-weighted MRI in patient with proven multiple sclerosis showing only minimal cord widening. (b) T2 image showing the area of demyelinating plaque (arrow).

paucity of objective deficits, is more difficult. Many patients are unwilling to risk neurological deterioration when their symptoms are minor and they have no significant functional impairment. In this situation it may not be unreasonable to follow the patient closely for the appearance of additional symptoms or the appearance of objective deficit. Frequently once patients realize that their symptoms have progressed as predicted, they are more prepared psychologically to face the risks of operative treatment.

The aims of operative management are total tumour removal with preservation or improvement of neurological function. These goals are not always achieved as certain tumours of the spinal cord infiltrate adjacent neural structures, making total removal impossible without incurring unacceptable loss of function. Even when tumours are clearly delineated from normal spinal cord, removal may result in a permanent increase in neurological deficit.

The patients should be commenced on steroid therapy 48 hours prior to surgery to minimize the risk of swelling. The solid portion of the tumour is the only portion of the lesion which must be removed, and its extent should be marked by intraoperative radiology to ensure that only the relevant laminae are removed.

After the laminectomy has been completed, intraoperative ultrasonography is used to locate the solid portion of the tumour precisely (Fig. 30.6). The use of ultrasonography during the operation means that the procedure should be performed in the prone position. This allows the irrigating solution necessary for ultrasonography to remain in the wound. It also reduces the risk of cerebral hypoperfusion which may occur if damage occurs to the cervical cord resulting in severe hypotension in the sitting position.

The use of ultrasonography prior to opening the dura permits accurate localization of the solid portion of the tumour. It may also aid the surgeon by indicating the nature of the lesion. Astrocytomas are relatively isodense with the spinal cord on ultrasound, and are identified by their adjacent cysts. Occasionally, microscopic foci of calcification may make them

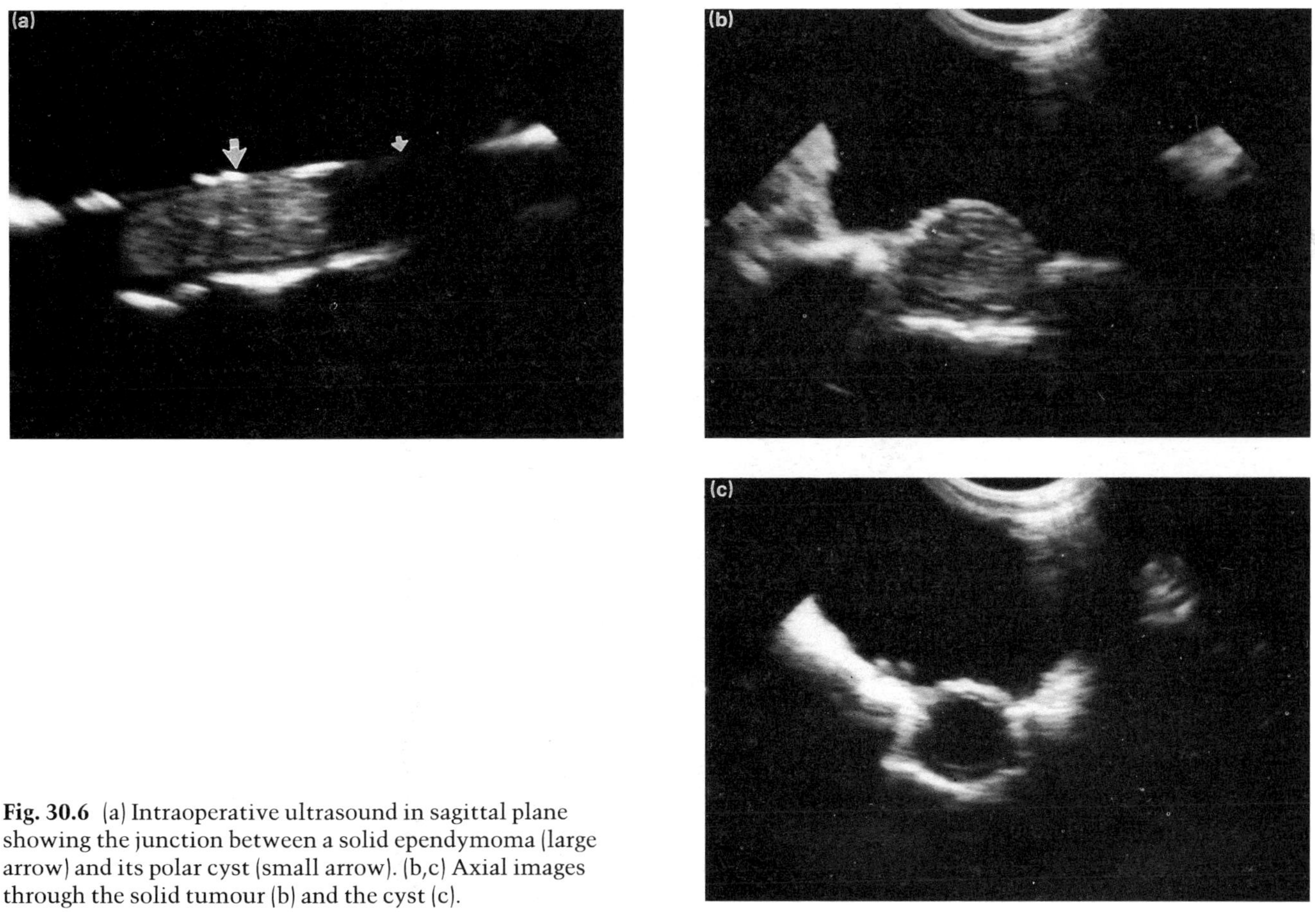

Fig. 30.6 (a) Intraoperative ultrasound in sagittal plane showing the junction between a solid ependymoma (large arrow) and its polar cyst (small arrow). (b,c) Axial images through the solid tumour (b) and the cyst (c).

hyperdense. In contradistinction, ependymomas are normally hyperdense to the cord on ultrasound. The use of ultrasound in the transverse plane will also show the relationship of tumour to the cord, with astrocytomas frequently being asymmetrical.

Once the solid portion of the tumour has been localized, the dura is then opened. A dorsal myelotomy placed exactly in the midline over the solid tumour is made. It is sometimes difficult to be absolutely certain of the exact midline because the spinal cord may be rotated or distorted asymmetrically by the tumour. An asymmetric laminectomy or an apparently midline blood vessel on the posterior surface of the spinal cord may give a false impression of the midline. It is therefore essential that both the left and right dorsal roots be identified, as the midline will be located midway between the left and right dorsal roots.

The myelotomy must not be placed in a paramedian location, in order to avoid a midline vein on the dorsal surface of the spinal cord. Such a manoeuvre is almost guaranteed to result in joint position sense loss. In such a situation the midline veins or arteries can be cauterized, using the bipolar cautery at a low setting. The pia-arachnoid and dorsal surface of the spinal cord are then incised sharply to a depth of 2–3 mm over the length of the spinal cord occupied by the solid tumour. This may also be achieved by the carbon dioxide laser coaxial to the operating microscope and sharply focused at a setting of less than 5 W. The laser must be used at low power and with a pinpoint-focused beam. The surgical laser is an undiscriminating tool and will readily vaporize neural tissue as well as tumour. It must therefore be used with great care.

The myelotomy is carefully deepened until the posterior surface of the tumour is encountered, and then exposed over the entire length of the solid tumour. In the presence of an astrocytoma with polar cysts the myelotomy should be commenced over the midpoint of the tumour where the depth of the covering spinal cord will be at its minimum. It is then extended towards the poles but stopping some 1 cm short of the tapered ends of the tumour. This is because it is the least voluminous part and the area of greatest risk of causing neurological damage as the myelotomy is deepened. The pia-arachnoid and dorsal surface of the spinal cord are held apart by passing a 6–O atraumatic suture through the pia-arachnoid at intevals of 1 cm on either side of the midline (Fig. 30.7). Traction is placed on the ends of the sutures with light haemostats. This has the effect of opening the centre of the spinal cord for further dissection.

Following myelotomy the tumour may on occasion bulge out of the cord and seem to deliver itself (Fig. 30.8). If the lesion is an ependymoma the plane between the tumour and cord should be identified and dissected. If the lesion is small it can occasionally be removed in one piece, but it is normally safer to initially debulk the tumour. If the ependymoma is particularly vascular, its size can be reduced by shrinking the capsule with bipolar cautery. As astrocytomas have no cleavage plane, attempts at an *en-bloc* removal are not indicated. The astrocytoma must be removed from the inside of the tumour.

The tumour is debulked using the ultrasonic aspirator. This instrument utilizes high-frequency sound to fragment the tumour. The irrigating fluid then creates a suspension with the microfragments of tissue, which are then sucked away by the suction pump. This procedure represents a major technical advance, and has greatly enhanced the surgeon's ability to

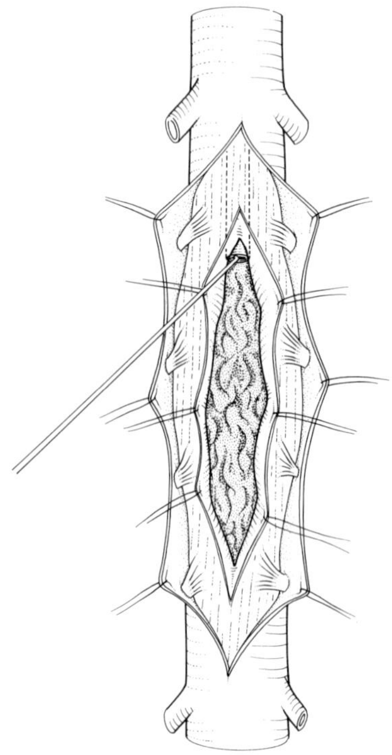

Fig. 30.7 Diagram of exposure of tumour by the use of pial traction sutures following myelotomy. The probe has entered the rostral cyst.

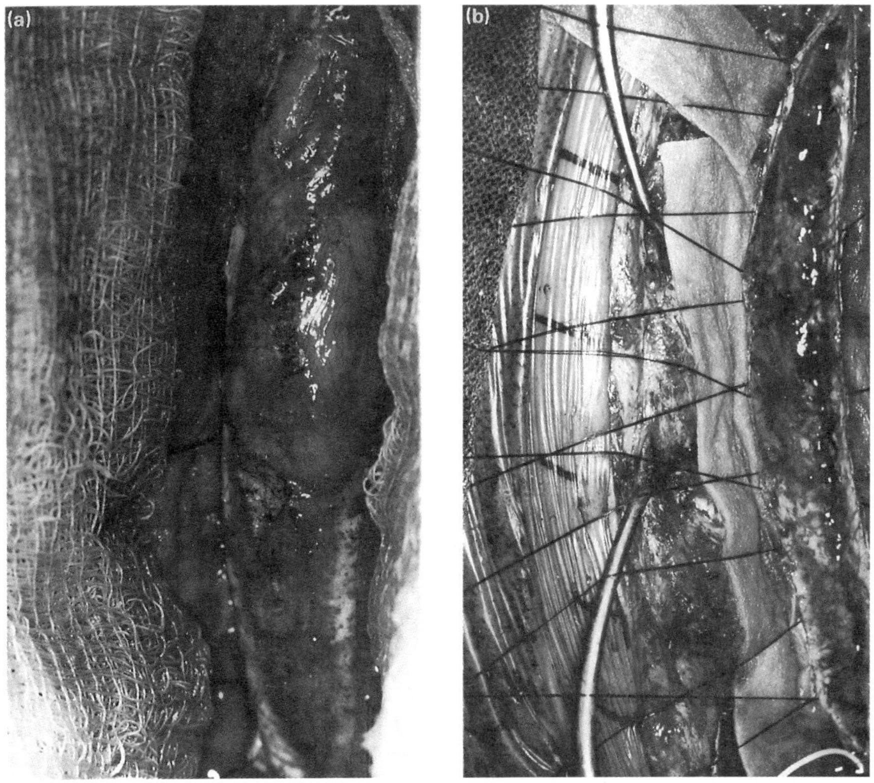

Fig. 30.8 (a) A large astrocytoma bulges out of the cord following myelotomy. (b) The tumour cavity following its removal.

remove intramedullary lesions without unnecessary traction or manipulation of the spinal cord. It should be used with the lowest power setting which will allow tumour fragmentation. Hard tumours are more safely removed by the use of laser vaporization.

Ultrasonic dissection continues from within the tumour itself, initially progressing towards the poles. The interface between the pole of the tumour and an adjacent cyst represents the only area in an astrocytoma where a 'plane' exists. Once the cyst has been entered, the contents drain into the wound and the cyst collapses. It is unnecessary to remove the glial lining of the cystic cavity, and such a manoeuvre should not be attempted. Tumour removal continues until the interface between the cord and the tumour becomes indistinguishable. Some authorities then treat the resultant cavity with the defocused laser in an attempt to vaporize any remaining tumour cells. However, it is likely that microscopic residual tumour is left behind (Guidetti *et al.*, 1981). This is especially so with astrocytomas, although Garrido & Stein (1977) felt that astrocytomas were no more difficult to remove than ependymomas.

As the tumour removal progresses anteriorly it is not uncommon for the surgeon to be uncertain in terms of the anterior extent of the tumour removal as compared to the anterior surface of the cord and the anterior spinal artery. It may often appear that most of the tumour has been removed when in fact a large volume of neoplasm remains. Again, the intraoperative use of the ultrasound to assess the transverse image allows accurate interpretation of the situation and encourages full removal of the tumour.

Certain other intramedullary tumours demand a different surgical technique. Intramedullary haemangioblastomas may occur as isolated lesions or in association with other haemangioblastomas in the posterior cranial fossa or elsewhere in the spinal cord. They are immediately apparent on the dorsal surface of the spinal cord along with a profusion of vessels which supply and drain the lesion. They range in size from a few millimetres in diameter to the size of a large grape, and are well defined from the surrounding spinal cord.

No attempt should be made to enter the tumour until its vascular supply is totally interrupted as these tumours are highly vascular. The arterial supply, part of which is visible on the dorsal surface of the spinal cord, is coagulated and cut, and the tumour is very slowly reduced in size by coagulating it with the bipolar cautery. When this is done the tumour may be more easily dissected from the adjacent spinal cord exposing additional vascular supply which is progressively interrupted allowing total removal. Haemangioblastomas are curable tumours, but may recur as a result of the growth of residual tumour or, as is more commonly the case, growth of additional tumours which were clinically silent or radiographically unapparent at the time of the first surgery.

Lipomas of the spinal cord also require an alternative approach. They are most commonly seen at the level of the conus medullaris in association with spinal dysraphism and a tethered spinal cord. The management of such lipomas is discussed in Chapter 14. Less commonly, isolated lipomas occur more rostrally in the thoracic and cervical spinal cord. Histologically identical to normal fat, these tumours are located on the dorsal surface of the spinal cord covered by little or no neural tissue.

Although distinct from adjacent spinal cord and non-invasive, they are densely adherent to normal spinal cord and total removal is not possible without incurring unacceptable neurological deficit (Greenwood, 1963). The most effective operative strategy consists of subtotal removal leaving a rim of tumour at the interface with the spinal cord. The laser is ideal for removal of lipomas as the fibrous interstices of the lesion make removal with the ultrasonic aspirator difficult. These are slowly growing lesions but recurrence may take place as a result of continued growth of residual tumour.

Other tumours include gangliogliomas, oligodendrogliomas, epidermoids and intramedullary neurofibromas. These tumours are rare and the problems they present to the surgeon are similar in nature to the tumours discussed above.

The development of spinal deformity following the removal of an intramedullary tumour in children is a common problem. Scoliosis may develop or progress but the major problem is the development of postlaminectomy kyphotic deformity (Haft *et al.*, 1959; Doubousset *et al.*, 1973; Yasouka *et al.*, 1981, 1982; Lonstein, 1988) (Figs 30.9 & 30.10). Postlaminectomy kyphosis in adults is rare unless there is pre-existing vertebral body disease or both facet joints are removed. However, children who undergo laminectomy must be carefully followed by regular radiology so that the development of a kyphosis can be diagnosed at an early stage, and treated by anterior or combined anterior and posterior fusion.

Postoperative bracing does not prevent the development of postlaminectomy kyphosis but intertransverse fusion performed at the time of laminectomy in the cervical or cervicodorsal spine does seem to be effective at limiting the development of deformity (G.F.G. Findlay, personal communication). In an attempt to prevent deformity many patients have had an osteoplastic laminectomy with replacement of all the bony elements on closure of the dura. While this has resulted in excellent bony union of the laminoplasty, it has not prevented progressive postoperative spinal deformity. This is because the elasticity of the posterior musculoligamentous structures are still lost, and their loss produces abnormal stresses on the growing spine. It may also be related to the loss of anterior horn cells caused by the tumour.

There has been much debate about the use of intraoperative spinal cord monitoring during these procedures (see Chapter 9). Monitoring is usually that of the somatosensory evoked response (SSEP). Unfortunately the currently available SSEP monitors are not always of use to the surgeon. Patients with profound preoperative sensory deficits will have either absent SSEP or potentials which are so abnormal that meaningful recordings cannot be obtained. Depending on the exact machine, there is a delay of 10–60 s for averaging from the time that an injury to the cord occurs to the time it is displayed on the monitor. In addition, the surgical manipulation of the dorsal columns necessary to remove the tumour will frequently distort the SSEP and may tend to confuse the surgeon, possibly leading to less than adequate tumour removal. SSEP monitoring also provides no evidence of motor tract function. Although the proximity of the motor pathways to the sensory ones may allow changes to be observed, this is not invariably so. Currently, intraoperative motor pathway monitoring is under investigation in many units.

Because of these problems, intraoperative spinal cord monitoring is beset with significant difficulties of both overestimating and sometimes underestimating any cord damage which may occur during the removal of a spinal cord tumour. The situation is totally different from that of scoliosis surgery, where the cord is reasonably normal to start with and a change in the SSEP may be reacted to by reducing the degree of correction obtained. There is no statistically

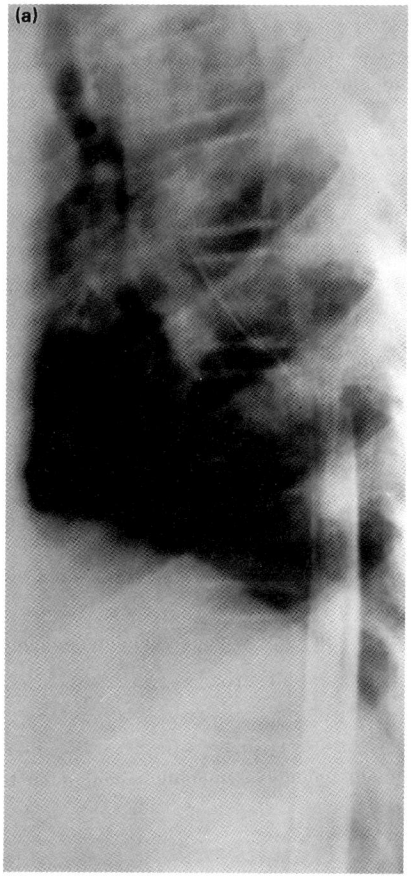

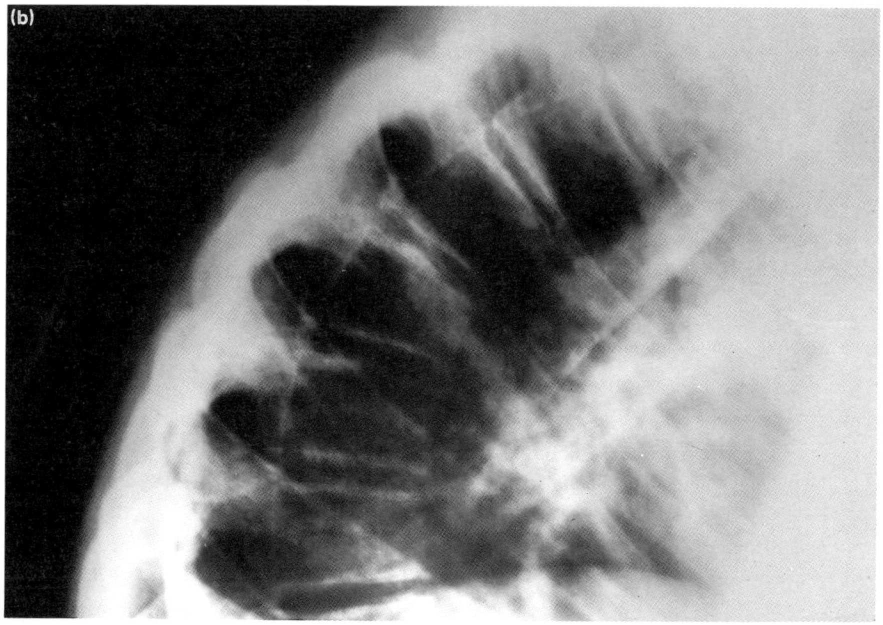

Fig. 30.9 (a) Myelogram of a seven-year-old child with an extradural neuroblastoma. (b) Lateral thoracic film of the same child, three years after a three-level laminectomy to remove the tumour. Severe kyphotic deformity has been allowed to develop.

valid evidence that the use of any electrophysiological monitoring technique improves the outcome of patients undergoing surgery for an intramedullary tumour.

Adjunctive therapy

No study has been performed demonstrating a beneficial effect of radiation therapy on neurological function or survival in patients with glial tumours of the spinal cord. Guidetti *et al.* (1981) found no consistent benefit from radiation therapy. Others have reported improvement or disappearance of deficits after irradiation, but none of these studies was controlled and there is no proof that the radiation treatment itself resulted in improvement (Woltman *et al.*, 1951; Wood *et al.*, 1954; Stein, 1979; Kopelson *et al.*, 1980). Moreover, the efficacy of radiation therapy is difficult to determine as the natural history of low-grade astrocytomas is unpredictable and long-term survival without radiation may occur (Reimer & Onofrio, 1985). Nevertheless it has been our policy to irradiate all adult patients with spinal cord astrocytomas regardless of the surgeon's impression of the completeness of removal or the histological grade of the tumour. The treatment consists of 4500 Gy given in divided doses to the region of the tumour. Garcia (1985) noted an improved outcome in patients treated with 4000 Gy compared to those treated with smaller doses. Marsa *et al.* (1975) used doses greater than 5000 Gy but such treatment is not recommended because of the risk of radiation myelopathy.

Because of the detrimental effect of radiation therapy on development in children, and the possibility that low-grade astrocytomas in children are potentially curable by surgery, treatment is deferred in paediatric patients who are thought to have had a gross total resection of their tumours. It is essential, however, that these patients be followed frequently with MRI to detect any evidence of tumour recurrence.

Patients with ependymomas who are thought to have had a complete removal are not irradiated

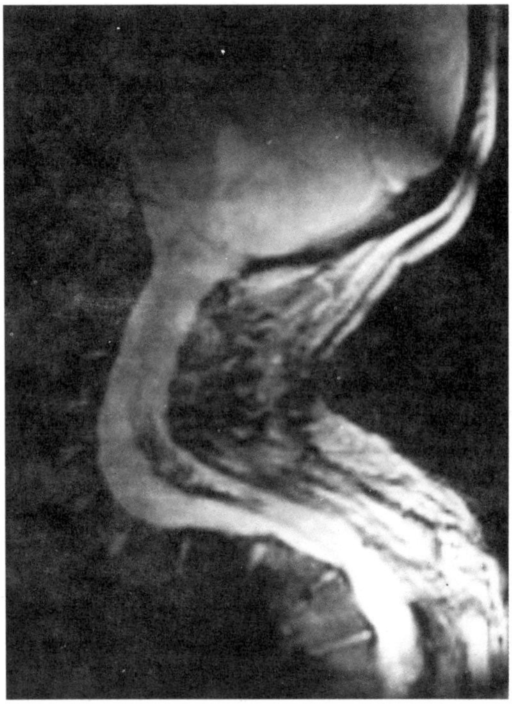

Fig. 30.10 Severe swan-neck deformity secondary to cervicodorsal kyphotic deformity presenting 20 years following C6–T2 laminectomy for intramedullary lipoma.

(Greenwood, 1963; Fischer & Mansury, 1980). They are followed closely with frequent MRI and treated with reoperation or radiation if recurrence becomes apparent. When removal is incomplete patients should be treated with local radiation to the area of residual tumour.

RESULTS

Whether the new surgically more aggressive approach described above will result in the cure of these patients is not clear. Particularly, with the benign astrocytomas, growth is slow and following a radical removal it may take years for a tumour to recur. What is clear, however, is that it is possible to radically remove most intramedullary neoplasms. Following some procedures there has been no increase in the neurological function, though more commonly there is a temporary derangement of proprioception function. Patients with the most severe preoperative motor deficit have the greatest chance of sustaining further neurological injury following resection. The frequency of neurological deterioration does not seem to be related to the histological type of the tumour or the extent of the surgical resection. Overall, some 20% of our adult patients have shown some degree of permanent increase in their neurological deficit following tumour removal. The different nature of childhood tumours means that there is less likelihood of producing increase in the deficit but, in any case, these figures have to be compared with the 100% rate of neurological deterioration which will occur if the tumour is only decompressed.

Long-term survival and neurological function are related to tumour histology, the patient's preoperative neurological status and extent of tumour resection. The prognosis for patients with malignant astrocytomas is remarkably similar to that of patients with the same tumours located intracranially, and no patients in this series survived longer than one year. Although the outlook for patients with low-grade astrocytomas is better, slow progression of tumours in the cervical region can result in death from respiratory paralysis. Other complications of quadriplegia—such as pulmonary embolus, sepsis and pneumonia—will also shorten the lives of these patients, making this anything but a benign lesion. Degeneration of low-grade tumours into malignant ones may occur with time, and will further adversely affect outcome.

Fortunately the long-term survival of patients with ependymomas is less bleak than is the case for patients with astrocytomas. Unlike astrocytomas, the outcome of patients with ependymomas does not appear to be related to histological grade (Rawlings *et al.*, 1988). Although ependymomas can seed in the subarachnoid space this method of spread seems to be the exception rather than the rule.

Haemangioblastomas are benign tumours which are curable if totally removed. As such they should have little effect on long-term survival. In practice haemangioblastomas are frequently found in multiple locations, and outcome is determined by the behaviour of tumours located elsewhere in the nervous system. Other varieties of tumours found within the spinal cord are encountered too infrequently to make a definitive statement regarding their effect on longevity.

Neurological outcome in the immediate postoperative period is most closely related to the patient's immediate preoperative neurological state. Patients who have no motor function may on rare occasions regain some small amount of function after operation, but it is unlikely that they will be able to walk or stand as a result of tumour resection. Similarly patients who cannot stand prior to surgery do not often regain the ability to walk in the postoperative period.

Looking at neurological function in adults in the longer term shows significant problems. The combination of increased neurological deficit from operation and progressive growth of residual tumour leaves a high percentage of patients with considerable neurological impairment in the years following operation. Almost one-half of all patients available for follow-up examination were worse than they were prior to the time of operation by one or more neurological grades (Cooper, 1989).

In spite of a number of advances in the past decade, tumours of the spinal cord continue to present a challenge to neurosurgeons. While advances in imaging, and in particular the advent of the MRI, have eliminated much of the uncertainty in diagnosis these tumours remain a particularly difficult entity to treat surgically.

From a conceptual point of view it has become clear that radical removal can be achieved by experienced surgeons with minimal morbidity. However, most spinal cord astrocytomas in adults are infiltrative and not totally resectable, and recurrence is frequent. This is especially true for the malignant astrocytomas which behave in a fashion similar to their counterparts located intracranially, and rapid neurological deterioration and death are the rule. For many ependymomas surgical cure is possible, but for infiltrating ependymomas and other spinal cord tumours of glial origin improved management awaits a greater understanding of the biology of these lesions.

REFERENCES

Ammerman, B.J. & Smith, D.R. (1975) Papilloedema and spinal cord tumours. *Surg. Neurol.*, **3**, 55–57.

Anderson, F.M. & Carson, M.U. (1953) Spinal cord tumours in children. A review of the subject and representation of twenty-one cases. *J. Paediatr.*, **43**, 190–207.

Arseni, C., Horvath, L. & Illiescu, D. (1967) Intraspinal tumours in children. *Psychiat. Neurol. Neurochir.*, **70**, 123–133.

Chigasaki, H. & Pennybacker, J.B. (1968) A long follow-up study of 128 cases of intramedullary spinal cord tumours. *Neurol. Medico-Chirurg.*, **10**, 25–66.

Cooper, P.R. (1989) Outcome after operative treatment of intramedullary spinal cord tumours in adults. Intermediate and long-term results in 51 patients. *Neurosurgery*, **25**, 855–859.

Cooper, P.R. & Epstein, F. (1985) Radical resection of intramedullary spinal cord tumours in adults. Recent experience in 29 patients. *J. Neurosurg.*, **63**, 492–499.

Doubousset, J., Guillamat, J. & Mechi, J.F. (1973) In Roujerie J. (ed.) *Les compression medullaires non traumatique de l'enfant.* Masson, Paris.

Epstein, F. & Epstein, N. (1981) Surgical management of 'holocord' intramedullary spinal cord astrocytomas in children. *J. Neurosurg.*, **54**, 829–932.

Fischer, G. & Mansury, L. (1980) Total removal of intramedullary ependymomas: follow-up study of 16 cases. *Surg. Neurol.*, **14**, 243–249.

Garcia, D.M. (1985) Primary spinal cord tumours treated with surgery and postoperative irradiation. *Radiat. Oncol. Biol. Phys.*, **11**, 1933–1939.

Garrido, E. & Stein, B.M. (1977) Microsurgical removal of intramedullary spinal cord tumours. *Surg. Neurol.*, **7**, 215–219.

Goy, A.M.C., Pinto, R.S., Raghavendra, B.N., Epstein, F.J. & Kricheff, I.I. (1986) Intramedullary spinal cord tumours: MR imaging with emphasis on associated cysts. *Radiology*, **161**, 381–386.

Greenwood, J. (1963) Intramedullary tumours of the spinal cord. A follow up study after total surgical removal. *J. Neurosurg.*, **20**, 665–668.

Guidetti, B., Mercuri, S. & Vagnozzi, R. (1981) Long term results of the surgical treatment of 129 intramedullary spinal gliomas. *J. Neurosurg.*, **54**, 323–330.

Haft, H., Ransohoff, J. & Carter, S. (1950) Spinal cord tumours in children. *Paediatrics*, **23**, 1152–1159.

Hardison, H.H., Packer, R.J., Rorke, L.B., Schut, L. & Sutton, L.N. (1987) Outcome of children with primary intramedullary spinal cord tumours. *Childs Nerv. Syst.*, **3**, 89–92.

Kopelson, G. & Linggood, R.M. (1982) Intramedullary spinal cord astrocytoma versus glioblastoma. *Cancer*, **50**, 732–735.

Kopelson, G., Linggood, R.M., Kleinman, G.M., Doucette, J. & Wang, C.C. (1980) Management of intramedullary spinal cord tumours. *Radiology*, **135**, 473–479.

Lonstein, J. (1988) Spinal stability after tumour resection by laminectomy. In Akbamia, B.A. (ed.) *Spinal Tumours.* Hanley & Belfus, Inc.

Marsa, G.W., Goffinet, D.R., Rubinstein, L.J. & Bagshaw, M.A. (1975) Megavoltage irradiation in the treatment of gliomas of the brain and spinal cord. *Cancer*, **36**, 1681–1689.

Neau, J.P., Roualdes, G., Bataille, B., Boissonnot, L. *et al.* (1987) Hypertension intracranienne et hydrocephalie par tumeurs medullaires. A propos de trolis observations. *Neurochirurgie*, **33**, 216–219.

Rawlings, C.E., Giangaspero, F., Burger, P.C. and Bullard, D.E. (1988) Ependymomas: a clinicopathologic study. *Surg. Neurol.*, **29**, 271–281.

Reimer, R. & Onofrio, B.M. (1985) Astrocytomas of the spinal cord in children and adolescents. *J. Neurosurg.*, **63**, 669–675.

Stein, B.M. (1979) Surgery of intramedullary spinal cord tumours. *Clin. Neurosurg.*, **26**, 529–542.

Woltman, H.W., Kernohan, J.W., Adson, A.W. & Craig,

W.M. (1951) Intramedullary tumours of spinal cord and gliomas of intradural portion of filum terminale. Fate of patients who have these tumours. *Arch. Neurol. Psychiatry*, **65**, 378–395.
Wood, E.H., Berne, A.S. & Taveras, J.M. (1954) The value of radiation therapy in the management of intrinsic tumours of the spinal cord. *Radiology*, **63**, 11–24.
Woods, W.W. and Pimenta, A.A. (1944) Intramedullary lesions of the spinal cord. Study of sixty-eight consecutive cases. *Arch. Neurol. Psychiatry*, **52**, 383–399.

Index

SURGERY OF THE SPINE

To Andrea and Meg

SURGERY OF THE SPINE

A COMBINED ORTHOPAEDIC AND NEUROSURGICAL APPROACH

Edited by

GORDON FINDLAY
BSc MB ChB FRCS
Consultant Neurosurgeon
Department of Medical and Surgical Neurology
Walton Hospital, Liverpool

and

ROBERT OWEN
DL, MB BS MCh(Orth) FRCS
Emeritus Professor of
Orthopaedic and Trauma Surgery
University of Liverpool

With an Introduction by

HENK VERBIEST

IN TWO VOLUMES

VOLUME 2

OXFORD
BLACKWELL SCIENTIFIC PUBLICATIONS
LONDON EDINBURGH BOSTON
MELBOURNE PARIS BERLIN VIENNA

Editorial offices:
Osney Mead, Oxford OX2 0EL
25 John Street, London WC1N 2BL
23 Ainslie Place, Edinburgh EH3 6AJ
3 Cambridge Center, Cambridge
Massachusetts 02142, USA
54 University Street, Carlton
Victoria 3053, Australia

Other editorial offices:
Librairie Arnette SA
2, rue Casimir-Delavigne
75006 Paris
France

Blackwell Wissenschafts-Verlag
Meinekestrasse 4
D-1000 Berlin 15
Germany

Blackwell MZV
Feldgasse 13
A-1238 Wien
Austria

First published 1992

Set by Excel Typesetter Ltd, Hong Kong
Printed and bound by Kin Keong, Singapore

DISTRIBUTORS

Marston Book Services Ltd
PO Box 87
Oxford OX2 0DT
(*Orders*: Tel: 0865 791155
Fax: 0865 791927
Telex: 837515)

USA
Blackwell Scientific Publications, Inc.
3 Cambridge Center
Cambridge, MA 02142
(*Orders*: Tel: 800 759-6102
617 225-0401)

Canada
Times Mirror Professional Publishing, Ltd
5240 Finch Avenue East
Scarborough, Ontario M1S 5A2
(*Orders*: Tel: 800 268-4178
416 298-1588)

Australia
Blackwell Scientific Publications
(Australia) Pty Ltd
54 University Street
Carlton, Victoria 3053
(*Orders*: Tel: 03 347-0300)

A catalogue record for this book
is available from the British Library

ISBN 0–632–03021–6 (The Set)
0–632–03246–4 (Vol. 1)
0–632–03247–2 (Vol. 2)

Contents

List of Contributors

G.M. BEDBROOK, Kt, OBE, OStJ, MS(Melb), HonMD(WA), HonFRCS(Ed), HonDTech(Curtin), FRCS, FRACS, DPRM(Syd), HonFCRM, *Emeritus Orthopaedic Surgeon, Royal Perth Rehabilitation Hospital, Perth, Australia*

S.H. BIGNER, MD, *Professor of Pathology, Duke University Medical Center, PO Box 3712, Durham, NC 27710, USA*

L.D. BLUMHARDT, BSc, MD, FRACP, *Reader in Clinical Neurology, Department of Neurological Science, Faculty of Medicine, Liverpool University; Honorary Consultant Neurologist, Walton Centre for Neurology Walton Hospital, Rice Lane, Liverpool, L91AE, UK*

H.H. BOHLMAN, MD, FACS, *Professor and Vice Chairman of Orthopaedics, Case Western Reserve University School of Medicine, Department of Orthopaedics, University Hospitals of Cleveland, 2074 Abington Road, Cleveland, Ohio 44106-2602 USA; Chief, Spinal Cord Injury Service, Department of Veterans Affairs, 10701 East Blvd., Cleveland, OH 44106, USA*

M.J. BOLESTA, MD, FACS, *Assistant Professor of Orthopaedics, Case Western Reserve University School of Medicine, Department of Orthopaedics, University Hospitals of Cleveland, 2074 Abington Road, Cleveland, Ohio 44106-2602, USA; Administration Chief, Spinal Cord Injury Service, Department of Veterans Affairs, 10701 East Blvd., Cleveland, OH 44106, USA*

R.E.M. BOWDEN, OBE, MB, BS, DSc, FRCS, *Emeritus Professor of Anatomy, University of London; formerly Sir William Collins Professor of Humanities and Comparative Anatomy, Department of Anatomy, Royal College of Surgeons of England, Lincoln's Inn Fields, London WC2A3PN, UK*

D.R. BOWSHER, MA, MD, Ph.D, MRCP(Ed), MRCPath, *Director of Research, Pain Research Institute, Walton Hospital, Liverpool L91AE, UK; Honorary Consultant Neurologist, Mersey Regional Centre for Pain Relief*

I.M. BOYD, FFARCS, MB, BS, BSc, DCH, *Consultant Anaesthetist, Department of Anaesthesia, Royal Liverpool Children's Hospital, Alder Hey, Eaton Road, Liverpool L122AP, UK; Honorary Lecturer, Liverpool University*

R. BRAAKMAN, MD, PhD, *Professor of Neurosurgery, Department of Neurosurgery, Erasmus University Rotterdam, University Hospital Rotterdam-Dijkzigt, Dr. Molewaterplein 40, 3015 GD, The Netherlands*

M. BROCK, MD, *Professor and Chairman, Department of Neurosurgery, Universitaetsklinikum Steglitz/Free University of Berlin, Hindenburgdamm 30, W-1000, Berlin 45, Germany*

R.G. BURWELL, BSc, MD, FRCS, *Professor of Human Morphology and Experimental Orthopaedics, Department of Human Morphology, University of Nottingham, Queen's Medical Centre, Nottingham NG72UH; Honorary Consultant in Orthopaedics, Nottingham Health Authority*

H. CARTY, FRCPI, FRCR, *Consultant Radiologist and Lecturer in Radiodiagnosis, Department of Radiology, Royal Liverpool Children's Hospital, Alder Hey, Eaton Road, Liverpool L122AP, UK*

V. CHACKO, MB, BS, MS(Orth), *Consultant Orthopaedic Surgeon, 'Illampallil, Tiruvalla-689 101, Kerala, India; Formerly Director/Professor and Head of Orthopaedics, Kasturba Medical College, Manipal; President of Indian Orthopaedic Association*

R.C.M. COOK, MA, BM, BCh, FRCS, *Consultant Paediatric Surgeon, Royal Liverpool Children's Hospital, Alder Hey, Eaton Road, Liverpool L122AP, UK*

P.R. COOPER, MD, *Professor of Neurosurgery, Department of Neurosurgery, New York University Medical Center 550 1st Avenue, New York, USA*

R.A. COWIE, BSc, MB, ChB, FRCS(Ed), FRCS(Ed) (SN), *Consultant Neurosurgeon, Department of Neurosurgery, Hope Hospital, Eccles Old Rd., Salford M68HD, UK; Department of Neurosurgery, Royal Manchester Children's Hospital, Hospital Road, Pendlebury, Swinton, Manchester M271HA, UK*

H.A. CROCKARD, FRCS(Ed), FRCSE, *Consultant Neurosurgeon, Department of Surgical Neurology, The National Hospital for Neurology and Neurosurgery, Maida Vale, London W91TL, UK; Honorary Senior Lecturer, Institute of Neurology*

P.H. DANGERFIELD, MD, *Lecturer in Human Anatomy and Cell Biology, Clinical Lecturer in Orthopaedic Surgery, Department of Human Anatomy and Cell Biology, University of Liverpool, PO Box 147, Liverpool, L693BX, UK*

J. DOVE, FRCS, *Director, Stoke-on-Trent Spinal Service, 31 Quarry Avenue, Hartshill, Stoke on Trent ST47EW, UK*

J. DVORAK, MD, *Head of Neurology Department, Spine Unit, Schuethese Hospital, 8008 Zurich, Switzerland*

M.A. EDGAR, MA, M.Chir, FRCS, *Consultant Orthopaedic Surgeon, 149 Harley St., London W1N2DE, UK; The Middlesex and University College Hospital, London W1; The Royal National Orthopaedic Hospital, Stanmore, Middlesex, UK; Civilian Consultant Adviser in Orthopaedics to the RAF*

R.H.T. EDWARDS, BSc, PhD, MB, FRCP, *Professor of Medicine, Director of Magnetic Resonance Research Centre, Director of Muscle Research Centre, Department of Medicine, University of Liverpool, PO Box 147, Liverpool L693BX, UK*

S.M. EISENSTEIN, MB, BCh, PhD, FRCS(Ed), *Director, Centre for Spinal Studies, Department for Spinal Disorders, The Robert Jones and Agnes Hunt Orthopaedic Hospital, Oswestry Hospital, Oswestry, Shropshire SY107AG, UK*

F.J. EPSTEIN, MD, *Director of Pediatric Neurosurgery, Professor of Neurosurgery, Department of Neurosurgery, New York University Medical Center, 550 1st Avenue, New York, USA*

J.A. EPSTEIN, MD, FACS, *Professor of Neurosurgery, Cornell University Medical College, 410 Lakeville Road, Ste #100, New Hyde Park, NY 11042, USA; Associate Clinical Professor of Neurosurgery, Albert Einstein College of Medicine; Attending Neurosurgeon, North Shore University Hospital and Long Island Jewish Medical Center*

N.E. EPSTEIN, MD, FACS, *Associate Clinical Professor of Neurosurgery, Cornell University Medical College, 410 Lakeville Road, Ste #100, New Hyde Park, NY 11042, USA; Assistant Attending Neurosurgeon, North Shore University Hospital and Long Island Jewish Medical Center*

H.S.Y. FANG, CBE, MB, BS, MCh(Orth), LLD(Hon), HKU, CUHK, FRCSE, FFACS, FACS, FRCPE, JP, *Consultant Orthopaedic Surgeon, Room 306, TakShing House, 20 Des Voeux Road, Hong Kong*

G.F.G. FINDLAY, BSc, MB, ChB, FRCS, *Consultant Neurosurgeon, Department of Neurosurgery, Walton Hospital, Rice Lane, Liverpool L91AE, UK*

P.M. FOY, MB, CHB, FRCS, *Consultant Neurosurgeon, Mersey Regional Department of Medical and Surgical Neurology, Department of Neurosurgery, Walton Hospital, Liverpool L91AE, UK; Clinical Lecturer, University of Liverpool*

R.D. FRASER, MB, BS, MD, FRACS, *Head of Spinal Unit, Department of Orthopaedic Surgery and Trauma, Royal Adelaide Hospital, Adelaide 5000, South Australia; Senior Clinical Lecturer, University of Adelaide*

C.S.B. GALASKO, MSc, MB, ChM, FRCS(Eng), FRCS(Ed), *Consultant Orthopaedic Surgeon, Department of Orthopaedic Surgery, Clinical Sciences Building, Hope Hospital, Eccles Old Road, Salford M68HD, UK; Consultant Orthopaedic Surgeon, Royal*

Manchester Children's Hospital; Professor of Orthopaedic Surgery, University of Manchester

A.D.H. GARDNER, MB, BS(Lond), FRCS(Eng), *Consultant Orthopaedic Surgeon, Basildon Hospital, Nethermayne, Basildon, Essex S16SNL, UK and Black Notley Hospital, Braintree, Essex*

M. GLANTZ, MD, *Assistant Professor of Neurooncology, University of Minnesota, Box 295, 420 Delaware Street, South-East Minneapolis, MN 55455, USA*

D.I. GRAHAM, MB, BCh, PhD, FRCPath, *Professor of Neuropathology, The University of Glasgow; Department of Neuropathology, Institute of Neurological Sciences, Southern General Hospital, Glasgow G514TF, UK*

R.D. GRIFFITHS, BSc, MD, MRCP, *Muscle Research Centre, Department of Medicine, University of Liverpool, PO Box 147, Liverpool L693BX, UK*

K.B. HEITHOFF, MD, *Medical Director, Center for Diagnostic Imaging(CDI), 2800 Chicago Avenue, Minneapolis, MN 55407, USA; CDI 5775 Wayzata Blvd., St Louis Park, MN 55416; 910 Sibley Memorial Highway, St Paul, MN 5518; CDI, 9247 North Meridian Street, Indianapolis, IN 46260, USA; Abbott Northwestern Hospital, 28th and Chicago Avenue, Minneapolis, MN 55407, USA*

N.J. HENDERSON, BM, BCh, FRCS, *Consultant Orthopaedic Surgeon, Stoke Mandeville Hospital, Aylesbury, Bucks HP218AL*

R.J. HERZOG, MD, *Medical Director, San Francisco Neuroskeletal Imaging Center, 1850 Sullivan Avenue, Suite 100, Daly City, California 94015, USA; Assistant Clinical Professor, Musculoskeletal Section, Department of Radiology, University of California, San Francisco*

E.K.W. HO, MB, BS, FRCSG, FRACS, *Senior Lecturer, Department of Orthopaedic Surgery, University of Hong Kong; Medical Director, The Duchess of Kent Children's Hospital, 12 Sandy Bay Road, Hong Kong*

H.J. HOFFMAN, MD, BScMed, FRCSC, FACS, *Neurosurgeon-in-Chief, The Hospital for Sick Children, 555 University Avenue, Toronto M5G1X8, Canada; Professor of Surgery, University of Toronto*

P.R.D. HUMPHREY, DM, FRCP, MA, BM, BCh, *Consultant Neurologist, Mersey Regional Department of Medical and Surgical Neurology, Walton Hospital, Rice Lane, Liverpool L91AE, UK*

M.I.V. JAYSON, MD, FRCP, *Professor of Rheumatology and Director of University Centre for Study of Chronic Rheumatism, Rheumatic Diseases Centre University of Manchester, Hope Hospital, Salford M68HD, UK*

T.E. JEFFREYS, FRCS(Ed), FRCS(Eng), *Emeritus Consultant Orthopaedic Surgeon, The Robert Jones and Agnes Hunt Orthopaedic Hospital, Oswestry, Shropshire SY107AG, UK*

J.R. JOHNSON, MB, BS, FRCS(Eng), *Consultant Orthopaedic Surgeon, Department of Orthopaedic Surgery, St Mary's Hospital and Medical College, Praed Street, London W2, UK*

R.A. JOHNSTON, BSc, MD, FRCS, *Consultant Neurosurgeon, Department of Neuorosurgery, Institute of Neurological Sciences, Southern General Hospital, Glasgow G514TF, Scotland, UK*

J.A. KANIS, MD, FRCP, *Professor in Human Metabolism and Clinical Biochemistry, World Health Organisation Centre for Metabolic Bone Disease, University of Sheffield Medical School, Sheffield S102DU, UK*

J.P. KOSTUIK, MD, FRCS(C), *Professor, Departments of Orthopaedics and Neurosurgery, Chief, Division of Spinal Surgery (Orthopaedics), John Hopkins Hospital, John Hopkins University, Baltimore, Maryland, USA*

J.C.Y. LEONG, FRCS, FRCSE, FRACS, *Professor and Head, Department of Orthopaedic Surgery, University of Hong Kong, 5/F Professorial Block, Queen Mary Hospital, Hong Kong*

M.C. LYNCH, MB, ChB, MChOrth, FRCS, *Consultant Orthopaedic Surgeon, Broadgreen Hospital, Liverpool L143LB, UK*

J.A. McCULLOCH, MD, FRCSC, *Professor of Orthopaedics, North-eastern Ohio Universities, College of Medicine, 75 Arch Street, 501 Akron, Ohio 44304, USA*

M.J. McMASTER, MD, FRCS, *Consultant Orthopaedic Surgeon, Princess Margaret Rose Orthopaedic Hospital, Edinburgh EH107ED, Scotland, UK*

T. McSWEENEY, MB, BCh, BAO(NUI), MCh, MChOrth, FRCS(Eng), FACS, *Emeritus Consultant Traumatic and Orthopaedic Surgeon, The Robert Jones and Agnes Hunt Orthopaedic Hospital, Oswestry, Shropshire SY107AG, UK*

H.M. MAYER, MD, *Assistant Professor, Department of Orthopaedic Surgery, Free University of Berlin, Oskar-Helene-Heim, Clay Allee 229, W-1000, Berlin 33, Germany*

P. MERTENS, MD, DSc, *Department of Neurosurgery, University of Lyon, Hospital Neurologique, 59 Blvd. PINEL, 69003 Lyon, France*

J.B. MILES, MB, ChB, FRCS, *Consultant Neurosurgeon, Walton Hospital, Rice Lane, Liverpool L91AE, UK*

R.M. MORAN, MCh(Orth), FRCSI, *Consultant Orthopaedic Surgeon, Beaumont Hospital, Beaumont Road, Dublin 9, Ireland*

R.C. MULHOLLAND, MB, BS, FRCS(Eng), *Consultant Orthopaedic Surgeon, Harlow Wood Orthopaedic Hospital, Mansfield; Queen's Medical Centre, Nottingham University Hospital, Nottingham, UK*

J.W. OGILVIE, MD, *Associate Professor, Department of Orthopaedic Surgery, University of Minnesota; Director, Twin Cities Scoliosis Spine Center, 2737 Chicago Ave So. LL-200, Minneapolis, Minnesota, USA*

A.K. OMMAYA, MA, MD, FRCS, FACS, *Professor of Neurosurgery, George Washington University, 8006 Glenbrook Road, Bethesden Md. 20814, Washington DC, USA*

O.L. OSTI, MD, PhD, *Orthopaedic Registrar, Royal Adelaide Hospital, Adelaide 5000, South Austrailia*

R. OWEN, DL, MB, BS, MChOrth, FRCS, *Emeritus Professor of Orthopaedic and Trauma Surgery, University of Liverpool, UCD Block, 4th floor, Royal Liverpool Hospital, Prescot Street, Liverpool L693BX, UK*

K.F. PARSONS, MB, ChB, FRCSE, FRCS, *Consultant Urological Surgeon and Director of Urological Studies, The 92 Link Unit, University of Liverpool, Royal Liverpool Hospital NHS Trust, Prescot Street, Liverpool L78XP, UK; Mersey Regional Spinal Injuries Centre, Town Lane, Kew, Southport*

R.W. PORTER, MD, FRCS, FRCSE, *Professor of Orthopaedics, Aberdeen University, University Medical Buildings, Foresterhill, Aberdeen A392ZD, Scotland, UK*

R.G. PRINGLE, FRCS, *Consultant Orthopaedic Surgeon, The Robert Jones and Agnes Hunt Orthopaedic Hospital, Oswestry, Shropshire SY107AG, UK; Consultant Orthopaedic Surgeon to Midlands Spinal Injury Unit and Royal Shrewsbury Hospital*

A.O. RANSFORD, BA(Hons), MB, BChir(Cantab), FRCS(Eng), *Orthopaedic Department, University College Hospital, 107 Harley Street, London W1, UK; Royal National Orthopaedic Hospital, Brockley Hill, Stanmore, Middlesex*

R. REID, BSc, MB, ChB, MRCPath, *Senior Lecturer in Osteoarticular Pathology and Honorary Consultant Pathologist, Osteoarticular Unit, University Department of Pathology, Western Infirmary, Glasgow G116NT, Scotland, UK*

E.B. RISKA, MD, *Professor and Head, Orthopaedic Department, Dextra Medical Centre, Rumantie La, 00350 Helsinki, Finland; Associate Professor, Department of Orthopaedics and Traumatology, Helsinki University Central Hospital, Helsinki, Finland*

T. RUSSELL, BSc(Hons), MB, ChB, FRCS(Ed), FRCS(Glas), *Consultant Neurosurgeon (Lothian Health Board), Department of Clinical Neurosciences, Western General Hospital, Crewe Road, Edinburgh EH42XU, Scotland, UK; Part-time Senior Lecturer in Neurosurgery, University of Edinburgh*

R.A. SAVAGE, MCSP, BSc, PhD, *Magnetic Resonance Research Centre, University of Liverpool, PO Box 147, Liverpool L693BX, UK*

S.C. SCHOLD, MD, *Professor of Neurology, Duke University Medical Center, PO Box 3963, Durham, NC 27710, USA*

R.J. SCOTHORNE, BSc, MD(Leeds and Chicago), FRCS(Glas), FRS(Ed), *Regius Professor of Anatomy (Emeritus), Department of Anatomy, University of Glasgow, G128QQ, Scotland, UK*

J.R. SILVER, MB, BS, FRCP(Ed and Lond), *Consultant Physician in Spinal Injuries, National Spinal Injuries Centre, Stoke Mandeville Hospital, Mandeville Road, Aylesbury, Bucks HP218AL, UK*

M.P. SINDOU, MD, DScBiol, *Professor of Neurosurgery, Department of Neurosurgery, University of Lyon, Hospital Neurologique, 59 Blvd PINEL, 69003 Lyon, France*

E.T.S. SMITH, MB, ChB, DMRD, FFR, RCSI, FRCR, *Consultant Radiologist, Walton Hospital, Rice Lane, Liverpool L91AE, UK*

M.F. SULLIVAN, MA, MB, BChir, FRCS, *Consultant Orthopaedic Surgeon, Royal National Orthopaedic Hospital, Bolsover Street, London W1, UK; Consultant Orthopaedic Surgeon, Institute of Orthopaedics, University of London; President of the European Spinal Society*

J.F. TAYLOR, MD, MChOrth, FRCS, DTM&H, *Consultant Orthopaedic Surgeon, Royal Liverpool Children's Hospital, Alder Hey, Eaton Road, Liverpool L122AP, UK*

M.J. TORRENS, BSc, MB, BS, MPhil, ChM, FRCS, *Consultant Neurosurgeon, Department of Neurosurgery, Iatriko Kentro (Athens Medical Centre), Maroussi, Athens, Greece*

N.J. TREBLE, MChOrth, FRCS, *Consultant Orthopaedic Surgeon, Department of Orthopaedics, North Devon District Hospital, Raleigh Park, Barnstaple, Devon UK; Consultant Orthopaedic Surgeon, Princess Elizabeth Orthopaedic Hospital, Wonford Road, Exeter, Devon*

H. VERBIEST, MD, PhD, Hon FRCS(Eng), *Emeritus Professor, Utrect University, Wilhelminapark 32, 3581 NH Utrecht, The Netherlands*

J.K. WEBB, FRCS, *Consultant Orthopaedic Surgeon, Harlow Wood Orthopaedic Hospital, Mansfield, Nottingham, UK*

A.I. WEIR, BSc, MSc, MB, ChB, FRCP(Glas), *Consultant Clinical Neurophysiologist, Department of Clinical Neurophysiology, Institute of Neurological Sciences, Southern General Hospital, Glasgow G514TF, Scotland, UK; Honorary Senior Clinical Lecturer, University of Glasgow*

J.C.D. WELLS, MB, ChB, FFRACS, *Director, Centre for Pain Relief, Walton Hospital, Liverpool L91AE, UK*

B. WILLIAMS, MD, ChM, FRCS, *Midland Centre for Neurosurgery and Neurology, Holly Lane, Warley, W. Midlands B677JX, UK*

S.J. WILLIAMS, FRCP, *Consultant Physician, Chest Unit, Stoke Mandeville Hospital, Mandeville Road, Aylesbury, Bucks HP21 8AL, UK*

P.J. WITHEROW, MB, ChB, FRCS, *Consultant Orthopaedic Surgeon, United Bristol Healthcare Trust, Bristol Royal Hospital for Sick Children, St Michael's Hill, Bristol BS28BJ, UK*

P.M. YEOMAN, MA, MB, BChir, MD, FRCS, *Consultant Orthopaedic Surgeon (Hon), The Royal National Hospital for Rheumatic Diseases, Bath BA1 1RL, UK*

Preface

The history of spinal surgery as we know it today extends back to the early years of this century when Sir Robert Jones established the surgical practice of Orthopaedics in Liverpool and Britain. In the years that followed, interest in all aspects of the human spine caught the imagination of many specialities, though the majority of developments occurred in the fields of orthopaedics and neurosurgery. However, it was regrettable that those disciplines showed a tendency to develop in relative isolation. Fortunately, in recent years the gap between these two specialities has begun to close with reference to the spine.

Cooperation between orthopaedists and neurosurgeons has been developing in many centres around the globe. In some of these units, the level of involvement may be restricted to certain areas but in others all aspects of spinal disease are cared for by multidisciplinary teams. These teams have arrived from different paths of training; be it orthopaedics, neurosurgery, radiology, rheumatology, rehabilitation or other allied disciplines. However, it is clear that spinal surgery has become established as a speciality in its own right and is here to stay.

With the growing interest in spinal surgery many textbooks have been published. The vast majority deal only with specific areas, such as the cervical or lumbar spine, within the greater compass of the many diseases which afflict the spine. Very few have attempted to address all those disease processes from a truly multidisciplinary approach.

For several years, we have run an annual instructional training programme which has brought together eminent orthopaedic surgeons and neurosurgeons in equal numbers from across the world to teach on the programme. The syllabus has been designed to cover every aspect of spinal disease in detail on the premise that the increased knowledge and awareness which this gives to individuals heightens their ability to practice in whatever sphere of spinal surgery is their chosen area. It also helps to lay the foundations for the training of the true spinal surgeons of the future.

The origins of this textbook of spinal surgery lie in this programme. Therefore, within this book will be found a truly comprehensive account of the most current thoughts on the nature of all conditions which affect the spinal column and its neurological contents, including their surgical management. Each chapter is written by an acknowledged expert in that field, many of whom have been actively involved in the Liverpool Spine Course over the years. To them we express our most grateful thanks, not only for their outstanding contributions but also for their continuing friendship.

GORDON FINDLAY
ROBERT OWEN
Liverpool

SIR GEORGE BEDBROOK

It was with great regret that the news of the death of Sir George Bedbrook in October of 1991 was received. One of the great pioneers of both the treatment and rehabilitation of spinal disorders, he will be sadly missed by his friends, colleagues and his many grateful patients.

SECTION 7
SPINAL INFECTION

31 · Spinal Osteomyelitis

By E.K.W. HO and J.C.Y. LEONG

PYOGENIC SPONDYLITIS

Epidemiology

Although an ancient disease, it is only during the past century or so that spinal osteomyelitis as a distinct entity has been recognized. Advances in medical knowledge and diagnostic techniques, and possibly the advent of antibiotics, have brought this about. Further clarification has come from experimental works of various authors including studies of iatrogenic disease (Nelaton). Because of lack of early treatment in the early days, many cases were diagnosed at post-mortem examination, while subclinical cases were missed. A recently reported series indicated that spinal osteomyelitis constitutes about 4% or less of all osteomyelitis (Kulowski, 1936; *Lancet*, 1985). As spinal osteomyelitis often originates from a primary focus elsewhere, a diligent search for such lesions is necessary. Numerous series report that males are affected more commonly, and the reason for this is obscure. Patients of all ages can be affected, though a recent series (Eismont *et al.*, 1983) indicated that more than 70% of patients were aged 50 years or over. Patients suffering from diabetes mellitus are prone to this condition.

All levels of the spine can be affected. Single or multiple vertebral bodies can be destroyed depending on the stage and severity of the disease. The lumbar and the dorsolumbar junction are the most frequent sites, while the cervical spine is least affected. With early diagnosis and the introduction of chemotherapy the mortality rate has dropped significantly from 70% to 25–30%.

Causative agent

Virtually all the most important Gram-positive and Gram-negative organisms have been incriminated. Although Gram-negative organisms are increasingly reported the most important sole agent is still *Staphylococcus aureus*. When non-staphylococcal infection is present some predisposing source of infection or condition may be suspected. *Escherichia* or *Proteus* infection suggest a genito-urinary tract origin, while *Pseudomonas* infection may be associated with mainliner drug addiction. Patients on renal dialysis may be predisposed to staphylococcal epidermidis infection. Syphilis may also be a causative agent (Johns, 1970). Invasive diagnostic procedures, e.g. genito-urinary instrumentation, prostatectomy and needle biopsy of the spine, can lead to direct or indirect bacterial contamination of the spine.

Pathology

Spinal osteomyelitis is generally reckoned to be a secondary manifestation of a primary infection elsewhere in the body, which may not be always obvious. The routes of bacterial spread are controversial. Batson (1940) advocated venous spread but Wiley & Trueta (1959) favoured the arterial route.

The possible anatomical sites that may be involved are:

1 vertebral body—especially the subchondral bone area;

2 intervertebral disc—because of the avascular nature of the disc it is rapidly destroyed;

3 posterior elements, rarely—may be due to posterior

extension from the cancellous bone of the vertebral body;
4 a combination.
Spread of infection to adjacent vertebral bodies is possible via the nearby arterial system.

In contrast, involvement of the intervertebral disc is a separate entity and can be either:
1 primary in adults (Kemp *et al.*, 1973);
2 paediatric discitis (Menelaus, 1964; Scoles & Quinn, 1982)—a more benign disease;
3 after discectomy (Sullivan *et al.*, 1958).
(Please refer to Chapter 33.)

With infective destruction of anterior structures, segmental spinal instability ensues, usually with accompanying kyphosis. Hyperostotic reaction sometimes appears when infection is less virulent. With effective control of the infection, spontaneous bony fusion is sometimes seen. Neural involvement may supervene because of either mechanical compression (by bone fragment, disc or abscess) or direct infective involvement of the neural tissue or meninges, thus leading to meningitis together with its sequelae. Autopsy studies in these paraplegic patients show intrinsic damage with cystic degeneration of the spinal cord (Eismont *et al.*, 1983).

Uncontrolled infection results in abscess formation that dissects along the plane of least resistance. The location and level of vertebral involvement dictates the siting of the abscess produced:
1 cervical region—retropharyngeal abscess later draining into the posterior triangle of the neck;
2 thoracic region—paraspinal abscess or subcutaneous masses lateral to the erector spinae muscle;
3 lumbar region—psoas abscess draining into the flank or the groin.
Subcutaneous abscesses pointing over these respective regions may thus appear.

Clinical presentation

This may be acute or chronic. Symptoms and signs are variable and often modified by prior treatment with antibiotics.

GENERAL

Fever, malaise, weight loss, dehydration and other signs of septicaemia may be present. Anorexia and vomiting in a child can also occur. Antibiotic treatment sometimes modifies these presentations and thus the diagnosis may be difficult. Symptoms may present either in an acute form or insidiously, depending on the virulence of the organism and the immunological resistance of the patient.

LOCAL

Localized spinal pain (Kulowski, 1936) is the hallmark of the acute disease. The pain is typically unrelieved by rest and may be aggravated by movement. Pain may be referred because of irritation of peripheral nerves. Tenderness is present on deep palpation or percussion of the spinous processes. Spinal movement is limited because of pain and muscle spasm. Straight leg raising limitation may be present.

Abscess formation can be superficial or deep. If superficial it may rupture spontaneously or can be surgically drained, sometimes resulting in a persistent discharging sinus. A deep paravertebral abscess may be difficult to diagnose. Physical signs such as hip contracture produced by a psoas abscess may lead to a suspicion of this and other diagnoses. Chronic cases may present with spinal deformity, notably a sharp kyphosis.

NEUROLOGICAL

About 15% of cases develop some form of neurological involvement, especially if the disease is acute. The possible causes of paraplegia are multiple. Direct compressive agents include a tense abscess and spinal instability from bone destruction. An indirect cause is septic thrombosis compromising the blood supply to neurological tissue. Epidural abscess may be localized or diffuse. If the abscess penetrates the dura, meningomyelitis ensues. The rapidity of onset and the extent of neurological deficit is variable. The most common level where spinal sepsis is complicated by neurological deficit is the cervical region. Mortality is higher if neurological involvement is present. Senile patients, patients with diabetes mellitus or those on systemic steroid therapy and rheumatoid arthritics all have a higher chance of paraplegia, especially if *Staphylococcus aureus* infection is present. Cervical or thoracic level involvement is most likely to produce paraplegia (Eismont *et al.*, 1983).

Laboratory investigation

Except for a positive blood culture, which is only likely during the septicaemic episodes, and a positive spinal biopsy none of the other investigations are confirmatory. The erythrocyte sedimentation rate (ESR) is usually elevated (Garcia & Grantham, 1960) and is helpful in monitoring the response to therapy. The white blood cell count may be raised, usually in the acute stage. Rising antibody titres to specific organisms or antigens are sometimes helpful (Digby & Kersley, 1979). The urine should be cultured if concomitant urinary tract infection is suspected as the primary infective source. Routine cerebrospinal fluid culture is not advocated. Superficial discharging sinuses provide a chance for bacterial culture and identification. However, contamination is frequent leading to a mixed growth. Usually a negative tuberculin test excludes tuberculous infection. Needle biopsy of the diseased vertebrae may yield useful material for culture and histology, but the success rate is variable ranging from 20% to 100% (Eismont *et al.*, 1983; Otolenghi, 1969). This technique is best performed under fluoroscopy or computerized tomography (CT) scan guidance.

Radiography

It is imperative to X-ray the whole spine with at least AP and lateral views. Abnormalities can be present in the early or late stages.

EARLY ABNORMALITIES

The very early radiographs are normal. After one to three weeks there may be loss of delineation of subchondral bone and bone destruction at adjacent vertebral bodies. There may be a decrease in intervertebral disc height (see Fig. 31.2a). Such a decrease may be absent in vertebral osteomyelitis of infancy (Eismont *et al.*, 1982). Bone destruction may increase with time. Soft tissue swelling due to oedema or an abscess may appear early, usually adjacent to the bony lesion (see Fig. 31.1a).

LATE ABNORMALITIES

After two to three months bony regeneration may be visible as sclerosis or eburnation. An osteosclerotic response is more suggestive of pyogenic than tuberculous osteomyelitis, whereas large calcified soft tissue abscesses without bony eburnation are usually indicative of tuberculous infection. Soft tissue swellings are usually more marked and extensive with the spread of abscesses. Sometimes when the infection is controlled early and effectively a radiodense vertebra is visible, with or without osteophytosis or bony bridging. Significant spinal deformity may result if the disease is allowed to progress. In general, the radiological changes of pyogenic spondylitis appear more rapidly as compared to the tuberculous counterpart; moreover there is less osteoporosis. Other radiological investigations that are sometimes necessary include tomography and myelography, particularly if neurological symptoms and signs are present. Serial X-rays taken at intervals are helpful in documenting progress.

CT scan

This is useful (Brant-Zawadzki *et al.*, 1983) in the diagnosis and management of spinal osteomyelitis. The examination can be performed with or without contrast material; preferably without. It will show the extent of bony and disc destruction at the affected site and the presence of intraspinal involvement. Adjacent abscesses will also be evident (Jeffrey *et al.*, 1980). The healing phase is heralded by a decrease in the size of soft tissue abscesses. The scan also affords guidance for fluid or tissue aspiration.

Magnetic resonance imaging

MRI is useful in the early diagnosis of this disease (Modic *et al.*, 1985). The infected bone and disc show a decrease in T1-weighted images and the reverse on the T2-weighted images. Paravertebral soft tissue involvement is also demonstrated (Lee & Glazer, 1986).

Bone scan

A bone scan is capable of showing early disease before the radiographic changes appear. Technetium and gallium scans are useful, especially when combined, with a sensitivity approaching 100% (Haase *et al.*, 1980). The indium-labelled leucocyte scan has not established itself as a useful diagnostic tool at the early stage of the disease.

Diagnosis

A high index of suspicion is mandatory if early diagnosis is to be achieved. The clinical, serological and radiological features give very important clues to a presumptive diagnosis, but the final answer depends on bacteriological examination of the pus and infected tissue obtained by needle or open biopsy. The identification of the organism responsible, and its antibiotic sensitivity, is *sine qua non* for successful treatment. If a positive blood culture is obtained, biopsy of the lesion may, however, not be necessary.

DIFFERENTIAL DIAGNOSIS

In the acute stage, when the main complaint is pain, other causes of discomfort such as malignant deposits in the spine must be considered. The nature of the pain and the absence of systemic complaints tend to rule out an infective cause. Retroperitoneal organic disease may cause referral of pain posteriorly mimicking spinal pain. Meningitis from other causes may be wrongly diagnosed if spinal infection is associated with neurological involvement. In the chronic stage the main problem is spinal deformity with or without a discharging sinus, in which case all causes of angular kyphosis have to be considered.

Management

Early diagnosis is absolutely essential in order to avoid morbidity and mortality. Treatment can be conservative or operative.

During the acute stage the aim is to identify the causative organism and its antibiotic sensitivity. Blood culture and needle biopsy of the spine (Fig. 31.1) are important investigations, also bone scan. Spinal pain is relieved by bed rest or immobilization of the affected region by orthosis. After taking blood for culture, immediate intravenous broad-spectrum antibiotic therapy (covering both Gram-positive and Gram-negative organisms) is started. This regime is continued if clinical response is favourable. Appropriate adjustment of antibiotics according to the result of bacterial culture is made later. The exact duration of antibiotic treatment is debatable. At least six weeks

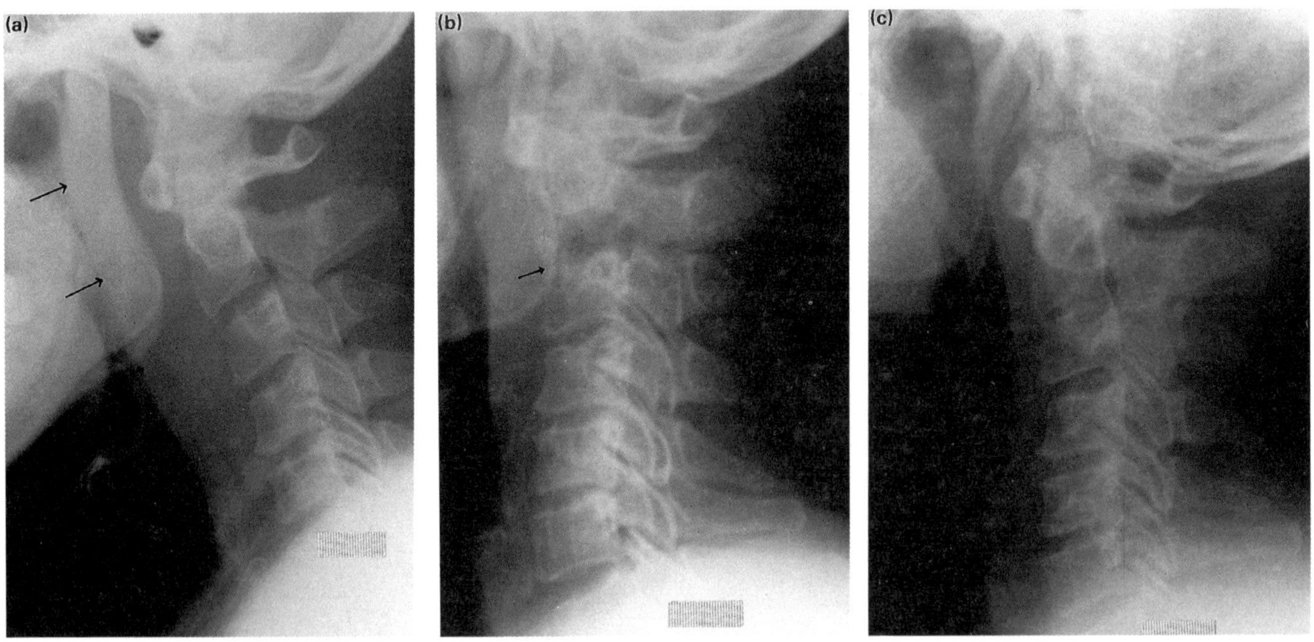

Fig. 31.1 (a) Radiograph of a 42-year-old man presenting with intense neck pain for three months. Tenderness was localized to the upper cervical area. There was marked restriction of neck movement because of pain. A huge prevertebral abscess was present but missed initially (arrowed). There was no obvious bony lesion. (b) Radiograph two months after presentation showed destruction of lower part of C2 body with narrowing of the C2–C3 disc. Bony erosion of C2–C3 facet was present. A transoral biopsy of C2 was performed under fluoroscopic guidance. Culture of tissue showed *Streptococcus*. Histology confirmed a chronic inflammatory lesion. He was treated with intravenous antibiotics for three months together with a neck collar. (c) Radiograph six years after conservative treatment showed spontaneous fusion of anterior and posterior element of C2–C3. His neck movement was only slightly limited but he remained pain-free. There was no clinical recurrence of his infection.

of intravenous therapy followed by another six weeks per oral route is the minimum recommended. Adequate blood levels of antibiotics require serum bactericidal level monitoring. The intravenous route ensures a high blood level of antibiotics while systemic upset, e.g. vomiting and malabsorption, makes the oral route unreliable. The total duration of antibiotic treatment is governed by the clinical, radiological and haematological response. This may last three months or more.

The indications for operative intervention include:

1 failure of adequate conservative treatment;
2 as a means of obtaining tissue for bacterial identification when needle biopsy fails;
3 drainage of abscess when evident, especially if pressure on neural elements supervenes;
4 gross bony destruction leading to spinal instability, especially in the cervical spine;
5 uncertain diagnosis.

Serial ESR measurement is helpful in monitoring the success with conservative treatment. Increased toxaemia, spinal pain, onset or worsening of neurological deficits and the appearance of subcutaneous abscess all indicate progression of the disease. Serial radiographs showing progressive bony destruction, increased spinal deformity and the appearance of soft tissue swellings indicate a bad prognosis.

The surgical approach to the diseased area is usually by the anterior route, either for abscess drainage, debridement, concomitant surgical stabilization or open biopsy (Fig. 31.2). The posterior approach is applicable only if the disease is localized to the posterior elements. This carries the danger of further destabilizing the spine. With adequate spinal debridement and antibiotic treatment, bone grafts used for stabilization purposes usually survive; indeed a fusion rate of about 93% is achievable (Fang *et al.*, 1990).

Postoperative external immobilization is important for pain relief and protection of the implanted bone graft. Results of treatment are usually good provided early diagnosis and prompt therapy is given.

However, in some cases of chronic pyogenic vertebral osteomyelitis, spinal deformity is due to continued vertebral destruction, even though the organism may be of low virulence. These patients are difficult to treat and the surgeon should be fully

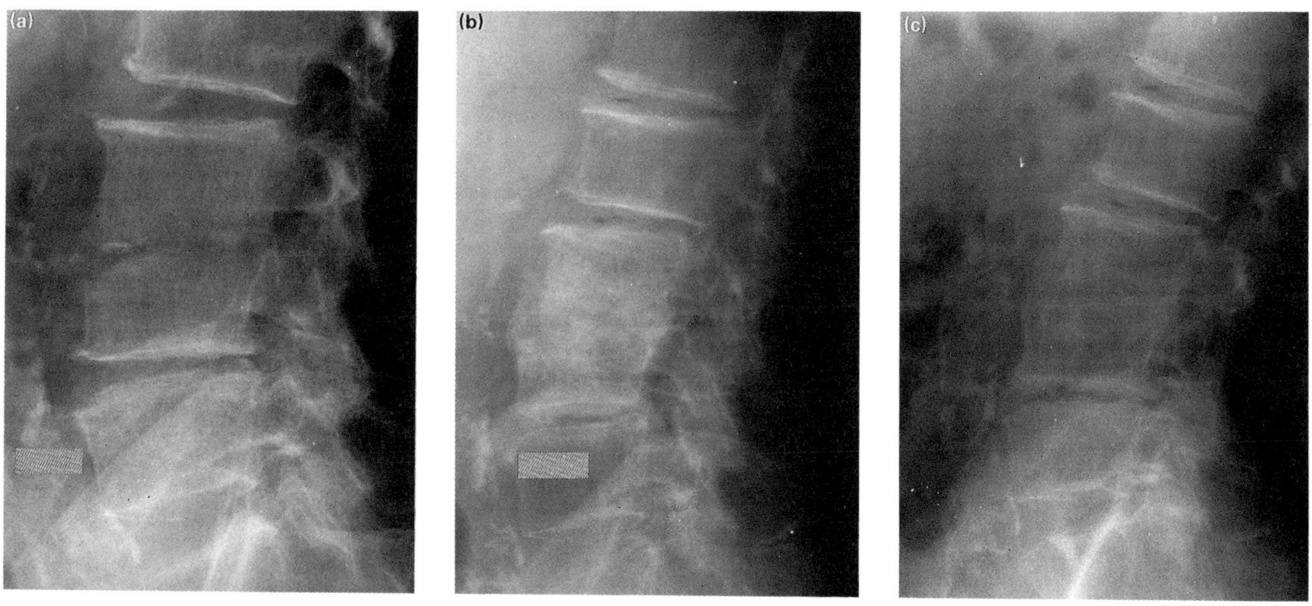

Fig. 31.2 (a) Preoperative radiograph of 60-year-old woman with low back pain for four months. A paradiscal lesion affecting L3–L4 level with narrowing of the intervening intervertebral disc was present. Needle biopsy of the lesion was negative. Her symptoms failed to respond to cloxacillin. (b) Exploration via an anterior spinal approach revealed a small prevertebral abscess and abundant granulomatous tissue. A debridement and fusion using iliac crest graft was performed. Culture of the debride showed *Pseudomonas aeruginosa* sensitive to gentamicin. A full three-month course of antibiotic was given. This radiograph showed the status at completion of the antibiotic treatment. (c) Postoperative radiograph at three years showing good surgical fusion without angular deformity. There was no recurrence of infection.

equipped with the surgical skill of anterior spinal surgery and stabilization techniques (see section on tuberculous spondylitis).

UNCOMMON INFECTIONS

Reports of spinal involvement by *Brucella* (Lifeso *et al.*, 1985), *Actinobacillus actinomycetemcomtans* (Muhle *et al.*, 1979), *Nocardia* (Yanoff *et al.*, 1983) and *Cryptococcus* infection (Litvinoff & Nelson, 1978) are rare (see Chapter 34).

TUBERCULOUS SPONDYLITIS

Spinal tuberculosis was first recorded by Hippocrates (450 BC) but for centuries the nature of this disease remained unclear. The first well-illustrated clinical description of a kyphotic spinal deformity in association with paraplegia was by Pott (1779). He also performed autopsies on patients affected by the disease.

A major impact on the management of tuberculous spondylitis was the development of surgical expertise in anterior approaches to the spine. Japanese authors (Ito *et al.*, 1934) and others subsequently, have reported on anterior surgery in spinal tuberculosis. Hodgson & Stock (1956), in particular, popularized anterior spinal surgery in the management of spinal tuberculosis. The other significant impact on management of this disease was, of course, the advent of specific antituberculous chemotherapy in 1954.

Opinions have been divided as to the best mode of treatment of spinal tuberculosis. Should one support the conservative school of chemotherapy with full ambulation, or the radical school of surgical excision of the disease focus and bone grafting as practised in Hong Kong? Such divergence of views stimulated a series of studies by the British Medical Research Council's Working Party (MRCWP Reports, 1973a,b, 1974a,b, 1976, 1978, 1982, 1985) (see later).

Epidemiology

This disease is still prevalent in Third World countries. In countries with good public health services, spinal tuberculosis usually presents early, but in view of its rarity diagnosis may be a problem. It should thus be considered in the differential diagnosis of all spinal disorders of all age groups.

A wide spectrum of disease manifestations is seen in developing nations. These vary from the early stage with minimal bony destruction, but with abscess formation, to end-stage with grotesque spinal deformity when the disease may still be active. Neurological complications may also be present, prognosis being correspondingly worse. Any age group may be affected in these endemic areas.

In a review of 1000 consecutive cases of bone and joint tuberculosis in Hong Kong (1957–59), 58.7% had spinal involvement. Of these 587 cases the most commonly affected vertebra was L1 and adjacent segments. The disease affects the male sex predominantly, and in countries where prevalence is high, disease in children is common. In advanced countries the disease affects the elderly and undernourished—including chronic alcoholic, and drug abusers. The 'childhood' type is distinguished clinically from the 'adult' type (Hsu & Leong, 1984) disease in being more malignant in its clinical course, except that it has less association with paraplegia.

Causative agent and pathology

Mycobacterium tuberculosis is the main causative agent of tuberculous spondylitis. It is usually a secondary infection, the primary lesion being in the lung, genito-urinary or alimentary tract. These primary lesions can be quite small or remain undetectable despite active search. Sometimes the spine may become involved by direct extension from adjacent structures. Experimental work by Hodgson (1975) showed that the venous plexus of Batson acts as a bypass for blood to flow from the pelvis and abdomen to the spine, especially when the inferior vena cava is blocked. Such venous plexus communication may explain the possible association between primary intrapelvic or intra-abdominal foci and the secondary spinal lesion. In contrast with pyogenic osteomyelitis, where the spine is involved in less than 5% (Kulowski, 1936), the incidence of spondylitis in tuberculous osteomyelitis is much higher. Such a difference in incidence may be due to a different pathway of bacterial spread. The pyogenic spinal infection is more often haematogenous (arterial) in origin, while the tuberculous counterpart probably spreads via the veins.

Pathology depends on the stage of the disease. The pre-pus phase is characterized by proliferative granulation tissue, Langhan giant cell, epithelioid and round cells. This is followed by paraspinal abscess formation, signifying an active disease process (Figs 31.3a & 31.4a). The pus is fluid initially but later

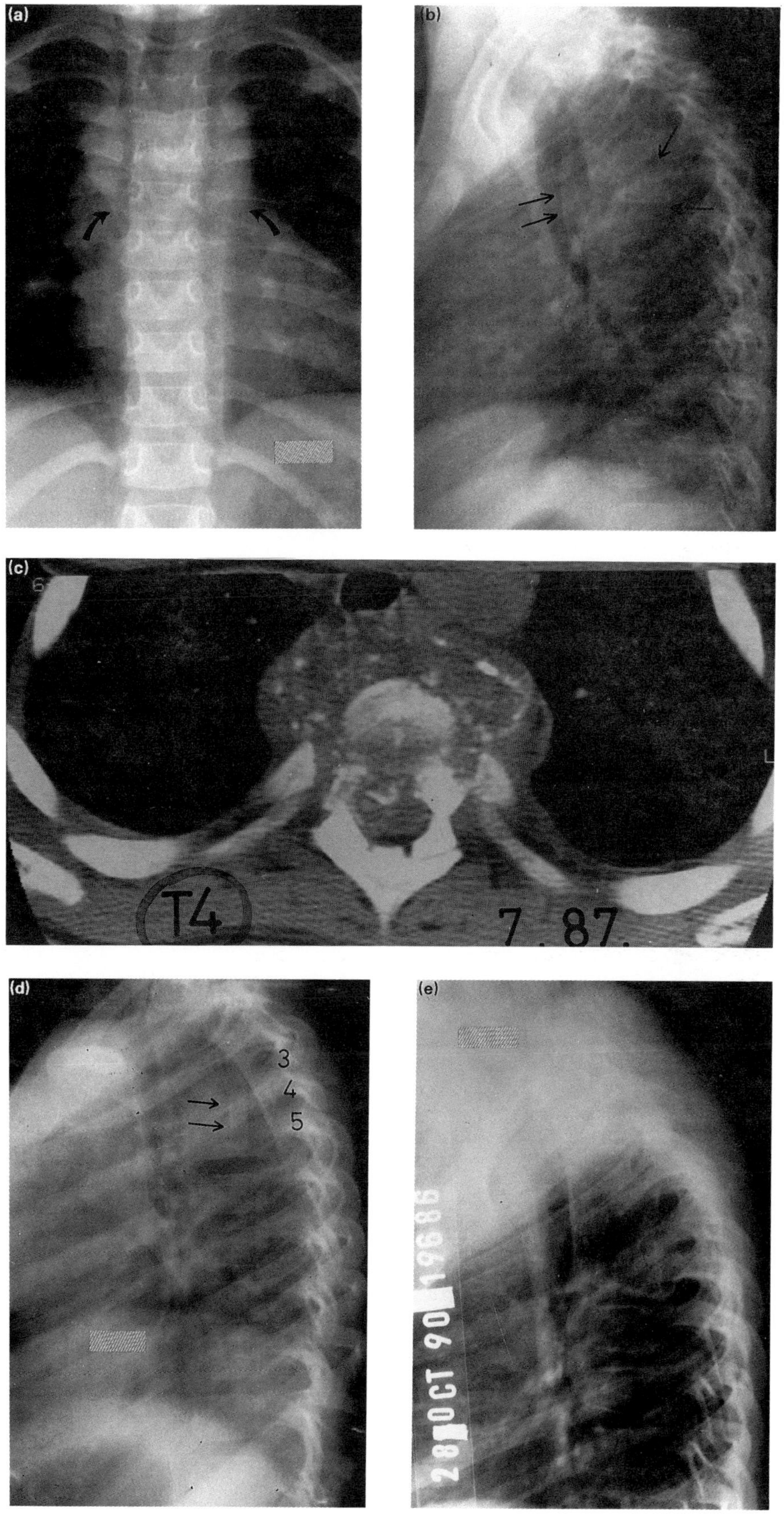

Fig. 31.3 (a,b) Preoperative radiographs of a six-year-old girl with tuberculous involvement of T4–T5. She presented with one week rapid onset of paraparesis. The paraspinal abscess (arrowed) has caused forward displacement of the trachea (arrowed). (c) Preoperative CT scan at T4 showed gross soft tissue involvement anteriorly, with bony destruction of the corpus and speckles of calcification in the abscess. There was also anterior cord compression by the abscess. The posterior element was not involved. (d) Radiograph immediately after decompression and fusion from T3 to T5. Neurological recovery was complete within one week postoperatively. Two block iliac crest grafts were used. A supplementary posterior fusion was performed two months later. (e) Radiograph three years postoperatively showed solid fusion. There was no evidence of recurrence of disease or angular deformity. The patient had complete neurological recovery.

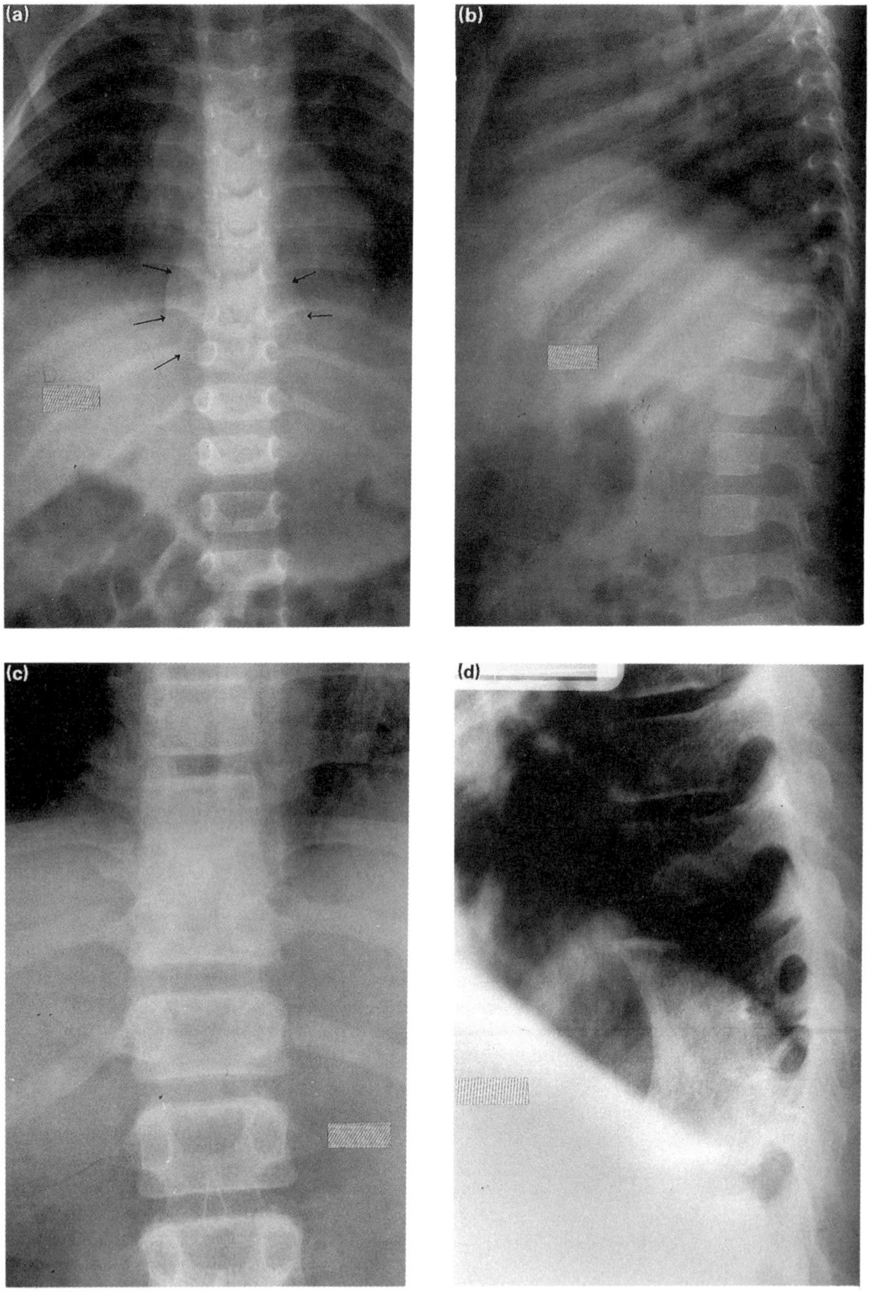

Fig. 31.4 (a,b) Preoperative radiographs of a five-year-old girl with tuberculous spondylitis destroying the body of D10 and upper part of D11. A globular abscess is present (arrowed) together with a mild kyphos. (c,d) Postoperative radiographs 10 years after the Hong Kong operation. Close-up view shows solid fusion and minimal kyphos.

becomes caseous and white in colour. As the abscess pressure increases the paravertebral ligaments and periosteum are elevated, thus impeding blood flow to the vertebral body with consequent sequestra formation. Sometimes the sequestra are retropulsed into the spinal canal, causing neurological deficit. With continued increase in pressure from abscess content, circumferential destruction, especially of the superficial portion of the vertebral body, supervenes. The aneurysmal syndrome (Ghormley & Bradley, 1928) may follow (Fig. 31.5a), usually in the thoracic or cervical spine, seen radiologically as anterior scalloping of the vertebral body. Another possible complication arising from increasing pressure in an abscess is rupture into adjacent organs. The lung is usually involved (Yau & Hodgson, 1968) in about 10% of cases. Other organs where penetration has been recorded include the trachea, oesophagus, bronchus,

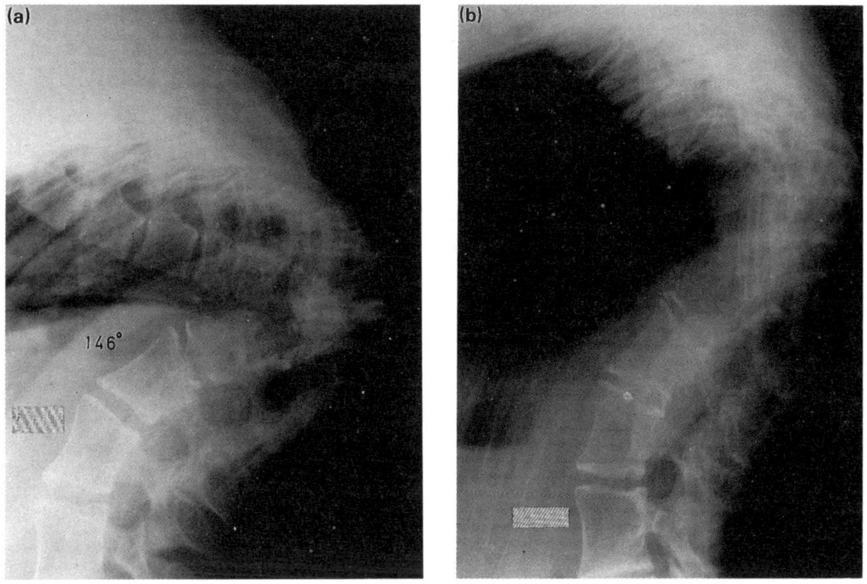

Fig. 31.5 (a) This 20-year-old lady had a significant kyphos affecting the thoracolumbar junction due to chronic tuberculous spondylitis. There is significant compensatory lordosis above and below. There were marked sclerotic changes of the remaining diseased vertebrae. She had a full course of antituberculous therapy. Myelogram showed a mild extradural compression anteriorly but there was no neurological deficit. (b) The patient had correction by anterior and posterior osteotomy and halopelvic distraction, followed by circumferential fusion. Good correction was achieved and maintained at 11 years follow-up. She had no neurological deficit.

mediastinum and aorta. The intervertebral disc is essentially avascular except at the periphery, and early disc narrowing occurs because of lack of nutrition via the subchondral bone. Gross disintegration of the disc is a late phenomenon, the detached disc lying free in the abscess. Rarely the disc may calcify, and progressive weakening of a vertebral body results in a concertina type of segmental collapse. With healing the granulation tissue becomes fibrous or calcified and may strangulate the cord; neurological deficit ensues. During the revascularization stage the bone progressively reossifies. Histological section shows a mixture of dead and new bone embedded in thick lamellae. Calcification of paravertebral ligament eventually leads to bony bridging.

Other interesting spinal changes include the vertebra within a vertebra phenomenon (O'Brien, 1969), which is essentially a manifestation of arrested bone growth. Lateral deviation of the spine is probably due to unilateral destruction of the spinal column, which usually occurs in the lower thoracic and lumbar segments. Due to significant kyphosis, normal weight-bearing in the lumbar spine is disturbed and the shape of the vertebral bodies, normally wider than taller, is reversed, especially if the infection has occurred in the growing child (Fig. 31.5a). This is due to a pressure-relieving effect leading to growth stimulation according to the Heuter–Volkmann law.

Classically the anterior elements of the spine are involved but sometimes the posterior structures are affected (Arthornthurasrok & Chongpieboonpatana, 1990). Classification of the disease involving the cervical spine into 'child' and 'adult' types is useful (Hsu & Leong, 1984), the difference being mainly due to the relatively low immunity of the child as compared with the adult.

Hodgson classified neural involvement in tuberculous spondylitis (Pott's disease) into paraplegia of 'active disease' or 'healed disease' (Hodgson *et al.*, 1967).

Active disease

Active disease, causing neurological deficit, is due to pressure from pus, granulation tissue, bony sequestra, intervertebral disc, vertebral collapse and bony subluxation or dislocation. Direct penetration of dura by pus causes tuberculous meningitis or meningomyelitis (Hodgson *et al.*, 1967).

Healed disease

Healed disease, causing the neurological disorder, is due to an internal bony ridge or fibrous tissue constriction.

The prognosis for neurological recovery after surgical decompression is much better in those patients with active disease.

Clinical presentation

This depends largely on the stage of presentation. Patients coming from underdeveloped or developing countries tend to have more advanced disease on presentation.

General features include symptoms and signs of infection in the form of fever, malaise and weight loss. Rarely there are features of septicaemia. These symptoms and signs may be masked by prior antibiotic treatment. Evidence of tuberculous involvement in other organs may be present. Neurological manifestations in the extremities or signs of meningitis may be obvious, sometimes making ambulation difficult. The patient may walk with a limp because of psoas abscess irritation. Respiratory embarrassment may be present even at rest, when gross kyphotic deformity affects the thoracic spine, or when a high thoracic lesion associated with a paraspinal abscess causes bronchial compression (Fig. 31.3b), irritation and rupture.

Other manifestations include localized spinal pain in the early stage, followed by spinal deformity (usually kyphosis) later, with or without a discharging sinus. Muscle spasm is common with limited spinal movements. Rest pain is present and is aggravated by movement. With the presence of kyphotic deformity adjacent segments in the spine develop compensatory lordosis. Such excessive lordosis may be a source of pain later, especially if the lesion is at the lumbosacral junction (Pun *et al.*, 1990).

Diagnosis

The systemic response is essentially the same as in pyogenic spinal osteomyelitis except that frank septicaemia is uncommon; indeed the clinical features may occasionally be mild. Radiological changes are well illustrated in a monograph by Hodgson *et al.* (1969). Myelographic study confirming neural compression is helpful when clinical features of such are present. Computerized tomographic scan will define the extent of the paraspinal abscess and calcification, together with bony destruction and sometimes neural encroachment (Fig. 31.3c). Similarly posterior element involvement will be evident on CT scan (Arthornthurasrok & Chongpieboonpatana, 1990). These radiological studies will assist in the differential diagnosis from other types of infective spondylitis and tumour infiltration. Sometimes healed tuberculous infection may closely resemble congenital fusion of vertebrae (Figs 31.4c & 31.4d).

Elevated erythrocyte sedimentation rate (ESR) is the rule, and serial readings serve to indicate the degree of activity of the disease. The tine skin test may be useful in the later stages of the disease in a non-endemic area where the chances of previous subclinical exposure are low.

The definitive diagnosis depends on a combination of clinicoradiological features, and in particular positive culture and histology of specimens obtained at operation. Ziehl–Nielsen staining is helpful, but in one study (MRCWP, 1974a,b) was positive only in 49 out of 103 histologically proven specimens. Of these 49 positive specimens only 42 yielded a positive culture for the mycobacterium. Of the remaining 54 specimens only 47 yielded a positive culture for the mycobacterium. A positive bacterial culture is thus indicative but not absolutely essential for a firm diagnosis of spinal tuberculosis. Bacterial diagnosis is easy during the active stage, but during the healing or chronic stage bacterial culture may be negative, thus confirmation of the diagnosis can be difficult.

Management of active disease

A complete course of antituberculous chemotherapy still remains the basis of treatment for all forms of active spinal tuberculosis. The routine 'three drug' regime forms the basis of 'first line' treatment consisting of:

1 Streptomycin sulphate 20 mg/kg body weight (maximum 1 g/day) for the initial two to three months. Symptoms of ototoxicity should be looked for.

2 Isoniazid 10 mg/kg body weight (maximum 400 mg per day) for a maximum of nine months. Hypersensitivity reactions may occur.

3 Rifampicin 15 mg/kg body weight (maximum 600 mg/day) for a total of nine months. Thrombocytopenia may occur. Rifampicin has now replaced para-aminosalicylic acid (PAS). Both rifampicin and isoniazid have to be administered for at least six months.

If there is a poor clinical response or continued elevation of the ESR, the second line drug regime may be necessary. Either ethambutol or pyrazinamide is needed to reinforce the 'first line' drugs.

Similarly 'second line' drugs may be required if there is demonstrable resistance of the bacillus at culture to the first line drugs. Close liaison with physician colleagues in this field is advisable.

Chemotherapy should preferably be commenced a week before surgery, although no added morbidity has been observed when started postoperatively.

Debate on whether surgery is indicated at all in spinal tuberculosis led to the British Medical Research Council trials in Korea, Rhodesia and Hong Kong (MRCWP, 1973a,b, 1974a,b, 1976, 1978, 1982, 1985). In essence, the trials showed that spinal tuberculosis can be managed successfully by either conservative or surgical methods. The treatment groups consisted of:

1 chemotherapy with immobilization in bed or in a plaster cast;
2 chemotherapy and ambulation;
3 limited surgical debridement and chemotherapy;
4 chemotherapy followed by the Hong Kong operation.

Criteria of a favourable outcome were:

1 return to full physical activity;
2 healed disease—clinically and radiologically;
3 no abscesses or sinuses;
4 no central nervous system involvement.

At five years such favourable status was obtained in 100% of patients in the chemotherapy and Hong Kong operation group (4), but was only achieved in 89% of patients with chemotherapy alone (no surgery, no external immobilization, no bed rest) (2). Nevertheless, these two groups yielded the best overall result. Bony fusion rate was 92% in the Hong Kong operation group, but only 50% in the chemotherapy-alone group, both at five years. Kyphotic deformity was not evident with the Hong Kong operation group compared to an increase of 10 degrees in kyphosis in the non-surgical group at five years follow-up. The debridement and chemotherapy group (3) was inferior to groups (2) and (4). At 10 years, patients in group (4) showed a mean *decrease* in kyphosis of 1.4 degrees in the thoracic and thoracolumbar region, and 0.5 degree in the lumbar region, compared to an *increase* in group (3) of 9.8 degrees and 7.6 degrees respectively (MRCWP, 1982). In the conservative treatment group an increase in kyphosis of 17.8 degrees of 5.2 degrees respectively occurred (MRCWP, 1985). Of the 160 patients assessed in the conservative group 52 increased their kyphosis between 11 and 30 degrees, 27 between 31 and 50 degrees, and nine between 51 and 70 degrees (MRCWP, 1985). Such deformity may well be a significant problem later in life.

The Hong Kong operation essentially consists of excision of the disease focus and strut graft fusion. Provided the appropriate expertise and facilities are available this procedure is worthwhile for the following reasons. The operation will yield ample material for bacteriological confirmation of the disease. Abscess evacuation will very often rapidly alleviate pain and improve the clinical condition of the patient. Surgical decompression of the abscess prevents further propagation of the abscess itself and its possible rupture into adjacent organs. Alleviation of pressure on neural tissue will enhance early neurological recovery, this being an absolute indication for surgery. The thorough debridement and placement of graft material under compression will enhance early fusion. Late recurrence is very uncommon once solid fusion has been achieved. Because of early fusion, increased deformity is prevented, thus late paraplegia arising from bony bars is also prevented. Some degree of kyphosis correction can sometimes be achieved during operation.

In our practice the absolute indication for the Hong Kong operation is paraplegia of 'active disease' (Fig. 31.3a–e). The operation will produce rapid relief of pressure on neural elements, especially in the cervical spine (Hsu & Leong, 1984).

The indications for non-surgical management are confined to patients with confirmed early disease having minimal bone involvement. Patients with medical contra-indications to surgery are also excluded.

Management of tuberculous spondylitis in special regions of the spine will not be discussed here. Readers interested should refer to articles concerning affection of the upper cervical spine (Fang *et al.*, 1983) and the lumbosacral junction (Pun *et al.*, 1990).

HONG KONG OPERATION

The two elements of this operation (Fig. 31.4a–d) are:

1 Eradication of the disease focus (pus, sequestrated disc, bony fragments and granulation tissue) down to vascular bone. This part of the operation must be thorough.
2 Anterior strut graft fusion. A slightly oversized graft is put under compression by springing open the kyphosis during insertion, using either rib removed during thoracotomy, or iliac crest grafts. After placing

the first piece, the rest of the graft (five or six pieces) are packed firmly in the adjacent defect. Supplementary staged posterior spinal fusion is necessary if the anterior graft spans two or more vertebral bodies, especially in a child (Jenkins *et al.*, 1975).

Approaches to the spine

A detailed knowledge of anterior approaches to the spine is essential in dealing with tuberculous spondylitis, as the disease focus is usually anteriorly situated. The most important approaches popularized by Hodgson and his co-workers will be described in detail.

THE TRANSORAL APPROACH TO C1 AND C2 (Fang & Ong, 1962)

There are no important anatomical structures anterior to the C1–C2 area. Preoperative infection in the oropharyngeal cavity should be treated, and a plaster shell to keep the head and neck in extension is prefabricated before surgery. Tracheostomy is usually necessary. The neck is extended and, after packing the hypopharynx, the anterior tubercle of atlas is palpated and an anterior midline incision is made below the anterior tubercle. Mucosal flaps are raised and stay-sutured, then dissection continues down to bone. The vertebral vessels are at the lateral edge of the wound and are safeguarded. The prevertebral abscess, if present, is thus drained and surgical fusion is undertaken by creating a slot for inlay grafts on both sides of the midline. When a concomitant C1–C2 subluxation/dislocation is present, gentle hyperextension of the head often reduces the displacement, but this must be undertaken with great caution, as the neuraxis is most vulnerable. Operative damage to the vertebral vessels is the only other important possible complication.

THE TRANSTHYROHYOID APPROACH TO C2–C4 (Fang & Ong, 1962)

The head and neck region is hyperextended. A transverse incision between the hyoid and thyroid cartilage is made. Cutting the platysma, sternohyoid and thyrohyoid muscles exposes the thyrohyoid membrane, which is also incised transversely at the superior attachment. Incising the mucosa of the exposed vallecula followed by retraction exposes the posterior pharyngeal wall. A direct midline incision will expose the C2–C4 region. The wound needs layer closure afterwards. The indications for this approach are few.

THE SOUTHWICK AND ROBINSON APPROACH C2–C7 (Southwick & Robinson, 1957)

The head is turned slightly to one side. A right-sided approach is preferable but not essential. A transverse skin incision is cosmetically superior but limits exposure. A vertical incision in front of the sternocleidomastoid muscle may be necessary if an extensive exposure over multiple levels is needed. The platysma muscle is incised and the sternocleidomastoid muscle retracted laterally. The cervical fascia thus exposed is divided, and the omohyoid muscle identified and either retracted or divided. The carotid sheath is retracted laterally and the oesophagus and trachea retracted medially. The prevertebral fascia is incised in the midline and retracted bilaterally, taking care not to damage the cervical sympathetics and the vertebral artery. The longus colli muscle is elevated from the vertebral body and intervertebral disc. These structures fall together easily after surgery, and are approximated in layers and a drain inserted.

THE POSTERIOR TRIANGLE APPROACH (Hodgson, 1965)

Hodgson developed this approach as tuberculous pus of diseased cervical vertebrae often tracks into the posterior triangle of the neck. Either the left- or right-sided approach is applicable. Theoretically the right side avoids the thoracic duct while the left has less chance of damaging the recurrent laryngeal nerve. A collar incision at the level of the diseased vertebrae is made, after which the platysma is cut in the same line. The external jugular vein is ligated and divided. Sometimes the suprascapular nerve is encountered and mobilized. The sternocleidomastoid muscle is divided at its posterior half to improve the operative field and to ease retraction. The fat pad in the posterior triangle is identified and mobilized. The sympathetic trunk and a muscle branch of the second part of the vertebral artery are important structures to avoid. The carotid sheath is identified and retracted forward, exposing the prevertebral fascia covering the cervical vertebral bodies. The rest of the procedure is identical to the Southwick and Robinson approach.

APPROACH TO THE CERVICODORSAL JUNCTION

This is a difficult area to approach. When a single vertebra is involved access can be either through the neck or the chest. With multiple vertebral involvement together with significant kyphosis, a split sternum approach is advocated. Readers need to refer to details described by Cauchoix & Binet (1957). An alternative is to excise or elevate the medial corner of the manubrium, the sternoclavicular joint and the medial half of the clavicle on a pedicle of the sternocleidomastoid muscle (Birch *et al.*, 1990; Sundaresan *et al.*, 1984).

APPROACH TO C7–T12

A thoracotomy approach, usually right-sided for lesion from C7 to T4 and left-sided for lesion from T4 to T12 is preferred. On the left side the aorta is a useful landmark and is less liable to be damaged as compared to the vena cava on the right. The favoured side is also dependent on such factors as pointing of a unilateral abscess or associated complications such as empyema or lung penetration. The patient is put in a full lateral position, usually with a sandbag or the bridge of the table under the involved vertebrae. Such a manoeuvre enables later impaction of the anterior bone graft when the spine is realigned. The rib to be excised is usually two levels or more higher than the centre of the vertebral lesion. Adjacent additional ribs may be osteotomized or excised for better exposure. To excise the upper ribs the scapula may need to be mobilized by cutting the scapulothoracic muscles. After excising the rib subperiosteally the parietal pleura is incised throughout its length. Special care is necessary if adhesions are present. Often the rib head is markedly curved, and is best removed within the chest cavity. Having retracted the lung forwards the interval between the great vessel (aorta or vena cava) and the abscess (if present) is developed. If there is no abscess the great vessels are mobilized from the vertebral body by incising the parietal pleura. The intercostal vessels need to be ligated or diathermized, then divided as near. If many spinal levels are involved, the anatomy of the vessels may be distorted because of crowding at the apex. The hemiazygos vein and branches of splanchnic nerve, if encountered, may be sacrificed to complete the exposure.

APPROACH TO THE THORACOLUMBAR JUNCTION D11–L2

The standard approach is through a left thoracotomy removing the ninth rib, although a right-sided approach is also feasible. The pleural cavity is entered through the ninth rib bed and the aorta mobilized. The retroperitoneal space is entered, usually at the costal cartilage of the ninth rib. The parietal peritoneum is mobilized from the undersurface of the diaphragm and retracted antero-inferiorly. The diaphragm is then cut circumferentially with diathermy, leaving a 1 cm edge so that approximation is possible during wound closure. The affected vertebra is identified easily by palpating the relevant rib as it articulates with the superior border of the corresponding vertebral body. An alternative is to identify the uppermost attachment of the psoas muscle at the body of the D12 vertebra. The psoas muscle needs to be mobilized laterally by gently separating it from the vertebral column; similarly the crus of the diaphragm. Any psoas abscess is drained, flaps raised and stay-stitched and the vertebral lesion exposed through the abscess.

Access to the upper lumbar area can be achieved through the eleventh rib bed, and to L2 vertebra through the twelfth rib bed.

APPROACH TO LUMBOSACRAL SPINE (L2–S1)

A left-sided approach is preferred because the arterial structures are easier to deal with than the venous counterpart. Even so, access from the right side is also possible. A full lateral position is used, as described previously. An oblique incision is made posteriorly starting at the midpoint between the iliac crest and the costal margin extending to the midpoint between the umbilicus and the anterior superior iliac spine. Having cut the abdominal musculature the retroperitoneal space is entered by stripping the parietal peritoneum from the posterior and lateral abdominal wall. The ureter and kidney are reflected medially with other abdominal contents. Division of the anterior or posterior rectus sheath will enhance exposure. In approaching the lumbosacral junction, the common and external iliac vessels are mobilized. The ascending and/or iliolumbar vessels need to be identified and sometimes ligated. The lumbar segmental vessels are usually thrombosed. The lumbosacral nerve trunk must be protected. The sympathetic chain, if damaged or cut, does not give rise to any permanent deleterious effects. If there is no psoas abscess the psoas muscle is mobilized and its origin detached, reflected, and stay-stitched. After thorough debridement and grafting the bridge is lowered, thus impacting the grafts.

COSTOTRANSVERSECTOMY

The reader should refer to the original work by Menard (1900), or its modifications.

Postoperative management

Besides the usual postoperative routine special precautions relating to the Hong Kong operation include the following. It is important to drain the wound. Most patients are nursed in bed although Stryker bed nursing may be necessary in paraplegic or quadriplegic patients. Most children need a protective prefabricated shell before cast application. Plaster immobilization is necessary for at least the initial three months. A collar or a halocast/Minerva jacket type of immobilization is needed for the cervical spine, depending on the stability and length of the graft. A pantaloon type of cast is necessary for fusion at the lumbosacral junction.

Surgical complications

INTRAOPERATIVE

These arise from damage to vascular, visceral or neural structures.

Vascular

This depends on the approach and anatomy of the area involved. Minor vascular tears can be repaired, or the vessel can be ligated if it is dispensable. Major vascular accidents may occur if the anatomy is grossly distorted and fibrosis so marked that normal dissection is difficult. A vascular surgeon's assistance may be necessary if such major complications occur.

Visceral

The lung and ureter are the endangered structures. The lung could be punctured during freeing of adhesions. An air leak calls for repair, but if it is minimal insertion of a chest drain will suffice. The ureter could be involved if retroperitoneal scarring is present; if damaged, every attempt at repair must be made, to prevent leakage or fistula postoperatively.

Neural

Dural tears require closure, otherwise a fistula and/or cerebrospinal fluid accumulation will occur. If repair fails the leakage will nevertheless still heal, but may take a few months to do so. Direct injury to the neural tissue in the canal is always possible especially with lack of experience in decompressing the healed but kyphotic patient. The lumbar plexus overlying a fibrotic psoas muscle may also be damaged during drainage of an abscess or mobilization of the muscle.

EARLY POSTOPERATIVE COMPLICATIONS

Visceral

Possible post-thoracotomy complications include pleural effusion, haemothorax, lung collapse and pneumonia. These can be prevented by good postoperative care of the drains and chest physiotherapy. Retroperitoneal dissection in the dorsilumbar and lumbar region often results in transient paralytic ileus.

Neural

Minor neurological complications include transient Horner's syndrome due to cervical sympathetic damage. Damage to the lumbar sympathetics results in a warm leg, but this condition is also transient. Major neurological complications include most importantly a worsening of the paraparesis/tetraparesis. This is probably due to either spinal cord concussion or neurapraxia intraoperatively, or significant slippage of graft impinging on the spinal cord. In the former, a short course of steroids may be helpful. In the latter repositioning of the graft surgically is necessary.

Vascular

Anterior spinal artery spasm or damage may produce permanent paraplegia.

LATE POSTOPERATIVE COMPLICATIONS

Progressive kyphosis may occur due to resorption of the grafts, the main reason being uncontrolled or recurrent infection. Adjustment of chemotherapy is necessary, depending on the results of further bacterial culture, usually at two to three months postoperatively. Continued external spinal support is necessary to prevent further kyphosis. Even when both ends of the graft are incorporated into the recipient beds, stress fracture of the midsegment of a long graft may occur at about one year postoperatively. This may be asymptomatic, but is best treated by immobilization till healing occurs, lest further kyphosis develops. Non-union even in the presence of infection should be treated conservatively unless there is increasing kyphosis or uncontrollable infection with adequate chemotherapy, in which case restabilization is necessary.

Management of paraplegia of healed disease

The prognosis of paraplegia associated with healed disease, even when adequate decompression has been achieved, is not good. Recovery at best is prolonged and often incomplete. The two main causes for such paraplegia are firstly an impingement on the cord by the hard anterior and retropulsed bony bridge arising from multiple-level vertebral destruction with bone softening and collapse into kyphosis, and secondly fibrosis arising from the maturing granulation tissue strangulating the spinal cord.

These two factors may be present simultaneously, lessening the chances of neurological recovery.

In dealing with patients with paraplegia of late onset and appreciable kyphosis, the anterior approach to the spine is preferred, although when the kyphosis is extreme and anterior surgery is not feasible, the alternative of costotransversectomy is to be recommended. Laminectomy alone is strongly contraindicated (Griffiths *et al.*, 1956).

Anterior access to the internal kyphos entails tracing a nerve root proximally to the intervertebral foramen. The bony ridge and fibrous tissue in front is carefully removed and the dura at the apex adequately exposed and protected. The dura should be observed to pulsate at the end of the decompression and also to be displaced forwards. Fusion should then be performed inserting rib grafts into cancellous bone in the two limbs of the kyphos. Should correction of the angular kyphus be required the halopelvic apparatus is useful after surgical decompression but prior to formal fusion.

In a long-term review of 22 patients with paraplegia of late onset (Hsu *et al.*, 1988), 14 patients had active disease. Because of abscess formation the approach to the front of the spinal cord was much easier in these patients. The approach to the inner bony kyphos in the remaining eight patients was difficult and fraught with complications (two cases of neurological deterioration, two cases with cerebrospinal fluid fistulae and four with cord neurapraxia). Thus in Pott's paraplegia of late onset the surgeon should define first whether active disease is still present. If so, prognosis for neurological improvement is much better. The surgical approach to both types of late onset paraplegia is essentially the same. However, a patient with proven active disease should be prescribed another full course of chemotherapy. This is not necessary when the disease is quiescent.

Surgical correction of severe kyphotic deformity

Severe kyphotic deformity is common when a significant number of vertebral bodies are destroyed; indeed there is good correlation between them (Rajasekaran & Shanmugasandaram, 1987). The worst deformities occur in the dorsolumbar and midthoracic region and least in the cervical and lumbar region. Besides the cosmetic problem and short stature, kyphosis of more than 90° at midthoracic region may cause impairment of pulmonary function. Thus surgical correction is sometimes part of the treatment of paraplegia when the disease is quiescent.

Surgical correction is often a lengthy procedure, usually undertaken in stages. The development of the halopelvic distraction apparatus has made such correction less dangerous and more successful. The device is fitted with a strain gauge to register the tension acting on the spine. Gradual distraction is necessary, and complications arising from overdistraction have to be detected early (O'Brien *et al.*, 1971). The maximum safe distraction force is about 40 lb (18 kg) or half the body weight of the patient. The stages of correction include:

1 fitting of the halopelvic distraction apparatus;
2 anterior spinal osteotomy and decompression of the spinal cord;
3 spinal distraction;
4 posterior osteotomy (and fusion);

5 further spinal distraction;
6 following maximum correction anterior spinal fusion;
7 posterior spinal fusion;
8 immobilization in halopelvic apparatus and later in a body cast.

Such a regime is tedious and not without risks; indeed the surgeon may encounter complications at any stage during the procedure (Yau *et al.*, 1974) (Fig. 31.5a,b). Good preoperative assessment is essential, including baseline neurological charting followed by monitoring changes throughout the whole procedure. A lateral cervical spine X-ray is mandatory in all patients prior to halopelvic traction. Myelography may be necessary if a preoperative neurological deficit is present. The halopelvic apparatus application possesses its own complications, and these will not be discussed here (O'Brien *et al.*, 1971). Distraction of the spine may precipitate paraplegia when prior anterior osteotomy is not done. As mentioned previously, costotransversectomy is sometimes preferred to thoracotomy if there is poor lung function or extensive pleural adhesion necessitating an extrapleural approach. Removal of the apex of the internal kyphos may be dangerous by any route, as neurapraxia of the spinal cord or dural tear resulting in cerebrospinal fluid fistula may develop. Thus, during distraction, diligent monitoring of the force acting through the spine, of neurological integrity and the amount of correction attained at the kyphos is essential.

These technical details must be adhered to carefully. The average correction of kyphosis in Yau's series approached 30%; however, three deaths were reported. There was improvement in cosmesis and pulmonary function, but loss of correction achieved may occur finally. This procedure should be done only in specialized spine centres, with staff and equipment appropriate for correction of such deformities. Furthermore, because of potential difficulties the halopelvic apparatus is currently not used as often as in the past.

REFERENCES

Arthornthurasrok, A. & Chongpieboonpatana, A. (1990) Spinal tuberculosis with posterior element involvement. *Spine*, **15**, 191–194.

Batson, O.V. (1940) The function of the vertebral veins and their role in the spread of metastases. *Ann. Surg.*, **112**, 138.

Birch, R., Bonney, G. & Marshall, R.W. (1990) A surgical approach to the cervicothoracic spine. *J. Bone Jt. Surg.*, **72B**, 904–907.

Brant-Zawadzki, M., Burke, V.D. & Jeffrey, R.B. (1983) CT in the evaluation of spine infection. *Spine*, **8**, 358–364.

Cauchoix, J. & Binet, J.P. (1957) Anterior surgical approaches to the spine. *Ann. Roy. Coll. Surg. Engl.*, **21**, 237.

Digby, J.M. & Kersley, J.B. (1979) Pyogenic non-tuberculous spinal infection. *J. Bone Jt. Surg.*, **61B**, 47–55.

Eismont, F.J., Bohlman, H.H., Soni, P.L. *et al.* (1982) Vertebral osteomyelitis in infants. *J. Bone Jt. Surg.*, **64B**, 32.

Eismont, F.J., Bohlman, H.H., Soni, P.L. *et al.* (1983) Pyogenic and fungal vertebral osteomyelitis with paralysis. *J. Bone Jt. Surg.*, **65A**, 19.

Fang, H.S.Y. & Ong, G.B. (1962) Direct anterior approach to the upper cervical spine. *J. Bone Jt. Surg.*, **44A**, 1588–1604.

Fang, D., Leong, J.C.Y. & Fang, H.S.Y. (1983) Tuberculosis of the upper cervical spine. *J. Bone Jt. Surg.*, **65B**, 47.

Fang, D., Remedios, I. & Leong, J.C.Y. (1992) Pyogenic spondylitis: results of anterior excision and anterior spinal fusion. *J. Bone Jt. Surg.* (Submitted).

Garcia, A. & Grantham, S.A. (1960) Hematogenous pyogenic vertebral osteomyelitis. *J. Bone Jt. Surg.*, **42A**, 429.

Ghormley, R.K. & Bradley, J.I. (1928) Prognostic signs in the X-rays of tuberculosis spines in children. *J. Bone Jt. Surg.*, **10**, 796–803.

Griffiths, D.L., Seddon, H.J. & Roaf, R. (1956) *Paraplegia.* Oxford University Press, London.

Haase, D., Martin, R. & Marrie, T. (1980) Radionuclide imaging in pyogenic vertebral osteomyelitis. *Clin. Nucl. Med.*, **5**, 533.

Hodgson, A.R. (1965) An approach to the cervical spine (C3–7). *Clin. Orthop. Rel. Res.*, **39**, 129–134.

Hodgson, A.R. (1975) Infectious disease of the spine. In Rothman & Simeone (eds) *The Spine*, 1st edn, pp. 567–598.

Hodgson, A.R. & Stock, F.E. (1956) Anterior spinal fusion. *Br. J. Surg.*, **44**, 266.

Hodgson, A.R. & Yau, A. (1967) Pott's paraplegia: a classification based upon the living pathology. *Paraplegia*, 5.

Hodgson, A.R., Skinsnes, O.K. & Leong, J.C.Y. (1967) The pathogenesis of Pott's paraplegia. *J. Bone Jt. Surg.*, **49A**, 1147.

Hodgson, A.R., Wong, W. & Yau, A.C.M.C. (1969) *X-ray Appearances of Tuberculosis of the Spine.* Charles C. Thomas, Springfield, IL.

Hsu, L.C.S. & Leong, J.C.Y. (1984) Tuberculosis of the lower cervical spine (C2–7): a report on forty cases. *J. Bone Jt. Surg.*, **66B**, 1.

Hsu, L.C.S., Cheng, C.L. & Leong, J.C.Y. (1988) Pott's paraplegia of late onset. *J. Bone Jt. Surg.*, **70B**, 534–538.

Ito, H., Tsuchiya, J. & Asami, G. (1934) A new radical operation for Pott's disease. *J. Bone Jt. Surg.*, **16**, 499.

Jeffrey, R.B., Callen, P.W. & Federle, M.P. (1980) Computed

tomography of psoas abscesses. *J. Comput. Assist. Tomogr.*, **4**, 639.

Jenkins, D.H.R., Hodgson, A.R., Yau, A.C.M.C. *et al.* (1975) Stabilization of the spine in the surgical treatment of severe spinal tuberculosis in children. *Clin. Orthop. Rel. Res.*, **110**, 69.

Johns, D. (1970) Syphilitic disorders of the spine. *J. Bone Jt. Surg.*, **52B**, 724.

Kemp, H.B.S., Jackson, J.W., Jeremiah, J.D. *et al.* (1973) Pyogenic infections occurring primarily in intervertebral discs. *J. Bone Jt. Surg.*, **55B**, 698.

Kulowski, J. (1936) Pyogenic osteomyelitis of the spine. An analysis and discussion of 102 cases. *J. Bone Jt. Surg.*, **28**, 343–364.

Lancet (1985) Pyogenic infections of the spine. *Lancet*, **1**, 619–620.

Lee, J.K.T. & Glazer, H.S. (1986) Psoas muscle disorders: MR imaging. *Radiology*, **160**, 683.

Lifeso, R.M., Harder, E. & McCorkell, S.J. (1985) Spinal brucellosis. *J. Bone Jt. Surg.*, **67B**, 345–351.

Litvinoff, J. & Nelson, M. (1978) Extradural lumbar cryptococcosis. *J. Neurosurg.*, **49**, 921–923.

Medical Research Council Working Party (1973a) Tuberculosis of the spine: a controlled trial of ambulant outpatient treatment and inpatient rest in bed in the management of tuberculosis of the spine in young Korean patients on standard chemotherapy: a study in Masan, Korea. *J. Bone Jt. Surg.*, **55B**, 678–697.

Medical Research Council Working Party (1973b) Tuberculosis of the spine: a controlled trial of plaster-of-paris jackets in the management of ambulant outpatient treatment of tuberculosis of the spine in children on standard chemotherapy: a study in Pusan, Korea. *Tubercle*, **54**, 261–282.

Medical Research Council Working Party (1974a) Tuberculosis of the spine: a controlled trial of debridement and ambulatory treatment in the management of tuberculosis of the spine in patients on standard chemotherapy. *J. Trop. Med. Hyg.*, **77**, 72–79.

Medical Research Council Working Party (1974b) Tuberculosis of the spine: a controlled trial of anterior spinal fusion and debridement in the surgical management of tuberculosis of the spine in patients on standard chemotherapy: a study in Hong Kong. *Br. J. Surg.*, **61**, 853–866.

Medical Research Council Working Party (1976) Tuberculosis of the spine: a five-year assessment of controlled trials of inpatient and outpatient treatment and of plaster-of-paris jackets for tuberculosis of the spine in children on standard chemotherapy: studies in Masan and Pusan, Korea. *J. Bone Jt. Surg.*, **58B**, 399–411.

Medical Research Council Working Party (1978) Tuberculosis of the spine: five-year assessments of controlled trials of ambulatory treatment, debridement and anterior spinal fusion in the management of tuberculosis of the spine: studies in Bulawayo (Rhodesia) and in Hong Kong. *J. Bone Jt. Surg.*, **60B**, 163–177.

Medical Research Council Working Party (1982) Tuberculosis of the spine: a ten-year assessment of a controlled trial comparing debridement and anterior spinal fusion in the management of tuberculosis of the spine in patients on standard chemotherapy in Hong Kong. *J. Bone Jt. Surg.*, **64B**, 393–398.

Medical Research Council Working Party (1985) A 10-year assessment of controlled trial of inpatient and outpatient treatment and of plaster-of-paris jacket for tuberculosis of the spine in children on standard chemotherapy. Studies in Masan and Pusan, Korea. *J. Bone Jt. Surg.*, **67B**, 103–110.

Menard, V. (1900) *Etude practique sur le mal de Pott.* Masson et Cie, Paris.

Menelaus, M.B. (1964) Discitis—an inflammation affecting the intervertebral disc in children. *J. Bone Jt. Surg.*, **46B**, 16.

Modic, M.T., Feiglin, D.H., Piraino, D.W. *et al.* (1985) Vertebral osteomyelitis; assessment using MR. *Radiology*, **157**, 157.

Muhle, I., Rau, J. & Ruskin, J. (1979) Vertebral osteomyelitis due to *Actinobacillus actinomycetemcomitans. J. Am. Med. Assoc.*, **241**, 1824–1825.

O'Brien, J.P. (1969) The manifestation of arrested bone growth. The appearance of a vertebra within a vertebra. *J. Bone Jt. Surg.*, **51A**, 1376–1378.

O'Brien, J.P., Yau, A.C.M.C., Smith T.K. *et al.* (1971) Halo pelvic traction. *J. Bone Jt. Surg.*, **53B**, 217–229.

Otolenghi, E.C. (1969) Aspiration biopsy of the spine. *J. Bone Jt. Surg.*, **51A**, 1531.

Pott, P. (1779) *Remarks on that kind of palsy of the lower limbs which is frequently found to accompany a curvature of the spine.* J. Johnson, London.

Pun, W.K., Chow, S.P., Luk, K.D.K. *et al.* (1990) Tuberculosis of lumbosacral junction: longterm follow-up of 26 cases. *J. Bone Jt. Surg.*, **72B**, 675–678.

Rajasekaran, S. & Shanmugasundaram, T.K. (1987) Prediction of the angle of gibbus deformity in tuberculosis of the spine. *J. Bone Jt. Surg.*, **69A**, 503–509.

Scoles, P.V. & Quinn, T.P. (1982) Intervertebral discitis in children and adolescents. *Clin. Orthop. Rel. Res.*, **162**, 31–36.

Southwick, W.O. & Robinson, R.A. (1957) Surgical approaches to the vertebral bodies in the cervical and lumbar regions. *J. Bone Jt. Surg.*, **39A**, 631–644.

Sullivan, C.R., Bickel, W.H. & Svien, H.J. (1958) Infection of the vertebral interspaces after operations on intervertebral disks. *J. Am. Med. Assoc.*, **166**, 173.

Sundaresan, N., Shah, J., Foley, K.M. & Rosen, G. (1984) An anterior surgical approach to the upper thoracic vertebrae. *J. Neurosurg.*, **61**, 686–690.

Wiley, A.M. & Trueta, J. (1959) The vascular anatomy of the spine and its relationship to pyogenic vertebral osteomyelitis. *J. Bone Jt. Surg.*, **41B**, 796.

Yanoff, D.B. & Church, McG.L. (1983) Nocardial vertebral osteomyelitis. *Clin. Orthop. Rel. Res.*, **175**, 223–226.

Yau, A.C.M.C. & Hodgson, A.R. (1968) Penetration of the lung by the paravertebral abscess. *J. Bone Jt. Surg.*, **50A**, 243–254.

Yau, A.C.M.C., Hsu, L.C.S., O'Brien, J.P. *et al.* (1974) Tuberculous kyphosis: correction with spinal osteotomy, halo-pelvic distraction and anterior and posterior fusion. *J. Bone Jt. Surg.*, **56A**, 1419–1434.

32 · Intraspinal Infection

By R.A. JOHNSTON

Intraspinal abscesses are conditions which occur infrequently, in which the diagnosis is often delayed and the consequences are frequently devastating to the patient. The most common intraspinal infection is the extradural abscess followed much less frequently by subdural abscess and intramedullary abscess. The medical literature contains references to intraspinal abscesses dating back to the 18th and 19th centuries (Morgagni, 1796; Dandy, 1926). From more recently published series the relative infrequency of this condition can be appreciated (Heusner, 1948; Hulme & Dott, 1954, Hancock, 1973, Baker *et al.*, 1975; Hakin *et al.*, 1979; Statham & Gentleman, 1989). In total, these six series comprise 162 cases of extradural abscess over a period of 121 years. Because of this infrequency and the dire consequences to the patient of late treatment it is important that clinicians involved in the early management of this condition maintain their diagnostic vigilance. Many authors note the fact that inappropriate management will result in permanent spinal cord damage or the death of the patient. Heusner in 1948 said 'delay in diagnosing epidural sepsis is more often attributable to a failure to give it consideration than to any other cause. . . . Bad results are usually traceable to the mistaking of these disorders for more everyday ailments until paralysis is complete and neurological damage irreversible.' Intraspinal abscess, and in particular extradural abscess, is an eminently treatable infection from which patients can make a full recovery provided that appropriate treatment is commenced without delay.

PATHOPHYSIOLOGY

The thoracic spine is the most frequent location for extradural abscess, and this could be expected given the relative size of the thoracic spine. However, the predilection for this region seems to exceed that which would be expected pro rata, and it might be surmised that there are anatomical reasons favouring the development of purulent infection in this part of the spine. Dandy (1926) gave a concise description of the anatomical relationships of the spinal extradural space, and indicated that the size of the space varies inversely with the diameter of the spinal cord. In the thoracic spine and lower lumbar regions the extradural space is at its most generous, while being least obvious in the cervical spine and the lumbar cord expansion.

Unlike the double layer of dura mater which is present in the cranium, the dura surrounding the spinal cord is a single layer. The endosteal cranial dura stops at the foramen magnum, leaving the inner or meningeal layer to continue over the spinal cord. The endosteal layer of dura in the spine is replaced by the periosteum lining the vertebral canal and is separated from the inner layer of dura by the extradural space. Immediately it can be seen that an extradural lesion in the head lies outside two layers of dura, while in the spine it is separated from the intradural contents by only a single layer of dura. The ventral surface of the spinal dura is adherent to the posterior surfaces of the upper cervical vertebra and also attached loosely to the posterior longitudinal ligament (Gray, 1967). Dandy (1926) indicated that the extradural space begins to appear at the lower cervical region, and that it is only in the lower lumbar region that the space extends significantly ventrally.

This anatomical configuration correlates with the clinical findings that the great majority of extradural abscesses, not directly associated with vertebral osteomyelitis, are found in the dorsal thoracic extradural space. Ventral infections are almost always secondary to a spread from a vertebral body infection. Of the 39 cases described by Baker *et al.* (1975) only seven were located in the ventral extradural space. Hakin *et al.* (1979) reported that the majority of extradural abscesses occurred in the midthoracic region and Statham & Gentleman (1989) found 12 of 17 abscesses in either the thoracic or lumbar region. Each of those series recorded one patient with two separate abscesses in the cervical and lumbar regions.

Dandy indicated in 1926 that abscesses of the extradural space arose either by direct extension of a contiguous infection or by haematogenous dissemination, and this has been supported by subsequent authors. Heusner (1948) divided the clinical presentation into two types, called either an 'acute metastatic syndrome' or an 'acute osteomyelitic syndrome'. The latter is in fact a more slowly progressive chronic type of infection in which the extradural abscess derives from adjacent vertebral body osteomyelitis. Baker *et al.* (1975) reported 19 of 39 patients presenting with a chronic extradural abscess, at least seven of which cases appeared to be associated with vertebral osteomyelitis. Other sources of direct spread include local, but non-vertebral abscesses, extradural catheters and serial lumbar puncture which has been implicated as a cause of lumbar extradural abscess with osteomyelitis (Bergman *et al.*, 1983).

Most authors report other associated, but distant, infections as the probable source of abscess reaching the extradural space via the circulation. These include pyelonephritis, furuncles, carbuncles, respiratory infections, dental abscesses, etc. Baker *et al.* (1975) reported that two of their 39 patients were intravenous drug abusers, and this was recognized in one of the patients reported by Statham & Gentleman (1989). Associated spinal trauma, usually of a relatively minor nature, was present in 12 of the 39 cases reported by Baker *et al.* (1979) and in six of the 17 reported by Statham & Gentleman. Hulme & Dott (1974) suggested that in nine of 25 patients trauma was a probable aetiological factor. It is difficult to know whether this is just a coincidental finding since trivial back injuries are so common. However, it is possible that in the presence of distant infection such minor trauma may produce local damage or local haematomas which provide a focus for any disseminating bacteria. Postoperative extradural abscesses are distinctly rare, although one is reported by Baker *et al.* (1975) as probably developing from an infected operation wound. Local infections following spinal surgery are for the most part wound infections, occasionally spreading into the vertebra. It is exceptional to find liquid pus in the extradural space although, if the infection has reached the vertebra, granulation tissue may be found in the extradural space.

Penetrating wounds of the spine lead to a surprisingly low rate of extradural abscess formation. These are relatively common injuries in South Africa but Lipschitz & Block (1962) found only two such abscesses in 130 stab wounds of the spine.

Pyogenic extradural abscesses are most frequently caused by *Staphylococcus aureus*. This was found to be present either alone or in combination in 87.5% of Statham & Gentleman's series, and in 58% by Baker *et al.* (1975). Other likely organisms include *Streptococcus*, *Escherichia coli*, *Pseudomonas*, *Propionibacterium* and *Bacteroides*. The latter, however, usually comprise only single cases in most series. Unusual organisms such as *Salmonella* causing extradural abscess have been reported (Rana *et al.*, 1985). Tuberculosis is a rare cause of extradural abscess in Western countries. However, extradural tuberculous abscesses are found in those countries where tuberculous infection is still common. Babhulkar *et al.* (1984) reported 10 such cases without radiological evidence of vertebral body or neural arch tuberculosis.

More exotic granulomatous infections occur, and because of their rarity the reports usually comprise individual cases. *Actinomyces israelii*, and *Coccidioides immitis* (Kannangara *et al.*, 1981; Delaney & Niemann, 1982) most characteristically cause vertebral body infection with secondary extradural abscess formation. Similarly *Aspergillus* will usually cause primary vertebral body infection with secondary extradural abscess formation (Byrd *et al.*, 1982; Wagner *et al.*, 1985). These infections are more likely to occur in patients who are immunosuppressed, which until recently was usually due to drug therapy following renal transplant or chemotherapy for malignant disease. With the spread of acquired immunodeficiency syndrome an increase in the number of exotic extradural abscesses can reasonably be expected.

How does the extradural infection lead to spinal cord damage? The two mechanisms which have been postulated are mechanical compression and ischaemia. Heusner (1948) suggested that compression was the most obvious mechanism, but that this would not explain all of the clinical observations. Baker *et al.* (1975) suggested that the neurological damage produced by extradural abscess can be more extensive than would otherwise be accounted for by mechanical compression alone, and postulated the additional hazard of spinal cord ischaemia. The possibility of some form of local circulatory disturbance was addressed by Browder & Meyers (1941) in describing patients who came to autopsy following extradural abscess. However, they found little confirmatory evidence to suggest that local spinal cord blood vessels were compromised by the compression or by the inflammation.

Thrombosis of spinal cord vessels has reasonably been suggested to occur secondary to the inflammatory process. Despite the fact that there is a significant mortality associated with extradural abscess, histopathological evidence of such medullary angiopathy is surprisingly scant. A laboratory model of extradural abscess was devised by Feldenzer *et al.* (1987) in rabbits, in an attempt to resolve the mechanical compression and/or vascular basis of spinal cord damage. The spinal cords of the animals were investigated by microangiographic techniques and by histopathological examination. They found that the grey matter of the spinal cord was relatively well preserved compared with axonal damage. There was no microscopic evidence of thrombosis or inflammation of major blood vessels, and it was only when compression was extreme that small perforating arteries became occluded. Their conclusions from these data, which suggest that the cord damage is primarily mechanical in nature, have obvious implications for speedy surgical decompression.

One could suppose that the mechanism of damage produced by subdural pus is similar. This condition is considerably less common than extradural abscess and histopathological data are not available. Perhaps the anatomical proximity of purulent material to subarachnoid blood vessels makes inflammatory thrombosis more likely. Pus in the substance of the spinal cord is rare nowadays, but Dutton & Alexander (1954) cited literature reporting 20 cases of haematogenous spread and 36 cases of direct spread of infection to the spinal cord. Many of these were terminal-stage illness infections, and virtually all occurred in the pre-antibiotic years. The pus does not seem to encapsulate easily, although this may reflect early surgical drainage. Like slowly advancing intramedullary tumours, the infective process, once begun, seems to enlarge by displacement of fibre tracts rather than their destruction. Infecting organisms include staphylococci, streptococci, pneumonococci, *Escherichia coli* and *Bacteroides fusiformis*. The abscess usually extends for about three cord segments, although in autopsy specimens extensive and multiple-level abscesses are seen. Given the absence of recent reports on this infection it would seem that its incidence has declined.

CLINICAL PRESENTATION

The age range of patients with extradural abscess reported by Statham & Gentleman (1989) was 16–70 years with a mean of 40 years. Hakin *et al.* (1979) reported a younger and narrower age spread between 12 years and 37 years with a mean age of 22 years, probably reflecting the selection of patients referred to the spinal injuries unit from which the report originated.

Infection in the extradural space produces severe spinal pain; in addition there may be a radicular component exacerbated by movement. Frequently there is exquisite local spinal tenderness to percussion. Spinal pain of this nature is the initial presenting feature of the condition and it is characteristic of extradural abscess just as sudden onset of severe headache is the classic presentation of subarachnoid haemorrhage. In all the reported series, spinal pain is the herald of neurological deterioration, and it is at this time that, if the diagnosis is made, the infection can be eradicated without significant spinal cord damage. However, such is the prevalence of back pain in our society that the diagnosis is seldom considered until the patient displays neurological deterioration. It is not difficult for neurosurgeons to diagnose an extradural abscess in a patient with spinal pain, local tenderness, plus paraparesis. However, this must be considered an end-stage diagnosis and a failure of the system to recognize the condition at the proper time. Patients presenting with thoracic spinal pain should not be assumed to have a degenerative condition or soft tissue damage without considering the possibility of more serious pathological lesions.

Spinal pain is almost a constant initial feature and may be present for a variable time before neurological symptoms develop. It may well be accompanied by a general malaise with pyrexia. The systemic features of infection were present in 75% of Statham & Gentleman's series (1989), and in an even higher percentage of those reported by Baker *et al.* (1975). Clinical progession culminating in neurological deterioration is well recognized, both in textbooks and in published series. Hakin *et al.* (1979) reported an average interval between the onset of spinal pain and complete paralysis of 5.5 days, whereas Baker *et al.* observed the progression from spinal pain to limb weakness to be 7.5 days.

In the early stages of presentation intraspinal abscess is frequently misdiagnosed. Statham & Gentleman (1989) found that the initial hospital diagnosis before referral to the neurosurgical service was correct in only three cases. Five patients were thought to have meningitis and the remainder a variety of diagnoses. Hakin *et al.* (1979) noted an incorrect prehospital diagnosis in every case. It is perhaps reasonable for a non-specialist not to diagnose an intraspinal infection as such, but it is very important that spinal pain and the possibility of cord damage is appreciated and appropriate early referral made.

That the diagnostic delay is not due to late presentation by the patient is shown by Hakin *et al.* (1979), who found that almost 90% of their patients presented to medical staff between 24 and 48 hours following onset of symptoms. In a review of causes of delay in the diagnosis of spinal cord compression from diverse causes Maurice-Williams & Richardson (1988) highlighted the potentially avoidable delays in transit of patients to neurosurgical units. The proportion of patients with complete spinal cord lesions rose from 1.5% to 28% during the referral process. Such delays are, of course, unacceptable and their elimination, while probably a counsel of perfection, should nevertheless be sought. Earlier diagnosis, before neurological deterioration, will result in more patients walking after treatment of intraspinal infection.

The very uncommon spinal subdural abscess presents in a similar fashion, although there are relatively few reported cases in the literature. Fraser *et al.* (1973) drew attention to the main difference between subdural and extradural spinal abscess. The predisposing factors, the organisms causing infection and the clinical presentation are all remarkably similar with the exception of local spinal tenderness, which is absent in a subdural abscess.

Dutton & Alexander (1954) described the intramedullary abscess as a pyosyrinx which produces a progressive and usually painless paraparesis over a variable period. In their own case the myelopathy developed over four weeks, although in most of the 11 other cases cited progression was more rapid.

RADIOLOGICAL DIAGNOSIS

Where the abscess is secondary to vertebral osteomyelitis evidence of the latter will be seen as bone erosion with involvement of adjacent disc space, vertebral collapse or paravertebral abscess. Otherwise plain films are not helpful in diagnosing intraspinal infection.

The mainstay of radiological diagnosis has been contrast myelography, and in spite of computerized tomography (CT) imaging techniques this is likely to continue to be the case as CT cannot readily provide the sagittal screening information which yelography supplies. In all cases partial or complete block to the flow of contrast is demonstrated (Figs 32.1 & 32.2). It is important, as in other cases of complete obstruction, to know both the upper and

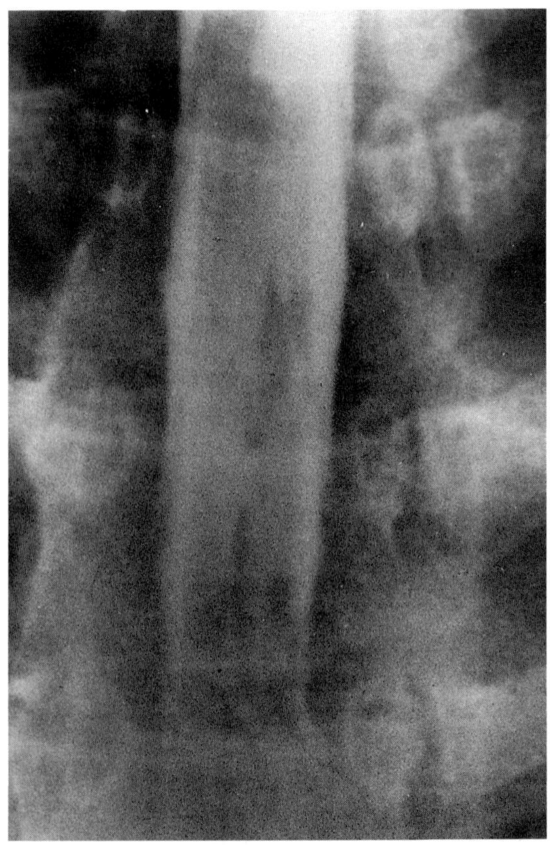

Fig. 32.1 Myelogram by cisternal puncture; extradural abscess causing obstruction at T2 level.

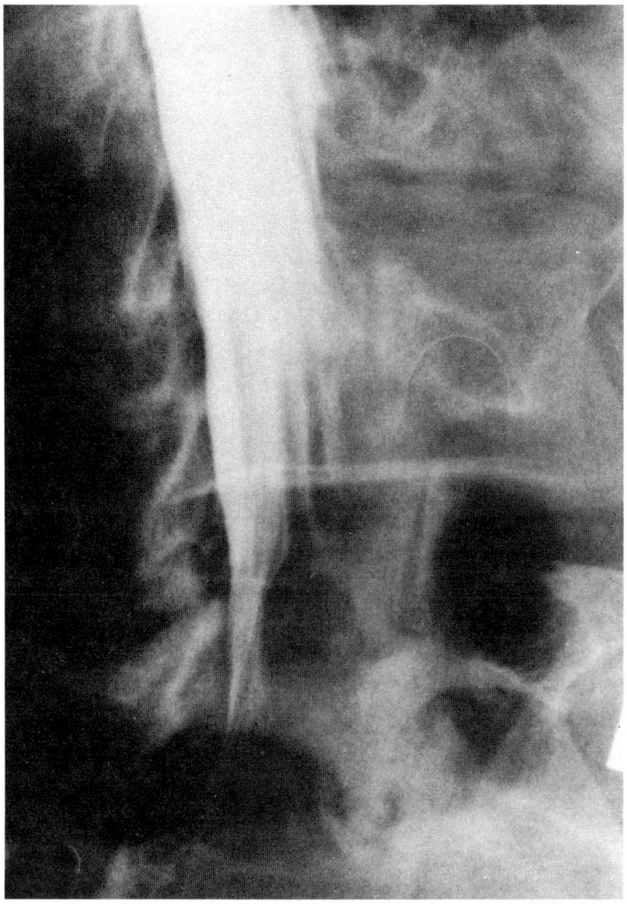

Fig. 32.2 Extradural abscess. Myelogram showing a filling defect at the lower lumbar level caused by extradural infection.

lower limits of the lesion, and this can be achieved by combining cisternal and lumbar myelography. Passing a lumbar puncture needle through an infected extradural space into cerebrospinal fluid (CSF) may lead to meningitis, though this complication fortunately seems to be uncommon. Occasionally the abscess may be tapped directly, in which case the CSF compartment should be approached by cisternal puncture. Some units recommend cisternal puncture alone (M. du Trevou, personal communication). Specimens of CSF obtained at myelography usually reveal a pattern suggestive of parameningeal infection with a variable leucocytosis and elevated protein level.

Myelography will usually distinguish extradural pus from subdural pus, and will demonstrate cord enlargement when an intramedullary abscess is present. It may again be necessary to carry out both lumbar and cisternal punctures to determine both lower and upper limits of infection or the presence of skip abscesses. CT scan is particularly helpful in vertebral osteomyelitis where it demonstrates the amount of bone destruction and paravertebral extension. The information provided in cases of pure extradural infection is of limited value, unless performed immediately following myelography.

Magnetic resonance imaging (MRI) is likely in the near future to replace myelography in the diagnosis of intraspinal infection as it improves in resolution and becomes more widely available (Fig. 32.3). To date there is no information available which compares MRI with standard radiological techniques in intraspinal infection. Extradural abscess is well demonstrated using T1- and T2-weighted spin echo studies, and the upper and lower extremities of the

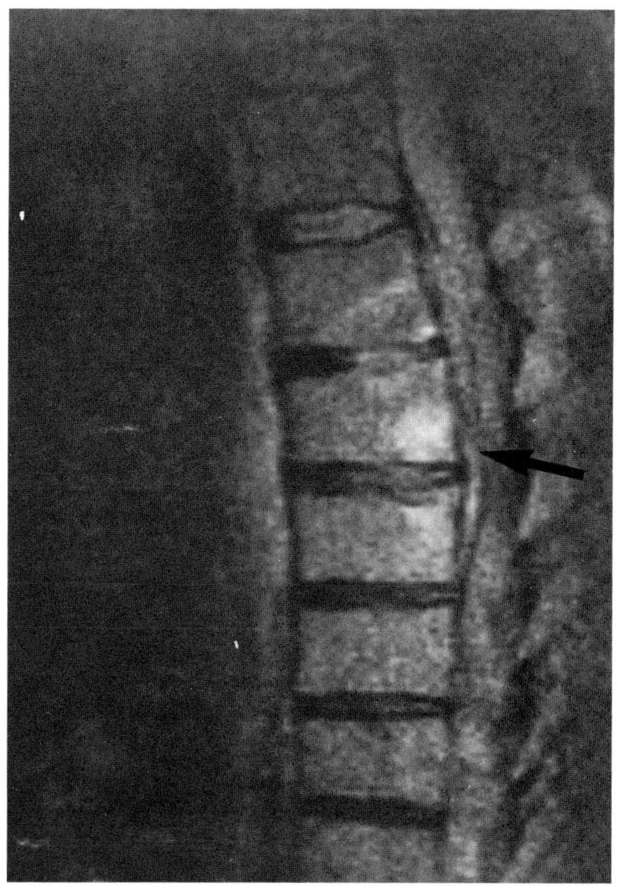

Fig. 32.3 Magnetic resonance imaging. Osteomyelitis with extradural abscess. Bright signal from vertebral bodies indicating osteomyelitis. Arrow points to ventral extradural pus.

abscess are also seen (Ross, 1989). It is possible to distinguish pus from haematoma in the extradural or subdural compartments using MRI (M.D.M. Hadley, personal communication) but this would be very difficult or impossible by myelography.

OPERATIVE TREATMENT

Because intraspinal abscess is likely to present with a combination of pain and progressive neurological deficit there is no place for non-operative management of this condition. The aims of surgery are (a) to confirm the diagnosis, (b) to obtain infected material from which antibiotic sensitivities can be established, (c) to decompress the spinal cord and (d) when relevant to leave the patient with a stable spine when the infection has been eradicated.

In the majority of cases the abscess is located in the thoracic or thoracolumbar region with purulent material lying dorsal to the spinal dura. The most commonly required surgical procedure is therefore a laminectomy. However, should the abscess be secondary to osteomyelitis of the vertebral body, laminectomy in that situation is contra-indicated. The management of such a condition is discussed in Chapter 31. The abscess may extend for a variable length along the spine, but a laminectomy comprising four or five lamina is usually adequate to decompress the majority of cases. Removal of infected material following adequate mechanical decompression is the endpoint of the operation, but sometimes traces of the infection can be seen at the extremities of the laminectomy. Whether more laminae are removed in order to reach 'clean' dura is an intraoperative decision to be made by the surgeon. If there is no significant compression and the infected material is minimal in volume it seems reasonable to allow this to be dealt with by appropriate antibiotic therapy. Also, if liquid pus, rather than more tenacious granulomatous material is found, then a limited decompression is often sufficient. The upper and lower levels of the obstruction should be known from the preoperative radiological investigations. This is important because extradural abscess can occur simultaneously at different levels, requiring separate laminectomy procedures. For very long abscesses judicious use of laminectomies at differing levels can be considered in order to avoid removing a large number of lamina (M. du Trevou, personal communication).

Removal of liquid purulent material is not difficult, although granulation tissue in the more chronic type of extradural infection is adherent to the dura. Obviously breach of the dura is to be avoided to prevent contamination of the intradural spaces. The use of extradural 'wound drains' for instillation of antibiotics probably has more basis in its hereditary passage through various descriptions of surgical technique than in any factual evidence which shows it to make any significant difference to recovery. Even the most 'complete' surgical clearance of pus/granulation tissue leaves behind some infected tissue which is dealt with by appropriate antibiotic therapy.

In the unlikely event of finding a normal extradural space all experienced spinal surgeons will automatically reconfirm the level of their surgical approach, by X-ray on the operation table. The dura should then be opened and the subdural space inspected. The intradural exposure must also be appropriate to the length of the abscess, and the removal of pus carried out by gentle blunt dissection and suction techniques. Fortunately pus in the subdural space is usually of a liquid type. It is not confined by the ventral attachments of the dura and may spread laterally and ventrally around the spinal cord, making complete evacuation more difficult. Gentle lavage with warm saline should be carried out. The spinal cord must not be manipulated to obtain access to the ventral regions. Once a clearance has been obtained the dura should be closed.

Intramedullary abscesses require a midline myelotomy to evacuate the contents of the abscess. This is usually liquid pus, and removal by gentle blunt dissection with careful suction is the method of choice. Intraoperative ultrasound can be useful in locating pus either within the spinal cord or ventral to it (Feldenzer *et al.*, 1986).

Some intraspinal abscesses develop secondary to dysraphic conditions where there is patent sinus track running from the skin surface to the intraspinal compartment. The sinus track must be excised along with the removal of the abscess.

In the uncommon event when tuberculosis is found in the extradural space removal of the granulation tissue should be carried out as for pyogenic infections. A preoperative diagnosis of this type of extradural spinal abscess is unlikely to be considered in the UK, due to the low frequency of tuberculous infections. It is likely to be mistaken for extradural tumour or haematoma. In South Africa, where tuberculosis is still common, tuberculous extradural abscesses are often recognized early and managed by chemotherapy without surgery (M. du Trevou, personal communication). The other granulomatous infections, including *Coccidioides*, *Aspergillus* and *Actinomyces*, frequently involve the extradural space secondary to vertebral body osteomyelitis. In general, where there is vertebral body osteomyelitis and anterior instability, a laminectomy will only further reduce the stability of the spine. Such extradural abscesses are frequently found in the ventral extradural space and may be drained through anterior or anterolateral approaches which are used to deal with the vertebral body infection.

The main problem in treating intraspinal infections is delivering correct management at an early stage. Once the diagnosis has been made appropriate management consists of relevant and adequate antibiotic therapy and immediate surgical decompression. There is no indication in the literature to support medical treatment alone for intraspinal abscess presenting with neurological deficit. In Dandy's series, compiled in the early part of the century when antibiotic treatment was not available, the mortality rate was over 90%. Subsequent authors have not deviated from the regime of early surgical decompression. In the majority of infections the organism is *Staphylococcus aureus*, and the antibiotics of choice are flucloxacillin and fucidin. The clinical combination of these two agents is satisfactory, and flucloxacillin should be delivered initially in adequate doses intravenously. Fucidin is best tolerated when given orally. Bone penetration is good, and this is especially relevant when the infection is secondary to vertebral osteomyelitis.

Once purulent material has become available for bacteriological analysis the initial antibiotic regime is altered as necessary. In the unlikely instance of a methicillin-resistant *Staphyloccus*, flucloxacillin will be of no value. In this situation the use of rifampicin and vancomycin is recommended. For less common organisms appropriate sensitivities will dictate the ultimate antibiotic treatment. For the fungal granulomatous infections amphotericin B intravenously is recommended, preferably under the guidance of a bacteriologist.

The practice of leaving a drain in the epidural space for the purposes of instilling antibiotics has little scientific basis. With adequate surgical decompression and correct antibiotic therapy this practice is redundant. Furthermore, such drains as these may well become colonized by coagulase-negative staphylococci which may, at least in theory, lead to a substitute infection of the wound or even of the intraspinal compartment.

OUTCOME

The mortality rate from this condition has improved dramatically since the early series reported by Dandy, which included reports from the late nineteenth century and some cases of non-pyogenic infections. However, the mortality rate is still substantial despite the advantages of powerful modern chemotherapeutic agents, better methods of radiological diagnosis and the accumulated medical knowledge of the past 60 years. Heusner (1948), who reported one of the earliest series in the antibiotic age, described a mortality rate of 20% which was not bettered by Statham & Gentleman's series 40 years later. Fortunately, however, the rate of paraplegia has apparently steadily dropped from the 25% reported by Heusner (1948) and 20% reported by Hulme & Dott (1954) to the 10% achieved by Baker *et al.* (1975) and the 6% achieved by Statham & Gentleman (1989). Obviously the use of antibiotics has improved the outcome of management of these conditions and the decreasing rate of paraplegia is encouraging (Table 32.1). The

Table 32.1 Outcome of management of spinal extradural abscess (percentages)

Source	Dandy, 1927 (n = 25)	Heusner, 1948 (n = 20)	Hulme & Dott, 1954 (n = 25)	Baker *et al.*, 1975 (n = 39)	Statham & Gentleman, 1989 (n = 17)
Complete recovery	8	55	44 (complete recovery and weak but walking combined)	59	37
Weak but walking				13	31
Paraplegic		25	20	10	6
Dead	92	20	36	17	25

persistently high mortality from this condition probably reflects a failure of management due to late diagnosis. This can be rectified only by raising awareness of these uncommon, potentially fatal, but highly treatable conditions.

REFERENCES

Babhulkar, S.S., Tayade, W.B. & Babhulkar, S.K. (1984) Atypical spinal tuberculosis. *J. Bone Jt. Surg.*, **66**B, 239–242.

Baker, A.S., Ojemann, R.G., Swartz, M.N. & Richardson, E.P. (1975) Spinal epidural abscess. *N. Engl. J. Med.*, **293**, 463–468.

Bergman, I., Wald, E.R., Meyer, J.D. & Painter, M.J. (1983) Epidural abscess and vertebral osteomyelitis following serial lumbar punctures. *Paediatrics*, **72**, 476–480.

Browder, J. & Meyers, R. (1941) Pyogenic infections of the spinal epidural space: a consideration of anatomic and physiologic pathology. *Surgery*, **10**, 296–308.

Byrd, B.F., Weiner, M.H. & McGee, Z.A. (1982) *Aspergillus* spinal epidural abscess. *J. Am. Med. Assoc.*, **248**, 3138–3139.

Dandy, W.E. (1926) Abscesses and inflammatory tumors in the spinal epidural space (so called pachymeningitis externa). *Arch. Surg. Chicago*, **13**, 477–494.

Delaney, P. & Niemann, R. (1982) Spinal cord compression by *Coccidioides immitis* abscess. *Arch. Neurol.*, **39**, 255–256.

Dutton, J.E.M. & Alexander, G.L. (1954) Intramedullary spinal abscess. *J. Neurol. Neurosurg. Psychiatry*, **17**, 303–307.

Feldenzer, J.A., Waters, D.C., Knake, J.E. & Hoff, J.T. (1986) Anterior cervical epidural abscess: the use of intraoperative spinal sonography. *Surg. Neurol.*, **25**, 105–108.

Feldenzer, J.A., McKeever, P.E., Schaberg, D.R., Campbell, J.A. & Hoff, J.T. (1987) Experimental spinal epidural abscess: a pathophysiological model in the rabbit. *Neurosurgery*, **20**, 859–867.

Feldenzer, J.A., McKeever, P.E., Schaberg, D.R., Campbell, J.A. & Hoff, J.T. (1988) The pathogenesis of spinal epidural abscess: microangiographic studies in an experimental model. *J Neurosurg.*, **69**, 110–114.

Fraser, R.A.R., Ratzan, K., Wolpert, S.M. & Weinstein, L. (1973) Spinal subdural empyema. *Arch. Neurol.*, **28**, 235–238.

Gray's Anatomy Descriptive and Applied, 34th edn, p. 1126. D.V. Davies & R.G. Coupland (eds) Longmans, London.

Hakin, R.N., Burt, A.A. & Cook, J.B. (1979) Acute spinal epidural abscess. *Paraplegia*, **17**, 330–336.

Hancock, D.O. (1973) A study of 49 patients with acute spinal extradural abscess. *Paraplegia*, **10**, 285–288.

Heusner, A.P. (1948) Non tuberculous spinal epidural infections. *N. Engl. J. Med.*, **239**, 845–854.

Hulme, A. & Dott, N.M. (1954) Spinal epidural abscess. *Br. Med. J.*, **64**, 64–68.

Kannangara, D.W., Tanaka, T. & Thadepalli, H. (1981) Spinal epidural abscess due to *Actinomyces israelii*. *Neurology*, **31**, 202–204.

Lipschitz, R. & Block, J. (1962) Stab wounds of the spinal cord. *Lancet*, **i**, 169–172.

Maurice-Williams, R.S. & Richardson, P.L. (1988) Spinal cord compression: delay in the diagnosis and referral of a common neurosurgical emergency. *Br. J. Neurosurg.*, **2**, 55–60.

Morgagni, G.B. (1796) *De sedibus et causis morborum per anatomem indagatis. Epist X Art.* 13 (Transl.).

Rana, P.V.S., Ragunath, D., Parakkal, K.U., Biswas, S. & Prakash, S. (1985) Spinal epidural abscess due to Salmonella Group C Monophasic 1,5. *J. Neurosurg.*, **62**, 942.

Ross, J. (1989) Inflammatory disease. In Modic, M., Masaryk, T. & Ross J. (eds) *Magnetic Resonance Imaging of the Spine*, pp. 167–182. Year Book Medical Publishers, Chicago, IL.

Statham, P. & Gentleman, D. (1989) Importance of early diagnosis of acute spinal extradural abscess. *J. R. Soc. Med.*, **82**, 584–587.

Wagner, D.K., Varkey, B., Sheth, N.K. & DaMert, G.J. (1985) Epidural abscess, vertebral destruction and paraplegia caused by extending infection from an aspergilloma. *Am. J. Med.*, **78**, 518–522.

Wright, R.L. Surgical management of intracranial and intraspinal infections. In Schmidek, H.H. & Sweet, W.H. (eds) *Operative Neurosurgical Techniques*, pp. 220–222. Grune & Stratton, New York.

33 · Discitis

By R.D. FRASER and O.L. OSTI

Discitis is a term which was first used by the late Dr Eric Price of the Melbourne Children's Hospital (Menelaus, 1964; Ryan & Taylor, 1987) to describe a self-limiting spinal disorder in children characterized by back pain, loss of intervertebral disc height and increased erythrocyte sedimentation rate (ESR).

Although the term discitis is commonly used to indicate an infectious process involving the intervertebral disc it should be more correctly reserved only for primary disc infections.

In the adult an initial infectious focus in the intervertebral disc space is invariably due to contamination following surgery, or investigative procedures which may violate the disc, such as discography. Current evidence suggests that spontaneously occurring spinal infections in adults involving the intervertebral discs are due to osteomyelitis of the vertebral body, probably starting in the bony endplate (Ryan & Taylor, 1987).

In children, however, because of the existing vascularity of the outer annulus fibrosus, primary haematogenous bacterial spread may occur into the intervertebral disc independent of a focus in the vertebral body. As will be debated in the section on childhood discitis, some authors have considered this condition to be secondary to vertebral osteomyelitis as for adults (Wenger *et al.*, 1978; Ryan & Taylor, 1987). Schmorl & Junghanns (1971) reported on the pathological sequence of disc space infection, which according to them would develop following small abscesses in the endplate region of the vertebral body with subsequent breach of the bony endplates and extension into the avascular intervertebral disc. The pathology of spinal osteomyelitis and its treatment are quite different from iatrogenic discitis and are discussed in Chapter 31.

Based on the above definition three types of true discitis may be recognized: iatrogenic discitis following surgery, iatrogenic discitis following percutaneous disc procedures, and childhood discitis.

IATROGENIC DISCITIS

Possible causes of iatrogenic discitis comprise bacterial contamination of the intervertebral disc after surgical removal of disc material, discography, chemonucleolysis, lumbar puncture, percutaneous nucleotomy, myelography, angiography and chemical sympathectomy.

Historically discitis was thought to be rare following discography (Collis & Gardner, 1962; Massie & Stevens, 1967; Gresham & Miller, 1969; Simmon & Segil, 1975; McCulloch & Waddell, 1978) with some authors attributing it to a chemical or aseptic process (Wiltse *et al.*, 1975; McCulloch, 1977; Brodsky & Binder, 1979; Crock, 1983). More recently it has been suggested that discitis is more common with an incidence as high as 6% (Fraser, 1984; H. Crock, unpublished data, 1986; Fraser *et al.*, 1989).

Following chemonucleolysis the radiographic evidence of discitis has been reported in as many as 2% of patients, and was attributed in the past to a chemical or aseptic process (J. McCulloch, unpublished data, 1985). In a review of 29,075 patients treated in the United States, Agre *et al.* (1984) reported an incidence of 22 patients with discitis. In nine of these, bacterial infection was confirmed by culture. The remaining patients were considered to have aseptic discitis on the basis of negative cultures, and some were treated with steroid therapy. McCulloch and McNab (1983) reported an incidence of discitis in less than 1% of over 6000 treated patients.

They felt that this apparent low incidence was due to the bactericidal effect of the enzyme.

The reported incidence of discitis following standard discectomy varies from 0% to 2.8% (Pilgaard, 1969; Lindholm & Pylkkanen, 1982; Kirkaldy-Willis, 1983; Graf *et al.*, 1984; Fernand & Lee, 1986). Recent reports analysing the long-term results of discectomy performed through the operating microscope suggest a slightly higher rate of discitis with this technique (J. McCulloch, unpublished data, 1985; Kho & Steudel, 1986).

Aetiology

The evidence for iatrogenic discitis being the result of bacterial contamination and not a chemical, allergic or other aseptic reaction is based both on clinical and experimental grounds.

In two clinical studies (Fraser *et al.*, 1987; Osti *et al.*, 1990) where the case records and radiographs of more than 500 patients who had undergone lumbar discography were reviewed there was an incidence of discitis of 2.7% in 222 patients where discography was performed without stilletted needles. When stilletted needles and a two-needle technique was employed the incidence dropped to 0.7%. In 127 patients where radiographic contrast was mixed with cephazolin (a first-generation cephalosporin) prior to discography as a prophylactic measure against bacterial contamination, no patient developed clinical or radiographic signs of discitis (Table 33.1).

In seven patients with discitis after discography that underwent anterior discectomy and fusion for back pain, bacteria were isolated from the discs of the three patients who had had surgery less than six weeks after discography. The histopathological findings in all patients were of a chronic inflammatory process. The prophylactic effect of the antibiotics and the histopathological findings suggest that bacteria are initiators but not promoters of the pathological process.

In a series of experimental studies using a sheep model (Fraser *et al.*, 1986, 1987, 1989; Osti *et al.*, 1990), where multiple-level lumbar discography was performed under direct vision using a retroperitoneal approach, the injection of contrast material, or chymopapain only, never resulted in the development of discitis. When as few as five bacteria (colony-forming units of *Staphylococcus epidermidis*) were injected together with radiographic contrast or chymopapain, however, discitis always developed (Table 33.2). The radiographic and pathological changes at six weeks were strikingly similar to those observed in humans. Bacteria could be isolated at one and two weeks after injection, but usually not after three weeks. In most cases endplate lesions developed at the three-week stage and no evidence of bacteria could be found at post mortem. By using intravenous or intradiscal cephazolin at the time of inoculation of bacteria, discitis never developed. Varying doses of intravenous or intradiscal cephazolin as early as one day following inoculation of bacteria, however, did not affect the sequence of pathological changes typical of discitis. This was irrespective of the dose used, length of treatment and time interval between inoculation of bacteria and commencement of antibiotic treatment. The results of these studies strongly suggest that discitis is due to contamination of the intervertebral disc by bacteria, and that antibiotics, whilst effective

Table 33.1 Incidence of discitis in 559 patients investigated by discography

Series (dates)	Number of patients	Levels examined (average per patient)	Patients with discitis		Discs involved	
			Number	Percentage	Number	Percentage
Open needle technique (1978–80)	222	463 (2.0)	6	2.7	6	1.4
Closed needle technique (1981–July 1983)	149	283 (1.9)	1	0.7	1	0.4
No antibiotics (August 1983–August 1984)	61	134 (2.2)	3	4	4	3.0
Prophylactic antibiotic (May 1986–January 1989)	127	337 (2.5)	0	0	0	0

Table 33.2 Data on 16 sheep treated with intradiscal injection of Conray 280 and chymopapain with and without *Staphylococcus epidermidis*

Series	Number of animals	Levels injected	Animals with discitis		Discs involved	
			Number	Percentage	Number	Percentage
Conray 280 only	4	12	0	0	0	0
Chymopapain only	4	12	0	0	0	0
Conray 280 + bacteria	4	12	4	100	9	75
Chymopapain + bacteria	4	18	4	100	18	100

prophylactically, would seem to have no effect on the development of the typical disc lesion once the condition is established.

Pathology

The typical pathological changes seen in human discs operated following the development of discitis comprise: (1) extensive vascularization with mature granulation tissue formation in both disc and vertebral body; (2) breaching of the bony and cartilage endplate with vertical disc protrusion and (3) occasional presence of acute inflammatory cells in addition to chronic inflammation.

In the sheep model, where observations were made from as early as two days after inoculation of bacteria, the earliest change seen is the presence of granulation tissue in the vertebral body confined to the zone close to the bony endplate. Once the bony and cartilage endplates are breached herniation of nuclear material into the vertebral body develops. The extruded nuclear material shows marked 'capping' by polymorphs but the granulation tissue generally contains only few acute inflammatory cells. Extensive replacement of bone by granulation tissue is commonly seen even in regions where the endplates and nucleus are normal. At six weeks disc material is replaced by vascular fibrous tissue and new bone forms at the periphery of the lesion in the vertebral body (Figs 33.1–33.3). Occasionally an area of microabscess formation is seen within the granulation tissue.

Based on the observation of the sheep model the following stages in the development of discitis have been determined:

1 Bacteria are introduced into the disc, and multiply with no initial apparent damage to the disc or endplate structure.

2 Progressive thinning of the endplate occurs with immature granulation tissue forming on the vertebral side of the endplate at one week.

3 At three weeks the endplates are breached and nuclear material herniates into the vertebral body. A more marked vascular response is seen and at this stage bacteria are destroyed.

4 At six weeks new bone is formed and disc material

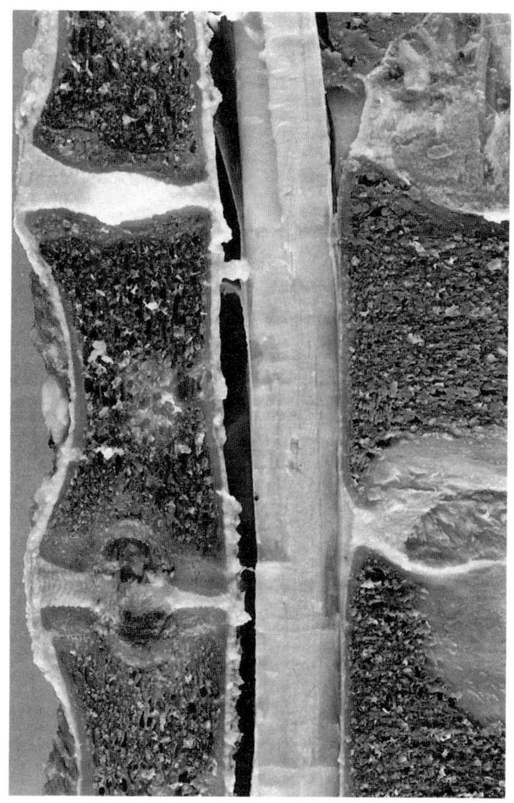

Fig. 33.1 Macroscopic view (midsagittal section) of sheep lumbar spine. The upper intervertebral disc appears normal. The lower intervertebral disc demonstrates the typical appearance of central discitis with bilateral endplate destruction.

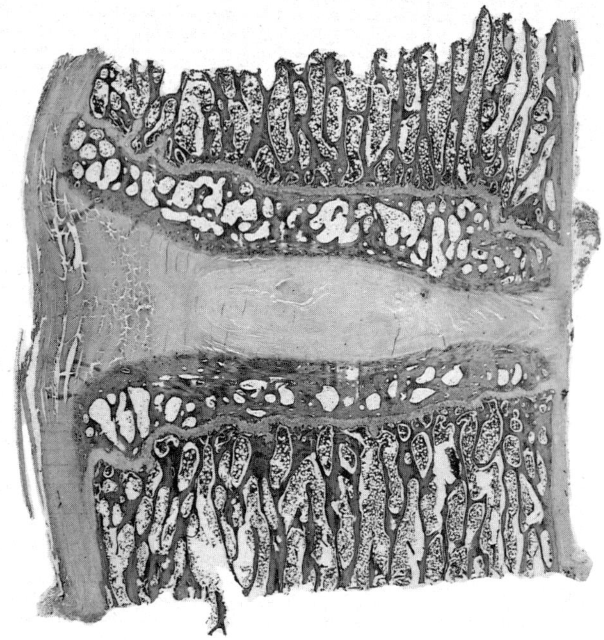

Fig. 33.2 Low-power micrograph of a sheep lumbar intervertebral disc. Normal appearance.

is extensively replaced by granulation tissue. Bacteria have generally been eradicated. In a few cases the lesion may lead to vertebral osteomyelitis.

Presentation and clinical course

Although presentation may vary, the most typical clinical feature of discitis is severe disabling back pain. Postoperative or postinjection pain persists and gradually increases in severity. The pain is usually intense, not relieved significantly by rest and only partially relieved by narcotics. Back pain is increased by movement and is associated with muscle spasm, which in the ambulating patient produces a characteristically hyperlordotic lumbar posture similar to that described in childhood discitis. Straight leg raising is generally limited on both sides by back pain. Pyrexia may be present and this has been described more commonly in association with postoperative discitis (Lindholm & Pylkkanen, 1982; Fernand & Lee, 1986). In the majority of patients with discitis following closed procedures such as discography or chemonucleolysis the patients remain afebrile. In some cases back pain may develop insidiously and may slowly subside over many months. Because of the extreme variation in the clinical presentation of patients with low back pain, and due to the recent procedure (investigative or surgical), the diagnosis of iatrogenic discitis is commonly overlooked. Hyper-reaction to operative or postinjection pain and functional overlay may be considered responsible in some patients for the exacerbation of symptoms.

The natural course of iatrogenic discitis is for slow spontaneous resolution over a period of several weeks to many months. Whilst a self-limiting infectious process is typical of discitis occasional cases have been described progressing to vertebral osteomyelitis with possible extension of the abscess to the epidural

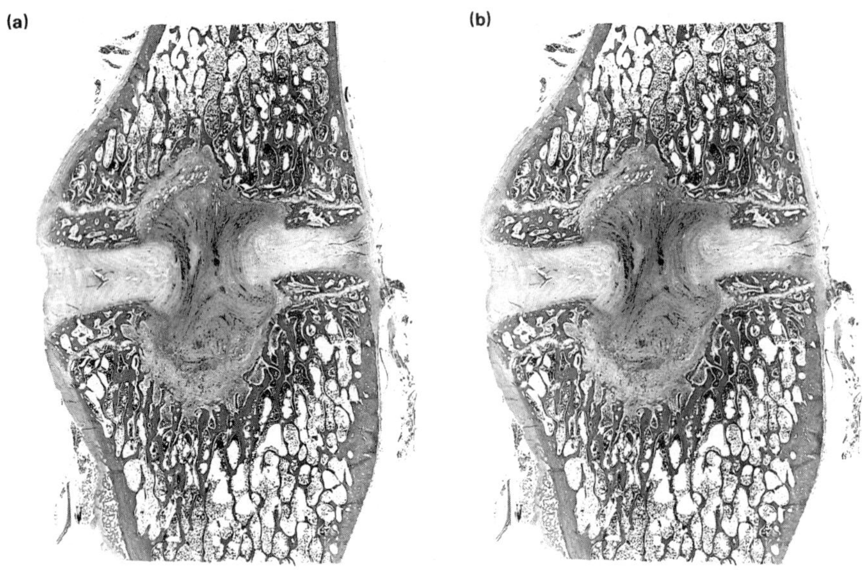

Fig. 33.3 Low-power micrograph of the lower disc shown in Fig. 33.1 (central discitis). There is extensive replacement of nuclear material by highly vascular granulation tissue.

space (H. Crock, unpublished data, 1986). Lindholm & Pilkkanen (1982), in their report on 33 patients with postoperative discitis, described an average duration of 7.4 months (range 1.5 months to 2 years). Long-term radiographic assessment revealed a spontaneous fusion at the level of discitis in approximately 50% of the cases.

Investigation

In iatrogenic discitis the erythrocyte sedimentation rate (ESR) is typically elevated, but following closed intradiscal procedures, such as discography or chemonucleolysis, it may take up to two weeks for the ESR to become significantly raised. Values as high as 90 mm/h are not uncommon.

The raised ESR is generally accompanied by a normal white cell count. Leucocytosis is more common in discitis following open procedures and is probably due to the surgical intervention. Blood cultures are frequently negative. As will be discussed in childhood discitis, according to Wenger *et al.* (1978) blood cultures may be positive only within the first six weeks after the onset of symptoms.

Plain radiographic appearance is generally normal in the early phases of the process, but narrowing of the intervertebral disc space would be evident in some cases as early as two weeks after the onset of symptoms. The narrowing which is generally marked once the process is well established is accompanied by loss of definition of the bony endplates usually seen on both sides. Vertebral body erosions related to the endplate lesion are much more difficult to appreciate on plain radiographs. Lateral tomography is invaluable in demonstrating the extent of the bony lesion (Fig. 33.4). Bony endplate erosions would generally be seen between the third and sixth week following the onset of symptoms, and their development parallels that of the animal model developed by the authors. Computerized tomographic (CT) scanning with sagittal reconstruction generally provides the same information obtained by lateral tomography.

Technetium bone scanning is of value in identifying and supporting the diagnosis of discitis following closed procedures, such as discography or chemonucleolysis, but is of less significance following surgery because of the increased uptake in the area of the operation. It must be said, however, that in our experience a minority of patients with proven discitis had negative bone scans. It would seem that magnetic resonance imaging (Mulholland *et al.*, 1986) with standard sagittal T1- and T2-weighted images is the procedure of choice for the radiographic confirmation of clinically suspected discitis. Because the process involves the bone marrow of the affected vertebra early in the course this would be clearly identified in the change of signal at MRI.

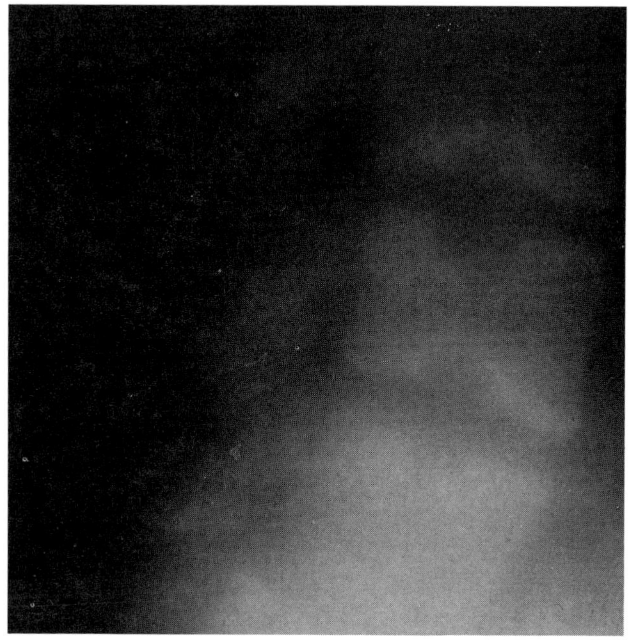

Fig. 33.4 Lateral tomography of lumbosacral spine showing bilateral endplate erosions at L4–L5 and L5–S1, consistent with central discitis. The patient had undergone discography 12 weeks prior to radiography. Plain X-ray had been reported as normal.

Treatment

Based on the results of our clinical and experimental studies it seems clear that prophylaxis is of prime importance. Great care should be taken in following a strict aseptic technique for any intradiscal procedures. Wide and thorough skin preparation with drapes firmly fixed to the patient is essential. Sedation with neuroleptic anaesthesia, to avoid sudden and uncontrolled movement of the patient, is also extremely useful to avoid contamination. A double-stilletted needle technique should be always used to avoid contamination of the disc with skin cores. The handling of needles is also of importance, as the operator should not touch the needle shaft, and in particular the tip, whilst separate needles should be used for separate skin punctures.

One of the most significant findings of our experimental study using the sheep model was the effectiveness of broad-spectrum antibiotics administered at the time of the procedure to prevent the development of discitis (Fraser *et al.*, 1989; Osti *et al.*, 1990). Multiple-level lumbar discography was carried out in nine mature sheep with radiographic contrast containing *Staphylococcus epidermidis* at various concentrations. In four animals antibiotic was added to the intradiscal suspension. In the remaining five sheep intravenous antibiotic was administered 30 min prior to the intradiscal inoculation of bacteria. At six weeks no sheep had developed any radiographic, macroscopic or histological signs of discitis with all intervertebral disc cultures being negative. In contrast with this in previous studies in which the same sheep model was employed an estimated five or more *Staphylococcus epidermidis* inoculated into lumbar intervertebral discs produced discitis with endplate erosions after two weeks in every instance.

The results obtained with the experimental model have been more recently confirmed by a prospective study (Osti *et al.*, 1990) on 127 patients undergoing lumbar discography for the investigation of low back pain. In all patients the radiographic contrast injected contained cephazolin in the concentration of 1 mg of antibiotic per 1 ml of contrast. At follow-up none of the patients developed clinical and radiographic signs consistent with the diagnosis of discitis. This is in contrast with an incidence of discitis as high as 4.9% observed in 1987 in a series of 61 consecutive patients in whom discography was performed without antibiotic by the same radiologists and using the same technique employed in the more recent study (Fraser *et al.*, 1987).

Based on the results of this study it is strongly recommended that a suitable broad-spectrum antibiotic in a single prophylactic dose should be used whenever the intervertebral disc is violated. In procedures such as discography the antibiotic can be suitably mixed with the radiographic contrast. In chemonucleolysis, however, a single intravenous dose of antibiotic at the time of the procedure is recommended.

In contrast with the effectiveness of prophylactic antibiotics, very little evidence exists to support the efficacy of antibiotics in the treatment of established discitis (Taylor & Dooley, 1978; Fraser *et al.*, 1989). Pilgaard (1969) found that antibiotics made no difference to the outcome of disc space infection following laminectomy. Gibson *et al.* (1987) failed to retrieve antibiotics from intervertebral discs of patients undergoing anterior spinal surgery following intravenous administration of high doses of cephalothin. The authors conducted a series of experiments to assess the intradiscal penetration potential of cephazolin and the effect of intravenous and intradiscal antibiotics following the inoculation of bacteria into the intervertebral disc. Six sheep had 1 g of cephazolin administered intravenously at various intervals between 30 and 120 min prior to death. At the time of death venous blood samples were obtained to determine the serum cephazolin levels. Two adjacent lumbar intervertebral discs were harvested and assayed for cephazolin content. Cephazolin could be detected in the discs of sheep killed 30 min after the administration of antibiotics, with the amount detected being approximately 1% of the serum level. No antibiotic could be detected in the sheep killed at 45, 60 and 120 min. In a separate experiment (Fraser *et al.*, 1989) intravenous cephazolin was administered 30 min prior to bacterial inoculation in 46 discs of nine sheep. In five animals the bacterial suspension contained radiographic contrast and in four sheep it contained reconstituted chymopapain. No evidence of discitis was found at any level, six weeks later, at post-mortem.

In an experiment to evaluate the therapeutic effect of antibiotics eight sheep were treated with intravenous cephazolin, commencing one, two and three weeks following bacterial intradiscal inoculation and for periods up to 21 days. All inoculated discs developed discitis and the lesions appeared to be similar, irrespective of time interval between inoculation and the commencement, duration and dosage of antibiotic therapy. In an additional three sheep intravenous antibiotics were commenced one, two and three days after intradiscal inoculation of bacteria. As in the previous group all discs developed discitis. These studies support the use of a suitable broad-spectrum antibiotic during any surgical procedure which invades the intervertebral disc. Antibiotics, however, are unable to arrest the progression of discitis once the condition is established. Where iatrogenic discitis leads to secondary vertebral osteomyelitis, however, antibiotics may have a therapeutic role, although this is not proven. It is because of this that an attempt at an early stage to isolate the bacteria by blood cultures and needle biopsy of the affected discs would seem reasonable in order to prescribe the appropriate antibiotic.

Symptomatic treatment comprises the use of plaster casts or polypropylene spinal jackets. External support may need to be prolonged for up to six months. Some authors have reported good relief of pain by injecting the affected disc with steroids (Crock, 1983). Because of the initiating role of bacteria, steroids should be considered only in the late phase of the process when both the clinical picture and radiographic finding would exclude the presence of active infection.

Discitis should be considered in broad terms as a self-contained and slowly resolving process, and the therapeutic approach should therefore be along conservative lines. In cases of persistent severe pain, however, which does not respond to appropriate vigorous conservative measures, surgical anterior disc clearance and interbody fusion may be considered.

If patients with disabling low back pain investigated by discography as part of a preoperative work-up develop discitis at either an abnormal and typically symptomatic level or at an adjacent disc it may be appropriate to treat the patient by anterior disc clearance and interbody fusion once the diagnosis has been confirmed, rather than wait for the natural resolution of the symptoms which in most cases would at best only return the patient to his preinjection status.

In view of the long-term disability reported by Lindholm & Pilkkanen (1982) with discitis following surgery, with a majority of patients still complaining of disabling back symptoms at an average follow-up of 7.5 years, anterior disc clearance and interbody fusion would have to be considered as an option of management if little or no relief of symptoms follows appropriate conservative measures.

CHILDHOOD DISCITIS

Childhood discitis has traditionally been labelled as a benign disease of unknown aetiology characterized by back pain, intervertebral disc space narrowing as seen on plain X-rays and resolution of symptoms with rest. Although no definite figures are available, based on the review of the literature it appears that this condition should be regarded as uncommon. In the series reported by Menelaus (1964) from the Children's Hospital in Melbourne, 35 children were included during a 16-year period. In 1978 Wenger *et al.* reported on 41 children admitted to the Hospital for Sick Children in Toronto with the diagnosis of discitis in a 24-year period (1950–74). Spiegel *et al.* (1972) reported on 48 children with the diagnosis of discitis admitted to the Children's Hospital of Los Angeles between 1951 and 1970.

Clinical picture

The age at onset ranges in the various reports (Menelaus, 1964; Smith & Taylor, 1967; Spiegel *et al.*, 1972; Wenger *et al.*, 1978) between six months and 15 years, with the average age varying between three and seven years. In children who are able to communicate, the commonest complaint is back pain which sometimes radiates to the buttocks and the thighs. Parents of very young children may observe that the child shows difficulty in sitting up or walking. In a minority of children the onset of back pain is associated with or preceded by fever, malaise or more specific complaints such as tonsillitis or respiratory tract infection. Trauma seems to be a very uncommon feature of the patient's history.

On examination significant limitation of motion of the back is usually noticed with, typically, in the case of a lesion in the thoracolumbar or upper lumbar spine, a hyperlordotic posture and severe muscle spasm. Straight leg raising may reveal marked hamstring spasm.

Investigative procedures

The ESR is generally elevated, with the highest values recorded in Menelaus' series of 58 mm in the first hour. White cell count may be normal but in a minority of patients is raised. Blood cultures in the series from Wenger *et al.* (1978) were positive in 10 of 22 patients. Based on Wenger *et al.*'s series it would appear that after six weeks from the onset of symptoms organisms are not isolated from blood cultures. Needle biopsies lead to a bacteriological diagnosis only in a minority of patients. Due to the rapid destruction of bacteria in the intervertebral disc once the endplates are breeched, only in the first few weeks of the process would isolation of organisms from intervertebral disc tissue be likely. Other serological tests are almost invariably negative.

The radiographic appearance at onset may be considered normal. According to Menelaus (1964), initial intervertebral disc narrowing can be seen as early as three weeks. The development of discitis follows the pattern seen in our animal model with progressive endplate lesions and marked erosion into the vertebral body as seen with tomography (Figs 33.5–33.7). In the Menelaus series progressive narrowing occurred in just over half of the patients. Only three of the 27 children included in his series showed clear evidence of bony fusion at the time of follow-up. In the remaining patients Menelaus often observed very little residual disc narrowing. CT scanning with sagittal reconstruction confirms the finding at tomography with visualization of the vertebral body erosions which are not appreicated on plain X-rays. As mentioned earlier MRI (T1- and T2-weighted images) is becoming the investigation of choice whenever discitis is suspected (Mulholland *et al.*, 1986). Based on the pathological sequence of changes it is postulated that an abnormal signal from the bone marrow adjacent to the endplate of the disc affected would be appreciated before intervertebral disc narrowing occurs.

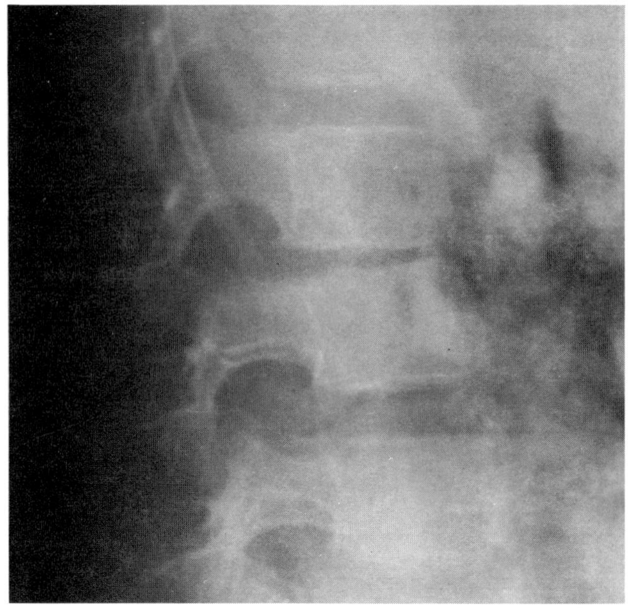

Fig. 33.5 Lateral radiograph of a six-year-old girl investigated for back pain. There is narrowing at the L2–L3 intervertebral disc space. Courtesy of Dr Lloyd Morris, Adelaide Children's Hospital.

Principles of treatment

Uniform agreement exists on the need for rest as the main modality of treatment. According to Menelaus (1964) rest in bed should continue until there is no pain or limitation of movement, and until the ESR is normal. His experience showed that when these guidelines were not followed readmission and a further period of bed rest was always necessary. Other authors after an initial period of bed rest would allow earlier mobilization with external support (TLSO brace).

The role of antibiotics is still quite controversial. Menelaus reserved antibiotic treatment only for children with pyrexia. Wenger *et al.* (1978) advocated early antibiotic treatment and stated that this, despite negative blood cultures, usually resulted in rapid decrease of symptoms within two to three days. In their series intravenous antibiotics were continued until the patient was ambulating and comfortable. This was followed by an oral antibiotic regime for an additional three-week period. Because of the striking similarities existing between childhood discitis and iatrogenic discitis after closed intradiscal contamination, it would seem that the rationale of antibiotic treatment could at least be questioned. However, in the presence of positive

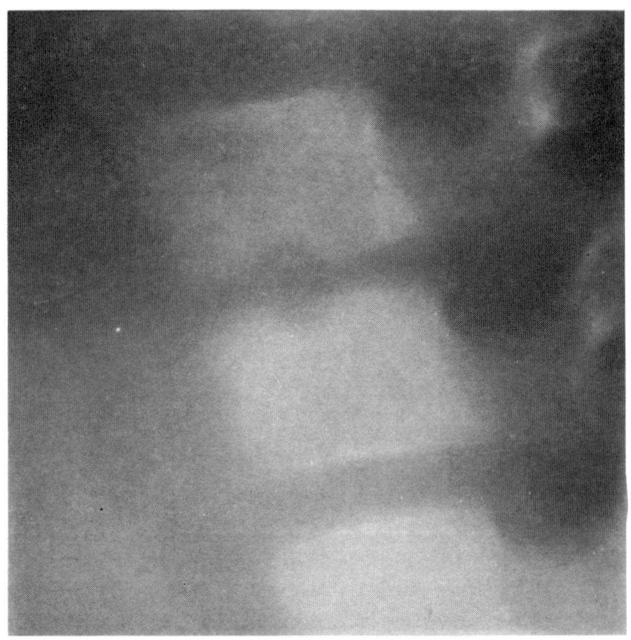

Fig. 33.6 Lateral tomograms in the same patient as Fig. 33.5, showing bilateral endplate erosions of L2–L3 consistent with central discitis. Cultures from specimen obtained by needle biopsy were negative. Courtesy of Dr Lloyd Morris, Adelaide Children's Hospital.

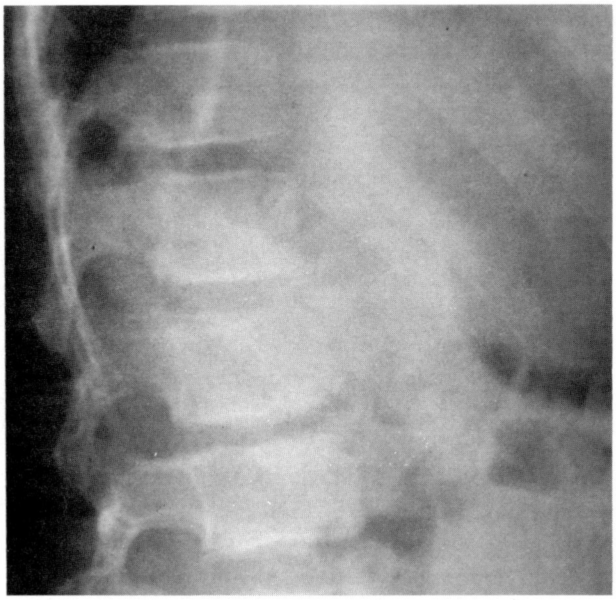

Fig. 33.7 The same patient two years later. There has been no further narrowing of the intervertebral disc space. Some sclerosis of the mid and anterior part of the endplates bilaterally is evident, accompanied by erosions of the anterior corners of the upper and lower endplate of L2–L3. The patient is asymptomatic. Courtesy of Dr Lloyd Morris, Adelaide Children's Hospital.

blood cultures, or isolation of bacteria from needle biopsy of the affected intervertebral disc and when the radiographic features indicate progressive destructive changes of the vertebral body, antibiotic treatment should be considered mandatory to limit the extent of secondary spinal osteomyelitis. However, progressive vertebral destruction is most uncommon in children and epidural extension is extremely rare.

SUMMARY

The term discitis should be reserved only for primary intervertebral disc infection which in the adult is invariably iatrogenic. The condition is due to bacterial contamination of the intervertebral disc, with *Staphylococcus aureus* the most likely organism responsible. Typically discitis is a self-contained and naturally resolving condition that, however, may run a prolonged course. Whilst plain X-rays and bone scans are useful lateral tomography and MRI scans are the investigations of choice. Needle biopsies are seldom successful in identifying the responsible organism. Principles of treatment comprise bed rest and external support. It is debatable whether appropriate intravenous antibiotics in the absence of secondary osteomyelitis would be of any value. Because of the limitations of treatment every attempt should be made to prevent this highly disabling condition by strict aseptic technique and by the administration of prophylactic antibiotics whenever the intervertebral disc is violated.

REFERENCES

Agre, K., Wilson, R.R., Brim, M. & McDermot, D.J. (1984) Chymodiactin: post-marketing surveillance: demographic and adverse experience data in 29,075 patients. *Spine*, **9**, 479–485.

Brodsky, A.E. & Binder, W.F. (1979) Lumbar discography—its value in diagnosis and treatment of lumbar disc lesions. *Spine*, **4**, 110–120.

Collis, J.S. & Gardner, W.J. (1962) Lumbar discography: an analysis of one thousand cases. *J. Neurosurg.*, **19**, 452–461.

Crock, H.V. (1983) *Practice of Spinal Surgery*. Springer-Verlag, Vienna.

Fernand, R. & Lee, C.K. (1986) Post laminectomy disc space infection: a review of the literature and a report of three cases. *Clin. Orthop. Rel. Res.*, **209**, 215–218.

Fraser, R.D. (1984) Chymopapain for the treatment of intervertebral disc herniation: the final report of a double-blind study. *Spine*, **9**, 815–818.

Fraser, R.D., Osti, O.L. & Vernon-Roberts, B. (1986) Discitis following chemonucleolysis: an experimental study. *Spine*, **11**, 34–43.

Fraser, R.D., Osti, O.L. & Vernon-Roberts, B. (1987) Discitis after discography. J. *Bone Jt. Surg.*, **69B**, 26–35.

Fraser, R.D., Osti, O.L., and Vernon-Roberts, B. (1989) Iatrogenic discitis: the role of prophylactic antibiotics in prevention and treatment. *Spine*, **14**, 1025–1032.

Gibson, M.J., Karpinsky, M.R.K., Slack, R.C.B., Cowlishaw, W.A., & Webb, J.K. (1987) The penetration of antibiotics into the normal intervertebral disc. *J. Bone Jt. Surg.*, **69B**, 784–786

Graf, R., Reinhardt, H. & Gratzl, O. (1984) Prolapses in adolescents of lumbar intervertebral discs: I—Clinical observations. *Neurochirurgia*, **27**, 12–15.

Gresham, J.L. & Miller, R. (1969) Evaluation of the lumbar spine by discography and its use in selection of proper treatment of the herniated disc syndrome. *Clin. Orthop. Rel. Res.*, **69**, 29–41.

Kho, H.C.H. & Steudel, W.I. (1986) Comparison between lumbar microdiscectomy and standard discectomy in lumbar disc herniations: a retrospective analysis of 267 cases. *Neurochirurgia*, **29**, 181–185.

Kirkaldy-Willis, W.H. (1983) Complications of disc surgery—discitis. *Orthop. Trans.*, **7**, 110.

Lindholm, T.S. & Pylkkanen, P. (1982) Discitis following removal of intervertebral disc. *Spine*, **7**, 618–622.

Massie, W.K. & Stevens, D.B. (1967) A critical evaluation of discography. *J. Bone Jt. Surg.*, **49A**, 1243–1244.

McCulloch, J.A. (1977) Chemonucleolysis. *J. Bone Jt. Surg.*, **59B**, 45–52.

McCulloch, J.A. (1980) Chemonucleolysis: experience with 2,000 cases. *Clin. Orthop.*, **146**, 128–135.

McCulloch, J.A. & MacNab, I. (1983) *Sciatica and Chymopapain*, p. 203. Williams & Wilkins, Baltimore, MD.

McCulloch, J.A. & Waddell, G. (1978) Lateral lumbar discography. *Br. J. Radiol.*, **51**, 498–502.

Menelaus, M. Discitis. *J. Bone Jt. Surg.*, **46B**, 16–23.

Mulholland, R., Gibson, M., Buckley, J. & Worthington, B. (1986) The changes in the intervertebral disc after chemonucleolysis shown by MRI. Presented at the Annual Meeting of the International Society for the Study of the Lumbar Spine, Dallas, 28 May–2 June.

Osti, O.L., Fraser, R.D. & Vernon-Roberts, B. (1990) Discitis after discography: the role of prophylactic antibiotics. *J. Bone Jt. Surg.*, **72B**, 271–274.

Pilgaard, S. (1969) Discitis (closed space infection) following removal of intervertebral disc. *J. Bone Jt. Surg.*, **51A**, 713–716.

Ryan, M.D. & Taylor, T.K.F. (1987) Septic discitis—a misnomer. *Med. J. Austral.*, **147**, 415.

Schmorl, G. & Junghanns, H. (1971) *The Human Spine in Health and Disease*, 2nd US edn. transl. by E.F. Besemann. Grune & Stratton, New York.

Simmon, E.H. & Segil, C.M. (1975) An evaluation of discography in the localization of symptomatic levels in discogenic disease of the spine. *Clin. Orthop.*, **108**, 57–69.

Smith, R.F. & Taylor, T.K.F.C. (1967) Inflammatory lesions of intervertebral discs in children. *J. Bone Jt. Surg.*, **49A**, 1508–1520.

Spiegel, P.G., Kengla, K.W., Isaacson, A.S. & Wilson, J.C. (1972) Intervertebral disc-space inflammation in children. *J. Bone Jt. Surg.*, **54A**, 284–296.

Taylor, T.K.F. & Dooley, B.J. (1978) Antibiotics in the management of post-operative disc space infections. *Austr. N.Z. J. Surg.*, **48**, 76–77.

Wenger, D.R., Bobechko, W.P. & Gilday, D.L. (1978) The spectrum of intervertebal disc-space infection in children. *J. Bone Jt. Surg.*, **60A**, 100–108.

Wiltse, L.L., Widell, E.H. & Yuan, H.L. (1975) Chymopapain chemonucleolysis in lumbar disc disease. *J. Am. Med. Assoc.*, **231**, 474–479.

34 · Parasitic Infections of the Spine

By V. CHACKO

Parasitic infestation of the human body in endemic areas is common. However, involvement of the skeletal system is rare. In the present era of migrating populations one should not be surprised to see a suspected spinal tumour, turning out to be cord compression due to any of the parasitic diseases such as hydatid cyst or the Guinea-worm abscess. Suspicion of human spinal parasitic infestation is based upon probable epidemiological exposure, although this may have been several years prior to onset of symptoms. The commonest infestation of the skeletal system is by *Echinococcus*, which produces hydatid disease. Such infections represent focal lesions of a more generalized disease and may present with one or more focal lesions in the spine producing spinal cord compression. These include:

1 Larval cestodes

(a) *Echinococcus* (hydatid)

(b) Cysticercosis (*Taenia solium*)

(c) *Multiceps* (coenurus).

The most common among these is hydatid disease affecting the vertebral body and causing cord compression. Cysticercosis usually presents with focal epilepsy but cord compression can occur.

2 Ectopic trematodes

(a) *Paragonimus*

(b) *Schistosoma*

Schistosoma haematobium and *S. mansoni* localize in the lower part of the spinal cord or cauda equina, causing transverse myelitis. This area is reached through paravertebral veins. *Heterophyes* and *Fasciola hepatica* are very rarely found in the spinal cord.

3 Migrating nematodes

(a) *Loa*

(b) *Gnathostoma*

(c) *Dracunculus medinensis* (Guinea-worm).

Gnathostoma larvae produce injurious tracts in neuronal tissue and the spinal cord is sometimes affected. *Loa loa* (microfilaria) are confined mostly to the brain. *Dracunculus medinensis* or Guinea-worm is another rare cause of paraplegia.

4 Protozoa

(a) *Entamoeba histolytica*

(b) Toxoplasmosis.

Amoebae, though very common pathogens, rarely produce cerebral abscesses. Spinal cord involvement is unreported, but possible. Toxoplasmosis is another infestation mainly confined to the brain.

The rarity of these conditions make parasitic infestations of the spine a presumptive diagnosis prior to surgery. Most infestations of the bone are slow-growing, produce very little inflammatory reaction and hence remain painless before much or all of the vertebral body is involved. A collapse of the vertebra or a pathological fracture of the bone unmasks the lesion. The morbidity of parasitic infestation is compounded by the late diagnosis. It is often complicated by secondary infection leading to chronic sinuses. Extirpation is often incomplete and difficult. Fatal anaphylaxis, especially with hydatid disease, can occur.

This chapter is compiled on the basis of case reports and experiences of several authors derived from the treatment of over 60 cases of hydatid disease of the spine, four cases of Guinea-worm abscesses causing cord compression, one of spinal cysticercosis and 20 cases of bilharzial paraplegia.

HYDATID DISEASE OF THE SPINE

The larval forms of *Echinococcus* infest the spine. Hydatid disease—though common among the sheep-rearing community in Australia, New Zealand, parts of India such as Kurnool and Punjab—is however ubiquitous. About 0.5–2% of all hydatid disease involves bone; 50% of the patients who have skeletal disease have spinal involvement.

Parasitology

Hydatid disease is caused by a cestode, *Echinococcus granulosus*, which requires a carnivorous and a herbivorous mammal to complete its life cycle. The adult worms inhabit the small intestine of the dog, and the ova are shed in its excreta. The ova when swallowed by sheep, cattle, swine, goats, camels, horses or humans, enter the portal venous system and are filtered first by the liver (75%) and next by the lung (15%); only 10% has any chance of dissemination beyond that. Bone may be infected either through the arterial route, after passing through the liver and lung, or through protovertebral venous shunts. Cysts are formed in various parts of the body, containing worm heads or scolices which proliferate. When they are swallowed by dogs the adult worm develops and the cycle is completed.

Pathology

Hydatid infestation of bone is nearly always primary. Secondary erosion from surrounding soft tissue may, however, occur. Growth of the scolex in the bone is slow. The slow growth and the small cysts produced are due to the resistance of the bone to the growth of the parasite. The cyst wall is made up of a laminated membrane which insinuates itself between trabeculae, but may slowly erode through the cortex into surrounding tissues. Larger cysts then form. Pathological fractures are common. Rupture of a cyst into muscular tissue is followed by a crop of secondary hydatid cysts originating from daughter cysts, scolices and brood capsules.

Owing to the peculiar structure and the resistant nature of bone, true hydatid disease in bone differs from hydatid disease elsewhere in two respects, namely exogenous vesiculation occurs and there is no adventitious layer, the ectocyst. As the embryo grows, bony resorption occurs very slowly. The parasite grows along the line of least resistance, along bony canals, to form a diverticulated type of cyst. The diverticula may become separated from the parent cyst—the so-called 'beading-off' of secondary cysts. When the cysts occur in or near the vertebral column the spinal cord may be compressed either by a cyst whose primary situation is in the spinal canal or by cysts arising from primary disease of the vertebrae or paraspinal tissues which have secondarily invaded the extradural space.

It is to be noted that, unlike cysticercosis, only one larva undergoes expansion into a hydatid cyst and daughter cysts form within (Fig. 34.1). The lack of inflammatory reaction is also quite characteristic.

Five types of hydatid disease of the spine have been recognized (Mills, 1956).

1 Primary cyst in the spinal cord: no cases have been reported though it is theoretically possible.

2 Intradural cyst: though primary cysts are rare, secondary cysts can occur and are common.

3 Extradural cyst: the primary cyst originates in the loose areolar extradural tissue and elongates by expansion upwards and downwards.

4 Hydatid disease of the vertebra: this is the commonest form of hydatid disease causing paraplegia. The disease may begin in the body, pedicle or lamina, and spreads in cancellous tissue. It may remain stationary, but eventually extraosseous extension into paravertebral muscles and extradural space gives rise to cord compression.

5 Paravertebral hydatid: extending into the spinal canal. The cyst which is primarily in the mediastinum, retroperitoneal tissues, or paraspinal muscles may erode vertebrae by pressure or may extend and rupture into extradural tissues through intervertebral foramina. The theoretical consideration of whether the extradural lesion is primary or secondary can be

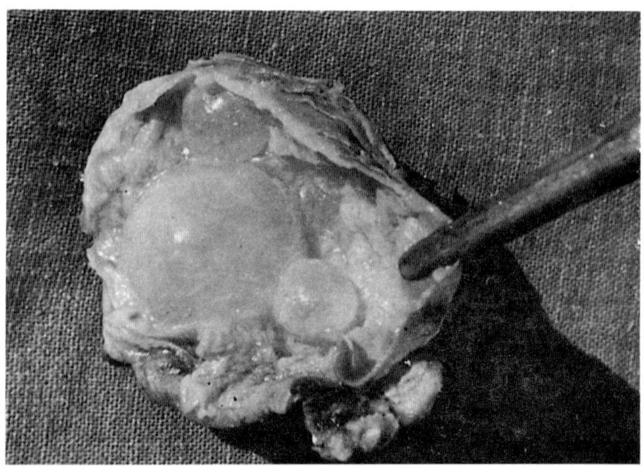

Fig. 34.1 Excised hydatid cyst of the spine showing the daughter cysts.

resolved by the size and position of the cyst and the time of onset of symptoms compared to the onset of neurological deficit.

Clinical features

Hydatid disease of the spine has an indolent course with infection often occurring in early childhood, but presenting in adults. The slow progress of the lesion precludes any major symptoms except pain and stiffness of the back. The dorsal spine is most commonly involved. The increasing severity of the pain and progressive paravertebral swelling denotes extension of the lesion. Paraplegia of varying degrees of severity may sometimes be the presenting feature. The paravertebral swelling itself is non-tender, fluctuant and a characteristic thrill may be present.

Investigation

In early stages a cystic area may arouse suspicion of a primary or secondary neoplasm. Angiomas, aneurysmal bone cyst, giant-cell tumour, fibrous dysplasia and tuberculosis of the spine form the differential diagnosis.

In late stages the areas of translucency in the affected vertebrae are partly masked by reactive sclerosis. Following a break in the cortex the paraspinal extension presents as soft tissue shadow, so-called 'ossifluent abscess' (Bellini, 1946) (Fig. 34.2). The heads of the adjacent ribs may be involved. Oblique views may show involvement of laminae—an important differentiating point from tuberculosis, besides the preservation of the intervertebral disc space unless secondary infection takes place. It is more difficult to differentiate hydatid cyst from plasmacytoma, which is very similar in gross appearance except that no marginal sclerosis is seen in plasmacytoma. Lung involvement and the presence of rounded transluscent shadows practically confirm hydatid disease.

Haematological assessment reveals an eosinophilia of around 25% as seen in all parasitic infestation. The Casoni test is an immediate hypersensitivity skin test. Intradermal injection of 0.2 ml of a fresh sterile hydatid fluid (sterilized by Seitz filter) produces, within half an hour, in all positive cases, a large wheal (5 cm in diameter) with multiple pseudopodia; it fades within an hour. Sterile normal saline, 0.2 ml, is injected in the other arm for control. It is now considered that the complement fixation test is more specific and sensitive. Other diagnostic methods include: flocculation test, indirect flourescent antibody test and immunoelectrophoresis.

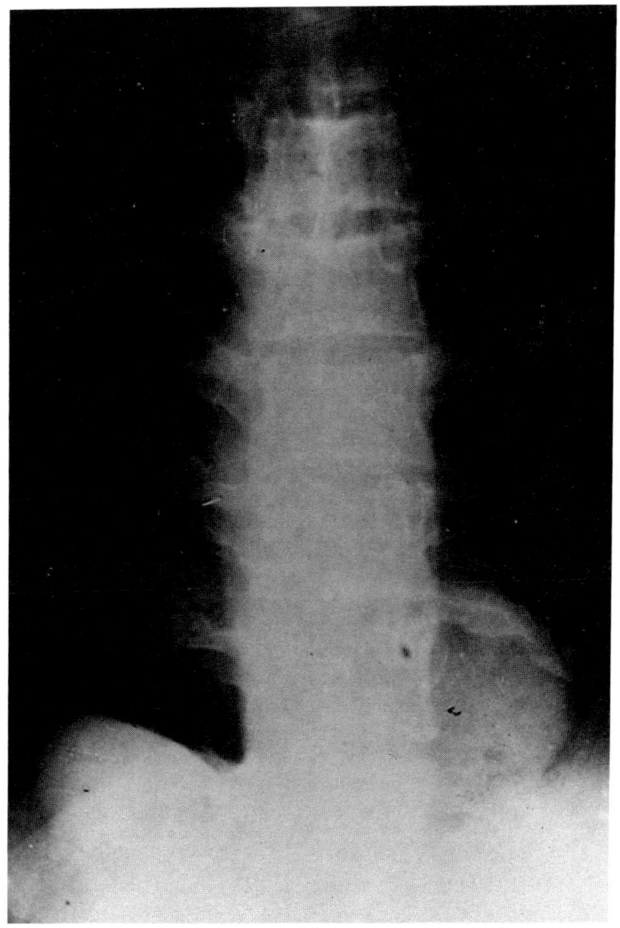

Fig. 34.2 Involvement of L4–L5 vertebrae with paravertebral shadow—'ossifluent abscess'.

Aspiration of the cyst will reveal the presence of scolices and is diagnostic. Great caution should be taken while aspirating. Rupture of the cyst or spillage leading to anaphylactic shock should always be anticipated, and should be urgently treated.

Early diagnosis has been helped by the use of computerized axial tomography. The cystic changes are visualized as irregular erosion of spongy bone. The margins of the lesion may be well defined in some and not so well defined in others, and they reflect the multivesicular infiltration of bone. The cortex may be eroded but no subperiosteal reaction or bony enlargement of the vertebra is seen. In late cases the whole vertebral body itself may be replaced by a soft tissue parasitic mass. Cysts in the spinal canal can be visualized, but it can be difficult to differentiate extradural from intradural pathology. The paraspinal extensions are, however, well visualized. The cysts show up as hypodense or isodense areas with a hyperdense margin.

Magnetic resonance imaging delineates compression of the spinal cord at different levels, and the extent of the lesion is mapped out more accurately than with computerized axial tomography.

Treatment

Though no chemotherapeutic agent has yet taken the place of surgery, as an adjuvant, mebendazole (a benzimidazole derivative) in high doses of up to 4.5 g/day for three weeks combined with surgical extirpation has given good results in selected cases. Complete surgical extirpation is, however, curative. Curettage and formalization and deep X-ray therapy are ineffective, when symptoms of vertebral disease occur, extraosseous extension has usually taken place and eradication is more difficult. Anterior destruction of the vertebral body leads to progressive kyphosis, instability and neurological deficit.

Extraspinal cysts should be dealt with by radical excision, and the cavities swabbed out with 5% formalin to kill any live parasitic tissue. However, as formalin cannot be used on neural tissue, 20% hypertonic saline has been used as a scolicide with variable results. Efficacy of the action of scolicides can be expected to occur only when there has been free opening-up of the primary bony foci.

Case reports

A few illustrative case reports bring out salient points in diagnosis and treatment.

1 *Pritam Das of Lucknow, India (1957) reported on a 28-year-old male presenting with difficulty in micturition and defaecation for nine months. Progressive loss of sensation and weakness of both lower limbs was present, resulting in an incomplete paraparesis. X-ray had shown laminar erosion of L5 and deficient upper sacrum.*

Multiple laminectomies L3–L4 and L5, done initially, had to be extended since the subdural cysts had extended up to D5. A suction catheter was used to evacuate the cysts. The primary cysts were found in the presacral space, several cysts had ruptured and the patient developed anaphylaxis. No improvement of neurological deficit was noted even after six months. In this report several points of interest are to be noted.

(a) The presacral lesion can only have occurred with rupture or spillage from a liver lesion which the patient probably had.

(b) The high level to which the hydatid had ascended was due either to proliferation and pressure from below or to repeated ruptures.

(c) Anaphylactic shock, a complication, has always to be anticipated.

A preoperative diagnosis was not made as a rectal examination was not done and a degree of suspicion was missing.

2 *Ramana Rao of Kurnool, India (personal communication, 1988) reports on a 15-year-old female patient who had symptoms for one year and paraplegia for six months. She had received antituberculous treatment for nine months. Examination showed a kyphos at D9 with X-rays revealing destruction of D9 with a paravertebral soft tissue shadow. She had a complete spastic paraplegia.*

With a presumptive diagnosis of Pott's paraplegia, an anterior decompression was performed. At surgery the typical hydatid cysts were found and excised. Oral mebendazole therapy for three weeks was added. Computerized axial tomography done later showed extension of the lesion (Fig. 34.3). The patient succumbed six months later.

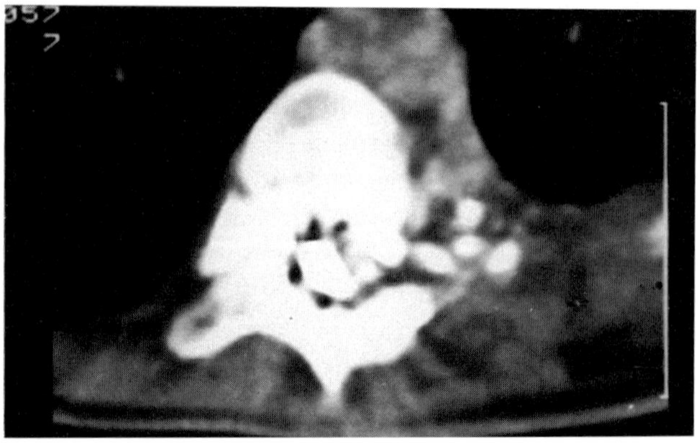

Fig. 34.3 CT scan of the spine showing the involvement of the pedicle, part of the body and the paravertebral extension.

3 *Hakim, of Bombay (1988) (personal communication) reports on a 30-year-old farmer with symptoms of backache for 10 months and paraplegia of three months duration. A soft paravertebral swelling at D9–D10 was found. Erosion of D10 body with involvement also of the 10th rib was noted (Figs 34.4 & 34.5). The cyst was excised along with a pedicle and the rib. A recurrence required further surgery. Despite this, the neurological status improved only marginally.*

The last two cases highlight the difficulties of complete extirpation and hence poor prognosis.

Adequate treatment requires extensive debridement of the necrotic material by anterior and posterior routes if necessary. Laminectomy may give transient relief of symptoms; however, it causes an increase in the kyphotic deformity and progressive neurological impairment.

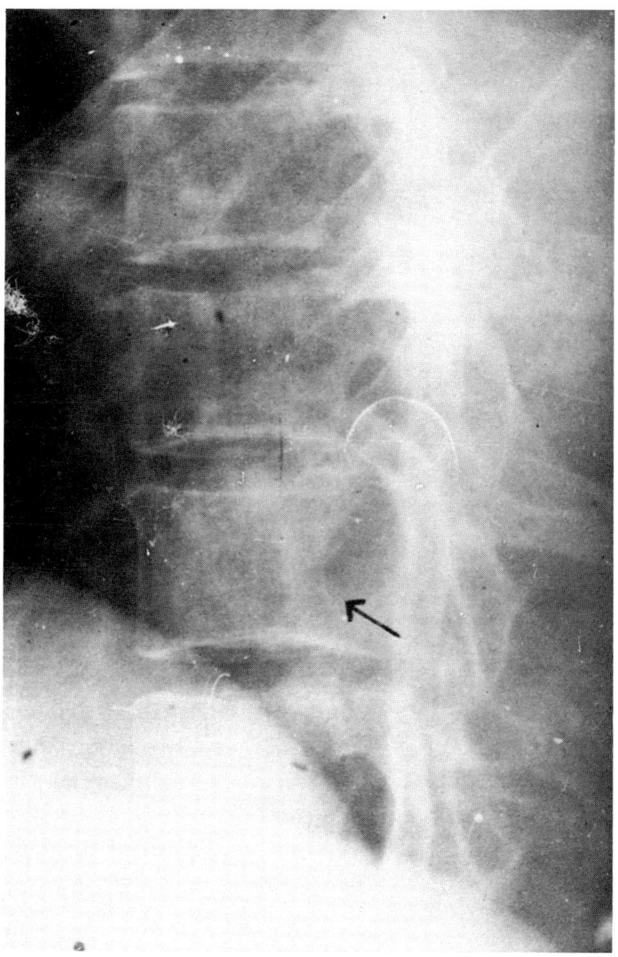

Fig. 34.4 X-ray showing the extraosseous extension of the cyst into the spinal canal.

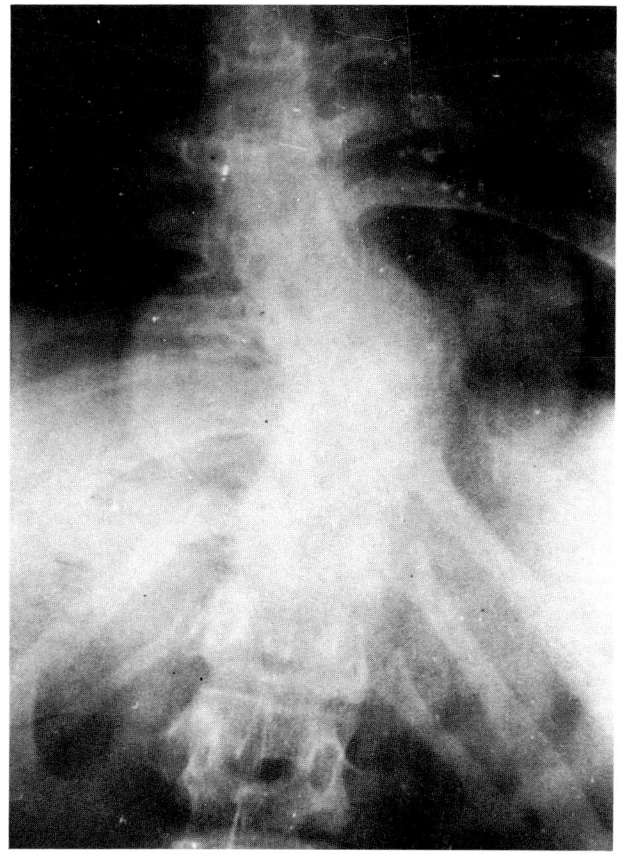

Fig. 34.5 X-ray showing involvement of D9 and D10 showing the scoliotic deformity and paravertebral abscess.

Duran (1978) was the first to report use of Harrington instrumentation in the treatment of spinal hydatid with instability.

Hodgson & Stock (1956) demonstrated the value of anterior decompression in the management of tuberculosis as it allows direct visualization of the pathology and an opportunity to exercise the diseased vertebra and decompress the cord. It is equally useful in hydatid disease.

Anterior spinal distraction devices and the use of fibular strut grafting obviates the need for subsequent surgery to correct kyphotic deformity.

The role of high-dose mebendazole for up to two months, starting before and continued after surgery, has recently been found to be effective (Fiennes & Thomas, 1982). This drug has been found to be lethal on secondary cysts. The drug may have more of a preventive role rather than curative effect in humans. Acute allergic phenomena and early recurrence are prevented. Thus mebendazole and surgery really play complementary roles.

The surgical principles involved in the management of hydatid disease of the spine were summarized by Dott in 1955.

1 A high degree of suspicion is essential in the diagnosis; no test gives conclusive proof of diagnosis.

2 Knowledge of gross pathology to recognize the disease at surgery is vital.

3 Careful draping: gentle and meticulous removal of cysts; judicious use of suction to prevent dissemination is imperative.

4 Careful and prolonged follow-up is essential to monitor evidence of hydatids developing elsewhere.

Review of the case reports from various parts of the world gives, in general, a poor prognosis for vertebral disease. Early radical excision combined with mebendazole therapy has given encouraging results in recent times. However, paraplegia recovers incompletely, slowly, or not at all. Epidural disease has a better prognosis as removal of the cysts in the loose areolar tissue is easy and vertebral erosion and invasion less common. Early vertebral drainage prevents extension to soft tissues and skin. Should a sinus form it avoids compression of the spinal cord but secondary staphylococcal osteomyelitis is inevitable. Nevertheless the sclerosis which follows makes further surgery safer (Fitzpatrick & Hamilton, 1965).

BILHARZIAL PARAPLEGIA

Involvement of the spinal cord is very uncommon. Some cases have been reported occasionally in the literature (Gamac & deSa, 1946, Pepler & Lombaard, 1956).

Between 1890 and 1952 12 cases with cord involvement had been reported. Six of these were caused by *Schistosoma haematobium*, five by *Schistosoma mansoni* and one by *Schistosoma japonicum*. Barnett (1965) found only 15 histologically proven cases of paraplegia due to bilharziasis. Bird (1965) reported eight cases which he treated in two years; three of these were proved histologically at operation.

Three types of spinal complication are described. Firstly, transverse myelitis, as in the cases reported by Abott & Spencer (1953) and Hutton & Holland (1960). Some of these were proved only at necropsy. Secondly, a bilharzial granuloma with compression of the cord was described by Gamac & deSa (1946), Ross *et al.* (1952) and Pepler & Lombaard (1956). Some of these cases were proved by biopsy. The third possible type is radiculitis affecting chiefly the cauda equina, as suggested by Bird (1964, 1965). Bird proved the disease histologically at operation: bilharzial ova were found in the centre of necrotic and cellular areas in the cord, roots and meninges. *Schistosoma haematobium* tends to produce diffuse lesions, while *Schistosoma mansoni* tends to produce a localized granuloma and shows an obstructive lesion on myelography (Hutton & Holland, 1960).

The route of infection is not certain. The adult worm is believed to gain access to the spinal canal through branches of pelvic veins, which anastomose with the vertebral venous plexus (Barnett, 1965). The possibility of the ova being disseminated as arterial emboli from a gravid worm after reaching the pulmonary blood stream is only speculation (Bird, 1964, 1965).

In all cases in which the diagnosis was confirmed by histological examination the paraplegia affected the lower thoracic or upper lumbar segments. Eight out of the 10 patients of whom details were given had abnormalities in the cerebrospinal fluid (CSF), ranging from a mild pleocytosis to a markedly elevated CSF protein. However, the complement fixation test is probably the most reliable diagnostic test for bilharziasis.

In endemic areas bilharziasis has to be considered as a possible diagnosis in cases of paraplegia of rapid onset with severe sensory and sphincteric disturbances affecting the lower thoracic and lumbar levels.

Treatment

The larval stages are not affected by antimony preparations. Only the worms are destroyed by these. Treatment is begun four to six weeks after infestation is suspected. This is indicated by generalized itching over the body, i.e. 'swimmer's itch'. Antimony preparations prevent the further production of ova. Spontaneous clinical improvement may occur as the inflammatory process subsides. Steroids are usually advisable in cases with neurological symptoms, to counteract the inflammatory reaction and to minimize the chance of side-reactions to antimony compounds (Bird, 1964, 1965).

The following drugs have also been found useful: tartar emetic (potassium antimonyl tartarate); a freshly prepared 1% solution of 8 mg in 10 cm^2 normal saline or 5% glucose is administered intravenously three times a week for three weeks. Fouadin (stibophen or neo-antimosan)—4 cm^3 of a 6.3% sterile isotonic solution which is injected three times a week for six weeks.

SPINAL CYSTICERCOSIS WITH PARAPLEGIA

Involvement of the brain and meninges is far more common than involvement of the spinal cord. The rarity of involvement of the spinal cord is stressed by the fact that Dixon & Lipscomb (quoted by Aggarwal & Singh, 1962) found that only one out of 450 cases of cysticercosis showed progressive tetraparesis as a result of spinal cord involvement. Paraplegia is extremely rare, and is likely to be missed unless calcification of cysticercosis meningeal cysts is found on routine radiological examination.

Treatment requires the radical excision of the cysts allowing decompression of the spinal cord. Corticosteroid medication intraoperatively prevents adverse reactions if the cyst ruptures during the operation.

GUINEA-WORM ABSCESS OF SPINE

Dracunculus medinensis is a freshwater migrating nematode seen in Rajasthan and the eastern coast of India. Spinal compression caused by a Guinea-worm abscess is also very rare; only four cases have been reported. The nematode causes a granulomatous lesion, which is highly vascular. Greenish-yellow pus is seen if it is an abscess due to Guinea-worm. The abscess wall on histopathology shows fibrofatty tissue with round-cell infiltration and foci of calcification. Myelomalacia at the site of compression may be the reason for absence of motor recovery following treatment. Radical excision and decompression of the spinal cord is treatment of choice.

Case report

James & Thomas, of Miraj, India (1961) reported on a 35-year-old male presenting with pain and stiffness of the neck of four months duration. Weakness of right upper limb developed three weeks prior to admission to hospital, and weakness of lower extremities 11 days later. He had lancinating pain down both lower limbs and poor bladder control. Examination revealed an almost complete quadriplegia and restriction of neck movements. A Guinea-worm ulcer was present over the left leg. The CSF showed a slight increase in protein. Myelography via cisternal puncture showed a complete block at C2. A laminectomy from C4 to occiput was performed. An abscess extending from C3 to the foramen magnum was found, from which thick yellow pus was drained. A Guinea-worm of 51 cm length was extracted. The abscess wall was excised and the patient made an uneventful recovery.

Spinal involvement complicating parasitic infestation is fortunately rare. A better understanding of preventive measures and pathology was developed. Newer diagnostic techniques such as computerized axial tomography and magnetic resonance imaging help to demarcate the extent of the lesion. Surgical methods have also been evolved to stabilize the spine and thereby prevent collapse and neurological deterioration. Provided that the diagnosis is made early, allowing radical extirpation of the infective lesions followed by appropriate chemotherapy, an improved prognosis can be achieved.

ACKNOWLEDGEMENTS

It is with pleasure that I record my gratitude to numerous of my surgical colleagues in India, who have supplied details of cases and material for the preparation of this chapter.

REFERENCES

Abbott, P.H. & Spencer, H. (1953) Transverse myelitis due to ova of *Schistosoma mansoni*. *Trans. R. Soc. Trop. Med. Hygiene*, **47**, 221.

Aggarwal, N.D. & Singh, H. (1962) Hydatid cyst—a cause of cauda equina lesion. *Indian J. Surg.*, **24**, 553–557.

Barnett, A.M. (1965) Bilharzial granuloma of spinal cord. *S. Afr. Med. J.*, **39**, 699.

Bellini, A.M. (1946) Osteohydatidosis: its radiological features. *Radiology*, **47**, 569.

Bird, A.V. (1964) Acute spinal schistosomiasis. *Neurology*, **14**, 647.

Bird, A.V. (1965) Spinal cord complications of bilharziasis. *S. Afr. Med. J.*, **39**, 158.

Das, P. (1957) Subdural spinal hydatids. *Indian J. Surg.*, **16**, 85–86.

Dott, N.M. (1955) As quoted by Mills, T.J. in Paraplegia due to hydatid disease. *J. Bone Jt. Surg.*, **38B**, 884–891.

Duran, H. (1978) Osseous hydatidosis. *J. Bone Jt. Surg.*, **60A**, 685–690.

Fiennes, A.G.T.W. & Thomas, D.G.T. (1982) Combined medical and surgical treatment of spinal hydatid disease: a case report. *J. Neurol. Neurosurg. Psychiatry*, **45**, 927–931.

Fitzpatrick, S.C. (1965) Hydatid disease of the lumbar vertebrae. *J. Bone Jt. Surg.*, **47**(**B**), 286–291.

Gamac, deSa, and deSa, J.M. (1946) Schistosomiasis of spinal cord. *Trop. Dis. Bull.*, **43**, 936.

Hutton, P.W. & Holland, J.T. (1960) Schistosomiasis of the spinal cord. *Br. Med. J.*, **2**, 931.

James, R.D., Thomas, A.A. & Miraj, (1961) *J. Bone Jt. Surg.*, **43A**, 197–198.

Mills, T.J. (1956) Paraplegia due to hydatid disease. *J. Bone Jt. Surg.*, **38B**, 884–891.

Pepler, W.J. & Lombaard, C.M. (1956) Spinal cord granuloma due to schistosoma haematobium. *J. Neuropathol. Exp. Neurol.*, **17**, 656.

Pritam Das (1957) Subdural spinal hydatid. *Indian J. Surg.*, **19**, 350–354.

Ross, G.L., Norcross, J.W. & Horrax, G. (1952) Spinal cord involvement by *Schistosoma mansoni. N. Engl. J. Med.*, **246**, 823.

SECTION 8
LUMBAR DEGENERATIVE DISEASE

35 · Anatomical and Physiological Aspects of Back Pain

By J.F. TAYLOR

A painful back is usually the result of stimulation of sensory nerve endings in the spine or associated structures. In some patients, however, the pain results from a disturbance within the substance of the afferent nerves, their ganglia or the spinal cord. Alternatively, as referred pain, it may originate in tissues of which the innervation is segmentally related to the spine or sacrum (Table 35.1). Pain is always subjective, but only on rare occasions is a psychological disorder the only reason for a patient having backache. However, pain perception is very dependent on the physical and psychological attributes of the individual.

Commonly the patient with backache has arthropathy at many spinal segments or in the intersegmental joints. Obvious examples are the facet joint arthropathy of rheumatoid disease, or the muscular strain and facet subluxation associated with kyphosis or scoliosis. Modern investigational techniques may then reveal so much disordered anatomy that it is difficult to provide a simple solution to the patient's disease. This chapter will consider the causes of primary back pain as if they arose at one segmental level. Consideration will be given to the nerves, the intervertebral joint composed of the disc and two facet joints, and to the associated muscles and ligaments. These structures are interrelated. Thus flexion or rotational injury may lead to annular degeneration, and consequent disc prolapse and neurological damage. Alternatively diminution of disc height may produce facet joint subluxation and lateral canal stenosis. Conversely facet joint arthropathy, capsular laxity and hypermobility may predispose towards disc disruption. Disorders of the spinal cord relevant to backache are discussed in Chapter 36.

ANATOMY OF THE LUMBAR NERVES

Afferent fibres are found in the posterior and anterior rami of each lumbar nerve and also in the sympathetic nerves. The posterior ramus carries sensory information from the facet joints. The dorsal rami of lumbar nerves 1–4 divide into two or three branches in the intertransverse space. The lateral branch runs across the subjacent transverse process, and supplies the iliocostalis lumborum and overlying skin (Bogduk & Long, 1979). An intermediate branch supplies longissimus thoracis, forming intersegmental loops within the muscle. The medial branch lies in a groove on the transverse process, between the accessory process and the mamillary process. Posteriorly it divides into rostral and caudal branches to supply the facet joints of two or three segments (Fig. 35.1).

Each facet joint is therefore innervated by two or three segmental nerves, the superior part of each facet from above, the inferior from below (Paris, 1983). Denervation of a facet can be achieved only by a circumferential lesion around the joint or by the precise destruction of the appropriate articular nerves (Bogduk & Long, 1979).

The meningeal branches of spinal nerves (sinuvertebral nerves) have been described by Pedersen *et al.* (1986). Each arises from the segmental nerve with, or near the origin of, the ramus communicans (Fig. 35.2) and entering the spinal canal runs towards the midline on the posterior longitudinal ligaments. Some filaments ascend towards the disc above, others past the disc below. They may anastomose across the midline. Branches terminate in the ligament, periosteum, blood vessels of the epidural space and dura mater. As with posterior rami each nerve contains fibres destined for, and having cell

Table 35.1 Some sources of backache

Primary
The pathology is within the vertebrae, or spinal muscles and ligaments affecting nociceptive receptors
Myofascial: trauma, spasm, fatigue, inflammation
Ligamentous
Articular: facet joint arthropathy, spinal stenosis
Disc degeneration and prolapse
Osseous: Paget's disease, infection, tumours, spondylosis
Vascular
Dural: epidural abscess; arachnoiditis

Secondary
The pathology is within the nerve, nerve root, spinal cord or brain
Neural inflammation, compression and fibrosis
Nerve root and ganglionic pathology
Central nervous system dysfunction

Referred backache
From organs of the genito-urinary system and other viscera

Psychosomatic backache

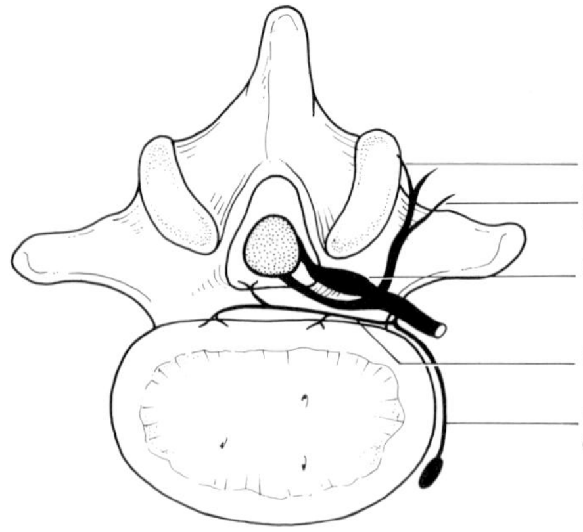

Fig. 35.2 Relationship between the lumbar nerve and ganglion, and the intervertebral foramen. The sinuvertebral nerve enters the foramen to supply the dura and posterior longitudinal ligament.

bodies within, both the segmental spinal nerves and in the sympathetic system.

The posterior part of the annulus fibrosus is supplied by sensory nerve fibres from the sinuvertebral nerve. The afferent fibres from the anterior longitudinal ligament and anterior annulus arise from the rami communicantes near their origin from the sympathetic trunk. The lateral surface of the disc is innervated by a branch from the ventral ramus and two branches from the rami communicantes.

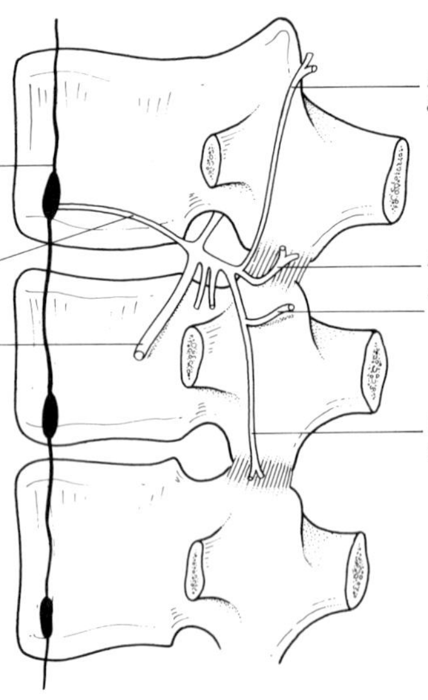

Fig. 35.1 A diagram of a lumbar nerve to illustrate the posterior ramus dividing into three branches. The medial branch, which lies in the transverse process, supplies branches to the facet joint at the same level, and also the adjacent joints.

Foerster (1933) defined a dermatome as the cutaneous area from which sensory fibres travelled to a particular segmental nerve. Kellgren (1938, 1939), however, noted that stimulation of connective tissue structures such as muscles and ligaments produced pain which was referred to areas which did not coincide with, and were more imprecise than, the dermatomes. He called such areas sclerotomes. Confirmation of the concept of 'referred' pain comes from the work of Mooney & Robertson (1976). These authors found that 3 ml of hypertonic saline injected into a facet joint produced pain in the low back, lateral thigh and occasionally in the calf. This probably relates to the multisegmental innervation of the discs and facet joints from both spinal and sympathetic nerves. However, there is considerable overlap of referred pain following provocative injections into the upper and lower spine, and McCall *et al.* (1979) noted that the intensity and radiation of the pain varied with the volume of fluid injected.

It has been thought that the afferent fibres gain access to the spinal cord in the dorsal root. However, the demonstration of afferent fibres in the ventral root (reviewed by Coggeshall, 1980) may explain the failure of rhizotomy in the relief of pain. A further possible cause of such failure are the sensory fibres travelling within the sympathetic nervous system.

Neurological relationships within the intervertebral foramen

The lateral root canal is considered to have three zones. Considering an efferent nerve Lee *et al.* (1988) named the intervertebral foramen the exit zone. For afferent fibres it is the entrance. Anteriorly is the vertebral body, but posteriorly the lateral aspect of the facet joint and the lateral edge of the ligamentum flavum. Osteophytes from the latter can therefore compress the lumbar nerve which is formed at the foramen by the fusion of the anterior and posterior roots. The midzone lies between that part of the lamina called the pars interarticularis and the vertebral body. Contained within this zone are the dorsal root ganglion and the ventral nerve root, covered by an extension of dura. The cephalad (or entrance) zone of the lateral lumbar canal (lateral recess, subarticular gutter) is bounded anteriorly by the intervertebral disc, laterally by the pedicle and posteriorly by the superior facet and attached ligamentum flavum. Stenosis here may also be due to hypertrophic arthrosis of the joint.

Narrowing of the canal may be dynamic or static. In spinal extension there is dynamic narrowing as the superior facet moves superiorly and anteriorly in relation to the inferior facet of the vertebrae above. The ganglion in the midzone is then compressed between vertebral body and displaced ligamentum flavum (Fig. 35.3). Structural stenosis results from annular bulging consequent upon disc disruption or even from disc prolapse. Alternatively osteophytic ridges may develop at the posterolateral region of the inferior endplate. In spondylosis such ridges project posteriorly and superiorly such that the ganglion and the nerve may be encroached upon by sclerotic bone (Fig. 35.4).

Radicular symptoms may also be produced by disproportion between neural structures and the canal produced by congenital abnormalities of the nerve and nerve roots (Kikuchi *et al.*, 1984). These take the form of conjoined roots such that two roots share the same root pouch. In some patients a separate furcal nerve may arise, commonly from the L4 root and exit through the L4–L5 foramen giving branches to the lumbosacral trunk, femoral and obturator nerves. Such irregularities are seen in many sensory fibres but rarely involve motor roots.

A complex network of fibrous bands (Hofmann ligaments) attaches the emerging nerve root to the

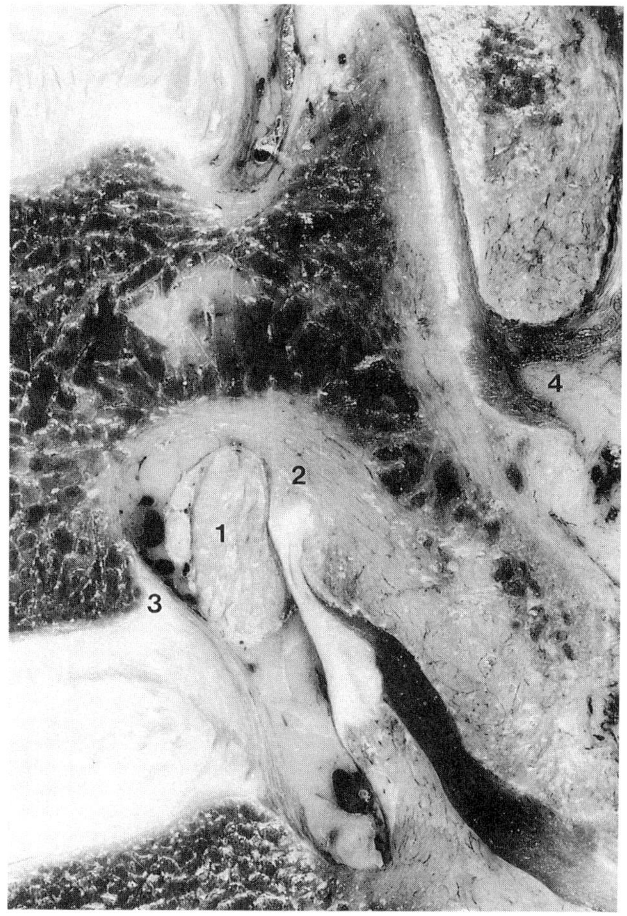

Fig. 35.3 A sagittal section through the L5–S1 root canal. The ganglion (1) and two motor roots lie between the vertebral body anteriorly and the pars interarticularis (2) and attached ligamentum flavum posteriorly. The outer fibres of the annulus (3) insert beyond the level of the apophyseal rim. A meniscoid synovial fold is seen in the L4–L5 facet joint (4). The author is greatly indebted to Dr W. Rauschning, who provided Figs 35.3, 35.4 & 35.7. They appear in his article of 1987, and are published by kind permission of the author and the publishers of *Spine*.

vertebra and posterior longitudinal ligament. The ganglion is anchored to the foramenal boundary by a foramenal complex of fibrous bands, with extensions to the joint capsule and subjacent pedicle (Sunderland, 1974). On straight leg raising the normal lower lumbar roots descend in the foraminae by as much as 1 cm (Goddard & Reid, 1965); however, this is not entirely due to the nerve and roots sliding within the foramen—it is also brought about by passive deformation of the nerve. When relaxed the axis cylinders are folded like an accordion within the

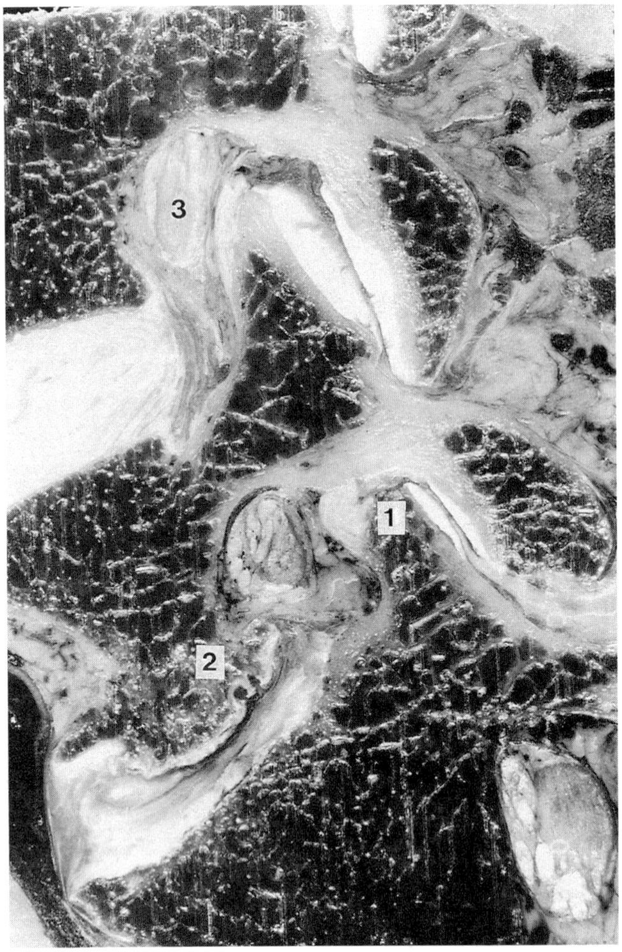

Fig. 35.4 A sagittal section through the extended spine of an elderly man, by courtesy of Dr W. Rauschning. As a consequence of disc resorption at L5–S1 the superior sacral facet (1) is in contact with the pedicle of L5. An osteophytic ridge (2) on L5 partly encloses the fifth lumbar nerve. The capsular ligamentum flavum at L4–L5 is displaced anteriorly and compresses the L4 ganglion (3).

perineurium, but straighten on extension (Breig, 1960).

The microanatomy of the nerve root and trunk

The nerve root differs in structure and function from the peripheral nerve trunk, such that the root is more likely to be a source of chronic pain. Each fascicle within a peripheral nerve is surrounded by perineurium which is lined by perilemma. The perineurium resists tensile force, but it is absent from nerve roots. Thus longitudinal distraction (as in brachial plexus injury) is more likely to produce axonal damage in the nerve root than in the peripheral nerve.

Free nerve endings within the endoneurium are thought to be sensory receptors. Their impulses are carried by branches from the axons passing through the nerve (nervi nervora) and also by a plexus of fibres which run on the vasa nervora. Such fibres run from the anterior nerve root to the sinuvertebral nerve, but from the posterior nerve root and ganglion they run to all bodies within the ganglion (Murphy, 1977). This system of sensory receptors may partly explain why an inflamed nerve (root) can become sensitive to light touch.

The distribution of spinal nociceptive receptors

The term 'nociception' arose from the conclusions of Sherrington (1906) in relation to stimuli capable of compromising the integrity of the organism. In animals such stimuli produce reflex responses such as tachycardia, and in humans they can cause pain. A full discussion of nociception and neurotransmitters is found in Chapter 56.

The nociceptive receptors of the facet joints are principally contained within the joint capsule as a plexus of unmyelinated fibres. Encapsulated endings respond to both dynamic and static loading. The articular cartilage contains no nerve endings, but in severe spondylosis erosion of articular cartilage may rarely expose pain receptors in the subchondral bone.

The posterior longitudinal ligament is innervated by fine free fibres and complex unencapsulated endings (Wyke, 1987) which contain the transmitter substances calcitonin gene-related peptide (CGRP), substance P (SP), and vasoactive-intestinal peptide (VIP) (Konttinen *et al.*, 1990; Liesi *et al.*, 1983; Weinstein, 1986). It is thought that the pain produced by a protruding or degenerate disc depends largely on excitation of these neural elements. Unmyelinated free fibres are also seen, but to a lesser extent, in the interspinous and flaval ligaments. Much of the support for the spine is due to passive elastic tension within these ligaments.

The ligamentum flavum has a unique elastic quality and serves to assist the subject standing upright after forward bending. It also exerts a constant pull on the anterior facet capsule. Instability leading to excessive vertebral displacement may thus stimulate ligamentous pain receptors.

There are neither sensory receptors nor nerves in

the normal nucleus pulposus, but unmyelinated fibres are found in the outer 1–2 mm of the annulus fibrosus. VIP and CGRP have been demonstrated in the outer annular fibres of the disc and also in the supraspinous and interspinous ligaments. The dorsal root ganglion serves as a warehouse for these peptides which may modulate pain as it relates to each motion segment (Malinsky, 1959; Bogduk *et al.*, 1981; Weinstein, 1986). In the degenerate disc clefts may develop in the annulus, permitting ingrowth of granulation tissue capillaries and associated sympathetic nerve fibres from the sinuvertebral nerve. Shinohara (1970) found such granulation tissue and free nerve endings in the nucleus pulposus and inner annulus of some degenerate discs, but this was not confirmed by Yoshizawa *et al.* (1980).

Neural inflammation

The structure of the nerve root is responsible for it being more liable to chronic inflammation than the nerve trunk. The arterial blood supply arises via the foramen from the segmental vessel. Nutrient arteries enter the epineurium within which they form a plexus from which branches enter the fasciculi. On each nerve root the proximal arteriolar supply is from the anterior spinal artery and vasa corona. Distally branches ascend from the epineurial plexus on the ganglion. Between the two is an area of relative hypovascularity in the midregion of the root (Murphy, 1977). The endoneurial blood vessels of the dorsal root ganglion and spinal nerve roots are more permeable to protein tracers than elsewhere (Olsson, 1971). In the ganglion this is due to lack of an endothelial cell barrier. Thus compression injury produces excessive protein loss at these sites, which in rodents persists over many months.

The perilemma acts as a diffusion barrier, and prevents chemical irritants penetrating the fasciculi of nerves (Olsson & Kristensson, 1973). Toxins and infectious agents more easily enter nerve roots where the perilemma is lacking. Tissue spaces within nerve root endoneurium do permit movement of fluid outside the fasciculi; however, such spaces do not communicate with the lymphatics. An inflammatory exudate within the endoneurial space is therefore cleared with great difficulty, predisposing to invasion by fibroblasts and to intraneural fibrosis. Thus nerve root tension secondary to prolapse, or nerve and ganglion compression within the intervertebral foramen, lead to vascular damage and the accumulation of protein within the epineurium. Microscopy reveals perivascular infiltration of leucocytes, fat granules in the Schwann cells, and fatty degeneration of the myelin sheaths. Subsequent infiltration of fibroblasts produces fibrosis (Irisigler, 1951).

The stages of neural inflammation and fibrosis have been classified by Burton (1978):

1 Radiculitis: inflammation of the pia arachnoid with hyperaemia and swelling of the nerve roots. There is a fibrinous exudate, and deposition of collagen strands between nerve roots and the pia arachnoid.

2 Arachnoiditis: progressive fibrosis and collagen deposition with adherence of nerve roots to the pia arachnoid.

3 Adhesive arachnoiditis: increased collagen deposition and proliferation of the pia arachnoid leads to a diminished vascular supply and atrophy (Figs 35.5 & 35.6).

Arachnoiditis is more common in cigarette smokers (Pountain *et al.*, 1986). The incidence of smoking is greater than normal among patients with low back pain, and smoking is associated with a defect in fibrinolytic activity. Such a defect has been demonstrated in low back pain patients (Jayson *et al.*, 1985). It is postulated that in some patients a failure to remove fibrin deposited during the inflammatory response may be important in the pathogenesis of radiculitis and arachnoiditis.

CHEMICAL AND IMMUNOLOGICAL 'NEURITIS'

Trauma and mechanical injury can account for symptoms in only about 30% of patients with disc disease. Irritation of the arachnoid by radiological contrast media is not a feature of patients at first presentation, and it has been suggested that a chemical or an autoimmune process may be responsible for the neurological damage (Naylor, 1962). In 1965 Bobechko & Hirsch showed that it was possible to produce a cell-mediated response to nucleus pulposus in the rabbit. Nachemson (1969) recorded a low pH in degenerate discs, and an inflammatory reaction in nerve roots adjacent to such discs, and postulated that metabolites could leak through the annulus to cause endoneurial inflammation.

Back pain patients with neurological lesions, with or without abnormal radiographs, have been found to have delayed hypersensitivity reactions to proteoglycans, and also to cellular extract from their own

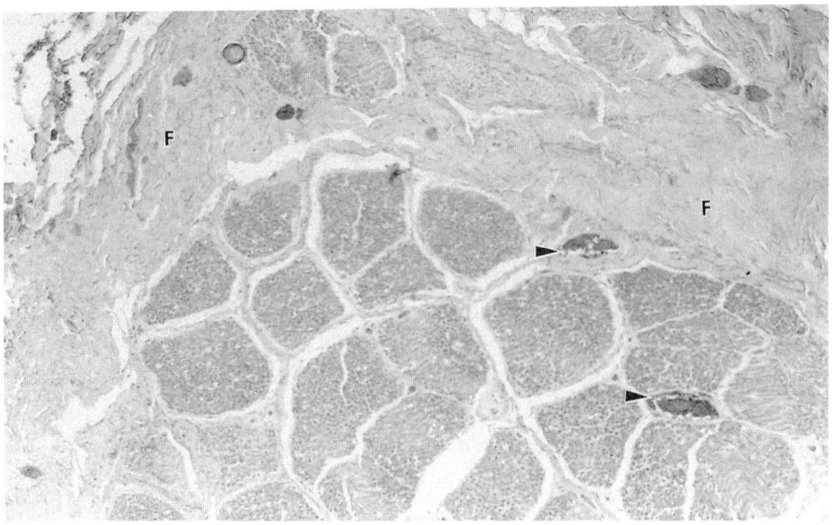

Fig. 35.5 A transverse section of a nerve root showing perineural fibrosis (F). There is only a small amount of interfascicular fibrosis. The intraneural blood vessels (arrowed) are dilated and have an amorphous subendothelial layer. The author is greatly indebted to Professor M.I.V. Jayson and Drs A.J. Freemont and J. Hoyland for preparing Figs 35.5 and 35.6, and for their permission to publish them here.

discs (Bisla *et al.*, 1976). Such results must be interpreted with caution as Gertzbein *et al.* (1976) found no evidence of such a response in patients with disc degeneration and no prolapse. Moreover, the proteoglycans of disc and articular cartilage from other joints are closely related, so that hypersensitivity to proteoglycans might develop in patients with arthrosis outside the axial skeleton. However, intraneural fibrosis is seen more frequently in nerves adjacent to degenerate discs (Holt, 1966), and it appears likely that an immune process contributes to the symptoms where there is no mechanical injury.

FIBROSIS OF NERVE AND ROOT

Within the spinal canal a prolapsed disc produces tension in the overlying nerve root; however, in the intervertebral foramen the nerve may be compressed by disc, joint capsule, ligamentum flavum (Fig. 35.3) or vertebral osteophytes (Fig. 35.4). Obstruction of epineurial venules and the subsequent endoneurial oedema and fibrosis renders the nerve inelastic. Whereas compression of a normal nerve causes a painless sensory and/or motor deficit, lightly touching an inflamed lumbar nerve produces low back

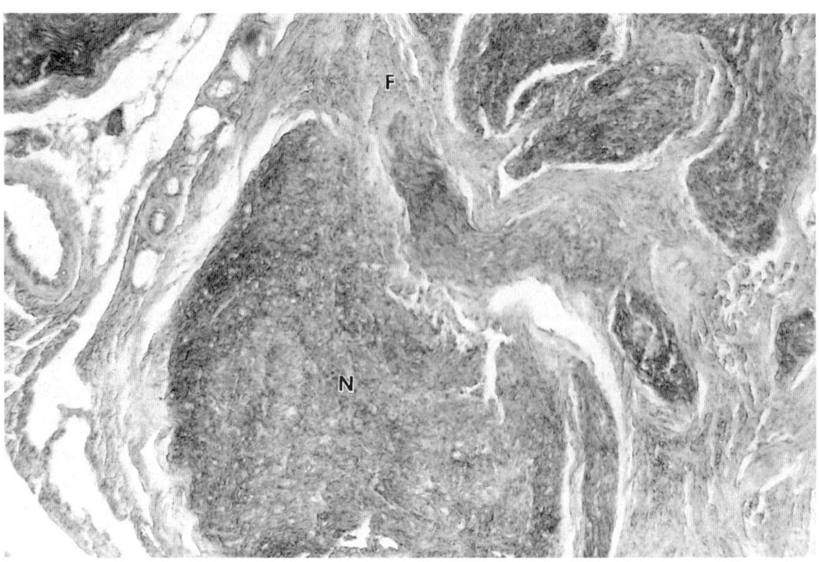

Fig. 35.6 A photomicrograph of a nerve in which dense intraneural fibrosis (F) is associated with atrophy of the neural elements.

pain and referred pain to the hip and thigh (Smyth & Wright, 1958). Similarly tension on inelastic or inflamed nerves produces radicular pain, with motor or sensory deficits if the tension is severe.

Back pain resulting from neural inflammation or fibrosis may be due to:

1 Stimulation of the intraneural sensory endings by compression, tension or the products of an inflammatory response.

2 A lowering of the excitation threshold of the afferent nerves.

3 A decrease in the afferent supply consequent upon interruption of impulses due to pressure, anoxia or atrophy. In such deafferentation the patient perceives pain due to an abnormal distribution of sensory supply. Tasker *et al.* (1980) defined deafferentation pain as 'discomfort arising once the flow of afferent impulses has been partly or completely interrupted'. It may be caused by lesions of nerves, dorsal roots, spinal cord, brain stem or cerebral cortex, and is further discussed in Chapter 56.

4 By artificial synapses between afferent and efferent nerves (Richards, 1951; Murphy, 1977). The myelin sheath normally acts as an insulator; however, in areas of compression or fibrosis the insulation may be lost. An ischaemic neuritis may be produced by multiple artificial synapses provoked by a defective neural blood supply.

Spinal stenosis and lateral canal entrapment

Compression of the nerve roots in the central canal, or the ganglion and nerve in the lateral canal, may be dynamic or due to fixed deformity. The pain is produced by similar mechanisms in either case, but is intermittent with dynamic compression. Central canal stenosis may be brought about by disc herniation, osteophytic enlargement of the facet joints or hypertrophy of the laminae or ligamentum flavum. Back pain is common but not invariable, the patients presenting with aching in the back and thighs which is worsened by walking. The source of these symptoms is uncertain, but they may be secondary to inadequate oxygenation of the cauda equina (Porter, 1987).

A reduction of the dimensions of the lateral nerve root canal may be brought about by diminution of vertical disc height, and bulging of the posterior annulus. The inferior facet of the upper vertebra is displaced downwards and backwards (retrospondylolisthesis), the superior facets of the lower vertebra riding up into the foramen. In the 'superior facet syndrome' the nerve may thus be compressed between the superior facet and the pedicle, or between facet and dorsal aspect of the vertebra (Fig. 35.2).

Computerized tomography reveals that the narrowing of the lateral canal is worsened by extension (Penning & Wilmink, 1987). As with the unstable phase of facet and disc disease, pain may arise from any of the soft tissues around the joints. In addition intraneural pain receptors may be stimulated in the segmental nerve or ganglion, to produce back pain and sciatica, the latter worsening at night (Porter, 1987).

The facet joints

These di-arthrodial joints have a well-defined capsule and synovium, the superior aspect of the superior facet lying in close relationship to the segmental nerve in the intervertebral foramen. The capsules have a superior and inferior recess (Fig. 35.7). Small meniscoids extend from the capsule into the joint (Fig. 35.3) (Bogduk & Engel, 1984). The junctional region of meniscoid and capsule is vascular, and it may well be that entrapment of a meniscoid within the joint is responsible for the pain of an acutely locked back.

The alignment of the lumbar joints permits flexion and extension, and resists rotation. Putti & Logroscino (1938) found that facetal arthrosis increased with age, being rare in patients aged less than 30. In older patients, asymmetry correlated with signs of arthrosis including capsular oedema and adhesions, synovial hypertrophy, detached cartilaginous bodies and fibrillation or erosion of the articular cartilage. In a later study Horal (1969) found that, though torsional forces play a role in disc degeneration, patients with facet asymmetry did not have a greater incidence of back pain. The relationship between joint asymmetry and symptomatic degenerative change in the motion segment remains unproven.

A spectrum of degeneration is seen in these joints, commencing with synovitis. Chondromalacia leads to cartilaginous fibrillation and erosion, the thinning of articular cartilage leading to capsular laxity and instability. Subsequently osteophytes develop around the articular processes which hypertrophy. Those osteophytes on the superior articular process protrude anteriorly and medially to narrow the lateral recess

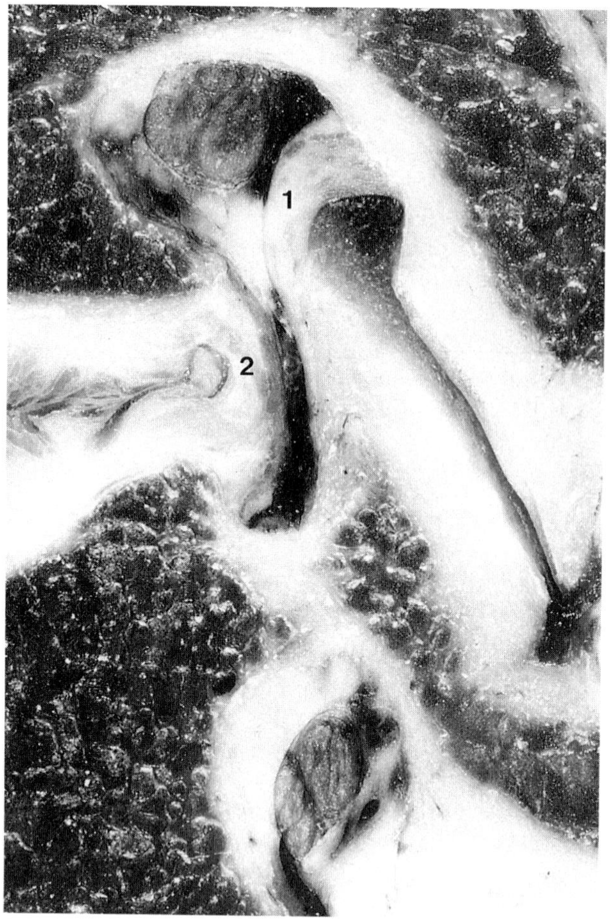

Fig. 35.7 A sagittal section through the L4–L5 facet joint and root canal, by courtesy of Dr W. Rauschning. An apparent effusion in the facet joint has caused the ligamentum flavum (1) to bulge anteriorly. Radial horizontal tears in the midsubstance of the L4–L5 posterior disc have left some peripheral annular lamellae intact (2).

of the spinal canal. The osteophytes on the inferior articular process bulge into and narrow the central canal. Degeneration of cartilage by itself is not a cause of pain, and exposure of pain receptors in subchondral bone is probably rare; however, painful stimuli may arise in these patients whose degenerative joints develop microfractures (Sims-Williams *et al.*, 1978).

The facet joints take some 20% of the axial load (Lorenz *et al.*, 1983), this proportion increasing with hyperextension. Lynch & Taylor (1986) investigated patients whose low back pain had been present for longer than six months, was exacerbated by hyperextension and was associated with focal paraspinal tenderness. Finding the disorder three times more common in women, they postulated that this was due to the greater lumbar lordosis in the female.

Computerized tomography has shown that, in a series of patients with low back pain, 20% had disc herniation and 40% had facet arthrosis (Carrera *et al.*, 1980). Facet arthropathy can therefore occur independently of any disc disorder and vice-versa. Kirkaldy Willis (1988) has emphasized that a disorder of any one component of the motion segment is likely to be followed by degenerative change in all of the three-joint complex (Fig. 35.8). Straining the joints leads to muscle spasm and synovitis, and this joint dysfunction predisposes to an unstable phase with erosion of articular cartilage and subluxation of the joint. Such instability predisposes to disc degeneration, just as primary disc disease, with a reduction in disc height, leads to increased wear of the posterior joints. The patient's pain may emanate from receptors in the joint capsules, paraspinal muscles or ligaments, or those in the outer annulus, all of which are subjected to unusual tension. Much later spontaneous stabilization occurs with osteophyte formation and increasing fibrosis.

The intervertebral joint

Spinal pain is normally precipitated or worsened by movement at several motion segments. At each of these, nociceptive impulses may arise in the components of the intervertebral joint, and from the surrounding tissues. Chronic disorders in any part of the three-joint complex will subsequently produce degenerative changes elsewhere at the same intervertebral level and at adjacent motion segments (Kirkaldy Willis, 1988).

DISORDERS OF THE INTERVERTEBRAL DISC AND POSTERIOR LONGITUDINAL LIGAMENT

The disc is strong and painless if the annulus is intact. Annular damage may occur with shearing or torsional forces. Shear forces are generated by flexion and extension; shear and torsion being produced by lateral flexion (Rabischong *et al.*, 1978). Torsional injury can also be produced by voluntary rotation, or may result from involuntary uncontrolled contraction of postural muscles. Such contraction is thought to arise from emotional disturbances (Kirkaldy Willis, 1988).

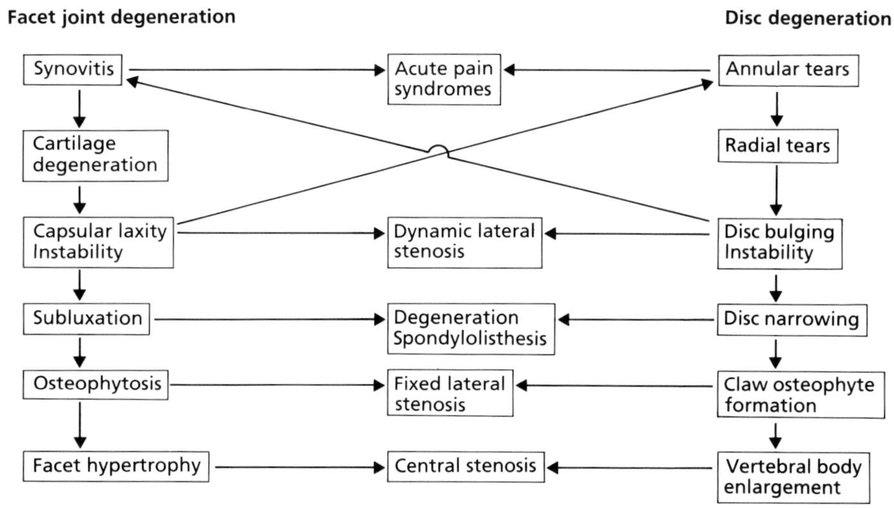

Fig. 35.8 A scheme of the pathophysiology of progressive segmental lumbar degenerative disease. Modified from Kirkaldy Willis (1988).

If the annulus is intact, the disc is stronger than the adjacent vertebral body (Brown, 1969). Lifting of an excessively heavy load will fracture the vertebra before rupturing the disc. However, at the lumbosacral joint the intradiscal force during lifting is only 70% of that derived by calculation, due to contraction of abdominal musculature and the increase of intra-abdominal pressure. Thus symptoms from a disorder of the intervertebral joint may be minimized if the abdominal musculature is efficient.

The demonstration of osteophytes (spondylophytes) at the margin of the vertebral body may lead to the conclusion that they are a source of pain, or that they indicate a painful motion segment. The fibres of the annulus form lamellae and the innermost run obliquely into the vertebral body. That part of the outer lamellae which runs parallel to the longitudinal ligaments is connected by a calcified zone to the margin of the vertebral body, and the claw osteophyte develops at this site with ageing. This has been differentiated from the traction spur or osteophyte which is more horizontal, situated 3–4 mm from the vertebral edge, and which is said to develop due to traction on the anterior longitudinal ligament (McNab, 1971). On the basis of an autopsy study Pate *et al.* (1988) suggested that in fact the claw osteophyte was only an advanced stage of the traction osteophyte. Quinnel & Stockdale (1982) found that the claw osteophyte was more commonly associated with normal discograms. We therefore accept McNab's view that the traction osteophyte is a radiological sign of instability at the intervertebral joint, and that there may be associated pain.

Intervertebral disc disease

The descriptions of disc disorders are based primarily on radiological findings (McCall, 1987). They cannot be differentiated on the basis of pain unless nuclear extrusion produces localizing signs.

Internal annular disc disruption

Circumferential or radial tears of the annulus (Fig. 35.7) do not involve the outer layers (Crock, 1970). Because the nucleus pulposus is not extruded through the annulus, the sensory nerve endings in the outer annulus are not mechanically stimulated. Nevertheless the patient has a dull, deep backache (McCall, 1987). This may arise from the effect on surrounding tissues of the initial hypermobility (Akkerveeken *et al.*, 1979). In more advanced degeneration mobility is reduced with synthesis of Type III collagen (Ayad & Weiss, 1987). Alternatively the pain may arise from stimulation of annular ligamentous or vertebral nociceptive receptors by diffusion of catabolites or neuropeptides. Intradiscal compression can pump fluid containing neuropeptides from the disc into adjacent vertebral bodies (Weinstein, 1986). Discography and concordant pain permits confirmation of the symptomatic disc (Blumenthal *et al.*, 1988).

Radial annular rupture

Complete radial tears may follow acute trauma either to previously normal discs or to those affected by internal annular disruption (Fig. 35.7). They are described in young adults with severe backache but no abnormal neurological signs. Mechanical disruption of the outer annular collagen fibres may stimulate the free sensory nerve endings (Rabischong *et al.*, 1978). Evidence to support the concept of direct irritation of the annular sensory nerve endings is found in the works of Lindblom (1951) and Perey (1951) who produced sciatica and backache by injecting contrast into diseased discs, the pain being prevented if local anaesthetic was injected simultaneously. Fraser *et al.* (1983) found that symptom reproduction was most frequent if contrast bulged into the spinal canal, leading to the conclusion that sensory endings in the posterior ligament may also be activated. Autoimmune 'neuritis' may also play a role, for those patients having annular disruption sufficient to permit the ingrowth of vascular granulation tissue show an immune response to products of the nucleus pulposus (Gertzbein *et al.*, 1976).

Disc prolapse

Extrusion of nuclear material, or laxity of the fibres of the posterior annulus, permits a mechanical disturbance to the posterior longitudinal ligament, epidural veins, dura and nerve roots. As demonstrated by Edgar & Park (1974), irritation of structures posterior to the annulus is associated not only with back pain but with a variable extent of back pain dependent on which structures are involved. Intense sciatica develops with tension in, or compression of, the emergent nerve roots.

Intraosseous nuclear extensions

Abnormal flexion/extension stress to the adolescent spine may produce intraosseous herniation at the anterior third of the disc (McCall, 1987). The pain is exacerbated by discography, which probably stimulates intraosseous pain receptors. However, in addition to any mechanical stimulation there may be an autoimmune component to the pain, as elevated levels of immunoglobulin M have been reported in patients with Schmorl's nodes (Bisla *et al.*, 1976).

Disc degeneration

The normal nucleus is contained within a hydrostatic pressure vessel, contains 80% water, a high content of proteoglycan and little collagen. With ageing there is reduced hydration and the development of clefts. Degeneration of the nucleus and annulus is accompanied by focal necrosis of cartilage and pulposal cells, and an infiltration of lymphocytes and mononuclears. Breakdown products or instability may be responsible for stimulation of sensory endings in the degenerate annulus. Increasing disc collapse produces facet joint subluxation and stenosis of the intervertebral foramen. These findings at one motion segment, and in the absence of disc prolapse, were termed 'isolated disc resorption' by Crock (1981); however, the degenerative process subsequently progresses to involve the facet joints equally.

Spondylolisthesis

The unstable phase of advancing degeneration may produce spondylolisthesis. At the L4–L5 motion segment the L5 nerve is then trapped between the inferior articular facet of L4 and the body of L5. Farfan (1980) has shown that in autopsy specimens there is usually associated vertebral rotation of the upper vertebra on that below, such that traction is applied to a nerve root by unilateral medial and forward pedicular displacement. In this situation, as with the superior facet syndrome, pain receptors are stimulated both in the paraspinal soft tissues and those in the disordered nerve root and dura.

Patients with spondylolytic spondylolisthesis and little displacement frequently present with symptoms due to reflex hamstring spasm. Following prolonged forward bending, resumption of the upright posture may be accompanied by severe back pain and transient weakness in the legs. These symptoms may be due to traction on the fibrous tissue in the defect producing afferent stimuli in the sympathetic fibres of the associated blood vessels. In more advanced spondylolysis at, for instance, L5–S1 the L5 nerve may be trapped in the foramen between the body of the sacrum and the pars interarticularis just cranial to the defect. In this condition the facet joints are essentially undisturbed, and pain production must be from the fibrous tissue in the defect, from the stretched ligament around the disc or from compressed dura, nerve roots or nerves.

Myofascial pain

The lumbodorsal fascia, sacrospinalis and multifidus muscles are supplied by branches from the posterior primary rami, with overlap of segmental innervation. Free nerve endings supply both myelinated and non-myelinated afferents. It is thought that stimuli arising in the muscle may produce muscular pain, and dysfunction that then leads to secondary changes in the joints (Fig. 35.9). It is also likely that disorders within the central nervous system, particularly the cord, can cause pain perceived to be in muscle. The patient with muscular pain may therefore have local and/or central pathology.

The muscles

Trigger points are tender areas in skeletal muscles which, when stimulated, produce muscle spasm, local fasciculation and pain referred to a wider or distant area. Iggo (1974) and Travell & Simons (1983) believe that trigger points commence with a muscular strain and become a site of reduced circulation and hypersensitive nerves. The referred pain is described as dull and aching. The trigger point and the referred pain frequently lie within the territory of one segmental nerve. The concept that the primary pathology is in the muscle is supported by the similarity of the pain to that produced by Kellgren (1938) when he injected hypertonic saline into skeletal muscle. Moreover, biopsies from trigger points may reveal loss of cross-fibrillar striation, variable staining intensity and/or replacement of muscle by fibrous tissue (Awad, 1973).

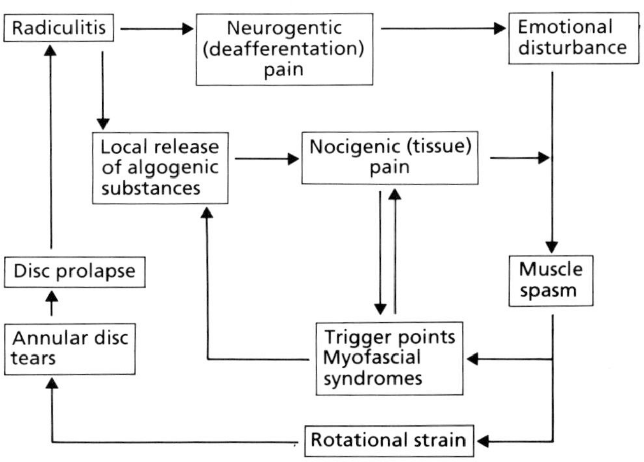

Fig. 35.9 The relationship between the central nervous system, muscle spasm and muscle pain. Radiculitis secondary to disc prolapse may be responsible for deafferentation pain, for the pain induced by stimulation of intraneural receptors, and for muscle pain consequent upon the peripheral release of algogenic substances.

If the disorder originates in the muscles, the mechanism producing referred pain is uncertain. Sensory afferent stimuli from the reference zone may be facilitated sufficiently by visceral activity so as to be interpreted as pain (convergence–facilitation—Ruch (1965). The efferent nerves are also involved. Motor neurones within the area of referred pain have reduced stimulation threshold (Travell *et al.*, 1944), and electromyography (EMG) studies may reveal spontaneous motor unit activity. The associated autonomic disturbances may be due to a reflex release of nociceptive substances such as substance P within the zone of referred pain (Procacci & Zoppi, 1981). Alternatively they may depend on an axon reflex similar to that causing a cutaneous flare around the site of a localized injury (Lewis, 1942).

Though patients with trigger points may suffer insomnia and fatigue suggestive of depression (Simons, 1976), the search for a correlation between anxiety and muscle tension has been generally unsuccessful; however, there is better evidence that spinal cord dysfunction produces 'muscular pain'. Ten per cent of patients with brachial plexus avulsion suffer paroxysms of 'burning' or 'electrical shooting' pain. Such pain may be produced by touching trigger zones on skin supplied by segmental nerves adjacent to that injured. It is thought that the traumatic deafferentation has produced abnormal neural communication leading to heightened activity in the sensory neurones of adjacent normal segments of the spinal cord (Nashold, 1988). Deafferentation can be produced by many compressive lesions already discussed; therefore an alteration in central neurophysiology may play a role in pain which is perceived to be in skeletal muscle (Fig. 35.9).

Kirkaldy Willis (1988) has said that uncontrolled spasm in the multifidus may lead to facet joint injury and tears of the annulus; also that, as part of a vicious circle, pathology in the joints may produce protective spasm in the overlying muscles and that long-standing spasm produces contracture in the spine extensors and weakness of the abdominal muscles, leading to a relatively greater load being applied to each facet joint. Whilst this may well apply in some patients, it has not been possible to produce EMG evidence to support the concept of reflex muscle spasm in chronic back pain (Cohen *et al.*, 1986). It therefore appears that the primary pathology in chronic low back pain is degenerative joint disease, but that of myofascial syndrome remains uncertain.

SUMMARY

Back pain is usually due to the stimulation of sensory receptors and the transmission of impulses to the sensory ganglion and spinal cord. Pressure applied to sensory nerve axons, whether by stenosis or disc protrusion, produces depolarization and an action potential, and subsequent axonal block. After the onset of symptoms a quiescent period is followed by a crescendo of secondary pain, ascribed to sensitization, and to lowering of nerve thresholds. Inflammation in the disordered tissue, and the release of substances such as histamine, increase the peripheral stimuli. Antidromic impulses or autonomic reflexes may be responsible for trigger points, and myofascial pain such as seen in the sacroiliac and trochanteric areas (Rosomoff & Rosomoff, 1987). Associated contraction produces a restricted range of motion; immobilization will then contribute to the overall disability. For this reason patients with back pain require prompt diagnosis and treatment of the primary source of nociceptive impulses, and encouragement to maintain moderate mobility.

REFERENCES

Akkerveeken, P. van, O. Brien, J.P. & Park, W.M. (1979) Experimentally induced hypermobility in the lumbar spine. *Spine*, **4**, 236–241.

Awad, E.A. (1973) Interstitial myofibrosis: hypothesis of the mechanism. *Arch. Phys. Med.*, **54**, 440–453.

Ayad, S. & Weiss, J.B. (1987) Biochemistry of the intervertebral disc. In Jayson, M.I.V. (ed.) *The Lumbar Spine and Back Pain*, 3rd edn, pp. 100–137. Churchill Livingstone, London.

Bisla R.S., Marchisello, P.J., Lockshin, M.D., Hart, D.M., Marcus, R.E. & Granda, J. (1976) Auto-immunological basis of disc degeneration. *Clin. Orthop. Rel. Res.*, **121**, 205–211.

Blumenthal, S.L., Baker, J., Bassett, A. & Selby, D.K. (1988) The role of anterior lumbar fusion for internal disc disruption. *Spine*, **13**, 566–569.

Bobechko, W.T. & Hirsch, C. (1965) Auto-immune response to nucleus pulposus in the rabbit. *J. Bone Jt. Surg.*, **47B**, 574–580.

Bogduk, N. & Engel, R. (1984) The menisci of the lumbar zygapophyseal joints. *Spine*, **9**, 454–460.

Bogduk, N. & Long, D.M. (1979) The anatomy of the so-called articular nerves and their relationship to facet denervation in the treatment of low back pain. *J. Neurosurg.*, **51**, 172–177.

Bogduk, N., Tynan, W. & Wilson, A.S. (1981) The nerve supply to the human lumbar intervertebral discs. *J. Anat.*, **132**, 39–56.

Breig, A. (1960) *Biomechanics of the Central Nervous System*. Year Book Medical Publishers, Chicago, IL.

Brown, M.D. (1969) The pathophysiology of the intervertebral disc. Anatomical physiological and biomedical considerations. MD thesis, Philadelphia Medical College.

Burton, C.V. (1978) Lumbosacral arachnoiditis. *Spine*, **3**, 24–30.

Carrera, G.F., Williams, A.L. & Naughton, V.M. (1980) Computed tomography in sciatica. *Radiology*, **137**, 433–437.

Coggeshall, R.E. (1980) Law of separation of function of the spinal roots. *Physiol Rev.*, **60**, 716–755.

Cohen, M.J., Swanson, G.A., Naliboff, B.D., Schandler, S.L. & McArthur, D.L. (1986) Comparison of electromyographic response patterns during posture and stress tasks in chronic low back pain patterns and control. *J. Psychom. Res.*, **30**, 135–141.

Crock, H.V. (1970) A re-appraisal of intervetebral disc lesions. *Med. J. Aust.*, **1**, 983–989.

Crock, H.V. (1981) Normal and pathological anatomy of the lumbar spine nerve root canals. *J. Bone Jt. Surg.*, **63B**, 487–490.

Edgar, M. & Park, W.M. (1974) Induced pain patterns on passive straight-leg raising in lower disc protrusion. *J. Bone Jt. Surg.*, **56B**, 658–667.

Farfan, H.F. (1980) The pathological anatomy of degenerative spondylolisthesis. *Spine*, **5**, 412–418.

Foerster, O. (1933) The dermatomes in man. *Brain*, **56**, 1–39.

Fraser, J., McCall, I.W., Park, W.M. & O'Brien, J.P. (1983) Discography in degenerating disc disease. *Orthop. Trans.*, **7**, 466.

Gertzbein, S.D., Tait, J.H. & Devlin, S.R. (1976) The stimulation of lymphocytes by nucleus pulposus in patients with degenerative disc disease of the lumbar spine. *Clin. Orthop. Rel. Res.*, **123**, 149–153.

Goddard, M.D. and Reid, J.D. (1965) Movements induced by straight leg raising in the lumbo-sacral roots, nerves and plexus, and in the intra pelvic section of the sciatic nerve. *J. Neurol. Neurosurg. Psychiatry*, **28**, 12–17.

Holt, S. (1966) Cervical spondylosis and nerve-root lesions. *J. Bone Jt. Surg.*, **48B**, 407–423.

Horal, J. (1969) The clinical appearance of low back disorders in the City of Gothenburg, Sweden. *Acta Orthop. Scand.*, Suppl. 118.

Iggo, A. (1974) Pain receptors. In: Bonica, J.J., Procacci, P. & Pagni, C.A. (eds), *Recent Advances in Pain*, pp. 24–25. Charles C. Thomas, Springfield, IL.

Irisigler, F.J. (1951) Mikroscopische Befunde an den Rückenmarkwurzeln beim lumbalen und lumbosakralen Diskuprolaps. *Acta Neurochir.*, **1**, 478–516.

Jackson, H.C., Winkelmann, R.K. & Bickel, W.H. (1966) Nerve endings in the human lumbar spinal column and related structures. *J. Bone Jt. Surg.*, **48A**, 1272–1281.

Jayson, M.I.V., Keegan, A.L., Million, R. & Tomlinson, I. (1985) A fibrinolytic defect in chronic back pain syndromes. *Lancet*, **2**, 1186–1187.

Kellgren, J.H. (1938) Observations on referred pain arising from muscle. *Clin. Sci.*, **3**, 175–190.

Kellgren, J.H. (1939) On the distribution of pain arising from deep somatic structures with charts of segmental pain areas. *Clin. Sci.*, **4**, 35–46.

Kikuchi, S., Hasue, M., Nishiyama, K. & Tsukasa, I. (1984) Anatomic and clinical studies of radicular symptoms. *Spine*, **9**, 23–30.

Kirkaldy Willis, W.H. (1988) The three phases of the spectrum of degenerative disease. In Kirkaldy Willis, W.H. (ed.), *Managing Low Back Pain*, pp. 117–132. Churchill Livingstone, New York.

Konttinen, V.T., Grönblad, M., Antti-Poika, I., Seitsalo, S., Santavirta, S., Hukkanen, M. & Polak, J.M. (1990) Neuroimmunohistochemical analysis of peridiscal nociceptive neural elements. *Spine*, **15**, 383–386.

Lee, C.K., Rauschning, W. & Glenn, W. (1988) Lateral lumbar spinal canal stenosis: classification, pathological anatomy and surgical decompression. *Spine*, **13**, 313–320.

Lewis, T. (1942) *Pain*. Macmillan, New York.

Liesi, P., Gronblad, M., Korkale, O., Karaharaju, E. & Rusanen, M. (1983) Substance P: a neuropeptide involved in low back pain. *Lancet*, 1328–1329.

Lindblom, K. (1951) Technique and results of diagnostic disc puncture and injection (discography) in the lumbar region. *Acta Orthop. Scand.*, **20**, 315–326.

Lorenz, M., Patawardhan, A. & Van Derby, R. (1983) Load bearing characteristics of lumbar facets in normal and surgically altered spinal segments. *Spine*, **8**, 122–130.

Lynch, M.C. & Taylor, J.F. (1986) Facet joint injection for low back pain. *J. Bone Jt. Surg.*, **68B**, 138–141.

McCall, I.W. (1987) Radiological investigation of the intervertebral disc. In Jayson, M.I.V. (ed.) *The Lumbar Spine and Back Pain*, 3rd edn, pp. 235–268. Churchill Livingstone, London.

McCall, I.W., Park, W.M. & O'Brien, J.P. (1979) Induced pain referral from posterior lumbar elements in normal subjects. *Spine*, **4**, 441–445.

MacNab, I. (1971) The traction spur. *J. Bone Jt. Surg.*, **53A**, 663–670.

Malinsky, J. (1959) The ontogenetic development of nerve terminations in the intervertebral discs of man. *Acta Anat.*, **38**, 906–1113.

Mooney, V. & Robertson, J. (1976) The facet syndrome. *Clin. Orthop.*, **115**, 149–156.

Murphy, R.W. (1977) Nerve roots and spinal nerves in degenerative disc disease. *Clin. Orthop.*, **129**, 46–60.

Nachemson, A. (1969) Intradiscal measurements of pH in patients with lumbar rhinopathies. *Acta. Orthop. Scand.*, **40**, 23–42.

Nashold, B.S. (1988) Deafferentation pain in man and animals as it relates to the DREZ operation. *Canad. J. Neurol.* Sci., **15**, 5–9.

Naylor, A. (1962) The biophysical and biochemical aspect of intervertebral disc herniation and degeneration. *Ann. R. Coll. Surg. Engl.*, **31**, 91–114.

Olsson, Y. (1971) Studies on vascular permeability in peripheral nerve. *Acta Neuropathol.*, **17**, 114–126.

Olsson, Y. & Kristensson, K. (1973) The perineurium as a diffusion barrier to protein tracers following trauma to nerves. *Acta Neuropathol.*, **23**, 105–111.

Paris, S.V. (1983) Anatomy as related to function and pain. *Orthop. Clin. N. Am.*, **14**, 475–490.

Pate, D., Goobar, J., Resnick, D., Hoghighi, P., Sartoris, D.J. & Pathria, M.N. (1988) Traction osteophytes of the lumbar spine: radiographic–pathologic correlation. *Radiology*, **166**, 843–846.

Pedersen, H.E., Blunck, C.F.J. & Gardner, E. (1986) The anatomy of lumbosacral posterior rami and meningeal branches of spinal nerves. *J. Bone Jt. Surg.*, **38A**, 377–391.

Penning, L. & Wilmink, J.T. (1987) Posture dependent bilateral compression of L4 or L5 nerve roots in facet hypertrophy. *Spine*, **12**, 488–500.

Perey, O. (1951) Contrast medium examinations of the intervertebral discs of the lower lumbar spine. *Acta Orthop. Scand.*, **20**, 327–334.

Porter, R.W. (1987) Spinal stenosis in the central and root canal. In: Jayson, M.I.V. (ed.), *The Lumbar Spine and Back Pain*, pp. 383–400. Churchill Livingstone, London.

Pountain, G.D., Keegan, A.L. & Jayson, M.I.V. (1986) Impaired fibrinolytic activity in defined chronic back pain syndromes. *Spine*, **12**, 83–86.

Procacci, P. & Zoppi, M. (1981) Pathophysiology and clinical aspects of visceral and referred pain. *Pain*, Suppl. **1**, 1–57.

Putti, V. & Logroscino, D. (1938) Anatomica dell artritismo Vertebrale Apofisario. *Chir. d. Organi di Movimento*, **23**, 317–353.

Quinnell, R.C. & Stockdale, H.R. (1982) The significance of osteophytes on lumbar vertebral bodies in relation to discographic findings. *Clin. Radiol.*, **33**, 197–203.

Rabischong, P., Louis, R., Vignaud, J. & Massare, C. (1978) *Anat. Clin.*, **1**, 55–64.

Rauschning, W. (1987) Normal and pathologic anatomy of the lumbar root canals. *Spine*, **12**, 1008–1019.

Richards, R.L. (1951) Ischaemic lesions of peripheral nerves, a review. *J. Neurol. Neurosurg. Psychiatry*, **14**, 76–87.

Rosomoff, H. & Rosomoff, R.S. (1987) Non-surgical aggressive treatment of lumbar spinal stenosis. In Hopp, E. (ed.), *Spinal Stenosis*, pp. 383–400. Hanley-Belfus, Philadelphia, PA.

Ruch, T.C. (1965) Pathophysiology of pain. In Ruch, T.C. & Patton, H.D. (eds), *Physiology and Biophysics*, pp. 357–358. W.B. Saunders, London.

Schaible, H.G. & Schmidt, R.F. (1983) Activation of groups iii and iv sensory units in medial articular nerve by local mechanical stimulation of knee joint. *J. Neurophysiol.*, **49**, 34–44.

Sherrington, C.S. (1906) *The Integrative Action of the Nervous System*. Yale University Press, New Haven, CT.

Shinohara, H. (1970) Lumbar disc lesions with special reference to the histological significance of nerve endings of the lumbar discs. *J. Jap. Orthop. Assoc.*, **44**, 553–570.

Simons, D.G. (1976) Muscle pain syndromes. Part II. *Am. J. Phys-Med.*, **55**, 15–42.

Sims-Williams, H., Jayson, M.I.V. & Baddley, H. (1978) Small spinal fractures in back-pain patients. *Ann. Rheum. Dis.*, **37**, 262–265.

Smyth, M.J. & Wright, V. (1958) Sciatica and the intervertebral disc. *J. Bone Jt. Surg.*, **40A**, 1401–1418.

Sunderland, S. (1974) Meningeal–neural relations in the intervertebral foramen. *J. Neurosurg.*, **40**, 756–763.

Tasker, R.R., Organ, L.W. & Hawrylyshyn, P. (1980) Deafferentation and causalgia. In Bonica, J.J. (ed.) *Pain*, pp. 350–379. Raven Press, New York.

Travell, J.G. & Simons, D.G. (1983) *Myofascial Pain and*

Dysfunction. The Trigger Point Manual. Williams & Wilkins, Baltimore, MD.
Travell, J., Berry, C. & Bigelar, N. (1944) Effects of referred somatic pain on structures in the reference zone. *Fed. Proc.*, **3**, 49.
Weinstein, J.N. (1986) Mechanisms of spinal pain: the dorsal root ganglion and its role as a mediator of low back pain. *Spine*, **11**, 999–1001.
Wyke, B.D. (1987) The neurology of low back pain. In Jayson, M.I.V. (ed.), *The Lumbar Spine and Back Pain*, pp. 56–59. Churchill Livingstone, London.
Yoshizawa, H., O'Brien, J.P., Smith, W.T. & Trumper, M. (1980) The neuropathology of intervertebral discs removed for low back pain. *J. Pathol.*, **132**, 95–104.

36 · Assessment of Low Back Pain

By J.R. JOHNSON

And I place the interrogation of the patient first, since in this way you can learn how far his mind is healthy or otherwise; also his physical strengths and weaknesses, and you can get some idea of the part affected. (Rufus of Ephesus, AD 100)

The assessment of low back pain has been attempted for centuries. While the need for treatment has not changed, thoughts about the causes of low back pain have changed considerably over the past 60–70 years, and methods of assessment have had to alter as a result. In 1926 Osler listed nine causes of back pain, the last of which was traumatic. Sciatica was not even thought of as being traumatic in origin. Indeed in World War I backache was hidden in the American Army diagnostic category of 'muscular rheumatism' and occurred in only 13% of soldiers. By World War II back pain accounted for 40% of hospital admissions for rheumatic disorders and had become a major issue in the army. Since then it has continued as a major cause of time off work in industry.

In the USA Kelsey & White (1980) have found that back pain is the most frequent cause of limitation of activity in people under the age of 45 years, and ranks only third after heart disease and arthritis in the 45–65-year-old age group. Why this change?

Part of the cause must be due to the classic paper by Mixter & Barr in 1934, ascribing a cause for backache and sciatica to prolapse of the intervertebral disc. More than this, they referred to this prolapse both in the paper and, indeed, in the title, as a 'rupture'. This term immediately suggests injury; thus backache changed from being an 'illness' to being the result of an injury.

As a result, backache has become one of the commonest causes of disability in the UK. Twelve million working days are lost by 300 000 people per year, and such figures do not include people not in work such as housewives and pensioners.

According to Waddell (1982), about 1.1 million patients consult their general practitioner, 0.3 million are referred to hospital, 30 000 are admitted to hospital and 5000 end up with an operation on the back. There are 80 000 people in the UK permanently disabled by backache. These statistics gave a total annual cost of backache in the UK of £1000 million in 1982.

Although four out of five people suffer from low back pain at some time in their life, 80–95% of patients having an acute attack recover within three months, and in 80% of patients no objective cause for the pain can be found after a thorough examination. The prognosis for those patients whose back pain persists for longer than six months is dismal (Campbell *et al.*, 1989). Less than 50% ever return to work, and if the time off work exceeds two years the rate of return to work is negligible.

The size of the problem seems to be increasing. In the USA between 1971 and 1981 the number of people registered disabled with low back pain increased by 168%, while the population only increased by 12.5%. This may also be due to a change in attitude with more patients complaining of 'an injury to their back' rather than backache, perhaps with compensation in mind.

Assessment of low back pain in degenerative disease still largely depends on the history and physical examination. However, because of problems in reliability and reproducibility of clinical findings in low back pain, many attempts have been made to make the assessment of low back pain more scientific. Thus interest has been drawn to measuring disability, to psychological testing, to more accurate methods of measuring impairment on examination and, more recently, there have been advances in computer-aided diagnosis, and in the use of machines to test trunk strength in a more objective manner.

The purpose of this chapter is to explore these various methods of assessment and to try and produce a comprehensive evaluation of the patients suffering with low back pain due to degenerative disease.

HISTORY

Despite all attempts to make this process more efficient by using questionnaires, computers and other techniques, there is no substitute for the taking of a careful history which gives an overall picture. Obviously some direct questioning will be needed, but there is much to be gained by listening to the patient and assessing the order of importance of symptoms. Pain is the predominant symptom, and this will be explored in more detail.

Pain

Pain is often the only symptom of degenerative spinal disease and it is difficult to identify precisely in the spine, because the pain is often not specific.

Over the years various attempts have been made to make the assessment of pain more scientific. However, in this part of the assessment the main object is to separate the low back pain into three main categories:

1 non-spondylogenic back pain;
2 back pain associated with leg pain or other symptoms with nerve root irritation;
3 mechanical or spondylogenic back pain.

Non-spondylogenic back pain

In a proportion of cases the cause of the low back pain lies outside the spine and may derive from the kidneys, pelvic viscera, retroperitoneal tumours, or from the vascular system. Low back pain is a common complaint in patients with vascular disease, and the differentiation between intermittent and neurogenic claudication may be difficult. Spinal tumours, although rare, may also present with low back pain and sometimes sciatica. Frequently they can be distinguished from symptoms due to mechanical low back pain, as the pain is not relieved by rest, is continuous and, especially in children, worse at night. However, spinal tumours may present exactly as do cases of degenerative disease, and full radiological evaluation of the lumbar canal to the conus is necessary (Ker & Jones, 1985). Generally all these causes of low back pain can be differentiated from mechanical low back pain because of other symptoms associated with a particular disorder, and can be confirmed by specific investigations.

Back pain associated with leg pain

The main purpose of this part of the history is to elicit the difference between pain arising from nerve root compression and referred pain from the back. Not all leg pain is due to nerve root compression, and the pain is not necessarily caused by a prolapsed intervertebral disc. Work by Kellgren (1977) and others has shown that by using percutaneous needle stimulation, or by injecting hypertonic saline solutions, referred pain from the back can spread into the buttock and thighs, but rarely spreads distal to the knees. Root pain is generally sharper, is more accurately localized, tends to follow the course of the sciatic nerve and is often associated with other neurological symptoms such as paraesthesia, numbness or weakness. If the leg pain is thought to be referred pain then it should be classified with the spondylogenic mechanical type of back pain. Waddell (1982) showed that 70% of new patients referred from general practitioners to an orthopaedic clinic with back trouble have leg pain, but most of this is referred pain, and only 23% had a primary nerve root presentation. Neurological symptoms associated with back pain together with leg pain are usually mild, and gross symptoms of numbness or weakness are unusual.

Mechanical low back pain

There are usually many pointers in the history suggesting mechanical low back pain—a history of trauma, and features making the pain better or worse. The relationships to various activities, e.g. standing, sitting and walking, are also useful indicators.

In an attempt to make the assessment of pain more scientific, various techniques such as pain drawings and pain questionnaires have been introduced. The site of the pain in the low back is important, but because many spinal structures are inaccessible to examination it is difficult to localize precisely the anatomical source of the pain. A subjective localization by the patient may be obtained using a pain drawing (Ransford *et al.*, 1976) (see Fig. 36.1) This is useful for showing both the site and distribution of the pain. It also has a particular part to play in the psychological assessment of pain. The pain drawing may be supplemented by the use of pain questionnaires. The simplest way to try and measure pain on an objective 'scale' is by using a visual analogue pain scale allowing the patient to grade the pain on a percentage scale. This technique has been refined in various questionnaires such as the Dallas pain questionnaire which has been developed over a six-year period (Lawlis *et al.*, 1989) (see Table 36.1). It is a compact questionnaire designed to provide a maximum amount of information regarding the subjective impact of chronic pain. The Dallas pain questionnaire is graded on a percentage scale of 0–100%, and 16 questions have been developed. Each question was formulated to avoid discrepancies and four basic categories were developed. Categories one and two reflect the patient's perception of physical activity. Categories three and four reflect the subjective perception of the emotional component of the pain. Category one (i.e. Sections I–VII), described as daily activities, measures the amount of disability the patient experiences in personal care, lifting, walking, sitting, standing and sleeping. Category two (i.e. Sections VIII–X) relates to vocational ability. Category three (i.e. Sections XI–XIII), labelled anxiety and depression, measures loss of emotional control. Finally the last section, category four (i.e. Sections XIV–XVI), measures social interest and social skills affected by pain. The results suggest that the Dallas pain questionnaire has the shortcomings of any self-report measure, i.e. that it cannot distinguish malingering from earnest assessment. However, it can be used together with physical assessment and systematic observation of pain behaviour. It was found that when categories 1 and 2 were over 50%, and categories 3 and 4 were less than 50%, medical intervention was effective. However when categories 1 and 2 were less than 50% and categories 3 and 4 were over 50% there was obviously a behavioural problem.

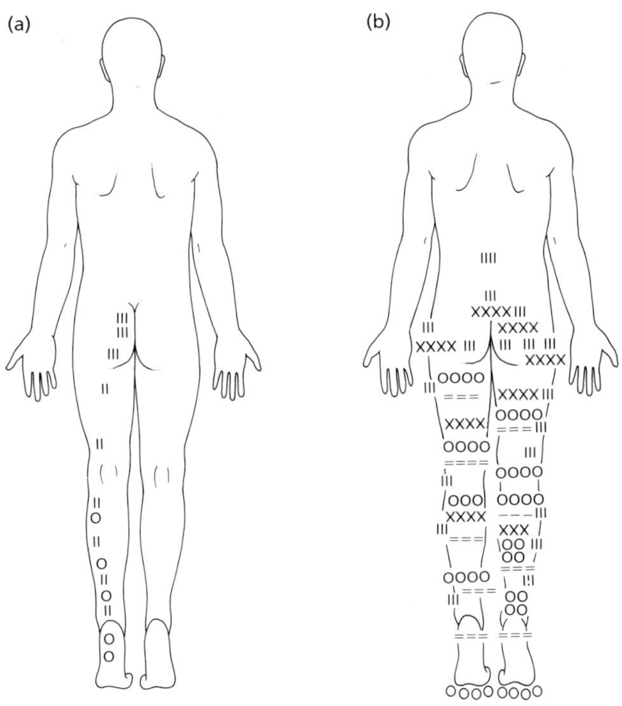

Fig. 36.1 Pain drawing: patient (a) describes the physical pattern of an S1 sciatica from a disc prolapse; patient (b) with a simple backache is communicating distress.

The McGill pain questionnaire (MPQ) was developed by Richard Melzack (1983), and again is a self-administered questionnaire consisting of 20 sets of adjectives from which the patient is asked to pick the words best describing the pain. In addition to this there is the pain line drawing of the body to show the distribution and character of the pain, a rating of present pain intensity. As in other tests there is a scoring system. It has the advantage of being quickly administered, often taking only as little as five minutes to complete, and most patients find the questions relevant. From a clinical point of view this test is more a descriptive test of pain, rather than aiming to be diagnostic. Recently there have been criticisms of this questionnaire since the results are hard to reproduce; in addition some workers feel that pain ratings are not good for assessing chronic pain.

Disability

Another approach in the quest for a more scientific assessment of patients with low back pain has been to try to measure disability. Disability is defined as the limitations of a patient's performance in a range of daily activities compared with those of a fit person. There is now general agreement, both in the USA and in the UK, that disability is probably the best method of assessment in low back disorders (Fairbank *et al.*, 1980; Roland & Morris, 1983; Frymoyer & Cats-Baril, 1987).

Table 36.1 Dallas pain questionnaire

Name ____________ Date of birth ____________
Today's date ____________ Occupation ____________

Please read: This questionnaire has been designed to give your doctor information as to how your pain has affected your life. Be sure that these are your answers. Do not ask someone else to fill out the questionnaire for you. Please mark an 'X' along the line that expresses your thoughts from 0 to 100 in each section.

Section I: Pain and intensity
To what degree do you rely on pain medications or pain relieving substances for you to be comfortable?
None — Some — All the time

0% (____:____:____:____:____:____) 100%

Section II: Personal care
How much does pain interfere with your personal care (getting out of bed, teeth brushing, dressing, etc.)?
None (no pain) — Some — I cannot get out of bed

0% (____:____:____:____:____:____) 100%

Section III: Lifting
How much limitation do you notice in lifting?
None (I can lift as I did) — Some — I cannot lift anything

0% (____:____:____:____:____:____) 100%

Section IV: Walking
Compared to how far you could walk before your injury or back trouble, how much does pain restrict your walking now?
I can walk the same — Almost the same — Very little — I cannot walk

0% (____:____:____:____:____:____) 100%

Section V: Sitting
Back pain limits my sitting in a chair to:
None (pain same as before) — Some — I cannot sit at all

0% (____:____:____:____:____:____) 100%

Section VI: Standing
How much does your pain interfere with your tolerance to stand for long periods?
None (same as before) — Some — I cannot stand

0% (____:____:____:____:____:____) 100%

Section VII: Sleeping
How much does pain interfere with your sleeping?
None (same as before) — Some — I cannot sleep at all

0% (____:____:____:____:____:____) 100%
(Sum × 3 = ________ % Daily activities interference)

Section VIII: Social life
How much does pain interfere with your social life (dancing, games, going out, eating with friends, etc.)?
None (same as before) — Some — No activities total loss

0% (____:____:____:____:____:____) 100%

Section IX: Travelling
How much does pain interfere with travelling in a car?
None (same as before) — Some — I cannot travel

0% (____:____:____:____:____:____) 100%

Section X: Vocational
How much does pain interfere with your job?
None (no interference) — Some — I cannot work

0% (____:____:____:____:____:____) 100%
(Sum × 5 = ________ % Work/leisure activities interference)

Section XI: Anxiety/Mood
How much control do you feel that you have over demands made on you?
Total (no change) — Some — None

100% (____:____:____:____:____:____) 0%

Section XII: Emotional control
How much control do you feel you have over your emotions?
Total (no change) — Some — None

100% (____:____:____:____:____:____) 0%

Section XIII: Depression
How depressed have you been since the onset of pain?
Not depressed significantly — Overwhelmed by depression

0% (____:____:____:____:____:____) 100%
(Sum × 5 = ________ % Anxiety/depression interference)

Section XIV: Interpersonal relationships
How much do you think your pain has changed your relationships with others?
Not changed — Drastically changed

0% (____:____:____:____:____:____) 100%

Section XV: Social support
How much support do you need from others to help you during this onset of pain (taking over chores, fixing meals, etc.)?
None needed — All the time

0% (____:____:____:____:____:____) 100%

Section XVI: Punishing response
How much do you think others express irritation, frustration or anger toward you because of your pain?
None — Some — All the time

0% (____:____:____:____:____:____) 100%
(Sum × 5 = ________ % Social interest interference)

Assessment of disability is made by specific questioning on a variety of activities likely to be affected by low back pain. Waddell & Main (1984) suggest the following activities.

1 Bending and lifting. Disability here means that help is required with heavy lifting, for example a heavy suitcase, or that heavy lifting is avoided by the patient.

2 Sitting. Sitting in an ordinary chair is limited to less than 30 minutes at a time.

3 Standing. This is limited to less than 30 minutes at a time.

4 Walking. This is limited to less than 30 minutes, or one to two miles at a time.

5 Travelling. Travelling for more than 30 minutes at a time is uncomfortable.

6 Social life. Patient regularly misses or has to curtail social activities (excluding sports).

7 Sleep. This is regularly disturbed, i.e. two or three times per week by low back pain.

8 Sexual activity. Frequency of sexual activity is diminished.

9 Footwear. Help is regularly required with footwear in terms of dressing, putting on socks, shoes, etc.

These types of questions have been formally incorporated into various disability questionnaires, for example the Oswestry Disability Questionnaire (Fairbank *et al.*, 1980), and tests have shown good short-term repeatability.

Psychological testing

Psychological factors are crucial in the successful assessment and treatment of low back disorders. All too often the outcome of conservative management or surgery is less successful than predicted because of a failure to assess the patient's psychological state. Nowadays a more holistic view of the patient is required if treatment is to be successful.

The assessment of pain has already been discussed. Chronic pain is very different from acute pain. With chronicity, patients may develop signs of psychological distress. How patients cope with their pain may be more important than tests of inappropriate behaviour. Another important factor is stress, and many patients admit that their level of back pain is affected by the level of stress. The psychological tests have been evolved in an attempt to distinguish organic symptoms and signs from those with psychological overlay. These tests should be regarded as complementary to the history-taking part of the assessment, and not as an alternative to taking a full history.

Most tests are in the form of self-administered questionnaires which are then scored by the clinician. They have the advantage of being unbiased and reproducible, but are limited by the specific questions asked. Bearing in mind these reservations, common tests in current use are described below.

The Minnesota multiphasic personality inventory (MMPI)

The MMPI is the best-known and most widely used test in the psychological assessment of patients with low back pain. However, it was designed for psychiatric patients to assess their character and was not designed for patients with low back pain. Secondly, it is very long and therefore time-consuming (it may take three hours to fill in). Thirdly it was designed by Americans for Americans, and is therefore phrased in a vocabulary which is not always familiar to patients of different nationalities, and there are cultural differences which make assessment difficult. In addition, several studies have found an unacceptable overlap between 'functional' and 'organic' groups of patients. Because of these problems various other questionnaires have evolved.

The Millon behavioural health inventory (MBHI)

This test has been designed to assess the psychological functioning of medical patients. Because it was designed specifically for medical rather than psychiatric patients it is more readily accepted by the patient, and the questions appear to be more relevant as a result. The test consists of 150 true/false items which can be completed in 20 minutes, even by a patient with relatively poor reading skills. It is divided into four parts: the first assesses basic coping skills; the second assesses stress levels and attitudes towards them; the third part correlates specific symptoms with those of other patients with similar disorders; and the final category attempts to assess the likelihood of the individual to respond to treatment and gives some form of prognostic index.

The major value of this test is that the data obtained are relatively clear and concise. Validity and reliability are well documented (Millon *et al.*, 1979) but it has not as yet been widely used in clinical trials and is not as well known as the MMPI.

The modified somatic perception questionnaire (MSPQ)

This test basically assesses distress (see Table 36.2), and was developed by Main (1983). Recently its relevance in back pain was reviewed by Deyo *et al.* (1989); they felt that it successfully distinguished between normal patients and those with back pain, and between mild and severe low back pain, but beyond this is was not very specific. Both this and the Zung depression inventory (see below) are completed by the patient on an unscored form.

The Zung depression inventory

Main, again, has adapted this to give an assessment of the patient's depressive symptoms. These last two tests can be taken together with inappropriate symptoms and signs to give an idea of the abnormal illness behaviour behind the patient's low back pain.

EXAMINATION

Examination of the spine has already been covered in Chapter 4; however, in the assessment of low back pain there are specific problems. Clinical examination is really an assessment of a particular patient's impairment at a particular moment. Many of the tests are subjective observations by the examiner. Recording is often vague and variations between examiners may be widespread (Nelson *et al.*, 1979).

Some attempts have been made to assess severity in low back pain. Most of these are based on the overall diagnosis and therefore are often biased towards one particular sign or symptom. For example, McBride's (1963) classification is very much orientated to subjective assessments. Waddell (1982) makes the distinction between organic manifestations and behavioural patterns, and has tried to suggest ways in which our examination techniques might be improved and standardized. The aim is to ensure reproducibility between examiners and to have specific objective tests of lumbar impairment. Obviously there is usually no argument over the standard neurological part of the examination.

Lumbar flexion

In order to avoid confusion between back movement and hip movement or hamstring tightness, the skin

Table 36.2 The modified somatic perception questionnaire (MSPQ) with scores

Please describe how you have felt during the *past week* by making a check mark (√) in the appropriate place. Please answer all questions. Do not think too long before answering.

	Not at all	A little/ slightly	A great deal/ quite a bit	Extremely/ could not have been worse
Heart rate increase				
Feeling hot all over	*0	1	2	3
Sweating all over	*0	1	2	3
Sweating in a particular part of the body				
Pulse in neck				
Pounding in head				
Dizziness	*0	1	2	3
Blurring of vision	*0	1	2	3
Feeling faint	*0	1	2	3
Everything appearing unreal				
Nausea	*0	1	2	3
Butterflies in stomach				
Pain or ache in stomach	*0	1	2	3
Stomach churning	*0	1	2	3
Desire to pass water				
Mouth becoming dry	*0	1	2	3
Difficulty swallowing				
Muscles in neck aching	*0	1	2	3
Legs feeling weak	*0	1	2	3
Muscles twitching or jumping	*0	1	2	3
Tense feeling across forehead	*0	1	2	3
Tense feeling in jaw muscles				

* Only these 13 items are scored.

marking technique (Fig. 36.2) or goniometer system (Mayer *et al.*, 1984) should be used. For the skin marking technique a mark is made on the skin on the midlower level of the dimples of Venus, approximately L5; a second mark is made 10 cm above, and a third mark 5 cm below, the initial mark. The patient is then asked to bend forwards with the knees straight and to reach as far as possible towards the toes. The increase in distance between the upper and lower marks is then taken as a measure of lumbar flexion. Waddell (1982) has shown that 90% of asymptomatic normal people can flex at least 5 cm, and this value may be even higher in young adults. An alternative is to use goniometric measures; however, these cannot easily discriminate between hip movement and spinal movement component, and the danger with these tests is that they may give the clinician a false sense that the test methods are objective and reproducible. Pain on extending from the flexed position has been associated with segmental instability or facet arthropathy. A sciatic tilt on forward flexion suggests a prolapsed disc.

Other spinal movements

A decrease in extension with pain suggests a facet arthropathy or spinal stenosis. It is normally also routine to measure decreases in lateral flexion and rotation; however, Waddell found that no other signs, apart from lumbar flexion, were helpful in assessing the level of impairment.

Straight leg raising

Restriction of straight leg raising suggests root irritation. It should be performed passively and may be repeated with distraction of the patient if exaggeration is suspected. Pain in the opposite leg, i.e. cross-leg pain, is highly suggestive of a prolapsed intervertebral disc.

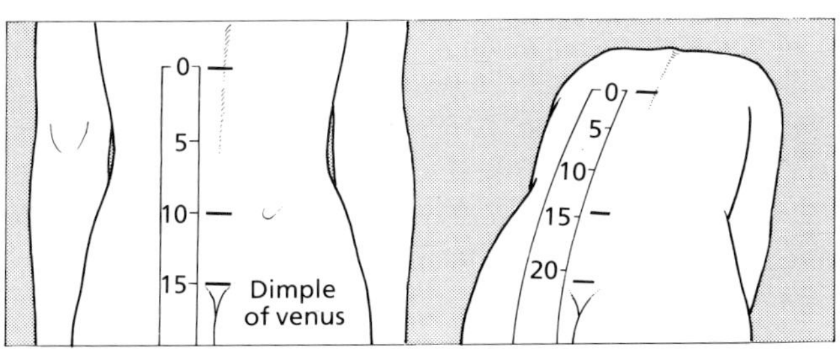

Fig. 36.2 The skin marking technique of measuring lumbar flexion.

Nerve compression signs

The standard neurological examination is performed. Usually any sensory, motor or reflex deficit will be confined to a single root origin and correspond to an exact anatomical distribution. Whole leg pain, or whole leg weakness and/or stocking anaesthesia, suggests a non-organic cause.

Unfortunately observer error is present to a greater or lesser extent in all these assessments, particularly in the examination. As Nelson *et al.* (1979) have shown, it is particularly high in some measured tests such as straight leg raising; however, the measurement of lumbar flexion does seem to be reproducible.

Illness behaviour

Although physical signs that appear to have a non-organic basis have long been recognized, it was Waddell *et al.* (1980) who took a group of non-organic physical signs and standardized them to review their value in the assessment of patients with low back pain. A standard group of five types of physical signs were used.

Superficial and non-anatomical tenderness (Fig. 36.3)

To elicit superficial tenderness the skin is lightly pinched (the pinch test) over a wide area of the lumbar skin. Non-anatomical tenderness is deep tenderness over a wide area, not localized to one specific structure.

Axial loading (Fig. 36.4)

If low back pain is reported on vertical loading of the patient's skull by the examiner's hand this test should be regarded as positive for an inappropriate response. Similarly rotation of the shoulders and pelvis together in the same plane, while a patient stands relaxed, should not cause back pain.

Distraction (Fig. 36.5)

The patient may be distracted in many ways during the examination. One of the most useful distraction tests is that of straight leg raising. There may be gross

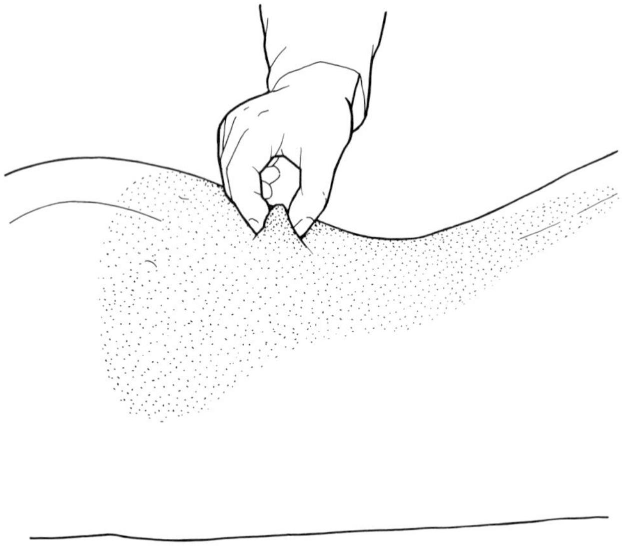

Fig. 36.3 Non-organic tenderness showing technique of testing superficial skin tenderness and area (shaded) frequently involved in widespread non-anatomical tenderness.

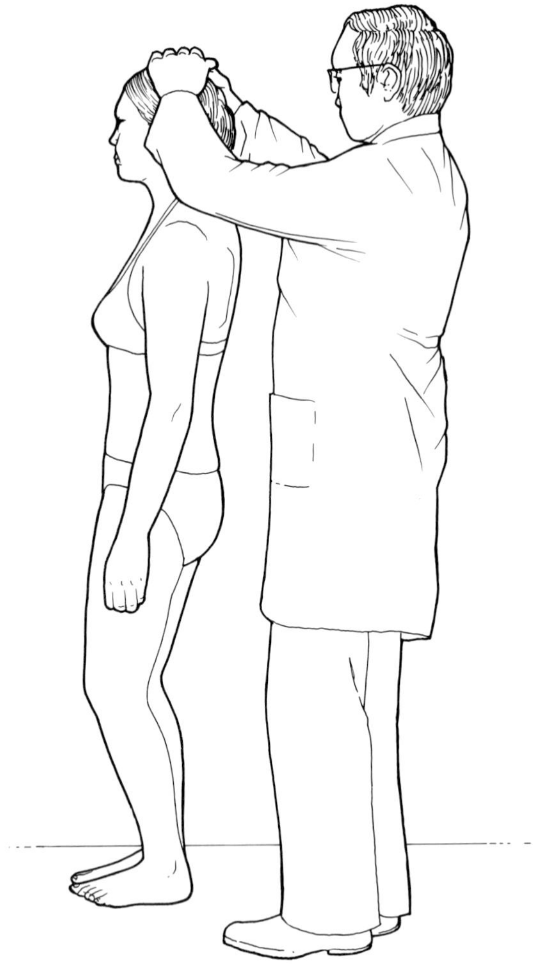

Fig. 36.4 Axial loading: back pain on vertical loading on the standing patient's head.

apparent loss of straight leg raising in the supine position, but if the patient is distracted and is made to sit up on the couch with the legs extended in front, then obviously there is an inappropriate response. In America this is called the 'flip test'.

Regional disturbances (Fig. 36.6)

These are motor or sensory deficits that do not fit with the normal anatomical pathways. For example, weakness may be shown as a cogwheel type of jerky giving-way of the knee or foot which cannot be explained neurologically. In similar vein are regional sensory disturbances of a stocking type which do not fit any particular dermatomal pattern.

Over-reaction (Fig. 36.7)

Over-reaction can take many forms, but muscle spasms, tremor, collapsing while being examined, etc., are all part of a complex behavioural pattern.

Waddell *et al.* (1980) found that over-reaction was the single most important non-organic sign, but it is also the sign most influenced by observer interpretation. Taken together, McCulloch (1977) has found the tests to be of major value in predicting the results of chemonucleolysis for prolapsed intervertebral disc, and the early results of more recent trials in surgery suggest that these tests do help in the identification of patients likely to have a poor result from surgery. Waddell has shown that the non-organic signs are more useful than the non-organic symptoms in identifying abnormal illness behaviour.

The first suggestion that psychological factors might influence the results of surgery was postulated by Wilfling *et al.*, in 1973. A small series of patients about to undergo spinal fusion had an MMPI etc., in addition to a clinical assessment, and were then assessed postoperatively. It was found that the 'poor' and 'fair' groups rated high in the hypochondriacal scale of the MMPI.

In 1975, Wiltse & Rocchio used psychological testing as a predictor of the success of chemo-

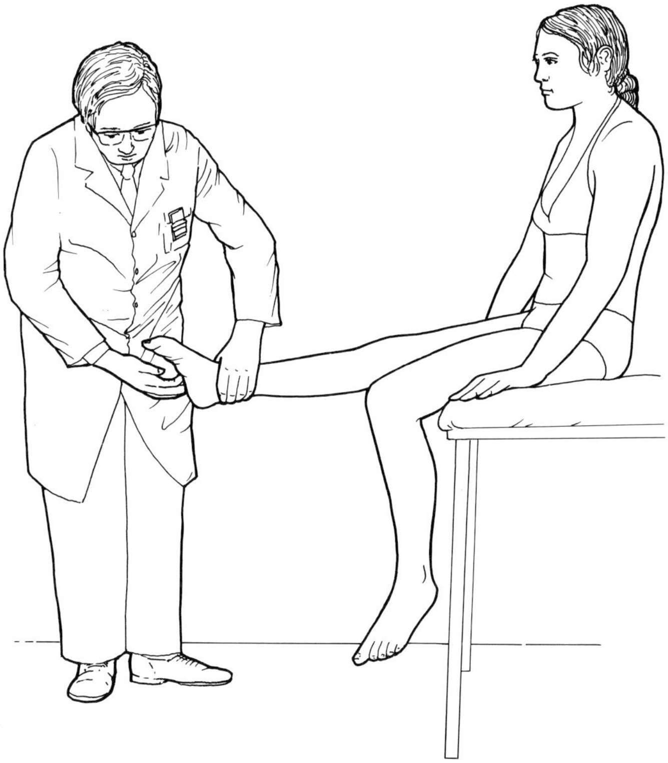

Fig. 36.5 Straight leg raising improving with distraction; as when testing the plantar reflex in the sitting position.

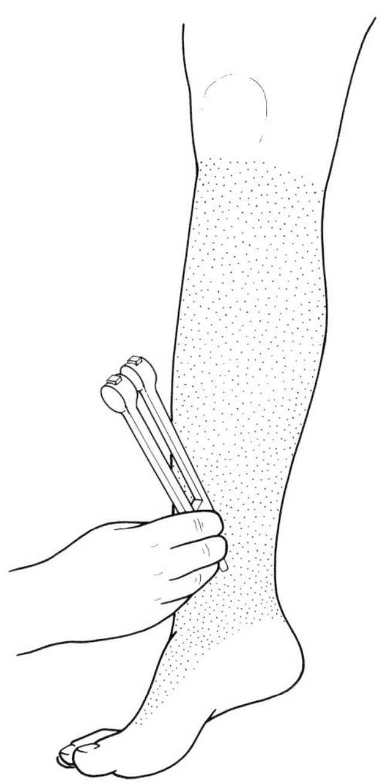

Fig. 36.6 Non-anatomical sensory alteration in a 'stocking' distribution affecting light touch, pin-prick, and sometimes other modalities.

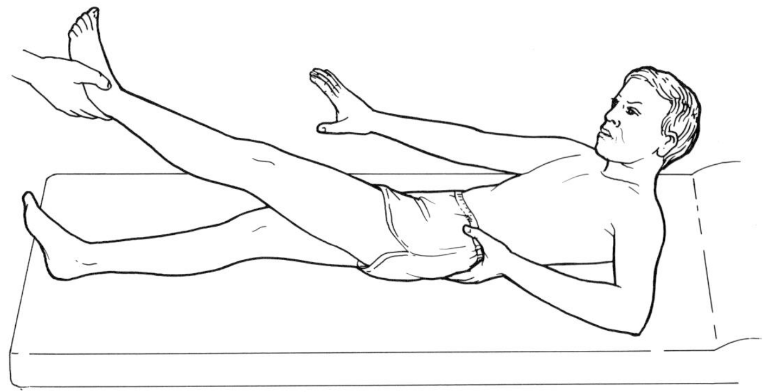

Fig. 36.7 Over-reaction to examination: disproportionate verbalization, facial expression, muscle tension and tremor, collapsing or sweating.

nucleolysis and came to similar conclusions. They found that when MMPI hysteria and hypochondriacal scores were low there was a 90% chance of obtaining a 'good' or 'excellent' result from surgery, assuming that the patient had objective findings which justified surgery.

However, in 1979, Pheasant *et al.* raised certain doubts about MMPI profiles being used as a predictor of surgical outcome. They suggested that MMPI scores should be used only as an adjunct to other clinical and psychological data.

A large series of patients about to undergo surgery were reviewed by Oostdam *et al.* in 1981. They investigated a mixed group of patients due to have either disc surgery, disc and lateral canal decompression or fusion for spondylolisthesis, and correctly predicted the results at follow-up in 79.4% of cases. They concluded that psychological investigation can contribute to the appropriate selection of patients for whom surgical treatment is likely to be successful.

In 1984, Dzioba & Doxey reviewed 116 patients submitted to a battery of clinical and psychological tests preoperatively. The psychological testing included the MMPI, a pain drawing and McGill pain questionnaire. Their group all had back problems following industrial injury, but none had had previous surgery. At follow-up, at three years, they had correctly predicted the results of surgery in 82% of cases. Interestingly, they found five main predicting factors from their preoperative assessment. Firstly, proficiency in English: many of their patients were migrant workers with a poor command of English and presumably this affected their assessment of the patients because of difficulties with the history and difficulties in explaining the procedure to the patients. Secondly, if any two or more of Waddell's non-organic signs were positive the result was not likely to be good. Thirdly, the results were much more likely to be favourable if leg pain rather than back pain was the predominant symptom. Fourthly, they confirmed the relationship with a hyper-chondriacal scale on the MMPI scoring. Finally, they found the pain drawing significant, and that it was complementary to the MMPI rather than a replacement. Overall, they concluded that the clinical prognosis by the orthopaedic surgeon was usually good, but not as good as when taken with these five psychological factors.

Waddell *et al.* (1986) published the results of a prospective study of 185 patients about to undergo surgery or chemonucleolysis. Patients were followed up for an average of two years postoperatively. Waddell *et al.* found that the physical outcome was almost entirely determined by physical factors: for example, the accuracy of the diagnosis, the operative findings, the surgical procedure, and the avoidance of complications. The most important psychological disturbances were distress and abnormal illness behaviour. Disability tends to result from a combination of the physical disorder together with the distress and illness behaviour. Unfortunately medical decisions tend to be based on distress and illness behaviour, and they therefore found that the symptoms of illness behaviour needed to be clearly distinguished from those of physical disease. Not only does inappropriate illness behaviour lead to inappropriate surgery, it also affects the subjective assessment of pain by the patient. These workers concluded that psychological disturbances appear to be secondary to physical disorders, and therefore tend to improve or deteriorate with successful or failed treatment, respectively.

From this type of simplified examination a fairly accurate measure of the degree of physical impairment can be made. In the attempt to measure physical impairment more accurately, attention has turned to the use of various machines to test trunk strength.

Trunk strength testing

Machines to test flexion/extension are now commercially available, and can assess isometric, isotonic or isokinetic trunk strength in both the sagittal plane, and now more recently in the axial plane. Techniques now exist for documenting effort, and have been built into the computer programs. The purpose of these machines is to isolate the thoracolumbar portions of the spine by stabilizing the shoulder blades above the level of the thoracolumbar segment, and the pelvic and lower extremity below the thoracolumbar segment (Fig. 36.8). A second device is used for rotation. Both devices allow measurement of trunk strength in multipositioned isometric (i.e. static) and multispeed isokinetic modes. A computerized numerical and graphic display shows the torque curve. Curve variability gives a measure of repeatability, which in turn correlates with patient effort.

Mayer *et al.* (1984) observed that the trunk strength measurement has to take into account the general fitness of the patient; therefore the aerobic capacity and general fatigue of the lower extremities is assessed by bicycle ergometry so that this can be taken into account in the assessment of trunk strength.

FINAL ASSESSMENT AND EVALUATION

The assessment of low back pain will ultimately depend on a reason for the assessment. Although the clinical information is gathered in the same way for every type of assessment, the way in which this information is used varies. One of the ways in which the various types of assessments can be correlated to give a final evaluation has been in the field of computer-aided diagnosis.

There have been several recent studies made of the diagnostic performance of clinicians against that of a computer. With the advent of new computer programs using artificial intelligence techniques there are now recent studies suggesting that in the assessment of low back disorders the computer can sometimes outperform the clinician. Computer-aided diagnostic systems are classically of two types; the older systems calculated the relative likelihood of different diagnoses for individual items on a probability basis.

The more recent method is the use of artificial intelligence or rule-based systems. In a recent study Mathew *et al.* (1988) attempted to break down the diagnostic categories of pain into four groups, namely: simple low back pain, root pain, spinal pathologies such as infection and malignancy, and illness behaviour. The computer used a mathematical theorem

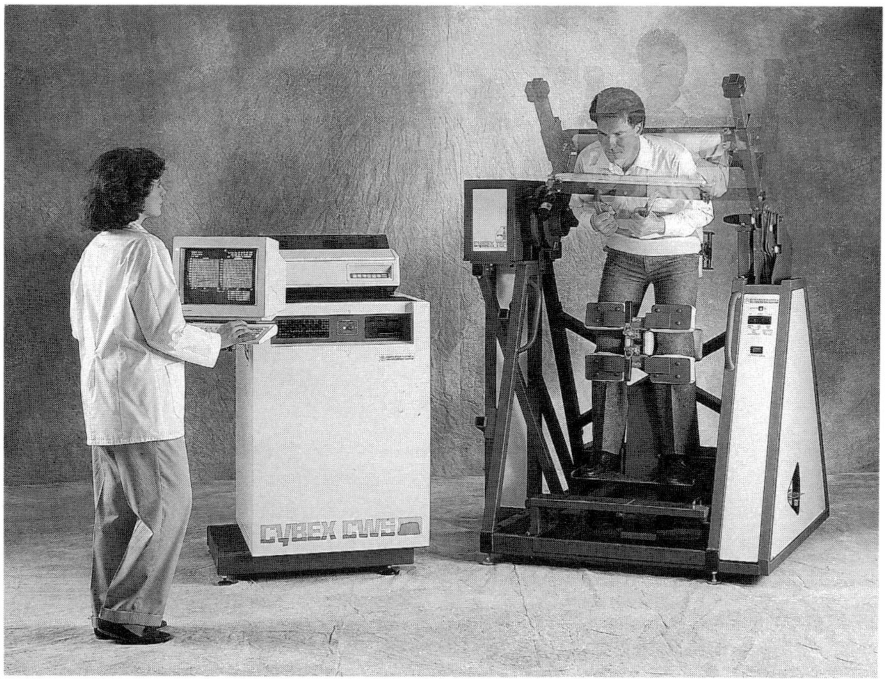

Fig. 36.8 Cybex trunk extension/flexion strength testing unit.

that mimics the human ability to learn from example. This theorem is based on 'fuzzy logic', which better models the uncertainties found in biological systems. Basically the computer looks for symptoms that are or are not representative of the four general diagnostic categories. This method had previously been validated in several different areas, including the acute abdomen. Using this method Mathew *et al.* looked at 200 patients comprising 50 from each of the four diagnostic categories. They found that the computer outperformed the clinicians even though its patient database was relatively small. This confirmed the importance of the symptomatic history, which was shown by the fact that the clinicians and the computer were equally accurate in the clinical assessment and the symptomatic assessment. Once this technique has been refined it is feasible that, in the future, this type of system could be used by family doctors for initial screening of patients. This would then help to discriminate between those who require hospital referral and those who are likely to get better with time.

The final evaluation will depend on whether the clinician is assessing an acute attack of low back pain, an exacerbation of chronic low back pain, an assessment of a patient with chronic impairment for a medicolegal report or an assessment of the results of surgery. For example, the long-term outcome of

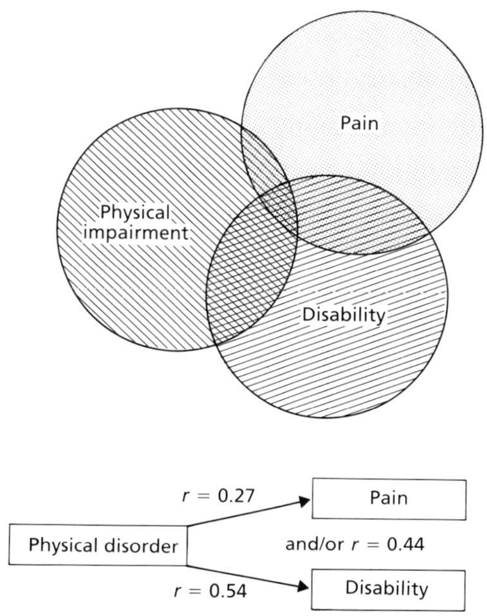

Fig. 36.9 The relationship between pain, disability and impairment showing the correlation and overlap between them. r is the correlation coefficient where 0 = no correlation and 1 = complete identity.

surgery cannot be assessed accurately in under one to two years, and this type of evaluation would be rather different from that for somebody with chronic low back pain due to a work injury.

In patients with low back problems the pain, disability and physical impairment are all related, and when those elements are taken together with work loss they provide a comprehensive evaluation and assessment of the degree of severity of the impairment in the individual (Fig. 36.9).

Although there have been many advances in the objective methods of assessment of low back pain, in the final analysis it is the careful history and examination that still provides the clinician with his main clinical information. The methods described serve to make the clinical examination more accurate and more reproducible between different observers and on different examinations.

REFERENCES

Campbell, D., Goss, E. & Eisenstein, S. (1989) The natural history of low back pain: 5-year study of a rural population. *Neuro-orthopaedics*, **7**, 32–35.

Deyo, R., Walsh, N., Schoenfeld, L. & Ramamurthy, S. (1989) Studies of the modified somatic perceptions questionnaire (MSPQ) in patients with back pain: psychometric and predictive properties. *Spine*, **14**, 507.

Dzioba, R.B. & Doxey, N.C. (1984) A prospective investigation into the orthopaedic and psychologic predictors of outcome of the first lumbar surgery following industrial injury. *Spine*, **9**, 614–623.

Fairbank, J.T., Davies, J.B., Couper, J. & O'Brien, J.P. (1980) The Oswestry low back pain disability questionnaire. *Physiotherapy*, **66**, 271.

Frymoyer, J. & Cats-Baril, W. (1987) Predictors of low back pain disability. *Clin. Orthop. Rel. Res.*, **221**, 89.

Kellgren, J.H. (1977) The anatomical source of back pain. *Rheumatol. Rehabil.*, **16**, 3.

Kelsey, J.G. & White, A.A. III (1980) Epidemiology and impact of low back pain. *Spine*, **5**, 133.

Ker, N. & Jones, C. (1985) Tumours of the cauda equina: the problem of differential diagnosis. *J. Bone Jt. Surg.*, **67B**, 358–362.

Lawlis, G.S., Cuencas, R., Selby, D. & McCoy, C.E. (1989) The development of the Dallas Pain Questionnaire: an assessment of the impact of spinal pain on behaviour: *Spine*, **14**, 511–515.

Main, C.J. (1983) The modified somatic perception questionnaire (MSPQ). *J. Psychosom. Res.*, **27**, 503–514.

Mathew, B., Norris, D., Hendry, D. & Waddell, G. (1988) Artificial intelligence in the diagnosis of low-back pain and sciatica. *Spine*, **13**, 168.

Mayer, T., Tencar, A., Kristoferson, S. & Mooney, V. (1984) Use of noninvasive techniques for quantification of spinal range of motion in normal subjects and chronic low back dysfunction patients. *Spine*, **9**, 588.

McBride, E.D. (1963) *Disability Evaluation*, 6th edn. J.B. Lippincott, Philadelphia, PA.

McCulloch, J. (1983) Chemonucleolysis. *J. Bone Jt. Surg.*, **59B**, 45–52.

Melzack, R. (1983) The McGill Pain Questionnaire. In Melzack, R. (ed.), *Pain Measurement and Assessment*. Raven Press, New York.

Millon, T., Green, C. & Meagher, R. (1929) The MBHI: A new inventory for the psychodiagnostician in medical settings. *Professional Psychol.*, **10**, 529.

Mixter, W.J. & Barr, J.S. (1934) Rupture of the intervertebral disc with involvement of the spinal canal. *N. Engl. J. Med.*, **211**, 210.

Nelson, M.A., Allen, P., Clamp, S.E. & De Bomber, F.T. (1979) Reliability and reproducibility of clinical finding in low back pain. *Spine*, **4**, 97–101.

Oostdam, E.M.M., Duivenvoorden, H.J. & Pondaag, W. (1981) Predictive value of some psychological tests on the outcome of surgical intervention in low back pain patients. *J. Psychosom. Res.*, **25**, 227–235.

Osler, W. (1926) *The Principles and Practice of Medicine*, 10th edn. Appleton, New York.

Pheasant, H., Gilbert, D., Goldfarb, J. & Herron, L. (1979) The MMPI as a predictor of outcome in low-back surgery. *Spine*, **4**, 78–84.

Ransford, A.O., Cairns, D. & Mooney, V. (1976) The pain drawing as an aid to the psychological evaluation of patients with low back pain. *Spine*, **1**, 127–134.

Roland, M. & Morris, R. (1983) A study of the natural history of back pain. Pt 1. Development of a reliable and sensitive measure of disability in low back pain. *Spine*, **8**, 141–144.

Waddell, G. (1982) An approach to backache. *Br. J. Hosp. Med.*, **28**, 201.

Waddell, G. & Main, C.J. (1984) Assessment of severity in low back disorders. *Spine*, **9**, 204.

Waddell, G., McCulloch, J., Kummel, G. & Venner, R. (1980) Non-organic physical signs in low-back pain. *Spine*, **5**, 117.

Waddell, G., Morris, E.W., DiPaola, M.P., Bircher, M. & Finlayson, D. (1986) A concept of illness tested as an improved basis for surgical decisions in low back disorders. *Spine*, **11**, 712–719.

Wilfling, F.J., Klonoff, H. & Kokan, P. (1973) Psychological, demographic and orthopaedic factors associated with prediction of outcome of spinal fusion. *Clin. Orthop. Rel. Res.*, **90**, 153–160.

Wiltse, L.L. & Rocchio, P.D. (1975) Preoperative psychological tests as predictors of success of chemonucleolysis in the treatment of the low-back syndrome. *J. Bone Jt. Surg.*, **57A**, 478–483.

37 · Soft Tissue Injury of the Lumbar Spine

By R.W. PORTER

Soft tissue injury of the spine is an important cause of back pain but, because of diagnostic difficulties, the size of the problem is uncertain. Back pain diagnoses which had favour in a previous generation, such as 'lumbago', 'fibrositis' or 'back strain', inferred a soft tissue pathology; but they have largely been discarded in favour of more easily identifiable disorders of the intervertebral disc and the spinal column. Nevertheless, disease of the musculoligamentous structures of the lumbar spine must be considered as a source of back pain.

Certain studies have given a better understanding of the soft tissue anatomy (Macintosh & Bogduk, 1987) and the biomechanics (Myklebust *et al.*, 1986) of the spine, an improvement in diagnostic skills, and better soft tissue imaging (Tracy *et al.*, 1989). These may show that many acute episodes of back pain are the results of soft tissue injury, which may precede disc and segmental disorders.

BIOMECHANICAL DEFINITION OF STRESS AND STRAIN

Stress is an internal force generated in a material in response to an external load. Strain is the change that develops in the material as a result of that stress; it may be an axial change in length, or a tortional or angular change. If the strain is within the elastic limit (Fig. 37.1) the material will return to the predeformed state. The elastic limit in biological tissues varies with the speed of the applied stress, the duration of the load, and its frequency. It is reached sooner if the force is applied rapidly, and if the tissue is fatigued by repetitive loading (Fig. 37.2).

Plastic deformation occurs when the tissues are strained beyond the elastic limit. The tissue fails to return to the predeformed state. Under further stress the tissues fail by disruption. This applies to all the soft tissues of the spine, muscles, tendons, fascia, ligaments, annulus, nerves, vessels, fat and skin. These tissues will be particularly vulnerable to strain beyond the elastic limit when fatigued by high-frequency repetitive loading, and then stressed by a fall, with the resulting failure of the protective reflexes.

Clinical definition of strain

A strain is an injury to muscle, tendon or fascia beyond the elastic limit (Baker, 1984). It will produce plastic deformation with irreversible axial stretching

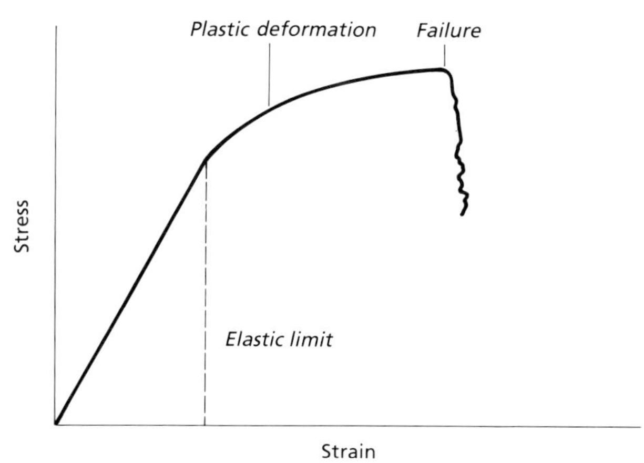

Fig. 37.1 Material is deformed with increasing stress, returning again to the predeformed state until the elastic limit is reached, when plastic deformation occurs. The material will be permanently deformed when the stress is reduced. The material will eventually fail with further stress.

and then, with increased stress, complete disruption of the tissues. The musculotendinous units repair by formation of fibrous tissue and, according to the amount of tissue damage, leave some reduction in function. Marked fibrosis of muscle can impair recovery from muscle injury (Lehto *et al.*, 1989). In practice, however, this reduced function is not apparent clinically; it reduces power, but does not significantly affect joint function.

Muscle rupture, disruption at a musculotendinous junction, or avulsion of ligamentous attachments, are probably just as common in the spine as in the limbs, but because of the inaccessibility of the spinal structures, isolated muscle injury is less easily diagnosed. It may be suspected, however, in a young athlete or an individual suddenly experiencing unusually high stress, whose tenderness is localized away from the midline. Discomfort is experienced when the muscle involved is stretched, or when movement is resisted. Tenderness above the posterior iliac crest in a young footballer, with pain extending into the buttock—whose pain is aggravated by spinal flexion and adduction of the hip, or resisted spinal extension or resisted abduction of the hip—probably results from musculotendinous injury rather than a mechanical disturbance of the lumbar spine.

Clinical definition of sprain

A sprain is an injury to the ligaments of a joint; they are either stretched by plastic deformation or disrupted, perhaps both types of injury occurring in one ligament. By contrast to muscle injury, fibrous repair is a poor substitute for a ligament. The repaired ligament is an inefficient restrainer of the joint and, depending on the degree of the injury, a sprain carries a poor prognosis.

Isolated disruption of spinal ligaments is a difficult diagnosis to prove, except in the combined bony ligamentous injury of unstable fracture and fracture–dislocation of the spine (Nicoll, 1949). Adams & Hutton (1982) suspected that interspinous ligament failure may be the precursor of the disc injury, by permitting an unacceptable degree of segmental flexion, subsequently overloading the disc. Disruption of the interspinous and supraspinous ligaments may also precede degenerative spondylolisthesis (Newman, 1963).

The orientation of the fibres of the interspinous ligament is interesting from a functional aspect,

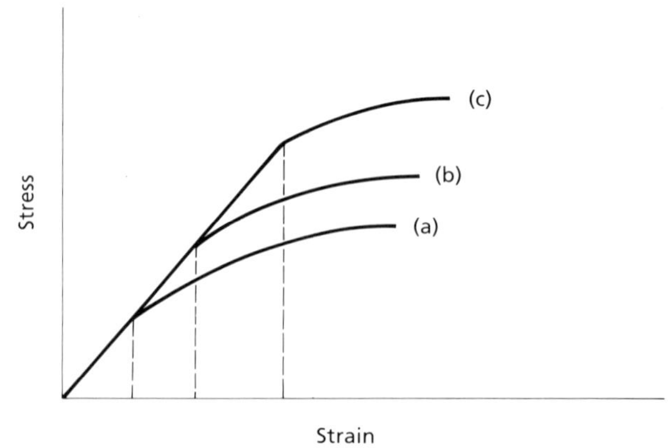

Fig. 37.2 In biological tissues, if the stress is applied rapidly (a) the elastic limit is reached at a lesser stress than if applied more slowly, (b) and (c). It is also reached at a lesser stress if the stress is applied frequently (a) compared with less frequent repetition (b) and (c).

passing obliquely from the spinous process above to be attached more anteriorly to the spinous process below (Heylings, 1978, 1980). This permits a controlled arc of forward flexion of the adjacent vertebrae (whilst a vertical orientation would permit no flexion at all). Disruption interferes with smooth restrained forward flexion and extension, increasing the demands on other restraining structures. This has been challenged recently by Hukins *et al.* (1990).

DIAGNOSIS OF SOFT TISSUE INJURY OF THE SPINE

By definition a muscle strain or a ligamentous sprain is the result of injury. The history at the onset of pain is therefore important (Nicholas & Reilly, 1985). Whilst the first symptoms of a disc protrusion may initially be mild, and then steadily increase over a few hours or days, a muscle, ligament or fascial injury will be most painful immediately, and gradually improve (Fig. 37.3). The events surrounding the onset of the pain are highly relevant. If the patient was hit by an object, or fell against a surface and contact was made with contusion, this is more likely to have caused muscle or fascial injury than ligamentous damage. An indirect injury, however—a slip, trip or fall—could produce ligamentous injury as well as a musculotendinous strain.

The mechanism of injury has important medico-legal consequences. A blunt injury, though very painful initially, is less likely to result in ligamentous

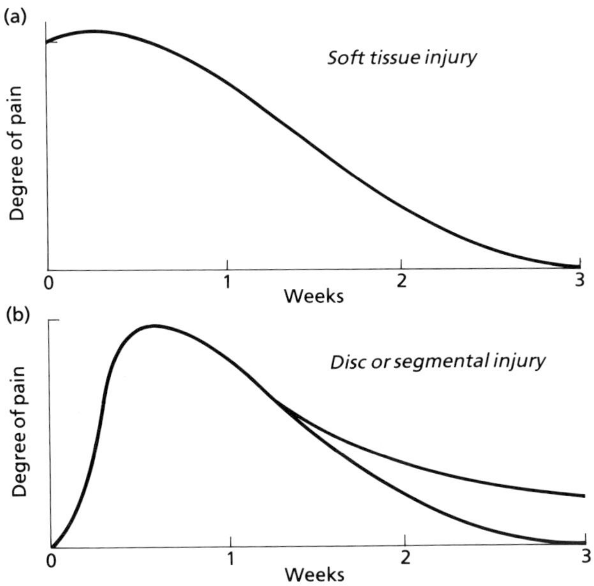

Fig. 37.3 (a) The pain from a soft tissue injury is initially severe, and slowly resolves over a few weeks. (b) The pain from disc or segmental injury can take several hours or days to develop, and although most patients improve in the following days or weeks, a few have persisting symptoms.

or disc damage than an indirect strain, and it carries a better prognosis.

The diagnosis of soft tissue injury is also a process of elimination. Soft tissue injury is excluded when pain below the knee in a root distribution suggests disc protrusion, root canal degeneration, spinal stenosis or vascular disturbance of the root. However, proximal pain in the lower limb can be referred from soft tissues in the back. Criteria of disc protrusion, even without leg pain—a list, pain aggravated by coughing, some reduction of straight leg raising, recurrent episodes of pain—would be unusual with soft tissue injury. Symptoms of inflammatory causes of back pain also have typical features—stiffness after rest, pain referred to one or other side alternately and variable in degree. The presence of a spondylolysis or spondylolisthesis is no reason for excluding soft tissue injury. Such a defect occurs in 5% of the population and may be an incidental finding (Roche & Rowe, 1951).

Abrasions or bruising of the back favour a diagnosis of soft tissue injury. Tenderness is more likely to be lateral to the midline, and sacral or sacroiliac tenderness is suggestive of contusion rather than segmental injury. Lateral flexion of the spine, which is usually well preserved in disc or segmental lesions, may be affected unilaterally with soft tissue injury. Resisted lateral flexion to the ipsilateral side is likely to be painful. Serious disruption of the interspinous ligament can be recognized by a palpable gap between the adjacent spinous processes.

Surgery provides a model of the natural history of musculotendinous injury to the spine. After discectomy many patients make a full recovery, and within a few months have no troublesome symptoms in the back. A traditional operation, with fenestration, stripping muscle from the laminae and spinous processes, and fairly strong retraction on the sacrospinalis muscles, is compatible with a full functional recovery. We have yet to discover if more restricted surgery by microdiscectomy confers any long-term benefits to soft tissues, but in practice it seems that the spine can recover from moderate musculotendinous trauma. It is reasonable to assume that closed soft tissue injury to muscle, tendons and fascia, though painful initially, carries a good long-term prognosis. Symptoms which continue beyond three months must have another explanation.

Contusion, fracture of transverse process, visceral injury

Severe blunt contusion to the loin will produce not only bruising to the soft tissues, but frequently avulsion of the lumbar transverse processes through the attachment of the lumbar fascia and the quadratus lumborum. There are usually abrasions of the skin and deeper bruising, associated with severe pain. Radiographs show avulsion of one or more transverse processes on the side of the injury. It is the possible association with visceral complications—kidney, liver, spleen or lung—that should concern the clinician.

Macroscopic or microscopic haematuria suggests the possibility of serious renal injury, and investigation is essential. Most patients with blunt renal trauma, no shock and only microscopic haematuria, have contusion to the kidney alone. They should be admitted for observation but about 1% will have severe renal injury, such as a laceration, rupture or renal pedicle injury which would not be diagnosed without further investigation (Cass *et al.*, 1986). The renal area should first be examined by ultrasound, which will generally identify a rupture (Furtschegger *et al.*, 1988). Urography, however, probably remains the best method to exclude significant renal injury. Dynamic computerized tomography (CT) is useful to assess parenchymal injury, and angiography to identify renal artery damage (Lang *et al.*, 1985; Bretan *et al.*, 1986). Sometimes avascularity on early angiography can mimic a tumour (Wiechen & Muller, 1986).

The liver can be damaged by blunt trauma in the region of the twelfth thoracic and first lumbar vertebrae, and the spleen, with its lower border along the eleventh rib and its lower pole at the level of the first lumbar vertebra, is at risk from injury in the left loin. Injuries to the thoracolumbar region can rupture the diaphragm and contuse the lung. These more serious visceral complications usually declare themselves with abdominal and chest symptoms and signs. Though uncommon, the visceral complications of blunt trauma to the lumbar region must always be considered because they are life-threatening. The prognosis regarding the musculoskeletal injury, however, is excellent. Full function is generally restored whether or not the transverse processes unite. The patients benefit from the assurance of a full recovery and they should begin to mobilize after a few days.

Local haematomas usually resolve over three weeks, with no continuing disability. The application of ice can hasten recovery time, probably by the vasoconstrictor effect, and haemostasis from histamine release; oedema and microhaemorrhage is reduced.

Chronic expanding haematoma (cystic haematoma)

On rare occasions a haematoma will slowly expand, forming a pseudo-capsule, with a gradual collection of central serous fluid (Friedlander & Bump, 1968; Sterling *et al.*, 1977; Vecchione, 1977; Reid *et al.*, 1980). This can occur in any muscular compartment, including the paraspinal tissues. It may be difficult to exclude sarcoma, even with sonography, and CT or magnetic resonance imaging (MRI) may be necessary to ensure there is no solid tissue within the pseudo-capsule. The capsule of the cystic haematoma is composed of dense fibrous tissue with haemosiderin deposits and iron-laden macrophages, with an inner lining of granulation tissue and fibrin with capillary ingrowth. The causation of the cystic formation is not well understood. Blood breakdown products can create an osmotic gradient causing fluid to be imbibed into the centre of the haematoma; a process enhanced by the inflammatory reaction (Labadie & Glover, 1976). Animal experiments have shown that cystic formation is more likely the larger the amount of blood injected. A cycle may develop, where blood breakdown and liquefaction activates vasoactive substances, and induces capsule formation, and continued inflammation produces effusion and new bleeding from damaged capillaries (Lewis & Johnson, 1987).

If the diagnosis is not in doubt the cystic haematoma can be left to resolve spontaneously. It may take many months, but a conservative approach is preferable to surgical excision, which is often followed by a recurrence of the lesion.

Contusion and pathology within the vertebral canal

The contents of the vertebral canal are singularly well protected from the effects of contusion, because of the bony ligamentous anatomy, and the protective cerebrospinal fluid in the envelope of the dura. There are records, however, of neurological concussion and neuropraxia from injury to the thoracolumbar region, without vertebral damage. Predisposing factors are spinal stenosis or pre-existing segmental instability (Bigio & Johnson, 1989). Extradural spinal haematomas are uncommon but can occur after injury with underlying blood dyscrasia, and occasionally in the absence of coagulation disorders (Combelles *et al.*, 1983). Spinal haematoma can occur in patients with ankylosing spondylitis.

Chronic compartment syndrome in the erector spinae muscle

Spinal muscle compartment syndrome has been suggested as an occasional cause of low back pain (Carr *et al.*, 1984; Peck *et al.*, 1986). Criteria for suspecting this syndrome are paravertebral low back pain induced only by exercise which is relieved by rest and no lower limb neurological deficit. It might be expected to occur in athletic subjects. Of 12 patients with these criteria, investigated by Styf & Lysell (1987) only one had raised intramuscular pressure which did not normalize with 20 minutes rest. Fasciotomy normalized the pressure in this patient and relieved the exercise-induced pain. Though a genuine cause of low back pain, it is extremely uncommon.

Painful muscle spasm

Spinal muscles may fail to relax voluntarily, and be in reflex spasm. This is frequently observed in patients with lower lumbar disc protrusion. Asymmetrical spasm produces the deformity of a list, sometimes described as a 'wind-swept spine'. This characteristic distinguishes the list from a structural scoliosis. It is affected by gravity (Porter & Miller, 1984). It is present only when the patient stands, and is abolished by lying down, or hanging from a bar. The list may be apparent only when the patient flexes forwards, and when the spasm is symmetrical there may be a loss of lumbar lordosis.

Spasm associated with an osteoid osteoma and with spinal infection is not abolished by lying down. An osteoid osteoma will produce a painful scoliosis with marked spasm, as distinct from the painless idiopathic scoliosis. It is not known, however, whether the muscle spasm is painful of itself. If the underlying condition producing the spasm is the pain source, pharmaceuticals to relieve the spasm would not be appropriate.

Some believe that anxiety and fear can produce increased muscle tension with resultant ischaemia, and a nociceptive stimulus from accumulation of metabolites, much like the muscular pain of intermittent claudication. Relaxation, biofeedback and the Alexander technique (Gelb, 1981) which train for poise, posture and balance are recommended. There is, however, no good evidence that muscle tension is a cause of low back pain.

Fibrositis–fibromyalgia

This is a diagnosis without any objective evidence of pathological change. Smythe (1985) believed that¨he pain source was neither in muscle nor fascia, but was a disturbance of pain modulation in the central nervous system. Patients complained of vague pain and tenderness in the muscles of the back, which was said to be more common with sleep disturbance, and after sleep deprivation in healthy subjects. They had backache, muscle tenderness and stiffness, especially in the mornings, sometimes associated with headaches. They complained of fatigue during the day, and symptoms were said to be affected by the weather. Symptoms may extend to other parts of the spine and limbs, and the condition is more common in tense, compulsive, energetic individuals (Cailliet, 1988). Unfortunately there are no laboratory tests to confirm the organic nature of such a condition. Biopsies of tender tissue are negative. Those who believe in this condition recommend coping strategies: improving sleep patterns, applying heat or ice, massage, relaxation, biofeedback and a functional rehabilitation programme; in the absence of objective diagnostic criteria, however, the benefits of treatment are not easily assessed.

Polymyalgia rheumatica produces similar symptoms, but the erythrocyte sedimentation rate (ESR) is raised, usually above 50 mm/h. Acute infective polyneuritis (Guillaine–Barré syndrome) may produce back pain, with weakness and aching in the limbs, headaches and vomiting; the protein level in the cerebrospinal fluid is usually raised.

Tender soft tissue nodules are not uncommon in patients with back pain. They have attracted interest from clinicians over many years (Froriep, 1843; Granhan, 1912; Steindler & Luck, 1938; Travell, 1942). They are circumscribed tender masses of connective tissue, sometimes infiltrated with lymphocytes. Pressure on these tissues can produce distal referred pain, and they are called 'trigger zones'. Spraying the overlying skin with coolant, stretching the tissue or injection with local anaesthetic and/or steroid is said to relieve the pain, though there are no adequate scientific studies.

Contusion to the buttock can cause ischaemia to the subcutaneous fat with atrophy and fibrosis and depression of the soft tissue contour. This is a cosmetic problem only.

Piriformis syndrome

The piriformis muscle leaves the pelvis through the greater sciatic foramen. The sciatic nerve lies anterior to the muscle, and passes inferiorly between the muscle and the superior gemellus of the obturator internus muscle to lie posterior to obturator internus. Sciatic pain is said to result from entrapment of the nerve deep and inferior to the piriformis muscle. The piriformis muscle arises from the front of the sacrum, the margin of the greater sciatic notch, and from the upper part of the anterior surface of the sacrotuberous ligament. In 15% of individuals the sciatic nerve leaves the pelvis between two bellies of this muscle rather than below its inferior surface. Entrapment is believed to be more common in women, and is associated with dyspareunia. The lumbar spine has a full range of motion, straight leg raising is reduced, and internal rotation of the leg at the limit of straight leg raising is said to increase the pain in this syndrome. However, Brieg & Troup (1979) showed that this test is positive whenever straight leg raising is limited by increased root tension, and it would not appear to be specific to this syndrome. Piriformis, being an external rotator of the hip, is stretched by internally rotating the hip, externally rotating the extended hip; resisting internal rotation should therefore increase the pain in this condition. The piriformis is also an abductor of the flexed hip; thus resisted abduction of the legs in the seated patient should be painful and reduced in power in this syndrome. Relief of pain by injection of local anaesthetic into the piriformis is said to be diagnostic.

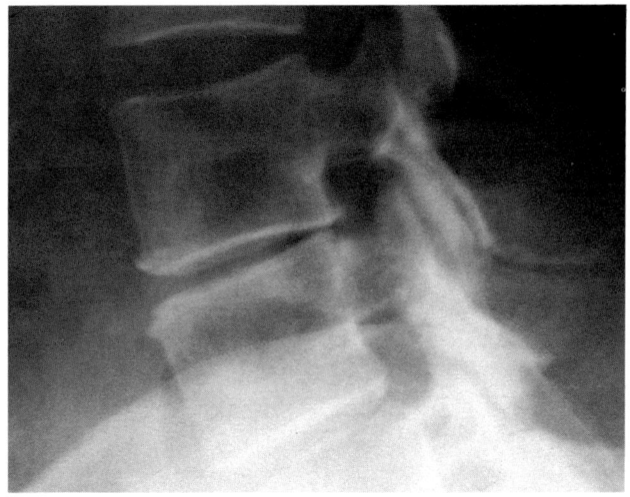

Fig. 37.4 Lateral radiograph showing traction spurs a few millimetres from the adjacent margins of the vertebral bodies, suggesting segmental instability.

Soft tissue injury: a precursor to instability

Although there is no universal agreement about the term spinal instability (Nachemson, 1985), a segment is probably unstable if it moves beyond its normal bounds of restraint, and returns again to its predeformed position (Farfan & Gracovetsky, 1984). Some unstable segments are not painful at all, and when an unstable segment is painful it is not easy to identify the source of pain. Instability in the presence of a small vertebral canal will compromise the neural elements, producing root pain or neurogenic claudication. This will occur in degenerative spondylolisthesis at L4–L5 level with forward or rotational displacement of a vertebra, an intact neural arch and spinal stenosis. However, when the canal is wide, as in an isthmic spondylolisthesis from a pars defect at L5, the vertebra displaces forwards, leaving the arch behind, and symptoms are probably those of fatigue in the structures that restrain shear (Porter, 1986; Roy *et al.*, 1989).

Various methods have been used to measure normal and unnatural segmental movement by serial radiological images of the spine (Pearcy *et al.*, 1984; Seligmen *et al.*, 1984; Ogston *et al.*, 1986; Stokes & Frymoyer, 1987). Attention has been focused on the vertebrae and discs, with little interest in the soft tissues. There are, however, a number of features about the instability syndromes that suggest a study of the soft tissues would be rewarding. It is possible that soft tissue injury is the precursor to an unstable lumbar segment.

MacNab (1971) described traction spurs arising a few millimetres from the adjacent margins of the vertebral bodies, as a sign of instability (Fig. 37.4). It is generally thought that disc degeneration produces unnatural segmental movement, and that the anterior longitudinal ligament is strained at the vertebral attachment, causing small osteophytes to grow into the ligament. However, discs between vertebrae with traction spurs are not inevitably degenerate and may be well hydrated on MRI scan. An alternative hypothesis is that a soft tissue ligamentous injury is the primary pathology, and it no longer prevents the normal restraint on the segment; the disc is normal, and instability, not disc degeneration, is responsible for the spurs. The very large claw spurs that develop on adjacent vertebrae may sometimes result from a soft tissue injury (Fig. 37.5). These also are quite compatible with a normal discogram.

The posterior spinal soft tissues are important restraining structures. The load on the spine is balanced between the moment in front of the axis of rotation and that behind (Fig. 37.6). The distance between the axis of rotation and the posterior muscle attachments, being shorter than from the axis of rotation to the centre of gravity, implies a very large stress on the posterior soft tissues of the spine. A deficiency in the neural arch, from a spina bifida occulta, will adversely affect the load-bearing properties of the spine, because the anomalous muscle and ligamentous attachments will be closer than normal to the axis of rotation. It is not surprising, therefore, that spina bifida occulta

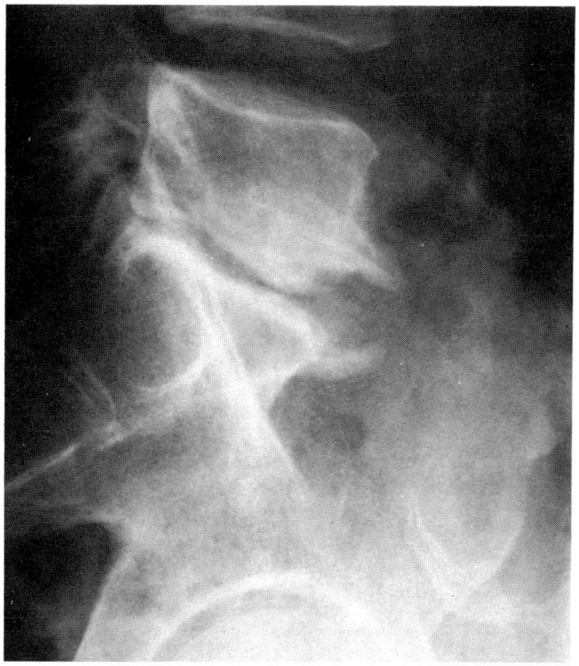

Fig. 37.5 Lateral radiograph showing large claw spurs at L5–S1, in a 56-year-old man. He recollects a road accident 30 years before, when he injured his spine and was admitted to hospital. The history is compatible with a soft tissue injury at the lumbosacral level, with instability.

is a common association of symptomatic isthmic spondylolisthesis (Fredrickson *et al.*, 1984). A 37% incidence of spina bifida occulta has been described in patients with instability symptoms but no spondylolisthesis or pars defect (Porter, 1990). This does suggest that the posterior anatomy and the integrity of the posterior soft tissues is important for spinal stability.

The hormone relaxin, which increases in the last trimester of pregnancy, may increase not only the elasticity of the pelvic ligaments, but also the laxity of spinal ligaments, and may be responsible for back pain which begins in pregnancy and then continues as a chronic instability problem. More patients with instability symptoms believe that pregnancy was responsible for the onset of their pain than do patients with other back pain syndromes (Porter & Jiang, 1990).

Some patients may have primary disc degeneration with subsequent instability which stresses the ligaments, causing lengthening, disruption and fibrous repair. Others, however, may have primary ligamentous injury which causes an unstable segment, and insignificant disc pathology.

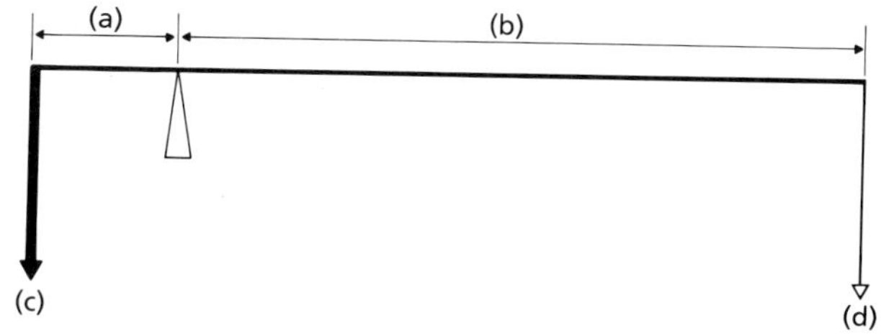

Fig. 37.6 Diagram to show the considerable stress on the posterior spinal soft tissues required to balance the anterior turning moment on the spine say at L3–L4 level; (d) is the body weight acting from the centre of gravity at a distance (b) from the L3–L4 disc, and (c) is the force through the posterior soft tissues at a short distance (a) from the L3–L4 disc.

In the appendicular skeleton ligamentous injury will produce an unstable joint. There is no reason why the axial skeleton should be the exception. If soft tissue injuries are suspected clinically, there are now available new imaging techniques to help in diagnosis, and it may well be found that these injuries have been seriously underestimated in the past.

REFERENCES

Adams, M.A. and Hutton, W.C. (1982) Prolapsed intervertebral disc—a hyperflexion injury. *Spine*, **7**, 184–191.

Baker, B.E. (1984) Current concepts in the diagnosis and treatment of musculo-tendinous injuries. *Med. Sci. Sports Exercise*, **16**, 323–327.

Bigio, M.R. and Johnson, G.E. (1989) Clinical presentation of spinal cord concussion. *Spine*, **14**, 37–40.

Brieg, A. & Troup, J.D.G. (1979) Biomechanical considerations in the straight leg raising test. *Spine*, **4**, 242–250.

Bretan, P.N., McAninch, J.W., Federle, M.P. & Jeffrey, R.B. (1986) Computerised tomographic staging of renal trauma: 85 consecutive cases. *J. Urol.*, **136**, 561–565.

Cailliet, R. (1988) *Soft Tissue Pain and Disability*, 2nd edn. F.A. Davis, Philadelphia, PA.

Carr, D., Frymoyer, J.W., Krag, M.H. & Pope, M.H. (1984) The lumbo-dorsal fascial compartment. *Transam. Orthop. Res. Soc.*, **9**, 252.

Cass, A.S., Luxenberg, M., Gleich, P. & Smith, C.S. (1986) Clinical indications for radiculographic evaluation of blunt renal trauma. *J. Urol.*, **136**, 370–371.

Combelles, G., Blond, S., Lesoin, F., Bousquet, C., Rousseaux, M. & Christiaens, J.L. (1983) Hematomes extra-duraux rachidiens sans lesion osseuse traumatique. A propos de 9 cas. *Neurochirurgie*, **29**, 417–422.

Farfan, H.F. & Gracovetsky, S. (1984) The nature of instability. *Spine*, **9**, 714–719.

Fredrickson, B.E., Baker, D., McHolick, W.J., Yuan, H.A. &

Lubicky, J.P. (1984) The natural history of spondylolysis and spondylolisthesis. *J. Bone Jt. Surg.*, **66A**, 699–707.

Friedlander, H.L. & Bump, R.G. (1968) Chronic expanding haematoma of the calf. *J. Bone Jt. Surg.*, **50A**, 1237–1241.

Froriep, H. (1943) *Ein Beitrag zur Pathologie und therapie des rheumatismus.* Weimar, Germany.

Furtschegger, A., Egender, G. & Jakse, G. (1988) The value of sonography in the diagnosis and follow up of patients with blunt renal trauma. *Br. J. Urol.*, **62**, 110–116.

Gelb, M. (1981) *Body Learning—an Introduction to the Alexander Technique.* Aurum Press, London.

Granhan, M. (1912) Uberden anatomeschon Bofience bel einem Fall von myositis Rheumatica. Doctoral dissertation, Cassel, Weber, Weidemeyer.

Heylings, D.J.A. (1978) Supraspinous and interspinous ligaments of the human lumbar spine. *J. Anat.*, **125**, 127–131.

Heylings, D.J.A. (1980) Supraspinous and interspinous ligaments in dog, cat and baboon. *J. Anat.*, **130**, 223–228.

Hukins, D.W.L., Kirby, M.C., Sikoryn, J.A., Aspdon, R.M. & Cox, A.J. (1990) Comparison of structure, mechanical properties, and function of lumbar spinal ligaments. *Spine*, **15**, 787–795.

Labadie, E.L. & Glover, D. (1976) Physiopathogenesis of subdural haematomas: I. Histological and biochemical comparisons of subcutaneous haematoma in rats with subdural haematoma in man. *J. Neurosurg.*, **45**, 382–392.

Lang, E.K., Sullivan, J. & Frentz, G. (1985) Renal trauma: radiological studies. Comparison of urography, computed tomography, angiography and radionuclide studies. *Diag. Radiol.*, **154**, 1–6.

Lehto, M., Hurme, M., Alaranta, H., Einola, S., Falak, B., Jarvinen, M., Kalimo, H., Mattila, M. & Paljarvi, L. (1989) Connective tissue changes of the multifidus muscle in patients with lumbar disc herniation. *Spine*, **14**, 303–309.

Lewis, V.L. & Johnson, P.E. (1987) Chronic expanding haematoma. *Plast. Reconstr. Surg.*, **79**, 465–467.

Macintosh, J.E. & Bogduk, N. (1987) The morphology of the lumbar erector spinae. *Spine*, **12**, 658–668.

MacNab, I. (1971) The traction spur. *J. Bone Jt. Surg.*, **53A**, 663–670.

Myklebust, J.B., Pintar, F., Yoganandan, N., Cusick, J.F., Maiman, D., Myers, T.J. & Sances, A. (1986) Tensile strength of spinal ligaments. *Spine*, **13**, 526–531.

Nachemson, A. (1985) Lumbar spine instability: a critical update and symposium summary. *Spine*, **10**, 290–291.

Newman, P.H. (1963) The etiology of spondylolisthesis. *J. Bone Jt. Surg.*, **45B**, 139–159.

Nicholas, J.A. & Reilly, J.P. (1985) Orthopaedic problems in athletes. *Compr. Ther.*, **11**, 48–56.

Nicoll, E.A. (1949) Fractures of the dorso-lumbar spine. *J. Bone Jt. Surg.*, **31B**, 376–394.

Ogston, N.G., King, G.J., Gertzbein, S.D., Tile, M., Kapasouri, A. & Rubenstein, J.D. (1986) Centrode patterns in the lumbar spine: baseline studies in normal subjects. *Spine*, **11**, 591–595.

Pearcy, M., Portek, I. & Shepherd, J.E. (1984) Three dimensional xray analysis of normal movement in the lumbar spine. *Spine*, **9**, 294–297.

Peck, D., Nicholls, P.J., Beard, C. & Allen, J.R. (1986) Are there compartment syndromes in some patients with idiopathic back pain? *Spine*, **11**, 468–475.

Porter, R.W. (1986) *Management of Back Pain.* Churchill Livingstone, London, p. 123.

Porter, R.W. (1990) The significance of spina bifida occulta in patients with low back pain. Presented to the International Society for the Study of the Lumbar Spine, Boston.

Porter, R.W. & Jiang, B. (1990) Pregnancy and chronic back pain. Presented to the International Society for the Study of the Lumbar Spine, Boston.

Porter, R.W. & Miller, C. (1984) Gravity induced list. Presented to the International Society for the Study of the Lumbar Spine, Montreal.

Reid, J.D., Kommareddi, S. & Lankerani, M. (1980) Chronic expanding haematomas, a clinicopathologic entity. *J. Am. Med. Assoc.*, **224**, 2441–2442.

Roche, M.B. & Rowe, G.G. (1951) The incidence of separated neural arch and coincident bone variation: a survey of 4200 skeletons. *Anat. Rec.*, **109**, 233–252.

Roy, S.H., De Luca, C.J. & Casavant, D.A. (1989) Lumbar muscle fatigue and chronic lower back pain. *Spine*, **14**, 992–1001.

Seligman, J.V., Gertzbein, S.D., Tile, M. & Kapasouri, A. (1984) Computer analysis of spinal segment motion in degenerate disc disease with and without axial loading. *Spine*, **9**, 566–573.

Smythe, H.A. (1985) Fibrosis and the referred pain syndromes. *Rheumatol. Forum*, vol. 3, no. 1.

Steindler, A. & Luck, J.V. (1938) Differential diagnosis of pain in the low back. *J. Am. Med. Assoc.*, **110**, 106–113.

Sterling, A., Butterfield, W.C., Bonner, R. & Quigley, W. (1977) Post-traumatic cysts of soft tissue. *J. Trauma*, **17**, 392–396.

Stokes, I.A.F. & Frymoyer, J.W. (1987) Segmental motion and instability. *Spine*, **12**, 688–691.

Styf, J. & Lysell, E. (1987) Chronic compartment syndrome in the erector spinae muscle. *Spine*, **12**, 580–582.

Tracy, M.F., Bibson, M.J., Szypryt, E.P., Rutherford, A. & Corlett, E.N. (1989) The geometry of the muscles of the lumbar spine determined by magnetic resonance imaging. *Spine*, **14**, 186–193.

Travell, J. (1942) Pain and disability of shoulder and arm: treatment by intramuscular infiltration with procaine hydrochloride. *J. Am. Med. Assoc.*, **121**, 417.

Vecchione, T.R. (1977) Persistent post-traumatic pseudosheath formation secondary to a moveable organised blood clot. *J. Traumatol.*, **17**, 481–482.

Wiechen, P.J. & Muller, W. (1986) The contused kidney, an angiographic picture. *Diagn. Imaging Clin. Med.*, **55**, 270–272.

38 · Conservative Management of Lumbar Degenerative Disease

By R.W. PORTER

Low back pain occurs commonly in the adult population. It is often a self-limiting disease or can usually be managed satisfactorily by non-operative methods. Although 400 000 patients are referred to British hospitals with back pain each year, only 7500 have surgery (Jayson, 1981; Nelson, 1982). A general practitioner will see approximately 200 patients each year with low back pain but, on average, only one will require an operation (Fig. 38.1) (Drinkall *et al.*, 1984).

Patients with mechanical back pain are a heterogeneous population and the first priority is to identify a back pain syndrome. Not only do these patients appreciate an attempt to identify the pain source, but unless the underlying syndrome is recognized, the clinician can only treat symptomatically. The syndromes where the diagnosis is not in doubt are those when root pain extends below the knee. However, greater controversy surrounds the diagnosis when there is only back pain or referred pain. If there are sufficient criteria to identify a back pain syndrome, the natural history can be explained as can ways of reinforcing a resolution of the problem, and the patient may need no active treatment.

LUMBAR DISC HERNIATION

McCulloch (1977) defined the essential criteria necessary for the diagnosis of a lumbar disc herniation. They are:

1 Unilateral leg pain in a typical sciatic root distribution, including discomfort below the knee, worse than or equal in severity to the back pain. If the roots of the femoral nerve are involved, the pain affects the front of the thigh.

2 Specific neurological symptoms incriminating a single nerve, i.e. symptoms to the big toe or outer foot.

3 Straight leg raising reduced to less than 50°, or cross-leg pain, or pain made worse by the bow-string test (in the early stages or when recovering, the straight leg raising is less affected).

4 Abnormal neurological signs—muscle wasting, muscle weakness, sensory change, hyporeflexia (these signs may be absent).

5 A positive myelogram, computerized tomography (CT) or magnetic resonance imaging (MRI) scan.

A gravity-induced list is further supportive evidence of a disc protrusion (Porter & Miller, 1986). Clinical signs which suggest that there is a complete annular tear rather than a protrusion with some intact peripheral annular fibres, are cross-leg pain (Khuffash & Porter, 1989) and diurnal changes in straight leg raising (Porter & Trailescu, 1990).

Most patients with a protrusion (as distinct from an extrusion or sequestration when the annulus is completely torn) (Fig. 38.2) will have recurrent episodes of pain which settle down with conservative management. If the pain is severe then patients have no choice but to rest in bed; they should, however, mobilize as soon as possible to avoid the deleterious effects of disuse. They need counselling about prognosis and rehabilitation, which may best be reinforced in the Back School. For most the prognosis is good (Saal & Saal, 1988).

When there are clear criteria of disc protrusion with straight leg raising less than 50°, enforced bed rest for as much as two weeks can allow a resolution in symptoms and signs.

Discectomy, either percutaneous or by open operation, is reserved for those patients with a protrusion whose symptoms do not resolve. Those with a com-

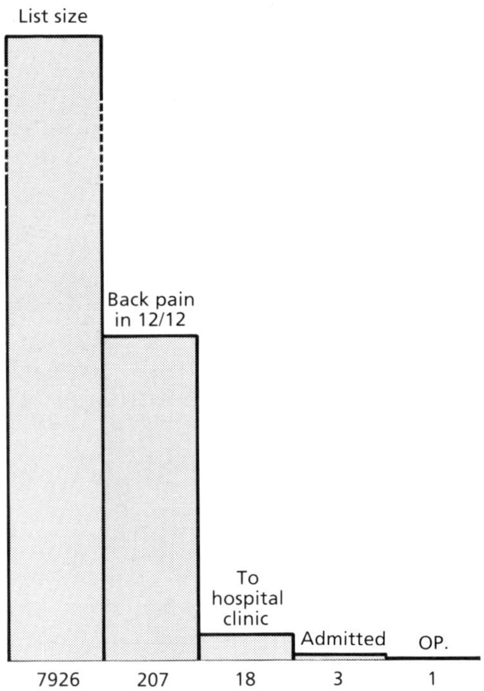

Fig. 38.1 Histogram showing the number of patients attending a general practice in one year complaining of low back pain, and the number referred to hospital.

plete annular tear need open discectomy, otherwise sequestrated nuclear disc material will compromise the vertebral canal indefinitely.

BONY ENTRAPMENT OF THE NERVE ROOT

Patients with root pain due to bony compression by stenosis in the lateral recess or nerve root canal have pain in a similar distribution to those with disc

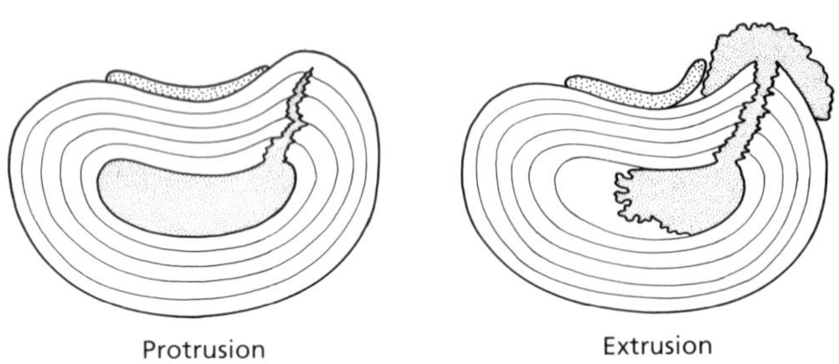

Fig. 38.2 Diagram to show an annular fissure allowing protrusion of the nucleus pulposus lateral to the posterior longitudinal ligament, and extrusion of the nucleus if the annular tear is complete.

protrusion, but with different features. They do not have a list, pain is not aggravated by coughing, the symptoms are not affected by diurnal changes (i.e. difficulty with socks in a morning); sitting for long becomes painful and straight leg raising is not severely limited. These patients are usually an older age group, and there are radiological features of degenerative change. A myelogram is generally negative, unless there is lateral encroachment from apophyseal joints at one segmental level. A CT scan will show bony and/or ligamentous encroachment into the lateral recess of the central canal, or into the root canal. MRI studies are positive with an absence of epidural fat (Crawshaw *et al.*, 1984). There may be rotational or sagittal vertebral displacement.

Treatment initially should be conservative, because most patients recover (Porter *et al.*, 1984). They require counselling about the mechanism of the pain, and the prognosis. Some with severe pain benefit from an epidural injection and the support of the Pain Clinic.

Surgical decompression is indicated when a short period of conservative management is unproductive, and when there is no natural resolution of symptoms.

An isthmic spondylolisthesis, either bilateral or unilateral (Porter & Park, 1982; Porter & Hibbert, 1984) can be associated with root entrapment syndrome when degenerative change compromises the adjacent nerve root. Once established, the symptoms fail to settle down without surgical intervention. A fusion rather than decompression is generally sufficient to abolish the dynamic effects of instability and relieve root symptoms.

Neurogenic claudication

Patients with neurogenic claudication due to nerve root entrapment experience pain or discomfort in both legs above and below the knees, limiting the walking distance. This is relieved by a short period of rest and if the spine is not too rigid (Dong & Porter, 1989) by stooping forwards. There is always radiological evidence of spinal stenosis on myelogram, CT or MRI. There may be partial, subtotal or complete occlusion of the metrizamide column at one or several levels. The diagnosis cannot be made in the presence of a normal myelogram. The critical cross-sectional area of the cauda equina is 100 mm (Bolender *et al.*, 1985) and this is further reduced by the dynamic changes of sagittal or rotational instability. In addition to the spinal pathology, there may be associated peripheral vascular disease (Johanssen *et al.*, 1982).

Symptoms of neurogenic claudication rarely resolve, but once established there is no evidence that increasing deterioration occurs. Major neurological damage is unusual.

Many patients accept their disability after explanation of the pathology and the likelihood that symptoms will not increase. They modify their lifestyle and avoid surgery. A course of calcitonin is worthwhile (Porter & Hibbert, 1983; Porter & Miller, 1988)—100 units subcutaneously four times a week for four weeks. If there is no improvement at four weeks, then a response is unlikely. Some, however, will obtain a dramatic improvement in their walking distance and avoid surgery.

PAINFUL UNSTABLE SPONDYLOLYSIS OR SPONDYLOLISTHESIS

It is not easy to be sure of the pain source for the patient with back pain alone. There is, however, less controversy about the diagnostic criteria for an unstable spondylolithesis than for other causes of back pain. Isthmic spondylolisthesis occurs in approximately 5% of the Caucasian population, with a greater incidence in athletes and gymnasts (Roche & Rowe, 1951; Kono *et al.*, 1975; Troup, 1975; Jackson *et al.*, 1976; Murray Leslie *et al.*, 1977; Bird *et al.*, 1980; Hitoshi, 1980). The pars defect can become unstable and a source of pain, but because the defect is common and frequently symptomless, it is important to exclude other causes of back pain (Fig. 38.3).

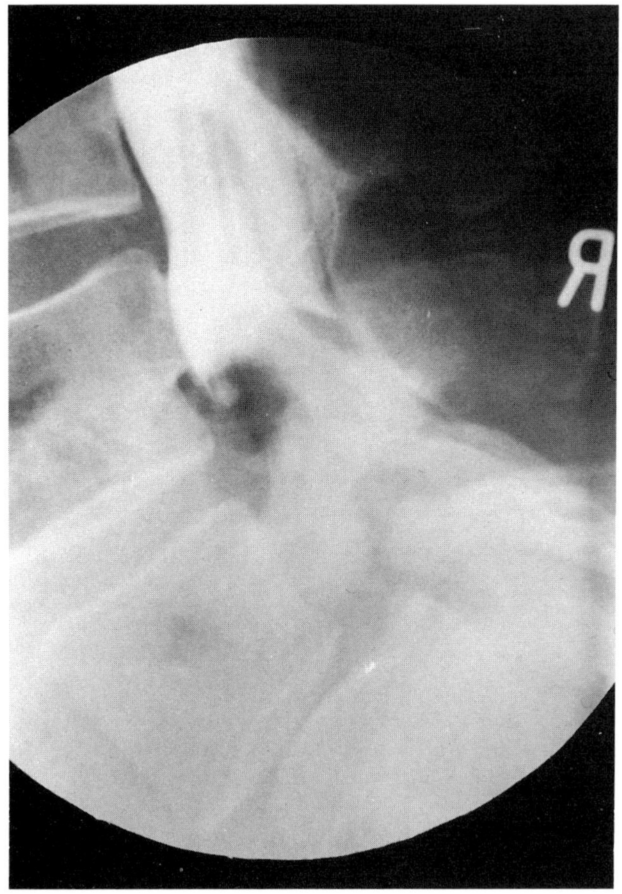

Fig. 38.3 A radiculogram prior to a proposed spinal fusion for a 37-year-old woman with severe low back pain and an isthmic spondylolisthesis. The well-circumscribed filling defect proved to be a rare paraganglioma.

Pain from an unstable spondylolisthesis often radiates into the buttocks and round the pelvis. It is aggravated by walking, shopping and driving, and partially relieved by lying down. There is sometimes a precipitating injury often many years before, and many women date their first symptoms to pregnancy (Porter & Hibbert, 1984).

Although the results of fusion are good, not every patient with spondylolisthesis requires an operation. A slight increase in the displacement is possible over a few decades of adult life but this may not produce symptoms (Porter, 1986; Postacchini, 1989). Many patients have instability symptoms in early adult life, with no discomfort thereafter (Fig. 38.4), and some develop strong bony stability.

The young adolescent with spondylolisthesis and the first attack of back pain may have a stress fracture apparent on a scintiscan. Immobilization in a half-spica may allow the defect to unite. An acute episode of pain in adult life requires a lumbar corset, help in the Back School and dietary advice.

One can expect excellent results from a spinal fusion, but it is indicated only when acute severe symptoms are not resolving naturally, when chronic symptoms are unacceptable, and when the quality of working and sporting life is significantly curtailed by back pain.

CHRONIC LOW BACK PAIN

There is considerable disagreement about the causation and the pain source in chronic low back pain. Some look for certain criteria to incriminate an un-

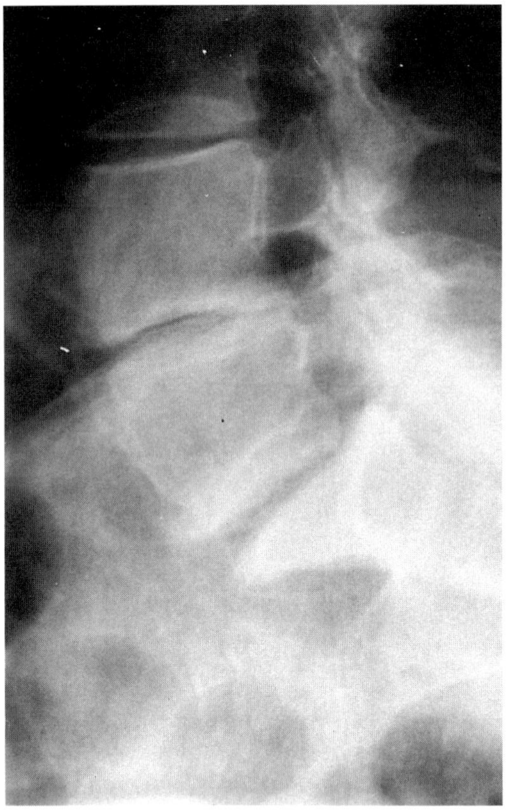

Fig. 38.4 Lateral radiograph of a 74-year-old woman with isthmic spondylolisthesis at L5–S1 and disc degeneration at L4–L5. She gave a history of back pain 40 years previously, but had no current back or root pain.

stable intervertebral segment (Farfan & Gracovetsky, 1984; Nachemson 1985); others describe facet joint pain (Rashbaum, 1983; Helbig & Lee, 1988). Some authorities attempt to make a specific soft tissue diagnosis such as sacroiliac, gluteus maximus or piriformis syndromes purely on clinical diagnosis (Kirkaldy Willis, 1988). It is not yet possible to establish the credibility of these syndromes when the symptoms have not been correlated with demonstrable pathology. If the pain is sufficiently disabling, and it is possible to identify the intervertebral segment responsible for the pain, then it is reasonable to hope that the prevention of movement at this level by surgical fusion will relieve the pain. Indications for fusion are more fully discussed in other chapters of this book, but random fusion for low back pain is not very successful. This is probably because patients with chronic low back pain are a heterogeneous population with different pathologies.

If fusion is being considered for a patient with chronic low back pain, most would agree that it should be preceded by an adequate trial of conservative management. This includes counselling, attending the Back School, functional rehabilitation, and assessment for a behavioural disorder. Some would offer short-term tricyclic antidepressant therapy (Ward, 1986).

Once an attempt has been made to come to a diagnosis and to identify the source of the pain, only rarely is it necessary to progress directly to surgical treatment. There are a multitude of conservative approaches available, and the most commonly used will be discussed.

TREATMENT

Counselling

Patients with back pain have two main areas of concern: What is wrong? Can it be cured? They are often troubled most by the former. The surgeon's role is to allay fears that there is serious underlying desease, that it is not a crippling condition, it will not result in paralysis or a spreading rheumatism, and that it is not a tumour. It is erroneous to believe that patients with back pain consult surgeons only for an operation.

It generally requires no more than an adequte history and examination supported by basic radiology and investigation to decide that the pain is of mechanical origin and not due to an inflammatory disorder or more sinister pathology. There may be sufficient criteria to identify one of the specific back pain syndromes, allowing an explanation of the pathology and probable source of pain, which is a great relief to an anxious patient. Failure to receive an adequate explanation of the back pain problem is a major source of patient dissatisfaction (Deyo & Diehl, 1986).

Half of the patients with an acute episode of back pain resolve within a week, 80% in two weeks, and only a minority are still in pain at the end of a month. Reassurance is therefore important at the start of an acute episode. For the patient whose pain is more persistent, counselling and advice on self-management can be as productive as active therapy. In the long term, many patients find that their back pain becomes less of a problem in later life and they need to know that age is kindly to the spine (Porter, 1987) (Fig. 38.5). It is not necessary to 'do something' for every patient; what is said may be more important.

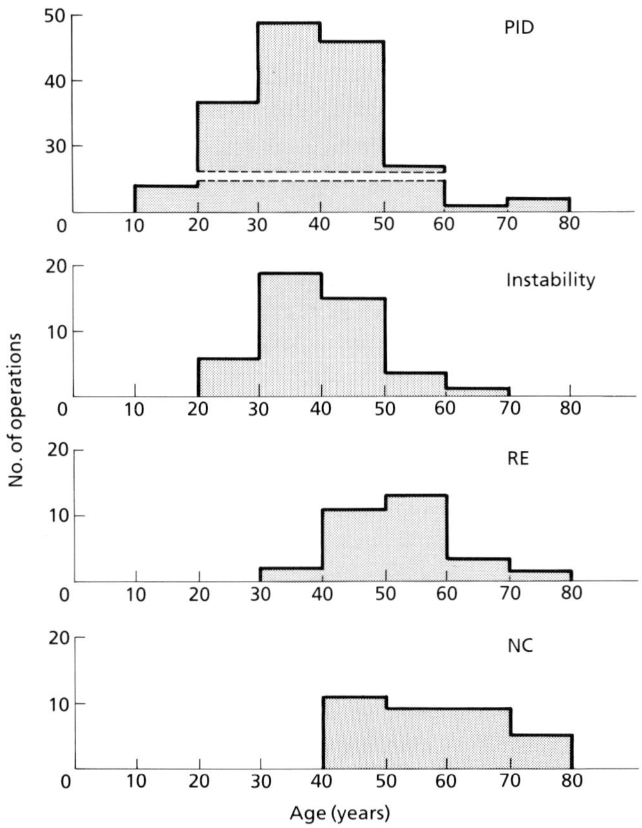

Fig. 38.5 Incidence of patients requiring spinal surgery during each decade of life for discectomy (PID), fusion for instability, decompression for root entrapment (RE) due to lateral stenosis, and decompression for neurogenic claudication (NC). The need for surgery decreases in later life, except in neurogenic claudication. From Porter (1987a).

Bed rest

There are times when the patient can do no other than rest in bed, but once the most acute symptoms have settled, mobilization should be encouraged. Recumbency has adverse effects on many systems including the spine. Whilst in bed it is immaterial whether the patient lies supine or on the side. A pillow beneath the knees can be helpful. Bed rest need not be total as personal hygiene may be more difficult to achieve in bed than out of bed. Analgesics are necessary at first round the clock, but they should be reduced as soon as possible.

There is no good evidence that tranquillizers hasten recovery (Weber, 1980). Anti-inflammatory drugs, however, do appear to be effective in relieving back pain if started within two days of the onset of an attack (Amlie *et al.*, 1987), and the early use of anti-spasmodic drugs also has benefit (Basmajian, 1989).

In the presence of nerve root tension signs, two weeks of bed rest is useful (Weber, 1983). With severe back pain only, two days of bed rest appears to produce results equivalent to seven days of rest in bed (Deyo *et al.*, 1985) whilst an earlier study demonstrated that 10 days of bed rest produces a better recovery and a faster return to work than no rest (Wiesel *et al.*, 1980).

If is agreed that too much rest in bed is counter-productive. Not only does recumbency weaken the musculoskeletal system, delaying recovery, but the anxious patient may become distressed by the fear of pain, and develop abnormal pain behaviour. Many a chronic disability could have been avoided by timely advice and early mobilization. Rest, though beneficial in the short term, should be kept to a minimum.

Spinal orthoses

Lumbar supports have been widely used for relief of back pain, but there is no documented evidence that they reduce the period of disability. Fidler & Plasmans (1983) showed that a canvas corset reduced the angular movement of the lumbar spine by one-third, but there are times when it will actually increase movement at the lumbosacral junction (Norton & Brown, 1957; Lumsden & Morris, 1968). A support within the corset gives better relief than the same canvas without support (Million *et al.*, 1981). Besides limiting lumbar mobility (Willner, 1985), an orthosis can decrease intradiscal pressure (Nachemson, 1985) and provide relief perhaps by local warmth and by stimulation of mechanoreceptors. However, compliance is often poor.

Back School

Starting in Scandinavia, the Back School concept has spread across the industrialized world (Zachrisson-Forsell, 1972). It is a structured intervention programme for a group of individuals, and provides patients with information about back pain of mechanical origin, about the types of stress that can injure the spine, how this knowledge can be applied in day-to-day activities, and how the spine can be strengthened by improving fitness. They are informed about self-management for the acute attack and how these generally get better without active treatment, how to manage recurrent and chronic back pain, and how to reduce the incidence of attacks. Back School programmes have been shown to be a better use of resources and time than other unproven therapeutic methods (Bergquist-Ullman & Larson, 1977; Williams, 1977; Attix & Tate, 1979; Aberg, 1982; Fisk *et al.*, 1983; Moffett *et al.*, 1986; Berwick *et al.*, 1989). The clinician can discuss the problem, the present management and prognosis during the first consultation, but he cannot spend two or three hours with the patient explaining and demonstrating the correct use of the spine. This is the role of the Back School.

Back Schools have no rigid structure, but each department offers instruction tailored to the needs of its own community (Pawliki *et al.*, 1982), with variation in content, duration and class size. It is helpful to discuss first spinal anatomy and function, with appropriate demonstrations. Disc protrusion and degeneration are described, and the vulnerability of the nerve roots in later life. If the probable cause of the patient's pain is known to the physiotherapist, she or he asks the patient if the pain mechanism explained by the doctor has been understood.

Relaxation is demonstrated and lifting techniques are practised. Advice is offered about posture and how everyday activities can be accomplished with minimal spinal stress. Dialogue is encouraged. Some Back Schools incorporate exercises into their programme (White, 1983). Exercises can be dynamic, with active contraction of a muscle group to bring about a change in length and cause articular movement, or static, producing a voluntary contraction without change in length or joint movement. Certainly subjects with improved fitness and endurance are less prone to back problems (Mayer *et al.*, 1987) but dynamic exercises may increase the intradiscal pressure.

Back School education does seem to make good sense; it seems to meet the needs of many patients seeking medical help; patients realize for the first time that management is in their own hands; it drops the anxiety level of many bewildered patients who have suffered with back pain for a long time without an explanation of their problem.

Functional rehabilitation

Many patients fail to recover from an acute episode of back pain because they have been led to believe that they should treat their back with great caution. Any activity that produces back pain is noted and avoided, more because of anticipated pain and suffering rather than the actual experience of pain (Fordyce *et al.* 1982; Linton, 1985). It has been suggested, however, that avoidance behaviour is as unproductive in reducing pain as it is in reducing fear (Philips & Hunter, 1981).

Not only does passive avoidance lead to psychological reinforcement of the invalidity status, but it also has adverse physical effects. Joints become stiff, soft tissues weak, and protective reflexes are impaired. This is further complicated by wearing corsets and jackets, and the injudicious use of analgesics. An acute episode of back pain which would be expected to resolve within a short period may therefore persist as chronic disability, with psychological disturbance and physical disuse phenomena.

Functional rehabilitation attempts to reverse this situation. It aims to improve physical fitness and influence low back pain by improving disc nutrition, assisting healing of connective tissues and increasing endorphins. Several studies have shown a correlation between fitness and recovery from back pain (Cady *et al.*, 1979; Mellin, 1986). Good isometric endurance of the back muscles may prevent the first-time occurrence of back pain (Biering Sorensen, 1984) and hard work may protect against disc protrusion (Porter, 1987; Porter & Adams, 1989).

The programmes vary, but have a common content of increasing activity and restoration of function, through vigorous physical exercise. Pain does not limit the activity; rather the concept of activity being detrimental to chronic low back pain is challenged (Nachemson, 1983a,b; Waddell, 1987). The activity programme is carefully monitored, with feedback to encourage the patient.

Patients with chronic back pain, for whom surgery has no place, and for whom traditional therapies have had little to offer, have frequently responded to a programme of functional rehabilitation, developing a new quality of life and with many returning to work (Mayer *et al.*, 1987; Hazars *et al.*, 1989).

Similarly, patients who have been off work for more than eight weeks with an acute episode of back pain, and who are treated with a vigorous exercise regime, not only return to work more quickly than an untreated control population, but they are also significantly better than the control group at one year (Lindstrom *et al.*, 1989).

'School for Bravery'

Those patients whose chronic disability has a large non-organic component of abnormal pain behaviour respond well to functional rehabilitation. Our own programme, designed by Mrs J. Williams (Porter *et al.*, 1989) is called 'School for Bravery'; entry is possible for those with considerable courage. Patients join the programme who have many inappropriate symptoms and signs, and who have had a full but unrewarding investigation for treatable pathology. They spend all day in the department, five days per week, wearing track-suit and trainers. Their disability is monitored on video, and their goals agreed. Pain is not discussed. They enter a demanding vigorous exercise programme. Improved performance is rewarded with praise, and illness behaviour ignored. Initially they have individual management, graduating into group activity, with the encouragement of others who are further advanced.

Those who respond convert suddenly to wellness behaviour in a few days, much earlier than can be explained by improved physical fitness. They are initially unstable for a few days, until healthy function becomes established. A new video is taken, and most patients are surprised to see how gross was their original degree of disability. They are assured that by their own efforts they have achieved a new quality of life, and they usually vow never to return to their previous state. The experience of pain may not be diminished but illness behaviour is abandoned.

Manipulation

The role of manipulative treatment for mechanical low back pain is uncertain and controversial, and a literature review provides only limited empirical support (Ottenbacher & Difabio, 1985). Many different techniques are practised with little agreement about when it is indicated, what is being treated, what happens when it is effective, and what are the short- and long-term results.

An osteopath will identify the level of the lesion, and relax the muscles by careful stretching and manipulation of the part. The patient usually lies on the side with the trunk twisted so that some joints are believed to be locked and others free. Using lever techniques on the pelvis and other parts, a high-velocity thrust is applied, often with audible cracks and clicks. Hadler *et al.* (1987) were able to demonstrate benefits in a controlled trial.

The chiropractor will manipulate the individual vertebrae with a rapid but not very powerful thrust. He decides which type of thrust is appropriate, and applies it with precision.

Some surgeons will manipulate a patient with chronic back pain under general anaesthesia, but the effects are generally less effective with time. The analgesic benefits from spinal manipulation do not appear to be mediated by increased endorphin production (Christian *et al.*, 1988).

Physiotherapists, though they may use different manipulative techniques, frequently practise the method described by Maitland. Oscillatory movements are applied to the spinous processes at the affected level, rotating away from the pain. A comparison of Maitland mobilization with placebo shows that (a) most episodes of back pain settle with or without treatment, (b) those likely to be helped with manipulation have only limited benefit with little long-term effect, and (c) although some patients are immediately improved after manipulation, many other patients have similar improvement after a placebo session (Sims-Williams *et al.*, 1978). The personal attention and interest of a physiotherapist probably plays a great part in hastening recovery (Jayson, 1986).

Other techniques often accompany manipulation therapy. Cryotherapy with the application of ice, or ice and water, with ice wrappings or compresses, aims to reduce oedema and pain, but except in spinal contusion it has not been demonstrated as efficacious. Neither have the benefits of the local application of superficial or deep heat, the use of diathermy, ultrasound, infrared rays, warm fomentations, heating pads or hydrotherapy been shown to be effective. Deep or superficial massage of the soft tissues is useful in controlling pain, but it has not been supported in a controlled study. The elevation of endorphins in the central nervous system may explain some of the beneficial effects (Kosierlitz *et al.*, 1977; Terenius & Wahlstrom, 1979).

Spinal traction, intermittent or continuous, manual or mechanical, has been widely used on the spine, but studies comparing different methods have not demonstrated their value (Weber *et al.*, 1985; Zylbergold & Piper, 1985).

The McKenzie treatment

This is designed for patients with mechanical low back disturbance (McKenzie, 1981). Three groups of patients are defined. Those with a 'postural syndrome' are young adults who have intermittent episodes of pain believed to be the result of prolonged stress on the soft tissues around the lumbar spine. They have no deformity and full movements, and they are treated by postural advice.

The second group have a 'dysfunctional syndrome'. They are older patients who are believed to have had trauma or a postural problem producing adaptive shortening of the soft tissues. Pain is triggered by overuse. Posture is poor, movements are restricted, and the pain is felt at the end of the range. They are given postural advice, and gentle stretching exercises to the limit of a little pain.

The third group have a 'derangement syndrome' of the lumbar intervertebral disc, with a kyphotic deformity, or a list when standing or stooping. Seven stages are described, and treatment is designed to move patients up to stage one, when they can manage themselves. After test movements the deformity is manually corrected, attempting to centralize the pain and produce a situation whereby the patients can care for themselves with extension activity, maintain a lumbar lordosis, and subsequently perform flexion exercises to obtain a functional recovery.

The goal of the technique is to introduce the patient to a self-care programme, eventually avoiding the help of therapists or clinicians.

Posture

Frederick Matthias Alexander was born in Tasmania in 1869. He had a precarious acting career until he discovered how to improve his voice by correcting his posture. The teachers of the technique that bear his name (Gelb, 1981) believe that poor posture can affect function and produce musculoskeletal pain; as a result of 'imbalance' some tissues suffer overuse and fatigue, and others disuse and atrophy. The Alexander technique is popular with musicians and athletes, who because of poor posture may underperform and suffer pain. It is also suggested that inefficient use of the spine accounts for much backache.

The teachers of the technique seek to inhibit unnecessary tension and produce 'poise and harmony, balance and coordination'. They describe 'pause before action and stillness in activity'. Their approach is also holistic, believing that a distorted posture produces distorted perceptions, that poise affects personality. A good posture certainly is attractive and it makes sense. There are many followers of the technique, but it has yet to be assessed scientifically.

The pain clinic

The advent of pain treatment as a clinical specialty has provided a new method of management for patients with back pain. Where surgery or further surgery is not indicated, and where intractable pain is a problem, the pain clinic which attempts to modify the patient's perception of pain has much to offer. Most patients have received counselling, and Back School advice; they have had manipulative therapy and exercise programmes, and still pain remains. If they exhibit inappropriate symptoms and signs of abnormal pain behaviour, they are unlikely to respond to pain-relieving procedures in the pain clinic. Further invasive procedures will only be counter-productive and will reinforce illness behaviour. However, for patients with back or leg pain when the non-organic component is small, the pain clinic may be the only source of help.

Many patients with intractable pain suffer from excessive medication. The clinician in the pain clinic is probably best fitted to review the drug regime, evaluate and prescribe appropriate analgesics, anti-inflammatory drugs, antidepressants and hypnotics. Too often these drugs have lost their efficacy, they have become addictive, and are producing side-effects. Patients can be weaned from habit-forming drugs, by prescribing a cocktail of increasing dilution.

Severe root entrapment pain from lateral canal stenosis or root canal stenosis can be helped by one or more epidural injections of 40 ml saline, with Marcaine and hydrocortisone. Although clinical trials to confirm its efficacy are still awaited, there is no doubt that many individual patients are supported through a stressful time with an occasional epidural injection. This regime is sometimes proposed for the root pain of a disc protrusion, to economize on bed rest. If one believes that extradural scarring can produce pain after a discectomy or decompression, then an epidural injection may help by breaking down adhesions and reducing inflammatory change. It can be useful therapy when postoperative recovery is slow, but it has not been scientifically assessed. The value of epidural injection is still controversial (Snoek *et al.*, 1977; Bourne, 1984; Cuckler *et al.*, 1985).

Similarly, without clear evidence of its efficacy, trigger points and fibrositic nodules are often injected with local anaesthetic and steroid, giving temporary relief. Superficial injection into a tender sacroiliac joint can be helpful, but in the absence of a controlled trial one cannot be sure that these procedures are successful by their placebo effect. They will be counterproductive for the patient with abnormal pain behaviour.

The apophyseal joint may be an important pain source. It can be examined by percutaneous injection of local anaesthetic into the joint under radiographic control (Lippitt, 1984). Relief of symptoms may convince the clinician that this is an important pain source, and the joint can then be denervated by radiofrequency block (Mehta & Sluijter, 1979). The critics rightly remind us that it is difficult to place a needle accurately into a small joint, and local anaesthetic will diffuse widely into the root canal and epidural space, making interpretation of pain relief difficult (Fig. 38.6) (Moran *et al.*, 1988). Denervation can also produce a Charcot joint with subsequent problems. The facet joint syndrome is still controversial (Jackson *et al.*, 1988).

Transcutaneous electrical nerve stimulation (Pike, 1978; Melzack *et al.*, 1983) probably involves the endorphin system. The analgesic effect is blocked by naloxone. The peripheral nerves are stimulated by an electric current transmitted transcutaneously, and this can relieve low back pain in some patients. It has the advantage that the patient can position the electrodes on the back for best effect, and can regulate the intensity of the stimulus. In the short term, percutaneous dorsal column stimulators can also help patients with chronic back pain (Racz *et al.*, 1989).

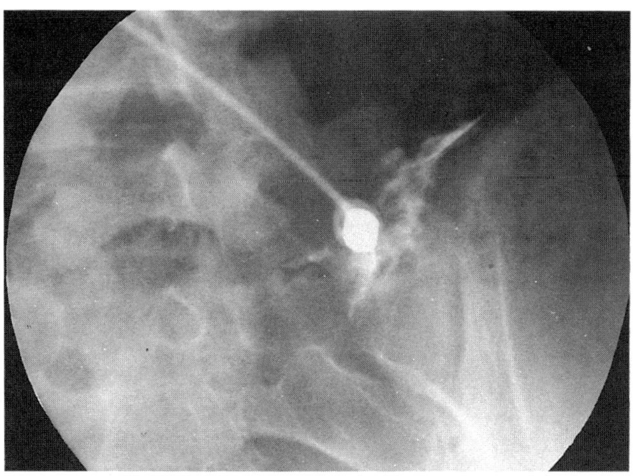

Fig. 38.6 Arthrogram of hemiarticulation of sacralized L5. Instillation of local anaesthetic did relieve back pain for a few days, but the pain source is uncertain, because of wide dissemination of opaque medium from the joint.

Biofeedback (electromyography, EMG) transposes the physiological activity of the muscle response into a visual or auditory signal, enabling the patient to modify that response. It is designed to inhibit excessive or unbalanced muscle activity, but although sometimes used in patients with chronic back pain, there is no scientific study demonstrating its benefit.

Acupuncture can relieve low back pain for some patients, but it is not possible to predict success. It has proved difficult to design satisfactory trials in order to judge its value (Lewith & Machin, 1983; Lewith, 1984). Two controlled double-blind trials suggest that acupuncture can be superior to placebo (Man & Baragar, 1974; Matsumoto *et al.*, 1974). On the other hand, five trials found no difference (Lee *et al.*, 1975; Gaw *et al.*, 1975; Moore & Berk, 1976; Mendelson *et al.*, 1983). The counter-irritant effect of stimulating the skin in a noxious manner with subcutaneous acupuncture needles was found to be superior to placebo dummy surface electrodes on both subjective and objective assessment of back pain (MacDonald *et al.*, 1983).

Not all the methods used in the pain clinic are of proven value, but many patients with severe pain for which no remedy has been found are grateful that someone is still prepared to try.

The management of patients with low back pain stretches the clinical judgement of the spinal surgeon as perhaps in no other field of medicine. Only a minority of the patients require surgery. Good results require judicial patient selection—which means an understanding of the back pain syndromes and their natural history, careful patient assessment, understanding the conservative options, and having the facilities available for the new methods of non-operative management.

REFERENCES

Aberg, J. (1982) Evaluation of an advanced back pain rehabilitation programme. *Spine*, 7, 317–318.

Amlie, E., Weber, H. & Holme, I. (1987) Treatment of acute low back pain with Piroxicam: results of a double-blind placebo-controlled trial. *Spine*, **12**, 473–476.

Attix, E.A. and Tate, M.A. (1979) Low Back School: a conservative method for the treatment of low back pain. *Mississippi State Med. Assoc.*, **20**, 4.

Basmajian, J.V. (1989) Acute back pain and spasm; a controlled multicentre trial of combined analgesic and anti-spasm agents. *Spine*, **14**, 438–439.

Berquhist-Ullman, M. & Larson, V. (1977) Acute low back pain in industry. *Acta Orthop. Scand.*, Suppl. 170.

Berwick, D.M., Budman, S. & Feldstein, M. (1989) No clinical effect of back school in an HMO; a randomised prospective trial. *Spine*, **14**, 338–344.

Biering Sorensen, F. (1984) Physical measurements as risk indicators for low back trouble over a one year period. *Spine*, **9**, 106–109.

Bird, H.A., Eastmond, C.J., Hudson, A. & Wright, V. (1980) Is generalised joint laxity a factor in spondylolisthesis? *Scand. J. Rheumatol.*, **9**, 203–205.

Bolender, N.F., Schonstrom, N.S.R. & Spengler, D.N. (1985) Role of myelography and computerised tomography in the diagnosis of central spinal stenosis. *J. Bone Jt. Surg.*, **67A**, 240–246.

Bourne, I.H.J. (1984) Treatment of chronic back pain comparing corticosteroid lignocaine injections with lignocaine alone. *Practitioner*, **228**, 333–338.

Cady, L.D., Bishoff, M.P.H., O'Connell, M.S., Thomas, B.A. & Allan, J.H. (1979) Strength and fitness and subsequent back injuries in firefighters. *J. Occup. Med.*, **21**, 269–272.

Christian, G.F., Stanton, G.J., Sisson, D., How, H.Y., Jamison, J., Alder, B., Fullerton, M. & Funder, J.W. (1988) Immunoreactive ACTH, β-endorphin, and cortisol levels in plasma following spinal manipulative therapy. *Spine*, **13**, 1411–1417.

Crawshaw, C., Kean, D.M., Mulholland, R.C., Worthington, B.S., Finlay, D., Hawkes, R.C., Gyngell, M. & Moore, W.S. (1984) The use of nuclear magnetic resonance in the diagnosis of lateral canal entrapment. *Spine*, **9**, 195–197.

Cuckler, J.M., Bernini, P.A., Wiesel, S.W., Booth, R.E. Jr, Rothman, R.H. & Pickens, G.T. (1985) The use of epidural steroids in the treatment of lumbar radicular pain. *J. Bone Jt. Surg.*, **67A**, 63–66.

Deyo, R.A. & Diehl, A.K. (1986) Patient satisfaction with medical care for low back pain. *Spine*, **11**, 28–30.

Deyo, R.A., Diehl, A.K. & Rosenthal, M. (1985) How much bed rest for backache? A randomised clinical trial (abstract). Conference of the American Federation for Clinical Research, Dallas, TX.

Dong, G.X. & Porter, R.W. (1989) Cycling and walking tests in neurogenic and intermittent claudication. *Spine*, **14**, 965–969.

Drinkall, J.N., Porter, R.W., Hibbert, C.S. & Evans, C. (1984) The value of ultrasonic measurement of the spinal canal diameter in general practice. *Br. Med. J.*, **288P**, 121–122.

Farfan, H.F. & Gracovetsky, S. (1984) The nature of instability. *Spine*, **9**, 714–719.

Fidler, M.W. & Plasmans, C.M.T. (1983) The effect of four types of support on the segmental mobility of the lumbosacral spine. *J. Bone Jt. Surg.*, **65A**, 943–947.

Fisk, J.R., DiMonte, P. & Courington, S.McK. (1983) Back schools: past, present and future. *Clin. Orthop. Rel. Res.*, **179**, 18–23.

Fordyce, W.E., Shelton, J.L. & Dundore, D.E. (1982) The modification of avoidance learning pain behaviour. *J. Behav. Med.*, **4**, 405–414.

Gaw, A.C., Chang, L.W. & Shaw, L.C. (1975) Efficacy of acupuncture on osteoarthritic pain. *N. Engl. J. Med.*, **293**, 375–378.

Gelb, M. (1981) *Body Learning—an introduction to the Alexander Technique*. Aurum Press, London.

Hadler, N.M., Curtis, P., Gillings, D.B. & Stinnett, S. (1987) A benefit of spinal manipulation as adjunctive therapy for acute low back pain: a stratified controlled trial. *Spine*, **12**, 703–706.

Hazars, R.G., Fenwick, J.W., Kalisch, S.M., Redmond, J., Reeves, V., Reid, S. & Frymoyer, J.W. (1989) Functional restoration with behavioural support: a one year prospective study of patients with chronic low back pain. *Spine*, **14**, 157–161.

Helbig, T. & Lee, C.K. (1988) The lumbar facet syndrome. *Spine*, **13**, 61–64.

Hitoshi, H. (1980) Spondylolysis in athletes. *Phys. Sports Med.*, **8**, 75–79.

Jackson, D.W., Wiltse, L.L. & Cirincone, R.J. (1976) Spondylolysis in the female gymnast. *Clin. Orthop.*, **117**, 68–73.

Jackson, R.P., Jacobs, R.R. & Montesano, P.X. (1988) Facet joint injection in low back pain; a prospective statistical study. *Spine*, **13**, 966–971.

Jayson, M.I.V. (1981) *Back Pain: The Facts*. Oxford University Press, New York.

Jayson, M.I.V. (1986) A limited role for manipulation. *Br. Med. J.*, **293**, 1454–1455.

Johansson, J.E., Barrington, T.W. & Ameli, M. (1982) Combined vascular and neurogenic claudication. *Spine*, **7**, 150–158.

Khuffash, B. & Porter, R.W. (1989) Cross leg pain and trunk list. *Spine*, **14**, 602–603.

Kirkaldy-Willis, W.H. (1988) The site and nature of the lesion. In Kirkaldy-Willis, W.H. (ed.), *Managing Low Back Pain*, 2nd edn, pp. 135–154. Churchill Livingstone, Edinburgh.

Kono, S., Hayashi, N., Kashahara, G., Akimoto, T., Keneko, F., Suguira, Y. & Harada, A. (1975) A study on the aetiology of spondylolysis with reference to athletic activities. *J. Jpn. Orthop. Assoc.*, **49**, 125–131.

Kosierlitz, H.W., Hughes, J., Law, J.H. & Waterfield, J.A. (1977) Encephalins, endorphines and opiate receptors. *Nerosci. Symp.*, vol. 2, Society for Neuroscience, pp. 291–307.

Lee, P.K., Andersen, T.W., Modell, J.H. & Saga, S.A. (1975) Treatment of chronic pain with acupuncture *J. Am. Med. Assoc.*, **232**, 1133–1135.

Lewith, G.T. (1984) Can we assess the effects of acupuncture? *Br. Med. J.*, **288**, 1475–1476.

Lewith, G.T. & Machin, D. (1983) The evaluation of the clinical effects of acupuncture. *Pain*, **16**, 111–127.

Lindstrom, L., Ohlund, C., Eek, C., Peterson, L.E. & Nachemson, A. (1989) Work return and LBP disability. Presented to the Society for the Study of the Lumbar Spine, Kyoto, Japan.

Linton, S.J. (1985) The relationship between activity and chronic back pain. *Pain*, **21**, 289–294.

Lippitt, A.B. (1984) The facet joint and its role in spine pain: management with facet joint injections. *Spine*, **9**, 746–750.

Lumsden, R.M. & Morris, J.M. (1968) An *in vivo* study of axial rotation and immobilization at the lumbo sacral joint. *J. Bone Jt. Surg.*, **50A**, 1591–1602.

McCulloch, J.A. (1977) Chemonucleosis. *J. Bone Jt. Surg.*, **59B**, 45–52.

MacDonald, A.J.R., Macrae, K.D., Master, B.R. & Rubin, A.P. (1983) Superficial acupuncture in the relief of chronic low back pain. *Ann. R. Coll. Surg. Engl.*, **65**, 44–46.

McKenzie, (1981) Spinal Publications Ltd. PO Box 2, Waikanae, New Zealand.

Man, S.C. & Baragar, F.D. (1974) Preliminary clinical study of acupuncture in rheumatoid arthritis. *J. Rheumatol.*, **1**, 126–129.

Matsumoto, T., Levy, B. & Ambrus, O.V. (1974) Clinical evaluation of acupuncture. *Am. Surg.*, **40**, 400–405.

Mayer, T., Gatchel, R.J., Kishino, N., Keeley, J., Capra, P., Mayer, H., Barnet, J. & Mooney, V. (1985) Objective assessment of spine function following industrial injury. *Spine*, **6**, 482–493.

Mayer, T.G., Gatchel, R.J., Mayer, H., Kishino, N.D., Keeley, J. & Mooney, V. (1987) A prospective two year study of functional restoration in industrial low back injury. *J. Am. Med. Assoc.*, **258**, 1763–1767.

Mehta, M. & Sluijter, M.E. (1979) The treatment of chronic pain. A preliminary survey of the effect of radiofrequency denervation of the posterior vertebral joints. *Anaesthesia*, **34**, 768.

Mellin, G. (1986) Chronic low back pain in men 54–63 years of age. Correlations of physical measurements with degree of trouble and progress after treatment. *Spine*, **11**, 421–426.

Melzack, R., Vetere, P. & Finch, L. (1983) Transcutaneous electrical nerve stimulation for low back pain; a comparison of TENS and massage for pain and range of motion. *Phys. Therapy*, **63**, 489–493.

Mendelson, G., Selwood, T.S., Kranz, H., Kidson, M.A. & Scott, D.S. (1983) Acupuncture treatment of chronic back pain: a double blind placebo controlled trial. *Am. J. Med.*, **74**, 49–55.

Million, R., Nilsen, K.H., Jayson, M.I.V. & Baker, R.D. (1981) Evaluation of low back pain and assessment of lumbar corsets with and without back supports. *Ann. Rheum. Dis.*, **40**, 449–454.

Moffett, J.A.K., Chase, S.M., Portek, I. & Ennis, J.R. (1986) A controlled prospective study to evaluate the effectiveness of a back school in the relief of chronic low back pain. *Spine*, **11**, 120–122.

Moore, M.E. & Berk, S.N. (1976) Acupuncture for chronic shoulder pain. *Ann. Intern. Med.*, **84**, 381–384.

Moran, R., O'Connell, D. & Walsh, M.G. (1988) The diagnostic value of facet joint injections. *Spine*, **13**, 1407–1410.

Murray Leslie, C.F., Lintott, D.J. & Wright, V. (1977) The spine in sport and veteran military parachutists. *Ann. Rheum. Dis.*, **36**, 332–342.

Nachemson, A. (1983a) Work for all. *Clin. Orthop. Rel. Res.*, **179**, 77–85.

Nachemson, A. (1983b) Work for all, for those with back pain as well. *Clin. Orthop.*, **179**, 177–182.

Nachemson, A. (1985) Lumbar spine instability; a critical update and symposium summary. *Spine*, **10**, 290–291.

Nelson, M. (1982) *Orthopaedic Surgery*. Proceedings of International Symposium of the Low Back Pain Association, London.

Norton, P.L. & Brown, T. (1957) The immobilizing efficiency of back braces. Their effect on the posture and motion of the lumbosacral spine. *J. Bone Jt. Surg.*, **39A**, 111–138.

Ottenbacher, K. & Difabio, R.P. (1985) Efficacy of spinal manipulation/mobilisation therapy. *Spine*, **10**, 833–837.

Pawlicki, R.E., Gil, K.M., Jopling, C.A., Bettinger, R. & Stevenson, J.M. (1982) The Low Back School: A new palliative approach to low back pain. *West Virginia Med. J.*, **78**, 249–251.

Philips, H.C. & Hunter, M. (1981) Pain behaviour in headache sufferers. *Behav. Anal. Modif.*, **4**, 256–266.

Pike, P.M.H. (1978) Transcutaneous electrical nerve stimulation. *Anaesthesia*, **33**, 165–171.

Porter, R.W. (1986) *Management of Back Pain*. Churchill Livingstone, Edinburgh, p. 51.

Porter, R.W. (1987a) Should one operate on the elderly spine? In Hukins, & Nelson, M. (eds), *The Ageing Spine*, pp. 79–93. Manchester University Press, Manchester.

Porter, R.W. (1987b) Does hard work prevent disc protrusion? *Clin. Biomech.*, **2**, 196–198.

Porter, R.W. & Adams, M.A. (1989) Physical activity and the strength of the spine. *Spine*, **14**, 201–203.

Porter, R.W. & Hibbert, C. (1983) Calcitonin treatment for neurogenic claudication. *Spine*, **8**, 585–592.

Porter, R.W. & Hibbert, C. (1984) Symptoms associated with lysis of the pars interarticularis. *Spine*, **9**, 755–758.

Porter, R.W. & Miller, C.G. (1986) Back pain and trunk list. *Spine*, **11**, 596–600.

Porter, R.W. & Park, W. (1982) Unilateral spondylolysis. *J. Bone Jt. Surg.*, **64B**, 344–348.

Porter, R.W. & Miller, C.G. (1988) Neurogenic claudication and root claudication treated with calcitonin: a double blind trial. *Spine*, **13**, 1061–1064.

Porter, R.W. & Trailescu, F. (1990) Diurnal changes in straight leg raising. *Spine*, **15**, 103–106.

Porter, R.W., Ellingworth, C., Hughes, T. & Trailescu, F. (1989) Assessment of a 'School for Bravery'—modification of abnormal pain behaviour. In Roland, & Jenner, (eds) *Back Pain*, pp. 157–165. Manchester University Press, Manchester.

Porter, R.W., Hibbert, C. & Evans, C. (1984) The natural history of root entrapment syndrome. *Spine*, **9**, 418–421.

Postacchini, F. (1989) Progression of spondylolysis in spondylolisthesis in adulthood. Presented to the International Society for the Study of the Lumbar Spine, Kyoto, Japan.

Racz, G.B., McCarron, R.F. & Talboys, P. (1989) Percutaneous dorsal column stimulator for chronic pain control. *Spine*, **14**, 1–4.

Rashbaum, R.F. (1983) Radiofrequency facet denervation: a treatment alternative in refractory low back pain with or without leg pain. *Orthop. Clin. N. Am.*, **14**, 569–575.

Roche, M.B. & Rowe, G.G. (1951) The incidence of separated

neural arch and coincident bone variation. A survey of 4200 skeletons. *Anat. Rec.*, **109**, 233–252.

Saal, J.A. & Saal, J.S. (1988) Nonoperative treatment of herniated lumbar intervertebral disc with radiculopathy; an outcome study. *Spine*, **13**, 431–437.

Sims-Williams, H., Jayson, M.I.V., Young, S.M.S., Baddeley, H. & Colins, E. (1978) Controlled trial of mobilisation and manipulation for patients with low back pain in general practice. *Br. Med. J.*, **ii**, 1338–1340.

Snoek, W., Weber, H. & Jorgensen, B. (1977) Double blind evaluation of extradural methyl prednisolone for herniated lumbar discs. *Acta Orthop. Scand.*, **48**, 635–641.

Terenius, L. & Wahlstrom, A. (1979) Endorphines and clinical pain: an overview. *Adv. Exp. Med. Biol.*, **116**, 261–277.

Troup, J.D.G. (1975) Classical factors in spondylolisthesis and spondylolysis. *Clin. Orthop. Rel. Res.*, **117**, 59–67.

Waddell, G. (1987) A new clinical model for the treatment of low back pain. *Spine*, 7, 632–644.

Ward, N.G. (1986) Tricyclic antidepressants for chronic low back pain: mechanisms of action and predictors of response. *Spine*, **11**, 661–665.

Weber, H. (1980) Comparison of the effect of diazepam and levomepromazine on pain in patients with acute lumbago-sciatica. *J. Oslo City Hosp.*, **30**, 65–68.

Weber, H. (1983) Lumbar disc herniation: a controlled prospective study with ten years of observation. *Spine*, **8**, 131–140.

Weber, H., Ljunggren, A.E. & Walker, L. (1985) Traction therapy in patients with herniated lumbar intervertebral discs. *J. Oslo City Hosp.*, **34**, 61–70.

White, A.H. (1983) *Back School and Other Conservative Approaches to Low Back Pain.* C.V. Mosby, St Louis.

Wiesel, S.W., Cucker, J.M., Deluca, F., Jones, F., Zeide, M.S. & Rothman, R.H. (1980) Acute low back pain: an objective analysis of conservative therapy. *Spine*, **5**, 324–330.

Williams, S.J. (1977) Back School. *Physiotherapy*, **63**, 90.

Willner, S. (1985) Effects of a rigid brace on back pain. *Acta Orthop. Scand.*, **56**, 40–42.

Zachrisson-Forsell, M. (1972) *Low Back Pain School.* Danderyds Hospital, Sweden.

Zylbergold, R.S. & Piper, M.C. (1985) Cervical spine disorders: a comparison of three types of traction. *Spine*, **10**, 867–871.

39 · Surgical Management of Lumbar Disc Prolapse

By J.A. McCULLOCH

It is common knowledge that the rate of surgical intervention for lumbar disc prolapse in the United States is 10 times greater than that in the United Kingdom. It is unlikely that there is any true pathological difference in disc prolapses, but there do exist wide differences not only in surgical indications but also in the demand, facilities and workload of both patients and doctors in the two countries. It is likely that, particularly due to improved imaging techniques, the diagnosis and treatment of lumbar disc prolapses around the world will become more uniform.

Prior to embarking on surgery for a lumbar disc prolapse it should be recalled that the long-term natural history for such a patient is likely to be good and that many radiologically proven discs may become or remain asymptomatic (Hitselberger & Witten, 1968, Wiesel *et al.*, 1984; Bowden *et al.*, 1989). Moreover, when Hakelius (1970) compared the outcome of surgical therapy for lumbar disc prolapse as compared to conservative therapy, he found that at six months there was no statistical difference between the two groups. By seven years of follow-up the surgically treated group had fared better, but only in that they had had less episodes of low back pain and had lost less time from work. In a similar study, Weber (1983) found that at one year the surgical group had fared much better, with 92% good results as compared with 60% in the non-surgical group. However, at both four- and 10-year follow-up there was again no statistical difference between the two groups. It does seem, therefore, that many lumbar disc problems ameliorate eventually, and that the role of surgery may serve only to achieve that improvement more quickly than can nature.

SURGICAL PATHOLOGY

It is essential that any surgeon performing a lumbar discectomy clearly understands the exact surgical anatomy of the lumbar disc prolapse which is to be removed. Discal herniations present as one of three consecutive stages (Fig. 39.1). A simple disc protrusion (sometimes described as a contained herniation) consists of a bulging disc where the degenerate nuclear material remains contained by the annulus. The posterior longitudinal ligament is a flimsy structure in the lower lumbar spine; the annulus acts as the main container of nuclear material. This normally progresses in a posterolateral direction, thereby easily compressing the nerve root. A non-contained herniation occurs once the nucleus protrudes through the torn annulus. This is described as an extruded disc, and may be either subligamentous or transligamentous but the nuclear fragment remains in contact with the interior of the disc space. A sequestered disc fragment is where part of the degenerate disc has separated from the disc space and has moved through the torn posterior longitudinal ligament. Such a sequestered disc lies free in the spinal canal and may migrate away from the disc space.

The relationship of the disc prolapse within the spinal canal is of obvious importance. A vertebral body along with the disc immediately below it can be considered to resemble a three-storey house (Fig. 39.2). The first storey corresponds to the intervertebral disc. Dividing the vertebral body by a line drawn along the inferior borders of the pedicles produces the upper two storeys. The nerve root which exits the canal by passing under the pedicle and out through the 'second storey' is assigned the same

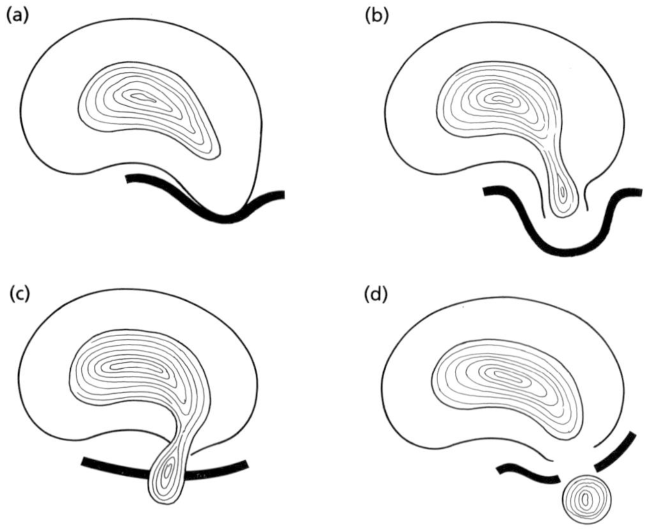

Fig. 39.1 Types of lumbar disc herniation: protrusion (a), extrusion—subligamentous/transligamentous (b,c), sequestered (d).

number as the pedicle beneath which it passes. It should be noted that it is only the nerve root of the segment below that vertebral level which actually traverses the disc space itself. Continuing the analogy of the house, the bony anatomy of the spine produces two 'windows' on each side of the spine through which the disc space can be reached (Fig. 39.3). The most commonly used 'window' is the interlaminar space, but occasionally the intertransverse 'window' may be used.

A contained discal protrusion will lie at the level of the disc space in the first storey of the house (Fig. 39.4). A sequestered fragment or an extruded disc with a long pedunculated tail may extend upward from its disc into the second storey and come to lie

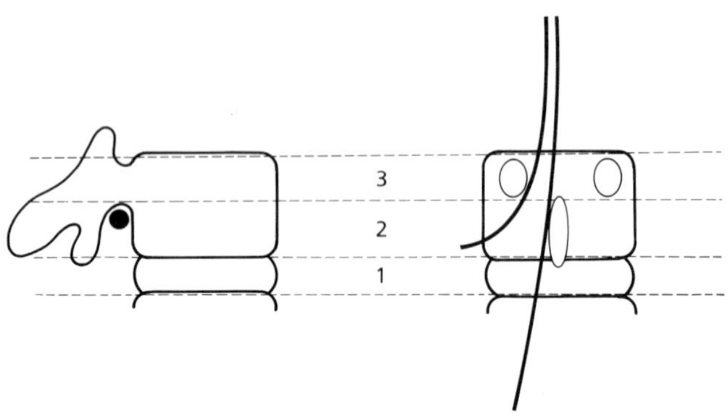

Fig. 39.2 Diagrammatic representation of vertebral body and the disc immediately caudal to it, showing the three-storey analogy.

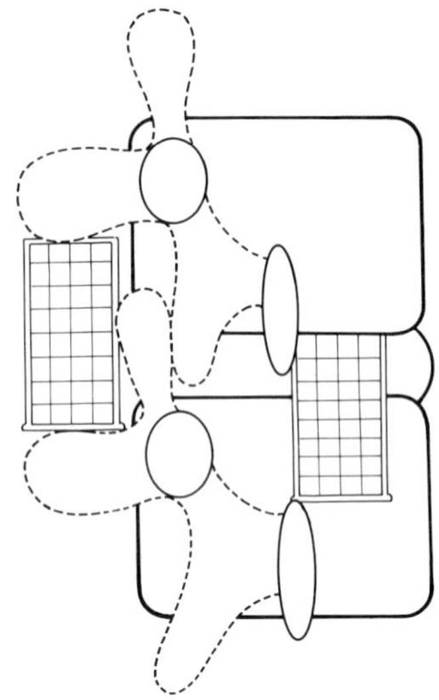

Fig. 39.3 Schematic posterior view to show the two 'windows' permitting access to the disc space.

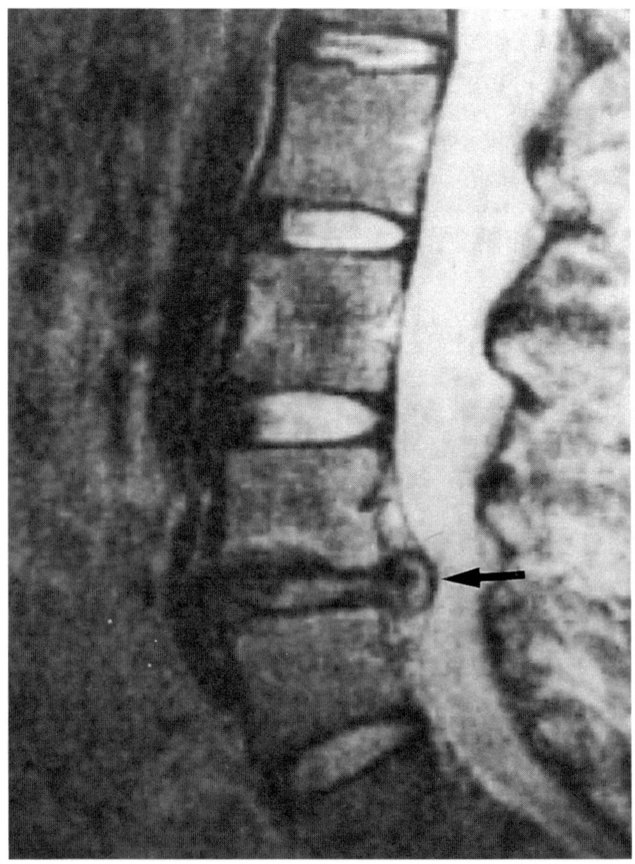

Fig. 39.4 MRI scan showing disc protrusion lying in the 'first storey' of L4.

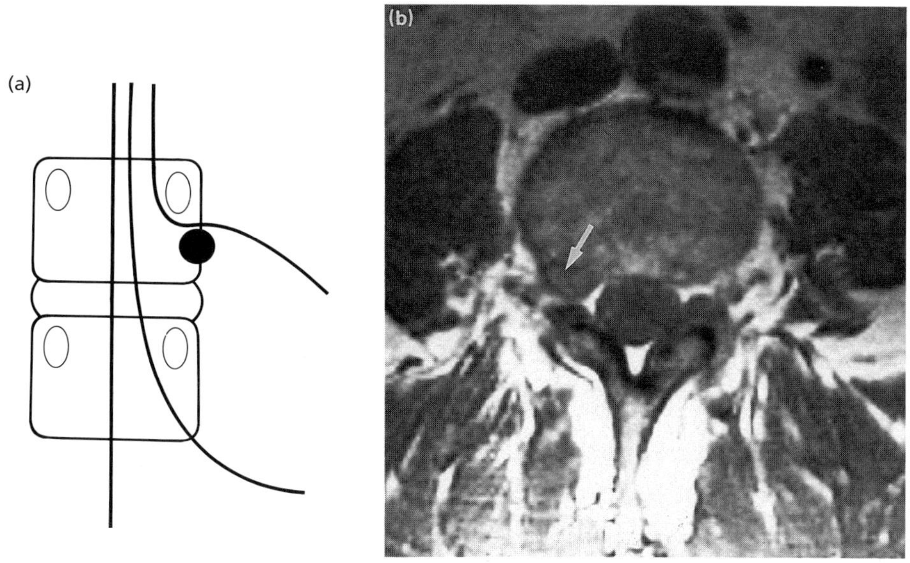

Fig. 39.5 A 'second-storey' foraminal disc shown schematically (a) and by MRI (b).

in the nerve root foramen (Fig. 39.5). Alternatively, Fig. 39.6 shows an extruded disc extending into the third storey of the segment below from the disc or first storey of the level above. Using such an approach when analysing radiology allows the surgeon to predict exactly where in the spinal canal the disc protrusion will be found at operation.

DIAGNOSIS AND INDICATIONS FOR SURGERY

Once a discal herniation has occurred it may result in nerve root compression producing the symptom of sciatica. The clinical features produced by lumbar disc disease and their assessment have been discussed in Chapter 32. Having made a clinical diagnosis of lumbar disc prolapse, that diagnosis must be confirmed by appropriate radiology. It is essential that the entire lumbar canal is imaged. This is best achieved by magnetic resonance imaging (MRI) scanning. As shown in Figs 39.4, 39.5 & 39.6, MRI scanning provides exquisite detail of the anatomy of a lumbar disc prolapse. The only other investigation required is plain radiography, as abnormalities such as abnormal lumbosacral segmentation or spondylolysis may not be appreciated on the MRI scan.

If MRI scanning is not available, computerized tomography (CT) scanning should always be accompanied by radiculography. Only by performing the dual investigation can the entire lumbar canal be assessed, and hence the uncommon situation of the sciatica being due to an intradural lesion of the conus or cauda equina be excluded. Both MRI and CT scanning are so sensitive that they frequently may show degenerative changes which may be asymptomatic (Bowden *et al.*, 1989). The scans must therefore always be interpreted carefully in the light of the clinical findings.

McCulloch (1977), refining the earlier work particularly of Macnab (1971), showed that four factors were important in diagnosing a lumbar disc herniation. They were: a dominant complaint of radicular rather than low back pain; signs of root tension such as limited straight leg raising; signs of root compression, such as changes in reflexes, sensation or power; and positive confirmatory radiology. When at least three of these factors were definitely present he found that a lumbar disc herniation was always found. The distribution of radicular pain is a most important criterion as the performance of a discectomy can be successful only if radicular pain is present. Discectomy performed for low back pain with or without referred pain is usually unsuccessful. Compression of L5 or S1 roots results in pain which radiates down the back of the leg below the knee and usually into the ankle or foot. However, it is important to note that, especially in adolescent patients, radicular pain may occasionally only produce buttock and thigh pain, but the quality and precise distribution of the pain allow its differentiation from referred pain. Compression of roots higher in the lumbar plexus by the less common midlumbar dis-

(a)

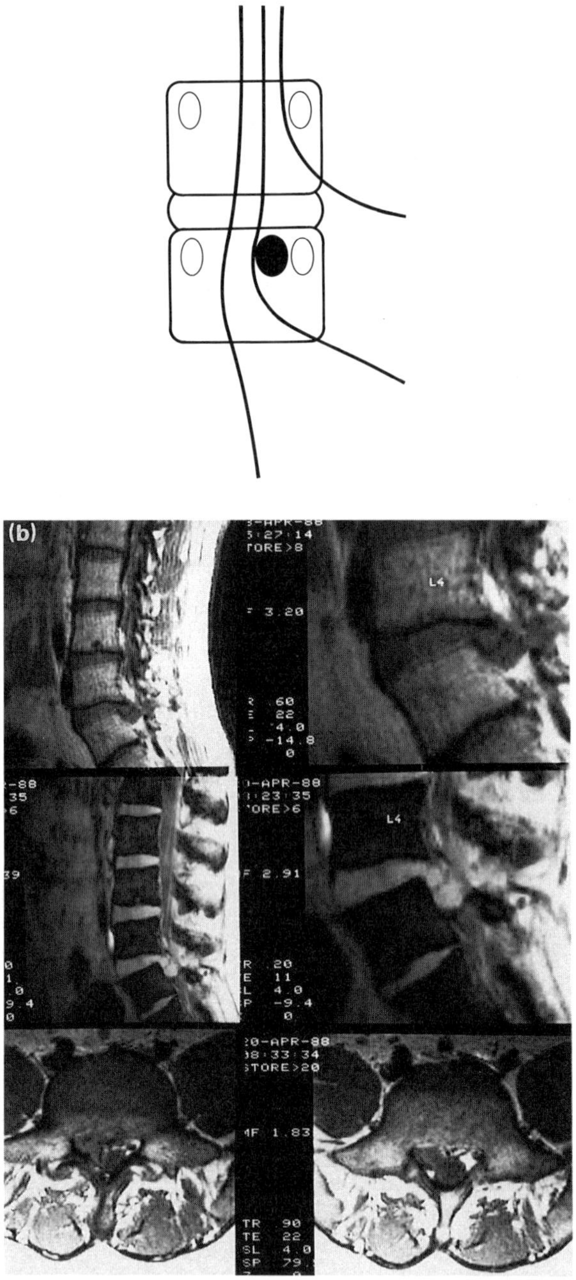

Fig. 39.6 A disc extrusion lying in the 'third storey' at the level of the pedicle shown schematically (a) and by MRI (b).

cal herniation produces radicular pain in the front of the thigh.

Surgical removal of a lumbar disc herniation is indicated in several differing clinical situations. Immediate surgical intervention is mandatory in the acute massive disc herniation presenting with bladder and bowel paralysis. Except in situations where marked spinal stenosis exists, a huge sequestered fragment will be found severely compressing the roots of the cauda equina. An immediate open operation with bony decompression to allow the removal of the sequestered fragment is required but, even when performed without delay, the results of sphincteric recovery can be very disappointing (O'Laire *et al.*, 1981; Kostuik *et al.*, 1986).

Where lesser degrees of neurological deficit are present, surgery should also be considered. Patients presenting with loss of an ankle jerk, numbness or even mild motor deficit may reasonably be treated conservatively. However, repeated neurological assessment is necessary as, if the deficit increases or fails to improve, then surgery is indicated.

The most frequent indication for surgical intervention is the failure of conservative treatment. Ideal conservative treatment is treatment that occurs over at least six weeks and not more than three months, and which results in improvement in the patient's symptoms and signs. The details of conservative therapy are discussed in Chapter 38. The key to measuring the success of conservative treatment is not only the patient's relief of leg pain but also the improvement in straight leg raising ability. If a patient goes to bed with appropriate medication for three to five days, and there is no improvement in leg pain and/or straight leg raising ability, then it is likely that the patient is going to follow a protracted conservative course, for which surgical intervention may be indicated. It is proposed that surgical intervention in the acute radicular syndrome should occur before three months of symptoms, to try to avoid the chronic pathological changes that can occur within a nerve root (Weber, 1983).

Conservative therapy may also fail where the patient experiences recurring attacks of sciatica. Ninety per cent of patients experiencing their first attack of sciatica will become better with conservative therapy, and the vast majority will remain better. Of those in their second episode of sciatica, again 90% will become better but 50% will go on to have further attacks. Most patients having their third or greater attack will still recover from that episode, but almost all will have further recurrent episodes. The knowledge of such prognostic data will allow discussion of the future course of the patient's illness and a surgical approach may quite reasonably be considered to attempt to prevent further episodes. It is, however, appropriate also to counsel the patient regarding the longer-term effects of a lumbar disc protrusion as described by Hakelius (1970) and Weber (1983), so that fully informed consent is obtained prior to surgery. The only absolute indication for surgical intervention is the presence of marked neurological deficit as described earlier. The remaining indication for surgery is where the patient, in full possession of the facts discussed above, decides that he or she can no longer cope with the activities of daily living because of the radicular pain, or when the certainty of future attacks is unacceptable.

The existence of compensation claims or significant non-organic components such as 'illness behaviour' reduce the success rate of surgery (Waddell *et al.*, 1980). The presence of a non-organic component does not, however, 'immunize' a patient against a disc herniation, but surgery should proceed only following careful patient counselling and with psychological support. Fortunately, relatively few people with a disc rupture exhibit such a non-organic component as it is much more commonly associated with low back pain.

SURGICAL TECHNIQUES

The satisfaction of a successfully completed surgical procedure, which is then followed by a poor result, quickly gives way to the realization that surgical outcomes are far more dependent on patient selection than on surgical technique. Obviously, a poorly done operation carries with it a greater risk of failure; but, given competent surgical expertise, there is little difference in outcome between the various approaches to surgical disc excision (Loew, 1986). The surgical options available are:

1 open surgery
 (a) standard fenestration/discectomy
 (b) microsurgical discectomy
 (c) anterior discectomy (only rarely performed for a simple disc herniation);

2 closed surgery
 (a) chemonucleolysis
 (b) percutaneous discectomy (see Chapter 40).

Open surgery

The aim of surgery for a lumbar disc herniation is to leave the affected nerve root free of encroachment by disc, ligament or bone and to maintain the stability of the spinal segment. Surgery may be carried out under general, spinal or local anaesthesia. The most expedient anaesthetic agent is general, although there are surgeons who believe that the procedure is best accomplished under either spinal or local anaesthesia. Most surgeons agree that having the patient in a kneeling position is best for the surgeon and the patient. This position allows for a free abdomen, removing pressure from the inferior vena cava and decreasing venous flow through Batson's plexus, in turn reducing bleeding during surgery. Great care is essential whilst positioning the patient, to avoid damage due to pressure or due to traction on peripheral nerves.

The standard surgical approach for a laminectomy or a microdiscectomy has been outlined in many articles (Scoville & Corkilig, 1973; Caspar, 1977; Williams, 1978). It is important to open the correct disc space. Once within the laminar opening it is necessary to find the lateral border of the nerve root and reflect the nerve root and cauda equina sheath medially to expose the lesion. It is sometimes necessary to remove some bone to see the lateral border of the nerve root, especially at the L4–L5 level and higher. This may require removal of the medial edge of the superior facet of the anatomical segment below. The attempt to find the lateral border of the lumbar nerve root has a few potential pitfalls. The first problem is a nerve root that has been displaced laterally by an axillary disc herniation. A second pitfall is the posterior displacement of a nerve root that occurs because of the location of the disc herniation, placing the nerve root in jeopardy when the ligamentum flavum is being opened. It is important to remove all the offending lesion, not to miss any extruded or migrated disc fragments, and not to leave behind bony nerve root encroachment.

Ninety-five per cent of exposures for lumbar disc herniations occur at either L4–L5 or L5–S1, with the former tending to be in the older patient and the latter tending to be in the younger patient. Five per cent of exposures occur at other levels (laterally at the L4–L5 level and at higher lumbar levels, such as L3–L4 and L2–L3). Exposure of more than one level is rarely indicated. The acute radicular syndrome caused by a ruptured disc is almost always single-level disease, and the routine exposure of a second level, searching for a 'shadow' on CT or MRI, should be discouraged.

It is important to be aware of root anomalies which by their nature reduce nerve root mobility (Helms *et al.*, 1982; Postacchini *et al.*, 1982; Neidre & Macnab, 1983). Very small disc herniations can cause major sciatic symptoms in a patient with an anomalous root. At the time of surgery those anomalies lead to a very immobile nerve root, and difficulty in reaching the disc pathology lying ventral to the root.

The place of the microscope in discectomy

It is the author's belief that the introduction of the microscope into lumbar disc surgery is a major advance. The microscope provides superior magnification, illumination, three-dimensional vision and comfort as compared to the use of headlight and loupes. These advantages enhance the ability to see the nerve root and deal with pathology, to coagulate epidural veins safely, and to distinguish between scar tissue and nerve root in reoperations. The use of the microscope also greatly facilitates the instruction of a surgical trainee.

A hidden benefit of the microscope is the more disciplined thinking it forces on the surgeon. The moment that a surgical incision is limited the more imperative it becomes for the surgeon to know exactly where to position the incision, and exactly what is to be found at the time of exposure. This forces the surgeon to look more critically at the patient and the imaging investigation. No longer can the surgeon seek and find; the pathology to be found, and its exact location, must be precisely known before the limited skin incision is made.

The increased surgical precision afforded by the use of the microscope allows the procedure to be performed through a much smaller incision. The actual length of the incision is of only cosmetic importance, but the size of the wound and the degree of soft tissue damage caused is significant. The longer the paraspinal incision, the greater will be the wound haematoma and the muscle damage resulting in terminal scar being laid down (Peacock, 1967). Larocca and Macnab (1974), in developing their hypothesis for a laminectomy membrane, observed that 'the fibrous response was always more marked when a wide operative exposure was employed'. It is every surgeon's intention to have clean wounds heal by primary intention. This is easy to accomplish when vascularized skin edges, clean and free of contamination, are apposed; it is virtually impossible to achieve when the deep portions of the wound fill with haematoma. The longer the paraspinal incision, the greater the paraspinal muscle dissection, the larger the dead space left behind, and the greater the haematoma. Haematoma can heal only by secondary intention through removal of necrotic debris and fibrin secondary to the inflammatory reaction. The end-result is scar. The greater the dead space, the greater the haematoma, the greater the inflammation response needed, the greater the scar. The reverse is also true. The less muscle dissection that occurs, the less potential dead space there is for haematoma. This can be achieved with a limited wound incision and microsurgical technique, reducing the requirement for healing by secondary intention and, in the end, resulting in less scar formation.

A further disadvantage of a longer incision is the denervation that occurs in paraspinal tissues. This was documented by Macnab *et al.* (1977) in a clinical study of 113 patients, showing some measure of denervation of the paravertebral muscles on electromyography (EMG) in 96% of the cases. Denervation was shown to persist for many years following surgery, and reinnervation was only partial.

Clinical support for the reduced morbidity of a microsurgical paraspinal wound came from the study of Kahonovich *et al.* (1989) comparing a group of patients who had a standard laminectomy to a group of patients who had a microsurgical exposure. In terms of surgical outcome the results of the two groups were identical, except that the patients who underwent a microsurgical approach had a much-reduced postoperative morbidity and a much shorter hospital stay.

Although the microscope has many advantages, in the author's opinion, there are certain disadvantages which also must be overcome. The limited field of vision encountered requires that exact positioning of both the microscope and the incision are necessary. The operator must become accustomed to altering the angle of view of the microscope to ensure that the entire nerve root area is seen, to ensure that fragments of disc or bony entrapment are not missed. Similarly, the microscope produces a relatively limited field in which to work. This demands a high standard of manipulative skills and certain specially designed instruments which must be used precisely to avoid damage to the root. The microsurgical approach results in a significantly decreased amount of haemorrhage. Nevertheless, any haemorrhage which does occur must be precisely controlled with bipolar coagulation so as to ensure that the operative field does not become obscured. Fortunately, the microscope greatly improves the visualization of epidural veins, allowing their careful coagulation. Wilson & Harbaugh (1981) and Dauch (1986) have reported an increased rate of disc space infection following microsurgery. This is most likely because of the presence of the microscope directly over the wound. Although the microscope is sterilely draped, there are parts of the microscope that are exposed (eyepieces) which have the potential to contaminate the wound. The limited operating space between the microscope and the wound also introduces another element of potential break in proper surgical technique that can result in wound contamination. Again, very detailed technique is required to minimize this risk.

Technical aspects of microdiscectomy

It is essential that the correct level is exposed. The potential for exploring an incorrect level rises dramatically as the size of the incision diminishes. Microdiscectomy demands radiological confirmation of the correct level. This may be achieved by using the image intensifier to provide an on-table lateral view with a lumbar puncture needle to identify the disc space. It is essential that the needle marks the inferior edge of the relevant disc space to avoid slipping cephalad on the lamina into the disc space above (Fig. 39.7).

A limited subperiosteal incision of the paraspinal muscles allows exposure of the interlaminar space. Exposure of the adjacent lamina is not normally required. With the knowledge of the exact location of the disc hernia available from the preoperative radiology, the lesion can be precisely exposed. A 'first-storey' herniation merely requires the spinal canal to be entered through the ligamentum flavum without any bone removal. On the other hand, 'second-storey' and 'third-storey' protrusions require partial removal of the cephalad and caudal hemilamina, respectively.

Once the spinal canal has been entered, the lateral edge of the nerve root must be identified by blunt dissection in order to allow its retraction medially to expose the herniation. Should it prove impossible to identify the lateral edge of the root, it is likely that there is either an anomalous nerve root or that the herniation is presenting in the axilla of the nerve root. The presence of lateral recess stenosis will also obscure the lateral edge of the root and such bone must be carefully nibbled away.

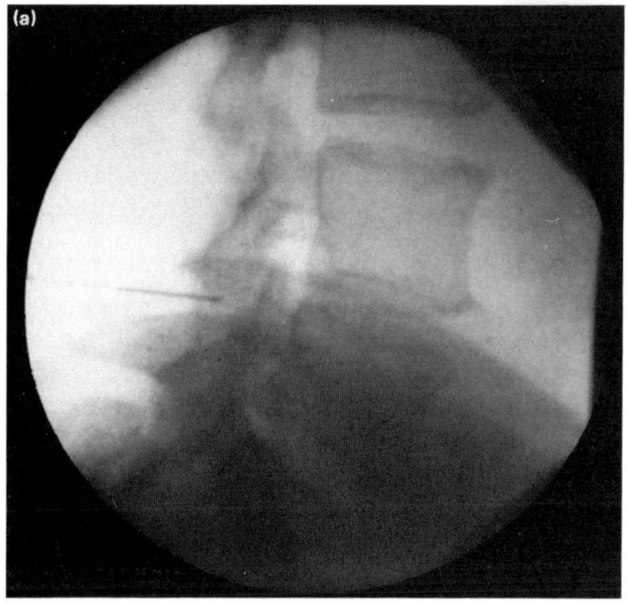

(b)

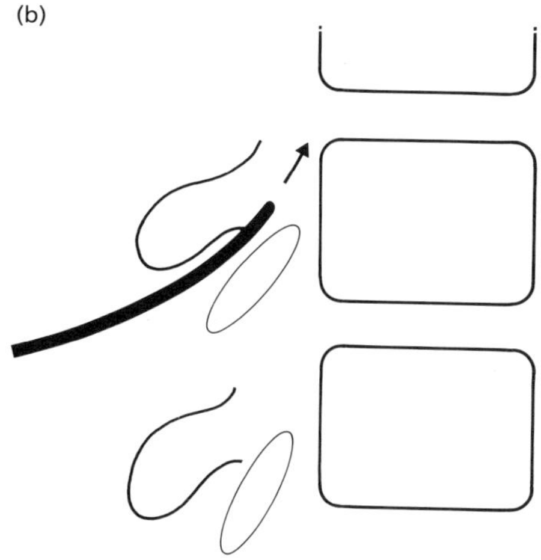

Fig. 39.7 (a) Lateral radiograph showing marking needle identifying the inferior edge of the L4–L5 disc space. (b) Diagram showing how the marking needle (and surgical instruments) can slip cephalad to the next level if not directed to inferior margin of disc.

The object of the surgical procedure is to leave a freely mobile nerve root. This requires removal of the obvious portion of the ruptured disc, but also includes a diligent search of the canal, along with probing of the foramen, for residual disc fragments or bony pathology. Classical teaching demands the removal of as much disc as possible from the interspace, a procedure facilitated by focusing down into the space with the microscope. However, it is clearly not possible to remove the entire disc, and over-vigorous attempts so to do may result in damage to the endplates and nerve roots and even vascular structures lying anterior to the disc space (Capana *et al.*, 1981). Radical removal of the disc may also produce abnormal degrees of postoperative disc space narrowing leading potentially to increased low back pain and root canal narrowing related to overriding of the facets. Some series, such as that of Scoville & Corkilig (1973), have suggested that radical disc clearance decreases the incidence of recurrent herniation. However, other series, such as that of Spengler (1982), refute this assumption. It seems essential, therefore, to remove the offending portion of the disc and then reasonable to remove any loose or lightly attached material from within the disc space.

Prevention of epidural scar formation is an ideal objective. The use of a small incision, a limited entry into the spinal canal, precise surgical manipulation and avoidance of haemorrhage all help to limit scar formation. LaRocca & Macnab (1974), Mayfield (1980) and Van Akkerveeken *et al.* (1986) all felt that the use of a fat graft decreased interlaminar scar formation. Although there are several animal studies which support this concept, there is no controlled series in the literature to prove its effectiveness (Martin-Ferrer, 1989); moreover, both Prusick *et al.* (1988) and Mayer & Jacobsen (1989) reported serious morbidity with cauda equina compression due to free fat grafts.

Complications of disc surgery

Obviously any patient undergoing a surgical procedure for a lumbar disc herniation may be subject to the general complications of surgery such as pulmonary embolus. Wound infection may occur but correct operative technique should limit this complication to less than 0.5% of cases. Deep-seated wound infection may occasionally be complicated by the development of extradural or even subdural abscess formation, which can result in serious neurological morbidity. Postoperative disc space infection is fully discussed in Chapter 33. Penetration of the anterior annulus with resultant injury to the aorta and/or vena cava is a well-recognized but fortunately rare complication.

Two complications which should be uppermost in the surgeon's mind at the time of operation are intervention at the incorrect level and failure adequately to decompress the nerve root, either by missing a fragment of disc or failing to identify bony compression of the root and to rectify it at the time of operation. Both have already been discussed.

Dural injury should be avoided by careful attention to surgical technique. Several factors increase the risk of dural injury, but probably the most important is inexperience on behalf of the surgeon. The use of oversized bone punches and rongeurs is also of relevance. Dural injury is much more likely in the presence of an axillary protrusion or of an conjoint nerve root. The latter may occur in as many as 5% of patients and such roots are virtually immobile until a wide bony decompression has been performed. The S1 root at L5–S1 often lies quite laterally in the canal and is at risk of damage if, on opening the canal, the S2 root is mistaken for it. Finally, in segmentation anomalies at the lumbosacral junction, the ligamentum flavum at the lowest mobile level may be very thin, permitting dural injury on incision. Should dural injury occur it should be repaired by suturing or by fibrin glue where possible. Attempts to repair a ragged laceration, however, may only result in greater dural damage.

Results of microdiscectomy

Feldman & McCulloch (1990) reported the results in 257 patients undergoing microsurgery for lumbar disc disease. The average length of follow-up was 19 months with 249 (97%) available for assessment. Of those 249, a total of 119 presented with a virgin herniated disc. Twenty-four had lateral recess stenosis and in 26 a fusion was added to the microdiscectomy. Eighty of the patients had had previous surgery, though in 70 of those the surgery had been a chymopapain procedure.

In patients with a virgin disc herniation an 84% success rate was achieved with 95% returning to work (Table 39.1). As can be seen, the results of patients with a discal herniation who also were making a compensation claim were predictably worse. Less acceptable results were also obtained in patients who had had a previous surgical procedure, and especially disappointing in patients with lateral recess stenosis. It was found in the latter group that the addition of a fusion to the microsurgical procedure improved the success rate from 50% to 90%, but the numbers in that group were small.

Analysis of the results in this series for virgin disc herniations shows no appreciable difference from

Table 39.1 Results of microdiscectomy (percentages) (n = 249)

Diagnosis	Satisfactory	Unsatisfactory
Virgin disc protrusion	84	16
Disc protrusion and compensation claim	66	34
Previous surgery/chymopapain	70	30
Lateral recess stenosis	50	50

the reported results for standard open fenestration. However, the patients had a much shorter hospital stay (average 2.3 days) and returned to work earlier. An overall complication rate of 10% was found, but serious complications such as postoperative discitis or increased neurological deficit were found in only 1.5%. Dural laceration occurred in six patients and the wrong level was explored in a further six. The fact that the wrong level had been explored was identified and corrected at the time of the surgery, and the incidence of both these complications decreased with increasing experience. It is too early yet to comment on the recurrence rate, but other series report recurrence with the same frequency as open operation.

Other types of disc herniation

The foraminal type of disc herniation occurs when a sequestered, or occasionally extruded, fragment migrates caudally into the nerve root foramen. They occur in approximately 3–10% of disc herniations (Abdullah *et al.*, 1974; Postacchini & Montanaro, 1979; Zindrick *et al.*, 1987; Abdullah *et al.*, 1988) and by migrating superiorly and laterally they come to lie in Macnab's hidden zone (Fig. 39.8). They compress the nerve root which exits the canal through that foramen (Fig. 39.9). Attempts to remove such a herniation through the standard interlaminar window may result in the complete removal of the adjacent facet joint.

Foraminal herniations usually occur at the L4–L5 and L3–L4 levels, affecting the L4 and L3 roots respectively. They tend to occur in older patients (average age 50) and from wide disc spaces rather than degenerative (narrow) disc spaces. The onset is usually sudden and the result is severe anterior thigh pain, interfering with all functions except sitting. Sleep patterns are grossly disrupted because the positive femoral stretch test does not allow the patient to lie on the back or in the prone position with the thigh extended. Neurological examination, especially the sensory examination, will usually give a clue as to which level is involved. Often, these disc ruptures do not respond to conservative care, or the pain is so severe that the patient is not prepared to accept too long a conservative treatment programme.

The foramen has no bony roof, and the best way to approach the region for a full view of the pathology, and without sacrificing the facet joint, is through the intertransverse window. This requires a paraspinal

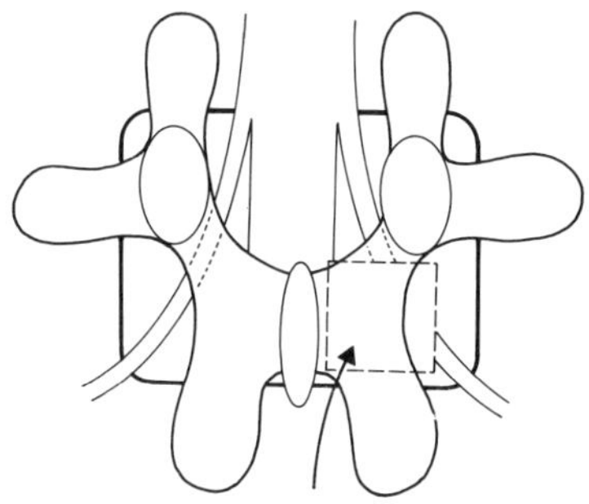

Fig. 39.8 Macnab's 'hidden-zone' which will obscure a foraminal disc herniation.

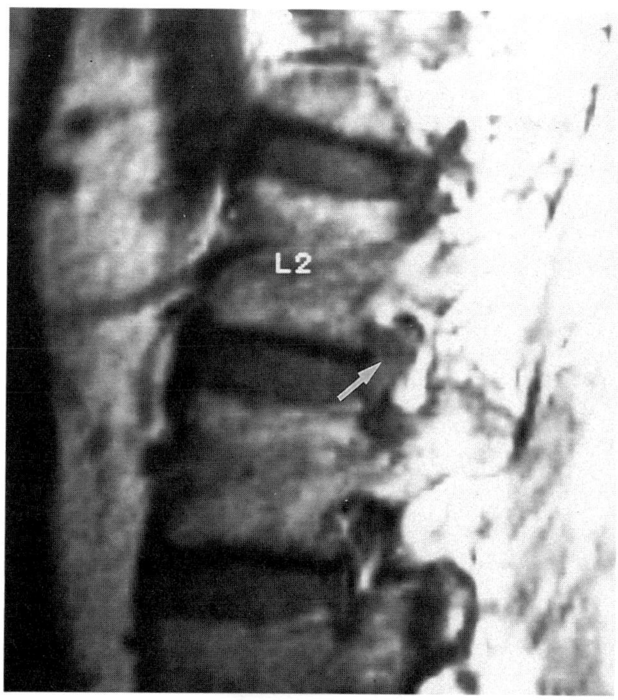

Fig. 39.9 A foraminal herniation at L2–L3 clearly showing compression of the L2 nerve root within the foramen.

approach exposing the lateral border of the pars and then dividing the arcuate ligament running between the adjacent transverse processes to gain access to the disc fragment and the lateral border of the disc (Wiltse *et al.*, 1968; Zindrick *et al.*, 1987). This approach allows removal of the disc without sacrificing the pars or the facet joint (Fig. 39.10).

Disc herniation in association with spondylolisthesis is a not-uncommon occurrence. The herniation may occur at the level above the slip and may be dealt with in a standard manner by microdiscectomy. Where the prolapse occurs at the level of a lytic spondylolisthesis, the potential for increased slip following discectomy demands that a fusion also be performed. However, the author feels that in older patients (over 35 years) there is enough established stability within the spondylolisthetic segment to allow simple microdiscectomy. Disc herniation occurring with degenerative spondylolisthesis and in spinal stenosis is discussed in Chapter 43. Adolescent disc prolapse is discussed in Chapter 42.

Recurrent discal herniation occurs in up to 5% of patients who have a successful discectomy. Recurrence may occur rarely within one or two weeks of surgery. Re-exploration in these patients will often show a major sequestered fragment, and it seems unlikely that such a fragment could have been overlooked at the time of operation. Most recurrences happen within the first 18 months of surgery, and in that situation usually the recurrence is at the same level. When recurrence occurs years after the discectomy it is common to find that a new level is involved.

Where recurrence occurs at the same level and on the same side as before diagnosis between true disc recurrence and epidural scarring can be very difficult. Investigations such as CT discography and MRI scanning with gadolinium-DTPA are most helpful. With gadolinium-enhanced MRI the contrast agent highlights the scar leaving a recurrent disc fragment unenhanced lying as a dark area within the brightly enhancing scar (Fig. 39.11). The epidural scarring present tends to bind the root to the posterior surface of the disc; hence even a small amount of recurrent disc material may cause significant radicular pain. However, the scar does tend to prevent migration of a new disc fragment and it is therefore normally found at the level of the disc space.

Surgical treatment can be difficult, and complications such as missed fragments, dural laceration and neurological damage are more common. To prevent this, most surgeons advise wide bony decompression allowing the identification of normal dura prior to root mobilization as, in any event, lateral recess stenosis is commonly present in a patient with a recurrence. However, Goald (1986) has shown that microsurgical techniques can again be used.

Lumbar microdiscectomy has now an established place in the management of lumbar disc herniations of all types. It has been shown beyond doubt that it allows: earlier and better postoperative mobilization, decreased hospitalization and possibly earlier return to work. It achieves these major early improvements and yet produces long-term results comparable to conventional open fenestration (Yasargil, 1977; Williams, 1978; Wilson & Kenning, 1979; Goald, 1980; Wilson & Harbaugh, 1981; Hudgins, 1983; Merli *et al.*, 1984; Ebeling *et al.*, 1986; Sachde, 1986; Williams, 1986; Abernathey & Yasargil, 1990; Caspar, 1990; Williams, 1990; Young, 1990).

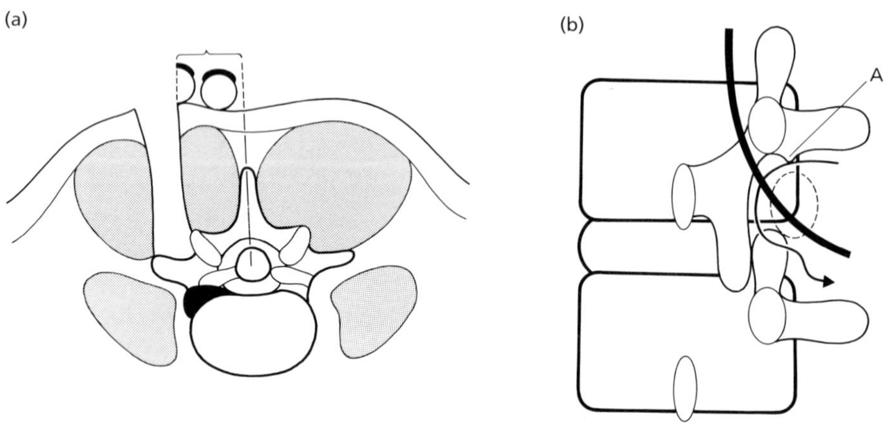

Fig. 39.10 Diagrammatic axial (a) and AP (b) views showing the paraspinal muscle splitting approach to the intertransverse 'window'.

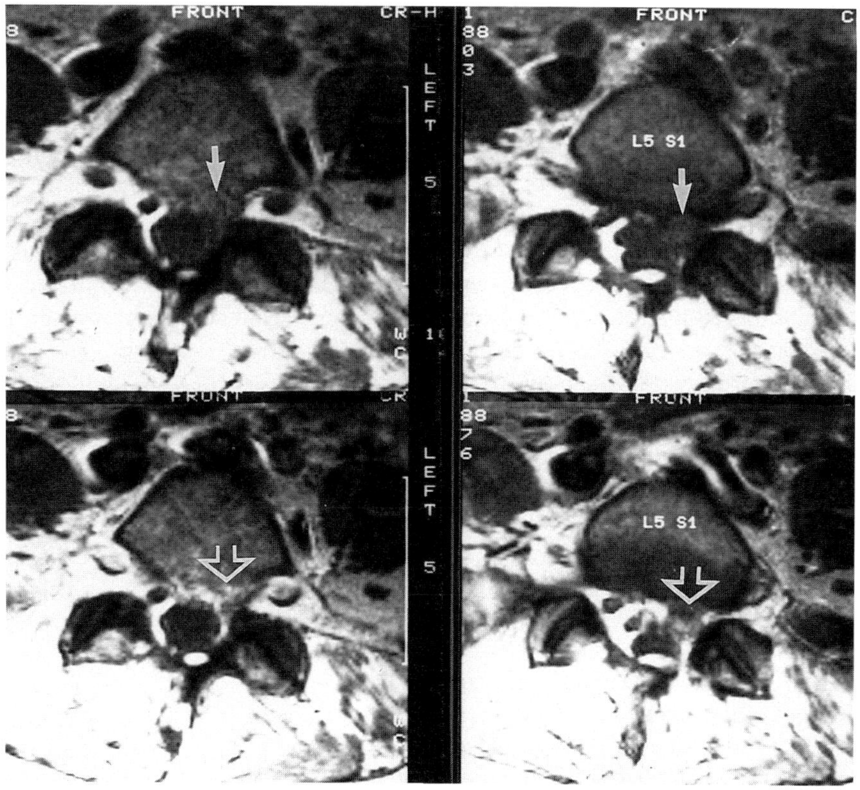

Fig. 39.11 Recurrent disc protrusion. Unenhanced MRI (*top*) and MRI with gadolinium enhancement (*bottom*). The lower right frame shows the typical appearance of the non-enhancing fragment surrounded by enhancing scar. The lower left frame shows enhancing scar and no recurrent HHP.

Closed surgery

The usage of differing percutaneous techniques in the treatment of lumbar disc herniation is discussed in Chapter 40.

Chymopapain

Smith (1964) was the first to report the clinical use of chymopapain in the treatment of lumbar disc herniations. Since that time it has followed a chequered course to clinical acceptance and its use throughout the world is quite variable. In America its use was somewhat limited because of a double-blind study published in 1976 by Schwetschenau *et al.* questioning the efficacy of chymopapain and a subsequent study by Agre *et al.* (1984), that described rather devastating complications with the use of chymopapain in the United States. Subsequent double-blind studies by Javid *et al.* (1983) and Fraser (1982), plus continuing clinical experience since Agre's published results, do support the use of chymopapain for the treatment of well-selected patients with lumbar disc ruptures.

Chymopapain is an extract of latex of the tropical fruit, papaya. Chymopapain is the most specific of the proteolytic enzymes in papaya and is a foreign protein capable of causing allergic reactions in humans. After injection into the disc space it is a classic enzyme in that it is immediately spent and little residual chymopapain can be found immediately after injection.

The cartilage connective tissue of nucleus pulposus contains cartilage cells, collagen, and proteoglycan/water complexes. It is the proteoglycan/water complexes that are broken down by the chymopapain enzyme, deflating the distended disc rupture. This relieves the hydrostatic pressure within the disc protrusion that is causing root compression, which is turn relieves sciatic discomfort. Since chymopapain is injected directly into the centre of the disc space cavity it will affect only discal tissue that is within reach and is histologically sensitive. Thus, the collagenous masses of extruded and sequestered disc fail to respond to chymopapain injection. The key to the use of chymopapain is to exclude those patients with extruded and sequestered discs.

Except for subarachnoid injection, chymopapain

enjoys a wide margin for safety between the effective therapeutic dose and the toxic dose. Because chymopapain has no effect on structures such as bone, ligaments, muscle, nerve and epidural tissue, it is very safe and has virtually no complications when properly injected. Rydevik *et al.* (1976) reported adverse effects on nerve tissue in rabbit tibial nerves, but this has not been borne out with clinical work.

Chymopapain is very dangerous when injected into the subarachnoid space. It dissolves the membrane of the pia arachnoid vessels, resulting in subarachnoid haemorrhage. This haemorrhage can cause a local phenomenon, such as arachnoiditis and cauda equina syndrome, or it can spread to the entire cerebrospinal fluid (CSF) space and cause a serious subarachnoid haemorrhage (Bouillet, 1983).

In addition, there seems to be some sinister, albeit iatrogenic, delayed possibility of a hypersensitivity effect of chymopapain in a subarachnoid space that has caused a few cases of transverse myelitis in humans. In over 7000 cases the author has had one subarachnoid haemorrhage that resolved in a few days with no permanent sequelae.

There is only one indication for the use of chymopapain, and that is in the patient with a protruded disc rupture. It is of no use in those patients who have extruded or sequestered fragments, and is of no use in patients with significant disc space narrowing, osteophyte formation and/or spinal canal stenosis.

Chymopapain is contraindicated in patients who are sensitive to chymopapain, in patients with disc herniations at cord levels, in patients with neurological lesions of unknown aetiology, in pregnant women and in patients with non-organic spinal pain.

Prior to chymopapain injection it is recommended that patients undergo a skin test to decide if the potential for an anaphylactic reaction exists. In untested patients anaphylaxis occurs in approximately one in 300 patients (Hall & McCulloch, 1983). Using the skin test, anaphylaxis has been eliminated as a complication in this author's practice.

It is essential that the patient have the procedure under local neuroleptic anaesthesia. An awake patient is better able to respond to errant needles trying to get into the disc space and is better able to report the immediate occurrence of complications, such as an allergic reaction.

The posterolateral approach to the disc space is mandatory. Under no circumstances should the needle introducing chymopapain into the disc space violate the subarachnoid space. Violation of the subarachnoid space is obviously avoided by using the posterolateral rather than the midline approach. In addition, a non-stiletted needle should be advanced into the disc space so that puncture of the CSF space will be immediately met with a backflow of CSF through the open lumen of the needle. Once within the disc space it is essential to take check X-rays to verify needle tip position. The dose of chymopapain to be injected is 1 ml or less.

There is an increased amount of pain following chemonucleolysis compared to the patient who has undergone microdiscectomy. However, this increased discomfort usually settles within a few days to a few weeks, and there is ultimately no difference in the recovery rate or the postoperative regime for a patient who has chemonucleolysis compared to microsurgery.

REFERENCES

Abdullah, A.F., Ditto, E.W., Byrd, E.B. & Williams, S.R. (1974) Extreme lateral lumbar disc herniations: clinical syndrome and special problems of diagnosis. *J. Neurosurg.*, **41**, 229–234.

Abdullah, A.F., Wolber, P.G.H., Warfield, J.R. & Gunadi, I.K. (1988) Surgical management of extreme lateral lumbar disc herniations: review of 138 cases. *Neurosurgery*, **22**, 648–653.

Abernathey, C.D. & Yasargil, M.G. (1990) Results of microsurgery. In Williams, R.W., McCulloch, J.A. & Young, P.H. (eds), *Microsurgery of the Lumbar Spine*, pp. 223–226. Aspen, Rockville.

Agre, K., Wilson, R.R., Brim, M. & McDermott, D. (1984) Chymodiactin postmarketing surveillance. *Spine*, **9**, 479–485.

Bouillet, R. (1983) Complications of discal hernia therapy. Comparative study regarding surgical therapy and nucleolysis by chymopapain. *Acta Orthop. Belg.* (Suppl. 1), **49**, 48.

Bowden, S., Davis, D., Dina, T., Patronas, N. & Wiesel, S. (1989) The incidence of abnormal lumbar spine MRI scans in asymptomatic patients. Presented at International Society for the Study of the Lumbar Spine. Kyoto, Japan, May.

Capana, A.H., Williams, R.W., Austin, D.C., Darmody, W.R. & Thomas, M.L. (1981) Lumbar discectomy. Percentage of disc removal and detection of anterior annulus perforation. *Spine*, **6**, 610–614.

Caspar, W. (1977) A new surgical procedure for lumbar disc herniation causing less tissue damage through microsurgical approach. *Adv. Neurosurg.*, **4**, 74–79.

Caspar, W. (1990) Results of microsurgery. In Williams, R.W., McCulloch, J.A. & Young P.H. (eds), *Microsurgery of the Lumbar Spine*, pp. 227–231. Aspen, Rockville.

Dauch, W.A. (1986) Infection of the intervertebral space following conventional and microsurgical operation on the herniated lumbar intervertebral disc. *Acta Neurochir. (Wien)*, **82**, 43–49.

Ebeling, U., Reichenberg, W. & Reulen, H.J. (1986) Results of microsurgical lumbar discectomy. *Acta Neurochir. (Wien)* **81**, 45–52.

Feldman, R. & McCulloch, J.A. (1990) Microsurgery for lumbar disc disease. In McCulloch, J.A. (ed.) *Principles of Microsurgery for Lumbar Disc Disease*. Raven Press, 1990.

Fraser, R.D. (1982) Chymopapain for the treatment of intervertebral disc herniation. *Spine*, **7**, 608.

Goald, H.J. (1980) Microlumbar discectomy: follow-up of 477 patients. *J. Microsurg.*, **2**, 85–10.

Goald, H.J. (1986) A new microsurgical reoperation for failed lumbar disc surgery. *J. Microsurg.*, **7**, 63–66.

Hakelius, A. (1970) Prognosis in sciatica: a clinical follow-up of surgical and non-surgical treatment. *Acta Orthop. Scand.*, **129** (Suppl.), 1–76.

Hall, B.B. & McCulloch, J.A. (1983) Anaphylactic reactions following the intradiscal injection of chymopapain under local anesthesia. *J. Bone Jt. Surg.*, **65A**, 1215.

Helms, C.A., Dorwart, R.H. & Gray, M. (1982) The CT appearance of conjoined nerve roots and differentiation from a herniated nucleus pulposus. *Radiology*, **144**, 803–807.

Hitselberger, W. & Witten, R. (1968) Abnormal myelograms in asymptomatic patients. *J. Neurosurg.*, **28**, 204–208.

Hudgins, W.R. (1983) The role of microdiscectomy. *Orthop. Clin. N. Am.*, **14**, 589–603.

Javid, M.J., Nordby, E.J., Ford, L.T., Hejna, W.J., Whisler, W.W., Burton, C., Millett, K., Wiltse, L.L., Widell, E.H., Boyd, R.J., Newton, S. & Thisted, R. (1983) Safety and efficacy of chymopapain (chymodiactin) in herniated nucleus pulposus with sciatica. *J. Am. Med. Assoc.*, **249**, 2489.

Kahanovich, N., Viola, K. & McCulloch, J.A. (1989) Limited surgical discectomy and microdiscectomy: a clinical comparison. *Spine*, **14**, 79–81.

Kostuik, J.P., Harrington, I., Alexander, D., Rand, W. & Evans, D. (1986) Cauda equina syndrome and lumbar disc herniation. *J. Bone Jt. Surg.*, **68A**, 386–391.

LaRocca, A. & MacNab, L. (1974) The laminectomy membrane. *J. Bone Jt. Surg.*, **56B**, 545–550.

Loew, F. (1986) Different operative possibilities for treatment of lumbar disc herniations. *Neurosurg. Rev.*, **9**, 109–111.

McCulloch, J.A. (1977) Chemonucleolysis. *J. Bone Jt. Surg.*, **59B**, 45–52.

Macnab, I. (1971) Negative disc exploration. *J. Bone Jt. Surg.*, **53A**, 891–903.

Macnab, I., Cuthbert, H. & Godfrey, C. (1977) The incidence of denervation of the sacro-spinales muscles following spinal surgery. *Spine*, **2**, 294–298.

Martin-Ferrer, S. (1989) Failure of autologous fat grafts to prevent postoperative epidural fibrosis in surgery of the lumbar spine. *Neurosurgery*, **24**, 718–721.

Mayer, P.J. & Jacobsen, F.S. (1989) Cauda equina syndrome after surgical treatment of lumbar spinal stenosis with application of free autogenous fat graft. *J. Bone Jt. Surg.*, **71A**, 1090–1093.

Mayfield, F.H. (1980) Autogenous fat transplants for the protection and repair of the spinal dura. *Clin. Neurosurg.*, **27**, 349–361.

Merli, C.A., Angiari, P. & Tonell, C. (1984) Three years experience with microsurgical technique in treatment of the protruded lumbar disc. *J. Neurosurg.*, **28**, 25–31.

Neidre, A. & MacNab, I. (1983) Anomalies of the lumbosacral nerve roots. Review of 16 cases and classification. *Spine*, **8**, 294–299.

O'Laoire, S.A., Crockard, H.A. & Thomas, D.G. (1981) Prognosis for sphincter recovery after operation for cauda equina compression owing to lumbar disc prolapse. *Br. Med. J.*, **282**, 1852–1854.

Peacock, E.E. (1967) Dynamic aspects of collagen biology, Part 1, Synthesis and assembly. *J. Surg. Res.*, **7**, 433–445.

Postacchini, F. & Montanaro, A. (1979) Extreme lateral herniations of lumbar discs. *Clin. Orthop.*, **138**, 222–227.

Postacchini, F., Urso, S. & Ferro, L. (1982) Lumbosacral root anomalies. *J. Bone Jt. Surg.*, **64A**, 721–729.

Prusick, V.R., Lint, D.S. & Bruder, W.J. (1988) Cauda equina syndrome as a complication of free epidural fat grafting. A report of two cases and a review of the literature. *J. Bone Jt. Surg.*, **70A**, 1256–1258.

Rydevik, B., Branemark, P., Nordborg, C., McLean, W.G., Sjostrand, J. & Fogelberg, M. (1976) Effects of chymopapain on nerve tissue. *Spine*, **1**, 137–148.

Sachde, V.P. (1986) Microsurgical lumbar discectomy: a personal series of 300 patients with at least 1 year follow-up. *J. Microsurg.*, **7**, 55–62.

Schwetschenau, P.R., Ramirez, A., Johnston, J., Wiggs, C. & Martins, A.N. (1976) Double-blind evaluations of intradiscal chymopapain for herniated lumbar discs. Early results. *J. Neurosurg.*, **45**, 622.

Scoville, W.B. & Corkilig, G. (1973) Lumbar disc surgery: Technique of radical removal and early mobilization. *J. Neurosurg.*, **39**, 265–269.

Smith, L. (1964) Enzyme dissolution of nucleus pulposus in humans. *J. Am. Med. Assoc.*, **187**, 137.

Spengler, D.M. (1982) Lumbar discectomy: Results with limited disc excision and selective foraminotomy. *Spine*, **7**, 604–607.

Van Akkerveeken, P., Van de Kraan, W. & Muller, J.W.T. (1986) The fate of the free fat graft. *Spine*, **11**, 501–504.

Waddell, G., McCulloch, J.A., Kummel, E.G. & Venner, R.M. (1980) Non-organic physical signs in low back pain. *Spine*, **5**, 117–125.

Weber, H. (1983) Lumbar disc herniation: a controlled prospective study with 10 years of observation. *Spine*, **8**, 131–140.

Wiesel, S.W., Tsourmas, N., Feffer, H.L., Citrin, C.M. & Patronas, N. (1984) A study of computed assisted tomography: Part I: The incidence of positive CAT scans in an asymptomatic group of patients. *Spine*, **9**, 549–551.

Williams, R. (1978) Microlumbar discectomy. A conservative surgical approach to the virgin herniated lumbar disc. *Spine*, **3**, 175–182.

Williams, R.W. (1986) Microlumbar discectomy: a 12-year

statistical review. *Spine*, **11**, 851–852.

Williams, R.W. (1990) Results of microsurgery. In Williams, R.W., McCulloch, J.A. & Young, P.H. (eds), *Microsurgery of the Lumbar Spine*, pp. 211–214. Aspen, Rockville, MD.

Wilson, D. & Harbaugh, R. (1981) Microsurgical and standard removal of protruded lumbar disc. A comparative study. *Neurosurgery*, **8**, 422–427.

Wilson, D.H. & Kenning, J. (1979) Microsurgical lumbar discectomy: Preliminary report of 83 consecutive cases. *Neurosurgery*, **4**, 137–140.

Wiltse, L.L., Bateman, J.G., Hutchinson, R.H. & Nelson, W.E. (1968) The paraspinal sacrospinalis-splitting approach to the lumbar spine. *J. Bone Jt. Surg.*, **50A**, 919–926.

Yasargil, M.G. (1977) Microsurgical operations for herniated lumbar disc. *Adv. Neurosurg.*, **4**, 81–82.

Young, P.H. (1990) Results of microsurgery. In Williams, R.W., McCulloch, J.A. & Young, P.H. (eds), *Microsurgery of the Lumbar Spine*, pp. 215–222. Aspen, Rockville, MD.

Zindrick, M.R., Wiltse, L.L. & Rauschning, W. (1987) Disc herniations lateral to the intervertebral foramen. In White, A.H., Rothman, R.H. & Ray, C.D. (eds), *Lumbar Spine Surgery*, pp. 195–207. C.V. Mosby, St Louis, MI.

40 · Percutaneous Disc Surgery

By H.M. MAYER and M. BROCK

The surgical treatment of herniated lumbar discs began in the first half of the twentieth century. The 'classic' work of Mixter & Barr in 1934 is widely recognized as the very beginning of disc surgery. However, Adson & Ott (1922), Stokey (1928) and Dandy (1929) had described the surgical removal of 'chondromas' or 'cartilaginous tumors' from the spinal canal which probably were unrecognized discal herniations. The access to the spinal canal was usually through a laminectomy at one or several levels.

Since then, due to the enormous sociomedical implications, the significance of surgical disc treatment has increased tremendously, mainly in industrialized countries (Waddell *et al.*, 1984; Waddell & Main, 1984; Quebec Task Force Study Group, 1987; Wickstroem & Haenninen, 1987). Improvement in imaging techniques has refined the diagnosis of lumbar disc herniation (Chafetz *et al.*, 1983; Bell *et al.*, 1984; Bosacco *et al.*, 1984; Grubb *et al.*, 1987; Sachs *et al.*, 1987; Schneiderman *et al.*, 1987). These techniques provide detailed information concerning the localization, extent and morphology of the protruded, extruded or sequestrated disc.

Surgical methods have become less traumatic and sophisticated, and have led to the standardized procedure of lumbar microdiscectomy (Yasargil, 1977; Williams, 1978; Gilsbach *et al.*, 1979; Wilson & Kenning, 1979; Goald, 1981; Seeger, 1982; Wilson & Harbaugh, 1982; Caspar, 1986). Microdiscectomy has improved the postoperative results and decreased the complication rates. However, the incidence of recurrent disc herniation did not decrease significantly (Oldenkott, 1979; Wilson & Harbaugh, 1982; Ebeling & Reulen, 1988).

The surgical procedures for lumbar disc removal have, in common, that the disc herniation is approached through a paramedian, interlaminar route, which implies dissection of paraspinal muscles, flavectomy sometimes with removal of bone and entry into the spinal canal. Surgical trauma to these structures, as well as epidural scarring and reherniation of the nucleus pulposus through the (created) perforation in the posterolateral annulus fibrosus, are important factors in the genesis of the postoperative 'failed back syndrome' (Williams, 1978; Burton, 1981; Wilkinson, 1983; Cauthen, 1985).

THE HISTORY OF PERCUTANEOUS DISC SURGERY

The search for alternative approaches to the lumbar intervertebral space is nearly as old as the conventional surgical procedures themselves.

In 1935 Robertson & Ball described a posterolateral approach to the spine which allowed percutaneous biopsies of uncertain pathological processes. This technique was further refined in the 1950s and since has been optimized by the introduction of computerized tomography (CT)-guided biopsy (Ottolenghi, 1955; Craig, 1956; El-Khoury *et al.*, 1983; Cserhati, 1986).

Erlacher (1952) introduced lumbar discography through a posterolateral approach, and this technique soon found acceptance in the radiological diagnosis of disc disease (Collis & Gardner, 1962; Day, 1969; McCulloch & Waddell, 1978).

In 1964 Lyman Smith described a method of enzymatic dissolution of nucleus pulposus. The procedure was soon introduced into clinical usage under the term 'chemonucleolysis'. The enzyme (chymopapain) was injected into the disc space through a cannula introduced via a posterolateral access (McCulloch & McNab, 1983). In fact, chemonucleolysis was the first therapeutic procedure for disc herniations through a posterolateral approach. The ups and downs of this method are well documented in the literature; however, despite the more or less qualified criticism, the success rates in long-term follow-ups have mostly been in an acceptable range of between 70% and 80% (Nordby, 1986; Sutton, 1986).

In 1975, Hijikata was the first to describe the method of 'percutaneous nucleotomy'. Due to the fact that chymopapain was not licensed in Japan, the author was looking for an alternative procedure (S. Hijikata, 1988, personal communication). Through a small cannula with an outer diameter of 2.6 mm introduced into the disc space through a posterolateral approach, parts of the nucleus pulposus could be removed with modified pituitary forceps. A similar method had been performed before by Hoppenfield in 1974, but had not been published at that time (Hoppenfield, 1989). In 1980, Kambin introduced percutaneous removal of the nucleus pulposus and published his first results in 1983 (Kambin & Gellman, 1983). Using modified Craig instruments, and introducing flexible forceps into the disc space, he was able to remove nucleus pulposus even from the posterior half of the disc space. The procedure was called 'percutaneous lateral discectomy'. At the same time, Suezawa developed a bilateral approach to the lumbar disc space and introduced endoscopic ('discoscopic') control of the procedure (Suezawa & Ruettimann, 1983). This method (also called 'percutaneous nucleotomy') was further improved and refined in following years (Suezawa & Jacob, 1986; Schreiber *et al.*, 1988; Leu, 1990). Attempts to reach the disc space through a far lateral, percutaneous access, as described by Friedman in 1983, failed due to severe complications.

In 1985 Onik *et al.* described the method of automated percutaneous lumbar discectomy (APLD). With this technique, the nucleus is removed by a Nucleotome® (Surgical Dynamics, USA), which is a small instrument similar to arthroscopic shaver systems operating with a suction, guillotine mechanism. Shepperd was the first to describe a percutaneous lumbar interbody fusion technique (Shepperd, 1986). In an attempt to further improve the removal of nucleus pulposus from the 'critical parts' of the disc space (namely in the dorsal third), percutaneous endoscopic laser discectomy is the most current innovation (Mayer *et al.*, 1991).

ANATOMICAL AND PATHOPHYSIOLOGICAL BACKGROUND

Lumbar disc herniations can be divided into 'contained' and 'non-contained' lesions. 'Contained' means a disc protrusion with an intact annulus fibrosus. However, the term 'non-contained' disc can include a variety of different morphological aspects. The disc can be prolapsed into the subligamentous space (annulus fibrosus ruptured, longitudinal ligament intact) or into the epidural space (annulus fibrosus ruptured, longitudinal ligament ruptured). In addition each form of 'non-contained' disc can have fragments migrating behind the cranial or caudal posterior surface of the adjacent vertebrae. Migration of large, perforated parts of nucleus pulposus can happen even without sequestration. In rare cases the herniation can also perforate the thecal sac. The location of a disc herniation can be in the midline, paramedian (between the midline and the medial border of the pedicle), intraforaminal (within the boundaries of the foramen) or extraforaminal (lateral to the outer border of the pedicle).

The morphology of lumbar disc herniations, as well as their location, are the parameters which determine the choice of the surgical technique. Due to technical reasons, percutaneous discectomy should be performed only in 'contained' discs (protrusion) or in small 'non-contained' (subligamentous) prolapse. 'Small' means that the herniated parts of the nucleus pulposus should be within the level of the disc space and should extend not more than one-third into the sagittal diameter of the spinal canal (Table 40.1).

Table 40.1 Indications for percutaneous endoscopic discectomy

Clinical findings	Morphology
Discogenic radicular symptoms Sciatica Sensory deficits Paresis (IV°—III°) Reflex—difference	Protrusion Subligamentous prolapse at the level of the disc space <⅓ of sagittal diameter of spinal canal
Conservative therapy unsuccessful	L1–S1

The aim of percutaneous discectomy is to decompress a compressed lumbar spinal nerve. This can be achieved by a selective removal of the protruded parts of the nucleus pulposus. The fact that the disc herniation is approached from within the intervertebral space implies several technical challenges. Since the disc space is reached at an angle of 50–60° to the sagittal plane, the working range of straight, rigid instruments can cover only a limited area, including the centre of the disc. Nucleus pulposus can be removed from this part of the intervertebral space, thus achieving an 'intradiscal decompression'. However, to achieve the selective removal of nucleus pulposus from the area where it leads to the compression of the nerve root implies the use of reverse opening, or flexible and adjustable, forceps. In addition, loose parts of the nucleus pulposus can be sucked from the dorsal region and excised by a high-powered vacuum coupled to automated shavers and cutters.

'Open' and percutaneous surgical procedures differ in the approach, the method and the amount of nucleus removed. In conventional techniques, including lumbar microdiscectomy, the disc space is reached through a paramedian, interlaminar access. This technique includes the dissection of paraspinal muscles, resection of the yellow ligament and sometimes extension of the approach by a more or less extensive laminotomy. The nerve root is exposed in the epidural space and must be separated from epidural fat and the venous plexus. These vulnerable and often congested venous plexuses tend to bleed and require bipolar coagulation or the application of gel foam pads. The nerve root has to be mobilized and the annulus fibrosus must be incised in cases of contained herniations. The nucleus pulposus is removed from the intervertebral space with rigid and angled forceps. It is customary to remove as much nucleus pulposus material as possible, to prevent reherniation through the perforation in the annulus fibrosus.

In percutaneous techniques the intervertebral space is approached through a posterolateral access bypassing the spinal canal. Trauma to paraspinous muscles is negligible and there is no need to resect ligamentous structures. The compromised spinal nerve root is not altered and the annulus fibrosus is perforated in the lateral, extraforaminal region. The removal of nucleus pulposus is limited for the following technical reasons: the working cannula allows a degree of freedom of 10° in each direction. The disc space is reached at an angle of between 50° and 60° to the sagittal plane. Even with specialized instrumentation the subligamentous area cannot always be reached within the working range of the instruments. Nucleus pulposus dislocated behind the cranial or caudal vertebral body cannot be reached. On the other hand, the radical removal of nucleus pulposus is not necessary. Herniation of remaining parts of the nucleus through the posterolateral perforation in the annulus is on the one hand part of the 'self-sealing-behaviour' of the disc (Markolf & Morris, 1974), and on the other hand part of the decompressive effect of percutaneous discectomy.

INDICATIONS FOR PERCUTANEOUS DISCECTOMY

Patient selection for percutaneous endoscopic discectomy is performed according to clinical and morphological criteria. It is the method of choice for patients with minor to moderate radicular symptoms due to a 'contained' or small 'non-contained' lumbar disc herniation (Table 40.1). Clinical symptoms should include sciatica with dermatomal distribution, as well as sensory deficits like dysaesthesias or hypoaesthesia and reflex differences. Patients with motor deficits worse than grade III (Seddon, 1972) are excluded from the procedure, as are patients with cauda equina syndrome and/or rapidly progressive neurological deficits. Since decompression of the nerve root cannot be visually controlled during the operation, the postoperative judgement of success or failure exclusively relies on clinical assessment. Thus there might be a significant postoperative time-loss in patients with severe neurological symptoms in a case of failure of percutaneous endoscopic discectomy.

Since percutaneous endoscopic discectomy is a surgical procedure, adequate conservative therapy (at least three months on an outpatient basis or two weeks in the hospital) must have been unsuccessful.

Percutaneous endoscopic discectomy is contraindicated in all patients with severe and rapidly progressive neurological deficits, as well as in patients with sequestrated or large 'non-contained' disc herniations. There is still controversy as to whether patients with the association of a 'contained' disc herniation with spinal stenosis or a narrow lateral recess should be included in the indications for percutaneous discectomy (Schreiber *et al.*, 1989).

The indication for percutaneous endoscopic disc-

Table 40.2 Imaging techniques for the diagnosis of lumbar disc herniation

Spinal CT scan
Magnetic resonance imaging
Discography
Disco–CT
Myelography
Myelo–CT

ectomy depends on the *in vivo* imaging of disc morphology. Table 40.2 shows the imaging techniques currently used in the diagnosis of lumbar disc herniations. The role of discography and postdiscographic CT scan is paramount in preoperative diagnosis. These methods have the highest reliability in proving or disclosing perforation of the annulus fibrosus and/or posterior longitudinal ligament in lumbar disc herniations (see Fig. 40.3b).

THE TECHNIQUE OF PERCUTANEOUS ENDOSCOPIC DISCECTOMY (Mayer & Brock, 1989a; Schreiber *et al.*, 1989)

The posterolateral approach to the disc space is used in all percutaneous techniques (Nazarian, 1985; McCulloch, 1989). The operation is performed under sterile conditions in an operating theatre. General anaesthesia is contra-indicated, to avoid nerve root injury, and because the patients have to cooperate with the surgeon during the procedure. However, an anaesthesiologist should always be available to monitor vital parameters and, if necessary, to provide the patients with analgesics or sedative medication. The patient is placed in a prone, comfortable position on a radiolucent operating table. The level of the lumbar disc to be treated is marked on the skin under fluoroscopic control. The instruments are introduced at 9–11 cm from the midline in the level of the disc. Local anaesthesia with lidocaine 1% is applied to the skin and subcutaneous tissue with a 21G cannula. An 18G cannula is advanced under fluoroscopic guidance into the lumbar intervertebral space. The tip of the cannula is placed into the geometric centre of the disc (Fig. 40.1). If the anatomical conditions allow a more lateral advancement of the instruments, they can be placed in the dorsal part of the disc space. This facilitates the removal of nucleus pulposus from the herniated region of the intervertebral disc (Fig. 40.2). Discography is then performed with a water-soluble contrast agent as it is essential during percutaneous discectomy to have a clear picture of the morphology of the herniated lumbar disc (Fig. 40.3). There should be no leakage of contrast medium into the epidural space, since such a finding cannot preclude a sequestered fragment. The contrast medium should accumulate in the posterior annulus fibrosus and should prove the disc herniation. However, a small leakage beneath the posterior longitudinal ligament is not necessarily a sign of sequestration and does not exclude percutaneous discectomy.

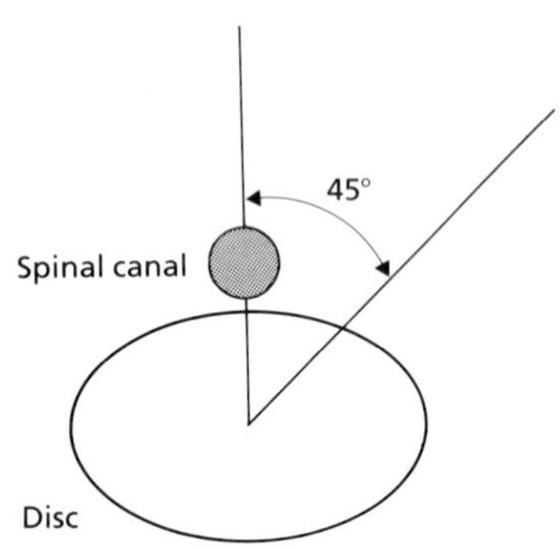

Fig. 40.1 Approach to the centre of the disc. Angle to sagittal plane 45°.

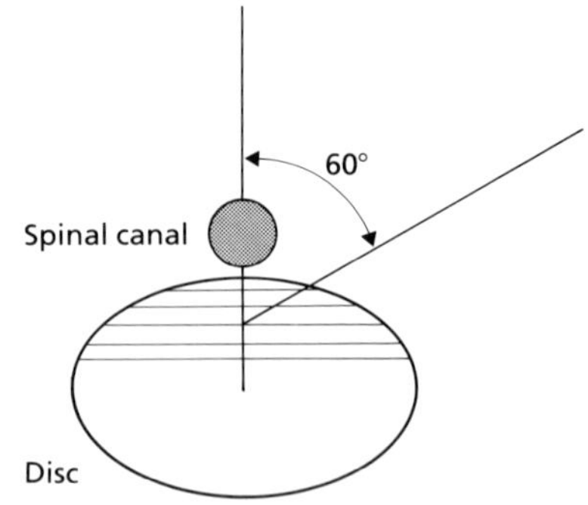

Fig. 40.2 Approach to the dorsal area of the disc space at an angle of 60° to the sagittal plane.

Following discography, a guidewire is introduced and the cannula is removed. A skin incision of 5–6 mm is performed at the entry point of the wire and a blunt trocar with an outer diameter of 4.5 mm is advanced to the posterolateral border of the disc space using the wire as a guide. The trocar itself serves as a guide for the working cannula (OD 5.5 mm). The latter is placed tightly on the outer annulus fibrosus and fixed with one hand. The trocar is then removed and the annulus fibrosus is perforated consecutively with small (OD 3 mm) and large (OD 4.5 mm) an-

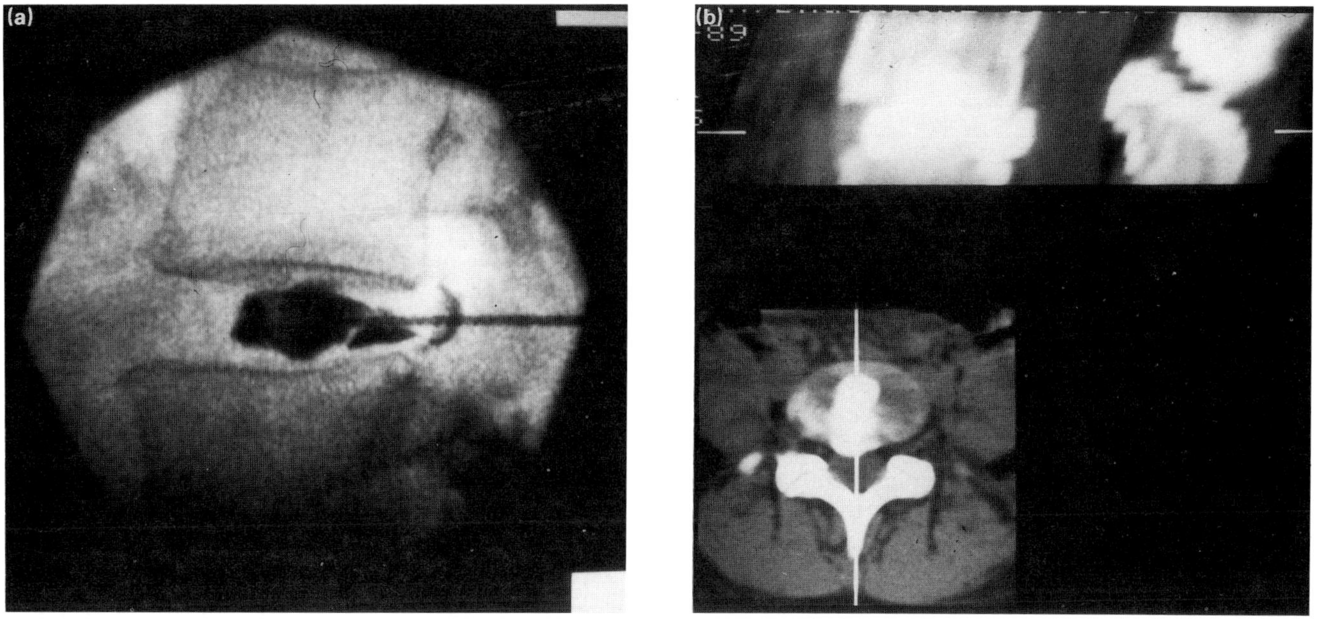

Fig. 40.3 (a) Discography at L4–L5 showing a disc protrusion with accumulation of contrast medium in the outer part of the annulus fibrosus. (b) Postdiscographic CT scan with sagittal reconstruction demonstrating no leakage of contrast medium.

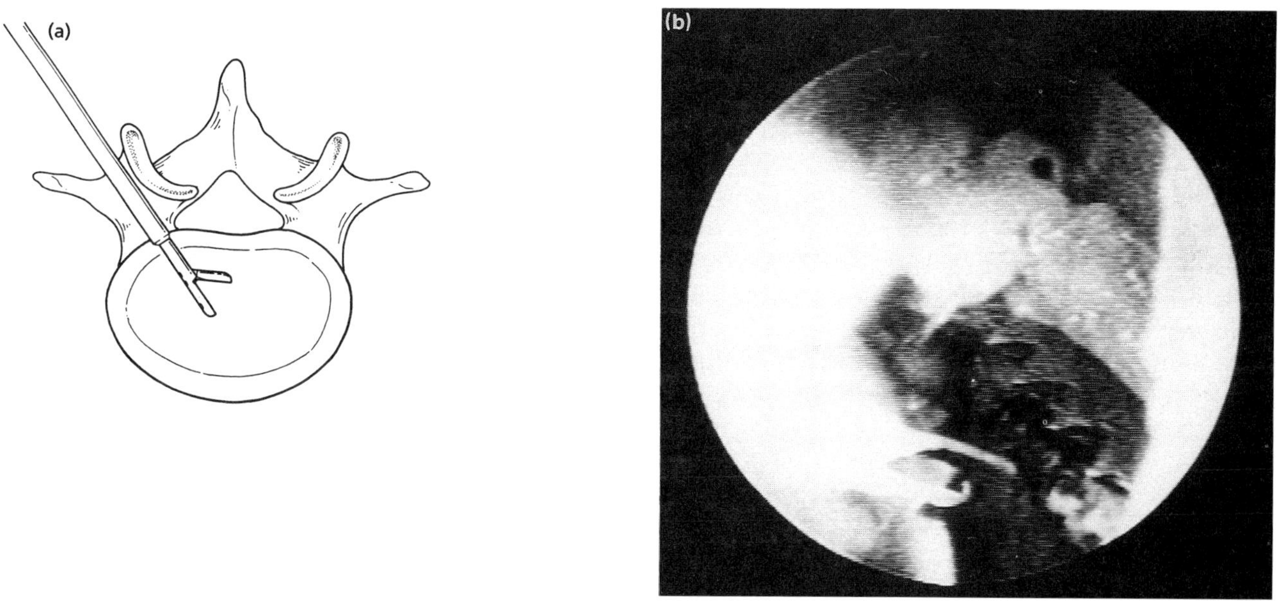

Fig. 40.4 (a) Straight forceps introduced into the intervertebral space. (b) Endoscopic control of nucleus pulposus removal from the contralateral side.

nulus trephines. Thus, access to the intervertebral space is completed. The trephines and the guidewire are removed and the working cannula is advanced 2–3 mm into the outer annulus fibrosus to stabilize its position.

Nucleus pulposus is then removed from the centre of the disc using straight and rigid forceps (Fig. 40.4a). In cases of large midline disc herniations we routinely use a second approach from the contralateral side. This has the advantage of allowing permanent endoscopic control (with a 3.5 mm angled endoscope—30° or 70°) of the disc removal (Fig. 40.4b). In the case of a unilateral approach, intermittent video-endoscopic control provides information on the removal process, as well as on the remaining amounts of nucleus pulposus. In addition, it gives information on further loose nuclear fragments within the disc space which can be moved by provocation tests, such as the Valsalva manoeuvre of pressing and coughing. Since the patient has to perform these tests it is mandatory to be able to keep verbal contact with him or her.

Removal of nucleus from the centre of the disc should be limited, since it serves only to create an access for larger or flexible instruments which reach the posterior third of the disc space. On the other hand it is necessary to remove a certain amount of nucleus to introduce the endoscope.

The surgical goal of percutaneous discectomy, namely to decompress the nerve root from the disc herniation, is achieved with other instruments:

Cutter systems

Automated cutters which have been modified from arthroscopic surgery are used to remove the nucleus pulposus from the dorsal part of the disc space (Mayer & Brock, 1989b; Schreiber & Leu, 1989). The cutters have a side opening and are coupled to a high-powered surgical suction device. The system was adopted from plastic surgery where it was used for lipectomy of abdominal fat tissue. It is able to apply a 99% vacuum to the disc space, and thus to remove nucleus pulposus from areas remote from the centre of the disc.

Reverse-opening forceps

These forceps reach the posterior aspect of the intervertebral space from the lateral border of the pedicle to the midline (Fig. 40.5a). They can also be used to remove intraforaminal herniations (Fig. 40.5b). When introduced through a bilateral approach, the total dorsal circumference of the disc can be covered by the working range of this instrument (Fig. 40.5c).

Flexible forceps

To remove small particles of nucleus pulposus at the end of the discectomy procedure, flexible forceps can be used. They can be directed to various angles by adjustable deflectors.

When no more nucleus pulposus material can be obtained with the described instruments, and when there is no evidence of remaining loose parts of nucleus in the provocation tests, the procedure is completed. The cannula is removed and the stab incision is closed with a single suture.

The patients are mobilized six hours following percutaneous discectomy and are allowed to leave the hospital between the second and third postoperative day.

CONCLUSION

The introduction of percutaneous discectomy into the surgical treatment of lumbar disc herniations is a further step to so-called 'minimal invasive surgery' of the spine. Thus, this technique should be regarded as

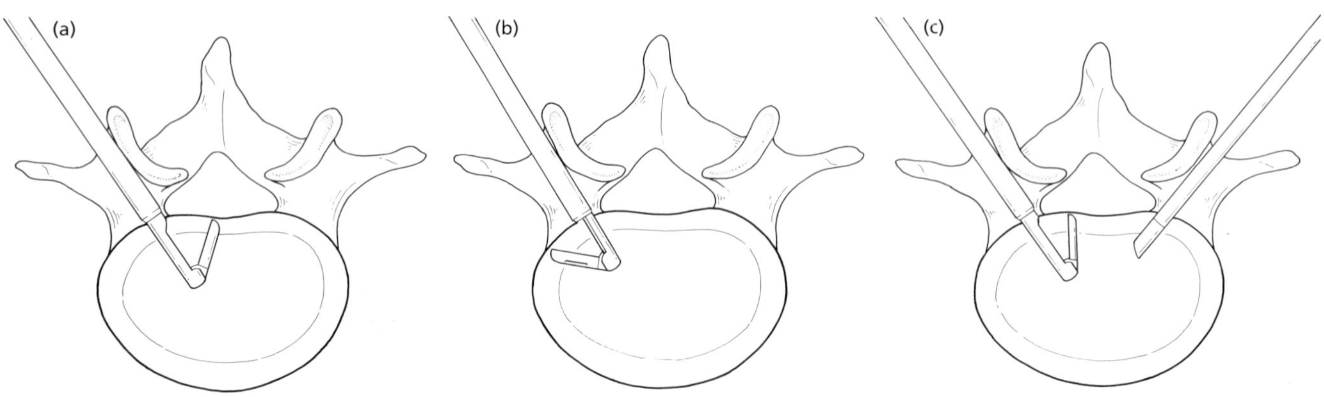

Fig. 40.5 (a) Reverse-opening forceps introduced into the intervertebral space. (b) Reverse-opening forceps for removal of intraforaminal parts of nucleus pulposus. (c) Endoscopic control of nucleus pulposus removal with reverse-opening forceps.

a starting point for further technical improvements. Currently there are two major innovations which are undergoing experimental development: percutaneous lumbar interbody fusion with bone grafts and percutaneous endoscopic laser discectomy.

Percutaneous interbody fusion was described in 1986 by Shepperd. Meanwhile the technique of percutaneous removal of the intervertebral disc and the introduction of bone graft from the iliac crest has been refined by Schreiber *et al.* (1989), Shepperd (1989), Shepperd *et al.* (1989) and by Leu (1990). This technique has been used in a preliminary clinical study in patients with spondylolisthesis (Leu, 1990). However, it seems to be essential that percutaneous interbody fusion is preceded by the percutaneous application of an external fixation system (*fixateur externe*) to achieve distraction, realignment and immobilization of the lumbar motion segment.

In 1989 percutaneous endoscopic laser discectomy was introduced into a first clinical trial (Mayer *et al.*, 1991). The use of laser light, which can be transmitted by flexible quartz fibres, improves the removal of the herniated parts of the nucleus pulposus. Different laser systems such as Nd:Yag, Er:Yag or Excimer lasers have been used under experimental and clinical conditions (Ascher, 1988; Leu, 1990; Mayer *et al.*, 1990, 1991). The main advantage of the use of lasers in addition or instead of mechanical instruments is the possibility of a permanent endoscopic control of the removal process, which is enabled by the small size of the light-transmitting quartz fibres (Mayer *et al.*, 1991). Moreover, the laser light can be applied in different modes so that shrinking and coagulation, as well as carbonization and vaporization of nucleus pulposus tissue, are possible.

Percutaneous endoscopic discectomy seems to be a reasonable surgical alternative for patients with 'contained' or slight 'non-contained' lumbar disc herniations. Provided that patients are selected according to the described selection criteria, the reported success rates range between 72% and 87.5% (Hijikata, 1989; Hoppenfield, 1989; Kambin & Schaffer, 1989; Schreiber *et al.*, 1989; Shepperd *et al.*, 1989; Stern, 1989; Mayer *et al.*, 1991). The results of percutaneous discectomy, however, are only preliminary, since there are only a few series with long-term follow-up. It should be emphasized that percutaneous endoscopic discectomy is a surgical procedure which should be performed only following adequate preoperative conservative therapy. The overall complication rate is less than 3% and thus comparable to other surgical procedures.

According to these criteria between 10% and 15% of patients for lumbar disc surgery are candidates for this method. Further technical improvements in endoscopy, laser systems, automated and manual instruments might explore new fields of indication for percutaneous disc surgery.

REFERENCES

Adson, A.W. & Ott, W.O. (1922) Results of the removal of tumors of the spinal cord. *Arch. Neurol. Psychiatry*, **8**, 520–538.

Ascher, W.P. (1988) Laser in der Neurochirurgie. In Walter, W. & Krenkel, W. (eds) *Jahrbuch der Neurochirurgie*, 101–119.

Bell, G. R., Rothman, R.H., Booth, R.E. & Cuckler, J.M. (1984) Comparison of metrizamide myelography and CT in the diagnosis of herniated lumbar disc and spinal stenosis. *Spine*, **9**, 552–556.

Bosacco, S.J., Berman, A.T., Garbarino, J.L. & Teplick, J.G. (1984) A comparison of CT-scanning and myelography in the diagnosis of lumbar disc herniation. *Clin. Orthop. Rel. Res.*, **190**, 124–128.

Burton, C.V., Kirkaldy-Willis, W.H., Yong-Hing, K. & Heithoff, K.B. (1981) Causes and failure of surgery on the lumbar spine. *Clin. Orthop. Rel. Res.*, **157**, 191–197.

Caspar, W. (1986) *Die mikrochirurgische OP-Technik des lumbalen Bandscheibenvorfalls. Empfehlungen zum Operationsablauf.* Aesculap AG, Tuttlingen.

Cauthen, J. (1985) How to avoid the failed back surgery syndrome. In Cauthen, J. (ed.) *Lumbar Spine Surgery*, pp. 204–215. Williams & Wilkins, Baltimore, MD.

Chafetz, N.I., Genant, H.K., Moon, K.L. & Helms, C.A. (1983) Recognition of lumbar disc herniation with NMR. *Am. J. Radiol.*, **141**, 1153–1156.

Collis, J.S. & Gardner, W.J. (1962) Lumbar discography; an analysis of one thousand cases. *J. Neurosurg.*, **19**, 452–461.

Craig, F.S. (1956) Vertebral body biopsy. *J. Bone Jt. Surg.*, **38A**, 93–102.

Cserhati, M.D. (1986) Die Wertigkeit der Stanz- und Punktionsbohrbiopsie in der Diagnostik der Spondylitis-Tbc. *Z. Orthop.*, **124**, 79–88.

Dandy, W.E. (1929) Loose cartilage from intervertebral disk simulating tumor of the spinal cord. *Arch. Surg.*, **19**, 660–672.

Day, P.L. (1969) Lateral approach for lumbar diskogram and chemonucleolysis. *Clin. Orthop. Rel. Res.*, **67**, 90–93.

Ebeling, U. & Reulen, H.J. (1988) Mikrochirurgische Technik bei lumbalen Bandscheibenoperationen: Ist sie der konventionellen Methode überlegen. In *Handbuch der Neurochirurgie 1988*, pp. 143–160. Regensberg & Biermann, Münster.

El-Khoury, G.Y., Terepka, R.H., Mickelson, M.R., Rainville,

K.L. & Zaleski, M.M.S. (1983) Fine-needle aspiration biopsy of bone. *J. Bone Jt. Surg.*, **65A**, 522–525.

Erlacher, P.R. (1952) Nucleography. *J. Bone Jt. Surg.*, **34B**, 204–210.

Friedman, W.A. (1983) Percutaneous discectomy: an alternative to chemonucleolysis? *Neurosurgery*, **13**, 542–547.

Gilsbach, J., Eggert, H.R. & Seeger, W. (1979) *Microsurgical Operation for Herniated Lumbar Disc*. Aesculap AG, Wiss. Informationen, Tuttlingen.

Goald, H.J. (1981) Microlumbar discectomy: follow-up of 477 patients. *J. Microsurg.*, **2**, 95–100.

Grubb, S.A., Libscomb, H.J. & Guilford, W.B. (1987) The relative value of lumbar roentgenograms, metrizamide myelography and discography in the assessment of patients with low back syndrome. *Spine*, **12**, 282–286.

Hijikata, S. (1989) Percutaneous nucleotomy—a new concept technique and 12 years' experience. *Clin. Orthop. Rel. Res.*, **238**, 9–23.

Hijikata, S., Yamagishi, M., Nakayama, T. & Oomori, K. (1975) Percutaneous nucleotomy: a new treatment method for lumbar disc herniation. *J. Toden Hosp.*, **5**, 39–46.

Hoppenfield, S. (1989) Percutaneous removal of herniated lumbar discs. *Clin. Orthop. Rel. Res.*, **238**, 92–97.

Kambin, P. & Gellman, H. (1983) Percutaneous lateral discectomy of the lumbar spine—a preliminary report. *Clin. Orthop. Rel. Res.*, **174**, 127–132.

Kambin, P. & Schaffer, J.L. (1989) Percutaneous lumbar discectomy—review of 100 patients and current practice. *Clin. Orthop. Rel. Res.*, **238**, 24–34.

Leu, H.J. (1990) Von der Perkutanen Nukleotomie mit Diskoskopie bis zur perkutanen Spondylodese: Ein neues Konzept zeichnet sich ab. *Z. Orthop.*, **128**, 266–275.

Love, J.G. & Walsh, M.N. (1938) Protruded intervertebral discs: report of 100 cases in which operation was performed. *J. Am. Med. Assoc.*, **111**, 396–400.

Markolf, K.L. & Morris, J.M. (1974) The structural components of the intervertebral disc. *J. Bone Jt. Surg.*, **56A**, 675–684.

Mayer, H.M. & Brock, M. (1989a) Percutaneous lumbar discectomy—the Berlin technique. In Mayer, H.M. & Brock, M. (eds) *Percutaneous Lumbar Discectomy*, pp. 107–117. Springer Verlag, Berlin.

Mayer, H.M. & Brock, M. (1989b) Discectomie percutanée avec systèmes Shaver. *Rev. Med. Orthop.*, **15**, 24–26.

Mayer, H.M., Brock, M., Sedlmaier, B., Berlien, H.P., Müller, G.J. & Dörschel, K. (1990) Ultrastructure of human nucleus pulposus following application of Erbium: Yag 2940 nm-laser. *Laser Med. Surg.*, **6**, 190–197.

Mayer, H.M., Brock, M., Berlien, H.P. & Müller, G. (1991) Preliminary experience with the Neodymium: YAG 1064 nm cw — laser for percutaneous endoscopic laser discectomy (PELD). *Neurochirurgia* (accepted for publication).

McCulloch, J.A. (1989) The posterolateral approach. In Mayer, H.M. & Brock, M. (eds) *Percutaneous Lumbar Discectomy*, pp. 16–30. Springer Verlag, Berlin.

McCulloch, J.A. & McNab, I. (1983) *Sciatica and Chymopapain*. Williams & Wilkins, Baltimore, MD.

McCulloch, J.A. & Waddell, G. (1978) Lateral lumbar discography. *Br. J. Radiol.*, **51**, 498–502.

Mixter, W.S. & Barr, I.S. (1934) Rupture of intervertebral disc with involvement of spinal canal. *N. Engl. J. Med.*, **211**, 210–215.

Nazarian, S. (1985) Anatomical basis of intervertebral disc puncture with chemonucleolysis. *Anat. Clin.*, **7**, 23–32.

Nordby, E.J. (1986) Eight- to 13-year follow-up evaluation of chemonucleolysis patients. *Clin. Orthop. Rel. Res.*, **206**, 18–23.

Oldenkott, P. (1979) Mikrochirurgische Behandlung lumbaler Wurzelkompressionssyndrome. *Med. Welt*, **30**, 1687–1691.

Onik, G., Helms, C.A., Ginsberg, L., Hoaglund, F.T. & Morris, J. (1985) Percutaneous lumbar diskectomy using a new aspiration probe. AJNR **6**, 290–293.

Ottolenghi, C.E. (1955) Diagnosis of orthopedic lesions by aspiration biopsy: results of 1061 punctures. *J. Bone Jt. Surg.*, **37A**, 443–464.

Quebec Task Force on Spinal Disorders (1987) Scientific approach to the assessment and management of activity-related spinal disorders. *Spine*, **12** (Suppl. 1).

Robertson, R.C. & Ball, R.P. (1935) Destructive spine lesions. Diagnosis by needle biopsy. *J. Bone Jt. Surg.*, **17**, 749–758.

Sachs, B.L., Vanharanta, H., Spivey, M.A. & Guyer, R.D. (1987) Dallas discogram description—a new classification of CT/discography in low-back disorders. *Spine*, **12**, 287–293.

Schneiderman, G., Flannigan, B., Kingston, S. & Thomas, J. (1987) Magnetic resonance imaging in the diagnosis of disc degeneration. *Spine*, **12**, 277–281.

Schreiber, A. & Leu, H.J. (1989) Réstabilisation intervertébrale et arthrodèse intersomatique percutanée: possibilités aujourd'hui. *RACHIS*, **1**, 173–179.

Schreiber, A., Suezawa, Y. & Leu, H.J. (1988) Therapie des Bandscheibenprolaps. *Dtsch. Med. Wochenschr.*, **113**, 1482–1485.

Schreiber, A., Suezawa, Y. & Leu, H.J. (1989) Does percutaneous nucleotomy with discoscopy replace conventional discectomy? *Clin. Orthop. Rel. Res.*, **238**, 35–42.

Seddon, H.J. (1972) *Surgical Disorders of the Peripheral Nerves*. Livingstone, Edinburgh.

Seeger, W. (1982) *Microsurgery of the Spinal Cord and Surrounding Structures*. Springer Verlag, Vienna.

Shepperd, J.A.N. (1986) Postero-lateral percutaneous surgery to the lumbar spine. A preliminary report. *Alt. Spinal Surg.*, **3**, 4.

Shepperd, J.A.N. (1989) The possibilities of percutaneous lumbar disc surgery. In Mayer, H.M. & Brock, M. (eds) *Percutaneous Lumbar Discectomy*, pp. 181–186. Springer Verlag, Belin.

Shepperd, J.A.N., James, S.E. & Leach, A.B. (1989) Percutaneous disc surgery. *Clin. Orthop. Rel. Res.*, **238**, 43–49.

Smith, L. (1964) Enzyme dissolution of nucleus pulposus in humans. *J. Am. Med. Assoc.*, **187**, 137–140.

Stern, M.B. (1989) Early experience with percutaneous lateral discectomy. *Clin. Orthop. Rel. Res.*, **238**, 50–55.

Stokey, B. (1928) Compression of spinal cord due to ventral extradural chondromas; diagnosis and surgical treatment. *Arch. Neurol. Psychiatry*, **20**, 275–291.

Suezawa, Y. & Jacob, H.A.C. (1986) Percutaneous nucleotomy—an alternative to spinal surgery. *Arch. Orthop. Trauma Surg.*, **105**, 287–295.

Suezawa, Y. & Ruettimann, B. (1983) Indikation, Methodik und Ergebnisse der perkutanen Nukleotomie bei lumbaler Diskushernie. *Z. Orthop.*, **121**, 25–29.

Sutton, J.C. (1986) Chemonucleolysis in the management of lumbar disc disease—a minimum six-year follow-up evaluation. *Clin. Orthop. Rel. Res.*, **206**, 56–60.

Waddell, G. & Main, C.J. (1984) Assessment of severity in low back disorders. *Spine*, **9**, 204–208.

Waddell, G., Main, C.J., Morris, E.W., Di Paola, M. & Gray, I.C.M. (1984) Chronic low-back pain, psychologic distress and illness behavior. *Spine*, **9**, 209–213.

Wickstroem, G. & Haenninen, K. (1987) Determination of sciatica in epidemiologic research. *Spine*, **12**, 692–698.

Wilkinson, H.A. (1983) *The Failed Back Syndrome.* Harper & Row, New York.

Williams, R.W. (1978) Microlumbar discectomy: a conservative surgical approach to the virgin herniated lumbar disc. *Spine*, **3**, 175–182.

Wilson, D.H. & Harbaugh, R. (1982) Lumbar discectomy: A comparative study of microsurgical and standard technique. In Hardy, R.W. (ed.) *Lumbar Disc Disease*, pp. 147–156. Raven Press, New York.

Wilson, D.H. & Kenning, J. (1979) Microsurgical lumbar discectomy: preliminary report of 83 consecutive cases. *Neurosurgery*, **42**, 137–140.

Yasargil, M.G. (1977) Microsurgical operation of herniated lumbar disc. In Wüllenweber, R., Brock, M. *et al.* (eds) *Advances in Neurosurgery*, vol. 4, pp. 81–82. Springer Verlag, Berlin.

41 · Lumbar Spinal Stenosis

By J.A. EPSTEIN and N.E. EPSTEIN

Spinal stenosis in the lumbar region is a ubiquitous disorder possessed of many forms and clinical manifestations. For a full understanding of this condition it is necessary to be conversant with the configuration not only of the lumbar spinal canal, but also of its lateral recesses, foramina and their various dimensions. In its most common form, stenosis essentially involves the sagittal diameter of the spinal canal. It may occur as a generalized, multiple-level disorder, or as a segmental lesion involving only one or two adjacent vertebrae. The narrowing can also be confined to the lateral recesses and foraminal areas, and is usually asymmetrical, accounting for symptoms often being unilateral (Verbiest, 1987).

PATHOPHYSIOLOGY

The anatomy of the lateral recess and the changes of spinal stenosis are shown in Fig. 41.1A and 41.1B. In Fig. 41.1A the diagram of an axial view through the sacrum (A) shows the trefoil nature of the spinal canal (SC) with narrowing of the lateral recesses (a,b). The vertical arrows show the difference in depth, the left (a) being of normal configuration whilst the right (b) is stenotic. The shaded portions of the superior articular facets (c,d) in the horizontal plane (g,h) provide cover for the nerve root (N) which is compressed on the right side of the diagram. Facet tropism producing altered joint alignment (e,f) may explain in some degree why the entrapment is often unilateral and associated with a more vertical orientation of the posterior facets. In (b) of Fig. 41.1A the posterior aspects of the L5 vertebra and sacrum are shown. The hypertrophied facet joint on the right covers the dura laterally as well as the nerve root, which could be exposed only by medial facetectomy. Part C of the figure shows the operative decompression necessary to expose the root by removal of the overhanging portions of the lamina and facet joint with liberal decompression of the roof of the nerve root canal but with preservation of the pars. The position of the pedicle (P) is shown. Fig. 41.1B shows cranial, axial views of L3, L4 and L5 (a,b,c). The typical trefoil canal of spinal stenosis is well shown at L4 and L5. The nerve roots would lie closely opposed to the bone of the lateral recesses (open arrows) beneath the medially overhanging portions of the superior facets and the contiguous lamina more distally.

The historical development of spinal stenosis since its first recognition has been described by Verbiest (1976, 1987) and by Ehni (1977). It is of interest that Verbiest, only after a comparative study of four patients with sciatica and a myelographic block in whom surgical exploration revealed no particular source of compression, concluded that abnormal narrowness of the vertebral canal caused the symptoms and signs. The vertebral canal in these patients was shallow, the laminae were abnormally thickened and supported enlarged articular facets which reached the mid-sagittal plane with an acute interlaminar angle. Since there was no apparent congenital malformation or abnormality in growth, Verbiest used the phrase 'developmental stenosis' to describe the narrowing, indicating that it was due to both a prenatal and postnatal growth disturbance. It was improbable that the hypertrophy of bone was already present at birth since the first manifestations occurred only in the adult. The narrowed midsagittal diameters were usually found at L3 and L4, with the L5 level rarely being compromised. The lowest value of the midsagittal diameter was 10 mm or less, and in these

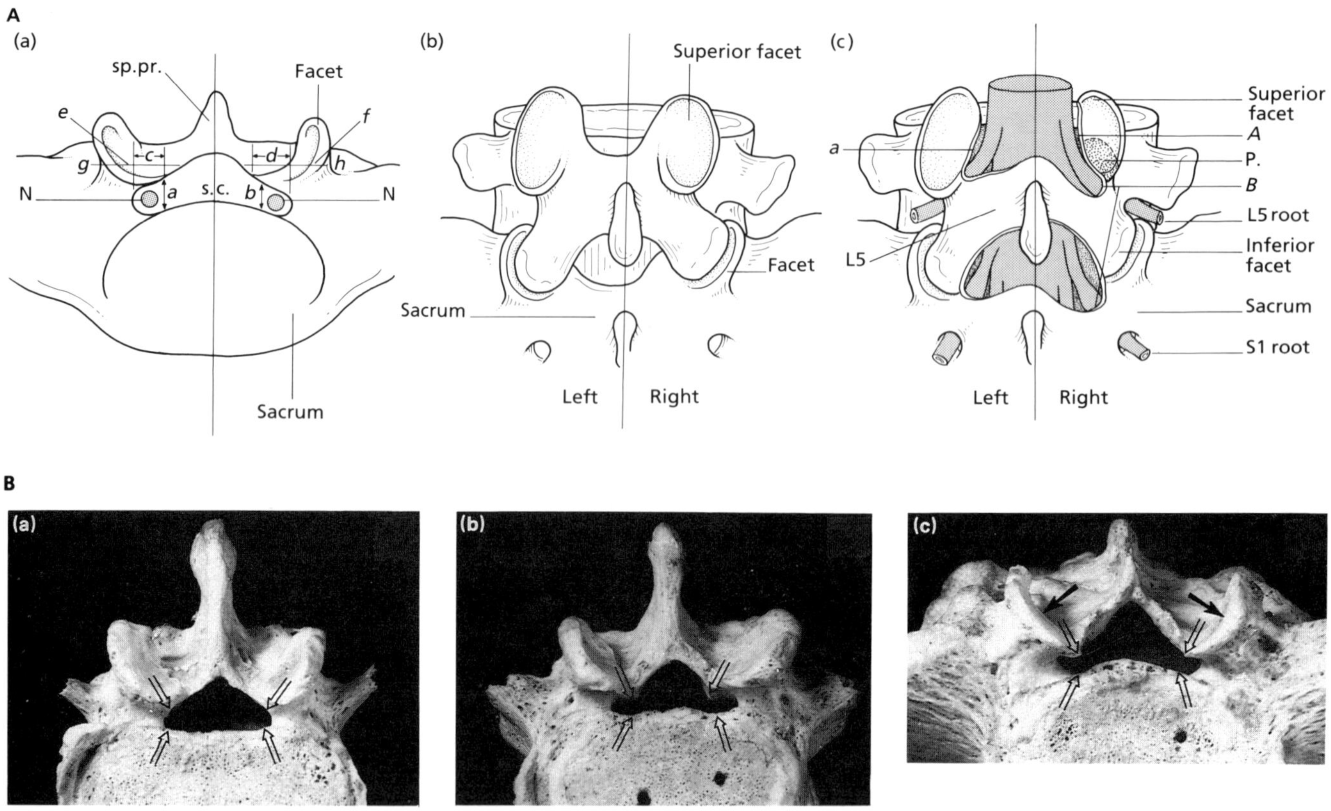

Fig. 41.1 Diagrammatic (A) and skeletal (B) views of lateral recess entrapment. See text for details.

circumstances compression of the neural content in the absence of other agents occurred. This he referred to as 'absolute stenosis'. The term 'relative stenosis' included all cases with midsagittal diameters between 10 mm and 12 mm, both measurements being approximate at best. The reserve capacity of the canal being quite small, minor intrusions such as spondylotic bars or hypertrophied facets and ligamenta flavum could further narrow the canal to a critical state with the onset of symptoms.

Acquired stenosis in a previously normal canal is the result of intrinsic and extrinsic alterations related to trauma, degenerative changes relative to ageing, or surgical procedures. Such changes have to be quite extensive before neural compression can occur, since the normal depth of the lumbar canal is 22–25 mm. In the majority of cases of previously asymptomatic stenosis, symptoms occur because of the development of spondylosis, arthrosis, and protrusion or herniation of intervertebral discs which exceed the critical reserve space for the caudal nerve roots. Verbiest considered stasis in the epidural venous plexus and increased cerebrospinal fluid pressure below a complete subarachnoid block in the upright posture important factors influencing the clinical picture. In his review of 195 cases with spinal stenosis, the extent varied between one and all five lumbar vertebrae, with involvement of two or three vertebrae occurring most frequently, namely in 49%. The maximum extent of pure relative stenosis involved only one or two vertebrae, occurring in 97% of such patients. Unfortunately, nothing is known about the frequency of absolute stenosis (Verbiest, 1980). It is reassuring, however, that the majority of patients with relative stenosis may remain asymptomatic for long intervals of time.

It is evident that there are mixed forms of narrowing of the spinal canal that rarely exist in a pure state, and all fall into the category of developmental stenosis. Measurements alone are unimportant if not associated with relevant clinical findings.

For the most part symptoms occur during the fifth

and sixth decades of life, except for the achondroplastic dwarf or the rare individual in the second or third decade of life who was born with an early congenital tendency towards the development of absolute stenosis (Epstein & Malis, 1955).

The only pure form of congenital stenosis exists in the achondroplastic dwarf, and the entire concept of stenosis cannot be fully appreciated without understanding the unique anatomical changes found in this disorder (Epstein & Malis, 1955; Verbiest, 1987). In such individuals the vertebral bodies are diminished in height and the caudal and cephalic surfaces of the vertebrae are enlarged and mushroomed. The vertebrae are trapezoidal in shape, and there is an acute lumbosacral angle. The growth of the neural arch is limited by premature fusion of the cartilaginous neurocentral synchondroses, while increased periosteal bone formation results in thickening of the lamina with the characteristic formation of the short, squat pedicles typical of this disorder. The result is a markedly diminished anteroposterior diameter of the canal and foramina producing severe compression of the nerve roots and cauda equina. Early disc degeneration with a complicating spondyloarthrosis gradually diminishes the reserve space available for the confined neural structures, which are of normal size and configuration. Such individuals are therefore devastated by the sudden herniation of an intervertebral disc, which can result in paraplegia, usually irreversible, even after adequate decompression has been achieved. The varieties of stenosis seen in the general population all possess some of the features seen in the achondroplastic spine, especially the thick, short pedicles and prominent articular facets. The abnormally large inferior facets often approach the spinous processes medially, making it extremely difficult to perform a laminectomy without removing portions of the facets. The shingling and hyperlordosis found in these individuals further contribute to the clinical problems or difficulties encountered during surgical decompression. Fortunately, only the true achondroplast shows disproportionate skeletal growth (Verbiest, 1987).

In young individuals, especially those in their teens and 20s, absolute spinal stenosis in the lumbar region usually covers the major portion of the lumbar spine excluding the lowermost interspace (Epstein *et al.*, 1988). While it may be associated with backache which can be treated conservatively, even a minor discal herniation can precipitate a dense radicular deficit including cauda equina syndromes and even paraplegia. Fortunately, this complication is quite rare.

The appreciation of stenosis involving the lateral recesses and subarticular areas only was described as a distinct clinical entity by Epstein *et al.* (1972, 1973) and by Getty *et al.* (1981). Epstein and his associates reviewed 15 patients with intense sciatic pain in whom surgical exploration disclosed no signs of a herniated disc, but in whom evidence was found of acute neural entrapment in an extremely narrow lateral recess beneath the lamina adjacent to the pedicle and extending underneath the superior articular facet in a trefoil canal. The central dorsoventral and transverse diameters of the canal were normal. The lateral recesses were cup-shaped and tightly embraced the nerve roots, where minor intrusions such as thickening of investing ligaments and discal protrusions could precipitate symptoms. Spondyloarthrotic changes further reduced the available space, contributing to the radicular pathology. Root decompression may be achieved by either fenestration, coronal hemilaminectomy or full laminectomy in severe cases (Fig. 41.2).

Degenerative spondylolisthesis with an intact neural arch is a frequent cause of acquired stenosis and usually occurs at the L4–L5 interspace (Cauchoix *et al.*, 1976; Epstein *et al.*, 1976, 1983; Fitzgerald, 1976; Alexander *et al.*, 1985; Lombardi *et al.*, 1985; Wiltse, 1987). It is prevalent more often in women than in men, with a ratio that varies from 2 : 1 to as much as 10 : 1. The huge arthrotic posterior facets ubiquitous to this disorder limit the anterior dislocation of the suprajacent vertebral segment as it moves forward, so that it is rare to find more than 1–1.5 cm of ventral subluxation (Fig. 41.3).

Watanabe & Parke (1986) presented the only postmortem study of a typical case of degenerative spondylolisthesis in a patient with a classical five-year history of intermittent neurogenic claudication. The nerve roots were constricted at the site of the olisthesis to less than 25% of their original diameter. The radicular venous system was more affected by the compression than were the arteries which, nonetheless, were severely compromised. There was an obvious loss in the number of large-calibre neurones with numerous empty axons and various degrees of demyelinization, pia-arachnoid adhesions, interstitial fibrosis and thick-walled congested veins. The patient showed no neurological deficit except for absent

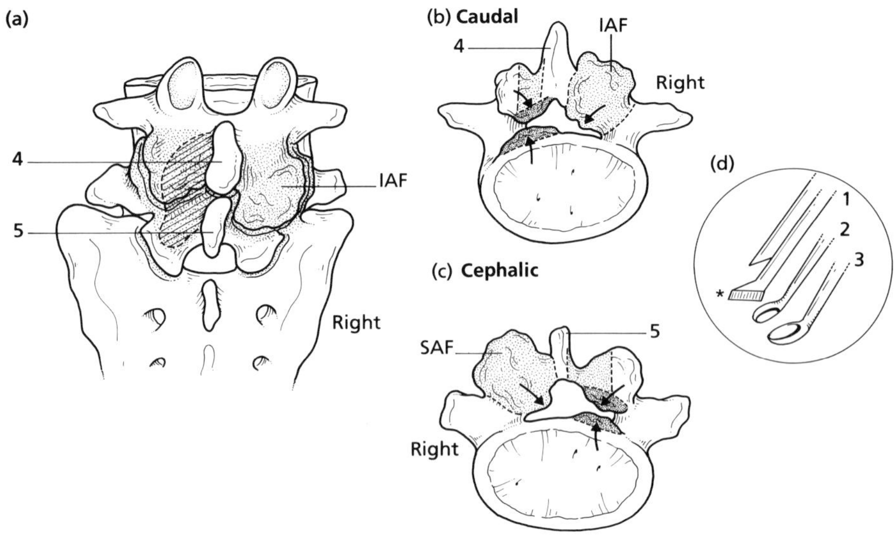

Fig. 41.2 Diagrammatic representation of acquired stenosis. The hypertrophied inferior articular facets (IAF) approximate the midline obliterating the interlaminar space. The amount of bone which typically must be removed to decompress the root is shown by the hatched area on the left of (a) and the dotted lines in (b) and (c). The curettes and modified punch used in root decompression are also shown (d).

ankle reflexes. The claudicant symptoms were attributed to ectopic neural impulse discharges elicited by rapid changes in the blood supply to the cauda equina following exertion. The minimal neural deficit was attributed to neuronal plasticity that permitted functional compensation to develop during the slow acquisition of the chronic nerve root pathology.

In younger individuals, especially women in their 40s and 50s, a pre-existing lumbar stenosis and hyperlordosis contributes to the early occurrence of symptoms. In these individuals the space within the vertebral canal is already limited. The scissoring effect associated with olisthesis and the intrusion of enlarged arthrotic posterior facets gradually eradicates the reserve space for the nerve roots and the cauda equina. In patients with large canals this degree of olisthesis can well be asymptomatic. Retrolisthesis, unless extreme, rarely diminishes the available space significantly. The clinical findings in degenerative spondylolisthesis do not differ remarkably from those found in the primary form of spinal stenosis. The step between the spinous processes at the level of olisthesis can often be palpated.

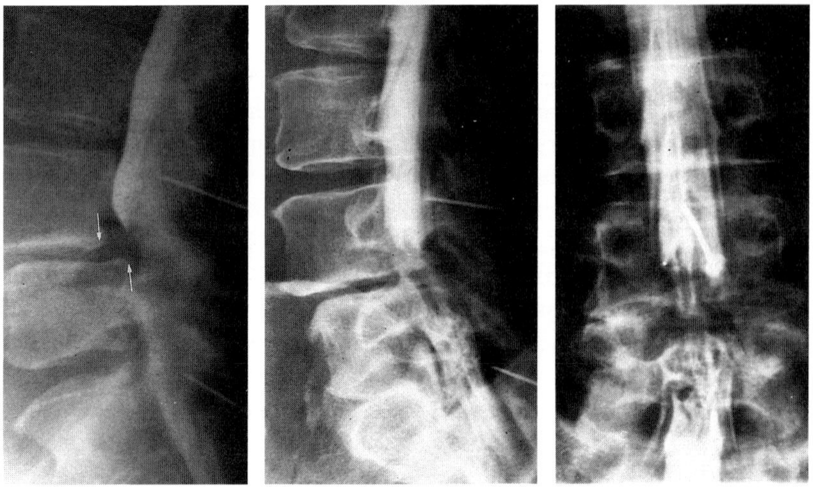

Fig. 41.3 Radiculogram showing degenerative spondylolisthesis with a block which could not be completely overcome by forward flexion. Double needles were used to completely display the canal.

CLINICAL FEATURES

In the majority of patients with symptomatic developmental spinal stenosis the neurological examination may be quite normal. Careful evaluation, however, will often show weakness of the extensor hallucis longus and peroneal muscle groups greater on one side than on the other, the patient often being completely unaware of such changes. Absent ankle reflexes are not uncommon in older individuals, as are findings suggestive of a peripheral neuropathy, particularly in those with a history of diabetes or a background of alcoholism. In older patients, evidence of impaired peripheral vascular perfusion may be a common coexistent problem.

While straight leg raising is commonly normal in patients with spinal stenosis, any deviation from the usual structural changes results in a higher frequency of a positive sign. Verbiest (1976) found the Lasegue sign to be negative in approximately 60% of cases of pure absolute stenosis and in 43% of patients with mixed stenosis. The finding of a positive or negative sign was not linked to the presence or absence of soft disc herniations or osteophytes. Symptoms of neurogenic claudication were noted in 142 out of 195 patients, occurring in about 80% of the pure, absolute, and mixed stenosis, and in 55% of those with pure relative stenosis. While radicular pain was a frequent symptom in patients with spinal stenosis, the motor deficit was most evident during episodes of claudication. Verbiest concluded that much remained to be explained regarding the unique symptoms found with this disorder, since he found no direct correlation between the presence or absence of neurogenic claudication, the degree of narrowing of the vertebral canal, or the presence or absence of additional compressive agents. He considered stenosis to be only one of the causes of neurogenic claudication, the other causes residing in individual differences in the anatomical structure of the nerve roots, constitutional variables in the resistance of the nerve roots to pressure or ischaemia and to changes due to ageing and chronic stress. Compression and traction on the nerve roots in the area of stenosis during various changes in body position and activity may be additional factors in determining the presence of claudication (Verbiest, 1976, 1980, 1987).

Backache is a common finding with varying radiation down the lower extremities since the vast majority of these patients have degenerative changes in the spinal column. The backache is rarely disabling and is usually responsive to conservative measures, especially when evidence of a myofascial syndrome contributes to the pain pattern (Rosomoff & Rosomoff, 1987).

A common finding in more than half of such patients is the presence of intermittent neurogenic claudication, and the initial description of this syndrome by Verbiest (1976) remains relevant to this day. Symptoms appear when the patient assumes any position which accentuates the lumbar lordosis, such as standing and walking. They are relieved quickly by sitting down or by recumbency. The ability to walk becomes rapidly compromised over a period of time, and the distance traversed becomes progressively shorter, though it can vary from day to day. Simply standing still is difficult, and these patients cannot wait in line without being forced to bend forward or to look for the nearest seat. The reverse is true for patients with vascular insufficiency.

Disability increases as the time for symptoms to occur decreases. There is a constellation of complaints such as low back pain and pain in the buttocks spreading diffusely down the lower extremities with numbness followed ultimately by weakness and a tendency for the limbs to collapse. This is the most common pattern, although numerous variations and asymmetries can exist. Under certain circumstances pain is not the dominant factor while numbness and weakness are most evident. Rarely is sphincter function compromised. The patient with neurogenic claudication can drive a car without difficulty and can play tennis with little restriction. In riding a bicycle, as patients lean over the handlebars, opening the lumbar canal, they can pedal away without difficulty. However, when sitting upright or leaning backward the lordotic curve is accentuated and the canal narrows, with symptoms increasing in severity. The patient eventually may assume the forward-flexed or simian posture in the course of ambulation.

In the presence of a herniated disc the symptoms of entrapment resemble those of a typical discal extrusion, but are usually extremely severe, accounting for the positive Lasegue sign found in such patients (Epstein *et al.*, 1968, 1972, 1974, 1988).

The claudication time varies directly with the oxygen availability, suggesting a relative ischaemia of the cauda equina during exercise (Evans, 1964). Compression of the nerve roots inhibits the normal vasodilatation and greater blood supply resulting from the demands of increasing activity, precipitating symptoms of ischaemic neuritis. Since these changes are reversible by postural alterations which open the spinal canal, it explains why so few neurological abnormalities occur. By terminating any activity that causes symptoms, and by reducing or reversing the lordotic posture, any neurological deficit which occurred resolves rapidly. Typical of ischaemic neuritis is the development of sensory signs and symptoms before changes in motor power are evident (Evans, 1964).

Differential diagnosis

The major differential diagnosis in spinal stenosis is that of ischaemic claudication, and the situation may be complicated by both ischaemic and neurogenic claudication being present in the same individual. Ischaemic cases localize the leg pain to the muscles of the posterior calf, whereas neurogenic claudication presents with the development or increase of radicular pain. If the onset of leg pain on walking is followed by the development of sensory loss or weakness and dragging of the leg, then a neurogenic cause is likely. Whilst merely standing still will rapidly resolve ischaemic calf pain, it is necessary to flex the lumbar spine by stooping or sitting to allow neurogenic pain to ease.

Whilst the presentation of specific radicular pain exacerbated by walking and relieved by sitting is highly suggestive of a diagnosis of spinal stenosis, other conditions may mimic the disorder. Lesions of the conus, especially of a vascular nature, not infrequently may present with exercise-related exacerbation in the early stages; it is thus essential to screen the entire lumbar canal either by radiculography or magnetic resonance imaging (MRI). Computerized tomography (CT) scanning of the lower lumbar levels alone is inadequate. The onset of sphincteric disturbance is unusual in spinal stenosis, and should suggest the possibility of an alternative diagnosis.

Tumours of the lumbar spinal column and intradural tumours of the cauda equina rarely produce claudicating symptoms. However, patients with spinal stenosis frequently complain of low back pain and persistent radicular pain, and in that clinical situation these lesions must be excluded. Peripheral neuropathy may pose diagnostic problems but can readily be assessed electrophysiologically.

One specific problem area is that of the patient with cervical as well as lumbar stenosis (Epstein *et al.*, 1984). It may be very difficult to determine how much of a gait problem is due to the cervical myelopathy and how much to the lumbar stenosis. It is usual in cases of doubt to decompress the cervical canal first but, if the lumbar spine is operated upon initially, great care with neck positioning under anaesthesia must be taken.

INVESTIGATION

In cases where there is suspicion of peripheral vascular disease, assessment of the patient's cardiovascular status will be necessary. In patients where clinical assessment suggests a diagnosis of spinal stenosis, complete radiological assessment of the spine is the prime investigation. Electrophysiological tests can be helpful and it may be necessary to exclude a peripheral neuropathy. Elderly patients may have gait difficulties due to hip or knee arthritis which require additional assessment.

Despite modern imaging techniques it remains necessary to obtain conventional AP and lateral radiographs of the lumbar spine supplemented by stress films, at least in the sagittal plane. Evidence of congenital canal narrowing or the development of a degenerative spondylolisthesis may well be found. MRI scanning serves to exclude unsuspected intradural lesions at the conus and, in patients with long tract signs, should include the whole spine as cervical stenosis is not uncommonly associated with lumbar stenosis (Epstein *et al.*, 1984). In the absence of high-quality MRI, radiculography or myelography is mandatory; assessment by plain X-ray and plain CT alone is inadequate due to the high false-positive rate associated with degenerative changes seen on CT, especially in the older age group.

Whilst MRI gives great detail regarding discal pathology and soft tissue changes within the spinal canal and foramina (Masaryk & Modic, 1988), bony detail is inferior to that provided by CT. As a result of this the 'gold standard' of investigating patients with spinal stenosis remains the combination of radiculography followed by CT scanning whilst the contrast remains within the intradural space (Figs 41.4 & 41.5). If a complete block to the flow of contrast is found, flexing the lumbar spine forward in the seated position will often open the canal and allow the contrast to pass through. If this manoeuvre does not relieve the block, then the remainder of the as yet unseen spinal canal must be examined by a further lumbar puncture beyond the block.

The abnormalities found by CT-radiculography may range from single- to multiple-level pathology, and from compression of a single root to complete obliteration of the cauda equina. The existence of multiple-level disease does not necessarily imply that surgery should be directed at all the abnormal levels. In all cases the radiological findings must be carefully correlated with the clinical situation. Finally, it should be stressed that degenerative disease in the lumbar spine may occur without producing clinical problems. It is essential that the patient is fully assessed both clinically and radiologically to avoid diagnostic error.

MANAGEMENT

Patients with symptoms due to spinal stenosis are not easy to treat non-surgically. Physiotherapy, nerve blocks, etc. seem to have a relatively unsuccessful role in improving the symptoms of exercise-induced root pain. However, Rosomoff & Rosomoff (1987) did report improvement in patients treated without operation but with an aggressive multidisciplinary team approach using physical, behavioural and rehabilitational techniques. In patients who do not respond, but who are stable, a choice may be made between surgical treatment and merely living with the disability. In those who have neurological deficit or whose walking distance is reducing, however, surgery is mandatory.

The operative procedure is best performed with the patient in the crouch or salaam position with the hips well elevated and a wide 80–90° angle at the hip and

A

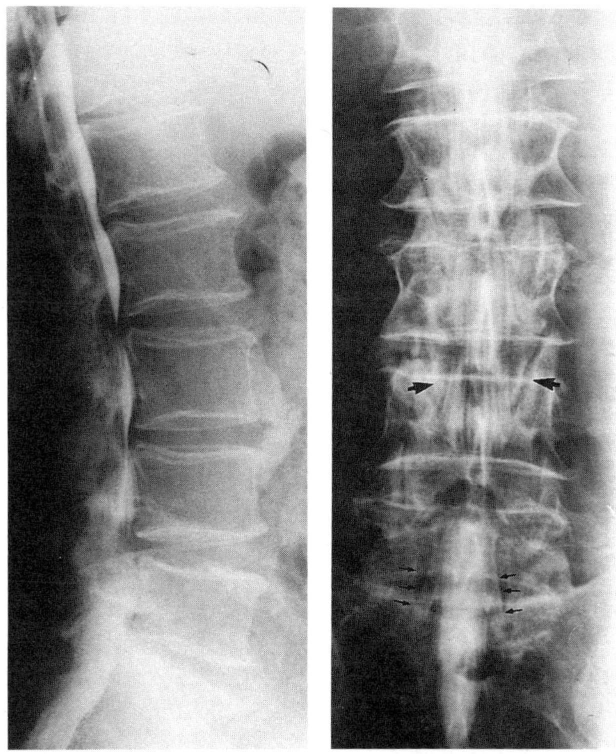

B

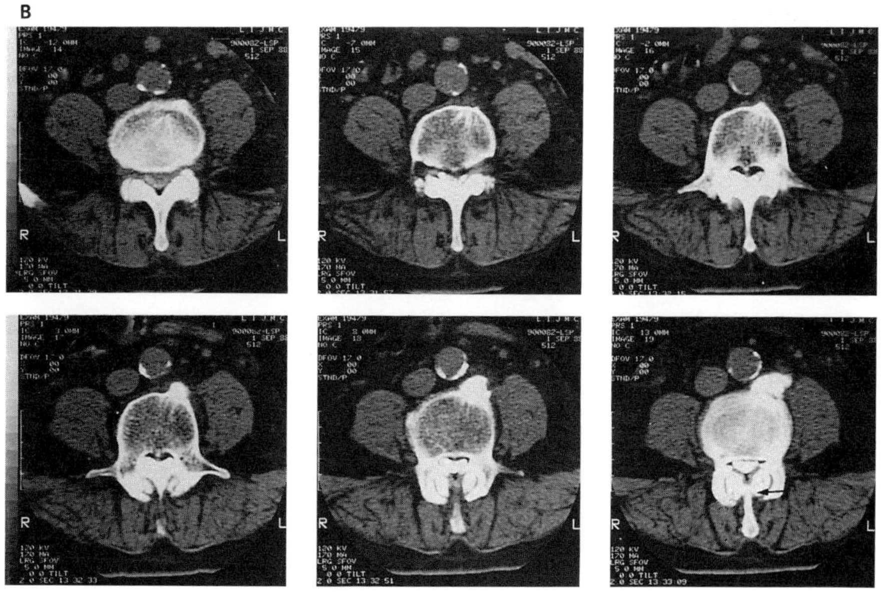

Fig. 41.4 CT radiculogram of a 71-year-old man showing evidence of both developmental and acquired spinal stenosis. There is canal narrowing over multiple levels but excluding L5–S1, where the roots fill well on the radiculogram (small arrows, A). The arthrotic articular facets converge particularly at L3–L4 on the left and to a lesser degree at L4–L5 (large arrows, A). The CT scan shows marked canal narrowing with marked overgrowth of the inferior articular facets which approach the midline (arrow, B). The facets are large and the pedicles are short and squat, indicating the coexistence of a degree of congenital stenosis.

knee to prevent any unusual pressure on the thigh or calf. The arms are extended at right angles to the trunk with the elbows flexed at approximately 90° and maintained forward on arm supports. Care must be taken to avoid hyperextending the cervical spine in positioning the patient. The major weight is supported by the buttocks. This position opens the spinal canal and spreads the laminar and spinous processes. The abdomen and chest are under no pressure, resulting in collapse of the epidural vessels with minimal operative blood loss and no need for transfusion.

The major purpose of the surgical procedure is to enlarge the spinal canal. The most important feature is to ensure that the lateral recesses and the nerve root foramina are decompressed, as well as the more central parts of the canal. Where the midline dimensions of the canal are reasonably well preserved, and the stenotic process is mainly sited laterally, the nerve roots may often be decompressed via a fenestration procedure (Lin, 1982; Epstein *et al.*, 1988; Young *et al.*, 1988). However, where the entire sagittal diameter of the canal is reduced, or where the inferior articular processes are so enlarged that they encroach upon the midline, laminectomy is necessary. It is also prudent to perform laminectomy in cases with marked neurological deficit, but the laminectomy must always be performed in conjunction with decompression of the lateral recesses as decompression of only the central part of the canal will not decompress the roots.

Where laminectomy is performed it should be achieved by an *en-face* technique. It is mandatory to preserve the pars interarticularis and the majority of the weight-bearing surfaces of the facets. This is best achieved by using an undercutting technique to remove the portion of the joint which intrudes into the canal whilst preserving the articular surfaces. Figure 41.6 is a diagram of a unilateral three-level exposure allowing decompression of both the dural tube and the roots. By carefully following the path of each individual nerve only those medial parts of the facets which actually impinge on the root are undercut and the pars is preserved. In order not to injure the nerve root during decompression, sharp up-biting curettes and 30° angled Kerrison punches

A

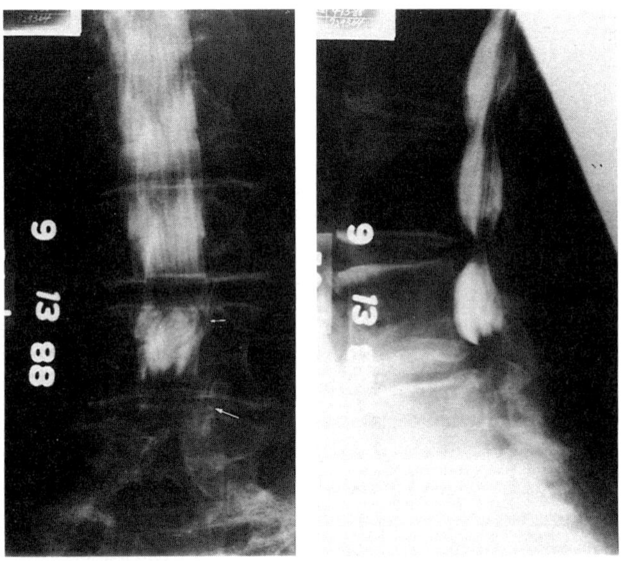

B

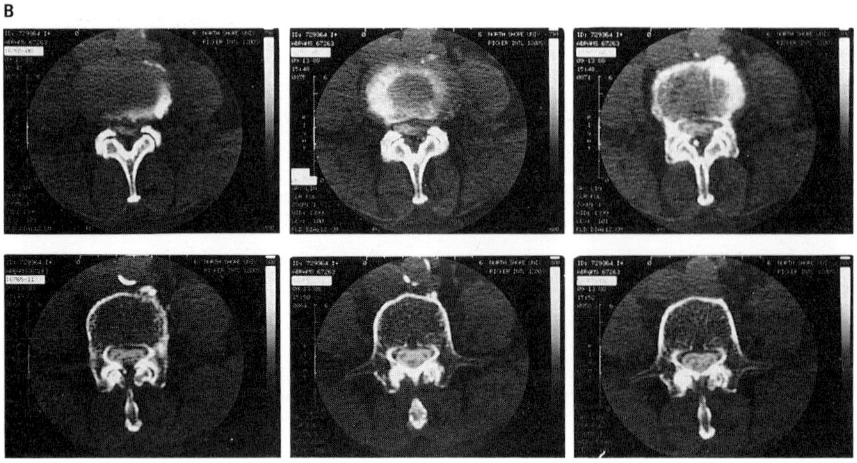

Fig. 41.5 CT radiculogram showing severe stenosis with an early degenerative spondylolisthesis at L4–L5. There is a partial block at L3–L4 and a complete block at L4–L5. The prominent articular facets at L4–L5 are clearly evident (large arrow, A). Redundant nerve roots are seen above the block (small arrow, A). The severe degree of stenosis is best appreciated on the upper three frames of the CT scan. There is marked hypertrophy of the articular facets with narrowing of the lateral recesses on both sides.

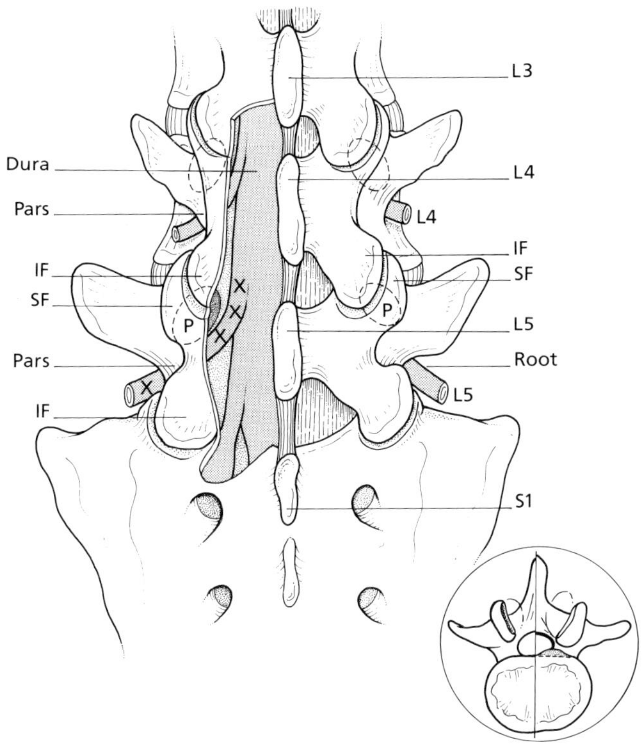

Fig. 41.6 Diagrammatic representation of a unilateral decompression over three levels. The first three '×s' indicate the point of most critical root compression. IF, inferior facet; SF, superior facet; P, pedicle.

with filed-down sole plates are used (Fig. 41.2). It is often not necessary to remove osteophytes if adequate lateral recess decompression has been achieved. Large osteophytes arising from the vertebral bodies are best tamped down and flattened with a small-bore punch.

In patients with degenerative spondylolisthesis, almost invariably at the L4–L5 level, where severe stenosis can occur with an attendant arthrotic degeneration of the facets, a two-level laminectomy may be indicated. This may be extended to an additional level if required. It is important that the L5 nerve root be explored well laterally with liberal foraminal decompression using an undercutting technique. The nerve root is followed from its axillary origin as it winds laterally over the ledge formed at the level of subluxation towards the foramen. At times this ledge may need to be tamped down if it distorts the nerve root. Portions of the pedicle may also be removed if kinking is present (Fig. 41.7). If the findings are most evident on one side, only limited decompression need be done on the opposite side, to facilitate stability. This allows more generous decompression on the involved side. It is not uncommon to find that the involved vertebrae have been fused by the spondylotic process. Severe arthrotic abnormalities in the facets may add further support so that more generous decompression can be performed if indicated. Coronal hemilaminectomy may suffice if the lesion is limited and amenable to this approach.

Appropriate flexion and extension X-ray studies are indicated preoperatively should there be a suggestion of abnormal mobility that would require fusion. If there is an acute radicular syndrome with signs of entrapment, exploration should include a search for a herniated and possibly sequestrated disc. The nerve roots at the level above may also require decompression if adjacent levels are involved by the stenotic process.

In 1967, Epstein *et al.* described a simple type of bilateral interlaminar laminotomy and foraminotomy with undercutting of the opposing lamina and facets decompressing the subarticular areas and lateral recesses. This exposure is especially helpful in patients with segmental disease at only one level, as is often found in degenerative spondylolisthesis. It can also be employed in younger individuals with absolute or relative stenosis over multiple levels where decompression can be achieved without sacrificing any of the major supporting structures of the spine. This procedure has been further refined by Lin (1982) and by Young *et al.* (1988).

Getty *et al.* (1981) described partial undercutting facetectomy with preservation of the pars interarticularis in 78 patients with entrapment of the nerve roots caused by degenerative changes in the posterior facets with lateral recess and subarticular stenosis. Lasting relief of pain was achieved without spinal stabilization. The superior articular facet was a major factor compressing the nerve root against the vertebral body. This was further emphasized by Kirkaldy-Willis *et al.* (1978), in describing the pathology and pathogenesis of lumbar spondylosis with stenosis. These authors demonstrated, in anatomical specimens, just where and how the cauda equina and the lumbar spinal nerves become entrapped, enabling the surgeon to formulate a rational type of therapy. They emphasized the fact that sacrifice of essential supporting structures must be avoided as well as iatrogenic trauma in the confines of a stenotic neural canal (Kirkaldy-Willis & Farfan, 1982).

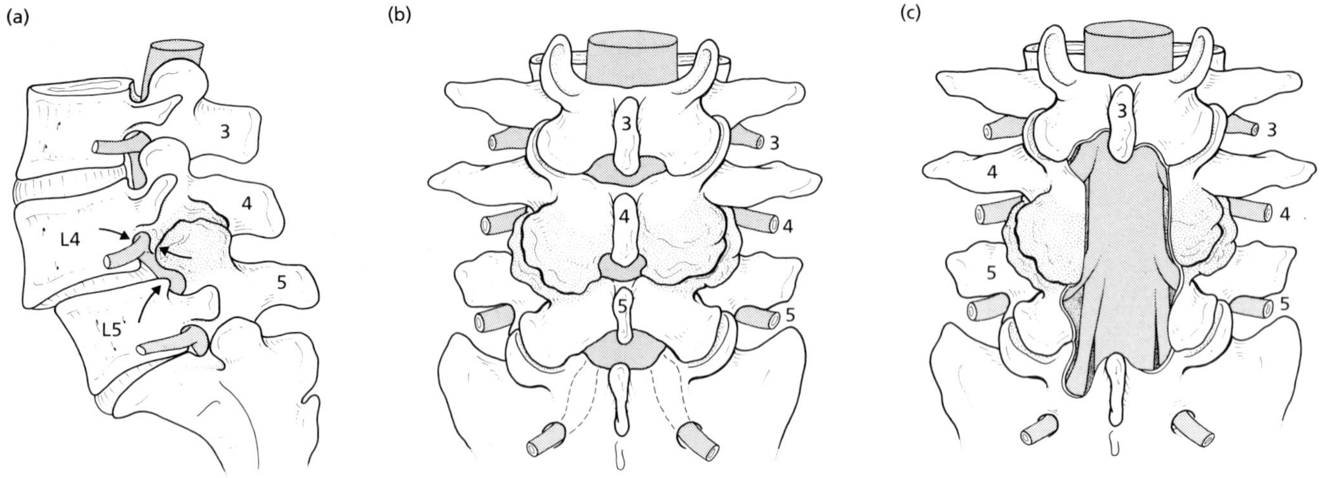

Fig. 41.7 Degenerative spondylolisthesis at L4–L5 with marked hypertrophy of the L4–L5 facets. A decompression by two-level laminectomy and undercutting facetectomy is shown in (c), preserving the major part of the L4–L5 joints to prevent the development of increased instability.

In degenerative scoliosis, stenosis may occur in the lateral recess in the concave side of the spine beneath enlarged, arthrotic facets where the foramina are further narrowed by approximation of the pedicles (Epstein *et al.*, 1974; Simmons & Jackson, 1979; San Martino *et al.*, 1983). These alterations can effectively cause neural compression with the appearance of radiculopathic signs (Fig. 41.8). Surgical decompression of the lateral recesses, by means of hemilaminectomy and foraminotomy, will effectively decompress the nerve root or roots and relieve radicular complaints.

The occurrence of discal herniation in conjunction with spinal stenosis and degenerative spondylolisthesis was reported by Alexander *et al.* (1985) and by Hall *et al.* (1985). Alexander *et al.* noted an incidence of 20% in 50 patients with degenerative spondylolisthesis, while Hall *et al.* found a 15% incidence of disc herniation in 68 patients with spinal stenosis. However, Tsou and Hopp (1987) found disc herniation or recurrence to occur in only 4.3% of their patients. Particularly in spondylolisthesis, the discal herniation often occurred at the level cephalad to the abnormal level.

While satisfactory results of approximately 80–85% may be expected following an initial operative procedure for spinal stenosis, this drops significantly in the authors' experience when second procedures are performed for recurrent symptoms. In that situation, those who fare best are individuals who have at the subsequent operation a discal herniation, particularly extrusion or sequestration. Of 26 patients undergoing reoperation, only 15 (58%) showed significant improvement, and they primarily had evidence of acute neural entrapment secondary to discal herniation.

The place of fusion in the management of spinal stenosis and, in particular, degenerative spondylolisthesis, remains highly controversial. Whilst the presence of biomechanical abnormalities causing an instability type of low back pain may require instrumentation and fusion, in many patients the spondylotic changes are sufficiently advanced to provide adequate stability after appropriate decompression. Many such patients have coped adequately with back pain for many years and seek medical attention only with the onset of radicular symptoms.

Johnsson *et al.* (1986) discussed postoperative instability after decompression for lumbar spinal stenosis in 45 patients, and observed that evidence of olisthesis after surgery was consistent with a poor result. In degenerative spondylolisthesis the risk of postoperative slipping was much higher yet, surprisingly, did not influence the quality of recovery. Of significance was that these patients underwent extensive laminectomies and facetectomies both partial and total. There was no correlation between postoperative slipping and the number of decompressed levels.

The incidence of symptomatic slippage described

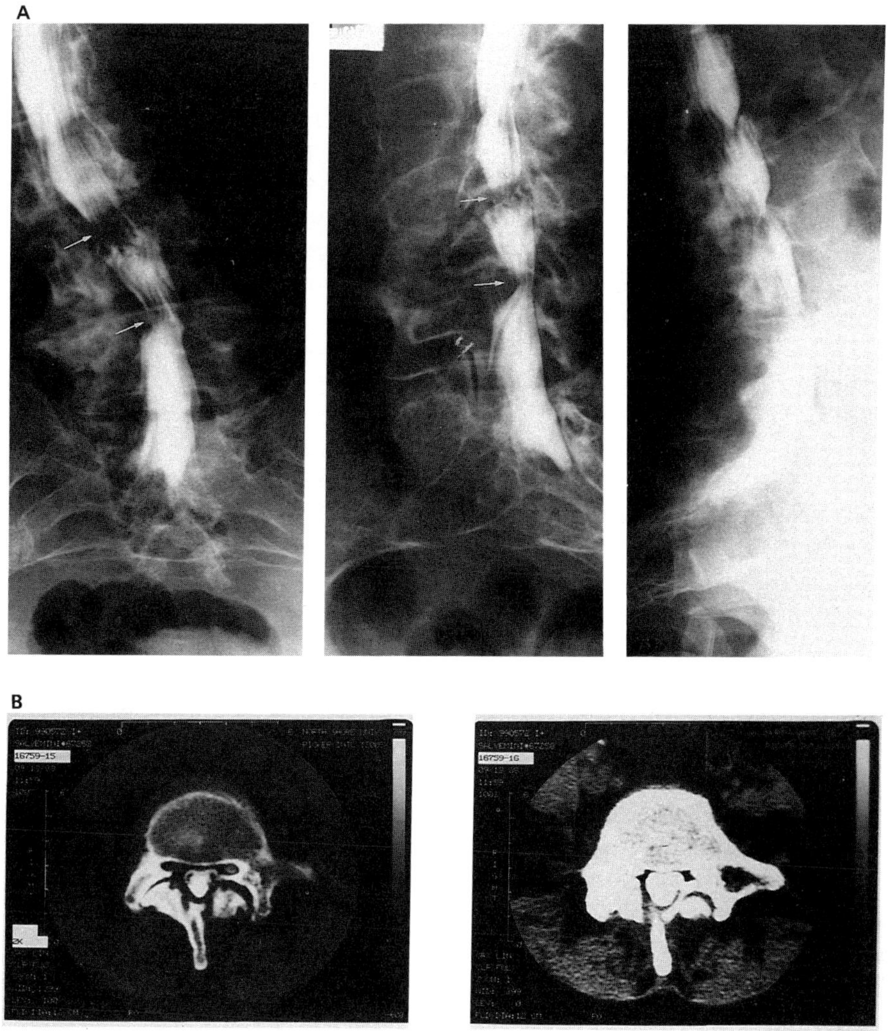

Fig. 41.8 CT radiculogram showing degenerative scoliosis; (A) shows marked radicular compression on the concave side (arrows); (B) confirms the compromise of the lateral recesses. The nerve root fills with contrast on one side only.

by Tsou and Hopp (1987) after decompressive procedures for spinal stenosis was 4.6% in 342 patients. Sixteen developed olisthesis and worsening of symptoms postoperatively requiring secondary stabilization. In reviewing the literature, these authors found a variation of from 2% to as much as 20% with the degree of olisthesis relating to the degree of facet removal. They advocated limited posterolateral fusion at the time of the primary decompressive laminectomy in selected cases.

Lee (1983), in performing extensive laminectomy and fusion in 22 patients, found that the incidence rate of pseudarthrosis was high (27.3%). Concomitant spinal fusion was not routinely indicated, since it was not effective in the prevention of olisthesis. However, the procedure used included the removal of all or most of the posterior spinal stabilizing structures and the fusion failed to prevent further olisthesis in four (18%) patients.

Rosomoff & Rosomoff (1987) performed extensive facetectomies along with complete laminectomies in 50 patients with lumbar stenosis, 36 of whom had had prior surgery. Only one (2%) required a postoperative fusion. Similarly, Shenkin & Hash (1979) studied 59 patients for three years following multilevel laminectomy and inferior facetectomy for spinal stenosis. Although six (10%) radiographically demonstrated postoperative spondylolisthesis, only two (3.3%) required fusion. The incidence of olisthesis increased with the number of lamina removed. This was 15% where three or more levels had been decompressed and 6% for two or fewer levels. They considered intertransverse fusion for olisthesis justified only after complete facet removal.

The role that prophylactic fusion plays in the management of spinal stenosis remains controversial. Based on the low incidence of olisthesis observed even in the presence of radical facet removal, it would not appear to be warranted at the initial procedure.

The success rate after surgical decompression for degenerative spondylolisthesis with an intact neural arch and stenosis should fall within the 80–85% range. In Alexander's series of 50 patients with degenerative spondylolisthesis treated over 11 years by means of wide decompressive laminectomy, medial facetectomy and foraminotomy, 91% exhibited a good response for three years, diminishing to 87% at six years (Alexander *et al.*, 1985). Hall's series of 68 patients showed an 84% good to excellent result after four years (Hall *et al.*, 1985).

Lombardi *et al.* (1985), in reviewing three surgical approaches for the treatment of degenerative spondylolisthesis, found that a midline decompression and preservation of the articular processes with an added intertransverse process fusion achieved a 90% good to excellent result. Those without fusion but with a similar operation had 80% equivalent results after two years. Patients with a wide decompression sacrificing the articular processes had good to excellent results in only 33% of the cases. While the 10% difference in good results in patients after this floating type of fusion may justify the added time and effort, in the high-risk patient one should seriously consider whether or not this added procedure is justified.

Cauchoix *et al.* (1976) reported on 26 patients with degenerative spondylolisthesis in whom only six (23%) required fusion: three at the first operative procedure and three for postoperative progressive olisthesis.

Alexander *et al.* (1985) reported 50 patients with degenerative spondylolisthesis treated with wide decompressive laminectomy and medial facetectomy, of whom only four were fused at the primary procedure. Two of these had undergone prior surgical procedures, and the remaining two were considered to be unstable at the time of surgery. Of the remaining 46 patients who were not fused, only two (4%) showed increased postoperative olisthesis but only one, who had developed spondylolisthesis one level above the site of prior surgery, had to be fused. Fager (1988), in a reviewer's comment upon the paper by Young *et al.*, reported 50 patients with L4–L5 degenerative spondylolisthesis treated by laminectomy and undercutting facetectomy, and found further subluxation in only two patients. He felt that excision of the disc at the spondylolisthetic level was an important cause of the postoperative instability in those patients.

The question of the place of spinal fusion in the management of degenerative spondylolisthesis is far from settled. This conflict is especially evident in the conservative attitude adopted by most neurosurgeons, and a more aggressive approach by orthopaedists who tend to favour fusion with varied instrumentation. Fusion in elderly patients, often obese, hyperlordotic, frequently diabetic with arteriosclerotic cerebrovascular and cardiovascular disease, is not to be contemplated lightly. Overall, provided the decompressive technique used preserves the pars and the majority of the facetal complex, as has been described, it seems that supplementary fusion is rarely required to maintain stability. However, review of the literature in addition to those papers already quoted indicates that indiscriminate removal of facets, the pars interarticularis and interruption of the annulus and the posterior longitudinal ligament in the absence of a significant discal herniation is to be avoided (Epstein *et al.*, 1962; Brodsky, 1976; Spengler, 1987). Preservation of the spinous processes and interspinous ligaments in coronal hemilaminectomy, although not proven to be helpful, does in part tend to restore a more anatomical state for muscular reattachment (San Martino, 1974; Jason & McCormick, 1987; Young *et al.*, 1988).

However, in certain situations fusion at the time of primary surgery may have to be considered. For example, in the case of a younger patient with a degenerative spondylolisthesis showing marked movements on preoperative flexion/extension X-rays, or a patient who has had both facet joints removed and who has relatively little in the way of other degenerative spondylosis at that segment, fusion may have to be considered especially in the presence of severe back pain.

Several differing techniques for fusion have been described. In patients undergoing surgical intervention for the relief of radicular pathology or even degenerative spondylolisthesis, there seems little place for anterior fusion, as the roots and spinal canal cannot be adequately decompressed. Reference has already been made to the use of bilateral intertransverse fusion at the time of decompression by several authors (Lee, 1983; Lombardi *et al.*, 1985; Tsou & Hopp, 1987). Wiltse, who was the senior author in Lombardi's paper, reported in 1987 the techniques of instrumentation to supplement a posterolateral fusion. He felt that the effect of facetal decompression, particularly in regard of rotational stability, demanded a supplementary fusion at the time of the primary surgery.

Cloward (1987) presented a most thorough evaluation of the treatment of spinal stenosis and its various manifestations by means of posterior lumbar interbody fusion. He described an effective method to provide a stable spine capable of meeting all functional demands. While not recommended as the treatment of choice for all forms of lumbar stenosis, he indicated that posterior lumbar interbody fusion when followed precisely is capable of addressing situations considered impossible to correct by other methods. His aim was to remove the causes of symptoms and to restore the spine to more normal anatomical contours and alignment by means of stabilization. Fortunately, he also discussed the formidable complications, indicating that a unique versatility and skill is required to perform this procedure properly.

The hazards of pedicle screw fixation were discussed by Weinstein *et al.* (1988), based upon the reliability and validity of roentgenogram assessment and the surgical technique. The overall failure rate for the accurate placement of the pedicle screw in cadaver specimens was approximately 21%, 92% of which resulted in cortical perforations within the spinal canal. The success rate was independent of surgical technique and was not significantly related to approach, surgeon experience, screw size or spine levels. Roentgenograms were found to produce unacceptably high rates of false-positive and false-negative evaluations. Pedicle screw placement is even more difficult in cases of degenerative spondylolisthesis.

Following fusion, the motion segment cephalad to the fusion in time becomes compromised, resulting in spondylotic and arthrotic changes in the posterior facets contributing to the development of stenosis. The threat of olisthesis increases. Such changes in the integrity of the segment above an area of fusion are of increasing importance now that a great variety of pedicular screws and plates have evolved for purposes of stabilization and the creation of block vertebrae. A 5% incidence of olisthesis following operations for spinal stenosis would scarcely seem to justify the use of prophylactic spinal fusion (Tsou & Hopp, 1987).

Review of the literature shows that using the techniques described in this chapter in carefully selected cases, 80–85% of patients achieve satisfactory results with improvement in radicular pain, neurological deficit and neurogenic claudication. Immediate improvement in the severity of claudicating symptoms when ambulation is resumed is a most encouraging sign.

The satisfactory results of surgery are also maintained in the long term. In the series of 50 patients treated over an 11-year period reported by Alexander *et al.* (1985), 91% showed a good outcome at three years only falling to 87% at six-year follow-up. Hall *et al.* (1985) also showed an 84% good or excellent outcome at four years.

REFERENCES

Alexander, E., Kelly, D.L., Davis, C.H., McWhorter, J.M. & Brown, W. (1985) Intact arch spondylolisthesis: a review of 50 cases and description of surgical treatment. *J. Neurosurg.*, **63**, 840–844.

Brodsky, A.E. (1976) Post-laminectomy and post-fusion stenosis of the lumbar sine. *Clin. Orthop. Rel. Res.*, **115**, 130–139.

Cauchoix, J., Benoist, M. & Chassaing, V. (1976) Degenerative spondylolisthesis. *Clin. Orthop. Rel. Res.*, **115**, 122–129.

Cloward, R.B. (1987) Spinal stenosis: treatment by posterior lumbar interbody fusion. In Hopp, E. (ed.), *Spine: State of the Art Reviews*, vol. 1, no. 3, pp. 457–516. Hanley & Belfus, Philadelphia, PA.

Ehni, G. (1977) Historical writings on spondylotic caudal radiculopathy and its effects on the nervous system. In *Lumbar Spondylosis: Diagnosis, Management and Surgical Treatment*, Chapter 1. Year Book Medical Publishers, Chicago, IL.

Epstein, J.A. & Malis, L.I. (1955) Compression of spinal cord and cauda equina in achondroplastic dwarfs. *Neurology*, **5**, 875–881.

Epstein, J.A., Epstein, B.S., Carras, R. & Lavine, L.S. (1968) The diagnosis and management of discogenic and related disorders of the lumbar spine in geriatric patients. *Proceedings of the Rudolph Virchow Medical Society in the City of New York*, vol. 26 (Suppl.), pp. 116–136. F. Berger Horn, Austria.

Epstein, J.A., Epstein, B.S. & Lavine, L.S. (1962) Nerve root compression associated with narrowing of the lumbar spinal canal. *J. Neurol. Neurosurg. Psychiatry*, **25**, 165–176.

Epstein, J.A., Epstein, B.S. & Lavine, L.S. (1974) Surgical treatment of nerve root compression caused by scoliosis of the lumbar spine. *J. Neurosurg.*, **41**, 449–454.

Epstein, J.A., Epstein, B.S., Lavine, L.S., Carras, R. & Rosenthal, A.D. (1976) Degenerative lumbar spondylolisthesis with an intact neural arch (pseudospondylolisthesis). *J. Neurosurg.*, **44**, 139–147.

Epstein, J.A., Lavine, L.S., Epstein, B.S. & Carras, R. (1967) Herniated disks and related disorders of the lumbar spine: surgical treatment in the geriatric patient. *J. Am. Med. Assoc.*, **202**, 115–118.

Epstein, J.A., Epstein, B.S., Rosenthal, A.D., Carras, R. & Lavine, L.S. (1972) Sciatica caused by nerve root entrapment in the lateral recess: the superior facet syndrome. *J. Neurosurg.*, **36**, 584–589.

Epstein, J.A., Epstein, B.S., Rosenthal, A.D., Carras, R. & Lavine, L.S. (1973) Lumbar nerve root compression at the interverebral foramina caused by arthritis of the posterior facets. *J. Neurosurg.*, **39**, 362–369.

Epstein, N.E., Epstein, J.A. & Carras, R. (1988) Spinal stenosis and disc herniation in a 14-year-old male. *Spine*, **13**, 938–941.

Epstein, N.E., Epstein, J.A., Carras, R. & Lavine, L.S. (1983) Degenerative spondylolisthesis with an intact neural arch: a review of 60 cases with an analysis of clinical findings and the development of surgical management. *Neurosurgery*, **13**, 555–561.

Epstein, N.E., Epstein, J.A., Carras, R., Vishnubhakat, S.M. & Hyman, R.A. (1984) Coexisting cervical and lumbar spinal stenosis: diagnosis and management. *Neurosurgery*, **15**, 489–496.

Evans, J.G. (1964) Neurogenic intermittent claudication. *Br. J. Med.*, **2**, 985–987.

Fager, C. (1988) Comments (article by Young *et al.*, 1988), *Neurosurgery*, **23**, 262.

Fitzgerald, J.A.W. (1976) Degenerative spondylolisthesis. *J. Bone Jt. Surg.*, **58B**, 184–192.

Getty, C.J.M., Johnson, J.R., Kirwan, E.O.G. & Sullivan, M.F. (1981) Partial undercutting facetectomy for bony entrapment of the lumbar nerve root. *J. Bone Jt. Surg.*, **63B**, 330–335.

Hall, S., Bartleson, J.D., Onofrio, B.M., Baker, H.L., Okazaki, H. & O'Duffy, D. (1985) Spinal stenosis: clinical features, diagnostic procedures, and results of surgical treatment in 68 patients. *Ann. Intern. Med.*, **103**, 271–275.

Jason, R.M. & McCormick, K.J. (1987) Preservation of the supraspinous ligament for spinal stenosis. *Neurosurgery*, **21**, 420–422.

Johnsson, K.-E., Willner, S. & Johnsson, K. (1986) Postoperative instability after decompression for lumbar spinal stenosis. *Spine*, **11**, 107–110.

Kirkaldy-Willis, W.H. & Farfan, H.F. (1982) Instability of the lumbar spine. *Clin. Orthop. Rel. Res.*, **165**, 110–123.

Kirkaldy-Willis, W.H., Wedge, J.H., Yong-Hing, K. & Reilly, J. (1978) Pathology and pathogenesis of lumbar spondylosis and stenosis. *Spine*, **3**, 319–328.

Lee, C.K. (1983) Lumbar spinal instability (olisthesis) after extensive posterior spinal decompression. *Spine*, **8**, 429–433.

Lin, P.M. (1982) Internal decompression for multiple levels of lumbar spinal stenosis: a technical note. *Neurosurgery*, **11**, 546–549.

Lombardi, J.S., Wiltse, L.L., Reynolds, J., Widell, E.H. & Spencer, C. (1985) Treatment of degenerative spondylolisthesis. *Spine*, **10**, 821–827.

Masaryk, T.J. & Modic, M.T. (1988) The lumbar spine. In Stark, D.D. & Bradley, W.G. (eds), *Magnetic Resonance Imaging*, pp. 666–682. CV Mosby, St Louis, MO.

Rosomoff, H. & Rosomoff, R.S. (1987) Nonsurgical aggressive treatment of lumbar spinal stenosis. In Hopp, E. (ed.), *Spine: State of the Art Reviews*, vol. 1, no. 3, pp. 583–400. Hanley & Belfus, Philadelphia, PA.

San Martino, A. (1974) Lumbar radicular syndrome in stenosis of the spinal canal (Epstein's syndrome): clinical diagnosis and treatment. *Chir. Organ. Mov.*, **LIII**, 273–278.

San Martino, A., D'Andria, F.M. & San Martino, C. (1983) The surgical treatment of nerve root compression caused by scoliosis of the lumbar sine. *Spine*, **8**, 261–265.

Shenkin, H.A. & Hash, C.J. (1979) Spondylolisthesis after multiple bilateral laminectomies and facetectomies for lumbar stenosis. *J. Neurosurg.*, **50**, 45–47.

Simmons, E.H. & Jackson, R.P. (1979) The management of nerve root entrapment syndromes associated with the collapsing scoliosis of idiopathic lumbar and thoracolumbar curves. *Spine*, **4**, 533–541.

Spengler, D.M. (1987) Current concepts review: degenerative stenosis of the lumbar spine. *J. Bone Jt. Surg.*, **69A**, 305–308.

Tsou, P.M. & Hopp, E. (1987) Postsurgical instability in spinal stenosis. In Hopp, E. (ed.), *Spine: State of the Art Reviews*, vol. 1, no. 2, pp. 533–550. Hanley & Belfus, Philadelphia, PA.

Verbiest, H. (1976) *Neurogenic Claudication—with Special Reference to Stenosis of the Lumbar Vertebral Canal.* North-Holland American Elsevier, New York.

Verbiest, H. (1980) Stenosis of the lumbar vertebral canal and sciatica. *Neurosurg. Rev.*, **3**, 75–89.

Verbiest, H. (1987) Introduction: spinal stenosis. In Hopp, E. (ed.), *Spine: State of the Art Reviews*, vol. 1, no. 3, pp. 361–368. Hanley & Belfus, Philadelphia, PA.

Watanabe, R. & Parke, W.W. (1986) Vascular and neural pathology of lumbosacral spinal stenosis. *J. Neurosurg.*, **64**, 64–70.

Weinstein, J.N., Spratt, K.F., Spengler, D., Brick, C. & Reid, S. (1988) Spinal pedicle fixation: reliability and validity of roentgenogram-based assessment and surgical factors on successful screw replacement. *Spine*, **13**, 1012–1018.

Wiltse, L.L. (1987) Salvage of failed lumbar spinal stenosis surgery. In Hopp, E. (ed.), *Spine: State of the Art Reviews*, vol. 1, no. 3, pp. 421–450. Hanley & Belfus, Philadelphia, PA.

Young, S., Veerapen, R. & O'Laoire, S. (1988) Relief of lumbar canal stenosis using multilevel subarticular fenestrations as alternative to wide laminectomy: preliminary report. *Neurosurgery*, **23**, 628–633.

42 · Adolescent Disc Disease

By M.F. SULLIVAN

What is a prolapsed intervertebral disc in an adolescent? The semantics of the word adolescence seems to pose the biggest single problem in diagnosis and hence treatment and results. Most authors seem to define adolescence as being under the age of 20 years (Grobler *et al.*, 1979; Leong *et al.*, 1982; Gibson *et al.*, 1987). Why this arbitrary age has been decided upon no authors seem to explain. If this age is accepted then three quite distinct pathologies need to be described: the vertebral rim fracture (Techakapuch, 1981; Ehni & Schneider, 1988); the young adult disc prolapse; and the true adolescent disc prolapse. All three present in much the same way and give very much the same neuroradiographic picture. However, the pathology and surgical treatment are somewhat different.

PATHOLOGY

The vast majority of so-called adolescent disc prolapses are in fact young adults similar in pathology to older patients. The internal architecture of the disc is deranged as seen on discography (Figs 42.1 & 42.2) or magnetic resonance imaging (MRI). These young people seem to have some abnormality in the disc proteoglycan. Gibson *et al.* (1987) reported a series of 20 adolescent patients with lumbar disc prolapse. Of these, 75% had multiple-level disc abnormality on MRI scan. In a different series (C. Sutton, personal communication) in which adolescent disc patients were treated by chymopapain, multiple-level disc degeneration was also seen to be common on discography. In the same way that Scheuermann's disease in adolescence often shows multiple endplate damage this does not mean that these radiographic abnormalities are symptomatic. In the control group of Gibson *et al.* (1987), 20% had disc abnormality on MRI scan, but had never had any lumbar spine symptoms.

In the posterior rim fracture there is a shear of the endplate with displacement of the attached annulus. The bone fragment can be seen on plain radiography and on computerized tomography (Fig. 42.3). Takata *et al.* (1988) reported a series of 29 patients with 31 vertebral rim or limbus fractures. They defined Type I lesions as simple separation of the posterior cortical margin. Type II and Type III lesions were more severe injuries consisting of central avulsion fractures extending into cancellous bone (Type II) and 'tear-drop' fracture frequently associated with proliferative callus (Type III). The Type I lesions have the potential to cause disc displacement causing an adolescent disc syndrome. Epstein *et al.* (1989) and Epstein & Epstein (1990) described a fourth type of limbus fracture which affected the entire length and breadth of the posterior vertebral body, causing marked compromise of the spinal canal. Reigel (1985) felt that between 8% and 20% of children with disc herniations had an associated limbus vertebral fracture.

The true adolescent disc prolapse is an intermediate between these two conditions. The child presents with all the signs and symptoms of a disc prolapse which is confirmed on neuroradiology but is normal on discography, but yet at surgery there is an obvious disc prolapse. On opening the disc the nucleus appears normal. This appears to be some sort of disc shear without any endplate involvement.

The importance of the latter two groups is that at surgery if one simply enucleates the disc the patient will have a poor result. The results of chemonucleolysis are also poor in such patients.

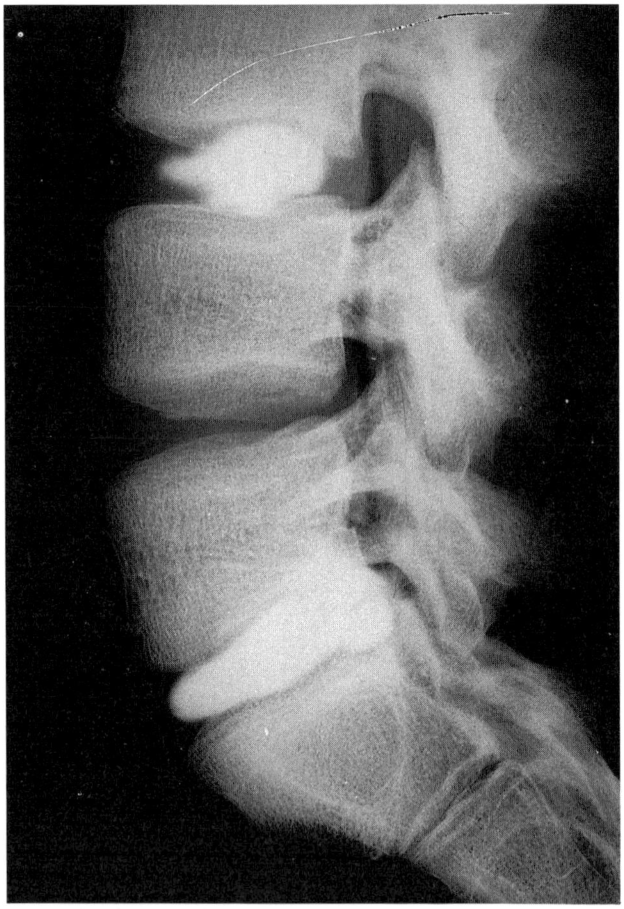

Fig. 42.1 Discography showing a normal L3–L4 disc but an abnormal L5–S1 disc in a teenager.

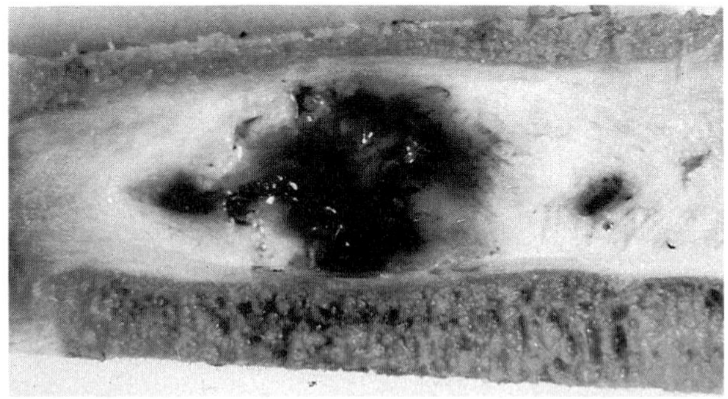

Fig. 42.2 Post-mortem study of a young L3–L4 disc. The nucleus has been injected with methylene blue, and spread of the dye along fissures in the annulus is clearly seen.

CLINICAL FEATURES

Under the age of 16 years girls are affected twice as frequently as boys; but between 16 and 20 the ratio is reversed, boys being affected twice as commonly as girls. This is probably because of the earlier maturity of girls. Also the period of active sporting activity is younger in girls than boys. There may of course be different pathologies, but that is unlikely. In general true adolescent discs are more common in younger girls, and boys tend to have the young adult type of disc degeneration.

Some patients with radiological evidence of disc degeneration will present with only back pain. However, patients with any of the three types of disc abnormality described above will also have sciatica (Grobler *et al.*, 1979). In these young people the sciatic pain often does not radiate as far distally as it does in older patients.

The most prominent physical finding is profound paravertebral and hamstring muscle spasm. Forward flexion is very limited (Fig. 42.4) but lateral flexion is not much affected. Scoliosis is present in 80% and especially in girls who are very aware of it.

An abnormal gait is always present to some extent due to the muscle spasm. The spasm may be so severe that the patients walk on tiptoe, and it may take many months for the spasm to settle following surgery.

All patients show marked limitation of straight leg raising which is normally bilateral, but cross-leg pain is unusual. Forty per cent of patients have a motor loss which is usually weakness of dorsiflexion in L5 root lesions. A further 40% will have a diminished or

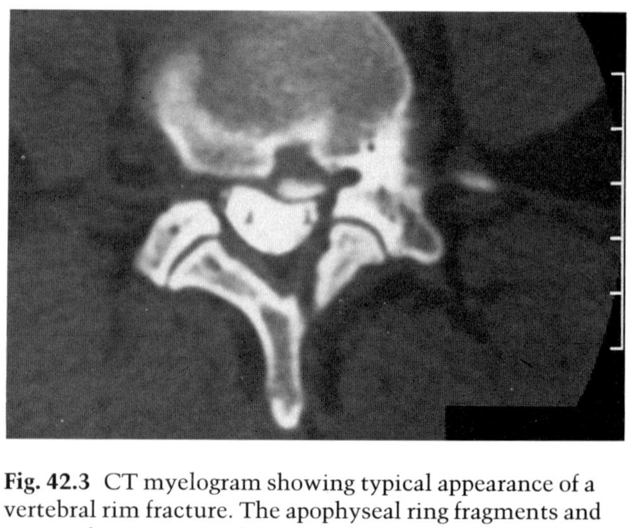

Fig. 42.3 CT myelogram showing typical appearance of a vertebral rim fracture. The apophyseal ring fragments and 'stripped-up' posterior longitudinal ligament is clearly seen.

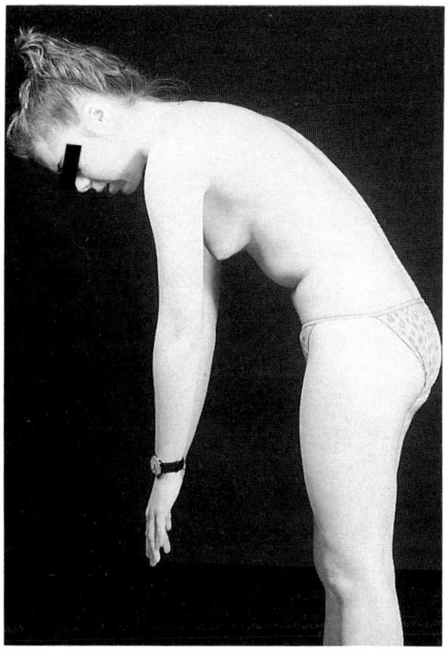

Fig. 42.4 Severe paravertebral and hamstring muscle spasm in a 14-year-old girl.

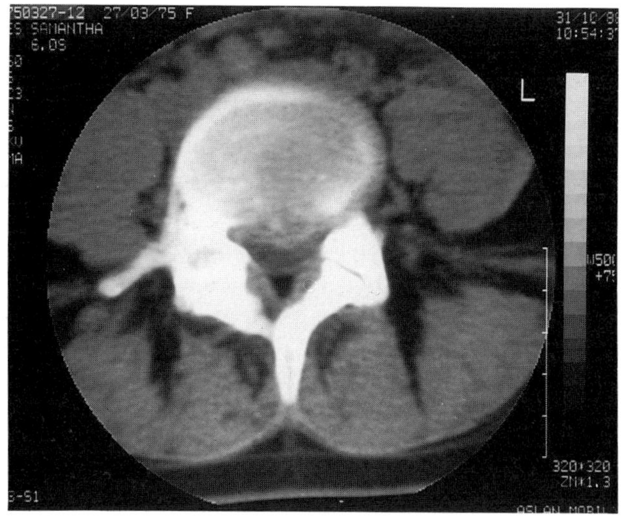

Fig. 42.5 CT scan showing a typical diffuse disc bulge.

absent ankle jerk, and 50% some sensory loss in the L5 or S1 root distribution. Bladder involvement can occur (Grobler *et al.*, 1979) but is rare.

Plain radiographs are unhelpful except in the vertebral rim fractures. Spina bifida, transitional vertebrae, and minor disc narrowing occurs in some of the patients but is not really significant and is unhelpful in diagnosis.

Myelography or MRI must be done to exclude a spinal tumour. If MRI is used the temptation to treat multiple levels must be resisted. There is only ever one significant pathological level. Discography should not be used as a diagnostic investigation. CT scanning will show a diffuse disc bulge (Fig. 42.5). If myelography, CT and MRI are normal the child does not need surgery.

Differential diagnosis

Spondylolisthesis of the dysplastic type commonly occurs in this age group with very similar symptoms. The lesion is easily seen on a plain radiograph. A spondylolysis can be more difficult to see, but can be confirmed on isotopic bone scanning.

An isotopic bone scan is very useful in investigating back and leg pain in children. It will not only confirm a spondylolysis but also will confirm an osteoid osteoma, and frequently confirms infectious disease of bone. In many parts of the world, spinal tuberculosis is still very common in childhood. The lesion is usually visible on plain radiology and can be confirmed by needle biopsy.

The most important differential diagnosis is with intraspinal tumours. If myelography or MRI are used routinely these will not be missed. Similarly the tethered spinal cord and diastematomyelia will be picked up on myelography. CT scanning alone will fail to diagnose the presence of such lesions.

TREATMENT

The efficacy of conservative treatment is very difficult to assess. There must be a small number of patients that have small disc prolapses that resolve over a few weeks and are never seen in specialist clinics. However, conventional conservative therapy should always be tried prior to considering surgery, unless there is major neurological deficit. Rest and analgesics are as likely to succeed as any other conservative therapy. Physiotherapy is uniformly unsuccessful due to the intense muscle spasm. If there has been no improvement at all by three months it is likely that the clinical course will be very protracted, and surgery should be considered.

The time from the start of symptoms to surgery averages nearly a year in most series. There is a natural reluctance to operate on the back of young patients. Certainly the symptoms improve markedly with bed rest, but rapidly regress when the patient becomes ambulant. The other reason for persevering with conservative treatment is that these children are remarkably stoic and uncomplaining even with severe disability.

Chemonucleolysis has been advocated as the treatment of choice for the adolescent disc; but this is not uniformly accepted. The ideal patient for chemonucleolysis is the young adult disc prolapse with positive neurological signs, and a positive myelogram. In a 10-year follow-up of the author's cases treated by chemonucleolysis, the 18–25-year age group had a success rate of 80%. It therefore seems reasonable to treat patients with the young adult type of prolapse who are in the late teenage group with chemonucleolysis.

Younger patients, and those with either vertebral rim fractures or true adolescent discs, should be treated surgically. Leong *et al.* (1982) advocated the anterior approach with total excision of the affected disc combined with an anterior interbody fusion. The majority of series, however, recommend a conventional posterior approach. It is quite unnecessary to do a formal laminectomy. An interlaminar approach should be used. In the true adolescent disc material cannot, by definition, be sequestrated. The annulus should be opened and if there is degenerative disc material, this should be cleared. If the nerve root is clear nothing further needs to be done.

Leong *et al.* (1982), reporting anterior disc excision combined with fusion, found a 90% success rate. Similarly Grobler *et al.* (1979) had 90% success simply doing posterior disc excision.

Ehni & Schneider (1988) reported two cases of vertebral rim fracture and reviewed the other 20 cases which had been reported at that stage. Trauma occurred in many of the cases and it was postulated that it caused disruption of the cartilaginous attachments of the apophyseal ring which then displaced posteriorly carrying the annulus with it. Reviewing the literature, they found that most had been treated by full laminectomy, discectomy and removal of the bony ridge. However, Ehni & Schneider felt that a more limited approach by a fenestration with discectomy and medial facetectomy without removal of the bony ridge was effective. Epstein & Epstein (1990) also felt the laminectomy was not always necessary, but they did stress the necessity for performing a generous decompression of the lateral recess, and felt that removal of the displaced vertebral rim was indeed necessary.

It is very easy to fool oneself into believing that a good result has been obtained. As previously stated, these children do not complain of much pain. It is easy to see the patient at follow-up, ask about pain and assume the continuing stiffness is just postoperative stiffness, and will wear off.

REFERENCES

Ehni, G. & Schneider, S.J. (1988) Posterior lumbar vertebral rim fracture and associated disc protrusion in adolescence. *J. Neurosurg.*, **68**, 912–916.

Epstein, N.E. & Epstein, J.A. (1990) Limbus vertebral fractures of the lumbar spine and spinal stenosis in five adolescents with further evaluation of Type III fractures. *Neur. Orthop.*, **9**, 33–52.

Epstein, N.E., Epstein, J.A. & Mauri, T. (1989) Treatment of limbus vertebral fractures and spinal stenosis in 4 adolescents and 5 young adults. *Neurosurgery*, **24**, 595–604.

Gibson, M.J., Szypryt, E.P., Buckley, J.H., Worthington, B.S. & Mulholland, R.C. (1987) Magnetic resonance imaging of adolescent disc herniation. *J. Bone Jt. Surg.*, **69B**, 6990–6703.

Grobler, L.J., Simmons, E.H. & Barrington, T.W. (1979) Intervertebral disc herniation in the adolescent. *Spine*, **4**, 267–278.

Leong, Y.C.Y., Hooper, G., Fang, D. & Chun, S.Y. (1982) Disc excision and anterior spinal fusion for lumbar disc protrusion in the adolescent. *Spine*, **7**, 623–626.

Reigel, D.H. (1985) Slipped lumbar apophyseal ring. *Concepts Paediatr. Neurosurg.*, **5**, 34–40.

Takata, K., Inove, S., Takahashi, K. & Ohtsuka, Y. (1988) Fracture of the posterior margin of lumbar vertebral body. *J. Bone Jt. Surg.*, **70A**, 589–594.

Techakapuch, S. (1981) Rupture of the lumbar cartilage plate into the spinal canal in an adolescent. *J. Bone Jt. Surg.*, **63A**, 481–482.

43 · Lumbar Spondylolisthesis

By R.C. MULHOLLAND

Slipping of the fourth or fifth lumbar vertebra over its inferior neighbour was mentioned by Herbineaux, a Belgian obstetrician in the latter part of the 18th century, and Rokitansky in 1839; Kilian in 1954 described the pathological findings. But it was Neugebauer in the 1880s who drew attention to its clinical importance, especially as a cause of obstructed labour, and spinal deformity (Neugebauer, 1888). He looked at many pathological specimens and it was clear that some had a defect in the pars interarticularis, a spondylolysis. This defect allowed the vertebra to slide forwards and was a cause of the slip in some patients. But there were other causes, and in 1963 Newman presented the first clear classification of the disorder. This classification was modified by Newman in conjunction with Wiltse and McNab in 1973, and is now the one that is generally accepted (Wiltse *et al.*, 1976).

CLASSIFICATION (Fig. 43.1)

1 Dysplastic. In this type there are congenital abnormalities of the upper sacrum and the arch of L5. This is commoner in girls, approximately three girls to two boys, and severe slip is commoner in females.
2 Isthmic. The lesion is in the pars interarticularis (this type is more common in males). Three types can be recognized.
  (a) lytic–fatigue fracture of the pars,
  (b) elongated but intact pars,
  (c) acute fracture.
3 Degenerative. Due to segmental failure both in the disc and in the facet joints, leading to degenerative osteoarthritis of the facet joints.
4 Traumatic. Due to fractures in areas of the bony hook other than the pars.
5 Pathological. There is generalized or localized bone disease.

Types 3, 4 and 5 are clearly different pathologies, but Types 1 and 2 are the same underlying disorder although clinically the presentation may be very different. The secondary effects of slip make further slip more likely. As the defect in the pars is used to define Type 2, and yet may be present in Type 1, the distinction between these first two types at the earliest stage of the disorder (minimal or no slip) is blurred, and it has not been possible to identify any features at this stage which will predict slip, although the presence of a spina bifida, and poor facet joints, suggest the likelihood of progression. Both the dysplastic and lytic varieties of spondylolisthesis have a genetic element in their causation; this is more marked in the dysplastic type. There may also be a greater flexibility or looseness at the L5–S1 segment in those children in whom the spondylolysis is subsequently associated with major slip (Wiltse *et al.*, 1975; Albanese & Pizzutillo, 1982).

Dysplastic

There is merit in regarding all major spondylolisthesis, those over 30%, as being dysplastic, because lytic spondylolisthesis does not slip further than this. Slip occurs soon after the development of the lysis, and in the adolescent growth spurt. Once slip is over 30% then the concern is whether it is likely to continue to slip. The development of various secondary bony changes described below is a result of the slipping, rather than a genetically determined abnormality; but this may be a factor in causing that slip to continue. There is evidence to suggest that once a spondylolisthesis exceeds 50% there are

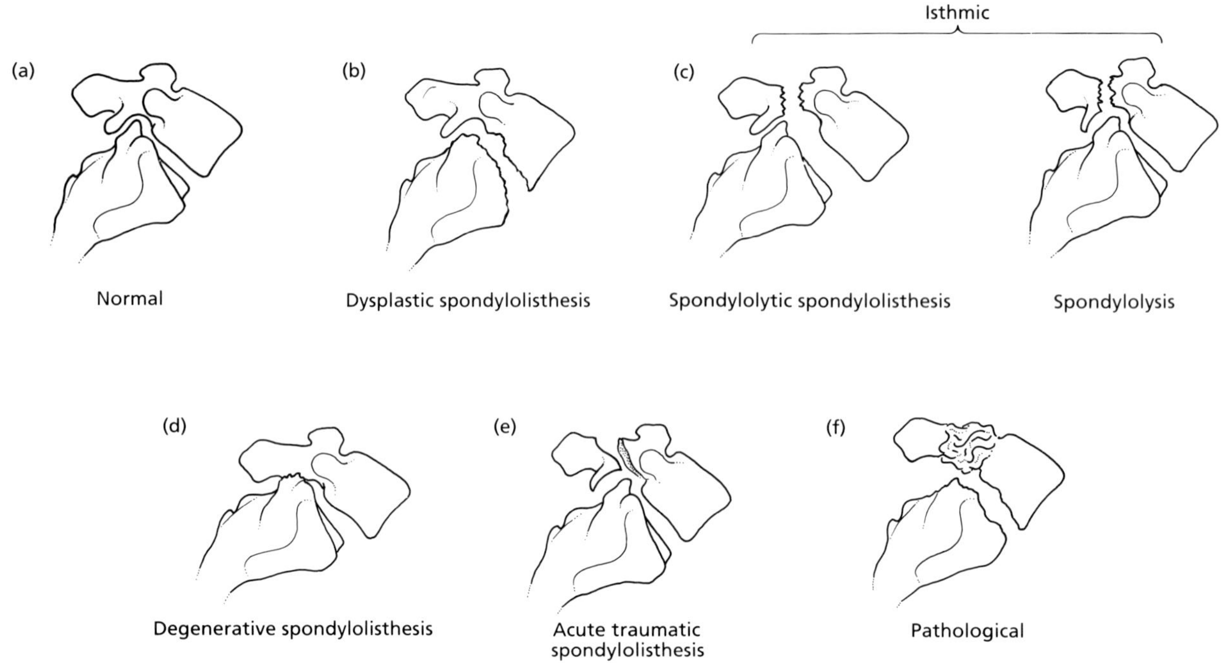

Fig. 43.1 Classification of lumbar spondylolisthesis. Modified from Wiltse *et al.* (1976).

dynamic and anatomical factors in the growing child which encourage further slip (Blackburn & Velikas, 1977; Bradford, 1983; Frederickson *et al.*, 1984; Saraste *et al.*, 1984b).

MEASUREMENT OF DEFORMITY

Various anatomical measurements can be made to assess the degree of deformity all of which express numerically the extent of the deformity.

Degree of slip

The two favoured methods to define slip are:

1 Meyerding method. This divides the anteroposterior diameter of the superior surface of the first sacral vertebra into quarters and assigns a grade of I, II, III or IV to slips of one, two, three or four quarters, respectively.

2 Taillard method (modified by Boxall). This signifies the percentage slip. The amount of slipping is calculated by measuring the distance from a line parallel to the posterior portion of the first sacral vertebra to a line drawn parallel to the posterior portion of the fifth lumbar vertebra. This is divided by the anteroposterior dimension of the inferior surface of the fifth lumbar vertebra, and the resulting figure is multiplied by 100.

Sacral inclination

This is the angle formed between a line drawn parallel to the back of the sacrum, and a vertical line drawn in a standing radiograph.

Angle of slip

This measures the degree of forward tilting or gibbus present. The angle is formed by a line drawn parallel to the inferior surface of the fifth vertebra, and a line drawn perpendicular to the posterior aspect of the first sacral vertebra. A particular method of doing this measurement (Speck *et al.*, 1984) is to draw one line parallel to the top of the fifth lumbar and one line along the inferior and undeformed surface of the first sacral segment. Normally this line should converge dorsally (a positive value). With a kyphosis it converges ventrally (a negative value). It will be appreciated that this latter measurement gives the angle of kyphosis or angulation forward of the spine.

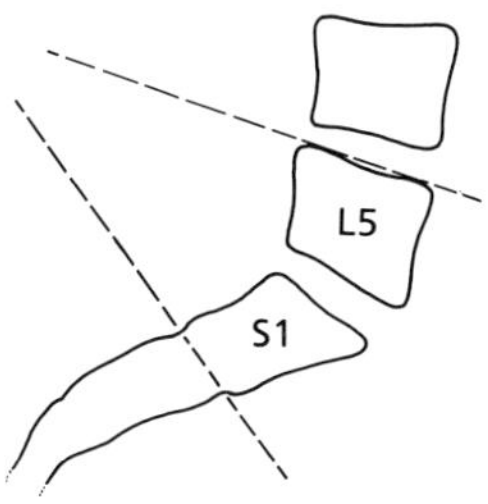

Fig. 43.2 The angle of kyphosis. Positive value in lordosis. After Speck (1984).

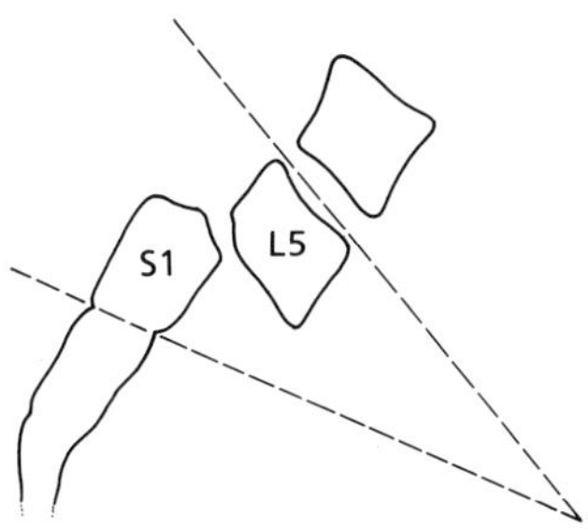

Fig. 43.3 The angle of kyphosis. Negative value in kyphosis. After Speck (1984).

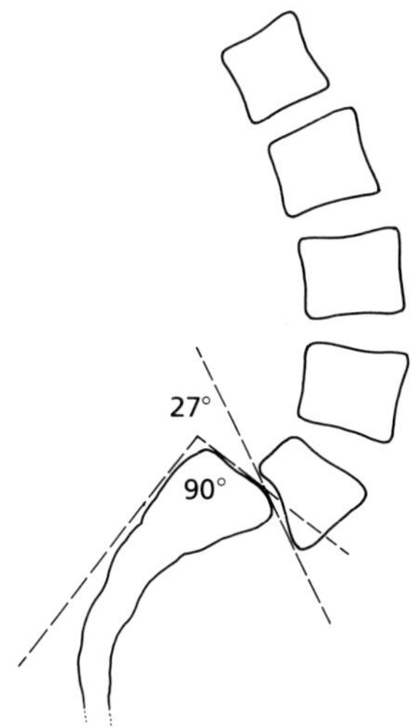

Fig. 43.4 Slip angle.

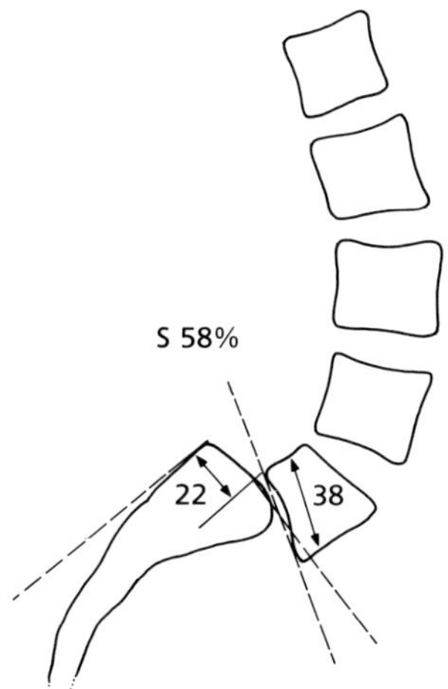

Fig. 43.5 Percentage slip. Taillard method. Modified from Boxall *et al.* (1979).

Measurements can be made of the degree of deformity of the fifth vertebra, its trapezoidal shape, and the rounded top of the first sacral vertebra. In fact all these indices and angles worsen as the degree of slip increases, but the most important is the slip angle. It is what produces a cosmetic deformity and is the one measurement that seems to be related to the liability of further slip (Boxall *et al.*, 1979; Wiltse & Winter, 1983; Speck *et al.*, 1984).

The classic clinical presentation is in a young girl, between the ages of 10 and 18 years, with a rigid back, tight hamstrings, a scoliosis and often a curious limp. There may not be a lot of pain, and this 'crisis' is thought to be due to cauda equina irritation, initiated by a sudden increase in a slip which may still be minimal. The scoliosis is due to spasm, although a few patients have a true structural curve which is always quite small (Libson *et al.*, 1984b). Occasionally there is so little discomfort in the back that the limp or curious gait may be the reason the patient consults the doctor. Significant neurological compromise is unusual despite the rather alarming appearances on radiography. If the pars does not fracture or lengthen as slip occurs, proportionately to the degree of slip, then the posterior elements become a compressing factor, so that S1 root problems and a cauda equina lesion may occur. If the pars fractures or lengthens appropriately then there is no risk of a cauda equina lesion, but the L5 root can be irritated (Buirski *et al.*, 1984).

Further significant slip does not occur once growth has ceased, so that if, as can sometimes occur, a child with a dysplastic spondylolisthesis remains asymptomatic throughout adolescence, or has minimal symptoms which it is felt do not justify intervention, then he or she is likely to remain either asymptomatic or only have minimal symptoms for some years (Harris & Weinstein, 1987).

MANAGEMENT

If an adolescent presents with symptoms and has a slip of over 50% then surgical treatment is indicated. Although adults, as mentioned above, may have a major slip and be asymptomatic, they do not usually give a history of problems in adolescence which subsequently resolved.

In a lesser degree of slip, under 50%, pain and disability are the indications for surgical treatment rather than the deformity itself. It is therefore appropriate in such cases to have a period of bracing, but unless this causes a complete resolution of symptoms and allows a return to full function, operation is required. Excellent results of bracing have been reported with even some degree of correction in some patients and no further slip in any patient. But this has been achieved only by a thoracolumbar sacral brace applied for 23 out of the 24 hours a day, for up to two years. This prolonged period of bracing covers the adolescent growth spurt period, when slip is particularly likely to occur. Whether this is a more 'conservative' treatment than operation is arguable. It seems likely that the natural stability which patients have developed during the period of bracing is as satisfactory as the stability achieved in those patients with a similar degree of slip who either do not present clinically, or become asymptomatic with a much shorter period of bracing. It is, however, not established whether in the long term they will do as well as a patient who has had a fusion without reduction (Edelmann, 1984; Bell *et al.*, 1988). The more usual practice is to use a brace for a shorter period, and wean the patient from it gradually when the acute episode has settled. If the symptoms recur surgical treatment is proceeded with.

Operative treatment

Fusion without reduction

The reason for reduction of a spondylolisthesis is to increase the height of the patient and improve the appearance of the back. In slips of under 50% (usually associated with a slip angle of under 30°) the cosmetic deformity is minimal and reduction is not indicated, having regard to the potential complications of reduction. A posterolateral fusion from L5 to S1 is most appropriate. But clearly a posterior fusion alone, to succeed, would have to include L4, as there would be no merit in fusing a loose posterior element unconnected to the body of L5, which is all that a posterior fusion of L5 to S1 would achieve. In slips of over 50% L4 is in any event included in the fusion, the transverse process of L5 being too far forward and too close to the ala of the sacrum to allow a mechanically sound fusion to develop.

Many series report a significant incidence of non-union (up to 16%) and also an incidence of postoperative slip (19%). These are more likely if the preoperative (slip) is over 50%. Treating the patient after operation in recumbency in a pantaloon cast for some two months, and the application of a Boston type brace (thoracolumbosacral) worn for a further period until fusion is solid, significantly reduces these complications. However, as in lesser degrees of slip (under 50% and a low slip angle) non-union and a slight slip postoperatively is compatible with a very satisfactory clinical result, it would seem reasonable to restrict the use of recumbency and prolonged postoperative bracing to the more major slips, and those with a high slip angle (kyphotic angle) (Turner & Bianco, 1981; Johnson & Kirwan, 1983; Pizzutillo *et al.*, 1986; Seitsalo *et al.*, 1988).

Anterior fusion (without reduction) is an alternative to posterolateral fusion, but the morbidity of this procedure is somewhat higher and there is no clear advantage. At the L5–S1 level if there is a slip of over 50% the approach has to be transperitoneal. However, with lesser degrees of slip the approach may be retroperitoneal through a left loin incision. The transperitoneal exposure may injure the presacral nerve in the male, leading to retrograde ejaculation and sterility. This is probably very rare but the possibility is alarming to the surgeon, the parents and the patient (Freebody *et al.*, 1971; Flynn & Priae, 1984).

Although patients with a major slip, who have a posterolateral fusion complicated by non-union and some degree of postoperative slip, are frequently asymptomatic, a few may have disabling symptoms, especially if they are adults when the operation is done. Anterior fusion in this postsurgical symptomatic group is a valuable salvage procedure, on occasion supplemented by re-fusion posterolaterally (Bradford & Gotfried, 1987; Jones *et al.*, 1988).

Decompression in dysplastic spondylolisthesis

Despite the rather alarming radiculographic appearance, neural decompression is seldom necessary in children and adolescents. Patients who have objective neurological abnormalities (clearly defined sensory loss, motor weakness, and reflex changes) should be appropriately decompressed, as well as fused. Patients with radicular pain without objective signs can be safely fused without decompression and symptoms of root irritation will resolve as the fusion becomes solid (Johnson *et al.*, 1988).

Excision of the whole of the loose posterior element alone adequately decompresses the cauda equina (Gill *et al.*, 1955). But this is not an appropriate procedure for children or adolescents, as it may be followed by further slip. However, it may be appropriate for the adult presenting much later who has a dysplastic spondylolisthesis, but who has only radicular symptoms, and no backache. It is a much lesser procedure than a fusion, and although in the young adult it may occasionally be followed by an increase of the slip, this is not necessarily associated with a clinical failure (Gill & White, 1965; Amuso *et al.*, 1970; Gill, 1984).

A posterolateral fusion alone, without root decompression, can be successful in relieving root pain, even when preoperative investigations suggest evidence of root compression supported clinically by reflex changes (but no objective motor changes). This is important because it is realized that root decompression of a major slip in an adult may destabilize a spondylolisthesis (especially if it needs to be more extensive than just excision of the loose posterior lamina), and therefore will need, in any event, to be combined with a fusion. If an extensive decompression is required, this might need to be an anterior fusion, the patients therefore requiring two operations (Peek *et al.*, 1989).

Reduction and fusion

An adolescent with a major slip, especially if presenting with a 'crisis', has a very obvious deformity made more obvious by the presence of tight hamstrings and frequently a scoliosis. It is reasonable to assume that restoration of the normal anatomy at the lumbosacral level will reduce the abnormal stresses on the spine above. Although there is no clear evidence that spondylolisthesis produces disc injury above the level of the slip (Henson *et al.*, 1987) it is natural that in the circumstances reduction of the deformity should be considered. It is also true that, as stated above, there is a significant incidence of postoperative slip and non-union after a posterolateral fusion alone; so possibly repositioning the vertebrae in a more normal position might be expected to improve the fusion rate. The success of Harrington instrumentation in the management of scoliosis encouraged its use in dealing with major degrees of spondylolisthesis. However, disappointingly there was an unacceptable rate of failure of the implants, and therefore over the past few years a wide variety of alternative implants have been used. It is now clear that if reduction is carried out then fusion anteriorly must be achieved. Stabilization with an implant is required posteriorly, and hence a posterolateral fusion is also carried out. Although when an open reduction is carried out the neural elements are protected, such reduction carried out even by very experienced surgeons is associated unfortunately in some patients with neurological complications, often minor and transient but some serious and permanent. It seems likely that some of the cosmetic deformity complained of by the adolescent with a major spondylolisthetic slip is a consequence of the spasm alluded to, producing the rather curious gait. This disappears when the fusion is solid, which may be one reason why fusion *in situ* of major slips seems to produce an acceptable cosmetic result in the great majority of patients. When one considers the modest disability the untreated disorder produces, then it would seem inappropriate to carry out the major surgery associated with reduction, especially as this may be associated with neurological complications (Snijder *et al.*, 1976; Harrington *et al.*, 1976; Boxall *et al.*, 1979; Dewald *et al.*, 1981; Sijbrandij, 1983; McQueen *et al.*, 1986; Matthiass & Heine, 1986; Noack & Raetzel, 1988; Dick & Schnebel, 1988; Steffee & Sitkowski, 1988).

It has been suggested that an early posterior operation in the growing child may produce a tether effect which may lead to an improvement in the kyphotic angle with continued vertebral growth anteriorly. Recent long-term studies of patients with a high-level slip treated by a posterolateral fusion without reduction have shown a high degree of patient satisfaction, and very little complaint concerning spinal cosmesis (Johnson, 1983; Harris *et al.*, 1987; Seitsalo *et al.*, 1988; Freeman & Donate, 1989).

More recently Freeman & Donate (1989), in a long-term follow-up, have shown that posterior and intertransverse fusion without reduction was associated in 10 out of 12 patients with an acceptable cosmetic result; indeed there had been no further slip of the spondylolisthesis after surgery.

Closed reduction with open fusion

A more recent development is to undertake a closed reduction after fusion, aiming only to correct the kyphotic angle (the principal cosmetic deformity) (Bradford, 1988). In this technique a posterolateral fusion is carried out, usually L4 to S1 (the fourth vertebra is included because with the higher degrees of slip the transverse process of L5 is so far forward that the fusion mass would be under a constant shear stress). Reduction is carried out postoperatively, using traction and a Risser table. Traction may be used preoperatively, and some form of external fixation (wires in the spinous processes or pelvic pins incorporated in the plaster may be used). A plaster spica is applied and worn for some months. This technique corrects the angle of slip (kyphotic angle), producing a degree of cosmetic improvement. However, of 22 patients so treated, one required an anterior fusion because of loss of correction and two patients had a transient radiculopathy (Bradford, 1988).

The present position regarding reduction of spondylolisthesis would appear to be that there is no indication in lesser degrees of slip because these do not present a significant cosmetic problem. It is misguided to aim for a reduction of a 50% displacement to a 25% displacement, because to achieve that it is necessary either to significantly destabilize any natural anterior stability or, if these tissues are stretched only, then an unacceptable degree of stress is placed on the internal fixation device. Even with such partial reductions neurological complications may occur.

In patients with a kyphotic angle over 55°, usually they have displacement of over 70% (Boxall *et al.*, 1979) then reduction of the kyphotic angle certainly produces an improved appearance, and this can be achieved by posterior surgery alone combined with internal fixation. It would seem wise to combine internal fixation with rigid external bracing until fusion is assured, even if one is only correcting the angle of kyphosis. The disadvantage of aiming to significantly reduce the slip as well is that fusion has to be achieved anteriorly and posteriorly, with or without internal fixation. There is a significant risk of some neurological injury and also a risk of fusion failure and some loss of reduction. Indeed this is as high a risk as with a posterolateral fusion without reduction. Unlike fusion without reduction, where failure of fusion is not infrequently asymptomatic, fusion failure after major reduction is likely to be symptomatic and further operation may be required.

SPONDYLOLYTIC OR ISTHMIC SPONDYLOLISTHESIS

This is a far commoner type of disorder than the dysplastic variety, presenting clinically if at all in the late teens and early 20s. The core abnormality of this group is the presence of a spondylolysis; yet this can, of course, be present in the dysplastic group. It is the fact that this is present with normal facet joints, and a lack of dysplasia of the posterior elements, that means that in this group slip is never more than 30%, hence there is no need to consider reduction in this group of patients and spinal deformity is not a consideration. A number of longitudinal studies of this disorder have added to our understanding of the natural history, and therefore allow for more logical management.

In a long-term follow-up of 500 children, none of whom had the dysplastic variety, over a 25-year period (Frederickson *et al.*, 1984) the authors came to the following conclusions. The incidence at the age of six of spondylolysis with or without spondylolisthesis was 4.4% compared with 6.5% in adults. The male : female ratio was 2 : 1. Slipping could occur up to the age of 16, but usually was demonstrated at the same time that the spondylolysis was first detected radiologically. This confirmed an earlier report (Blackburn & Velikas, 1977) that if at presentation a slip was less than 30% then a slip to over 30% was unlikely. Two-thirds of the children with spondylolysis had a spondylolisthesis. This was never more than a 30% slip in this series. The shape of the fifth vertebra is a result of slip, and not the cause. Not all 500 children were followed to adulthood, although once a defect was found the patient was observed. Of the 27 patients with a spondylolysis or spondylolisthesis, only four developed backache as an adult, and only one underwent surgery to deal with a disc protrusion at the level above that of the defect. The authors conclude that a child with a spondylolysis or spondylolisthesis can be permitted to enjoy a normal childhood without restriction of activities, if he or she is asymptomatic. If a child on presentation has a slip of under 30% and there is no spina bifida or obvious dysplasia, then that child belongs to the lytic group, rather than the dysplastic group, and there would seem little merit in serial X-rays throughout adolescence (Oakley & Carty, 1984). However, even if such a case were asymptomatic, but had evidence of dysplasia and a slip over 30%, the child should be considered to be in Group I or dysplastic group and then serial X-rays should be done, especially during the adolescent growth spurt, as a slip to over 50% may be asymptomatic. If progressive slip is occurring then, despite the child being asymptomatic, it would seem wise to fuse at a stage where a posterolateral fusion alone is likely to succeed, rather than having to deal with a high-level slip.

The genetic element in spondylolysis has been confirmed in a number of studies. If the frequency of the defect is 5–6% in the normal Caucasian population, it increases up to 35% in families where one member has a spondylolysis or spondylolisthesis. This genetic effect, however, is more marked in the dysplastic group (Wiltse, 1975; Wynn-Davies & Scott, 1979; Pfeil *et al.*, 1987).

Pregnancy and spondylolysis

A recent study indicated that pregnancy did not lead to progression of the disorder, or to increased problems after pregnancy compared with women who had not been pregnant who had the disorder. Despite the historical association between spondylolisthesis and labour complications, in this particular study spondylolisthesis did not lead to obstetric problems (Saraste, 1966).

Stress or sport and spondylosis

The considerably higher incidence of the defect in special groups of adolescents, such as gymnasts and American football players, would suggest that the development of the defect in adolescence may be related to a stress fracture (Jackson *et al.*, 1976; Letts *et al.*, 1986). In a group of mature college freshmen, all very keen sportsmen, entering college on sports scholarships, the incidence of spondylolysis was 15.2% which, despite their continuing sports activities, only rose by a further 2% (McCarroll *et al.*, 1986). It is of interest that there is also an increased incidence in helicopter pilots, apparently related to vibrational stress (Froom *et al.*, 1984).

From these studies it is clear that the spondylolytic defect is a stress fracture in a genetically vulnerable population. It seems that if slip or spondylolisthesis is going to occur it occurs fairly early in the disorder, probably in the first year after the fracture, or during the adolescent growth spurt. It is clear that major slip does not occur in Type II spondylolysis because of the well-formed facet joints and the absence of associated dysplasia.

Clinical features

The young patient presenting with back pain due to a spondylolysis is found to have minimal restriction of spinal movement, but with pain at extremes especially on forward flexion and hyperextension. There will be pain after activity, but only occasionally sciatica. Usually spinal stiffness is a feature of discogenic disorder, and its absence should alert the doctor to the possibility of a spondylolysis being present, the disc being normal.

Radiological and other investigations

As well as coned anteroposterior and lateral views of the lumbosacral area, obliques must be taken as some 20% of lytic defects will be missed if only the standard anteroposterior and lateral films are relied on (Gehweiler & Daffner, 1983; Libson *et al.*, 1984a). There may be some merit in doing a technisium bone scan if there is a suggestion of a recent injury. A hot scan at the site of a lysis would indicate a degree of bone activity and suggest a propensity for healing (Lowe *et al.*, 1984; Collier *et al.*, 1985; Papanicolaou *et al.*, 1985; Elliott *et al.*, 1988; Van-den Oever *et al.*, 1987).

Although computerized tomography can show a lysis, unfortunately if the axial cut is above or below the defect it will not be demonstrated. However, it does show the rather curious appearance of the disc area when a spondylolisthesis has occurred, the so-called pseudo-bulging of the disc (Teplick *et al.*, 1986). If a spondylolisthesis is not recognized this peculiar appearance may be misinterpreted as a true disc protrusion. Oblique tomography is the most effective method of demonstrating a lysis if there is doubt after ordinary oblique films have been taken. This is of especial importance in demonstrating a unilateral lysis (McAffee & Yuan, 1982; Porter & Park, 1982).

Management

There are five clinical situations we may meet in the management of isthmic spondylolisthesis at the lumbosacral level in the young person under 25 years.

1 The adult or adolescent found to have a lytic defect but who has no symptoms. In the under 20-year-old it would seem wise to keep under review for a year or so, and in the younger adolescent to advise against taking up sports such as gymnastics, fast bowling, netball and those sports involving hyperextension or shear forces across the pars (Wiltse *et al.*, 1975; Farfan *et al.*, 1976; Troup, 1976). However, if they were already heavily involved in such sports, then they should be permitted to continue, pointing out to them that there was some risk of aggravation, and if they got back symptoms they would have to stop those particular sports. But once over 20 years it seems likely that the spine is sufficiently stable for the patient to lead a normal life, and no career restraints should be imposed.

2 The adolescent or young adult with a lysis and a degree of slip, but also with no symptoms. Such patients do not need surgical treatment but there should be some career advice as certainly the back is vulnerable. There is some evidence that disc failure is more likely at the level of a spondylolisthesis than at a normal level (Szypryt, 1989). However, it is important to emphasize to the patient that there is no risk in the adult of further significant slip. There may be some forward displacement throughout life as the disc fails, and such people have a somewhat higher risk of backache than a normal person, but the doctor should be judicious in his advice, and not cause such anxiety about the future that the person becomes unduly concerned about his or her back.

3 The adolescent presenting with backache, who is found to have a spondylolytic defect, but with no slip. This is best treated with a period of support with a brace, to allow the stress fracture to heal or stabilize. If a bone scan is positive, the probability of healing is greater. If the spondylolysis is unilateral the probability of it healing with bracing is much greater than if it is bilateral. If symptoms subside after a few months whether the lysis heals or not the patient should be encouraged to lead a full and normal life.

4 The adolescent or young adult who presents with backache and is found to have a lysis but whose symptoms do not settle with a period of rest and the use of a lumbar support, or recur when they return to normal activity. If the patient is under 25 years it is likely that the back pain is due to the lysis (McNab, 1977). Myelography (radiculography) is indicated only if there is radicular pain, to exclude the presence of a coincidental disc protrusion, or if it is feared that a spinal tumour may be present. If the disc at the level of the spondylolysis is normal (as shown either by discography or MRI scan), then repair of the lysis is appropriate. If the disc is already abnormal then local fusion of the segment is to be preferred.

5 The adolescent with a spondylolysis and a slip and persistent symptoms, this group merits fusion.

Lytic spondylolysis and spondylolisthesis in the older person

A person over 35 years may present with backache and a lysis may be found. Backache is a common disability and some 50% of people at some stage will consult their doctor regarding the pain. Spondylolysis is a cause of back pain and is present in 4% of the population. Hence in the person over 35 years the two may coexist without there being any relationship between them, whereas under 25 years a spondylolysis is probably the cause of back pain. Between 25 and 35 years there is clearly a greater likelihood that the cause of the backache is the lysis, but over 35 years one should carefully seek for other causes (McNab, 1977). Injury may cause a previously asymptomatic lysis to become symptomatic. The development of magnetic resonance imaging (MRI) allows imaging at one sitting of all the lumbar discs, and therefore allows one to detect whether any other disc could be a source of low back pain. A useful investigation is to inject an anaesthetic into the lysis area under radiological imaging, confirming placement with contrast. It is usually the case that the anaesthetic also anaesthetizes the associated facet joints, but at least relief of pain indicates the segmental cause of the pain. Generally one should be reluctant to assume that a spondylolysis without any slip in the over-35-year-old is a cause of back pain. Such an assumption is probably why the result of fusion for spondylolysis in the older person is less successful clinically in relieving back pain.

However, if there is an associated spondylolisthesis it is somewhat more likely that back pain is from that

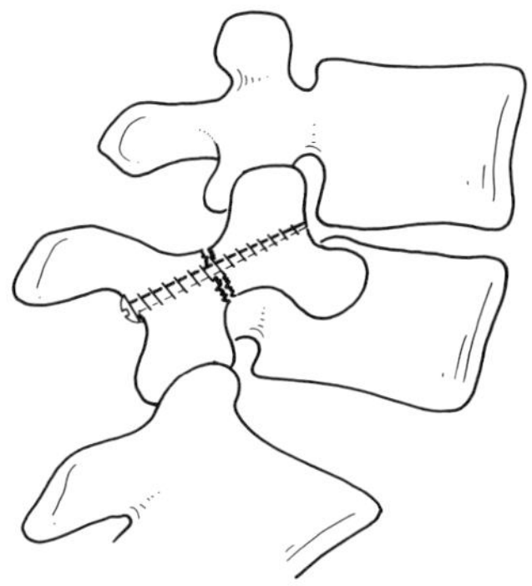

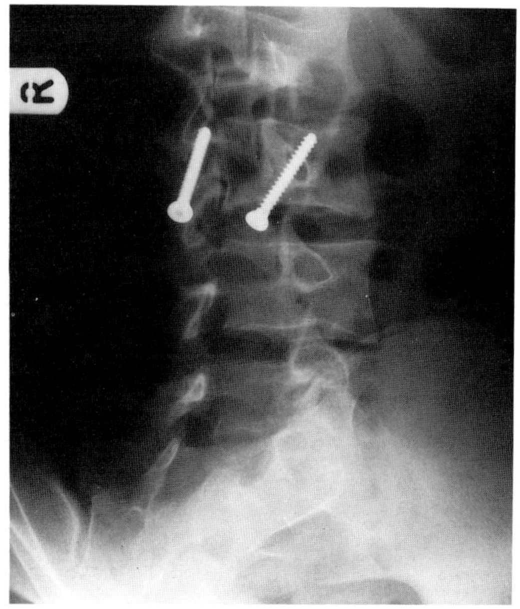

Fig. 43.6 Buck repair.

segment. There is, however, a higher degree of disc failure associated with a spondylolysis, and pain may be from segmental failure due to the combination of disc disturbance and the failure of the posterior elements.

In some patients the exuberant bone from the area of the lysis may impinge on the L4–L5 facet joint and be a cause of pain in extension, and produce complaints of something catching in the back on certain movements.

Spondylolysis, spondylolisthesis and sciatica

The most important late complication of a lysis, almost invariably associated with some degree of spondylolisthesis, is the development of sciatica. This may be due to the root being entrapped beneath the lysis (L5 root at a L5–S1 lysis) or it may be due to a disc protrusion. A disc protrusion at the L5–S1 level, that is at the level of the lysis, will produce symptoms and signs of an S1 root entrapment. However a protrusion at the L4–L5 level will produce signs of an L5 root lesion, and thus mimic root entrapment due to the lysis. Hence it is important to carry out a radiculogram or equivalent investigation (CT or MRI) in a patient with sciatica and a spondylolysis. If it is established that the cause of the sciatica is due to the lysis and there is no discogenic cause, then unilateral removal of the loose posterior element is appropriate. Clearly if the patient has a bilateral radiculopathy associated with and shown to be caused by the lysis, then excision of the whole of the loose element is appropriate.

Surgical treatment

There are three methods of repair of the lysis.

1 Buck repair. In this technique the defect is screwed together and bone slip graft applied around it. This is appropriate when there is a minimal defect (Buck, 1970).

2 Scott repair (Nicol & Scott, 1986). In this technique a wire is passed around the transverse processes and then around the spinous process of the affected vertebra making a figure of eight. The wire is tightened to approximate the posterior element to the root of the transverse processes, thereby closing the gap. Bone graft can be placed within the gap and around it. This has the great advantage that it can be used when there is a size of gap that is too large for the Buck technique. It allows graft to be placed within the gap rather than having much of the gap filled by a screw. If, as occasionally occurs, the transverse process breaks or is very thin, then a hole can be drilled in the base of the process and wire passed through it. A hook and screw system has also been developed, again approximating the lysis and applying graft around it (Morscher, 1984).

3 Louis repair (1977). Louis & Maresca hold the view that any repair that closes the gap interferes

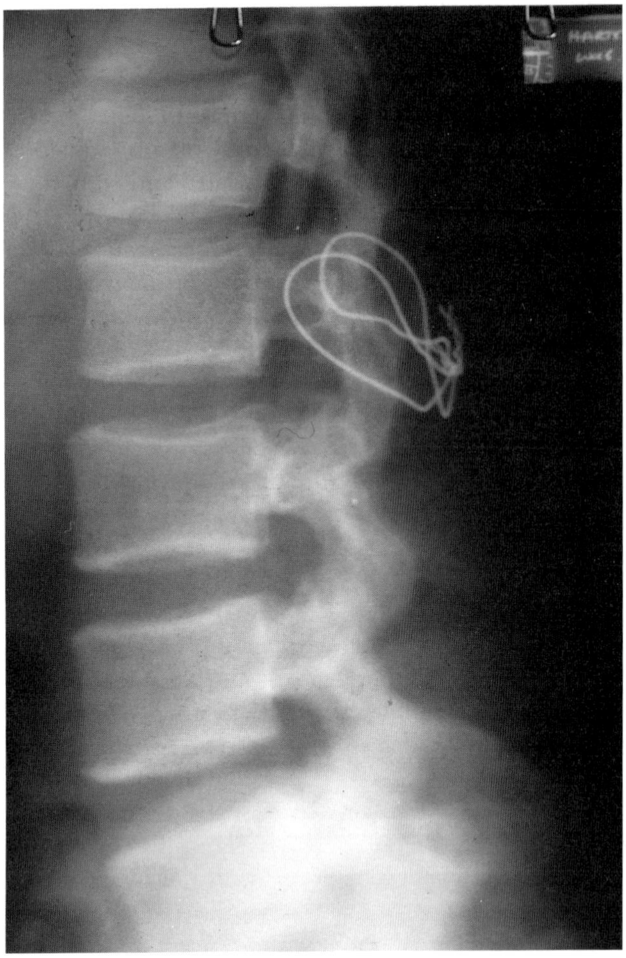

Fig. 43.7 Scott repair.

with the facet joint between L5 and S1, as inevitably it subluxes to the extent that the gap is closed, as clearly when the two elements are approximated the loose lamina is the one that moves, not the body of L5. Louis first of all removes the loose posterior element and ensures that the site of the defect is cleared of fibrous tissue and that there is no root entrapment of L5. He then replaces the loose fragment and places grafts around and within the defect. He then applies a butterfly-shaped plate with pedicular screws in L5 and S1, to stabilize the whole segment while the lysis heals. Some six months later, when the lysis is healed, the plate is removed. This is a very logical approach as clearly in all the other methods the lysis area is transmitting body loads whilst healing; with this technique it is protected. However, all techniques seem to be associated with a similar success rate, so the Louis approach seems rather complicated, although very logical (Louis & Maresca, 1977).

Fusion

When the disc has failed, especially likely when a degree of spondylolisthesis is present, then local fusion is appropriate if symptoms merit it, and one is confident that the causes of the symptoms are indeed due to segmental failure at that level. Posterior fusion alone clearly would have to be over two levels in the presence of a spondylolytic defect at L5–S1 as there would be little achieved fusing the loose segment to the sacrum, as it is not attached to the body of L5. An intertransverse fusion, in which the transverse processes and the side of the pedicle of L5 are fused to the ala of the sacrum, appears to produce a satisfactory clinical result. This may be done through the midline posteriorly, reflecting the muscles laterally and filling what has been described as the 'lateral gutter', the space behind the ala and transverse processes, with bone taken from the iliac crests. Alternatively the approach can be made through the muscles directly (Wiltse *et al.*, 1968). This may be done with two parallel skin incisions, or a single skin incision and parallel incisions in the sacrospinalis fascia. Anterior fusion is another alternative approach, with the theoretical advantage that the back muscles remain undisturbed. This may be done transperitoneally, but this has the disadvantage in the male of occasionally injuring the presacral nerve, and producing retrograde ejaculation. Alternatively an approach can be made retroperitoneally, the presacral nerve is at much less risk, but there is some hazard of vascular injury to the iliac vessels, and the approach is difficult if there is a significant degree of slip.

Unilateral spondylolysis

This may be a cause of acute back pain in young people experiencing repetitive stresses to their backs, shearing, hyperextension, or rotational (Froom *et al.*, 1984; Letts *et al.*, 1986).

Clearly there may on occasion be a bilateral lesion, and one side heals; this can occasionally be observed when open repair of a supposed bilateral lesion is carried out. On other occasions the lesion may only be unilateral, and as one might expect if this is the case it is more likely to heal. If the diagnosis is made soon after injury or onset of symptoms then use of a thoracolumbar orthosis may encourage healing (Letts *et al.*, 1986).

Spondylolysis at levels other than L5–S1

A spondylolytic defect can occur at levels other than the L5–S1; indeed it may occur at multiple levels. However, when it occurs at the penultimate mobile segment, usually L4–L5, then it presents a rather different clinical problem.

If it presents at a later age, usually in the early 30s, it is more likely to present with sciatica. If backache is a problem then it does less well with fusion than spondylolytic spondylolisthesis at the L5–S1 level. Whereas a symptomless L5–S1 lysis may be ignored, a lysis at L4–L5 (if this is the penultimate mobile segment) should be dealt with even if asymptomtic because of the poorer prognosis once slip has occurred (Jackson *et al.*, 1978; Saraste, 1986; Deburge & Lassalle, 1984; Lowe, 1987).

DEGENERATIVE SPONDYLOLISTHESIS

This was initially described by Junghanns in 1929, who called it pseudo-spondylolisthesis, as he felt that spondylolisthesis necessarily implied a pars defect. However, as we have seen, even in dysplastic spondylolisthesis the pars may be intact, and as the reason for this type of spondylolisthesis is degenerative change in the facet joints it seems more appropriate to call it a degenerative spondylolisthesis. It is important to appreciate that the slip is not a dislocation, or even a subluxation, but a progressive remodelling of the facet joints due to arthritic change, so that the facet joints of the superior facet of the lower vertebra progressively move ventrally on the pedicle towards the body. This explains two important features of the disorder: firstly the slip can never be more than some 20%, as the joint would reach the back of the body, and secondly the root emerging below the level of the spondylolisthesis is caught by the joint as the latter migrates down the pedicle. Hence a L4–L5 degenerative spondylolisthesis presents with an L5 root lesion, whereas an L4–L5 lytic spondylolisthesis presents with a L4 root lesion (Rosenberg, 1976).

It is a disorder that is more common in women, by a factor of about 4:1. It may present with root pain, either mimicking a disc protrusion, or more commonly presenting as a lateral canal spinal stenotic

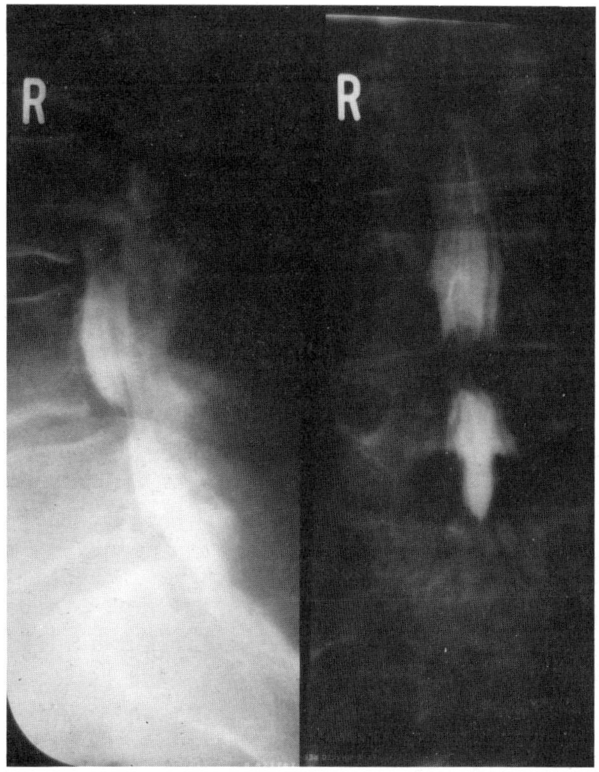

Fig. 43.8 Degenerative spondylolysthesis producing spinal stenotic syndrome.

syndrome. In this syndrome the radicular pain is brought on by activity and is not associated with any tension signs; that is the straight leg raising test is normal. The radicular pain may be bilateral.

It may also present with a central canal stenotic syndrome in which the patient complains of a weakness or deadness of the legs, again brought on by walking, and relieved by bending forwards or sitting. Careful enquiry in this group of patients may elicit subtle alteration in the control of micturition, either a poorer stream or some urge incontinence. As these symptoms are not uncommon in the older woman, due to a degree of prolapse, their neurological source may not be appreciated. The patient may have a varying degree of backache which has the features of osteoarthritic pain elsewhere, relieved by rest and analgesics, and aggravated by activity, and associated with stiffness after rest such as in the morning. It is important to distinguish the leg pain from that which may be due to vascular insufficiency. Indeed the two may well coexist. The altered gait produced by central canal stenosis may also of course be due to cervical spondylosis. Although in lateral canal stenosis there may be no objective neurological signs, in those patients presenting with a central canal stenotic picture there is usually reduction or absence of the ankle jerks. Indeed if these are brisk then the cause of the gait abnormality is likely to be cervical spondylosis, or a demyelinating disorder. On occasion a major disc protrusion may occur at the level of the degenerative spondylosis, and the patient may present with an acute cauda equina lesion.

A curious but important symptom is groin pain, when the lesion is at L4–L5 (which is the most common site). As these patients may have associated osteoarthritis of the hips, on occasion hip replacement has been done in the mistaken belief that the groin pain was due to hip osteoarthritis. Indeed the two disorders may not only coexist but indeed may both be productive of symptoms. If there is doubt then a local injection of marcaine into the hip joint may clarify the true source of the pain. However, on occasion both disorders may contribute to the patient's disability, and in this situation joint replacement should be carried out first.

Unilateral degenerative change in a facet joint can also lead to a forward subluxation of the joint. This leads to a rotation of the vertebra around the intact joint. The diagnosis is not easily made on the plane films, because in the lateral film no forward slip may be apparent. The degree of rotation is so slight that translocation of the spinous processes is not very obvious, and the degenerate joint may not look too unusual. The patient may present with a radiculopathy alone, associated with a lateral canal stenosis. A marked asymmetry of the transverse processes in the anteroposterior films will alert the surgeon to the possibility of this diagnosis. This asymmetry is due to the foreshortening of the process on one side due to the rotation, associated with an apparent lengthening of the contralateral process.

Management

The management of degenerative spondylolisthesis depends on the presenting symptom complex, the age of the patient and the degree of disc narrowing that has occurred at the site of the spondylolisthesis. In those patients that present with backache alone, conservative management is appropriate; the use of a support, control of obesity, and a physiotherapy programme to improve abdominal and back musculature. Those patients that present with unilateral radicular pain should initially be treated non-operatively, as there is a high spontanous remission rate. On occasion traction may produce dramatic relief, but it is important that it is carried out with the hips and knees flexed to ensure that the spine, when being pulled, is itself in flexion. Good results have been claimed from the use of calcitonin (Porter & Park, 1982). It is believed that this drug alters the distribution of the blood supply to the bone so that more is available to the neurological elements. The basis for its use was the observation that, in Paget's disease presenting with paraparesis, it produced rapid improvement which was clearly not due to an alteration in bone size (Ravichandran, 1979). However, if time does not produce relief of the radicular pain then surgical intervention is appropriate. Once again one must emphasize that the root compressed in a degenerative spondylolisthesis is the one existing at the level below the listhesis. As it is perfectly possible that a spondylolisthesis may be asymptomatic, and the patient may have another cause for the radicular pain, it is important that appropriate preoperative investigations are carried out to confirm the diagnosis. A CT scan may confirm that there is no other site of root entrapment, but if it is ambiguous then a radiculogram should be done and, on occasion, a root block should be carried out to confirm that the symptoms complained of are indeed due to entrapment of that root. A symptomatic root should be decompressed, ensuring that the spinal stability is not compromised, preserving at least half the joint, and undercutting the subarticular canal to achieve adequate decompression. Whereas in a normal spine one may remove a joint, and forward slip may not necessarily follow, one can be certain in this group of patients that if the joint is removed the disc has already failed and inevitably further slip will occur. If adequate root decompression can be achieved only by excision of the joint then a decision has to be made as to whether fusion should be done also. In making this decision certain facts have to be considered. If the disc space is already extremely narrow then further slip may be very slight, and further slight slip may be entirely asymptomatic. If decompression has been restricted to one side, the contralateral joint provides a degree of continued stability. Preoperative investigations (CT and radiculogram) commonly show root entrapment bilaterally, although symptoms are unilateral. The temptation to decompress prophylactically on the asymptomatic side should be carefully considered, as the bilateral decompression makes the need for fusion much more likely.

Excellent results are claimed for anterior fusion alone without decompression, but with some correction of deformity and disc height. Such surgery, however, cannot decompress the subarticular element of the root entrapment, which is due to the actual remodelling of the superior facet joint on the pedicle. But it does increase the cross-sectional area of the spinal canal if reduction either complete or partial is achieved, and may therefore be particularly suitable for central spinal stenosis where the compressing agents are the back of the inferior vertebra, and the trailing edge of the lamina of the upper vertebra (Inoue *et al.*, 1988).

However, the relief of root pain is presumably achieved by stopping all movement. The ability of fusion alone to stop radicular pain without decompression has also been observed in the management of dysplastic spondylolisthesis (Peek *et al.*, 1989). However, excellent results have been claimed following extensive decompression alone, despite the development of some postoperative slip (Epstein *et al.*, 1983). The worst course is to do an inadequate decompression, trying to maintain stability, and combine this with an inadequate fusion. The main reason for not always doing a fusion is that a very satisfactory degree of relief of stenotic symptoms will be achieved in the great majority of cases by doing a decompression alone (Deburge *et al.*, 1983). A fusion procedure is a much more major operation than a decompressive one, and commonly these patients are elderly and infirm. A few patients will have an increase in their degree of listhesis, but this may be asymptomatic. Unfortunately, a few will have increased back pain with decompression alone.

It would therefore appear reasonable that at all ages isolated radicular pain due to root compression beneath the degenerative joint, not associated with backache, should be treated by root decompression alone. In fit patients, whatever their age, if they present with back pain and root pain then decompression and fusion should be carried out. The fact that a fusion is being done should not encourage an excessively destructive decompression. Trimming the superior edge of the lamina and removal of all flaval tissue provides adequate central decompression, and decompression of the lateral recesses can be achieved by uncutting the facet joints, as well as excising the medial half of the joints. A posterolateral fusion may then be done. There may be some merit in using pedicular fixation if it is felt that the decompression has of necessity compromised the stability of the facet joints (Hanley, 1986; Kaneda *et al.*, 1986). When decompression is followed by slip in those patients who have a stenosis not associated with a degenerative spondylolisthesis, such a slip is much more likely to produce disabling back pain (Johnsson *et al.*, 1986).

If it is elected to carry out a fusion posteriorly when doing a root decompression, the choice lies between a posterolateral fusion alone or combined with fixation. The necessary posterior decompression, which may involve a laminectomy, may mean that pedicular fixation alone is possible. If the surgeon is experienced in this technique this probably provides the most secure option. It does permit an attempt at reduction to be carried out, but the rigidity of the anterior structures means any reduction done from behind alone is minimal. However, posterolateral fusion alone may provide sufficient security against further slip.

TRAUMATIC SPONDYLOLYSIS AND SPONDYLOLISTHESIS

There are a number of documented cases where, following fairly modest injury, a lysis is found to be present in the pars, and fortuitously previous radiological examination has shown no abnormality (Klinghoffer & Murdoc, 1982). It seems likely that these do represent stress fractures; they are not associated with acute spondylolisthesis. On other occasions following major trauma, of a type which may well have caused a fracture of the pars bilaterally, a spondylolysis is found to be present. As it may have been present before the injury, one cannot be confident that the injury caused it, or merely made a pre-existing spondylolysis symptomatic. This type of pars defect, although discovered following injury, is a stable injury and behaves like a lysis, discovered fortuitously in an adult where there is no history of injury. The diagnosis of a traumatic spondylolysis or traumatic spondylolisthesis is now restricted to fractures, in the posterior elements, other than at the pars, either through the joint or pedicle. Based on this definition traumatic spondylolisthesis in the lumbar spine is of course much less common, as very major injury is required to damage all three columns of the spine and allow forward subluxation to occur. Fractures that allow this subluxation will involve both the posterior elements and the body of the vertebra, as the healthy disc is such a strong structure, a shearing of the top of the vertebra may occur rather than through the disc. A spondylolisthesis produced by major trauma is likely to be a very unstable injury; that is to say it may displace further with minor force. There may be associated neurological compromise, either a single root problem or a major cauda equina injury.

In the presence of the latter, early reduction and stabilization is necessary. The recent development of pedicular fixation systems makes operative reduction easier as the pedicle screws can be used to achieve the reduction during the operation, the cauda equina being visualized during the reduction, and indeed using pedicular fixation a laminectomy can be done to ensure adequate decompression without compromising the stability of the fixation. It also allows the affected segment alone to be reduced and held. Previous techniques relying on laminar fixation usually meant a number of segments had to be fixed, especially if a laminectomy had to be done at the level of the spondylolithesis. Methods of stabilizing a reduction relying on spinous processes not only involved stiffening many levels but were quite ineffective in holding an unstable segment, unless the patient was in fact treated in bed until union had occurred. It was these very ineffective methods of fixation that invited criticism of surgical stabilization of spinal fractures (see Chapters 44 & 61).

In patients in whom there is no neurological compromise then some degree of postural reduction can be achieved, treating the patient supine in bed for some weeks. Because there is usually considerable bony injury the segment will stabilize and bony union will occur. In the absence of the necessary specialist surgical skills, or in an environment unsuitable for their use, such a conservative or non-surgical approach is acceptable. It has the advantage that there is no further muscle injury produced by the surgeon. However, it does require a high degree of nursing skill and a patient patient.

PATHOLOGICAL SPONDYLOLISTHESIS

Destruction of the pedicles and posterior elements by tumour, either primary or secondary, may cause

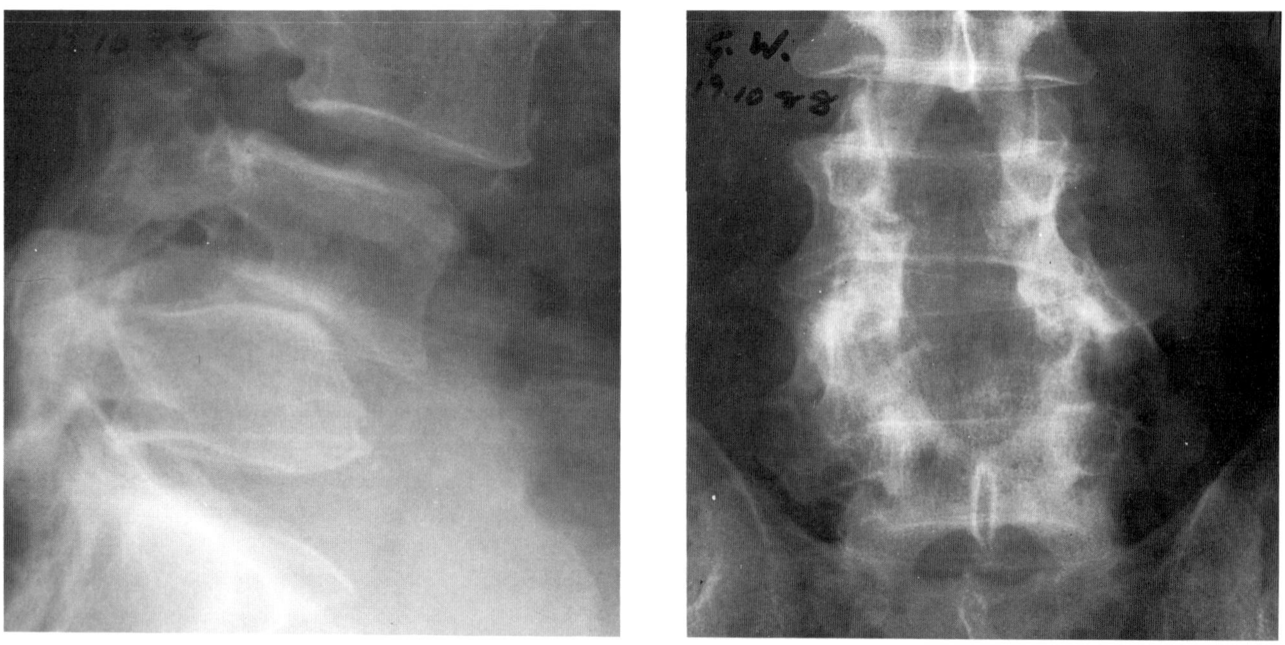

Fig. 43.9 Iatrogenic spondylolysthesis following wide laminectomy.

a spondylolisthesis. This is not very frequent as metastases usually arise in the body rather than the posterior elements. The patient may present with severe back pain, a very rigid spine, and very acute focal tenderness. There may be major neurological compromise. This latter complication may require urgent surgery to decompress the cauda equina and roots. If this is necessary then stabilization of the segment using rigid internal fixation will be required (see Chapters 27 & 28). However, there may be no neurological compromise despite an alarming radiological appearance. In this situation it is justifiable to establish a tissue diagnosis by means of needle biopsy, and if the tumour is one amenable to local or systemic treatment, then to treat. However, on occasion, despite control of the tumour and in the absence of neurological abnormalities, severe pain persists. This is due to continued mechanical instability, and rigid internal fixation is very rewarding in terms of pain relief. If pedicular fixation is used, and the quality of the bone of the body of the vertebrae is poor, polymethacrylate cement may be put down the pedicle to reinforce screw hold.

Infection may cause spondylolisthesis. Disc infection after operative treatment of a disc protrusion is the most frequent cause. However, whether spondylolisthesis or retrospondylolisthesis occurs depends on the continued integrity of the posterior joints. If these are not involved by the infection, and have not been injured surgically, then forward displacement will not occur (Wynne & Southgate, 1986).

Bone disease other than neoplasm may lead to failure of the hook mechanism holding each vertebra in place, that is the pars, pedicle, and the facet joints. Examples of such disorders are:

1 Albers Schönberg disease (osteopetrosis) (Szappanos *et al.*, 1988). In this disorder fractures of the pars are frequent, they heal and spondylolisthesis is very uncommon.

2 In a variety of arthrogryposis, called Kuskokwim disease, a number of pedicles may be elongated, and may produce a true spondylolisthesis at the lumbosacral level (Petajan *et al.*, 1969).

3 Paget's disease rarely may be associated with lengthening of the pedicles allowing forward slip of the vertebra.

4 Syphilis producing a gumma of the articular process has caused a spondylolisthesis (Karaharjii & Hunnuksella, 1973).

Spondylolysis or spondylolisthesis aquisita

This is a pathological fracture through the pars, occurring either above a spinal fusion or following a lumbar root decompression in which the pars has been unduly thinned or stripped of its blood supply so that it fractures in the postoperative period. It is, of course, a particular risk when a root is being decompressed towards the root exit where the pars forms the posterior margin. However, it can also be produced by too aggressive and too lateral a removal of the lamina proximally when performing a fenestration. It may be fractured during operation, or so weakened that it subsequently fractures. However, it is not usually followed by a spondylolisthesis, unless it is produced bilaterally (Brunet & Wiley, 1984).

REFERENCES

Albanese, M. & Pizzutillo, P.D. (1982) Family study of spondylolysis and spondylolisthesis. *J. Pediatr. Orthop.*, **2**, 496–499.

Amuso, S., Neff, R., Coulson, D. & Laing, P. (1970) The surgical treatment of spondylolisthesis by posterior element resection. *J. Bone Jt. Surg.*, **52A**, 529–536.

Bell, D.F., Ehrlich, M.G. & Zaleske, D.J. (1988) Brace treatment for symptomatic spondylolisthesis. *Clin. Orthop.*, **236**, 192–198.

Blackburn, J.S. & Velikas, E.P. (1977) Spondylolisthesis in children and adolescents. *J. Bone Jt. Surg.*, **59B**, 490–494.

Boxall, D., Bradford, D.S., Winter, R.B. & Moe, J.H. (1979) Management of severe spondylolisthesis in children and adolescents. *J. Bone Jt. Surg.*, **61A**, 479–495.

Bradford, D.S. (1983) Management of spondylolisthesis. *Inst. Course Lecture (IFC)*, **32**, 151–162.

Bradford, D.S. (1988) Closed reduction of spondylolisthesis: An experience in 22 patients. *Spine*, **13**, 580–587.

Bradford, D.S. & Gotfried, Y. (1987) Staged salvage reconstruction of Grade IV and V spondylolisthesis. *J. Bone Jt. Surg.*, **69A**, 191–202.

Brunet, J.A. & Wiley, J.J. (1984) Acquired spondylysis after spinal fusion. *J. Bone Jt. Surg.*, **66B**, 720–724.

Buck, J.E. (1970) Direct repair of the defect in spondylolisthesis. *J. Bone Jt. Surg.*, **52B**, 432.

Buirski, G., McCall, I.W. & O'Brien, J.P. (1984) Myelography in severe lumbosacral spondylolisthesis. *Br. J. Radiol.*, **B28**, 1067–1072.

Collier, A.T., Johnson, R.P., Carrera, G.F., Meyer, G.A, Schwab, J.P., Flatley, T.J., Isitman, A.T., Hellman, R.S., Zielonka, J.S. & Knobel, J. (1985) Painful spondylolysis or spondylolisthesis studied by radiography and single photon emission computed tomography. *Radiology*, **154**, 207–211.

Deburge, A. & Lassale, B. (1984) Isthmic spondylolisthesis with spontaneous development in adults. Apropos of 8 cases. *Rey. Chir. Orthop.*, **70**, 147–149.

Deburge, A., Lassale, B., Benoist, M. & Cauchoix, J. (1983) The surgical treatment of lumbar stenosis and its results. A series of 163 operated cases. *Rev. Rheum. Mal. Osteoartic.*, **50**, 47–54.

Dewald, R.I., Faut, M.M., Tadonio, R.F. & Neuwirth, M.G. (1981) Severe lumbosacral spondylolisthesis in adolescents and children. *J. Bone Jt. Surg.*, **63A**, 619–626.

Dick, W.T. & Schnebel, B. (1988) Severe spondylolisthesis reduction and internal fixation. *Clin. Orthop.*, **232**, 79–79.

Edelmann, P. (1984) Conservative therapy of spondylolisthesis using body braces. *Z. Orthop.*, **122**, 152–154.

Elliott, S., Hutson, M.A. & Wastie, M.L. (1988) Bone scintigraphy in the assessment of spondylolysis in patients attending a sports injury clinic. *Clin. Radiol.*, **39**, 269–272.

Epstein, N.E., Epstein, J.A., Carras, R. & Lavine, L.S. (1983) Degenerative spondylolisthesis with a intact neural arch: A review of 60 cases with an analysis of clinical findings and the development of surgical management. *Neurosurgery*, **13**, 555–561.

Farfan, H., Osteria, V. & Lamy, C. (1976) The mechanical etiology of spondylolysis and spondylolisthesis. *Clin. Orthop.*, **117**, 40–58.

Flynn, J.C. & Price, C.T. (1984) Sexual complications of anterior fusion of the lumbar spine. *Spine*, **9**, 489–492.

Fredrickson, B.E., Baker, D., McHolic, W.J., Yua, H.A. & Lubicky, J.P. (1984) The natural history of spondylolysis and spondylolisthesis. *J. Bone Jt. Surg.*, **66A**, 699–707.

Freebody, D., Bendall, R. & Taylor, R.D. (1971) Anterior transperitoneal lumbar fusion. *J. Bone Jt. Surg.*, **53B**, 617.

Freeman, B. & Donate, N. (1989) Spinal arthrodesis for severe spondylolisthesis in children and adolescents. A long term follow up. *J. Bone Jt. Surg.*, **71A**, 594–599.

Froom, P., Froom, J., Van Dyke, D., Caine, Y., Ribak, J., Margaliot, S. & Floman, Y. (1984) Lytic spondylolisthesis in helicopter pilots. *Aviat. Space Environ. Med.*, **55**, 556–557.

Gehweiler, J.A. & Daffner, R.H. (1983) Low back pain: The controversy of radiological evaluation. *Am. J. Rheumatol.*, **140**, 109–112.

Gill, G. (1984) Long term follow up evaluation of a few patients with spondylolisthesis treated by excision of the loose lamina with decompression of the nerve roots without spinal fusion. *Clin. Orthop.*, **182**, 215–219.

Gill, G.G. & White, H. (1965) Surgical treatment of spondylolisthesis without spine fusion. *Acta Orthop. Scand.* **85** (Suppl.).

Gill, G.G., Manning, J.G. & White, H.C. (1955) Surgical treatment of spondylolisthesis without spine fusion. Excision of the loose lamina with decompression of the nerve root. *J. Bone Jt. Surg.*, **37A**, 493–520.

Hanley, E.N. Jr (1986) Decompression and distraction-derotation arthrodesis for degenerative spondylolisthesis. *Spine*, **11**, 269–276.

Harrington, G.R. & Dickson, J.H. (1976) Spinal instrumentation in the treatment of severe progressive spondylolisthesis. *Clin. Orthop.*, **117**, 157–163.

Harris, I.E. & Weinstein, S.L. (1987) Long term follow up of patients with grade III and IV spondylolisthesis. Treatment with and without posterior fusion. *J. Bone Jt. Surg.*, **69A**, 960–969.

Henson, J., McCall, I.W., O'Brien, J.P. (1987) Disc damage above a spondylolisthesis. *Br. J. Radiol.*, **B28**, 69–72.

Inoue, S., Watanabe, T., Goto, S., Takahashi, K. & Sho, E. (1988) Degenerative spondylolisthesis pathophysiology and results of anterior interbody fusion. *Clin. Orthop.*, **227**, 90–98.

Jackson, A.M., Kirwan, E. & Sullivan, M. (1978) Lytic spondylolisthesis above the lumbosacral level. *J. Bone Jt. Surg.*, **60B**, 439.

Jackson, D., Wiltse, L. & Circincione, R. (1976) Spondylolysis in the female gymnast. *Clin. Orthop.*, **117**, 68–73.

Johnson, J.R. & Kirwan, E.O. (1983) The long term results of fusion *in situ* for severe spondylolisthesis. *J. Bone Jt. Surg.*, **65B**, 43–46.

Johnson, L.P., Nasca, R.J. & Dunham, W.K. (1988) Surgical management of isthmic spondylolisthesis. *Spine*, **13**, 93–97.

Johnsson, K.E., Willner, S. & Johnsson, K. (1986) Postoperative instability after decompression for lumbar spinal stenosis. *Spine*, **11**, 107–110.

Jones, A., McAfee, P., Robinson, R., Zinreich, S. & Wang, H. (1988) Failed arthrodesis of the spine for severe spondylolisthesis salvage by interbody fusion. *J. Bone Jt. Surg.*, **70A**, 25–30.

Junghanns, H. (1929) Spondylolisthesis 30 pathologisch-anatomisch untersuchte Falle. *Bruns Beitr. Klin. Chir.*, **158**, 554.

Kaneda, K., Kazama, H., Satoh, S. & Fujiya, M. (1986) Follow up study of medial facetectomies and posterolateral fusion with instrumentation in unstable degenerative spondylolisthesis. *Clin. Orthop.*, **203**, 159–167.

Karaharjii, E., & Hunnuksela, M. (1973) Possible syphilitic spondylitis. *Acta Orthop. Scand.*, **44**, 289.

Klinghoffer, L. & Murdoc, M.G. (1982) Spondylolysis following trauma. A case report and a review of the literature. *Clin. Orthop.*, **166**, 72–74.

Letts, M., Smallman, T., Afanasiev, R. & Gouw, G. (1986) Fractures of the pars interarticular in adolescent athletes: a clinical-biomechanical analysis. *J. Pediatr. Orthop.*, **6**, 40–46.

Libson, E., Bloom, R.A., Dinari, G. & Robin, G.C. (1984a) Oblique lumbar spine radiographs: importance in young patients. *Radiology*, **151**, 89–90.

Libson, E., Bloom, R.A. & Shapiro, Y. (1984b) Scoliosis in young men with spondylolysis or spondylolisthesis. A comparative study in symptomatic and asymptomatic subjects. *Spine*, **9**, 445–447.

Louis, R. & Maresca, C. (1977) Stabilization chirurgicale avec reduction des spondlysis et des spondylolisthesis. *Int. Orthop.*, **1**, 215.

Lowe, J., Schachner, E., Hirshberg, E., Shapiro, Y. & Libson, E. (1984) Significance of bone scintigraphy in symptomatic spondylolysis. *Spine*, **9**, 653–655.

Lowe, J., Libson, E., Ziv, I., Nvska, M., Floman, Y., Bloom,

R.A. & Robin, G.C. (1987) Spondylolysis in the upper lumbar spine. A study of 32 patients. *J. Bone Jt. Surg.*, **69B**, 582–586.

Matthiass, H.H. & Heine, J. (1986) The surgical reduction of spondylolisthesis. *Clin. Orthop.*, **203**, 34–44.

McAfee, P.C. & Yuan, H.A. (1982) Computed tomography in spondylolisthesis. *Clin. Orthop.*, **166**, 62–71.

McCarroll, J.R., Miller, J.M. & Ritter, M.A. (1986) Lumbar spondylolysis and spondylolisthesis in college football players. A prospective study. *Am. J. Sports Med.* **14**, 404–406.

McNab, I. (1977) *Backache*. Williams & Wilkins, Baltimore, MD.

McQueen, M.M., Court-Brown, C. & Scott, J.H. (1986) Stabilization of spondylolisthesis using Dwyer instrumentation. *J. Bone Jt. Surg.*, **68B**, 185–188.

Morscher, E., Gerber, B. & Fasel, J. (1984) Surgical treatment of spondylolisthesis by bone grafting and direct stabilization of spondylolysis by means of a hook. *Arch. Orthop. Trauma Surg.*, **103**, 175–178.

Neugebaur, F.L. (1888) Reprinted in English in *Clin. Orthop. Rel. Res.* **117**, 4–22 (1988).

Nicol, R.O. & Scott, J.H. (1986) Lytic spondylolisthesis repair by wiring. *Spine*, **11**, 1027–1030.

Noack, W. & Raetzel, G. (1988) Treatment of spondylolisthesis in adults using the dorsal approach with the fixateur interne and a special repositioning device. *Z. Orthop.* **126**, 205–210.

Oakley, R.H. & Carty, H. (1984) Review of spondylolisthesis and spondylolysis in paediatric practice. *Br. J. Radiol.*, **57**, 877–885.

Papanicolaou, N., Wilkinson, R.H., Emans, J.B., Trevas, S. & Micheli, L.J. (1985) Bone scintigraphy and radiography in young athletes with low back pain. *Am. J. Rheumalol.*, **145**, 1039–1044.

Peek, R., Wiltse, L., Reynolds, T.J., Gwyer, D. & Widell, E.H. (1989) *In situ* arthrodesis without decompression for Grade III and IV isthmic spondylolisthesis in adults who have severe sciatica. *J. Bone Jt. Surg.*, **71A**, 62–68.

Petajan, J., Manberger, G., Aase, J. & Wright, D.G. (1969) Arthrogryposis syndrome (Kuskokwim Disease) in the Eskimo. *J. Am. Med. Assoc.*, **209**, 1481.

Pfeil, J., Niethard, F.U. & Cotta, H. (1987) Pathogenesis of paediatric spondylolisthesis. *Z. Orthop.*, **125**, 526–533.

Pizzutillo, P.D., Mirenda, W. & McEwan, G.D. (1986) Posterolateral fusion for spondylolisthesis in adolescents. *J. Pediatr. Orthop.*, **6**, 311–316.

Porter, R.W. & Park, W. (1982) Unilateral spondylolysis. *J. Bone Jt. Surg.*, **64B**, 344–348.

Ravichandran, G. (1979) Neurological recovery of paraplegia following use of salmon calcitonin in a patient with Paget's disease of the spine. *Spine*, **4**, 37–40.

Rosenberg, N. (1976) Degenerative spondylolisthesis. *Clin. Orthop.*, **117**, 112–120.

Saraste, H. (1966) Spondylolysis and pregnancy: a risk analysis. *Acta Obstet. Gynaecol. Scand.*, **65**, 727–729.

Saraste, H., Brostrom, L.A. & Aparisi, T. (1984a) Prognostic radiographic aspects of spondylolisthesis. *Acta Radiol. (Diagn.) (Stockh.)*, **25**, 427–432.

Saraste, H., Nilsson, B., Brostrom, L.A. & Aparisi, T. (1984b) Relationship between radiological and clinical variables in spondylolysis. *Int. Orthop.*, **8**, 163–174.

Seitsalo, S., Osterman, K. & Poussa, M. (1988) Scoliosis associated with lumbar spondylolisthesis. A clinical survey of 190 young patients. *Spine*, **13**, 899–904.

Sijbrandij, S. (1983) Reduction and stabilization of severe spondylolisthesis. A report of three cases. *J. Bone Jt. Surg.*, **65B**, 40–42.

Snijder, J., Seroo, J., Snijder, C. & Schijvens, A. (1976) Therapy of spondylolisthesis by repositioning and fixation of the olisthetic vertebra. *Clin. Orthop.*, **117**, 149–156.

Speck, G., McCall, I. & O'Brien, J.P. (1984) Spondylolisthesis: the angle of kyphosis. *Spine*, **9**, 659–660.

Steffee, A.D. & Sitkowski, D.J. (1988) Reduction and stabilization of grade IV spondylolisthesis. *Clin. Orthop.*, **227**, 82–89.

Szappanos, L., Szepesi, K. & Thomazy, V. (1988) Spondylolysis in osteopetrosis. *J. Bone Jt. Surg.*, **70B**, 428–430.

Szypryt, E.P. (1989) The value of magnetic resonance imaging in disc space infection and patients with neural arch defects. Meeting of the International Society for Study of the Lumbar Spine, Miami, 1988.

Teplick, J.G., Laffey, P.A., Berman, A. & Haskin, M.E. (1986) Diagnosis and evaluation of spondylolisthesis and/or spondylysis on axial CT. *Am. J. Neuroradiol.*, **7**, 479–491.

Troup, J.D.G. (1976) Mechanical factors in spondylolisthesis. *Clin. Orth. Rel. Res.*, **117**, 59–67.

Turner, R.H. & Bianco, A.J. (1981) Spondylolysis and spondylolisthesis in children and teenagers. *J. Bone Jt. Surg.*, **53A**, 1298–1306.

Van-den Oever, M., Merrick, M.V. & Scott, J.H. (1987) Bone scintigraphy in symptomatic spondylolysis. *J. Bone Jt.* Surg., **69B**, 453–456.

Wiltse, L.L., Bateman, J.G., Hutchinson, R.H. & Welson, W.E. (1968) The paraspinal sacrospinalis-splitting approach to the lumbar spine. *J. Bone Jt. Surg.*, **50A**, 919.

Wiltse, L.L., Widell, E. & Jackson, D.W. (1975) Fatigue fracture: the basic lesion in isthmic spondylolisthesis. *J. Bone Jt. Surg.*, **57A**, 17.

Wiltse, L.L., Newman, P.H. & McNab, I. (1976) Classification of spondylolysis and spondylolisthesis. *Clin. Orthop.*, **117**, 23–29.

Wiltse, M.D. & Winter, R. (1983) Terminology and measurement of spondylolisthesis. *J. Bone Jt. Surg.*, **65A**, 768–772.

Wynne, A.T. & Southgate, G.W. (1986) Discitis causing spondylolisthesis. A case report. *Spine*, **11**, 970–972.

Wynne-Davies, R. & Scott, J.H.S. (1979) Inheritance and spondylolisthesis: radiographic family survey. *J. Bone Jt.* Surg., **61B**, 301–305.

44 · Surgery for Low Back Pain

By J. DOVE

The joints of each lumbar motion segment are the disc in front and the two facet joints behind. This chapter considers surgery for chronic low back pain resulting from degenerative change within those joints. The question of surgery for other specific causes of chronic low back pain, such as spondylolisthesis, is dealt with elsewhere in this volume.

Selection of patients

The selection of patients for chronic low back pain surgery is highly controversial. There is an existing dogma which states that following appropriate investigation there is a place for surgery for leg pain secondary to low back problems but that there is not a place for surgery for chronic low back pain alone. This dogma is partly based on the very poor reputation of low back pain fusions with a high pseudarthrosis rate (Shaw & Taylor, 1956; Prothero *et al.*, 1966; Nelson, 1968).

However, since the era that gave rise to that dogma the quality and range of investigations have improved greatly, as have surgical techniques, in particular with the introduction of effective means of internal fixation of the lumbosacral spine. As a result there is a small group of patients who are disabled by chronic low back pain, who have an identifiable localized organic cause for that pain and in whom surgery can produce very worthwhile and rewarding results. The first part of this chapter discusses how to identify those patients who are likely to benefit from low back pain surgery and, perhaps more importantly, to predict those who will have a poor result from surgery.

There are two aspects governing the selection of patients for chronic low back pain surgery: the selection of the appropriate patient and the selection of the appropriate surgery.

Selection of appropriate patients

Serious efforts are being made to put the selection of patients for chronic low back pain surgery on a proper scientific basis (Mathew *et al.*, 1988). Until such methods are widely accepted and proven each surgeon must work out for himself what method of selection suits his or her own practice best. The author makes no apology for the fact that what follows in this section is both empirical and idiosyncratic.

History

Nowhere is a detailed and accurate history more important than in chronic low back pain. This chapter will draw attention to one or two important aspects of the history which are frequently neglected in patients referred to the author's service.

One needs to know how long the patient has been troubled, and specific enquiry must be made into precisely how the pain started. It is quite inadequate, for example, in a complex low back pain problem to dismiss the history in a few words such as '16 years of low back pain'. It is essential to establish whether the pain developed gradually in the natural course of events or whether there was a clearly identifiable injury. If there has been a specific injury then knowledge of the mechanism of injury may give a clue to a specific type of spinal lesion.

In addition detailed enquiry must be made as to whether the patient is involved in any form of litigation or claim in relation to an injury. This may not come to light unless specific enquiry is made. The fact that a patient is involved in a claim does not mean that he or she does not have a genuine low back problem, but as will be outlined below, it does mean that patient is not a suitable candidate for surgery.

The history must also include details of any treatment the patient has undergone, and must state whether or not that treatment was effective and, if effective, for how long the patient was relieved. This is particularly true of any previous operations, in which case a copy of the original operation notes will be required.

Examination

A full examination of the back and lower limbs is carried out. It may be just as important to observe the manner in which the patient dresses and undresses as to pay attention to the clinical findings once the patient is undressed.

Although one carries out a full neurological examination it is only infrequently in patients with chronic low back pain that the examination reveals any specific important signs. Much more important in chronic low back pain is to establish whether or not 'inappropriate' or 'non-organic' signs are present (Waddell *et al.*, 1980). The presence of such non-organic signs does not mean the patient does not have a genuine back pain problem, but it does mean that he or she is unlikely to be a suitable candidate for surgery.

The author believes it is important to note and record apparently subsidiary features of the examination such as whether or not the patient is accompanied by their spouse or partner. If the patient has prepared a written list of complaints this should also be noted. Such features are important in establishing how a patient and the family have reacted to a particular back pain problem. Patients who react 'inappropriately' to attacks of back pain may react equally 'inappropriately' to back surgery.

Independent patient assessment

A detailed history and examination of a patient with a complex back problem takes considerable time. To circumvent this problem in our centre we have developed a detailed protocol for complex spinal cases which includes a back pain disability questionnaire and a pain drawing. The patient is admitted overnight for this assessment. On successive days a detailed history is taken and a full examination and functional assessment are carried out by physiotherapists experienced in dealing with spinal cases. In addition the patient is observed by the ward staff. At the conclusion of 24 hours the assessment is summarized by the surgeon and a plan of management is formed. An alternative approach to the problem of a lengthy and detailed assessment is the recent introduction of computerized interview (Gardner *et al.*, 1986; Thomas *et al.*, 1989).

As part of the primary assessment plain radiographs of the lumbar spine are taken, but until such time as a decision regarding the appropriateness of the patient for surgery has been made, more specialized investigation is not appropriate (see below).

Criteria for surgery

At this point following the preliminary assessment a decision must be made as to whether or not the patient is a suitable candidate for surgery. The criteria that such a patient must satisfy are listed in Table 44.1. Most of these criteria are self-explanatory but the fourth needs a little explanation. There are many patients who are severely incapacitated by low back pain, who have a structural low back problem apparently suitable for surgery and who say that they would undertake any risk in the hope of relieving their back pain problem. However, their life has become so intricately involved in a complex physical and psychological manner with their low back problem that not only do they obtain no relief from surgery, they also become successively more disabled with each well-intended operation.

Prediction of bad results from surgery

It is important to identify those patients who can be predicted to have a bad result from surgery. In our own centre an independent review was carried out of a number of our surgical cases which identified four factors that consistently predicted bad results from surgery (Frish *et al.*, 1988). The four factors were litigation, being off work for more than 12 months prior to surgery, an abnormal pain drawing and the presence of inappropriate or non-organic signs on examination. However sympathetic the surgeon may feel towards such a patient, if all four of these features are present there is no point in offering back pain surgery. It should be noted that in our study previous low back pain surgery did not in itself necessarily predict a bad result from further surgery. If a detailed assessment in a patient who has had previous back surgery shows that the original cause of the pain remains unclear, and if each of the operations was carried out without there being a specific diagnosis and without providing any worthwhile relief, then the prognosis for further surgery is extremely poor.

However, if, for example, a patient had established lumbar instability and then had surgery with a view to stabilizing the spine, but the attempted stabilization was unsuccessful, then it may well still be worth considering further surgery to provide a structurally secure spine.

At this point, following a complete and thorough assessment, a definite decision has to be made. Unless the patient satisfies the criteria in Table 44.1 there is no point in going ahead with the specialized investigations needed for surgery. Either the patient does not satisfy those criteria, in which case he or she must be offered an alternative solution outside the scope of this chapter, or he or she does satisfy those criteria, and one can then proceed to further investigation. To put matters in proportion the great majority of patients referred for back pain surgery do not satisfy the criteria in Table 44.1. In our service only 2.3% of the 1388 patients that were referred in 1988 because of low back pain satisfied the criteria and went ahead to surgery. In other words in our own service for 97.7% of patients a solution other than surgery had to be found.

Selection of appropriate surgery

Investigations

In the small proportion of patients that satisfy the criteria for surgery, specialized investigations now play their invaluable part in helping plan that surgery.

Those patients who will have the best results from surgery are those who happen to have a one-level, or at the most a two-level, low back problem. The point of the investigations is to establish the cause for the patient's pain and to discover whether that patient does indeed have a localized problem amenable to surgery.

Within the terms of reference of this chapter the point of investigation is to identify whether or not the patient's main pain source is arising from the disc in front, from the facet joints behind or from a combination of the two (see also Chapters 4, 35 & 36).

In a few cases the relevant joints may be clearly identified from a clinical examination and plain X-rays. Sometimes, however, the plain X-rays will be relatively normal, and one may have to identify features in the history which help suggest the pain source; for example pain on extension, worse at night and in the early morning may suggest facet joint pain (Eisenstein & Parry, 1987) whereas pain brought on by sitting and worse later in the day may be anterior discogenic pain.

Table 44.1 Criteria for surgery for chronic low back pain

Pain that has been bad enough and has gone on for long enough
Pain that is no better or worse despite thorough conservative treatment
Pain that is significantly interfering with the patient's lifestyle
Pain that the patient genuinely wants to lose
Absence of litigation
A realistic appraisal of what surgery has to offer

Anterior pain source

As a first step a magnetic resonance imaging (MRI) scan will show whether there is a loss of signal from any of the lumbar discs, and whether this loss of signal is localized to one or two levels or whether it is more diffuse. Such a scan will show if there is loss of signal from a disc but it will not indicate whether that disc is or is not a pain source. If the MRI scan shows that the anterior problem is restricted to one or at the most two levels, then a pain provocation discogram is carried out in order to establish whether or not the relevant levels constitute a pain source.

Posterior pain source

If it is thought that the main pain source is posterior then, in the absence of root symptoms and signs, a diagnostic facet joint injection is carried out under X-ray control to identify which joints are giving rise to pain. If there are root symptoms and signs then a contrast-enhanced computerized tomography (CT) scan neatly demonstrates the anatomy and defines any specific nerve root problems. In patients who have had previous surgery, who have lumbar instability with degenerative change, and who have significant leg pain we have found selective nerve blocks to be helpful (Knight & Dove, 1985). In such cases electromyography may also be helpful (Leyshon *et al.*, 1981).

Preoperative planning

Following the initial assessment and subsequent investigations one may well not have identified a clear-cut cause for the patient's pain, in which case that patient should not be offered surgery. If investigations have revealed a degenerative basis for the patient's pain then this may be either a one- or two-level problem, or several levels throughout the lumbar spine may be involved. If the problem is diffuse and involves more than two levels, we dissuade the patient from surgery as in our experience in such cases the results are less satisfactory. If a one- or two-level degenerative low back problem has been established then the patient may be a straightforward candidate for surgery, or the surgeon may still have reservations. If there is any doubt then a trial of a plaster spica may be helpful. A plaster body jacket or brace alone are not satisfactory in that they do not sufficiently immobilize the lumbosacral junction (Fidler & Plasmans, 1983). The patient is immobilized for six weeks in a plaster spica, including one thigh. If the patient tolerates such an awkward device and has worthwhile but only temporary relief of pain, then it is reasonable to consider a surgical fusion. A more accurate means of assessing a patient's suitability for a fusion with a more precise identification of levels may be provided by the use of an external fixator (North *et al.*, 1989).

Preoperative advice

If, following a thorough assessment, the surgeon is happy that the patient satisfies the criteria for surgery and a localized one- or two-level problem has been found, then the patient must be counselled. It is our practice to tell patients that if they are going to have surgery, then the only reason for an operation is pain relief. We regard it as being the place of the surgeon to tell the patient whether or not an operation can be considered, but it must be the patient who makes the final decision as to whether or not an operation is carried out.

The patient is encouraged not to make too ready a decision regarding surgery. Any specific risk involved in the surgery is discussed and the patient is warned that there can be no guarantee that the surgery will relieve the pain to the extent that is desired. In addition the patient is handed an advisory pamphlet (Fig. 44.1). This pamphlet is used in addition to and is no substitute for the standard consent procedure. The use of this pamphlet derives from a similar advisory pamphlet issued by the British Scoliosis Society for patients undergoing spinal deformity surgery. Following the consultation we write to patients confirming the details of the advice and we also send them an explanatory leaflet about the type of surgery involved (copies of our leaflets are available from the author on request). The advice is copied to patients' general practitioners and where appropriate to the referring surgeon, and it is then left to patients to decide whether or not they wish to proceed with surgery.

It will thus be clear that the assessment, investigation, planning and counselling of a patient undergoing surgery for chronic low back pain are lengthy and involved, but nonetheless are an essential preamble to surgery in this very complex area.

Philosophy of surgery: to fuse or not to fuse?

We believe that the principle in low back pain surgery is firstly to identify a localized pain source. The surgery should then be designed to remove that pain source and if in the process of so doing the spine is rendered unstable then it should be stabilized or fused. If the spine is to be stabilized then this should be supplemented with internal fixation to obtain a more reliable fusion rate. It is a basic principle of spinal deformity surgery that in order to obtain a reliable fusion the facet joints should be excised and the spine should be internally fixed. These principles have been traditionally ignored in surgical fusions for low back pain so perhaps it is no surprise that traditional techniques that leave the facets intact and do not involve internal fixation have a high reported pseudarthrosis rate, and their proponents are now reporting their experience of internal fixation systems (Shaw & Taylor, 1956; Wiltse & Bateman, 1965; Prothero *et al.*, 1966; Horowitch *et al.*, 1989).

Certainly a surgical fusion imposes an increased load on the immediately adjacent spinal levels, which may then at some time in the future give

ADVICE FOR THOSE CONSENTING TO SPINAL SURGERY

You (or in the case of minors the parent or legal guardian) should read this pamphlet carefully and sign it once you have read it and understood it. It should then be handed to the doctor when you are admitted to hospital.

This pamphlet has been prepared by the Stoke-on-Trent Spinal Service

The advice in this pamphlet is in addition to that advice which your surgeon has already given you regarding the need for an operation on your spine. Your surgeon will have advised you as to why in his opinion an operation is necessary in your particular case.

Spinal surgery is major surgery and no major surgery is without risk. The main worry in spinal surgery is the risk of paralysis with loss of use of the legs and loss of control of the bladder and bowels. Despite very careful precautions such a risk can never be completely eliminated but in straightforward spinal surgery this risk is extremely small.

If your particular case is a difficult or complex one with an increased risk of such weakness then your surgeon will advise you accordingly.

If you have any further questions or worries then you should raise them with your surgeon before the operation. He will be pleased to advise you.

I ____________________

of ____________________

In the case of minors

I ____________________

of ____________________

being the parent/legal guardian of

____

agree that I have read and understood the contents of this pamphlet.

Signed .... Date ....

I confirm that I have explained the details of the surgery and its risks.

Signed .... Date ....

Fig. 44.1 Three-page pamphlet giving advice for those consenting to spinal surgery.

rise to secondary problems. It is because of this that firstly as far as possible the initial surgery must be designed so that the levels adjacent to the fusion are normal, and at present a MRI scan is the most sensitive way of determining this. Secondly, because a surgical fusion may give rise to secondary problems at a later date the surgeon must be quite sure that the patient is presently sufficiently disabled for there to be no alternative to back pain surgery.

Designing surgery

In the lumbar spine degenerative change may begin in the disc anteriorly and result in secondary subluxation and degenerative change in the lumbar facet joints, or the process may begin in the lumbar facet joints and involve the disc secondarily. Such degenerative change may occur primarily or secondarily, but it is not the remit of this chapter to discuss the aetiology. As far as designing surgery is concerned, if the degenerative change is primarily in the anterior column and the spinal canal and lumbar facet joints are essentially normal then we prefer an anterior approach with an anterior disc excision and fusion. If the primary problem is posterior with degenerative change in the lumbar facets and secondary bony compromise of the lateral recess with a fairly normal disc in front, then we prefer a posterior approach only. In an advanced case where the whole motion segment is affected, then we believe that a combined anterior and posterior approach is required (O'Brien & Speck, 1987).

Surgery

The basic principles of the different types of surgery will now be discussed, but it is not the place of this chapter to provide technical details of the different internal fixation techniques, which can be found in the references.

Surgery of anterior column

The lumbar spine can be approached anterolaterally by a retroperitoneal approach, and this is the preferred approach particularly if more than one level is to be tackled. However, if only the L5–S1 level is involved, this is sometimes awkward to reach through a standard retroperitoneal approach and in such cases we prefer a transperitoneal approach through a Pfannenstiel incision, which provides a speedy, straightforward and a 'face-on' approach to the lumbosacral disc (Freebody *et al.*, 1971).

The classical technique, particularly for a one-level anterior disc excision and fusion, is a thorough excision of the disc together with curettage of the endplates down to cancellous bone and then large blocks of corticocancellous graft from the iliac crest are inserted across the disc space (Sacks, 1965). These tricortical grafts do, however, leave a defect in the iliac crest which can be a cause of significant morbidity (Summers, 1989). This morbidity can be avoided by the use of a dowel system (Crock, 1982). Because of donor site morbidity there is intense interest in bone graft substitutes such as blocks of titanium mesh (Yau, 1989).

A disc excision and fusion can be carried out from behind by placing blocks of bone graft across the disc space from a posterior approach, a posterior lumbar interbody fusion or PLIF (Cloward, 1963). This is a difficult technique but it does place the grafts in the biomechanically most suitable place.

If a more than one-level anterior disc excision and fusion is to be performed then without internal fixation there is a risk of pseudarthrosis, particularly at the upper level. In such cases the surgeon may prefer to supplement the anterior fusion with internal fixation using, for example, a standard AO fracture plate. Alternatively the surgeon may prefer to use a system specifically developed for this purpose (Ryan *et al.*, 1986; Kostuik & Thomas, 1986). One of the problems of an anterior disc excision without internal fixation is that even if a solid fusion occurs there may be collapse of the graft with loss of disc height which can result in important secondary changes in the posterior column. In order to avoid this we have developed a device, the Hartshill horsehoe, that incorporates a central bone graft or bone graft substitute and which is screwed into place in the disc space to act as a spacer (Valentine *et al.*, 1989b). More recently an attempt is being made at the same time to excise an anterior discogenic pain source and yet preserve segmental movement with a prosthetic disc replacement (Büttner-Janz *et al.*, 1987).

Surgery of posterior column

It is not within the terms of reference of this chapter to consider the relief of back pain by minor percutaneous procedures such as electrocautery or closed rhizolysis. However, in a few carefully selected cases open rhizolysis of the lumbar facet joints can be useful in early degenerative change in sportsmen. From time to time a keen or professional sportsman will be troubled by facet joint pain which is relieved by injection under X-ray control. If after a time the injections fail to have sufficiently lasting benefit, and if the patient's sport is sufficiently important to him, then an open rhizolysis of the relevant facet joints may allow him to continue his sport. This is particularly so if only one facet joint is affected. The relevant joint is exposed through a very short midline incision and thorough diathermy of the whole of the visible capsule of the joint is carried out. Whatever the physiological mechanism, this procedure can produce very worthwhile results in this small demanding group of patients. The benefit may be only temporary, but is may allow the patient to continue to compete in his sport at the highest level.

Posterior surgery is normally carried out through a midline approach except for certain specific instances such as a bilateral intertransverse fusion (Wiltse & Bateman, 1965).

A surgical fusion with internal fixation can be performed by a screw fusion of the facet joints (Boucher, 1959; Andrew *et al.*, 1986). This technique addresses the question of pain arising from the facet joints themselves, but the internal fixation is insubstantial and the problem of the narrow lateral recess remains unresolved.

If as a result of hypertrophic degenerative change of the lumbar facet joints there is narrowing of the lateral recess and bony nerve root compression (Crock, 1981), then there may be a place for the surgical procedure of undercutting facetectomy (Getty *et al.*, 1981). This allows a bony decompression of the nerve root without destabilizing the spine, and addresses the problem of leg pain but does not solve the problem of back pain arising from the degenerative facet joints themselves.

If the patient has significant degenerative changes in the lumbar facet joints then we believe the surgery should consist of a wide excision of the relevant facets supplemented by a fusion with internal fixation. For a one-level stabilization at L5–S1 it is still probably reasonable to perform a bony intertransverse fusion alone without internal fixation, but if more than one level is involved, or if one is above L5, then internal fixation should normally be used. There is now a wide choice of available internal fixation systems to supplement a posterior lumbosacral fusion (Cotrel & Dubousset 1984; Dove, 1986; Kaneda *et al.*, 1986; Krag *et al.*, 1986; Louis, 1986; Luque, 1986; Roy-Camille *et al.*, 1986; Selby, 1986; Steffee *et al.*, 1986; Zielke and Strempel, 1986; Dick, 1987; Horowitch *et al.*, 1989; Puno *et al.*, personal communication, 1989). Each system has its advantages and disadvantages. Most methods provide adequate stabilization of the lumbar spine but the problem common to all systems is adequate fixation to the sacrum, which remains an unresolved problem. It is not appropriate to provide here a detailed biomechanical comparison of the different fixation devices. Suffice it to say that the basic requirements of an internal fixation for the back of the lumbosacral spine are that it should provide secure fixation, it should not be too bulky, it should allow preservation of the normal lumbar lordosis, it should be inexpensive, it should be adaptable (incorporating the facility both for sublaminar wiring and pedicle screw fixation as appropriate) and finally in order to provide torsional stability there should be crosslinks. Each surgeon must select the internal fixation which suits him or her best, and should learn the technique either from the originator or from someone with considerable practical experience of the relevant device.

Any internal fixation may be supplemented by a bony fusion. Through a midline approach one can split the transverse process via an osteotomy through the upper facet of the relevant vertebra, allowing one easily to place the graft in a rich cancellous bed; the intratransverse fusion technique (Dove, 1986). There is, however, no reason why the surgeon should not combine his internal fixation with a traditional intertransverse fusion should this be desired (Wiltse & Bateman, 1965).

Combined anterior and posterior surgery

If there is advanced degenerative change of the whole motion segment then it may be necessary to stabilize both the anterior and posterior columns. Certainly it is well established that if there is significant anterior degenerative change then even a solid posterior fusion with internal fixation will not exclude all movement of the anterior column, and the patient may still suffer from anterior discogenic pain (Weatherley *et al.*, 1986). In such circumstances we believe that anterior and posterior surgery should be combined.

If there is significant deformity, especially a severe congenital spondylolisthesis, then we would first carry out an anterior disc excision and fusion and then under the same anaesthetic would perform a posterior approach with fusion and internal fixation (O'Brien & Speck, 1987).

However, if there is no deformity we now prefer to carry out the whole of the surgery through the posterior approach. The relevant disc space is exposed, and on each side the dura retracted medially and a dowel of disc and bone removed. A dowel of bone graft or bone graft substitute is then hammered into place across the disc space from behind both from right and left to form a modified posterior lumbar interbody fusion. This is then combined with a facet joint excision and fusion with internal fixation at the same level to give a very secure fixation of both columns (Mulnier, 1989).

The future

However sophisticated modern internal fixation systems may be, an extensive back pain fusion with internal fixation is a crude approach to the problem of back pain. Nowadays increasing attention is being paid to the prevention of back pain, but it is unlikely that this will reduce the workload of back pain surgery in the immediately foreseeable future. Currently techniques to allow a percutaneous lumbar fusion are being developed (Shepperd, 1989). Certainly this is an interesting development and in the long-term prevention of back pain, together with

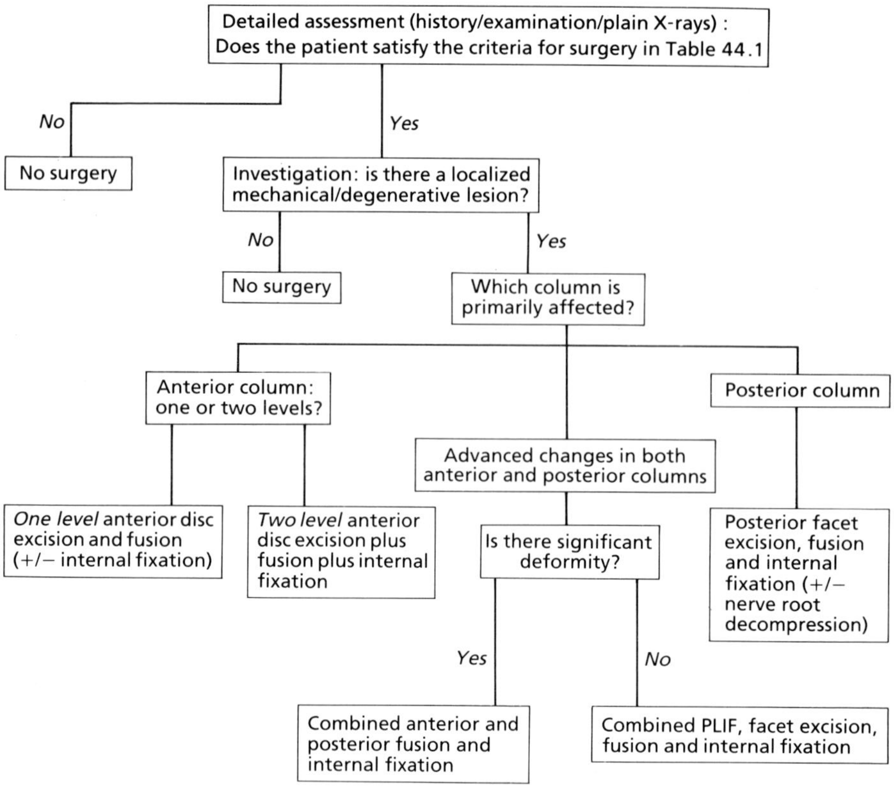

Fig. 44.2 Scheme of management of chronic low back pain.

the development of better-designed and less invasive surgery, is the ideal.

Summary

We emphasize that the type of surgery for low back pain described in this chapter is appropriate only to a very small number of patients presenting with chronic low back pain (Karl Hirsch, 'Do not hide your ignorance of the back behind a large spinal fusion'). In other words there is no point in carrying out an extensive back pain fusion merely because the surgeon feels sorry for a particular patient. However well-intentioned, an extensive low back fusion carried out as a last resort without any clear indication frequently produces disastrous results.

We believe that traditional posterior surgical techniques have had limited success because they have been performed through a limited access. This was because of trying to perform a sufficient bony decompression without at the same time destabilizing the spine. Now that suitable internal fixation systems are available we believe that there should be a wide surgical approach with a wide excision of the relevant degenerate facets supplemented by a bony fusion and secure internal fixation.

In a small group of patients disabled by chronic low back pain, and who have an identifiable localized mechanical cause for their pain, modern techniques of back pain surgery can revolutionize their lives. Given the confusing multiplicity of techniques available, what in January 1990 (the time of writing) should be the approach of the surgeon who wishes to use tried and tested techniques for the relief of chronic low back pain?

The essentials are (Fig. 44.2).

1 The surgeon must satisfy him- or herself based on the criteria in Table 44.1, that the patient's back pain is bad enough to need surgery.

2 Investigations should be carried out with a view to identifying a localized one- or two-level mechanical or degenerative problem.

3 If the main problem is anterior discogenic pain and the posterior structures are essentially normal, then an anterior disc excision and fusion should be performed.

4 If the problem is in the posterior structures and the disc in front is essentially normal then a posterior procedure with facet excision fusion and internal fixation should be carried out.

5 If there are major changes in both the anterior and posterior columns then if there is significant deformity combined anterior and posterior surgery should be carried out, and if there is no such deformity then both anterior and posterior columns should be stabilized through a posterior approach by a posterior lumbar interbody fusion, together with facet excision, fusion and internal fixation.

REFERENCES

Andrew, T.A., Brooks, S. & Piggott, H. (1986) Long-term follow up evaluation of screw and graft fusion of the lumbar spine. *Clin. Orthop. Rel. Res.*, **203**, 113–119.

Boucher, H.H. (1959) A method of spinal fusion. *J. Bone Jt. Surg.*, **41B**, 248–259.

Büttner-Janz, K., Schellnack, K. & Zippel, H. (1987) Eine alternative Behandlung Strategie beim lumbarhen Bandscheibenschaden mit der bandscheibenendoprothese Mondulartyp SB Charite. *Z. Orthop.*, **127**, 1–6.

Cloward, R.B. (1963) Lesions of the intervertebral discs and their treatment by interbody fusion methods. *Clin. Orthop.*, **27**, 51.

Cotrel, Y. & Dubousset, J. (1984) Nouvelle technique d'osteosynthese rachidienne segmentaire par voie posterieure. *Rev. Chir. Orthop.*, **70**, 489–495.

Crock, H.V. (1981) Normal and pathological anatomy of the lumbar spinal nerve root canals. *J. Bone Jt. Surg.*, **63B**, 487.

Crock, H.V. (1982) Anterior lumbar interbody fusion. *Clin. Orthop.*, **165**, 157.

Dick, W. (1987) The 'fixateur interne' as a versatile implant for spine surgery. *Spine*, **12**, 882–900.

Dove, J. (1986) Internal fixation of the lumbar spine: the Hartshill rectangle. *Clin. Orthop. Rel. Res.*, **203**, 135–140.

Eisenstein, S.M. & Parry, C.R. (1987) The lumbar facet arthrosis syndrome: clinical presentation and articular surface changes. *J. Bone Jt. Surg.*, **69B**, 3–7.

Fidler, M.W. & Plasmans, C.M.T. (1983) The effect of four types of support on the segmental mobility of the lumbosacral spine. *J. Bone Jt. Surg.*, **65A**, 943.

Freebody, D., Bendall, R. & Taylor, R.D. (1971) Anterior transperitoneal lumbar fusion. *J. Bone Jt. Surg.*, **53B**, 617.

Frish, E., Hoyle, M.D. & Dove, J. (1988) The Hartshill system for osteoarthritis of the lumbar facet joint: an independent review. Presented at the annual meeting of the International Society for the Study of the Lumbar Spine, Florida.

Gardner, A.D., Pursell, L.M., Murty, K. & Smith, D.G. (1986) The management of the clinical problem of spinal pain with the assistance of a micro-computer. In Hukins, D.W.L. & Mulholland, R.C. (eds), *Back Pain*, pp. 24–41. Manchester University Press, Manchester.

Getty, C.J.M., Johnson, J.R., Kirwan, E.O'G. & Sullivan, M.F. (1981) Partial undercutting facetectomy for bony entrapment of the lumbar nerve root. *J. Bone Jt. Surg.*, **63B**, 330–335.

Horowitch, A., Peek, R.D., Thomas, J.C., Widell, E.H., Dimartino, P.P., Spencer, C.W., Weinstein, J. & Wiltse, L.L. (1989) The Wiltse pedicle screw fixation system. *Spine*, **14**, 461–467.

Kaneda, K., Kazama, H., Satoh, S. & Fujiy, M. (1986) Follow-up study of medial factectomies and posterolateral fusion with instrumentation in unstable degenerative spondylolisthesis. *Clin. Orthop. Rel. Res.*, **203**, 159–167.

Knight, C.L. & Dove, J. (1985) Can selective lumbosacral nerve tests help your difficult back pain patients? Presented at the Intractable Pain Society Meeting, Bristol.

Kostuik, J.P. & Thomas, J.E. (1986) Techniques of internal fixation for degenerative conditions of the lumbar spine. *Clin. Orthop. Rel. Res.*, **203**, 219–231.

Krag, M.H., Beynnon, B.D., Pope, M.H., Frymoyer, J.W., Haugh, L.D. & Weaver, D.L. (1986) An internal fixator for posterior application to short segments of the thoracic, lumbar or lumbosacral spine. *Clin. Orthop. Rel. Res.*, **203**, 75–98.

Leyshon, A., Kirwan, E.O.G. & Wynne-Parry, C.B. (1981) Electrical studies in the diagnosis of compression of the lumbar root. *J. Bone Jt. Surg.*, **63B**, 71–75.

Louis, R. (1986) Fusion of the lumbar and sacral spine by internal fixation with screw plates. *Clin. Orthop. Rel. Res.*, **203**, 18–33.

Luque, E.R. (1986) Interpedicular segmental fixation. *Clin. Orthop. Rel. Res.*, **203**, 54–57.

Mathew, B., Norris, D., Hendry, D. & Waddell, G. (1988) Artificial intelligence in the diagnosis of low back pain and sciatica. *Spine*, **13**, 168–172.

Mulnier, J.J.H. (1989) Posterior lumbar interbody fusion plus Hartshill fixation. Presented at Recent Advances in Spinal Surgery meeting, London. August.

Nelson, M.A. (1968) A long-term review of posterior spinal fusion. *Proc. R. Soc. Med.*, **611**, 558–559.

North, A.D., Roberts, A.P., Wilde, G.P., Pembleton, C.J., Mulholland, R.C. & Webb, J.K. (1989) The Harlow Wood external fixator. *Proc. Inst. Mech. Eng.*, pp. 63–66.

O'Brien, J.P. & Speck, G.R. (1987) Simultaneous combined anterior and posterior fusion of the lumbar spine. *J. Bone Jt. Surg.*, **69B**, 164.

Prothero, S.R., Parkes, J.C. & Stinchfield, F.E. (1966) Complications after low back pain fusion in 1000 patients: a comparison of two series one decade apart. *J. Bone Jt. Surg.*, **48A**, 57–65.

Roy-Camille, R., Saillant, G. & Christian, M. (1986) Internal fixation of the lumbar spine with pedicle screw plating. *Clin. Orthop. Rel. Res.*, **203**, 7–17.

Ryan, M.D., Taylor, T.K.F., Phil, D. & Sherwood, A.A. (1986) Bolt-plate fixation for anterior spinal fusion. *Clin. Orthop. Rel. Res.*, **203**, 196–202.

Sacks, S. (1965) Anterior interbody fusion of the lumbar spine. *J. Bone Jt. Surg.*, **47B**, 211.

Selby, D. (1986) Internal fixation with Knodt's rods. *Clin. Orthop. Rel. Res.*, **203**, 179–184.

Shaw, E.G. & Taylor, J.G. (1956) The results of lumbosacral

fusion for low back pain. *J. Bone Jt. Surg.*, **38B**, 485.

Shepperd, J. (1989) Current possibilities of percutaneous disc surgery. *Percutaneous Lumbar Discectomy*, pp. 185–187.

Steffee, A.D., Biscup, R.S. & Sitkowski, D.J. (1986) Segmental spine plates with pedicle screw fixation. *Clin. Orthop. Rel. Res.*, **203**, 45–53.

Summers, B.N. (1989) Donor site pain from the ilium. *J. Bone Jt. Surg.*, **71B**, 677–680.

Thomas, A.M.C., Fairbank, J.C.T., Pynsent, P.B. & Baker, D.J. (1989) A computer based interview system for patients with back pain. *Spine*, **14**, 844–846.

Valentine, N.W., Sell, P.J., Hastings, G. & Dove, J. (1989a) Development and assessment of a device for anterior spinal fusion: the Hartshill horsehoe. Presented at Combined Meeting of Scoliosis Research Society and European Spinal Deformity Society, Amsterdam, September.

Valentine, N.W., Aziz, R., Sell, P.J. & Dove, J. (1989b) A pedicle screw bridge modification of the Hartshill system. Presented at the Combined Meeting of the Scoliosis Research Society and European Spinal Deformity Society, Amsterdam, September.

Waddell, G., McCulloch, J.A. & Kummel, E.D. (1980) Non-organic physical signs in low back pain. *Spine*, **5**, 117–125.

Weatherley, C.R., Prickett, C.F. & O'Brien, J.P. (1986) Discogenic pain persisting despite solid posterior fusion. *J. Bone Jt. Surg.*, **68B**, 142–143.

Wiltse, L.L. & Bateman, J.G. (1965) Experience with transverse process fusion of the lumbar spine. *J. Bone Jt. Surg.*, **47A**, 848–849.

Yau, A.C.M.C. (1989) Anterior spinal fusion: the Hong Kong experience. Presented at Recent Advances in Spinal Surgery Meeting, London, August.

Zielke, K. & Stempel, A.V. (1986) Posterior lateral distraction spondylodesis using the twofold sacral bar. *Clin. Orthop. Rel. Res.*, **203**, 151–158.

SECTION 9
CERVICAL AND THORACIC DEGENERATIVE DISEASE

45 · Cervical Disc Disease

By M.J. TORRENS

An expanded version of the title might read 'Degenerative disorders of cervical intervertebral discs and their associated joints'. It is not possible to separate out disc degeneration from the secondary changes occurring at the uncinate process and in the facet joints. The majority of clinical problems occurring in the neck are related to such degenerative disease and the following account will relate primarily to this, though in the process of diagnosis every effort must be made to exclude other conditions such as infection, tumour and occult trauma.

PATHOLOGICAL ANATOMY OF DISC DEGENERATION

The nucleus pulposus up to puberty is of a globular shape and holds the vertebral bodies well apart. The uncinate process at this time is separated from the body by the neurocentral synchondrosis and the area above the uncinate processes contains only vessels and connective tissue with no synovium.

Between the ages of 20 and 30 years the nucleus pulposus becomes flatter and the lamellae of the annulus fibrosus become orientated outwards. Between these lamellae clefts form starting laterally above the uncinate processes and gradually extending medially towards the centre of the nucleus. In these clefts the surface of the annulus may become smooth and undergo hyaline metamorphosis but there is no true synovial joint formation in this area which is sometimes called the neurocentral joint (of Lushka). The process of cleft formation starts at the most mobile disc (usually C5–C6) and then occurs subsequently at the spaces above and below this.

The nucleus gradually desiccates and becomes less resilient. Through the clefts or through fractures in the annulus pieces of the nucleus may dislocate. Although a deficiency in the annulus is common in the posterior central region, where the annulus is concave forwards, the disc prolapse seldom projects centrally into the spinal canal due to the presence of the strong posterior longitudinal ligament. Because of this ligament the fragments tend to migrate laterally and protrude posterolaterally, immediately posterior to the uncinate process in relationship to the nerve root.

As the nucleus gradually desiccates and disappears the joint surfaces come closer together and osteophytes begin to form, particularly from the uncinate processes and also elsewhere around the disc margin. As age advances the fibrocartilage disappears and there is further narrowing of the joint space. The uncinate processes become more horizontal and the osteophytes here may themselves impinge upon the nerve roots. There is thickening and sclerosis of the vertebral bone adjacent to the disc space. Eventually the joint becomes relatively immobile. This then passes the stress of movement on to the next joint, which may either accelerate the same degenerative changes or cause a pathological subluxation.

At the same time that the disc joint is becoming narrower, an additional stress is being passed on to the facet joints, which themselves may hypertrophy and produce osteophytes. However, this pathological process is not as common in the cervical spine as in the lumbar spine. This is probably because, as the disc spaces collapse, the anterior surfaces come to lie closer together than the posterior surfaces, producing a reversal of the cervical lordosis and protecting the posteriorly sited facet joints. In fact, facet arthrosis seems to be more prevalent in the higher cervical joints, perhaps associated with the increased mobility in this region following relative immobility in the lower cervical joints which are the first to deteriorate.

There are thus a number of pathological processes associated with disc degeneration which may cause clinical syndromes. Nerve root or spinal cord compression may be caused by simple disc protrusion or by the extrusion or sequestration of a nuclear or annular fragment. In addition to cervical disc prolapse, neural compression may result from the development of osteophytes arising from the posterior margins of the vertebral body, the region of the uncinate process, or from facet joints causing in that case compression from posteriorly. Osteophytes arising in a lateral direction may cause nerve root compression distal to the nerve root foramen or may compress the vertebral artery (see Chapter 46). Hypertrophy of the ligamentum flavum may cause posterior compression of the spinal cord. Finally, degenerative subluxation of cervical vertebrae may cause cord compression.

A considerable proportion of the axial rotation in the cervical spine takes place at the atlanto-axial joint (Penning, 1979). This joint alone provides 40–50% of the axial rotation with the lower cervical spine in total contributing the remaining 50–60%. In contrast flexion, extension and lateral flexion are more or less evenly distributed between all the intervertebral levels. The C5–C6 level, which is very often the earliest to degenerate, does have a slightly greater range of mobility in flexion and extension than the other joints (White & Panjabi, 1978). Indeed, abnormal ranges of cervical mobility may have pathological significance. Barnes & Saunders (1984) found that an abnormally increased range of cervical mobility was an adverse factor in the prognosis of cervical spondylotic myelopathy.

Another important factor in the development of clinical problems as a consequence of cervical spondylosis is the role of cervical canal stenosis. Payne & Spillane (1957) were the first to observe that patients with cervical spondylotic myelopathy frequently had a constitutionally narrow cervical canal, allowing the effects of degenerative disease to be exaggerated. Their study was performed on autopsy material but has been confirmed by many authors. Normal ranges for the sagittal diameter of the cervical canal have been established radiologically and the clinical role of cervical stenosis in the aetiology of cervical myelopathy is well established (Nurick, 1972, 1975; Veidlinger *et al.*, 1981).

CLINICAL DIAGNOSIS

Cervical disc disease may present in various ways. It may be evident as an asymptomatic finding on plain radiography at any age but such a finding is increasingly common with increasing age. It may present by producing neck pain alone. More severe problems arise when either radiculopathy or myelopathy result, with combinations of these two problems being common. A rare presentation results when the cervical spondylosis produces vertebral artery disease.

Neck pain

Pain in the neck, which may radiate into the paraspinal muscles, the interscapular area, the shoulder and sometimes the occipital region, is extremely common and usually self-limiting. It may arise in relationship to trauma, or spontaneously.

Neck pain after trauma, commonly and usually imprecisely described as a whiplash injury, is very often considered to be an entirely benign process. A small proportion of cases, however, have a traumatically disrupted disc as a basis of their continuing complaints. If the pain does not resolve progressively in the expected fashion, and is associated with very focal tenderness over one or two cervical spinous processes on examination then it may be due to a disc prolapse even in the absence of radicular signs and symptoms. It is therefore not unreasonable to consider investigation such as magnetic resonance imaging to screen such patients. The problem of soft tissue injuries of the cervical spine is fully discussed in Chapter 63.

The spontaneous onset of neck pain may be associated with a reduced range of movement, paraspinal muscle spasm and tenderness and occasionally an acute torticollis. Examination is directed mainly to identifying evidence of any neurological involvement and also to determining whether there is any particular focus for the pain. Tenderness over the occipital nerve or over the rotator cuff in the shoulder may indicate a separate lesion, though both 'occipital neuralgia' and the rotator cuff syndrome are common in association with neck disorders. White count, sedimentation rate or plasma viscosity, C-reactive protein and creatine phosphokinase may be performed to exclude any form of specific inflammatory or infective process. If an infection is suspected then radiological investigation of this should proceed forthwith. Every severe neck pain should also be assessed radiologically if there is no rapid resolution, otherwise a trial of conservative treatment is usually appropriate.

Brachial neuralgia

When brachial neuralgia is accompanied by a neuropathy the commonest cause is some form of nerve root compression. In the more usual situation where brachial neuralgia is not accompanied by any objective neurological signs, the differential diagnosis is less simple. If the brachial neuralgia is associated with neck pain or increased by neck movement (particularly lateral flexion away from the side of the pain or rotation towards the pain) then nerve root involvement is likely. The dermal distribution of the paraesthesiae in the appropriate nerve root territory also suggests a nerve lesion but other features, including the distribution of pain, are relatively less helpful.

The differential diagnosis of brachial neuralgia is wide. A neurofibroma may occur in the intervertebral foramen or more peripherally; this tends to produce relatively more sensory loss than pain. The intervertebral foramen may be widened on plain X-ray. Other lesions involving the brachial plexus, such as a Pancoast tumour, may mimic cervical root entrapment; the association of Horner's syndrome should lead one to suspect this lesion. So-called neuralgic amyotrophy usually affects the C5 region producing severe pain with weakness and wasting in the shoulder muscles. There is usually no disturbance of the neck and relatively little sensory abnormality. The neurological deficit may be severe but usually appears as the severe pain starts to settle. The pain of angina may radiate down the arm and into the neck but is usually easy to distinguish. Focal pain in the shoulder with weakness of abduction may be due to the rotator cuff syndrome. There is usually focal tenderness over the area of tenosynovitis and a painful arc syndrome where abduction becomes painful after about 30°. There are various so-called pseudo-radicular syndromes which may be some form of non-compressive neuritis. Their pathological nature is unclear. Polymyalgia rheumatica may produce pain similar to brachial neuralgia but not associated with focal motor deficit, although there may be some generalized weakness. More peripherally median and ulnar nerve entrapment syndromes may be confused initially, but should be easily identified clinically by the pattern of the neurological deficit and confirmed if necessary by neurophysiological studies.

Myelopathy

Spinal cord compression in degenerative disease of the neck may be due to acute cervical disc prolapse, to a chronic osteophytic compression at one or more levels or to compression associated with vertebral subluxation. Hypertrophy or buckling of the ligamentum flavum may exacerbate this, and any patient with relative spinal stenosis is more vulnerable to the effects of degenerative disease.

The actual pathophysiological mechanism which results in the production of myelopathy from cervical spondylosis remains unclear. Many people who survive with severe radiological disease of the cervical spine never develop myelopathy. The actual cause of myelopathy is likely to be multifactorial, with factors such as chronic ischaemia due to compromise of the radicular arteries in association with obstruction to venous drainage and actual compression of the spinal cord by disc or osteophytes being the main causative factor. Other factors of importance are: trauma—either on one occasion or repetitive, traction on cord and roots, excessive cervical mobility, and absolute or relative canal stenosis.

The onset of myelopathy may be acute and the symptoms initially may be relatively non-specific, the patient complaining of neck pain associated with rather vague symptoms of weakness and disturbed sensory function in the rest of the body which is not always easy to confirm on neurological examination. These patients should be taken seriously. Every year a small number of cases fail to be diagnosed and progress to a more serious degree of quadriparesis or quadriplegia. The acute onset of complaints of paraesthesiae or electrical feelings through the body associated with neck movement is an important symptom to elicit.

The more chronic presentation is very typical. Lower cervical levels tend to produce a spastic paraparesis with a typical unsteady scuffing gait associated with hyperreflexia and extensor plantar responses. If there is a significant degree of posterior column deficit then some element of posterior compression of the spinal cord should be suspected. Micturition may be disordered with frequency and urgency, but this occurs relatively less commonly than in other spinal cord disorders and is usually a late finding in cervical spondylotic myelopathy.

At higher cervical levels, the likelihood of impaired hand function is greater. At the C3–C4 level the typical presentation is the numb, clumsy hands syndrome (Good *et al.*, 1984) and this may occur without much in the way of symptoms of dysfunction in the legs. An alternative cause of disordered function in the arms and hands may be multiple nerve compression from narrowed intervertebral foraminae. This should be distinguishable from the hand dysfunctions associated with spinal cord compression by virtue of the fact that the signs in the arms should be of a lower motoneurone nature. The situation, however, is seldom as clear-cut as this and the co-existence of upper and lower motoneurone features in the hands is common. The relative distribution of such neurological signs is an important factor to take into account when planning the exact details of operative treatment.

Differential diagnosis in myelopathy is less extensive and usually easier to distinguish radiologically. Multiple sclerosis does not always present with additional cerebral features but commonly presents with bladder disturbance before any paraparesis. Intramedullary spinal tumour may be indistinguishable on a clinical basis. Extramedullary spinal tumours may well show some degree of lateralization of the signs but this can be mimicked by a unilateral osteophyte and a Brown–Sequard syndrome is not uncommonly due to cervical spondylosis. Syringomyelia is usually associated with a more profound, and sometimes a suspended spinothalamic, sensory loss. The paraparesis is usually later and often more obvious in one leg. Subacute combined degeneration due to vitamin B_{12} deficiency seems extremely uncommon now. This affects the posterior columns more profoundly than the rest of the spinal cord but is a differential diagnosis to consider when the myelopathy appears to be mainly posteriorly based. There is probably also a myelopathy which is primarily associated with vascular insufficiency. It seems that this may be associated with features of brain stem disorder such as dysarthria. Diffuse cerebrovascular disease may also produce a gait disorder (*marche à petits pas*) which at first sight may be mistaken for a myelopathic gait. Close assessment of the gait, and the fact that such patients usually have features other such as emotional lability, allows the correct diagnosis to be made.

CONSERVATIVE TREATMENT

Degenerative disease of the cervical spine is extremely common and only a very small proportion of cases warrant consideration for surgery. Conservative treatment therefore has a significant part to play in managing minor non-specific problems, those without neurological deficit or where the neurological deficit is stable or improving, or cases where radiological diagnosis is entirely normal. In the vast majority of cases the acute exacerbations of pain are self-limiting and much of the conservative management is to support the patient whilst the situation settles down of its own accord.

Neck pain is usually mechanical and not neurogenic; treatment is therefore somewhat empirical, ranging from strict immobilization on the one hand to active mobilization on the other. Immobilization is frequently by a soft cervical collar which produces very little support to the neck and virtually no restriction of movement except perhaps flexion. Some types of hard or specially moulded collars are more effective but seldom reduce movement by more than about 70%. In acute cases bed rest with the head supported appropriately by pillows is probably the best technique, as this removes the effect of gravity.

Alternatively physiotherapeutic manoeuvres such as heat, massage, vibration, traction and manipulation may be employed. It is probably reasonable to try the effect of each technique on a short-term basis and continue the treatment only if it is showing benefit. In any case with mechanical joint pain it is appropriate to try analgesic and anti-inflammatory drugs which work better in mechanical disorders than in neurogenic pain.

Thus often in chronic pain problems the techniques of a pain clinic may be appropriate. These include injections of anaesthetic, steroid or neurolytic agents into or around tender areas, facet joints and the occipital nerves. Transcutaneous nerve stimulation is seldom effective in the cervical area.

RADIOLOGICAL DIAGNOSIS

The quality of radiology has improved so much that no patient should be operated upon without a definite anatomical diagnosis and surgical strategy worked out largely on the basis of the radiological investigations.

Plain X-rays

Recently patients have been proceeding directly to more sophisticated investigations. Plain X-rays, however, are important in all cases and should include *routinely* good-quality oblique foraminal views and flexion/extension lateral films. Such a series of films is needed for an overview of the area. The extent of degenerative disease and relative mobility influence the choice of treatment. On the lateral film the relative size of the spinal canal can be judged from comparing its depth to that of the vertebral bodies (normally approximately 1 : 1). The pedicular height and laminar obliquity can also be assessed; the latter by measuring the space between the back of the facet joints and the anterior (intracanalicular) surface of the vertebral spine. Incipient degenerative subluxation is important to discover. It may be the site of symptoms even if other adjacent levels show more osteophytic outgrowth and such subluxation will progress rapidly after adjacent fusion.

Myelography and computerized tomography

Water-soluble, non-ionic, contrast media greatly improved the investigation of radiculopathy in the past decade, and the addition of computerized tomography (CT) adds further information about the transverse spatial relationships within the spine. CT should be performed immediately following the myelogram as the combined examination provides enhanced information, especially in cases where lateral canal osteophytes or disc prolapses are suspected. Plain CT alone is an insufficient means of assessing the cervical spine.

It is not enough to inject intrathecally a low dose of contrast medium and then scan by CT alone. Myelography has the benefit of screening the whole spine and the foramen magnum area, and reducing the time and radiation exposure of subsequent CT by selecting the appropriate area to scan. The flow characteristics of the contrast medium are significant, as is the degree of obstruction that occurs on extension of the neck. CT myelography (Fig. 45.1) is currently the best overall single investigation for cervical spinal disorders. This may change with better resolution and faster acquisition times from magnetic resonance imaging (MRI).

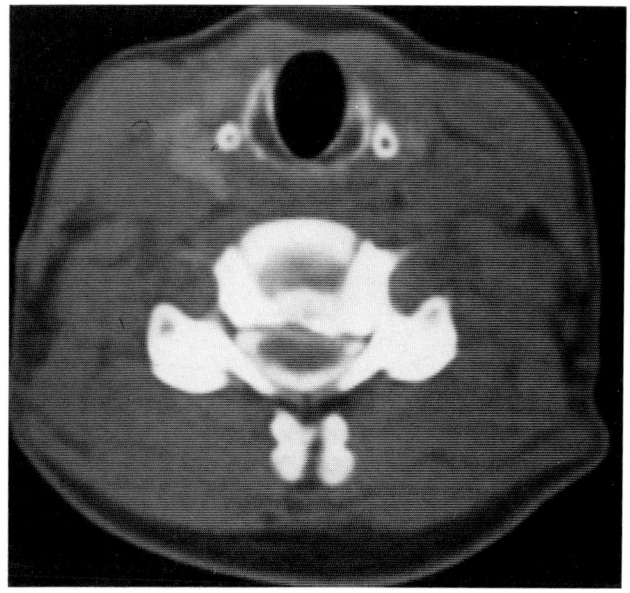

Fig. 45.1 CT myelography showing a predominantly unilateral osteophyte indenting the spinal cord and narrowing the intervertebral foramen on one side.

Magnetic resonance imaging

MRI is the most versatile investigation for cases of myelopathy (Ullrich, 1989). Intrinsic cord pathology can be visualized and a dynamic view of compression obtained by flexion/extension sagittal images. Bone is not well shown and the extent of the compression needs to be judged from deformation of the spinal cord (Fig. 45.2). Deformation of the dura can be seen on T2-weighted images using movement artifact suppression techniques (MAST). These are performed by gating the acquisitions with reference to the ECG to remove pulse flow artifacts in the CSF (Fig. 45.3). This tends to overemphasize the extent of compression with respect to myelography.

MRI can image disc material well if the water content is high (Figs 45.4 & 45.5). Osteophytes may not be well seen unless they displace epidural fat

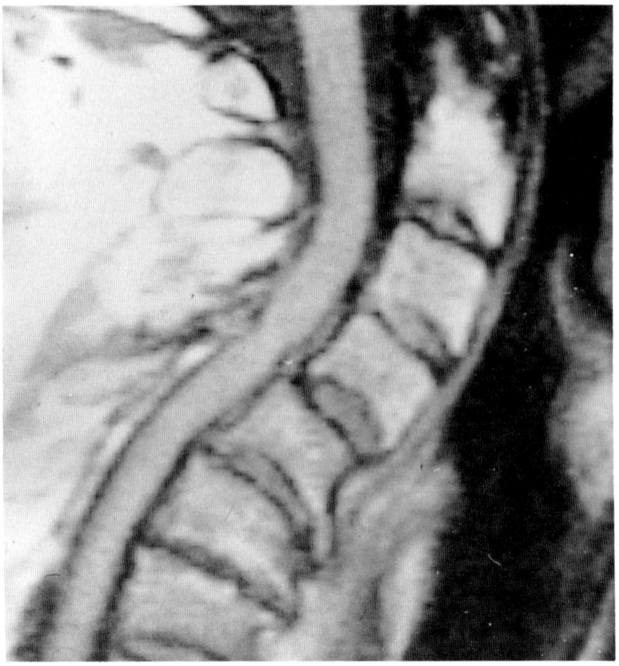

Fig. 45.2 Midsagittal cervical MRI (T1) showing spinal cord compression from anterior and posterior elements at C4–C5 due to hypermobility and incipient subluxation at the level above the relatively fused lower cervical motion segments.

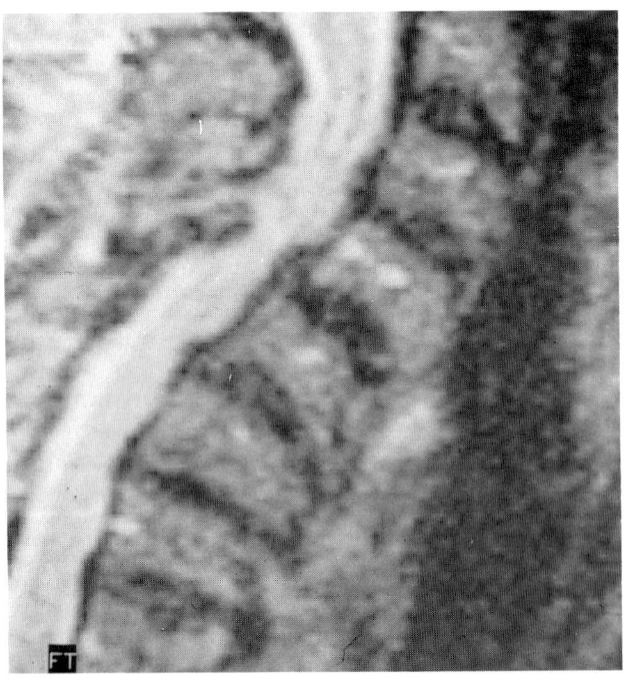

Fig. 45.3 MRI (T2 MAST) of the case in Fig. 45.2 showing the indentation of the dura at C4–C5. The detail of the cord is lost and the compression is slightly overemphasized.

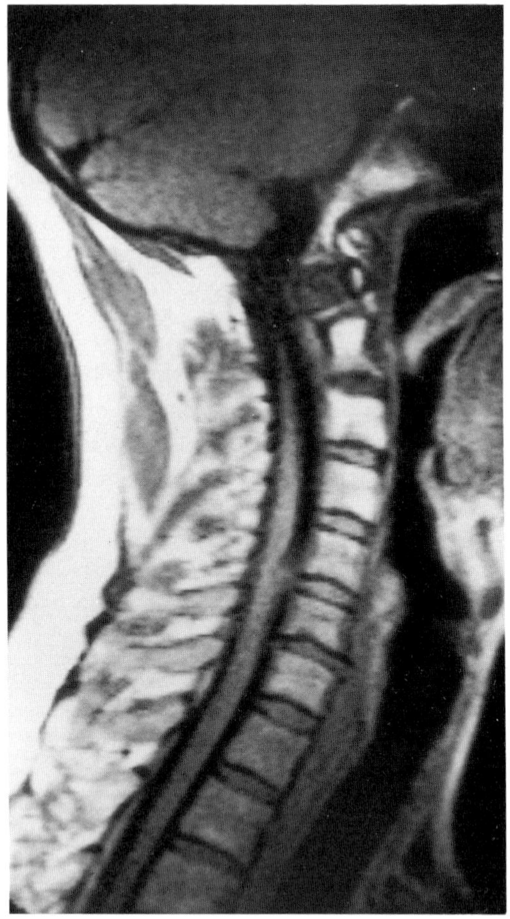

Fig. 45.4 Sagittal MRI (T1) showing disc material at C5–C6 indenting the spinal cord.

or unless a high-quality MAST image is obtained (Fig. 45.6). In my experience a significant number of cervical spondylosis patients investigated by MRI require subsequent CT·myelography. Very few CT myelograms require to be supplemented by MRI.

Discography

Cervical discography has been justly criticized and is relatively seldom used, for good reasons. The test is painful (deliberately) and the majority of discs injected in patients over the age of 30 will show 'degenerative' changes as might be expected from the anatomical description given above. Experience in needle placement centrally in the disc is necessary. A positive discogram is one that reproduces exactly the patient's symptoms during the injection of dye and demonstrates extrusion of dye on one side and at

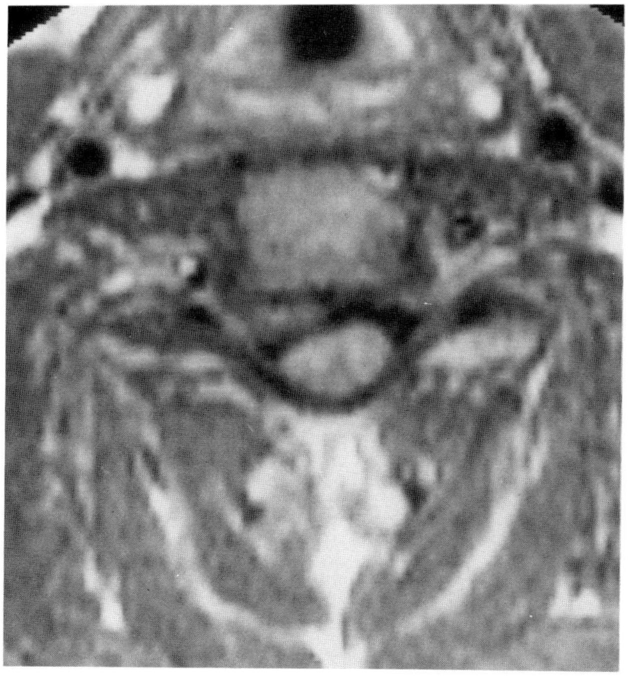

Fig. 45.5 Transverse MRI (T1) showing a lateral disc prolapse rotating and flattening the spinal cord.

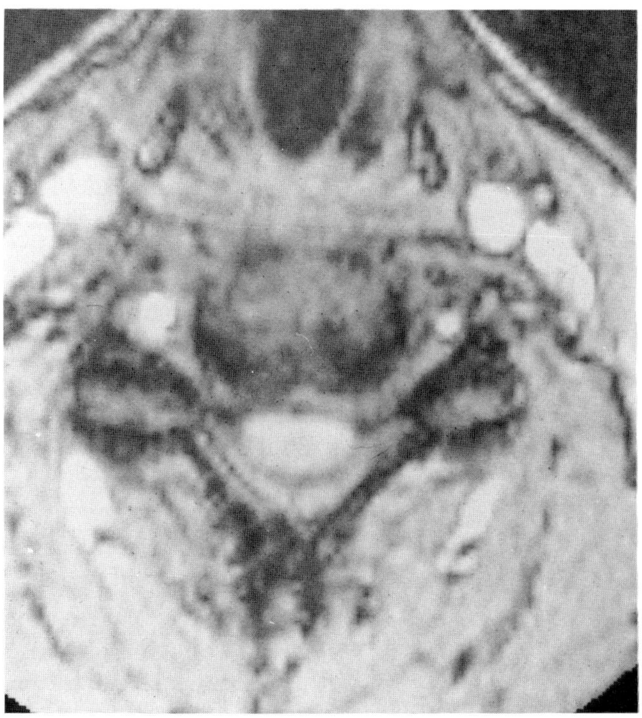

Fig. 45.6 Transverse MRI (T2 MAST) showing a lateral osteophyte touching but not displacing the spinal cord.

one level corresponding to the clinical features. The indications therefore are in young patients with a very typical clinical picture of disc prolapse but otherwise negative investigations. As noted earlier, the occasional case of 'whiplash' can be shown to be due to a single focally disrupted disc and cured by its surgical treatment.

CHOICE OF SURGICAL APPROACH

In general the approximate maxim is that anterior problems should be approached from anteriorly and posterior problems from posteriorly. The way to design an optimum decompressive procedure may become obvious after good-quality radiology. The various surgical approaches which may be utilized are illustrated in Fig. 45.7. Various large series operated by one approach, either anterior or posterior and then compared (Epstein & Epstein, 1989) show very little difference in the comparative rates of success. This would suggest that future improvements may come not from the acquisition of great skill in one partic-

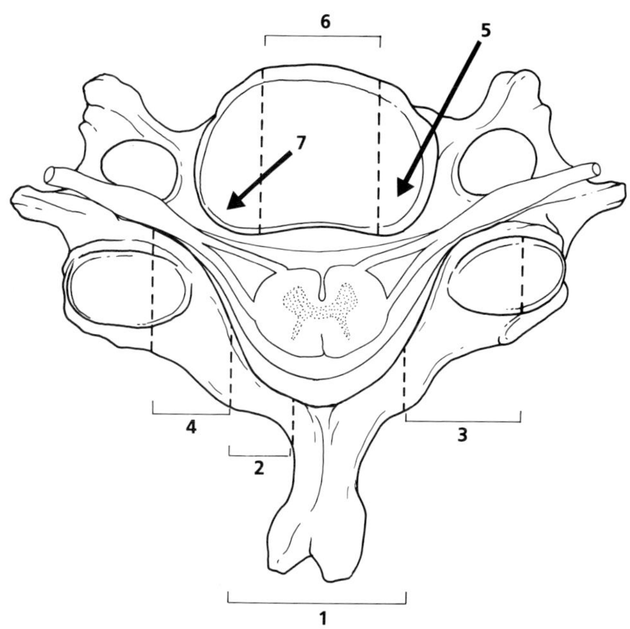

Fig. 45.7 Transverse section of the cervical spine illustrating the various surgical approaches: (1) laminectomy, (2) microsurgical laminotomy, (3) extended foraminal decompression (potentially destabilizing), (4) microsurgical proximal foraminotomy, (5) anterolateral foraminal approach, (6) anterior transcorporal approach, (7) lateral extension of the anterior approach to form an anterior foraminotomy.

ular technique, but by developing a range of different approaches for differing clinical entities.

The factors which influence the choice of approach will be briefly discussed. Laminectomy—with or without laminoplasty—remains the preferred option for cases with absolute or relative canal stenosis. It is also best for cases of myelopathy due to multiple-level disease, but in such cases where there is one predominant, large compressive lesion due either to disc prolapse or osteophytosis, it is often safer to perform an anterior approach at that level. Subsequent laminectomy can then be performed if there is insufficient clinical improvement. Laminectomy is also appropriate where myelopathy is mainly due to posterior compression such as is produced by buckling and thickening of the ligamentum flavum. Occasionally, laminectomy is necessary where it proves impossible to exclude the presence of a spinal tumour despite full radiological assessment.

Hemilaminectomy is particularly appropriate in cases of lateral canal disc prolapse, especially where an anterior approach would be difficult, as it can be at the extremes of the cervical spine. Posterior foraminotomy is indicated when there is radiculopathy at multiple levels. It is also of use where the intervertebral foramen is narrowed by facetal osteophytes. The latest approach, described by Verbiest in 1968 (see Chapter 46), is indicated for radiculopathy caused by far lateral disc extrusions, osteophytes or where there is vertebral artery compression.

The anterior transcorporal approach combined with fusion described by Cloward (1958, 1988) and by Smith & Robinson (1958) is indicated where central or posterolateral discal or osteophytic compression of nerve roots or the spinal cord exists. These procedures are also of use in the presence of localized ossification of the posterior longitudinal ligament. Anterior discectomy without fusion may be combined with an anterior foraminotomy in similar situations where a distractible disc space remains present.

Finally, a technique which has been termed 'trench vertebrectomy' may be appropriate to deal with cases where there is multiple-level anterior compression or ossification of the posterior longitudinal ligament. It is also of use where relative collapse of the vertebral bodies and their intervening discs has produced a focal stenosis or kyphotic deformity.

The place of fusion as an integral part of anterior cervical surgery has been debated for years. For one- or two-level disease the addition of a fusion seems to result in little overall benefit. Fusion is essential, however, when dealing with multiple levels or a single level where instability is clearly shown by the presence of subluxation or where a previous laminectomy has been performed. Where a single-level simple discectomy is performed, solid fusion will normally result provided the cartilaginous end-plates are removed. Such fusion does, however, take longer than if a bone graft is used, and may result in a minimal degree of kyphosis. This is not normally of clinical significance. As the adjacent bodies are not distracted following simple discectomy, it is essential that the foramen is enlarged at the time of surgery by the removal of any osteophytes from the uncal area. Fusion is seldom performed following posterior decompression but is necessary if preoperative subluxation is present or if facetectomies are performed at multiple levels.

Choice of operated levels

Multiple-level disease is a very common in cervical spondylosis whether causing radiculopathy or myelopathy. Unless an extended posterior decompression is to be performed, some decision has to be made as to the number of levels which require surgical intervention. In most cases it is possible to decide which single level is most responsible for the disease, or at least to narrow it down to two, or occasionally three, levels, if adjacent levels are also severely affected. This process is achieved mainly by close comparison of which levels seem to be clinically affected and comparing them with the most severely affected levels radiologically.

However, Phillips (1975) showed that both in myelopathy and, less frequently, in radiculopathy the radiologically involved level is often between one and three segments cranial to that which would be anticipated from the clinical findings. One reason for this is that a central anterior osteophyte may press on the anterior root exit zone of the cord and result in local demyelinization of the motor fibres. The level of the root exit zone is usually at least one vertebra above the intervertebral foramen for that root. Such compression may cause radiculopathy without myelopathy despite the cord compression. A similar explanation resulting from the discrepancy between cord and bony segmental levels accounts for cases of myelopathy where the clinical and radiological levels differ. Every case, therefore, requires detailed and careful analysis.

In some cases the extent of the disease may be so widespread that a single responsible level cannot be identified with any degree of certainty. This is particularly likely in cases with absolute or relative canal stenosis. In such a situation all abnormal levels require decompression and this will, therefore, frequently demand a posterior approach. Some authorities would advocate surgical treatment of all radiological levels even if thought to be asymptomatic at the time, in order to prevent future deterioration. The time-course of the progression of cervical spondylosis is so long and variable that such a course is difficult to justify, and it does seem entirely justifiable to ignore mild to moderately affected levels which are felt to be asymptomatic. However, where there is an asymptomatic level which is severely affected radiologically adjacent to a segment which is to be fused, then it is reasonable to prophylactically treat that adjacent level. This is because of the excessive stress which will be applied to the adjacent level by the fused segment which will accelerate the degenerative process. This is particularly likely if the adjacent asymptomatic level already shows signs of radiological instability.

Surgical techniques

A comprehensive description of technique is not appropriate here, and the main principles only will be outlined. For more surgical detail the reader is referred to works on operative surgery (Jung *et al.*, 1974; Sherk *et al.*, 1989; Torrens & Dixon, 1991).

Laminectomy

Early results from laminectomy reported by Nurick (1972) showed rates of improvement in myelopathy of 56%, little better than the rate of spontaneous resolution with conservative treatment of 40%. A significant number of patients were made worse by operation, emphasizing that surgical manipulation within a narrow spinal canal can be disastrous. Subsequent modifications of the technique have produced rates of improvement up to 85% (Epstein & Epstein, 1989).

The emphasis is on careful handling of the patient. Positioning must take place without unreasonable extension or manipulation of the neck. Fixing the head in a Gardner pin head rest protects against inadvertent movement and allows the head and neck to be elevated, thus reducing epidural venous pressure when the prone position is used. The blood pressure must be maintained. The laminectomy technique must avoid the insertion of instruments into the canal. One good method is to perform the laminectomy using a high-speed drill. This is employed at the junction of lamina and pedicles to produce a gutter (Fig. 45.8). The contents of the spinal canal are protected by the ligamentum flavum. When the spines and laminae are loose the area of decompression can be removed en bloc by cutting through the ligaments. If foraminotomies (see below) are also required these should be drilled first while the lamina remains as an extra protection.

Instability following laminectomy is very uncommon except in cases of spinal tumour where the local musculature may be adversely affected. The strength in the spine is not reduced until more than 50% of the facet joint has been removed bilaterally (Raynor *et al.*, 1985).

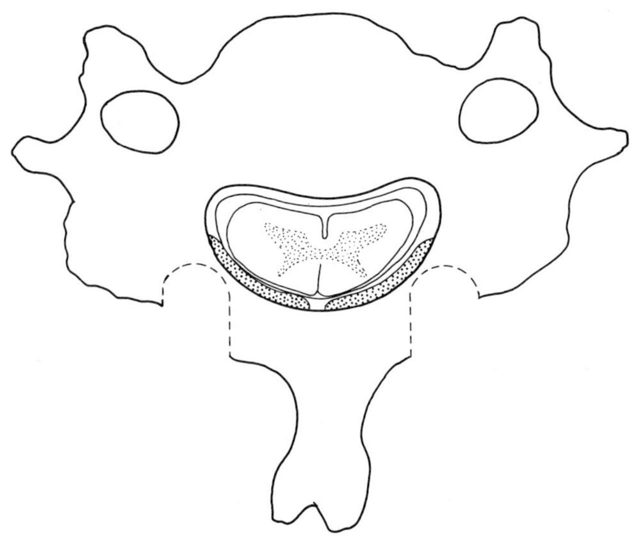

Fig. 45.8 Transverse section of a cervical vertebra demonstrating the position of the lateral troughs to be produced during drill laminectomy. Correct positioning at the junctions of the laminae and lateral mass means that the troughs are away from the spinal cord, and sudden deep penetration of the drill is prevented by the bone of the pedicle. When the spinal canal is entered the ligamentum flavum will usually be between the trough and the dura.

Laminoplasty

Full-depth drilling on one side and partial drilling only on the other side allows 'hinged' or 'open-door' laminoplasty. This has been a popular approach for the treatment of ossification of the posterior longitudinal ligament in Japan. It produces only a very small increase in the canal diameter but this is enough in these very chronic cases to reduce the ischaemia of the spinal cord and avoids the risks of deterioration inherent in a more radical anterior decompression and excision. The laminoplasty is held open by suturing the vertebral spines to the ligament nuchae or contralateral facet or by inserting a bone graft. The laminoplasty technique tends to reduce the range of cervical spine movement postoperatively by partial fusion. This reduces the rate of growth of the ossified longitudinal ligament (Hirabayashi *et al.*, 1989).

Microsurgical laminotomy

The original operation for cervical disc prolapse described by Scoville *et al.* (1951) remains popular, and is eminently suitable for employing a restricted microscopic approach as in lumbar microdiscectomy. X-ray guidance to the correct interspace is necessary. The lumbar microdiscectomy retractor (Williams type, Codman Shurtleff) can be used. The 1 cm laminotomy can be performed with a high-speed air drill or with a small Kerrison-type punch having a thin footplate. It is necessary to be sure of the diagnosis of a laterally placed soft disc prolapse in order to avoid manipulation or damage to the cord. The removal of osteophytic spurs anterior to the cord and roots has been described, but the use of chisels, curettes and drills on the other side of the spinal canal is unnecessarily complicated and dangerous when the procedure can be accomplished more safely from an anterior route.

Microscopic posterior cervical foraminotomy

Posterior foraminal decompression was described by Frykholm (1951). Foraminal narrowing can be dealt with either from anterior or posterior, and it is reasonable to approach an anterior problem from the front and a posterior problem from the back. However, a transdiscal exposure would produce some degree of rigidity of that motion segment which may aggravate adjacent degenerative processes. There is some evidence that the compressive effects of an anterior foraminal osteophyte can be relieved by posterior decompression even when the anterior osteophyte is not itself removed (Williams, 1983). Indeed, anterior osteophytes probably should *not* be removed from a posterior route because their removal is often difficult and causes trauma to the nerve root which may mean the results are poor even if the operation is technically successful.

The levels to choose for foraminotomy are indicated by clear evidence of foraminal narrowing combined with radicular symptoms and signs. It is probably more important to concentrate on the segmental clinical evidence of neuropathy than on the radiological changes. In particular, care should be taken in interpreting transverse CT scans which appear to show foraminal narrowing because some CT cuts may be too thick to show the cervical foramina properly and the narrowed appearance may be due to partial volume artifact. The microscopic surgical approach is conducted as noted in the section above, but a little more lateral. Bone is removed with the high-speed drill at the junction of the lamina and lateral mass going down through the medial half of the facet joint until the bone over the root is of eggshell thickness. This can then be removed safely with curettes or a 1 mm Kerrison-type punch.

Anterolateral foraminotomy

Verbiest (1968) described an approach to the intertransverse space paraspinally that can be extended medially into the disc space and spinal canal to remove osteophyte and disc fragments. This is seldom employed currently but deserves a place in the surgeon's repertoire. It covers exactly the far lateral area which is most difficult to approach by a transdiscal or Cloward technique (see Chapter 46).

Anterior transcorporal approach

A transdiscal or transvertebral approach to decompress the spinal cord has been described by Robinson & Smith (1955), Smith & Robinson (1958), Cloward (1958, 1988). In most cases of cervical spondylosis where decompression is required, the disc space cannot be distracted easily enough to allow a transdiscal approach without the removal of bone in some way. Indeed, violent attempts to distract the vertebrae may cause spinal cord damage. It is therefore appropriate to use the Cloward drill centred on the disc space or to cut a transverse trough through at the level of the disc space using a high-speed drill or a special horizontally cutting osteotome (Collis type, Baxter Healthcare). This is very carefully deepened posteriorly until the remaining cortical bone is of eggshell thickness and can be broken off with a curette.

The advantage of the Cloward drill technique is that there is a large central exposure which can be directed slightly to one side or the other if the position of the offending osteophyte is known. It is, however, relatively easy to misdirect the drill and therefore not to remove completely the compressing elements. On the other hand the advantage of the Smith–Robinson technique is that a full-width decompression can be performed and orientation to the anatomy of the vertebra is more simple. However, with a transverse trough it is less easy to remove any thickened posterior longitudinal ligament and if the osteophytes spread up and down the vertebral body, or there is ossification of the posterior ligament, this may be inaccessible.

A failure to complete an adequate lateral decompression is the commonest technical failure in Cloward's procedure. Certainly a lateral extension can be difficult, especially on the right side for a right-sided approach and vice-versa. The disc spaces should be cleaned and explored laterally and the upper curve of the uncinate processes identified on each side. Decompression should then be continued laterally removing the uncinate process until the lateral edge of the vertebra is running anteriorly. Venous bleeding here often means that the vertebral venous plexus has been reached.

If the posterior longitudinal ligament is floppy and bulges back into the decompression it can be left alone. If it is thick it should be removed and the dura exposed. A narrow sharp Kerrison punch is useful for performing this. CSF leaks are, in fact, extremely rare. Primary repair by stitching is not feasible. Usually they can be left alone and will cause no trouble, otherwise they can be repaired with a patch using fibrinogen glue (Tisseel, Immuno).

Because of inconsistencies in selection and variations in technique the results of anterior surgery are difficult to compare. Operation earlier in the course of the disease produces better results. Myelopathy existing for over two years is less likely to respond. In brachial neuropathy Phillips (1975) recorded that arm pain was relieved in 82%, motor loss in 69% and sensory loss in 49%. Neck pain is relieved in 68% (Weber, 1974). In myelopathy that was already very severe Senegas *et al.* (1985) report a cure in 27%, improvement in 46% and no change in 27%. These reports seem to represent the average expectation from surgery although excellent outcomes in brachial neuralgia with abolition of pain in as many as 96% of the cases had been reported (Gorge & Sepic, 1984).

Anterior cervical discectomy

A focal disc prolapse in the absence of significant osteophyte formation and with normal intervertebral foraminae can be treated by anterior discectomy alone (Wilson & Campbell 1977).

The relevant space, identified radiologically, can be opened up using an instrument such as the Cloward vertebral spreader (Codman, Shurtleff). Complete discectomy is relatively easy, and usually a hole in the posterior ligament is revealed posteriorly which can be enlarged to remove the prolapsed disc fragments. Careful assessment of the X-rays and scans is necessary to ensure that no free epidural fragments have migrated out of the reach of a transdiscal exposure.

No graft or prosthesis is necessary in the disc space unless there is already foraminal narrowing, in which case the foraminal size needs to be preserved or increased. In fact postoperative MRI often shows very little narrowing or anatomical disturbance after discectomy. However, mobility at the level is reduced by fibrous union and the disc space may fuse with time. It is typical for there to be interscapular pain for about three months postoperatively, and the patient can be reassured that this will settle down. With the correct selection of patients the rate of relief for brachial neuralgia should be greater than 90%.

Trench vertebrectomy

In cases where multiple level anterior compressing elements are present, and especially when these are so large that a posterior decompression would still mean they were indenting the spinal cord, a radical multiple-level anterior decompression is required. This may also be the case in patients with cervical kyphosis and in some cases of fixed subluxation. It also applies to cases of hypertrophy or moderate ossification of the posterior longitudinal ligament.

The optimal decompression is made by removing the central part of several adjacent vertebrae.

Because of the extent of bone resection the insertion of a graft is probably appropriate to prevent kyphosis. It is important that this is prepared and cut in a way that it is unlikely to dislocate. Some surgeons hold the graft in place with a plate or other metal device. Alternatively the graft can be cut in a keystone fashion, with undermining of the upper and lower vertebral edges so that, after the graft has been inserted in distraction, it is held securely. This applies to an iliac crest graft. The same principle can be used if a fibula strut graft is employed and this is generally rather stronger. If a transverse notch is cut across the end of the fibula leaving the main triangular width posterior this slot can be organized to wrap around the anterior cortical edge of the vertebrae at the top and bottom of the exposure.

The place of elective fusion

One of the disadvantages of the anterior approach is that the resultant fusion of a motion segment may transfer stress to adjacent joints. These may already be showing signs of degeneration and therefore the increased stress will provoke pain or further neurological problems at a later date. Many anterior approaches will eventually fuse, whether or not a bone graft is used. The choice of whether or not to perform an elective fusion therefore depends on other concurrent circumstances. If there is any suggestion of instability then a posterior approach is best avoided and an anterior approach should incorporate an elective fusion and bone graft. If neck pain from arthrogenic rather than discogenic causes is a prominent part of the syndrome then again fusion may alleviate this. It is sometimes difficult, however, to discover exactly from which joint the pain arises.

Extensive bone removal may tend to provoke vertebral collapse and kyphosis. This can be counteracted by an insertion of a bone graft provided the graft itself is of adequate quality and can withstand the compression forces and is not affected by osteoporosis. If the bone is inadequate then some other form of support needs to be considered, either anterior plating, posterior prosthetic insertion or long-term immobilization externally.

Occasionally there is a need to improve or maintain the vertebral height in order to open up the intervertebral foraminae or correct the cervical kyphosis. Under these circumstances a strong bone graft is required and the use of a tibial strut graft may well be considered.

What to use for fusion remains controversial. There is no doubt that the patient's own iliac crest bone, when of good quality, provides a rapid and secure form of fusion. If stronger bone is required then fibula may be used, as noted above, but this does not fuse so rapidly and needs external fixation for three months. Cadaveric bank bone (Cloward, 1988) and processed animal bone (Surgibone, Hymed) are available. Both of these fuse more slowly, and the total process may take over six months. The eventual incorporation rate of animal bone is almost certainly less than that of autogenous bone. Cadaveric or animal bone avoids the morbidity and pain of a separate iliac incision but this is counteracted by the need for longer external support to encourage fusion.

Recent opinion suggests that no graft insertion of any sort is necessary in many cases, stability being maintained by the lateral masses of the vertebrae (Senegas *et al.*, 1985). The final decision about grafting probably depends on the number of levels being operated, the extent of resection and the preoperative rigidity, and no rigid guidance is appropriate.

Cervical disc operations are common and occur at the rate of 8 per 100 000 population per annum (Gleista *et al.*, 1977). These figures for Minnesota, USA, correspond exactly with the frequency observed at Frenchay Hospital, Bristol, and are equivalent to the number of operations performed on all brain tumours.

The various conditions respond well to surgery, which can be designed to be minimally invasive. Progressively improved results may come from a high level of experience in what is technically a very demanding surgical technique, and also from elaborating a repertoire of operations that may be tailored to each patient's requirements.

REFERENCES

Barnes, M.P. & Saunders, M. (1984) The effect of cervical mobility on the natural history of cervical spondylotic myelopathy. *J. Neurol. Neurosurg. Psychiatry*, **47**, 17–20.

Cloward, R.B. (1985) The anterior approach for removal of ruptured cervical disc. *J. Neurosurg.*, **15**, 602–617.

Cloward, R.B. (1988) The anterior surgical approach to the cervical spine: Cloward procedure: past, present and future. *Spine*, **13**, 823–827.

Epstein, J.A. & Epstein, N.E. (1989) The surgical management of cervical spinal stenosis, spondylosis and myeloradiculopathy by the means of a posterior approach. In Cervical Spine Research Society (eds) *The Cervical Spine*, 2nd edn, pp. 635–641. Lippincott, Philadelphia, PA.

Frykholm, R. (1951) Cervical nerve root compression resulting from disc degeneration and root sleeve fibrosis: a clinical investigation. *Acta Chir. Scand.* (Suppl.), **160**, 1–147.

Gleista, G.G., Miller, R.H., Kurland, L.T. & Jereczek, M.L. (1977) Neurosurgical procedures in Olmsted County, Minnesota, 1970–1974. *J. Neurosurg.*, **46**, 46–51.

Good, D.C., Couch, J.R. & Wacaser, L. (1984) 'Numb, clumsy hands' and high cervical spondylosis. *Surg. Neurol.*, **22**, 285–291.

Gorge, D.R. & Sepic, S.B. (1984) Anterior cervical fusion for degenerated or protruded discs. A review of 146 patients. *Spine*, **9**, 667.

Hirabayashi, K., Satomi, K. & Sasaki, T. (1989) Ossification of the posterior longitudinal ligament in the cervical spine. In Cervical Spine Research Society (eds) *The Cervical Spine*, 2nd edn, pp. 678–692. Lippincott, Philadelphia, PA.

Jung, A., Kehr, P., Magerl, F. & Weber, B.G. (1974) *The Cervical Spine*. Hans Huber, Vienna.

Nurick, S. (1972) The natural history and the results of surgical treatment of the spinal cord disorder associated with cervical spondylosis, *Brain*, **95**, 101–108.

Nurick, S. (1975) Cervical spondylosis and the spinal cord. *Br. J. Hosp. Med.*, **14**, 668–676.

Payne, E.E. & Spillane, J.D. (1957) The cervical spine. *Brain*, **80**, 571–596.

Penning, L. (1979) Normal movements of the cervical spine. *Am. J. Roentgenol.*, **130**, 317.

Phillips, D.G. (1975) Upper limb involvement in cervical spondylosis. *J. Neurol. Neurosurg. Psychiatry*, **38**, 386–390.

Raynor, R.B., Pugh, J. & Shapiro, I. (1985) Cervical facetectomy and its effect on spine strength. *J. Neurosurg.*, **63**, 278.

Robinson, R.A. & Smith, G.W. (1955) Anterolateral cervical disc removal and interbody fusion for cervical disc syndrome. *Bull. Johns Hopkins Hospital*, **96**, 223–224.

Scoville, E.W.B., Witcomb, B.B. & McLaurin, R. (1951) The cervical ruptured disc: report on 150 operative cases. *Trans. Am. Neurol. Assoc.*, **76**, 222.

Senegas, J., Guerin, J., Vitol, J.M., Duplan, R. & Dols, J.M. (1985) The treatment of myelopathy in cervical spondylosis by extensive anterior decompression of the cord. *Rev. Chir. Orthop.*, **71**, 291–300.

Sherk, H.H., Dunn, E.G., Eismont, F.J. *et al.* (eds) (1989) *The Cervical Spine*. Lippincott, Philadelphia, PA.

Smith, G.W. & Robinson, R.A. (1958) The treatment of certain spine disorders by anterior removal of the intervertebral disc and interbody fusion. *J. Bone Jt. Surg.*, **40A**, 624–626.

Torrens, M.J. & Dixon, R. (1991) *Operative Spinal Surgery*, Churchill Livingstone, Edinburgh.

Ullrich, C.J. (1989) Magnetic resonance imaging of the cervical spine and spinal cord. In Cervical Spine Research Society (eds). *The Cervical Spine*, 2nd edn, pp. 157–175. Lippincott, Philadelphia.

Veidlinger, O.F., Colwill, J.C., Smyth, H.S. & Turner, D. (1981) Cervical myelopathy and its relationship to cervical stenosis. *Spine*, **6**, 550–552.

Verbiest, H. (1968) A lateral approach to the cervical spine: technique and indications. *J. Neurosurg.*, **28**, 191.

Weber, B.G. (1974) Anterior midline cervical operations: the Cloward procedure. In Jung, A., Kehr, P., Magerl, F. & Weber, B.G. (eds) *The Cervical Spine*, pp. 113–120. Hans Huber, Vienna.

White, A.A. & Panjabi, M.M. (1978) The basic kinematics of the human spine: a review of past and current knowledge. *Spine*, **3**, 12.

Williams, R.W. (1983) Microcervical foraminotomy, a surgical alternative for intractable radicular pain. *Spine*, **8**, 708–716.

Wilson, D.H. & Campbell, D.D. (1977) Anterior cervical discectomy without bone graft. A report of 71 cases. *J. Neurosurg.*, **47**, 551–555.

46 · Pathologies of the Cervical Intertransverse Space

By H. VERBIEST

The concept of the cervical intertransverse space was introduced by Verbiest in 1981, who described it as an entity that forms the lateral continuation of the cervical intervertebral foramen. In previous years several different anatomical definitions of the intervertebral foramen in the cervical spine had been described. The reason for these varying anatomical descriptions probably lies in the complicated nature of the Gestalt of the foramen as discussed in the introductory chapter of this book. A short review of the history of the cervical intervertebral foramen may give an insight to the problem and explain the significance of the intertransverse space as a separate entity.

No mention of the intervertebral foramen is found in the *Corpus Hippocraticum*, although other vertebral structures were carefully described in the book on the articulations. The authors of the Hippocratic books ignored the nature of the nerves. Galen, during his stay at the Alexandrian medical school, was instructed there about the theories of motor and sensory nerve function, developed by Erasistratos and Herophilos. Through these functions his attention became focused on the exits of the spinal nerves from the vertebral canal, resulting in the first description of the intervertebral foramen. In Galen's definition the foramen is determined by the inferior and superior notches of the vertebral pedicles.

In Galen's view the posterolateral joints had two functions. Apart from permitting movement between vertebrae these joints provided protection for the spinal nerves. This part of the history shows how discovery of nerve function drove the attention to the Gestalt of the intervertebral foramen, whereas according to Galen's teleological thinking the posterolateral joints had a different function.

Nothing new happened until Gowers, in 1893, in a chapter on diseases of the spinal articulations, wrote: 'The articular processes, it will be remembered, form one side of the intervertebral foramina, which are thus encroached on by any enlargements of the bones.' With the development of radiology, arthritic narrowing of the foramen could be visualized in cases presenting with signs of compression of the spinal nerve roots or ganglia.

In the well-known descriptions of Forestier (1922) different participations of the cervical, thoracic and lumbar vertebral bodies in forming the anterior foraminal walls were described, but the posterior wall of these foramina was invariably described as being formed by the superior articular process of the vertebra below and the superior border of the interarticular joint. It was Epstein *et al.* (1972) who reported compression of nerve roots inside the lumbar vertebral canal by the superior articular process, so drawing attention to the fact that a medial portion of the superior lumbar articular process participates in the formation of the posterior wall of the lumbar vertebral canal and thus does not belong to the walls of the lumbar intervertebral foramina.

Further discussion will be limited to the evolution of ideas concerning the cervical intervertebral foramen. Many anatomists and clinicians, even now, consider the entire articular processes as the posterior boundary of the foramen. This is the result of failing to analyse the parts of its Gestalt, as may be demonstrated with the following examples.

Poirier & Charpy (1899), when describing the foraminal boundaries, considered that: the inferior vertebral body formed the anterior border; the entire superior articular process of the inferior vertebra formed the posterior wall; the roof was formed by the transverse process and the inferior incisura of the pedicle of the vertebra above; and the floor by the pedicle and neural groove of the transverse process of the vertebra below. Although the internal entry zone of the foramen is evident in this description the situation of its exit zone is not clear at all, and was not described.

Forestier (1922) followed Poirier's definition of the foramen but added, in an effort to make its form more comprehensible, that it has the form of a 'double sac' (*bissac* in French), whose largest axis runs obliquely in a postero-inferior direction. The narrowing in the double sac was, in his view, caused by the uncinate process. The use of the word '*bissac*' was a metaphor that removed the concept of the foramen still more from reality. Definitions that include the entire superior articular process as the posterior boundary lead to the inevitable conclusion that the vertebral artery is situated inside the foramen, but no-one would accept such a conclusion.

Radiological visualization of the cervical intervertebral foramen revealed that the direction of the axis of the interpedicular portion was different from that of the axis of the space between the transverse processes, so that radiological visualization of both portions required another direction of the X-ray beam and positioning of the film. Pichler (1955) therefore dropped the name and replaced it by the term 'cervical intervertebral canal'. In his description there is no clear definition of the anterior wall and the lateral exit of the intertransverse portion of the cervical intervertebral canal. The surgical approaches to the lateral portions of the cervical spine led to different views on nomenclature. The first direct approach to the cervical transverse processes was described by Henry (1957), based on studies upon anatomical specimens. Hardin (1960, 1965) was the first to use Henry's approach in living beings, for relieving the vertebral artery from osteophytic compression. Jung (1963) and Jung & Vierling (1965) described the resection of the uncus for relieving osteophytic compression of the vertebral artery or intraforaminal osteophytic nerve root compression with the use of Henry's approach.

On the basis of their experience with this method, Jung and his co-worker Kehr (1972) described new Gestalten in the area of the cervical transverse processes, which they called 'the intertransverse canal' and 'the unco-arterial-radicular crossroad'. They divided the foramen into an interpedicular and an inter-unco-artericular portion; that is the space between the posterolateral joints and the uncus. The latter forms the anterior wall of the medial portion and the medial wall of the lateral portion of the foramen. It is similar to Forestier's definition.

The crossroad comprises, according to Jung & Kehr (1972), posteromedially the foramen occupied by a spinal nerve and its anterior and posterior branches. The floor is formed by the neural groove of the transverse process of the inferior vertebra and its roof by the inferior surface of the transverse process above. The anterior wall is constituted by the posterior aspect of the uncovertebral joint and the anterior intertransverse muscles, and the posterior wall is formed by the articular processes and the transverse neck muscles. Even when accepting the principles of this definition the posterior wall should be described as being formed by the anterior surface of the superior articular process of the inferior vertebra and by the posterior intertransverse muscles. But the principle of the definition is wrong, because the authors do not describe a crossroad but only an intersection of two tubular spaces. The real roads are formed by the spinal nerve on the one hand and the vertebral artery and veins on the other hand. They do not have a common intersection as crossroads have, but cross independent of each other. The transport along these roads, nerve impulses and blood respectively, would not be compatible with a common intersection.

This concept is an audacious metaphor that does not promote insight into its clinical significance. Jung & Kehr did not formulate their purpose, when proposing this difficult, complex and rather unreal Gestalt pattern. When Verbiest (1968, 1970a,b,c) developed a new technique of lateral approach to the cervical spine, it appeared that, with the diagnostic means involved, particular abnormal findings and technical surgical experience were a reason to consider a new Gestalt; namely, the cervical intertransverse space as a separate entity (Verbiest, 1978a,b, 1981a,b).

THE ANATOMY OF THE CERVICAL INTERTRANSVERSE SPACE

A most striking anatomical detail in this region is that the inferior articular process of C2 and both superior and inferior articular processes of the third through the seventh cervical vertebrae are situated on about the medial two-thirds of the transverse processes and on the posterior ends of the pedicles. The exits of the cervical spinal nerves from the vertebral canal to the extraspinal space in the area between C2 and C7 are rather large canals formed by an intervertebral foramen and an intertransverse space in continuity. It is because of the composite structure of the cervical transverse processes, in contrast to the transverse processes at lower vertebral levels, that notable intertransverse spaces exist only at cervical levels. At thoracic and lumbar levels the transverse processes and the intertransverse muscles are situated only behind the spinal nerves. The true cervical transverse processes arise at the posterior ends of the pedicles. They are connected with rudimentary rib elements, originating from the cervical vertebral bodies at the same level, through the costotransverse lamellae.

The cervical spinal nerves run over the neural grooves of the transverse processes between the anterior intertransverse muscles anteriorly and the anterior surface of the superior articular process and the posterior intertransverse muscles posteriorly. The C1–C2 intertransverse space differs from all others between C2 and C7 in that it projects more laterally. There is no C1–C2 foramen. The only bordering bony wall of the C1–C2 space is situated medially, being formed by the articular facet joints. There is no uncus of C2. The C2 spinal nerves pass medially to the facet joints, leaving the spinal canal posteriorly between the posterior arches of C1 and C2 through openings in the atlanto-axial ligament. The only important contents of the C1–C2 intertransverse space are the vertebral artery and vein, and the vertebral nerve. Narrowing of this C1–C2 intertransverse space by osteophytes might theoretically occur only at the external border of the lateral facet joints, but such osteophytes have never been encountered in our cases.

The only surgical indications for exposing the C1–C2 intertransverse space are tumours and extremely rare cases of symptomatic kinking of the vertebral artery produced by atlanto-axial dislocation.

Because of the minor role of the C1–C2 intertransverse space in pathology and its great differences with respect to the spaces between C2 and C7, the discussion in this chapter will be limited to the latter. There is no intertransverse space at C7–T1 because the transverse process of T1 is connected only with the posterior intertransverse muscles to the transverse process of C7. In addition the vertebral artery runs in front of the transverse process of C7. The author found reason to introduce the spaces between C2 and C7 as separate entities distinct from the foramina because they have their own specific pathology, requiring a specific diagnostic approach. A definition of these intertransverse spaces first requires a definition of their borderlines with the intervertebral foramina. Since the extents of the bony elements forming the anterior and posterior walls of the foramina vary with the cervical, thoracic, lumbar and sacral regions, the pedicles form the sole constant parameters, that change only in thickness. In this sense the foramen is determined by the superior and inferior incisures of the pedicles above and below respectively. The pedicles are smallest in their middle portion and fan out anteriorly and posteriorly. Accordingly the depth of the foramen as part of a canal is determined by two planes placed tangentially to the lateral and medial surfaces of the smallest central portion of the pedicles (Fig. 46.1). The anterior and posterior boundaries of the foramina are determined by the portions of the superior articular process, uncus and vertebral body situated between the intersections of both planes with these structures.

The tunnel between the vertebral canal and the extravertebral space is constituted by the cervical intervertebral foramen delimited by lanes X and Y in Fig. 46.1 and the cervical intertransverse space whose floor is hatched on the left in the figures. The space of the foramen is determined by two planes, both passing tangentially along the external and internal surfaces, respectively, of the pedicles forming the floor and roof of the foramen where their cross-sections are smallest. These points of tangency are at the same time the intersections of the coordinates of both planes; one coordinate connects the respective external or internal tangency points of the pedicles in the floor and the roof of the foramen, and the other coordinate parallels the longitudinal axes of these pedicles. A slight possible difference in orientation of the axes of the pedicles above and below the foramen is disregarded. In biplanar images the sections through the planes limiting the foramen are represented by the X and Y lines along the pedicle forming the floor of the foramen examined.

The floor of the intertransverse space is formed by the neural groove of the transverse process of the vertebra below, and its roof by the inferior surface of the transverse process of the vertebra above. The posterior wall is formed medially by the lateral two-thirds of the anterior surface of the superior articular

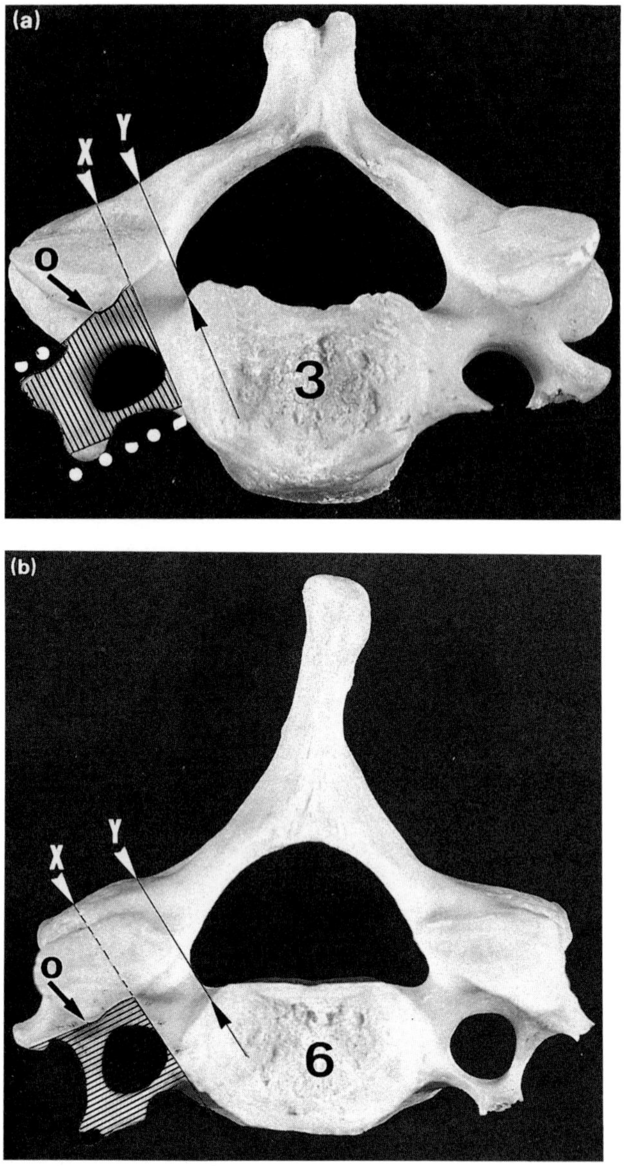

Fig. 46.1 Superior views of C3 and C6 to show the intervertebral foramina and the intertransverse spaces.

process of the vertebra below and the superior border of the interarticular joint, and laterally by the posterior intertransverse muscles. The anterior wall is formed by the anterior intertransverse muscles reinforced by the overlying longus capitis and longus colli muscles. The hatched areas in Fig. 46.1 indicate the floor of the intertransverse space. The arrows (O) point to the neural groove behind the transversarial foramen and vertebral blood vessels. The larger portion of the superior articular facet forms the major portion of the posterior wall of the space that is completed by the posterior intertransverse muscles. The anterior wall of the space is completely muscular, and the extent of the muscular walls is indicated by white dotted lines in the figure.

The capacity of the intertransverse space is small so that minor space-occupying lesions may readily compress its contents. The contents of the intertransverse space are vascular and neural structures. The vascular contents comprise the segmental portions of the vertebral artery and its accompanying venous plexus with the radicular arteries and veins. The neural contents are the segmental portions of the vertebral nerve and the spinal nerve with its anterior and posterior rami. The posterior ramus leaves the intertransverse space lateral to the superior articular process, and the anterior ramus leaves through the lateral exit situated at the end of the neural groove posterior to the anterior tubercle of the transverse process.

As the neural content of the medial two-thirds of the intertransverse space is the same as the neural content of the foramen, pathological processes in both regions may produce identical signs and symptoms. Thus, for example, transuncal extrusion of disc material directly into the intertransverse space produces signs and symptoms as observed with radicular compression inside the foramen, but myelography may be completely normal. If the presence of a transuncal disc extrusion is not recognized but the myelogram indicates simultaneous nerve root compression inside the vertebral canal or the foramen, only the latter will be removed. The failure of such an operation may be listed as failed nerve root surgery, whereas it really is failed spinal nerve surgery. A transuncal disc extrusion may, however, be recognized in the vertebral artery angiogram, showing occlusion or displacement of the artery at the level of the transuncal extrusion.

ANTERIOR AND LATERAL APPROACHES TO THE CERVICAL SPINE

Operations upon the lateral structures of the cervical spine can be performed by means of an anterior or a lateral approach. As regards the anterior approaches, uncal osteophytes inside the foramen can be removed via a central hole in the spinal column drilled with the Cloward technique. Bakay & Leslie (1965) applied a bore-hole with the Cloward technique sited laterally, and were able to remove lateral osteophytes compressing the vertebral artery. The description of details of their technique is, however, not very clear. Gortvai (1964) resected the superior lateral quadrant of a vertebral body by means of an anterior approach, removing anterior intraforaminal osteophytes.

Initially, Verbiest & Paz y Geuze (1966) removed posterior spurs of the vertebral body and/or of the uncus anteriorly via an emptied disc space. This approach has been abandoned because the anterior introduction of small chisels or osteotomes for removing posterior osteophytes carried the risk of transmitting mechanical energy to the compressed spinal cord and/or nerve roots. Transdiscal removal of the uncus for removal of lateral osteophytes compressing the vertebral artery is a blind procedure as the vertebral artery is exposed only after removal of the uncus. Since the artery may be adherent to the lateral osteophyte, the artery may be torn during removal of the uncus.

Henry (1957) devised an anterior approach for exposure of the second portion of the vertebral artery inside the transversarial foramina. He interrupted the medial attachments of the longus colli and longus cervicis muscles and retracted these muscles laterally, exposing the anterior borders of the transversarial foramina. Resection of the anterior borders of these foramina and of the anterior intertransverse muscles exposed the vertebral artery. The exposure was limited to performing safe resection of lateral uncal osteophytes or for surgery of the artery itself. The exposure by means of a lateral approach provided more freedom in these respects.

The differences in the author's technique from that of Henry's procedure are as follows. Firstly, the lateral attachments of the longus colli and capitis muscles are interrupted, and these muscles are retracted medially, allowing resection of the anterolateral borders of the transversarial foramina and resulting in easier access to the vertebral artery and the spinal nerve.

The lateral approach to the area C2–C7

Apart from preliminary clinical examination of the patient with respect to pathology, the lateral approach to the intertransverse space requires preoperative vertebral angiography. One of the initial steps in the exposure of the space is medial retraction of the longus capitis and longus colli muscles. Usually the vertebral artery leaves its course through the transversarial foramina below C6, but exceptionally it may be situated at the front of the transverse processes at higher cervical levels (Fig. 46.2) so that the surgeon, who is unaware of this abnormality, may damage the artery during medial retraction of the muscles. Digital subtraction angiography is not desir-

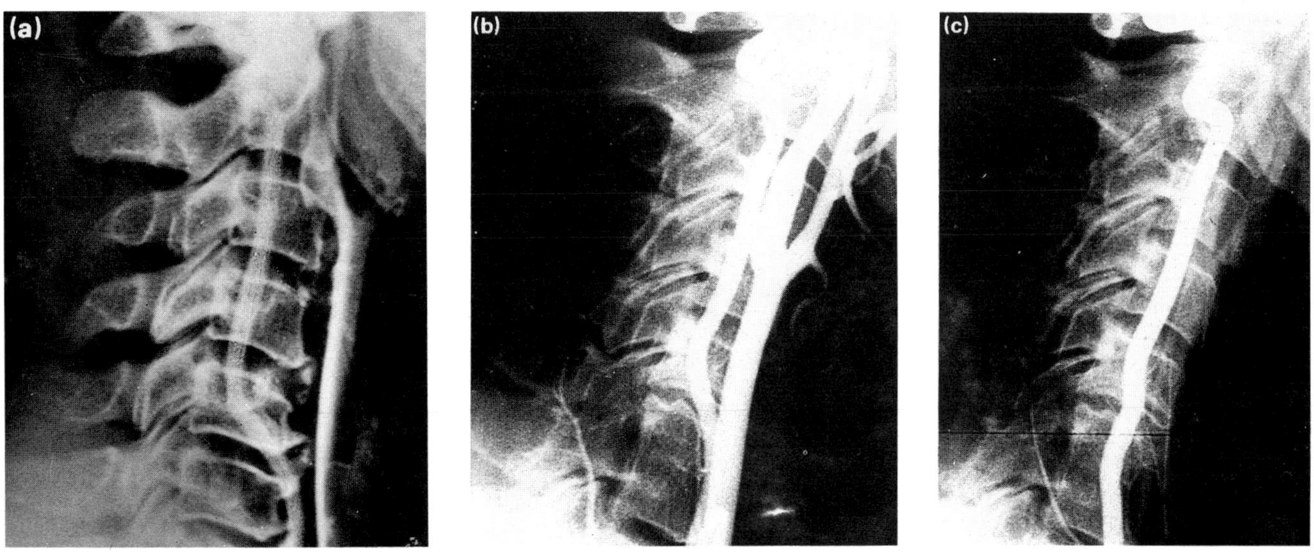

Fig. 46.2 (a) Lateral view showing the vertebral artery leaving the transversarial foramen of C5 and passing in front of the transverse process of C6. (b) The right vertebral artery leaves the transversarial foramen at C5, above the block vertebrae C6–C7. (c) The left vertebral artery has a normal course.

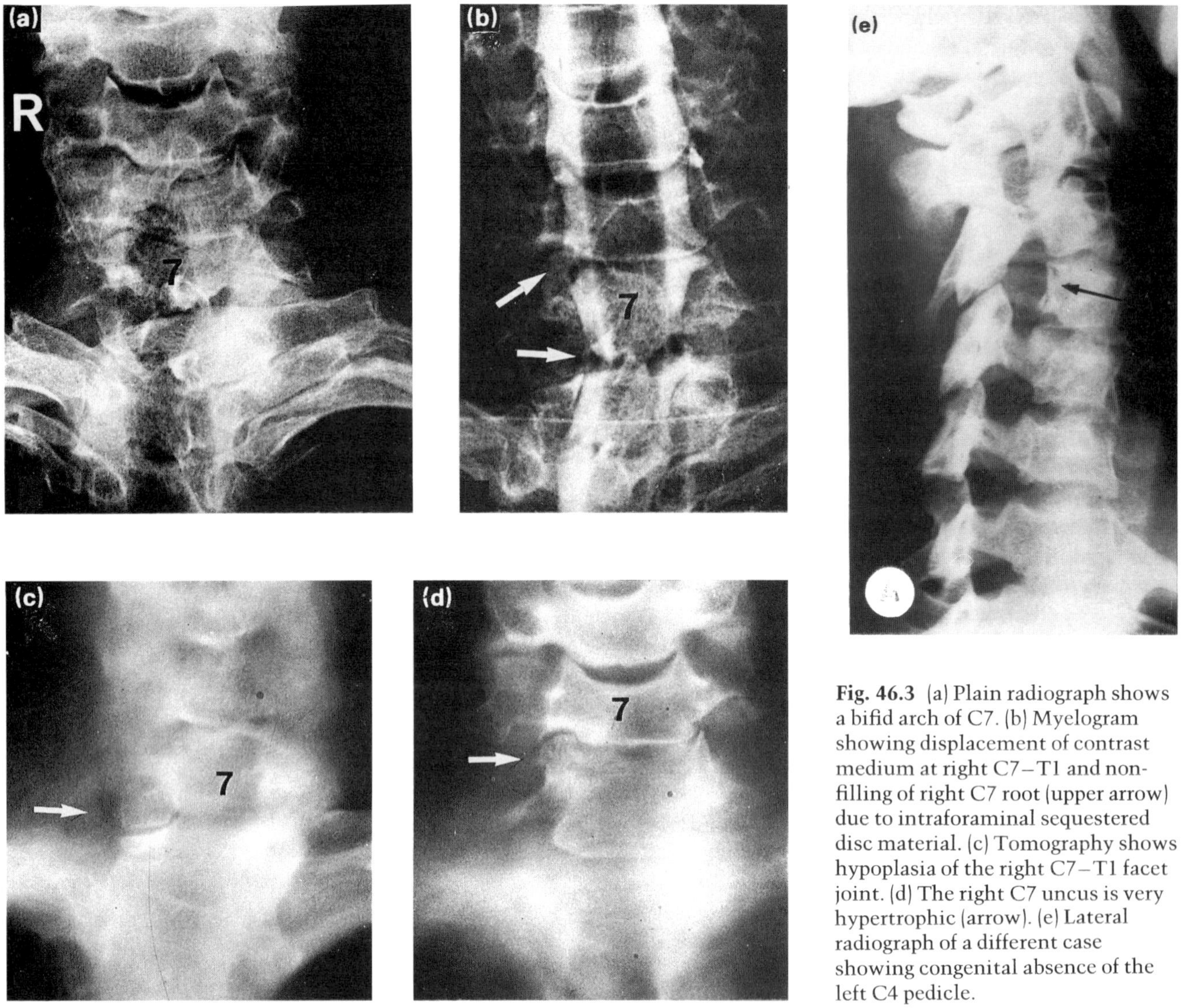

Fig. 46.3 (a) Plain radiograph shows a bifid arch of C7. (b) Myelogram showing displacement of contrast medium at right C7–T1 and non-filling of right C7 root (upper arrow) due to intraforaminal sequestered disc material. (c) Tomography shows hypoplasia of the right C7–T1 facet joint. (d) The right C7 uncus is very hypertrophic (arrow). (e) Lateral radiograph of a different case showing congenital absence of the left C4 pedicle.

able for this purpose, since visualization of the spatial relations of the vertebral artery with the vertebral structures is essential. Simultaneous bilateral retrobrachial high-pressure angiography results, in most cases, in perfect visualization of the second portions of both vertebral arteries. On the left side only the vertebral artery is visualized, since the retrograde current of the contrast medium does not reach the origin of the left common carotid artery from the aortic arch. In rare cases of the left vertebral artery originating from the aortic arch, retrograde brachial angiography will not result in filling the vertebral artery, so that Seldinger vertebral arteriography is required. On the right side, retrograde brachial angiography usually results in filling of both vertebral and carotid arteries, because the origin of the subclavian and common carotid artery form a bifurcation of the brachiocephalic trunk.

Particular attention should be given to plain radiographs of the cervical spine as regards the presence of congenital anomalies of the cervical spine in the vicinity of the intertransverse space (Fig. 46.3). Exceptionally cervical nerve root sleeves containing cerebrospinal fluid (CSF) may project outside the foramen, so that damage to the root during surgical exploration of the intertransverse space may rupture such sleeves, with a resultant CSF leak. Particular attention should be paid to this aspect in the preoperative myelograms.

The operation is performed with the patient's head

in the neutral position. Slight cervical lordosis may facilitate the procedure, depending on the body-build of the patient. At the same time lordosis results in more relaxation of the spinal cord (Breig, 1978).

A transverse skin incision in the target area is the most cosmetic. If more than one intertransverse space has to be explored a bow-shaped skin incision gives good access and better cosmetic results than a straight incision along the anterior border of the sternocleidomastoid muscle. Splitting the fasciae, and lateral retraction of the muscular–vascular bundle, is performed as with the anterior approach to the cervical spine. When operating upon the left side in the area of the scalenovertebral trigonal space (Waldeyer's trigone) damage to the thoracic duct should be avoided. Damage to the thoracic duct produces lymphorrhoea, but the duct can be ligated without problems. When leakage is not recognized it may produce postoperative swelling of the wound area. When exposing the intertransverse space of C2–C3 or C3–C4 it may be necessary to separate the sternocleidomastoid muscle from the mastoid process, followed by eversion of this muscle. In that case care should be taken not to injure the accessory nerve. Identification of the vertebral level can be readily achieved following Chassaignac's advice, given in 1834, when describing the anterior tubercles of the cervical transverse processes. He stressed that the anterior tubercle of the sixth cervical transverse process is the most prominent, and that it can be most easily identified when gliding a finger over the anterior tubercles from the most superior one downward. The abrupt loss of contact with these turbercles indicates that the finger has just passed the sixth one. Among the many uses of this sixth anterior tubercle, Chassaignac reported that it was of great help in identifying the segmental level of the cervical spinal nerves during autopsy. This manoeuvre can be used to identify the level of cervical intervertebral discs, the C5–C6 disc being situated in a plane immediately above that through the cephalad border of the anterior tubercle of C6. The anterior tubercle of C6 covers the exit of the C5–C6 space, so that it may serve as a reference for determining the anterior tubercle of the space to be surgically exposed.

The phrenic nerve is very sensitive to damage, so that great care must be taken with surgical manipulations in the area of the third to fifth spinal nerves. In a few cases a temporary diaphragmatic weakness on the operative side at lower cervical levels has been observed, which may be due to the well-known variation in diaphragmatic innervation. Although diaphragmatic weakness recovered rapidly in all of the few cases observed, a lateral approach on both sides of the neck should never be performed during the same operation.

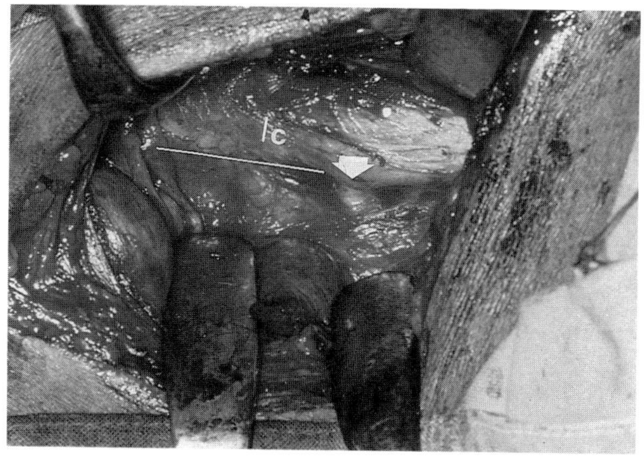

Fig. 46.4 Light downward pressure on the muscles lateral to the transverse processes makes the anterior tubercle of C6 more obvious (arrow); lc is the longus colli muscle. The white line is drawn medial to the anterior tubercles of the transverse processes above C6. This is a right-sided approach with the cranial end of the exposure at the left of the photograph.

The first step in obtaining surgical access to the intertransverse space is interruption of the lateral attachments of the longus colli and longus capitis muscles from the anterior tubercles and anterior rims of the transverse processes of the space to be exposed and of, at least, the spaces above and below. These muscles are retracted medially so that the anterior aspects of the transverse processes are exposed. The next step is resection of the anterior tubercle covering the exit of the spinal nerve that exits the space to be opened. Light finger pressure immediately lateral to the anterior tubercle makes the tubercle more prominent (Fig. 46.4). All muscular attachments to this tubercle are then sectioned. One small bite of a rongeur is inserted behind and in close contact to the posterior surface of the anterior tubercle, because the spinal nerve lies immediately beneath (Fig. 46.5). After removal of the anterior tubercle a small portion of the anterior aspect of the anterior ramus of the spinal nerve is left exposed (Fig. 46.6). This nerve serves as a guide in the identification of the intertransverse space and the foramen to be exposed.

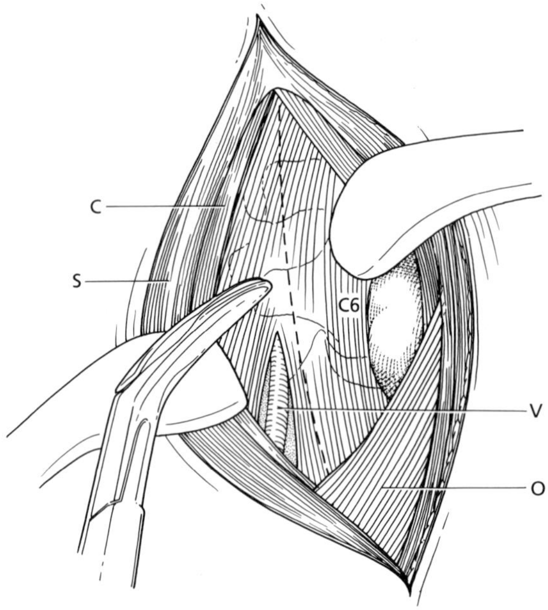

Fig. 46.5 Position of forceps for detaching the anterior tubercle from a C6 transverse process. C, carotid sheath; S, sternocleidomastoid; V, vertebral artery; O, omohyoid.

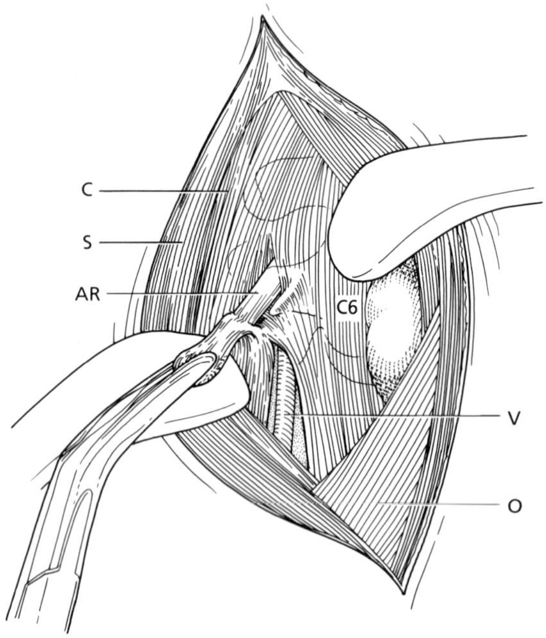

Fig. 46.6 The detached anterior tubercle is pulled laterally by means of the forceps, exposing the underlying portion of the cervical spinal nerve. AR, anterior ramus.

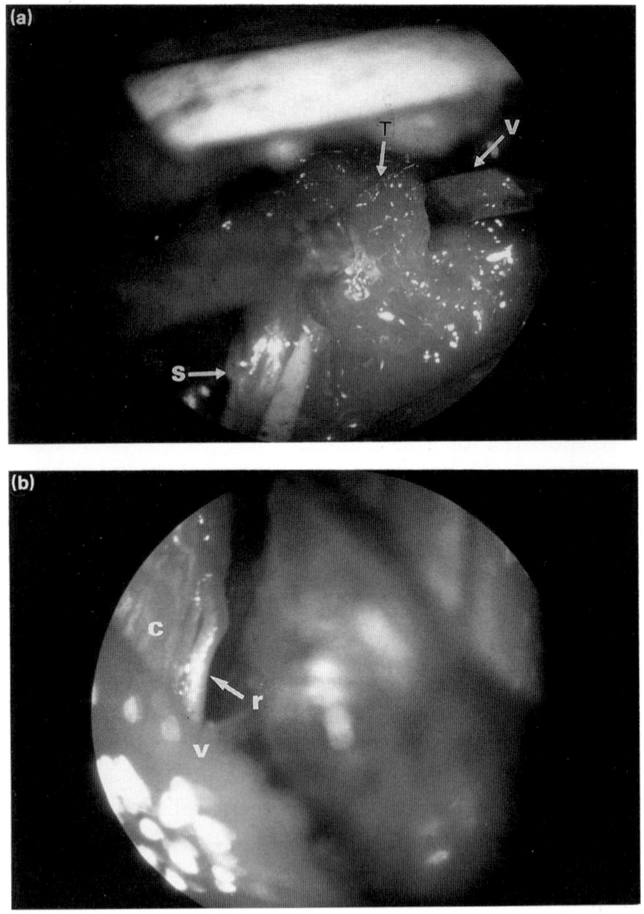

Fig. 46.7 (a) View through the surgical microscope of a right-sided approach with the head to the right of the photograph. Arrow T points to the exposed lateral and anterior borders of the transversarial foramen. Arrow V points to the vertebral artery where the anterior intertransverse muscles have been removed. Arrow S points to the spinal nerve distal to the exposed intertransverse space. (b) A radicular artery (r) is seen running along the cervical nerve root (c).

Next, the anterior intertransverse muscles of the space to be exposed and of the space below are resected (Fig. 46.7a). The anterior rim of the transversarial foramen, forming the floor of the space to be exposed, is resected. The periarterial vertebral venous plexus (or, more rarely, two distinct vertebral veins) and veins covering the spinal nerves are exposed. The veins may be very dilated because of increased venous pressure. The anaesthetist should be requested to avoid or reduce this increased pressure because rupture of the veins inside the space produced by surgical manoeuvres may result in abundant haemorrhage. For this reason perivertebral veins have to be removed in the exposed area. This can be achieved with minor blood loss by rapidly stripping the veins from the vertebral artery up to the intact transversarial foramina and tamponing these veins by plugging gelfoam inside these foramina.

The further surgical steps are made with the aid of the microscope. Radicular arteries should be protected (Fig. 46.7b). In the earliest years some patients, after a postoperative interval of two to seven days, developed very painful cramps in the arms over a period of one or more weeks. This complication was also reported by Jung & Kehr (1972), who attributed these cramps to intraoperative retraction of, or pressure upon, the cervical spinal nerves. In our experience avoiding this retraction or pressure did not prevent these painful cramps. During this period the vertebral artery was often retracted during surgical manipulation inside the space. After retraction of this artery was avoided, and the artery protected by a thin blade during surgical activities in its immediate vicinity, the postoperative painful cramps no longer occurred. Possibly retraction of the vertebral artery produced distension of its radicular branches in some patients, resulting in hypoxia of spinal nerves. Resection of the lateral border of the transversarial foramen and of the covering proximal portions of the anterior scalene muscle allows extension of the surgical procedure to the extravertebral portion of the spinal nerves or to the brachial plexus.

PATHOLOGICAL PROCESSES IN THE CERVICAL INTERTRANSVERSE SPACE

Pathological processes within the cervical intertransverse space may affect either its contents or its walls. The surgical approach described above allows access to deal with pathology within the intertransverse space, or by extension into the vertebral bodies or the discs.

Posterolateral sequestered discs

Sequestered disc fragments may leave the spinal canal and can then migrate through the foramen into the intertransverse space. Such sequestration is characterized clinically by the onset of acute cervical pain followed after a few hours to a few days by acute pain radiating into the arm. It may be accompanied by early or late signs of radicular deficit.

Ruth Jackson (1966) felt that posterolateral disc extrusions could not occur because of the cupped posterior portions of the uncus which serve as barriers preventing discal extrusions in this area. She stressed, in addition, that the cervical spinal nerve roots in their course inside the vertebral canal do not pass over intervertebral discs. Therefore cervical disc extrusions would produce compression of the spinal cord rather than nerve root compression. In her opinion posterolateral disc extrusions occurred rarely, cervical compressive radiculopathy being usually the consequence of osteophytes inside the foramen. She admitted, however, that hypoplasia of the uncus of C6 and C7 might account for posterolateral disc extrusions reported in this area. Jackson felt that extruded sequesters might migrate between the deep and superficial layers of the posterior longitudinal ligament to below the ventral portion of a nerve root, but even then radiculopathy would be associated with signs of spinal cord compression. Our experience obtained through exposure of the intertransverse space in cases of acute radiculopathy caused by extruded disc material shows that it certainly does occur without any associated spinal cord deficit. Should spinal cord compression be present, it is invariably unilateral and limited to exaggerated tendon reflexes, a positive Rossolimo and, exceptionally, pathological plantar reflexes. No loss of power of the legs and no Brown–Séquard syndromes have been encountered. The radicular disturbances in these patients were segmental hypoaesthesia accompanied by radicular pain. Patients presenting with radicular motor deficit and muscular atrophy rarely showed signs of spinal cord compression.

Elvidge & Luh (1950) described sensory disturbances in the trigeminal area attributed to compression of the spinal descending trigeminal tract in a case of medial disc protrusion at C4–C5. These disturbances disappeared after decompressive laminectomy. Keuter (1970) described disturbances of protopathic sensation in the trigeminal area delimited according to Solders lines in seven cases of lower cervical spinal lesions. Two of these patients with disc protrusions, compressing the C6 and C7 nerve roots respectively, had diminished sensation of pain and temperature in the ipsilateral trigeminal area and the C2–C3 dermatomes with the exception of the perioral region. The ipsilateral corneal reflex was also reduced in one of these two patients. Following removal of these protrusions sensation recovered in the first patient but follow-up of the second patient was not mentioned.

Similar trigeminal disturbances were encountered in three out of our 56 cases of posterolateral disc extrusions at C5–C6 and in one out of 46 cases of posterolateral extrusions at C6–C7. Complete recovery of these trigeminal disturbances was noted in all four cases following removal of the disc extrusions. For a tentative explanation of these trigeminal disturbances the reader is referred to Keuter's paper (1970).

In all cases of cervical compressive radiculopathy the corresponding spinal nerve exposed in the intertransverse space showed hyperaemia of its sheath. In cases of more than one month's duration the epineurium of these nerves was surrounded by proliferous connective tissue, that in cases with many years' history had formed a non-transparent layer over the nerve(s). In cases of a first episode operated on within one month after its onset, the access to the foramen was not occluded, and the sequester could be extracted via the foramen by means of curved tweezers (Fig. 46.8).

Another new finding following the adoption of these surgical approaches was the migration of disc sequesters outside the foramen and along the vertebral artery or the spinal nerve. They have been found adherent to the vertebral artery at 2 cm distance from the foramen. Sequesters of long standing become desiccated and calcified. They may occlude the foramen by agglomeration and encapsulation, and bulge outward from the foramen (Fig. 46.9a). This outward bulging may be visualized in the AP vertebral arteriogram (Fig. 46.10); it closely resembles lateral displacement of the vertebral artery by uncal osteophytes (Fig. 46.11) but in contrast to the osteophytes the displacing agent is usually radiotranslucent. A defect of a root pouch in the myelogram and lateral displacement of the vertebral artery at the same level is a strong indication of the presence of migrated disc sequesters. A large mass of migrated sequesters may produce kinking of the vertebral artery that may also be seen in the lateral arteriogram (Figs 46.9b, 46.12b & d). The surgical removal of long-standing sequestered material occluding the foramen must be performed in piecemeal fashion to avoid injury to the spinal nerve and requires, in addition, preliminary removal of small portions of the surrounding anterior, upper and lower bony boundaries of the foramen.

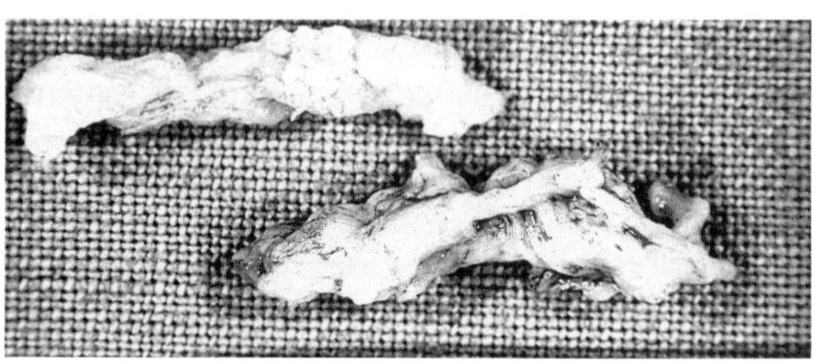

Fig. 46.8 Sequestered disc fragments removed from the foramen via the intertransverse space in a case of acute radiculopathy.

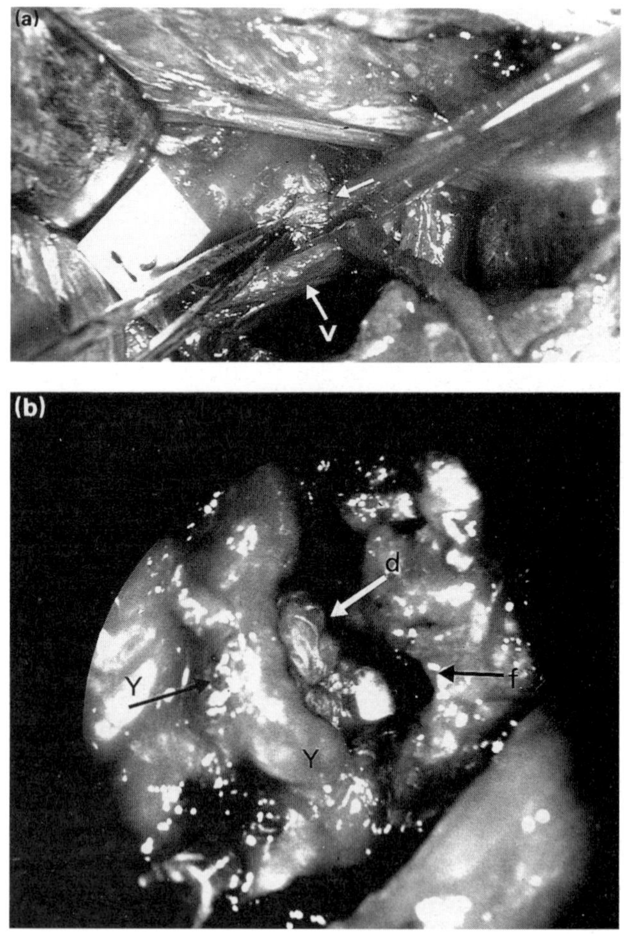

Fig. 46.9 (a) Surgical exposure showing long-standing sequester which has migrated out of the foramen into the intertransverse space (arrow at end of sucker). It is producing displacement of the vertebral artery (V). (b) View through surgical microscope after removal of a large sequestered disc. The dura is visible through the foramen (f) as an area of reflected light. Arrow (d) points to some residual disc adjacent to and distorting the vertebral artery (Y). (See also Figs 46.12b & d.)

Migration of disc sequesters outside the foramen may be accompanied by migration of sequesters inside the vertebral canal, usually along the anterolateral surface of the dura. The myelogram may not show the full extent of this migration in the PA view with the patient in ventral decubitus, but becomes obvious when the patient is slightly rotated from this position towards the side of the lesion (Fig. 46.13). Removal of these migrated sequesters may necessitate the resection of a vertebral pedicle (Fig. 46.14).

Initially this procedure was limited to the removal of the sequestrated disc material, but further degeneration of the remaining disc resulted in some

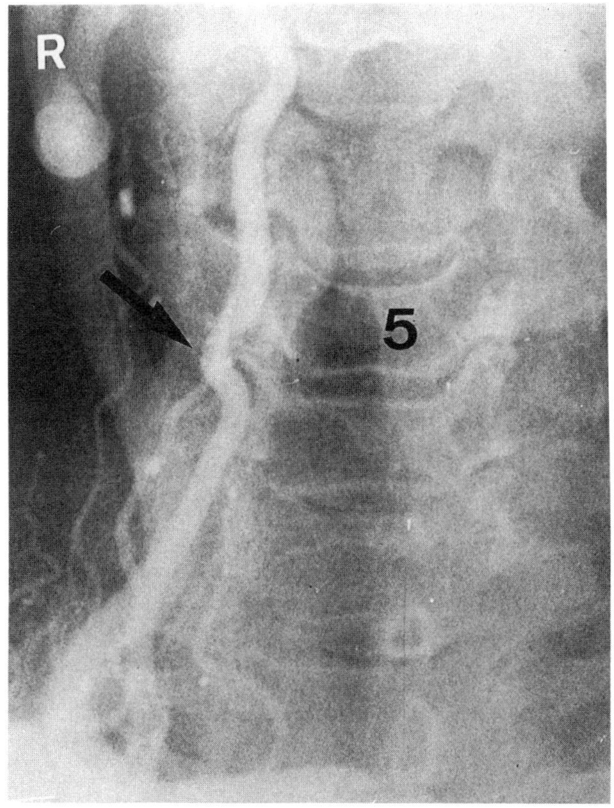

Fig. 46.11 Local outward bending of vertebral artery produced by right lateral uncal osteophyte at C6 does not show a translucent space as seen in Fig. 46.10.

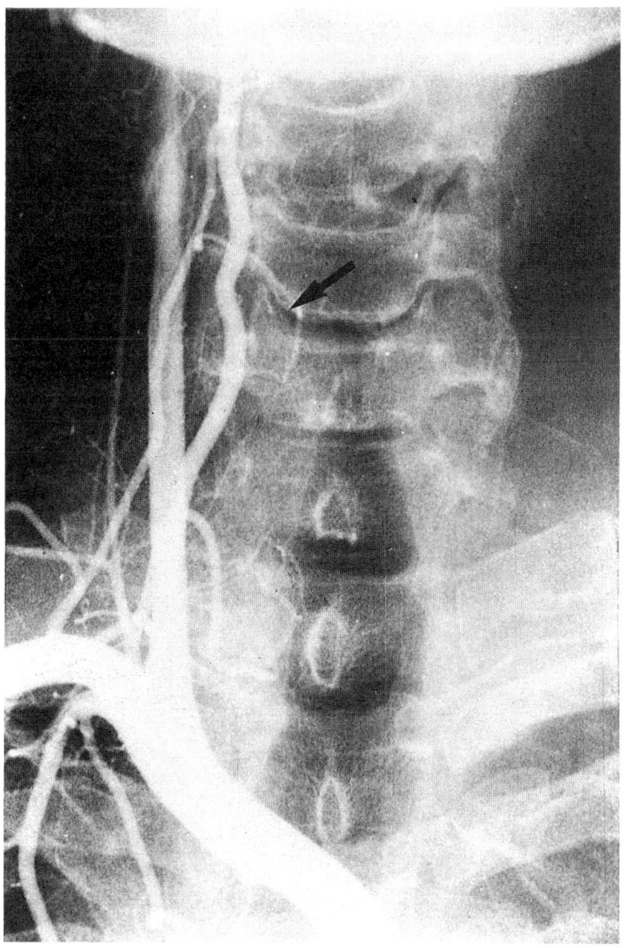

Fig. 46.10 AP view of right vertebral angiogram. Between the lateral aspect of the right uncinate process of C6 and the local lateral outward bend of the artery at this level there is a translucent space produced by organized migrated disc material protruding through the C5–C6 foramen. The arrow points to the uncovertebral joint.

of the cases in osteophytic narrowing of the opposite foramen. For this reason the residual intervertebral nucleus pulposus was also removed, after uncusectomy, by means of a lateral transdiscal approach.

The lateral approach has led to the discovery of so far unknown aspects of migration of posterolateral disc extrusions and changes in the spinal nerves distal to the site of compression. The extruded sequesters may become asymptomatic either through extraspinal migration or through resorption. It is our policy not to operate immediately upon patients developing acute painful radiculopathy in the absence of obvious signs of radicular deficit or of spinal cord compression. In a number of these cases the pain subsides gradually and eventually disappears. Increasing pain, chronic pain and/or early or late development of neural deficit are indications for surgery by means of a lateral approach. Tables 46.1 and 46.2 give a survey of the distribution of 108 posterolateral disc ex-

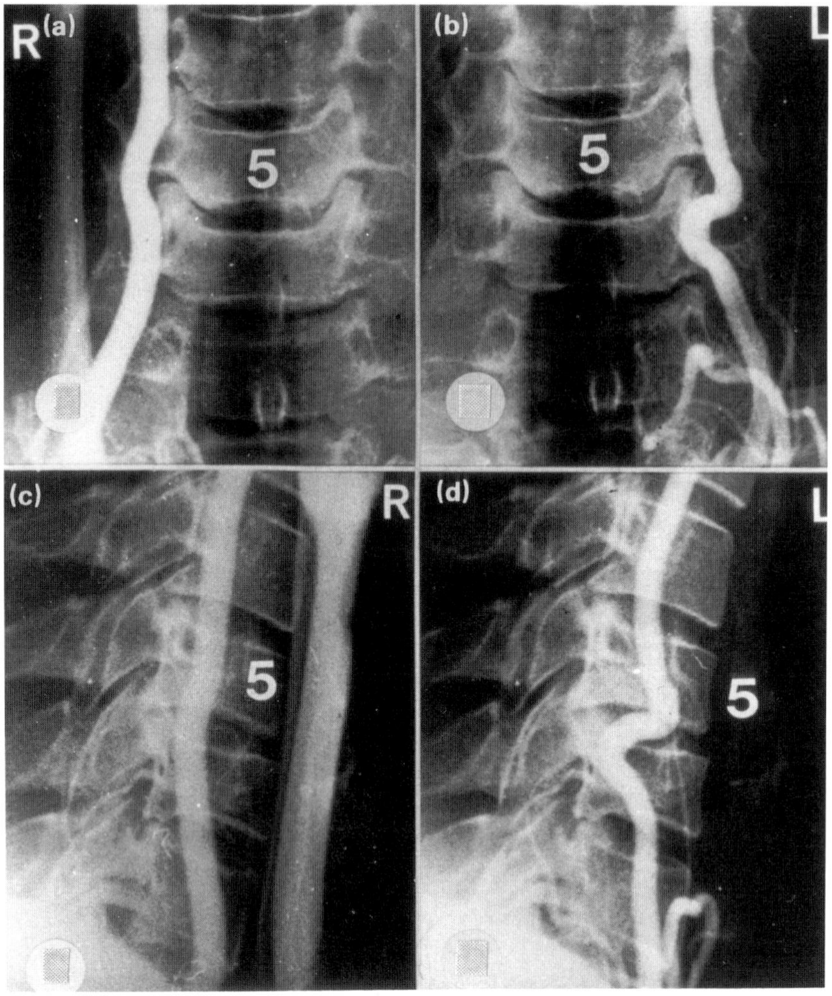

Fig. 46.12 (a,c) Anterior and lateral right vertebral angiograms show minor lateral and posterior local displacement of the artery caused by uncal osteophyte. (b,d) Left anterior and lateral vertebral angiograms of same patient show kinking of the artery produced by large mass of sequestrated disc material inside the intertransverse space C5–C6 (see also Fig. 46.9b).

trusions removed in 101 patients by means of a lateral approach.

Transuncal disc extrusions

The posterolateral disc extrusions described above all occur secondary to a posterolateral annular rupture with migration of fragments to the intertransverse space via the intervertebral foramen. However, the development of the lateral approach to the intertransverse space led to the discovery that disc extrusion could occur directly into the intertransverse

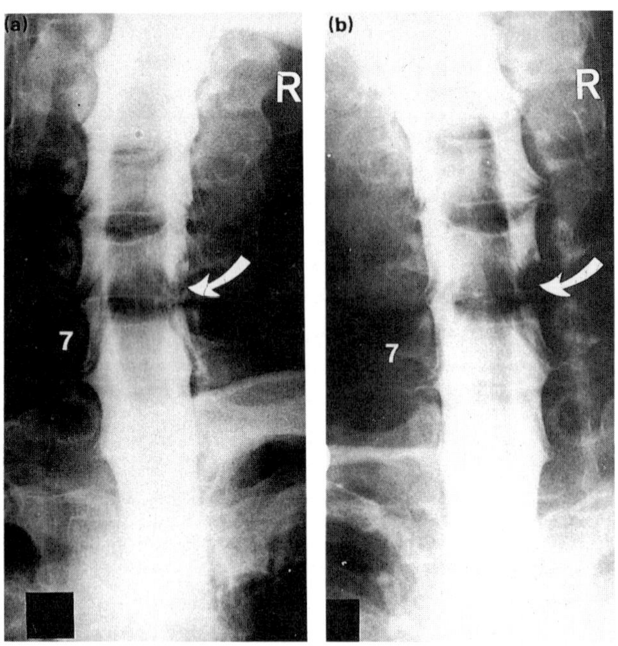

Fig. 46.13 (*Left*) (a) PA myelogram with the patient in ventral decubitus shows interruption of the contrast on the right at C6–C7. (b) Slightly rotating the patient's cervical spine with the right side downward results in a larger interruption of the contrast medium on the right at C6–C7.

Table 46.1 Relationship of posterolateral disc sequesters and osteophyte formation at 134 levels in 115 patients

	Levels		Number of patients	
Disc sequesters only, normal foramina	C4–C5		2	
	C5–C6		37	
80 patients	C6–C7		33	
	C7–T1		1	
	C4–C5 and C5–C6		2	
	C5–C6 and C6–C7		5	
			80 cases	80 cases
Osteophytes only, foraminal narrowing	C5–C6		4	
	C6–C7		1	
14 patients	C4–C5 and C5–C6		3	
	C5–C6 and C6–C7		6	
			14 cases	14 cases
Osteophytes and disc sequesters at same level	C5–C6		9	
13 patients	C6–C7		4	
			13 cases	13 cases
	Level of sequester	Level of osteophyte		
Osteophytes and disc sequesters at different levels	C4–C5	C5–C6	1	
	C5–C6	C6–C7	2	
	C5–C6	C5–C6 and C6–C7	1	
	C6–C7	C5–C6	2	
	C6–C7	C5–C6 and C6–C7	2	
			8 cases	8 cases
	Total 134 levels			*Total* 115 cases

Table 46.2 Levels involved by the intraforaminal sequesters and intraforaminal uncal osteophytes in the 115 patients presented in Table 46.1

Levels	Sequesters	Osteophytes
C4–C5	5	3
C5–C6	56	28
C6–C7	46	16
C7–T1	1	–
	108	47

In 66 (61.1%) of the 108 sequesters part of the material had migrated along the nerves and/or the vertebral artery.

space through a transuncal route (Fig. 46.15). It is a rare phenomenon, and the author has seen only six cases. Five of these six cases had a traumatic onset and the sixth was associated with torticollis. Four of the cases were at C5–C6 with the remaining two at C6–C7 but, more importantly, five of the cases had abnormally hypoplastic uncovertebral joints, thereby facilitating extrusion by the transuncal route.

In two cases the extrusion was sufficiently large that it occluded the vertebral artery at the level of the extrusion, though more distal vertebral filling occurred due to collaterals from the ascending and deep cervical arteries. The traumatic incident in both these cases was severe enough to produce vertebral fractures. One case showed significant right-sided subluxation at C6–C7 with a transuncal herniation

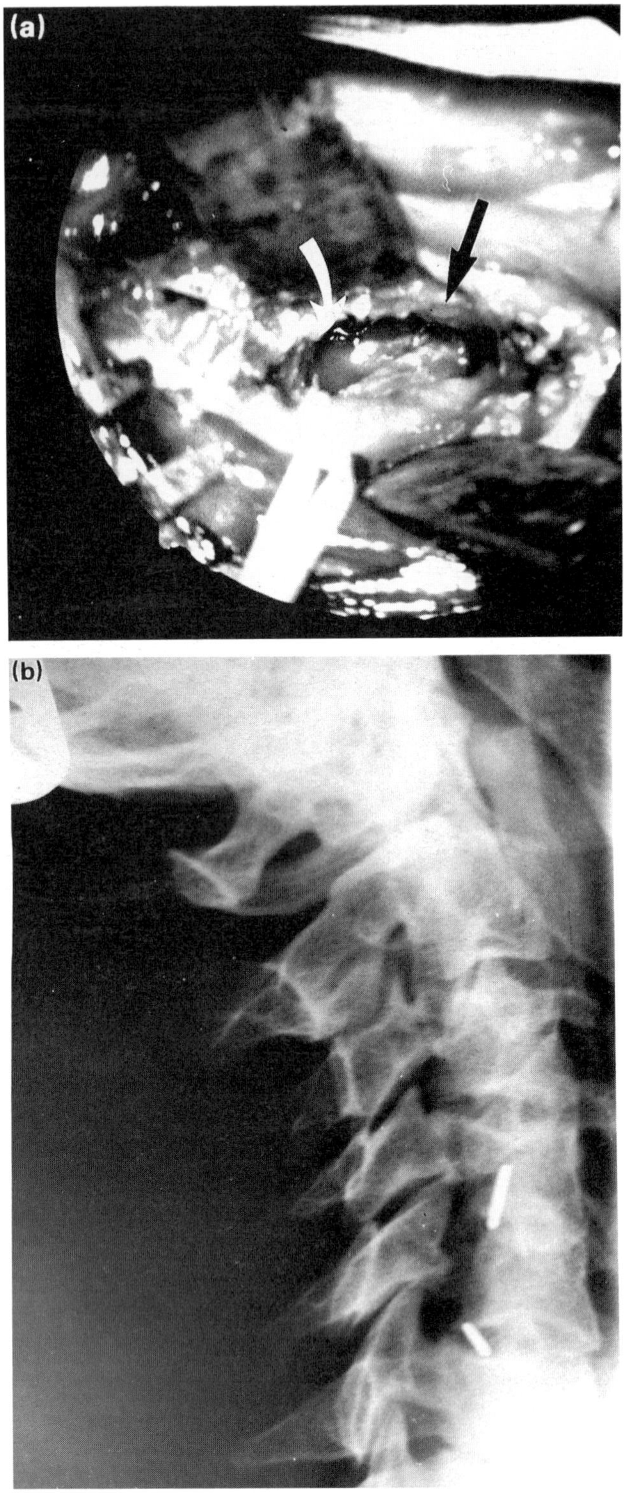

Fig. 46.14 (a) A very large partly intraspinal sequestered disc has necessitated the removal of the adjacent pedicle for exposure. The arrows indicate the enlarged dural exposure achieved. (b) Postoperative radiograph showing the extent of pedicle removal.

at the same level, but on the left side. At operation, sequestered disc material protruded below the medial attachments of the longus colli muscle in front of the vertebral column. The other patient had a fracture of the articular processes at C5–C6 with transuncal sequestration at the same level and side (Figs 46.16(a)–(c), 46.16(d)–(f) & 46.17). In the other patients traumatic transuncal disc extrusion was not accompanied by vertebral fractures. The vertebral angiogram showed only displacement without total occlusion of the artery. The diagnosis of transuncal extrusion could be made during operation only, when disc material could be followed through a cleft above the uncus (Fig. 46.18). Following removal of the extruded fragments the remaining disc was cleared and replaced by a wedge-shaped graft of cortical bone in all cases.

Dumbbell tumours

Certain neurofibromas may present as dumbbell tumours extending outside the spinal canal. Those whose anatomy shows only a small intraspinal

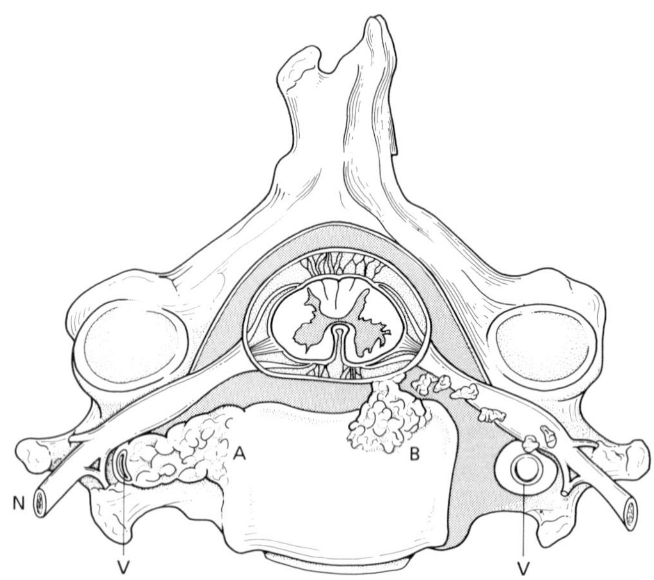

Fig. 46.15 The diagram illustrates the differing routes taken by a posterolateral disc extrusion (B) and by a transuncal extrusion (A). In the former, the annulus ruptures in its posterolateral part and disc fragments migrate through the foramen into the intertransverse space. In the latter, the disc extrudes directly into the intertransverse space and may occlude the vertebral artery (V) as shown.

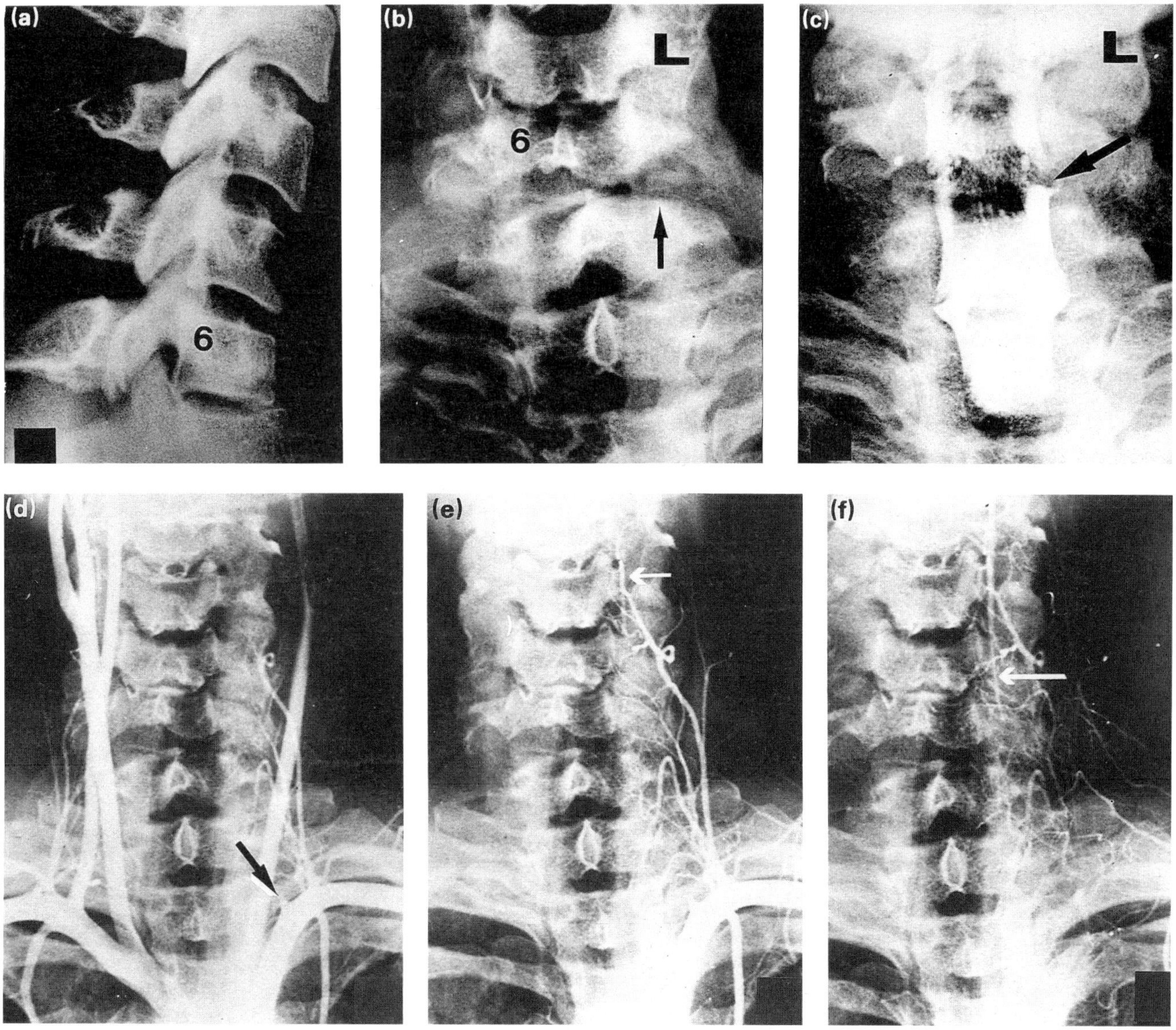

Fig. 46.16 (a)–(c) Case of left transuncal disc extrusion at C6–C7. The patient had had a traumatic lateral dislocation of C6 to the right, that had been almost completely reduced. (a) Normal alignment in lateral view. (b) There is some residual right lateral displacement of the spinous process of C6. Arrow points at hypoplastic left uncus of C7. (c) The myelogram shows a left lateral interruption of the contrast medium at the level of the C7 nerve root pouch. The patient had left triceps muscle weakness and reduced left triceps tendon reflex. (d) Arrow points at obliteration of the left vertebral artery at its origin from the subclavian artery. (e) and (f) show collateral circulation through the deep and ascending cervical arteries to the patent upper portion of the vertebral artery.

proportion but a large extraspinal portion extending via an enlarged foramen into and beyond the intertransverse space can be totally excised via the lateral approach. Attempts to remove such lesions via a laminectomy approach often result in subtotal removal of the extraspinal portion, or result in a total facetectomy. Computerized tomography (CT) and magnetic resonance imaging (MRI) scanning show the anatomy of the tumour in graphic detail, but vertebral angiography is essential to show the site and degree of arterial displacement.

After the tumour has been exposed within the

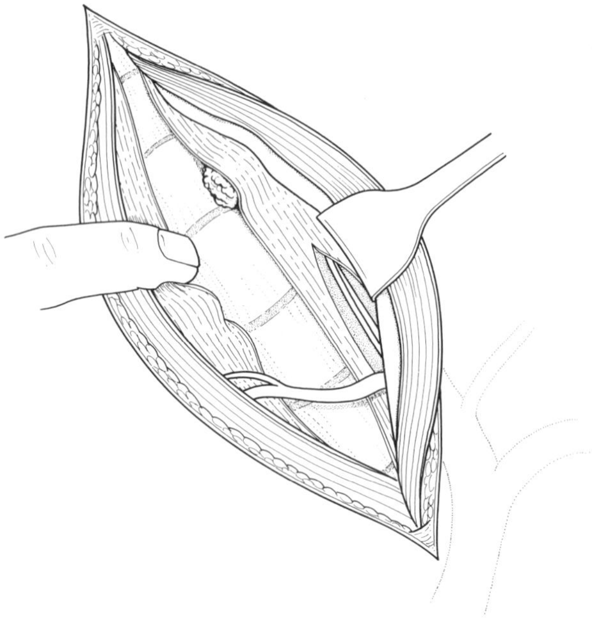

Fig. 46.17 Diagrammatic representation of operative findings in the case shown in Fig. 46.16. A large transuncal extrusion is seen elevating the muscles lying anterior to the cervical intertransverse space.

cervical intertransverse space the vertebral artery should be identified. No attempts should be made to free the vessel from the tumour at this stage. The capsule of the tumour should be incised and as much of the internal tumour substance should be removed as possible. Only then is the collapsed capsule and residual tumour removed, with the dural opening being closed with sutures or clips (Fig. 46.19).

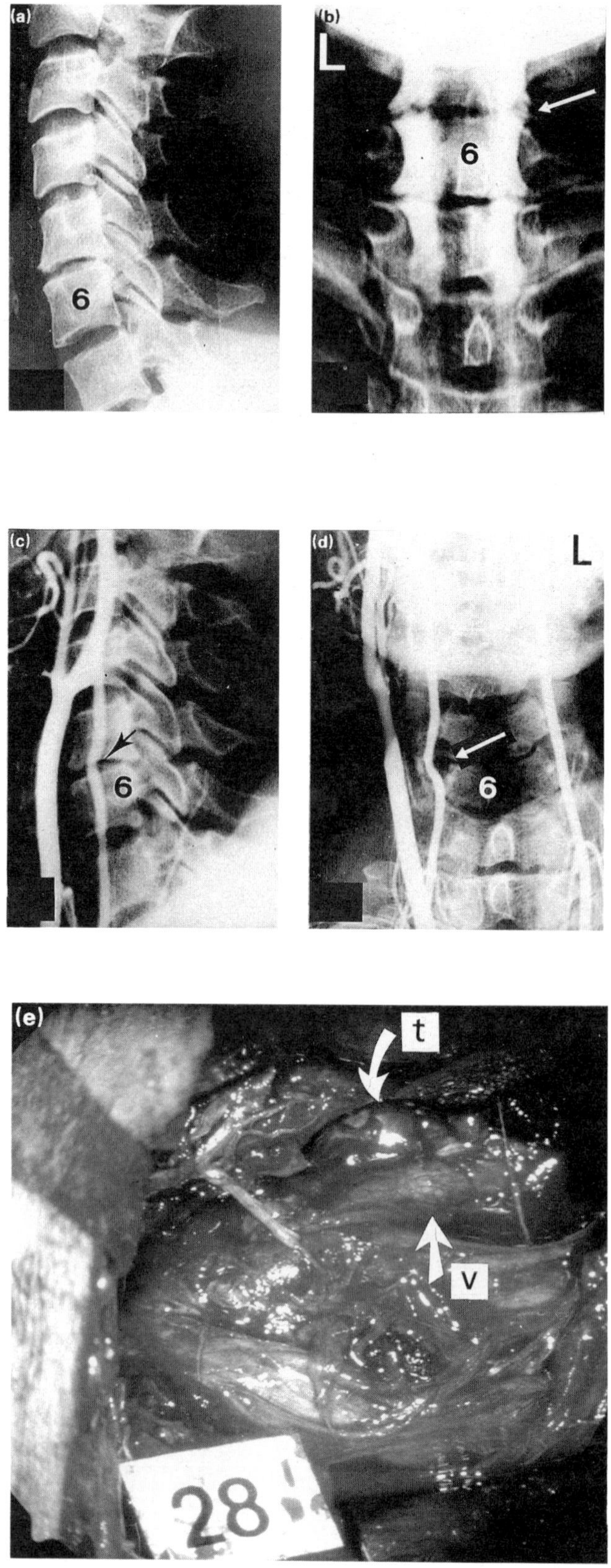

Fig. 46.18 Case of small traumatic transuncal disc extrusion in the right C5–C6 intertransverse space. No fracture or dislocation. (a) Narrowed C5–C6 disc space. (b) Myelogram shows minor deformity of right nerve root pouch (arrow) as compared with the left side. (c) Lateral view of right vertebral arteriogram showing anterior kinking of the artery at the level of the narrowed disc. (d) The AP view of the bilateral retrograde brachial vertebral angiogram showing lateral displacement of the right vertebral artery at the level of C5–C6. Note radiotranslucent area between the lateral bend of vertebral artery and the lateral borders of the vertebral bodies C5 and C6. Note absence of right uncus C6 and presence of left C6 uncus. (e) Intraoperative view. Two interspaces have been exposed. Arrow (t) points to transuncally sequestrated disc material situated at the medial aspect of the vertebral artery (v) (compare with (d)).

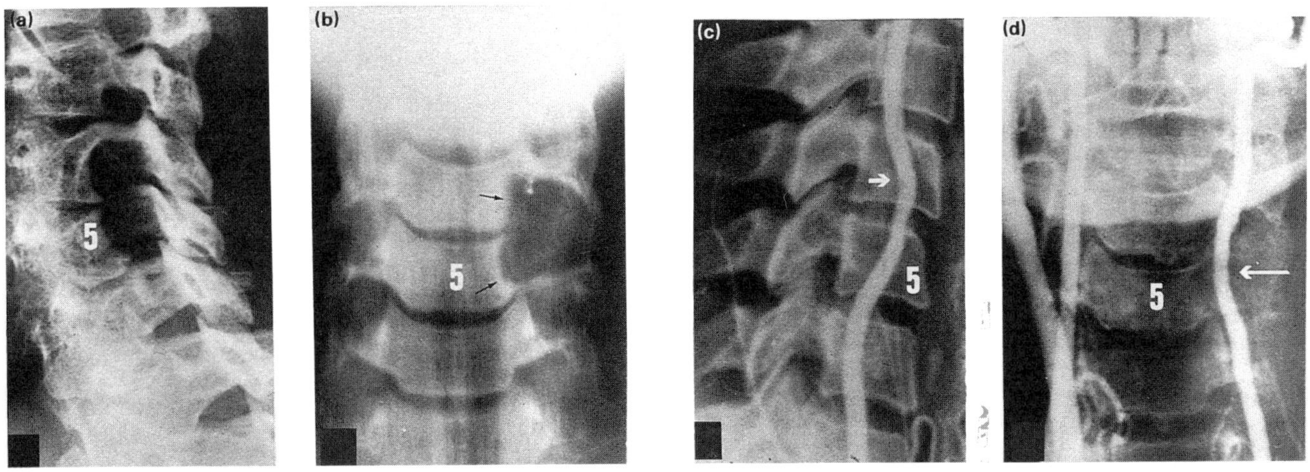

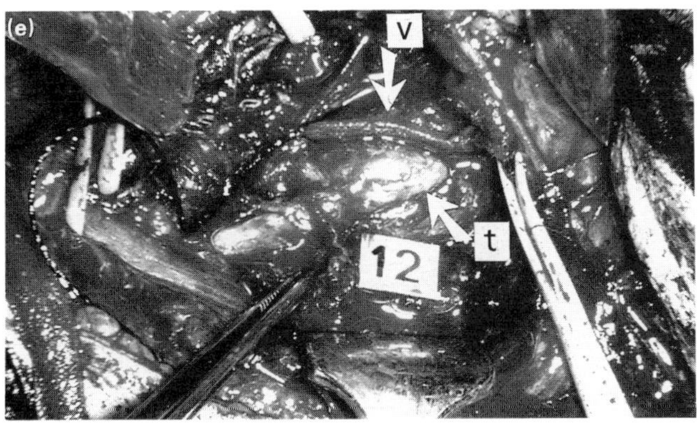

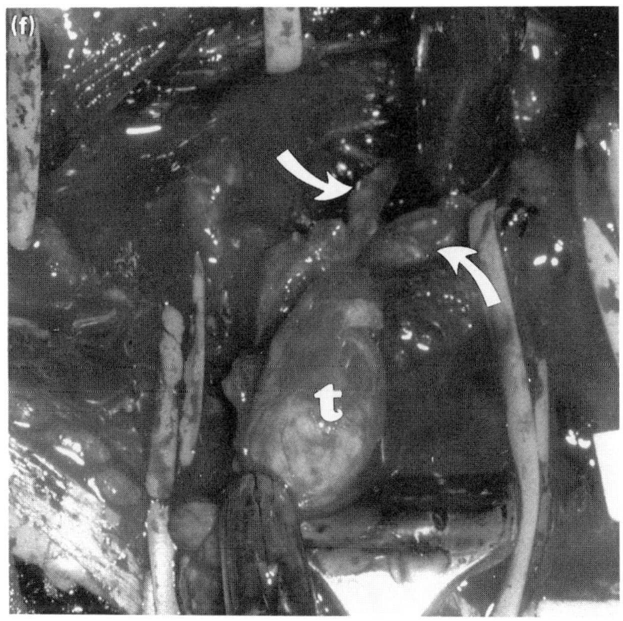

Fig. 46.19 Dumbbell neurofibroma. (a) Enlargement of the foramina of C4–C5 and C5–C6 by a dumbbell tumour that also has eroded the pedicle of C5. (b) AP view shows destruction of the floor of the C4 intertransverse space that also forms the roof of the C5 space. (c) The vertebral artery is dislocated forward and (d) medially by the portion of the dumbbell tumour inside the intertransverse spaces of C4–C5 and C5–C6. (e) Exposure of the dumbbell tumour (t) inside the intertransverse spaces C4–C5 and C5–C6. Arrow (v) points at the anteriorly displaced vertebral artery. (f) After removal of part of the tumour its portion lying inside the foramen and vertebral canal is exposed and will be removed. Arrows point at the anterior and posterior nerve roots thickened as a consequence of ingrowth of the tumour. Nerve roots and tumour could be completely removed by means of this lateral approach.

Traction injuries of the brachial plexus

During injury to the brachial plexus the lateral extremity of the transverse processes may act as a fulcrum, thereby limiting lesions to the vicinity of the intertransverse space. When the brachial plexus is explored in order to attempt neural repair, the resection of the anterior border and costotransverse lamella at the level of the intertransverse space involved permits resection of the traumatic neuroma up to the foramen. Following the resection of neuromas in this region, the removal of the floor of the intertransverse space reduces the gap between the nerve ends by some 2 cm, thereby facilitating repair. If nerve grafting is required, the exposure of the intertransverse space allows the proximal suture line to be very close to the foramen (Fig. 46.20).

PATHOLOGICAL PROCESSES IN THE WALLS OF THE INTERTRANSVERSE SPACE

In practical terms the pathologies which affect the walls of the intertransverse space are limited to the bony walls; namely, the articular processes, the pedicles, the uncus and the lateral part of the vertebral body.

Lateral uncal osteophytes

Lateral uncal osteophytes may compress the vertebral artery, especially during rotation of the head along one of its three coordinates, and may result in drop attacks and/or signs of cerebral or brain stem insufficiency. It has been suggested that this type of compression cannot be responsible for causing cerebral or brain stem signs and symptoms, since the second portion of the artery can be ligated without producing any disturbances in most cases. Yet considerable improvement has been observed following resection of the lateral uncal osteophytes.

The following experience may provide an explanation of this fact. A 57-year-old female suffered from drop attacks when rotating the head, and she suffered from vertigo. Vertebral angiography showed lateral displacement of both vertebral arteries by bilateral uncal osteophytes at C6. Rotation of the head to the left produced arrest of the angiographic contrast medium in both vertebral arteries. The lateral right and left uncal osteophytes were removed in two

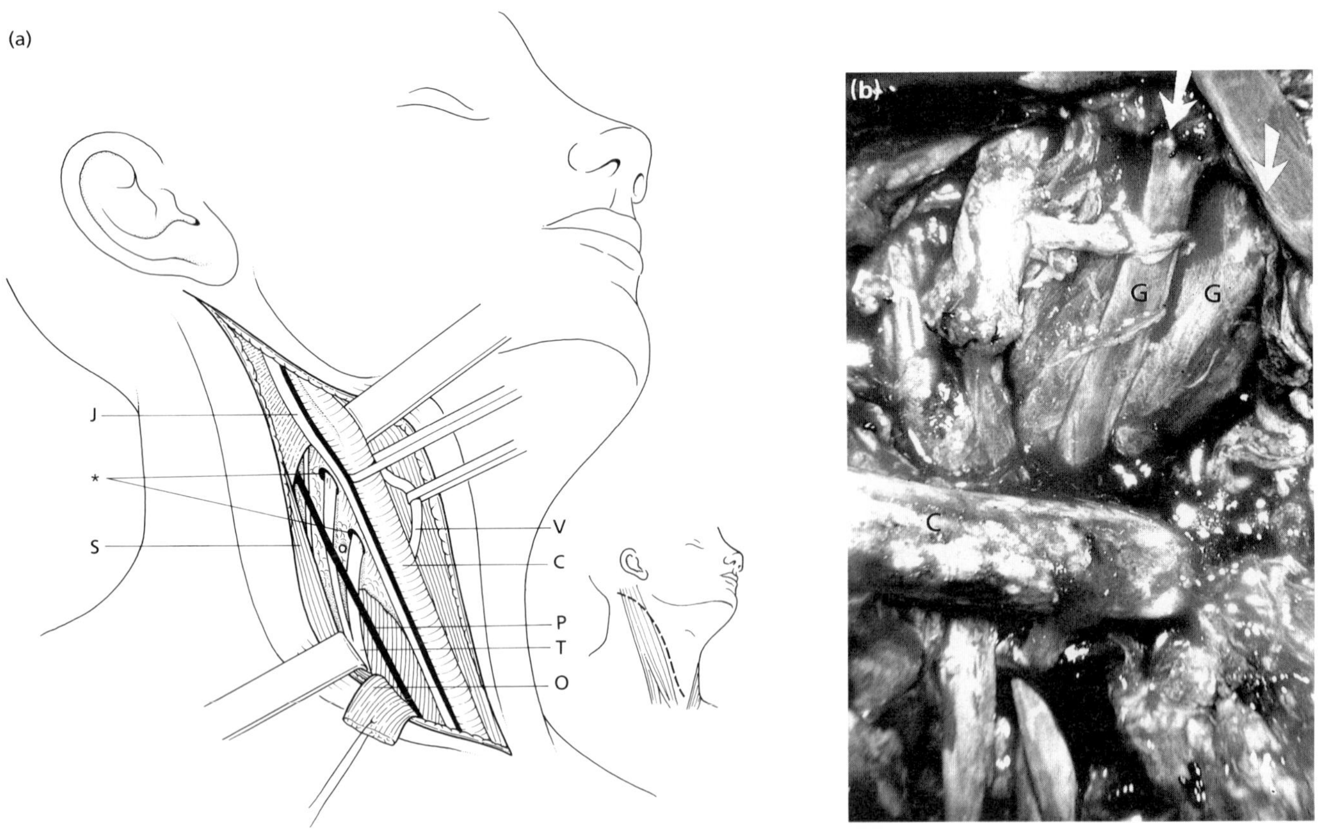

Fig. 46.20 (a) Exposure of branches of the brachial plexus in the intertransverse space results in a gain in access to these branches of about 2 cm (*). J, Jugular vein; S, retracted sternocleidomastoid muscle; T, beginning of a trunk of the brachial plexus; O, divided omyhoid muscle; P, phrenic nerve; C, carotid artery and vagus nerve; V, vertebral artery is retracted to show its position. This artery is never retracted during operation. (b) Repair of traction lesion of brachial plexus by grafting. Two of the grafts (G) were sutured, after resection of the underlying transverse processes, to the spinal nerves at the exit from the foramen.

stages. During decompression of the left vertebral artery its medial wall at the site of the lateral uncal osteophyte appeared to be very thin, and it ruptured during the surgical procedure. An end-to-end anastomosis was performed. Since the right vertebral artery was very small a postoperative bilateral retrobrachial vertebral control angiography was performed, and disappointingly both vertebral arteries appeared to be occluded but collateral circulation to the upper portions of both vertebral arteries was visualized. Since the operation, however, the patient is completely free from drop attacks and vertigo up to the present time, 20 years after the operation. The explanation may be that before the removal of the uncal osteophytes the circulation through the vertebral arteries was very unstable under the influence of head movements. Resection of the uncal osteophytes may stabilize the circulation through patent vertebral arteries or, if it results in obstruction in the vertebral arteries, it may encourage the development of collateral circulation, as in the present case.

The wall of the vertebral arteries is often very thin at the site of compressive lateral uncal osteophytes as a consequence of turbulence of echo waves in the blood flow through this area. This explained our early experience of efforts to liberate the wall of the artery from the osteophyte resulting in its rupture. The procedure was therefore modified by separating the portion of the osteophyte that is adherent to the wall of the artery from the main mass of the osteophyte by means of a small sharp osteotome. The separated small portion, that is adherent to the artery, is not removed, while the other larger portion of this osteophyte is removed from the uncus. No vascular rupture has been observed since (Fig. 46.21).

Posterior uncal osteophytes

These osteophytes narrow the foramen, producing compressive radiculopathy. They may extend into the vertebral canal and their extent must be checked with CT. The posterior intraforaminal uncal osteophytes are separated by means of small osteotomes directed in a plane parallel to the anterior surface of the spinal nerve (Figs 46.22 & 46.23). This technique prevents iatrogenic damage to the nerve, which is a real danger when removing the intraforaminal osteophyte via an anterior approach.

Anterior articular osteophytes

The role of cervical spondylotic disease in producing symptoms such as dizziness and drop attacks has often been questioned. There is little doubt that, in many patients, the cause of such symptoms lies

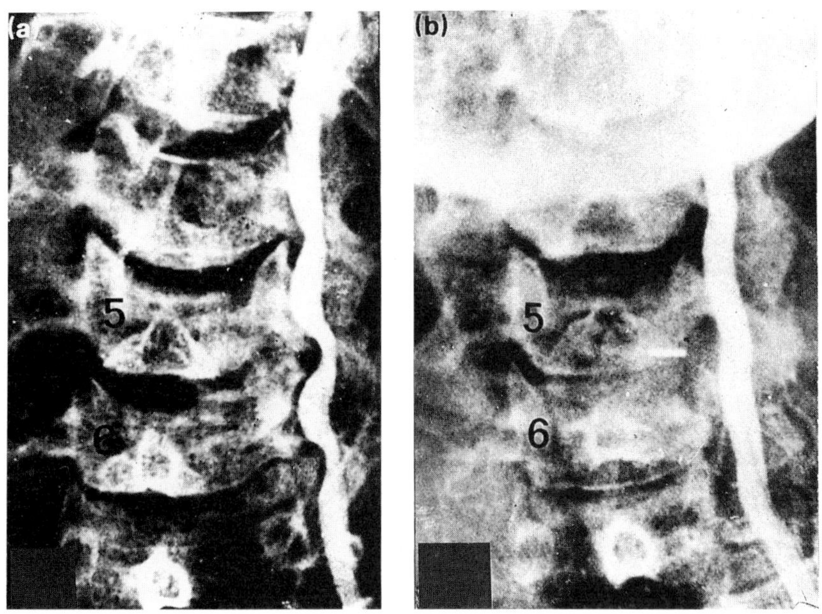

Fig. 46.21 (a) Osteophytic narrowing of left vertebral artery by lateral uncal osteophytes. (b) Narrowing of the artery relieved following resection of uncal osteophytes via the respective intertransverse space.

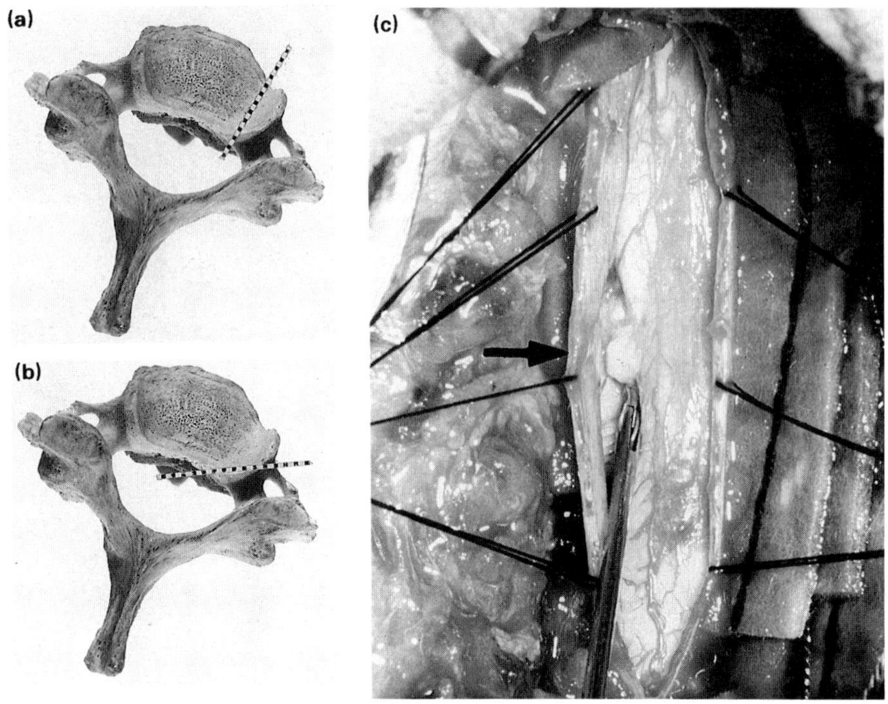

Fig. 46.22 (a) For removal of intraforaminal posterior uncal osteophytes the entire uncus is removed by means of an osteotome. (b) In addition, a second plane of section is directed inward and slightly beyond the foramen, because (c) the intraforaminal uncal osteophyte may reach inside the vertebral canal (black arrow).

in an abnormal psychological over-reaction to their underlying pain syndrome. However, osteophytes arising from the superior articular processes may occlude the vertebral artery during marked extension of the head resulting in sudden drop attacks or vertigo. Previously such osteophytes could be removed only by means of complete facetectomy, but the development of the lateral approach with exposure of the intertransverse space allows their removal with preservation of the joint.

Fig. 46.24 illustrates a case of a patient who developed acute vertigo and dysbasia every time the neck was hyperextended. The patient had sustained a diving injury with a fracture of C6 without neurological deficit 13 years earlier, and had been treated with a C4–T1 posterior fusion. Figure 46.24(c) shows osteophytic occlusion of the left C3–C4 foramen in extension. The left lateral vertebral angiogram (Fig. 46.24(e)) shows a fusiform dilatation of the artery at C3 and, in extension, the artery immediately proximal to this dilatation becomes narrowed (Fig. 46.24(f)). Following removal of the osteophytes by exposure of the C3–C4 intertransverse space, the contour of the left vertebral artery is restored to

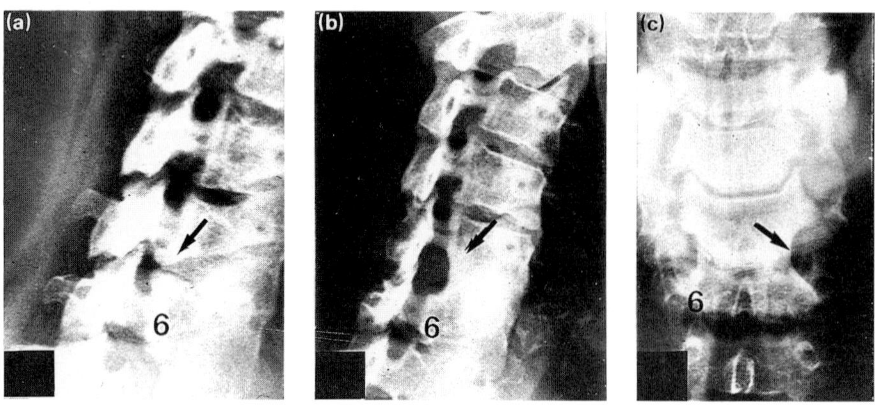

Fig. 46.23 (a) C5–C6 foraminal narrowing due to osteophytosis. (b) Enlarged C5–C6 foramen following removal of uncal osteophytes by a lateral approach. (c) Typical AP view of changes produced by opening the intertransverse space at C5–C6 (arrow). The anterior and lateral borders of the transversarial foramina of C5 and C6 have been removed.

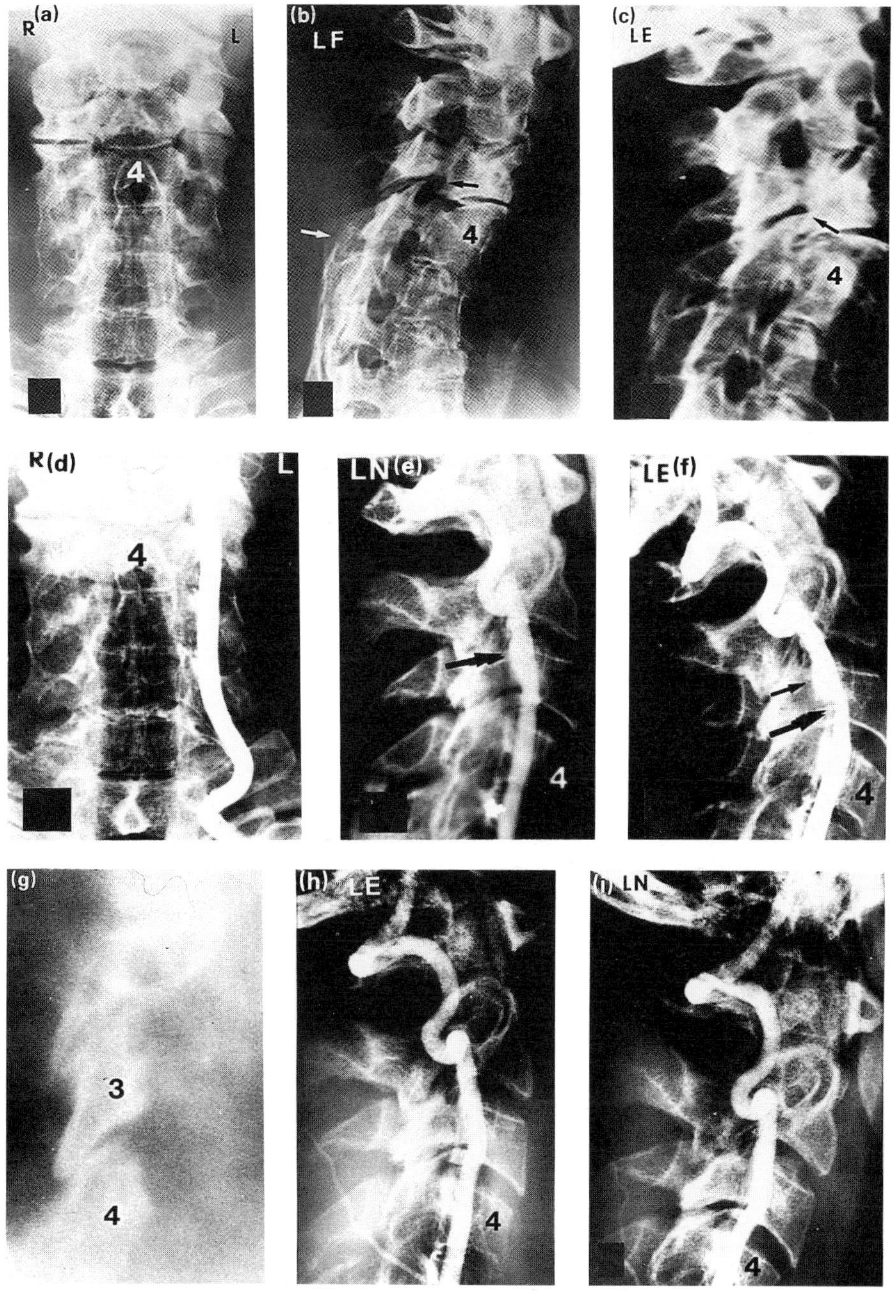

Fig. 46.24 (a) AP plain radiograph. (b) Left oblique views in flexion, showing posterior C4–T1 fusion (white arrow). The black arrow points to the left inferior articular process of C3 and no narrowing of the C3–C4 foramen is evident. (c) The same view as in (b), but with the neck in extension. The left C3–C4 foramen is now occluded (arrow) by osteophytes. (d) Left vertebral angiogram is normal in AP view. (e) Lateral view shows fusiform dilatation of vertebral artery at C3. (f) In extension there is constriction of the artery immediately proximal to the dilatation (large arrow). (g) Tomograms showing the removal of the osteophytes of the left C3–C4 joint following the exposure of the intertransverse spaces at C2–C3 and C3–C4. (h) Left lateral vertebral angiogram showing resolution of the fusiform dilatation and (i) the constriction of the artery in extension.

normal, with complete relief of symptoms (Fig. 46.24(g)–(i)).

Locked facets

Traumatic locking of the facet joints, either on one or both sides, following traumatic subluxation produces foraminal narrowing. Such locking should be urgently reduced, but on occasions reduction proves to be impossible or the diagnosis is made only at a delayed stage when manipulative reduction is impossible due to the formation of callus. In the long term this may produce radiculopathy either by narrowing of the foramen by the subluxed inferior articular process or by its tip which may compress the spinal nerve in the intertransverse space, where the nerve lies in the neural grove of the transverse process of the vertebra below the luxated one, as was originally reported by

Malgaigne (1855). In addition, anterior displacement of a vertebra produces forward displacement of the vertebral artery by the transversarial foramen of the dislocated vertebra. It results in anterior compression and kinking of the artery by the anterior rim of the transversarial foramen below, and may be a cause of vertebrobasilar artery insufficiency (Fig. 46.25).

The oldest method of reducing persistent locked facets consisted of the removal of the superior tips or a greater portion of the superior articular processes of the vertebra below by means of a posterior approach (Rogers, 1942; Suechting & French, 1955). Because of the resulting instability of the spine it had to be fused during the same posterior operation. Unlocking of the articular facets by means of an anterior transdiscal approach below the dislocated vertebra was described by Cloward in 1961. He inserted a levering instrument into the emptied disc space, using the anterior superior border of the vertebral body below as a fulcrum and rotating the lever arm inside the disc space upwards. At the same time digital backward pressure had to be applied to the anterior surface of the dislocated vertebral body for reduction when the facet joints had been unlocked by the movement of the levering instrument. In our experience this manoeuvre was usually ineffective because it resulted in forward rotation of the dislocated vertebra (Fig. 46.26) while digital backward pressure was ineffective. Cloward (1973) replaced his original manoeuvre himself, and developed a special device, called a 'cervical dislocation reducer', that replaced digital backward pressure; it necessitated the excision of two discs. In addition the new method, as did the previous one, meant that reduction was effected under flexion of the dislocated vertebra, which, as Breig (1978) demonstrated, produces traction on, and forward movement of, the spinal cord, pressing it against the posterior superior rim of the vertebral body below the dislocated one. Verbiest (1968) described the insertion of a wedge-shaped cortical bone graft in the emptied disc space below the luxated vertebra, which produced separation between the locked facets and retroflexion of the dislocated vertebral body, resulting in reduction. He therefore reversed Cloward's manoeuvre by using the anterior inferior border of the dislocated vertebral body as a fulcrum and moving the extradiscal lever arm upwards (Fig. 46.26). This resulted in reduction in 28 out of 30 cases of old bilateral locking of articular processes, irreducible by skull traction alone. No digital pressure was needed, and moving the lever arm required only little force. Through the backward rotation of the dislocated vertebra during this manoeuvre the spinal cord is not subject to traction forces, but slackens and moves away from the protruding rim of the vertebral body below the dislocated one.

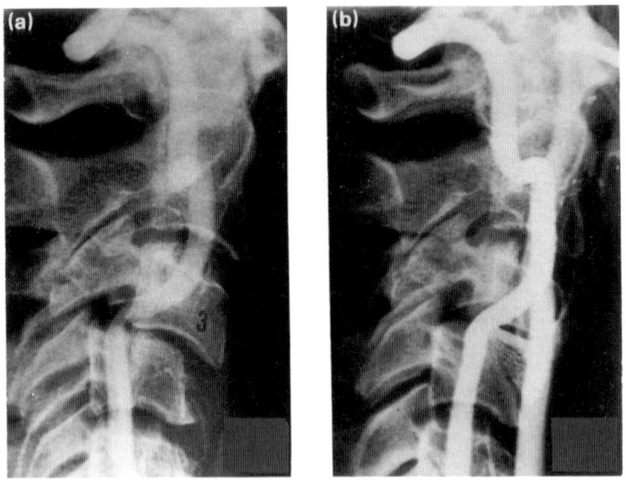

Fig. 46.25 (a) Case of old unilateral locking of articular processes C3–C4. Symptomatic pronounced narrowing of vertebral artery caused by its kinking and narrowing above the anterior rim of the transversarial foramen of C4.
(b) Decompression of the vertebral artery by resection of the anterior rim of the transversarial foramen of C4 and freeing the artery from constricting fibrous tissue resulted in relief of narrowing of the artery. Displacement of the vertebral artery remains, as the locking was not reduced because of absence of spinal cord and nerve root deficit. Symptoms of vertebrobasilar insufficiency disappeared after the vertebral artery was decompressed.

This manoeuvre failed in two cases. In earlier years the wound had to be closed in such cases and the patient had to be placed in the prone position for sectioning the superior articular processes, that prevented reduction, by a posterior approach. With the exposure of the intertransverse space, the superior portion of the superior articular process can be removed via the same anterior approach, when the manoeuvre described above fails to reduce the facet locking. After reduction has been achieved interbody fusion is performed.

The exact operative procedure performed depends on the clinical situation. In very rare instances, longstanding facetal locking will produce vertebrobasilar arterial insufficiency alone. In such a situation,

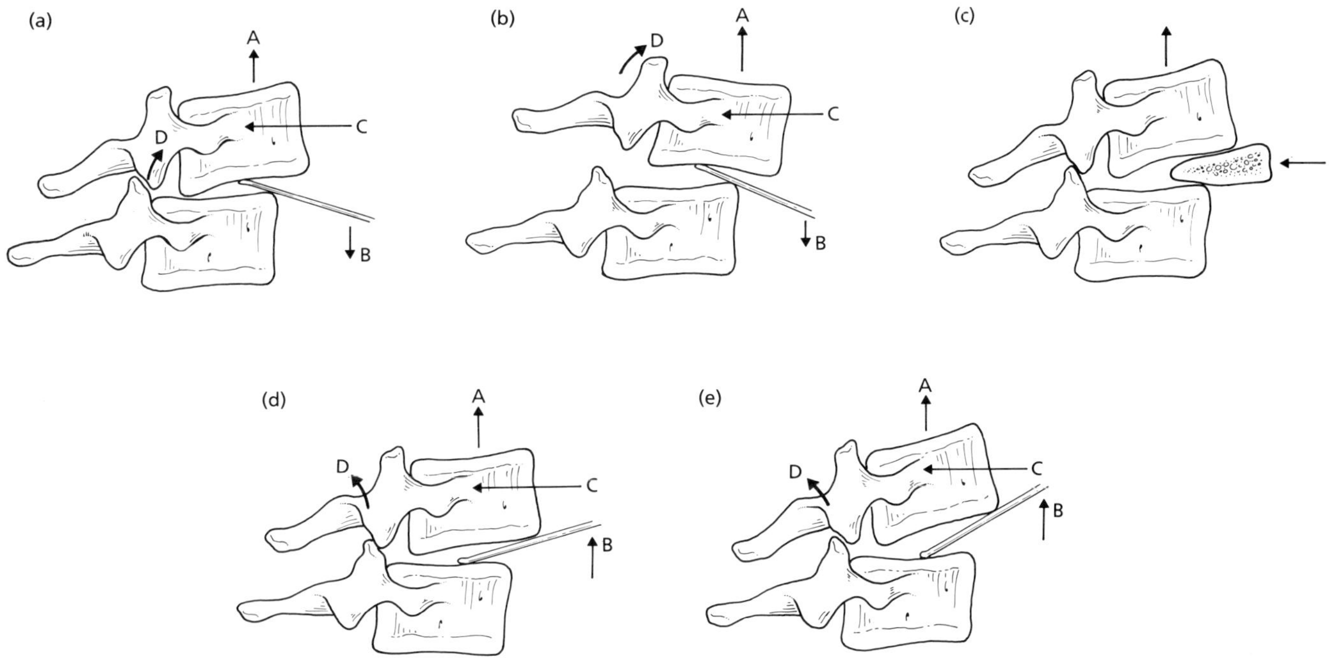

Fig. 46.26 Diagrams (a) and (b) show result of Cloward manoeuvre for reducing locked facet joints. The lever instrument in the emptied disc space moves the overlying vertebral body upward and forward so that great pressure must be applied to the front of this body for obtaining reduction. Diagram (c) shows our experience of the introduction of a wedge-shaped cortical graft, introduced below the luxated vertebra, producing upward and backward rotation of that body resulting in complete reduction. Diagrams (d) and (e) show the reason for the performance of the reverse Cloward procedure for reducing locked facet joints. Light pressure on the anterior aspect of the luxated vertebral body may be helpful to achieve reduction when the tips of the inferior articular during the reverse Cloward manoeuvre have arrived in the overriding position upon the tips of the underlying superior articular processes.

decompression of the vertebral artery by resection of the compressing anterior border of the transversarial foramen inferior to the dislocated vertebra may relieve the arterial narrowing and kinking. In long-standing cases the osseous decompression must be followed by arteriolysis of the vertebral artery from the constricting fibrous scar at the level of compression (Verbiest, 1970a,b,c).

Where there is unilateral irreducible locking in association with radiculopathy, the nerve root must be freed by unlocking through resection of the tip of the superior articular process that prevents reduction (Verbiest, 1978a,b,c). The interspace at the level of the locked facets is exposed by a lateral approach and a small long osteotome is introduced in an antero-posterior direction, immediately lateral to the vertebral artery (Fig. 46.27). The superior articular process of the caudal vertebra is interrupted just below the tip of the locked inferior articular process in front. Penetrating too far posteriorly is not dangerous because the osteotome will encounter muscular tissue only. In some cases this section must extend into the foramen. The removal of the tip of this process allows reduction to be performed. After reduction of the rotated vertebral body the underlying disc is removed by means of a lateral transdiscal approach and interbody fusion is performed. The reduced articular processes may ankylose after reduction.

Occasionally, unilateral locking is accompanied by marked rotation of the subluxed vertebra and the forward rotation of its transverse process may result in compression of the spinal nerve as it leaves the intertransverse space of the level above the subluxation (Fig. 46.28) (Verbiest, 1978a). Such a mechanism may be anticipated in the presence of nerve root deficit indicating a higher segmental level of involvement, although it may also be an expression of segmental variation and be caused by compression at the level of locking. It is, however, an indication also

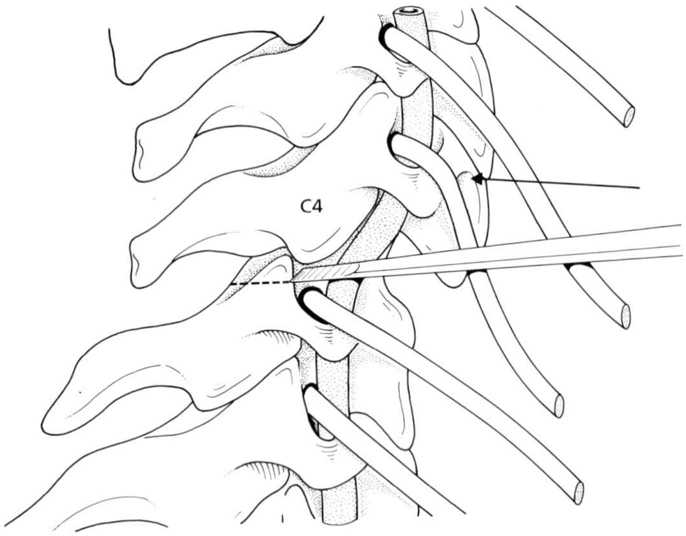

Fig. 46.27 Diagram of unilateral locking of C4–C5. To achieve reduction an osteotome is introduced lateral to the vertebral artery into the intertransverse space. The tip of the superior articular process of the caudal vertebra is sectioned, allowing reduction.

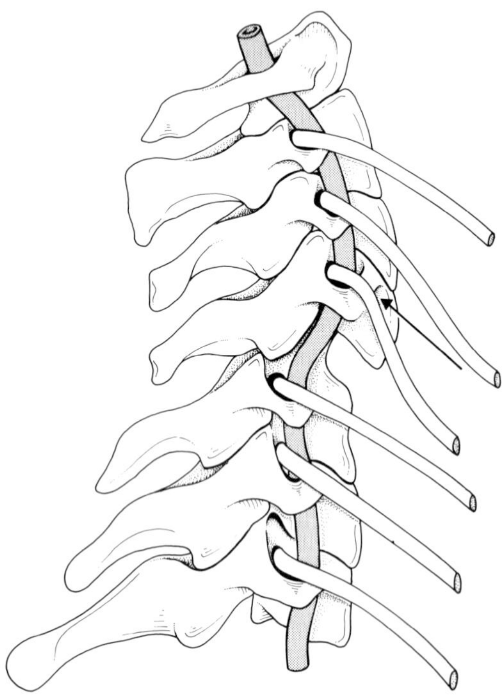

Fig. 46.28 Diagrammatic representation of unilateral facet locking at C4–C5 with marked rotation of C4 causing compression of the spinal nerve exiting through the C3–C4 intertransverse space by the transverse process of C4.

to explore, during the lateral approach, the nerve at the exit of the intertransverse space above.

Tumours of the walls of the intertransverse space

This subject has been extensively reviewed by the author (Verbiest, 1970a,b,c, 1989). Malignant tumours confined to the walls of the intertransverse space have not been encountered. The only tumours seen which are limited to the intertransverse space have been cartilaginous exostoses, hyperostoses, osteomas and benign osteoblastomas. Their total excision can be achieved easily by means of the lateral approach. Other tumours such as aneurysmal bone cysts, intraosseous neurofibromatosis, eosinophylic granulomas, giant-cell tumours and haemangiomas can all affect the intertransverse space, but normally also involve the midline structures of the spine.

Such tumours which involve the articular processes and extend into the adjacent lamina can be removed via the cavity created by their removal from the articular process. The same holds for tumours extending through the lateral surface of a cervical vertebral body into its centre. In that case repair of the vertebral body has to be performed with autologous bone grafts.

THE ROLE OF THE INTERTRANSVERSE SPACE IN ACCESS TO DISEASED CERVICAL DISCS AND VERTEBRAL BODIES

The use of this approach provides an alternative to the anterior approach and may be useful in certain circumstances.

Removal of the cervical disc and posterior corporeal osteophytes by a lateral approach

This procedure may be applied for the removal of central disc protrusions and sequestrated disc material situated inside the vertebral canal. Massive central extrusion of disc material into the vertebral canal is a dramatic occurrence. The patient suddenly develops a complete or incomplete transverse lesion of the spinal cord. With the approach through the intertransverse space, removal of such large protrusions is the most rapid and safe procedure (Fig. 46.29).

The lateral transdiscal approach begins with removal of the anterior and lateral borders of the

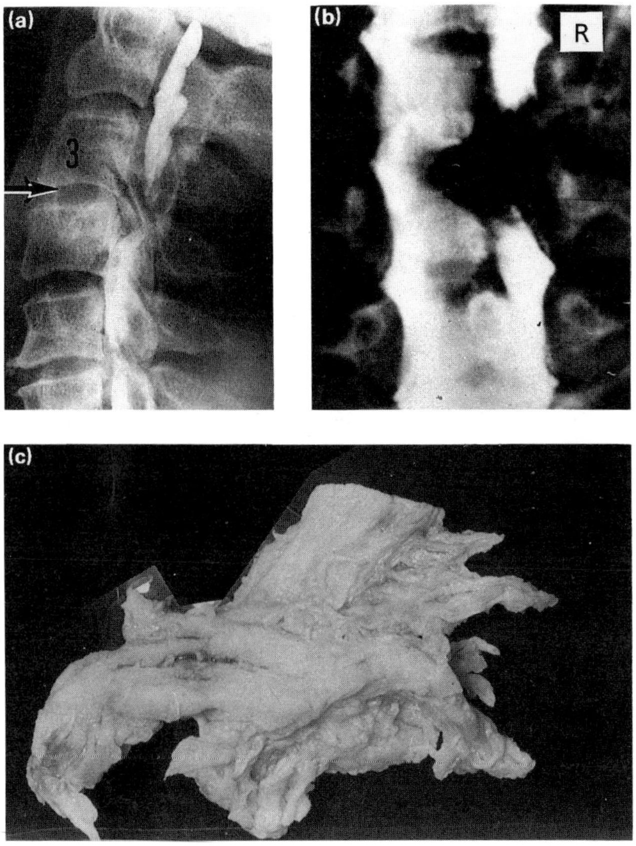

Fig. 46.29 Case of acute massive C3–C4 disc sequestration. (a) Lateral myelogram showing near-total block. (b) AP view showing a large central to right-sided disc fragment. (c) Large (×4 magnification) disc sequester removed by lateral transdiscal approach.

transversarial foramen. The anterior two-thirds of the uncus are removed by interrupting its continuity with the vertebral body by means of an osteotome, and the posterior portion of the uncus is removed by means of a rongeur with fine bites, care being taken not to injure the spinal nerve or ganglion (Fig. 46.30). The intervertebral disc is then removed piecemeal and the cartilaginous endplates are detached from the cortical endplates of the vertebral bodies by hand-driven osteotomes. Extruded disc sequesters are first carefully pulled back into the emptied disc space and, subsequently, pulled outward. The anterior annulus fibrosus and the anterior longitudinal ligament remain intact, so that this approach presents no risk of producing instability of the spine. Additional complete evacuation of residual discal material inside the intervertebral space is important for avoiding the production or recurrence of osteophytosis at that level, and promotes interbody fusion. No interbody grafting for fusion is needed. The emptied disc space flattens in the course of weeks without being accompanied by anterior angulation of the spine. In earlier years, a wedge-shaped cortical graft was inserted through the lateral access into the emptied disc space, the smallest height of this graft facing posteriorly to prevent its dislocation into the vertebral canal.

The lateral approach is the safest procedure for the removal of such protruding or extruded disc material. It replaces the more hazardous laminectomy and necessary intradural retraction of the spinal cord.

The theory that anterior transdiscal disc removal followed by insertion of an autologous bone graft results in spontaneous resorption of posterior osteophytes of the vertebral bodies involved (Smith & Robertson, 1958) is not true in most cases. If they are resorbed it takes months, which is of no use when the surgical indication is based on the need for rapid relief of symptomatic spinal cord compression. Verbiest and Paz y Geuze (1966) were the first to report anterior transdiscal removal of posterior vertebral and uncal osteophytes by means of an anterior transdiscal

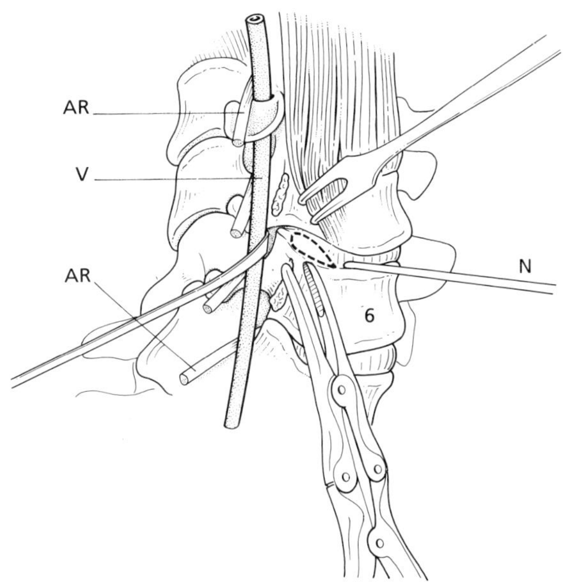

Fig. 46.30 Lateral transdiscal approach. The uncus is exposed via the intertransverse space and its anterior two-thirds are removed by a small osteotome (N); see also Fig. 46.22. The anterior root (AR) and vertebral artery (V) are protected during this manoeuvre and the subsequent enlargement of the access through the uncal area with fine rongeurs. The intervertebral disc is then excised through the dotted area of access indicated in the figure.

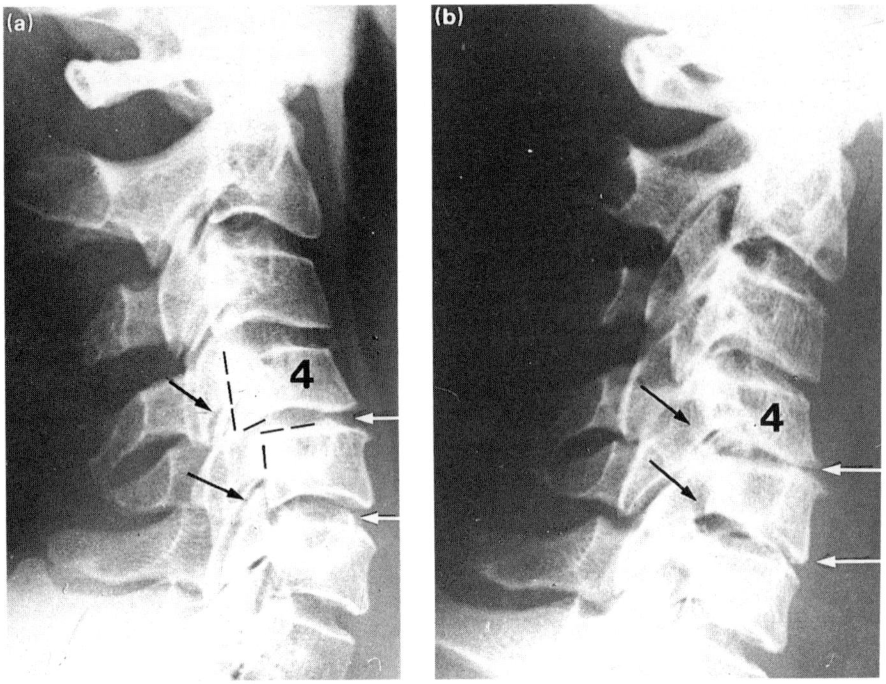

Fig. 46.31 (a) Degenerative retrolisthesis at C4–C5 producing narrowing of the cervical canal. Less marked changes at C5–C6. (b) The postero-inferior rims of C4 and C5 have been removed by the lateral transdiscal approach, restoring the canal diameter to normal.

approach. This procedure, however, carried a risk of transmitting mechanical surgical energy to the cord, nerve roots and vertebral artery, the more so since these structures become visible only after the compressive osteophytes have been removed. The lateral transdiscal approach permits the removal not only of disc sequesters but also of posterior vertebral body osteophytes by driving a small osteotome parallel to the anterior aspect of the dural theca along a plane of cleavage between these osteophytes and the vertebral body, under direct visual control of the movements of the osteotome with respect to the dura (Fig. 46.31). In addition to the removal of posterior osteophytes causing narrowing of the cervical canal, all other osteophytes (articular, lateral, uncal) can be removed by means of the lateral approach under direct vision of the compressed vertebral artery and spinal nerve, so that this approach is much more inclusive and safer than the anterior transdiscal procedure, and is far safer than removal of facet joints by means of a posterior approach.

The lateral approach in surgery of the vertebral body

There is only one indication for the use of the lateral approach alone for surgery of the vertebral body proper; that is for removing its posterior portion. Verbiest (1973) published the problems experienced in two cases of neglected treatment of traumatic kyphotic vertebral deformity of C3–C4, that had fused. The vertebral canal was narrowed at the site of the kyphosis. Both patients developed late myelopathy. In one of these patients the kyphotic traction on the cord had caused descending motor unit deficit, resulting in atrophy of the thoracic muscles, thoracic paralytic scoliosis and a flail chest. There was diaphragmatic weakness and the vital capacity was so poor that the patient had to take a breath after every spoken word. The other patient showed a similar picture. Complete removal of the kyphotic and fused vertebral bodies and their replacement by bone grafts posed major problems in the postoperative care of respiration, and both patients succumbed to respiratory failure. Following this experience the author felt that such patients should not be operated on, until he was confronted by two further patients with the same problem. Again, both patients were victims of neglected treatment of traumatic vertebral deformities resulting in kyphotic block vertebrae in the midcervical region, accompanied by cord compression at that level. Both patients were paraplegic since the injury, but in

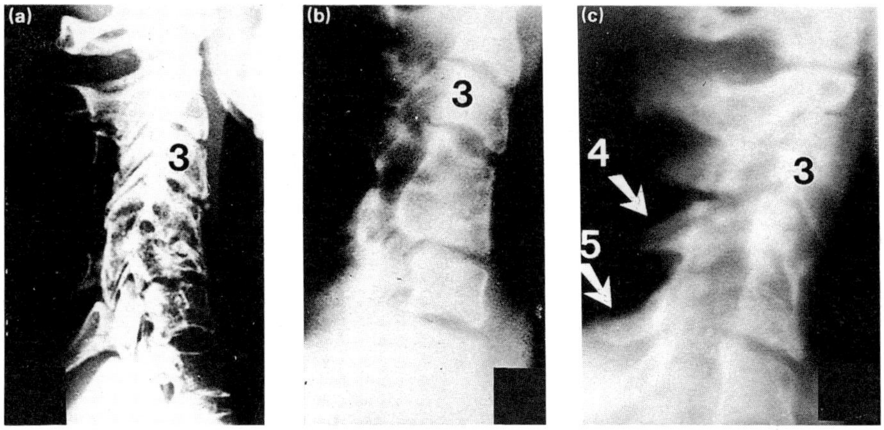

Fig. 46.32 Old kyphotic deformity due to fusion of C4 and C5 as a late complication of trauma producing severe myelopathy. (a,b) Plain radiograph and tomogram showing severe canal narrowing due to the kyphotic deformity. (c) Postoperative tomogram showing removal of the posterior portions of the fused vertebral bodies with restoration of the sagittal canal diameter.

later years developed ascending neural deficit mainly characterized by respiratory insufficiency. They again had to take a breath after speaking one word and their vital capacity of respiration was much reduced. Because of more experience with the lateral approach the author decided to remove the posterior portion of the traumatic kyphotic block vertebrae leaving its anterior portion intact so that the patients could be mobilized immediately after the operation (Fig. 46.32).

The procedure was as follows. One lateral aspect of the kyphotic block at C4–C5 was exposed via the intertransverse space. The posterior half of its cortex was removed followed by removal of the cancellous bone of the posterior portion of the vertebral block, while leaving the posterior cortex and contralateral cortex intact. Next, the thin posterior and contralateral cortex could be easily pulled away and removed. Both patients survived with marked respiratory improvement. Intervertebral fusion was not necessary. Whilst it is true that this case could have been treated by anterior partial vertebrectomy, such a procedure would require excision of the C3–C4 and C5–C6 discs, with a resultant anterior keystone graft from C3 to C6. In addition, the dura and spinal cord are seen only once the excision has been achieved, and are therefore at increased risk of damage. With the lateral approach through the intertransverse spaces the dura can be decompressed under direct vision, and fusion is not necessary.

Complete corporectomy

Complete removal of the vertebral bodies from C3 through C7 because of severe traumatic deformity or tumour involvement is more safely performed by means of a combined anterior and lateral approach than by an anterior approach alone (Verbiest, 1973, 1978b,c, 1989) due to the greater protection of the spinal cord and the vertebral artery. The latter may be greatly displaced by tumour extension or vertebral body dislocation. Vertebral artery displacement by the tumour may be relieved by means of the lateral approach. If complete corporectomy must be performed the anterior and lateral aspects of the target body are exposed by means of an anterolateral approach. The longus colli and longus capitis muscles are completely detached from at least the vertebra above and below the target body and retracted medially or laterally depending upon the site of surgical activity.

The floor of the intertransverse space at the level of the vertebral body to be removed is resected in the sequence indicated in Fig. 46.33. Initially, the anterior tubercle is removed, followed by the anterior and lateral border of the transversarial foramen. Next, the ipsilateral uncinate process of the vertebral body to be removed and the intervertebral discs above and below that body are excised, leaving the posterior longitudinal ligament intact. The opposite uncinate process is left intact at this stage. The ipsilateral pedicle of the body to be removed is then resected. Next, the vertebral body is removed in piecemeal fashion with a rongeur up to its opposite lateral cortical layer. The opposite longus colli and longus capitis muscles are retracted laterally and the residual bone of the vertebral body is carefully resected down to the opposite transverse process. The anterior rim of its transversarial foramen is resected. A thin blade is introduced between the vertebral artery and the last remaining

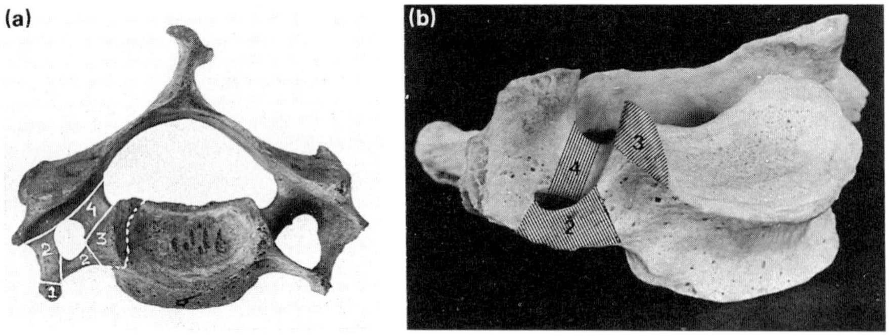

Fig. 46.33 The sequential steps necessary during an anterolateral approach prior to corporectomy to allow initial access for the complete removal of the vertebral body including the walls of the intertransverse space.

lateral cortex of the body, so that the latter can be safely resected. It is not the aim of this chapter to discuss the methods of vertebral body replacement, but an appropriate reconstruction must be performed.

A particular problem may be presented by cases of old traumatic bilateral vertebral luxation with late onset of signs of spinal cord compression. If in such cases the articular processes are fixed in a overriding position by a callus mass, it is not advisable to try to reduce this luxation, but it is safer to remove the vertebral body below the dislocated one by means of a combined anterior and lateral approach and to replace that body by a bone graft. The ankylosed tips of the overriding articular processes provide sufficient immobilization so that the patient can be rapidly mobilized with a cervical collar (Fig. 46.34).

COMPLICATIONS AND RESULTS

Some of the indications for the lateral approach described above are uncommon conditions such as the tumours described and the transuncal disc extrusion. The lateral approach not only extends and simplifies the surgery involved in dealing with such conditions, but in many cases provides a safer option than anterior and certainly posterior approaches.

The most common reason for performing the approach to the intertransverse space has been to deal with posterolateral disc extrusions or intraforaminal osteophytes. The author has explored 123 levels in 115 patients for these conditions (Table 46.1). During the development of the technique, many patients complained of severe cramp-like pains in the arms

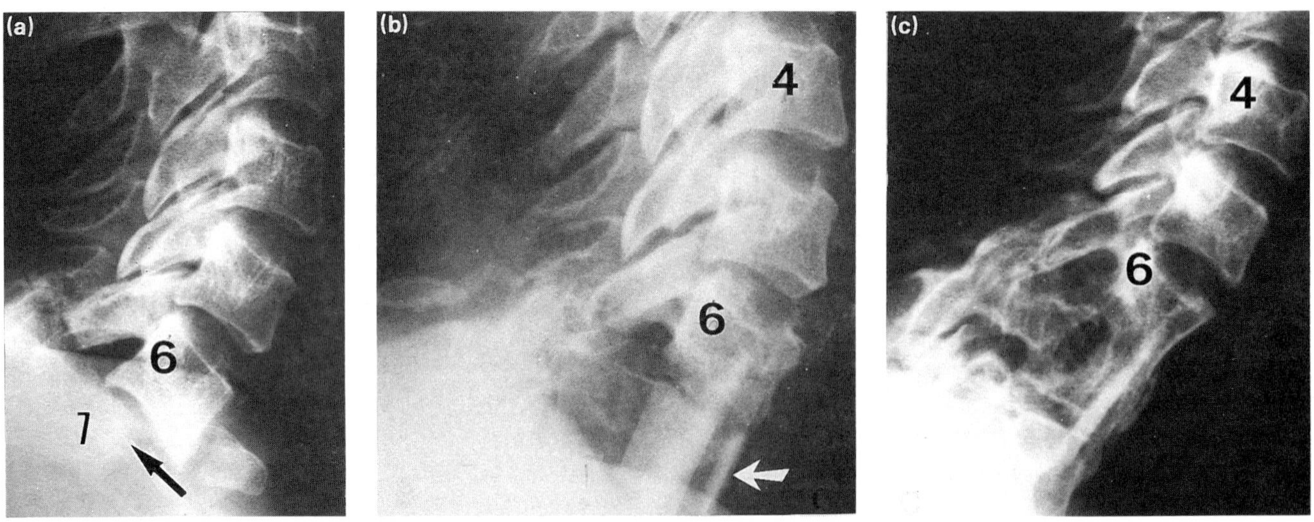

Fig. 46.34 Case of old bilateral irreducible locking of articular processes C6–C7 and late onset of compressive myelopathy. (a) Before operation. Arrow points to body of C7 protruding with its superior posterior portion into the vertebral canal. (b) Immediate postoperative radiograph showing total removal of the body of C7 with reconstruction by a tibial graft inserted into C6 and T1 through their endplates. (c) Late view showing solid fusion. Total neurological recovery resulted.

after the operation. Once the technique was modified to avoid retraction of the vertebral artery this complication disappeared. Motor deficit was seen in only two patients following the removal of intraforaminal uncal osteophytes, and it was permanent in only one of those patients. Spinal cord injury did not occur with this approach.

Recovery or near-total recovery from radicular pain was seen in almost all cases of disc extrusion. In patients whose radicular pain was due to osteophytic compression, total relief of pain was achieved in 50%. A further 40% achieved a major reduction in pain.

The developments of the concept of the cervical intertransverse space and the surgical approach to it have enlarged the understanding of cervical spine pathology, particularly with reference to radicular disorders. The rare but important discovery of lateral transuncal disc extrusion was made only by this approach. It also led to the understanding that disc sequesters could migrate through the foramen into the intertransverse space, not only compressing the spinal nerve in its extraspinal course but also sometimes distorting and occluding the vertebral artery.

The clinical features of root compression in the intertransverse space are virtually identical to those of the more commonly seen compression within the spinal canal or intervertebral foramen. This understanding should prompt the search for intertransverse compression in patients with symptoms and signs of cervical radiculopathy but in whom myelography is normal. In the search for such compression, high-quality plain radiography and tomography is essential in showing not only the uncal anatomy but also the presence of osteophytes arising from the uncus or superior articular process, or facet abnormalities such as undiagnosed locking.

Vertebral angiography remains indispensable as a means of indicating pathology in the intertransverse space. It may be the only means of indicating the presence of significant disc extrusion into the intertransverse space in the presence of root cut-off on the myelogram. Conventional angiography remains the ideal investigation in that it clearly shows the relationship of any abnormality to the bony anatomy, but digital subtraction angiography is the best method to assess the vascular pattern of tumours in this area.

The role of CT and MRI scanning in this area is as yet unclear. The production and interpretation of high-quality axial images in this area is difficult due to the complex anatomy. Three-dimensional reconstruction does not solve these problems. CT scanning is an ideal method for showing fractures of the vertebral bodies. However, visualization of locked facets by CT is time-consuming, and oblique conventional tomography produces superior images. The visualization of cervical disc extrusions with CT is vastly inferior to CT in the lumbar spine, and CT fails entirely to show extruded disc material in the intertransverse space. CT is, however, indispensable for demonstrating the shape and situation of vertebral osteophytes anterior to the dura if they are to be removed by a lateral approach through the intertransverse space. It is also useful in the assessment of the nature and extent of vertebral tumours.

MRI is an excellent medium for displaying intraspinal disc extrusions, provided that the correct imaging parameters, surface coils and a sufficiently powerful magnet is used. However, as in CT, it does not give adequate imaging of soft tissues in the intertransverse space, and is much worse than CT in imaging osteophytes. MRI is a helpful tool in assessment of tumours. Only the most modern MRI machines give adequate images of intraspinal nerve roots in the axial and coronal planes. In the absence of this quality MRI, myelography remains essential to assess the intraspinal nerve roots up to their foramina and to exclude intradural pathology. For the evaluation of the lateral extent of pathology into the intertransverse space, neither CT nor MRI is, as yet, sufficiently accurate to replace the use of plain radiology, tomography and vertebral angiography, as has been discussed in this chapter.

The refinement of Henry's original operation (1957) into the lateral approach described by the author means that the cervical spine can now be approached from all its sides. The lateral approach allows the exposure of the cervical nerve roots from their exit from the dural sac to their continuation as spinal nerves. The surgical field can be extended to the supra- and infraclavicular portions of the brachial plexus, if necessary, allowing surgery of complex brachial plexus lesions and large dumbbell tumours. When used for the surgery of cervical root compression due to disc extrusions or osteophytes, the lateral approach allows decompression of the nerves under direct observation. It preserves the integrity of the spine, leaving not only the posterior bony structures, joints, ligaments, and muscles intact but also the anterior bony structures, the anterior longitudinal ligament and the anterior annulus.

When combined with the anterior approach for vertebral corporectomy, the lateral approach enlarges the access to the body that must be removed, and improves the safety of the procedure in that again the dura is visualized by this approach allowing decompression under direct vision. The lateral approach permits the resection of a bony kyphosis causing dural compression without compromising stability and avoiding the necessity of bone grafting or other spinal reconstruction. Finally, the lateral approach is the only means available for dealing with vertebral artery pathologies, lateral uncal osteophytes and transuncal disc extrusions.

REFERENCES

Bakay, L. & Leslie, E.V. (1965) Surgical treatment of vertebral artery insufficiency caused by cervical spondylosis. *J. Neurosurg.*, **23**, 596.

Breig, A. (1978) *Adverse Mechanical Tension in the Central Nervous System.* Almqvist & Wiksell, Stockholm; John Wiley & Sons, New York.

Chassaignac, E.P.M. (1834) Extrait d'un mémoire sur quelques points d'anatomie, de physiologie et de pathologie de la colonne vertébrale. *Arch. Gén. Méd. IIe série* **IV**, 458.

Cloward, R.B. (1961) Treatment of acute fractures and fracture dislocations of the cervical spine. *J. Neurosurg.*, **18**, 201.

Cloward, R.B. (1973) Reduction of traumatic dislocation of the cervical spine with locked facets. *J. Neurosurg.*, **38**, 527.

Elvidge, A.R. & Luh, L.Ch. (1950) Central protrusion of cervical intervertebral disk involving descending trigeminal tract. *Arch. Neurol. Psychiatry, Chicago*, **68**, 455.

Epstein, J.A., Rosenthal, A.D., Carras, R. & Levine, S.L. (1972) Sciatica caused by nerve root entrapment in the lateral recess: the superior facet syndrome. *J. Neurosurg.*, **36**, 584.

Forestier, J. (1922) *Le Trou de Conjugaison vertébral et l'Espace épidural.* Jouve, Paris.

Gortvai, P. (1964) Insufficiency of vertebral artery treated by decompression of its cervical part. *Br. Med. J.*, **2**, 233.

Gowers, W.A.A. (1893) *Manual of Diseases of the Nervous System*, Vol. I, 2nd edn., pp. 263–264 (reprinted 1970, Hafner).

Hardin, C.A., Williamson, W.P. & Steegmann, A.T. (1960) Vertebral artery insufficiency produced by cervical osteoarthritic spurs. *Neurology*, **10**, 855.

Hardin, C.A. (1965) Vertebral artery insufficiency produced by cervical osteo-arthritic spurs. *Arch. Surg. Chicago*, **90**, 629.

Henry, A.K. (1957) *Extensile Exposure*, 2nd edn. Livingstone, Edinburgh.

Jackson, R. (1966) *The Cervical Syndrome*, 3rd edn. Charles C. Thomas, Springfield, IL.

Jung, A. (1963) Résection de l'articulation unco-vertébrae et ouverture du trou de conjugaison par voie antérieure dans le traitement de la névralgie cervico-brachiale. Technique opératoire. *Mém. Acad. Chir.*, **89**, 361.

Jung, A. & Vierling, J.P. (1965) Nouveaux résultats et compléments de technique de uncusectomie dans le traitement de complications radiculaires et artério-vertébrales des cervicarthroses. *Rev. Chir. Orthop. Rep. Appl. Mot.*, **51**, 605.

Jung, H. & Kehr, P. (1972) *Pathologie de l'artère vertébrale et des racines nerveuses.* Masson, Paris.

Keuter, E.W. (1970) Vascular origin of cranial sensory disturbances caused by pathology of the lower cervical spine. *Acta Neurochir.*, **23**, 229.

Malgaigne, J.F. (1855) *Traité des fractures et des luxations*, Tome II: *Luxations*, p. 371. Baillière, Paris.

Pichler, A. (1955) Anatomische und röntgenologische Studien über die intervertebrale Kanäle der Halswirbelsäule. *Fortschr. Röntgenstr*, **83**, 638.

Poirier, P. & Charpy, A. (1899) *Traité d'Anatomie Humaine.* Masson, Paris.

Rogers, W.A. (1942) Treatment of fracture dislocation of the cervical spine. *J. Bone Jt. Surg.*, **24A**, 245.

Smith, G.W. & Robertson, H.A. (1958) The treatment of certain cervical-spine disorders by anterior removal of the intervertebral disc and interbody fusion. *J. Bone Jt. Surg.*, **40A**, 607.

Suechting, R.L. & French, L.A. (1955) Posterior inferior cerebellar artery syndrome following a fracture of the cervical vertebra. *J. Neurosurg.*, **12**, 187.

Verbiest, H. (1968) A lateral approach to the cervical spine: technique and indications. *J. Neurosurg.*, **28**, 191.

Verbiest, H. (1969) Anterolateral operations for fractures and dislocations in the middle and lower parts of the cervical spine. *J. Bone Jt. Surg.*, **51A**, 1489.

Verbiest, H. (1970a) La chirurgie antérieure et latérale du rachis cervical. *Neurochirurgie*, **16** (Suppl. 2), Ch. III, 91–122.

Verbiest, H. (1970b) La chirurgie antérieure et latérale du rachis cervical. *Neurochirurgie*, **16** (Suppl. 2), Ch. IV, 123–170.

Verbiest, H. (1970c) La chirurgie antérieure et latérale du rachis cervical. *Neurochirurgie*, **16** (Suppl. 2), Ch. V, 171–203.

Verbiest, H. (1973) Anterolateral operations for fractures and dislocations of the cervical spine due to injuries or previous surgical interventions. *Clinical Neurosurgery*, **20**, 334–366. Williams & Wilkins, Baltimore, MD.

Verbiest, H. (1976) L'Ostéophytectomie par voie latérale. *Rev. Chir. Orthop.*, **62** (Suppl. II), 32.

Verbiest, H. (1978a) Lesions of the cervical spine: a critical review. In Carrea, R. (ed.), *Neurological Surgery*, Int. Congr. Series, 433, pp. 374–383. Excerpta Medica, Amsterdam.

Verbiest, H. (1978b) From anterior to lateral operations on

the cervical spine. *Neurosurg. Rev.*, **1**, 47.

Verbiest, H. (1978c) De l'abord antérieur à l'abord latéral du rachis cervical. *Cahiers d'enseignement de la SOFCOT*, **8**, 45–64 (Expansion Scientifique Française, Paris, 1978).

Verbiest, H. (1981a) Some particular aspects of soft cervical disc herniation. Verspyck Lecture in Paris. *Rev. Int. Rhumatol*, **52**, 115.

Verbiest, H. (1981b) The cervical intertransverse space: anatomy, pathology and surgical treatment. *Orthop. Trans. J. Bone Jt. Surg.*, **5**, 124.

Verbiest, H. (1989) Benign cervical spine tumors: clinical experience. In Cervical Spine Research Society (eds), *Cervical Spine*, 2nd edn, pp. 723–774. Lippincott, Philadelphia, PA.

Verbiest, H. & Paz y Geuze, H.D. (1966) Anterolateral surgery for cervical spondylosis in cases of myelopathy or nerve root compression. *J. Neurosurg.*, **25**, 611.

47 · Thoracic Intervertebral Disc Protrusion

By T. RUSSELL

Herniation of a thoracic intervertebral disc is relatively uncommon, and is not recognized as often as herniations of the cervical and lumbar discs. In addition, the various clinical features occurring with thoracic disc herniations are not characteristic and can lead to a delay in diagnosis. Disc herniation in this region is of particular importance because of the serious disorders of function which result from anterior compression of the spinal cord: early diagnosis and prompt surgical treatment are imperative because of the progressive and serious neurological deficit which results from delay. Experience with decompressive laminectomy has proved disappointing, and other operative approaches have been advocated, e.g. transthoracic, transpleural, posterolateral and transpedicular.

INCIDENCE

There have been various estimates of the incidence of thoracic disc protrusion. Love & Kiefer (1950) estimated that for every 100 cases of intervertebral disc herniations seen only two or three were in the thoracic region. Logue (1952) reported a 4% incidence of thoracic disc herniation, but Love & Schorn (1965) placed the incidence at 0.5% of all disc ruptures. The most recent and largest report, by Russell (1989), indicates an incidence of approximately one case per million population per year. There is little doubt that it is an uncommon, but probably underdiagnosed, entity: a postmortem study by Haley & Perry (1950) revealed two thoracic disc herniations in 99 cases. Modern investigative methods coupled to a greater tendency to investigate patients presenting with unexplained myelopathy is likely to result in improved diagnosis. Findlay (1991) reported a series of 23 patients encountered in only five years.

The lower incidence of disc protrusions of the thoracic as compared to the lumbar and cervical area has been attributed to the limited motion in the thoracic spine, which is a consequence of the small size of the thoracic intervertebral disc, the restraints of the rib cage and sternum and the anteroposterior direction of the apophyseal joints.

PATHOPHYSIOLOGY

An understanding of the anatomical relationships in the thoracic spine helps to explain the clinical symptoms due to thoracic disc herniation. The thoracic spinal canal is small, and little leeway exists between the thoracic disc and the spinal cord. The cord is restrained from backward displacement by the dentate ligaments (Kahn, 1947). Circulation to the lower dorsal and lumbar segments of the spinal cord is precarious, since these regions may be supplied largely or totally by a single unilateral medullary artery, the artery of Adamkiewicz, which arises between T8 and L4 on the left side in over 60% of cases (Doppman & DiChiro, 1968). Occasionally the artery may originate as high as T5, as reported by Faure *et al.* (1967). Mechanical trauma and vascular compression, either separately or combined, can damage the thoracic spinal cord. Neurological deficit due to vascular compromise has been reported in the monkey by Yoss (1950) and by Doppman & Girton (1976). Carson *et al.* (1971), in three patients, observed indirect signs of ischaemia of the cord caused by protruded discs that compressed the artery of Adamkiewicz.

A myelopathy arising from compression of the cord

between a modest protrusion of the disc in front and a buckled and hypertrophic ligamentum behind has been reported (Carson *et al.*, 1971; Love & Schorn, 1965). The combination of mechanical and vascular damage to the cord may account for the severe neurological symptoms that sometimes seem disproportionate to the size of the protrusion, and also for the poor recovery that sometimes follows complete removal of the ruptured disc (Reeves & Brown, 1968). Vascular damage may account for symptoms that seem inappropriately rostral for the level of the rupture (Hawk, 1936; Arseni & Nash, 1960; Jefferson, 1975).

The role of trauma in the aetiology of thoracic disc protrusion has occasioned much debate, and has been variously reported by Love & Keifer (1950), Abbott & Retter (1956), Tovi & Strang (1960), Jefferson (1975), Reif *et al.* (1983), Sekhar & Jannetta (1983), Arce & Dohrman (1985), and Chin *et al.* (1987). The two largest reported series (Love & Schorn, 1965 and Russell, 1989) both indicate that trauma played a role in approximately 25% of cases. Detailed analysis of the latter report revealed a bimodal incidence in terms of age in males only. The incidence of trauma in males under the age of 40 years was 53%, whereas the incidence of trauma in the remainder of the study (men and women) was much lower at 17%. However, it should be borne in mind that all studies reported are relatively small, and definitive data are not available on many aspects of thoracic disc herniation.

Although herniated thoracic discs have been reported at every level (Love & Schorn 1965; Alberico *et al.*, 1986; Kumar & Buckley, 1986) and with unusual symptomatology (Gelch, 1978; Hann, 1980; Lloyd *et al.*, 1980; Tahmouresie, 1980; Michoury *et al.*, 1984), the majority occur below T8, with disc protrusion at T11 being the most frequent (Love & Schorn, 1965; Singounas & Karvounis, 1977; Otani *et al.*, 1982; Sekhar & Jannetta, 1983; Maiman *et al.*, 1984; Arce & Dohrman, 1985). It has been suggested that the more frequent occurrence in the lower thoracic spine is due to the proximity of the thoracolumbar junction which places increased torsional strain on those discs (Arseni & Nash, 1960; Tovi & Strang, 1960; Pansini & Conte, 1974), and in lesions at higher levels a significant association has been noted, with kyphosis secondary to Scheuermann's disease (Zielke, 1943).

Single disc herniations are the rule, but multiple thoracic disc protrusions have been described by Svien & Karvatis (1954), Van Landingham (1954), Abbott & Retter (1956), Bhole & Gilmer (1984), Chin *et al.* (1987), and Shikata *et al.* (1988).

The majority of herniated thoracic discs are extradural, but intradural free fragments have been reported (Wang & Zamani, 1986; Chowdhary, 1987), and Patterson & Arbit (1978) reported a case with a free fragment impacted into the cord.

CLINICAL FEATURES

An accurate diagnosis of this disease based on clinical features is, for all practical purposes, impossible. Pain and myelopathy, either alone or in combination, are the major presenting features of this disease. Unfortunately, neither is diagnostic and a 'high index of suspicion' in thoracic myelopathies is required in order to focus the clinician's attention on the appropriate investigations leading to a definitive diagnosis. Early diagnosis and treatment is imperative, especially when symptoms develop rapidly because the subsequent neurological deficits appear to be much more severe (Love & Schorn, 1965; Reeves & Brown, 1968).

The majority of patients describe a dull dorsal pain which may have been present for some years; others describe unilateral or bilateral radicular pain which varies greatly in its duration. Rarely is the pain 'unbearable' in severity. Pain may, however, be absent and the disease may simulate a demyelinating disease such as multiple sclerosis (Love & Kiefer, 1950; Hulme, 1960; Carson *et al.*, 1971; Benson & Byrnes, 1975; Sekhar & Jannetta, 1983; Russell, 1989).

Pain, however, is not the usual presenting feature, and most patients seen by neurological surgeons have some evidence of spinal cord dysfunction. In general, motor symptoms and signs of myelopathy predominate and it is extremely unusual that a patient will have sensory manifestations without any motor component. The history may be a progressive one with the development of weakness, spasticity and numbness, but it frequently may have a step-wise development. In the latter case the periods where the deficit seems static may lead to an erroneous diagnosis of demyelinating disease. Although the disc lesion lies anteriorly, posterior column dysfunction is not uncommon. The resultant proprioceptive loss may produce a markedly ataxic gait even when motor power is relatively well preserved. Spinothalamic loss produces numbness and a sensory level which is usually fairly symmetrical, but even a Brown–Sequard pattern may be seen. Problems of sphincteric and sexual dysfunction are uncommon, and usually occur only in the later stages of the disease (Love & Kiefer, 1950; Arseni & Nash, 1960; Love & Schorn, 1965; Maiman *et al.*, 1984; Russell, 1989).

Most studies indicate that the commonest age for thoracic disc protrusion is between the third and fifth decade (Epstein, 1954; Love & Schorn, 1965; Benson & Byrnes, 1975; Singounas & Karvounis, 1977; Otani *et al.*, 1982; Sekhar & Jannetta, 1983; Arce & Dohrman, 1985; Russell, 1989), but the study by Russell (1989) suggested that two peaks occurred. One was in the 30–40-year group in men primarily, in whom there may be a strong relationship with trauma and the main peak affected both sexes between the ages of 50 and 60 years. Thoracic disc herniation has been described in children (Brennan *et al.*, 1987), but this must be viewed as excessively rare.

In most series, men are more commonly affected than women (Hawk, 1936; Jefferson, 1975; Albrand & Corkhill, 1979; Otani *et al.*, 1982; Sekhar & Jannetta, 1983; Maiman *et al.*, 1984). However, such series are small, and larger series would seem to indicate that men and women are almost equally affected (Love & Kiefer, 1950; Love & Schorn, 1965; Russell, 1989). The actual male-to-female ratio is difficult to ascertain, because of the relatively small size (in statistical terms) of all series, but summation of the available data indicates an almost equal male and female incidence.

Thoracic spinal pain with or without radicular radiation can be caused by thoracic disc herniation as well as by a variety of other pathologies. Other possibilities include rheumatoid arthritis, ankylosing spondylitis, tumours (benign or malignant), disc space infection, fractures and subluxations.

A number of intrathoracic and intra-abdominal conditions can also be confused with thoracic disc herniation. Peptic ulceration, pancreatitis, retroperitoneal tumours, gallbladder disease, myocardial ischaemia, urinary tract disorders and aortic aneurysms can all mimic thoracic disc protrusion.

If the clinical picture is that of myelopathy without pain, then the demyelinating diseases must be considered.

INVESTIGATION

The approach to investigation is that of investigating a myelopathy, as described in Chapter 4. Radiology provides the mainstay of investigation. The traditional role of plain X-rays of the thoracic spine was to detect calcification within the disc space and canal. Logue (1952) described disc calcification in 70% of plain spine films of prolapsed thoracic disc compared with a 4% incidence in a series of control patients. Similar figures have been reported by both Love & Schorn (1965) and McAllister & Sage (1976). In contrast, Baker *et al.* (1965) indicated that disc calcification was not a useful sign, and in only 12% of cases did it help to diagnose thoracic disc herniation. Less than 50% of offending discs demonstrated radiological calcification in the report by Russell (1989). The conclusion to be drawn is that plain radiology of the thoracic spine is not a satisfactory screening examination, and that a 'normal' plain X-ray of the thoracic spine does not exclude a thoracic disc protrusion.

The success rate of plain radiology can be increased by the use of sagittal tomography, but the technique is less popular than hitherto because of the increasing availability of computerized tomography (CT) and magnetic resonance imaging (MRI).

Experience with myelography is better than that with plain radiology. Thomson (1966) reported 10 cases in which myelography was diagnostic, and similar results have been reported by others (Baker *et al.*, 1965; McAllister & Sage, 1976; Maiman *et al.*, 1984; Russell, 1989). Myelography is diagnostic in approximately 95% of cases and would appear to be the standard investigation against which other investigations are measured (Fig. 47.1). However, it cannot be stressed too highly that incomplete examinations are to be avoided (Cohen & Tucker, 1985).

There are numerous reports indicating that CT scanning is as effective as myelography in establishing the diagnosis of thoracic disc protrusion with the advantage of non-invasiveness (Hochman *et al.*, 1980; Bhole & Gilmer, 1984; Chin *et al.*, 1987; Wang & Zamani, 1986; Russell, 1989). In view of the high incidence of myelopathy, however, CT scanning as a first investigation has the disadvantage that it would be impractical to scan the whole thoracic spine and some localization, either clinical or radiological, is required. In the presence of radicular pain, CT scanning of one or two levels is probably preferable to myelography. Performing the CT scan in the presence of intrathecal contrast allows exact delineation of the anatomical relationship between the disc and the spinal cord (Fig. 47.2). This information is required

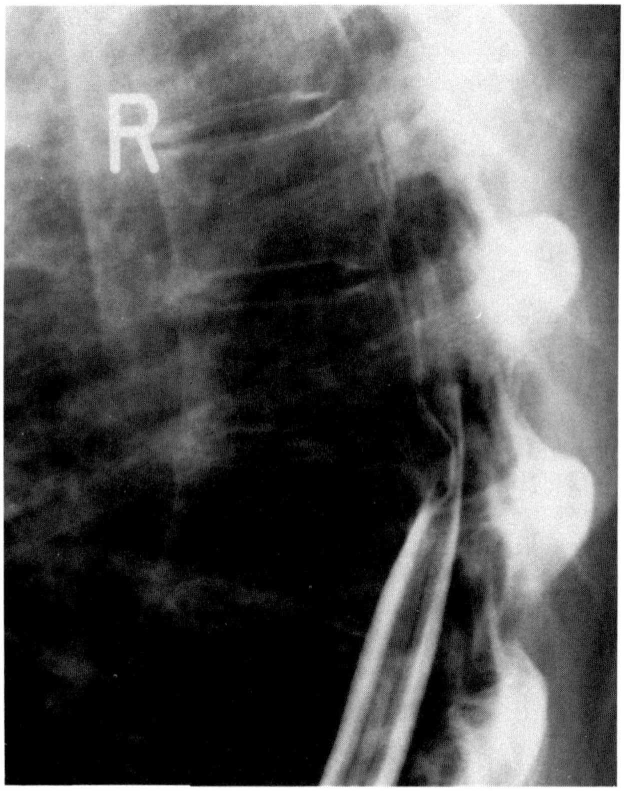

Fig. 47.1 Myelogram showing severe cord compression due to a large, partially calcified T8–T9 disc lesion. Note the presence of calcification within the disc space.

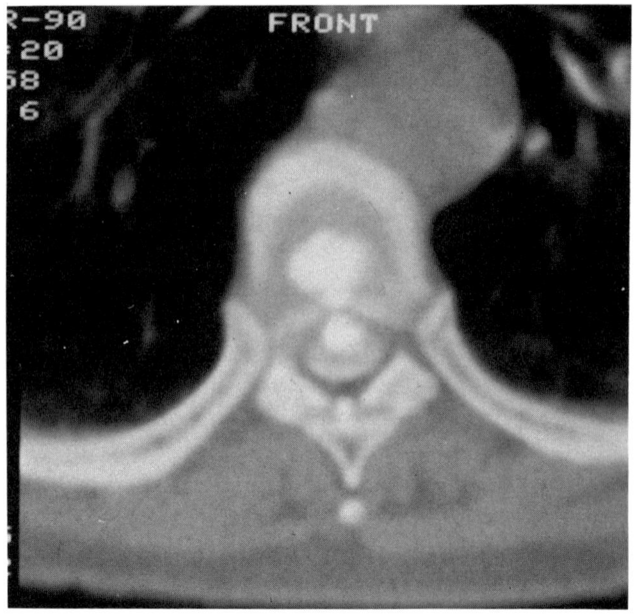

Fig. 47.2 CT myelogram of the same patient as in Fig. 47.1. The intradiscal calcification is clearly seen. It is separate from the intraspinal calcified disc protrusion which is causing severe deformation of the cord.

when considering which surgical approach should be utilized.

There are few reports in the literature concerning the role of MRI in thoracic disc protrusion. A recent report by Maiman *et al.* (1988) of six cases found that MRI was extremely useful, and suggests that it should be performed in all suspected cases of herniated thoracic disc. It is likely that MRI will replace other methods of imaging, although the production of high-quality axial images may be hampered by cardiac and respiratory movements.

TREATMENT

'The grave sequelae following operations on protruded thoracic intervertebral discs have cast a pall over those attempting surgery for the relief of this disorder' (Epstein, 1954). This quote summarizes the attitude towards this disorder from the first report of a case of thoracic disc herniation by Middleton & Teacher (1911) until the 1960s, when advances in technique completely altered the outcome. Elsberg (1931) was the first to remove these lesions surgically, but at that time they were referred to as 'chondromas', and it was not until 1934 that Mixter & Barr introduced the concept of intervertebral disc herniation.

Patients presenting only with pain may be helped by conservative measures such as transcutaneous nerve stimulation and nerve blocks. However, the majority present only once neurological deficit has become established, and then surgical intervention is mandatory. Various surgical approaches have been suggested. The first operative approach for herniated thoracic discs was laminectomy. However, this approach produced such disastrous results that interest in alternative approaches was stimulated. In 1960, Hulme reported four cases treated with a lateral approach and costotransversectomy (a similar approach had been used in tuberculous spinal disease for some time): three of his patients were cured and one showed improvement. This approach had the advantage of producing a more oblique approach to the disc, and avoiding entering the thoracic canal until a space had been created in the disc space into which the intracanalicular disc fragments could be safely pulled.

A similar approach through the pedicle was described by Patterson & Arbit in 1978. The spine is exposed via a midline incision and the paravertebral muscles are reflected on one side to expose the facet joints: the facets and the pedicle of the vertebra inferior to the disc are removed. The disc space is entered and disc material is removed from the centre of the disc space. When a cavity has been created in the disc space, disc material is removed from adjacent to the canal. If an intradural disc fragment is suspected, the dura can be opened and the fragment removed under direct vision.

That technique is probably better than that described in 1971 by Carson *et al.*, in which a 'T'-shaped incision was used to approach the disc from the lateral aspect after removal of the lamina, transverse process and pedicle: the need for laminectomy and a transverse incision through the paravertebral muscles is usually accompanied by greater morbidity. Other variations on this general approach have been published by Capener (1954) and Garrido (1980).

Anterolateral excision of a thoracic disc protrusion was described in 1958 by Crafoord *et al.*, and encouraging results were reported in 1969 by Perot & Munro, and by Ransohoff *et al.* (1969) in a total of five patients operated upon by a transpleural approach via a thoracotomy. Many authors have described similar approaches. A standard thoracotomy incision is made. The rib is followed to the appropriate intervertebral foramen, the pleura resected from the head of the rib and vertebral bodies and the pedicles removed. The disc is then identified and the anterior two-thirds removed before any attempt is made to remove the intracanalicular fragment. When this is complete, chest drains are placed and the chest is closed. Although spinal fixation has been advocated by Lobosky *et al.* (1984), this additional procedure is not commonly performed and spinal instability is not a problem. Findlay (1991) described a more radical transthoracic approach suitable for large, central disc protrusions.

Reviews describing the relevant anatomy and surgical approaches have been published by Weiss *et al.* (1975), Safdari & Baker (1985) and Findlay (1991). It cannot be overemphasized that positive identification of the correct disc space is essential, and intraoperative radiology is obligatory prior to disc removal.

Whatever approach is used, it is imperative that no instrument should be introduced into the canal prior to decompression, as there is no space for an instrument in the presence of a herniated thoracic disc. This comment is of particular importance if the thoracic disc protrusion coexists with canal stenosis as described by Ungersbock *et al.* (1987).

Despite modern radiology it sometimes happens that a herniated thoracic disc is discovered at operation, usually via a routine laminectomy. If this is the case, probably the best procedure is to remove the inferior pedicle and enter the disc space laterally, as described previously.

RESULTS

The results of operative intervention in protruded thoracic disc should be examined in relation to the operative procedure performed.

Posterior approach

The generally poor outcome from this approach has been alluded to earlier, and this depressing state of affairs has been described by many authors over a considerable time span. Elsberg (1931), Hawk (1936), Love & Kiefer (1950), Muller (1951), Logue (1952), Epstein (1954), Abbott & Retter (1956), Kite *et al.* (1957), Arseni & Nash (1960), Tovi & Strang (1960), Love & Schorn (1965), Reeves & Brown (1968), Perot & Munro (1969) and Benson & Byrnes (1975) have all reported unacceptable results using this approach.

Of Muller's four patients, three were paraplegic after operation (Muller, 1951); reports from Love & Kiefer (1950) and from Logue (1952) presented equally dismal results, with all of Logue's patients being neurologically worse postoperatively and only four showing eventual improvement. Perot & Munro (1969) collected 91 cases from the literature: 40 of the patients were not improved by laminectomy, and 16 were rendered paraplegic. Central disc herniation and an advanced preoperative deficit carry the most ominous prognosis for laminectomy (Perot & Munro, 1969). Despite the bad experience reported by most, laminectomy continues to be used (Singounas & Karvounis, 1977; de Tribolet *et al.*, 1982). Singounas & Karvounis reported that a carefully performed laminectomy was safe in their hands but the case reported by de Tribolet *et al.* had a poor outcome. The difficulty of attempting to decompress an anteriorly placed mass in the thoracic canal has been well demonstrated by Doppman & Girton (1976), who showed in experimental material that laminectomy failed to decompress the cord as judged by angiographic displacement and clinical results. Similar work by Bennett & McCallum (1977) demonstrated that laminectomy in cats with an anterior mass resulted in worsening of somatosensory evoked potentials and outcome. It is difficult to remove a mass (frequently calcified) anteriorly without manipulating the cord to some extent, which might be sufficient to produce mechanical damage and which might also interfere with the blood supply (Ravichandran & Frankel, 1981; Terry *et al.*, 1981; Sekhar & Jannetta, 1983).

It may be argued that these results were obtained two to three decades ago, and that recent developments in surgical technique, in particular the use of the operating microscope, and improvements in radiology with more accurate preoperative diagnosis, make comparison iniquitous. However, the more recent reports of the results of laminectomy by Singounas & Karvounis (1977), de Tribolet *et al.* (1982) and Russell (1989) suggest that these recent developments have not resulted in any significant alteration in the outcome.

In view of the unacceptable results from this approach, the general consensus is against the use of laminectomy in known thoracic disc herniation.

Posterolateral approach

The results from this approach are better than those from laminectomy. The technical variations in this technique discussed earlier do not result in any significant difference in outcome, and personal preference and experience should dictate which one is used. The early results of Hulme (1960), Carson *et al.* (1971) and Patterson & Arbit (1978) have been supported by more recent reports from Young *et al.* (1989) and Russell (1989), with 70–75% of patients being either normal or improved.

The approach is certainly less traumatic than the anterior transthoracic approach, and while the field of view may be inferior to that in the more extensive anterior procedure, the posterolateral approach should certainly be considered as an option, particularly in cases of disc herniation where the fragment is not central or at the thoracolumbar junction. It may, indeed, be the approach of choice in patients who are elderly or who have contraindications to thoracotomy.

Anterior approach

This is the most major of all the approaches, and carries the risks of thoracotomy in addition to the risks of the spinal procedure. In view of these increased risks and morbidity, some authors do not advocate such an approach (Sekhar & Jannetta, 1983; Maiman *et al.*, 1984; Lesoin *et al.*, 1986).

Against this, however, must be balanced the excellent results reported by Ransohoff *et al.* (1969), Otani *et al.* (1977, 1982), Sekhar & Jannetta (1983), Fidler & Goedhart (1984), Bohlman & Zdeblick (1988), Russell (1989) and Findlay (1991); where overall results were approximately 85% of patients either normal or improved.

In summary, thoracic disc herniation is a relatively uncommon event which is probably underdiagnosed. Although the sex distribution is fairly equal, and trauma plays only a minor role in the aetiology, there may be a subgroup with predominantly younger males in which trauma has a major role. The diagnosis should be considered in all cases of myelopathy.

MRI is the investigation of choice if available, but CT remains the most widely available investigation and provides excellent localization.

The surgical procedure of choice should be either the posterolateral or anterior one; laminectomy is contraindicated.

The role of intraoperative monitoring of spinal sensory evoked potentials in this condition is unknown, but is worthy of investigation in an attempt to minimize neural trauma and improve the eventual outcome of surgery for this uncommon but benign condition.

REFERENCES

Abbott, K.H. & Retter, R.H. (1956) Protrusions of thoracic intervertebral discs. *Neurology*, **6**, 1–10.

Alberico, A.M., Sahni, K.S., Hall, J.A. Jr & Young, H.F. (1986) High thoracic disc herniation. *Neurosurgery*, **19**, 449–451.

Albrand, O.W. & Corkhill, G. (1979) Thoracic disc herniation: treatment and prognosis. *Spine*, **4**, 41–46.

Arce, C.A. & Dohrman, G.J. (1985) Herniated thoracic discs. *Neurol. Clin.*, **3**, 383–392.

Arseni, C. & Nash, F. (1960) Thoracic intervertebral disc protrusion. *J. Neurosurg.*, **17**, 418–430.

Baker, H.L., Love, J.C. & Uhlein, A. (1965) Roentgenologic features of protruded thoracic intervertebral discs. *Radiology*, **84**, 1059–1065.

Bennett, M.H. & McCallum, J.E. (1977) Experimental decompression of spinal cord. *Surg. Neurol.*, **8**, 63–67.

Benson, M.K.D. & Byrnes, D.P. (1975) The clinical syndromes and surgical treatment of thoracic intervertebral disc prolapse. *J. Bone Jt. Surg.*, **57B**, 471–477.

Bhole, R. & Gilmer, R.E. (1984) Two level thoracic disc herniation. *Clin. Orthop. Rel. Res.*, **190**, 129–131.

Bohlman, H.H. & Zdeblick, T.A. (1988) Anterior excision of herniated thoracic discs. *J. Bone Jt. Surg.*, **70A**, 1038–1047.

Brennan, M., Perrin, J.C., Canady, A. & Wesolowski, D. (1987) Paraparesis in a child with herniation of a thoracic disc. *Arch. Phys. Med. Rehabil.*, **68**, 806–808.

Capener, N. (1954) The evolution of lateral rachotomy. *J. Bone Jt. Surg.*, **28**, 103–107.

Carson, J., Gumpert, J. & Jefferson, A. (1971) Diagnosis and treatment of thoracic intervertebral disc protrusions. *J. Neurol. Neurosurg. Psychiatry*, **34**, 68–77.

Chin, L.S., Black, K.L. & Hoff, J.T. (1987) Multiple thoracic disc herniations: case report. *J. Neurosurg.*, **66**, 290–292.

Chowdhary, U.M. (1987) Intradural thoracic disc protrusion. *Spine*, **12**, 718–719.

Cohen, H.C.M. & Tucker, W.S. (1985) Pitfalls of incomplete myelography with thoracic spinal lesions. *Can. J. Neurol. Sci.*, **12**, 121–124.

Crafoord, T.C., Hierton, T., Lindblom, K. & Olsen, S.E. (1958) Spinal cord compression caused by a protruded thoracic disc: report of a case treated with anterolateral fenestration of the disc. *Acta Orthop. Scand.*, **28**, 103–107.

de Tribolet, N., Schnyder, P., Livio, J.J. & Boumghar, M. (1982) L'abord transthoracique des hernies discales dorsales. *Neurochirurgie*, **28**, 187–193.

Doppman, J.L. & DiChiro, G. (1968) The arteria radicularis magna. Radiographic anatomy in the adult. *Br J. Radiol.*, **41**, 40–45.

Doppman, J.L. & Girton, M. (1976) Angiographic study of the effect of laminectomy in the presence of acute anterior epidural masses. *J. Neurosurg.*, **45**, 195–202.

Elsberg, C.A. (1931) The extradural ventral chondromas (echondromas), their favorite sites, the spinal cord and root symptoms they produce and their surgical treatment. *Bull. Neurol. Inst. NY*, **1**, 350–388.

Epstein, J.A. (1954) The syndrome of herniation of the lower thoracic intervertebral discs with nerve root and spinal cord compression: a presentation of 4 cases with a review of the literature, methods of diagnosis and treatment. *J. Neurosurg.*, **11**, 525–538.

Faure, C., Debrun, G. & Djindjian, R. (1967) La vascularisation arterielle normale et pathologique du renflement lombaire de la moelle epiniere chez l'enfant: l'artere d'Adamkiewicz. *Ann. Radiol. (Paris)*, **10**, 129–140.

Fidler, M.W. & Goedhart, Z.D. (1984) Excision of prolapse of thoracic intervertebral disc. *J. Bone Jt. Surg.*, **66B**, 518–522.

Findlay, G. (1991) Transthoracic approach for thoracic disc and kyphectomy. In Torrens, M. & Dickson, R. (eds), *Operative Spinal Surgery*. Churchill Livingstone, London.

Garrido, E. (1980) Modified costotransversectomy: a surgical approach to ventrally placed lesions in the thoracic spinal canal. *Surg. Neurol.*, **13**, 109–113.

Gelch, M.M. (1978) Herniated thoracic disc at T1–2 level associated with Horner's syndrome. *J. Neurosurg.*, **48**, 128–130.

Haley, J.C. & Perry, J.H. (1950) Protrusions of intervertebral discs. Study of their distribution, characteristics and effects on the nervous system. *Am. J. Surg.*, **80**, 394–404.

Hann, E.C. (1980) Experience with ruptured T1–2 discs. *J. Indiana State Med. Assoc.*, September, pp. 598–599.

Hawk, W.A. (1936) Spinal compression caused by echondrosis of the intervertebral fibrocartilage: with a review of the recent literature. *Brain*, **59**, 204–224.

Hochman, M.S., Pena, C. & Ramirez, R. (1980) Calcified herniated thoracic disc diagnosed by computerized tomography. *J. Neurosurg.*, **52**, 722–723.

Hulme, A. (1960) The surgical approach to thoracic intervertebral disc protrusion. *J. Neurol. Neurosurg. Psychiatry*, **23**, 133–137.

Jefferson, A. (1975) The treatment of thoracic intervertebral disc protrusions. *Clin. Neurol. Neurosurg.*, **78**, 1–9.

Kahn, E.A. (1947) Role of dentate ligaments in spinal cord compression and syndrome of lateral sclerosis. *J. Neurosurg.*, **4**, 191–199.

Kite, W.C. Jr, Whitfield, R.D. & Campbell, E. (1957) The thoracic herniated disc syndrome. *J. Neurosurg.*, **14**, 61–67.

Kumar, R. & Buckley, T.F. (1986) First thoracic disc protrusion. *Spine*, **11**, 499–501.

Lesoin, F., Rousseaux, M., Autrique, A., Villette, L., Clarisse J. & Jomin, M. (1986) Thoracic disc herniations: evolution in the approach and indications. *Acta Neurochirurg.*, **80**, 30–34.

Lloyd, T.V., Johnson, J.C., Paul, D.J. & Hunt, W. (1980) Horner's syndrome secondary to herniated disc at T1–2. *Am. J. Radiol.*, **134**, 184–185.

Lobosky, J.M., Hitchon, P.W. & McDonnell, D.E. (1984) Transthoracic anterolateral decompression for thoracic spinal lesions. *Neurosurgery*, **14**, 26–30.

Logue, V. (1952) Thoracic intervertebral disc prolapse with spinal cord compression. *J. Neurol. Neurosurg. Psychiatry*, **15**, 227–241.

Love, J.G. & Kiefer, E.J. (1950) Root pain and paraplegia due to protrusions of thoracic intervertebral discs. *J. Neurosurg.*, **7**, 62–67.

Love, J.G. & Schorn, V.G. (1965) Thoracic disc protrusions. *J. Am. Med. Assoc.*, **191**, 627–631.

Maiman, D.J., Larson, S.J., Luck, E. & El-Ghatit, A. (1984) Lateral extracavitary approach to the spine for thoracic disc herniation: report of 23 cases. *Neurosurgery*, **14**, 178–182.

Maiman, D.J., Daniels, D. & Larson, S.J. (1988) Magnetic resonance imaging in the diagnosis of lower thoracic disc herniation. *J. Spinal Disord.*, **1**, 134–138.

McAllister, V.L. & Sage, M.R. (1976) The radiology of thoracic disc protrusion. *Radiology*, **27**, 294–299.

Michoury, S.D., Rappaport, H.Z., Shaked, I., Yellin, A. & Sahar, A. (1984) Thoracic disc herniation associated with papilloedema. *J. Neurosurg.*, **61**, 1132–1134.

Middleton, G.S. & Teacher, J.H. (1911) Injury of the spinal cord due to rupture of an intervertebral disc during muscular effort. *Glasgow Med. J.*, **76**, 1–6.

Mixter, W.J. & Barr, J.S. (1934) Rupture of the intervertebral disc with involvement of the spinal canal. *N. Engl. J. Med.*, **211**, 210–215.

Muller, R. (1951) Protrusion of thoracic intervertebral disc with compression of the spinal cord. *Acta Med. Scand.*, **139**, 99–104.

Otani, K., Nakai, S., Fujimura, Y., Manzoku, S. & Shibasaki, K. (1982) Surgical treatment of thoracic disc herniation using the anterior approach. *J. Bone Jt. Surg.*, **64B**, 340–343.

Otani, K., Manzoki, S., Shibasaki, K. & Nomachi, S. (1977) Surgical treatment of thoracic and thoracolumbar disc lesions using the anterior approach. *Spine*, **2**, 266–275.

Pansini, A. Lo Re & Conti, P. (1974) L'ernia discale del tratto inferiore dorsale. *Boll. Soc. Tosco-umbra Chirurg.*, 233–254.

Patterson, R.H. Jr & Arbitt, E. (1978) A surgical approach through the pedicle to protruded thoracic discs. *J. Neurosurg.*, **48**, 768–772.

Perot, P.L. & Munro, D.D. (1969) Transthoracic removal of midline thoracic disc protrusions causing spinal cord compression. *J. Neurosurg.*, **31**, 452–458.

Ransohoff, J., Spencer, F., Siew, F. & Gage, L. Jr (1969) Transthoracic removal of thoracic disc: report of 3 cases. *J. Neurosurg.*, **31**, 459–561.

Ravichandran, G. & Frankel, H.L. (1981) Paraplegia due to intervertebral disc lesions: a review of 57 operated cases. *Paraplegia*, **19**, 133–139.

Reeves, D.L. & Brown, H.A. (1968) Thoracic intervertebral disc protrusion with spinal cord compression. *J. Neurosurg.*, **28**, 24–28.

Reif, J., Gilsbach, J. & Ostheim-Dzerowycz, W. (1983) Differential diagnosis and therapy of herniated thoracic disc. *Acta Neurochirurg.*, **67**, 255–265.

Russell, T. (1989) Thoracic intervertebral disc protrusion: experience of 67 cases and review of the literature. *Br. J. Neurosurg.*, **3**, 153–160.

Safdari, H. & Baker, R.L. (1985) Microsurgical anatomy and related techniques to an anterolateral transthoracic approach to thoracic disc herniations. *Surg. Neurol.*, **23**, 589–593.

Sekhar, L.N. & Jannetta, P.J. (1983) Thoracic disc herniation: operative approaches and results. *Neurosurgery*, **12**, 303–305.

Shikata, J., Yamamuro, T., Iida, H. & Kashiwagi, N. (1988) Multiple thoracic disc herniations: case report. *Neurosurgery*, **22**, 1068–1070.

Singounas, E.G. & Karvounis, P.C. (1977) Thoracic disc protrusion. *Acta Neurochirurg.*, **39**, 251–258.

Svien, H.J. & Karvatis, A.L. (1954) Multiple protrusions of intervertebral discs in the upper thoracic region: report of a case. *Proc. Staff Meet. Mayo Clin.*, **29**, 375–378.

Tahmouresie, A. (1980) Herniated thoracic intervertebral disc—an unusual presentation: case report. *Neurosurgery*, **7**, 623–625.

Terry, A.F., McSweeney, T. & Jones, H.W.F. (1981) Paraplegia as a sequela to dorsal prolapse. *Paraplegia*, **19**, 111–117.

Thomson, J.L.G. (1966) Myelography in dorsal disc protrusion. *Acta Radiol. Diagn. (Stockh.)*, **5**, 1140–1146.

Tovi, D. & Strang, R.R. (1960) Thoracic intervertebral disc protrusion. *Acta Chir. Scand. Suppl.*, **267**, 1–41.

Ungersbock, K., Perneczky, A. & Korn, A. (1987) Thoracic vertebrostenosis combined with thoracic disc herniation. Case report and review of the literature. *Spine*, **12**, 612–615.

Van Landingham, J.H. (1954) Herniation of thoracic intervertebral discs with spinal cord compression in kyphosis dorsalis juvenilis (Scheuermann's disease): case report. *J. Neurosurg.*, **11**, 327–329.

Wang, A.M. & Zamani, A.A. (1986) Intradural herniation of a thoracic disc. *Comput. Radiol.*, **10**, 115–118.

Weiss, M.H., Heiden, J.S., Apuzzo, M.L.J. & Kurze, T. (1975) Anterior decompression of the thoracic and thoracolumbar spine. *Bull. Los Angeles Neurol. Soc.*, **40**, 112–115.

Yoss, R.E. (1950) Vascular supply of the spinal cord. The production of vascular syndromes. *Univ. Mich. Med. Bull.*, **16**, 333–345.

Young, S., Karr, G. & O'Laoire, S.A. (1989) Spinal cord compression due to thoracic disc herniation: results of posterolateral costotransversectomy. *Br. J. Neurosurg.*, **3**, 31–38.

Zielke, H. (1943) Scheuermannsche Krankheit, Brandscheibenprolaps und Tuberkulose. *Der Chirurg.*, **15**, 542–548.

SECTION 10
VASCULAR DISEASES OF THE SPINE

48 · Acute Spinal Haematoma

By R.A. COWIE

Acute spinal haemorrhage is a rare clinical event which usually presents with acute back pain, followed within a short time by symptoms and signs of loss of function of the spinal cord or its nerve roots. Haematomas may develop in the extradural, subdural or subarachnoid spaces and produce a pattern of clinical events which can be difficult to distinguish from other more common causes of cord compression. Some cases are associated with trauma to the spine, others with congenital vascular lesions or tumours. Haemorrhage which occurs within the spinal cord itself, and which is large enough to produce a solid haematoma, is termed a haematomyelia, though this is much less common than the haemorrhagic contusions commonly seen after spinal trauma.

SPINAL EXTRADURAL HAEMATOMA

This is a rare clinical entity, and according to Bruyn & Bosma (1976) only 180 cases had been reported since the mid 19th century. These authors record, in an authoritative review of the condition, that the first description of intraspinal haemorrhage was given by Du Verney in 1688 before the Parisian Royal Academy of Sciences. The true incidence of spontaneous extradural haematoma is not clear, though most neurosurgical centres will see occasional cases, especially those related to anticoagulant therapy.

Thirty-three cases have been reported to date in children under 18 years of age, the youngest being at four months. There is a slight male predominance. Of the 148 cases reported in adults up to 1973, 101 were in men and 47 in women. The peak incidence is in the fourth and fifth decade, respectively. In male patients the haematomas are situated most frequently in the lower cervical and thoracolumbar regions, whereas they predominate in the lower thoracic region in females.

Trauma is an important cause of extradural haemorrhage, though this complication occurs only rarely after spinal injury. Holzer & Kloss (1962) recorded a 3.8% incidence of extradural haematoma in 94 fatal spinal injuries. However, spinal extradural haematoma is more common in neonates, and Towbin (1968) estimated that 10% of all neonatal deaths are due to spinal haemorrhage. Some cases follow iatrogenic trauma, such as lumbar puncture or epidural anaesthesia (Gingrich, 1968); some complicate primary or secondary coagulopathies, such as haemophilia, leukaemia, polycythaemia rubra vera, anticoagulant therapy and liver disease. A third group occur in primary vascular anomalies of the epidural space or vertebra, or tumours of the spinal canal (Harris *et al.*, 1978). Other cases have complicated Paget's disease (Stuart Lee *et al.*, 1988) and pregnancy (Yonekawa *et al.*, 1975).

However, a large number of cases have been reported where the haematoma has occurred during activities of normal life, such as coughing, straining, etc., and where no predisposing cause has been shown. The source of bleeding in such cases of spontaneous epidural haematoma is not clear, though most authors have concluded that it is of venous origin. This is because there is a complex venous network within the spinal canal, composed of large-calibre longitudinal veins mainly in the ventrolateral extradural space, which are linked anteriorly and posteriorly to the dura by transversely running anastomoses. The extradural plexus, in turn, anastomoses through the segmental veins to the external vertebral plexus and thence to the inferior vena cava and azygos and hemiazygos veins. An important connection with the basilar plexus and the cranial dural sinuses allows this system to act as a major pathway for cerebral blood to leave the head when in the erect position (Dilenge & Perey, 1973). The lack of venous valves allows blood to pass cephalad and caudad, and for the vessels to act as capacitors, regulating volume, pressure and flow of blood between chest, abdomen and the craniospinal system (Bruyn & Bosma, 1976). This reversal of flow probably protects the spinal cord from sudden surges of pressure. It has been suggested, however, that excessive surges of pressure may be the explanation of spontaneous haemorrhage within the extradural space, arising from rupture of the venous plexuses.

On the other hand, Beatty & Winston (1984) suggest that this mechanism is inadequate to explain the source of extradural spinal haematoma. They observed that the pressure of blood within extradural veins is always less than the cerebrospinal fluid pressure at the same level. In addition, the distended dural sac tamponades perioperative bleeding from extradural veins. They argue that the speed of development of cord compression and its location within the epidural space is consistent with haemorrhage of arterial origin. An arterial network within the extradural fat arises from the lateral spinal arteries, which divide into three branches: radicular arteries; posterior central branches supplying the ventral half of the extradural space and dura; and a prelaminar ramus which supplies the dorsal half of the space. These vessels anastomose with rami from the vertebral body arteries. Two types of small arteries on the spinal dura have been described by Lazorthes & Manelfe (1970). The first are of the spiral type which run longitudinally and which are concentrated in the cervical and lumbar regions; the second are a cluster type situated posteriorly in the thoracic region. Beatty & Winston (1984) hypothesized that excessive axial movement of the spinal dura may rupture any of the extradural arteries and precipitate an acute extradural haematoma.

Patients with spontaneous extradural haematoma generally present with the acute onset of back pain localized at the level of the lesion, quickly followed in some patients by radicular pain. Signs of compression of the spinal cord rapidly develop in most cases. However, a subacute or chronic mode of onset has been recorded in some patients (Boyd & Pear, 1972).

The clinical presentation mimics those disorders which cause acute back pain, together with nerve root or spinal cord dysfunction. Spinal extradural abscess is sometimes associated with the clinical features of sepsis and pyrexia. Vertebral and metastatic tumours usually have a history of pre-existing back pain. Vascular disease, involving the arterial supply of the spinal cord, particularly with subarachnoid haemorrhage, may present a similar picture. However, the cerebrospinal fluid is usually clear in extradural haemorrhage with no increase in cell content, though the protein concentration may be elevated. Only in coagulopathies or coincident haemorrhage in the subdural space or spinal cord is blood present in the cerebrospinal fluid.

After initial clinical evaluation, urgent investigation is required to confirm the presence of cord compression and locate its site. There is a poor prognosis for motor recovery if paralysis is present for longer than 36 hours (McQuarrie, 1978).

Plain X-rays of the spine are usually normal unless a vertebral angioma, Paget's disease or some other lesion is identified. Urgent myelography usually reveals a complete extradural block, though occasionally an incomplete block or irregular indentation of the dye column can be encountered. Further information can be obtained using computed tomographic scanning after myelography. Magnetic resonance imaging of patients with spinal cord symptoms (Larsson *et al.*, 1988; Servadei *et al.*, 1987) may reveal an extradural haematoma and avoid the need for myelography and its associated risk of neurological deterioration.

Treatment of the condition is a neurosurgical emergency and prompt decompressive laminectomy is required. The laminectomy should be ample to evacuate the haematoma and restore pulsation to the dura. If this cannot be achieved, then the dura should be opened to see if an associated intradural lesion is present.

The prognosis for recovery is related to the speed of diagnosis and decompression of the spinal cord. Less than 50% of patients with paralysis of greater than 36 hours duration at the time of surgery regained useful motor function (McQuarrie, 1978). Delay in diagnosis and treatment of the condition can cause ischaemic myelomalacia and cord necrosis. The prognosis in the group of patients presenting with lumbar and radicular symptoms is far better than where compression of the spinal cord has occurred. If the compression is above the fifth cervical segment there is a much poorer prognosis, because of associated respiratory depression.

SPINAL SUBDURAL HAEMORRHAGE

This condition is much less common than extradural haematoma of the spine. Since the report by Schiller *et al.* (1948) only approximately 25 cases of spontaneous subdural haematoma have been reported. Many have occurred in association with bleeding disorders, such as haemophilia, anticoagulant therapy or with thrombocytopenia (Edelson, 1976).

A literature survey by Russell & Benoit (1983) found 58 cases of subdural haematoma and confirmed that 19 cases were associated with anomalies of coagulation. In 11 of these the haemorrhage occurred after lumbar puncture. This investigation may have caused the haematoma in seven others. Subdural haematoma complicating trauma to the spine is very unusual, and only 10 cases have been reported. Two cases have followed rupture of an arteriovenous malformation and two followed previous spinal surgery.

Of the reported cases the female to male ratio is 2.1 : 1. The age ranges from four months to 80 years, with an average of 41 years. The thoracic and thoracolumbar regions are most frequently involved, though the haematoma may extend over many spinal segments.

The clinical presentation was acute in 29 cases, with a sudden onset of severe back pain, followed by radicular pain radiating into the arms, trunk or legs. Sensorimotor impairment, ranging from mild loss of function to complete paraplegia and incontinence, followed within a short time, sometimes immediately. Some patients had accompanying headache and meningism. In 12 of the patients there was a subacute or chronic presentation, sometimes fluctuating in severity, where painless cord compression was diagnosed (Khosla *et al.*, 1985).

The source of bleeding leading to the development of a subdural haematoma is not clear. The subdural space is traversed by small vessels (Djindjian *et al.*, 1970), which may be the source of the bleeding, particularly if sudden surges of intravascular pressure occur. However, the pathogenesis of chronic subdural haematoma remains obscure, though inflammation of the arachnoid may be responsible for the fluctuant course.

Myelography in these patients may be difficult if a 'dry' tap is encountered. In most cases a complete block will be seen, and the majority will have blood-stained cerebrospinal fluid with a high protein content. Computed tomography and magnetic resonance imaging should be employed where available.

Thirty-six of the reported cases were treated by laminectomy and drainage of the haematoma. At operation the dura was found to be tense and purple, and a semiliquid clot could be removed by suction and irrigation. In patients with a chronic haematoma a well-defined membrane enclosing a fluid-filled cavity has been encountered. Treatment of the bleeding disorder requires close cooperation with a haematologist. The prognosis for recovery is better in those patients whose neurological function is preserved before operation; in paraplegic patients complete recovery is rare.

SPINAL SUBARACHNOID HAEMORRHAGE

Less than 1% of all cases of spontaneous subarachnoid haemorrhage arise in the spine (Walton, 1953). The varied clinical presentation and the frequent absence of segmental spinal cord and nerve root signs means that delay in diagnosis is common.

The typical presentation is of a sudden low back or neck pain, described as *coup de poignard* by Michon (1928), followed by radicular pain and meningism. Sometimes bilateral sciatica and opisthotonus may follow. Headache, nausea, vomiting and photophobia occur when blood extends into the cranial cavity, though coma is seen only rarely. The majority of patients do not have major neurological signs, unless an associated intramedullary haematoma develops. Cord compression from a subarachnoid haematoma is very rare, as blood is diluted by cerebrospinal fluid. Recurrent episodes may occur before the diagnosis is made.

The most common source of bleeding is from an arteriovenous malformation (Chapter 49). Spinal arterial aneurysms also occur, either independently or in association with arteriovenous malformations. However, spinal tumours, particularly those in the cauda equina or conus, can cause spinal subarachnoid haemorrhage. This occurs most frequently from an ependymoma, though neurofibroma, haemangioblastoma, meningioma, astrocytoma, sarcoma and spinal endometriosis have been implicated. Collagen vascular disorders such as polyarteritis nodosa, systemic lupus erythematosus, Sjögren's syndrome and pseudoxanthoma elasticum can cause isolated cases of subarachnoid haemorrhage. Spinal trauma only rarely causes subarachnoid haemorrhage, except for patients with bleeding disorders and in the perinatal period.

The diagnosis depends upon sampling cerebrospinal fluid, though lumbar puncture can fail if there is a solid subarachnoid haematoma. Subsequent myelography generally using the cisternal route may show small subarachnoid clots which can mimic an intradural or intramedullary tumour. Magnetic resonance imaging can reveal the characteristic filling defects of a spinal arteriovenous malformation, or an extra- or intramedullary tumour.

If at decompressive laminectomy the source of the haematoma is not found, then myelography and magnetic resonance imaging should be repeated in the postoperative period. Spinal angiography is not generally undertaken prior to urgent decompressive surgery, but should be carried out if the source of the haemorrhage is not clear.

SPINAL INTRAMEDULLARY HAEMORRHAGE

The majority of cases of intramedullary haemorrhage occur after trauma, following compression or contusion of the cord. Generally petechial haemorrhages are seen and large intramedullary collections are less common. Spontaneous haematomyelia was reviewed by Jellinger (1972), who defined it as primary non-traumatic intramedullary haematoma which usually follows rupture of abnormal blood vessels. It is most often associated with arteriovenous, venous or cavernous angiomas, or from rupture of spinal aneurysms. However, syphilis, spinal arteriosclerosis, hypertension and blood dyscrasias have also been implicated. Secondary haemorrhage into the cord can occur from myelitis and arachnoiditis, and from primary intramedullary tumours. It may also follow compressive lesions of the cord, such as extramedullary tumours, spondylosis or intervertebral disc protrusion (Jellinger, 1972). Acute haemorrhage can occur into a pre-existing syringomyelic cavity (Gowers, 1903), possibly resulting from the rupture of abnormal vascular channels in the cavity walls.

The haematoma within the cord causes expansion of it which resembles an intramedullary tumour on myelography. However, the investigation of choice, when available, is magnetic resonance imaging. Decompressive surgery and release of the intramedullary haematoma through a dorsal midline myelotomy accompanied by the removal of any associated lesion such as a vascular malformation is indicated. The prognosis for recovery, however, is poor.

REFERENCES

Beatty, R.M. & Winston, K.R. (1984) Spontaneous cervical epidural haematoma. *J. Neurosurg.*, **61**, 143–148.

Boyd, H.R. & Pear, B.L. (1972) Chronic spontaneous spinal epidural haematoma; report of two cases. *J. Neurosurg.*, **36**, 239–242.

Bruyn, G.W. & Bosma, N.J. (1976) Spinal extradural haematoma. In Vinken, P.J. & Bruyn, G.W. (eds) *Handbook of Clinical Neurology*, vol. 13, pp. 1–30. Elsevier, Amsterdam.

Dilenge, D. & Perey, B. (1973) An angiographic study of the meningorachidian venous system. *Radiology*, **108**, 333–337.

Djindjian, R., Hurth, M., Houdart, R. *et al.* (1970) *Angiography of the Spinal Cord.* University Park Press, Baltimore, MD.

Edelson, R.N. (1976) Spinal subdural haematoma. In Vinken, P.J. & Bruyn, G.W. (eds) *Injuries of the Spine and Spinal Cord*, pt. II, *Handbook of Clinical Neurology*, vol. 26, pp. 31–38. Elsevier, Amsterdam.

Gingrich, T.F. (1968) Spinal epidural hematoma following continuing epidural anesthesia. *Anesthesiology*, **29**, 162–163.

Gowers, W.R. (1903) Syringeal haemorrhage into the spinal cord. *Lancet*, **1**, 993.

Harris, D.J., Fornasier, V.L. & Livingstone, K.E. (1978) Haemangiopericytoma of the spinal canal. Report of three cases. *J. Neurosurg.*, **49**, 914–920.

Holzer, F.J. & Kloss, K. (1962) Todliche Wirbelsaulenverletzungen. *Wien. Klin. Wochenschr.*, **74**, 125–129.

Jellinger, K. (1972) Traumatic vascular disease of the spinal cord. In Vinken, P.J. & Bruyn, G.W. (eds) *Vascular Diseases of the Nervous System*, pt. II, *Handbook of Clinical Neurology*, vol. 12, pp. 556–630. Elsevier, Amsterdam.

Khosla, V.K., Kak, V.K. & Mathuriya, S.N. (1985) Chronic spinal subdural haematomas. *J. Neurosurg.*, **63**, 636–639.

Larsson, E.M., Holtas, S. & Cronqvist, S. (1988) Emergency magnetic resonance examination of patients with spinal cord symptoms. *Acta Radiol.*, **29**, 69–75.

Lazorthes, G. & Manelfe, C. (1970) La vascularisation arterielle de la duremere raclidienne. Les arteres spinales et les pelotons vasculaires. *C.R. Acad. Sci. (Paris)*, series D, **271**, 88–91.

McQuarrie, I.G. (1978) Recovery from paraplegia caused by spontaneous spinal epidural hematoma. *Neurology*, **28**, 224–228.

Michon, P. (1928) Le coup de poignard rachidien symptome initial de certaines hemorrhagies sous-arachnoidiennes. Essai sur les hemorrhagies meningees spinales. *Presse*

Med., **36**, 964–966.

Russell, N.A. & Benoit, B.G. (1983) Spinal subdural hematoma. *Surg. Neurol.*, **20**, 133–137.

Schiller, F., Neligan, G. & Budtz-Olsen, O. (1948) Surgery in hemophilia: A case of spinal subdural hematoma producing paraplegia. *Lancet*, **2**, 842–845.

Servadei, F., Trevisan, C., Bianchedi, G. & Padovani, R. (1987) Spontaneous dorsal epidural haematoma: usefulness of magnetic resonance imaging and importance of operative treatment even in cases with complete paraplegia. *Acta Neurochir. (Wien)*, **89**, 137–139.

Stuart Lee, K., McWhorter, J.M. & Angelo, J.N. (1988) Spinal epidural hematoma associated with Paget's disease. *Surg. Neurol.*, **30**, 131–134.

Towbin, A. (1968) Spinal injury related to the syndrome of sudden death ('crib-death') in infants. *Am. J. Clin-Pathol.*, **49**, 562–567.

Walton, J.N. (1953) Subarachnoid haemorrhage of unusual aetiology. *Neurology*, **3**, 517–543.

Yonekawa, Y., Mehdorn, H.M. & Nishikawa, M. (1975) Spontaneous spinal epidural hematoma during pregnancy. *Surg. Neurol.*, **3**, 327–328.

49 · Spinal Arteriovenous Malformations

By A.K. OMMAYA

Vascular malformations of the spinal canal and its contents are essentially hamartomatous in nature, and variously termed arteriovenous malformations or angiomas. In clinical practice, lesions such as cavernous angiomas and telangiectasia are usually not included in the discussions of such lesions (Ommaya, 1984a). Because cavernomas of the spinal cord are an unusual variant, only a brief mention will be made (see Rees-Cosgrove *et al.*, 1988). The usual abbreviation 'AVM' for arteriovenous malformation is probably the most suitable appellation, because it describes succinctly the abnormal connection between arteries and veins without the intervening capillaries that is the essence of this entity. Apart from the anatomical constraints of the spinal canal and the unique neurobiology of the spinal cord structures, spinal arteriovenous malformations are comparable to vascular lesions in the brain, with only minor differences. Whereas much of our understanding of neural anatomy, physiology and pathology has followed a path from spinal cord to brain, knowledge of arteriovenous malformations has come first from the brain and only later from the spinal cord. Although angiography of the brain began in 1927 with the work of Moniz, it was not until 1969 that the first monograph on selective angiography of the spinal cord was published by the group at the National Institutes of Health (Doppman *et al.*, 1969). The first angiographic demonstration of an aneurysm of the spinal cord described as part of an arteriovenous malformation was reported in 1962 by Djindjian, who with his colleagues M. Hurth and R. Houdart in Paris, summarized their early experience in a monograph published in 1970. Knowledge of the diagnostic and therapeutic aspects of spinal cord arteriovenous malformations has gradually increased since that time, with significant continuing contributions by the two pioneering groups in France and the USA, in addition to others (DiChiro *et al.*, 1967, 1971; Ommaya, 1973; Djindjian, 1975; Yasargil *et al.*, 1975; Aminoff, 1976; Kendall & Logue, 1977; Pia, 1978; Ommaya, 1984; Symon *et al.*, 1984; Yasargil *et al.*, 1984; Rosenblum *et al.*, 1987).

The first report which drew attention to the pathological features of arteriovenous malformation was that of Foix and Alajouanine in their paper, 'La myelite necrotique subaigue' (Foix & Alajouanine, 1926). Two patients were described who developed a progressive ascending paralysis and loss of sensation, leading to death within two years of the onset of the initial clinical syndrome. The pathological findings were predominantly in the lower thoracic, lumbar and sacral parts of the spinal cord, and essentially consisted of marked areas of necrosis with macroscopically striking enlargement and thickening of the extramedullary and intramedullary vessels of the spinal cord, chiefly involving the veins.

The authors described these vascular changes as 'endomesovasculitis' and postulated that there might be a toxic or infective agent. Subsequently, this syndrome was further described by Scholtz & Manuelidis in 1951. In 1962 Antoni clarified these earlier observations, and described the pathological findings as being related to a spinal arteriovenous malformation, the terms 'aneurysm' or 'fistula' being also introduced for the first time. Subsequent case reports have reviewed the condition in detail (Ansari, 1965; Jellinger, 1966, 1978). A case of Foix–Alajouanine disease diagnosed clinically and confirmed radiologically and at surgery has been reported by Wirth *et al.* (1970).

Apart from the excellent publications of

McCormick, there have been few detailed descriptions of the pathological features of such lesions. (McCormick, 1966; McCormick & Nofzinger, 1966). Burger & Vogel (1976) attempted to simplify the situation as seen in the following quotation: 'To tackle the literature that describes the pathological features of spinal arteriovenous malformations is to become as ensnarled as the lesions themselves. Simplicity and practicality dictate description of only two large groups.' They go on to describe these two groups as follows: firstly, aggregates of thin-walled vessels, contained entirely within the substance of the cord, ranging as a compacted lesion with a honeycomb appearance, or dispersed through the parenchyma with calibres ranging from cavernous to capillary. The authors note that such malformations are prone to produce symptoms by haemorrhage, rather than by compression, and very few surgical specimens have been available in the literature. The second group, described as being much more common, is characterized by large, redundant, serpentine vascular channels in the leptomeninges, usually accompanied by smaller, hyalinized vessels in the underlying parenchyma. These lesions, which are more extramedullary than the first type, are much more likely to produce their effects by pressure or ischaemia. Some pathologists have attempted to subclassify arteriovenous malformations as venous, arterial or arteriovenous; however, this classification may well be misleading because of the marked abnormalities that occur in the venous channels and the fact that such channels may well be hybrids of arteries and veins.

In the latest edition of *Greenfield's Neuropathology* (Hume, 1984) a very important point is made regarding the diagnostic importance of the macroscopic appearances of different types of arteriovenous malformation, which are remarkably uniform as compared to the complexity of the microscopic changes. This is probably why, to the best of our knowledge, there has been no clear-cut correlation of the detailed microscopic neuropathology with each type of arteriovenous malformation as described currently in the clinical literature, on the basis of angiographic and surgical data. Most often the usual histological description at post mortem describes an unusual form of incomplete necrosis in the spinal cord, involving both grey and white matter, particularly in the central part of the cord. Histological changes are noted to be more advanced in the caudal portions of the spinal cord, particularly in the lumbosacral enlargement, with many capillaries and thick-walled channels, suggesting abnormal alterations in these vessels. Recent thromboses are common within the intermedullary vessels, and the changes seen are indicative of repeated episodes of thrombosis. Large extramedullary veins also may show such thrombosis. As in cerebral arteriovenous malformations, the large abnormal vessels show changes indicating the structure of arterialized veins.

APPLIED ANATOMY OF THE SPINAL CORD CIRCULATION

The first publication on the vessels of the human spinal cord was by Thomas Willis, in his book *Cerebri Anatome* (1664). The drawings of Willis were not improved upon until the late eighteenth century, by the work of von Haller. The classic publications of Adamkiewicz (1882), and his pupil, Kadyi (1889), laid the foundations for our understanding of the blood supply of the human spinal cord. More recent publications, both in animals and humans, include the work of Bolton (1939), Herren & Alexander (1939), Suh & Alexander (1939), Sahs (1942), Corbin (1961), Lazorthes *et al.* (1958), Jellinger (1966), Hughes (1967, 1971), Dommisse (1975) and Aminoff (1976).

The fetal segmental vascular supply to the spinal cord is replaced by the adult pattern as early as six months after gestation. A series of lateral spinal arteries supply branches to paravertebral muscles, dura and vertebrae, as well as radicular and radiculomedullary branches which form the blood supply to the spinal cord. Radicular and radiculopial branches enter each level and supply both anterior and posterior segments of the spinal canal content, but the true supply of the cord itself is via certain anterior and posterior radiculomedullary vessels, entering only at certain levels, which varies among individuals. The single median anterior spinal artery thus receives three to 12 feeding arteries at intermittent and irregular levels of its course. Thus, anywhere from zero to six branches enter at the cervical levels, two to four in the thoracic zone, and one or two in the lumbar region on each side. Similar posterior radiculomedullary branches to the paired posterior spinal arteries are more numerous, that is, between 10 and 23. These vessels provide contributions to their respective posterior spinal artery, usually at the same segmental level as the anterior radiculo-

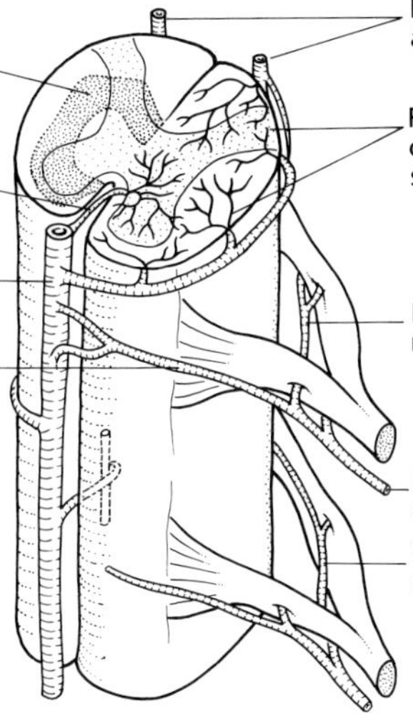

Fig. 49.1 Arterial supply to spinal cord.

medullary arteries. The anatomical arrangement of the arterial supply is shown in Fig. 49.1, where it should be noted that the anterior spinal artery lies within the pia, and when approached through a myelotomy is often obscured by its central or sulcal commissural branches supplying the central grey matter, but not including the posterior horns.

The venous drainage of the spinal cord is depicted in Fig. 49.2. The direction of blood flow in the medullary veins is outward to the intervertebral veins, passing through the intervertebral foramena, and draining into the interconnected epidural and paravertebral plexus. This venous plexus drains into the vertebral, posterior, intercostal, lumbar and lateral sacral veins.

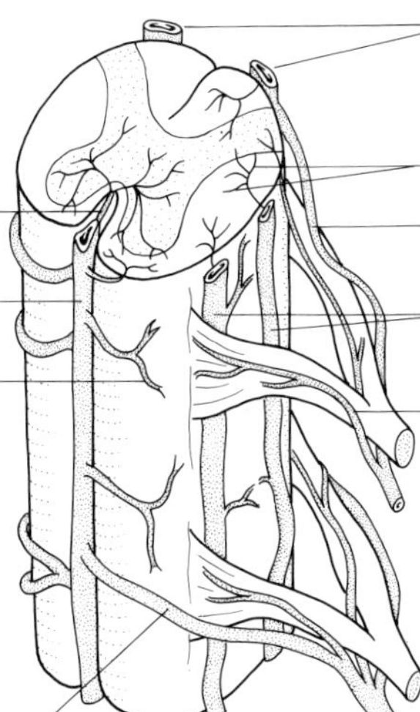

Fig. 49.2 Venous drainage of spinal cord.

TERMINOLOGY AND CLASSIFICATION

The terms 'angioma' and 'arteriovenous malformation of the spinal cord' are interchangeable, essentially describing congenital abnormal clusters of blood vessels formed as a developmental anomaly of the spinal circulation. In his work on the development of the spinal vascular system, Turnbull has described four stages. It is at the end of the second stage, between three and six weeks, that maldevelopment can lead to the persistence of thin-walled tortuous vessels with poorly developed media and elasitica, primitive capillary and precapillary channels, and abnormal arteriovenous shunts typical of those seen in arteriovenous malformation (Turnbull *et al.*, 1966). Such lesions were first described in reports by Hebold in 1885, and by Gaupp (1887), who picturesquely called them 'haemorrhoids of the pia mater' and recognized them as a source for subarachnoid haemorrhage.

It was not until the advent of selective spinal angiography by our group at the National Institutes of Health in the United States, and by Djindjian and his group in France, that attempts at clinical classification of arteriovenous malformations could be developed (Doppman *et al.*, 1969; Djindjian *et al.*, 1970). Our preliminary radiological classification of arteriovenous malformations recognized three basic types: the single-coiled unbranched Type I lesion, commonly seen in adults, and not in teenagers or children; the less common compact plexus or 'glomus' Type II lesion; and a variable, rapid-flow, Type III lesion with multiple feeding arteries often seen in younger patients, and hence termed the juvenile type. The majority of Type I lesions are now recognized as being essentially dural arteriovenous malformations (Kendall & Logue, 1977; Ommaya, 1984a,b).

From a surgical point of view, a division of all spinal cord arteriovenous malformations into low-flow and high-flow lesions is a simple rubric to separate the surgically easy, mainly extramedullary and dural slow-flow cases, from the surgically difficult, and often intermedullary, high-flow lesions. High-flow arteriovenous malformations are completely visualized by selective angiography in less than five seconds, whereas low-flow arteriovenous malformations require much longer times for contrast clearance. A current classification is summarized in Table 49.1.

Michael Djindjian (1976) following in the footsteps of his illustrious father, has analysed the angiographic results in 150 cases of spinal arteriovenous malformations, and found the following regional distribution: cervical (C1–T1), 14%; thoracic (T2–T6), 22%; thoracolumbosacral (T7–cauda equina), 64%. He showed also that in intradural lesions the posterior arteries supply the main feeders to the arteriovenous malformation in 48% of cases, with a supply from both anterior and posterior vessels in the remainder. More rostral arteriovenous malformations obtain more of their blood supply from the anterior spinal artery than do more caudally placed arteriovenous malformations.

In addition to the regional and surgical classifications discussed above, there is also an angiographic classification of arteriovenous malformations which breaks down the angiomas into four categories.

1 Retromedullary, with the main supply from the posterior spinal artery sources.

2 Intramedullary, from primarily anterospinal artery sources.

3 Extramedullary, with medullary venous drainage (subclassified as either arteriovenous malformations with a dural supply, and arteriovenous malformations with a perimedullary blood supply). Merland and his colleagues have named this second subtype the intrathecal perimedullary arteriovenous fistulas, fed by medullary arteries (Merland *et al.*, 1980).

4 Extradural with extramedullary drainage.

The value of an angiographic classification becomes particularly significant when surgical treatment by direct excision of the nidus is difficult, and preliminary or definitive treatment by embolization is required. A simplified angiographic classification has also been proposed by Thron *et al.* (1988) which is similar to that proposed by Vuia & Alexaniu (1969) and by Bradac *et al.* (1984). They differentiate arteriovenous malformations into three types.

1 Intradural arteriovenous malformations supplied by medullary feeding arteries, and drained by perimedullary veins. Location of the nidus is either intramedullary or in the perimedullary zone (or at both levels).

2 Dural arteriovenous malformations or fistulas supplied by radicular meningeal arteries not feeding the spinal cord, and drained by perimedullary veins.

3 Extradural arteriovenous malformations with possible intraspinal extensions, but supplied and drained exclusively by extradural vessels.

The radiological morphology of arteriovenous malformations may therefore range from a simple fistula, as seen typically in dural arteriovenous malformations, to a conglomeration of greatly dilated vascular masses. These latter types can involve soft tissues, bone, dura and the spinal cord. In the majority of published series the dural arteriovenous malformation or fistulas are the most frequent form of arteriovenous malformation, consisting of up to 80% of the cases.

Table 49.1 Spinal angiomas or arteriovenous malformations (AVM) of the spinal cord

Low-flow arteriovenous malformations	High-flow arteriovenous malformations
Synonyms	*Synonyms*
(a) Type 1 arteriovenous malformations[a]	(a) Type II (glomus)[a]
(b) Single-coiled vessel[a]	(b) Type III (juvenile)[a]
(c) Angioma racemosum venosum (Wyburn–Mason)	(c) Angioma racemosum arteriovenosum (Wyburn–Mason)
(d) Angioma racemosum (Krayenbuhl *et al.*)	(d) Arteriovenous malformation with multiple feeders
(e) Long dorsal malformation (Malis)	
Location of nidus	*Location of nidus*
(a) Extradural and/or dural	(a) Extradural and/or dural
(b) Subdural and subarachnoid (extramedullary)	(b) Subdural extra- and/or intramedullary
(c) Combined types	(c) Combined types
Usual level of arteriovenous malformations[b]	*Usual level of arteriovenous malformations*[b]
Thoracolumbar–sacral	Cervical–thoracolumbar

[a] Doppman *et al.* (1969).
[b] Levels are indicated in sequence of most to least common site.
NB: Type II (glomus) arteriovenous malformations occur mostly in the cervical cord or cervicomedullary junction.

AETIOLOGY AND PATHOPHYSIOLOGY

Rosenblum and his colleagues (1987) attempted to divide the aetiology of arteriovenous malformations into congenital and acquired categories, classifying dural arteriovenous malformations, which are more common in older people, as being acquired, as opposed to the congenital intradural arteriovenous malformations. This hypothesis is, however, not supported by any pathological or epidemiological evidence.

Thron *et al.* (1988) recommend the term 'dural arteriovenous anomaly or fistula,' rather than malformation or angioma, in order to counter assertions that dural arteriovenous malformations have either a congenital or acquired nature. They also suggest a possible morphological basis for the dural arteriovenous malformation in the arteriovenous anastomoses found in the dura in the vicinity of root sheaths as described by Vuia & Alexaniu (1969). Manelfe *et al.* (1972), in their study on the blood supply of the dura, have named such vascular clusters as the 'pelotons vasculaires'.

Although the two classes of arteriovenous malformation are indeed quite distinct clinically, it is probably premature at this stage of our knowledge to separate these essentially hamartomatous lesions into two categories. It is interesting to note that the posterior spinal cord circulation develops later than the anterior one, both circulations being completed later in caudal regions as compared to rostral zones. Aminoff (1976) suggested that the predilection of arteriovenous malformations for these regions of the spinal cord could therefore be related to the sequence of development.

If one correlates the angiographic data with findings at surgery, it is possible to suggest that most arteriovenous malformations are fed by one or more radiculopial vessel, with only a minority being supplied by radiculomedullary vessels, either in part or in whole. The majority of these feeders enter with the dorsal root, or in the region of the dorsal root when they are primarily dural in nature. The less common anterior feeders are found primarily in the cervical region.

The bulk of the arteriovenous malformation is usually constituted by the longitudinally disposed coronal veins, which are the vessels most commonly noted at myelography and at surgery as bulky varicosities. In the earliest attempts at surgical removal, excision of all such varicosities was commonplace. However, extensive coagulation or stripping of such components may further aggravate the myelopathy. With the greater understanding of the applied anatomy of spinal cord blood supply, as well as that of spinal arteriovenous malformations, made possible by the development of selective spinal angiography (Doppman *et al.*, 1969; Djindjian *et al.*, 1970), it has been recognized that it is necessary to excise only the actual arteriovenous fistula.

Five factors may be responsible for the signs and symptoms of spinal cord vascular malformations, namely: compression, vascular diversion ('steal'), haemorrhage, thrombosis, and increased venous pressure (Kaufman *et al.*, 1970). The role of the last factor has been well clarified by the work of Aminoff and others (Aminoff, 1976; Pia & Djinjian, 1978; Symon *et al.*, 1984). The consensus of opinion would point to a variable contribution of five factors, causing spinal cord ischaemia and necrosis. These include, in order of importance, increased venous pressure, subarachnoid haemorrhage, thrombotic episodes and mechanical distension by bulky arteriolized veins. The majority view is that steal is the least common mechanism to be effective in causing cord ischaemia, although it can have a role to play in some cases such as the recurrent postprandial paraplegia noted in two of our cases. A steal mechanism cannot play a role in a purely dural arteriovenous malformation, because of the absence of an intradural source of supply to the nidus.

The aetiology of thrombosis in an arteriovenous malformation is unknown, but that it occurs is unequivocally certain. The role of increased extramedullary venous pressure has been hypothesized by Aminoff (1976), who postulated a sequence of high venous back-pressure, causing a reduced intramedullary arteriovenous pressure gradient, which in turn causes a reduced blood flow, leading to spinal cord ischaemia either directly or indirectly via intravascular thrombosis. This mechanism, which has also been clearly elaborated by Aboulker *et al.* (1977), is supported by intraoperative measurements of vascular pressures in the draining veins of dural arteriovenous malformations, in which occlusion of the nidus can cause a drop in mean pressure of up to 30 to 40 mm of mercury (Aboulker *et al.*, 1977). Such a pressure measurement change was also found by Thron *et al.* (1988).

The clinical data which follow are based on two

series, one of 104 cases of arteriovenous malformations, culled from over 200 cases of non-traumatic myelopathy, referred between 1961 and 1980 to the clinical centre of the National Institutes of Health, and a second series between 1980 and the present at the George Washington University Medical Center. This series consists of 31 cases. Long-term follow-up has been completed in a total of 104 cases for the period between 1965 and 1981, and the figures that are presented are based on that series.

The incidence of spinal arteriovenous malformations is quite variable according to the published source, and in neurosurgical series this ranges from a low of 3.3% in the pre-angiography era, to a figure of up to 40% of all central nervous system vascular malformations after the introduction of selective angiography, according to Aminoff (1976). It would be accurate to state, therefore, that the true incidence is not known, because of the lack of adequate epidemiologic data. It has been estimated that at least 10% of vascular space-occupying lesions of the spinal cord will be arteriovenous malformations (Ommaya, 1984a). In most series the incidence of dural, or what has been termed 'low-flow', arteriovenous malformations is much higher than that of the high-flow arteriovenous malformations. In our own series high-flow arteriovenous malformations were approximately one-fourth of that of the low-flow lesions and low-flow lesions were much more common in individuals over 18 years of age. Seventy-nine per cent of the patients were male and the incidence by age group was approximately equal from the second to the sixth decade.

A number of authors have dismissed the role of mechanical compression in all arteriovenous malformations, but it is likely that bulky intramedullary arteriovenous malformations can act as space-occupying lesions. In an excellent monograph by Pia and Djindjian (1978), pathological evidence is clearly reviewed to show the possibility of both cord and root compression and distortion by such a mechanism.

CLINICAL FEATURES

It is likely that the clinical effects of an arteriovenous malformation are due to a combination of any or all of the above factors. Indeed, the variable contribution of those factors may explain the sometimes unpredictable response to embolization, a procedure which affects the compressive element less markedly.

Arteriovenous malformations of the spinal cord are not characterized by any specific syndrome. Indeed, the protean nature of its natural history makes early diagnosis, i.e. within six months of the first symptom, very difficult in the absence of haemorrhage. In 60% of our cases, two years or more had elapsed before the diagnosis was made. Increasing awareness of arteriovenous malformation as a cause of progressive non-traumatic myelopathy has, however, considerably improved recognition in the past decade. In our own series, of the first 45 of the 104 patients referred to us until 1981, only 17 were recognized within one year of the onset of symptoms, whereas 19 were not properly diagnosed until three to 15 years after the original symptoms began. Within the past 15 years, however, 50 patients were referred to us who had been diagnosed within two years of onset. The symptom of acute subarachnoid haemorrhage has not been described with dural arteriovenous malformations; therefore these do not present with the most pathognomonic features of an arteriovenous malformation of the spinal cord, i.e. a sudden onset of significant neurological deficit with associated severe back pain. This symptom, sometimes called *coup de poignard*, or 'blow of a knife', is typical of the presentation of a spinal arteriovenous malformation with subarachniod haemorrhage.

Difficulty of early diagnosis is often related to the insidious character of the onset of the initial symptoms and signs. The most common deficits to appear first are either motor or sensory, or both, in over 80% of cases. Pain is a frequent component in nearly half the patients. Disturbances of sphincteric and sexual function as initial signs are less common. The acute onset of any or all of these symptoms and signs (usually due to subarachnoid haemorrhage) occurred in only 11% of our cases. The clinical course is invariably progressive, but in a third of our cases the progressions displayed a fluctuating intensity, which is a characteristic feature of intramedullary lesions and well described by other authors (Aminoff, 1976; Kendall & Logue, 1977; Ommaya, 1984a,b; Yasargil *et al.*, 1984; Rosenblum *et al.*, 1987).

It is obvious from the above that there is no unique constellation of symptoms and signs that can characterize the spinal cord arteriovenous malformation. The shortest history in our series was a case with subarachnoid haemorrhage, producing sudden, severe back pain and paraplegia, the final diagnosis being established in less than one week from the first symptom. The longest delay between symptom onset and diagnosis was 16 years in a patient misdiagnosed as having motoneurone disease. Differential diagnosis includes all the disease categories listed in Table 49.2, which summarizes the discharge diagnosis of the 201 patients referred with myelopathy thought to be due to an arteriovenous malformation between 1965 and 1981.

The presence of a cutaneous angiomatous lesion may be of value in indicating and localizing spinal cord arteriovenous malformations, as found in 19% of our first series of 104 cases (Doppman *et al.*, 1969). Bruits over the region of the arteriovenous malformation in the spinal canal are rare, and we have observed this sign in only three patients, each of whom had extensive extradural and extraspinal components.

Occasionally, a temporary clinical deterioration can be seen after trauma, pregnancy, increase of body temperature, overeating, postural changes and muscular exertion, the latter being particularly significant for dural arteriovenous malformations. One of our patients, a successful fund-raiser whose work necessitated regular indulgence in large meals, presented to us with three episodes of postprandial transient paraplegia that spontaneously reversed four to six hours after the meal.

NEURORADIOLOGICAL DIAGNOSIS

Prior to the development of magnetic resonance imaging, the foundation of radiological identification of an arteriovenous malformation was the myelogram. It has been our experience that a completely negative myelogram, when done with a water-soluble medium carried throughout the extent of the spinal canal, is essential if the diagnosis of arteriovenous malformation is to be excluded. On the other hand, angiography has proved to be invariably useless as an exploratory procedure if the myelogram is indeed negative. The selective spinal angiogram, as developed by our work in Bethesda and the work of Djindjian and his colleagues in Paris, is indeed the foundation for the subsequent clarification of the nature of these lesions and their proper surgical management (Doppman *et al.*, 1969; Djindjian *et al.*, 1970). Plain X-ray films were only occasionally useful in our series, with only 6% being positive.

Table 49.2 Discharge diagnosis in 201 patients referred with myelopathy due to suspected arteriovenous malformations (1965–1981)

Spinal arteriovenous malformation	104
Non-traumatic myelopathy of unknown origin	34
Intradural spinal tumour	24
Astrocytoma	12
Ependymoma	4
Haemangioblastoma	4
Neurofibroma	4
Cervical or lumbar spondylosis or disc herniation	20
Syringomyelia	12
Motoneurone disease	2
Multiple sclerosis	2
Chronic arachnoiditis	2
Cholesteatoma of posterior fossa	1

The finding of bony erosions and widening of intervertebral foramena in patients with motosensory deficit in the lower extremities are the main diagnostic clues, but are relatively non-specific. Myelography was positive in 97% of cases and diagnostic for arteriovenous malformation in 86%, showing the characteristic serpiginous filling deficits. The necessity for a complete myelographic examination of the cord, including its dorsal aspect, has been repeatedly emphasized, not only for exact diagnosis, but also to provide the necessary localization of the arteriovenous malformation that precedes angiographic delineation of its vascular details. Thus, in dural arteriovenous malformations, one can often see the enlarged venous drainage beginning laterally close to the location of the dural nidus.

Without myelographic guidance, spinal angiography, as noted above, is tedious and usually futile. In our series, we have not had a single case in which a normal myelogram was found in an arteriovenous malformation case, and myelography of a total nature with normal findings is conclusive in ruling out an arteriovenous malformation. However, cases with non-specifically abnormal myelograms not clinically diagnosed as an arteriovenous malformation, but with clinical evidence of progressive neurological deterioration, should be examined by selective spinal angiography. The relative contributions of the three major modes of radiological investigation of arteriovenous malformation are summarized in Table 49.3.

The interpretation of angiograms, as well as of myelograms, must be based on a clear understanding of the normal intraspinal structure. Selective angiography was successful in demonstrating the lesion in 98% of our cases. An arteriovenous malformation that has been suspected both clinically and myelo-

Table 49.3 Radiological diagnosis

	Positive (%)	Negative (%)
Plain spine films[a]	6	94
Myelography[b]	97	3
Arteriography[c]	98	2

[a] Widening of interpedicular space and bone erosions.
[b] Six did not show typical serpiginous defects. Four had complete blocks. Two of the negative myelograms suggested arachnoiditis only, with subsequent positive angiography.
[c] Six studies were incomplete.

graphically, yet fails to be displayed by careful and repeated selective angiography, suggests a bad prognosis, indicating significant thrombosis within the lesion. Results of surgical removal of such 'non-filling' arteriovenous malformations in our series was not attended by any significant benefit to the patient. Spinal angiography is a time-consuming procedure, and a careful examination of the blood supply and vascular anatomy of a large arteriovenous malformation may require two, or even three, angiographic sessions. It is our practice to protect the patient during such investigations with dexamethasone. Recently we have also begun the use of spinal Wada tests in those cases in which a complex arteriovenous malformation has to be treated by preoperative embolization, and where critical feeders to the anterior spinal artery require functional management (Doppman *et al.*, 1986). This allows a physiological assessment of the importance of any cord supply arising from a feeding vessel.

MANAGEMENT

The methods available for use in the therapy of spinal arteriovenous malformations include: surgical exposure and ligation with partial resection of feeding arteries; definitive procedures for microsurgical total excision of the arteriovenous malformation nidus; and embolization with and without partial resection of arteriovenous malformation components. Embolization of the arteriovenous malformation nidus was used both as a preoperative manoeuvre and as a sole or supplementary mode of therapy. Each of these methods alone, or in combination, has to be utilized by the surgeon wishing to provide optimal management for spinal cord arteriovenous malformation.

The evolution of microsurgical techniques has resulted in a consensus that the true nidus, or shunt zone of the spinal cord arteriovenous malformation, has to be resected *in toto* whenever possible. In our own series dorsal, low-flow lesions with a primarily posterior blood supply—the majority of which have a dural nidus—as well as glomus-type high-flow lesions in the cervical and cervical medullary zones, were amenable to total resection, even where significant intramedullary extensions were present. Anteriorly placed intramedullary or combined lesions, invariably of the high-flow type, were not usually amenable to total resection, and partial resections and arterial ligations, with or without embolization, were alternative procedures undertaken. Intramedullary lesions of the non-glomus, or juvenile, type with the major supply from the anterior spinal arteries are not usually totally resectable. Partial resections in combination with embolization, however, may be quite useful in arresting neurological deterioration and causing neurological improvements in some patients whose onset of symptoms has been relatively recent (within one year.)

The results of the 104 treated cases, which have been followed up adequately, are summarized in Table 49.4. The patients have been divided into three groups, according to the type of therapy used as the primary method of management. Results shown are based on clinical evaluation at a minimum of two years after the primary procedure. The category of result described as 'unchanged' means that the previously progressive myelopathy was arrested, but not reversed. This effect on the pre-existing myelopathy was clear-cut in Group one patients, but often was temporary in Group two and Group three patients followed up for more than five years. Delayed resumption of progressive myelopathy was especially noted in patients over the age of 60 in whom all results were qualitatively less satisfactory. The best results were obtained in low-flow lesions situated over the dorsum of the spinal cord, where total resection and intradural or extradural obliteration of the nidus produced almost equally good results. In high-flow lesions, total resection achieved within the first year of lesion presentation produced similarly good results, especially in the cervical cord, provided the myelopathy was noted to be minimal, and present for less than six months. The worst results occurred

Table 49.4 Results of therapy

Group	Types of therapy	Total number of patients	Improved	Unchanged	Worse
1	Microneurosurgical total resection	64	50	12	2
2	Arterial ligation ± partial resection	28	16	8	4
3	Embolization	12	2	9	1
	Totals	104	68 (65.4%)	29 (27.9%)	7 (6.7%)

in patients in whom angiography failed to reveal the myelographically diagnosed arteriovenous malformation, as well as in patients with progressive myelopathy of more than 12 months duration, and patients with high-flow lesions in whom total resection of the nidus was not achieved. The critical role of symptom duration on the results of treatment was clearly shown in our group one patients, among whom 50 recovered almost completely after surgery was done within the first year of onset of symptoms (Ommaya, 1984a,b).

The course of recovery after surgical treatment can be very variable. Whilst many patients improve steadily following surgery, it is important to recognize that recovery can be very slow and delayed with some patients taking several years to achieve full recovery. It is also of importance to recognize that late deterioration can occur either due to recrudescence of the lesion from previously unrecognized vascular channels or due to arachnoiditis and progressive atrophy of the cord.

It is important to emphasize that the precise nature and operability of a spinal cord arteriovenous malformation is finally determined at the time of exposure during surgery. It is true to say, however, that, with the marked improvement over the past decade in the skill and precision of neuroradiological studies, the surgeon's task has been clarified and it is now possible to treat these lesions in a much more precise manner. The surgical approach to spinal cord arteriovenous malformations is always via laminectomy, and this basic procedure will not be described in any detail. Because of the marked change in the quantity and quality of manual exertion required between the laminectomy phase and the subsequent microneurosurgical phase for treatment of the arteriovenous malformation, it is advisable to allow an assistant to perform the laminectomy. The lateral extent of bone removal should allow wide exposure bilaterally, without disturbing the facet joints, and the length of the laminectomy should be limited to the exposure of the nidus. Preoperative indelible marking of the upper and lower levels of the arteriovenous malformation nidus zone is essential. It is not necessary to expose the extensive venous drainage, except in certain high-flow lesions with multiple feeders at different levels, which may be intertwined with venous components.

After exposure of the dura the microscope is introduced, and the dura is carefully examined, particularly in the lateral recesses and along the roots to assess the dural components of the arteriovenous malformation. A dural opening in the midline is then performed in such a manner as to preserve the arachnoidal layer and prevent the escape of cerebrospinal fluid (CSF) at this stage. Placing separate traction sutures on the dura and then opening the arachnoid, helps to keep the field clear of blood. In this way there is a marked reduction in the risk of premature injury to the arteriovenous malformation, and the overall anatomy of the arteriovenous malformation is seen more clearly when the arachnoid layer is opened in this step-wise manner. The bulging arachnoid is then carefully opened and split in the midline to allow its edges to be lifted up and tacked to the restrained edges of the previously opened dura, using small metal clips. Arachnoidal adhesions to the cord are divided with microscissors, so that the arachnoidal opening can be completed symmetrically so as to display the arteriovenous malformation as fully as possible.

Assuming that the opening has corresponded precisely to the preoperative, angiographically guided landmarks, the arteriovenous malformation should now be fully displayed. If dural feeders had been previously seen, the transdural and intradural components (if any) should be identified. Such extradural or dural feeders usually form single trunks intradurally. An entirely intradural arteriovenous malformation requires thorough examination under low magnification to make as much of a match as possible between the angiographic patterns and the operative findings. Only when this is completed should the actual resection procedures, as detailed below, be initiated. The surgical technique varies dependent upon the nature of the malformation.

Resection of a low-flow, intradural, extramedullary arteriovenous malformation

Typically, the major feeding arteries, which are rarely more than one or two, enter with the dorsal root and travel rostrally, forming a hairpin bend before entering the convoluted venous drainage, as seen in Fig. 49.3. The nidus is essentially subarachnoid and extrapial, and the resection need not extend significantly beyond the artery entering at the dura, and its first or second convolution. It is not uncommon to find multiple small vessels connecting the nidus to the subpial, intramedullary circulation. These are simply coagulated with the bipolar current, and divided at their pial entry. The main nidus is thus removed by a combination of blunt and sharp dissection, proceeding from the entering arterial feeder to the arterialized vein. Successful removal of the nidus should be followed by the onset of patchy pallor and vascular stasis in the residual venous varicosities. These should be carefully examined, and if an area of high-pressure veins remains, a persistent and separate feeder has most probably been missed, and should be searched for and removed. It is unusual to find true subpial, intramedullary extensions of the nidus in such low-flow arteriovenous malformations.

Resection of low-flow, dural arteriovenous malformations

This type of arteriovenous malformation, which is probably the most common arteriovenous malformation in adults, has the majority of its arterial inputs located outside or within the dura itself. Most commonly the intradural component is a single arterialized vein, which while entering with the dorsal root, does not usually form a hairpin bend prior to developing the thoracic venous varicosities, as shown in Fig. 49.4. The extent of nidus resection is shown extending into the critical dural zone. It is seldom necessary to resect dura itself, and careful examination of the extradural and dural components will enable elimination of the nidus with bipolar coagulation of thëdural feeding arteries. These vessels are often multiple and thin-walled. Resection of a significant length of the intradural arterialized vein is usually all that is required to thus permanently disconnect the nidus from its drainage into the intermedullary draining veins.

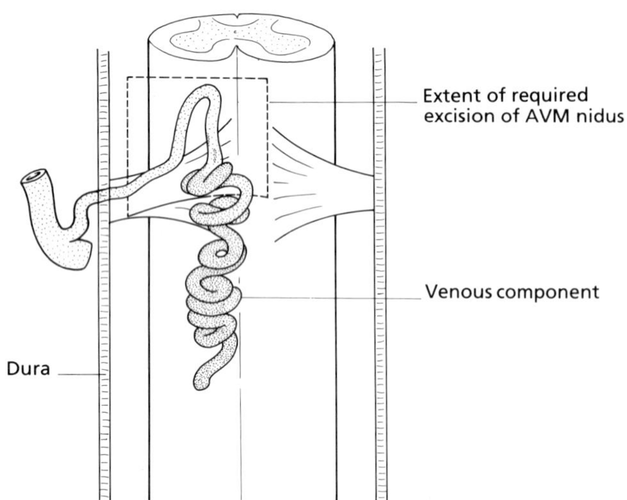

Fig. 49.3 Low-flow arteriovenous malformations (AVM), intradural nidus.

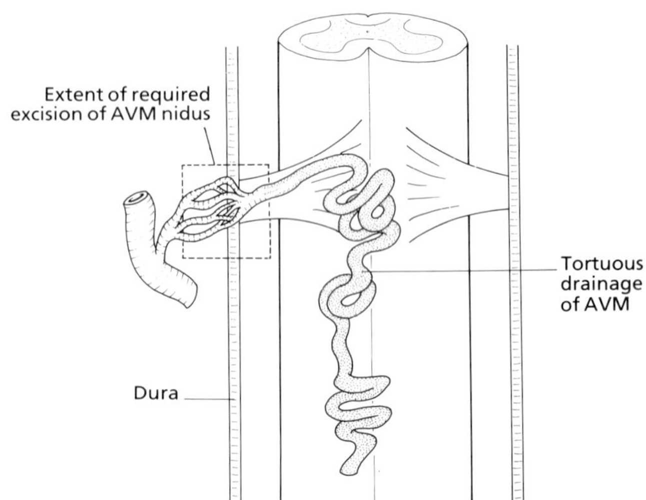

Fig. 49.4 Low-flow arteriovenous malformations (AVM), dural nidus.

Resection of high-flow, extramedullary and intramedullary arteriovenous malformations (juvenile type)

This type of arteriovenous malformation is the most difficult to treat, and radical resection is possible to a much lesser degree as compared to the other two groups described. The usual location is in the thoracolumbar zone and the incidence is in the younger age group, hence the term 'juvenile' given in the classification. The operative exposure in such cases is usually more extensive, and preoperative embolization with extraspinal ligation may be helpful in reducing the volume of the shunt as seen during surgery. The operative approach is identical to that previously described, with the significant difference being that the search for feeding arteries must include sources from the anterior spinal artery. Arachnoidal adhesions tend to be thicker, and more extensive, and sharp dissection is essential to identify vessels which enter lateral and anterolateral aspects of the arteriovenous malformation and spinal cord. Intramedullary extensions are always present, and deliberate myelotomy is often necessary to dissect out the extensive nidus component from within the spinal cord, as shown in Fig. 49.5. It is not uncommon to find radiculomedullary feeding arteries entering at the level of the nidus, and indeed at the level of the artery of Adamkiewicz. If branches from such a vessel are clearly seen to be entering the main nidus, they may be taken with impunity, but only at the level of the nidus, and never at more proximal or extramedullary zones. The main trunk should never be occluded prior to its contribution to the anterior spinal artery.

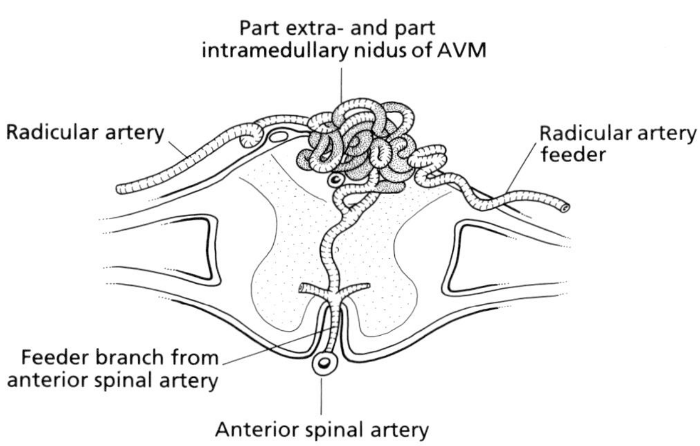

Fig. 49.5 High-flow arteriovenous malformations (AVM), juvenile type.

Complex juvenile arteriovenous malformations may surround and penetrate the cord *'en cuirasse'*, without any compact space-occupying components. In such cases surgical removal is precluded and only palliative results can be achieved.

Resection of high-flow, intramedullary arteriovenous malformation (glomus type)

This type of spinal arteriovenous malformation is often called a glomus angioma because of its compact habitus as compared to the juvenile type. It is most commonly found in the cervical cord, and is predominantly intramedullary, with associated extramedullary components being less significant. In spite of the comparative importance of this part of the spinal cord, total surgical removal of the glomus-like nidus is much more often feasible, as compared to the juvenile arteriovenous malformation lesion described above. The glomus type of lesion is illustrated in Fig. 49.6. Because feeding arteries to such lesions arise not only from radiculopial and radiculomedullary branches, but also directly from central branches of the anterospinal artery, a deliberate myelotomy is required. Dissection on either side of the nidus mass proceeds alternatively to isolate, coagulate and divide these anteriorly approaching vessels through the myelotomy, and removal of the arteriovenous malformation can be accomplished *in toto*. This technique has been very well described by Yasargil *et al.*

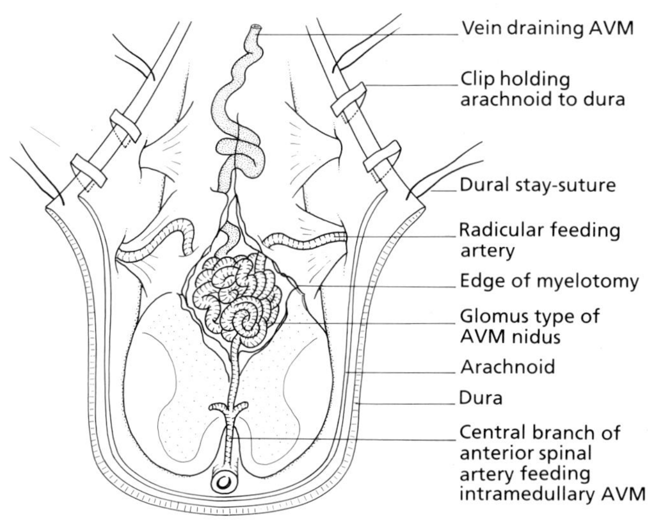

Fig. 49.6 High-flow arteriovenous malformations (AVM), glomus nidus.

(1975) and also by Pia & Djindjian (1978). In tackling intramedullary arteriovenous malformations the morphology of its intramedullary components, as described by Djindjian (1976) is an important guide. There are three basic types, with several subdivisions, and precise details of the microsurgical techniques required are given by Yasargil *et al.* (1984).

A key technical aspect is to maintain the dissection of an intramedullary arteriovenous malformation close to the lesion itself, exactly in the manner in which cerebral arteriovenous malformations are dissected. The gliotic cord tissue has to be gently separated, using blunt dissection with bipolar forceps, and the thin-walled vessels of the arteriovenous malformation have to be coagulated for significant distances of a few millimetres before partial division, recoagulation, and then full division. Clips are often required for vessels larger than 0.2–0.3 mm diameter. Temporary clips are required for vessels which are not clearly identified as being a feeding artery or a draining vein. Just as in the other types of arteriovenous malformation, the decrease in the turgor of the venous components will usually be the endpoint for resection. Excision of the draining veins is not necessary.

Increasing experience with these lesions has not eased the difficulties one faces with atypical variants of these highly variable lesions. Resection of a dorsally placed, low-flow, extramedullary lesion, whether dural or subdural, and with exact correspondence with angiographic and surgical anatomy, is usually quite easy and straightforward. However, the high-flow arteriovenous malformation, with major intramedullary and anteriorly placed components, often with dense cicatricial attachments to normal structure, remains a major challenge. Increasing experience frequently converts the impossible to the merely difficult case, but the hazards for the patient are, correspondingly, much greater.

The role of embolization

Embolization can be a very useful adjunct in the preoperative management of the difficult, high-flow arteriovenous malformation with multiple feeders, and significant anterior or intermedullary components. Recent advances in interventional neuroradiology using mini-balloon catheters, control-setting glues, and improved embolic materials have enabled much greater precision in occluding part, or occasionally all, of the arteriovenous malformation. Unless clinical indications contradict a further procedure it is recommended that laminectomy and exposure of complex intradural high-flow arteriovenous malformations for an attempt at radical removal should be carried out after embolization, or similar, shunt volume reductive procedures have been completed. The principal role of embolization may be summarized as the conversion of a high-flow arteriovenous malformation into a low-flow lesion more amenable to surgical removal of the nidus.

The first report on angiographic demonstration and embolization of an arteriovenous malformation was by Newton & Adams in 1968. Subsequent experiences with embolization were reported by Doppman *et al.* (1971) and by Djindjian (1975). The French school has been very active in this aspect of interventional neuroradiology, and embolization has been demonstrated to be an effective preoperative technique to facilitate surgical resection of difficult lesions (Riche *et al.*, 1983). It may also be the only recourse in patients with previous incomplete surgery with severe arachnoiditis, which makes further surgery hazardous. In low-flow cases with solitary feeders or with few feeders, embolization may well succeed in effectively occluding and delaying the vascularization of the lesion for significant periods of time, but the consensus now is that ultimately such lesions will recur (Hall *et al.*, 1989; Morgan & Marsh, 1989). In an experienced hand it may be considered as part of the angiographic session. Recent advances in catheter and embolic material technology have significantly contributed to the technique of embolization as well as to the improved diagnosis and management of vascular lesions of the spinal cord (Horton *et al.*, 1986). In particular, the use of controlled, intraoperative obliteration of flow in a complicated, high-low lesion with quick-setting polymers may be a very useful addition to our surgical armamentarium. Controlled-release balloon catheters have also been used to detect lateral networks not otherwise seen radiologically, as described by Riche *et al.* (1983). The use of sensory evoked potentials has also been tried by Berenstein and his colleagues (1984) to provide a functional index of the state of the spinal cord during embolization. However, although embolization (like arterial ligation or clipping) may be a useful expedient, it is not a definitive treatment.

REFERENCES

Aboulker, J., Bar, D., Mursault, L., Khoudja, F., Redondo, A., Gard, L. & Nahum, H. (1977) L'hypertension veineuse intra-rachidienne par anomalies multiples du systeme cave: une cause majeure de souffrance médullaire. *Chirugie*, **103**, 1003–1015.

Adamkiewicz, A. (1882) Die Blutgefässe des menschlichen Rückenmarkes. 2. Die Gefässe der Rückenmarksoberfläche. Sitzungsberichte der Akademie der Wissenschaften in Wien. *Mathematisch-naturwissenschaftliche Klasse*, **85**, 101–130.

Aminoff, M.J. (1976) *Spinal Angiomas* (with contributions by V. Logue and B.E. Kendall). Blackwell Scientific Publications, Oxford.

Ansari, F. (1965) Hämatomyelie bei arteriovenösem Hämangiom des Rückenmarks. Ein Betrag zur Pathogenese der Foix-Alajouanineschen Krankheit. *Beitr. Pathol. Anat.*, **131**, 137–161.

Antoni, N. (1962) Spinal vascular malformations (angiomas) and myelomalacia. *Neurology*, **12**, 795–804.

Benhaiem, N., Poirier, J. & Hurth, M. (1983) Arteriovenous fistulae of the meninges draining into the spinal veins. A histological study of 28 cases. *Acta Neuropathol.*, **62**, 103–111.

Berenstein, A., Young, W. & Ransohoff, J. *et al.* (1984) Somatosensory evoked potentials during spinal angiography and therapeutic transvascular embolization. *J. Neurosurg.*, **60**, 777–785.

Bolton, B. (1939) Blood supply of the human spinal cord. *J. Neurol. Psychiatry*, **2**, 137–148.

Bradac, G.B., Pöll, W. & Merland, J.J. (1984) Extradurale angiome mit venöser perimedullarer drainage. *Neurochirurgia*, **27**, 136–140.

Burger, P.C. & Vogel, F.S. (1976) *Surgical Pathology of the Nervous System and its Coverings*. Wiley, New York.

Corbin, J.L. (1961) *Anatomie et Pathologie Artérielles de la Moelle*. Masson, Paris.

DiChiro, G., Doppman, J.L. & Ommaya, A.K. (1967) Selective arteriography of arteriovenous aneurysms of spinal cord. *Radiology*, **88**, 1065–1077.

DiChiro, G., Doppman, J.L. & Ommaya, A.K. (1971) Radiology of spinal arteriovenous malformations. *Prog. Neurol. Surg.*, **4**, 329–354.

Djindjian, M. (1976) *Le traitement chirugical des angiomes intramedullaires*. Thesis, University of Paris.

Djindjian, R. (1975) Embolization of angiomas of the spinal cord. *Surg. Neurol.*, **4**, 411–420.

Djindjian, R., Hurth, M. & Houdart, R. (1970) *L'angiographie de la moelle épinière* (English extract by L. Kricheff). Masson, Paris.

Djindjian, R., Merland, J.J., Djindjian, M. & Stoeter, P. (1981) *Angiography of Spinal Column and Spinal Cord Tumors*. G. Thieme, Stuttgart.

Dommisse, G.F. (1975) *The Arteries and Veins of the Human Spinal Cord from Birth*. Churchill Livingstone, Edinburgh.

Doppman, J.L., DiChiro, G. & Ommaya, A.K. (1969) *Selective Angiography of the Spinal Cord*. Warren H. Green, St. Louis.

Doppman, J.L., DiChiro, G. & Ommaya, A.K. (1971) Percutaneous embolization of spinal cord arteriovenous malformation. *J. Neurosurg.*, **34**, 48–55.

Doppman J.L., Girton, M. & Oldfield, E.H. (1986) Spinal Wada test. *Radiology*, **161**, 319–321.

Doppman, J.L., Wirth, F.P. Jr, DiChiro, G. & Ommaya, A.K. (1969) Value of cutaneous angiomas in the arteriographic localization of spinal cord arteriovenous malformations. *N. Engl. J. Med.*, **281**, 1440–1444.

Foix, C. & Alajouanine, T. (1926) La myélite nécrotique subaigue. *Rev. Neurol.*, **33**, 1–42.

Gaupp, J. (1887) Casustische Beiträge zur pathologischen Anatomie des Rückenmarks und seiner Häute. *Beitr. Pathol. Anat.*, **2**, 510–524.

Hall, W.A., Oldfield, E.H. & Doppman, J.L. (1989) Recanalization of spinal arteriovenous malformations following embolization. *J. Neurosurg.*, **70**, 714–720.

Hebold, O. (1885) Aneurysmen der kliensten Rückenmarkgefässe. *Arch. Psychiatr. Nervenkr.*, **16**, 813–823.

Herren, R.Y. & Alexander, I. (1939) Sulcal and intrinsic blood vessels of human spinal cord. *Arch. Neurol. Psychiatry*, **41**, 678–687.

Horton, J.A., Latchaw, R.E., Gold, L.H. *et al.* (1986) Embolization of intramedullary arteriovenous malformations of the spinal cord. *Am. J. Neuroradiol.*, **7**, 113–118.

Hughes, J.T. (1967) *The blood supply and vascular disorders of the human spinal cord*. DPhil Thesis, University of Oxford.

Hughes, J.T. (1971) Venous infarction of the spinal cord. *Neurology*, **21**, 794–800.

Hume, Adams J., Corsallis, J.A.N. & Duchen, L.W. (eds) (1984) *Greenfield's Neuropathology*, 4th edn. Wiley, New York.

Jellinger, K. (1966) *Zur Orthologie und Pathologie der Rückenmarksdurchblutung*. Springer, Berlin.

Jellinger, K. (1978) Pathology of spinal vascular malformations and vascular tumors. In Pia, H.W. & Drindjian, R. (eds) *Spinal Angiomas: Advances in Diagnosis and Therapy*, pp. 47–59. Springer, New York.

Kadyi, H. (1889) *Ueber die Blutgefässe des nenschlichen Rückenmarkes*. Gubrynowicz & Schmidt, Lemberg.

Kaufman, H.H., Ommaya, A.K., DiChiro, G. & Doppman, J.L. (1970) Compression vs. 'steal': the pathogenesis of symptoms in arteriovenous malformations of the spinal cord. *Arch. Neurol.*, **23**, 173–178.

Kendall, B.E. & Logue, V. (1977) Spinal epidural angiomatous malformations draining into intrathecal veins. *Neuroradiology*, **13**, 181–189.

Lazorthes, G., Gouaze, A. & Djindjian, R. (1958) *Vascularization et pathologie vasculaire de la moelle épinière*. Masson, Paris.

Manelfe, C., Lazorthes, G. & Roulleau, J. (1972) Artères de la dure-mère rachidienne chez l'homme. *Acta Radiol.*, **13**, 829–841.

McCormick, W.F. (1966) The pathology of vascular ('arteriovenous') malformations. *J. Neurosurg.*, **24**, 807–816.

McCormick, W.F. & Nofzinger, J.D. (1966) 'Cryptic' vas-

cular malformations of the central nervous system. *J. Neurosurg.*, **24**, 865–875.
Merland, J.J., Riché, M.C. & Chiras, J. (1980) Les fistules arterio-veineuses intra-canalaires, extra-medullaires à drainage veineux médullaire. *J. Neuroradiol.*, **7**, 271–320.
Morgan, M.K. & Marsh, W.R. (1989) Management of spinal dural arteriovenous malformations. *J. Neurosurg.*, **70**, 832–836.
Newton, T.H. & Adams, J.E. (1968) Angiographic demonstration and nonsurgical embolization of spinal cord angioma. *Radiology*, **91**, 873–876.
Ommaya, A.K. (1973) Arteriovenous malformations of the spinal cord. In Youmans, J.R. (ed.) *Neurological Surgery*, 1st edn, pp. 852–862. Saunder, Philadelphia, PA.
Ommaya, A.K. (1984a) Arteriovenous malformations of the spinal cord. In Wilkins, R. & Rengachary, S. (eds) *Neurosurgery*, pp. 1499–1495. McGraw-Hill, New York.
Ommaya, A.K. (1984b) Surgery for arteriovenous malformations of the spinal cord (spinal angiomas). In J. Ransohoff (ed.) *Modern Techniques in Surgery*, vol. 34, *Neurosurgery*. Instalment VI, pp. 1–14. Futura, New York.
Ommaya, A.K., DiChiro, G. & Doppman, J. (1969) Ligation of arterial supply in the treatment of spinal cord arteriovenous malformations. *J. Neurosurg.*, **30**, 679–692.
Pia, H.W. & Djindjian R. (eds) (1978) *Spinal Angiomas: Advances in Diagnosis and Therapy*. Springer Verlag, Berlin, Heidelberg, New York.
Rees-Cosgrove, G., Bertrand, G., Fontaine, S. *et al.* (1988) Cavernous angiomas of the spinal cord. *J. Neurosurg.*, **68**, 31–36.
Riche, M.C., Melki, J.P. & Merland, J.J. (1983) Embolization of spinal cord vascular malformations via the anterior spinal artery. *Am. J. Neuroradiol.*, **4**, 378–381.
Rosenblum, B., Oldfield, E.H., Doppman, J.L. *et al.* (1987) Spinal arteriovenous malformations: a comparison of dural arteriovenous fistulas and intradural AVMs in 81 patients. *J. Neurosurg.*, **67**, 795–802.
Sahs, A.L. (1942) The vascular supply of the spinal cord in monkeys. *J. Comp. Neurol.*, **76**, 403–415.
Scholz, W. & Manuelidis, E.E. (1951) Myélite nécrotique (Foix-Alajouanine)-Angiodysgenetische nekrotisierende Myelopathie. *Dtsch. Z. Nervenheilk.*, **165**, 56–71.
Suh, T.H. & Alexander, L. (1939) Vascular system of the human spinal cord. *Arch. Neurol. Psychiatry*, **41**, 659–677.
Symon, L., Kuyama, H. & Kendall, B. (1984) Dural arteriovenous malformations of the spine. Clinical features and results in 55 cases. *J. Neurosurg.*, **60**, 238–247.
Thron, A.K., Rossberg, C. & Mironov, A. (1988) *Vascular Anatomy of the Spinal Cord Neuroradiological Investigations of Clinical Syndromes*. Springer-Verlag, Vienna.
Turnbull, J.M., Breig, A. & Hassler, O. (1966) Blood supply of cervical spinal cord in man; a microangiographic cadaver study. *J. Neurosurg.*, **24**, 951–965.
Vuia, O. & Alexaniu, M. (1969) Arteriovenous shunt in the spinal cord circulation. *Acta Neurol. Scand.*, **45**, 216–223.
Wirth, F.P. Jr, Post, K.D., DiChiro, G., Doppman, J.L. & Ommaya, A.K. (1970) Foix–Alajouanine disease: spontaneous thrombosis of a spinal cord arteriovenous malformation. *Neurology*, **20**, 1114–1118.
Wyburn-Mason, R. (1943) *The Vascular Abnormalities and Tumors of the Spinal Cord and its Membranes*. Kimpton, London.
Yasargil, M.G., DeLong, N.B. & Guarnuschelli, J.J. (1975) Complete microsurgical excision of cervical extramedullary and intramedullary malformations. *Surg. Neurol.*, **4**, 211–224.
Yasargil, M.G., Symon, L. & Teddy, P.J. (1984) Arteriovenous malformations of the spinal cord. In *Advances and Standards in Neurosurgery*, vol. II. Springer, Vienna.

50 · Occlusive Vascular Disease of the Spine

By P.R.D. HUMPHREY

In contrast to cerebral ischaemia, occlusive vascular disease of the spine is undoubtedly rare. There are no epidemiological figures concerning the incidence and a significant proportion is iatrogenic following aortic or cardiac surgery (Kim *et al.*, 1988).

The blood supply of the spinal cord has been described in Chapter 49. The regression of the paired embryological segmental vessels leaves a small but variable number of critical vessels which supply the anterior spinal arterial system and a somewhat greater number of vessels to the paired posterior systems. Certain of these persisting vessels, such as the artery of Adamkiewicz, provide a dominant role in the arterial supply of large regions of the spinal cord. Both the anterior and posterior systems may be relatively incomplete in certain regions, and flow may occur in either rostral or caudal directions. This creates areas where zones of potential ischaemia may exist, the so-called 'watershed zones', the most critical of which is in the upper thoracic region. Within the substance of the spinal cord itself there are no anastomotic channels and the vessels of supply become end-arteries.

Following obstruction of the subclavian and vertebral arteries the blood supply to the cervical cord comes from anastomoses between the occipital, thyroid, cervical and internal mammary arteries. In obstruction of the artery of Adamkiewicz, anastomoses can appear from the anterior and posterior lumbosacral radicular arteries. The venous drainage of the spinal cord is via the anterior and posterior spinal veins and thence into the radicular veins. These anastomose with epidural veins and thence into vertebral, intercostal, lumbar and sacral veins. Ultimately they drain into the jugular, azygos and pelvic venous systems.

The physiology of the spinal circulation is similar to the cerebral circulation with vasodilatation following CO_2 administration or hypoxia. Autoregulation maintains a constant blood flow through the normal range of blood pressure. There is a dense autonomic innervation of the blood vessels with adrenergic and cholinergic fibres which control constriction and dilatation (Peerless *et al.*, 1972).

PATHOGENESIS

A large number of causes of spinal infarction have been reported (Table 50.1). Ischaemia may follow embolic events from the heart or great vessels and primary atherothrombotic events in the aorta or its branches, analogous to cerebrovascular disease. Loss of perfusion pressure, which may be generalized or local especially as a result of disease or operative procedures on the aorta, is a particularly common cause of spinal infarction. Trauma to the aorta or dissection of its branches may also result in spinal cord infarction. Arteriovenous malformation (AVM) may result in spinal ischaemia due to thrombosis or steal, and spinal cord infarction may result from an AVM without evidence of haemorrhage. Arteritis due to collagen vascular disease or infection, forms an important aetiology as it may be treatable.

CLINICAL SYNDROMES

Anterior spinal artery syndrome

This is the most commonly recognized syndrome following ischaemia of the cord. It is usually of sudden onset with paraparesis or quadriparesis, spinothalamic sensory loss and sphincter involve-

Table 50.1 Causes of spinal cord ischaemia

Cause	References
Hypotension	Blumbergs & Byrne, 1980; Brown *et al.*, 1987
Cardiac arrest, saddle embolus	Silver & Buxton, 1974
Valvular heart disease	Whiteley *et al.*, 1979
Subacute bacterial endocarditis	Corbin, 1961
Atrial myxoma	Hirose *et al.*, 1979
Cardiomyopathy	Kochar *et al.*, 1987
Cardiac surgery	Puntis & Green, 1985
Atherosclerosis	Hughes & Brownell, 1966
Aortic dissection	El Toraei & Juler, 1979
Aortic and thoracic surgery	Ross, 1985
Aortic thrombosis, rupture, coarctation	Ross, 1985; Sumpio & Gusberg, 1987
Intra-aortic balloon	Harris *et al.*, 1986
Angiography	El Toraei & Juler, 1979
Therapeutic embolization	Gang *et al.*, 1977
Vertebral occlusion and dissection	Schneider & Schemm, 1961
Cervical sprain and dislocation	Grinker & Guy, 1927
Cervical spondylosis	Hughes & Brownell, 1964
Intervertebral disc embolism	Srigley *et al.*, 1981
Infection and granulomatous meningitis, tuberculosis, malaria, syphilis	Spiller, 1909
Collagen disease	
Polyarteritis nodosa	Whiteley *et al.*, 1979
Giant-cell arteritis	Gibb *et al.*, 1985
Takayasu	Nair *et al.*, 1985
Sickle cell anaemia	Rothman & Nelson, 1980
Plasmacytoma	Schott *et al.*, 1959
Reticulum cell sarcoma	Isrow *et al.*, 1976
Diabetes mellitus	Whiteley *et al.*, 1979
Phenol	Hughes, 1970
Sympathectomy	Hughes & MacIntyre, 1963

ment; dorsal column sensation is spared (Spiller, 1909). Rarely a single anterior spinal artery branch is affected, resulting in a Brown–Séquard syndrome with intact dorsal column sensation. Due to its acute onset, classical signs of spinal cord disease are often absent, the patient usually being hypotonic and areflexic (Henson & Parsons, 1967). The more classical upper motoneurone signs appear later. Occlusion of the origin of the anterior spinal artery may produce damage to the hypoglossal nucleus, medial lemniscus and pyramidal tract; there is thus contralateral pyramidal weakness with dorsal column loss and ipsilateral twelfth nerve palsy (Davison, 1937). Atrophy of the small hand muscles may appear in the long term if the insult is in the cervical region. Radicular, especially girdle, or ascending leg pain occasionally occurs.

More rarely the clinical picture evolves over hours, and a chronic form has been described by Marie & Foix in 1912 and by Hughes & Brownell, 1966. Here a painless progressive flaccid areflexic paraplegia with wasting of the legs may occur.

Transient spinal ischaemic episodes have also been described in coarctation of the aorta, aortic dissection and with anteriovenous malformations (Kendall & Andrew, 1972; Rosen, 1988). Other transient cases may follow embolic events from the heart or aorta. Infarction is most commonly in the upper to midthoracic region, where there is a watershed area and collateral supply is poorest.

Posterior spinal artery syndrome

This is rare: it results in dorsal column sensory loss below the level of the lesions with anaesthesiae. Tendon reflexes are lost. However, the clinical differentiation of anterior and posterior spinal artery syndromes is not always so clear-cut. Sphincter loss and weakness has been reported in some cases of posterior spinal artery occlusion (Hughes, 1970), although inspection of the individual case reports leaves doubt about the specificity of the lesions concerned.

Lacunar lesions

Fieschi *et al.* (1970) have described lacunar lesions in the spinal cord of elderly atherosclerotic subjects. They were mainly located in the lower cervical and mid-dorsal tracts in the grey matter and anterior horn cells. All of their patients had cerebral ischaemic lesions clinically.

Venous infarction

Venous infarction is also rare: it often follows venous thrombosis elsewhere as a result of malignancy of sepsis. There is back pain with progressive paralysis, sensory and sphincter loss coming on over hours to days. Venous infarction may be haemorrhagic or non-haemorrhagic (Kim *et al.*, 1984). Haemorrhagic infarction tends to be more sudden in onset and is often accompanied by more pain. In non-haemorrhagic infarction, Kim *et al.* (1984) described a case with a clinical story over one year. The prognosis is poor, and any part of the cord may be affected. The causes of venous infarction described by Kim *et al.* are shown in Table 50.2.

INVESTIGATION AND DIFFERENTIAL DIAGNOSIS

Spinal cord ischaemia is usually suspected if the deficit is of abrupt onset. The differential diagnosis includes viral myelitis, demyelinating and necrotizing meylitis, myelitis as a non-metastatic effect of malignancy, sarcoidosis, spinal cord compression, bacterial infection, radionecrosis and syringomyelia.

A full assessment of the vascular system is important, particular attention being paid to peripheral pulses and possible sources of emboli. Clearly a history of any preceding events may give a clue to the aetiology. Ultrasound of the abdomen may demonstrate aortic pathology.

All patients require full blood count, erythrocyte sedimentation rate (ESR), urea and electrolytes, serology for syphilis, blood sugar, chest X-ray, and electrocardiography. Some may require detailed cardiac assessment or more sophisticated haematological/vasculitic investigation. Plain X-rays of the spine, followed by myelography with cerebrospinal fluid (CSF) analysis and/or magnetic resonance imaging are necessary to exclude an acute compressive cause; however, myelography may show a swollen spinal cord after infarction. Investigation may also provide evidence of an AVM or infective cause. Cytology of the CSF may be useful and the CSF in spinal cord ischaemia may show a mild lymphocytic pleocytosis with a slightly raised protein.

Table 50.2 Causes of venous infarction

Haemorrhagic
Acute myelogenous leukaemia
Thrombophlebitis migrans
Pulmonary emboli
Furunculosis with thrombophlebitis
Spinal gliosarcoma
Orchidectomy
Tuberculosis
Pelvic infection with thrombophlebitis
Liver abscess
Non-haemorrhagic
Polycythaemia rubra vera
Thrombophlebitis migrans
Pulmonary emboli
Thrombosis leg veins
Decompression sickness
Chronic meningitis

TREATMENT

There is no specific treatment for spinal cord ischaemia. In view of the acute onset with frequent loss of sensation, care of bowel, bladder and skin is important. Treatment is aimed at finding a specific treatable cause (see Table 50.1). Identification of vascular risk factors such as hypertension, smoking, hypercholesterolaemia and diabetes mellitus is important to prevent further damage. Emergency aortic reconstruction may be necessary after dissection or trauma. If the cause is found to be embolic, then anticoagulant or antiplatelet drugs should be considered, especially if the deficit is progressing.

Experimental data have suggested that thiopentone, hypothermia, magnesium, opiate antagonists (naloxone) and the calcium channel blocker, nimodipine, may all be effective in reducing the neurological deficit after ischaemia or increasing spinal cord blood flow in animals; however, in all these cases it was given soon after the ischaemic insult, or in some cases before (Faden *et al.*, 1981; Vacanti & Ames, 1984; Robertson *et al.*, 1986; Guha *et al.*, 1987). There is no real evidence that these agents are useful in the clinical situation.

Prophylaxis

Rapid reduction in blood pressure has on several occasions resulted in spinal cord ischaemia: it is clearly important to be prudent when treating hypertension, particularly as an emergency (Brown *et al.*, 1987). Prophylaxis is most important when aortic surgery is being undertaken. This especially applies if the thoracic aorta is being repaired. Cross-clamping should whenever possible be for periods of less than 30 minutes: the higher the cross-clamp the more likely is spinal cord ischaemia. Cross-clamping increases the proximal blood pressure, which in turn increases the CSF pressure. This, combined with the reduced distal aortic pressure, is likely to reduce spinal cord perfusion. Some authors have advocated the use of either intrathecal drainage of CSF or intrathecal papaverine preoperatively to reduce CSF pressure and hence maintain the perfusion pressure to the cord.

Somatic sensory evoked potentials (SSEPs) may be useful to monitor spinal cord function to detect impending ischaemia in aortic surgery (Krieger & Spencer, 1985; Dasmahapatra *et al.*, 1987). However, such monitoring only assesses dorsal column function, which is likely to be unaffected by ischaemia.

Hypotension should be avoided during aortic surgery. Some surgeons have advocated the use of shunts; others argue that the increased morbidity and time associated with shunt insertion does not justify their routine use (Svensson & Hinder, 1987). Partial or total cardiopulmonary bypass may have a part to play in some cases (Laschinger *et al.*, 1987). Preservation of the branches of the aorta is important in protecting the spinal cord, particularly if there is backflow.

REFERENCES

Blumbergs, P.C. & Byrne, E. (1980) Hypotensive central infarction of the spinal cord. *J. Neurol. Neurosurg. Psychiatry*, **43**, 751–753.

Brown, P., Gross, M. & Harrison, M.J.G. (1987) Paraplegia following oral hypotensive treatment of malignant hypertension. *J. Neurol. Neurosurg. Psychiatry*, **50**, 104.

Corbin, J.L. (1961) *Anatomie et Pathologie Arterielles de la Moelle.* Masson et Cie, Paris.

Dasmahapatra, H.K., Coles, J.G., Taylor, M.J., Cass, D., Couper, G., Adler, S., Burrows, F., Sherret, H., Trusler, G.A. & Williams, W.G. (1987) Identification of risk factors for spinal cord ischaemia by the use of monitoring of somatosensory evoked potentials during coarctation repair. *Circulation*, **76** (Suppl. IIIK), 14–18.

Davison, C. (1937) Syndrome of the anterior spinal artery of the medulla oblongata. *Arch. Neurol. Psychiatry (Chicago)*, **37**, 91–107.

El-Toraei, I. & Juler, G. (1979) Ischaemia myelopathy. *Angiology*, **30**, 81–94.

Faden, A.I., Jacobs, T.P. & Holaday, J.W. (1981) Opiate antagonist improves neurological recovery after spinal injury. *Science*, **211**, 493–494.

Fieschi, C., Gottlieb, A. & De Carolis, V. (1970) Ischaemic lacunae in the spinal cord of arteriosclerotic subjects. *J. Neurol. Neurosurg. Psychiatry*, **33**, 138–146.

Gang, D.L., Dole, K.B. & Adelman, L.S. (1977) Spinal cord infarction following therapeutic renal artery embolization. *J. Am. Med. Assoc.*, **237**, 2841–2842.

Gibb, W.R.G., Urry, P.A. & Lees, A.J. (1985) Giant cell arteritis with spinal cord infarction and basilar artery thrombosis. *J. Neurol. Neurosurg. Psychiatry*, **48**, 945–948.

Grinker, R.R. & Guy, C.C. (1927) Sprain of the cervical spine causing thrombosis of the anterior spinal artery. *J. Am. Med. Assoc.*, **88**, 1140–1142.

Guha, A., Tator, C.H. & Piper, I. (1987) Effect of calcium channel blocker on post-traumatic spinal cord blood flow. *J. Neurosurg.*, **66**, 423–430.

Henson, R.A. & Parsons, M. (1967) Ischaemic lesions of the spinal cord. *Q. J. Med.*, **36**, 205–222.

Hirose, G., Kosoegawa, H. & Takado, M. (1979) Spinal cord ischaemia and left atrial myxoma. *Arch. Neurol.*, **36**, 439.

Hughes, J.T. (1970) Thrombosis of the posterior spinal arteries. *Neurology*, **20**, 659–664.

Hughes, J.T. & Brownell, B. (1964) Cervical spondylosis complicated by anterior spinal artery thrombosis. *Neurology*, **14**, 1073–1077.

Hughes, J.T. & Brownell, B. (1966) Spinal cord ischaemia due to arteriosclerosis. *Arch. Neurol.*, **15**, 189–202.

Hughes, J.T. & MacIntyre, A.G. (1963) Spinal cord infarction during thoracolumbar sympathectomy. *J. Neurol. Neurosurg. Psychiatry*, **26**, 418–421.

Isrow, L.A., Thomas, G.W. & Hadfield, M.G. (1976) Massive spinal cord infarction due to vascular invasion by reticulum cell sarcoma. *Va. Med.*, **103**, 213–217.

Kendall, B.E. & Andrew, J. (1972) Neurogenic intermittent claudication associated with aortic steal from the anterior spinal artery complicating coarctation of the aorta. *J. Neurosurg.*, **37**, 89–94.

Kim, R.C., Smith, H.R., Henbest, M.L. & Choi, B.H. (1984) Non-haemorrhagic venous infarction of the spinal cord. *Ann. Neurol.*, **15**, 379–385.

Kim, S.W., Kim, R.C., Choi, B.H. & Gordon, S.K. (1988) Non-traumatic ischaemic myelopathy. A review of 25 cases. *Paraplegia*, **26**, 262–272.

Kochar, G., Kotler, M.N., Hartman, J., Goldberg, S.E., Parry, W., Parameswaran, M.D. & Scanlon, M. (1987) Thrombosed aorta resulting in spinal cord ischaemia and paraplegia in ischaemic cardiomyopathy. *Am. Heart J.*, **113**, 1510–1513.

Krieger, K.H. & Spencer, F.C. (1985) Is paraplegia after repair of coarctation of the aorta due principally to distal hypotension during aortic cross-clamping? *Surgery*, **97**, 2–7.

Laschinger, J.C., Izumoto, H. & Kouchoukos, N.T. (1987) Evolving concepts in prevention of spinal cord injury during operations on the descending thoracic and thoracoabdominal aorta. *Ann. Thoracic Surg.*, **44**, 667–74.

Marie, P. & Foix, C. (1912) L'atrophie isolée non-progressive des petits muscles de la main. Frequence relative et pathogénie. Tephromalacie anterieure. Polyo-myélite, nérvite radiculaire au non radiculaire. *Nouv. Iconog. Salpêt.*, **25**, 353–363, 427–453.

Nair, K.R., Bhaskasran, R., Retrakumari, S. & Madhusoodanam, M. (1985) Ischaemic myelopathy in Takayasu's disease. *J. Assoc. Phys. India*, **33**, 735–736.

Peerless, S.J., Yasargil, M.G. & Kendall, M.J. (1972) The adrenergic and cholinergic innervation of the cerebral blood vessels. In Fusek, I. & Kune, Z. (eds) *Present Limits of Neurosurgery*, pp. 199–202. Avicenum, Prague.

Puntis, J.W.L. & Green, S.H. (1985) Ischaemic spinal cord

after cardiac surgery. *Arch. Dis. Childh.*, **60**, 517–520.

Robertson, C.S., Foltz, R., Grossman, R.G. & Goodman, J.C. (1986) Protection against experimental ischaemic spinal cord injury. *J. Neurosurg.*, **64**, 633–642.

Rosen, S.A. (1988) Painless aortic dissection presenting as spinal cord ischaemia. *Ann. Emerg. Med.*, **17**, 840–842.

Ross, R.T. (1985) Spinal cord infarction in disease and surgery of the aorta. *J. Canad. Sci. Neurol.*, **12**, 289–295.

Rothman, S.M. & Nelson, J.S. (1980) Spinal cord infarction in a patient with sickle cell anaemia. *Neurology*, **30**, 1072–1076.

Schneider, R.C. & Schemm, G.W. (1961) Vertebral artery insufficiency in acute and chronic spinal cord trauma. *J. Neurosurg.*, **18**, 348–360.

Schott, B., Cotte, L. & Tommasi, M. (1959) Ramollissement spinal posterieur en D7–D8 par my myelome ossenx plasmocytaire D_{11}–L_1. *Rev. Neurol.*, **101**, 16–27.

Silver, J.R. & Buxton, P.H. (1974) Spinal stroke. *Brain*, **97**, 539–550.

Spiller, W.G. (1909) Thrombosis of the cervical anterior median spinal artery. Syphilitic acute anterior poliomyelitis. *J. Nerv. Ment. Dis.*, **36**, 601–613.

Srigley, J.R., Lambert, C.D., Bilbao, J.M. & Pritzker, K.P.H. (1981) Spinal cord infarction secondary to intervertebral disc embolism. *Ann. Neurol.*, **9**, 297–301.

Sumpio, B.E. & Gusberg, R.J. (1987) Aortic thrombosis with paraplegia: an unusual consequence of blunt abdominal trauma. *J. Vasc. Surg.*, **6**, 412–414.

Svensson, L.G. & Hinder, R.A. (1987) Haemodynamics of aortic cross clamping: experimental observations and clinical applications. *Surg. Ann.*, **19**, 41–65.

Vacanti, F.X. & Ames, A. (1984) Mild hypothermia and Mg^{++} protect against irreversible damage during C.N.S. ischaemia. *Stroke*, **15**, 695–698.

Whiteley, A.M., Hauw, J.J. & Escourolle, R. (1979) A pathological survey of 41 cases of acute intrinsic spinal cord disease. *J. Neurol. Sci.*, **42**, 229–242.

SECTION 11
INFLAMMATORY DISEASES OF THE SPINE

51 · Chronic Inflammatory Diseases of the Spine

By M.I.V. JAYSON

The various forms of inflammatory arthritis produce a chronic inflammatory synovitis commonly localized to the joints and related structures. This produces progressive erosion of articular cartilage and joint damage. The initial pathology is predominantly chronic inflammatory swelling, but subsequent erosion and destruction of articular surfaces, tendons and ligaments leads to progressive deformity. These processes occur in the spine as well as in peripheral joints, and can give rise to a wide variety of forms of spinal damage.

The spine may be involved by a wide variety of forms of chronic inflammatory arthritis. The most common are rheumatoid arthritis and ankylosing spondylitis, together with related disorders. However, other problems may involve the spine. In assessing patients with chronic spinal damage it is important to determine the underlying diagnosis and to assess the severity and extent of damage to spinal structures. In particular it is important to distinguish symptoms and signs arising from inflammation, as distinct from the secondary mechanical damage, as this can dictate the optimum approaches to treatment.

RHEUMATOID ARTHRITIS

Rheumatoid arthritis is a systemic chronic inflammatory disorder in which the most obvious feature is a chronic, inflammatory, symmetrical, peripheral polyarthritis. The disease is usually associated with the presence of rheumatoid factor in the blood. The characteristic pathology lies in the synovium, which is thickened with chronic inflammatory cell proliferation and surface cell hyperplasia. As the disease progresses there is erosion of articular cartilage and bone. This, combined with inflammation of tendon sheaths, gives rise to the characteristic deformities seen in advanced disease.

Rheumatoid arthritis commonly affects the cervical spine. In particular disease at the atlanto-axial joint may lead to subluxation and neurological damage. In the lower cervical spine, instability may be followed by forward subluxation of the vertebrae, again producing neurological damage. Involvement of the lumbar spine is less well recognized. It may be followed by severe destructive changes with a kyphoscoliosis and back pain.

Atlanto-axial disease

The odontoid peg normally is held against the anterior arch of the atlas by the transverse ligament. Rheumatoid synovitis of the bursa between this ligament and the odontoid peg can lead to erosion of the odontoid peg (Fig. 51.1), weakening and rupture of the ligament and atlanto-axial instability. There is backward movement of the odontoid peg which may impinge on the upper cervical spinal cord and brain stem. Of particular importance in some patients is atlanto-axial instability during flexion of the neck. The atlas moves forward and the odontoid peg relatively backwards, with risk of severe neurological damage. In a proportion of patients ligamentous damage combined with erosion of the atlanto-axial joints may allow the cranium to settle on the cervical spine with apparent vertical subluxation of the odontoid peg which can become embedded in the brain stem and lead to severe neurological complications.

Subaxial cervical involvement

Rheumatoid inflammation may affect both the apophyseal joints and the tiny uncovertebral joints at

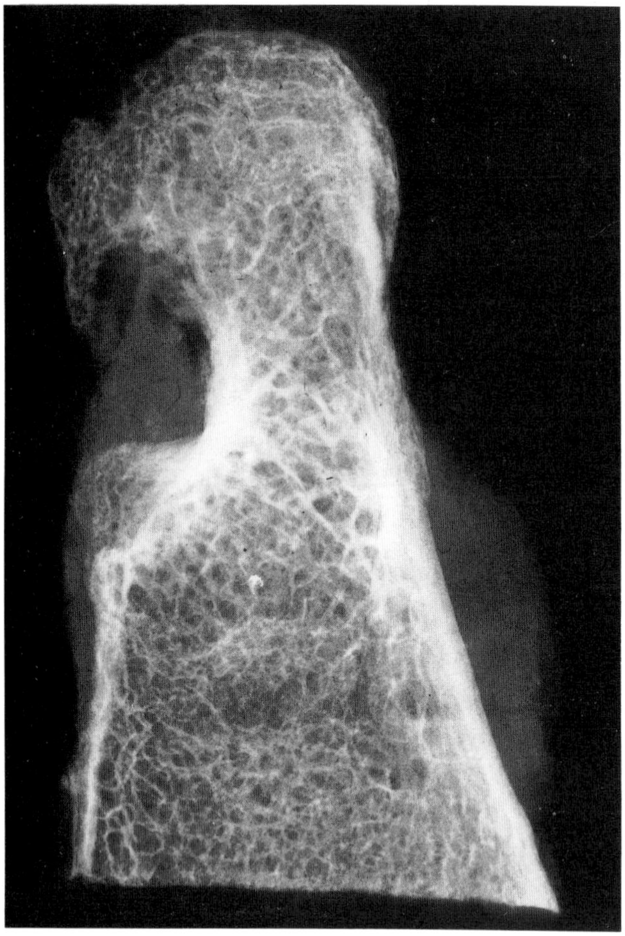

Fig. 51.1 Microradiograph of odontoid peg in rheumatoid arthritis showing posterior erosion. Courtesy of Dr A.J. Freemont.

the lateral margins of the intervertebral discs. There is progressive erosion of the apophyseal joint surfaces and destruction of the substance of the intervertebral disc with loss of disc height and lower cervical instability (Fig. 51.2a,b). This process predominantly occurs at C4, C5, C6 and C7, with the development of anterior subluxation of these vertebrae on top of each other. This process is aggravated by forward flexion of the neck, and there is risk of upper motoneurone damage to the cervical cord, and lower motoneurone damage to the cervical nerve roots.

Clinical features of cervical involvement

Rheumatoid involvement of the cervical spine is virtually always associated with severe peripheral arthritis. The clinical features of peripheral rheumatoid arthritis are obvious, and should alert the clinician to the possible risks of cervical involvement and instability. Patients requiring general anaesthesia are at particular risk even if their cervical disease is asymptomatic. In the patient with cervical instability the loss of protective reflexes, combined with unguarded movements of the neck and perhaps forcible neck movements during insertion of the endotracheal tube, may produce severe neurological damage. There have been a number of cases of patients undergoing general anaesthesia and suffering devastating neurological complications. The symptoms of rheumatoid involvement of the neck can be relatively mild, and may easily be ignored because of many more prominent features of the disease. Any patient with rheumatoid arthritis undergoing general anaesthesia should undergo routinely appropriate investigations including flexion/extension radiographs of the cervical spine. If there is any evidence of cervical instability the anaesthetist and other staff must be appropriately warned to protect the neck. The patients should wear a cervical collar when sent to theatre. This provides only minimal direct protection of the neck but does alert all staff to the presence of cervical problems so they ensure the neck is properly protected.

It is a characteristic of rheumatoid inflammation that symptoms are aggravated by rest. In particular patients commonly experience their symptoms at their worst when they first wake in the morning with severe stiffness, aching and pain, and there is a variable period of time which can last several hours until the symptoms ease up. Later in the day when the patient is tired there is often an exacerbation of aching and stiffness. Examination of the neck will show limitation of cervical movements with reproduction of symptoms. In particular forward flexion and extension may be limited, although not necessarily so. Lateral flexion is more severely affected than lateral rotation. It is possible to palpate the back of the pharynx with the finger and to assess the atlanto-axial joints and recognize instability during flexion of the neck. However, this examination is extremely unpleasant for the patient and commonly produces severe gagging. Careful palpation of the cervical spine with the patient lying prone and relaxed may reveal localized tenderness of the apophyseal joints and help to identify the particular joints which are affected.

The symptoms of cervical involvement are pain and stiffness in the back of the neck, commonly

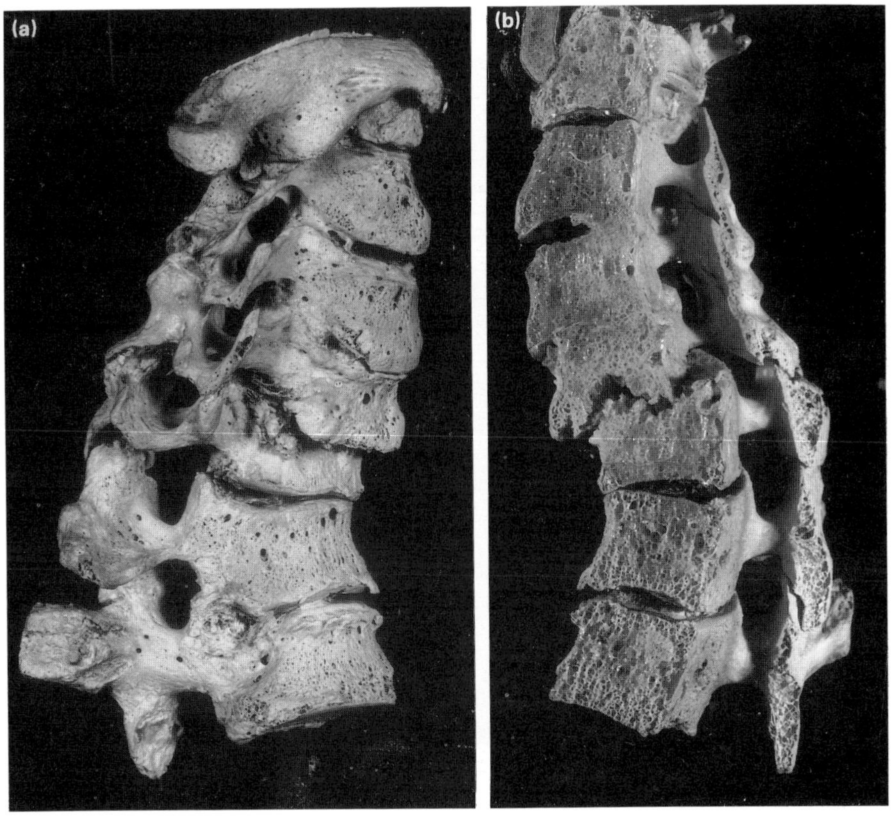

Fig. 51.2 Intact (a) and sagittal section (b) cervical spine in rheumatoid arthritis showing subaxial disease with erosion, subluxation and kyphotic deformity. Courtesy of Dr A.J. Freemont.

spreading to the occiput or into the shoulders depending on the level of involvement. Complaints of sensations of movement, clicking or crunching on movement are common. With atlanto-axial involvement the degree of occipital pain may be very severe. Patients with severe instability may actually support the head in the hands. Flexion deformity and torticollis are common in severe cases.

The severe occipital neuralgia seen in atlanto-axial disease is due to C2 root entrapment. Subaxial disease may cause root entrapment producing brachialgia. This appears to be more frequent in cases where the disease is still active, and true radiculopathy is surprisingly uncommon in cases with advanced disease. Radiculopathy is frequently transient and may respond to rest and anti-inflammatory therapy. Established neurological deficit due to root compression in those patients can be quite difficult to distinguish from the peripheral neuropathy which also occurs in rheumatoid patients.

The onset of myelopathy due to cord compression can be sudden or insidious. Deterioration of limb function is common in rheumatoid patients due to their peripheral disease. However, the onset of myelopathy produces a change in limb function which the patient can usually identify as being due to some factor other than changes in their peripheral disease. Complaints of tingling, numbness and clumsiness of the hands are common. The legs appear heavier and stiffer and the gait deteriorates with poor balance. Falls are frequent and dangerous.

Examination is very difficult. Assessment of weakness is impeded by the pain and deformity in the joints. Sensory loss other than due to peripheral neuropathy or nerve entrapment must be sought. A sensory level to pinprick can be identified, but in atlanto-axial disease this can be at the C2 level and will be identified only if sensation in the occipital and posterior cervical areas is examined. Loss of proprioceptive sensation in the fingers strongly suggests cord involvement. Examination of tendon reflexes is difficult due to joint deformity, and absent reflexes are not uncommon even in the presence of myelopathy. In severe cases with marked joint deformity, the mere persistence of an easily elicited tendon reflex suggests that it is exaggerated. Patients

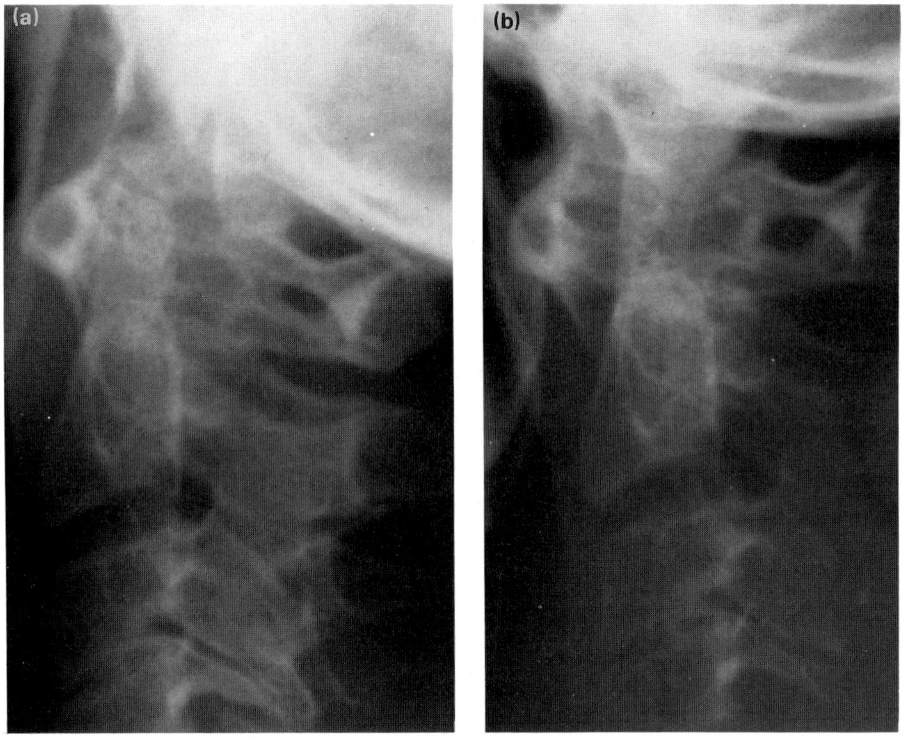

Fig. 51.3 Rheumatoid upper cervical spine. Radiographs in extension (a) and flexion (b) showing mobile atlanto-axial subluxation.

with cranial settling may show brain stem involvement with dysarthria, dysphagia and diplopia. Low cranial nerve palsies and nystagmus are commonly found.

Investigations

The diagnosis predominantly rests on radiological investigation of the cervical spine and lateral flexion/extension views are mandatory.

In atlanto-axial disease erosion of the odontoid peg may be seen particularly well in the per-oral view. This radiograph also shows the C1–C2 apophyseal joints and lateral subluxation can be identified.

On the lateral flexion/extension radiographs measurements are made of the distances between the posterior surface of the anterior arch of the atlas and the anterior border of the odontoid peg (Fig. 51.3a,b). Normally this should not exceed 3 mm. In atlanto-axial subluxation this may be increased in some cases up to 12 mm or more. When the amount of subluxation is greater in the flexion than the extension view this indicates instability of the odontoid peg during these movements, and a much greater risk of neurological damage. In the patient with vertical

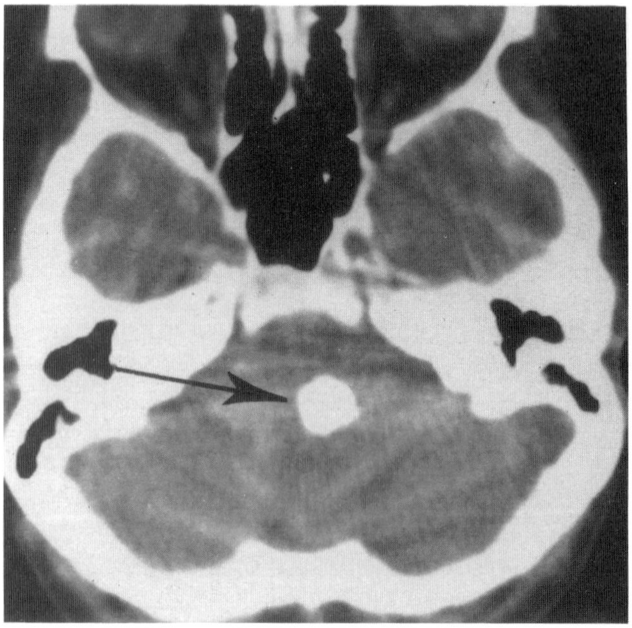

Fig. 51.4 Computerized axial tomographic scan in a rheumatoid patient with severe vertical atlanto-axial subluxation and cranial settling. The odontoid peg (arrowed) lies within the posterior cranial fossa severely compressing the brain stem. Courtesy of Mr G. Findlay.

subluxation the tip of the peg appears to migrate upwards above the occipitomental line (Fig. 5.14). In these circumstances there is particular risk of brain stem damage.

In the lower cervical spine the early radiographic features may be difficult to distinguish from cervical spondylosis. There may be loss of the cervical disc space but with relatively little or no osteophyte formation. Erosive changes may be seen. In more severe cases forward subluxation of the vertebrae becomes obvious and is accentuated by forward flexion (Fig. 51.5). The detailed radiological assessment of the rheumatoid cervical spine is discussed in Chapter 52.

Rheumatoid involvement of the lumbar spine

This is rarely recognized, as it is difficult to distinguish rheumatoid involvement of the lumbar spine from degenerative spondylosis. Rheumatoid synovitis affects the apophyseal joints. There may be rheumatoid destruction of the intervertebral discs, but it is uncertain whether this arises by spread by synovitis from the apophyseal joints or by inflammation of clefts in the discs which have become lined by synovium-like cells. There is progressive loss of disc substance and erosion of the intervertebral endplates. Commonly this is asymmetric and the patient develops a kyphoscoliosis with disc narrowing on one side and often erosion, sclerosis and sometimes osteophytes due to secondary spondylosis on the concave side (Fig. 51.6).

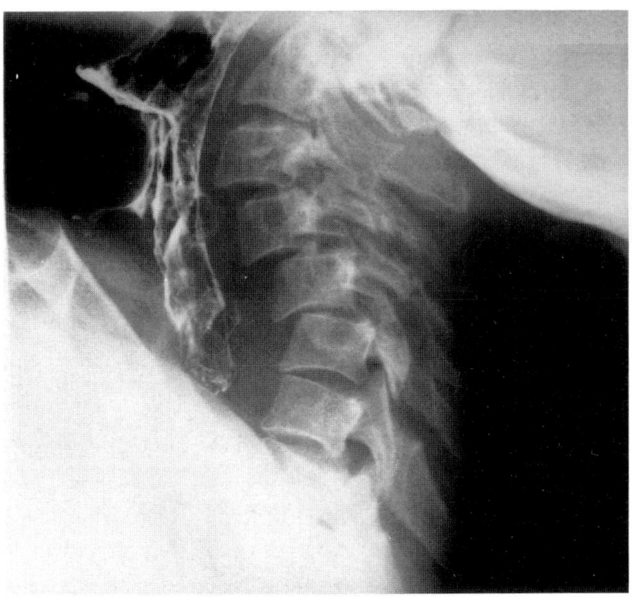

Fig. 51.5 Rheumatoid involvement of the midcervical spine with forward subluxation of the cervical vertebrae in this case causing dysphagia investigated by barium swallow.

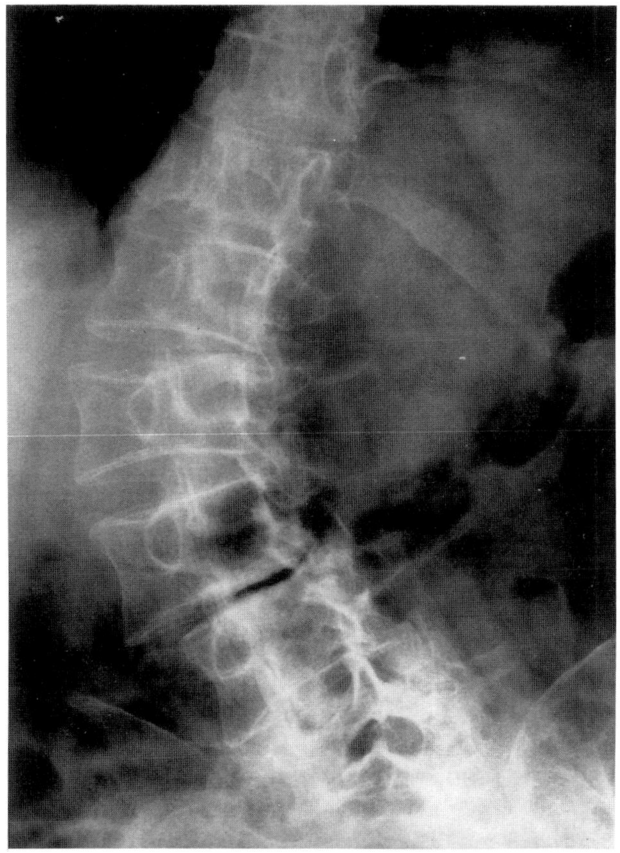

Fig. 51.6 Rheumatoid involvement of the lumbar spine with a severe kyphoscoliosis and destructive changes of the L4–L5 disc.

The problem may be compounded by osteoporosis and vertebral collapse. This is due to a combination of the rheumatoid disease itself, lack of physical activity with disuse osteoporosis, and often the use of systemic steroids.

The patient develops back pain and stiffness, with perhaps referred pain in the lower limbs depending on damage to nerve roots and other structures. The symptoms may follow the typical pattern of rheumatoid inflammation being aggravated by rest with marked morning stiffness, but also they are exacerbated by physical activity and towards the end of the day. The pain can be very severe and the patient very disabled.

Treatment of rheumatoid involvement of the spine

Each patient should be assessed individually to determine the activity of the rheumatoid arthritis and the relative contributions of chronic inflammation, erosive damage and secondary osteoarthritis of the joints, spine and other tissues. The presence of active synovitis will indicate the importance of medical measures to control chronic inflammation, whereas if mechanical problems predominate physical solutions will be required.

Anti-inflammatory analgesic drugs are in general use. These include drugs such as salicylates, ibuprofen, naprosyn, piroxicam, diclofenac and many others. They are effective at relieving pain and stiffness but do not alter the course of the disease. By careful analysis of the pattern of the symptoms, the type of anti-inflammatory drug and its timing can be chosen to provide optimum symptom control. In particular severe morning pain and stiffness may be controlled by a long-acting or slow-release agent given last thing at night. Unfortunately these drugs are prone to cause dyspepsia and peptic ulceration, particularly in older subjects, and appropriate care is needed. In the event of dyspepsia the non-steroidal anti-inflammatory drugs may have to be stopped and pure analgesics such as paracetamol, dihyrocodeine and others relied on for pain relief. Gastroscopy may be required and symptoms of peptic ulceration controlled with antacids and H_2 antagonists. Sometimes the non-steroidal anti-inflammatory drug is used as a suppository, although there is still some risk of dyspepsia and peptic ulceration. The risk appears less than when taken by mouth, probably because of lack of direct contact with the gastric mucosa and also slower absorption with more prolonged effect and lower drug levels in the blood.

The second-line antirheumatic agents such as chloroquine, sulphasalazine, gold and penicillamine, produce remissions of the underlying disease process. They usually take two to three months to exert their full effects. Despite apparent control of the disease it remains uncertain whether they prevent the long-term development of erosive changes. They all can produce important toxic reactions and require very careful monitoring. In more severe cases immunosuppressive agents such as azathioprine, cyclophosphamide or methotrexate may be necessary.

Steroids may be used and are very effective at relieving the symptoms of rheumatoid arthritis. However, in the long run they may lead to a wide variety of complications including osteoporosis and vertebral collapse. The decision to use steroids requires very careful consideration and should not be taken lightly.

The symptoms of neck and back pain may be relieved by local heat, ice or massage. Many patients use various rubifacients and recently a transcutaneous preparation of non-steroidal anti-inflammatory agents has been developed and may be helpful. Intermittent and forceful traction, mobilizing exercises and in particular manipulation of the neck must be avoided because of the risks of neurological damage.

Many patients use cervical collars. The common soft cervical collars, or even plastic collars, are very poor at limiting neck movements. However, they often provide relief, perhaps by making the patient conscious of the need to protect the neck, local warmth of the skin or even by stimulation of sensory receptors which may block the passage of nociceptive impulses. The only effective way of externally immobilizing the neck is with an occipitonatal or Minerva collar, but these are not acceptable for long-term use by the majority of patients.

In acute cervical pain, bed rest with the patient lying flat and light cervical traction in the neutral position will usually relieve symptoms within a few days. In severe deformity with neurological disability, traction with either excessive weight or incorrect direction may cause deterioration. These symptoms and signs may improve or even resolve completely. At the least rest and traction give time to plan appropriate surgical intervention but it should be realized that persisting neurological deterioration requires immediate surgery.

Specific treatment of the lumbar spine involvement by rheumatoid arthritis is extremely difficult. To minimize osteoporosis steroids should be reduced and perhaps substituted by second-line agents or immunosuppressive drugs. Mobility is encouraged but may aggravate the back pain. Long lumbar corsets and spinal jackets are sometimes prescribed to immobilize the back. Commonly they prove difficult to fit and are a constant source of problems. The limitation of back movements may exacerbate the predisposition towards osteoporosis. Spinal fusion is sometimes considered, but in most of these patients the bone is very osteoporotic so that grafts fuse poorly. Many of these lumbar spine problems prove insoluble.

ANKYLOSING SPONDYLITIS AND RELATED DISORDERS

This is a group of inflammatory forms of polyarthritis in which rheumatoid factor is not found, and which involves the spine in a characteristic fashion. The seronegative spondylarthritides include ankylosing spondylitis, reactive arthritis (Reiter's disease), psoriatic arthritis and the arthritis of ulcerative colitis and of Crohn's disease. There are commonly overlapping features between these disorders and sometimes it can be very difficult to classify any patient into one or other diagnosis.

Pathogenesis

There is a genetic predisposition towards this group of disorders. The human leucocyte antigen B27 (HLA B27) occurs in about 5–8% of the normal population. In contrast it is found in about 95% of patients with ankylosing spondylitis, 75% in reactive arthritis, 65% in psoriatic arthritis and about 55% in patients with the spondylitis of ulcerative colitis and Crohn's disease. In a patient with back pain and no other clinical problems in whom ankylosing spondylitis is suspected the presence of HLA B27 does *not* make the diagnosis, as it can be found in healthy individuals, but its absence would make this diagnosis unlikely. Examination of the tissue type HLA B27 is more useful when it is absent for excluding the diagnosis of ankylosing spondylitis, whereas its presence is not a diagnostic test for this disorder.

The development of tissue typing has led to immunogenetic studies of this group of disorders. Many patients have a family history of ankylosing spondylitis or one of the related disorders such as colitis, psoriasis, reactive arthritis or uveitis.

Infection may play an important role in initiating this disorder in predisposed individuals. Sexually acquired reactive arthritis (Reiter's syndrome) commonly follows a non-specific urethritis, perhaps due to *Chlamydia*, and enteric-acquired reactive arthritis may follow an episode of diarrhoea due to *Yersinia enterocolitica* and certain *Salmonella* and *Shigella* species. Pelvic inflammation and infection is, of course, common in ulcerative colitis and Crohn's disease, and in ankylosing spondylitis there is an increased incidence of prostatitis and of inflammation of the bowel. Positive faecal cultures for *Klebsiella aerogenes* have been reported.

The similarity of antigen receptors for the postulated invading organisms and the HLA B27 receptor has suggested a possible lack of the normal immune response to such infection, so predisposing towards chronic inflammation.

Ankylosing spondylitis

This disorder most commonly starts between the ages of 15 and 25 years, although it may develop in children or in other age groups. It is more common in males, the sex ratio usually being regarded as about 5 : 1. However, in surveys of very mild disease the sex incidence does appear much more evenly balanced. The prevalence of ankylosing spondylitis is usually quoted in epidemiological studies as around 0.5%; however, this may be a gross underestimate. One survey suggested that 20% of HLA B27-positive individuals may develop at least mild forms of the disease, indicating a prevalence of 1–1.5% of the population. In clinics dealing with young adult males, such as army recruits or university students, ankylosing spondylitis is a very common cause of back pain.

The characteristic pathological change is known as an enthesopathy (Fig. 51.7). This is inflammation of the insertion of tendons and ligaments into bone. This heals by fibrosis then ossification, so forming a small bony spur. The tip of this spur then becomes the enthesis so there is progressive ossification of tendons and ligaments. In the spine these bony spurs, known as syndesmophytes, may meet and fuse so that the vertebrae become joined by bone with severe

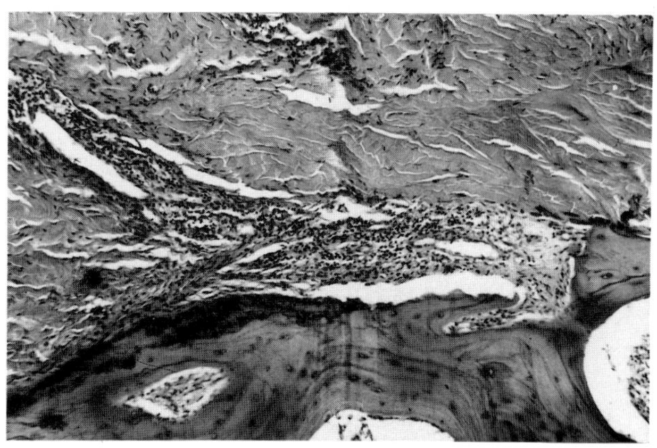

Fig. 51.7 The enthesopathy of ankylosing spondylitis—inflammation of the attachment of ligament to bone.

loss of movement. Peripherally the same process can cause plantar spurs, Achilles' tendinitis, etc., again with bony spurs to be seen on X-rays.

The commonest presenting feature is low back pain and stiffness. It is a characteristic that the symptoms are aggravated by rest and relieved by exercise. The patient will describe aching and stiffness across the low back, spreading down the backs of the thighs and up the lumbar and into the dorsal spine. The patient wakes in the early morning and often has to get up and perform physical exercises to obtain relief. By the time the patient is seen in the clinic he or she is often symptom-free and has a normal range of spinal movements.

As the condition advances the pain and stiffness become more extensive and long-lasting. There is gradual development of permanent limitation of spinal movements and of deformity. Eventually the patient may develop the characteristic posture with flattening of the lumbar spine, loss of the normal lordosis, an increase in the dorsal kyphosis and a protruded neck in an effort to look forwards rather than downwards. In contrast to mechanical problems in the spine, all lumbar movements, including not only extension and flexion but also lateral flexion and lateral rotation, become severely limited. In the advanced case all spine movements including the neck may be lost and the spine may become completely rigid (Figs 51.8a,b).

Involvement of the costovertebral joints may limit chest expansion. A peripheral arthropathy can occur. Most often this affects the lower limb joints and in particular the hip, knee and foot. Hip involvement is often accompanied by loss of hip movements and many patients develop flexion contractions of the hips and knees adding to their mobility problems.

Another characteristic musculoskeletal feature which often may be a presenting problem is inflam-

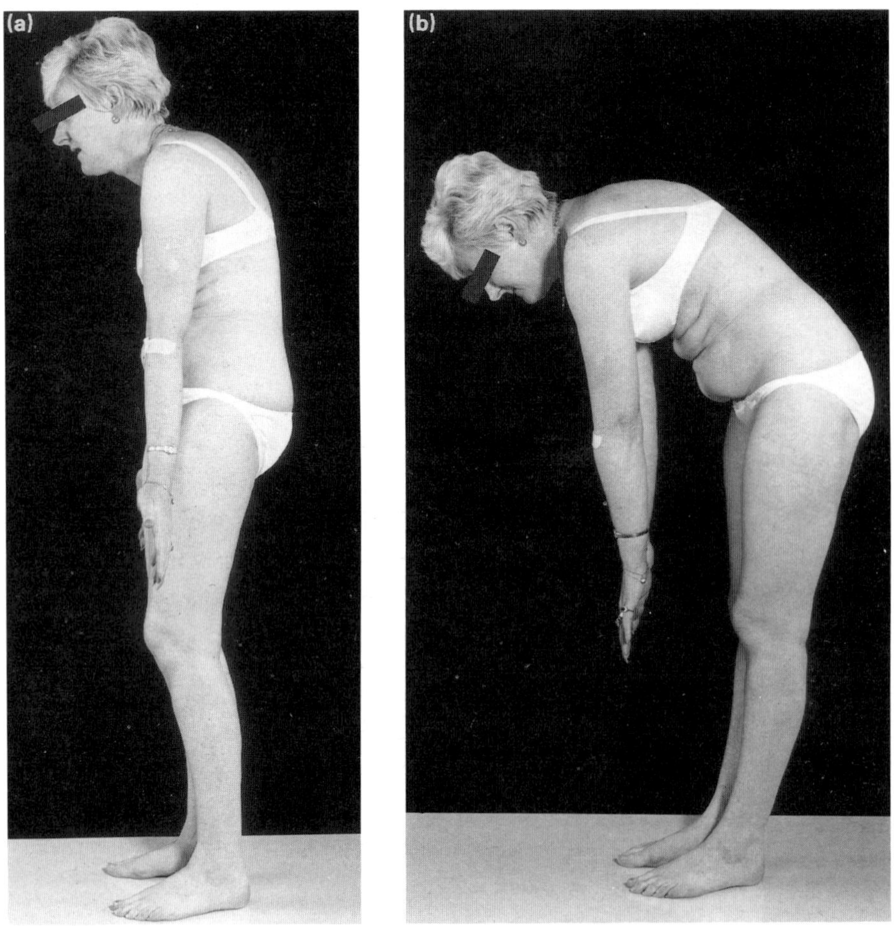

Fig. 51.8 Ankylosing spondylitis in a female subject. There is loss of lumbar lordosis, a smooth dorsal kyphosis and a protruded neck. Virtually all spine movement is lost during forward flexion. There is hip involvement with fixed flexion of the hips and knees when upright, and limitation of hip movements.

mation and pain at the sites of attachment of ligaments to bone—known as an enthesopathy. This may be manifest as plantar fasciitis with a plantar spur, Achilles' tendinitis, ischial bursitis, etc. These can all develop as idiopathic problems but when they complicate ankylosing spondylitis they are frequently resistant to treatment.

The spine becomes rigid in ankylosing spondylitis but is osteoporotic and weak. Fractures can develop in response to modest trauma. Most often this occurs in the cervical spine, perhaps due to a whiplash car injury. There is a major risk of quadriplegia and other severe neurological damage.

Another important problem occurs when there is one mobile segment in an otherwise ankylosed area. There may be a fracture of the posterior elements of the spine and severe erosive and destructive changes of the disc and of the vertebral endplates. These patients often give a history of long-standing back stiffness but with relatively little pain until the recent onset of acute symptoms localized to the area of abnormal movement. In contrast to early ankylosing spondylitis the pain is relieved by rest and aggravated by movements.

Iritis (anterior uveitis) occurs in 20–30% of ankylosing spondylitics. Often it is a recurrent problem. Sometimes it is the presenting feature of the disease and investigation of back pain in patients with iritis often reveals ankylosing spondylitis as the underlying cause. Iritis, if inadequately treated, can produce severe and permanent ocular damage. The development of an acute red eye in a patient with ankylosing spondylitis is an indication for immediate referral to an ophthalmologist for appropriate examination and treatment.

Fibrosis may develop in the upper lobes of the lungs. It is not clear whether this is a specific complication of ankylosing spondylitis or due to failure of ventilation and perfusion of the upper lobes due to poor chest expansion. In some patients infection may occur, and adds to the pulmonary problems. Aortic valve reflux and cardiac conduction defects are reported in the literature but are very rare. Amyloidosis also may occur in association with severe and extensive disease.

The earliest radiological changes may be seen in the sacroiliac joints with erosion and sclerosis of the joint margins. Sacroiliac fusion ocurs in more advanced cases (Fig. 51.9). Another early feature is new bone formation on the anterior aspects of the vertebral bodies, particularly in the dorsolumbar region. There is progressive ossification of the longitudinal ligaments with syndesmophytes which may meet and fuse, leading to appearances of a 'bamboo' spine. Destructive changes can develop, particularly at the anterior, superior and inferior margins of the vertebral bodies when there is a remaining mobile level between two rigid segments of the spine (Fig. 51.10).

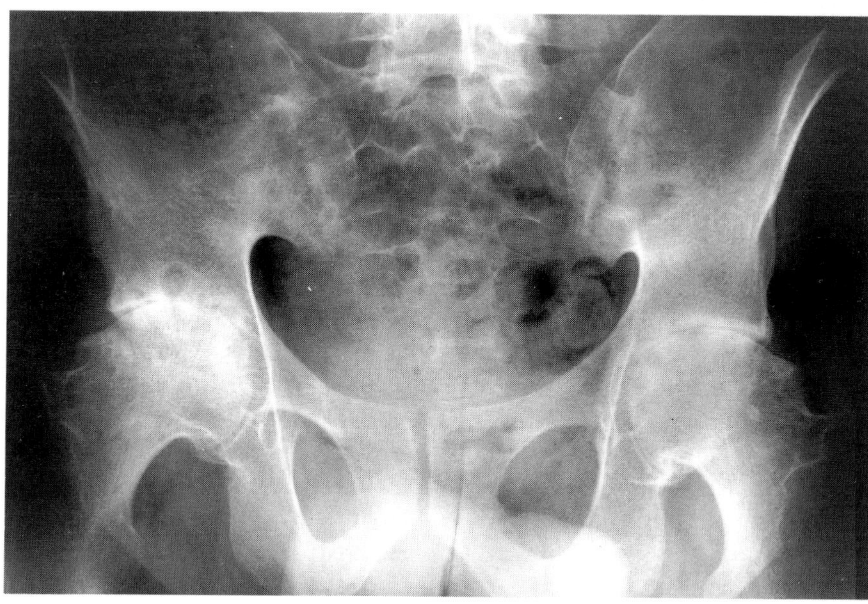

Fig. 51.9 Advanced ankylosing spondylitis with fusion of the sacroiliac joints and advanced hip involvement.

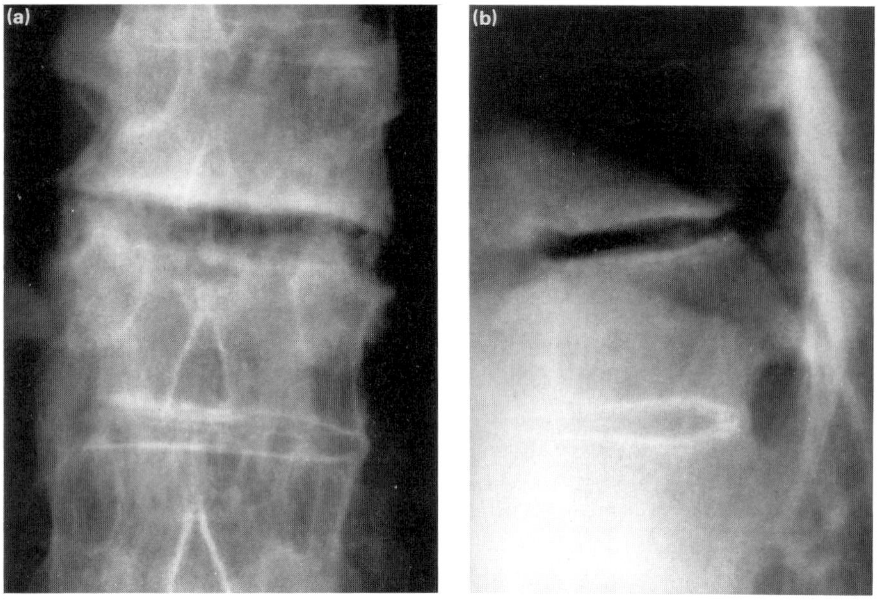

Fig. 51.10 AP and lateral radiographs showing a mobile segment with destructive changes in the vertebral bodies due to ankylosing spondylitis.

Psoriatic arthritis

Psoriasis is a persistent and recurrent skin condition with characteristic circumscribed raised erythematous lesions which produce fine scales when scratched superficially. They may occur in plaques anywhere on the body, but most often over the knees and elbows. In more severe cases diffuse generalized erythroderma of the skin may occur. The nails are often affected but the evidence sometimes may be minimal and show only as pitting of the nail surface. This can be the only evidence of psoriasis in patients presenting with typical psoriatic arthritis.

Psoriasis may be associated with several different patterns of joint disease. These are:

1 A chronic inflammatory asymmetric oligoarthritis. There is chronic inflammation affecting a small number of joints in a non-symmetrical distribution in contrast with rheumatoid arthritis.

2 Distal interphalangeal joint arthritis. This most often occurs in the fingers but also occasionally in the toes. There are usually psoriatic changes in the nails of the same fingers. These joints are rarely affected in rheumatoid arthritis.

3 Arthritis mutilans. This is a very severe destructive arthritis in which there is resorption of the epiphyses leaving flail but often painless joints. Most often this affects the small joints of the fingers.

4 Spine involvement. The patient develops changes in the spine very similar to, and often indistinguishable from, those of ankylosing spondylitis. In contrast with that disorder, however, the disease more often starts in the dorsal spine and neck rather than in the lumbosacral spine and sacroiliac joints. There can be excessive proliferation of new bone in the paravertebral region and some patients show a curious pattern of paravertebral ossification in which X-rays show a band of translucency separating these areas of new bone from the vertebral column. The clinical problems associated with psoriatic spondylitis are similar to those of ankylosing spondylitis.

Reactive arthritis

This refers to a pattern of arthritis which may develop following exposure to certain infective agents. It was originally recognized as a sexually acquired disorder and known as Reiter's syndrome. This is better termed sexually acquired reactive arthritis or SARA, and is believed to be due to persistent chlamydial antigen in predisposed individuals. This is to distinguish it from enteric-acquired reactive arthritis which may follow some dysenteric infections due to certain *Salmonella* or *Shigella* species or *Yersinia enterocolitica*. About 90% of patients with reactive arthritis are positive for the tissue type HLA B27. If a person with this tissue type develops an appropriate infection, the chances of developing reactive arthritis are several hundred-fold greater than those negative for HLA B27.

The classical syndrome is of a urethritis with a urethral discharge which is sterile on ordinary culture but which may be shown due to *Chlamydia*. This may be followed by conjunctivitis and then arthritis, with joint disease most often involving the lower limbs—the joints of the toes, tarsus and ankles and then other joints such as knees or elsewhere. There is acute synovitis which with appropriate treatment will remit, but with a significant risk of relapse. Other features of the disease include a rash which appears on the penis as circinate balanitis, a scaling rash on the soles of the feet and elsewhere, known as keratoderma blenorrhagica, and mucosal ulceration. The histology of the skin rash is identical with that of pustular psoriasis.

The arthritis will usually remit but often relapses and may proceed to destructive joint changes. With relapses and remissions there is progressive spine involvement with symptoms, physical findings and X-ray changes very similar to those of ankylosing spondylitis.

In the acute stage of Reiter's syndrome treatment is with rest and often a course of tetracycline or other antibiotics. If there is spine involvement the back is treated as for ankylosing spondylitis.

Treatment of ankylosing spondylitis

Management of this condition demands careful assessment of the extent and activity of the underlying disease and planning of a coordinated programme of long-term management. It is essential that patients are followed up regularly and in the long term. An understanding by the patient of the disease and of the slow deterioration that can take place is a great encouragement for cooperation in long-term management. Regular measurements of spinal movements must be made to assess progress, and in particular to identify any deterioration.

The most important aspect of treatment, particularly in early disease, is a regular, active programme of mobilizing exercises in order to retain full joint mobility. These should be practised daily and should involve mobilizing exercises for the neck, lumbar spine, shoulders, hips, peripheral joints and also breathing exercises. The patient should be encouraged to perform these exercises to the limits of his or her ability. It is usually possible to obtain major improvements in spinal function and to maintain this improved mobility. Repeated measurements of spinal movements will usually indicate whether or not the patient is regularly performing the exercise programme.

It is also important for the patient to make a conscious effort to try to avoid the stoop that commonly occurs in this condition. Careful instruction on posture by the physiotherapist, with regular checking, will help to prevent the development of the spondylitic posture.

Anti-inflammatory drugs are very effective at relieving the symptoms. Agents commonly in use include ibuprofen, piroxicam, diclofenac and indomethacin. Phenylbutazone is particularly effective for ankylosing spondylitis; unfortunately, however, it does carry a greater risk of gastric problems and can also produce blood dyscrasias. For these reasons its use generally has been curtailed, but because of its special value for ankylosing spondylitis it is still available for this condition.

Long-acting or slow-release anti-inflammatory drugs are often used and they may be given last thing in the evening, often with some milk in order to relieve night symptoms and early morning stiffness. For those with dyspepsia they may sometimes be acceptable as suppositories or with the addition of antiulcer treatment as for rheumatoid arthritis. Their pain-relieving effect can be supplemented with pure analgesics such as paracetamol, dihydrocodeine, dextropropoxyphene and others, as necessary. In addition sulphasalazine is believed to have a specific effect in controlling the underlying disease activity and is used as a second-line agent as in rheumatoid arthritis. Enteric coated sulphasalazine is given in doses up to 3 g per day, and in appropriate cases may lead to disease remission.

Steroids are required only rarely. The most common indication is the development of iritis. Steroids may be given locally as drops or occasionally systemically. Very rarely the drug is used for patients with severe spinal involvement, and pain and stiffness not controlled by more conservative means. For the peripheral enthesopathy such as plantar fasciitis or Achilles' tendinitis, steroids are often injected locally together with anaesthetic.

Although commonly used in the past there is very little indication for the use of radiotherapy today. It does not seem to halt the progress of the disease when used for the spine and appears to carry an increased risk of leukaemia. The only use is in tightly collimated doses given to an area of resistant peripheral enthesopathy such as Achilles' tendinitis or plantar fasciitis when it has not responded to other types of local treatment.

Surgical intervention is rarely required in ankylosing spondylitis. The principal indications are as follows.

Severe kyphosis

Surgical correction of the deformity can be performed in appropriately motivated individuals. There is a significant risk of neurological complications.

Mobile segments

In some patients there may be a remaining mobile segment between adjacent rigid segments of spine. Severe destructive changes and pain may occur at this level. Surgical fusion can be the only way of controlling the pain in such subjects.

Peripheral arthritis

Most often the hips become involved. In ankylosing spondylitis this often leads to severe loss of hip movements. Combined with spinal rigidity this can render the patient immobile. Hip replacement can be successful but early remobilization after operation is required as there is a great tendency for these hips to stiffen rapidly.

52 · Surgical Management of Rheumatoid Cervical Spine Disease

By H.A. CROCKARD and A.O. RANSFORD

The rheumatoid arthritic process characteristically exhibits 'flare-up' and remissions. The resultant joint destruction is more disabling in the weight-bearing joints of the lower limbs and surgery is soon requested. In the upper limbs and axial skeleton, appropriate conservative treatment delays the necessity for surgical intervention. Indeed, there is a reservoir of rheumatoid patients where 'interventionist' and potentially life-changing operations have been postponed for too long, for the immobilization techniques and some of the drugs used to control the acute inflammatory episodes have encouraged endstage osteoporosis. Paradoxically in the subaxial cervical spine, 'burnt-out' rheumatoid arthritis may result in spontaneous facetal ankylosis which may be symptom-relieving; unfortunately any unfused and less diseased neighbouring joints are then stressed to failure.

This panoply combines to produce neck pain, but, due to the proximity of neurological structures there may be in addition a radiculopathy or myelopathy alone or in combination. Occasionally with neural compression at the craniovertebral junction there may be brain stem signs. The instability produced by the disease may render the neuraxis liable to serious injury following trivial trauma.

The purpose of this chapter is to present the indications and surgical approaches in this condition as viewed by the authors. Clearly there may be alternative views, but all therapeutic regimens must be a compromise between the natural history of the disease, the risks involved and the expertise available on site.

In this condition particularly, the 'overall view' must be taken. For example, patients with widespread rheumatoid arthritis have a higher risk of cancer and a shorter life expectancy than comparable age- and sex-matched groups (Garrod, 1890; Symmons, 1988). Furthermore, as the surgery is usually restricted to one area of the cervical spine, the effects of the stabilization on the other neck joints must be considered.

THE RHEUMATOID PROCESS

In the long-term studies of rheumatoid patients by Boyle (1971) and Winfield *et al.* (1981), it was found that, while almost half of the patients developed problems at C1–C2, any cervical level could be involved to a greater or lesser degree (Fig. 52.1) from the occipito-atlantal level down to the cervicodorsal junction (see Fig. 52.2; see also Fig. 51.2). The exact pathology will vary; in some an acute synovitis will simply cause local acute pain, in others florid disease may produce pain with cord compression and neurological signs. In some the pannus is fibrous; in most it is the endstage disease of joint erosion and deformity which causes neuraxial distortion and compression. The actual pathological processes involved are of direct relevance to the surgeon and will be discussed in detail.

The pannus (Fig. 52.3a,b)

Set out in Table 52.1 are some of the pathological changes which may confront the surgeon. The role of the inflammatory tissue, still inappropriately called pannus in the cervical spine, is one which has received increasing attention since the advent of non-invasive scanning techniques, even though its compressive effect was first documented by Garrod in 1890. There is no doubt that an acute neuraxial com-

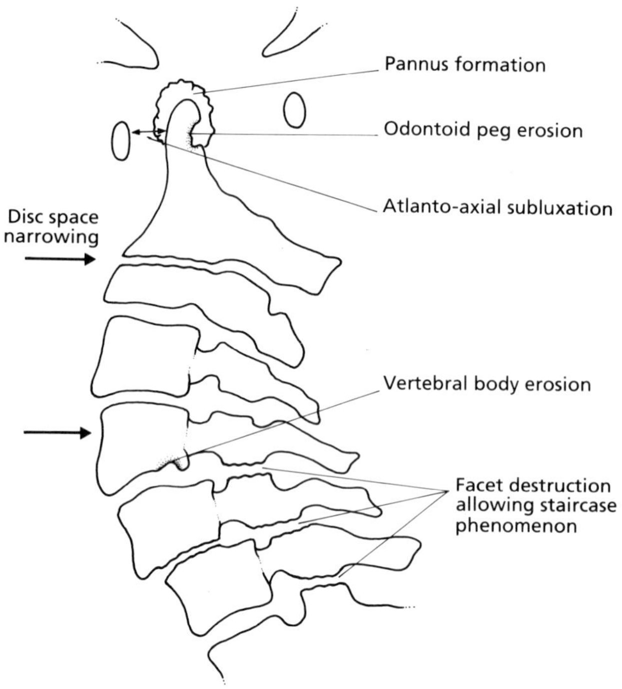

Fig. 52.1 Cervical spine changes in rheumatoid arthritis.

pression may be produced by a florid acute synovitis and periodontoidal bursitis (Fig. 52.3b). As at other joints temporary immobilization of the neck may permit resolution of the inflammatory tissue, but if the neuraxial compression persists the pannus needs to be excised or encouraged by some other treatment to disperse. In orthopaedic circles it is well known that stabilizing the neck will eventually result in regression of the pannus and neurological improvement. A simple posterior fusion has been undertaken with excellent results, but this is an extremely dangerous procedure in the presence of anterior compression. Brattstrom & Granholm (1976) reported resolution of the inflammatory mass with no significant morbidity, but this is an exceptional report (Hamblen, 1983).

Table 52.1 Some of the pathological changes which may occur in cervical rheumatoid disease

Pathology	Type	Effect
Pannus	Fluid Florrid Fibrous	Dural compression Irreducible luxation
Luxations	Occipital–C1 C1–C2 Midcervical Staircase	Intermittent compression Fixed compression
Bone erosion/ absorption	Odontoid peg Lateral mass C1 or C2 Vertebral body Facet joint	Luxation Translocation Kyphos/angulation Fracture
Ankylosis	Lateral mass Facet Vertebral	Stiffness Excessive wear other joints

While pannus is usually related to the synovial joints, there are occasions when it is found in a more remote situation. Occasionally it may encircle the dura and cause a fibrous constrictive ring. It must also be documented that the patient presenting with myelopathy due to the acute synovitis is rare; most of the patients presenting with myelopathy in this condition have endstage pathology with dense fibrous tissue replacing the acute synovitis. In such patients it is unlikely that the resolution of this tissue with external or internal immobilization would occur. The condition has 'burnt out' and there is little synovial tissue remaining; instead the compression is due to distorted, fragmented and crushed vertebral elements and any hypermobility associated with this. Immobilizing this situation may result in some clinical improvement but such fixation may be very dangerous in the presence of major irreducible compression of the spinal cord or lower brain stem.

Craniocervical junction

While dislocation of the odontoid process is the commonest finding, the other joints in the area may be affected. Disease at the atlanto-occipital joint has received scant attention generally, yet these diseases are involved in over 50% of patients with C1–C2 involvement. Only one joint may be affected and this, combined with destruction of the homolateral C1–C2 joint, may result in resorption or erosion of the lateral mass of C1 and a fixed torticollis.

Nearly half of the cervical rotatory movements occur at the atlanto-axial joint and, as a movement is executed, there is a slight associated up-and-down movement due to the sloping shoulders of the joint (Greenberg, 1968). With progressive joint erosion this movement can be exaggerated. As the lateral masses of C1 and C2 erode, the odontoid process moves into the foramen magnum. This upward herniation can be shown on static radiographs where it is variously termed 'upward migration', 'cranial settling' or 'translocation'. However, static views underestimate the amount of repetitive concussion to the brain

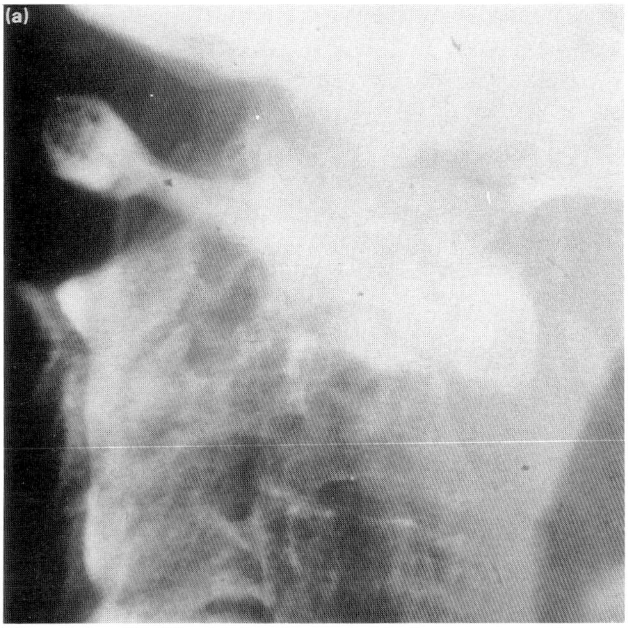

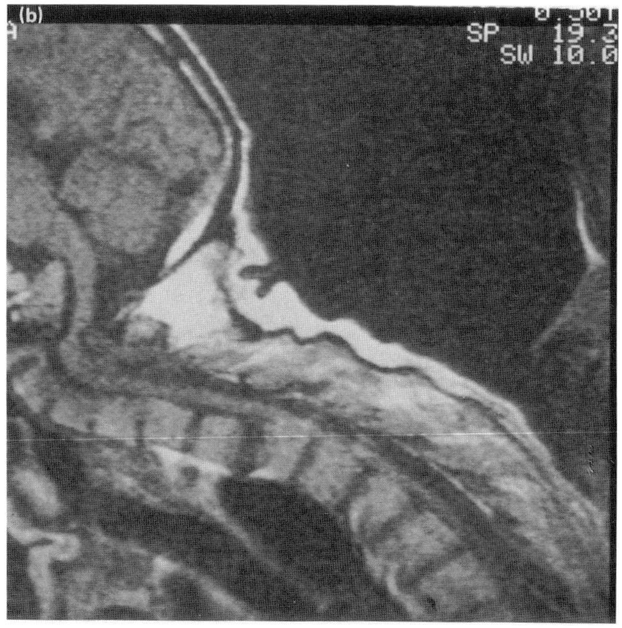

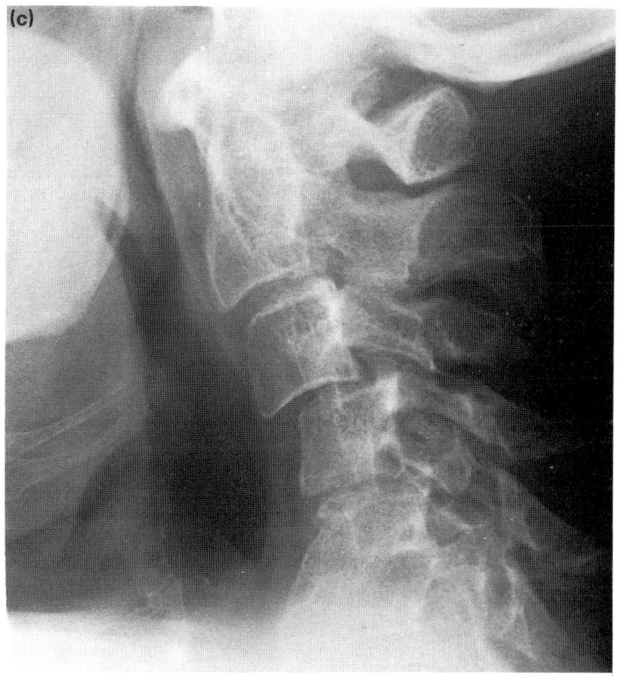

Fig. 52.2 Any joint may be affected but the most mobile or those adjacent to a fixed segment are most vulnerable. (a) Atlanto-axial destruction and anterior subluxation; (b) translocation due to lateral mass erosion and subaxial subluxation; (c) staircase phenomenon above a fused segment.

stem from below on each rotatory action, which is extremely harmful. The exact extent of the damage will depend on the length of surviving odontoid peg and the degree of neuraxial distortion.

Any pathological rotation or tilting of the atlas will affect the vertebral artery, and this has implications in anterior and posterior surgery. With progressive bone destruction there may be a fracture or combination of fractures in the region.

Subaxial spine

While any or all of the joints may be involved, the midcervical region bears the brunt of the destruction with crush erosion and fragmentation of C4, C5 and C6 causing anterior angulation, lordosis or a torticollis. There may be single-level instability or fixed luxation. Occasionally all the levels are, to some extent, involved, and a 'staircase' effect results (Figs

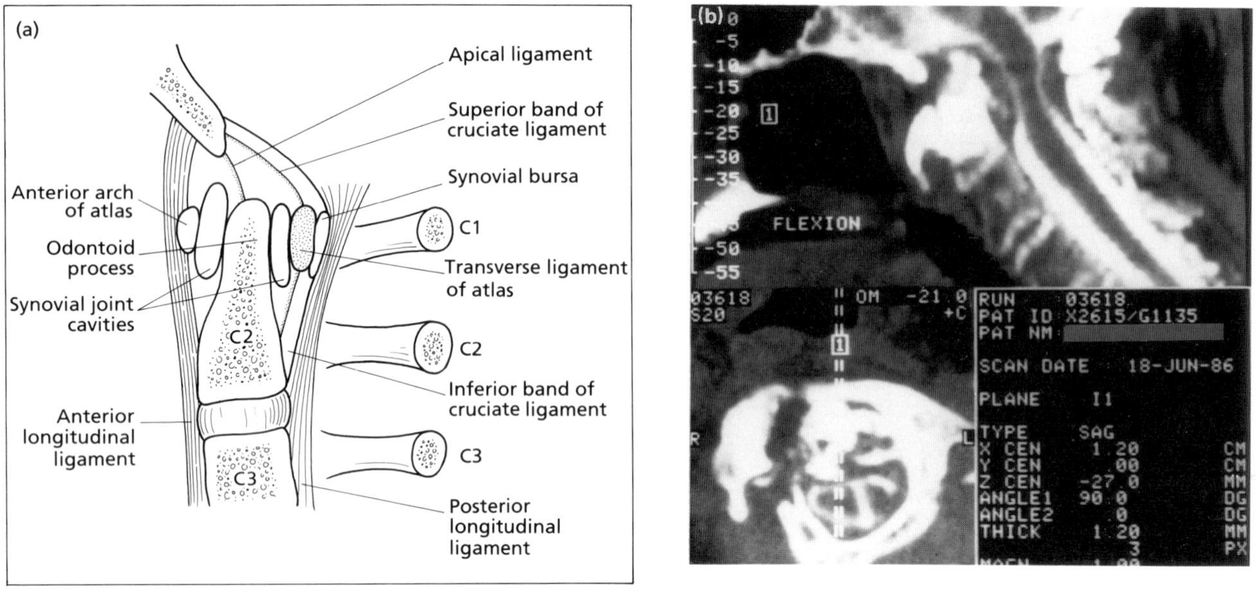

Fig. 52.3 (a) Pannus may originate in any or all of the synovial bursae shown but may extend and encompass the dural sac; (b) a CT myelographic reconstruction showing a translocated odontoid, but the actual cord compression is due to circumferential pannus.

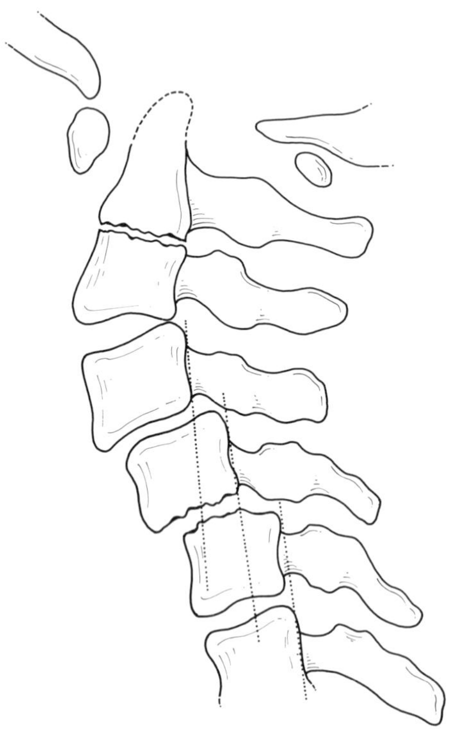

Fig. 52.4 An atlanto-axial subluxation may be associated with fixed or reducible subluxation in the subaxial spur. The so-called 'staircase' will be seen only in flexion views if the subluxation is mobile. A fixed subluxation may be relatively innocuous.

52.2c & 52.4). Very occasionally there may be an acute disc prolapse or compression by acute synovitis. In long-established disease there is often a degree of segmental ankylosis, and then gross instability and subluxation may occur between adjacent fixed segments.

RADIOLOGICAL INVESTIGATIONS

A simple lateral radiograph in flexion and extension is an extremely important screening, planning and follow-up investigation; but does not provide sufficient information to plan all the management decisions especially with regard to the type and extent of surgery. In cases with marked erosion or osteoporosis, conventional AP and lateral tomography may give added detail. Myelography is a difficult and uncomfortable procedure in these patients. Whichever radiological method is chosen, it is essential that an assessment of the effects of movement be obtained and dynamic imaging with flexion and extension views, or occasionally lateral rotation studies, is necessary to understand the neuraxial compression.

Magnetic resonance imaging (MRI) (Fig. 52.2b) provides magnificent evidence of the neuraxial distortion and the soft tissue element of compression. The bone structure is good but currently not up to the level of the information obtained from computerized tomography. At present distortions of the midline, with torticollis or scoliosis, are less easy to interpret and reformating facilities are still improving. Due to the shape of the imaging tunnel there is a high incidence of claustrophobia and resultant 'failed' investigations. All these current disadvantages are likely to be temporary and it will be the most widely used technique in the future. Dynamic images in flexion and extension may also be obtained.

Computerized tomography (CT) is the most reliable method of demonstrating the bony and joint changes, but requires the introduction of a few millilitres of water-soluble contrast into the theca to provide evidence of the state of the spinal cord and the soft tissue compression (Fig. 52.3b). Absolute measurement of translocation, cross-sectioned area of the cord and dural sac and neuraxial angulation mean that, for prospective research studies, it provides more information than MRI. The incidence of claustrophobia is significantly less, and machines are more widely available (Stevens *et al.*, 1986).

Three-dimensional reconstruction of MRI or CT imaging allows the clinician to view the pathology from a variety of vantage points enabling detailed planning of surgery. The effects of various components of the pathology may be selectively excluded. It is the technology used by the maxillofacial surgeons to plan complex facial bone procedures and it will have a real place in craniocervical surgery (Fig. 52.5).

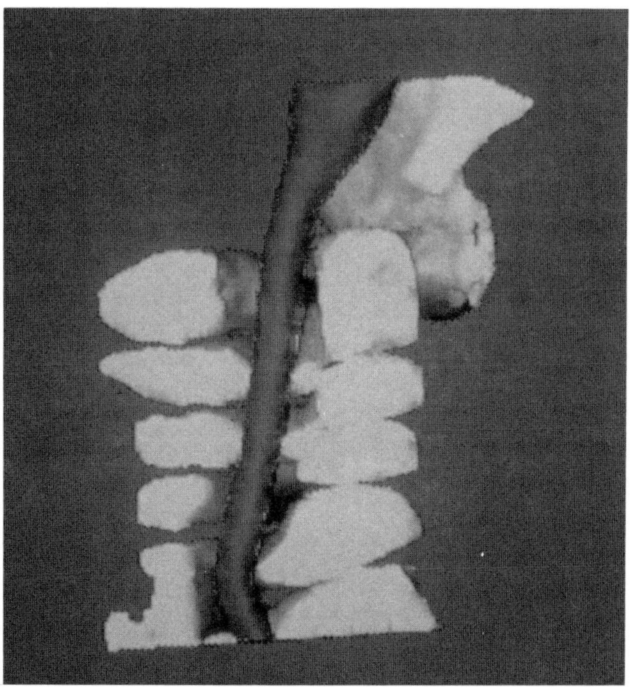

Fig. 52.5 Three-dimensional reconstructions of mid cervical kyphos causing neuraxial compression.

Vertebral angiography—the cervical distortion in rheumatoid arthritis may cause intermittent vertebrobasilar insufficiency and occasionally vertebral angiography is needed to demonstrate the vascular anatomy. Again, if there is a positional element in the symptomatology, a flexion, extension and rotation study is essential to evaluate effectively the potential vascular embarrassment.

TREATMENT OPTIONS (Fig. 52.6)

The management of the rheumatoid cervical spine is exceedingly difficult both for the patient and clinician. In one form or another it is a life-long problem; thus a variety of factors must be taken into account to arrive at the decision optimal for the individual patient at that point in his or her life. The patient with single-level disease with minimal systemic illness is a different management problem to an elderly subject with multijoint involvement and compromised respiratory and renal function. Specific management decisions arise, such as the young patient with asymptomatic atlanto-axial subluxation but rapidly deteriorating renal function in Felty's syndrome; in such patients surgery should be undertaken before dialysis becomes necessary.

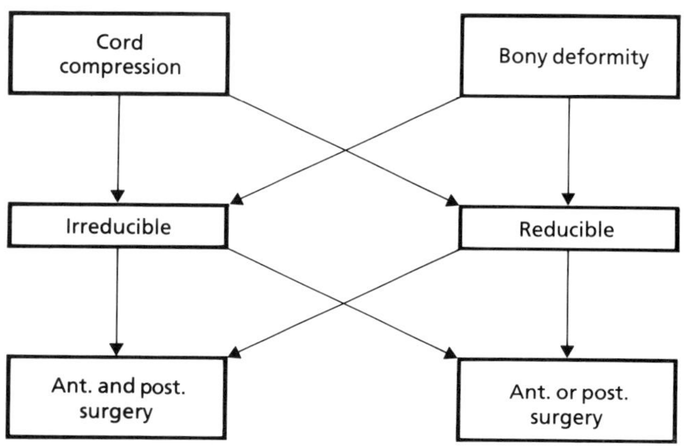

Fig. 52.6 A flowchart to illustrate the surgical decisions in rheumatoid cervical cord compression. Without anterior decompression in the irreducible condition there is a high risk of producing neurological damage by posterior surgery alone.

Another example is the patient with asymptomatic cervical subluxation who may require several corrective procedures for disease in other joints. Will the induction of anaesthesia for the limb surgery precipitate or unmask cervical myelopathy?

The skill and experience of the team undertaking the patient's care is also critical in decision-making; a group skilled in external stabilization techniques will have a differing approach to those practised in internal fixation systems. The point that must be made most firmly is that the overall management mortality and morbidity are the important points, not an operative mortality rate which only takes into account the first month after operation. An example of 'false' accounting is the effect of recumbency and skull traction for one to three months prior to surgery. Meijers *et al.* (1984) reported a relatively high rate of deep venous thrombosis and pulmonary embolism which, when added to the operative problems, produce a significant management mortality. Thus in this disease, the importance of clinical audit cannot be overemphasized.

In Table 52.2 some of the advantages and disadvantages of various management decisions are summarized. It follows that some form of objective evaluation is essential if difficult decisions are to be made with any reassurance to patient and clinician alike.

Evaluation of the patient

The clinical features of rheumatoid cervical spine disease have been discussed in Chapter 51. The full evaluation of the patient is a complex and time-consuming process which requires a team approach. The criteria may differ from centre to centre. The degree of cervical pain may be recorded, or a self-assessment linear analogue scale which has shown some reliability in other painful conditions may be used. The evaluation of the functional capacity of the patient may be recorded by one of the activities for daily living (ADL) classifications such as that described by Steinbrocker *et al.* (1949) or the health activity questionnaire (HAQ) (Kirwan & Reeback, 1986) which allows quantification and reproducibility in a prospective assessment. The Ranawat grading (Ranawat *et al.*, 1979) (Table 52.3) has been employed most widely in the evaluation of cervical spinal surgery but the classification is somewhat insensitive and takes no account of less obvious skills in the

Table 52.2 The advantages and disadvantages of various treatment options

	Advantages	Disadvantages
Cervical collar	Readily available A 'red flag' Relieves pain	Self-application difficult No real stability No effect on myelopathy May still need surgery
Traction	Easily applied Pain relief Improves myelopathy temporarily	Deep venous thrombosis/ pulmonary embolism Pressure sores Chest and urine problem Not a permanent solution May still need surgery
Halo body cuirasse	Improves myelopathy Pain relief	Expert team needed Constant readjustment Not a permanent solution May still need surgery
Surgery	Can decompress Can stabilize	Major surgery Skilled team necessary Systemic complications Local complications Late effects of surgery
No treatment		Myelopathy worsens Pain progresses Respiratory problems

Table 52.3 The Ranawat grading of disability is widely used; the categories, however, are too broad for detailed analysis of results

I	No neurological abnormality
II	Paraesthesiae, hyperreflexia
IIIa	Myelopathy, ambulatory
IIIb	Quadriparesis, bed-bound

already crippled patient, so that results are difficult to evaluate. Tests of manual dexterity such as Jebsen's hand function test (Jebsen *et al.*, 1969) may also be employed to quantify recovery or deterioration in that particular function.

The objectives of surgery might be summarized as aiming to:

1 decompress the neuraxis;
2 stabilize the spine;
3 relieve pain;
4 correct deformity;
5 allow as much movement as possible;
6 prevent further deterioration; and
7 prevent 'overloading' adjacent joints.

While this is a counsel to perfection, it is important to keep the goal in mind and not become devoted to technological achievement. In the following sections surgical correction of specific problems will be described; but before that the general principles of safe anaesthetic technique will be mentioned.

Airway management

Because many of these patients are grossly unstable it is absolutely imperative that expert airway management is planned before and after any surgery. There are a significant number of rheumatoid patients who date their neurological deterioration to their last hip or knee surgery, and it is reasonable to assume that inexpert handling may have caused that problem. In the best units all rheumatoid patients going for surgery have up-to-date cervical spine radiographs, including lateral flexion and extension views. These are carefully analysed and, if necessary, acted upon. If there is any doubt a soft collar is applied before proceeding to the anaesthetic room. At the very least this alerts everyone to a potential problem.

In those patients who have proven cervical instability it is essential to use the fibreoptic laryngoscope in intubation. This is introduced nasally and over it is passed an armoured nasotracheal tube. In those having transoral surgery the nasotracheal tube is maintained in position for two to five days postoperatively. Some anaesthetists depend on local mucosal anaesthetic and pass the instrument in the awake patient. This is fairly uncomfortable and requires a great deal of patient cooperation, but is one way of ensuring minimal risk of further damage to the

Table 52.4 Summary of surgical procedures in rheumatoid spine

Condition	Procedure
Craniocervical	
Atlanto-axial subluxation reducible	Laminar clamp C1–C2 Gallie C1–C2
Occipital–C1 instability and atlanto-axial subluxation reducible	Stabilize 0–1–2
C1 Lateral mass collapse	Stabilize 0–1–2
C1–C2 rotation subluxation	Stabilize 1–2
Fracture C1	Stabilize 0–1–2
Fracture C2	Stabilize 1–2–3
Anterior compression and atlanto-axial subluxation	One-stage transoral and posterior stabilization 0–1–2 (or more)
Translocation odontoid peg and anterior compression	One-stage transoral and posterior stabilization 0–1–2 (or more)
Subaxial	
Acute disc (good bone)	Smith Robinson/Cloward
Reducible subluxation (no anterior compression)	Laminar clamp/rectangle
Anterior compression and subluxation	One-stage anterior decompression and posterior fixation
Vertebral body collapse	One-stage Vertebrectomy Bone graft Posterior fixation
Combined axial and subaxial	
Atlanto-axial subluxation and subaxial subluxation	One-stage Subaxial anterior decompression Odontoidectomy Posterior stabilization 0–1–2 to T1 (as appropriate)

spinal cord. Calder (1987) has adopted a 'sleep' dose of orally inhaled gases while the nasotracheal tube is passed.

By and large, tracheostomy is not encouraged in these patients. Firstly, if the problem is subaxial the 'clean' and 'dirty' wounds in close approximation may cause problems, as will the holding tapes. Secondly, many of the more advanced rheumatoid patients have 'shortened' necks due to collapse and angulation, and in such patients the tracheostomy may be extremely difficult.

Surgical procedures

There are a wide variety of fixation and stabilization techniques, and it is inevitable that a personal bias will be presented. Set out in Table 52.4 is a summary of the various surgical choices. In this section the points of the main procedures will be described.

Positioning

For transoral surgery, whether or not combined with a posterior fixation, the patient is placed in the lateral position with the head held in the Mayfield Head Holder (Fig. 52.7) (Crockard *et al.*, 1990). It is essential, however, that the head is not overtly flexed forward on the cervical spine to improve the posterior exposure. Rather, the head should be held in gentle extension to ensure anatomical reduction during the posterior fusion once the odontoid has been excised. The advantage is that the blood, drill fragments and washings drain from the operative site, allowing clear visibility. The transoral procedure can therefore be carried out with the surgeon in the seated position. The lateral tilt facility on the operative table will allow access to the occipitocervical area for posterior fusion without moving a grossly unstable spine.

For patients requiring a posterior approach alone the prone position with the head in Mayfield skull fixation is used. For anterior midcervical procedures a supine posture with slight neck extension and intermittent halter traction allows access and distraction.

Bone grafts

Achieving a solid bony fusion can be very difficult in rheumatoid patients due to the poor osteoporotic quality of the bone in the cervical spine and the associated instability. Despite the fact that the patient's own iliac crest may also be osteoporotic, it is still best to use homologous bone as this has a higher

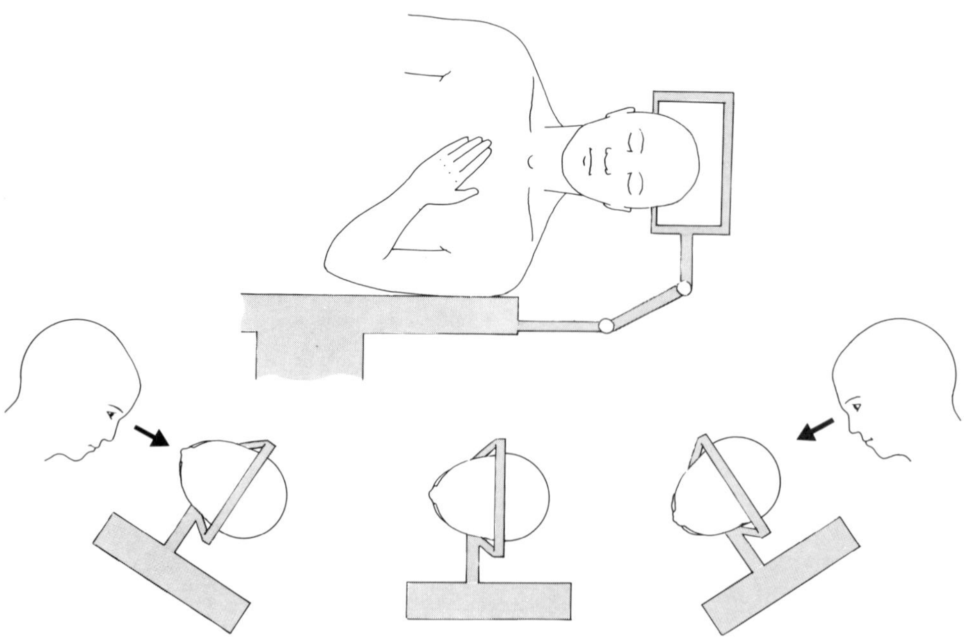

Fig. 52.7 Lateral positioning of the patient will enable anterior decompression and posterior stabilization without risk of movement during the combined one-stage procedure. The lateral tilt facility of the operating table will ensure adequate exposure.

union rate than allograft. Indeed, certain types of allograft material may be too hard for this situation and may produce pressure erosion of the surrounding softer bone in the host site of the rheumatoid spine.

For fusion in the subaxial spine or for a Gallie type C1–C2 block posterior fusion, appropriate dowels, blocks or struts can be fashioned from the iliac crests. For the supplementation of instrumented fusions, corticocancellous strips and chips of bone can easily be obtained from the posterior ilium. Fibular and tibial struts do not seem to provide any advantage to the rheumatoid patient.

The whole question of bone grafting in the segmentally instrumented rheumatoid cervical spine is at present open to question. In some patients who have not had a formal bony fusion as well as instrumentation, the dense fibrous reaction produced by the surgical process is remarkable. Perhaps in the elderly, severely affected rheumatoid, whose bones would fracture with any attempt at decortication, internal stabilization without bony fusion may be the best compromise. Clearly such an emotive subject awaits detailed evaluation.

Intraoperative radiographs

The vertebral anatomy in these patients may be so distorted that normal bony landmarks are obliterated. With subaxial lesions a confirmatory radiograph will add reassurance to a difficult operation and is virtually obligatory.

Transoral surgery offers particular problems in this regard, as the head holder may render any attempts fruitless. A radiotranslucent graphite head holder would improve the situation. The dangers of atlantal rotation must be stressed in transoral surgery and the operator must be sure of the position of the anterior tubercle on C1 and the vertebral artery before making the incision. In difficult cases tomography with a pharyngeal radio-opaque marker performed on the anaesthetized patient may clarify the situation.

The efficacy of a reduction should also be checked radiographically prior to tightening sublaminar wires or firming interlaminar hooks.

Choice of implant

While the type of implant used will vary with individual preference and availability, there are several points which are particularly important in patients with rheumatoid arthritis (Crockard & Ransford, 1990). Firstly, the vertebral bodies are often osteoporotic and the lamina thin. Screw-type fixation may be ineffective. Thus, only when there are very healthy lateral masses will the screw fixation described by Grob & Magerl (1987) be successful. Similarly, there are reservations about the value of anterior cervical spinal plating for the same reasons. Most surgeons favour the use of homologous bone for anterior fusion and instrumentation supplemented with bone for posterior fusion in all but the most healthy necks.

Many rheumatoid patients have atrophied neck muscles, and a large implant or acrylic mass may cause wound problems. In general terms a low-profile system fixed at multiple levels is to be preferred; this spreads the loading at any individual lamina and thus reduces the incidence of failure. Should there be a wound infection, the simpler and lighter the implant the more likely is eventual wound healing to occur without removing the implant.

Specific surgical procedures

Transoral odontoidectomy

The indications for this procedure are a significant irreducible anterior compressive mass. This may be bone, fibrous tissue or pannus, or a dislocated or translocated odontoid peg causing neuraxial compression or angulation. It is not required for reducible subluxations or when the translocation can be corrected by a short period of traction, e.g. 24–48 hours.

With the patient in the lateral position the operator can be comfortably seated and a microdissection carried out with the operating microscope. Using a mouth-gag and tongue retractor, specially designed for this procedure, it is usually possible to expose up to the anterior margin of the foramen magnum without division of the soft palate (Fig. 52.8). The tubercle on anterior arch of C1 is palpated. A 3 cm longitudinal midline incision will expose the arch of C1 and the base of C2. The high-speed air drill with cutting burr will remove a 1 cm segment of the anterior arch of the atlas centred on the central tubercle to expose the compressive mass. The pannus is excised with cutting monopolar diathermy or the laser. The bone of the odontoid is thinned using the cutting burr, and the diamond burr is employed for the final cortical thinning. If the peg is very mobile it is stabilized in position with a holding

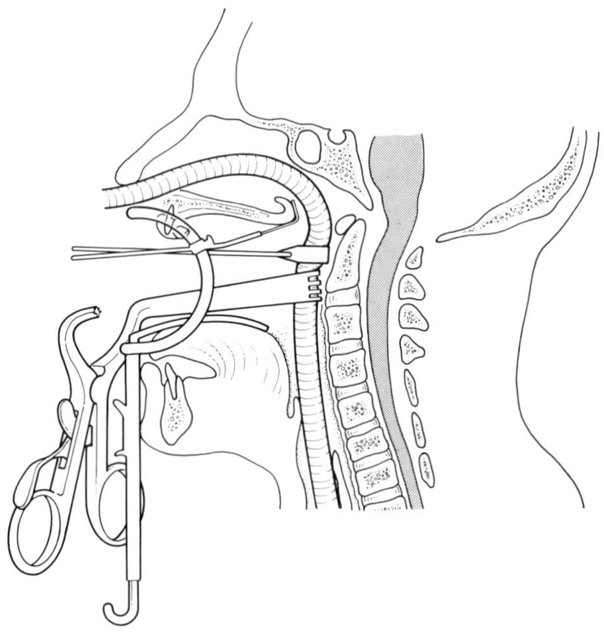

Fig. 52.8 The transoral approach allows direct access to the anterior craniocervical junction. With suitable retraction of the soft palate, light and microsurgery, there is no increased risk of infection.

instrument. If there is significant translocation the peg is osteotomized and the intracranial portion pulled downwards using grasping forceps. The remains of the alar and apical ligaments are then made taut and can be divided with knife, diathermy or laser. Occasionally the dens has already eroded through the dura and a cerebrospinal fluid (CSF) leak occurs. Should this happen, fibrin/thrombin glue, Surgicel, fascia and fat in association with continuous lumbar CSF drainage for five days will allow watertight closure.

The anterior decompression is continued until the dura is seen to pulsate freely, but every portion of fibrous tissue need not be excised. The pharyngeal wound is closed in two layers of interrupted absorbable sutures inserted with a long needle-holder and a 'J'-shaped needle.

Anterior midcervical decompression

The indications for this approach are significant anterior compression and angulation due to wedging and destruction of the midcervical region (Figs 52.7 & 52.9a; see also Fig. 51.2). It is not required in an anterior subluxation, which can be reduced on traction in extension.

The exposure may be exceedingly difficult as the neck is often foreshortened and the distance between the mandible and sternum only a few centimetres. A supine position is best and usually there is little help from attempting to extend the neck. The operating microscope is again an invaluable device for both illumination and magnification.

An anterior border of sternomastoid incision is made. This muscle and the carotid sheath are retracted laterally and medial displacement of the trachea and oesophagus will expose the anterior aspect of the vertebral column lying between the longus coli muscles, which are usually easily identified even with considerable spinal distortion. Because of the angle of approach, and the extent of the 'knuckle', it is usually necessary to remove the central portion of the body of the wedged vertebra and at least half of the vertebra above and below (Fig. 52.9a–c). The air drill, angled curettes and the small upcutting Kerrison rongeurs are necessary to these manoeuvres. As at the atlanto-axial level there may be marked dural constriction by fibrous tissue, and this requires division to allow the dura to pulsate adequately.

A bone block, cut to a template of the operative

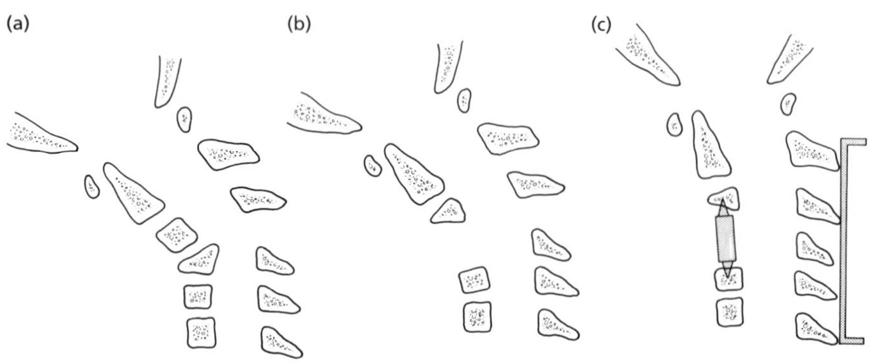

Fig. 52.9 The rheumatoid midcervical kyphos requires anterior decompression and posterior stabilization; the bone is usually not strong enough to allow anterior surgery alone. (a) A midcervical kyphus with C4 wedge; (b) anterior excision of wedge including adjacent areas of C3 and C5; (c) correction of deformity with anterior 'key' bone graft and posterior cervical loop (Ransford) held in place with sublaminar wires.

defect, is obtained from the iliac crest, impacted into position and stay-sutured from one side to another. Such an anterior fusion must be supplemented by a posterior fixation.

Sublaminar wiring

The passage of sublaminar wires requires a great deal of practice and careful surgical technique, otherwise significant neurological complications may occur. It is a very useful technique in the irregular spines of rheumatoid patients and it allows a specifically moulded metal implant to be held firmly in a segmental fixation, thus spreading the load and minimizing the risk of 'cut-out' or wire breakage. It provides instant stability and allows the rapid mobilization of these systemically ill patients. The technique is also useful for wiring in strut bone grafts, but the bone does not guarantee immediate stability and thus the patient may require external stabilization.

The laminae are dissected from the overlying muscle out to the facet joints. The spinous processes within the planned area of fixation may be trimmed, but above and below this the junctional spinous process and ligaments must be carefully preserved to prevent postoperative junctional instability.

The ligamentum flavum must be excised on either side to allow the free passage of the moulded wire. The choice of wire is very important. It should have some memory to retain the shape required for its passage. It must not be too stiff, however, or it may spring back against the dural sac during fixation and cause cord damage. If there is any resistance to the wire passage it suggests either that the space has been inadequately prepared or that the wire is not in the epidural space. The absence of cerebrospinal fluid, either through leakage or dural narrowing, removes the hydrostatic protection from the neuronal tissue. Cord concussion can occur when a wire is passed under a lamina and consequently, in these circumstances, even more care must be taken.

A useful adjunct is the use of a specially designed sublaminar dissector and wire guide (Fig. 52.10), which will aid the interlaminar dissection and pass the wire while protecting the dura. There is a specific model for C1 which has a unique shape (Fig. 52.11); the other levels have more in common. If the operator chooses to pull a guiding thread or the wire through the prepared space, the sublaminar guides have an

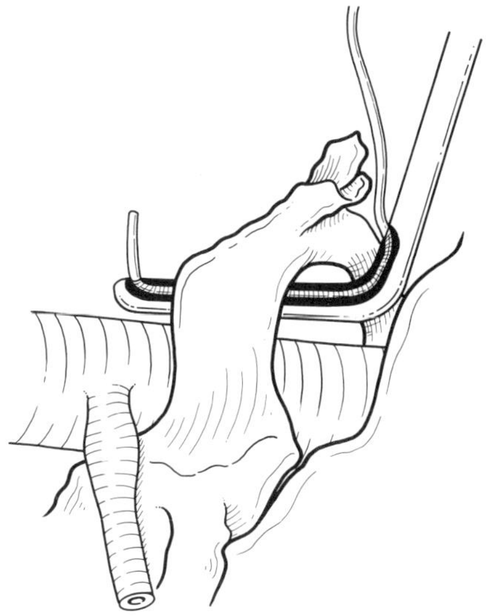

Fig. 52.10 A sublaminar wire guide which allows dissection of ligamentum flavum, a groove along which to pass the wire and prevent dural damage. This model is designed for C2–C7.

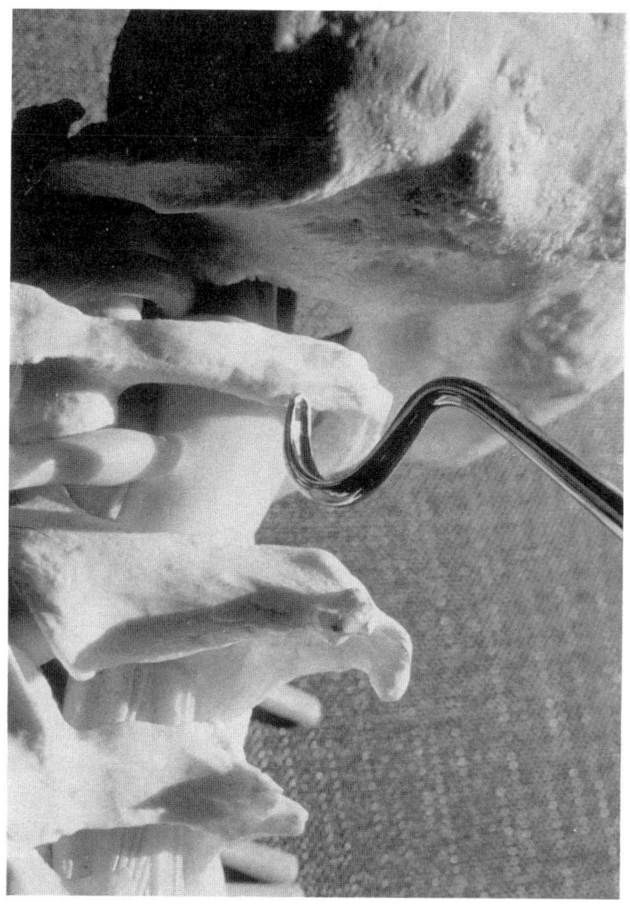

Fig. 52.11 A special shape of sublaminar wire guide is required for C1.

'eye' through which a malleable wire can be passed, to be pulled through underneath.

One of the great problems with the present wires and implants is that they are manufactured in stainless steel. While tried and tested over many years their major disadvantage is interference with follow-up imaging, and it is hoped that soon titanium implants and fixation techniques will be more generally available.

Wiring may be undertaken at each level in a segment of fused spine. In this situation the fused segment is wired segmentally by finding the ligamentum flavum by locally drilling away overlying bone. The 1 mm or 2 mm Kerrison upcutting instrument can then enlarge the interlaminal space enough to allow passage of the wires.

Ransford Hartshill loops

The advantage of preformed but adjustable loops held in place with sublaminar wires is that they require much less technical skill and back-up equipment than implants demanding the insertion of screws which, in the weak rheumatoid bone, would be difficult anyway. The multiple-level sublaminar fixation allows a spreading of the loading forces and minimizes the chances of wire or laminar fracture. The occipitocervical loop has been designed to be fixed via paired burr holes to the occipital bone, rather than at the foramen magnum which is a very difficult area to pass wires. There is a flare at C2 below which the C2 sublaminar wire should be fixed. As the C2 wires are tightened they should slip caudally off the flare, producing occipitocervical distraction and secure fixation (Crockard *et al.*, 1990).

For occipitocervical instability with erosions at occipito/C1 and C1–C2 a minimum six-point fixation is recommended (occiput, C1 and C2) but if the C1 lamina is weak then further laminae should be incorporated. If there is a 'staircase' phenomenon or ankylosed segments then further subaxial levels may be incorporated.

For subaxial levels the lumbar Hartshill rectangle has been used (Fig. 52.12), but these are quite bulky

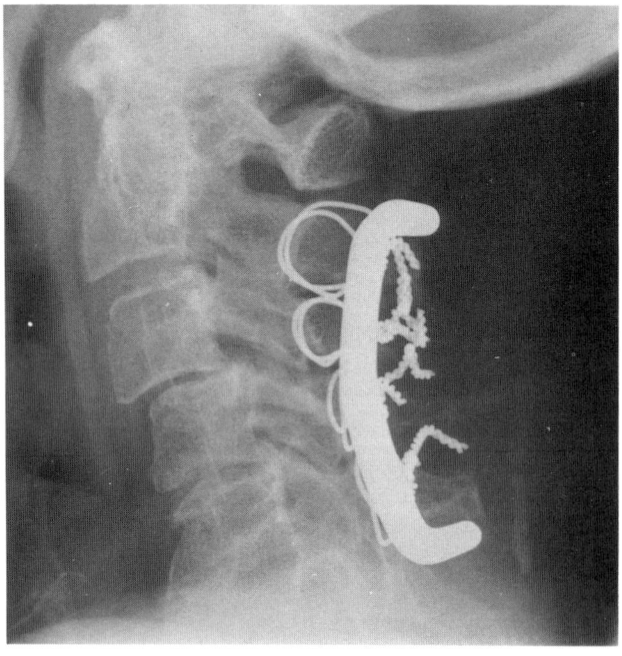

Fig. 52.12 The postoperative radiograph of the patient with a 'staircase' phenomenon seen in Fig. 52.2c.

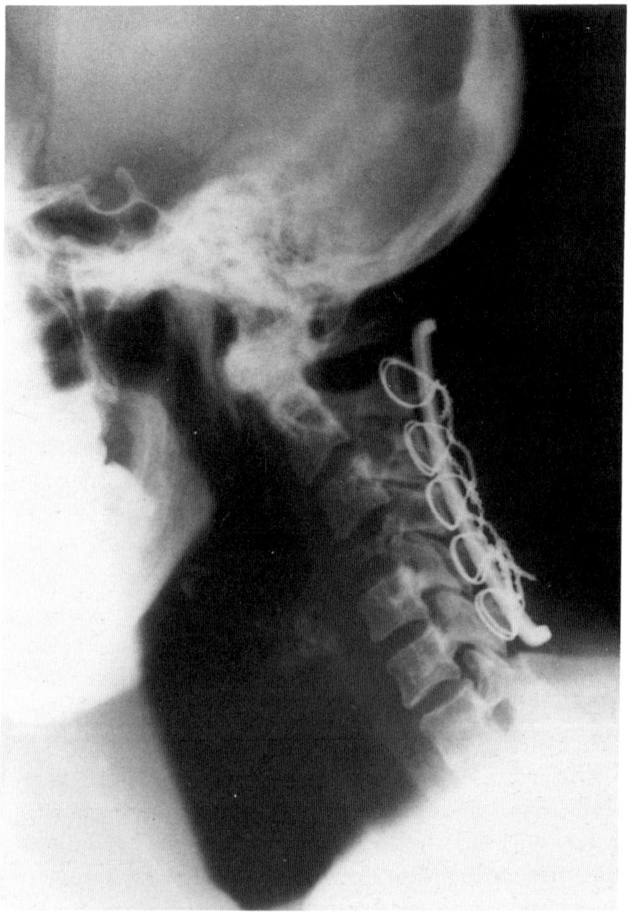

Fig. 52.13 A Ransford low-profile cervical loop to stabilize and correct deformity, held in position with sublaminar wire fixation.

and a modified low-profile cervical loop (Fig. 52.13) has been designed to overcome this problem. If two or three segments have ankylosed, each level should be used for sublaminar fixation. There is no point in 'fusing short' into a fused segment.

Laminar clamps

The advantage of this type of implant (e.g. the Halifax clamp) is that the dissection is limited to defining the laminae without removing the ligamentum flavum. It is particularly suited to single-level disease and not very useful in the 'staircase'-type deformity and not at all in occipitocervical subluxation. In uncomplicated reducible C1–C2 subluxation it is very useful. The technique involves selecting the appropriate-sized clamp for the individual lamina effecting reduction and fixation (Moskovich & Crockard, 1991) (Fig. 52.14).

Considering the systemic effects of this autoimmune disease and the profound side-effects produced by their long-term steroid intake, it is remarkable how well these patients tolerate such complex surgery. It must be emphasized, however, that the utmost care by a team of rheumatologists, anaesthetists, physicians, orthopaedic surgeons, neurosurgeons, nurses and therapists must be used to achieve best results. Such an approach, combined with the correct choice of surgical approach, allows successful surgery with very low morbidity and mortality. Impressive neurological recovery can be achieved in the majority of patients provided that the principle of obligatory anterior decompression in the presence of irreducible anterior cord compression is followed.

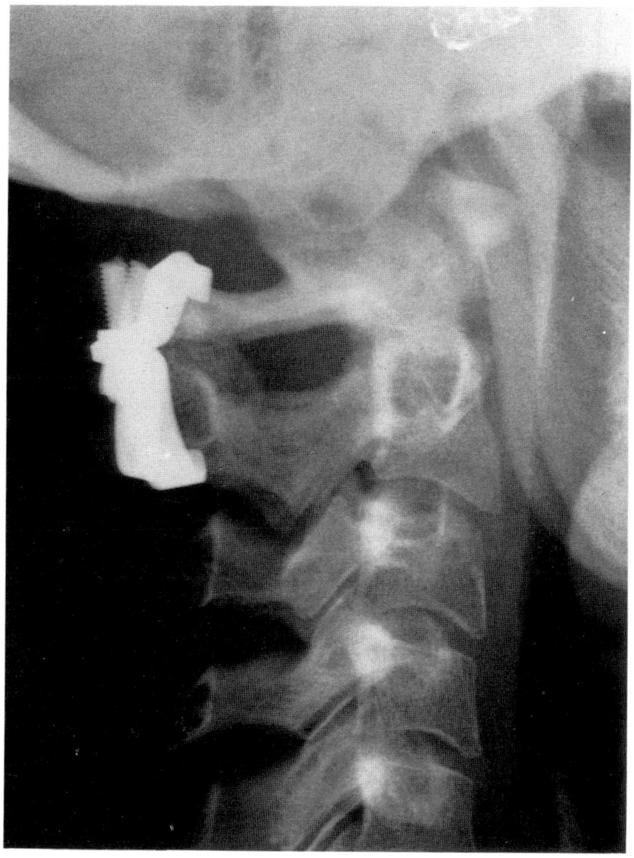

Fig. 52.14 A Halifax clamp fixation to correct and hold a rheumatoid atlanto-axial subluxation.

In the correct environment, complex cervical surgery is well tolerated in rheumatoid patients. The correction and stabilization of deformity or decompression of the neuraxis can greatly improve their quality of life. The lessons learnt in the treatment of major joint replacement now permit an equally active surgical approach to rheumatoid cervical spine disease. A nihilistic approach of supervised neglect is no longer tenable.

REFERENCES

Boyle, A.C. (1971) The rheumatoid neck. *Proc. R. Soc. Med.*, **64**, 1161–1165.

Brattstrom, H. & Granholm, L. (1976) Atlanto-axial fusion in rheumatoid arthritis. *Acta Orthop. Scand.*, **47**, 619–628.

Calder, I. (1987) Anaesthesia for transoral and craniocervical surgery. In Jewkes, D. (ed.) *Baillière's Clinical Anaesthesiology*, pp. 441–457. W.B. Saunders, London.

Crockard, H.A. & Ransford, A.O. (1990) Stabilization of the spine. In Symon, L., Calliauw, L., Cohadon, F., Guidetti, B., Loew, F., Nornes, H., Pasztor, E., Pertuiset, B., Pickard, J.D. & Yasargil, M.G. (eds) *Advances and Technical Standards in Neurosurgery*, vol. 17, pp. 159–188. Springer, Vienna.

Crockard, H.A., Calder, I. & Ransford, A.O. (1990) One stage transoral decompression and posterior fixation in rheumatoid atlanto-axial subluxation: a technical note. *J. Bone Jt. Surg.*, **72B**, 682–685.

Garrod, A.E.A. (1990) *A Treatise on Rheumatism and Rheumatoid Arthritis*, pp. 1–342. C. Griffith, London.

Greenberg, A.D. (1968) Atlanto-axial dislocations. *Brain*, **91**, 655–684.

Grob, D. & Magerl, F. (1987) Operative stabilisation in C1–2 fractures. *Orthopade*, **16**, 46–54.

Hamblen, D.L. (1983) *Postgraduate Textbook of Clinical Orthopaedics*, pp. 487–497. Wright, Bristol.

Jebsen, R.H., Taylor, N., Treischmann, R.B., Trotter, M.J. & Howard, L.A. (1969) An objective and standardised test of hand function. *Arch. Phys. Med.*, **50**, 311–319.

Kirwan, J.R. & Reeback, J.S. (1986) Stanford health assessment questionnaire modified to assess disability in British patients with rheumatoid arthritis. *Br. J. Rheumatol.*, **25**, 206–209.

Meijers, K.A.E., Cats, A., Kremer, H.P., Luyendijk, W., Onvlee, G.J. & Thomeer, R.T. (1984) Cervical myelopathy in rheumatoid arthritis. *Clin. Exp. Rheumatol.*, **2**, 239–245.

Moskovich, R. & Crockard, H.A. (1991) Atlanto-axial arthrodesis using interlaminar clamps: an improved technique. *Spine* (In press).

Ranawat, C.S., O'Leary, P., Pellicci, P., Tsairis, P., Marchisello, P. & Dorr, L. (1979) Cervical spine fusion in rheumatoid arthritis. *J. Bone Jt. Surg.*, **61A**, 1003–1010.

Steinbrocker, O., Traeger, C.H. & Batterman, R.C. (1949) Therapeutic criteria in rheumatoid arthritis. *J. Am. Med. Assoc.*, **140**, 659–662.

Stevens, J.M., Kendall, B.E., Crockard, H.A. (1986) The spinal cord in rheumatoid arthritis with clinical myelopathy: a computed myelographic study. *J. Neurol. Neurosurg. Psychiatr.*, **49**, 140–151.

Symmons, D.P.M. (1988) Neoplasia in rheumatoid arthritis. *J. Rheumatol.*, **15**, 1319–1321.

Winfield, J., Cook, D., Brook, A.S. & Corbet, M.A. (1981) A prospective study of the radiological changes in the cervical spine in early rheumatoid disease. *Ann. Rheum. Dis.*, **40**, 109–114.

53 · Surgical Management of Ankylosing Spondylitis

By P.M. YEOMAN

The genetic studies embracing the B27 antigen have provided an exceptional opportunity to consider the aetiology and epidemiology of ankylosing spondylitis (Brewerton, 1978). Not only are those people who possess HLA B27 antigens more likely to develop ankylosing spondylitis, but those who do not are likely to be spared. Ankylosing spondylitis is within the group of seronegative athropathies and the rheumatoid factor is therefore absent from the serum. At one time, and not very long ago, it was considered to be a condition almost confined to men in the ratio of 1 : 8; but now that ratio has been considerably adjusted to 1 : 2 and it has been suggested that there is no sex discrimination. There are certain predisposing factors; it is often associated with ulcerative colitis and occasionally with Crohn's disease. It was popular to incriminate low-grade infection, in particular in the intestinal tract where the *Klebsiella* organism was isolated (Isenberg *et al.*, 1987), but treatment directed towards clearing the infection made only transient benefit on the progress of the spinal condition.

Ankylosing spondylitis may provide lesions in the wrists and hands which are almost identical to those seen in rheumatoid arthritis, but that is about as far as a possible link is obtained, because the progress of the disease in the hips in young adults is not the same, and the pathological process in the spine is entirely different.

Clinical picture

The earliest symptoms of ankylosing spondylitis may arise in adolescence with pain and stiffness in the hip, or pain in the knee referred from the hip, or even local heel pain. The classical picture of low back ache is unusual before the age of 18, but it gradually increases and is associated with stiffness, worse on waking, and tends to pursue a relentless course. The rib cage may become involved via the costovertebral joints.

The active phase of the disease may be short-lived and rarely lasts later than the age of 35, but the entire spine may be involved so that if the relentless course of the disease is not checked the patient will be transformed not only into a solid pillar of bone from head to thigh but also into a flexed pillar.

There are other side-effects to be considered such as reduced vital capacity, loss of thoracic breathing which is replaced by abdominal breathing, occasional aortic stenosis and bundle branch block. In addition there may be associated intestinal problems from ulcerative colitis. The untreated clinical picture is thus a very despondent one resulting in a relatively young patient reduced to a complete cripple in a matter of 10–15 years. The diagnosis of ankylosing spondylitis is still delayed, and yet it should be in the forefront when assessing young men and girls who complain of back ache with no obvious radiological defect and no response from a reasonably short course of conventional treatment.

Management (non-surgical)

If the diagnosis is made correctly in the early stages of the disease much of the deformity of the spine can be prevented. The management is in the hands of an experienced team which includes rheumatologists, physiotherapists, occupational therapists and social workers. The team should be in a separate unit but preferably within a large district hospital, which in turn acts as a regional referral centre with reasonably easy access to a total body scanner and/or imaging with magnetic resonance.

Relief of pain is the patient's main concern, and non-steroidal anti-inflammatory agents are usually fairly effective.

Assessment

This is the next part of the team's work and involves not only measurement of the patient's physical ability in climbing stairs, walking, running and playing games but the posture has to be recorded in such a way that the patient can continue to be assessed at home by a relative or friend. There should be an assessment of the vital capacity and lung function. The social history should contain information about the patient's lifestyle, employment, ability to cope with a family, education and future prospects. This important set of details may take a few days to elucidate in hospital in order to prepare a baseline for management now and plans for the future. It will also serve as a reference for comparison with later assessments.

Exercise

Physiotherapy is the next stage in management. There is no doubt that group sessions are not only more effective but more enjoyable for the patients and the team. Competitive exercise, suitably graded as regards age and ability, provides a very important climate within the group, which in turn engenders an ability to win. Passive exercises are also performed, and there is no doubt that contractures of joints and poor postures can be improved (Bulstrode *et al.*, 1987). This regime can be taught to the patient and a near relative or friend so that the improvement can be maintained.

Finally, experience of this type of team work has proved successful in overcoming many of the serious problems in ankylosing spondylitis. It has provided a base for patients to contact when in trouble, and they return for further sessions at intervals of one year or less, depending on the severity of their condition. Indeed the patients themselves have formed a national association which has a well-informed newsletter, and regular scientific meetings are held which are well organized and very popular.

Management (surgical)

The indications for surgical correction of the spine in ankylosing spondylitis are flexed posture and pain. These two factors usually arise separately but may occur together. The most important is the correction of posture, and the reason for this is related to the cause of the symptoms.

Flexed posture (Fig. 53.1)

Prevention of this problem is obviously the best policy, but even today we are faced with patients who have either not heard of the exercise regime or have failed to respond. It is axiomatic that flexion contractures of the hips have been excluded in the first medical assessment. This is perhaps easier said than done, because the patient is usually lying or standing in a fixed flexed posture and the hips can be examined only if the patient is lying on his or her side. Mobile hips and suitably corrected hip contractures will undoubtedly improve the overall posture, thus reducing the need for surgical correction of the spine.

The greatest disability is the lack of forward vision, so that patients have difficulty walking in corridors or streets because they are continually bumping into people. They are unable to look at buildings or views more than a few metres ahead of them, and have difficulty in reading public notice-boards at stations or enjoying a picture gallery. These are a few of the many complaints gleaned from patients not only before surgical correction but also from comments expressed after correction.

Pain

Pain is due to three separate causes: the disease is still active, a stress fracture, an ordinary (straightforward) fracture.

THE DISEASE PROCESS

This may become quiescent and then flare up again in a similar manner to rheumatoid arthritis although this is not the usual pattern. Generally patients complain of relentless pain, hopefully relieved to some extent by drugs, but continuing its course during the active phase of the disease which may last until the patient is about 35 years old. Thereafter there should be a lull in the severity of the pain or it

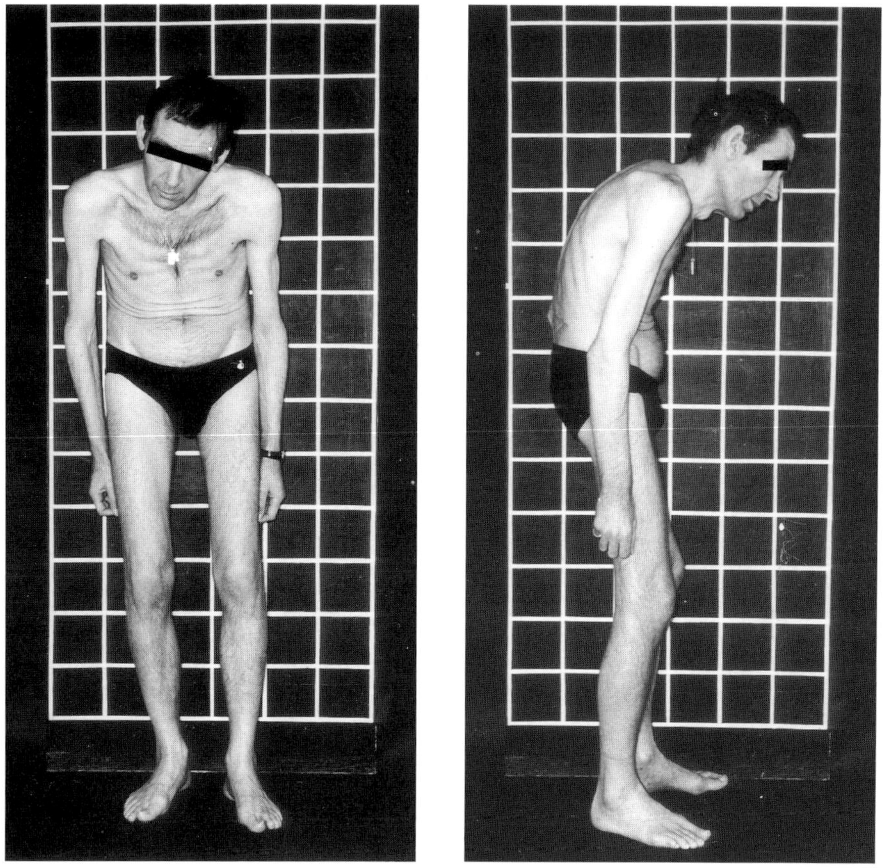

Fig. 53.1 The flexed posture.

may cease. It is in this later period when correction can be contemplated.

A STRESS FRACTURE

A stress fracture may arise at any time, but usually some months or years after the active phase has resolved. Variously described as a 'Romanus lesion' (Romanus & Ydén, 1955; Fig. 53.2) it is radiologically similar to a low-grade or chronic infection seen in tuberculosis or even brucellosis, and there lies the confusion. It has been proved by Yau & Chan (1974) from material found at anterior fusion that the so-called destructive lesion in the vertebral column is a pseudarthrosis resulting from an initial stress fracture in the posterior elements of a vertebra. The anterior lesion may occur across the body of the vertebra or between two vertebrae to give an appearance of discitis. The lesions may be single or multiple and most occur near the dorsilumbar region (Fang *et al.*, 1988).

The cause of these lesions is related to the points of mechanical stress arising from the uneven ossification (Ball, 1980) between the vertebrae, which in turn produces fused segments dispersed between mobile unfused portions. In the past it was always assumed that the bamboo appearance of the spine occurred in

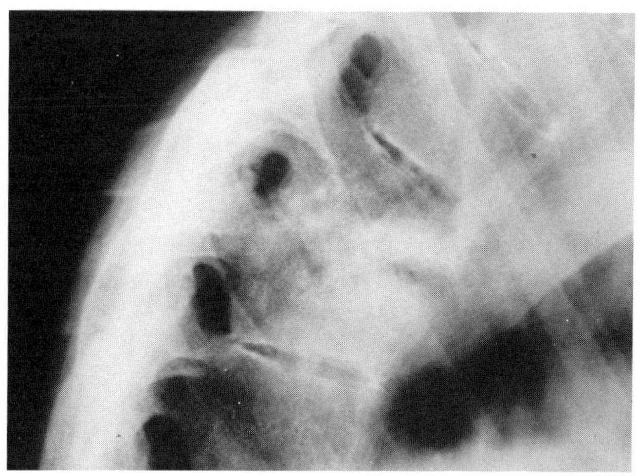

Fig. 53.2 A stress fracture D8–D9.

a uniform manner, and that one area was as strong as another, but this idea is no longer tenable.

The diagnosis of a stress fracture is made on the clinical history of pain in the back arising *de novo* many months or years after cessation of pain in the active phase of the disease, and confirmed by conventional X-rays, but now proved unequivocally by isotope bone scanning and even magnetic resonance imaging.

Healing of a stress fracture may be spontaneous and so a delay in treatment could be an advantage. Sadly, it is not possible to predict those who will proceed to spontaneous healing, and it may be necessary to advise a more active programme.

TREATMENT OF A STRESS FRACTURE (NON-SURGICAL)

A plaster jacket or spinal brace worn for three months may induce healing of the fracture, and the choice depends on the extent of the spinal deformity. The patient may not wish to proceed with a cumbersome support which will not provide any guarantee of success or prevent a recurrence. This is not the occasion to allow the patient to decide, but can be the basis of a reasoned argument to proceed to an operation.

TREATMENT OF A STRESS FRACTURE (SURGICAL)

Posterior fusion

Posterior fusion using metal fixation across the affected level of the fracture can be an effective method of relieving the pain and is recommended when the deformity is minimal. If the deformity has caused fixed flexion of the spine this method will fail.

Anterior spinal fusion

Anterior spinal fusion has been recorded as a very successful method (Yau & Chan, 1974; Fang *et al.*, 1988) but it has the disadvantage that it can be a formidable task in the lower dorsal and upper lumbar spine. Furthermore it fails to correct the deformity and thus the cause of the mechanical stress is not removed.

Osteotomy of the spine

The kyphosis has to be assessed not only on the radiographs but on the clinical photographs (Fig. 53.3) in order to decide on the optimum level for operative correction. The level will be either in the lumbar or cervical spine because any correction in the dorsal spine may be too hazardous for the spinal cord.

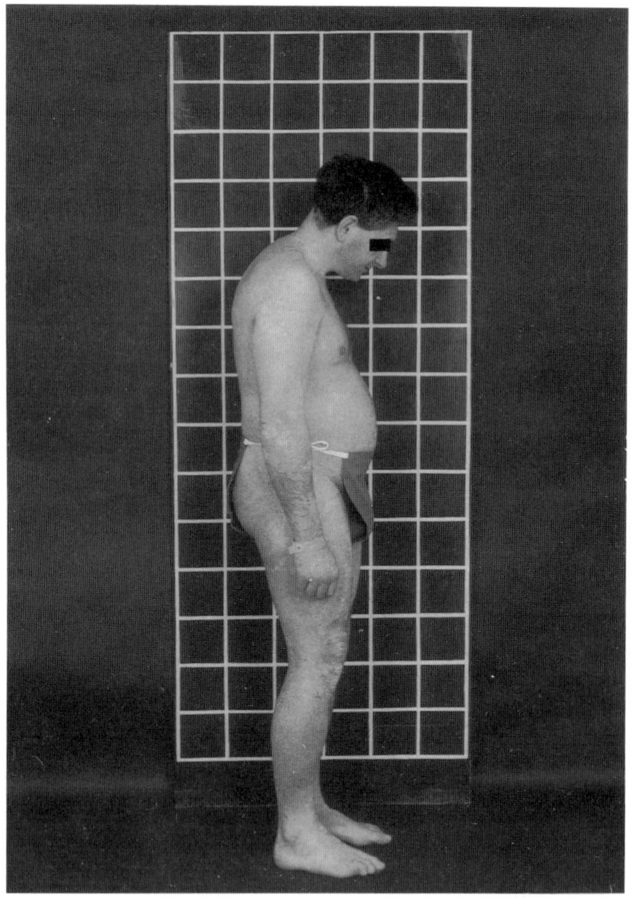

Fig. 53.3 Flexed spine—mainly cervicodorsal.

Osteotomy of the spine is not a new idea and it was well recorded by Smith-Petersen *et al.* (1945) followed by Law (1976). In the early years there was a fairly high mortality and morbidity related almost entirely to compression of the spinal cord. The operation was not always the main hazard because a patient with a rigid flexed neck presented the anaesthetist with an extremely difficult task. Correction of part of the flexed posture in the author's experience has altered the mechanical stress imposed over a wide segment, and allowed spontaneous healing of either one or two stress fractures between the middorsal and midlumbar areas.

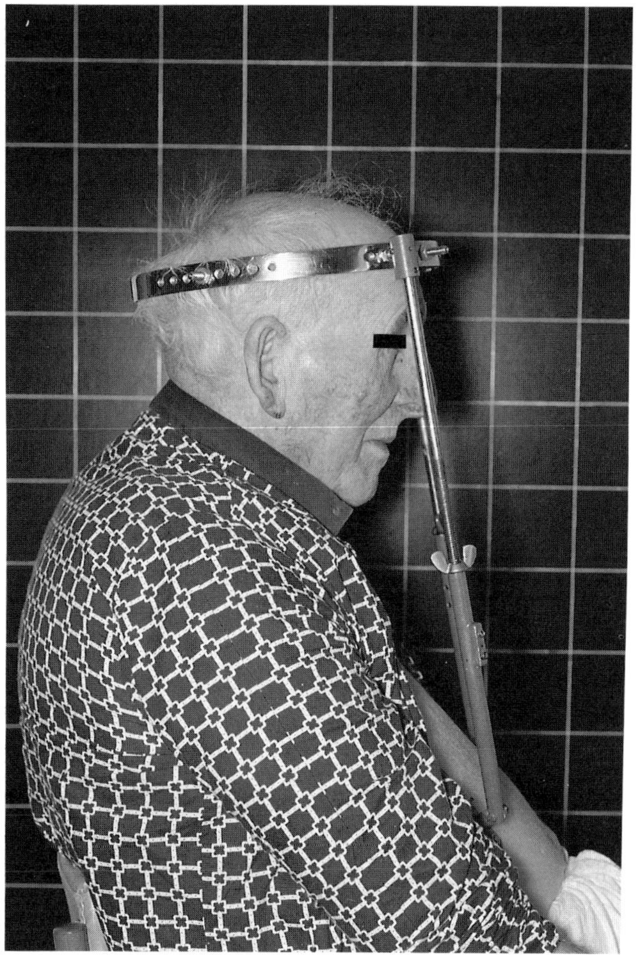

Fig. 53.4 Halovest correction without osteotomy for a fracture at C7.

FRACTURE OF THE SPINE

A fracture of the spine in ankylosing spondylitis is not unexpected; bearing in mind that the spine may be rigid from the head to the pelvis and contrary to previous teaching it may not be as strong as a normal vertebral column because of osteoporosis (Hanson *et al.*, 1971).

Pain developing immediately after a fall or any traumatic incident is due to a fracture. It is unlikely to be revealed on conventional radiographs and thus the fracture will be missed. In fact it can be stated with some confidence that a patient with burnt-out ankylosing spondylitis who complains of pain in the neck after a fall must have a fracture at the cervico-dorsal junction; a notoriously difficult area to define radiographically. Tomography was the accepted method and this would reveal the crush fracture of the body of the seventh cervical or first dorsal vertebra. A total-body scanner is now the accepted method. Other fractures arise lower down the spine after a fall down stairs or a traffic accident, and these usually involve the posterior elements of a vertebra; the fractured areas which may proceed to a pseudarthrosis and an anterior stress fracture.

Treatment of a simple fracture of the spine

It would initially appear to be an elementary exercise to manage an undisplaced fracture of the body of the seventh cervical or the pedicle of a second lumbar vertebra; indeed it is, because a supporting collar or special spinal support will probably allow the fracture to heal. A golden opportunity to correct at least part of the deformity will have been thrown away.

Some of the patients who have sustained fractures in the lower cervical spine have been too old, or ill in other ways, to withstand a major operation, but it was possible on five occasions to apply an external fixator and make a fair correction of the flexed posture.

The halovest apparatus was applied under local anaesthesia and simple threaded rods, bottle screws and universal joints were made in the hospital workshop. These were attached to either a plaster or Baycast vest (Fig. 53.4). Gradual extension of the spine was achieved over a period of three to four weeks, during which time the patient was mobile but had to be kept in hospital in order to keep a close eye on the apparatus. The apparatus was retained for a further three months but the patient was then at home and checked at intervals. Finally the halovest was replaced with a rigid collar for another three months.

PREPARATION FOR SPINAL OSTEOTOMY

This will be a major event for the patient, who is entitled to know at least some of the operative detail and the serious complications. Some will have heard the experience of other patients who have undergone the operation. They need to know the risk to the spinal cord, the mortality and their expectations. It is of some surprise to find that patients expect to regain a reasonable range of movement or to be able to take a more active part in games. It must be explained that the operation entails making a deliberate but controlled fracture across the spine and that the spine has to be supported (a) in the neck by an external fixator, that is, the halovest; (b) in the lower spine by a long spinal support. They require to know the approximate duration of stay in hospital, the length of time wearing any harness and the number of return admissions to hospital.

Anaesthesia

A fibreoptic bronchoscope is an essential piece of equipment and has virtually resolved the immense difficulty of performing endotracheal intubation in a patient with teeth, a restricted range of movement in the temporomandibular joints and a stiff flexed neck (Fig. 53.5). The patient needs to discuss the procedure with the anaesthetist, particularly if it is intended to embark on an 'awake' intubation, which appears to be a safe precaution.

Lumbar osteotomy

Surgical technique

The patient is placed prone on a suitably hinged and padded operating table. A longitudinal midline incision is made for the entire length of the lumbar spine, and the posterior aspect of the lumbar vertebrae and sacrum is exposed by sharp and/or diathermy dissection. A suitable level for the osteotomy is selected, usually between the third and fourth lumbar vertebrae, to allow sufficient room for the metal fixation. At the selected level the spinous process is removed and saved for bone graft. The exposure continues laterally with the aid of Cobb's elevators as far as the expected site of the facet joints; bleeding from the small lumbar vessels has to be controlled.

The base of the spinous process is nibbled away down to the dura, which provides the depth and direction for the removal of the laminae on each side. On the lateral margins the emerging nerve roots can be defined together with their accompanying vessels, and a generous chevron-shaped piece of bone is removed in order to allow not only sufficient room for the nerves, but stability when the bone gap is closed. All is now set for the correction, but it is an advantage to have exposed the bone covering the facet joints for three joints above and below the osteotomy site.

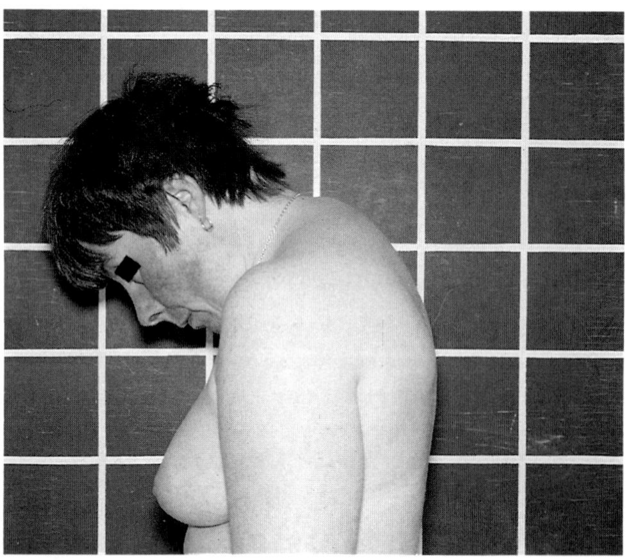

Fig. 53.5 A rigid flexed neck presenting a difficult problem for the anaesthetist.

Closure of the osteotomy

This has to be conducted as a controlled manoeuvre by gently straightening out the table and holding the spinous processes above and below the osteotomy site with large bone-holding forceps. It may be necessary to apply some body pressure on the spine to achieve 'osteoclasis' and closure of the osteotomy, but the nerves have to be seen in order to prevent their entrapment. The adjacent spinous processes may have to be trimmed to allow tidy apposition. On most occasions the bone is much softer than normal, which provides a bonus for the operator.

Internal fixation

A variety of methods have been tried, and discarded except for one which has met with approval. Interspinous fixation was perhaps the easiest technique, but encircling wires tended to break or cut through the soft bone and the more rigid plates and bolts avulsed the spinous processes. This was abandoned and replaced with interlaminar wiring and Luque rods or Hartshill rectangle but again the bone may either be too soft and weak to hold the position, or the introduction of the wires difficult because of the solid sheet of bone obscuring the laminae, although, surprisingly, the interlaminar spaces are often preserved even in apparently solid spines.

Interpedicle fixation seems to achieve the necessary

stability and although the Webb–Morley technique was developed for anterior interbody fixation during correction of scoliosis it has been found most successful in posterior stabilization. It is not always easy to find the pedicle in order to insert the large fixation screw, but the combination of a skeleton alongside for checking the anatomy and a small drill or awl make the task much easier. The wound is closed with drainage and a posterior carapace of plaster is made.

Postoperative regime

An indwelling catheter makes life more comfortable for female patients, but is used in males only when retention occurs. The patient is nursed in an ordinary bed and receives antibiotic cover for five days. On the second day the patient is turned and an anterior carapace of plaster is made so that the two plaster shells can be strapped together for turning on a regular basis. A paralytic ileus often develops, due in part to retroperitoneal bleeding from the osteotomy site, so it is necessary to continue intravenous fluid therapy until the bowel sounds have returned and any distension has begun to resolve.

During the third week the patient is allowed to sit out and stand with the support of the temporary plaster cast; later a definitive plaster jacket is applied. The patient returns home when the gait is steady and the plaster is satisfactory.

Three months later the patient is readmitted for a further X-ray check and a new plaster, which is retained for a further three months. Finally if there is evidence of union at the osteotomy site the plaster can be replaced with a long spinal support (Fig. 53.6).

Dorsal osteotomy

Correction at thoracic level is very rarely indicated, as in most patients a lumbar or cervical procedure will suffice. Occasionally, however, there is an angular kyphotic deformity in the mid-dorsal area when local correction should at least be considered.

One must approach this area with caution, however, as correction can be achieved only by a two-stage

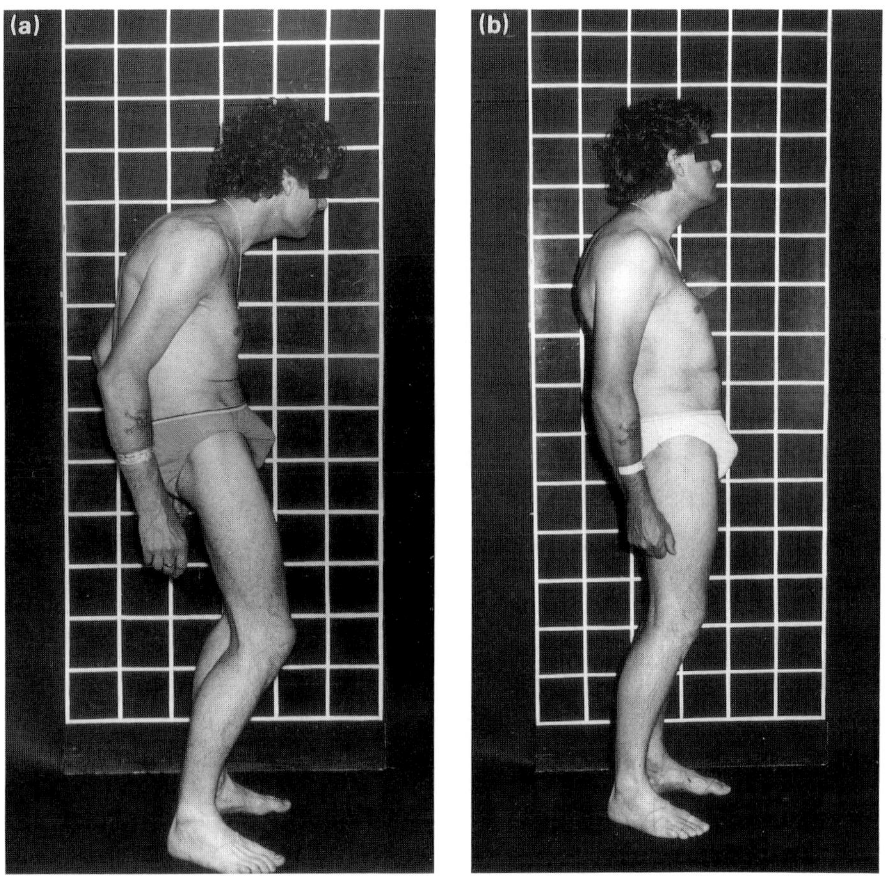

Fig. 53.6 (a) Preoperative posture—awaiting a lumbar osteotomy; (b) postoperative posture—after lumbar osteotomy.

procedure involving first a transthoracic approach to excise the disc spaces at the kyphos and rib grafting; secondly, a week later, proceed to posterior correction and fixation. Such surgery is not without potential dangers cardiopulmonary-wise and neurologically, as there is often depleted cardiac and pulmonary reserve.

Although the author has not had occasion to resort to such measures a few others have achieved correction successfully (Owen, 1990, personal communication).

Cervical osteotomy

This operation is technically more difficult than lumbar osteotomy because the spinal cord is vulnerable and the final stability depends more on external than internal fixation. Smith-Petersen (1945), Law (1976) and more recently Simmons (1972) described techniques of cervical osteotomy, but we also owe much to the halovest external fixator. The preparation of the patient and the anaesthetic problems are exactly the same as for lumbar osteotomy.

Surgical technique

As soon as the patient is fully anaesthetized the halo is secured to the skull with screws at a suitable angle to compensate for the proposed correction, and the patient is transferred to the operating table with separate head support (Fig. 53.7). The incision is vertically placed in the midline in order to allow more room for internal fixation, which is a sad change from the author's original transverse approach which gave better healing but not such good access.

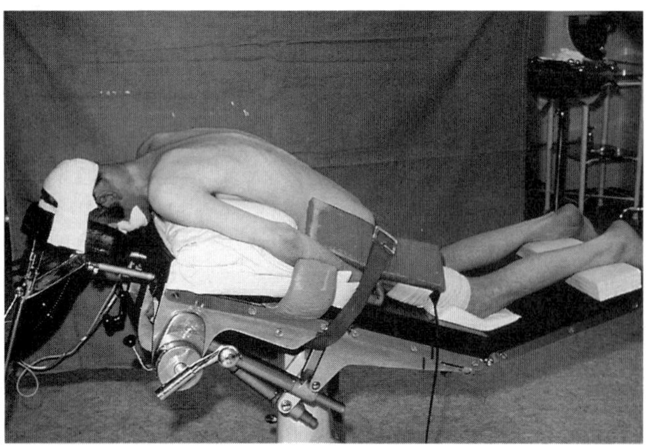

Fig. 53.7 Position on the padded operating table before cervical osteotomy.

The spinous processes, occiput and laminae are exposed by sharp and/or diathermy dissection until a complete sheet of bone is revealed.

The lateral margins of the dissection have to include the posterior site of the facet joints so that a reasonable exposure can be obtained of the emerging nerves at the osteotomy level. Venous haemorrhage can be troublesome at this stage, but with patience and skill it will be controlled. A spinous process is selected for the proposed level of the osteotomy, which is usually at the sixth cervical vertebra, and it is removed with bone nibblers. Ample bone removal continues until the dura is exposed and then it becomes easier to define a gap of approximately 1.5 cm which extends laterally to reveal the cervical nerves.

CLOSURE OF THE OSTEOTOMY

The anaesthetist will have to adjust the headpiece either as a means of closing the osteotomy or preferably after the surgeon has performed the correction by osteoclasis while gripping the halo through the towels. The control of the closure and correction is thus entirely and literally in the hands of the surgeon, but the assistant has to provide a clear view of the dura and emerging nerves in order to prevent any compression of these important structures.

FIXATION

There is limited space and a relatively small area of bone in the cervical spine for any extensive metal fixation, yet the strain imposed on the adjacant vertebrae after an osteotomy must be considerable. This factor is reflected in the need for the strongest possible internal fixation combined with a similar method of external fixation in order to provide a stable environment for sound fusion at the unstable osteotomy site. Unfortunately this cannot be achieved, and a compromise is the only solution.

The moulded Daap plate is secured to the four adjacent spinous processes and small pieces of the previously removed bone are packed loosely on the exposed sheet of bone, part of which can be lightly roughened with a powered burr.

The halo is attached to the padded vest with four supporting rods and the patient is transferred either to an intensive-care unit or special recovery area.

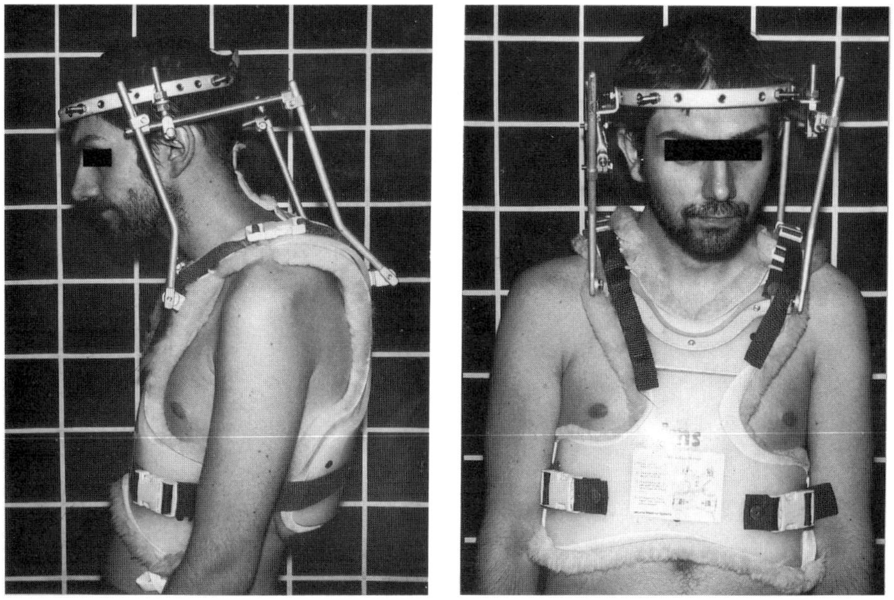

Fig. 53.8 Postoperative position to show halovest external fixator.

Antibiotic cover is provided for five days, during which time the patient receives breathing exercises. As soon as possible the patient is lifted into a sitting posture so that the halovest supports can be adjusted (Fig. 53.8).

POSTOPERATIVE MANAGEMENT

During the second week after the operation the patient should be able to walk within the hospital, and will return home when confident. A torque screwdriver is

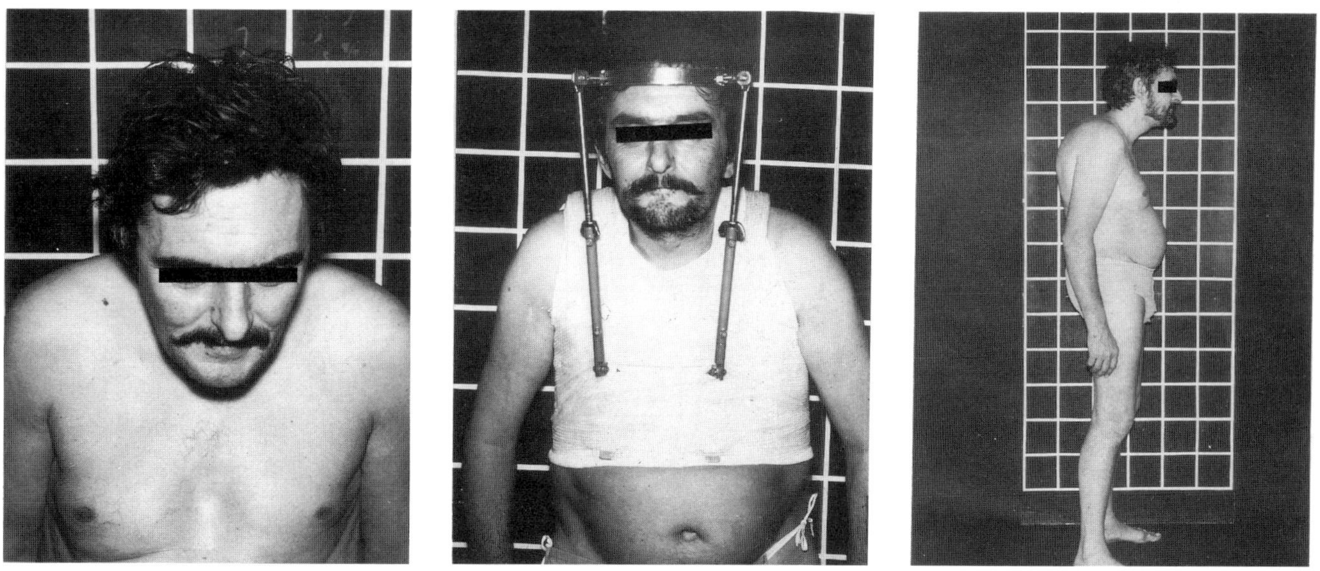

(a) (b) (c)

Fig. 53.9 (a) Preoperative posture—awaiting cervical osteotomy; (b) postoperative posture—immediately after cervical osteotomy; (c) postoperative posture to show final correction at six months.

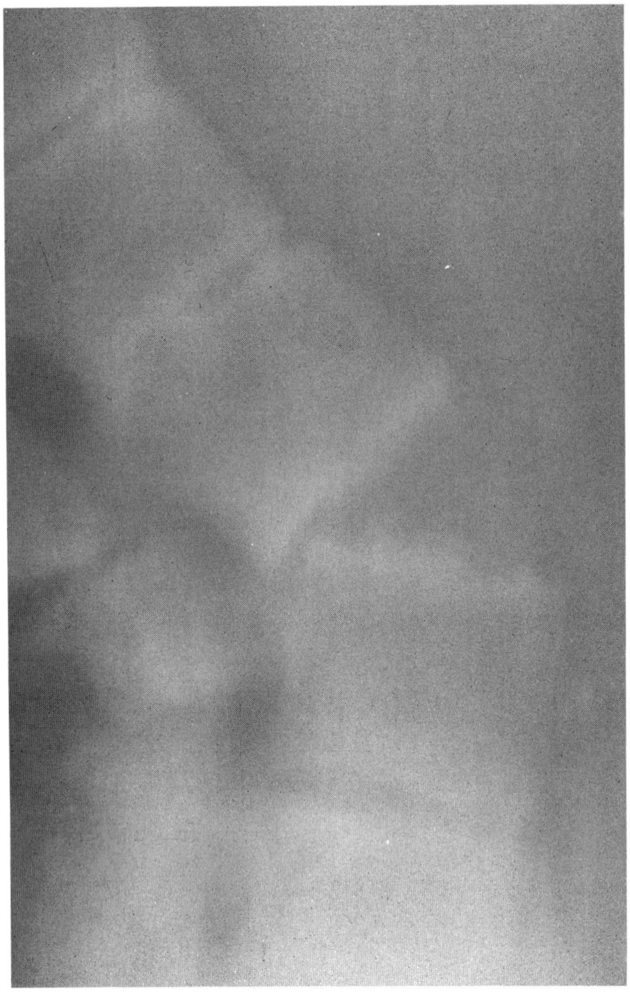

Fig. 53.10 Overcorrection beyond 45° has caused an unstable and potentially dangerous situation. Fortunately the osteotomy fused spotaneously without any complications.

part of the equipment. The patient, close relative or friend is instructed about its use because the skull fixation requires to be checked each week.

At three months further X-ray checks are made, but the halo is retained for six months. It is then replaced with a firm collar for another three months or longer depending on the X-ray assessment (Fig. 53.9).

Results

An average correction of 35° was achieved both in the lumbar and cervical spine. In the early stages 10° and occasionally more were lost, particularly in the lumbar spine due to inadequate internal fixation, but this problem was resolved by the use of pedicle anchorage.

Any ambitious correction exceeding 45° produces an alarming X-ray appearance (Fig. 53.10); indeed this was seen at operation on two occasions; one in the lumbar and the other in the cervical spine. A forward slip or spondylolisthesis is almost inevitable and

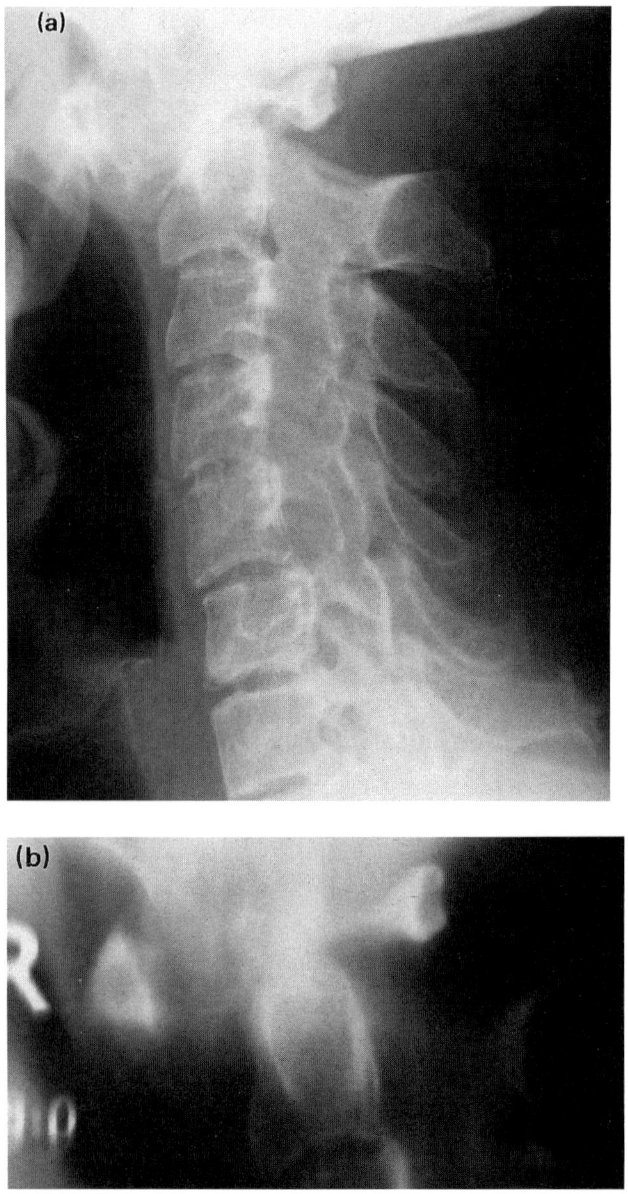

Fig. 53.11 Instability at C1–C2 causing spinal cord compression.

this cannot be corrected via the exposed posterior approach. It is better to accept a 30° correction than to endanger the vital nerve tissues.

Discussion

In addition to the corrective operations which have been described there are a few patients who develop instability either between the skull and atlas or between the atlas and axis (Fig. 53.11).

The symptoms mimic those seen in rheumatoid arthritis. A few can be corrected, at the upper cervical (atlanto-axial) level, by *gradual* halo extension followed by fusion posteriorly, but the author has performed successfully a posterior decompression and fusion at this level rather than the alternative anterior approach. In conclusion, it is evident that a limited number of patients require a spinal osteotomy with a good chance of producing worthwhile improvement in their posture. It can be expected that most of the patients will be over the age of 35, but a clear warning is given to avoid the operation in patients over 65, and to carefully consider methods of correction without an operation in all those with a fracture. In the future, centres of excellence might resolve the problem of spinal deformity in ankylosing spondylitis, preferably by prophylactic conservative means, and much less frequently by major surgery.

REFERENCES

Ball, J. (1980) Pathology and pathogenesis. In Moll, J.M.H. (ed.) *Ankylosing Spondylitis*, p. 96. Churchill Livingstone, Edinburgh.

Brewerton, D.A. (1978) Inherited susceptibility to rheumatic disease. *J. R. Soc. Med.*, **71**, 331–332.

Bulstrode, S.J., Barefoot, J., Harrison, R.A. & Clarke, A.K. (1987) The role of passive stretching in the treatment of ankylosing spondylitis. *Br. J. Rheumatol.*, **26**, 40–42.

Fang, D., Leong, J.C.Y., Ho, E.K.W., Chan, F.L. & Chow, S.P. (1988) Spinal pseudarthrosis in ankylosing spondylitis. *J. Bone Jt. Surg.*, **70B**, 443.

Hanson, C.A., Shagrin, J.W. & Duncan, H. (1971) Vertebral osteoporosis in ankylosing spondylitis. *Clin. Orthop.*, **74**, 59–64.

Isenberg, D.A., Feldman, R., Dudeney, C., Konikoff, F. *et al.* (1987) A study of antipolynucleotide antibodies, anti-Klebsiella [K30] antibodies and anti-DNA antibody idiotypes in ankylosing spondylitis. *Br. J. Rheum.*, **26**, 168.

Law, W.A. (1976) Ankylosing spondylitis and spinal osteotomy. *Proc. R. Soc. Med.*, **69**, 715–720.

Romanus, R. & Ydén, S. (1955) *Pelvospondylitis Ossificans: Rheumatoid or Ankylosing Spondylitis*. Munksgaard, Copenhagen.

Simmons, E.H. (1972) The surgical correction of flexion deformity of the cervical spine in ankylosing spondylitis. *Clin. Orth. Rel. Res.*, **86**, 132–143.

Smith-Petersen, M.N., Larson, C.B. & Aufranc, O.E. (1945) Osteotomy of the spine for correction of flexion deformity in rheumatoid arthritis. *J. Bone Jt. Surg.*, **27**, 1–11.

Yau, A.C.M.C. & Chan, R.N.W. (1974) Stress fracture of the fused lumbo-dorsal spine in ankylosing spondylitis. *J. Bone Jt. Surg.*, **56B**, 681–687.

SECTION 12
SYRINGOMYELIA

54 · Syringomyelia

By B. WILLIAMS

The presence of fluid cavities extending over several segments within the spinal cord is a pathological entity with many possible origins. Hindbrain herniation, paraplegia and intraspinal tumours are the three commonest causes. The clinical presentation may be very variable and the resemblance of the final clinical pictures is convergent because of the eventual widespread destruction of the cord. It is almost always a surgical condition, in the sense that the destructive forces are essentially those of fluid cutting into the tissues. Expeditious and careful surgery is often successful, particularly if practised early. However, the surgical management of the various problems is not easy. Established neurological losses are likely to be permanent as are orthopaedic problems such as Charcot's joints and kyphoscoliosis.

With the increasing use of magnetic resonance imaging (MRI) it is likely that increasing numbers of cases where syringomyelia comes to light as an unexpected finding will occur. In the management of those cases it should be borne in mind that neurological deficits, if they are allowed to develop, are likely to be irreversible and may permanently adversely affect the prognosis.

Syringomyelia is characterized by longitudinal cavities within the spinal cord. The collection of fluid within the cavities must have a cause and it is tempting to classify the cases by the presumed reason for the accumulation of the fluid. Thus the simplest division is into tumorous and non-tumorous cases. The cause of fluid collecting in and adjacent to tumours is presumably the same as those for tumour cysts in other parts of the neuraxis; since the fluid is proteinaceous, secretion from the substance of the tumour seems most likely. Management of tumour cystic cavities is linked to that of the tumour and covered in other parts of this book. Small cord cavities may occur with spinal injuries and cervical spondylosis. These cavities are the result of liquefaction or degeneration in the cord and are not so large as to produce pathology by their own enlargement. The fluid in larger cavities, excepting tumour cases, is almost always similar to cerebrospinal fluid (CSF) and the presence of an increasing collection of fluid within the spinal cord suggests a filling mechanism. The mechanisms which cause the syrinx are not necessarily those which maintain its existence, and therapy is only to a limited extent directed towards concepts of what caused the syringomyelia to develop.

Ollivier, who named this condition in 1827, understood that the process of cavitation followed the weaknesses along which fluid tracked through the grey matter of the spinal cord and carried out air injection to support this notion. A later concept was that the disease was due to degenerative changes in the supporting glia. The cavities become surrounded by gliosis, but Greenfield (1963), said that the cavities appeared to be due to tearing of tissues by the spread of fluid. Studies on human cadavers, subsequent to that of Ollivier, and also by injections of saline or CSF into the grey matter of living animals produced cavities mimicking syringomyelia (Williams, 1980). Syringomyelia may be reliably produced by kaolin-induced hydrocephalus in animal models (Williams & Bentley, 1980), but the relevance to the human condition is limited.

The relationship between abnormalities of the base of the brain which cause pressure differences between the head and the spinal subarachnoid space was noted by Gardner (1973). He suggested that the majority of cases have a communication from the fourth ventricle to the syrinx in the initial stages of syringomyelia.

Gardner showed that operative craniovertebral decompression was often accompanied by improvement in the patient's clinical state; and he produced a unified theory which attempted to explain spina bifida, anencephalus, iniencephalus, Dandy Walker cysts and syringomyelia, on the basis of failure of the fourth ventricle roof to perforate during embryogenesis. This concept now seems unsound, but has been of value in stimulating subsequent workers.

Cases related to abnormalities of the hindbrain have many causes, including tumours and arachnoiditis. It seems likely that the common descent of the tonsils through the foramen magnum, which is sometimes called the Chiari Type I malformation, is a herniation of the hindbrain. The term Arnold Chiari deformity is sometimes used to describe the severe deformities of the hindbrain and upper cord found in association with spina bifida and hydrocephalus. Such a situation is sometimes termed a Chiari Type II anomaly. The aetiology of both types is likely to be due to pressure differences (Williams, 1975, 1977b, 1981, 1989). The term hindbrain hernia will be used for both variants.

The classification of syringomyelia is thus not agreed upon, but a suggested classification with some idea of the frequency of instances is given in Table 54.1.

Table 54.1 Classification of syringomyelia (according to presumed cause)

Hindbrain-related syringomyelia (73%)
Hindbrain herniation
Idiopathic (Chiari Type I)
Secondary to birth injury
Secondary to head injury (non-perinatal)
Secondary to bony abnormality
Basilar invagination (idiopathic or birth injury)
Basilar invagination (genetic bone softening, acro-osteolysis, osteogenesis imperfecta, etc.)
Basilar invagination (acquired bone softening, rickets, Paget's disease, etc.)
Associated with hydrocephalus
Intracranial arachnoid pouches
Dandy-Walker cysts
Early-onset hydrocephalus (aqueduct stenosis)
Secondary to spina bifida (Chiari Type II)
Secondary to tumours of the posterior fossa
Arachnoiditis at the foramen magnum
Birth injury related
Post-traumatic (postnatal)
Infections
Non-hindbrain-related cases (17%)
In association with spinal tumours—mainly intramedullary
Dysraphism without hindbrain hernia (lipoma, tethered cord)
Archnoiditis of the spinal subarachnoid space
Postinflammatory
Tuberculous meningitis
Myodil (Pantopaque)
Post-traumatic (10%)

PATHOGENESIS

Hydrodynamic forces

The CSF within the neuraxis is in continual movement. Cardiac pulsation in the capillary bed of the brain is constant and transmitted throughout the nervous system. Of greater significance and power are the effects of the venous plexuses which have free connections through valveless veins present at each vertebra of the neuraxis and up to the head. Any increase in pressure in the abdominal and thoracic cavities is thus transmitted into the spine. Compression of the dura by venous distension of the epidural plexus produces rapid movements of CSF with concomitant pressure changes. Williams (1981), found that the pressures produced by a cough may exceed the pressures produced by cardiac pulsation by 100 times. The energy imposed upon the tissues of the neuraxis affects the formation and the maintenance of syringomyelia.

'Suck'

The first mechanism is the creation of pressure differences between CSF compartments by venous pulsation. If the patient has a spinal tumour, for example, energetic coughing will force fluid upwards past the tumour more efficiently than it can run back down again.

This leads to a collapsed theca below the tumour with a high protein content and a low pressure—Froin's syndrome. If fluid can find its way into the cord at the site of the obstruction then this may be the mechanism which gives rise to a syrinx. Common causes of this situation include tumour outside the cord, fracture, Pott's disease or other partial blockage of the subarachnoid spaces caused by the formation of pathological arachnoid adhesions.

The effects of such pressure differentials are magnified by the presence of a valve-like morphology. The production of a cerebellar cone or hindbrain hernia naturally forms a valvular configuration (Fig. 54.1). When a patient coughs or sneezes in the presence of such conical impaction in the foramen magnum, the CSF passes into the head easily because it lifts the cone out of the foramen magnum, but then the instant the cone drops back in again the fluid is trapped in the head. This gives rise to a period when the pressure is higher than that of the spine. This is evident in Chiari Type II malformation when a baby with a tight head may have a slack spina bifida at atmospheric pressure. Pressure on the head will not inflate the meningocele, but pressure on the meningocele can inflate the head. This was pointed out by Van Houweninge Graftjik (1932), and subsequent analysis of the behaviour in babies vindicates this view (Williams, 1975, 1977b, 1989).

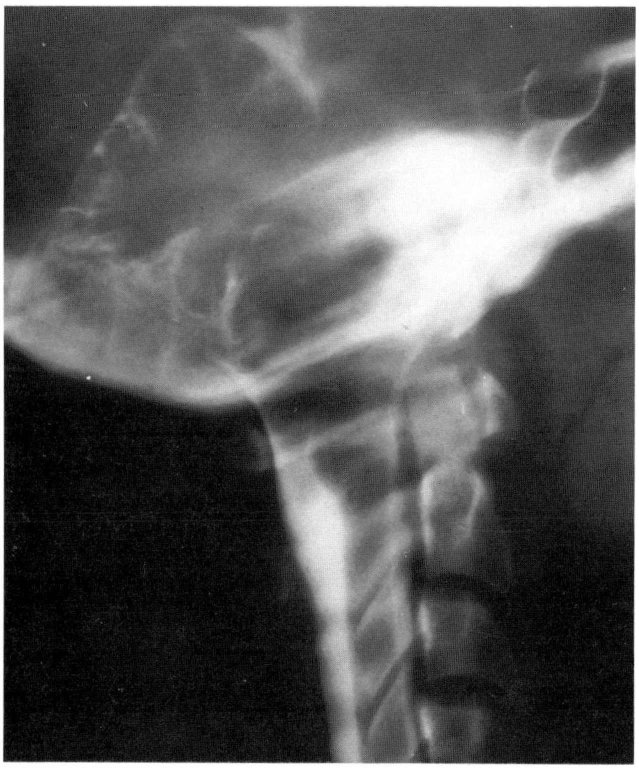

Fig. 54.1 Water-soluble myelography showing a hindbrain hernia. The moulding of the tonsils and hindbrain is clearly seen and narrowing of the subarachnoid space indicates the valvular morphology. Note that the cisterna magna is almost absent.

In the majority of adults with hindbrain-related syringomyelia, simultaneous measurement of both intracranial and intraspinal pressures at rest will show the pressures to be substantially equal in the head and the spine. When coughing and sneezing, the pressure in the lumbar sac rises higher, quicker and sooner than it does in the head. In the majority of patients with hindbrain hernia, however, the CSF is delayed in its return downwards past the foramen magnum. Figure 54.2 shows the ventricular and lumbar pressure traces during six coughs by a patient. Subtraction of the ventricular pressure from the lumbar gives a differential trace such that displacement of the pressure above the zero of the differential trace means an upward-acting force across the foramen magnum, and displacement downwards indicates a downward-acting force. Note that, after a sequence of coughs, the lumbar pressure becomes low and the arterial pulsation pressure is not visible. The baseline pressure in the ventricles rises at A, B and C, indicating that a pump-like action is at work pumping more CSF progressively into the head. When coughing ceases at D, there is a pressure difference of almost 22 mm of mercury, which takes over 12 seconds to return to normal, thereby sucking the hindbrain into the foramen magnum, distorting the hindbrain hernia and probably producing active filling of the syrinx in some cases.

In normal cases the half-life of the return of pressure differences to normal is less than 1/10 second. With Chiari Type I malformation the return of press-

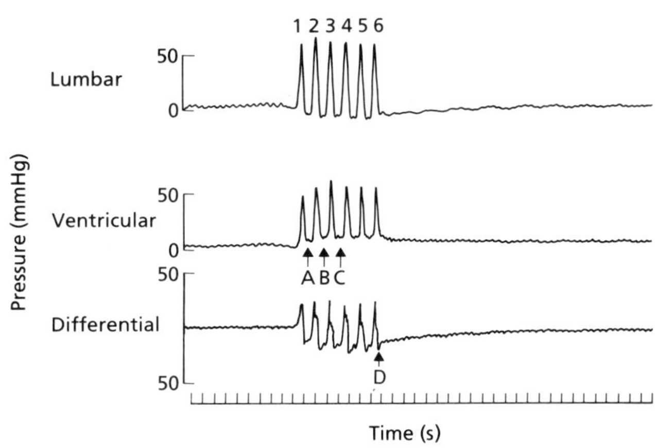

Fig. 54.2 Craniospinal pressure dissociation manifest after six coughs (see text for explanation).

ure may be delayed, sometimes with a half-life of over 30 seconds. During a post-Valsalva rebound after straining, the pressure across the foramen magnum may be high for a significant period. Such an abnormal pressure difference across the foramen has been termed craniospinal pressure dissociation (Williams, 1977b, 1981), but both that and the differences across the site of any obstruction lower in the neuraxis, may be conveniently described as 'suck'. This, of course, continues to mould the hindbrain hernia as well as being concerned with the pathogenesis of syringomyelia. Correction of the hindbrain hernia will commonly produce radiological and clinical improvement in the syringomyelia.

'Slosh'

Energy imposition upon the spine by manoeuvres which raise the intrathoracic and intra-abdominal pressure is probably the usual mechanism which maintains an established syrinx. Due to the resistance to movement from the dura, the pia, dentate ligaments, arachnoid strands, blood vessels and nerve roots outside the cord, the fluid within the cord is likely to move more readily than that outside. Fluid surging on the inside can stress the walls of the cord and lead to tearing of the tissues in the same way as injection of fluid. Pathological preparations showing the collapsed cord are misleading, as most syrinx cavities in life are partially if not tightly filled. It was stressed by Williams (1974), after creation of an analogue model, that cord fluctuations could be violent and the fluid inside is free to surge upwards and downwards in an undulating manner, imposing ballistic distending stresses which may be grouped together under the heading 'slosh' (Figs 54.3 & 54.4). If a cavity is being maintained by 'slosh' then it is likely that the natural shape of the cavity will be kept in existence by the diffusion of fluid through the walls of the cord. The cord is a porous structure with no tight junctions in the gliotic lining of the syrinx cavity, and fluid can enter readily, as may be seen from water-soluble contrast material in post-myelography computerized tomography (CT) scans. Septations commonly seen within the syrinx cavity, sometimes called haustrae, are of interest. They probably represent nodes or no-flow areas in the cord. The 'slosh' occurs in limited zones and the walls tend to heal at the site of septation. These septae are important inasmuch as they impede drainage, making it difficult for the surgeon to pass a drainage catheter, and sometimes even lead to persistence of a short section of syrinx after other parts of the cavity have been drained.

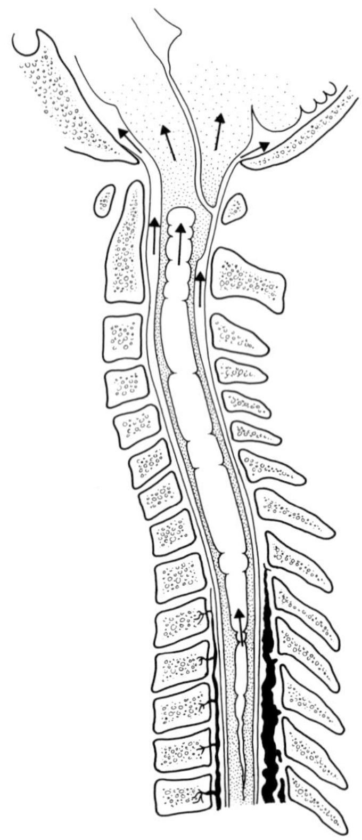

Fig. 54.3 Upward movement of CSF. The hindbrain is lifted up and the CSF pathways between the points of the brain and in the subarachnoid space are opened freely. Also upward movement occurs inside the syrinx; this is 'slosh' and is responsible for stressing the syrinx walls.

Other forces

The occurrence of an intracord haematoma at the time of injury may provide an initiatory cavity. Subsequent liquefaction of the clot may leave a cyst susceptible to 'slosh'.

The cord has zones of weakness which are susceptible to forces other than hydrodynamic. If there are tight adhesions between the pia, arachnoid and dura, and especially if the spinal canal is narrowed by the impingement of bone fragments after a fracture, then the cord may be directly stressed during hydrodynamic events or on spinal movement. Some such explanation seems called for when considering post-

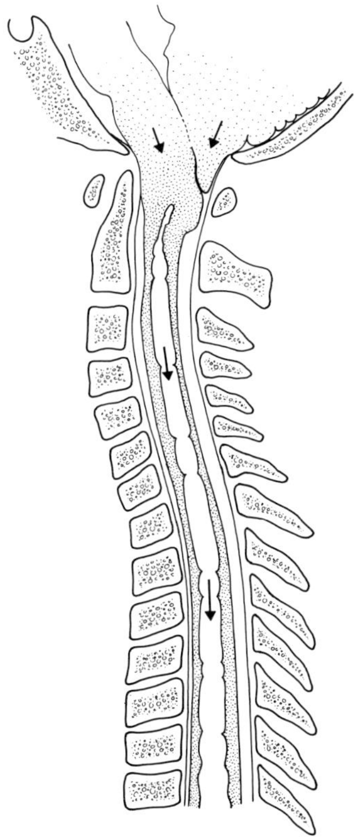

Fig. 54.4 When fluid attempts to move back into the low-pressure area of the spine, tight compression takes place at the foramen magnum and the low pressure in the spine sucks the tissues into the hole. 'Slosh' may rebound, causing transmission of energy in a downward direction.

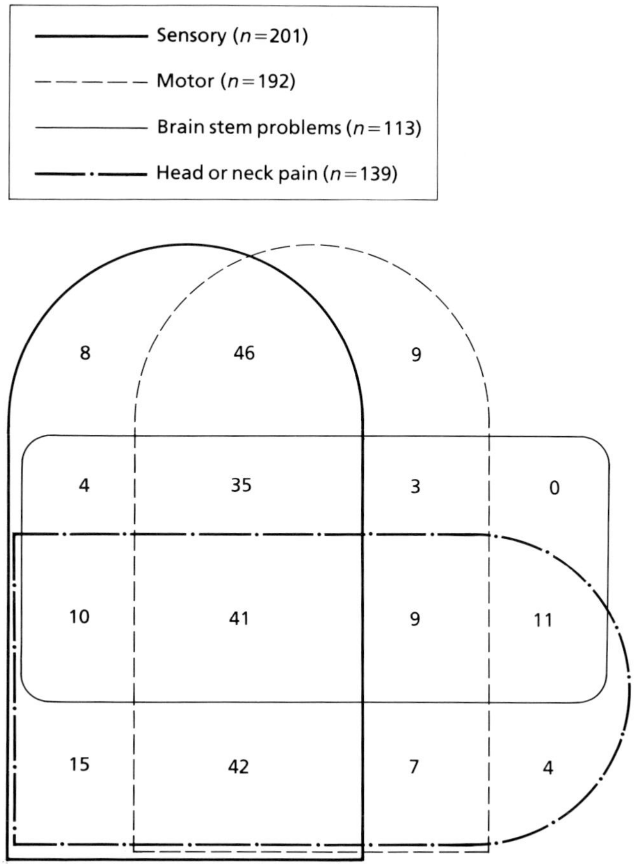

Fig. 54.5 Diagrammatic representation of the grouping of multiple symptoms in 244 cases of hindbrain-related syringomyelia. The top left '8' means that eight patients had sensory symptoms excluding pain, there were 15 patients with sensory symptoms including pain and the commonest presentation (46) was of motor and sensory limb problems but without pain or brain stem features.

inflammatory syringomyelia, which may occur after the development of extensive adhesions along several segments of the spine; but in which there was no past haematoma cord cavity such as may be proposed for post-traumatic cases.

CLINICAL PRESENTATION

The presentation is variable, and usually the symptoms are multiple. Figures 54.5 & 54.6 represent the unpublished clinical findings discovered in the analysis of patients with hindbrain-related syringomyelia as part of a larger group of 550 cases of syringomyelia of all causes. They show that the commonest presentations are of pain along with sensory, motor and structural damage. Patients may present with features of the hindbrain hernia rather than the syrinx. These include intracranial symptoms, pain, medullary symptoms such as vertigo, oscillopsia, or any complaint of lower cranial nerve involvement. These symptoms are often thought of as 'syringobulbia'. However, the majority of cases with brain stem signs have no actual cavities within the brain stem; only dysfunction due to compression of tissues in the foramen magnum or traction upon lower cranial nerves aggravated by suck.

The history is paramount. Taking a birth history in adult life is not common, since most birth-related injuries are diagnosed in paediatric practice. Hydrocephalus, epilepsy and syringomyelia are causes of late neurological presentation. Difficult birth is related to over half the cases of adult syringomyelia, and of those who have no other cause detectable

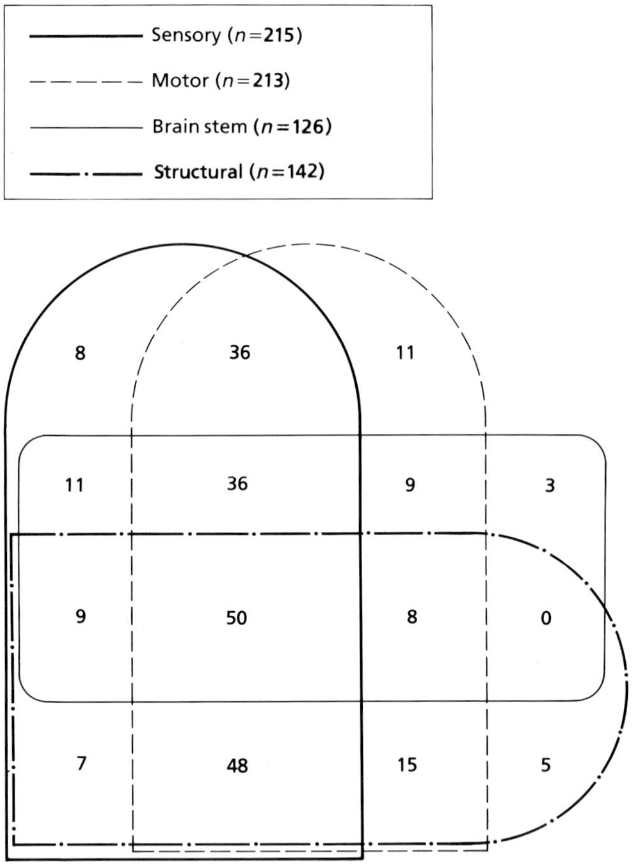

Fig. 54.6 Diagram similar to Fig. 54.5, showing the physical signs in 254 patients with hindbrain syringomyelia. Structural features include altered cervical canal dimensions, kyphoscoliosis, Charcot's joints, ulcers, scars, Morvan's syndrome and limb asymmetries.

it is probable that the majority are birth-related (Williams, 1977a).

Any manifestations of spinal cord symptoms may be the first symptom, including scoliosis, trophic, sensory or motor features (Barnett *et al.*, 1973). The upper limbs are the site of presentation of sensory changes in the majority; nevertheless stiffness in the legs was the commonest symptom reported by Barnett *et al.* (1973), and the presentation with leg symptoms alone is not uncommon. Pain occurs in the majority of patients and it is notable that most of them present to an orthopaedic surgeon before seeing a neurologist or neurosurgeon (Williams, 1979a). Pain may be associated with 'slosh'; for instance a sudden pain in the trunk or limbs after coughing or sneezing.

Patients who present with neurological deficits may have a history of head or neck pain particularly related to coughing and sneezing (Nightingale & Williams, 1987). This may not have been connected by the patient to the subsequent problems. Pain in the neck or areas of the body corresponding to cavities in either the cervical or lumbar enlargements surely suggests that central cord pain is commonly a problem (Williams, 1979b). There may also be pain from Charcot's joints or associated joint degeneration such as cervical spondylotic myelopathy.

Scoliosis is present in more than half of patients with hindbrain-related syringomyelia. It is correlated with early onset, and usually precedes other neurological features. The side and level of the cord cavity are not related to the curve. Paraplegia during correction of scoliosis may be the first declaration of syringomyelia.

Complaints such as giddiness, syncope, drop-attacks, sweating changes, transient double vision, swallowing difficulties, hypersalivation, stiffness of the legs and so on, may not be linked by the patient to the presenting complaint if that is a different type of symptom, such as pain or scoliosis. The characteristic dissociated sensory loss is often not present in the opening stages, but enquiry may include asking if an underarm deodorant feels the same on the two sides, and asking women if their hair rollers burn the backs of their necks, or if the drying of nail varnish on the nails feels different on the two sides.

On examination, scoliosis is often visible. Hemiatrophy, asymmetries of the face and upper limbs, wasting, Charcot's joints, trophic changes often with severe finger involvement, are all late manifestations. Slight trophic changes, such as burns or ulceration from brassiere straps, may precede the patients noticing that they have dissociated sensory loss.

Hindbrain herniation

Strain-related headache is the characteristic presentation. The pain is usually nuchal and bilateral, radiating into the occiput or vertex. It is usually pounding and brought on by suddenly rising from the lying or sitting position or by coughing and straining (Nightingale & Williams, 1987). This type of headache is, of course, the same as that found when patients have a hindbrain hernia due to a brain tumour, and that diagnosis must always be the first consideration in cases presenting in this way.

Cases associated with spinal tumours

In the situation of intramedullary cyst formation in association with a spinal tumour, the clinical picture is usually that of pain accompanied by sensory and motor changes distal to the tumour. Thus, the legs are more frequently involved than the arms. Kyphoscoliosis is a common presentation in childhood and, if associated with pain, stiffness and loss of use in the legs, then careful examination of the arms may reveal loss of tendon reflexes and wasting. Such cases merit full neuroradiological evaluation before treatment of scoliosis is instituted.

Post-traumatic and postarachnoiditic cases

Post-traumatic syringomyelia can be a late complication of paraplegia, either complete or incomplete. Extension of the syrinx may cause ascent of the neurological level; a factor of critical importance where upper limb function is so essential. Early symptoms are ascending pain sometimes followed by numbness. Often there is a zone of hyperaesthesia above the fracture level, which disappears as the cord is distended. The pain and numbness may ascend by segmental steps or may jump into the arm and the side of the neck leaving an area of the trunk uninvolved. Pain and sensory loss usually precede motor loss, and certainly it is best for the patients if surgical treatment precedes weakness. Loss of tendon reflexes occurs early. Changes in sweating, often below the level of the lesion, manifest most clearly as asymmetry, rather than either hyperhidrosis or hypohidrosis (Williams *et al.*, 1981; Rossier *et al.*, 1985; Williams, 1989) and are more common than in hindbrain-related cases.

RADIOLOGICAL ASSESSMENT

Plain radiographs

In hindbrain-related cases the X-ray findings may be rich and variable. Radiographs of the skull may show effects of hydrocephalus, platybasia, basilar invagination or evidence of bone dysplasia (Rice Edwards, 1982). There may be segmentation abnormalities of the skull base with fusion of the occiput and atlas or fusions of cervical vertebrae. Encephalocele or spina bifida are uncommonly seen. A small posterior fossa is not necessarily support for the concept of primary osseous dysplasia.

Some tumour cases may have had syringomyelia for sufficiently long, or at an early enough age, to have affected the growth of the bones. The diagnosis of syringomyelia from enlargement of the vertebral canal is not possible because intraspinal tumours without syringomyelia may also cause this, and it is also common in neurofibromatosis. Comparing the AP diameter of the canal and body at C5, there is a 25% chance of pathology if the canal is more than 4 mm bigger than the body, and a 98% chance of pathology if the difference is more than 6 mm (Williams, 1979a).

Computerized tomography and myelography

The ventricles should be scanned in the majority of cases, even those with a spinal presentation. Patients with walking difficulty, for example, may have vertex meningiomas or hydrocephalus. In around one-third of cases of syringomyelia there is some ventricular enlargement (West & Williams, 1980) and in 10% this is clearly hydrocephalus. Midbrain and posterior fossa tumours are known causes of syringomyelia, but tumours at the foramen magnum are more common and are sometimes missed on CT.

Water-soluble myelography is a valuable technique. Since the diagnosis of hindbrain hernia has been recognized to be more common than previously suspected, it has been recommended that in any mysterious neurological case the contrast agent should be run up to the cisterna magna, and the position of the tonsils and the IVth ventricle checked.

Postmyelography CT scanning is of value in showing hindbrain compression and tonsillar descent (Fig. 54.7). Convenient times for CT scanning are 1 hour after the myelogram, then at the end of the radiographer's working day, usually 4–6 hours postmyelography, and the following morning, about 20–24 hours after myelography. The cavity within the spinal cord may opacify, commonly at 6 hours. Occasionally it will enhance best at 24 hours. The great flexibility of the cord and its susceptibility to 'slosh' are readily demonstrated (Stevens *et al.*, 1985). These investigations have largely been supplanted by MRI.

Magnetic resonance imaging

This shows the ventricles, including the IIIrd and IVth, hindbrain descent and the spinal cord (Lee

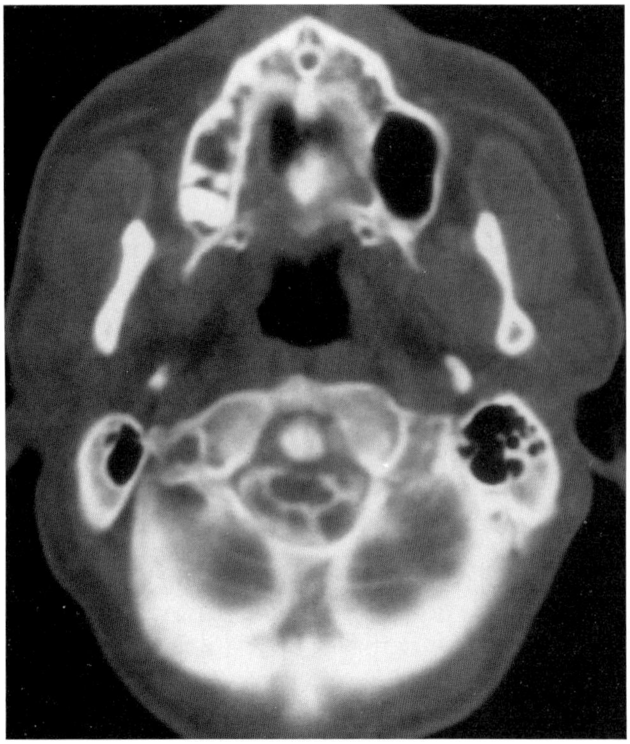

Fig. 54.7 CT myelogram of a case of basilar invagination and a high odontoid peg. Hindbrain distortion and tonsillar descent are clearly shown (cf. Fig. 54.1).

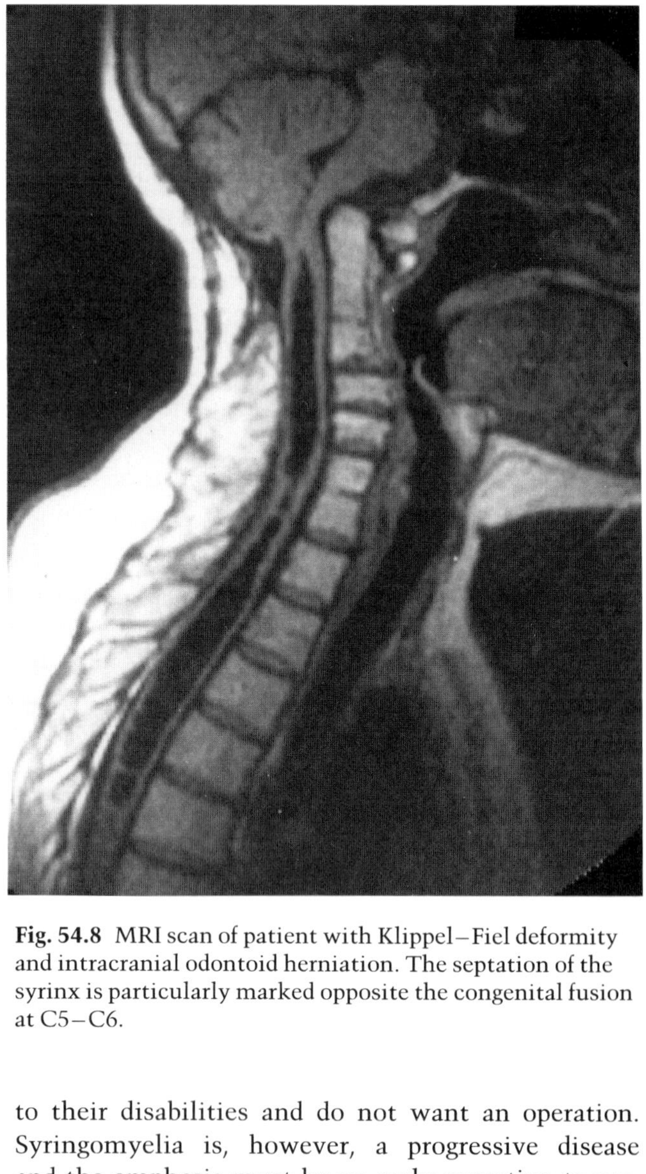

Fig. 54.8 MRI scan of patient with Klippel–Fiel deformity and intracranial odontoid herniation. The septation of the syrinx is particularly marked opposite the congenital fusion at C5–C6.

et al., 1985; Barkovich *et al.*, 1986, 1987; Sherman *et al.*, 1987; Grant *et al.*, 1987). Scanning patients with severe scoliosis may be difficult, and skill is required in interpretation. Platybasia is difficult to spot because the bony structures do not show well. Myelography may be dispensed with and also CT scanning, provided that the whole brain is imaged, but plain radiographs remain useful. The main value of MRI, apart from its non-invasive nature, is its ability to delineate the intramedullary lesion. Due to its CSF content a syrinx is readily differentiated from an intramedullary tumour provided that there is also no enhancement with gadolinium. The exact extent and anatomy of the syrinx is shown, including the presence of septation, which is of importance in shunting procedures (Fig. 54.8).

MANAGEMENT

Indications for operation

The progression of syringomyelia is often slow and in some cases the patients have become accustomed to their disabilities and do not want an operation. Syringomyelia is, however, a progressive disease and the emphasis must be on early operation to prevent the development of deficit. There is little doubt that the best results come from procedures performed in young patients at an early stage of their disease. Patients therefore require careful counselling of the risks involved, but surgical intervention should be considered the norm.

Early operation is ideal. Unfortunately many of the cases do not present until they are very disabled, and often it may be suspected that they are 'burnt out'. Fortunately, with MRI scanning it is quite possible to see cases with tonsils which no longer look as though they are impacted, and furthermore, when syrinx cavities have collapsed. If the syrinx cavity is small and occluded at several points along its length, and if there is no hydrocephalus and the hindbrain hernia is disimpacted, or if the wall of the cord is calcified in parts, then even recent neurological deterioration is not an indication for operation. If such a radiological result had been obtained by operation, then the surgeon would be well pleased and could not promise arrest of progression. This kind of decision is increasingly necessary now that MRI scanning can lead to the unsuspected diagnosis of hindbrain hernia with syringomyelia.

Sizeable hydrocephalus with neurological symptoms is an indication for correction usually by ventriculoventricle shunting; occasionally by hindbrain hernia decompression or removal of a tumour. Objective improvement of syrinx size may often be achieved merely by ventricular shunting, as well as sometimes improvement in limb function.

If there is a communication from the ventricles to the inside of the cord then such cases seem to do well after shunting, and such shunts seem sensible (Krayenbuhl, 1974). There is no proof that the communication is necessary for an improvement to result. The benefits of ventricular shunting are likely to be due to moving the patients to the left along the pressure–volume curve, that is to say, by reducing the overall volume of CSF and predistending the veins (Williams, 1974, 1986). Kruse *et al.* (1987) suggested that measurement of CSF conductance to outflow may be a predictor of cases which will benefit from shunting. This is a difficult technique, and hydrocephalus or a communication from the fourth to the syrinx are easier to see.

Indications for operation on hindbrain abnormalities include not only syringomyelia, but also the clinical hindbrain hernia features such as headache. Ideally, pressure studies should be performed to show craniospinal dissociation. Unfortunately, this is a demanding test in terms of manpower and apparatus, and has not proved to be a reliable predictor (Williams, 1981). It seems that many patients who still have 'suck' will not show it under test; also patients who have had a careful hindbrain hernia decompression with good clinical results may sometimes show persisting 'suck'. This is a salutary observation to someone practising craniovertebral decompression.

The question often arises as to whether a minor degree of hindbrain herniation might be contributing to a clinical problem. Cases with multiple sclerosis, for example, may present with nystagmus and cord signs, and if a sizeable hindbrain hernia is present it is tempting to decompress it even if there is no syrinx present. The degree of descent which is symptomatic is difficult to determine; looking at the shape of the herniation may help to decide if it seems likely to be responsible for 'suck'. Minor degrees of tonsillar herniation may be symptomatic if they are shaped so as to cause 'suck' or especially if there is some adhesive fibrosis present. Barkovich *et al.* (1986) noted that there is an association between the degree of descent of the tonsillar herniation, and suggested that 5 mm of descent below the foramen magnum may still be normal. In a group of patients with symptomatic hindbrain herniation they found the tonsils to be 3–29 mm below the foramen, with a mean descent of 13 mm.

When it is established that a hindbrain hernia requires decompression, how may that be best achieved? Occasionally, the hindbrain herniation may be in association with severe upward odontoid herniation causing marked anterior brain stem compression. In such a situation the odontoid process must first be removed by a transoral appoach (Dyste *et al.*, 1989). More commonly, a posterior procedure will suffice and this should be kept as simple as possible merely to abolish the mechanism of 'suck'. Combining the procedure routinely with procedures such as: obex plugging (Gardner, 1973); stents or wicks (Rhoton, 1976; Wissoff & Epstein, 1989); dural grafting; or terminal ventriculostomy (Williams & Fahy, 1983) serve only to increase the risks, and the individual contribution of such measures cannot be determined.

If there is significant hydrocephalus or features of raised intracranial pressure then a valved ventriculoatrial or ventriculoperitoneal shunt should be performed prior to hindbrain decompression. On the other hand, the temptation to shunt the syrinx as a primary procedure rather than deal with the hindbrain hernia should be resisted, as it may exacerbate the mechanism of 'suck'.

Hindbrain decompression

The objectives of operation vary with the surgeon's ideas of the pathogenetic mechanisms, which are not universally agreed. The main benefit is probably produced by decompressing tissues within the foramen magnum so that they no longer impact. This stops 'suck' and downward traction on the tonsils and the cranial nerves, preventing vascular loops being pressed into the medulla, and probably lessens or stops the flow into the syrinx in some cases.

The objective, therefore, is to provide a communication between all the normal CSF-containing spaces; the cisterna magna should be in communication with the subarachnoid spaces around the cord, the fourth ventricle and also the spaces alongside the upper medulla leading up to the cerebellopontine angles. The aim therefore is to provide a sizeable artificial cisterna magna by leaving the dura open and a deliberate cavity under the suboccipital musculature.

An additional benefit of leaving a large artificial cisterna magna is the provision of a reservoir into which fluid from the spine may move during pressure surges. The movements of fluid may be diverted there instead of washing past the lower cerebellum, and also the damping effect of the decompression provides a mechanism whereby the pressure is prevented from rising; the energy is dispersed in moving the occipital musculature, or lifting the cerebellum, which does no harm; instead of being imposed on more central structures. Minor degrees of hydrocephalus may sometimes be relieved by this decompression.

Blockage of the presumed communication is of doubtful value. The plug is likely to be dislodged by CSF movement in the postoperative period and there is a complication rate attached to fixing of tissue into the region of the obex (Williams, 1978; Matsumoto & Symon, 1989). Also the lack of a visible communication in MRI studies makes this manoeuvre less popular than it was in the past. Other procedures such as inserting a syringostomy drain (Rhoton, 1976) or a IVth ventricle drain (Wissoff & Epstein, 1989; Batzdorf, 1991) are also probably not helpful.

The comparison of results is of course difficult in such a complex disorder, but there is no proof that results are improved by obex blockage, drains or 'stents' as compared to simple hindbrain decompression alone.

The use of too large a decompression in the occipital bone may lead to 'slump' of the lower parts of the cerebellum in the wound (Williams, 1978; Lee *et al.*, 1985). This may be aggravated by the mechanisms of 'suck' persisting if the tissues reimpact around the edge of the decompression. Too small a decompression may lead to impaction of tonsils and postoperative respiratory arrest.

Following a vertical midline incision to expose the occiput and posterior lamina of the atlas, about 3–4 cm of occipital bone on each side and a similar amount above the foramen magnum, gives a good decompression without provoking 'slump'. The arch of the atlas is removed well laterally, taking thought about the vertebral arteries. In most cases it is possible to leave the spinous process of the axis in position with those muscles which run caudally from it still in position.

The incision in the dura should expose the inferior parts of the cerebellum but, at and below the foramen magnum, it should be taken well laterally to fully expose the impacted tonsils (Fig. 54.9). The central part of the dura may be hinged downwards above the arch of C2. It will conveniently reach to the spinous process of the axis to which it may be sutured, thus bringing the posterior surface of the posterior spinal subarachnoid space into alignment with the artificial cisterna magna planned for the closing stages. The dura at the sides is then gently sutured backwards. Thought should be given to the effect of slackening off the retractors at the end of operation procedure; if the dura is stitched to muscle away from the bone it may slacken and adhere to the cerebellum.

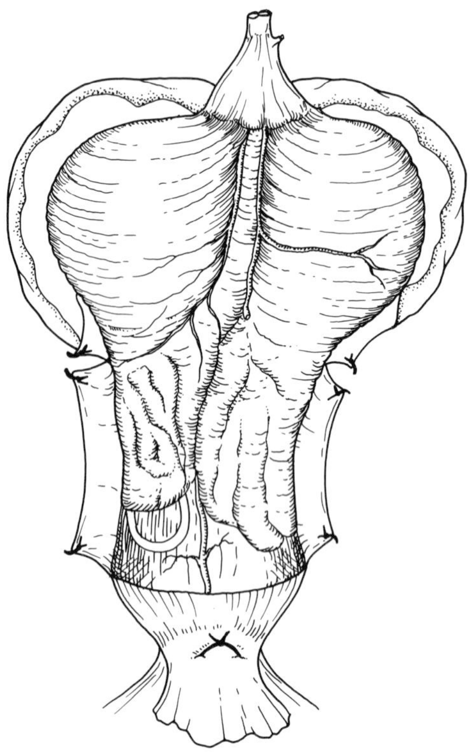

Fig. 54.9 Operative exposure necessary following wide opening of the dura to display the impacted hindbrain hernia.

Usually the arachnoid can be partly resected and partly sutured back. This is an important part of the operation; the arachnoid may look insubstantial, it may also lie down and appear to be out of the way. If it is left to float about in the CSF it tends to adhere to whatever it can, and then to thicken up. It is therefore important to stitch the arachnoid back at the bottom of the exposure to ensure permanent communication between the spinal spaces and the artificial cisterna magna. Leaving the arachnoid intact is sometimes advocated (Logue & Rice-Edwards, 1981) although correction of 'suck' is not so effective if this is done. It is important not to leave arachnoid with a small hole in it. If fluid can collect between the arachnoid and the inside of the artificial cisterna magna, then the arachnoid may be pressed against the back of the tonsils and form a dense adhesion here. If a small hole remains to link the main pathways to the artificial cisterna magna then fluid cannot pass through easily, and a tight cyst behind the cerebellum may act as a space-occupying lesion. Such features may destroy the benefits of operation.

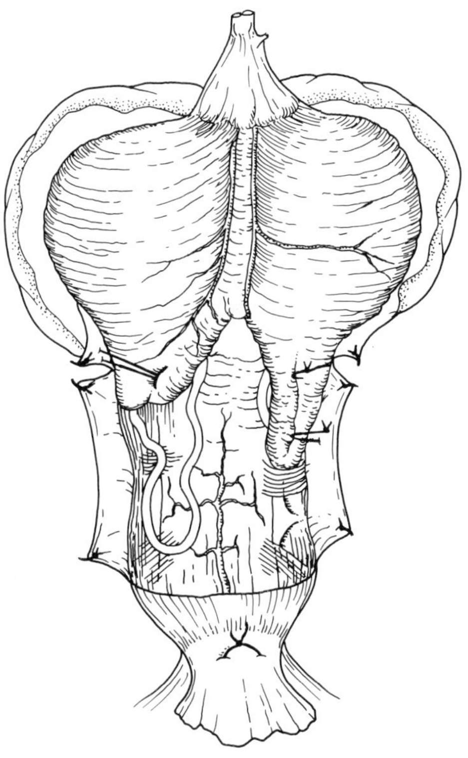

Fig. 54.10 Excision of the centre of the tonsils by suction allows them to be stitched sideways as shown on the right, or upwards and sideways as shown on the left. Free access for CSF can then be provided to all compartments.

The tonsils may be left alone but, if they are bound together and to the back of the medulla with arachnoid adhesions, then dissection may imperil vessels such as branches of the posterior inferior cerebellar arteries. In such situations it seems best to rely upon the opening up of the anterior CSF spaces and the artificial cisterna magna, and to leave the tonsils alone.

Usually the tonsils are not bound down and may be picked up, after division of a few strands of arachnoid, to expose the obex. Most commonly there is a patent foramen of Magendie. This is obscured by the tonsils dropping back when they are released. Under these circumstances it is tempting to remove part of the tonsils to ensure that the pathways are maximally opened up. In picking the tonsils up, the access to the lateral spaces is usually improved and the situation looks so much better that it is tempting to remove either the largest tonsil or else both. Light diathermy of the pia may make them shrink upwards. A vertical incision may allow most of the inside to be sucked out. Leaving some septa on the inside gives stronger tissue to stitch. The suture may be passed through the medial wall of the tonsil and its pia once or twice. The tissues should be pulled upwards, considering that the cerebellum will tend to move upwards after operation. The stitches should not be overtight or they may tear out if the tonsils develop postoperative swelling (Fig. 54.10).

The anterior spaces often open up well, but if there is a large cystic cord which collapses, the nerve roots, the dentate ligaments and the flattened cord all tend to separate the anterior subarachnoid space from the new, artificial cisterna magna. The upper part of the cord may be moved backwards and forwards by pulsation as fluid is forced in and out of the artificial cisterna magna. Under these circumstances the dentate ligament may be removed or stitched backwards.

Closure of the wound is an important part of the procedure to form the artificial cisterna magna. The muscle should not be tightly sutured close to the cerebellum. The spinous process of the axis gives a firm attachment point for resuturing, and the remainder of the upper part of the muscle may be closed so as to leave a sizeable artificial cisterna magna. The dura should be left open. If it is closed then the advantages of the operation are lost; to expose the patient to the risks of the procedure and then carefully reconstruct the valvular mechanism and reestablish 'suck' is a negation of present understanding of this disorder. Some surgeons like to graft the defect. The suturing cannot be watertight; therefore the graft may be pushed forwards against the back of the cerebellum with the artificial cisterna magna behind it instead of in front. Fascia lata graft will instigate a new blood supply for itself and may develop adhesions at that site, resulting in a constrictive arachnoiditis worse than the original. If a graft such as silastic is used, subsequent reopening shows a cavity, filled with CSF and lined with a membrane. The graft is usually curled up in this cavity, sometimes pressing on neural structures. The front membrane of the cavity may be dense fibrosis, tightly adherent to the cerebellum. A graft is not necessary; a membrane grows in the right place, away from the surface of the cerebellum. All that is required is that the muscle is closed in a reasonably watertight manner and not against the brain. If a CSF leak develops, or the decompression bulges, then the patient may need a valved shunt.

Spinal arachnoiditis and post-traumatic cases

The objectives are to establish a free flow of CSF up and down past the obstruction to abolish 'suck'. In the primarily spinal cases, however, it is reasonable to drain the syrinx when this is sizeable, further to lessen 'slosh' (Williams, 1989). Some authors believe that drainage is sufficient (Davis & Symon, 1990).

The advantages of an artificial meningocele are as for an artificial cisterna magna. The opening of the spaces into the artificial meningocele is more difficult than in the head because of the shortage of space. In cases of total paraplegia the principal area of cord damage may confidently be excised. This may be combined with insertion of a syringopleural shunt inserted into the transected cavity. In cases where some cord function remains, then the opening up of the spaces above and below the area of main damage is one objective. The adherent area is often diffuse and opening up of the anterior spaces is difficult. The lateral subarachnoid spaces are often obstructed by arachnoid adhesions, nerve roots, and also the dentate ligaments. When the primary lesion is arachnoiditis associated with late adhesions, rather than a fracture, such as in patients who have suffered tuberculous meningitis or myodil (Pantopaque) myelography, then the arachnoiditis may be widespread so that drainage of the syrinx may be all that is reasonable, especially if the paraplegia is partial.

Opening up the subarachnoid spaces so that they communicate with the artificial meningocele may be aided by leaving 'stents' in position, such as blocked-off silicone catheters, running from the subarachnoid space at the top and the bottom of the wound, through the meningocele and out through the skin. They may be removed after three days.

Myelotomy is one of the oldest operations for syringomyelia and is occasionally successful (Tator *et al.*, 1982). Syringosubarachnoid shunts (Barbaro *et al.*, 1984) and terminal ventriculostomy are sometimes advocated, but may be criticized (Williams & Fahy, 1983). The only reason that a syrinx should empty through a syringostomy, rather than fill through it, is when there is some residual elasticity in the wall. The majority of syrinxes which come to operation are too big to empty through their elasticity. The syringostomies, whether with an intraspinal drain or just left open, may allow fluid to enter the cavity. Additional to this is the consideration that it is probably preferable to substantially flatten all of the syrinx. If the syrinx is only partly drained, even if part of it may heal, then redissection may occur from another part, where a filling mechanism still exists (Fig. 54.11). Drainage to a low-pressure area outside the theca has been used latterly, both peritoneum (Suzuki *et al.*, 1986) and pleura (Williams & Page, 1987; Wissoff & Epstein, 1989).

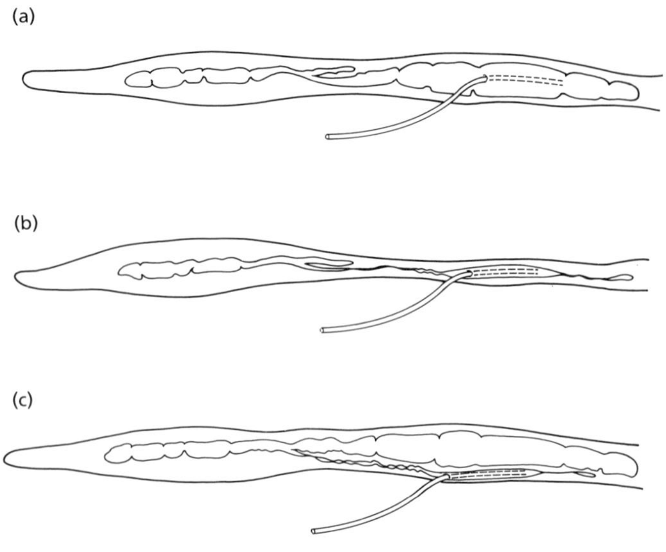

Fig. 54.11 No syringomyelia should be treated by drainage unless the filling mechanism has also been dealt with. The sequence of drawings suggests how, even should quite a large portion of syrinx collapse, a new syrinx cavity may cut alongside it.

A valve complicates the system and is designed to lower the CSF pressure to normal, so if the initial pressure was already normal, a likely state if there was no hydrocephalus, then a valve may stop the system from working. A simple system is therefore advocated. Care should be taken to close the pathways through which the CSF from outside the syrinx might enter the pleura. A lumbar drainage catheter is a convenient size; this is pulled through a small hole in the musculature, and the entry to the cord is patched. The closure should leave the pathways fully open from above to below so as to minimize 'suck'. The ideal result is outlined in Fig. 54.12. The artificial meningocele also performs a damping function, as does an artificial cisterna magna. Watertight closure is not always easy in this situation, but is essential.

COMPLICATIONS

Hindbrain-related syringomyelia

Many patients have a diminished respiratory reserve. There may be impaired function either of the phrenic nerves or of the respiratory centres. Matsumoto & Symon (1989) reported a mortality of two cases out of 22 after attempts to block the presumed communication at the obex. In their cases with craniovertebral decompression alone they had no mortality. They related their deaths to respiratory problems. Additional problems arise from damaged lower cranial nerves in many cases, sometimes with risk of inhalation. Careful preoperative selection is needed and then vigilant postoperative observation. Even so, sudden respiratory arrest is not unknown, and in cases where there is anxiety an apnoea alarm is justifiable. Physiotherapy, vigilant trials of drinking clear water before thick fluids or solids are tried and the use of tracheostomy all have their place. If inadequate amounts of occipital bone are removed, respiratory inadequacy or arrest may result. If the dura is sutured reimpaction may occur, and is likely to lead to progression of the neurology in later stages with persistent enlargement of the syrinx.

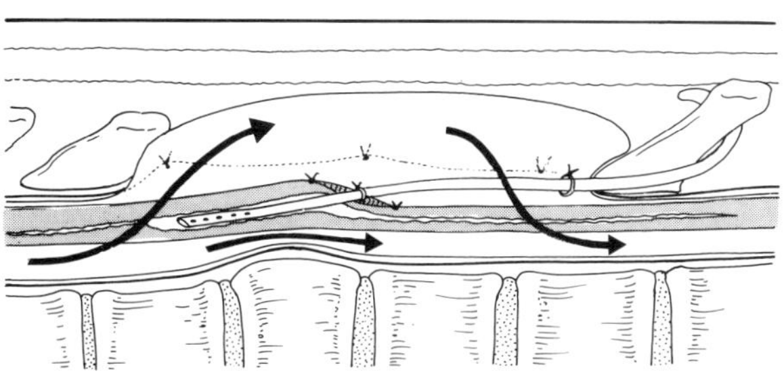

Fig. 54.12 Idealized situation after operation on paraplegia with secondary syringomyelia. The drainage tube should be well inside the syringomyelia and a muscle patch used to prevent entry from the subarachnoid space. The dura should remain stitched open; there should be a sizeable meningocele with free access of CSF from both ends. Decompression of the site of the fracture should allow fluid also to move ventral to the site of major cord damage. Note that the distal end of the tube should pass to a low-pressure cavity such as the pleura or the peritoneum.

Worsening of hydrocephalus is sometimes a problem; the ventricles may enlarge slowly and late after surgery. Hydrocephalus may cause subdural haematoma as an acute complication.

Overdecompression of the hindbrain with lack of support of the cerebellum may lead to its falling down into the decompression. This is more probable if 'suck' is not eliminated. The hitching up of emptied tonsils may help to prevent this, but the size of the decompression is primary. The commonest symptom of slump is headache. If there is no hydrocephalus there seems to be little further which can be done to remedy the situation.

Even after an adequate hindbrain decompression, the syrinx may persist. It is unlikely that success will follow a second attempt at dissection. The adhesions are commonly severe, the vessels are sometimes hidden and attempts to further free the 'suck' mechanisms may be dangerous. If the syrinx is still tightly full then the use of a syringopleural or peritoneal drain may be attempted. However, in the majority of cases the syrinx is present, but relatively slack; any attempt to get a drainage tube into such a cavity may encounter haustrae and healing of parts of the cavity, with difficulty in inserting the drainage tube (Barbaro *et al.*, 1984; Williams & Page, 1987).

Non-hindbrain-related syringomyelia

Deterioration of neurological features is uncommon, but not unknown. A drainage tube may press on the edges of the cord or it may be kinked and produce neurological problems or even haemorrhage. Overdrainage of the syrinx may occur with overflattening of the cord and kinking of the lateral margins. This is a theoretical rather than a proven point, but Carmel (1986) observes that in the patient with marginal cord function operation may appear to accelerate decline.

Pain may be exacerbated after the syrinx is deflated; this is possibly due to distortion, but recovery of function may allow the afferent tracts to conduct more sensory information, often of a dysaesthetic and unpleasant kind. This usually settles in time and is less common than improvement of pain problems (Williams, 1989).

The persistence of a tightly filling cavity at the site of the neurological deterioration, or below it, should signal an attempt at correction. It is probable that 'suck' and/or 'slosh' is still active. Revision of the operation may be required. The drain may sometimes need to be repositioned above the previous site. The presence of a full syrinx below the operation, even if the top is collapsed, means that there is a pump available so that the 'slosh' mechanism may project the fluid upwards. If there is a sizeable zone of filling then syringopleural shunting may be advisable (Williams & Page, 1987).

RESULTS

There are few reports on outcome. This is because of the relative rarity of cases and the fact that chronic neurological deficits are difficult to record objectively. Additionally, the placebo effects of operation are powerful, and the natural history may be long and uneventful.

The results of hindbrain hernia decompression are often pleasing. The symptoms which do best are those of the long tracts, pain—especially neck pain and headache—and bulbar features (Saez *et al.*, 1976; Logue & Rice-Edwards, 1981; Dyste *et al.*, 1989; Matsumoto & Symon, 1989; Wissoff & Epstein, 1989). Signs related to the cavity are not so favourably influenced; loss of tendon reflexes, muscle wasting and sensory loss seldom improve (Saez *et al.*, 1976; Dyste *et al.*, 1989).

Improvement after shunting arachnoiditic syringomyelia is seldom great. All major neurological deficits are permanent. The pain may be worse for a while as function returns to the pain pathways. The improvements are often quite impressive, however, and seem worthwhile (Barkovich *et al.*, 1987; Williams, 1989). The long-term results include a tendency to progression as the patients age (Aboulker, 1979; Matsumoto & Symon, 1989), but many of them become stable.

In patients showing late progression, reinvestigation to establish the state of the ventricles is sometimes rewarding and MRI is enormously helpful (Barkovich *et al.*, 1987). A completely collapsed cord and adequate hindbrain decompression is helpful in reassurance. It is sometimes tempting, on reviewing a patient with a persisting cord cavity and tonsils still jammed in an inadequately decompressed foramen magnum, to recommence surgery even years after the initial attempt, but the clinical progression may be equal in cases with a surgically perfect result and enthusiasm may need to be checked.

Patients with syringomyelia of almost all kinds often have to anticipate the problems of chronic and slowly progressive neurological disease, even if operation may have produced improvement. Patients with paraplegia, especially, may not regain such fundamental skills as transferring, and may need psychological and social support. In various countries, self-help associations exist which may be helpful for some patients and their families.

The problems of syringomyelia would be better prevented than cured; early diagnosis is best. The most obvious example of patients who might benefit by routinized imaging is the paraplegic population who have a high risk. Both complete and partial paraplegic patients should have investigation early in the illness, and then have periodic review (Sett & Crockard, 1991). Magnetic resonance imaging is the investigation of choice. The incidence and significance of small cavities remains to be worked out, but in complete paraplegics at least the likelihood is that early surgery, before the cavities become symptomatic, will pay dividends.

Children with 'idiopathic' scoliosis and all forms of dysraphism constitute another high-risk group for which early surgery may be helpful (Wissoff & Epstein, 1989).

The discovery that in hindbrain-related cases there is a strong association with difficult birth (Williams, 1977a, 1986; Newman *et al.*, 1981; Battersby & Williams, 1982) is interesting. It seems likely that a high proportion of cases without such an association being noted also came on at birth. There is a need to study the infantile hindbrain during labour and immediately afterwards. The moulding of the infant skull during normal birth suggests that the hindbrain is commonly forced into the foramen magnum. Crying and suckling may tend to hold this in place by 'suck'. This area is little explored, and the tool most likely to advance understanding is real-time ultrasound imaging. It may be that prophylactic measures against dysraphism, screening of other infants at risk from birth trauma and judicious surgery at an early stage may eliminate hindbrain-related syringomyelia, as well as that secondary to paraplegia, in developed societies in the future.

REFERENCES

Aboulker, J. (1979) La syringomyélie et la liquides intrarachidiens. *Neurochirurgie*, **25** (Suppl. 1).

Barbaro, N.M., Wilson, C.B. & Gutin, P.H. (1984) Surgical treatment of syringomyelia: favourable results with syringoperitoneal shunting. *J. Neurosurg.*, **61**, 531–538.

Barkovich, A.J., Sherman, J.L. & Citrin, C.M. (1987) Magnetic resonance of postoperative syringomyelia. *Am. J. Neuroradiol.*, **8**, 319–327.

Barkovich, A.J., Wippold, F.J. & Sherman, J.L. (1986) Significance of cerebellar tonsillar position on magnetic resonance. *Am. J. Neuroradiol.*, **7**, 795–799.

Barnett, H.J.M., Foster, J.B. & Hudgson, P. (1973) *Syringomyelia*. W.B. Saunders, London.

Batzdorf, U. (1991) Syringomyelia with craniovertebral junction abnormality. In Batzdorf, U. (ed.) *Syringomyelia, Current Concepts in Diagnosis and Treatment*, pp. 163–182. Williams & Wilkins, Baltimore, MD.

Battersby, R.D.E. & Williams, B. (1982) Birth injury: a possible contributory factor in the aetiology of primary basilar impression. *J. Neurol., Neurosurg. Psychiatry*, **45**, 879–883.

Carmel, P. (1986) The Chiari malformations and syringomyelia. In Hoffman, H.J. & Epstein, F. (eds) *Disorders of the Developing Nervous System: Diagnosis and Treatment*, pp. 133–151. Blackwell Scientific Publications, Oxford.

Davis, C.H.G. & Symon, L. (1990) Mechanism and treatment in post-traumatic syringomyelia. *Br. J. Neurosurg.*, **3**, 669–674.

Dyste, G.N., Menezes, A.H. & VanGilder, J.C. (1989) Symptomatic Chiari malformations, an analysis of presentation, management and long term outcome. *J. Neurosurg.*, **171**, 159–168.

Gardner, W.J. (1973) *The Dysraphic States*. Excerpta Medica, Amsterdam.

Grant, R., Hadley, D.M. & MacPherson, P. (1987) Syringomyelia: cyst measurement by magnetic resonance imaging and comparison with symptoms, signs and disability. *J. Neurol. Neurosurg. Psychiatry*, **50**, 1008–1014.

Greenfield, J.G. (1963) Syringomyelia and syringobulbia. In Blackwood, W., McMenemy, W.H., Myer, A., Norman, R. & Russell, D.S. (eds), *Greenfield's Neuropathology*, 2nd edn, pp. 306–312. Arnold, London.

Krayenbuhl, H. (1974) Evaluation of the different surgical approaches in the treatment of syringomyelia. *Clin. Neurol. Neurosurg.*, **77**, 110–128.

Kruse, A., Rassmussen, G. & Borgesen, S.E. (1987) CSF dynamics in syringomyelia: intracranial pressure and resistance to outflow. *Br. J. Neurosurg.*, **1**, 477–484.

Lee, B.C.P., Zimmerman, R.D. & Manning, J.T. (1985) Magnetic resonance imaging of syringomyelia and hydromyelia. *Am. J. Neuroradiol.*, **6**, 221–228.

Logue, V. & Rice Edwards, M. (1981) Syringomyelia and its surgical treatment—an analysis of 75 patients. *J. Neurol. Neurosurg. Psychiatry*, **44**, 273–284.

Matsumoto, T. & Symon, L. (1989) Surgical management of syringomyelia—current results. *Surg. Neurol.*, **32**, 358–365.

Newman, P.L., Terenty, T.R. & Foster, J.B. (1981) Some observations on the pathogenesis of syringomyelia. *J. Neurol. Neurosurg. Psychiatry*, **44**, 964–969.

Nightingale, S. & Williams, B. (1987) Hindbrain hernia headache. *Lancet*, **1**, 731–734.

Ollivier, C.P. (1827) *Traité de la Moelle Épinère et de ses Maladies*. Crevot, Paris.

Rhoton, A.L. (1976) Microsurgery of Arnold–Chiari malformation in adults with and without hydromyelia. *J. Neurosurg.*, **45**, 473–483.

Rice Edwards, M. (1982) Syringomyelia and its surgical management. In Rice Edwards, M. (ed.), *Topical Reviews in Neurosurgery*, pp. 161–184. Wright, Bristol.

Rossier, A.B., Foo, D. & Shillito, J. (1985) Post traumatic cervical syringomyelia. *Brain*, **108**, 439–461.

Saez, R.J., Onofrio, B.M. & Yanagihara, T. (1976) Experience with Arnold–Chiari malformation, 1960–1970. *J. Neurosurg.*, **45**, 416–422.

Sett, P. & Crockard, A.H. (1991) The value of magnetic resonance imaging in the follow up management of spinal injury. *Paraplegia*, **29**, 396–410.

Sherman, J.L., Citrin, C.M. & Barkovitch, A.J. (1987) M.R. Imaging of syringomyelia. *J. Comp. Assist. Tomogr.*, **11**, 407–411.

Stevens, J.M., Olney, J.S. & Kendal, B.E. (1985) Post-traumatic cystic and non-cystic myelopathy. *Neuroradiology*, **27**, 48–56.

Suzuki, M., Davis, C. & Symon, L. (1986) Syringo-peritoneal shunt for treatment of cord cavitation. *J. Neurol., Neurosurg. Psychiatry*, **48**, 620–627.

Tator, C.H., Meguro, K. & Rowed, D.W. (1982) Favourable results with syringosubarachnoid shunts for treatment of syringomyelia. *J. Neurosurg.*, **56**, 517–523.

Van Houweninge Graftdijk, C.J. (1932) *Over Hydrocephalus*, Thesis, University of Leiden.

West, R.J. & Williams, B. (1980) Radiographic studies of the ventricles in syringomyelia. *Neuroradiology*, **20**, 5–16.

Williams, B. (1974) A demonstration analogue for ventricular and intraspinal dynamics (DAVID). *J. Neurol. Sci.*, **23**, 445–461.

Williams, B. (1975) Cerebrospinal fluid pressure-gradients in spina bifida cystica, with special reference to the Arnold–Chiari malformation and aqueductal stenosis. *Dev. Med. Child. Neurol.*, **17** (Suppl. 35), 138–150.

Williams, B. (1976) Cerebrospinal fluid pressure changes in response to coughing. *Brain*, **99**, 331–346.

Williams, B. (1980) On the pathogenesis of syringomyelia. *J. R. Soc. Med.*, **73**, 798–806.

Williams, B. (1977a) On the pathogenesis of Chiari malformation. *Z. Kinderchirurg. Grenzgeb.*, **22**, 533–553.

Williams, B. (1977b) Difficult labour as a cause of communicating syringomyelia. *Lancet*, **2**, 51–53.
Williams, B. (1978) A critical appraisal of posterior fossa surgery for communicating syringomyelia. *Brain*, **101**, 223–250.
Williams, B. (1979a) Orthopaedic features in the presentation of syringomyelia. *J. Bone Jt. Surg.*, **61B**, 314–323.
Williams, B. (1979b) Subarachnoid pouches of the posterior fossa with syringomyelia. *Acta Neurochirurg.*, **47**, 187–217.
Williams, B. (1981) Simultaneous cerebral and spinal fluid pressure recordings. 2. Cerebrospinal dissociation with lesions at the foramen magnum. *Acta Neurochirurg.*, **59**, 123–142.
Williams, B. (1986) Progress in syringomyelia. *Neurol. Res.*, **8**, 130–145.
Williams, B. (1989) Cough headache due to craniospinal pressure dissociation. *Arch. Neurol.*, **37**, 226–230.
Williams, B. (1990) Post-traumatic syringomyelia, an update. *Paraplegia*, **28**, 296–313.
Williams, B. & Bentley, J. (1980) Experimental communicating syringomyelia in dogs after cisternal kaolin injection. *J. Neurol. Sci.*, **48**, 93–107.
Williams, B. & Fahy, G. (1983) A critical appraisal of 'terminal ventriculostomy' for the treatment of syringomyelia. *J. Neurosurg.*, **58**, 188–197.
Williams, B. & Page, N. (1987) Surgical treatment of syringomyelia with syringopleural shunting. *Br. J. Neurosurg.*, **1**, 63–80.
Williams, B., Terry, A.F. & Jones, H.W.F. (1981) Syringomyelia as a sequel to traumatic paraplegia. *Paraplegia*, **19**, 67–70.
Wissoff, J.H. & Epstein, F. (1989) Management of hydromyelia. *Neurosurgery*, **25**, 562–571.

SECTION 13
METABOLIC BONE DISEASE

55 · Metabolic Bone Disease

By J.A. KANIS

Like many terms, metabolic bone disease defies an accurate description. It traditionally comprises generalized disorders of bone such as osteoporosis and osteomalacia; but this framework is unsatisfactory for several reasons. It omits focal disturbances of bone such as Paget's disease of bone and neoplastic bone disease, which are of some importance since there have been marked advances in our understanding of their pathophysiology and treatment. Conversely, it includes many disorders where we lack any knowledge of pathophysiology or of treatment. This chapter reviews those disorders where our knowledge of cause or treatment is sufficient that orthopaedic surgeons or neurosurgeons should take account of the disorder in their management. The chapter focuses upon disorders of adulthood rather than those arising during growth, but the development of the spine is briefly reviewed. The skeleton is the major reservoir for calcium, and it is not surprising that metabolic bone disease is commonly associated with abnormalities of calcium homeostasis. It is difficult, therefore, to separate calcium homeostasis from skeletal homeostasis. Extracellular calcium homeostasis is not completely ignored in this chapter, but for a more detailed appreciation of the endocrinology of calcium metabolism and the associated disorders the reader is referred to the further reading list.

Whereas the treatment of metabolic bone disease is usually beyond the area of interest of surgeons, these disorders are important to recognize since the success of surgical intervention often depends on their medical treatment. Examples include osteomalacia and renal bone disease. In addition, the recognition and treatment of bone diseases may decrease the need for surgery. In this regard the effects of medical treatment of slowly progressive paraparesis due to Paget's disease are at least as good as those of surgery. It is not the intention of this chapter to suggest that bone disease should be managed by the surgeon, but rather to provide enough information to stimulate greater interest in the overall management of patients and to instil confidence in the investigation or at least the referral of affected patients.

THE COMPOSITION OF BONE

Bones and teeth are the only structures which depend upon their rigidity by virtue of calcification, and this rigidity is of obvious importance in providing structural stability to aid locomotion and protect internal organs. It is important to recognize, however, that the skeleton is not inert, and subserves a number of important metabolic functions. These include extracellular calcium homeostasis, but also the maintenance of skeletal integrity, since the turnover of bone ensures the self-repair of the skeleton and its ability to respond to physiological or pathological stress. The way in which bone disease arises is frequently through a disruption of the processes which normally maintain skeletal turnover.

Bone is specialized connective tissue that comprises an organic phase, a mineral phase and bone cells. The majority of the matrix is composed of collagen fibres, and collagen in bone accounts for 60% of total body collagen and 90% of skeletal weight in the adult. There are several types of collagen, but that of adult bone is Type I, which is laid down by osteoblasts in a highly structured arrangement. Each unit of collagen (tropocollagen) comprises a heterotrimer consisting of two $\alpha 1$ chains and one $\alpha 2$ chain encoded on chromosomes 17 and 7, respectively.

During the process of collagen synthesis, procollagen chains coil together, and during maturation undergo a number of transformations including cleavage of amino acid and carboxyterminal extension peptides, glycosylation and the formation of crosslinks with other tropocollagen macromolecules. Evidence of such activity can be measured in serum and urine (e.g. procollagen peptides, non-dialysable hydroxyproline), and provides non-invasive indices of skeletal metabolism in the investigation of metabolic bone disease.

The mineral of bone is laid within the collagen fibres in a highly organized manner since the latter are normally arranged as lamellae parallel to bone surfaces (Fig. 55.1). Where the turnover of bone is increased the assembly of collagen fibres is anarchic with a random arrangement of fibres, but mineralization also occurs in woven bone. The mineral phase of bone comprises mainly calcium phosphate and carbonate in the form of hydroxyapatite. Mineralization begins with the precipitation of amorphous calcium phosphate, and with time the mineral phase becomes progressively more crystalline. Crystals of hydroxyapatite are elongated hexagonal crystals which conform closely to the orientation of the collagen fibres.

Bone cells are found throughout skeletal tissue. These include osteoblasts, osteoclasts and osteocytes. The osteoblast is the cell responsible for the synthesis of collagen and the subsequent mineralization of the matrix. In addition, many other proteins are found in bone, many of which are also synthesized by osteoblasts. The osteoblast is rich in alkaline phosphatase and this enzyme may be important for the process of mineralization. Irrespective of its precise function, this ectoenzyme is shed from the osteoblast to the extracellular fluid and the measurement of its activity in serum provides one of the biochemical indices of skeletal metabolism widely used in clinical practice. Osteocalcin (bone gla protein) is another bone protein produced exclusively by osteoblasts. Measurement in serum of osteocalcin levels provides an indirect index of bone formation.

Osteocytes are osteoblasts which have been trapped within the bone matrix during the process of bone formation. The osteocytes are interconnected to osteoblasts and other osteocytes by fine intercellular projections running within bone canaliculae. The other major cell type found in bone is the osteoclast. This is a multinucleated cell which is responsible for bone resorption. Osteoclasts preferentially degrade fully mineralized bone by attaching onto a bone surface and secreting acids and lysosomal enzymes into the space provided between the osteoclast and the mineralized bone surface. The surface of the osteoclast at this interface is ruffled by cytoplasmic extensions that infiltrate the resorbing bone surface.

Growth and architecture of bone

All bones begin as mesenchymal condensations during the early embryonic period. Some of these condensations become fibrocellular and directly ossify to form the intramembranous bones. The spine, like

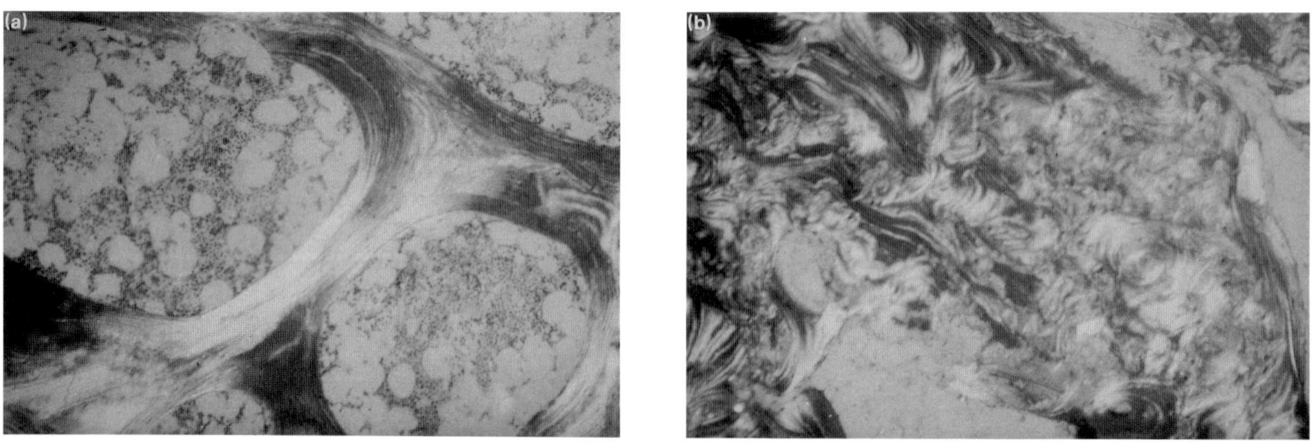

Fig. 55.1 Light microscopy of normal (a) and woven (b) bone. Note the neat lamellar organization of collagen normally laid down at trabecular bone in the long axis of the trabeculae. The panel on the right shows areas of lamellar bone, but most of the trabecular bone tissue comprises anarchic woven bone with a subsequent loss of normal architectural pattern.

most of the skeleton, is derived from the transformation of mesenchymal tissues into cartilage and its subsequent transformation into bone. In the spine, like the long bones, the cartilage model is transformed into bone in a series of phases. These include the formation of a primary bone collar by the conversion of the perichondrium into a periosteum, the calcification of cartilage at the hypertrophic region, the penetration of the bone collar by vascular tissue and the replacement of central cartilage by bone. These steps result in the formation of the diaphysis and metaphysis. Secondary ossification centres appear in the apophyses. In these respects the vertebral bodies are very comparable to long tubular bones of the appendicular skeleton.

In the spine, three primary centres of ossification occur in each vertebra, with the exception of C1, C2 and the sacrum. One is in each vertebral body and one in each neural arch. At birth, only small areas are still cartilaginous. Secondary areas of ossification are the ring apophyses, which begin to ossify in adolescence and may not completely ossify until the early 20s. The spinous and transverse processes are also secondary areas of ossification appearing during adolescence. Fusion of the epiphyseal ossification centre with the primary ossification centre begins by the age of 14–15, but may not be completed until the age of 25 in the lumbar spine. Horizontal growth may occur by subperiosteal apposition and by diametric growth of the apophysis. Vertical growth ceases when apophyseal fusion occurs with the centrum. The events which occur during the growth of bone are complex, and the mechanisms by which they are regulated are ill-understood. The sequence of events may be altered by many disorders which give rise to an alteration either in the shape or the composition of bone. The general shape of the spine is thus dependent on the normal development of the structures and their maintenance during later life.

The architectural features of the bones of the spine have features in common with all other bones. These include a cortical shell of compact bone that surrounds all external surfaces and a loosely meshed spongy cancellous bone within the cortical shell (Fig. 55.2). The cortical endplates of each vertebral body transmit compressive forces from the intravertebral discs to the trabeculae. The cortex is thicker centrally, up to 1 mm thick, and thins to 0.3 mm in areas towards the endplate. This outer shell not only transmits mechanical forces, but can carry much of the load itself. The skeleton as a whole is largely composed of compact bone (75–80%). In bones of the spine, however, the ratio of compact to trabecular bone is near unity. In the vertebral bodies themselves the majority of bone is trabecular. This means that the mechanical competence of the vertebral bodies is highly dependent upon the integrity of the trabecular meshwork and its organization. If all the trabeculae are removed from the lumbar vertebrae the cortical shell can carry over 50% of the normal peak load.

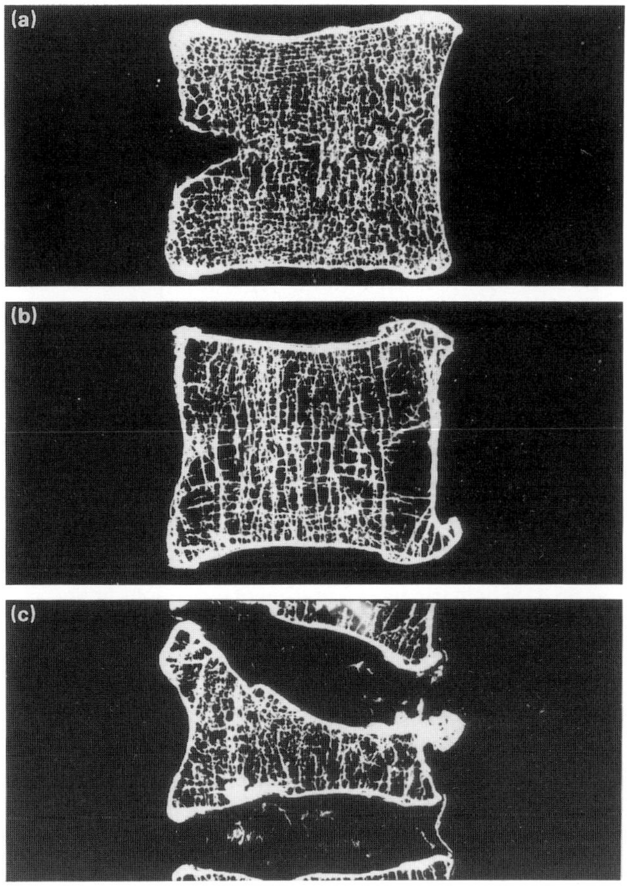

Fig. 55.2 Photograph of a lumbar vertebra at skeletal maturity (a), in postmenopausal osteoporosis (b), and following anterior vertebral collapse (c). Note that the osteoporotic bone has less bone, but this is largely associated to the loss of trabecular elements themselves.

X-rays of the vertebral bodies give the impression of longitudinal weight-bearing trabeculae and transverse stabilizing trabeculae. In fact throughout most of the vertebral body the trabeculae are transverse fenestrated plates of bone where each longitudinal trabecula arises from the corner of each fenestration

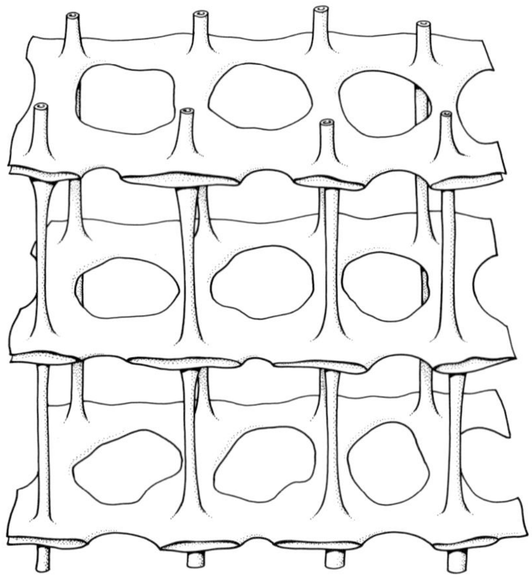

Fig. 55.3 Schematic representation of cancellous bone showing a series of perforated trabecular plates connected by trabecular rods.

(Fig. 55.3). The central portion of the vertebral body is much less uniform, in part related to the presence of the basivertebral vein. Thus, the disposition of the trabecular meshwork is far from random, and its structured arrangement is disposed to transmit forces applied to the bone in a highly efficient manner. This is an appropriate physiological design, but its efficiency makes the vertebral bodies paradoxically prone to mechanical failure when disease disrupts the connectivity of trabecular elements. The destruction of connectivity is a characteristic feature of some forms of osteoporosis, particularly that due to gonadal deficiency (see Fig. 55.2).

Bone remodelling

In the adult who is neither increasing nor decreasing in skeletal size the skeleton is in zero balance. Despite this equilibrium, bone is continuously being turned over. In the adult these changes in focal skeletal balance comprise modelling and remodelling events. Modelling refers to changes in the architecture or size of bones that result from unopposed formation or resorption of bone, and is a conspicuous feature of growth. In the adult the gradual increase in the diameter of some long bones with age is a form of modelling, but accounts for less than 5% of all skeletal turnover. Remodelling comprises the process of removing old bone by bone resorption, which is followed by new bone formation and accounts for more than 95% of skeletal turnover in the mature adult. The overall turnover of the skeleton is slow and on average takes nine to 11 years. Notwithstanding, turnover is extremely important for skeletal health since it provides a mechanism for self-repair of fatigue damage and adaptation to stress. All solid structures undergo fatigue damage and, without the capacity to self-repair, bone would be no exception. Indeed, if turnover is halted experimentally or clinically this may give rise to pathological fracture within one or two years, even without inducing any change in the amount of bone present.

The turnover of bone is predominantly a surface-based phenomenon, and several different types of bone surface are available in the skeleton. These include the trabecular and cortical endosteal surfaces and the vascular channels within bone. All these surfaces are covered by cells with distinct morphological and functional features. The majority of these cells are flat lining cells with a somewhat inert appearance, or inactive osteoblasts. It is thought that these cells are predominantly concerned with extracellular calcium homeostasis in concert with the osteocytes and their extensive cell processes lying in the canalicular network. It is on these bone surfaces that the processes of bone remodelling occur throughout life.

Compact bone, by its very nature, has a low surface to volume ratio, whereas the converse is true for trabecular bone. The surface to volume ratio is nearly 10 times higher in trabecular bone (Table 55.1). It is readily apparent from this consideration that the activity of bone remodelling is much greater at trabecular than cortical sites. This means that, when disorders of remodelling occur, they affect trabecular tissue earlier in their evolution: and the predominance of trabecular tissue at the spine makes this a vulnerable site for metabolic bone disease.

The principles of bone remodelling are similar for trabecular and cortical bone but differ in minor respects.

Trabecular bone remodelling

Bone remodelling is largely mediated by the activity of bone-forming cells (osteoblasts) and bone-resorbing cells (osteoclasts) and is a prominent feature of endosteal sites. At any one time such cells occupy the

Table 55.1 Some characteristics of the normal skeleton

Surface	m^2
Cortical bone	3.5*
Trabecular bone	9*
Osteocyte	90
Lacunar and canalicular	1200
Mass	**g**
Cortical bone	4000
Trabecular bone	1000
Total skeleton	5000
Surface* to mass ratio	**cm^2/g**
Cortical bone	8.75
Trabecular bone	90.0
Total skeleton	25.0

* Surface available for remodelling.

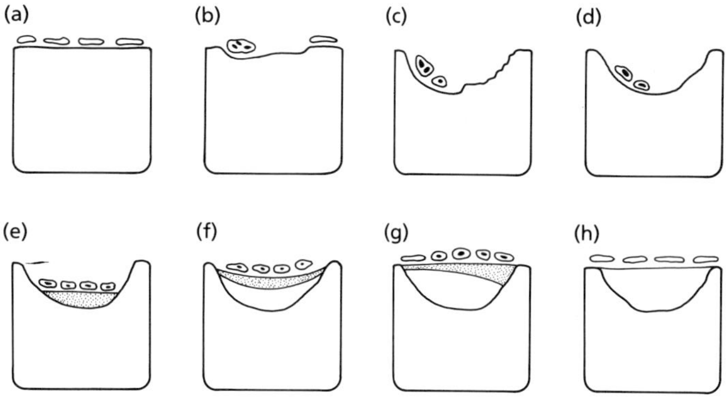

Fig. 55.4 Steps in the bone remodelling sequence of trabecular bone. Early in the remodelling sequence osteoclasts are attracted to a quiescent bone surface (a) and excavate a resorption cavity (b, c). Mononuclear cells smooth off the resorption cavity (d) which is a subsequent site for the attraction of osteoblasts (coupling) which synthesize an osteoid matrix (e). Continuous new matrix synthesis (f) is followed by calcification (g) of the newly formed bone. When complete, lining cells once more overlie the trabecular surface (h).

minority of the bone surface (10–15%), most of which is covered by quiescent lining cells. Bone turnover is a series of discrete cellular events organized both in time and space on this surface. The steps involved have been well characterized both in health (Fig. 55.4) and in disease, giving rise to a detailed knowledge of the pathophysiology of many skeletal disorders.

ACTIVATION

The first visible step of bone remodelling is the attraction of osteoclasts to the quiescent surface. Osteoclast precursors are, however, present for several days beforehand close to the quiescent surface. It is not known how or if this process is regulated, but fat tissue appears to slow turnover, and may decrease the availability of osteoclast precursors for activation. The origins of osteoclasts are still controversial but they can be formed from cells of the monocyte/macrophage lineage. The factors that determine the site for the focal attraction of a team of osteoclasts are not known, but it may be that fatigue damage to bone is a stimulus. Other structural and biochemical signals may also be important.

RESORPTION

Osteoclasts are mononucleated or more usually multinucleated cells capable of undertaking bone resorption by the secretion of acid and lysosomal enzymes beneath their ruffled borders, which become closely applied to bone tissue. A team of osteoclasts can cut a depth of up to 20 μm/day. Osteoclasts preferentially resorb fully mineralized bone, but may sometimes be found on osteoid when this is abundant. Osteoclasts are motile with a small geographical domain, and working in concert they create a resorption or erosion cavity in bone. In trabecular bone resorption cavities are completed in approximately 10 days and are 50 μm in depth. In cortical bone a team of osteoclasts tunnel parallel to the long axis of the osteon several hundred micrometres in length.

REVERSAL

Later in the process of bone resorption, multinucleate cells disappear and are replaced by mononuclear cells which appear to be capable of some resorption and smooth off the resorption cavity. Over the next 7–10 days a layer of cement substance is deposited which is rich in proteoglycans, glycoproteins and acid phosphatase, but poor in collagen. This is termed the reversal phase, and the bed of the resorption cavity can be identified as a reversal or cement line by histological techniques even after subsequent bone formation has infilled the resorption cavity (Fig. 55.5).

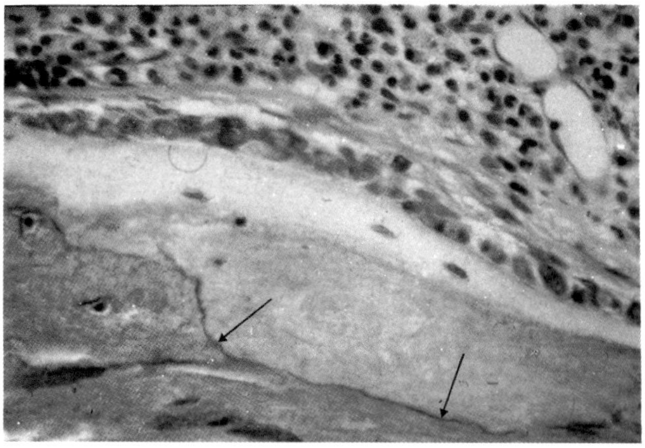

Fig. 55.5 Histological section to show the limits of an erosion cavity shown as the reversal or cement line (arrowed). New bone has formed within the erosion cavity which, under the influence of osteoblasts lining the bone surface, is undergoing mineralization. Note the osteocytes within the bone matrix which represent trapped osteoblasts (toluidine blue).

MATRIX SYNTHESIS

Once a resorption cavity is complete the process termed coupling attracts osteoblasts to the resorbed surface, which thereafter synthesize an osteoid matrix (see Fig. 55.4). The coupling signal is not known, but might be mediated by reversal cells within resorption cavities, the cement substance of the reversal surface or the exposure of chemotactic proteins within bone matrix such as collagen fragments or transforming growth factors. The factor which determine the number of osteoblasts recruited to the reversal surface is also not known, but may be critical in determining whether a resorption cavity is infilled adequately. The osteoblasts form a sheet of cells, beneath which they synthesize layers of osteoid matrix which comprise unmineralized bone tissue. The newly formed osteoid has a well-ordered lamellated arrangement of collagen bundles due to periodic changes in the orientation of bundles which are well visualized under polarized light (see Fig. 55.1). In cancellous bone the lamellae are usually parallel to the trabeculae. In cortical bone the lamellae are more frequently arranged as concentric rings around vascular channels formed in the erosion tunnel. There are, however, interconnections of collagen between lamellae which decrease the risk of slippage and increase, therefore, the mechanical competence of bone. It is clear that the construction of a lamellar sheet requires the concerted action of a team of osteoblasts but, as in the case of osteoclast teamwork, the processes which regulate this are not understood.

MINERALIZATION

A few days after the onset of matrix formation by osteoblasts, the newly formed osteoid undergoes mineralization. The time interval between the onset of matrix synthesis and the start of mineralization is about 10 days, when the osteoid seam width is 8–20 μm in depth. The delay accounts for the appearance of osteoid in normal bone; during this period maturation of collagen occurs, which involves the formation of collagen crosslinks and probably the incorporation of other bone proteins. The junction between mineralized bone and osteoid is sharply demarcated (the calcification front), indicating the rapidity of the initial rate of mineralization. It can be detected by stains such as toluidine blue under light microscopy (see Fig. 55.5) or by ultraviolet fluorescence of bone prelabelled with tetracyclines. Tetracycline is localized and bound by calcium salts at critical concentrations both *in vivo* and *in vitro*, and the administration of a short course of tetracycline (generally two to four days) permits the visualization of the extent of the bone surface undergoing mineralization at any one time. If two courses of tetracycline are given, but separated by a known time interval, both the extent and the rate of mineralization can be measured. The combined measurements can give an estimate of the rate of mineralized bone formation.

Some osteoblasts, perhaps 30% in trabecular and half as many in cortical bone, become buried within the osteoid matrix to become osteocytes within bone. The fate of the remaining cells is not known. Osteocytes have extensive canaliculi which form a network between osteocytes and surface osteoblasts. They probably function in mineral transport and the surrounding bone is less mineralized. When cell death occurs this gives rise to micropetrosis.

Osteoid mineralization occurs rapidly to begin with, and is three-quarters complete within a few days. In contrast, it takes many months to become fully mineralized. After three months osteoid is no longer visible as unmineralized bone on conventional staining, but further mineralization and maturation of the crystal phase may account for a further 10–20%

increase in bone mineral density over one or two years. The decreased bone mineral density of young bone can be detected by microradiography.

QUIESCENCE

When osteoblast synthesis of matrix is complete the morphology of osteoblasts changes. During mineralization they become flatter, and when this is complete the resting osteoblasts become flattened.

The sequence of resorption, formation and mineralization occurs on the minority of the bone surface, and at any one time 90% or so of available surfaces are inert. The moiety of bone, termed a bone structural unit (BSU) at its completion, takes several months to be synthesized and mineralized. In contrast, the process of osteoclastic bone resorption is nearly complete in three or four days. This explains why formation surfaces on bone are more abundant than resorption surfaces. The fact that bone formation rates can be measured by tetracycline labelling, as well as the surface extent of formation, means that the time period of all events on bone surfaces can be measured. For example, if the time taken to form a new BSU is four months, and these events occur on the minority of the bone surface (usually 10%), then the average quiescent interval on any bit of bone surface is 40 months.

Cortical bone remodelling

The remodelling sequence summarized in Fig. 55.4 for trabecular tissue is not dissimilar in cortical bone (Fig. 55.6). Cortical bone has a system of interconnecting canals orientated in a plane longitudinal to the long axis of osteons and long bones (Haversian canals) or perpendicular (Volkmann's canals). The canals contain blood vessels, lymphatics, nerves and connective tissue so that bone cells lie within 150 µm of the blood supply. Osteoclasts gather together and tunnel within a Haversian canal, to form a tunnel through the cortex at a rate comparable to that in trabecular bone (20 µm/day). Behind the advancing resorption cone the tunnel is infilled several days later by new unmineralized bone matrix arranged in concentric lamellae by osteoblasts and, as for trabecular bone, thereafter undergoes mineralization to create a long cylindrical bone structural unit termed an osteon. Interstitial lamellae in cortical bone represent the remnants of earlier osteons.

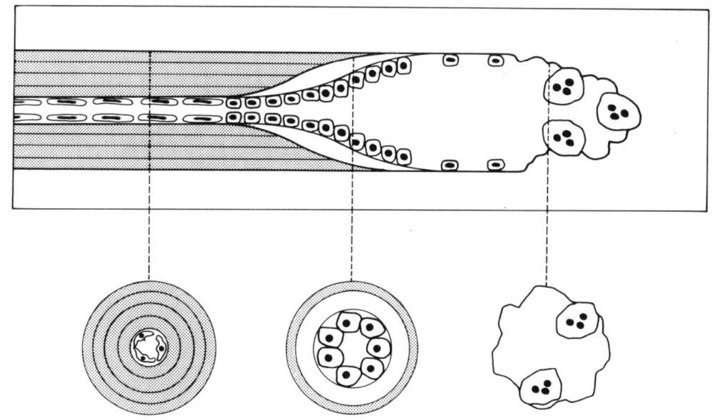

Fig. 55.6 Schematic diagram of a bone remodelling unit in cortical bone cut in its long axis with three transverse sections. Osteoclasts tunnel into the long axis of the cortex to create a cutting cone (right). The resorption cavity is smoothed off during the reversal phase; thereafter, osteoblasts synthesize an osteoid matrix in the form of concentric lamellae (centre) which infill a resorption cavity (left) leaving a new Haversian canal. Note that, unlike trabecular bone, the resorption cavity cannot be markedly overfilled.

BRUs and BSUs

The remodelling sequence thus involves an organized and focal series of cellular events which have been termed bone multicellular units or bone remodelling units (BRU). The completion of activity of a bone remodelling unit results in the creation of a bone structural unit (also termed a bone metabolic unit). In the case of cortical bone the BSU is a secondary osteon or Haversian system and is cylindrical in shape, 100–300 µm in diameter and several millimetres in length. In trabecular bone the BSU is flat, 40–60 µm thick with an area of 0.5 to 1 mm^2 (Table 55.2).

Thus, skeletal tissue comprises a series of BSUs which in the adult human have been estimated at 35 million in number, of which 40% are in trabecular bone. Where BSUs are in contact they are separated by the cement line or reversal surface which are not traversed by osteocytic canaliculi.

PATHOPHYSIOLOGY OF METABOLIC BONE DISEASE

Many generalized bone disorders represent abnormalities in the normal remodelling sequence. These include: accelerated bone turnover, as seen, for example, in renal bone disease, hyperparathyroidism and in Paget's disease; a delay in the mineralization

Table 55.2 Some characteristics of normal bone structural units (BSUs) and bone remodelling units (BRUs)

	Cortex	Trabecular bone	Cortical and trabecular bone
BSUs			
Number (millions)	21	14	35
Volume (mm^3)	0.065	0.025	0.048
Total volume (cm^3)	1365	350	1715
Total calcium	800	200	1000
Calcium (μg/BSU)	38	14	
BRUs			
Number (thousands)	280	1400	1680
Number (% BSUs)	1.3	10	4.8
Number (per cm^3 bone tissue)	205	4000	1000
Total resorption space (cm^3)	5.6	7.1	12.6
Resorption space (g calcium)	3.4	4.2	7.6
Resorption space (% total volume)	0.4	2.0	0.72

of bone giving rise to osteomalacia; and focal imbalances between formation and resorption, giving rise to changes in the amount of bone present (osteopetrosis or osteoporosis). Like many tissues, bone can respond to pathological and physiological insults in a limited manner, and typical responses are summarized below.

Changes in bone turnover

The events of bone remodelling occupy a minority of the bone surfaces. The proportion of bone surface involved in remodelling at any one time is a function of the number of remodelling units present, their size and also the duration of time between the onset of resorption and the completion of formation, i.e.

$$\text{prevalence} = \text{incidence} \times \text{duration.}$$

Most abnormalities of bone turnover are related to a change in the incidence of BRUs which may be increased or decreased. Both have clinical consequences for the mechanical competence of bone tissue which differ in some respects.

High bone turnover

Many disorders are associated with an increase in the incidence of bone remodelling units (termed an increase in activation frequency). These include Paget's disease of bone, hyperparathyroidism, hyperthyroidism and some forms of renal osteodystrophy. The disorder associated perhaps with the greatest turnover is Paget's disease of bone. The consequences of increased turnover are largely accounted for by abnormal new bone formation. As expected with an increase in activation frequency, all aspects of the remodelling sequence are found with greater frequency, so that up to 100% of the bone surface may be occupied by the active events of resorption, formation and subsequent mineralization.

In most disorders associated with accelerated bone resorption the numbers of osteoclasts are increased. In these disorders the size of the osteoclast also increases, as does the number of nuclei. In Paget's disease osteoclasts may reach 200 μm in diameter, with up to 100 nuclei per cell (termed giant osteoclasts). In many disorders of accelerated bone resorption the coupling mechanism is preserved, which dictates that osteoblasts are recruited to sites of previous resorption. Provided that the number and functional activity of osteoblasts is normal, resorption cavities will be infilled with an equal volume of bone. The fact that bone resorption precedes formation will dictate that bone mass is slightly decreased, even though the balance between formation and resorption may be intact (Fig. 55.7). This has minor clinical

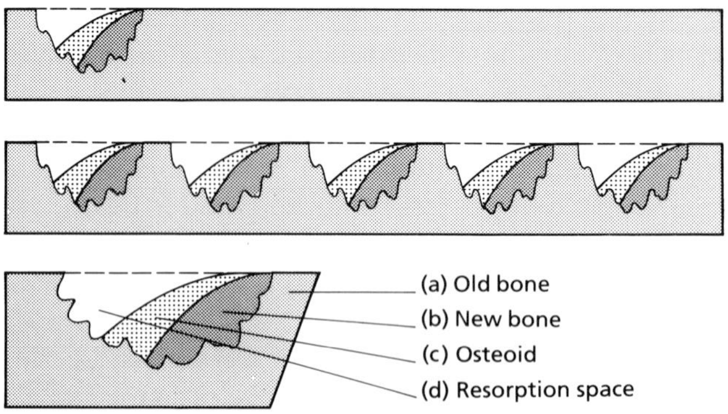

Fig. 55.7 Effect of skeletal turnover on bone calcium balance. The upper panel depicts a trabecular bone surface showing normal bone remodelling activity occurring on 15% of the surface. The resorption space (d) occupies 2% of the bone volume and a somewhat smaller amount is occupied by osteoid, accounting for 3.5% of bone volume. When the activation frequency is increased fivefold (centre panel) without affecting the balance between formation and resorption, the resorption and osteoid space is increased to 17.5% of bone volume.

significance since this bone deficit is reversible when bone turnover is decreased.

The major consequence of accelerated bone turnover is related to the production of woven rather than lamellar collagen. Woven bone is not normally present in the adult, except during fracture repair, but is found in many disorders associated with rapid rates of bone remodelling such as hyperparathyroidism, Paget's disease, renal bone disease and fluorosis. It is characterized by collagen fibres which are more randomly dispersed in contrast to the lamellar orientation of normal bone (see Fig. 55.1). It also has a lower and more variable mineral content. Thus, woven bone lacks much of the structural organization which gives it greater flexibility and hence less resistance to deformation. In addition, woven bone occupies more space; thus even when the balance between resorption and formation is unaffected, this would provide a mechanism for an increase in bone volume and a distortion of trabecular architecture. In those disorders associated with greatly accelerated bone remodelling (e.g. Paget's disease), most of the clinical features are due to anarchic bone formation.

When remodelling is accelerated all events on bone surfaces are increased. Thus, the surface coverage of bone with osteoid is also increased. This does not necessarily imply the presence of osteomalacia or a defect in the mineralization of bone. Where lamellar bone is being formed the mean osteoid seam width is not increased, and this forms a useful way of distinguishing osteomalacia from accelerated bone turnover. Of course the two may coexist and, for example, a simple vitamin D deficiency will not only cause osteomalacia, but also accelerate bone turnover due to secondary hyperparathyroidism.

Low bone turnover

The normal remodelling of bone is important for structural strength *in vivo*. In both clinical and experimental disorders the risk of pathological fracture increases if remodelling activity is substantially decreased. This is not due to a decrease in the amount of bone present, but due to the inability of the skeleton to undergo self-repair. A classic experimental example is the inhibition of bone turnover that can be attained experimentally with the use of very large doses of bisphosphonates. These decrease the activation frequency so that few remodelling sites are present at any one time. Animals which are treated in this way may show no changes in skeletal mass or bone mineral content, but develop pathological fractures after one or two years. An analogous situation is found in the aluminium toxicity which occurs in some patients maintained on dialysis treatment. The water used for dialysis may be contaminated with aluminium, which accumulates at the site of mineralization and impairs the activity of osteoblasts. In addition, aluminium inhibits the secretion of parathyroid hormone which is one of the major activators of bone remodelling. It is possible, but less certain, that decreased bone remodelling might contribute to increased skeletal fragility with advanced age.

Skeletal imbalance and uncoupling

It is useful to draw a distinction between skeletal balance and the coupling of bone formation to bone resorption. Uncoupling implies a dissociation of these two processes; either the creation of resorption cavities without subsequent attraction of osteoblasts, as is sometimes seen in neoplasia, or conversely, the deposition of new bone at sites other than sites of previous resorption. The latter occur conspicuously in various tumours such as prostatic bone disease and other cancers causing osteosclerotic metastases. In many other bone disorders a decrease or increase in bone mass is due to an imbalance between the amount of mineral and matrix removed during resorption and that subsequently incorporated into each resorption cavity. In advanced postmenopausal osteoporosis there is evidence to suggest that the imbalance between the amount of bone resorbed and that formed at each remodelling site is due to a decrease in the functional capacity of osteoblasts, or to a decrease in the recruitment of sufficient osteoblasts to resorption sites. Irrespective of the mechanism, a finite deficit of bone is the end-result of each remodelling sequence. If bone turnover is increased, the number of bone remodelling units present at any one time also increases. If the imbalance at each site remains constant, the result of increasing turnover will be to amplify the rate of bone loss. In the case of postmenopausal osteoporosis, oestrogen deficiency not only induces a focal imbalance of remodelling sites, but also increases the remodelling rate of bone. In this way bone loss is accelerated. Thus the coexistence of hyper-remodelling and focal skeletal imbalance will accelerate bone loss, and is one of the reasons why thyrotoxicosis and hyperparathyroidism, disorders associated with accelerated remodelling, also induce bone loss, particularly in elderly women who have other reasons for a focal skeletal imbalance.

It is likely that some forms of osteopetrosis are associated with focal positive balance at remodelling sites. This is certainly true in endemic fluorosis and a similar mechanism may operate in other forms of osteosclerosis acquired in adulthood (e.g. long-standing osteomalacia, some forms of renal bone disease, Paget's disease).

Architectural abnormalities of trabecular bone

The continual imbalance between formation and resorption in osteoporosis might be expected to result in a progressive decrease in the width of trabecular bone elements. This occurs in many forms of osteoporosis, but it is clear that in postmenopausal osteoporosis and after immobilization there is not only a decrease in trabecular width, but also a marked loss of trabecular elements themselves. Indeed, there is little evidence of trabecular thinning (see Fig. 55.3), so that the loss of trabecular elements must be partly a result of the generation of resorption cavities which transect or perforate the trabecular structures.

The disruption of trabecular architecture characteristic of postmenopausal vertebral osteoporosis has important implications for structural strength. The selective destruction of cross-bracing elements leads to a failure of the structure out of proportion to the amount of bone removed. Even though remnant trabeculae in postmenopausal osteoporosis can thicken, evident even radiographically, this cannot compensate adequately to prevent skeletal failure. Similarly, therapeutic manipulation of the remodelling process might be expected to thicken remnant trabecular structures without necessarily restoring trabecular continuity (Fig. 55.8). The finding of decreased trabecular elements early in postmenopausal osteoporosis suggests that not only is there focal skeletal imbalance, an acceleration of bone turnover, but that so too is the depth of resorption cavities increased. This contrasts with some other forms of osteoporosis (e.g. corticosteroid-induced osteoporosis) and osteoporosis of ageing where bony trabeculae are thin, but not decreased in number.

If a wave of bone resorption is sufficiently deep to transect a trabecular structure this destroys the bone surface on which subsequent attraction of osteoblasts can occur. Perhaps the most florid example is found

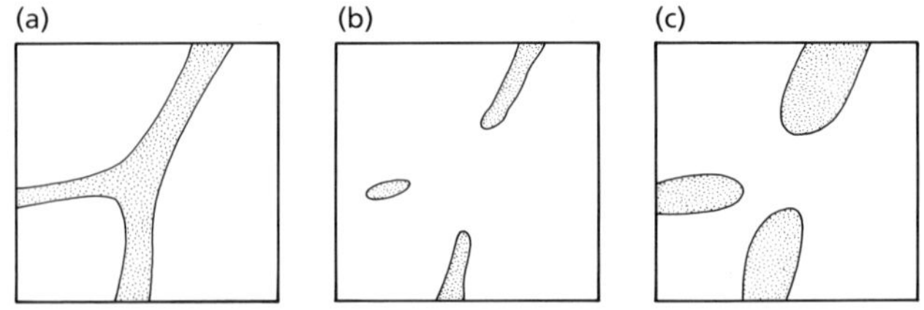

Fig. 55.8 Schematic representation of trabecular bone showing normal trabecular architecture (a) and the thinning and discontinuity of trabecular elements during postmenopausal osteoporosis (b). The surface deposition of bone by anabolic agents may thicken remnant structures (c), without necessarily restoring trabecular continuity.

in neoplasia, where products from tumour tissue or surrounding host cells activate focal osteoclasts which progressively resorb bone in the locality to give rise to an osteolytic metastasis with little evidence of bone formation. Where progressive osteolysis occurs without new bone formation scintigraphic uptake on bone scanning is low, and this is one of the reasons why the bone scan may be negative in myelomatosis, despite extensive focal osteolytic lesions. In disorders where coupling is more preserved, the bone scan is positive due to the focal deposition of the labelled polyphosphate or diphosphonate to sites of mineralization, or even to poorly mineralized osteoid (e.g. osteomalacia).

Some disorders are associated with an increase in trabecular numbers. Examples include breast cancer and prostatic cancer. The mechanism is due to the condensation of osteoblast cells within the marrow cavity rather than on bone surfaces. This is therefore uncoupled bone formation, probably due to focal production by tumour cells of osteoblast activating factors.

Osteomalacia

Osteomalacia implies a defect or delay in the mineralization of newly formed bone matrix (osteoid). The most common cause is a deficiency or a defect in the metabolism of vitamin D, but this is not invariably so. Osteoid is present in normal bone since osteoid must undergo a period of maturation before it begins to mineralize. In osteomalacia this period is exceeded, and in severe osteomalacia mineralization may be totally absent. This means that new bone formed never mineralizes, and the amount of osteoid present progressively increases. As mentioned previously, the amount of osteoid may increase in hyper-remodelling states due to an increase in the number of BRUs. Where this occurs the surface coverage by osteoid increases, but not the width, since mineralization proceeds normally. This is a useful distinction that can be made from the assessment of bone biopsies.

Osteoclasts normally resorb fully mineralized bone, though they are capable of resorbing osteoid. As the osteoid surface and thickness increases in the course of osteomalacia, progressively less mineralized surface is available for resorption. It is not uncommon, therefore, to see all the fully mineralized surface being occupied by a resorption. When osteoid occupies more than 90% of the bone surface, then osteoclasts can be seen to resorb osteoid. Thus, bone formation and resorption may proceed relatively normally despite the presence of a defect in one of the elements of bone remodelling.

TOOLS FOR THE ASSESSMENT OF BONE DISEASE

As in the diagnosis of most disorders, history and examination are central features of assessment. In addition, there are many biochemical indices which can be measured which are either the cause of skeletal disease (e.g. increased parathyroid hormone (PTH) levels in hyperparathyroidism) or the result of changes in skeletal metabolism (e.g. increased hydroxyproline excretion in the same disorder). In addition, there are a number of physical measurements which can be used to assess the amount of bone present, usually in restricted axial or appendicular sites. Bone biopsies are occasionally necessary, most notably in the assessment of osteomalacia and of renal bone disease. These are briefly reviewed below; their application, together with the major signs and symptoms of bone disease, is discussed subsequently.

Serum calcium

Since the skeleton is the major reservoir for calcium (Table 55.3), it is to be expected that serum calcium homeostasis is disturbed in a number of skeletal disorders. This is not invariably true, and for example in Paget's disease where bone remodelling is accelerated many-fold, disturbances in serum calcium are remarkably infrequent, related to the fact that bone formation and bone resorption rates are generally matched. The concentration of calcium in the extracellular fluid is maintained within a narrow range (Table 55.4), despite the large movements of calcium each day across gut, bone and kidney. Several hormones, including parathyroid hormone and the active form of vitamin D (1,25-dihydroxyvitamin D or calcitriol) appear to regulate the ionized fraction of plasma calcium, and in turn the production rate of these hormones is governed by the concentration of free calcium in the extracellular fluid.

Ionized calcium is distributed passively throughout the extracellular fluid, so that any change in its plasma concentration will affect all extracellular compartments. Within the plasma compartment, however, only approximately half of the calcium exists in the free ionized form; the other half is bound mainly to albumin and to a lesser extent to other proteins and anions. Automated techniques for the direct measurement of ionized calcium are not widely available, so that the total calcium concentration of plasma is usually measured. Because total calcium values are influenced by alterations in the quantity of protein present, most laboratories also report an adjusted

Table 55.3 Distribution of calcium in normal adults

	Calcium
Total body content (for 70 kg adult)	1000–1500 g
Skeleton	98%
Skeletal muscle	0.3%
Skin	0.08%
Liver	0.02%
Central nervous system	0.01%
Other tissues	0.6%
Extracellular fluid	1%

Table 55.4 Distribution of plasma calcium (percentages)

Ultrafilterable calcium (53%)	
Ionized calcium	47
Complexed calcium	
Phosphate	1.5
Citrate	1.5
HCO_3 etc.	3
Protein-bound calcium (47%)	
Albumin	37
Globulin	10
Total plasma calcium (2.12–2.6 mmol/l)	100

total plasma calcium, which is corrected to a specified normal value of serum albumin or total protein. The effect of protein binding on total plasma calcium is not negligible. Where there is an increase in protein concentration or the presence of abnormal proteins, the total calcium concentration may be spuriously high, so that hypercalcaemia is incorrectly diagnosed. Similarly, in hypoproteinaemic states (e.g. malnutrition, liver disease, disseminated carcinoma) the total calcium concentration may be low, when the ionized calcium is normal or even increased.

Serum phosphate

Serum phosphate is less well regulated than calcium. The major determinants of plasma phosphate include gastrointestinal sources and the setting of renal tubular reabsorption of phosphate. Several skeletal disorders are associated with hypophosphataemia, particularly osteomalacia due to vitamin D deficiency or due to a defect in renal phosphate transport. Because serum phosphate is highly dependent upon the dietary intake it is usual to assess serum phosphate after an overnight fast when contributions to serum phosphate from the gut are minimized. Under these conditions, chronic hypo- or hyperphosphataemia are usually due to changes in renal tubular reabsorption of phosphate, which in turn can be assessed by looking at the relationship between fasting serum phosphate and its fractional excretion in urine. Causes of chronic hyper- and hypophosphataemia are discussed subsequently, but it is important to note that phosphate is a major intracellular anion, and that transient changes in serum phosphate may be caused by transcellular shifts of phosphate (e.g. insulin, haemolysis, increased cell catabolism).

Biochemical indices of calcium metabolism

Indirect markers of skeletal metabolism provide a valuable tool for the diagnosis and assessment of patients, and also for the evaluation of treatment. The most commonly used measurement is the urinary excretion of calcium. The 24-hour urinary excretion of calcium is dependent upon the net flux of calcium across its major sites of exchange with the extracellular fluid. These sites comprise the gut, bone and kidney. These major movements of calcium (Fig. 55.9) determine the balance of calcium and an increase in the 24-hour urinary excretion of calcium

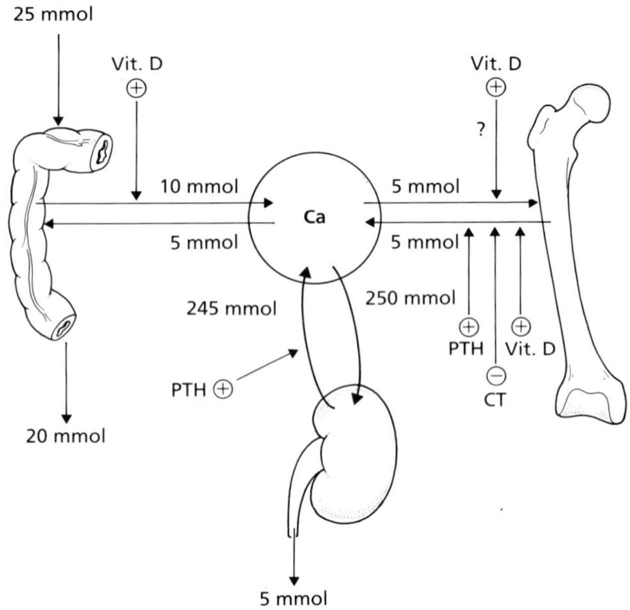

Fig. 55.9 Major fluxes of calcium (mmol per day) in a healthy adult. Exchange of calcium to and from the extracellular fluid occurs at the bones, gut and kidney. The net balance for calcium equals the net absorption minus the loss of calcium in faeces and urine, which in a healthy adult is zero. The major fluxes of calcium are regulated by the regulating hormones. PTH increases renal tubular reabsorption of calcium and bone resorption. The precise role of vitamin D in augmenting bone resorption and mineralization *in vivo* is not known.

is usually attributable either to an increase in intestinal absorption of calcium, an increase in bone resorption or both. There is not a close relationship between serum and urinary calcium. For example, in hypo- and in hyperparathyroidism, serum calcium is characteristically low or high respectively, but the 24-hour urinary excretion of calcium is usually normal. This is because intestinal absorption of calcium is only modestly increased or decreased, and because the balance between bone formation and bone resorption is not markedly impaired. The major mechanism for hyper- and hypocalcaemia in these disorders relates to the action of parathyroid hormone on renal tubular reabsorption of calcium.

As in the case for urinary excretion of phosphate, the study of urinary excretion of calcium under fasting conditions minimizes gastrointestinal sources. Urine is usually collected after an overnight fast, and the subsequent urine produced with continued fasting collected over a one or two-hour period. The urinary excretion can be expressed as a ratio to creatinine clearance (normally < 0.4 mmol/mmol creatinine). Under these conditions, increases in the fasting calcium/creatinine ratio suggest accelerated skeletal losses of calcium due to an increase in bone resorption, decrease in bone formation or both.

Because the fasting urinary excretion of calcium and phosphate are determined under relatively steady-state conditions, these measurements also provide an assessment of renal tubular reabsorption of calcium and phosphate, respectively, if serum concentrations of calcium phosphate and creatinine are measured concurrently. Nomograms or formulae are available to calculate both, but in clinical practice the renal tubular reabsorption of phosphate is the more commonly assessed. Phosphate reabsorption is increased by growth hormone, in hypoparathyroid conditions and in phosphate deprivation. It is diminished by calcitonin, in hyperparathyroidism and in several inherited or acquired renal tubular disorders. Renal tubular reabsorption of calcium is increased in hyperparathyroidism and in hypercalcaemia due to some malignancies.

Parathyroid hormone affects both the renal tubular reabsorption of calcium and phosphate, but the mechanisms are not fully elucidated. The action of PTH on the kidney is known to produce an increase in adenylate cyclase activity which increases the urinary excretion of cyclic adenosine monophosphate (cAMP). Urinary measurement of cAMP in response to PTH is commonly used in the assessment of hypoparathyroidism. In the clinical disorder of pseudohyperparathyroidism there is probably a defective receptor mechanism for PTH in kidney, so that the administration of PTH does not always produce the normal response of an increased excretion of phosphate and cAMP.

Hormone assays

The major calcium-regulating hormones include parathyroid hormone, the active metabolites of vitamin D (particularly calcitriol) and calcitonin. These are the so-called major regulating hormones because not only do they affect serum calcium, but the major stimulus to their production is a change in the serum concentration of calcium. Many other hormones affect skeletal metabolism (Table 55.5) but their secretion rate is determined predominantly by other factors.

Table 55.5 The major regulating endocrine hormones involved in plasma calcium homeostasis. The other hormones may indirectly influence calcium homeostasis, but their production is regulated by factors other than plasma calcium

Major calcium-regulating hormones
Parathyroid hormone
Vitamin D
Calcitonin
Influencing hormones
Oestrogen
Prolactin
Thyroxine
Growth hormone
Corticosteroids
Insulin

Parathyroid hormone

Parathyroid hormone is a major determinant of skeletal turnover. This is an 84 amino acid polypeptide, though the biological activity of the hormone resides in the first 34 amino acid residues. The hormone is cleaved in the circulation and radioimmunoassays using antibodies raised to circulating fragments are widely available for the assay of circulating PTH. However, the clearance of some fragments is largely renal (particularly carboxy terminal peptides) so that the interpretation of results is more difficult in the presence of renal failure. These problems have been partly overcome by the development of assays which detect the intact hormone, which are now increasingly used.

The major stimulus to the secretion of parathyroid hormone is a fall in serum calcium, and the target organ effects are to raise serum calcium (Table 55.6). It does this by accelerating bone turnover, increasing renal tubular reabsorption of calcium and stimulating the production of the active form of vitamin D, which in turn has effects on calcium metabolism. Thus, increased production of PTH induces hypercalcaemia, but hypocalcaemia will increase the secretion rate of PTH. There is often an overlap between PTH levels in health and various disorders. These considerations mean that PTH should be interpreted alongside values for serum calcium. High serum calcium in the presence of high or normal values of PTH indicate primary hyperparathyroidism, whereas a high or normal circulating level of PTH in the presence of hypocalcaemia denote an appropriate physiological

Table 55.6 Major effects of parathyroid hormone

Bone	
Increased bone remodelling	
Increased calcium transport from quiescent bone surfaces	
Kidney	
Increased urinary cAMP	
Increased renal tubular reabsorption of calcium	
Decreased renal tubular reabsorption of phosphate	
Decreased renal tubular reabsorption of bicarbonate	
Activation of 1-α-hydroxylase	
Gut	
Increased intestinal absorption of calcium indirectly (by activation of calcitriol synthesis)	

response to hypocalcaemia. In hypercalcaemic states, which are not mediated by PTH, PTH levels are commonly normal or suppressed.

Vitamin D

Vitamin D undergoes a series of metabolic transformations before becoming biologically active. Vitamin D is synthesized in the skin by the influence of ultraviolet (UV) radiation on 7-dehydrocholesterol, or acquired by the diet, mainly from dairy produce. The first step in its metabolism is the production of 25-hydroxyvitamin D (calcifidiol), a step which is not closely regulated. The assay of 25-hydroxyvitamin D provides the major assay used in the assessment of vitamin D nutritional status.

Before becoming fully biologically active, calcifidiol is hydroxylated in the 1-alpha position to give rise to 1,25-dihydroxyvitamin D (calcitriol). The major site of synthesis of calcitriol is the kidney, and this production is under close metabolic regulation. Assays for calcitriol are generally available only to specialized units, and may be used in the investigation of patients in whom the synthesis of calcitriol is impaired due to a renal lesion, or where there is target organ resistance to the action of vitamin D.

Calcitriol production is increased in disorders of calcium and phosphate privation, and is stimulated by hypocalcaemia and hypophosphataemia. In addition, a variety of hormones such as PTH, growth hormone, gonadal steroids and prolactin also increase the conversion of calcifidiol to calcitriol, related to the increased demands for calcium during pregnancy, growth and lactation.

Calcitonin

Calcitonin is a 32 amino acid peptide produced by the c-cells of the thyroid. Although calcitonin is classed as a major calcium-regulating hormone, its function in humans is still not known. Part of the reasons for this are that its absence (total thyroidectomy) or excess (medullary carcinoma of the thyroid) are not associated with major changes in serum calcium or skeletal homeostasis. Its assay has no place in the diagnosis or management of bone disease, and its clinical utility is confined to the diagnosis and follow-up of medullary thyroid cancer.

Indirect indices of skeletal metabolism

Plasma alkaline phosphatase is the most frequently used and probably the most useful biochemical marker for bone disease. Alkaline phosphatase is derived in part from osteoblasts, where it may be involved in calcium and phosphate transport in bone. Hypophosphatasia is a rare cause of osteomalacia where decreased amounts of alkaline phosphatase are found. In health, about half of the alkaline phosphatase measurable in plasma is derived from bone, the rest coming mainly from the liver. There may also be contributions to the plasma from the intestine and other tissues, including the placenta in pregnancy. These different isoenzymes may be measured by semiquantitative techniques based on electrophoresis, chemical or heat inactivation or by immunological methods.

In the absence of liver disease, serum activity of alkaline phosphatase provides a reasonable index of the number of functional osteoblasts. It is particularly useful in disorders associated with increased bone formation such as Paget's disease, severe hyperparathyroidism with bone disease, osteomalacia due to vitamin D deficiency and renal bone disease. Because of its non-specificity it is less satisfactory in the assessment of mild bone disease or in osteoporosis.

Measurements of hydroxyproline in urine provide the other major biochemical marker used to monitor bone disease. Collagen is rich in hydroxyproline, and following its degradation it is not reutilized. Most hydroxyproline is metabolized, but a proportion appears in the urine. Collagen is a major protein of bone and skin, and most hydroxyproline of endogenous origin probably comes from the turnover of collagen in these tissues. When bone turnover is increased, however, the relative skeletal contribution to total excretion is correspondingly increased. As in the case of alkaline phosphatase, values lying within the normal range do not exclude the presence of increased bone resorption.

A major difficulty in the use of hydroxyproline is that there are significant dietary sources in food products derived from animal sources. It is traditional to measure hydroxyproline, therefore, only after restricting the collagen and gelatin intake of patients. This can be avoided by collecting urine after an overnight fast, and expressing the excretion of hydroxyproline as a ratio to creatinine concentration.

Table 55.7 Biochemical markers of disease activity used in the assessment of metabolic bone disease

Measurement	Source	Changes in high bone turnover
Formation		
Alkaline phosphatase	Liver/bone/gut	Increased
Skeletal alkaline phosphatase	Bone: osteoblasts	Increased
Osteocalcin	Bone: osteoblasts	Increased
Non-dialysable hydroxyproline	Post-translational maturation of collage	Increased
Procollagen Type I	Bone: osteoblasts	Increased
Procollagen Type II	? fibrous tissue	Increased
Alpha$_2$ HS glycoprotein	Liver: incorporated into bone	Decreased
Resorption		
Hydroxyproline (dialysable)	Collagen degradation	Increased
Hydroxylysine and its glycosides	Collagen degradation	Increased
Glucosylgalactosyl/galactosyl hydroxylysine	Skin/bone collagen	Decreased
Acid phosphatase	? osteoclasts	Increased
3-Hydroxylysyl-pyridinolone	Collagen crosslinks	Increased
Proline iminopeptidase	? osteoclasts ? osteoblasts	Increased
Urinary or serum free Gla protein	Osteocalcin degradation	Increased

In disorders associated with increased bone turnover there is, as might be expected, a close correlation between serum alkaline phosphatase and urinary hydroxyproline, reflecting the balance between formation and resorption. In such disorders it is clearly not necessary to measure both indices, and activity of alkaline phosphatase is the preferred measurement since it is simpler to obtain samples and to analyse, and is more reproducible. Both measurements are useful when assessing responses to treatment and in disorders where imbalance or uncoupling are expected.

A number of other indices of bone turnover are utilized in the assessment of bone disease (Table 55.7). These are generally available only in specialized centres, but serum determination of osteocalcin is becoming more widely available. Like alkaline phosphatase this is an osteoblast marker, but is more specific and sensitive.

Assessment of bone mass

A variety of non-invasive techniques have been developed to assess bone mass, most usually measured as bone mineral content or density (Table 55.8). These provide estimates of skeletal mass, provided that osteomalacia does not coexist. Sequential measurements can be used to measure rates of bone loss and are widely used in the assessment of osteoporosis. The most widely used techniques are single-photon absorptiometry of the wrist, and more recently dual-energy X-ray absorptiometry of the spine or hip. The latter has the advantage of being capable of measuring bone mineral density at sites of biological relevance such as the spine and hip.

The risk of osteoporotic fracture increases progressively as bone density decreases, and measurements of bone mineral density provide an index of fracture risk. Their sequential use permits the assessment of bone loss and the efficacy of intervention. It is important, however, to recognize that the precision (reproducibility) of these techniques, when compared to rates of bone loss, encountered, for example, in osteoporosis, dictate that patients must be assessed over a long period of time. For example, single-photon absorptiometry at the wrist and dual-energy absorptiometry at the spine both have a reproducibility of between 1% and 2%. Since skeletal losses in established osteoporosis may be only 1–2% per annum, this means that patients may need to be

Table 55.8 Non-invasive techniques used in the assessment of bone mass and bone loss

Technique and site	Reproducibility (coefficient of variation %)
Neutron activation analysis	
Hand	2–4
Spine	2–10
Whole body	5–10
Single-photon absorptiometry	
Appendicular cortex	1–3
Appendicular trabecular	3–5
Dual-photon absorptiometry	
Appendicular	2–5
Axial (e.g. spine)	3–5
Dual-energy X-ray absorptiometry	
Spine	1–2
Whole body	2–4
Appendicular regions	1–2
Hip	2–4
Radiogrammetry	
Metacarpals	1–2
Ultrasound	
Velocity (patella)	1
Attenuation (heel)	3–6

followed over several years before one can be confident that a real change has occurred.

The radiological assessment of the skeleton is an extremely important aspect of the investigation of bone disease, and features are reviewed briefly with the disorders, subsequently. Other imaging techniques used in the investigation of bone disease include scintigraphy and more rarely computerized axial tomography.

Bone biopsy

Much of the information on the pathophysiology of bone disease has been obtained from bone biopsies and from detailed histomorphometric studies. The indications for biopsy are, however, limited in routine clinical practice. Bone biopsy may be the only way of excluding osteomalacia and this is the most common clinical indication outside of clinical research. Bone biopsies are also an important component in the assessment of renal osteodystrophy where many types of bone disease may coexist. In the case of metabolic bone disease, bone is usually taken by a transiliac trephine under local anaesthetic. Sections are stained without decalcification so that unmineralized osteoid can be clearly distinguished from mineralized bone. Biopsy may also be helpful in the assessment and diagnosis of some forms of osteoporosis (e.g. osteogenesis imperfecta, mastocytosis) and in some patients with focal bone disease such as Paget's disease, fibrous dysplasia, metastatic disease, bone tumour, etc., where these disorders are not widespread and a tissue diagnosis is required.

DISORDERS OF CALCIUM METABOLISM

Hyperparathyroidism

Hyperparathyroidism is defined as an increase in the circulating level of parathyroid hormone (PTH). It is classically divided into three clinical categories.

Primary hyperparathyroidism is an intrinsic disorder of the parathyroid glands, which results in an inappropriate increase in the secretion of PTH from the parathyroid cells, which gives rise to an increase in serum calcium.

In secondary hyperparathyroidism the increase in PTH secretion occurs secondary to a reduction in the plasma concentration of ionized calcium. It is most commonly observed in chronic renal failure and nutritional deficiency of vitamin D. The increased secretion occurs from all four parathyroid glands, and treatment of the underlying disorder (raising serum calcium) restores PTH secretion to normal; for example, the administration of vitamin D in nutritional osteomalacia.

In some cases of secondary hyperparathyroidism, prolonged stimulation of the parathyroid glands results in the development of an adenoma or irreversible hyperplasia with subsequent hypercalcaemia. This so-called tertiary hyperparathyroidism is most commonly observed in patients with chronic renal disease, especially after renal transplantation. The hypercalcaemia may have adverse effects on the function of the transplanted kidney, and is usually treated by subtotal parathyroidectomy.

Primary hyperparathyroidism is a common disorder affecting approximately 1 : 1000 of the general population. In the majority (85%), hypercalcaemia is associated with the presence of a single chief cell adenoma in one of the four parathyroid glands. Hyperplasia of all of the glands occurs less commonly, most notably in patients with multiple endocrine neoplasia syndrome (MEN Type I or IIa) or familial forms (autosomal dominant inheritance). Parathyroid cancer is a rare cause of primary hyperparathyroidism.

The mechanism by which parathyroid adenomas arise is unknown. Adenomatous parathyroid cells have a higher 'set-point' for plasma calcium about which the secretion of PTH is regulated. Thus, for a given value of plasma calcium, secretion of PTH is higher from these cells. Adenomatous cells are not truly autonomous, since their secretory rate is still determined by serum calcium concentrations, and secretion will be suppressed, for example, in the presence of hypercalcaemia due to other causes such as calcium infusion or malignancy.

Primary hyperparathyroidism occurs most commonly in women in the early postmenopausal years. This suggests that oestrogen and/or progestogen withdrawal is a contributing factor to its development or expression. Indeed, hormone replacement therapy may lower serum calcium levels in postmenopausal women with hyperparathyroidism. It is not known whether this is due to an effect of gonadal steroids on PTH secretion or on bone.

Hypercalcaemia and hypophosphataemia are the two classic features of primary hyperparathyroidism, reflecting the effects of PTH on bone and renal tubular reabsorption of calcium and phosphate (Table 55.9). A mild hyperchloraemic acidosis is usually also present. In most cases the serum alkaline phosphatase is normal or only slightly elevated, but may be moderately increased in those patients with clinical or radiographic manifestations of bone disease.

The increase in serum calcium is maintained in part by increased renal tubular reabsorption of calcium by PTH, and also by increased intestinal absorption of calcium. The 24-hour urinary excretion of calcium is often high, reflecting increased intestinal absorption of calcium by higher circulating levels of calcitriol. The hypophosphataemia is caused by a reduction in the renal tubular reabsorption of phosphate (estimated as the maximum tubular reabsorption rate of phosphate/glomerular filtration rate, Tm_p/GFR). Fasting urinary excretion of hydroxyproline is usually slightly increased, reflecting increased rates of bone resorption.

A large proportion of patients with primary hyperparathyroidism are detected on routine blood analyses, and are relatively asymptomatic. When symptoms are present these are usually due to hypercalcaemia (Table 55.10). Hypercalcaemic symptoms may be vague and non-specific; they include nausea, vomit-

Table 55.9 Biochemical features of primary, secondary and tertiary hyperparathyroidism; the features of secondary hyperparathyroidism are those seen in privational vitamin D deficiency

	Type of hyperparathyroidism		
	Primary	Secondary	Tertiary
Serum			
Calcium	High	Low	High
Phosphate	Low	Low	Low or normal
Alkaline phosphatase	Normal or high	High	High
Creatinine	Normal	High	Normal or high
Urine			
Calcium excretion (24 hours)	High	Low	High

Table 55.10 Clinical features of hypercalcaemia

Neurological
Lethargy and drowsiness
Confusion, coma
Emotional lability, depression
Cranial nerve palsies
Hypotonia and decreased deep tendon reflexes

Gastrointestinal
Anorexia, vomiting
Constipation
Peptic ulceration
Acute pancreatitis
Visceral calcification

Cardiovascular
Hypertension
Arrhythmias
Sensitivity to digoxin

Renal
Polyuria, polydipsia
Hypercalciuria and nephrolithiasis
Nephrocalcinosis
Impairment of glomerular filtration rate

Other tissues
Soft tissue calcification
Red-eye syndrome
Pseudo-gout
Pruritus

ing, fatigue and constipation. Hypercalcaemia induces a nephrogenic diabetes insipidus and the resulting polyuria causes dehydration and thirst. Increased calcium excretion may result in renal stone formation (in up to 40% of patients in some series), nephrocalcinosis and renal impairment. Mental disturbances are not uncommon, but may be subtle. Frank psychoses and cranial nerve lesions may occur in some cases. Abdominal pain may also occur. Peptic ulceration is present in 5–10% of patients, possibly due to calcium-induced increases in gastrin secretion. Primary hyperparathyroidism may present as an episode of acute pancreatitis. It should be borne in mind that calcium sequestration in the pancreas may result in normal or even low levels of serum calcium, thus masking the underlying diagnosis during the acute phase of the disease.

Bone pain is an uncommon presentation of primary hyperparathyroidism in all but the most severe cases, but increased bone turnover is commonly found in bone biopsies. Radiographic features include subperiosteal erosions classically seen on the radial borders of the middle phalanges (Fig. 55.10) and bone resorption in the skull (resulting in a mottled or 'salt-and-pepper' appearance), but occur in less than 2% of patients. Bone pain and radiographic changes are more florid in the secondary and tertiary hyperparathyroidism of chronic renal failure.

In the majority of patients the diagnosis of primary hyperparathyroidism is straightforward and depends on finding an inappropriately high circulating level of PTH in the presence of hypercalcaemia. Other causes of hypercalcaemia must be considered, however (Table 55.11). The distinction between hyperparathyroidism and hypercalcaemia of malignancy is the most frequent problem. The majority of patients with carcinoma and hypercalcaemia have disseminated osteolytic skeletal metastases, and are usually symptomatic. Some tumours, however, including those of the bronchus and kidney, are associated with the development of hypercalcaemia in the absence of skeletal metastases (humoral hypercalaemia of malignancy). The presence of hypophosphataemia and hypercalcaemia in patients with these tumours suggests a PTH-like effect, probably due to the production of PTH-related peptide (PTHrp) by such tumours. PTHrp does not cross-react with the antibodies to PTH used in most assays, and PTH concentrations are usually suppressed.

The hydrocortisone suppression test has in the past been widely used to distinguish primary hyperparathyroidism from other causes of hypercalcaemia. It is, however, of very limited value in discriminating between these disorders, and its value has been superseded by the development of specific assays for PTH. It is still of value in the investigation of hypercalcaemic patients in whom a cause is not readily apparent. Restoration of serum calcium occurs in multiple myelomatosis, vitamin D toxicity, some lymphomas and sarcoidosis, but the suppression of hypercalcaemia in solid tumours is incomplete. Variable responses occur in primary hyperparathyroidism.

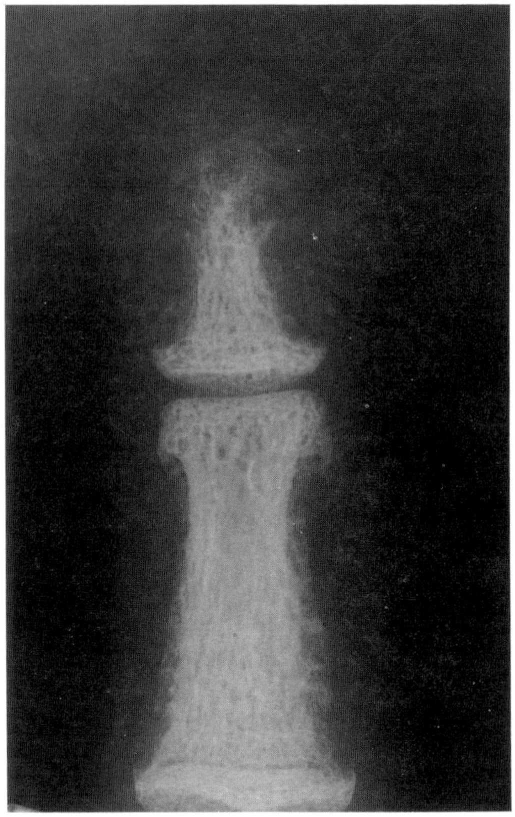

Fig. 55.10 Marked hyperparathyroidism of the middle and distal phalanx showing subperiosteal resorption most marked at the radial border of the middle phalanx and the tuft of the terminal phalanx.

In an asymptomatic patient with borderline hypercalcaemia, levels of PTH at or close to the upper limit of the reference range may be difficult to interpret. An asymptomatic patient may be followed but occasionally further investigation is required. The most common example encountered is in the investigation of calcium nephrolithiasis, where it is important to

Table 55.11 Causes of hypercalcaemia

Common
Primary hyperparathyroidism
Neoplasia
Vitamin D toxicity
Thiazide diuretics
Artifactual (prolonged venous stasis, hyperproteinaemia)
Infrequent
Immobilization
Tertiary hyperparathyroidism, especially in transplant recipients
Sarcoidosis (and other granulomatous diseases)
Hyperthyroidism
Rare
Diuretic phase of acute renal failure
Benign familial hypercalcaemia
Addisonian crisis
Phaeochromocytoma
Milk-alkali syndrome
Vitamin A toxicity
Aluminium toxicity
Parenteral nutrition (calcium and aluminium)
Silicon retention
Pseudo-hypercalcaemia (e.g. myeloma)

arrive at an accurate diagnosis. Such cases may demand further investigation such as localization studies. Another problem is primary hyperparathyroidism where the increase in serum calcium is attenuated by coexisting osteomalacia, a common but fortuitous association in the elderly.

It is important to distinguish primary hyperparathyroidism from benign familial hypercalcaemia. In the latter, urinary calcium is characteristically low. Recognition of this autosomally dominant inherited condition is important, since parathyroidectomy is of little benefit.

The treatment of choice in most patients with primary hyperparathyroidism is neck exploration and excision of the adenoma. In the hands of an experienced surgeon no further investigation is required. Several methods may be used to localize the adenoma before surgery. These include selective venous catheterization (for PTH levels), ultrasound scanning, computerized tomography and isotope (thallium/technetium) subtraction scanning. These procedures are most needed after a failed exploration when their sensitivity is least (due to the previous surgery). Rarely, failed neck explorations, or inability to localize a gland in the neck, may be due to the presence of a parathyroid adenoma in the mediastinum. Conservative management is advocated by some in elderly patients with mild, uncomplicated hypercalcaemia.

Medical management has its limitations. Gonadal steroids (such as norethisterone 5 mg daily) may be of value in postmenopausal women who refuse surgery, or who pose too great an operative risk. The diphosphonates can prevent progressive bone loss, but the effects on serum calcium are relatively short-lived, usually lasting only for some months.

Other causes of hypercalcaemia

Hypercalcaemia may result from a disturbance in any one of the fluxes of calcium between the extracellular fluid and the gut, bone and kidney. Normal homeostatic responses offset the effect of challenges to the extracellular calcium, and the development of hypercalcaemia often results from a combination of abnormalities. Hypercalcaemia exists if the total plasma concentration of calcium (adjusted for albumin) is higher than the upper limit of the reference range (usually > 2.6 mmol/l). The management of hypercalcaemia includes the diagnosis and/or treatment of the underlying disorder and, if necessary, specific treatment of the hypercalcaemia.

Mild, transient hypercalcaemia is relatively common and probably reflects a combination of analytical and biological variability. If the hypercalcaemia is sustained an underlying cause can be elicited in the majority of patients (Table 55.11) by a good clinical and drug history, in conjunction with the measurement of plasma calcium, phosphate, protein, erythrocyte sedimentation rate (ESR) and creatinine. Sensitive and specific assays for PTH are now widely available. Radiography or scintigraphy are useful for detecting the presence of asymptomatic skeletal metastases.

HYPERCALCAEMIA OF MALIGNANCY

Malignancy is the most common cause of sustained hypercalcaemia in hospitalized patients, accounting for 45–50% of cases, whereas primary hyperparathyroidism is the most frequent finding in the general population. Tumours of the lung, breast, urinary tract, head and neck, and oesophagus are the most common solid tumours associated with the development of hypercalcaemia, and myeloma is the most frequently encountered haematological malignancy. There is a wide variation in the prevalence of hypercalcaemia within different tumour types, with hypercalcaemia being observed in about 30% of patients with myeloma, but only in 1% of large-bowel cancers. Similarly, there is much variation in the presence and extent of skeletal metastases at the time of hypercalcaemia, reflecting the different mechanisms by which tumours may induce increases in extracellular calcium (Table 55.12). These mechanisms include increased bone resorption, increased renal tubular reabsorption of calcium, increased intestinal absorption of calcium and the effects of hypercalcaemia on renal function.

Increased bone resorption is the most common mechanism for the development of the hypercalcaemia of malignancy, and is usually associated with widespread osteolytic metastases. The increased bone resorption is often uncoupled and mediated by stimulation of normal osteoclasts by local factors such as prostaglandin E2, interleukins and procathepsin D, which are released from tumour cells or from normal host cells in response to the presence of tumour cells. Osteoclast-activating factors such as lymphotoxin (tumour necrosis factor) and interleukin-6 (IL-6) are released from myeloma cells, and cause lytic lesions and generalized osteoporosis which may give rise to pathological fracture and hypercalcaemia.

Osteoclasts may also be stimulated by systemic factors released into the circulation by solid tumours in the absence of skeletal metastases (humoral hypercalcaemia of malignancy). These factors include the PTHrp and more rarely, calcitriol in HIV-associated lymphoma. PTHrp is a 144-amino acid peptide in which eight of the first 15 amino-terminal amino acids are homologous with human PTH. It is a potent stimulator of bone resorption and, like PTH, also increases renal tubular reabsorption of calcium. In some patients this may be the major mechanism for the induction of hypercalcaemia, and this is one reason why such patients respond poorly to treatment with inhibitors of bone resorption. PTHrp is also present in a wide variety of normal adult and fetal tissues, but its physiological role is not yet known.

Table 55.12 Mechanisms for the induction of hypercalcaemia in haematological malignancy (myeloma), solid tumour with skeletal metastases (e.g. breast cancer) and humoral hypercalcaemia of malignancy (e.g. renal carcinoma)

	Bone resorption	Increased renal tubular reabsorption of calcium	Impaired glomerular filtration
Multiple myeloma	+++	−	+++
Breast carcinoma	+++	+	−
Renal carcinoma	+	+++	−

Even in the absence of specific hormones which alter renal handling of calcium, changes in renal function play a significant part in inducing or exacerbating hypercalcaemia. Chronic hypercalcaemia is associated with increased urinary sodium excretion and intravascular volume depletion. Volume depletion decreases renal blood flow and glomerular filtration, and thus impairs the ability to excrete a calcium load. Furthermore, calcium reabsorption in the proximal renal tubule is closely linked to that of sodium, so that increases in tubular reabsorption of sodium in the volume-depleted patients increase renal tubular reabsorption of calcium and exacerbate hypercalcaemia. Volume depletion and impaired renal function are therefore important contributory factors in the majority of patients with significant hypercalcaemia. It is for this reason that the first line of treatment is adequate volume expansion with isotonic saline.

More specific treatments to inhibit bone resorption are available for the management of hypercalcaemia (see below). Of these, the diphosphonates (also known as bisphosphonates) are of particular interest, not only in the management of hypercalcaemia but also in the management of increased osteolysis. The duration of effect of the diphosphonates appears to last for the duration of treatment and, for example, the use of clodronate (1600 mg by mouth daily) decreases the frequency of fracture, bone pain and recurrent hypercalcaemia in a substantial proportion of patients with osteolytic bone disease due to malignancy.

RARER CAUSES OF HYPERCALCAEMIA

Thiazide diuretics may cause mild hypercalcaemia, and further investigation is not necessary unless hypercalcaemia persists when treatment is stopped. Thiazides, unlike loop diuretics, increase renal tubular reabsorption of calcium. Hypercalcaemia secondary to immobilization is most frequently encountered in children and young adults, or in more elderly patients with increased bone turnover (Paget's disease, hyperparathyroidism, metastatic bone disease, renal osteodystrophy). Immobilization suppresses bone formation, whereas bone resorption is accelerated, so that the net efflux of calcium from bone is increased. The increase in plasma calcium may occur several weeks after the onset of immobilization.

A variety of endocrine disorders are associated with hypercalcaemia. Mild hypercalcaemia occurs in hyperthyroidism due to increased bone turnover with resorption predominating; it may respond to propranolol. Mild hypercalcaemia may occur in acromegaly, due to increased circulating levels of calcitriol or parathyroid hyperplasia. Addisonian crisis (acute adrenal insufficiency) and phaeochromocytoma are rare but important causes of hypercalcaemia.

The importance of milk alkali syndrome as a cause of hypercalcaemia has decreased with the increasing use of more specific peptic ulcer therapies. The diagnosis is made from the clinical history, and the finding of alkalosis, hypercalcaemia, hyperphosphataemia, renal impairment and ectopic calcification.

Rarely, in patients with myelomatosis or chronic liver disease with marked hypercalcaemia in the absence of symptoms, the increase in total serum calcium is due to increased calcium binding to an abnormal paraprotein. In such cases the ionized calcium concentration is normal (pseudo-hypercalcaemia).

The signs and symptoms of hypercalcaemia are shown in Table 55.10. Hypercalcaemia may be associated with multisystemic non-specific symptoms which vary in severity from those that are recognized only in retrospect, after treatment, to acute life-threatening events. The severity of symptoms may relate more to the rate of increase of serum calcium, rather than the absolute level. It is important to recognize that neurological sequelae may take several days to resolve following the correction of hypercalcaemia. This is important in the management of patients with hypercalcaemia of malignancy, where symptoms may be incorrectly attributed to metastatic disease. In these patients the severity of hypercalcaemia may be masked by the presence of hypoalbuminaemia, so that a high index of suspicion is appropriate.

The aims of treatment of hypercalcaemia are twofold; firstly, to identify and treat the underlying cause, and secondly, to reduce the plasma calcium. If a cause is readily apparent and the plasma calcium is only moderately elevated with minimal symptoms, then specific therapy for the cause may be all that is required, such as parathyroidectomy in primary hyperparathyroidism or effective chemotherapy in myelomatosis. Adequate intravascular volume expansion with saline is the mainstay of acute treatment. Several agents which inhibit bone resorption, including calcitonin and the diphosphonates, are effective in restoring normocalcaemia, but the success of such agents will be limited in the presence of increased renal tubular reabsorption of calcium. Calcitonin induces a rapid decrease in bone resorption and plasma calcium falls within hours of its administration (100–200 units six-hourly). Unfortunately, the calcium lowering effect is not usually sustained. The diphosphonates have a more durable action. They may be given by slow (2–4 hours) intravenous (i.v.) infusion. Typical regimens are etidronate 7.5 mg/kg i.v. for three to five days, pamidronate 30–45 mg i.v. as a single infusion and clodronate 300 mg i.v. for five days. Clodronate may also be given by mouth (1600 mg daily) and is suitable for long-term use to decrease osteolytic bone disease and its complications. The use of corticosteroids should be confined to sarcoidosis, myelomatosis and other haematological malignancies.

Hypoparathyroidism

Hypoparathyroidism is due to the absence or inappropriately low circulating levels of PTH in the presence of hypocalcaemia. It can result from any process which interferes with the production, secretion or peripheral action of PTH, but there are few causes (Table 55.13).

Transient hypoparathyroidism is relatively common following thyroid, parathyroid or laryngeal surgery. In those patients undergoing total thyroidectomy or laryngeal resection, hypoparathyroidism may be permanent and they require lifelong treatment. Idiopathic hypoparathyroidism in adults results from autoimmune destruction of parathyroid

Table 55.13 Causes of hypoparathyroidism

Postsurgical
Idiopathic
Magnesium deficiency
Pseudo-hypoparathyroidism
Infiltration—rare, e.g. thalassaemia
DiGeorge syndrome

tissue. There may be a positive family history, and it is occasionally associated with other autoimmune diseases including thyroid, adrenal and gonadal insufficiency, diabetes mellitus, pernicious anaemia, vitiligo and alopecia areata.

In children, idiopathic hypoparathyroidism is associated with retarded growth, malabsorption and osteomalacia. This disorder should be distinguished from neonatal hypoparathyroidism, which is a transient phenomenon due to suppression of fetal PTH secretion by maternal hypercalcaemia. Rarely, congenital hypoparathyroidism may result from complete absence of the parathyroid glands associated with thymic aplasia and a defect in cellular immunity (DiGeorge syndrome).

Severe hypomagnesaemia impairs both PTH secretion and the responsiveness of PTH receptors in the bone and kidney. It may arise in malabsorption syndromes, especially if associated with severe diarrhoea, for example Crohn's disease, bowel resection and during prolonged parenteral alimentation. The syndrome is important to recognize, since patients are refractory to treatment without restoration of magnesium levels.

Occasionally, hypocalcaemia and hyperphosphataemia are found in the presence of normal or high levels of PTH. This pseudo-hypoparathyroidism results from the resistance of kidney and/or bone receptors to stimulation by PTH. It is often associated with typical somatic features. Other family members may share this appearance, but have completely normal serum levels of calcium, phosphate and PTH. This is termed pseudo-pseudo-hypoparathyroidism. Patients with pseudo-pseudo-hypoparathyroidism may develop hypocalcaemia (pseudo-hypoparathyroidism) and vice versa, often during intercurrent infections or during stresses on calcium homeostasis (pregnancy, the contraceptive pill, etc.).

The distinction between hypoparathyroidism and other causes of chronic hypocalcaemia is usually straightforward (Table 55.14). The hypocalcaemia of hypoparathyroidism is caused by decreased renal tubular reabsorption of calcium and decreased intestinal absorption of calcium. The latter is due to decreased production of calcitriol, in turn due to the suppression of the renal 1-hydroxylase by the absence of PTH and hyperphosphataemia. Hyperphosphataemia is a direct result of increased renal tubular reabsorption of phosphate. The urinary excretion of cAMP is low.

Table 55.14 Distinguishing biochemical features of disorders associated with chronic hypocalcaemia

	Osteomalacia	Chronic renal failure	Hypoparathyroidism
Serum			
Calcium	Low	Low	Low
Phosphate	Low	High	High
Alkaline phosphatase	High	High	Normal*
Creatinine	Normal	High	Normal
PTH	High	High	Low*

* May be high in pseudo-hypoparathyroidism.

Infusion of PTH to patients with postsurgical or idiopathic hypoparathyroidism induces a decrease in serum phosphate (due to a decrease in Tm_P/GFR), an increase in calcium reabsorption and in urinary excretion of cAMP (Chase–Aurbach or Ellsworth–Howard test). Some or all of these responses are impaired in the several variants of pseudo-hypoparathyroidism.

The most frequent clinical manifestations of hypoparathyroidism are caused by hypocalcaemia (Table 55.15). Neurological sequelae of chronic hypocalcaemia include abnormal EEG patterns, papilloedema, and increased intracranial pressure, and these usually resolve following adequate treatment. Chronic hypocalcaemia in early life is associated with irreversible mental retardation, and the development of cataracts and soft tissue calcification (subcutaneous and basal ganglia). Additional features of idiopathic hypoparathyroidism include dry skin, malformations of teeth

Table 55.15 Clinical features of hypocalcaemia

Neurological
Neuromuscular irritability
  Paraesthesiae
  Tetany
Irritability
Convulsions
Intracranial calcification
Papilloedema

Eyes
Cataracts

Cardiovascular
Prolongation of QT interval
Resistance to digoxin

and nails (transverse grooves) and moniliasis of the nails.

Pseudo-hypoparathyroidism (and pseudo-pseudo-hypoparathyroidism) are associated with somatic features similar to those of Turner's syndrome. These include short stature, round face, and a short neck. Characteristically, there is shortening of the fourth and fifth metacarpals and metatarsals. Metacarpal shortening may be seen on clinical examination by the presence of dimples instead of a knuckle on clenching the fist (Fig. 55.11).

The treatment of acute hypocalcaemia is discussed below. The mainstay of chronic treatment is the use of calcium and/or vitamin D. Some patients respond to dietary supplements of calcium alone. Requirements vary from 500 mg to several grams daily, but many will require treatment will vitamin D. The requirements for vitamin D_2 or D_3 are very variable and may range from 1000 to 300 000 units daily because of the variable efficiency with which patients convert the vitamin to calcitriol. Calcitriol or its synthetic analogue, alfacalcidol, are preferred to vitamin D, since they bypass the renal hydroxylation step. Requirements range from 0.5 to 2 μg daily. One consequence of treatment is a relatively high 24-hour urinary excretion of calcium. Stone formation and renal impairment can be avoided by avoiding hypercalcaemia.

Other causes of hypocalcaemia

The most common causes of hypocalcaemia are shown in Table 55.16. The majority of cases are attributable to artifact (low serum albumin), vitamin D deficiency, chronic renal failure or hypoparathyroidism. These can readily be distinguished by simple biochemical investigations, and have been discussed previously (Table 55.14).

Neuromuscular irritability is the characteristic feature of hypocalcaemia, manifested as carpopedal spasm; paraesthesiae of the face, fingers and toes; and occasionally as abdominal cramps. Latent tetany may be detected by tapping the facial nerve at the angle of the jaw resulting in facial muscle contraction (Chvostek's sign—present in 5% of the normal population), or by occluding the arterial circulation in the arm leading to carpal spasm (Trousseau's sign). Other causes of tetany include hypomagnesaemia, hypokalaemia and alkalosis (e.g. hyperventilation syndrome).

Acute symptomatic hypocalcaemia requires the use of intravenous calcium (10–30 ml of 10% calcium gluconate in 500 ml of physiological saline). In some cases, particularly in those patients following parathyroidectomy for severe secondary hyperparathyroidism in chronic renal failure, continuous or frequent intermittent calcium infusions may be required until the patient is established on oral calcium and vitamin D supplements. The necessity for vitamin D supplements and the choice of agent to use depends on the underlying cause, and is discussed separately.

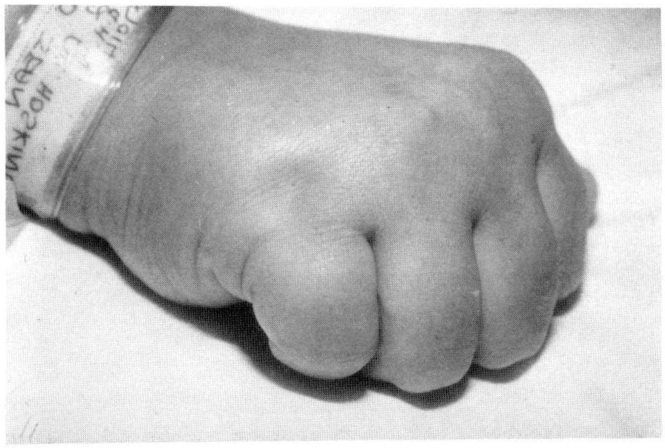

Fig. 55.11 Dimpling of the knuckle in the clenched fist of a patient with pseudo-hypoparathyroidism as a result of metacarpal shortening.

VITAMIN D DEFICIENCY SYNDROMES

Vitamin D deficiency may result from an abnormality at any one of several points in the availability, pro-

Table 55.16 Causes of hypocalcaemia

Common
Artifact (low albumin or haemodilution, e.g. liver disease)
Vitamin D deficiency
Chronic renal failure
Hypoparathyroidism
Infrequent
Hypomagnesaemia
Acute pancreatitis
Acute renal failure
Pseudo-hypoparathyroidism
Septicaemia
Drugs—calcitonin, diphosphonates, chemotherapy, citrate
Prostatic carcinoma
Rapid correction of metabolic acidosis
Respiratory alkalosis (hyperventilation syndrome)

Table 55.17 Disorders which give rise to vitamin D deficiency syndromes classified by their interference in the metabolic pathway of vitamin D

Privational
Poor diet
Dietary fads, e.g. vegans
Housebound elderly
Pigmented skin, e.g. Asian population
Malabsorption
Postgastrectomy
Coeliac disease
Cystic fibrosis
Blind loop syndrome
Chronic liver disease
Phytates, e.g. Eastern diet
Abnormal 25-OHD$_3$ metabolism
Anticonvulsants?
Chronic liver disease
Nephrotic syndrome
Decreased 1-hydroxylation
Chronic renal failure
Hypoparathyroidism
Oncogenic osteomalacia
Vitamin D-dependent rickets Type I
Target-tissue resistance to calcitriol
Anticonvulsants
Vitamin D-dependent rickets Type II
Intestinal disease, e.g. coeliac disease

duction, metabolism and action of vitamin D (Table 55.17). Vitamin D deficiency impairs the mineralization of bone, giving rise to osteomalacia in the adult and rickets in childhood. The other causes of osteomalacia and their skeletal consequences are discussed later. Vitamin D-related disorders are included here because of their significant impact on serum calcium.

Insufficient dietary intake is common in the elderly and in diets where there is a reduced intake of vitamin D rich foods such as dairy products and fish (e.g. vegans). Inadequate exposure to sunlight is also an important factor, especially in the housebound elderly and in the immigrant Asian population. In the latter, symptoms are frequently first noted at times of increased demand for vitamin D and calcium, such as during pregnancy or the adolescent growth spurt.

Osteomalacia may occur in diseases associated with long-standing malabsorption. These include coeliac disease, cystic fibrosis, Crohn's disease and blind loop syndromes. The mechanisms for vitamin D deficiency are complex and include malabsorption of the vitamin and of calcium, and disruption of the target tissues responsible for vitamin D-mediated calcium transport. Osteomalacia is also observed in some patients after total or partial gastrectomy, but the mechanism is unknown. Since vitamin D is a fat-soluble vitamin and 25-OHD$_3$ undergoes entero-hepatic circulation, its absorption may be decreased in chronic hepatobiliary disease and chronic pancreatitis, but these are only rarely associated with osteomalacia. The high intake of phytates in some Eastern diets (e.g. chapatis) decreases calcium absorption, and contributes to the development of osteomalacia.

Contrary to expectation, abnormal or decreased production of 25-OHD$_3$ is uncommon in chronic liver disease. A high alkaline phosphatase (liver disease), hypocalcaemia (due to hypoalbuminaemia) and a low serum phosphate (due to decreased renal tubular reabsorption) are common features of chronic liver disease and may erroneously suggest the presence of osteomalacia. The use of anticonvulsants which induce hepatic microsomal enzymes has been associated with the development of osteomalacia, possibly through increased hepatic catabolism of vitamin D metabolites. It is more likely, however, that they induce target-tissue resistance to calcitriol. Loss of vitamin D binding protein and 25-OHD$_3$ in the urine occurs in the nephrotic syndrome, and may lead to decreased intestinal absorption of calcium and hypocalcaemia.

Decreased activity of the renal 1-hydroxylase is most commonly observed in chronic renal failure. In the early stages of renal failure, decreased activity is secondary to phosphate retention which is augmented, since the kidney is the major regulator of serum phosphate. As the disease advances, decreased calcitriol production is due to the progressive destruction of renal tissue which is the site of the 1-hydroxylase enzyme. Rarely, defective 1-hydroxylation may occur in association with benign or malignant mesenchymal tumours (oncogenic osteomalacia), and a primary inherited defect in hydroxylase activity is also recognized (vitamin D dependent rickets Type I). Decreased 1-hydroxylase activity also occurs in hypoparathyroidism and pseudo-hypoparathyroidism, but is not commonly associated with defective mineralization of bone.

Several disorders are associated with target tissue resistance to vitamin D. Anticonvulsants may induce osteomalacia by impairing the sensitivity of gut and/or bone to calcitriol. In vitamin D-dependent rickets Type II, osteomalacia occurs despite high circulating concentrations of calcitriol, and does not respond even to pharmacological doses of calcitriol due to end-organ insensitivity to calcitriol.

Long-standing vitamin D deficiency induces hypocalcaemia due in part to decreased intestinal absorption of calcium. The stimulation of PTH secretion induces the expected changes of secondary hyperparathyroidism. These include hypophosphataemia due to decreased renal tubular reabsorption of calcium, and an increase in bone turnover. Bone disease may cause pain, fracture and, particularly in growing children, deformities such as genu valgum or varus. Proximal myopathy is a common feature. The radiographic features are reviewed in the next section.

Calciferol (vitamin D_2) or cholecalciferol (vitamin D_3) is quite adequate in the treatment of privational vitamin D deficiency (400–1000 units daily). In the elderly and in patients unlikely to be compliant, vitamin D may be given by intramuscular injection (for example 250 000 i.u. six-monthly). This route may also be necessary in some patients with malabsorption syndromes, but others appear to absorb calcitriol or alfacalcidol adequately. Some patients with coeliac disease do not respond to vitamin D since the intestinal villi responsible for vitamin D-dependent transport of calcium are destroyed by the disease.

In disorders associated with impaired renal hydroxylation of 25-OHD_3, large but variable doses of vitamin D are required, which increase the risk of toxicity. The reversal of toxicity is very slow. The 1-hydroxylated derivatives of vitamin D (calcitriol, alfacalcidol, dihydrotachysterol) have a more rapid onset of action, and are frequently used in patients with hypoparathyroidism or chronic renal failure. The daily maintenance dose for these derivatives is usually 0.5–2 μg for calcitriol or alfacalcidol, and 100–200 μg for dihydrotachysterol. Close monitoring is required of all patients on vitamin D supplementation. Drug interactions may occur, either to decrease (thiazide diuretics) or increase (anticonvulsants) the requirements of vitamin D.

VITAMIN D EXCESS

Increased renal synthesis of calcitriol is seen most commonly in primary hyperparathyroidism, and also occurs in tertiary hyperparathyroidism due to hypophosphataemia. Hypercalcaemia due to vitamin D is most commonly iatrogenic, but in a number of disorders there is evidence of unregulated extrarenal synthesis of calcitriol.

Iatrogenic vitamin D toxicity is common. It causes hypercalcaemia and hyperphosphataemia, and it prolongs bone loss. Symptoms and other features are those of hypercalcaemia. For this reason patients receiving treatment with pharmacological amounts of vitamin D or its analogues and metabolites require regular monitoring of serum calcium to detect and prevent the development of hypercalcaemia. Hypercalcaemia and hyperphosphataemia result from increased intestinal absorption and bone resorption. The presence of renal failure (due to renal disease or a consequence of hypercalcaemia, will decrease the ability to clear large phosphate and calcium loads. The speed of onset and resolution of the hypercalcaemia is dependent on the agent used. With parent vitamin D or 25-OHD_3 hypercalcaemia may develop many months or years after the start of treatment, but because of their long half-life and their storage in fatty tissues, plasma calcium may remain elevated for many months, sometimes for years, and may require treatment with corticosteroids. Increases in plasma calcium occur more rapidly with calcitriol and its analogues, and the shorter half-life of biological effect (three to five days) results in a more rapid reduction in plasma calcium to normal after stopping treatment.

Serum levels of calcitriol are not markedly increased in vitamin toxicity due to the parent vitamin, since the kidney can regulate its production. Hypercalcaemia is therefore due to the activation of vitamin D receptors by the parent vitamin or 25-OHD. There are, however, a number of disorders where the close regulation of the hydroxylase is impaired and hypercalcaemia occurs with modest challenges to vitamin D. Mild or transient hypercalcaemia occurs in approximately 10% of patients with sarcoidosis, and hypercalciuria is considerably more common due to increased intestinal absorption of calcium and excessive bone resorption. Plasma PTH is suppressed. The cause of hypercalcaemia is the increased production of calcitriol mediated by a 1-hydroxylase enzyme in sarcoid granulomatous tissue. Unlike the renal 1-hydroxylase this enzyme is not subject to metabolic control, so that patients are very sensitive to challenges with small amounts of vitamin D or ultraviolet light. The hypercalcaemia usually responds to treatment with corticosteroids, and suspected sarcoidosis is one situation where the hydrocortisone suppression test may be helpful in establishing the diagnosis. Long-term treatment with corticosteroids, in addition to more simple measures such as the use of barrier skin creams and a low-calcium diet, may be required to control the hypercalcaemia. Extrarenal synthesis of calcitriol also occurs more rarely in other granulomatous diseases including tuberculosis, berylliosis, coccidioidomycosis and histoplasmosis.

DISORDERS OF SKELETAL METABOLISM

Osteomalacia

Osteomalacia (literally soft bones) is characterized by defective mineralization of bone, resulting in an excess of non-mineralized osteoid. It may result from a number of hereditary and acquired metabolic disorders (Table 55.18). The most common cause is vitamin D deficiency or disorders associated with impaired metabolism or action of vitamin D. In much the same way as vitamin D deficiency, that is not always associated with osteomalacia (e.g. hypoparathyroidism), not all osteomalacia is caused by vitamin D deficiency syndromes.

Table 55.18 Some causes of osteomalacia

Vitamin D deficiency syndromes (see Table 55.17)
Renal tubular disorders
X-linked hypophosphataemia (vitamin D-resistant rickets)
Oncogenic osteomalacia
Renal tubular acidosis
Fanconi syndrome
Wilson's disease
Galactosaemia
Cadmium toxicity
Cystinosis
Chronic renal failure
Aluminium toxicity
Drugs
Anticonvulsants
Fluoride
Etidronate
Antacid abuse
Hypophosphatasia
Ureterosigmoidostomy (acidosis)
Axial osteomalacia

It has been recognized for many years that vitamin D deficiency impairs the mineralization of bone and that this is healed following its administration. There is still a great deal of uncertainty whether vitamin D has direct effects on bone to promote mineralization or whether this is achieved by the effects of the vitamin on the gut to increase the availability of calcium and phosphate. Certainly, both calcium deficiency and hypophosphataemia can cause osteomalacia. Furthermore, although hypocalcaemia and hypophosphataemia are commonly observed in disorders of vitamin D metabolism, it is possible that these secondary effects of D deficiency impair the mineralization of bone. This notion is strengthened by the finding that a number of disorders associated with chronic hypophosphataemia give rise to osteomalacia.

The most common abnormality in hypophosphataemic osteomalacia is impaired renal tubular reabsorption of phosphate. The most common disorder is familial or X-linked hypophosphataemic rickets (so-called vitamin D-resistant rickets; VDRR). Rarely, osteomalacia may occur secondary to a tumour-derived factor which reduces renal tubular phosphate reabsorption, and sometimes the synthesis of calcitriol production (oncogenic osteomalacia). The tumours are usually benign and most commonly of mesenchymal origin (for example sclerosing haemangiomas, non-ossifying fibromas). They may be very small but are important to identify since the bone disease is healed after excision. Hypophosphataemia may also occur in renal tubular acidosis and in disorders associated with a multiple renal tubular defects (Fanconi syndrome). Antacid abuse with aluminium hydroxide results in hypophosphataemia, due to the ability of this agent to bind phosphate in the gut and render it unavailable for absorption. This may also induce osteomalacia.

Hypophosphatasia is a rare cause of osteomalacia characterized by abnormally low levels of tissue non-specific alkaline phosphatase activity. The inheritance is variable. Recessive forms present with severe intrauterine skeletal abnormalities, whereas the autosomal dominant disorder presents in adulthood with relatively mild disease. The osteomalacia occurs due to increased levels of pyrophosphate, an inhibitor of mineralization. Urinary excretion of phosphoethanolamine is increased, and is used as a diagnostic test.

Several drugs are associated with the development of osteomalacia, including aluminium, fluoride and the diphosphonate, etidronate. Aluminium toxicity occurs most frequently in patients with chronic renal failure, where impaired renal excretion, the contamination of water used for dialysis and the use of aluminium salts as phosphate binders, results in accumulation of aluminium at the mineralization front which may cause osteomalacia. More commonly aluminium retention in renal failure induces a form of aplastic bone disease where rates of bone and mineral formation are both low. As previously mentioned, large doses of antacids which bind intestinal phosphate such as aluminium hydroxide may induce hypophosphataemic osteomalacia. The mechanism by which etidronate, commonly used in Paget's disease, induces impairment of mineralization remains unclear. It limits the duration for which etidronate can be prescribed, and its use should probably be avoided in patients with fissure fractures in Paget's disease. Fluoridation of the water supply is not associated with the development of osteomalacia. Endemic fluorosis, however, can result in severe skeletal disease, including osteomalacia, and is a common problem in certain areas, including the Punjab region of India. Oral fluoride taken in relatively high doses (10–30 mg daily) is used in the treatment of osteoporosis in several European countries, and may impair the mineralization of bone if vitamin D or calcium supplements are not concurrently taken.

Whatever the cause of osteomalacia, the characteristic histological appearance is an increased thickness (greater than four lamellae) of the osteoid seam. The mineralization rate, as assessed by *in vivo* tetracycline labelling, is delayed or absent. In the presence of hypocalcaemia it is also common to see PTH-mediated effects due to secondary hyperparathyroidism. These include an increase in the bone surfaces covered with osteoid, and increased numbers of osteoclasts and osteoblasts.

The characteristic features of osteomalacia associated with privational vitamin D deficiency are hypocalcaemia, hypophosphataemia and high serum alkaline phosphatase activity (see Table 55.14). The serum levels of 25-OHD_3 are low, and the 24-hour urinary excretion of calcium is low due to decreased intestinal absorption of calcium. Hypophosphataemia is also due in part to decreased intestinal absorption of phosphate, but the decrease in serum phosphate is further exacerbated by secondary hyperparathyroidism. Alkaline phosphatase activity is increased due to the effects of increased PTH secretion and its effects on bone turnover. The finding of hypoproteinaemia or anaemia may suggest the presence of malabsorption.

In osteomalacia due to hypophosphataemia, plasma calcium is normal, and serum alkaline phosphatase less markedly elevated. Plasma PTH is characteristically normal. Hypophosphatasia is characterized by very low levels of serum alkaline phosphatase activity.

Bone pain and proximal muscle weakness are the cardinal symptoms of osteomalacia due to vitamin D deficiency syndromes, but are rare in hypophosphataemic states. Muscle weakness may be manifest as a waddling gait, difficulty in rising from chairs or climbing stairs, and difficulty in combing hair or reaching overhead objects. Skeletal deformity may also occur, especially in children, and includes bowing of the long bones, enlargement of the costochondral junctions (rickety rosary) and radial epiphyses, and frontal bossing. If severe, a marked kyphosis and compression of the pelvis (triradiate pelvis) may result. In X-linked hypophosphataemic osteomalacia, marked bowing of the lower limbs occurs, and short stature is common, especially in males. Muscle weakness is not present.

Radiographic examination may reveal several abnormalities in osteomalacia. In rickets, widening of the growth plate and splaying of the metaphysis is noted at the ends of the long bones (Fig. 55.12). Translucent lines of unmineralized osteoid running perpendicular to the bone cortex (Looser's zones) (Fig. 55.13) are diagnostic features of osteomalacia in adults. They are often bilateral and symmetrical, occurring most commonly in the long bones at their concave border, and the pubic rami, ribs and scapulae. The vertebral bodies may become biconcave (codfish spine). In the vitamin D-related disorders there may be found radiographic features of secondary hyperparathyroidism. These include subperiosteal bone resorption of the phalanges (especially the radial aspect), pubic symphysis and the clavicles (outer third). Other changes include patchy osteosclerosis (such as 'rugger-jersey spine') and, in children, resorption of the metaphyses. In most patients radiographic abnormalities are not detected, and that is one of the reasons why a high index of suspicion is required and bone biopsy remains a useful adjunct to diagnosis.

Radiographic evidence of secondary hyperparathyroidism is lacking in untreated hypophosphataemic osteomalacia. There may be marked osteoscleosis,

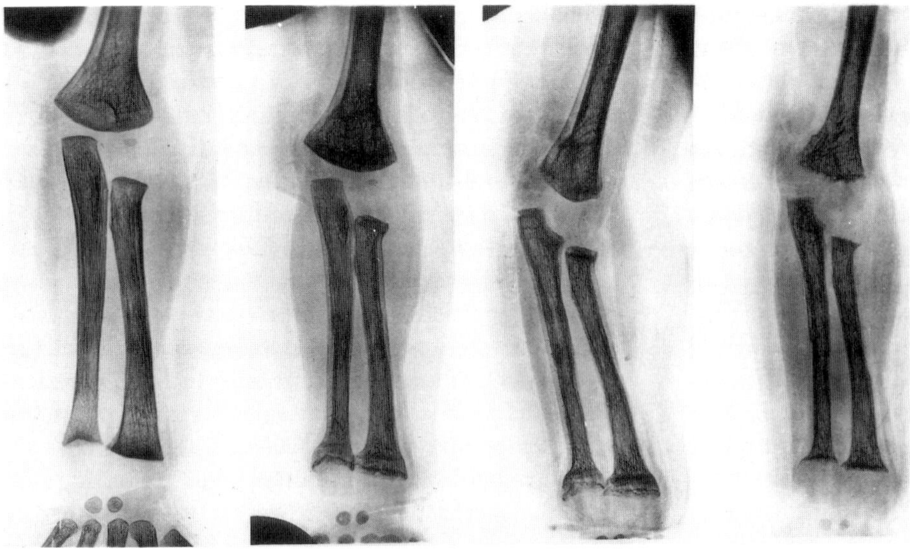

Fig. 55.12 Rickets at the wrist. In the untreated state (right-hand panel) there is an increase in the epiphyseal width and splaying and irregularity of the metaphyseal margins. Note the progressive resolution of these findings following treatment with vitamin D.

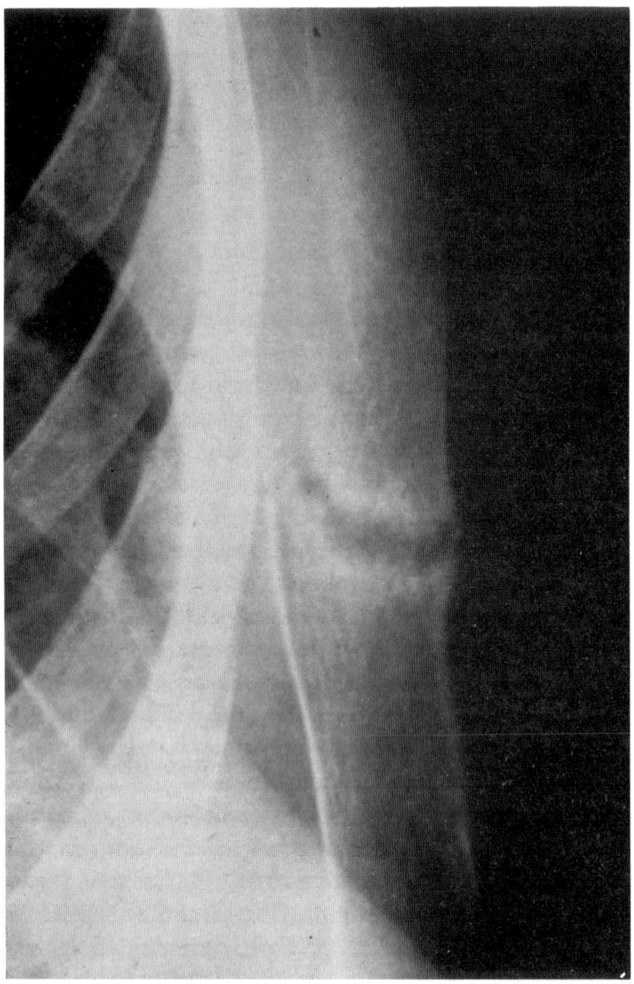

Fig. 55.13 A Looser's zone present at the margin of the scapula characteristic of osteomalacia.

however, due to an abundance of poorly mineralized osteoid. The Looser's zones of hypophosphatasia, unlike in vitamin D deficiency, are characteristically found on the convex surface of cortices.

The treatment of vitamin D deficiency syndromes has been discussed earlier.

In hypophosphataemic osteomalacia, supplementation with both calcitriol and phosphate is often required to promote healing of osteomalacia. Phosphate supplements should be given evenly spaced throughout the day (e.g. 0.5 g eight-hourly), but diarrhoea is a frequent side-effect and not all patients tolerate these doses. In patients with oncogenic osteomalacia the disorder is cured if the tumour can be identified and resected.

Osteomalacia associated with renal tubular acidosis usually responds well to correction of the acidosis with sodium bicarbonate.

Renal bone disease

Renal bone disease (renal osteodystrophy) is an important cause of morbidity in patients with end-stage renal failure, maintained on dialysis treatment. It is characterized by bone pain and/or tenderness, skeletal deformity and pathological fracture. It is a multifactorial disorder with a varied clinical and histological expression which may exist in isolation or in combination (Table 55.19). Knowledge of the disruption of normal calcium, phosphate and skeletal homeostasis in renal failure contributes to a better

Table 55.19 Features of renal osteodystrophy in chronic renal failure; each may occur in isolation, or a combination of several may occur in one individual

Osteomalacia and rickets
Osteitis fibrosa
Osteoporosis
Osteosclerosis
Osteonecrosis (avascular necrosis)
Amyloidosis
Extraskeletal calcification

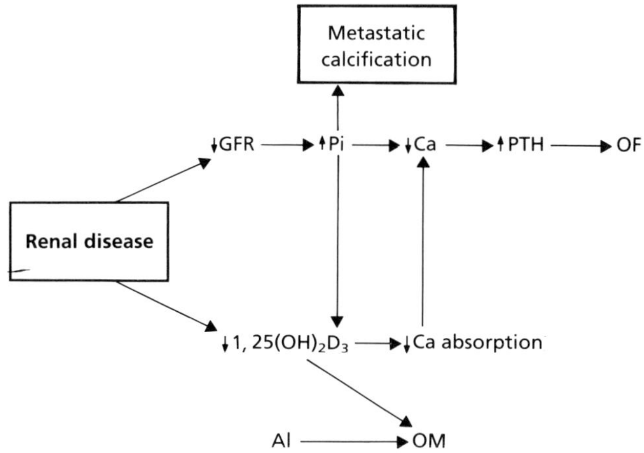

Fig. 55.14 A simple schema for the pathogenesis of renal bone disease. Progressive renal failure induces decrements in glomerular filtration rate (GFR) and synthetic capacity for calcitriol (1,25-$(OH)_2D_3$). An increase in plasma phosphate (Pi) due to the fall in GFR stimulates the secretion of PTH indirectly by decreasing plasma calcium values. During progressive renal failure, plasma calcium and phosphate tend to remain normal (because of the renal and skeletal effects of PTH) at the expense of an increasing secretion rate of PTH. When the compensatory abilities of the kidney are compromised by renal failure, hyperphosphataemia and hypocalcaemia prevail. Hyperphosphataemia may further inhibit synthesis of calcitriol and cause osteomalacia (OM). Malabsorption of calcium may contribute to secondary hyperparathyroidism. Aluminium retention (Al) has a direct effect on osteoblasts and may cause osteomalacia.

understanding of the mechanisms underlying the development of renal osteodystrophy.

The three major factors contributing to the development of renal bone disease are decreased synthesis of calcitriol, hyperparathyroidism, and aluminium accumulation (Fig. 55.14). The interaction of these factors, in combination with other effects—including age, the renal pathology and concomitant therapy—produces the heterogeneous osteodystrophy of chronic renal failure.

Calcitriol production is impaired early in the course of chronic renal failure, when the GFR falls below 50 ml/min. Initially, this reduction is probably due to inhibition of the renal 1-hydroxylase enzyme due to an increase in intracellular phosphate concentration, which is the result of impaired ability to excrete phosphate loads in the urine. At this stage dietary phosphate restriction may restore levels of calcitriol to normal. As renal disease progresses the destruction of renal tissue becomes a progressively more important factor in decreased production of calcitriol. Deficiency of calcitriol impairs intestinal absorption of calcium, and this and the hyperphosphataemia are the major factors which induce hypocalcaemia.

The role of calcitriol deficiency in the development of osteomalacia in chronic renal failure (CRF) remains unclear. Calcitriol deficiency in CRF usually leads to the development of secondary hyperparathyroidism and hyperparathyroid bone disease, rather than osteomalacia. In some instances, however, including the nephrotic syndrome and patients maintained on continuous ambulatory peritoneal dialysis (CAPD), loss of 25-OHD_3 is associated with florid osteomalacia. This suggests that 25-OHD_3 or other metabolites (e.g. 24,25-dihydroxyvitamin D) may play a direct role in mineralization.

Secondary hyperparathyroidism is a common feature of chronic renal failure. High concentrations of PTH are found even in the early stages of renal failure. This reflects a true increase in hormone secretion, but some assays may give very high values since they detect fragments which are not effectively cleared by the failing kidney. Hypocalcaemia is the main stimulus to the secretion of PTH in CRF, and early in the disease the increased secretion of PTH will partly offset the hypocalcaemia and hyperphosphataemia by its effects on renal tubular reabsorption of calcium and phosphate, but at the expense of hyperparathyroid bone disease. With progressive renal impairment, hyperparathyroidism fails to maintain these effects, and results in the development of marked hypocalcaemia and hyperphosphataemia. Correction of hypocalcaemia by calcitriol supplementation and/or calcium supplementation (for example, by using increased calcium concentrations in the dialysate fluid) is associated with suppression of PTH levels and improvement in hyperparathyroid bone disease. However, other factors are of importance in the development of parathyroid gland hyperplasia in CRF, as PTH secretion and bone disease will eventually recur despite maintenance of a normal plasma calcium.

PTH stimulates the turnover of bone. Histologically, this is characterized by an increase in the bone surfaces undergoing remodelling, and an increase in the number of both osteoclasts and osteoblasts. When turnover is markedly increased the normal lamellar bone is replaced by bone in which the collagen is deposited in a very chaotic pattern (woven bone). There is frequently an increase in unmineralized bone matrix or osteoid, reflecting both increased bone formation and impaired mineralization. Rapid bone resorption is associated with the development of marrow fibrosis (osteitis fibrosa).

The classical radiographic features of hyperparathyroid bone disease are subperiosteal erosions of the phalanges (see Fig. 55.10) and the distal ends of the clavicles (Fig. 55.15). Bone resorption in the skull gives rise to the classical 'salt-and-pepper' appearance. Osteosclerosis is common in the axial skeleton, especially in patients receiving calcitriol supplementation, due to the mineralization of abundant woven bone. Radiographic evidence of osteomalacia, including the presence of Looser's zones, is uncommon.

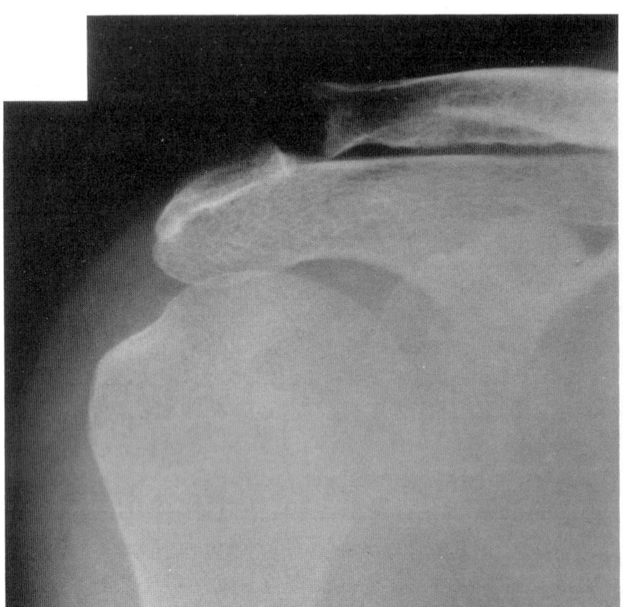

Fig. 55.15 Radiograph showing subperiosteal erosion of the distal end of the clavicle with erosion of the endplate. This is a common feature of secondary hyperparathyroidism due to renal failure, but rarely found in primary hyperparathyroidism.

Aluminium is normally excreted by the kidney, so that renal failure is associated with aluminium accumulation. It was first noted that patients on dialysis in areas of high water aluminium content developed an unusually florid bone disease. This was characterized by marked osteomalacia, decreased bone turnover and in particular decreased activity of osteoblasts. This 'aplastic' bone disease is due to a direct toxic effect of aluminium on osteoblasts, but aluminium also impairs the secretion of PTH from the parathyroid glands. Thus, in patients with aluminium overload, secondary hyperparathyroidism, as judged by the level of PTH and severity of parathyroid bone disease, may not be as marked as expected for the degree of renal failure. Mild hypercalcaemia is not uncommon in patients with aluminium bone disease, and this leads to further suppression of PTH. The hypercalcaemia is mediated by the inhibition of normal calcium fluxes across quiescent bone surfaces (that is surfaces not undergoing remodelling) by aluminium. For this reason these patients are very sensitive to treatment with calcitriol, and rapidly become hypercalcaemic. Other features of aluminium toxicity in renal failure include bone pain, pathological fractures, encephalopathy and anaemia.

The use of uncontaminated water has reduced the incidence of aluminium bone disease, particularly osteomalacia. Aluminium salts are, however, effective phosphate binders and are still widely used to control hyperphosphataemia in CRF. They act by binding dietary phosphate and rendering it nonabsorbable, but some aluminium is absorbed and gives rise to adynamic bone disease. It is common to observe hyperparathyroid and aluminium bone disease within the same individual, leading to problems in the management of their bone disease.

The major symptoms of renal bone disease are bone pain and muscle weakness. In patients with multisystem disease these symptoms may be noted retrospectively by the patient when treatment is started. Fractures are relatively uncommon except in aluminium-induced bone disease where spontaneous fractures may cause major problems. Deformities due to metaphyseal resorption of bowing of long bones often occurs in children, and may be very rapidly progressive.

In dialysis-treated patients retention of phosphate

and high serum phosphate levels are a major cause of extraskeletal calcification. This gives rise to symptoms which depend largely on the site. Common problems include itching (of eyes or skin), the red-eye syndrome and more rarely periarticular problems due to the deposition of large masses of amorphous calcium phosphates. Hypocalcaemia is usually present in advanced renal failure for the reasons discussed above. However, there may be great variation in serum calcium values depending on the underlying bone pathology. Thus osteomalacia is frequently associated with low or low–normal values, whilst severe hyperparathyroidism (so-called tertiary hyperparathyroidism), aluminium toxicity and treatment with calcitriol may be associated with hypercalcaemia.

In hyperparathyroid bone disease the serum activity of alkaline phosphatase is usually increased proportional to the increase in bone turnover. In aluminium bone disease, however, the activity is usually normal or only slightly elevated. Thus, measurement of the prevailing alkaline phosphatase may provide a pointer to the predominant underlying bone pathology.

High circulating levels of immunoreactive PTH are characteristic of secondary hyperparathyroidism. The magnitude of the increase depends to a large extent on the PTH fragment measured by the assay used. Thus, levels of the carboxy-terminal fragment of PTH, which is normally cleared by the kidney, may be 10 times higher than levels of the amino-terminal fragment or intact molecule. However, irrespective of the type of assay used, there is a good correlation between the level of PTH and the severity of hyperparathyroid bone disease. The level of PTH may be lower in patients with aluminium toxicity. The severity of aluminium toxicity may be assessed by measuring serum aluminium levels, and the sensitivity of this test can be improved by examining values of aluminium before and after infusion of the chelating agent, desferrioxamine. In aluminium overload the infusion of desferrioxamine is associated with an increase in serum aluminium detected over the following 48–72 hours. Aluminium staining at the mineralization front on iliac crest bone biopsies is also indicative of aluminium toxicity.

The major problems to be tackled are hyperphosphataemia and the control of secondary hyperparathyroidism. Control of extracellular phosphate is desirable for two reasons. Firstly, in early renal failure it may correct the hypocalcaemia and decrease PTH secretion. Secondly, hyperphosphataemia is a major risk factor for the development of extraskeletal calcification in chronic renal failure, and the risk is highest if the level is maintained above 2.4 mmol/l. It is important to realize that serum phosphate levels may rise during treatment with calcitriol, since it also increases intestinal absorption of phosphate.

Apart from dietary restriction and dialysis, the main method for reducing serum phosphate is the use of oral phosphate binding agents. Aluminium salts, e.g. aluminium hydroxide, are given approximately 30 minutes before meals for maximum effect. Calcium and magnesium salts are also used since they contain no aluminium. They are less effective, however, and magnesium salts frequently cause diarrhoea, whereas calcium salts (for example, calcium carbonate) may induce hypercalcaemia and extraskeletal calcification in patients also taking calcitriol.

Although an adequate dietary intake of calcium is important, further increases in dietary intake of calcium alone are an inefficient method of correcting the hypocalcaemia and suppressing hyperparathyroidism. In patients on dialysis the use of high-dialysate calcium concentrations can also suppress PTH secretion. The availability of calcitriol and other 1-hydroxylated derivatives has led to their widespread use in renal bone disease. The dose for calcitriol and alfacalcidol is usually 1–2 μg daily, and for dihydrotachysterol 100–200 μg. The dose should be titrated against the alkaline phosphatase activity, and reduced when this is restored to normal. Maintenance doses vary from 0.25 μg thrice weekly to 1 μg daily.

Subtotal parathyroidectomy is often required, especially in those patients with severe hyperparathyroidism (tertiary hyperparathyroidism). These patients are frequently hypercalcaemic, and are unable to tolerate treatment with calcitriol. Careful postoperative monitoring is required as these patients develop marked hypocalcaemia, due to the rapid uptake of calcium by the skeleton (hungry bones syndrome). Prolonged treatment with intravenous calcium may be required. Preoperatively, treatment with calcitriol or diphosphonates to decrease the rate of bone turnover may reduce the degree of hypocalcaemia. Severe extraskeletal calcification in the presence of hyperparathyroidism is another indication for parathyroidectomy, since this may reduce periarticular and small vessel calcification. Treatment of aluminium bone disease is aimed at reducing the aluminium burden. This is most successfully achieved by the chelating agent, desferrioxamine, which is usually given intravenously or intraperitoneally.

Osteoporosis

Osteoporosis, the most common metabolic disorder of bone, is characterized by fragility fractures due to a reduction in the amount of bone (bone mass). It may arise in the absence of other clinical disease (primary osteoporosis) or may be associated with a wide variety of acquired and inherited disorders (secondary osteoporosis) (Table 55.20). It is most frequently encountered in postmenopausal women, one in three of whom will sustain an osteoporotic fracture in their lifetime. Osteoporotic fractures occurring in the spine and wrist are associated with significant morbidity, but the most serious consequence occurs in more elderly patients, where femoral neck fracture has a high mortality (15–20%) and morbidity.

Table 55.20 Causes of osteoporosis

Primary osteoporosis
Postmenopausal*
Age-related (senile)*
Idiopathic
Juvenile
Secondary osteoporosis
Endocrine disorders
Hypogonadism, e.g. Klinefelter's, Turner's syndrome
Cushing's syndrome
Hyperthyroidism*
Hyperparathyroidism
Diabetes mellitus
Haemachromatosis
Anorexia/bulimia nervosa
Athletes—usually female, long-distance
Bone marrow disorders
Multiple myeloma*
Systemic mastocytosis
Carcinomatosis
Intestinal malabsorption
Postgastrectomy
Chronic liver disease, e.g. primary biliary cirrhosis
Severe malnutrition
Connective tissue disorders
Osteogenesis imperfecta*
Homocystinuria
Marfan's syndrome
Drug-related
Corticosteroids*
Thyroxine
Chronic heparin therapy
Alcohol*
Miscellaneous
Immobilization
Chronic respiratory disease*

* Most common causes.

The incidence of osteoporotic fractures increases with age, although a well-recognized idiopathic bone loss may occur in some children shortly before or around the time of puberty (juvenile osteoporosis) and in pregnancy. The major factors involved in the development of ageing-related osteoporosis are the peak bone mass attained in early adulthood, and the subsequent rate of bone loss. Other skeletal factors are also of importance in the development of fracture, which include trabecular connectivity and bone turnover. For any given bone mass the risk of fracture is higher in the elderly, because of an increased tendency to fall, and impaired protective neuromuscular responses to falls. These factors become important determinants of fracture risk in the elderly.

Bone mass is a major determinant of skeletal strength. Attention has focused on bone mass rather than other determinants of skeletal strength, largely because a variety of non-invasive techniques are available for the measurement of bone mineral content or density. Peak bone mass is attained at 30–35 years, with rapid increases occurring during the early years of life and the pubertal growth spurt. The peak bone mass is less in women than in men. There are several determinants of peak bone mass including genetic (parental bone mass) factors and the lifetime mechanical loading of the skeleton, related to physical activity. Controversy surrounds the role of nutritional factors, particularly dietary calcium intake, but some believe that inadequate calcium intake in the peripubertal years may result in a suboptimal peak bone mass, and predispose to the later development of osteoporosis. The risk of fracture in postmenopausal women will be highest in those with low peak bone mass, even if the subsequent rate of bone loss is low.

Age-related bone loss occurs in both sexes from middle age. The rate of loss is approximately 1% per annum in men, but any increase in this rate of loss will further increase the future risk of fracture. Higher rates of bone loss (2–4% per annum) occur in the first five to ten years following the menopause, and this is one of the main reasons for the increased incidence of fracture in women. Other diseases associated with increased bone turnover, such as primary hyperparathyroidism and hyperthyroidism, will also increase the rate of bone loss.

Loss of bone occurs if the balance between bone resorption and formation is not maintained. Within BRU this may result either from an increase in the amount of bone removed by osteoclasts or a decrease in the amount of new bone formed by osteoblasts. Whatever the nature of the imbalance, an increase in the rate of bone turnover, that is an increase in the number of remodelling units on the bone surface at any one time, will exacerbate the rate of loss and decrease trabecular bone width and increase the porosity of cortical bone.

Age-related osteoporosis in both sexes results from an age-dependent decrease in osteoblastic function. This defect leads to incomplete filling of resorption cavities with gradual thinning and eventual loss of trabecular elements. There is a proportionate loss of both cortical and trabecular bone, associated with an increased risk of vertebral and hip fracture. In women, postmenopausal bone loss is characterized by an increase in the rate of bone remodelling and an increase in the depth of resorption cavities, so that the amount of bone removed by resorption exceeds that replaced by osteoblasts during bone formation. The increased depth of resorption causes perforation of trabecular elements, so that no bone surface exists for subsequent formation (irreversible bone loss). Perforation and removal of trabecular elements contributes to structural weakening. The rate of bone loss is greatest at sites of predominantly trabecular bone, reflecting the greater surface area involved in bone remodelling. Fractures occur most commonly at the hip, distal forearm (Colles' fracture) and spine.

Several mechanisms have been proposed to explain the increase in bone loss following oestrogen withdrawal. These include impaired vitamin D activation and impaired calcium absorption, decreased secretion of calcitonin and increased skeletal sensitivity to PTH. A direct action of oestrogen on bone cells is also possible, and oestrogen receptors have recently been demonstrated on osteoblast-like cells.

The role of dietary calcium in the development of age-related bone loss remains controversial. Calcium absorption decreases in both sexes with ageing, especially after the age of 70 years. Possible mechanisms include reduced production of vitamin D (poor diet, inadequate sunlight exposure) and impaired renal conversion to calcitriol. It is unclear however, whether decreased calcium absorption contributes to increased mobilization of skeletal calcium and bone loss. It may represent an appropriate homeostatic response to increased calcium influx to the extracellular fluid from the skeleton.

Secondary osteoporosis

A secondary cause of osteoporosis can be identified in up to 20% of women and 40% of men presenting with osteoporotic fracture (see Table 55.20). Where possible, adequate treatment of the underlying disorder should be undertaken before considering the need for any specific therapy for the osteoporosis. In the elderly, myeloma and thyrotoxicosis are not uncommon, and routine investigations should include a full blood count; serum calcium, phosphate, alkaline phosphatase and liver function tests; thyroid function tests and a myeloma screen (erythrocyte sedimentation rate, serum immunoglobulins, and urinary Bence-Jones protein).

Primary gonadal dysfunction or agenesis is associated with an increased risk of osteoporosis, for example Turner's syndrome. Increased bone loss also occurs following artificial or premature menopause, and early bilateral oophorectomy is an important cause of secondary osteoporosis in young women. Functional hypogonadism associated with bone loss also occurs in anorexia/bulimia nervosa, and in female athletes. Hypogonadism is an important cause of male osteoporosis, as in Klinefelter's syndrome.

Iatrogenic glucocorticoid excess is a frequent cause of osteoporosis. It usually results from the use of pharmacological doses of corticosteroids in the management of chronic debilitating diseases such as asthma, chronic obstructive airways disease, dermatological disorders and rheumatoid arthritis. Spontaneous fracture is a not uncommon presentation of Cushing's disease, and may occur in the absence of other classical signs and symptoms. Glucocorticoids impair osteoblast function, and decrease intestinal calcium absorption. There is a gradual thinning of trabecular elements, similar to that in ageing-related osteoporosis. Vertebral fractures predominate and may be associated with excessive callus (pseudocallus) on X-ray.

Thyrotoxicosis increases bone turnover, but resorption exceeds formation. Other clinical features of thyrotoxicosis may not be obvious, especially in the elderly. Bone loss may also occur in patients receiving thyroxine replacement therapy. Regular monitoring of therapy should aim to maintain TSH in the upper normal range.

Myeloma is an important cause of generalized osteoporosis, which may occur in the absence of focal osteolytic lesions. Bone resorption is stimulated by myeloma cell-derived osteoclast activating factors (OAF) acting on normal osteoclasts. Fractures and bone pain are usually of recent onset, and may progress rapidly. Other systemic symptoms, including nausea, vomiting, thirst and polyuria, may indicate the presence of hypercalcaemia.

Heavy alcohol intake is associated with the development of osteoporosis, and is probably the most common cause of osteoporosis in young men. Cigarette smoking and chronic respiratory disease are also risk factors for the development of osteoporosis. The mechanism(s) by which alcohol and smoking reduce bone mass are not fully understood.

It is well known that gravitational stresses stimulate osteoblast function. Prolonged immobilization results in bone loss, due to continuing bone resorption in the presence of suppressed bone formation. Several prospective studies in postmenopausal osteoporosis have shown that patients undergoing regular exercise lose less bone than controls. Obesity appears to protect against bone loss. This may reflect increased mechanical loading of the skeleton, increased conversion of androgens to oestrogen by aromatase enzyme activity in adipose tissue, or both.

Some of the rarer causes of osteoporosis are shown in Table 55.20. It is important to note that patients with osteogenesis imperfecta may not necessarily have a history of childhood fracture, and may only experience problems when postmenopausal or age-related bone losses exacerbate the underlying weakness is bone strength.

Clinical features

Thin bones, or osteopenia, is asymptomatic. The clinical consequence of osteoporosis is, therefore, fracture. Osteoporosis is characterized by fractures which occur spontaneously or follow relatively minor trauma. Vertebral fractures are the most common, leading to back pain, loss of height and spinal deformity. Vertebral wedge fractures are frequently painless, and result in the characteristic thoracic kyphosis often referred to as a 'dowager's hump'. (Fig. 55.16). Total vertebral collapse, or crush fractures, tend to occur in young patients, and are associated with sudden severe pain which recedes over several weeks. It is not unusual for patients to lose between 10 and 20 cm in height, and in severe cases the rib cage may come to rest on the pelvic brim. Apart from girdle pain, neurological complications are very rare.

Fractures at the wrist tend to occur in relatively young postmenopausal women (50–60 years old), and characteristically are sustained by falling on the outstretched hand. The incidence is highest in the winter months. Most wrist fractures heal with relatively few long-term complications. Algodystrophy characterized by pain, stiffness, swelling and vasomotor disturbances of the hand, occurs commonly, but usually resolves within six months.

The incidence of hip fractures increases exponentially with age. They are twice as common in women as in men, and it has been estimated that one-third of women and one-sixth of men will experience a hip

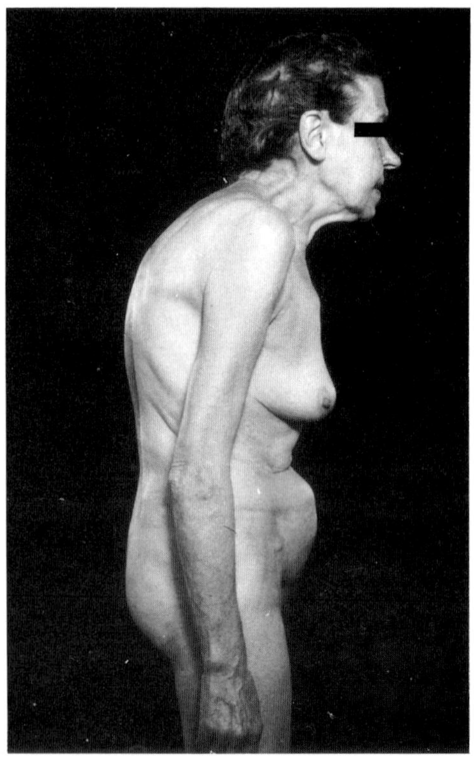

Fig. 55.16 Characteristic dowager's hump caused by multiple wedge fractures of the thoracic vertebrae in osteoporosis.

fracture if surviving to extreme old age. Fractures usually occur with relatively minor trauma. An increase in the frequency of falls, possibly related to drug therapy (such as postural hypotension with antihypertensives), visual deterioration and impaired mobility, and an impaired neuromuscular protective response to falls (such as Parkinson's disease) are probably of importance. In a minority of patients the fall is precipitated by the fracture. Hip fracture is the most serious consequence of osteoporosis, with a mortality of 12–20% in the first year following fracture. Much of this mortality is due to concomitant disabling illnesses. Fewer than half of the survivors fully recover function by one year, and up to 25% will require long-term care.

Apart from the findings associated with the causes of secondary osteoporosis, laboratory findings are not marked. Serum values of calcium, phosphate and alkaline phosphatase activity are usually normal. Increases in alkaline phosphatase occur in association with fractures and persist for several months. Fasting urinary levels of hydroxyproline and calcium, usually expressed as a ratio to urinary creatinine, provide indices of current rates of bone resorption and net skeletal calcium losses respectively. Both may be high in the early postmenopausal years due to increased osteoclastic activity (high-turnover osteoporosis), but the levels are frequently normal in more elderly patients, reflecting the predominance of age-related bone loss (low-turnover osteoporosis).

Radiographic abnormalities include a decrease in apparent bone density. Density cannot be judged by radiographic translucency and is diagnosed in the spine by the apparent prominence of the outer cortical shell of vertebral bodies (Fig. 55.17). Within the vertebral bodies the accentuation of vertical trabecular markings suggests hypogonadal bone loss, whereas a 'ground-glass' appearance is more characteristic of steroid-induced osteoporosis or age-dependent bone loss in men. At the hip there are characteristic patterns of trabecular markings which are progressively lost during the osteoporotic process. These can be scored semiquantitatively (the Singh score). Cortical bone loss can be evaluated most readily at the metacarpals and the radial and ulnar cortical width at the midpoint of the shaft of the second and fourth metacarpal should occupy two-thirds of the total width.

In the spine the most common vertebral deformity is a central collapse of the endplate, followed by anterior collapse and thereafter complete collapse. Deformities of the posterior height of the vertebral bodies without anterior collapse are rare (except at L4 and L5) and raise the suspicion of other coexisting disorders. Anterior vertebral deformities are not always due to osteoporosis, and the widespread nature of deformities may be due to apophysitis in youth. Focal deformities may be due to osteoarthrosis.

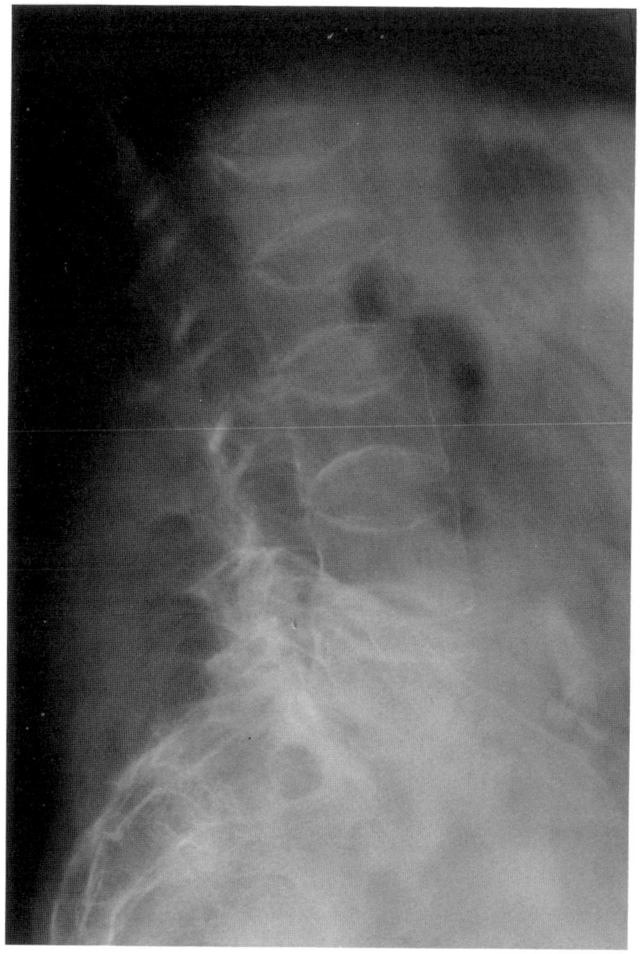

Fig. 55.17 Radiography of the lumbar spine in a patient with osteoporosis. Note the accentuation of the cortical margins of the vertebral bodies due to rarefaction of the trabecular bone and the multiple central deformities due to a reduction in central vertebral height.

Bone density can be measured non-invasively with a variety of techniques, including single- and dual-energy photon or X-ray absorptiometry. Sites commonly measured are the mid or distal radius, the spine, hip and os calcis. These techniques are of value in providing estimates of future fracture risk when

Table 55.21 Agents used in the prevention of osteoporosis and treatment of established osteoporosis

Agents which prevent or decrease bone loss
Oestrogens and progestogens
Calcitonins (salmon, porcine, eel)
Diphosphonates (etidronate, clodronate, pamidronate)
Calcium
Anabolic steroids (e.g. stanozolol, nandrolone)
Agents which may increase bone mass
Fluorides (sodium fluoride, monofluorophosphates)
Parathyroid hormone
Coherence therapy (e.g. phosphate and calcitonin)
Other factors
Exercise

Table 55.22 Oestrogens and progestogens which are commonly used in hormone replacement therapy. The progestogens are presently available in oral preparations and taken for the last 12 days of the cycle

Class of agent	Route	Name	Bone-sparing dose
Oestrogens	Oral	Conjugated equine oestrogens	0.625 mg/day
		Oestradiol valerate	2 mg/day
	Trans-dermal	17-β oestradiol	50 μg/day
Progestogens	Oral	Norethisterone	1–5 mg/day
		Norgestrel	150 μg/day

measurements are compared with age- and sex-matched values of an appropriate reference population. Sequential measurements are also of value in assessing the rate of change of bone density with time on treatment.

Management of osteoporosis

Management includes symptomatic treatment for pain, the use of exercise to maintain mobility and the prevention of falls. Broadly speaking the drug treatment of osteoporosis can be divided into prevention, primarily of postmenopausal osteoporosis, and the treatment of established osteoporosis (Table 55.21).

Oestrogen replacement therapy is effective in preventing the rapid loss of bone in the early postmenopausal period, and decreases the risk of vertebral and hip fractures. Bone loss is prevented for the duration of treatment (at least for 10 years) and for this reason many believe that it should be given for five years or more to have a significant impact on future risk of fracture. The optimal bone sparing dose for conjugated equine oestrogen, the most widely used oestrogen, is 0.625 mg daily (Table 55.22). Oestrogen replacement also ameliorates other menopausal symptoms, including hot flushes, sweating and vaginal dryness, but may do so with lower doses. The use of unopposed oestrogens appears to decrease the risk of ischaemic heart disease in postmenopausal women by up to 50%. However, there are potential risks and side-effects with replacement therapy. Unopposed oestrogens are associated with a three- to eight-fold increase in the risk of endometrial carcinoma. This increase is prevented by the concomitant cyclical use of progestogens, and oestrogens can be prescribed alone if the patient has had a hysterectomy. The effects of opposed treatment on cardiovascular risks are not known. There is some controversy concerning the risk of breast cancer from oestrogen therapy. If the risk is increased at all it is a small increase, and appears to be related to the duration of therapy and perhaps the type of oestrogen used. Other side-effects include headaches, weight gain, depression, breast tenderness and hypertension. The latter usually occurs as an idiosyncratic phenomenon within the first few months of treatment. In hypertensive patients exacerbation of the hypertension may be avoided by using transdermal oestrogens, as this avoids the hepatic first-pass metabolism of oestrogen which induces an increase in renin substrate. Some women find persistent menstruation a significant problem.

Exercise and physical activity also appear to be of some importance in preventing or slowing bone loss, and should be encouraged. However, the optimal type, duration and frequency of exercise remain unknown. Calcium in pharmacological doses (1–1.5 g daily) slows the rate of bone loss but, like exercise, it is not as effective as hormone replacement therapy. Several other agents inhibit bone loss at the time of the menopause. These include calcitonin and the diphosphonates, but their use for prophylaxis in the UK remains experimental.

The use of non-invasive techniques to measure bone mass at the time of menopause (including single- and dual-energy photon absorptiometry and dual-energy X-ray absorptiometry) provides a reasonably accurate prediction of future fracture risk. The use of biochemical markers to assess the rate of bone loss (such as fasting urinary calcium and hydroxyproline excretion) may also prove useful in the identification of those who might benefit from preventive measures.

When established, osteoporosis is very difficult to treat. Further bone loss can be stopped or delayed by all of the inhibitors of bone turnover (Table 55.21). Fluoride is known to increase trabecular bone mass (by up to 15% in one year). Trabecular bone mass can be restored but disrupted architecture persists, and its efficacy in preventing fracture is still questioned. The anabolic steroids prevent bone loss including cortical losses and improve general well-being and muscle function. They probably do not restore bone mass in the long term. They are a reasonable option in men and in more elderly women. Oral agents such as stanozolol (5 mg daily) are convenient, but side-effects include fluid retention, hypertension, an atherogenic lipid profile and abnormal liver function. These complications are less frequently seen with nandrolone (e.g. 50 mg three- or four-weekly i.m.) but androgenic effects such as hirsutism and voice changes are more frequent and also require that treatment is stopped in some patients. Many experimental drugs and combinations have been proposed in an attempt to manipulate the remodelling cycle to increase bone mass, but these require further evaluation.

Paget's disease of bone

Paget's disease of bone (osteitis deformans) is a focal, often multicentric, disorder of increased bone turnover. First described by Sir James Paget in 1876, it is estimated to affect about 750 000 people in Britain. Although cases in young people have been described, Paget's disease is much more frequent in the elderly, and slightly more common in men than in women. There are marked geographical and racial variations in incidence, both within countries (more common in northern industrial regions of England) and throughout the world. It is most common in Anglo Saxons, but rare in Scandinavians, Orientals and Africans.

The discovery of viral-like inclusion bodies in pagetic osteoclasts has led to the hypothesis that Paget's disease represents a response to a slow virus infection. The viral neuclocapsids appear to be paramyxoviridal and have been variously identified as respiratory syncytial virus (RSV), measles or canine distemper viruses. They may not, however, be specific for pagetic bone. There is also a genetic predisposition for Paget's disease. A positive family history is found in 10–15% of patients.

Osteoclasts in Paget's disease are much larger than normal, with an increased number of nuclei. Histologically, there is usually a combination of intense osteoclastic bone resorption (osteolysis) coupled with increased osteoblastic activity (sclerosis). The normal lamellar pattern of bone collagen is disrupted and the disposition of woven bone is a prominent feature. The resulting bone is often enlarged, deformed, and more vascular than surrounding normal bone. Bone strength is compromised with an increased risk of fracture.

Most patients (perhaps 90%) are asymptomatic, and the diagnosis is often an incidental radiographic or biochemical finding. The pelvis, lumbar spine, femora, tibiae and skull are common sites of involvement. The clinical features and complications which may arise in Paget's disease are shown in Table 55.23.

Bone pain is the most common presenting symptom, usually resulting from the Paget's disease or arthropathy in a joint involving pagetic bone. In the latter case, distinguishing between the two types of pain can be very difficult, although pagetic pain is classically described as greater at rest (often occurring during the night) in contrast to the mobility-associated discomfort of arthritis. Pain in the lower limbs exacerbated by weight-bearing may indicate the presence of fissure fractures (incomplete cortical fractures). Rarely, increasing pain may herald the development of sarcoma.

Bony enlargement and deformity are also frequent signs in Paget's disease. Enlargement is most striking in the skull vault, whereas bowing deformity characteristically occurs in the long bones, typically the femur and tibiae (Figs 55.18 & 55.19). The skin overlying pagetic bone often feels warm, due to increased vascularity of bone and overlying skin. Hyperdynamic cardiac failure is a complication of very extensive disease.

Neurological sequelae may result from neural compression. Deafness is a frequent finding with skull involvement. Rarely, blindness may result from compression of the optic nerve. Involvement of the skull base may lead to lower cranial nerve palsies, and platybasia may induce acute brain-stem lesions, long tract and vascular compression syndrome and internal hydrocephalus. The distribution of Paget's

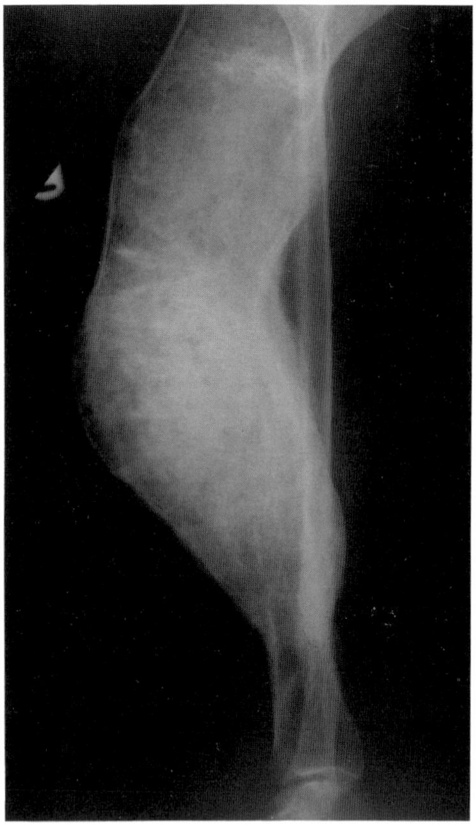

Fig. 55.18 Paget's disease of the tibia. Note the bowing deformity and presence of multiple fissure fractures. The distal end of the tibia is normal.

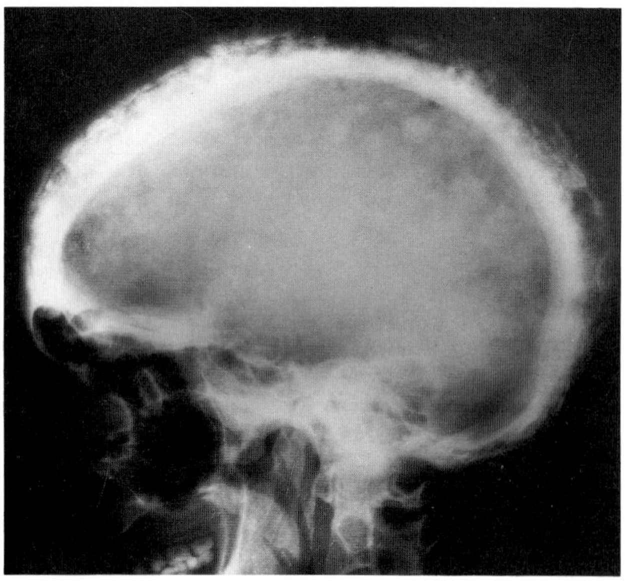

Fig. 55.19 Radiograph of the skull to show extensive involvement with Paget's disease. Note the platybasia and the increase in width of the skull vault.

Table 55.23 Clinical features and complications of Paget's disease

Asymptomatic (90%)
Pain
Pagetic
Secondary osteoarthrosis
Fissure fractures
Neurological compression syndromes
Vascular steal
Sarcoma
Deformity
Bowing (especially tibiae, femora)
Enlargement (e.g. skull)
Fractures
Cortical fissure
Complete
Avulsion
Increased vascularity
Increased local temperature
Perioperative bleeding
High-output cardiac failure
Vascular steal syndromes
Neurological
Deafness and cranial nerve compression
Spinal cord compression
Vascular steal syndromes
Hydrocephalus, brain-stem and cerebellar syndromes
Epidural haematoma
Metabolic disorders
Hypercalciuria and hypercalcaemia
Chondrocalcinosis
Valvular calcification
Osteosarcoma (less than 1%)

disease of the spine is striking and the prevalence of the disorder increases caudally (Fig. 55.20). The neurological syndromes associated with enlarged vertebral bodies are, however, more commonly associated with thoracic disease, perhaps related to the smaller diameter of the spine at this site. Vertebral Paget's disease may cause spinal cord, root or corda equina syndromes. This is commonly due to compression but is frequently associated with a vascular steal syndrome.

Pathological fractures are a frequent complication of Paget's disease. The most common sites are the vertebral bodies, femur and tibia. Most occur spontaneously or after apparently minor trauma. Localized pain and tenderness may precede the fracture by

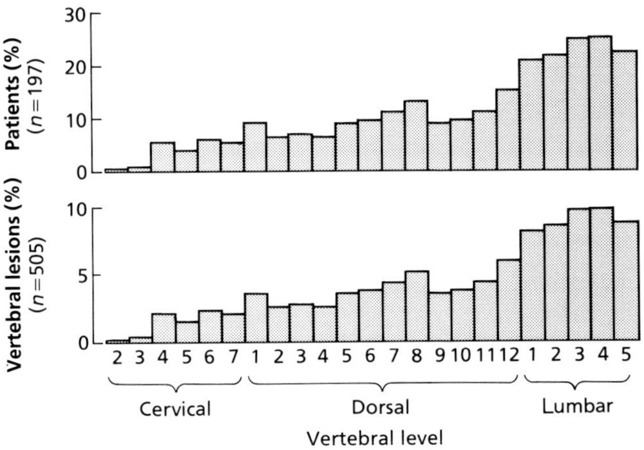

Fig. 55.20 Distribution of 505 vertebral lesions in Paget's disease assessed by scintigraphy in 197 patients. C1 is not shown since this vertebra was not readily assessed by scintigraphy in the presence of Paget's disease at the base of the skull.

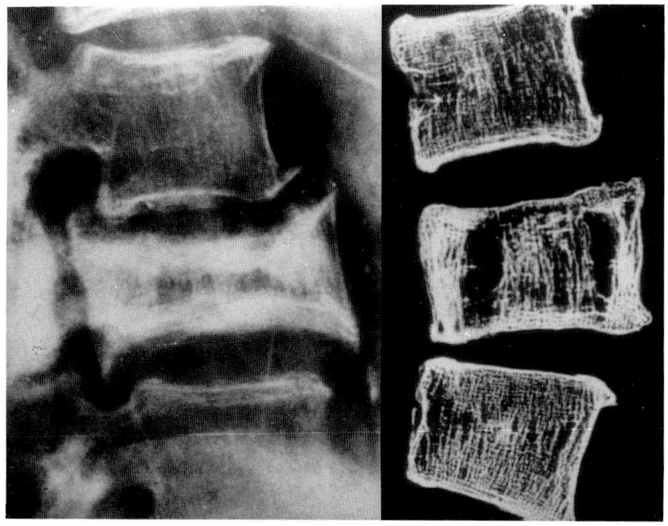

Fig. 55.21 Lateral radiograph of the spine to show a single vertebral body affected by Paget's disease. Note the marked enlargement in both the anterior and posterior aspect.

several weeks, coinciding with the extension of a fissure fracture at the site.

Osteosarcoma develops in less than 1% of patients, and is more frequent in men, particularly those with extensive disease. The humerus and femur are the most common sites involved. The prognosis is extremely poor, and less than 40% survive for longer than one year after diagnosis.

Bone biopsy shows characteristic features of increased bone remodelling and abnormally large osteoclast bearing viral inclusions. Biopsy is occasionally necessary for diagnosis in monostotic Paget's disease. More normally, the diagnosis is made by its characteristic radiographic and scintigraphic features. Scintigraphic uptake is high with homogeneous uptake at affected sites. This contrasts with the often multifocal uptake seen in skeletal neoplasia. Scintigraphy lacks specificity but is particularly useful in determining the extent of disease and for monitoring response to treatment and relapse.

The most characteristic findings in Paget's disease are observed on skeletal radiography (Figs 55.18, 55.19 & 55.21). Features include enlargement of bones (by periosteal or endosteal growth), coarse and accentuated trabecular markings, and patchy osteosclerosis and osteolysis. None of these features is specific for the disorder, but the combination is. The greatest difficulties arise in distinguishing monostotic disease, particularly in the spine where bone enlargement is not marked (Table 55.24).

Increased activity of serum alkaline phosphatase activity is the most characteristic biochemical abnormality. This reflects the increased production of the osteoblast-derived isoenzyme, and is a useful biochemical marker of the increased bone formation observed in Paget's disease. However, in 15% of patients, serum alkaline phosphatase is normal, usually in those with localized disease, perhaps involving only a single bone. Increased bone resorption is reflected by an increased fasting urinary excretion of hydroxyproline. Bone turnover usually remains in balance, so that serum calcium and fasting urinary excretion of calcium are characteristically normal. Hypercalciuria and more rarely hypercalcaemia occur, however, following immobilization due to pain or fracture.

Simple analgesics are the first step in the management of patients with bone pain. Non-steroidal anti-inflammatories may prove of most benefit in those with osteoarthritis secondary to Paget's disease. If this fails a trial of specific anti-pagetic therapy is worthwhile as this may either relieve the pain (if due to Paget's disease rather than arthritis) or decrease the bone vascularity prior to arthroplasty.

Calcitonin, usually salmon calcitonin, administered as 100 units daily or thrice-weekly, reduces bone turnover, and also has useful analgesic properties. At present it is administered by subcutaneous or intramuscular injection, side-effects including

Table 55.24 Some causes of focal bone sclerosis in adults

Common
Paget's disease of bone*
Renal bone disease
Osteosclerotic metastases*
Uncommon
Haemangioma
Hodgkin's disease
Osteomyelosclerosis*
Radiation necrosis*
Histiocytic lymphoma*
Chronic vitamin D poisoning
Lead poisoning
Fluorosis
Hypothyroidism
Coccidioidomycosis
Bone islands and primary benign tumours*
Hyperostosis interna
Pseudocallus*
Osteoarthrosis*
Osteomyelitis*
Fibrous dysplasia*
Melorheostosis
Pycnodysostosis
Osteopoikilosis
Osteopathia striata
Rare
Myelomatosis
Sarcoidosis*
Primary hyperparathyroidism
Osteopetrosis
Primary malignant bone tumours*

* May give rise to a solitary ivory vertebra.

nausea, vomiting and flushing are relatively common, and some patients cannot tolerate treatment. Preparations which are administered intranasally may become available. Relapse usually occurs soon after stopping therapy, and resistance to therapy can occur.

The diphosphonates are stable analogues of pyrophosphate which suppress bone turnover by inhibiting osteoclast-mediated resorption. One of these, etidronate, has been widely used in the treatment of Paget's disease. The recommended oral dose is 5 mg/kg per day, with treatment lasting up to six months. Intestinal side-effects do occur, but only rarely require withdrawal of therapy. The major side-effect of etidronate is that it inhibits the mineralization of bone, particularly at high doses (> 10 mg/kg per day) or with prolonged use. This may increase the risk of fracture, especially in those patients with fissure fractures or predominantly osteolytic Paget's disease. Careful examination of radiographs should be undertaken before treatment and this agent avoided if these features are present. Several newer diphosphonates which do not inhibit mineralization have been evaluated in Paget's disease; these include clodronate and pamidronate which are available in some countries. Like etidronate, even short intravenous courses of treatment may induce long-term suppression of disease activity, which not uncommonly persists for several years (Fig. 55.22).

Total hip arthroplasty is frequently required for secondary osteoarthritis. Multiple osteotomy may be used to correct bowing deformity, especially in the tibia. If large fissure fractures are present, prophylactic nailing of long bones may be undertaken since fissure fractures respond poorly to medical therapy. In contrast, slowly progressive pagetic spinal cord syndromes respond well to medical treatment (such as intravenous diphosphonates), without the risks of surgical decompression. This is probably because the treatments decrease the vascularity of bone and thereby improve the blood supply to the spinal cord.

Inherited disorders of collagen metabolism

Several inherited disorders of collagen metabolism may affect the skeleton (Table 55.25), but their discussion is beyond the scope of this chapter. The most common disorder of collagen which results in skeletal disease is osteogenesis imperfecta.

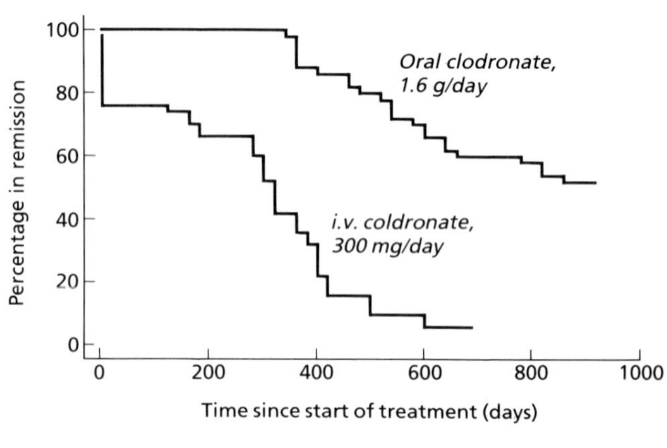

Fig. 55.22 Duration of biochemical responses following treatment with Paget's disease with two regimens (clodronate 1.6 g daily by mouth for six months or 300 mg intravenously for five days). Note the prolonged duration of remission which may persist for several years despite short courses of the diphosphonates.

Table 55.25 The most common inherited disorders of collagen which are associated with skeletal disease

Disorder	Defect	Features of skeletal disease
Osteogenesis imperfecta	Defective collagen gene(s)	Excessive bone fragility
Marfan's syndrome	Unknown	Tall, thin, arachnodactyly, osteoporosis, scoliosis, joint hypermobility
Ehlers–Danlos syndrome		
VI	Defective cross-linkages	Kyphoscoliosis
VII	Amino acid defect in procollagen	Short stature, joint dislocations
Homocystinuria*	Defective cystathionine synthetase activity—abnormal crosslinks	Similar to Marfan's syndrome
Alkaptonuria*	Deficient homogentissic acid oxidase	Blue–black discoloration of cartilage, tendons, ligaments; intervertebral disc calcification; early arthritis

* Primary disorders of amino acid metabolism, with secondary effects on collagen synthesis

Table 55.26 The genetic and clinical features of the four main types of osteogenesis imperfecta

Type	Inheritance	Clinical features
I	Dominant	Mild skeletal deformity, normal stature, blue sclerae, deafness, dentinogenesis imperfecta
II—	New mutations	Lethal in perinatal period, deep blue sclerae
III	Some recessive	Fractures at birth, kyphoscoliosis, normal sclerae, dentinogenesis imperfecta common
IV	Dominant	Short stature, fragile bones, normal sclerae in adults, dentinogenesis imperfecta

Osteogenesis imperfecta

Several defects of Type I collagen have been identified in osteogenesis imperfecta, usually resulting from a mutation within one or other of the two genes coding for the alpha chains. There are four main types of osteogenesis imperfecta, which are classified by the severity of the skeletal disease and other clinical features (Table 55.26).

Type I osteogenesis imperfecta is the most common form of the disease. Blue sclerae may be the only obvious abnormality. Severe bone deformity is rare, and the significance of fractures in the early years of life may not be appreciated. The diagnosis may not become apparent until later in life when postmenopausal bone loss increases still further the risk of facture. Deafness may occur due to deformity or fracture of the ossicles, and early loss of dentition arises from concomitant problems with dentine (dentinogenesis imperfecta). Joint hypermobility is often demonstrable.

In mild disease, radiographs may be normal apart from thinning of the cortices of the long bones, and the changes in the spine may be indistinguishable from simple osteoporosis. With increasing severity, bowing of the long bones occurs, with expansion of the ends of the long bones. The face may have a characteristic shield shape with a wide skull vault tapering to a relatively narrow mandible. Multiple small bones may be visible on radiographs of the skull, especially in the occipital area (Wormian bones).

There is as yet no simple biochemical test which is of use in the diagnosis of osteogenesis imperfecta, and the diagnosis is usually made from the clinical features, family history and radiographs. In young children the most important differential diagnosis is non-accidental injury, but distinguishing between the two is often very difficult.

Prenatal diagnosis of the more severe forms is possible using ultrasound at around 16 weeks and radiographs at 20 weeks. In dominantly inherited disease with prospective mildly affected parents with dominantly inherited disease, there is a 50% chance of any child being affected. However, if the disease in the parent is mild, reassurance should be given that the severity of the disease appears to remain constant across generations. In apparently spontaneous cases of osteogenesis imperfecta the maximum chance of a further affected child is 25% (1 in 4 recessive inheritance), but is probably much lower.

There is no effective medical treatment for osteogenesis imperfecta. Steps should be taken to minimize the effects of other factors on bone strength, including the provision of hormone replacement therapy to women with Type I disease at the time of menopause. Surgical intervention may be required to correct progressive skeletal deformity in more severe cases, but repeated operations are often necessary.

FURTHER READING

Albright, J.A. & Brand, R.A. (eds) (1979) *The Scientific Basis of Orthopaedics*. Appleton-Century-Crofts, New York.

Avioli, L.V. & Krane, S.M. (eds) (1990) *Metabolic Bone Disease*, 2nd edn. W.B. Saunders, Philadelphia.

Kanis, J.A. (ed.) (1990) *Calcium Metabolism. Progress in Basic and Clinical Pharmacology*, 4. Karger, Basle.

Kanis, J.A. (1991) *The Pathophysiology and Treatment of Paget's Disease of Bone*. Martin Dunitz, London.

Smith, R. (ed.) (1990) *Osteoporosis*. Royal College of Physicians, London.

SECTION 14
PAIN AND SPASTICITY

56 · Neural Mechanisms of Pain

By D.R. BOWSHER

Most experimental information about pain comes from the application of acute noxious stimulation to skin innervated by branches of plexuses formed by the anterior primary rami of spinal nerves. What least is known about are the mechanisms of painful sensation resulting from chronic insult to muscles and joints innervated by branches of posterior primary rami. Nothing is known about the extent to which the composition of nerves running in posterior primary rami differs from those in anterior primary rami; nor is it known whether the absence of plexuses made up by the merging of roots has any physiological significance. The account given below is perforce drawn mainly from available data on anterior ramus components, in the hope and belief that it will for the most part be relevant to problems of spinal pain. It should not, however, go unremarked that since pain is more common in the elderly, and peripheral branches of anterior primary rami are known to undergo changes in composition with age, the possibility of some association between backache and posterior primary ramus composition may be borne in mind.

Nociceptors

Nociceptors are sensory units responding specifically to damaging stimuli. They are as specific as rods and cones for light or Pacinian corpuscles for mechanical deformation. Pain is due to the activation of such nociceptors, and is not produced by the overstimulation of other types of receptor. Nociception is associated with the smaller categories of primary peripheral afferent axon: unmyelinated fibres conducting at 0.5–1.5 metres/s (1–2.5 m.p.h.), and the smallest myelinated (Aδ) axons conducting at 12–30 metres/s (25–60 m.p.h.). Tissue damage results in the release or formation of some substance which activates nociceptor terminals; prostaglandin E_2 is the most recently implicated (Taiwo *et al.*, 1987; Schaible & Schmidt, 1988). This means that, in accordance with their phylogenetic primitiveness, nociceptors are in fact chemoreceptors. Stimulation of nociceptors as a result of tissue damage due to trauma or disease gives rise, when impulses reach conscious level, to pain which may be called *nocigenic* (Table 56.1).

In rat/cat striated muscle two-thirds of unmyelinated (Group IV) and somewhat over half of small myelinated (Group III) afferent fibres respond only to high-intensity (noxious) stimuli; half of all these fibres also respond to close arterial injection of algogenic substances such as bradykinin, serotonin, histamine, or K^+ ions. A substantial proportion of Group IV fibres respond only to chemical stimulation, and some of these have been shown to be activated during ischaemic contraction (Mense & Stahnke, 1983). The rest of the small fibres respond to low-intensity (non-noxious) mechanical stimulation; some of them also respond to chemical stimulation. Mense (1982) has also shown that bradykinin-induced activity in nociceptive muscle afferents of Groups III and IV is reduced by aspirin—the first demonstration of a peripheral pharmacological effect on pain. More recently, morphine has also been shown to have a peripheral action which raises the threshold of nociceptor terminals (Russell *et al.*, 1987). Microneurographic studies so far in human volunteers have already implicated Group III fibres in muscle pain (Torebjörk *et al.*, 1984).

Afferents from the cat knee (Schaible & Schmidt, 1983) and rat ankle (Guilbaud *et al.*, 1985) joints have

Table 56.1 Nerve fibre types in mammalian nerves. (After Ganong)

Neurones	Numeral classification	Origin	Fibre diameter (nm)	Conduction velocity (metre/s)	Function
Aα	I	Muscle spindle and annulospiral ending and Golgi tendon organs	12–20	70–120	Proprioception
Aβ	II	Muscle spindle, flower spray efferent	5–12 3–6	30–70	Touch, pressure
Aγ	—			15–30	Motor to muscle spindle
Aδ	III	Pain and touch receptors	2–5	12–30	Pain, temperature, touch
B	Efferent	Preganglionic autonomic	3	3–15	Efferent autonomic
C Dorsal root	IV	Pain receptor, touch	0.5–1.2	0.5–2	Pain, reflex responses
Sympathetic	—	Postganglionic sympathetic efferent	0.3–1.3	0.7–2.3	Sympathetic efferent

recently been studied. The situation is similar to that in muscle in that small myelinated and unmyelinated fibres responding to both noxious (extreme rotation) and innocuous (angle and acceleration) mechanical stimulation have been identified. All unmyelinated joint afferents examined, both nociceptive and non-nociceptive, have been activated by bradykinin. However, the joint story can be carried further because joint afferents have been examined in animals with adjuvant-induced polyarthritis or carrageenin-induced monoarthritis, by the French and German groups respectively. Guilbaud and her collaborators have shown that afferents in acutely inflamed joints become sensitized, in that normally non-noxious stimuli, such as gentle handling (agonizing to the rheumatic patient), now activate small, normally high-threshold, fibres (Guilbaud *et al.*, 1987); in other words, inflammation *lowers* the threshold of nociceptors, so that they are activated at lower intensities of stimulation. As mentioned above, Russell *et al.* (1987) have demonstrated peripheral inhibition of fine afferent discharge from inflamed cat knee joint by morphine. It is therefore now no longer necessary to regard peripheral receptors (or at least nociceptors) as transducers with immutable properties, but rather as entities whose activation threshold may be modulated in either direction by pathological or pharmacological processes.

Posterior roots

Posterior roots exhibit two phenomena worthy of surgical note:

1 All unmyelinated afferent fibres, of course, have their cell bodies in the posterior root ganglia; but the proximal part of the axon, in some 30% of C (Group IV) neurones in humans, instead of entering the cord through the posterior root, doubles back to enter through the ventral root (Coggeshall *et al.*, 1975). If all or most of these small fibres—originating from skin, muscle, and viscera—are nociceptive (as some are known to be in non-human species), it may help to explain (in addition to the classical phenomenon of root overlap) the failure of posterior rhizolysis to relieve pain. It has, however, been suggested that they are chiefly concerned with blood pressure regulation (Shin *et al.*, 1986).

2 As the proximal portion of the posterior root approaches the spinal cord in humans and other primates, the fibres segregate into a lateral division containing the C and Aδ axons, and a medial division containing the large (Aβ) fibres (Sindou *et al.*, 1974).

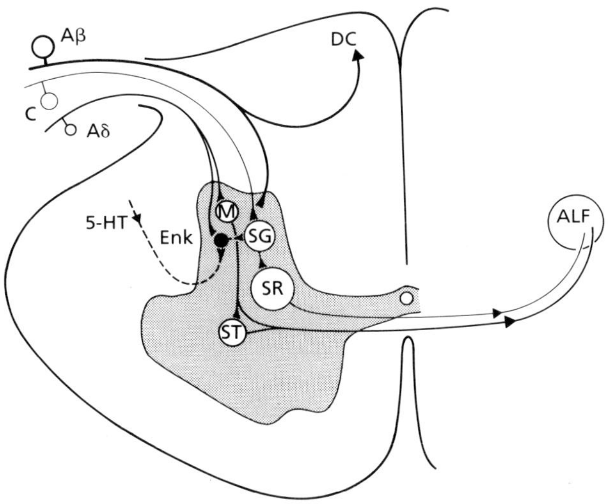

Fig. 56.1 The dorsal horn—this diagram demonstrates some of the components of the dorsal horn. Aδ peripheral afferents from pinprick receptors end on marginal zone (M) cells in lamina I and send axon branches to inhibitory enkephalinergic interneurones (Enk) on the lamina I–II boundary. Aδ fibres also reach lamina V; spinothalamic (ST) axons thus originate from laminae I and V. They cross to the other side of the spinal cord and ascend in the anterolateral funiculus (ALF) towards the ventrobasal thalamus. Polymodal nociceptors reach the spinal cord as primary afferent C fibres (C); their axons contain SP. Polymodal nociceptors from skin end in synaptic contact with cells in the substantia gelatinosa (SG) of lamina II (illustrated); those from deep tissues and viscera terminate on cells deeper in the dorsal horn (not shown). C fibre terminals are contacted presynaptically by collateral branches of large low-threshold cutaneous afferents (Aβ), whose main branches ascend in the ipsilateral dorsal columns (DC). SG and other polymodal nociceptor-receiving cells are also inhibited by the Enk interneurones whose cell bodies are situated on the lamina I–II border, in a naloxone-reversible fashion. Enk cells can be driven by peripheral Aδ afferents and by serotoninergic (5-HT) fibres descending in the dorsolateral white funiculus of the spinal cord. SG, and other dorsal horn cells receiving primary polymodal nociceptor (C) afferents, indirectly activate cells of origin of spinoreticular (SR) axons in laminae VII and VIII. SR axons, in company with ST fibres, ascend in the crossed ALF to end in the reticular formation and intralaminar thalamus.

This arrangement may permit (functionally) differential root section to be performed with the operating microscope.

Intraspinal termination

The intraspinal termination of primary afferent nociceptors (Fig. 56.1) is a matter of considerable practical as well as theoretical importance. In thick sections the spinal grey matter can be seen to be organized in a number of layers or *laminae* (Rexed, 1952), which are numbered postero-anteriorly. The dorsal horn consists of the first five or six laminae; lamina VII constitutes the intermediate spinal grey matter; the anterior horn is made up of laminae VIII and IX (the latter containing the anterior horn cells = lower motoneurones); while lamina X surrounds the central canal. There is little disagreement about the distribution of high-threshold Aδ (Group III) primary afferent axons within the spinal cord: they end in the superficialmost (marginal, Waldeyer) layer—lamina I—and to a lesser extent in the outer part of lamina II (substantia gelatinosa) of the spinal dorsal horn, the lateral part of lamina V in the neck of the dorsal horn, and in the dorsal part of lamina X, surrounding the central canal. These termininal sites have been demonstrated with intra-axonal tracers in primates (Light & Perl, 1979). It is equally agreed that low-

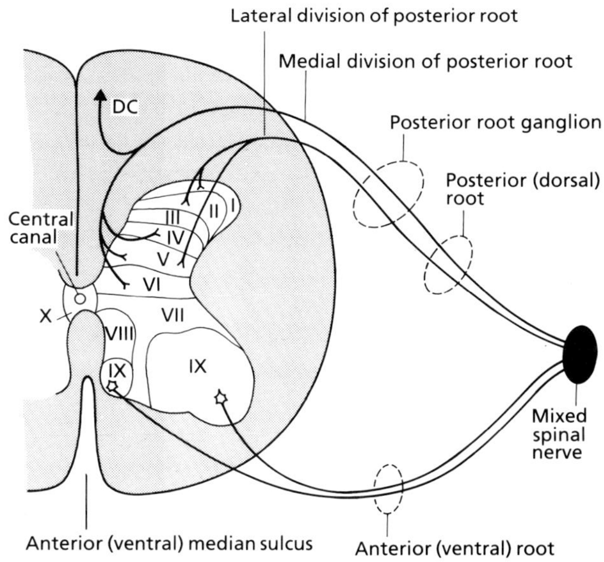

Fig. 56.2 Diagrammatic hemisection of spinal cord at lumbar level. The Rexed laminae of the grey matter are indicated by Roman numerals. The medial division of the posterior root contains large myelinated (Aβ) primary afferent fibres; in addition to terminations in the deeper layers of the posterior horn, unrelayed fibres pass directly upwards in the dorsal columns (DC) to the dorsal column (gracile and cuneate) nuclei in the medulla oblongata. The lateral division of the posterior root contains small myelinated (Aδ) and unmyelinated (C) primary afferent fibres, which terminate in the superficial layers of the posterior grey horn.

threshold mechanoreceptive primary afferent fibres end in deeper dorsal horn laminae—mainly III and IV.

Degeneration studies suggest that their principal site of termination of cutaneous polymodal nociceptors is the substantia gelatinosa (lamina II), with a possible extension into at least the deeper part of lamina I, and this has recently been confirmed by intra-axonal transport studies (Sugiura *et al.*, 1986). However, intra-axonal transport studies in the cat suggest that muscle afferents do not terminate in the substantia gelatinosa, but only in the marginal zone of Waldeyer (lamina I) and lamina V (Craig & Mense, 1983; Swett, 1983; Abrahams *et al.*, 1984). Since this also appears to be true of visceral afferents, one is left to ponder whether the substantia gelatinosa, the most intensely researched part of the nervous system in recent years, may not be merely a skin-related structure, and thus have little importance in the pathophysiology of pain arising in muscles, joints, and viscera.

Neurotransmitters and neuromodulators

In primary afferents these have also been a topic which has attracted much attention in recent years. Despite the ability to study small myelinated fibres by intra-axonal transport methods, very little is known of possible transmitter or modulator substances in Aδ (Group III) nociceptive primary afferents. Of the many amino acids and peptides whose presence has been detected in unmyelinated primary afferent neurones, the favoured candidate is substance P (SP), an undecapeptide originally described by von Euler & Gaddum in 1931. It is reported to be present in higher concentration in muscular than in cutaneous afferents in the rat. Immunocytochemical staining reveals its presence in high concentration in laminae I and II_0 of the monkey dorsal horn (de Lanerolle & LaMotte, 1983). In experimental animals (mainly but not exclusively the rat), SP concentration in the cord increases following noxious stimulation (Kuraishi *et al.*, 1985), and is also increased in the dorsal horn of the arthritic rat (Schoenen *et al.*, 1985). Perhaps more convincingly, SP concentration is reduced in lamina II of patients insensitive to pain (Pearson *et al.*, 1982). Nevertheless, none of this proves that SP is necessarily the pain transmitter or modulator; indeed, the fact that only 20% or fewer of unmyelinated primary afferents contain SP argues rather strongly against it.

Furthermore, dorsal rhizotomy only reduces the concentration of SP in the monkey cord by about 50% (LaMotte, 1977). Subsequent work has demonstrated the presence of SP in spinal interneurones and descending axons of supraspinal origin. This simply reinforces the perceived opinion that functionally system-specific transmitters (if SP *is* a transmitter) do not exist. However, it must be reported that anti-nociception has been obtained in mice by spinal intrathecal injection of an SP receptor antagonist (Post *et al.*, 1987).

The spinal grey matter

This contains numbers of different neurone types in each of its 10 laminae (Abdel-Maguid & Bowsher, 1985). However, from the point of view of nociception two functional types of neurone (see Besson *et al.*, 1982; Besson & Chaouch, 1987) are important (Fig. 56.3).

The first type of spinal neurone driven by noxious peripheral stimulation is the *convergent* or *wide-dynamic range* cell. These elements are usually found deep in the grey matter (laminae VII or VIII), and do not receive a monosynaptic input from primary afferents; they are activated by convergence through more superficially situated cord cells. As the name implies they are activated, but differentially, by a wide variety of non-noxious and noxious stimuli (Fig. 56.3a). They have large receptive fields, often covering a whole limb; in the spinal animal these receptive fields are frequently bilateral (Molinari, 1982), which means that in the intact animal there must be a tonic descending inhibitory system which suppresses upward transmission of the input from the (contralateral) half of the receptive field.

The second is the nociceptive-specific neurone (Fig. 56.3b), responding only to noxious stimulation in the periphery. Such cells typically have small receptive fields, and are commonly found in the marginal layer (lamina I) of the spinal dorsal horn. Many of them project to the contralateral ventroposterior thalamus (see below).

Segmental reflexes elicited by stimuli such as pinprick, which excite Aδ primary afferents and nocispecific cord cells, consist of (phasic) flexion withdrawal. The biological value of this reaction is to remove part or all of the organism from a source of potential tissue damage. Tissue damage such as inflammation or trauma, on the other hand, activates unmyelinated primary afferents and convergent cord

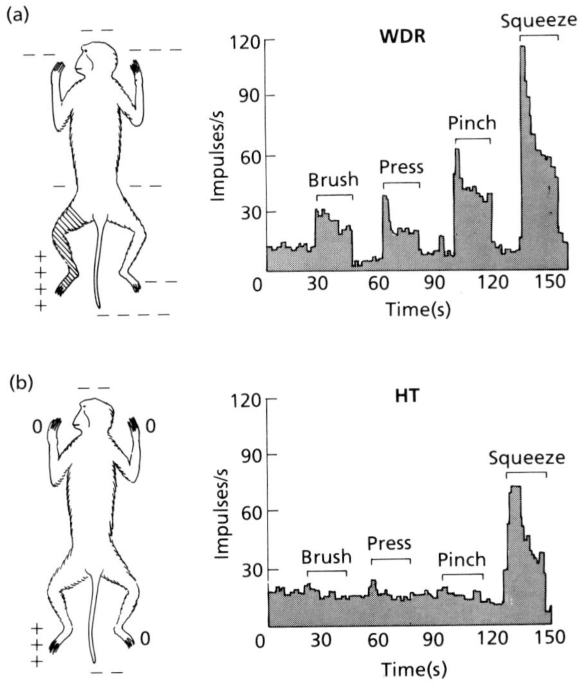

Fig. 56.3 Two types of nociceptive cell in the spinal dorsal horn. (a) WDR is a wide dynamic range or convergent cell which responds in a graded fashion to mechanical stimuli of all kinds; it fires maximally when the stimulus is noxious (squeeze = toothed forceps). Note that the receptive field is large, covering most of the leg; and that the cell can be inhibited from many body points outside the receptive field. (b) HT is a nocispecific or high-threshold cell, which responds only to high-intensity stimulation. Note the small receptive field on the foot, and lack of effect from stimulation of most body points outside the receptive field, except the crown of the head and the tip of the tail, from which the cell is inhibited. Based on Willis (1985).

cells. The reflex response to such stimulation is tonic muscle contraction—spasm, guarding, rigidity—resulting in local or even general immobilization, which allows the organism the best chance of recovering from and repairing such damage. A moment's reflection makes it obvious that these two mutually exclusive responses could not share the same reflex circuit.

The spinal white matter

This contains ascending axons from both nocispecific and convergent cells; both run together in the anterolateral funiculus of the cord (Fig. 56.4). In the monkey, retrograde transport of horseradish peroxidase (HRP) shows that cells projecting to the ventroposterior thalamus (the classical 'spinothalamic tract') are chiefly found in laminae I and V, and their axons are mainly crossed; while HRP injected into the medial thalamus or brain-stem reticular formation chiefly fills cells in laminae VII and VIII, together with a number in lamina V. The axons of these spinoreticular and 'palaeospinothalamic' neurones, running in the anterolateral funiculus in company with classical spinothalamic fibres, have a much larger uncrossed component than the latter (Willis *et al.*, 1979; Kevetter *et al.*, 1982).

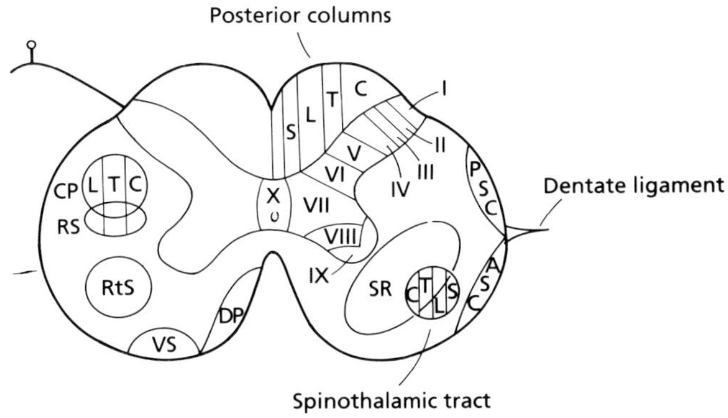

Fig. 56.4 CP, crossed pyramidal; RS, rubrospinal; RtS, reticulospinal; VS, vestibulospinal; DP, direct pyramidal; PSC, posterior spinocerebellar; ASC, anterior spinocerebellar; SR, spinoreticular; C, cervical; T, thoracic; L, lumbar; S, sacral. Laminae of spinal grey matter are shown in Roman numerals on the right.

Cells in the brain stem reticular formation with ascending axons project mainly to the medial thalamus (Fig. 56.3) and hypothalamus (Nauta & Kuypers, 1958; Scheibel & Scheibel, 1966). It has very recently been shown that there are also some direct spinohypothalamic connections (Burstein *et al.*, 1987), just as there are a number of direct spinomedial thalamic fibres; though in both cases the majority relay through the reticular formation.

Somewhat simplistically, then, two main components of the anterolateral funiculus may be distinguished (Fig. 56.5):

1 A spinothalamic pathway running directly to the ventroposterior thalamus. It is mainly crossed, and arises chiefly from nocispecific cells in lamina I, with an important contribution from neurones with their cell bodies in lamina V.

2 Fibres running mainly to the reticular formation (Bowsher, 1957), and thence relaying to the medial

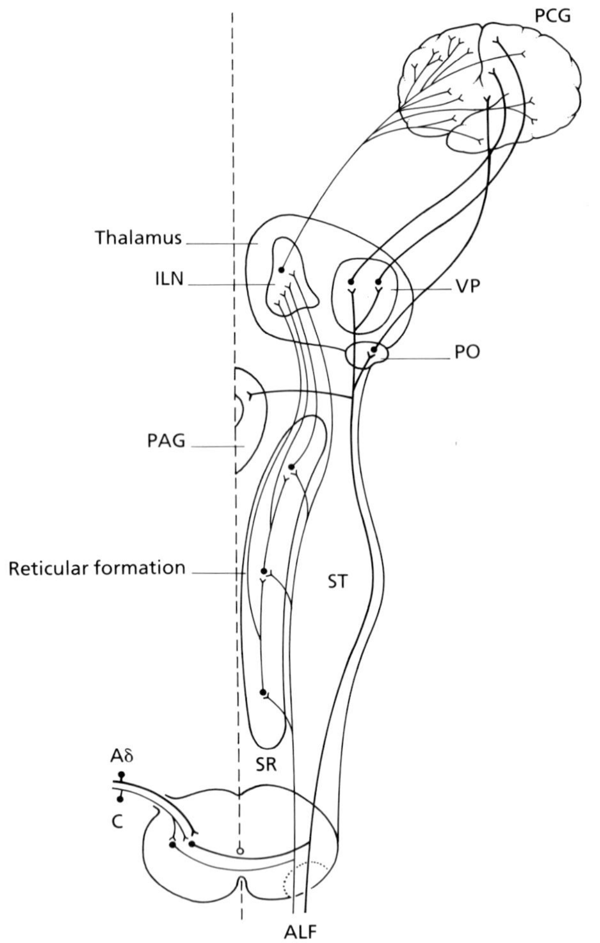

Fig. 56.5 Central pain pathways—the anterolateral funiculus (ALF) of the spinal white matter contains two kinds of long ascending fibres: spinothalamic (ST) axons, principally activated by Aδ (pinprick) peripheral afferents, and spinoreticular (SR) axons, activated mainly, but indirectly, by C (tissue damage) peripheral afferents. Above the spinal cord, ST fibres remain on the lateral border of the brain stem and, after giving off collaterals to the periaqueductal grey (PAG) in the midbrain, terminate in the ventrobasal thalamus. The ventrobasal thalamus has two parts: the ventroposterior nucleus (VP), which projects point-to-point to the first somatic sensory area in the postcentral gyrus (PCG), and the posterior group (PO) of cells, which project to the second somatic sensory area in the region of the insula and parietal operculum. In the brain stem, SR fibres swing medially and end at various levels of the reticular formation; the longest SR axons reach the intralaminar nuclei (ILN) of the thalamus. The reticular formation also projects to the ILN, which gives rise to the so-called 'diffuse' thalamocortical projection. This projection reaches all areas of the non-primary cortex, although with prefrontal predominance.

thalamus and hypothalamus; a minority of axons run directly from the spinal cord to these diencephalic destinations. The origin of this pathway is mainly from convergent (wide dynamic range) cells of deep spinal grey laminae VII and VIII, with a contribution from laminae V; many of their axons are crossed, but there is an important ipsilateral component.

The astute reader will not have failed to observe that both pathways receive contributions from lamina V. Physiological studies show that bifurcating axons from such cells may reach both lateral (ventroposterior) and medial thalamus, and that activity generated in wide dynamic range cells may be recorded in the lateral thalamus, and activity from nocispecific cells in the medial thalamus. Thus the two pathways are not as distinct, either anatomically or physiologically, as may have been suggested in the foregoing paragraphs; however, from a practical, clinical, point of view, the separation is pretty sharp.

The first anterolateral cordotomy for the relief of pain was reported by Spiller & Martin in 1912. For the first half-century and more, cordotomy was an open surgical procedure, but is now usually performed by a percutaneous electrocoagulation technique (Lipton, 1984). Loss of pain sensation following a lesion in the anterolateral quadrant of the spinal cord had first been observed in a case of localized tuberculoma by Spiller in 1905. Successful cordotomy not only abolishes the sensations of (tissue-damage) pain and pinprick on the opposite side of the body, but also temperature sensation, ticklishness, erotic sensation, and the ability to be startled by a sudden tactile stimulus (although the touch itself is perfectly normally felt).

It is salutary to consider the remarkable case described by Noordenbos & Wall (1976), in which a young woman had her whole spinal cord severed, with the exception of one anterolateral quadrant; the extent of the lesion was confirmed at operation. The preserved sensations included not only contralateral pinprick and thermal modalities; but touch-pressure and pain could be identified on both sides. Pain was in fact felt first contralaterally, but then 'spread' to the other side. This is presumably explained in the same way as contralateral mirror-image pain following cordotomy by the fact that the spinoreticular cells responsible for tissue-damage pain sensation have a bilateral receptive field, the ipsilateral side of which is suppressed by tonic descending influences in the intact cord (Bowsher, 1988a).

Opioid receptors

Opioid receptors, or binding sites, were discovered in 1973 (Pert & Snyder; Simon *et al.*; Terenius). They are parts of a (neuronal) cell membrane to which opioids bind and produce an effect (inhibition) in the underlying cell; they are usually, but not always, postsynaptic sites. Once existence of specific receptor sites had been established it was not long before members of each of the three families of naturally occurring opioids were discovered (met- and leu-enkephalins, Hughes *et al.*, 1975; β-endorphin, Bradbury *et al.*, 1976; dynorphin, Goldstein *et al.*, 1979). There are now known to be subgroups of receptors specific for each of the families of opioids: δ receptors for enkephalins, μ receptors for endorphins, and κ receptors for dynorphins. Morphine acts predominantly at μ receptors, to which naloxone also preferentially attaches itself; Table 56.2 shows the affinities of naturally occurring opioids, morphine, and naloxone to the various subclasses of receptor.

In considering pain mechanisms it is important to take account of the anatomical distribution of opioid receptors. Three points in particular should be noted in the present context:

1 Like putative transmitters, opioid receptors are not confined to a particular functional system concerned only with pain transmission. The presence of μ receptors in brain-stem respiratory centres (n. parabrachialis) explains the depressant effect of morphine on respiration, while the euphoriant effect is usually explained by the high concentration of receptors in the amygdala.

2 The high concentration of μ receptors in the superficial dorsal horn of the spinal grey matter accounts for the serendipitous fact that morphine introduced in low concentrations into the subarachnoid space, or even the epidural space, around the cord is able to produce analgesia without greatly affecting other functions (Wang, 1977). Many superficial spinal μ receptors are not postsynaptic, but are apparently situated on the intraspinal terminals of C fibres. Their biological function may be to bind circulating β-endorphin, since there are no β-endorphinergic nerve terminals in the adult human spinal cord. The superficial spinal grey matter also contains a high concentration of δ receptors as well as enkephalinergic interneurones.

3 At supraspinal levels, opioid receptors are found in relatively high concentration in the brain-stem reticular formation and intralaminar thalamic nuclei, but only in very low concentration in the ventroposterior thalamus (LaMotte *et al.*, 1978); while microinjection of morphine in the former but not the latter sites produces analgesia (Yaksh & Rudy, 1978). In other words, the spinoreticulodiencephalic pathway activated by tissue damage is morphine-sensitive, while the direct spinothalamopostcentral pathway is not. This is illustrated by the fact that while clinical nocigenic pain is relieved by therapeutic doses of morphine, subsequent pinprick sensations (e.g. needles used for injection) are felt normally (though not, of course, any tissue-damage pain which they might provoke).

Taking this datum together with the point made above about the different reflex circuits activated by pinprick and tissue damage, respectively, there appears a clear clinical (if not anatomicofunctional) separation between the classical 'spinothalamic' pathway associated with Aδ input, flexion withdrawal, and pinprick sensation, and a spinoreticulodiencephalic pathway associated with tissue damage-evoked C input, reflex muscle spasm, and pain sensation. The former is virtually of no clinical significance (except for the usefulness of its reflexes), while the latter is responsible for the pain, complaint of which is the starting point of 30% of all medical consultations. The fact that both pathways are inextricably mixed in the anterolateral quadrant of the spinal white matter has in the past given rise to much confusion; but if properly understood can be very useful in assessing the results of cordotomy or the site of spinal cord injury.

Table 56.2 Percentage binding affinity. From Kosterlitz & Paterson (1985)

Substance	μ	δ	κ
Met-enkephalin	9	91	0
Leu-enkephalin	6	94	2
β-Endorphin	53	45	2
Dynorphin	5	6	89
Morphine	97	2	1
Naloxone	85	6	9

Deafferentation and neurogenic pain

The foregoing has been concerned with *nocigenic* pain—the stimulation of nociceptor terminals by trauma or disease. There is, however, a totally different category of pain, presenting difficult clinical problems which may be classified under the general heading of *neurogenic* pain. Neurogenic pain is due to dysfunction within the peripheral or central nervous systems in the absence of nociceptor stimulation (or, in the many mixed cases due to trauma, in addition to nociceptor stimulation).

In orthopaedic and neurosurgical practice the most frequently encountered form of neurogenic pain consists of conditions such as (brachial) plexus avulsion, causalgia, and causalgia minor (reflex sympathetic dystrophy). Taking the first of these as an example (and it is in fact *partial* or *subtotal* avulsion), the following features may be distinguished (Bowsher, 1988b):

1 There is a (usually incomplete) sensory deficit (hence *deafferentation*).

2 Allodynia—the elicitation of pain by an innocuous tactile stimulus—may be present; and if so is pathognomonic. In fact allodynia is produced by the activation of only one category of large low-threshold cutaneous afferent, and that is the non-pacinian rapidly adapting (movement) receptor. Slowly adapting receptors, responding to maintained pressure, and pacinian receptors, responding to vibration, are not involved. Allodynia, though often described by patients by the term 'tenderness', is clinically easily distinguishable from true tenderness due to inflammation.

3 In most cases there is evidence of autonomic dysfunction. This is most frequently seen as an exacerbation of pain by physical (e.g. cold) or emotional (e.g. anxiety) stress. There may less commonly be local cutaneous vasoconstriction or vasodilation, measurable in terms of altered skin temperature.

4 Although the pain may be described in almost any of the innumerable terms of an apparently inexhaustible vocabulary, use of the term 'burning' occurs virtually exclusively in neurogenic pain, and 'shooting' almost so.

5 Although the patient may wake in agony, he or she is usually able to fall asleep as easily (or not) as premorbidly.

6 At the practical level, perhaps the most important feature of neurogenic pain is that it is resistant to narcotic analgesics. Since (for unknown reasons) neurogenic pain becomes more intractable the longer appropriate treatment is delayed, it is vitally important not to waste time attempting to control this easily recognized type of pain with analgesics. At a theoretical level this feature demonstrates better than any other that neurogenic pain does *not* involve the morphine-sensitive pain pathways described in preceding sections. This fact is also demonstrated by the failure of procedures such as posterior rhizotomy or anterolateral cordotomy to relieve these pains. Whatever the mechanism of neurogenic pain, it is not an aberrant setting-off of the same mechanisms as are activated by the stimulation of peripheral nociceptors. Indeed, Cassinari & Pagni (1969) have suggested that when neurogenic pain occurs as a result of central nervous system pathology, the lesion is always in the (classical) spinothalamic system or its cortical projection to the postcentral gyrus, with sparing of the more medially placed spinoreticular system and its upward projections. Thus in the spinal cord, postcordotomy dysaesthesia and neurogenic pain resulting from central spinal artery thrombosis or multiple sclerosis fit this pattern.

Deafferentation or neurogenic pain is sometimes also called sympathetic–dependent pain. This name at least recognizes the fact that the most encouraging forms of treatment to date are those which diminish peripheral sympathetic tone in absolute or relative terms. Thus drugs such as tricyclics (which reduce sympathetic outflow from the central nervous system) or peripheral sympatholysis by ganglion blockade or terminal depletion (i.v. guanethidine or reserpine) seem to offer the best chance of alleviation, particularly if instituted early. Shooting pains can be relieved by anticonvulsants—this is as true of acute sciatica as of trigeminal neuralgia, though it is hardly a recommended way of treating a mechanically curable condition!

In many instances, of course, there is coexistence of nocigenic (tissue-damage) and neurogenic pain. This is seen not only when, for example, a neoplasm involves a nerve or plexus as well as compressing and destroying non-neural tissue; a herniated intervertebral disc compresses nerve roots as well as causing mechanical disruption; and brachial plexus avulsion usually involves a great deal of damage to non-neural tissue. In these cases simultaneous but different therapies must be employed to treat both types of pain.

REFERENCES

Abdel-Maguid, T. & Bowsher, D. (1985) The grey matter of the dorsal horn of the adult human spinal cord, including comparisons with general somatic and visceral afferent cranial nerve nuclei. *J. Anat.*, **142**, 33–58.

Abrahams, V.C., Richmond, F.J. & Keane, J. (1984) Projections from C_2 and C_3 nerves supplying muscles and skin of the cat neck: a study using transganglionic transport of horseradish peroxidase. *J. Comp. Neurol.*, **230**, 142–154.

Besson, J-M. & Chaouch, A. (1987): Peripheral and spinal mechanisms of nociception. *Physiol. Rev.*, **67**, 67–186.

Besson, J-M., Guilbaud, G., Abdelmoumène, M. & Chaouch, A. (1982) Physiologie de la nociception. *J. Physiol., Paris*, **78**, 7–107.

Bowsher, D. (1957) Termination of the central pain pathway in man: The conscious appreciation of pain. *Brain*, **80**, 606–622.

Bowsher, D. (1988a) Contralateral mirror-image pain following anterolateral cordotomy. *Pain*, **14**, 10–18.

Bowsher, D. (1988b) Neurogenic pain: diagnosis and treatment. *Res. Staff Phys.*, **34**, 23–29.

Bradbury, A.F., Feldberg, W.F., Smyth, D.G. & Snell, C. (1976) Lipotropic C-fragment: an endogenous peptide with potent analgesic activity. In Kosterlitz, H.W. (ed.) *Opiates and Endogenous Opioid Peptides*, pp. 9–17. North-Holland, Amsterdam.

Burstein, R., Cliffer, K.D. & Giesler, G.J. (1987) Direct somatosensory projections from the spinal cord to the hypothalamus and telencephalon. *J. Neurosci.*, **7**, 4159–4164.

Cassinari, V. & Pagni, C.A. (1969) *Central Pain: A Neurosurgical Survey*. Harvard University Press, Cambridge, MA.

Coggeshall, R.E., Applebaum, M.L., Fazen, M., Stubbs, T.B. & Sykes, M. (1975) Unmyelinated axons in human ventral roots: A possible explanation for the failure of dorsal rhizotomy to relieve pain. *Brain*, **98**, 157–166.

Craig, A.D. & Mense, S. (1983) The distribution of afferent fibers from the gastrocnemius-soleus muscle in the dorsal horn of the cat, as revealed by the transport of horseradish peroxidase. *Neurosci. Lett.*, **41**, 233–238.

Euler, U.S. von & Gaddum, J.H. (1931) An unidentified depressor substance in certain tissue extracts. *J. Physiol.*, **72**, 74–87.

Goldstein, A., Tachibana, S., Lowney, I., Hunkapiller, M. & Hood, L. (1979) Dynorphin (1–13), an extraordinarily potent opioid peptide. *Proc. Natl. Acad. Sci. USA*, **76**, 6666–6670.

Guilbaud, G., Iggo, A. & Tegner, R. (1985) Sensory receptors in ankle joint capsules of normal and arthritic rats. *Exp. Brain Res.*, **58**, 29–40.

Guilbaud, G., Neil, A., Benoist, J.M., Kayser, V. & Gautron, M. (1987) Thresholds and responses to mechanical stimuli in the ventrobasal thalamus during carrageenin-induced hyperalgesic inflammation in the rat. *Exp. Neurol.*, **68**, 311–318.

Hughes, J., Smith, T.W., Kosterlitz, H.W., Fothergill, L.A., Morgan, B.A. & Morris H.R. (1975) Identification of the related pentapeptides from the brain with potent opiate agonist activity. *Nature*, **258**, 577–579.

Kevetter, G.A., Haber, L.H., Yezierski, R.P., Chung, J.M., Martin, R.G. & Willis, W.D. (1982) Cells of origin of the spinoreticular tract in the monkey. *J. Comp. Neurol.*, **207**, 61–67.

Kosterlitz, H.W. & Paterson, S.J. (1985) Types of opioid receptors: relation to antinociception. *Phil. Trans. R. Soc. Lond., B*, **308**, 291–298.

Kuraishi, Y., Hirota, N., Satoh, M. & Takagi, H. (1985) Antinociceptive effects of intrathecal opioids, noradrenalin, and serotonin in rats: mechanical and thermal algesic tests. *Brain Res.*, **326**, 168–171.

LaMotte, C.C. (1977) Distribution of the tract of Lissauer and the dorsal root fibers in the primate spinal cord. *J. Comp. Neurol.*, **172**, 529–562.

LaMotte, C.C., Snowman, A., Pert, C.B. & Snyder, S.H. (1978) Opiate receptor binding in rhesus monkey brain: association with limbic structures. *Brain Res.*, **155**, 374–379.

Lanerolle, N.C. de & LaMotte, C.C. (1983) Ultrastructure of chemically defined neuron systems in the dorsal horn of the monkey. III. Serotonin immunoreactivity. *Brain Res.*, **274**, 65–78.

Light, A.R. & Perl, E.R. (1979) Spinal termination of functionally identified primary afferent neurons with slowly-conducting myelinated fibers. *J. Comp. Neurol.*, **186**, 133–150.

Lipton, S. (1984) Percutaneous cordotomy. In Wall, P.D. & Melzack, R. (eds) *Textbook of Pain*, pp. 632–638. Churchill Livingstone, Edinburgh.

Mense, S. (1982) Reduction of the bradykinin-induced activation of feline group III and IV muscle receptors by acetylsalicyclic acid. *J. Physiol.*, **326**, 269–284.

Mense, S. & Stahnke, M. (1983) Responses in muscle afferent fibres of slow conduction velocity to contraction and ischaemia in the cat. *J. Physiol.*, **342**, 383–397.

Molinari, H.H. (1982) The cutaneous sensitivity of units in laminae VII and VIII of the cat. *Brain Res.*, **234**, 165–169.

Nauta, W.J.H. & Kuypers, H.G.J.M. (1958) Some ascending pathways in the brainstem reticular formation. In Jasper, H.H. *et al.* (eds) *Reticular Formation of the Brain*, pp. 3–30. Little, Brown, Boston, MA.

Noordenbos, W. & Wall, P.D. (1976) Diverse sensory functions with an almost totally divided spinal cord. A case of spinal cord transection with preservation of one anterolateral quadrant. *Pain*, **2**, 185–195.

Pearson, J., Brandeis, I. & Cuello, A.C. (1982) Depletion of substance P-containing axons in substantia gelatinosa of patients with diminished pain sensitivity. *Nature, London*, **295**, 61–63.

Pert, C.B. & Snyder, S.H. (1973) Opiate receptor: demonstration in nervous tissue. *Science*, **179**, 1011–1024.

Post, C., Freedman, J., Paulsson, I. & Hökfelt, T. (1987) Antinociceptive effects in mice after intrathecal injection of a substance P receptor antagonist, Spantide: lack of 'neurotoxic' action. *Regul. Pept.*, **18**, 243–252.

Rexed, B. (1952) The cytoarchitectonic organization of the spinal cord in the cat. *J. Comp. Neurol.*, **96**, 415–495.

Russell, N.J.W., Schaible, H-G. & Schmidt, R.F. (1987) Opiates inhibit the discharges of fine afferent units from inflamed knee joint of the cat. *Neurosci. Lett.*, **76**, 107–112.

Schaible, H-G. & Schmidt, R.F. (1983) Activation of groups III and IV sensory units in medial articular nerve by local mechanical stimulation of knee joint. *J. Neurophysiol.*, **49**, 34–44.

Schaible, H-G. & Schmidt, R.F. (1988) Excitation and sensitization of fine articular afferents from cat's knee joint by prostaglandin E_2. *J. Physiol.*, **403**, 91–104.
Scheibel, M.E. & Scheibel, A.B. (1966) Patterns of organization in specific and non-specific thalamic fields. In Purpura, D.P. & Yahr, M.D. (eds) *The Thalamus*, pp. 13–47. Columbia University Press, New York.
Schoenen, J., van Hees, J., Gybels, J., de Castro Costa, M. & Vanderhaegen, J.J. (1985) Histochemical changes of substance P, FRAP, serotonin and succinic dehydrogenase in the spinal cord of rats with adjuvant arthritis. *Life Sci.*, **36**, 1247–1254.
Shin, H.K., Kim, J., Nam, S.C., Paik, K.S. & Chung, J.M. (1986) Spinal entry route for ventral root afferent fibres in the cat. *Exp. Neurol.*, **94**, 714–725.
Simon, E.J., Hiller, J.M. & Edelman, I. (1973) Stereospecific binding of the potent narcotic analgesic ^{3}H-etorphine to rat brain homogenate. *Proc. Natl. Acad. Sci. USA*, **70**, 1947–1949.
Sindou, M., Quoex, C. & Baleydier, C. (1974) Fiber organization at the posterior spinal cord-rootlet junction in man. *J. Comp. Neurol.*, **153**, 15–26.
Spiller, W.G. (1905) The occasional clinical resemblance between caries of the vertebra and lumbothoracic syringomyelia, and the location within the spinal cord of the fibres for the sensations of pain and temperature. *Univ. Penn. Med. Bull.*, **18**, 147–154.
Spiller, W.G. & Martin, E. (1912) The treatment of persistent pain of organic origin in the lower part of the body by division of the anterolateral column of the spinal cord. *J. Am. Med. Assoc.*, **58**, 1489–1490.
Sugiura, Y., Lee, C.L. & Perl, E.R. (1986) Central projection of identified, unmyelinated (C) afferent fibers innervating mammalian skin. *Science*, **234**, 358–361.
Swett, J.E. (1983) Few C fibres from muscle terminate in lamina II of the spinal cord of the cat. *J. Physiol.*, **345**, 157*P*.
Taiwo, Y.O., Goetzl, E.J. & Levine, J.D. (1987) Hyperalgesia onset latency suggests a hierarchy of action. *Brain Res.*, **423**, 333–337.
Terenius, L. (1973) Stereospecific interaction between narcotic analgesics and synaptic plasma membrane fraction of rat cerebral cortex. *Acta Pharmacol. Toxicol.*, **32**, 317–320.
Torebjörk, H.E., Lamotte, R.H. & Robinson, C.J. (1984) Peripheral neural correlates of magnitude of cutaneous pain and hyperalgesia: Simultaneous recordings of sensory judgements of pain and evoked responses in nociceptors with C-fibers. *J. Neurophysiol.*, **51**, 325–339.
Wang, J.K. (1977) Analgesic effect of intrathecally administered morphine. *Reg. Anesth.*, **4**, 2–3.
Willis, W.D. (1985) *The Pain System*. Karger, New York.
Willis, W.D., Kenshalo, D.R. & Leonard, R.B. (1979) The cells of origin of the primate spinothalamic tract. *J. Comp. Neurol.*, **188**, 543–574.
Yaksh, T.L. & Rudy, T.A. (1978) Narcotic analgetics: CNS sites and mechanisms of action as revealed by intracerebral injection techniques. *Pain*, **4**, 299–359.

57 · Pathophysiology, Assessment and Management of Spasticity

By M.P. SINDOU and P. MERTENS

DEFINITION AND PATHOPHYSIOLOGY

Spasticity is a hallmark of an upper motor neurone disorder and may result from a variety of central nervous system diseases. As pointed out by Katz (1988), 'Spasticity is something easier to recognize than characterize, and perhaps more difficult to treat successfully.' In 1980 Lance proposed an operational definition: 'Spasticity is a motor disorder characterized by a velocity-dependent increase in tonic stretch reflexes (muscle tone) with exaggerated tendon jerks, resulting from hyperexcitability of the stretch reflex, as one component of the upper motor neuron syndrome.'

According to the classical concept, first proposed by Sherrington (1906), exaggerated reflexes are caused by a release from supraspinal inhibition, thus resulting in an imbalance in favour of an exaggerated excitatory state at the spinal level. This notion is derived from the observation that hypertonia is an immediate consequence of decerebration.

However, in most human cases of spasticity, increased tone and hyperreflexia develop gradually over months, after a period of depressed spinal activity. It is doubtful that such a slow time-course can be explained simply in terms of disinhibition of spinal circuits. Wiesendanger (1989) felt that it strongly pointed to profound reorganization of the denervated structures at the spinal level, in response to the degeneration of descending fibres. These compensatory reactions are characterized by long-term changes in the synaptic transmission. Primary collaterals sprout from intact stem fibres and occupy synaptic sites vacated in the course of degeneration (McGough *et al.*, 1958). Receptor supersensitivity of neurones occurs as a response to a loss of synaptic inputs. Both these mechanisms develop with a time-course compatible with the development of spasticity following an acute lesion.

CLINICAL AND NEUROPHYSIOLOGICAL ASSESSMENT

In acute spinal cord lesions the cord damage is followed by a period of spinal shock. Later, with a delay suggesting neural reorganization, a phase of increased intrinsic spinal activity with exaggeration of both proprioceptive and afferent flexor reflexes occurs. In spastic syndromes from spinal origin, hypertonia involves both lower limb flexors and extensors, together with the urethral striated sphincter. Noxious stimuli may exacerbate flexor reflex afferents, leading to flexor spasms and irreducible abnormal postures in flexion.

In order to adequately examine the patient with spasticity, it is essential to ensure that the patient is placed in a comfortable lying position. The tonic stretch reflex is described as the degree of resistance to manual passive stretching. Hyperactive tendon jerks—which manifest exaggerated phasic stretch reflexes—can be easily elicited by percussion of the tendon with a reflex hammer. Reinforcement manoeuvres—such as forceful closing of eyes, clenching of the jaw, making a fist, etc.—are useful for demonstration of any residual suprasegmental motor control.

Spasticity is detected by passively moving the limb segment and noting the resistance offered by the muscles. Only stretch at high velocity explores muscle tone. Limitation in passive movement at slow speed assesses only the degree of capsular and/ or musculotendinous retraction present. The most

Table 57.1 Evaluation of spasticity by measurement of the stretch reflex (Held)

Studying:

1 Its angle of appearance from the usual reference positions

2 Its intensity
- 0 no muscular contraction
- 1 visible muscular contraction
- 2 contraction with a short catch
- 3 contraction lasting a few seconds (or with transient clonus)
- 4 permanent clonus
- 5 rigidity without any possible passive mobilization

These measurements are performed at the three different velocities shown below:
- V1 slow stretching
- V2 velocity of gravity
- V3 fast stretching

sensitive scale to quantify spasticity clinically is Held's test, which measures the angle of appearance of the catch response to a high speed stretching and its intensity (Table 57.1). In very severely affected patients the most adequate tone scale to use is the spasticity grade (Ashworth's scale, Table 57.2) and the spasm frequency (Penn's scale, Table 57.3).

With the practical purpose of evaluating the degree of disability in patients affected with paraplegia, Millet *et al.* (1981) developed in Lyon University a 'functional disability score' which is detailed in Table 57.4. The score ranges from 0 to 4 for each of the five components, with a total of 20/20 indicating a bedridden and totally dependent patient. A score of 10/20 corresponds to the threshold between an acceptable and an unacceptable condition, and thus is the lowest position at which to consider surgery. A different functional disability score has been also developed for the upper limb (Table 57.5).

Table 57.2 Tone scale (Ashworth)

Grade	Degree of muscle tone
1	No increase in tone
2	Slight increase in tone, giving a catch during stretch
3	More marked increase in tone; but affected part easily mobilized
4	Considerable increase in tone; passive movement difficult
5	Rigidity without any possible passive mobilization

Table 57.3 Spasm frequency scale (Penn)

Grade	Frequency of spasms
0	No spasms
1	Mild spasms induced by stimulation
2	Infrequent full spasms occurring less than once per hour
3	Spasms occurring more than once per hour
4	Spasms occurring more than 10 times per hour

The most classical neurophysiological method to assess spasticity is based on measurement of the H-reflex, which is the electrically elicited equivalent of the tendon jerk, both being mediated through activation of motoneurones by the primary spindle afferents. The H_{max}/M_{max} ratio is a good indicator of spasticity, especially at the soleus level.

Measurements of withdrawal reflexes, although not included—strictly speaking—in the definition of spasticity, may be useful. Finally measurements using polyelectromyographs of motoneuronal overactivity, and of its fluctuation, as advocated by Dimitrijevic *et al.* (1981), is of prime importance.

MANAGEMENT

Basic nursing care and physical treatments

Much can be achieved by high-quality nursing care. Careful nursing and positioning of the patient will reduce the frequency and intensity of the noxious stimuli which may exacerbate hypertonia. It is also important to ensure the avoidance of pressure sores, muscular contractures and articular ankyloses; as well as the prevention of urinary tract complications, faecal impaction and venous thrombosis.

A daily stretching programme is also of prime importance for spasticity prevention. Bobath (1970), working on the principle that proprioceptive systems determine motor output, advocated a regular regime of positioning the limbs such as to inhibit the development of spasticity at an early stage in its evolution. He advocated extension to counterbalance the flexion patterns in the upper limbs, and flexion–abduction to

Table 57.4 Functional disability score for spastic lower limbs in paraplegic patients (Lyon University)

Pain

0 No pain
1 Infrequent pain and/or minor intensity without any consequence on daily life
2 Frequent pain, and/or moderate intensity
3 Very frequent pain and/or severe intensity, interfering with daily life
4 Permanent and unbearable pain

Spasms

0 No spasm
1 Infrequent spasms and/or minor intensity
2 Frequent spasms and/or moderate intensity, not affecting sitting or lying.
3 Very frequent spasms and/or severe intensity
4 Almost constant spasm

Wheelchair

0 No discomfort
1 Minor discomfort, not reducing significantly sitting time in wheelchair
2 Moderate discomfort, reducing sitting time in wheelchair
3 Strapping is required to maintain correct sitting position
4 Wheelchair impossible

Transfers

0 Easy, alone
1 Possible alone, but difficult
2 Need for one person helping
3 Possible but difficult with one person helping
4 Need for two persons helping

Washing and dressing

0 Easy, alone
1 Possible alone, but difficult
2 Need for one person helping
3 Possible but difficult with one person helping
4 Need for two persons helping

Table 57.5 Functional disability score for upper limb in hemiplegic patients (Lyon University)

Grade	Description
I	Good active mobility allowing a grasp in the hand and fingers
II	Slight, but useful voluntary motor function
III	Easy passive mobilization, but without any useful voluntary movements
IV	Absence of useful active motility

oppose the usual extension–adduction pattern in the lower limbs.

The use of physical agents may be helpful as temporary measures. Cold baths or topical applications of ice may be used on the basis that cold probably decreases nerve conduction. They may be effective for several hours. Functional electrical stimulation—the mechanisms of which are complex—is able to decrease spasticity temporarily. In addition it can relieve pain, especially when associated with algodystrophic complications. Negative biofeedback can be used to obtain antagonist relaxation during agonist contraction and splinting techniques can improve the range of motion in a joint in patients with harmful contractures.

Pharmacological treatment

There are three major drugs for the treatment of spasticity (Young & Delwaide, 1981). Their negative features versus their positive effects should be weighed before treatment is begun.

Baclofen (Lioresal) is an analogue of γ-aminobutyric acid (GABA), a neurotransmitter involved in presynaptic inhibition, which inhibits calcium influx into presynaptic terminals and suppresses release of excitatory neurotransmitters. Baclofen inhibits both monosynaptic and polysynaptic reflexes, and also reduces activity of the γ afferents. It is safe in long-term use and has a low incidence of side-effects. Sudden withdrawal may lead to hallucinations and/or seizures. It is the drug of choice for treatment of spasticity from spinal origin.

Diazepam (valium) has no direct GABA-mimetic effects, but exerts indirect effects only if GABA transmission is functional. Diazepam is well tolerated except for its sedative effect, intellectual impairment and motor coordination. Its main indication is in spastic hypertonia from spinal cord injury.

Dantrolene sodium (Dantrium) is the only drug which acts at a muscular rather than a segmental reflex level. It reduces muscle action potentials induced by calcium release into the sarcoplasmic reticulum. The most harmful side-effect is hepatotoxicity. Dantrolene is less likely to cause lethargy and/or cognitive disturbances than are baclofen and diazepam. It is preferred for cerebral forms of spasticity such as hemiplegia or cerebral palsy.

To overcome the obstacle of poor transfer of baclofen through the blood–brain barrier, Penn & Kroin (1985) introduced a new treatment of spasticity by direct spinal intrathecal administration of baclofen. The effectiveness of the method is linked with the presence of high concentration of GABA-B binding sites in the dorsal horn. This allows a decrease in dosage necessary from an average of 60 mg/day with the oral administration to an average of 100 µg/day intrathecally. To avoid daily injection by lumbar puncture, this method uses a programmable pump device implanted subcutaneously—consisting of a reservoir containing the drug which is refilled percutaneously every month, and a pump which provides the desired flow according to the programme.

This method is indicated in patients with severe spasticity from spinal cord origin, especially if there are painful spasms. There is a serious risk of overdose, which could be irreversible due to the lack of baclofen antagonists; therefore this technique requires great care. Other complications comprise mechanical catheter migration or occlusion, and also infection requiring revision or removal of the system, respectively. The essential advantage of the technique is the reversibility of the effects; but high cost, the necessity of periodic refilling and reprogramming, and geographic dependence, are serious limitations to this conservative method.

Chemical blocks

Nerve and motor point blocks offer a reduction in spastic tone on a temporary basis. Motor point infiltration, with 1–2 ml of 45% of pure alcohol, or 5% aqueous phenol solution—was proposed by Tardieu *et al.* (1975). They rely on a specific lytic effect on the fine γ fusimotor fibres, allowing a decrease in tone without provoking paralysis. The motor points are located on a reference map or determined after surface electric stimulation. The limits of the method are related to the small number of muscles that can be simultaneously infiltrated and the multiplicity of motor points within a single muscle. The effects are also only transient. The best candidates are patients with spasticity in the triceps or wrist and finger flexor muscles.

Never blocks with alcohol or 5% phenol require location of the nerve upon precise anatomical landmarks and percutaneous stimulation using a catheter sheathed with Teflon. The most commonly used blocks are the musculocutaneous nerve for flexion in the elbow; the median nerve for flexion of the wrist and fingers; the obturator nerve for flexion–adduction of the hip; the tibial nerve for the equinovarus foot and/or flexed toes. Immediate painful reactions can be reduced by combining the agent with local anaesthesia. The patients must be advised that dysaesthesias and causalgias may occur in 10% of cases. Implantable reservoirs can be used for repeated injection of local bupivacaine into the brachial plexus for severe spasticity in the upper limb (Keenan, 1987).

Neuroablative procedures

When spasticity cannot be successfully controlled by physical and pharmacological therapies, functional neurosurgery may provide some alternative solutions.

It is possible to modify excitability on the level of the segmental neural circuits, which are hyperactive after being deprived of their descending inhibitory influences (Dimitrijevic & Nathan, 1967a,b, 1968). The surgery should be performed so that excessive hypertonia is reduced without suppressing the useful muscular tone or impairing the residual motor and sensory functions. Therefore the neuroablative techniques must be as selective as possible. Such selective lesions can be implemented at the level of peripheral nerves, spinal roots, spinal cord, or the dorsal root entry zone.

Peripheral neurotomies

Peripheral neurotomies were introduced first for the treatment of localized spastic deformities of the foot by Stoffel (1913). More recently Gros *et al.* (1977) and Sindou & Mertens (1988) have advocated making neurotomies more selective by using microsurgical technique and intraoperative electrical stimulation for better identification of the function of the fascicles constituting the nerve. Neurotomies affect all the various types of motor and sensory peripheral nerve fibres.

In the management of spasticity of the lower limbs, neurotomies of the tibial nerve at the popliteal region (Fig. 57.1) and to a lesser extent of the obturator nerve are the most commonly used, respectively for the so-called spastic foot and for flexion–adduction deformity of the hip. Selective neurotomies of the branches to the knee flexors can also be performed, at the level of the sciatic trunk through a short skin incision in the buttock.

The technique of selective tibial neurotomy requires the exposure of the tibial nerve from the popliteal region down to the soleus muscular arcade (Fig. 57.1). Under general anaesthesia without curarization, all its branches are individualized and identified one by one using the operating microscope and bipolar stimulation. Each branch (or fascicle) considered as the support of the harmful spasticity is partially resected over a 5 mm length, in order to prevent regrowing of fibres. Conservation of one-third to one-fifth of the fibres of each branch is sufficient to avoid loss of motor function and amyotrophy. The branches to be operated on are determined preoperatively according to all components of the spastic disorders. For example, equinus deformity and/or ankle clonus require section of the soleus nerve(s), and if necessary of the two gastrocnemius branches. A varus deformity necessitates interruption of the posterior tibialis nerve. Tonic flexion of the toes needs section of the

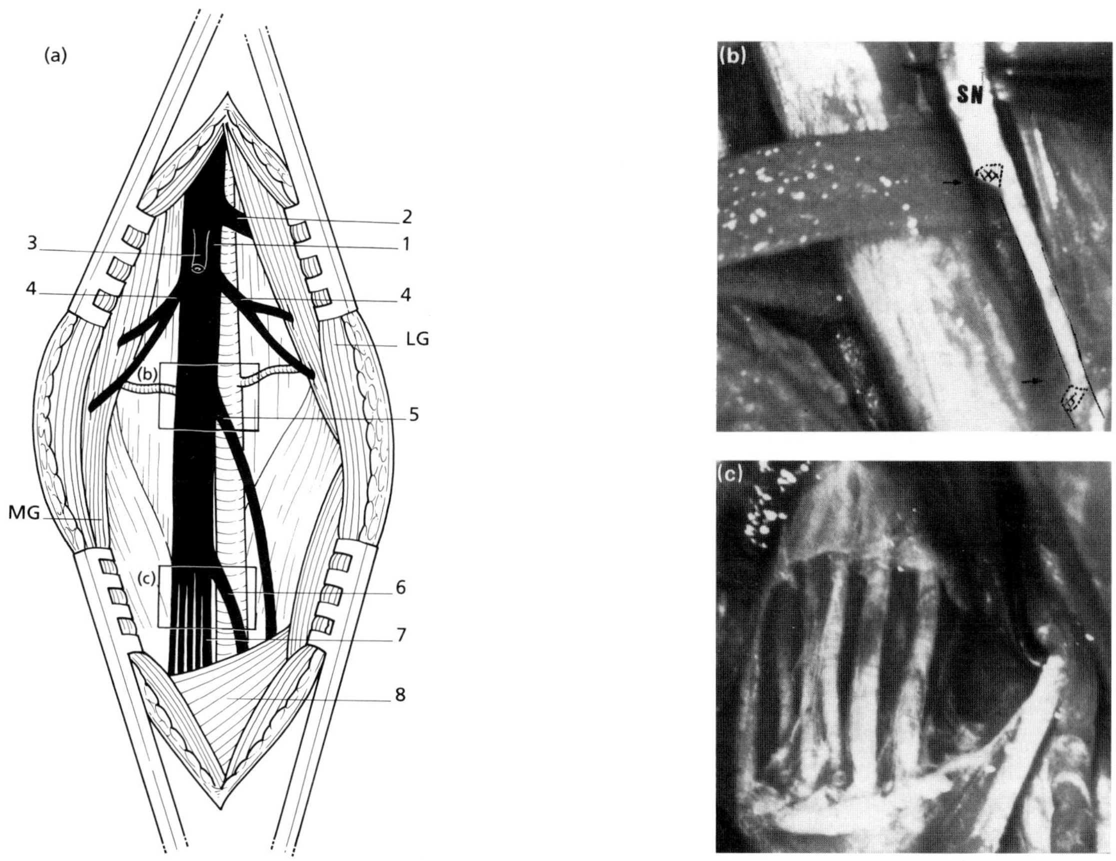

Fig. 57.1 Selective tibial neurotomy. (a) Dorsal view of the right popliteal region showing tibial (1) and peroneal (2) nerves, (sensory) sural nerve (3), medial and lateral gastrocnemius nerves (4), soleus nerve (5), posterior tibialis nerve (6). The distal trunk of the tibial nerve (7), just above the soleus arcade (8), contains five to eight fascicles, averaging 1 mm in diameter each; two-thirds are motor fascicles and one-third sensory. (b) Operative view of the resection, over 7 mm in length (between the two arrows), of two-thirds of the soleus nerve (SN). (c) Operative view of five dissected fascicles inside the distal part of the tibial nerve at the level of the soleus arch, after the epineural envelope has been opened.

flexor fascicles situated inside the distal trunk of the tibial nerve. Their precise identification, apart from the sensory fascicles, is of paramount importance to avoid hypoaesthetic and dysaesthetic disturbances, as well as trophic lesions of the plantar skin.

Surgery is generally able to obtain suppression of the disabling spasticity, total pain relief, and consequently improvement of the residual voluntary movements (by achieving a better balance between agonist and antagonist muscles). These beneficial effects are permanent. However, these procedures must be performed prior to the onset of contractures and fixed deformity.

In contrast to the lower limbs, neurotomies are seldom indicated for spasticity in the upper limbs. However, selective fascicular neurotomies—of the musculocutaneous nerve for spastic elbow flexion, of the median (and/or cubital) nerve for spastic hyperflexion of the wrist and fingers—can be performed, provided special care is taken with the sensory fascicles to avoid causalgic painful manifestations.

Anterior rhizotomies

Introduced by Monro (1945), extensive anterior rhizotomies can be applied to severe spastic paraplegias without residual voluntary movements, either in patients in whom posterior rhizotomies had failed or in patients with diffuse lesions of the interneurones in the spinal cord grey matter.

Anterior rhizotomies limited to a small number of rootlets have been recommended by Gros *et al.* (1981) in association with posterior rhizotomies, for instance to reduce hypertonia in the adductor muscles of the hip at the L2 level or in the flexor muscles of fingers and hand by lesions of some rootlets of C7–T1. Of course this can be done only if intraoperative stimulation of the corresponding anterior rootlets reproduces the existing disorders.

Posterior rhizotomies

Posterior rhizotomy was performed for the first time for the modification of spasticity by Foerster in 1908 (see Foerster, 1913), after Sherrington demonstrated in 1898 (see Sherrington, 1906) that decerebrate rigidity in the animal model was abolished by section of the dorsal roots. In spastic syndromes, posterior rhizotomy suppresses the afferent input to the monosynaptic stretch and polysynaptic withdrawal reflexes which are deprived from their suprasegmental inhibitory control. But its undesired effects on sensory and sphincter functions limit its application.

To diminish these disadvantages, several authors in the 1960s and 1970s made attempts to develop more selective operations, especially for the treatment of children affected with cerebral palsy.

POSTERIOR SELECTIVE RHIZOTOMY

In order to reduce the sensory side-effects of the original Foerster's method, Gros *et al.* introduced in 1967 a technical modification consisting of sparing one rootlet of the five of each root, from L1 to S1.

On similar principles Ouaknine (1980), a pupil of Gros, developed a microsurgical technique consisting of resecting from one-third to two-thirds of each group of rootlets of all the posterior roots, from L1 to S1.

SECTORIAL POSTERIOR RHIZOTOMY

In an attempt to reduce the side-effects on the postural tone in walking patients, Privat *et al.* (1976) and Gros (1979) proposed a topographic selection of the rootlets. The procedure is prepared by preoperative assessment of useful spasticity, related to postural tone (abdominal, quadriceps, gluteus medius), and harmful spasticity of hip flexors, adductors, hamstrings and triceps surae.

The first step of the method consists of a mapping of the evoked motor activity of the exposed rootlets, from L1 to S2, by direct electrostimulation of each posterior group of rootlets. Sections are decided according to the preoperative programme.

PARTIAL POSTERIOR RHIZOTOMY

In 1977, Fraioli & Guidetti reported on a procedure consisting of dividing the dorsal half of each rootlet of the selected posterior roots, a few millimetres before their entrance into the posterolateral sulcus.

The absence of patent sensory deficit was probably explained by the fact that partial section leaves intact a significant number of fibres of all kinds.

'JNCTIONAL POSTERIOR RHIZOTOMY

The neurological search for specially organized circuits responsible for spasticity led Fasano *et al.*

(1976) to propose the so-called functional posterior rhizotomy. The method is based on bipolar intra-operative stimulation of the posterior rootlets and analysis of the type of muscle responses by EMG recordings. Responses characterized by a permanent tonic contraction (disinhibition), with an after-discharge pattern and a large spatial diffusion to distant muscle groups, were considered to belong to spinal circuits responsible for spasticity. This procedure has also been used by other authors, especially for children with cerebral palsy or myelomeningocele (Peacock & Arens, 1982; Cahan *et al.*, 1987; Storrs, 1987; Abbott *et al.*, 1989).

Percutaneous thermorhizotomies and intrathecal chemical rhizotomies

Percutaneous radiofrequency rhizotomy was initially performed for the treatment of pain by Uematsu *et al.* (1974). Then Young & Mulcachy (1980) proposed percutaneous sacral rhizotomy for neurogenic detrusor hyperreflexia, followed by Kenmore (1983), Herz *et al.* (1983) and Kasdon & Lathi (1984) for spasticity in the limbs. This method has the advantage of being less aggressive than the open procedures in very debilitated patients. It seems more appropriate for spastic disturbances limited to a few muscular groups, corresponding to a small number of spinal roots. Although the effects are often only temporary, the procedure can be repeated.

Intrathecal injection of alcohol was introduced by Dogliotti in 1931 for relief of cancer pain, and later by Guttman (1953) for the treatment of hypertonia in patients with severe spastic paraplegia. In 1955, Maher replaced alcohol by phenol in hyperbaric solution as the neurolytic agent for pain relief, with the famous remark that 'it is easier to lay a carpet than to paper a ceiling'. Use of phenol for treatment of spasticity was then developed simultaneously by Nathan (1959) and Kelly & Gauthier-Smith (1959), because of a better selectivity than alcohol.

The best candidates for phenol intrathecal injections are paraplegic patients suffering from severe spasms, without useful residual motor, sensory or sphincteric capabilities below the level of the lesion.

Longitudinal myelotomy

Longitudinal myelotomy—introduced by Bischof in 1951—was made more selective by Pourpre (1960), and later by Laitinen & Singounas (1971). The procedure consists of a coronal separation between the posterior and anterior horns of the lumbosacral enlargement from T11 to S2. It is performed from inside the spinal cord after a posterior commissural incision reaching the ependymal canal. Longitudinal myelotomies are indicated only for spastic paraplegias with flexion spasms, when the patient has no residual useful motor control and no bladder and sexual function.

Surgery in the dorsal root entry zone (DREZ)

Selective posterior rhizotomy in the DREZ, also called microsurgical DREZ-tomy (MDT), was introduced in 1972 to treat intractable pain (Sindou, 1972; Sindou *et al.*, 1974a,b, 1976). Because of its inhibitory effects on muscular tone it has been also applied to patients with focalized hyperspasticity (Sindou *et al.*, 1982, 1985a,b, 1986; Sindou & Jeanmonod, 1989). This method aims at selectively interrupting the small nociceptive and the large myotatic fibres (situated laterally and centrally, respectively), whilst sparing the large lemniscal fibres which regroup medially. It also enhances the inhibitory mechanisms of Lissauer's tract and dorsal horn (Eccles *et al.*, 1961; Wall, 1974) (Fig. 57.2).

MDT consists of (2 mm deep and at 45° angle) microsurgical incisions and bipolar coagulations performed ventrolaterally at the entrance of the rootlets into the dorsolateral sulcus, along all the cord segments selected to be operated on.

For paraplegia the L2–S5 segments are approached through a T11–L2 laminectomy, while for the hemiplegic upper limb a C4–C7 hemilaminectomy with conservation of the spinous processes is sufficient to reach the C5–T1 segments. Identification of the metameric levels selected as supporting the harmful tonic mechanisms (and/or corresponding to the painful territories) is achieved by studying the muscle responses to bipolar electrical stimulation of the anterior and/or posterior roots. Then, the lateral aspect of the DREZ is exposed to perform the microsurgical lesions.

MDT is indicated for spasticity in the lower limbs in disabled patients with severe hypertonic paraplegia, especially when there are flexion spasms, irreducible abnormal postures and/or pain. A spastic bladder can be favourably influenced provided the detrusor is not fibrotic. MDT is also indicated in

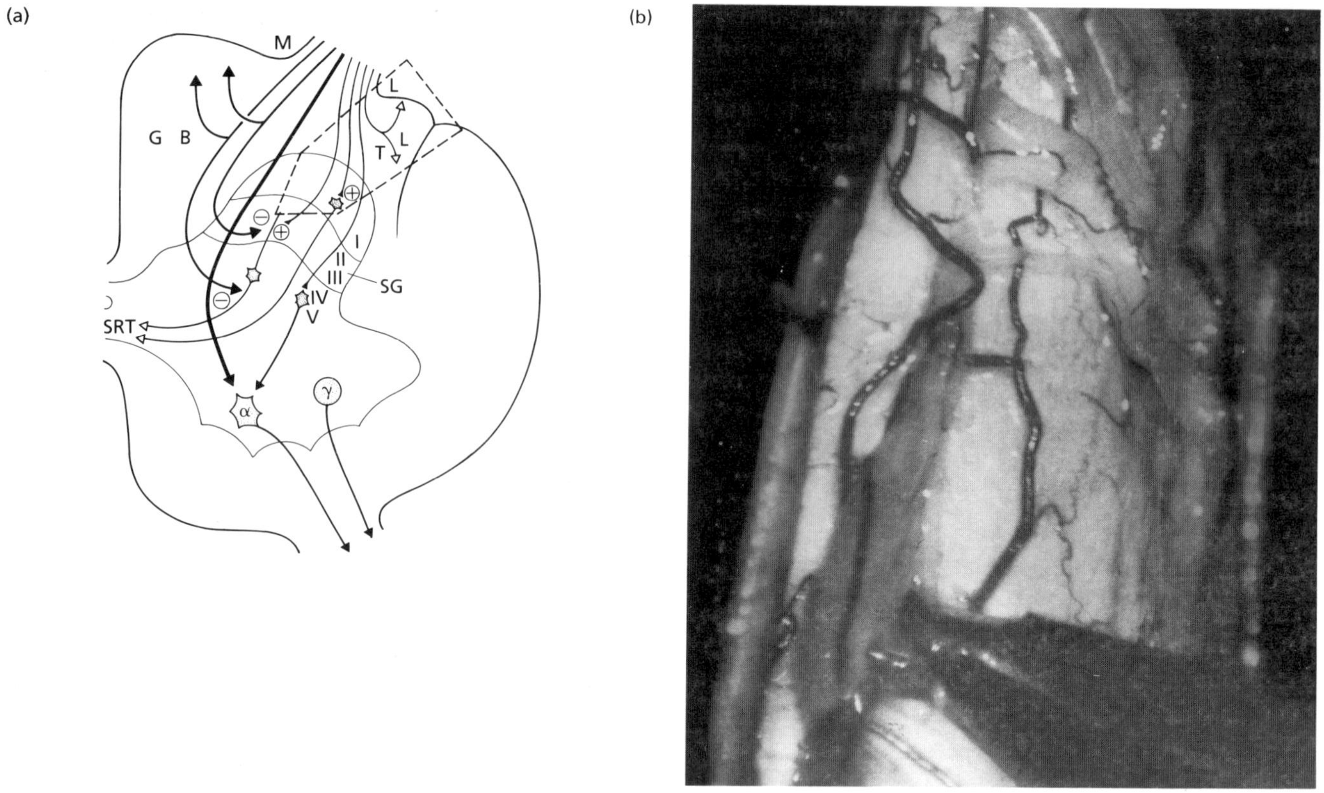

Fig. 57.2 (a) Organization of fibres at the DREZ in humans. The dashed lines shows the proposed extent of microsurgical-DREZ-tomy, i.e. the lateral and central bundles formed by the nociceptive and myotatic fibres, as well as the excitatory medial part of the tract of Lissauer (TL) and the upper layers of dorsal horn. (b) Technique of MDT. Example through a right cervical hemilaminectomy (the procedure for the lumbosacral roots is approximately the same). The right C6 posterior root has been retracted toward the inside to make the ventrolateral region of DREZ accessible. The incision is performed into the DREZ using a small piece of razor blade. This incision is 2 mm deep and makes a 45° angle. Then microcoagulations are performed down to the apex of the dorsal horn.

hemiplegic patients who have harmful spasticity in the upper limb.

By suppressing the excess of spasticity, correcting the abnormal postures and relieving the frequently associated pain, MDT allows physiotherapy to be resumed and sometimes the reappearance or improvement of useful voluntary motility.

Neuroaugmentative procedures

Developed in the 1970s on the basis of the 'gate control theory' of Melzack & Wall (1965) for the treatment of neurogenic pain, stimulation of the spinal cord (SCS) has shown some effectiveness in spastic syndromes such as those encountered in multiple sclerosis or spinal cord degenerative diseases (Cook & Weinstein, 1973; Siegfried, 1980; Gybels & Van Roost, 1987). The electrodes (usually bipolar electrodes) are implanted extradurally in the posterior extradural space, either through an interlaminar direct approach or percutaneously under local anaesthesia through a Tuohy puncture needle. For the latter method the electrodes are connected to a generator device implanted subcutaneously.

Most of the authors who tried SCS for spasticity due to lesions from spinal cord origin agree that the method is significantly effective only when spasticity is mild, and on the condition that the dorsal columns have sufficient functional fibres, as assessed by somatosensory evoked potentials.

The other methods of neurostimulation, such as deep brain stimulation or cerebellar stimulation—which have some positive results in dystonic or dyskinetic syndromes—are not significantly effective for the treatment of spasticity itself (Siegfried & Lazorthes, 1985).

Orthopaedic procedures

Orthopaedic procedures can act in reducing spasticity by means of muscle relaxation resulting from tendon lengthening and/or in restoring articular function when deformities have become irreducible.

Current techniques for correcting excessive shortness of the muscle tendon assembly are: muscular reinsertion, myotomy, tenotomy or lengthening tenotomy. Such techniques aim at obtaining a more functional position. Excessive lengthening can lead to a decrease in muscular strength.

Tendon transfer has a different goal: to normalize articular orientation when it has been deviated by muscular imbalance. Transfer of spastic muscles must be avoided. If necessary, suppression of spasticity must be achieved by a neurosurgical procedure prior to tendon transfer.

Osteotomies aim at correcting bone deformation due to a growth distortion in a child, or at treating stiffened joints. Articular surgery (arthrodesis) is indicated only when osteoarticular deformity cannot be corrected by osteotomy or tendon surgery alone. Arthrodesis must not be performed in children until end of growth.

In adults, orthopaedic surgery can be undertaken to increase comfort in the more severely affected patients, or to improve function in those who have recovered sufficient level of voluntary motricity.

Whatever the situation and aetiology may be, orthopaedic surgery must be considered only after spasticity has been reduced, by physical and pharmacological treatments first and, when necessary, by neurosurgical procedures if they are possible.

Finally, it must be said that the management of patients with severe spasticity is both a moving and potentially dangerous field. In order to deal adequately with these patients it is necessary to work with a multidisciplinary approach which allows rigorous methods of assessment along with great anatomical, physiological, pharmacological and surgical expertise. Such an approach can bring enormous benefit to the disabled person.

REFERENCES

Abbott, R., Forem, S.L. & Johann, M. (1989) Selective posterior rhizotomy for the treatment of spasticity. *Child. Nerv. Syst.*, **5**, 337–346.

Bischof, W. (1951) Die longitudinale Myelotomie. *Zentralbl. Neurochir.*, **2**, 79–88.

Bobath, B. (1970) *Adult Hemiplegia: Evaluation and Treatment*. Heinemann Medical Books, London.

Cahan, L.D., Kundi, M.S., McPherson, D., Starr, A. & Peacock, W.J. (1987) Electrophysiologic studies in selective dorsal rhizotomy for spasticity in children with cerebral palsy. *Appl. Neurophysiol.*, **50**, 459–682.

Cook, A.W. & Weinstein, S.P. (1973) Chronic dorsal column stimulation in multiple sclerosis. *N.Y. St. Med.*, **73**, 2868–2872.

Dimitrijevic, M.R. & Nathan, P.W. (1967a) Studies of spasticity in man: some features of spasticity. *Brain*, **90**, 1–30.

Dimitrijevic, M.R. & Nathan, P.W. (1967b) Studies of spasticity in man: analysis of stretch reflex in spasticity. *Brain*, **90**, 333–358.

Dimitrijevic, M.R. & Nathan, P.W. (1968) Studies of spasticity in man: analysis of reflex activity evoked by noxious cutaneous stimulation. *Brain*, **91**, 349–368.

Dimitrejevic, M.R., Dimitrijevic, M.M., McKay, W.B. & Sherwood, A.M. (1981) Supra-spinal influence on motor unit activity in paralysed muscles: effects of reinforcement maneuvers. *Arch. Phys. Med.*, **62**, 540.

Dogliotti, A. (1931) Traitement des syndromes douloureux de la périphérie par l'alcoolisation sous-arachnoïdienne des racines postérieures à leur émergence de la moelle épinière. *Presse Méd.*, **39**, 1249–1252.

Eccles, J., Eccles, R. & Magni, F. (1961) Central inhibitory action attributable to presynaptic depolarization produced by muscle afferent volleys. *J. Physiol.*, **159**, 147–166.

Fasano, V.A., Barolat-Romana, G., Ivaldi, A. & Sguazzi, A. (1976) La radicotomie postérieure fonctionnelle dans le traitement de la spasticité cérébrale. *Neurochirurgie*, **22**, 23–34.

Foerster, O. (1913) On the indications and results of the excision of posterior spinal nerve roots in men. *Surg. Gynecol. Obstet.*, **16**, 463–474.

Fraioli, B. & Guidetti, B. (1977) Posterior partial rootlet section in the treatment of spasticity. *J. Neurosurg.*, **46**, 618–626.

Gros, C. (1979) Spasticity: Clinical classification and surgical treatment. In Krayenbühl, H. (ed.), *Advances and Technical Standards in Neurosurgery*, vol. 6, pp. 55–97. Springer, Vienna.

Gros, C., Frerebeau, P., Benezech, J. & Privat, J.M. (1977) Neurotomie radiculaire sélective. In Simon, L. (ed.), *Actualités en Rééducation Fonctionnelle et Réadaptation*, série 2, pp. 230–235. Masson, Paris.

Gros, C., Ouaknine, G., Vlahovitch, B. & Frerebeau, P. (1967) La radicotomie sélective postérieure dans le traitement neurochirurgical de l'hypertonie pyramidale. *Neurochirurgie*, **13**, 505–518.

Gros, C., Privat, J.M., Frerebeau, P. & Benezech, J. (1981) Les radicotomies antérieures: leur place dans le traitement de la spasticité. In Simon, L. (ed.), *Actualités en Rééducation Fonctionnelle et Réadaptation*, série 6, pp. 63–70. Masson, Paris.

Guttman, L. (1953) The treatment and rehabilitation of patients with injuries of the spinal cord. *History of the Second World War*, vol. Surgery, pp. 422–516. HMSO,

London.

Gybels, J. & Van Roost, D. (1987) Spinal cord stimulation for spasticity. In Symon, L. (ed.), *Advances and Technical Standards in Neurosurgery*, vol. 15, pp. 63–96. Springer, Vienna.

Herz, D.A., Parsons, K.C. & Pearl, L. (1983) Percutaneous radiofrequency foraminal rhizotomies. *Spine*, **8**, 729–732.

Kasdon, D.L. & Lathi, E.S. (1984) A prospective study of radiofrequency rhizotomy in the treatment of post-traumatic spasticity. *Neurosurgery*, **15**, 526–529.

Katz, R.T. (1988) Management of spasticity. *Am. J. Phys. Med. Rehabil.*, **67**, 108–116.

Keenan, M.A.E. (1987) The orthopedic management of spasticity. *J. Head Trauma Rehabil.*, **2**, 62–71.

Kelly, R.E. & Gauthier-Smith, P.C. (1959) Intrathecal phenol in the treatment of reflex spasms and spasticity. *Lancet*, **2**, 1102–1105.

Kenmore, D. (1983) Radiofrequency neurotomy for peripheral pain and spasticity syndromes. *Contemp. Neurosurg.*, **5**, 1–6.

Laitinen, L.V. & Singounas, E. (1971) Longitudinal myelotomy in the treatment of spasticity of the legs. *J. Neurosurg.*, **35**, 536–540.

Lance, J.W. (1980) Pathophysiology of spasticity and clinical experience with baclofen. In Feldman, R.G., Young, R.R. & Koella, W.P. (eds), *Spasticity Disordered Motor Control*, pp. 185–203. Year Book Medical Publishers, Chicago, IL.

McGouch, G.P., Austin, G.M., Liu, C.N. & Liu, C.Y. (1958) Sprouting as a cause of spasticity. *J. Neurophysiol.*, **21**, 502–516.

Maher, R. (1955) Relief of pain in incurable cancer. *Lancet*, **1**, 18–20.

Melzack, R. & Wall, P.D. (1965) Pain mechanisms: a new theory. *Science*, **150**, 971–979.

Millet, M.F., Mortamais, J., Sindou, M., Eyssette, M., Boisson, D. & Bourret, J. (1981) Neurochirurgie dans les paraplégies spastiques et douloureuses de la sclérose en plaques. Résultats à moyen terme de la radicellotomie postérieure sélective dans 12 cas. In Simon, L. (ed.), *Actualités en Rééducation Fonctionnelle et Réadaptation*, série 6, pp. 76–85. Masson, Paris.

Monro, D. (1945) The rehabilitation of patients totally paralyzed below the waist: anterior rhizotomy for spastic paraplegia. *N. Engl. J. Med.*, **233**, 456–461.

Nathan, P.W. (1959) Intrathecal phenol to relieve spasticity in paraplegia. *Lancet*, **2**, 1099–1102.

Ouaknine, G. (1980) Le traitement chirurgical de la spasticité. *Union Med. Can.*, **109**, 1–11.

Peacock, W.J. & Arens, L.J. (1982) Selective posterior rhizotomy for the relief of spasticity in cerebral palsy. *S. Afr. Med. J.*, **62**, 119–124.

Penn, R.D. & Kroin, J.S. (1985) Continuous intrathecal Baclofen for severe spasticity. *Lancet*, **2**, 125–127.

Pourpre, M.H. (1960) Traitement neurochirurgical des contractures chez les paraplégiques post-traumatiques. *Neurochirurgie*, **6**, 229–236.

Privat, J.M., Benezech, J., Frerebeau, P. & Gros, C. (1976) Sectorial posterior rhizotomy. A new technique of surgical treatment of spasticity. *Acta Neurochir.*, **35**, 181–195.

Sherrington, C. (1906) *The Integrative Action of the Nervous System*, 2nd edn. Yale University Press, New Haven.

Siegfried, J. (1980) Treatment of spasticity by dorsal cord stimulation. *Int. Rehabil. Med.*, **2**, 31–34.

Siegfried, J. & Lazorthes, Y. (1985) La neurochirurgie fonctionnelle de l'infirmité motrice d'origine cérébrale. *Neurochirurgie*, **31** (Suppl. 1), 1–118.

Sindou, M. (1972) *Etude de la jonction radiculo-medullaire postérieure: la radicellotomie postérieure sélective dans la chirurgie de la douleur*. Med. Thesis, Lyon.

Sindou, M. & Jeanmonod, D. (1989) Microsurgical-DREZ-otomy for the treatment of spasticity and pain in the lower limbs. *Neurosurgery*, **24**, 655–670.

Sindou, M. & Mertens, P. (1988) Selective neurotomy of the tibial nerve for treatment of the spastic foot. *Neurosurgery*, **23**, 738–744.

Sindou, M., Fischer, G., Goutelle A. & Mansuy, L. (1974a) La radicellotomie postérieure sélective. Premiers résultats dans la chirurgie de la douleur. *Neurochirurgie*, **20**, 391–408.

Sindou, M., Fischer, G., Goutelle, A., Schott, B. & Mansuy, L. (1974b) La radicellotomie postérieure sélective dans le traitement des spasticités. *Rev. Neurol.*, **130**, 201–215.

Sindou, M., Quoex, C. & Baleydier, C. (1974c) Fiber organization at the posterior spinal cord-rootlet junction in man. *J. Comp. Neurol.*, **153**, 15–26.

Sindou, M., Fischer, G. & Mansuy, L. (1976) Posterior spinal rhizotomy and selective posterior rhizidiotomy. *Prog. Neurol. Surg.*, 7, 201–250.

Sindou, M., Millet, M.F., Mortamais, J. & Eyssette, M. (1982) Results of selective posterior rhizotomy in the treatment of painful and spastic paraplegia secondary to multiple sclerosis. *Appl. Neurophysiol.*, **45**, 335–340.

Sindou, M., Abdennebi, B. & Sharkey, P. (1985a) Microsurgical selective procedures in the peripheral nerves and the posterior root–spinal cord junction for spasticity. *Appl. Neurophysiol.*, **48**, 97–104.

Sindou, M., Pregelj, R., Boisson, D., Eyssette, M. & Goutelle, A. (1985b) Surgical selective lesions of nerve fibers and myelotomies for the modification of muscle hypertonia. In Sir Eccles, J. & Dimitrijevic, M.R. (eds), *Recent Achievements in Restorative Neurology: Upper Motor Neuron Functions and Dysfunctions*, pp. 10–26. Karger, Basel.

Sindou, M., Mifsud, J.J., Boisson, D. & Goutelle, A. (1986) Selective posterior rhizotomy in the dorsal root entry zone for treatment of hyperspasticity and pain in the hemiplegic upper limb. *Neurosurgery*, **18**, 587–595.

Stoffel, A. (1913) The treatment of spastic contractures. *Am. J. Orthop. Surg.*, **10**, 611–619.

Storrs, B. (1967) Selective posterior rhizotomy for treatment of progressive spasticity in patients with myelomeningocele. *Pediat. Neurosci.*, **13**, 135–137.

Tardieu, G., Got, G. & Lespargot, A. (1975) Indications d'un nouveau type d'infiltration au point moteur (alcool à 90°). Application clinique d'une étude expérimentale. *Ann.*

Med. Phys., **18**, 539–557.
Uematsu, S., Udvarhelyi, G.B., Benson, D.W. & Siebens, A.A. (1974) Percutaneous radiofrequency rhizotomy. *Surg. Neurol.*, **2**, 319–325.
Wall, P.D. (1974) Presynaptic control of impulses at the first central synapse in the cutaneous pathway. *Prog. Brain Res.*, **12**, 92–118.
Wiesendanger, M. (1989) Neurobiology of spasticity. In Emre, M. & Benecke, R. (eds), *Spasticity: The Current Status of Research and Treatment*, pp. 45–61. Parthenon, Lancashire.
Young, B. & Mulcachy, J.J. (1980) Percutaneous sacral rhizotomy for neurogenic detrusor hyperreflexia. *J. Neurosurg.*, **53**, 85–87.
Young, R.R. & Delwaide, P.J. (1981) Drug therapy: spasticity. *N. Engl. J. Med.*, **304**, 28–33.

58 · Pain and its Management

By J.C.D. WELLS and J.B. MILES

Pain is an important and complex human experience. The Taxonomy Committee of the International Association for the Study of Pain (Mersky, 1979) defined pain as 'an unpleasant sensory and emotional experience associated with actual or potential tissue damage, or described in terms of such damage'. Mersky went on to observe that pain is always subjective. Each individual learns the application of the word through experiences related to injury in early life. It is unquestionably a sensation in a part of the body, but it is also unpleasant, and therefore also an emotional experience. Many people report pain in the absence of tissue damage or any likely pathophysiological cause; usually this happens for psychological reasons. There is no way to distinguish their experience from that due to tissue damage, if we take this subjective report.

The Office of Health Economics in the United Kingdom (1985) indicated that back pain was the third most frequently described symptom in apparently normal healthy people. Twenty-one per cent of normal people complained of backache over a one-month period. About one-tenth of these consulted their general practitioner, resulting in an estimated 2.2 million consultations per year for back pain! There were 330 000 hospital referrals a year and 63 000 hospital inpatient treatments a year, averaging two weeks, for back pain. Sixty per cent of these patients have unspecified backache, still not diagnosed when discharged.

All surgeons who operate on the spine are sometimes confronted with the problem of a patient with chronic spinal pain which has persisted in spite of 'conventional' treatment. Forty per cent of patients referred to pain clinicians come into this category, and almost certainly this figure would be much higher should there be an open-door policy to pain clinics, or if the waiting time for being seen in such clinics could be reduced.

There is usually little doubt but that the pain originates from the spine, but its true causation or mechanism of perpetuation is often uncertain and may remain so.

ANALYSIS OF THE PROBLEM

The first responsibility of the specialist pain clinician will be to review the natural history of the condition and the treatment to date, and thereby to review or even challenge the diagnosis or diagnoses previously entertained. This throws a great responsibility on the doctor concerned, and this is best tolerated in a multidisciplinary group environment (Miles, 1989a). Conventional disease processes might still be active and capable of responding to conventional treatment (O'Brien, 1984). If still no diagnosis can be recognized, or if the condition has advanced beyond the range of available treatment, then measures directed specifically and exclusively to relieving the pain may be indicated.

With reference to the spine, it is not uncommon for patients to present at the pain clinic who are still suffering from a disease process which might be amenable to conventional therapy. Some of the more common examples of this are briefly discussed.

Patients with radicular pain may arrive in the pain clinic with an undiagnosed or inadequately treated lumbar disc prolapse or bony entrapment of the nerve root. A careful review of the history of the symptoms, such as the onset being associated with effort, with aggravating features such as coughing, and alleviation with lying down, may clearly suggest that a disc fragment may still be present, causing or aggravating the symptoms complained of. Modern radiological diagnosis will usually confirm this but exploration is still worthy of consideration, especially in patients having had previous surgery who have recurrent radicular pain, even when the most sophisticated modern diagnostic investigations have failed to confirm the presence of a disc.

The pain of instability of the spine is present on weight-bearing and on turning, and may be relieved by recumbency or splinting. Radiographs may show malalignment, subluxation or dislocation, but it is the clinical syndrome and particularly the description of the pain that establishes the diagnosis and the need for its treatment by some form of fixation or fusion. The assessment of patients for fusion is extremely complex and is discussed in detail in Chapter 44.

The so-called 'facetal syndrome' causes pain on movement, and specifically during a particular movement such as extension of the spine or rotation of the spine, or a combination of the two (Murley, 1978). A painful arc in the movement may be evident. Focal pressure on the appropriate joint may provoke the pain, including that part that might be radiating into a limb. Local anti-inflammatory treatment may prove therapeutic as well as diagnostic, but the syndrome may be or may become part of an instability of the whole segment (Mooney & Robertson, 1975).

Spinal stenosis may give rise to compression of neural elements and cause pain and neurological dysfunction. When the stenosis is in the cervical or thoracic region there should be evidence of persisting spastic weakness and/or sensory loss with a level, as it is the spinal cord that is being compressed. In the lumbar region when the roots of the cauda equina are compressed, pain is the dominant symptom, usually occurring only when the patient is in the standing position or when walking, while neurological dysfunction, motor or sensory, may not be recognized in the resting state.

Stenosis of the intervertebral nerve root canal may similarly cause intermittent symptoms of pain in a single nerve root distribution and, like stenosis of the vertebral canal, demands appropriate treatment in the form of surgical decompression.

These four recognizable conditions may coexist or contribute to a more complex pain syndrome that may still require their treatment as part of the overall management.

The most common tumour of the vertebral spine will be malignant (Findlay, 1987). The most common site will be in the vertebral body, whether the tumour is a primary or metastatic growth (Miles *et al.*, 1984).

The most common tumour pain will be that typical of an expansion of the bone and probably emanating from the periosteum. It will tend to constancy but being worse at night. When the bone morphology has been lost in weight-bearing or mobile bones, instability pain will supervene.

The symptoms may persist for months, and may often be attributed to other causes, such as trauma. Again, clinical awareness is paramount and there is definitely a place for repeating the radiographs, as the true nature of the condition may well not be disclosed by the first films. Scanning, especially by magnetic resonance, most clearly indicates tumour in bone; isotope bone scanning, although non-specific, is also important.

Of the intradural tumours neurofibromas will tend to cause a radiculopathy pain, especially from the cauda equina, while the extrinsic meningioma rarely, and the intrinsic astrocytomas or ependymomas more commonly, are likely to cause myelopathic, central, dysaesthetic pain syndromes. Their presence can be recognized only by constant vigilance and a sound neurological examination technique.

Congenital causes for chronic pain abound. Spinal dysraphism, particularly at the lumbosacral region, but also at any level, may be associated with occult dermoids, lipomas, tetherings and bony instabilities that can all have pain as a prominent feature, and all may have their presentation delayed into adulthood.

Ischaemic vascular accidents of the cord commonly give rise to central dysaesthetic pain. Arteriovenous malformations can suddenly bleed, but more commonly insidiously give rise to radiating radiculopathic pains or dysaesthetic myelopathic pain. If there has been no recognizable bleed then again neurological deficit is the clinical clue, and myelography or magnetic resonance imaging is the diagnostic investigation.

RECOGNITION OF PSYCHOLOGICAL FACTORS

The assessment of patients with low back pain is discussed fully in Chapter 36. It is obviously essential to assess the psychological factors involved in the maintenance of chronic back pain, before embarking on major therapeutic interventions. All too often patients are seen in the pain relief clinic who have been told that surgery will put things right, and when it hasn't, a referral letter is sent suggesting that they are psychologically or psychiatrically unstable. Surely this diagnosis needs to be made before the surgery and not afterwards! Fortunately, an understanding of illness behaviour and psychological techniques is becoming more and more recognized by surgeons managing back pain. Neither is it possible to label the patient as having psychogenic pain in the absence of known organic pathology. Specific factors must be identified in the history and lifestyle, in order to ensure that as yet undiagnosed physical pathology is not labelled as psychogenic (Main & Spanswick, 1991).

SPECIFIC TREATMENTS FOR PAIN

Drugs

These can be classified into four types. Firstly there are non-steroidal anti-inflammatory agents, secondly opioid derivatives, thirdly opioid agents themselves and fourthly novel compounds often used in pain relief units to reduce pain (Budd, 1983).

Non-steroidal anti-inflammatory agents are agents which work as prostaglandin synthetase inhibitors and may all produce gastrointestinal irritation (Huskisson, 1984). Their use is applicable wherever an inflammatory component is thought to contribute to the pain, when it can be given a therapeutic trial. It must be remembered that many patients will have taken, or will be taking, over-the-counter anti-inflammatory agents, and they must be questioned about this. Aspirin and paracetamol are as good as any others in their effect, the dose of aspirin being 300–900 mg every 4–6 hours, and paracetamol 0.5–1 g every 4–6 hours, to a maximum of 4 g per day. Naproxen 250 mg, one or two twice daily, or diflunisal, 250 mg, one or two twice daily, offer a dosage regime which may be more convenient to the patient and better-remembered.

Opioid derivatives such as codeine, dextropropoxyphene and dihydrocodeine can be used with great effectiveness for acute pain, but are not so useful for chronic pain. They were introduced because of the lesser incidence of side-effects compared with opioids, but in chronic usage these side-effects can become as frequent as those from opioids in acute pain. If they are effective, allowing the patient greater mobility and a significant increase in activity, then they can be continued. However, often the analgesic effect wears off, which can leave the patient with a drug habituation problem and side-effects such as constipation. None of these drugs should be used for more than six weeks without medical assessment, to ensure that they are not being abused. Pentazocine and buprenorphine are agonist–antagonist drugs which do not have the same incidence of addiction. However, they can be addictive and also cause proportionally more side-effects; neither are they well-tolerated by a significant number of patients. They are best avoided. Nefopam (Acupan) is a drug of which the mode of action is not fully understood. It is relatively weak.

Opioids are extremely useful for postoperative or cancer pain, but not for the management of chronic back pain. A significant number of chronic pain patients have been commenced on these drugs, become addicted, and often present an insurmountable problem. They need admission to hospital for weaning from their drug, often with a long-acting opiate such as methadone, before any sensible treatment can be commenced. They should be used only in the rarest of circumstances, and particularly have very little effect on neurogenic pain (Hardy, 1991).

Secondary analgesics are drugs which have pain-relieving properties, but which are marketed primarily for some other property (Wells, 1987). They can be classified according to the primary mode of action.

Psychoactive drugs

ANTIDEPRESSANTS

Patients with chronic pain are often depressed, either as a cause or consequence of their pain. In many patients who respond to treatment with these drugs, the pain and the depression may resolve equally. However, there are some in whom the depression will lift without affecting the pain, and others in whom there appears to be no evidence of depression, who nonetheless achieve benefit. Sometimes these patients get pain relief on doses well below that which would be expected to cause mood elevation. It has been suggested that the analgesic action of these drugs is caused by their action on neurotransmitter function, in reducing the amount of noradrenalin in the nerve terminals. Many trials have been carried out with conflicting evidence, and Monks (1981) found that amitriptyline 25 mg at night, increasing if tolerated, tends to improve sleep as well as mood, but reduces pain in only about one-quarter of patients. It is particularly useful whenever burning pain is described by the patient, or of course whenever there are signs of depression or sleep deprivation. Many patients complain of a dry mouth, constipation, fluid retention and weight increase, and there may also be problems with decreased visual accommodation. These drugs are contra-indicated in cardiovascular disease because of palpitations, and also urinary retention and aggravation of glaucoma may occur. Some of the more recent agents such as maprotiline, 25 mg at night, appear to have less side-effects, but may be even less effective as pain relievers. Antidepressants are now probably used too often for chronic back pain (Hanks, 1987; Wells & Miles, 1991).

Monoamine oxidase inhibitors have been used with success in certain intractable pain conditions, but their use is limited by their interactions with many other drugs and with foodstuffs. Phenelzine, 15 mg three times a day, is the agent most commonly used, and they are said to have a specific effectiveness in patients with hypochondriasis, pain and depression. Unfortunately many pain patients are reluctant to forgo their cheese and Bovril, let alone their chianti!

ANTICONVULSANTS

Pain of a lancinating or shooting nature is often due to nerve damage, and may respond to anticonvulsants. This has been widely recognized in the treatment of trigeminal neuralgia, since the use of carbamazepine for this condition in the 1960s (Crill, 1973). Although back pain itself is unlikely to respond to this treatment, postlaminectomy shooting pain and other nerve irritation pains may all respond to anticonvulsants (Bowsher, 1991). Sodium valproate, 200–500 mg three times a day, tends to be best tolerated. Carbamazepine can be used in doses of up to 400 mg four times a day, but all of the anticonvulsants may produce drowsiness, dizziness, skin rashes and blood dyscrasias.

TRANQUILLIZERS

Minor tranquillizers such as the benzodiazepines, and major tranquillizers such as phenothiazine derivatives and the butyrophenones, have all been used to try to control chronic back pain. The latter two compounds exhibit analgesic properties among their other effects. However, they also can produce bothersome side-effects, and all tranquillizers are potentially habit-forming. They must consequently be used with great caution. Many patients do have muscle spasm, but the long-term use of tranquillizers will not reduce this, and these patients are much better treated by teaching various relaxation techniques or self-hypnosis. These drugs can be used for short periods with effect, and in conjunction with other treatments aimed at improving mobility, and self-reliance.

Muscle relaxants

Nearly all patients with chronic back pain have increased muscle tone. Drugs such as orphenadrine, 30 mg three times a day, and methocarbamol, 1.5 mg daily, have been used, but results are generally disappointing. These drugs inhibit restive segmental interneuronal discharge in the cord, and may often be found in preparations in combination with simple analgesics. Severe muscle spasm, particularly associated with neurological syndromes, has been treated with baclofen (5 mg three times a day), and dantrolene (25 mg a day). This dosage is increased as tolerated, until a useful effect is achieved. Drowsiness, weakness and confusion can follow treatment, and in general these drugs are not well tolerated. Baclofen has a specific analgesic action, and has been used spinally to some effect.

Steroids

These may be used orally for short periods, especially in certain forms of degenerative disease. However, more often they are used by local injection into the epidural space. Injection into the joint spaces to reduce pain in the short term could accelerate the eventual degeneration of a joint in the long term.

Other drugs

Many other drugs are used in the management of chronic pain. These include enzyme-blocking drugs, such as delucine, transmitter precursors (L-tryptophan), and various peptides (Budd, 1983). Calcitonin has been used for Paget's disease and osteoporosis. Although some of these drugs show promise, as yet there is little general advice that can be given as to their usage, and they must remain as experimental agents to be further evaluated by pioneering units.

Nerve blocks

Pain can be alleviated during surgery by means of regional neurogenic blockade. This is done easily on a temporary basis, and usually with excellent results (McQuay *et al.*, 1988; Tverskoy *et al.*, 1990), and so it is tempting for the doctor to think that a more permanent block would achieve just as excellent a permanent result for chronic pain. Unfortunately permanent damage to the nerves generally leads to unpleasant sequelae (Wells, 1989). First of all there will often be damage to sensory and motor fibres, with an unpleasant lack of sensory input, or worse, lack of important movement. Secondly, even if weakness or paralysis can be avoided, damage to nerve tissue leads to instant and irreversible, and possibly progressive, central nervous system changes, which may sooner or later be evidenced as a neurological pain syndrome. Thus an unpleasant and disabling phantom pain is experienced in the original area, although the pain is now being generated centrally, and is largely untreatable.

The use of local anaesthetic blockade fulfils two functions. Firstly, by blocking off selected pathways there may be an indication as to which particular pathway is transmitting the pain, enabling the condition and its underlying cause to be more readily identified, or giving a prognostic indication as to the possible efficacy of a more permanent procedure. Secondly, in chronic pain the mere interruption of a pain pathway for a few hours can sometimes result in longer-term pain relief. Thus a patient with chronic back pain, with associated muscle spasm and possible psychosocial problems, may get long-term relief if the pain is eased for a short term and the muscle spasm allowed to settle.

The local anaesthetic can also be combined with a further therapeutic agent such as steroids, usually in a prolonged-release form such as Depo Medrone or Kenalog, in order to reduce any underlying inflammatory process. It may also be combined with guanethidine for sympathetic blockade. Other drugs may be injected spinally, into the epidural or subarachnoid spaces, in order to produce pain relief. These include clonidine, baclofen, opiates and benzodiazepines. However, their use is highly specialized and only within the remit of large, multidisciplinary pain centres.

Diagnostic blocks include paravertebral, intercostal, facet nerve and facet joint injections, local infiltration of trigger points, blockage of the lumbar sympathetic chain and also differential spinal blockade (Wilson, 1976). In this latter procedure, increasing concentrations of local anaesthetic are given into the cerebrospinal fluid to assess the patient's response to a placebo, sympathetic block, sensory and then motor blockade (Winnie & Collins, 1968). If pain is still present after this, and in a surprising number of patients it still is, it must be assumed that the pain is central, and not amenable to direct attacks upon the spine and soft tissues. Local anaesthetic can also be given intravenously; it is said to reduce the pain of nerve damage, and is supposed to carry a prognostic significance as to the efficacy of anticonvulsants and membrane-stabilizing drugs such as mexiletine. However, undoubtedly it also has an effect on psychogenic pain.

Epidural injections can be performed easily via the lumbar route, or via caudal injection through the sacral route. There is much conflicting evidence as to their efficacy, including whether or not steroids should be used, whether or not a manipulation of the spine should be carried out, and so on. Undoubtedly, as the management of back pain has involved more investigation, with possible referral to specialist surgeons, the use of epidural blocks has been greatly reduced. As they are relatively cheap, simple to perform and seem to have a very low incidence of side-effects, this is probably an appropriate treatment which is now being underutilized.

Many theories have been advanced to explain the possible beneficial effects. The pressure of the large volume of fluid injected may assist in freeing a nerve root stretched in some way, and the local anaesthetic would relieve pain from sensitive peridural structures which were inflamed in some way. Adhesions or scar tissue may also be weakened or reduced, and muscle spasm, which has been referred to previously, will be stopped, and a vicious cycle of pain and spasm may be removed. Steroids might be beneficial in relieving the inflammation and oedema of compressed nerve tissue, or inflamed and swollen peridural structures.

In the past three years, the authors have looked for filling defects in the epidural space by means of carrying out an epidurogram. The epidural injection is monitored using a C-arm image intensifier, and niopam or omnipaque is injected when the needle is in the correct position within the epidural space. This produces a classical appearance, with the nerve roots being seen to spread out in a symmetrical pattern on either side. If there is evidence of reduced filling, then this area can have the needle manipulated into it, and after injection of local anaesthetic, steroids and hyalase (1500 units), dye can be injected once more and the improvement monitored (Wells, 1991).

Degenerative changes in the intervertebral joints are accepted as a source of back pain in a significant number of patients. Indeed there are a number of structures in this area which may produce symptoms, not only the facetal joints. However, an injection of local anaesthetic and steroids, either within the joint or laid down near to it, may produce pain relief (Mehta, 1978). Attempts have been made to denervate the facet joints, but no control studies have been carried out to establish whether this is more effective than a local anaesthetic and steroid injection. Injection of the capsules of the facet joints, and infiltration with local anaesthetic in this area, if it does produce instant pain relief, may indicate that subsequent fusion procedures might be more likely to be effective.

Acupuncture

The oldest known book on acupuncture was written in 300 BC. Undoubtedly, however, the technique extends back much earlier than that. The name was coined by a Dutch physician, Willem ten Rhyne (1683) from 'acus', meaning a needle, and 'puncturo' meaning puncture. It has been used as a treatment for all sorts of conditions, but primarily for the relief of acute pain, and it has been possible to perform surgery under acupuncture analgesia, initially in China. It is now used widely by many clinicians, and of course by many non-medical practitioners, in the relief of chronic pain. It has achieved credibility with many previously doubting and unimpressionable scientists. There is a wealth of conflicting scientific data on its mode of action, influencing factors and the like, and of course there may be a significant placebo effect, but there is also some form of useful analgesia effected on some patients which lasts for a varying period of time (Kenyon, 1979; Kenyon *et al.*, 1983).

It is now generally accepted that stimulation of descending inhibitory pain pathways, with possible endorphin release, has a large part to play in acupuncture analgesia. As there is a very low incidence of side-effects it must deserve a place in the treatment of chronic pain, in particular for some patients for whom nothing else seems to be of benefit. It must be performed on a regular basis; like most treatments it does have a finite length of action and it does not cure the patient. At present it is almost impossible for patients to get regular treatment through the Health Service, and consequently they must turn elsewhere. This will only result in them getting into unskilled, and possibly unscrupulous, hands, and it seems a nonsense that this treatment is not more readily available throughout the Health Service on an outpatient basis. Over £6 million per year is spent on the use of corsets for back pain in the Health Service, without one iota of evidence that they do any good, but merely on the personal prejudice of the consultants concerned, and undoubtedly this money could be better spent on provision of acupuncture analgesia.

Electrical stimulation

Transcutaneous nerve stimulation (TNS) has its origins in the use of naturally generated electricity, such as in the *Torpedo* fish. It is reported to have been used to relieve chronic pain by the application of the fish, or more specifically the area of its electric organ, to the painful part of the patient. There it provoked a numbing sensation (torpor) and relieved the pain. Hand-generated electricity was extensively used to relieve pain and cure disease in the 19th century, but it received scientific credit only after the proposition of the gate control theory for pain and its relief, by Melzack & Wall (1965).

TNS can be used as a simple pair of electrodes or a more complex array of multiple electrodes, placed on the skin of the patient in the vicinity of the pain. The generated electricity must provoke paraesthesia in the area of pain, and for the best response the paraesthetic tingling must mix in with the pain and must in itself prove a pleasant substitute for the pain. TNS is thus readily applied to the painful neck, arm and leg, but with more difficulty to the wide areas of the back (Fig. 58.1). Still, with ingenuity, perseverance, and especially if assistance is available, patients with even widespread trunk pain due to degenerative

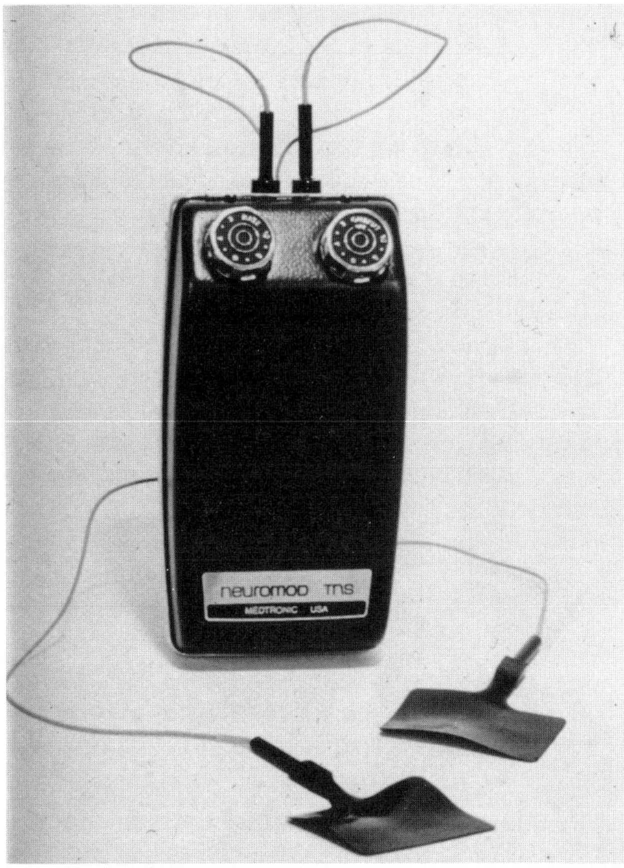

Fig. 58.1 Simple, single channel TNS machine.

disease can maintain a satisfactory degree of comfort for many years. The more the pain is somatic in origin, rather than neurogenic, the more likely is TNS to suppress it. If the deficit is so great that no paraesthesia will project into the painful area, then no relief will be obtained.

Conventional TNS is used at high (50–150) frequency and low output, while acupuncture, unlike TNS, is used at low (2–5) frequency and high output (the exact output will depend on tissue resistance, and therefore be determined by the area of the body being treated). Either form of electrical stimulation can relieve pain of spinal origin and therefore should be tried. Woolff (1989) has summarized the reported differential specificity for the two electrical modes.

Dorsal column stimulation (DCS) or spinal cord stimulation was applied to the human in pain within two years of the gate control theory, in 1967, by Shealy *et al.* It proved possible to design and manufacture electrical implants that could be induced into repeated and long-term activity, because of the progress already made in the production of cardiac pacemakers (Fig. 58.2).

Implanted stimulators were quickly tried for a wide range of pains due to both malignant and benign conditions. They have proved successful in almost all chronic pains, but only in a proportion of the sufferers. Pain relief from malignancy has often

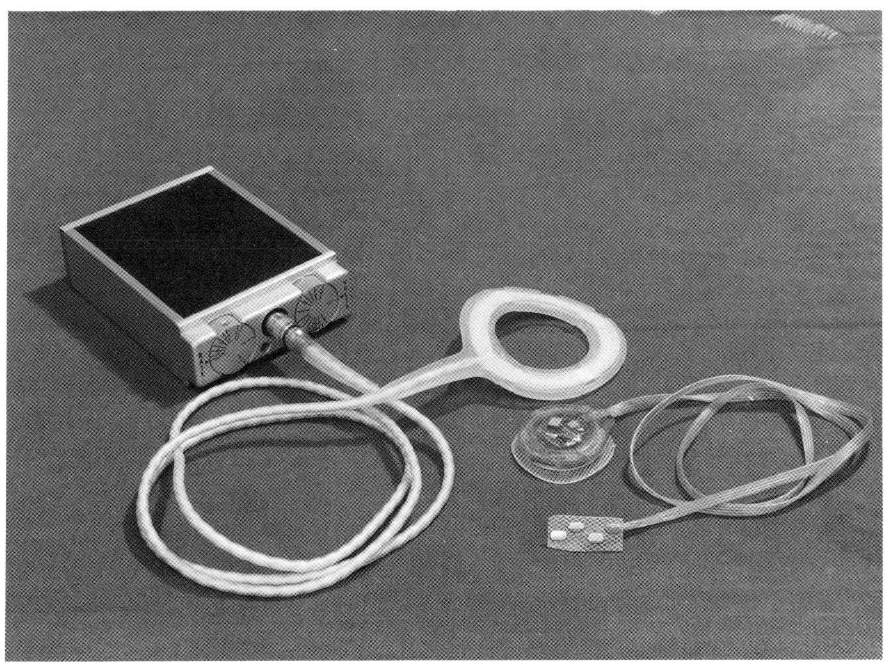
Fig. 58.2 Dorsal column stimulator. The implant is on the right and the transmitter is on the left.

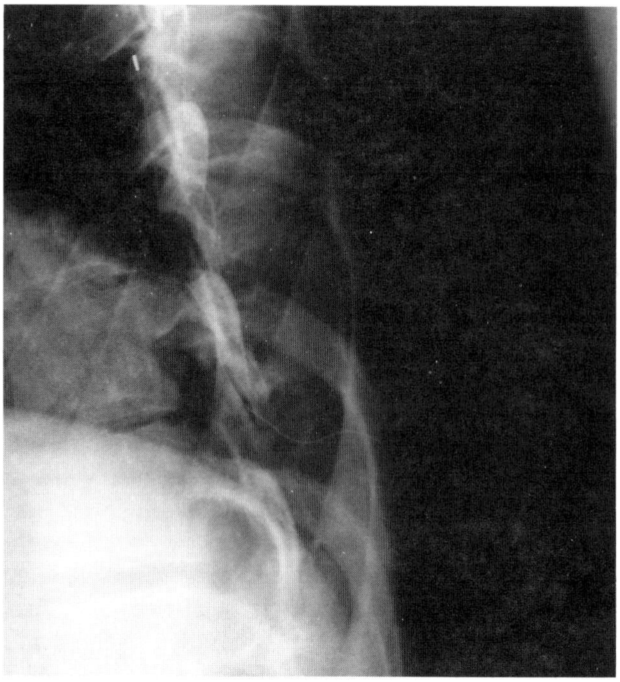

Fig. 58.3 Lateral view showing fine trial electrode inserted percutaneously via a Tuohy needle.

proved to be inadequate in degree, and the method has been more readily applied to chronic pains associated with non-malignant conditions. Many of the pains already described, such as those due to degenerative conditions of the spine, come into this category, but specifically not that of instability and those associated with major or total sensory loss.

Assessment as to suitability for this treatment is difficult but absolutely essential to attempt. The consequences of failure to relieve pain after surgical implantation are to further insult the already injured chronic pain patient—both psychologically and physically, and to have expended a great deal of expensive time and equipment to no avail.

The details of assessment are beyond the scope of this book, but must include intensive pharmacological, psychological and physiological scrutiny. Analysis of factors influencing the pain, on the basis that electrical stimulation is a form of counter-irritation, is most important (Miles, 1983). A trial period of percutaneous stimulation with an indwelling wire electrode is virtually obligatory (Fig. 58.3).

Patients with back and leg pain that has failed to respond to conventional surgery (failed back syndrome, arachnoiditis, etc.) constitute a potentially inexhaustible supply of candidates for this treatment. The more the pain is in the leg, rather than in the back, and the less there is obvious neurological deficit, the more likely is this treatment to work, but each patient requires individual and careful scrutiny. Pain relief from successful implants can reduce with time (Krainick & Thoden, 1980), but also has now been shown to be capable of persisting for more than 15 years (Meyerson, 1989; Miles, 1989b).

Radiculopathic and myelopathic pain syndromes due to slow-growing tumours, such as ependymoma, congenital abnormalities and vascular causes can undoubtedly prove treatable by spinal cord stimulation. As with TNS, the less the neurological deficit, the more it is possible to project the paraesthesiae into the painful regions and the more the pain will be relieved.

Surgical techniques

Deep brain stimulation (DBS) can also relieve pain of spinal, spinal cord and peripheral nerve origin. A similar implant circuit is used with an electrode designed for insertion into the brain (thalamus, or medial lemniscus tract) using stereotactic techniques. This method has proved popular and effective in many parts of North America even when necessitating bilateral implantation for bilateral leg pain. In Britain, patients are undoubtedly more resistant to the idea of cerebral implantation for non-life-threatening conditions.

Dorsal root entry zone (DREZ) destruction

Anterolateral cordotomy by either the open surgical or percutaneous radiofrequency method is no longer practised for benign persistent pain syndromes. It does not last long enough, and is increasingly prone to actually provoking new dysaesthetic pain. DREZ lesioning is used for some benign persistent pain syndromes, and amongst those affecting the spine perhaps the best treated is the boundary dysaesthetic pain syndrome sometimes encountered in paraplegic patients. The likelihood of total relief is high, while the added neurological deficit by performing this procedure over four to six segments, at the level of the paraplegia, provokes minimal additional loss. Why this further destruction does not provoke further pain, like much surgical logic, remains a mystery.

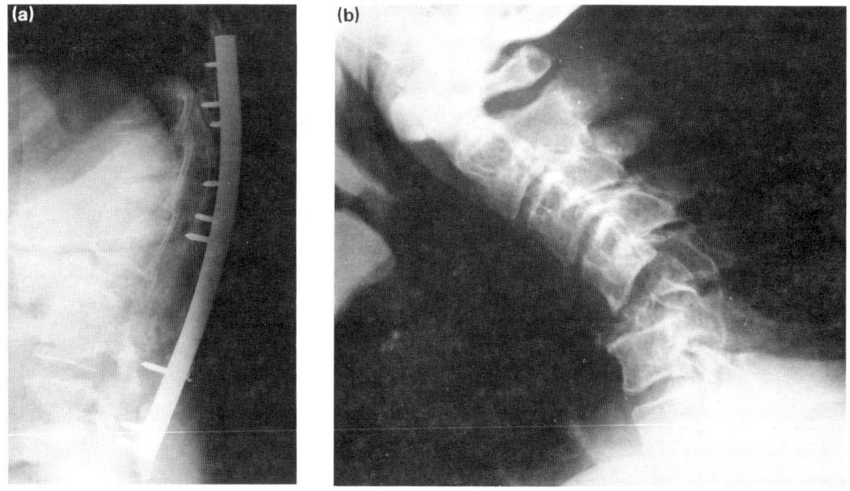

Fig. 58.4 (a) Posterior segmental fixation with a Banks–Dervir bar in a patient with severe pain due to multiple spinal metastases from carcinoma of the breast. (b) Severe kyphotic deformity due to metastasis from carcinoma of prostate.

Fixation of the spine in malignancy

There is a need to restate the case for surgical stabilization for the relief of instability pain in the patient with malignant tumour of the vertebral spine. None of the measures designed to attempt to suppress the tumour itself will relieve this type of pain, though they can and should be used in addition to fixation. When the tumour suggests a suitable degree of indolence in its natural history, and when the patient exhibits sufficient biological resilience, then radical surgical removal of the tumour with fusion, preferably using bone grafting, should be undertaken. However, the majority of patients by the time of presentation will not come into this category, and may still need, and benefit from, surgical fixation by the simplest secure method available (Figs 58.4 & 58.5).

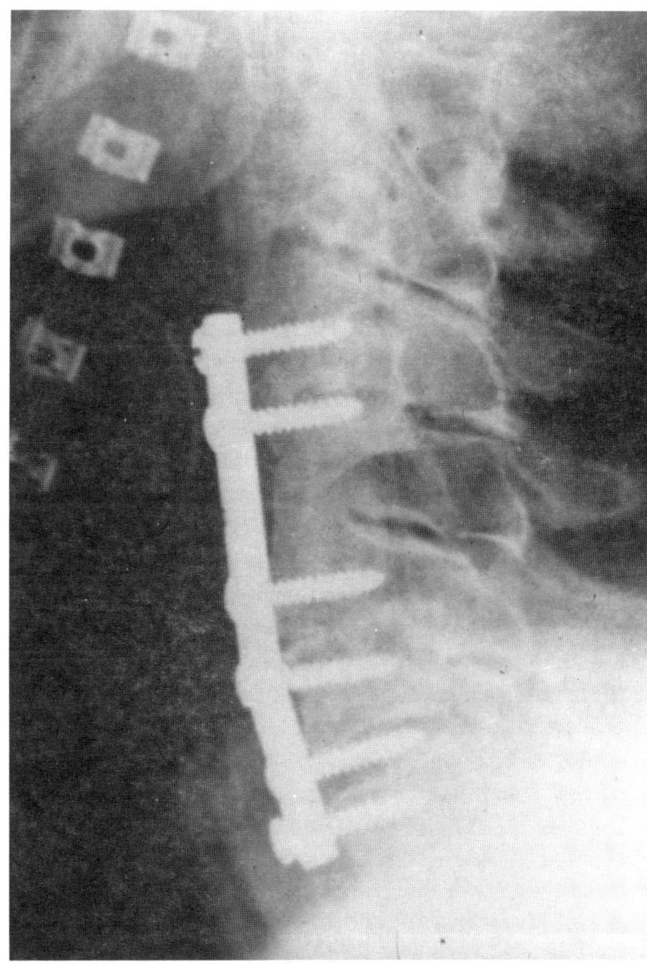

Fig. 58.5 Postoperative view of patient shown in Fig. 58.4b. The metastasis has been resected, grafted and stabilized by the anterior approach.

Psychological techniques

All injury or nociception produces an emotional response. This response modifies the pain perception itself. Whilst this is important in the appreciation of what happens in acute pain, it is even more important in patients with chronic pain. The original injury may have healed completely, but either some unknown neurobiochemical process, or an emotional or psychological response, or perhaps both, have allowed the pain to continue. Most patients will be both depressed and frustrated (Tyrer, 1985; Ward, 1990); indeed, if they are somewhat euphoric an element of hysteria may be suspected in the 'causation' of the pain. The mood changes may predate, or follow, the onset of the pain; however, this is usually impossible to determine (Main & Spanswick 1991).

Simple relaxation training, available from psychologists or occupational therapists, can help many chronic pain sufferers (Linton & Gotestan, 1984). Not only does it relax overtight muscles, but it also gives the patient a measure of self-control over the problem, rather than constantly seeking medical help for a condition which is not curable. The relaxation may be extended to meditation, hypnosis or biofeedback (Keefe *et al.*, 1981). More extensive psychological training, including behaviour modification therapy or operant conditioning, has been widely used for many years in the United States (Aronoff *et al.*, 1983). It is important to stress to these patients that the therapist believes in their pain and suffering, as all too often these patients have been told that they are mad, or that their pain is imaginary.

Specific psychiatric illnesses need to have careful evaluation by a psychiatrist with an interest in pain, rather than someone who just wants to fit patients into diagnostic categories such as schizophrenia or depression. The most useless interaction is involved with those psychiatrists who merely say 'well, if your pain was better you wouldn't be feeling so bad'. These doctors do not realize the multidimensional nature of pain (Turk & Flor, 1984), and do the patient a great disservice. Psychologists can be much more useful for the chronic back pain sufferer, particularly as patients are more readily able to accept seeing such a specialist, given the explanation that 'this is a paramedic who helps you to cope with your thoughts about your condition'.

In the pain centre at Walton Hospital, Liverpool, a multidisciplinary pain management programme is run for the rehabilitation of chronic pain sufferers, of which over 50% have back pain. This programme has been running since 1982, and started with the recognition of three major factors in the chronic pain sufferer for whom all other treatment had failed. First of all, psychological changes have taken place, so that the patient shows features such as depression, sleeplessness, inactivity, lack of fitness, excessive drug consumption, pain behaviours and cognitive dysfunction, which pattern has been labelled the 'chronic pain syndrome'. Secondly, patients have become apprehensive about movement, leading to further reduction in fitness, and compensatory muscle spasm whenever any activity is attempted. They have become wary of their pain, and are looking for it to come and then identifying it as a warning of ongoing tissue damage. Thirdly these patients have become very reliant on the medical profession, the Health Service, their family and friends and the state, for means of payments for their illness status (Wells & Miles, 1991).

Fordyce (1976) and Sternbach (1974) in the United States treated such patients in a behavioural setting. Using operant conditioning, they showed these patients that pain behaviour could be abolished, and their function improved. Subsequent work has added cognitive elements to these programmes, and the psychologists involved in our programme use both behavioural and cognitive techniques in order to influence the patients' perception of their pain, and their behaviours. Relaxation training, by means of intermittent tensing and relaxing of muscles, and also by means of a self-hypnosis technique, is used firstly to produce a reduction of muscle spasm and decreasing resting tone, and secondly to give the patients a sense of self-control and responsibility for their health and the management of their pain. Thirdly, a programme of exercises is carried out which builds up muscle tone, stretches up shortened tendons and ligaments and improves peripheral blood flow. It is aimed to increase activity by less than 10% every day, but on a long-term basis. Patients are retrained in correct posture and locomotion (Pither & Nicholas, 1991).

The Walton programme is a four-week one, with two new patients starting every week and joining a group which thus totals eight. Patients in their last week are expected to offer help to the new patients, not only explaining the timetable and what is done, but also giving positive reassurance that the course might be of benefit. Indeed, the impact of new pain sufferers seeing people who have made great improvements over the four weeks is perhaps a major reason for the success of the programme. Patients have a daily schedule of exercise, including dance, yoga and T'ai Chi, as well as physiotherapy. There are also individual targets and a speedwalk. Targets and goals are set in all aspects of the programme, not only in exercise but also in social skills and activities in the home. Thus the pain is not allowed to stop the patients from doing things; neither are they allowed to use the pain as an excuse for taking drugs. Another of the important factors involved in their rehabilitation is in them being within a group of other people, all striving for improvement in activities, rather than moaning about their discomfort. Many patients with chronic pain become socially isolated, and very dependent upon their families. Following completion of the programme they are encouraged to come back to a Self-help In Pain group, which has been set up by ex-patients, and which meets on a regular basis.

The programme has now been running for eight years, and over 800 patients have completed it. It is unusual for their pain to be greatly affected. A small percentage (17%) do have a 50% reduction long-term in their pain, but most improve slightly, or remain as uncomfortable. However, a very significant proportion (78%) improve their activities to a very significant degree during the four weeks. Even at six months, 47% show a great improvement in their activity. The patients' usage of chronic and possibly addictive drugs is also reduced, as also is their reliance on the health-care system, and their subsequent search for further treatment, particularly invasive treatment. Some 30% of patients in the job market manage to return to work, even though the mean time off work prior to the programme for this group was 2.4 years. This obviously represents a very significant saving in benefits, as well as being of great satisfaction to the pain sufferer and his or her family.

Back pain is a common condition which is difficult to treat. It is a significant economic load on the population and health resources, and a severe emotional and financial strain on many patients and their families. The cause is often multifactorial, with structural damage, myofascial pain (Travell & Simons, 1984), nerve damage (Bowsher, 1991) and psychological causes all playing a part to produce a condition which is extremely difficult to treat effectively. This leads to a great deal of frustration in some doctors, with the inappropriate dismissal of the patient as a malingerer, or as imagining the pain. Other doctors seize upon some simple and superficial organic explanation, and attack the patient with a dazzling amount of medical technology, heaping operation upon operation, or corset upon crutches and collar, and reinforcing the patient's disability in his eyes and those of his family. Only meticulous assessment of these patients with back pain, to understand the various factors involved in maintaining their illnesses, can lead to an effective treatment programme, which almost certainly needs a multidisciplinary approach. As yet, this type of management often remains poorly organized and underfunded. Until surgeons, rheumatologists, pain specialists and psychologists get together in a determined effort to tackle the problem of chronic back pain, and insist that appropriate resources are channelled into appropriate assessment and management units, then it is unlikely that any more than a small minority of the millions of people who have chronic back pain will receive effective and useful treatments.

REFERENCES

Aronoff, G.M., Evans, W.O. & Enders, P.L. (1983) A review of follow-up studies of multi-disciplinary pain units. *Pain*, **16**, 1–11.

Bowsher, D. (1992) Management of neurogenic pain and injured nerve. In *Pain Mechanisms and Management* (In press).

Budd, K. (1983) Analgesic drugs. In Williams, N.E. & Wilson, H. (eds) Pain and its management. *International Encyclopaedia of Pharmacology and Therapeutics*, Section 112, pp. 51–64. Permagon Press, Oxford.

Crill, W. (1973) Carbamazepine. *Ann. Intern. Med.*, **79**, 79–80.

Findlay, G.F.G. (1987) Compression and vascular disease of the spinal cord. In Miller, J.D. (ed.) *Northfields' Surgery of the Central Nervous System*, 2nd edn. Blackwell Scientific Publications, Oxford.

Fordyce, W.E. (1976) *Behavioural Methods for Chronic Pain and Illness*. C.V. Mosby, St Louis, MO.

Hanks, G.W. (1987) Antidepressants in chronic pain: a clinical perspective. In *The Pain Clinic*, vol. 2, pp. 93–108. VNU Science Press, Utrecht.

Hardy, P.A.J. (1991) Use of opiates in treating chronic benign pain. *Br. J. Hosp. Med.*, **45**, 257.

Huskisson, E.C. (1984) In Melzack, R. & Wall, P.D. (eds) *A Textbook of Pain*, pp. 505–537. Churchill Livingstone, Edinburgh.

Keefe, F.J., Bloch, A.R., Williams, R.B. & Serwitt, R.J. (1981) Behavioural treatment outcome of chronic low back pain: clinical outcome and individual differences in pain relief. *Pain*, **11**, 221–231.

Kenyon, J.N. (1979) Acupuncture in pain relief. In Lipton, S. (ed.) *Persistent Pain—Modern Methods of Treatment*, vol. 2, pp. 203–222. Academic Press, London.

Kenyon, J.N., Knight, C.J. & Wells, J.C.D. (1983) A randomised double-blind trial on the immediate effects of naloxone on classical Chinese acupuncture for chronic pain. *Acu. Electrother. Res., Int. J.*, **8**, 17–24.

Krainick, J.-U. & Thoden, U. (1980) Pain reduction in amputees by long-term spinal cord stimulation. *J. Neurosurg.*, **52**, 346–350.

Linton, S.J. & Gotestan, K.G. (1984) A controlled study of the effects of applied relaxation and operant procedures in the regulation of chronic pain. *Br. J. Clin. Psychol.*, **23**, 291–299.

McQuay, H.J., Carroll, D. & Moore, R.A. (1988) Post-operative orthopaedic pain—the effect of opiate premedication and local anaesthetic blocks. *Pain*, **33**, 291–295.

Main, C.J. & Spanswick, C. (1992) In Wells, J.C.D. & Woolff, C.J. (eds) *Pain Mechanisms and Management* (In press).

Mehta, M. (1978) Facet joints and low back pain. *Br. Med. J.*, **1**, 1624.

Melzack, R. & Wall, P.D. (1965) Pain mechanisms: a new theory. *Science*, **150**, 971–979.

Mersky, H. (1979) Pain terms: a list with definition and notes on usage. Recommendation by IASP Sub-Committee on Taxonomy. *Pain*, **6**, 249–252.

Meyerson, B. (1989) Long-term treatment by dorsal column stimulation. Proceedings of the combined meeting of Scandinavian Pain Society and Intractable Pain Society, Oslo, April.

Miles, J.B. (1983) Surgical procedures for the relief of pain. In *Pain and its Management*, Sect. 112, pp. 89–98.

Miles J.B. (1989a) The neurosurgeon in the pain clinic. *Br. J. Neurosurg.*, **3**, 231–629.

Miles, J.B. (1989b) Assessment for dorsal column stimulation. Proceedings of the combined Meeting of the Scandinavian Pain Society and Intractable Pain Society, Oslo, April.

Miles, J.B., Banks, A.J., Dervin, E. & Noori, Z.N. (1984) Stabilisation of the spine affected by malignancy. **47**, 897–904.

Mooney, V.T. & Robertson, J. (1984) The facet syndrome. *Clin. Orthop. Rel. Res.*, **115**, 149–156.

Monks, R.C. (1981) The use of psychotropic drugs in human chronic pain: a review. *VIth World Congress of the International College of Psychosomatic Medicine.* Montreal, Canada, September.

Murley, A.H.G. (1978) Facet joints and low back pain. *Br. Med. J.*, **1**, 1283; **2**, 125–126.

O'Brien, J.P. (1984) In Melzack, R. & Wall, P.D. (eds) *A Textbook of Pain*, pp. 240–251. Churchill Livingstone, Edinburgh.

Office of Health Economics–Wells, N. (1985) *Back Pain*, p. 28.

Pither, C.E. & Nicholas, M.K. (1992) Psychological and psychiatric management. In Wells, J.C.D. & Woolff, C.J. (eds) *Pain Mechanisms and Management* (In press).

Shealy, C.N., Mortimer, J.T. & Reswick, R.J. (1967) Electrical inhibition of pain by stimulation of the dorsal column: preliminary clinical Report. *Anaes. Analg.*, **46**, 489–491.

Sternbach, R.A. (1974) *Pain Patients: Traits and Treatment.* Academic Press, New York.

Travell, J.G. & Simons, D.G. (1984) Myofascial pain syndromes. In Melzack, R. & Wall, P.D. (eds) *A Textbook of Pain*, pp. 263–276. Churchill Livingstone, Edinburgh.

Turk, D.C. & Flor, H. (1984) Aetiological theories and treatments for chronic back pain. II: Psychological models and interventions. *Pain*, **19**, 209–233.

Tverskoy, N., Cozacov, C., Ayache, M., Bradley, E.L. & Kissen, I. (1990) Post-operative pain after inguinal herniorrhaphy with different types of anaesthesia. *Anaes. Analg.*, **70**, 29–35.

Tyrer, S. (1985) The role of the psychiatrist in the pain clinic. *Bull. R. Coll. Psych.* **9**, 135–136.

Ward, N.G. (1990) Pain and depression. In Bonica, J.J. & Bull, R. (eds) *The Management of Pain*, 2nd edn. Lee & Febiger, Philadelphia, PA.

Wells, J.C.D. (1987) The place of the pain clinic. *Baillières Clin. Rheumatol.*, **1**, 123–153.

Wells, J.C.D. (1989) The use of nerve destruction for the relief of pain in cancer: a review. *Palliative Med.*, **3**, 239–247.

Wells, J.C.D. & Miles, J.B. (1991) Pain clinics and pain clinic treatments. *Br. Med. Bull.*, **47**, 762–785.

Wilson, F. (1976) Some uses of local analgesics, phenol and alcohol in intractable pain. In Proctor, H.W. & Burns, P.S. (eds) *A Handbook of Treatment*, pp. 335–345. MTP Press, Lancaster.

Winnie, A.P. & Collins, V.J. (1968) The pain clinic. I: Differential neuronal blockade in pain syndromes of questionable aetiology. *Med. Clin. N. Am.*, **52**, 123.

Woolff, C.J. (1989) Segmental afferent fibre induced analgesia: transcutaneous electrical nerve stimulation (TENS). In Melzack, R. & Wall, P.D. (eds) *A Textbook of Pain*, 2nd edn, pp. 889–896. Churchill Livingstone, Edinburgh.

SECTION 15
SPINAL INJURY

59 · Mechanisms of Injury

By R. BRAAKMAN

Injuries to the spine may occur at any level of the spine, but the most common areas are the cervical spine and the thoracolumbar junction. They can be caused by an abnormal quantity of force, an abnormal quality of force, or a combination of the two (Kummer, 1987). In some cases these injuries are the result of direct impact, e.g. a falling object hitting the neck. Such direct injury differs biomechanically from the more common indirect injury mechanism. Most injuries are caused by indirect trauma, generated by forces applied to the head, shoulders, trunk or pelvis and resulting in movements of the spine beyond the physiological range (Stauffer, 1987). This range is determined by the intervertebral disc, by the shape and terminal positions of the intervertebral joints and is braced by the ligaments. As soon as the segment with the smallest range of motion reaches its end-position, this part of the spine becomes rigid (Kummer, 1987). A large amount of stress at the level of the junction with the still mobile part of the spine may produce a spinal injury at that site.

STABILITY OF THE SPINE

It would take too much space to present a review, or discussion of the controversies concerning the many definitions of (in)stability. The author prefers the definition by L. Penning (personal communication, 1989): 'stability of an articular structure is the ability to oppose in any position any attempt to change that position'.

This definition has, however, only limited practical applicability. In practice there are degrees and patterns of instability. For the purpose of this survey the distinction between mechanical and neurological instability, according to Denis (1983) is used. Denis distinguished instability of the first degree—mechanical instability—from instability of the second degree—neurological instability—and instability of the third degree—mechanical and neurological instability. Mechanical instability does not acutely threaten the neural elements. In neurological instability the neural elements are at risk as, for example, in burst fractures. A severe burst fracture or a fracture–dislocation usually is unstable in the third degree.

The two- and three-column concepts

Holdsworth (1970) subdivided the spine into an anterior and a posterior column. He considered that rupture of the posterior column was sufficient to cause mechanical instability of the spine. Additional studies, however, have demonstrated that instability appears only after additional rupture of the posterior longitudinal ligament and of the annulus fibrosus—neither of which belongs to the posterior column. Moreover, tears in the anterior longitudinal ligament and intervertebral disc may also result in marked instability (Louis, 1982; Bedbrook, 1985).

These facts induced Denis to replace the two-column concept by a new biomechanical three-column concept, in particular in relation to injuries of the thoracic and lumbar spine (Fig. 59.1). The anterior column is formed by the anterior longitudinal ligament, the anterior annulus fibrosus and the anterior part of the vertebral body, and the middle column by the posterior longitudinal ligament, the posterior annulus fibrosus and the posterior wall of the vertebral body. The posterior column is the same as the one described by Holdsworth and is formed by the posterior arch alternating with the posterior

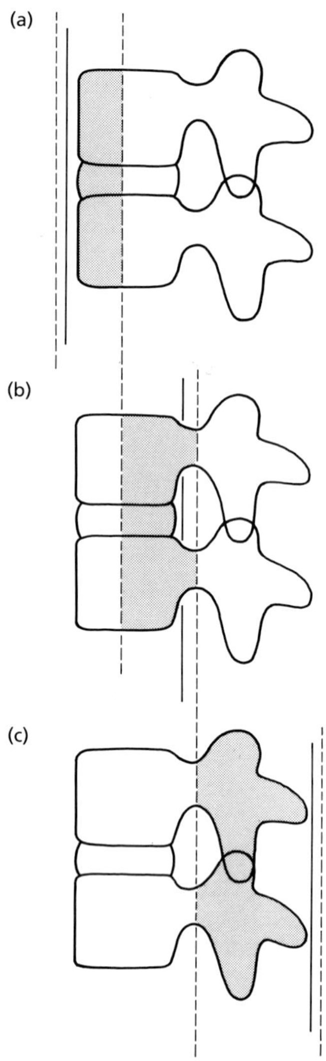

Fig. 59.1 The three columns of the spine according to Denis. (a) Anterior column, (b) middle column, (c) posterior column.

ligamentous complex (supraspinous ligaments, interspinous ligaments, capsules, and ligamentum flavum). This concept forms the basis of a classification of injuries of the thoracic and lumbar spine.

BIOMECHANICS OF INJURIES OF THE SPINE

Cervical spine

The cervical region is the most mobile part of the spine. Indirect injuries are commonly produced by acceleration or deceleration of the head with respect to the trunk or the trunk with respect to the head, as occurs in road traffic accidents, or as a result of a blow to the head or trunk (Braakman & Penning, 1971, 1976; Bohlman, 1979). Such forces cause lesions of the cervical spine due to movements which extend beyond the physiological range. The result is a distractive hyperanteflexion, hyperretroflexion (commonly also designated hyperextension), hyperlateroflexion or hyperrotation injury. For ease of usage a distractive hyperanteflexion injury is usually termed a 'hyperflexion injury' and a distractive hyperretroflexion injury a 'hyperextension injury'.

In addition, injuries may be caused by axial compression or distraction loads and by shear. Forces acting along the axis of the cervical spine may be compressive, approximating the skull and trunk; or distractive, separating them. They may be purely axial or may be part of, for example, a compressive hyperflexion or compressive hyperextension injury. Shear forces may displace the vertebrae more or less parallel to each other. Combinations of excessive movements, such as hyperflexion and hyperrotation, may also occur. Such combinations play a role in many injuries.

Sometimes a series of movements occurs, such as hyperflexion, followed by hyperextension. In this context 'whiplash' injuries should be mentioned which are discussed in detail in Chapter 63. Hyperflexion and hyperextension may also occur at the same time at different places. A hyperextension injury of the upper cervical spine, such as a fracture of the posterior atlantal arch, may be combined with a hyperflexion injury of the lower cervical spine, like interlocking of the articular facets. Rotational forces may play a contributory role in any kind of injury of the cervical spine. Intervertebral discs, joints and ligaments are highly vulnerable to rotation and horizontal shear forces. The atlanto-axial segment is particularly susceptible to hyperrotation injuries because it has less resistance to hyperrotation than the segments of the lower cervical spine. Lateral hyperflexion may cause injuries of the lower cervical spine. They often result in unilateral compression of an articular process and in lesions of the brachial plexus and spinal cord.

Classification

The three-column classification can also be applied to injuries of the lower cervical spine. Another classification of injuries of the cervical spine, based on the localization, the morphology and the causative mechanism of the lesion, is more popular and will be used here (Table 59.1) (Braakman & Penning, 1971, 1976; Allen *et al.*, 1982). The mechanism of injury can often be deduced from the study of radiographs post-injury. In such a classification, biomechanical concepts are deduced rather than demonstrated. The upper and lower cervical spine are anatomically dissimilar; therefore, preferably their classification should not be combined.

Table 59.1 Classification of injuries to the cervical spine

Distractive hyperflexion	Anterior subluxation, unilateral facet interlocking, bilateral facet interlocking
Compressive hyperflexion	Wedge compression fracture of vertebral body, teardrop fracture, hyperflexion fracture–dislocation
Distractive hyperextension	Hyperextension dislocation
Compressive hyperextension	Hyperextension fracture–dislocation

Specific types of injuries

UPPER CERVICAL SPINE

The most common lesions of the upper cervical spine are anterior atlanto-axial dislocation, atlas fracture, fracture of the odontoid process, fracture of the body of the axis and hangman fracture. Fracture of the posterior arch of the atlas is often due to a direct blow applied to the vertex of the head, forcing the occipital condyles downwards upon the atlas. Fractures of the axis may result from shear (Howorth & Petrie, 1964) but also from axial compression and from distraction or extension (Sances *et al.*, 1984; Mouradian *et al.*, 1985). In the upper cervical spine region the spinal canal is wide and consequently, neurological deficit is a relatively rare consequence of injury to this area. However, in the more severe injuries with combinations of fractures of the atlas and axis, marked deformation may occur during the impact, resulting in severe, even fatal, craniospinal cord lesions (Sances *et al.*, 1984; Dickman *et al.*, 1989).

In the past the hangman fracture—traumatic spondylolisthesis of C2—was the result of a hanging mechanism, when there was a drop of at least a few metres. It is a bilateral fracture through the neural arch of C2, with or without dislocation of the body of the axis, upon that of the third vertebra. The odontoid process and the transverse ligament remain intact. The lesion is nowadays usually the result of a road traffic accident (Fig. 59.2), the victim having caught his chin on the steering wheel or dashboard, produc-

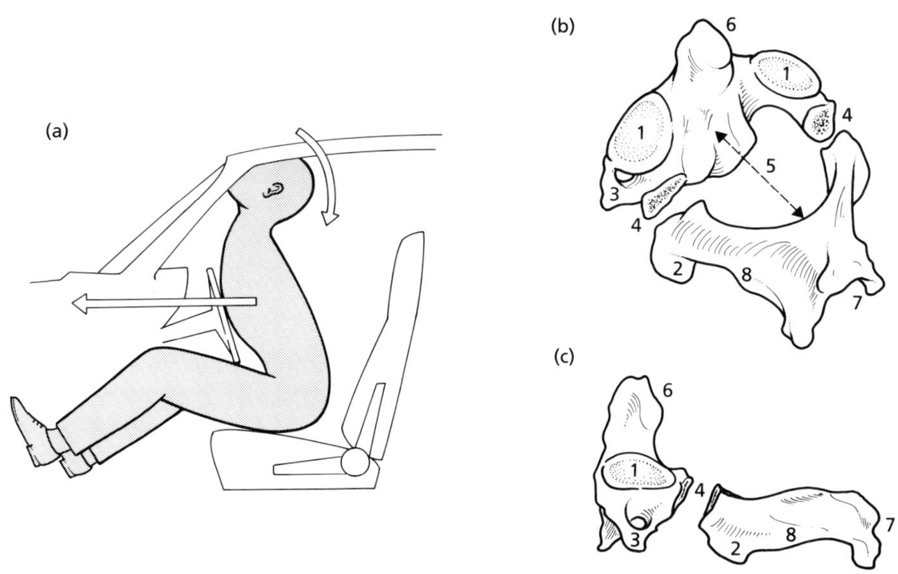

Fig. 59.2 The commonest mechanism producing a 'hangman fracture' today is shown in (a); (b) and (c) show superior and lateral views of the fractured C2. 1, superior facet C2; 2, inferior articular process; 3, transverse process; 4, fracture line; 5, increased sagittal diameter of spinal canal; 6, odontoid process; 7, spinous process; 8, laminar arch.

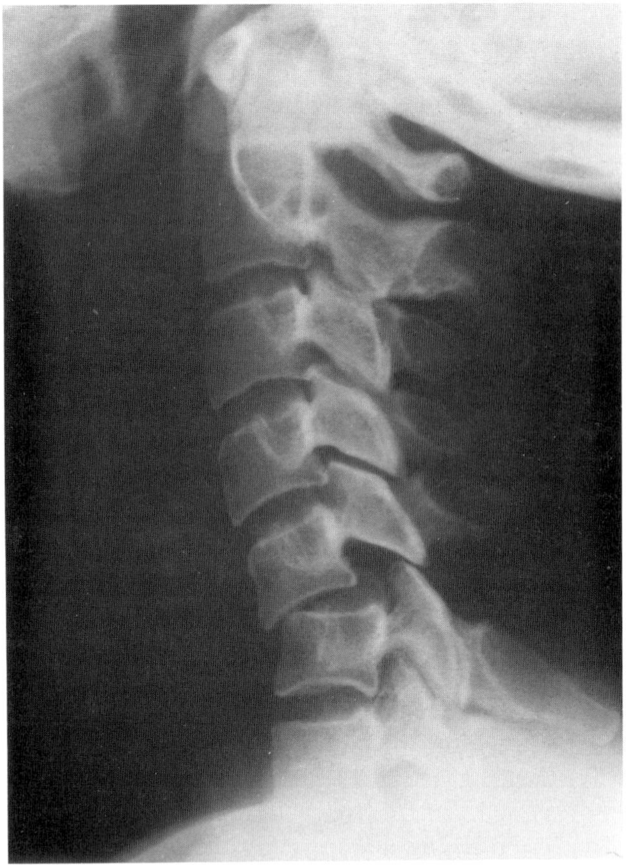

Fig. 59.3 Anterior subluxation = hyperflexion sprain. Note the characteristic kyphotic angulation. No overriding of articular facets and no reduction of the sagittal diameter of the spinal canal.

ing hyperextension. Because the sagittal diameter of the spinal canal is increased rather than reduced, neurological deficit is rare.

LOWER CERVICAL SPINE

In distractive hyperflexion, caused by an upward blow to the occiput, separation of the spinous processes with overstretching of the posterior ligaments is the predominant feature. As hyperflexion continues, the ligaments are torn at a certain level and a hyperflexion sprain (anterior subluxation) may ensue, with marked angulation of the spine, but as yet no interlocking of the articular facets.

Usually there is no cord involvement in a hyperflexion sprain, because the sagittal diameter of the spinal canal is not involved (Fig. 59.3). With greater force the articular facets may lose contact, override and then, as they spring back after injury, become

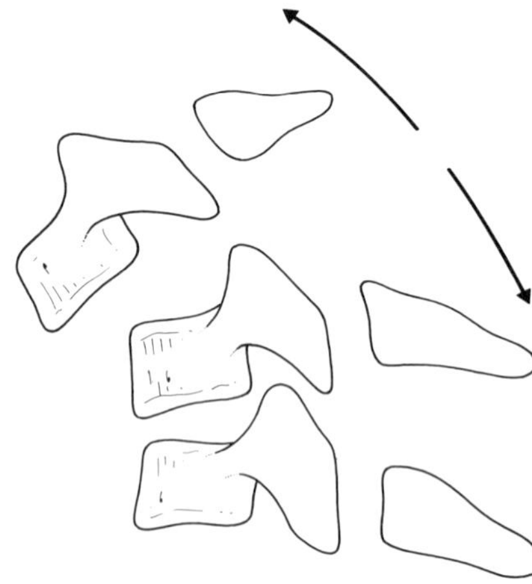

Fig. 59.4 Distractive hyperflexion. Pure distractive hyperflexion results in preservation of the vertebral bodies, but marked angular kyphosis due to rupture of the interspinous ligaments and joint capsules. The articular facets override. Instability of the third degree. The sagittal diameter of the spinal canal is often markedly reduced.

interlocked (bilateral facet interlocking) (Fig. 59.4). The sagittal diameter of the spinal canal is markedly reduced, commonly with serious cord involvement. If rotation occurs at the same time, the interlocking may be unilateral (Fig. 59.5). The site of the unilateral locked facet may be recognized because below it the spine is seen in a strictly lateral view with superimposition of both articular processes. However, cranial to the injury the articular processes appear oblique and separated. The tips of the articular processes may be broken off at the site of interlocking.

In compressive hyperflexion a blow to the back of the head is transmitted along the column of the vertebral bodies. A compression fracture of a vertebral body results in, for instance, a wedge-like compression, or a teardrop fracture or a fracture with marked backward displacement of the posterior part of the broken vertebral body into the spinal canal (hyperflexion fracture–dislocation) (Fig. 59.6). The sagittal diameter of the spinal canal is reduced, often resulting in a severe cord lesion.

Distractive hyperextension of the cervical spine, as in an upward blow to the chin, may result in rupture of the anterior ligamentous apparatus and of the intervertebral disc (Fig. 59.7). The portion of the cervical spine above the separation moves backwards, and pinches the spinal cord between the inferior posterior border of the dislocating vertebral body and the leading edge of the posterior arch of the vertebra

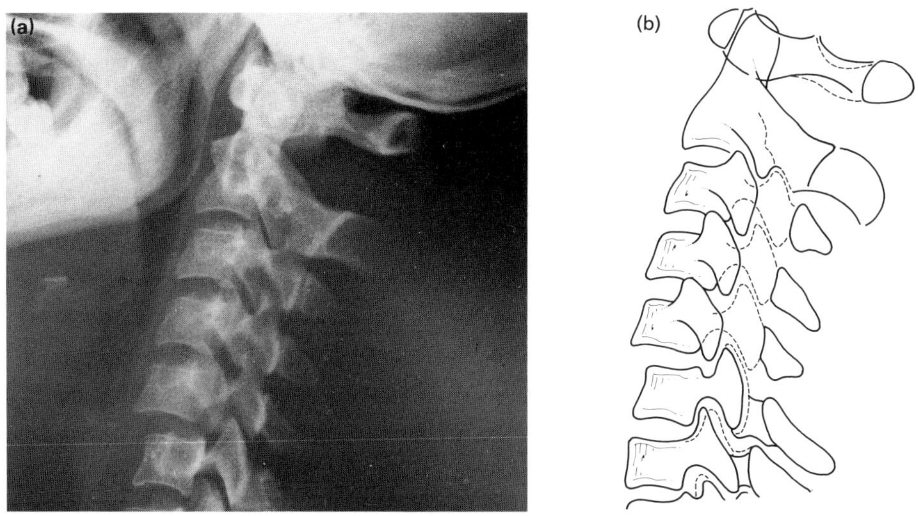

Fig. 59.5 Unilateral facet interlocking. (a) Unilateral facet interlocking C5–C6; (b) schematic drawing of the lateral projection of the cervical spine to elucidate the radiograph.

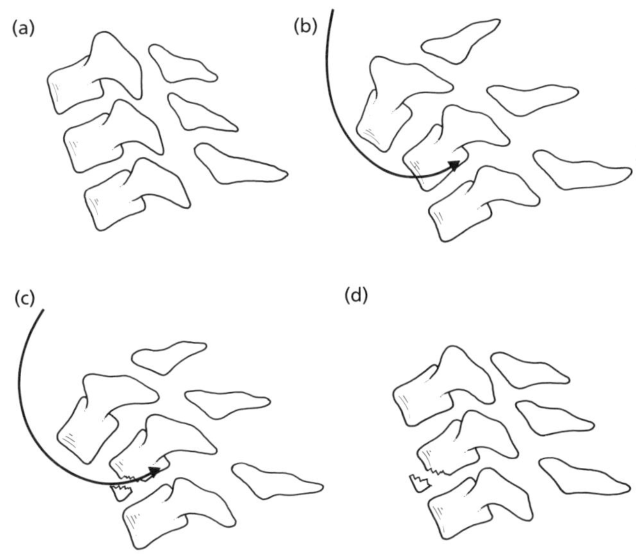

Fig. 59.6 Mechanism of injury in compressive hyperflexion, resulting in hyperflexion fracture–dislocation. (a) Before injury. (b) First stage of injury; the compressive hyperflexion force causes the spine to move through an arc, displacing the upper vertebra backward with respect to the lower and rupturing the intervertebral joint capsules. (c) Last stage of injury; marked widening of the intervertebral joint space. The posterior part of the intervertebral disc is disrupted, the antero-inferior margin of the upper vertebra has broken off, but maintains a normal relationship with the lower vertebra through the unsevered anterior part of the disc. (d) After injury.

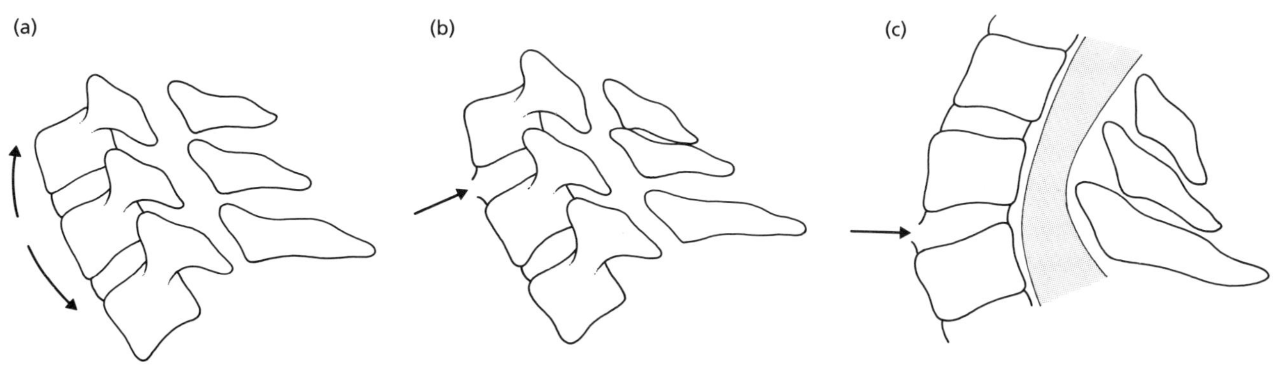

Fig. 59.7 Distractive hyperextension. (a) As a result of the force the anterior longitudinal ligament ruptures and the intervertebral disc is detached from the body of the upper vertebra (hyperextension–dislocation). (b) The upper vertebra commonly moves backwards and the cervical cord is subjected to pinching (c).

below it. When the traumatic force is removed there is a spontaneous reduction, usually to such a degree that radiographs taken subsequently appear normal. This type of injury is usually designated as hyperextension dislocation (Allen *et al.*, 1982) or hyperextension sprain (Braakman & Penning, 1971, 1976).

In compressive hyperextension, hyperextension is accompanied by compression along the axis of the spine. The compressive force, usually applied to the forehead, first forces the head and cervical spine into a position of hyperextension. The articular processes then fracture, and finally the body of the fractured vertebra is dislocated forwards, because the role of the articular processes in preventing this type of dislocation has been eliminated. The head moves through an arc (Fig. 59.8). This type of injury, simulating a hyperflexion injury, is called a hyperextension fracture–dislocation.

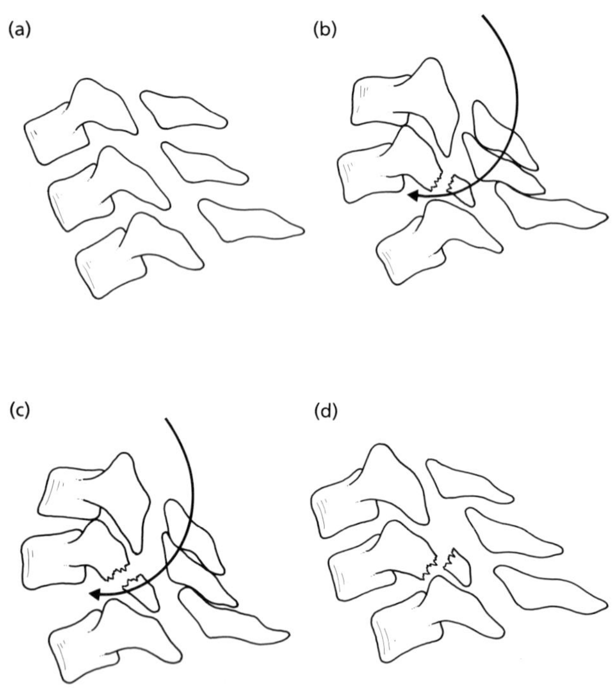

Fig. 59.8 Mechanism of injury in compressive hyperextension, resulting in hyperextension fracture–dislocation. (a) Before injury. (b) First stage of injury; the trauma forces the head backwards and downwards. The spine moves through an arc displacing the upper vertebra forwards with respect to the lower, and fracturing the articular processes. (c) Last stage of injury; marked widening of the intervertebral disc space with anterior displacement of the body of the upper vertebra and complete disruption of the disc. Note the dehiscence of the two parts of the articular processes. (d) After injury.

More detailed classifications, taking into account various stages of severity of these lesions, have been given by Braakman & Penning (1971, 1976) and by Allen *et al.* (1982). Almost all these injuries of the lower cervical spine are neurologically unstable, except the anterior subluxation, the wedge compression fracture and the hyperextension fracture–dislocation which are mechanically unstable.

Thoracic spine

In the thoracic spine, rotation and ventral bending are relatively unrestricted, as a result of the coronal configuration of the facets. Lateral and dorsal flexion, however, are restricted and the narrow spaces between the laminae and between the spinous processes limit dorsal flexion (Kummer, 1987).

Most injuries between T1 and T10 are generally quite stable, due to splinting by the rib cage and the sternum; this is in contrast to the thoracolumbar junction, where considerably more motion occurs. Consequently, most upper thoracic injuries do not need internal fixation and can be treated with external orthotic support. Early mobilization can be encouraged. In more severe injuries with additional shear forces, a complex fracture–dislocation occurs in which the vertebral body and the dorsal elements are fractured, allowing lateral or anterior translation of the upper trunk and upper vertebrae at the fractured segment. Such lesions usually require open reduction, internal fixation and spinal fusion or long-term bed rest immobilization to achieve stability (Bohlman *et al.*, 1985; Bedbrook, 1985).

Thoracolumbar spine

Injuries of the thoracolumbar junction are caused by combinations of flexion–rotation and axial load. The middle and posterior columns may also be subjected to distraction. As the chest is rotated and flexed the rib cage absorbs the flexion energy, because the thoracic, coronal facets allow rotation to occur, in particular at the lower thoracic level where the ribs are not attached to the sternum (Denis, 1983; Sances *et al.*, 1984).

From the thoracic spine downwards the facet joint angle changes abruptly at the thoracolumbar junction, usually at the dorsal element of T12. This vertebra has coronally shaped superior facets and sagittally shaped inferior facets. Therefore, according

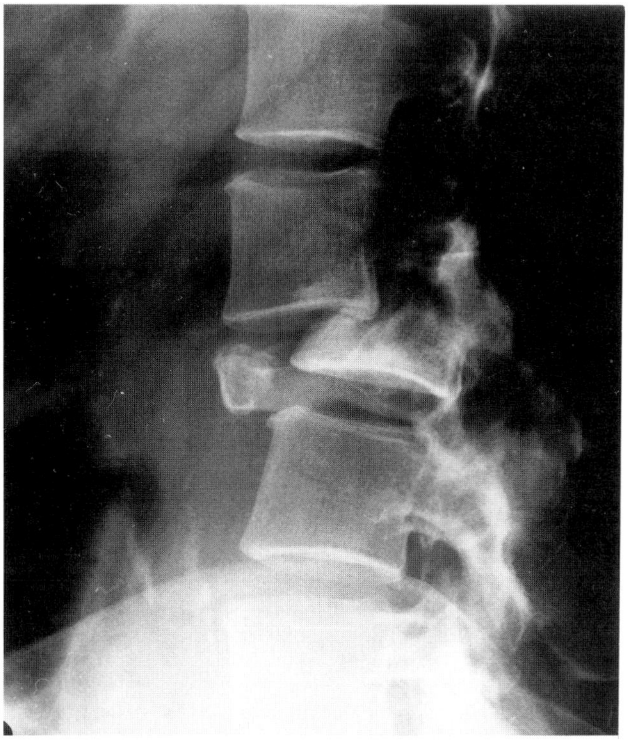

Fig. 59.9 Fracture–dislocation of the thoracolumbar spine, lateral view.

to Stauffer (1987), injuries centred at the T11–T12 level are often fracture–dislocations with a slice fracture through the upper portion of the T12 vertebral body (Fig. 59.9). At the T12–L1 level the superior sagittal facets of L1 block rotation, and the facet on the compression side suffers a fracture, which extends down through the superior aspect of the vertebral body of L1. The opposite facet on the distracted side commonly dislocates.

These fracture–dislocations are markedly unstable; to achieve stability, long-lasting bed rest immobilization in the horizontal position or surgical stabilization is required.

Lumbar spine

The lumbar spine is characterized by the freedom of dorsal and ventral flexion and by marked but restricted lateral flexion. The sagittal configuration of the facet joints limits rotation, except at the L5–S1 articulation (Sances *et al.*, 1984; Kummer, 1987).

Torsional movements primarily stress the intervertebral discs and the vertebral joints, producing ruptures of fibres of the annulus fibrosus as well as fractures of the articular processes. Lateral bending results in bending stress for the vertebral body, with compression on the concave side of the bend.

A specific injury to the lumbar spine occurs when a person is wearing a seatbelt and suffers a sudden deceleration in a car or aeroplane crash (Smith & Kauffer, 1969; Denis, 1983).

Classification of injuries of thoracic and lumbar spine

For injuries of the thoracic and lumbar spine the classification of Denis (Table 59.2) is currently the most widely used. He distinguished minor and major injuries. Minor injuries are represented by fractures of the transverse process, the articular process of the pars interarticularis and of the spinous process. The major injuries comprise compression fractures, burst fractures, fracture–dislocations and the seatbelt-type of injury. The basic modes of failure of the three columns in the four major types of spinal injury are indicated in Table 59.2. The compression fracture is a failure under compression of the anterior column. The middle column is completely intact and acts as a hinge. There may be a partial tension failure of the posterior column. This is the only major type of injury with an intact middle column.

The burst fracture results from failure of the vertebral body under axial load. This results in failure of the anterior and middle columns, both under compression. The burst fracture is differentiated from the compression fracture by the integrity of the vertebral ring in the latter. The vertebral ring in a burst fracture is fractured both anteriorly and posteriorly. A computerized tomography (CT) scan demonstrates the most important characteristic of the burst fracture: the break of the posterior wall of the vertebral body with marked retropulsion of bone into the canal causing partial obstruction of the canal (Fig. 59.10).

In fracture–dislocations there is a failure of all columns under compression, distraction, rotation or shear. Denis distinguished a flexion–rotation, a shear and a flexion–distraction type. In a seatbelt injury both posterior and middle columns are damaged under tension forces, generated by flexion and sometimes by additional distraction. The anterior part of the anterior column acts as a hinge. The result is a seat-belt fracture in which the superior and inferior fragments of the dorsal spinous process, lamina and vertebral body are separated. This type of fracture is relatively rare (Smith & Kauffer, 1969).

Table 59.2 Mechanisms of failure in the four major types of injury to the thoracic and lumbar spine. After Denis (1983)

Type of fracture	Column damage			Mechanism	Stability	Therapy
	Anterior	Middle	Posterior			
Compression	Compression	None	None or distraction (severe)	Compression axis: middle	Stable	Conservative
Burst	Compression	Compression	None or compression	Compression axis: posterior	Often unstable	Surgical decompression, distraction stabilization
Seatbelt type	None or compression	Distraction	Distraction	Distraction–flexion axis: anterior	Often unstable	Compression stabilization
Fracture–dislocation	Compression rotation shear	Distraction rotation shear	Distraction rotation shear	Translation + distraction, flexion, torsion axis: variable	Unstable	Decompression, instrumental stabilization

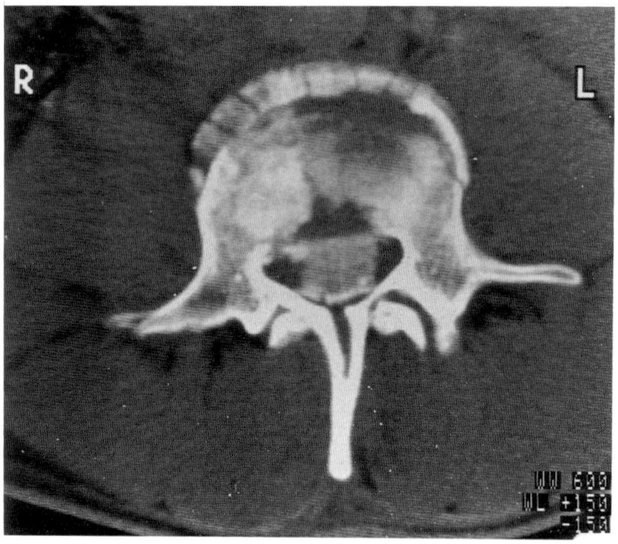

Fig. 59.10 CT scan of a patient with severe burst fracture of the lumbar spine. Note the many fracture lines in the vertebral body and the posterior displacement of a posterior part of the vertebral body into the spinal canal, producing marked compromise of the spinal canal.

In the very rare extension injuries, the anterior longitudinal ligament and the disc are torn. Due to the marked transverse instability there is usually severe cord involvement.

Minimal and moderate compression fractures with an intact posterior column are stable and may be treated by early ambulation with or without external immobilization, depending upon the degree of compression, the kyphosis and the age of the patient (Denis, 1983). Severe compression fractures and seatbelt injuries show mechanical instability, allowing buckling around the hinge of the middle column in the former and around the hinge of the anterior column in the latter type. External immobilization, and—in certain cases—open reduction and internal fixation, will be required. In burst fractures and in fracture–dislocations neurological instability is present.

INVOLVEMENT OF THE SPINAL CORD OR CAUDA EQUINA

Various factors may be held responsible for damaging the spinal cord or nerve roots in injuries of the spine (Table 59.3). The size of the spinal canal, and in particular the sagittal diameter, plays a decisive role in the development of spinal cord damage in spinal injuries. There is considerable interindividual variation in the constitutional size of the bony spinal canal. The midsagittal diameter of the spinal cord, however, varies only slightly.

Consequently, in patients with small canals less 'play' is available around the spinal cord. This means that an acquired or constitutional narrow canal predisposes to serious neurological damage which may, therefore, also occur in young people.

Cord involvement in upper cervical injuries is rare,

Table 59.3 Factors involved in producing injury to the spinal contents

Mechanism	Compressive agent
Pinching (compression from two sides)	Bone, ligaments?
'Contact pressure' (compression from one side)	Bone, intervertebral disc, haematoma, direct injury (vertebral arch)
Overstretching	
Secondary cord damage	Cord swelling, cord ischaemia, thrombosis of cord vessels, venous obstruction
Traumatic haematoma	

because the sagittal diameter of the spinal canal is markedly wider in the upper cervical spine than in the lower cervical spine.

It has been shown, in series of patients with injuries of the lower cervical spine, that a large sagittal diameter allows protection from neurological injury (Eismont *et al.*, 1984), and that patients without neurological deficit have significantly wider canals than those with deficit (Ersmark & Löwenhielm, 1988). The spinal canal is particularly narrow in the thoracic spine.

Injuries in which bony structures pinch the spinal cord sagittally are particularly likely to produce severe neurological damage: in facet interlocking the cord is pinched between the arch of the anterior displaced luxated vertebra and the superoposterior part of the vertebral body below it. Bony pinching of the spinal cord in a hyperextension dislocation between the vertebral body above the injured segment and the arch below it is illustrated in Fig. 59.7. It may, in addition, also be due to infolding of the flaval ligaments (Taylor & Blackwood, 1948).

The second common cause of cord involvement is contact pressure, compression of the cord (and roots) on one side. It is usually caused by displacement into the spinal canal of the posterior fragment of a broken vertebral body as in cervical hyperflexion fracture–dislocations (Fig. 59.6) and in burst fractures of the thoracolumbar spine (Fig. 59.10). This contact pressure is also the mechanism in direct injuries, e.g. by a vertebral arch being displaced into the spinal canal. Contact pressure may also be exerted by a traumatic disc prolapse. These prolapses are particularly observed in distractive and compressive hyperflexion injuries of the lower cervical spine. Moreover, contact pressure may be the mechanism in late myelopathy in cases with persistent marked angular kyphosis in cases of old, non-reduced facet interlocking or long-standing teardrop fracture (Schneider, 1955; Verbiest, 1973). In extremely rare cases compression of the spinal cord is exerted by an intramedullary or extramedullary haematoma.

Overstretching after an injury is rare, but may occur if excessive skull traction is used on a spine with extensive ligamentous damage.

Many cases of severe cervical cord damage have been described, even following a minor injury with no radiological sign of damage to the spine or sagittal narrowing of the bony spinal canal. The majority of these patients are elderly, and the sagittal diameter of the spinal canal is below average, either due to developmental narrowing or to cervical spondylosis. The damage can then be explained by the reduced 'play' of the cord within the spinal canal with consequent earlier pinching of the cord. Most of these injuries are hyperextension injuries, e.g. after a fall downstairs (Fig. 59.7). Many of these patients have wounds to their face, disclosing the mechanism.

Traumatic spinal cord damage without radiological abnormality is also seen in children (Pang & Wilberger, 1982). They found that this occurred in two-thirds of children between infancy and 16 years who presented with spinal cord injury. Over 50% of these children presented with a delayed onset of the major neurological injury, with the latent period ranging from 30 minutes to 4 days, with a mean of 1.2 days. They felt that the syndrome could result from either hyperextension or hyperflexion-type injuries with the former more likely in the lower cervical spine and the latter in the upper cervical spine. Severe neurological injury was more common in the younger children. When severe cord injury was present the prognosis for recovery was poor.

The mechanism of the cord injury was not clear, and probably multifactorial. They felt that the anatomical features of a child's spine would allow transient subluxation which could injure the cord but then revert to a normal configuration. The features responsible were: the increased elasticity of spinal ligaments and joint capsules, the horizontal orientation of the facet joints in a child, the presence of anterior wedging of the vertebral body increasing the likelihood of anterior displacement, the absence of uncinate articulation, and the proportionately increased mass of the head in children.

In order to explain the delayed onset of the neurological deficit, two possible mechanisms were described. Firstly, that the original transient subluxation produced instability which could be reactivated by further movement of the neck, causing multiple insults to the cord. Secondly, that the original injury triggered either ischaemic change or progressive destruction of neural tissue. Little objective evidence is available to support either explanation.

The narrower spinal canal in the thoracic spine allows less bone encroachment before neurological injury occurs (Bohlman *et al.*, 1985). This fact also explains why more than 80% of cases with traumatic involvement of the thoracic spinal cord have complete lesions.

In thoracic and lumbar injuries compression fractures and seatbelt injuries do not involve the sagittal diameter of the spinal canal. They are not directly responsible for any acute neurological damage. Patients with burst fractures, however, with sagittal narrowing of the spinal canal, may be neurologically intact but about 50% of these patients show partial or complete involvement of the spinal cord. In fracture–dislocations, and in the rare extension injuries with severe deformation of the spinal canal, about 75% of patients have severe, often complete, cord, conus or cauda lesions.

After the primary damage inflicted by the impact the secondary cord damage may develop. This damage is comparable to the secondary damage in traumatic brain injury. Cord swelling, ischaemia, thrombosis of small vessels and venous obstruction may all play a part. The exact role of these various contributing mechanisms is still disputed and is the subject of continuing investigation.

REFERENCES

Allen, B.L., Ferguson, R.L., Lehmann, T.H.R. & O'Brien, R.B. (1982) A mechanistic classification of closed indirect fractures and dislocations of the lower cervical spine. *Spine*, **7**, 1–27.

Bedbrook, G.M. (1985) Spinal injuries with tetraplegia and paraplegia. *J. Bone Jt. Surg.*, **67A**, 360–369.

Bohlman, H.H. (1979) Acute fractures and dislocations of the cervical spine—an analysis of three-hundred hospitalized patients and review of the literature. *J. Bone Jt. Surg.*, **61A**, 1119–1142.

Bohlman, H.H., Freehafer, A. & Dejak, J. (1985) The results of treatment of acute injuries of the upper thoracic spine with paralysis. *J. Bone Jt. Surg.*, **67A**, 360–369.

Braakman, R. & Penning, L. (1971) *Injuries of the Cervical Spine*. Excerpta Medica, Amsterdam.

Braakman, R. & Penning, L. (1976) Injuries of the cervical spine. In Vinken, P.J. & Bruyn, G.W. (eds), *Handbook of Clinical Neurology*, vol. 25, pp. 227–380. North-Holland, Amsterdam.

Denis, F. (1983) The three column spine and its significance in the classification of acute thoracolumbar spinal injuries. *Spine*, **8**, 817–831.

Dickman, C.A., Hadley, M.N., Browner, C. & Sonntag, V.K.H. (1989) Neurosurgical management of acute atlas–axis combination fractures. *J. Neurosurg.*, **70**, 45–49.

Eismont, F.J., Clifford, S., Holdberg, M. & Green, B. (1984) Cervical sagittal spinal canal size in spine injury. *Spine*, **9**, 663–666.

Ersmark, H. & Löwenhielm, P. (1988) Factors influencing the outcome of cervical spine injuries. *J. Trauma*, **28**, 407–411.

Holdsworth, F.W. (1970) Fractures, dislocations and fracture–dislocations of the spine. *J. Bone Jt. Surg.*, **52A**, 1534–1551.

Howorth, M.B. & Petrie, J.G. (1964) *Injuries of the Spine*. Williams & Wilkins, Baltimore.

Kummer, B. (1987) Biomechanics of the thoracic and lumbar spine. In Harris, P.H. (ed.), *Thoracic and Lumbar Spine and Spinal Cord Injuries. Advances in Neurotraumatology*, vol. 2, pp. 17–27. Springer, Vienna.

Louis, R. (1982) *Chirurgie du rachis. Anatomie Chirurgicale et voies d'abord*. Springer, Berlin.

Mouradian, W.H., Fietti, V.G., Crochran, G.V.B., Fielding, J.W. & Young, J. (1978) Fractures of the odontoid: a laboratory and clinical study of mechanisms. *Orthop. Clin. N. Am.*, **9**, 1985.

Pang, D. & Wilberger, J. (1982) Spinal cord injury without radiographic abnormalities in children. *J. Neurosurg.*, **57**, 114–129.

Sances, A. Jr., Myklebust, J.B., Maiman, D.J., Larson, S.J. & Cusick, J.F. (1984) The biomechanics of spinal injuries. *Crit. Rev. Biomed. Eng.*, **11**, 1–76.

Schneider, R.C. (1955) The syndrome of acute anterior spinal cord injury. *J. Neurosurg.*, **12**, 95–122.

Smith, W.S. & Kaufer, H. (1969) Patterns and mechanisms of lumbar injuries associated with lap seat-belts. *J. Bone Jt. Surg.*, **51A**, 239–254.

Stauffer, E.S. (1987) Clinical aspects of thoracic and lumbar spine and spinal cord injuries. In Harris, P. H. (ed.), *Thoracic and Lumbar Spine and Spinal Cord Injuries. Advances in Neurotraumatology*, vol. 2, pp. 27–39. Springer, Vienna.

Taylor, A.R. & Blackwood, W. (1948) Paraplegia in cervical injuries with normal radiographic appearance. *J. Bone Jt. Surg.*, **30B**, 245–252.

Verbiest, H. (1973) Antero-lateral operations for fractures or dislocations of the cervical spine, due to injuries or previous surgical interventions. *Clin. Neurosurg.*, **20**, 334–367.

60 · Effects of Injury on the Spinal Cord

By R.G. PRINGLE

Maoist parable

An old man was faced with two mountains which he wished to level to the ground. He set about these mountains with a shovel. His neighbours mocked him but he replied, 'If I and my son and his son and so on, each digs away part of these mountains they will be levelled to the ground.'

In the case of spinal cord injury the two mountains are those of vertebral stability and spinal cord damage. Important inroads have been made into the much smaller mountain of the spinal column, but in our understanding of spinal cord pathology, and particularly in our attempts to modify the response to injury, we are still in the foothills.

Clinical conjecture

The basic patterns of neurological deficit resulting from spinal cord injury are well established. Complete and incomplete lesions were documented 4000 years ago in the Edwin Smith papyrus (Hughes, 1988). More recently Dimitrijevic (1987) has defined a third category, 'discomplete' lesions, where there is neurophysiological evidence of residual motor function in patients who are clinically complete. The significance of this in functional and prognostic terms remains unclear at present.

The common syndromes of incomplete lesions—anterior and central cord, and Brown–Séquard—are equally well recognized, and good descriptions of them may be found in 19th-century literature (Bramwell, 1884; Thorburn, quoted by Braakman, 1976).

Nonetheless, and despite this long acquaintance with the problem, the patterns, behaviour, and progress of spinal cord injury remain infinitely variable and at times bizarre, commonly frustrating yet at times joyful, and in general resistant to active medical and surgical attempts to improve recovery. Early neurological deterioration, conversely, is common even in the best of hands, and in most cases is simply a reflection of the developing pathological process rather than the result of mismanagement. Toscano (1988) found evidence of deterioration between the time of the accident and arrival in a spinal injury unit in 25% of patients, and in the hospital environment it is not uncommon to see a complete lesion ascend one or two, or, less frequently, several segments within a day or two of injury. In most cases this occurs in the dorsal region and is of no functional significance, but occasionally it is seen at the midlumbar level where its importance is much greater. The loss of several segments is attributed to cord infarction and is irreversible. The reason for the loss of one or two segments is unclear. It may be related to oedema, or to haemorrhage in the cord, or ischaemia. In any event, spontaneous recovery of the affected segments not uncommonly takes place over a period of weeks or months, particularly in the younger patients, and there is no evidence that surgical or other intervention is helpful once deterioration has occurred.

EXAMPLE 1

A 22-year-old male sustained a 'stable' wedge compression fracture of D6 at a motor cross event (Fig. 60.1). He walked to the ambulance and had no neurological symptoms initially. He was positioned sitting in the ambulance, and over the next 20 minutes during transport to hospital in this position developed a paraparesis which on admission to hospital was complete.

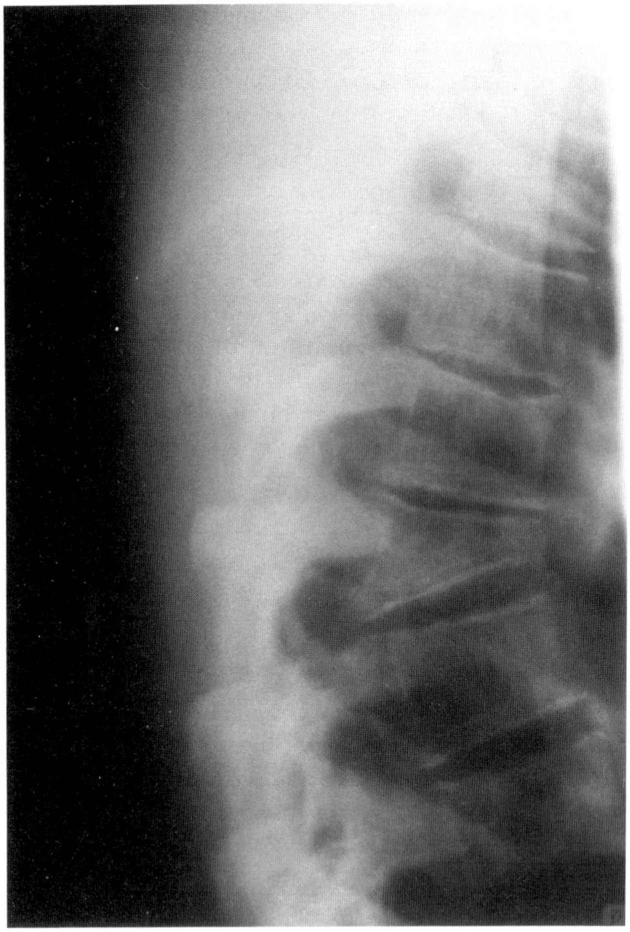

Fig. 60.1 Example 1: lateral X-ray on admission.

He was nursed in recumbency and developed significant sensory recovery overnight. Motor recovery commenced within a few days and after six weeks in recumbency he had power 4–5 in all lower limb groups. At this time he commenced inclining up in bed. Over the next few days as this process continued he developed increasing lower limb weakness, which was reversible on lying down. It was found to be associated with hypotension when he was tilted upwards beyond 40°, and the lower limb weakness produced by this was reversed by ephedrine.

He was therefore confined to bed for a further three weeks, after which his mobilization proceeded uneventfully, although initially with ephedrine cover when he was upright. No further episodes of weakness occurred and at the time of his discharge from hospital, four months after injury, he had made an almost complete sensory, motor and visceral recovery. At review two years after injury he was neurologically intact apart from reflex changes. No change in the radiological appearances of his spinal fracture took place at any time following the initial injury.

EXAMPLE 2

An elderly man with a relatively mild tetraparesis following cervical spine fracture in ankylosing spondylitis developed rapid-onset motor tetraplegia associated with an acute episode of hypotension caused by a bleeding peptic ulcer some weeks after injury. No useful recovery of function took place.

On clinical grounds, therefore, there would seem little doubt that the cord is vulnerable to hypotension and possibly hypoxia for many weeks following injury, yet the intact cord is unaffected by these phenomena unless they are so severe as to cause infarction. Why should this be?

Other questions posed by clinical observation also lack answers. Why may the cord be spared totally in some cases of severe spinal fracture or dislocation, yet suffer major damage in the apparent absence of spinal column injury at other times? Why is there frequently a poor correlation between the levels of column and cord injury? What are the causes of neurological deterioration—particularly the ascending lesion? What is the explanation of sacral sparing? Why has it such great prognostic significance? Why may neurological recovery continue for two to three years—often in a steplike fashion with episodes of important functional gain after long plateaus? Why may improvement occasionally occur many months after injury following such disparate measures as surgical decompression (Bohlman *et al.*, 1975), omental transposition (Goldsmith *et al.*, 1986) or a journey to Lourdes (H.W.F. Jones, personal communication, 1989)? What is the cause of post-traumatic syringomyelia? And most importantly, by what means may the clinician hope to obtain consistent improvement in the rate and extent of return of neurological function following injury?

Answers to these and other questions may come from studies in human and experimental pathology, and in spinal cord physiology and biochemistry.

Autopsy analyses

Hughes (1978) describes a sequence of events following injury, commencing with swelling of nerve fibres

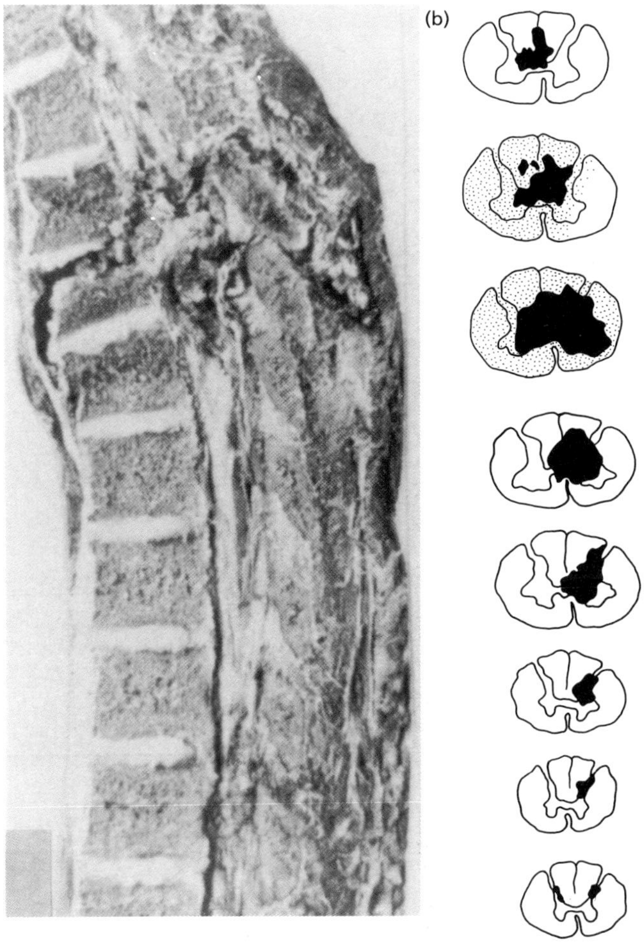

Fig. 60.2 Left: compression-burst fracture of C7. Right: diagram of the cord lesions between C5 and T4. After Jellinger (1976).

and disintegration of both axon material and myelin. Axonic changes vary from beading through the formation of droplets to 'dust' with increasing severity of injury. Associated with this is disruption of the cell bodies, or chromatolysis if the axonic damage is remote from the cell bodies.

An exudate in the cord forms from oedema, red cell diapedesis, and an inflammatory reaction best seen some distance from the main injury where they are obscured by haemorrhage and necrosis. The oedema may be slight and perivascular, but often affects the whole cord. Initial haemorrhage and later venous stasis occur and the cord becomes rounded and tense within the meninges, obliterating the subarachnoid and subdural spaces. Hughes emphasizes the fusiform extent of damage over one or more segments tapering off above and below the level of injury, commonly as a small round area in the posterior column (Fig. 60.2).

After two or three weeks the process of repair supervenes with phagocytosis, cyst formation and gliosis leading to a final stage of a connective tissue scar with evidence of regeneration from the cell bodies of the posterior root ganglia which, however, do not penetrate the scar or enter intact nervous tissue.

Kakulas & Bedbrook (1976) reports that in the first 24 hours reactive microscopic changes are minor or absent, but after that time there is necrosis, swelling, cellular infiltrate and breakdown products from neuronal degeneration. In 50 out of 67 clinically complete lesions examined at post mortem some neuronal continuity across the injured segments was observed (Kakulas, 1988).

Even when there has been massive bony injury Kakulas describes complete cord transection as rare, while the cord may appear macroscopically normal in the presence of severe bone damage. In his experience, from a large number of post mortem studies, bone fragments are rarely found to be causing cord compression.

The important features to emerge from these studies are that quite gross microscopic changes appear after 24 hours, but that neural tissue and particularly the long tracts may be preserved despite very severe injury, that major and particularly anterior spinal artery occlusion and major disc protrusion are rarely seen, that cord compression by bone is rare also, and that in the late stages there is evidence of regeneration of nerve fibres.

Post-mortem material and clinical experience both emphasize the fact that the cord lesion may be some distance from the site of bone injury, and indeed both the severity and site of damage are dictated by the directions and intensity of the causative force, and the physical state of the victim at the moment of impact (Jellinger, 1976).

Mammal models

In the 100 years since Schaus introduced the first recognized experimental model (Schaus, 1890, quoted by Goodkin, 1976) a variety of techniques including the weight-drop method, inflatable balloons, and compressive clips, have been employed to study the effects of spinal cord injury in animals.

There is obvious difficulty in establishing a standard limited spinal cord injury without using a method so artificial as to be of doubtful value when related to the crushing violence of the human injury. Furthermore, the neurological recovery of animals from incomplete spinal cord injury, commonly measured as ability to walk up an incline, bears little resemblance to the varied and complex stages of recovery in humans.

Nonetheless, a good deal of information has been gained on the pathology and pharmacology of spinal cord injury in animals from such experiments, while Panjabi & Wrathall (1988), in a biomechanical analysis of the weight-drop method, report that 'It is now possible to produce animals with a pre-defined amount of neurological deficit, and, therefore, to evaluate different treatment modalities against spinal cord injury.' While the original Allen weight-drop technique contained too many variables, they describe modifications of the technique which largely eliminate these.

Experimental evidence bears out clinical experience in that epidural, subdural and subarachnoid haemorrhage as a cause of cord compression are rarely seen, and the important changes take place in the cord itself.

The sequence of events in the first few hours following experimental spinal cord injury is summarized in Fig. 60.3. The first changes are seen in the grey matter, bearing out clinical experience that the central part of the cord is most severely affected in

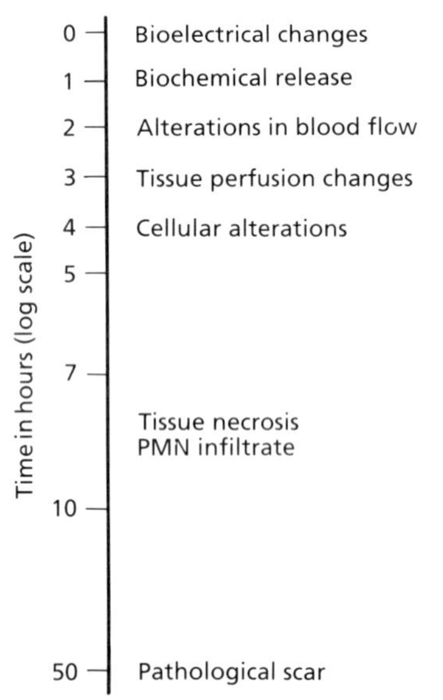

Fig. 60.3 Pathophysiological changes that take place as result of spinal cord injury. After Ducker (1976).

incomplete cord injuries of all types. Within five minutes the grey matter venules are distended, and between 15 and 30 minutes there is escape of red cells from venules and capillaries. Small haemorrhages in the grey matter appear within an hour, and within a few hours increasing vacuolation and swelling of the endothelium of these vessels takes place. After four hours there is evidence of central ischaemic change and haemorrhagic lesions followed by progressive grey matter necrosis.

Microscopic changes in the white matter commence three to four hours after injury, apart from occasional flame-shaped haemorrhages immediately following the original impact. The white matter pathology commences with oedema leading to disordered perfusion followed by progressive destruction of the white matter over a period of days. The oedema itself increases for up to five days and then regresses over the next 10. Both the amount of oedema and the total amount of tissue destruction are in general proportional to the severity of the initiating trauma (Ducker, 1976; Jellinger, 1976; De La Torre, 1981). However, the time sequence of events is uniform regardless of the forces involved (Fig. 60.4).

Vasomotor vicissitudes

The vasomotor reactivity of the involved segment is lost immediately after injury (Ducker, 1976) and impaired spinal cord blood flow and hypoxia are possibly the most important ensuing secondary features. The $P\text{O}_2$ commences falling after 30 minutes and there is persistent hypoxia after seven hours. Spinal cord blood flow (SCBF) falls progressively in the grey matter from one to four hours after injury. Initially up to four hours after injury it may increase in the white matter to twice normal, then decrease, until eight hours following injury it is again normal, at which level it remains. Major vascular occlusion is not seen, but there may be spasm or occlusion of small vessels in the cord, with stagnation of blood flow particularly in the postcapillary venules. The decrease in blood flow is a local phenomenon and independent of arterial blood pressure. There is evidence that the response in an irreversibly injured cord is ischaemic, while that in a cord that will recover becomes hyperaemic and hyperoxic (Ducker, 1976).

Less severe changes occur in adjacent segments also. Eleven hours after cord transection and four hours after impact injury axonic degeneration is seen

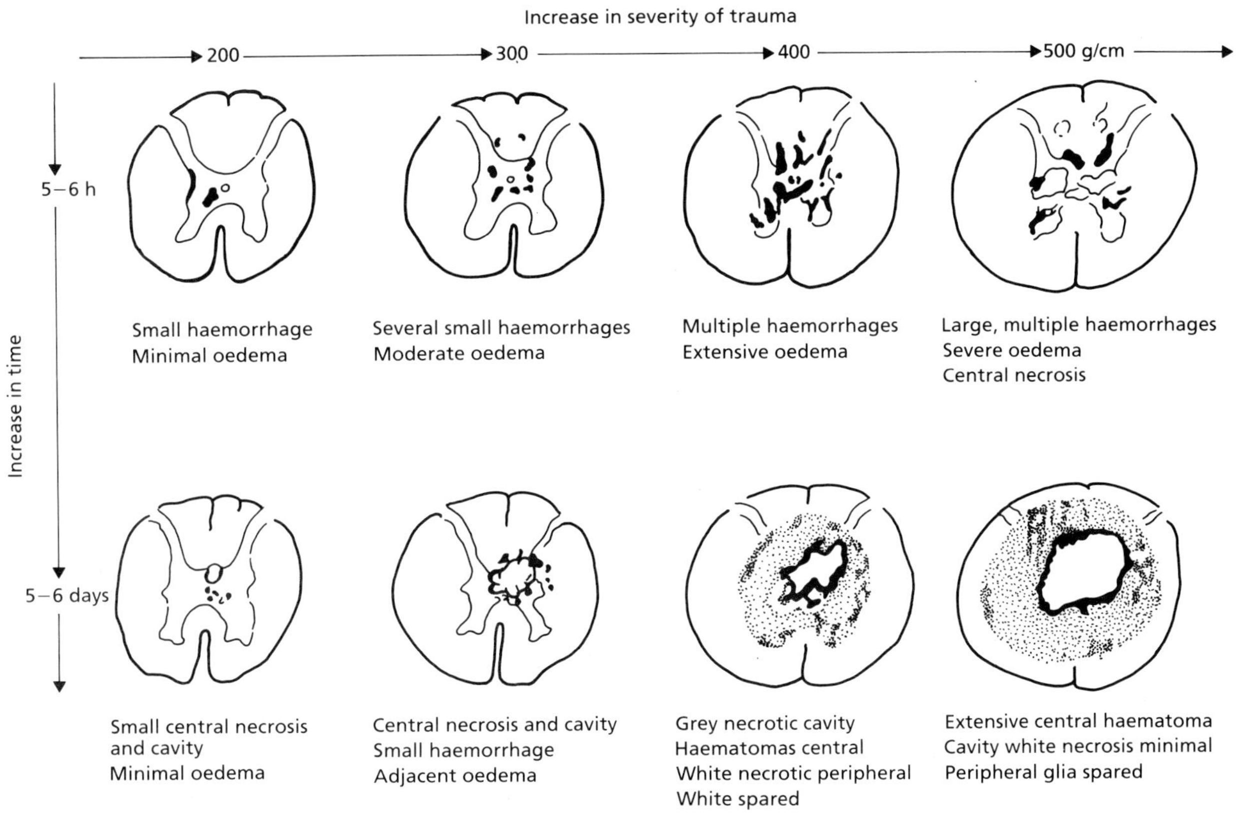

Fig. 60.4 The pathological picture as it relates to trauma and time. After Ducker (1976).

both proximal and distal to the lesion (Dohrmann, 1971, quoted by Jellinger, 1976), while areas of haemorrhage, necrosis, oedema and cord softening may be seen distally (Fig. 60.5).

The manner in which the early post-traumatic changes affect the grey matter predominantly with initial sparing of the white matter, particularly in incomplete injury, has led to speculation that therapy aimed at limiting the secondary response (especially ischaemia and hypoxia) to injury, may preserve the white matter and limit the ultimate neurological deficit. Hence much attention has been directed at the mechanisms which may affect the SCBF following injury and particularly biochemical changes.

Metabolic mayhem

A significant increase in tissue water and sodium concentration and decrease in potassium are seen three days following impact spinal cord injury (SCI) in cats. These changes occur up to 5 cm above and below the lesion. More importantly perhaps, significant falls in extracellular calcium levels with an influx of calcium to the cells result.

There is lasting reduction in oxygen and pyruvate, and marked increase in lactate levels, together with a great reduction in adenosine triphosphate and phosphocreatine, and a lesser reduction in tissue

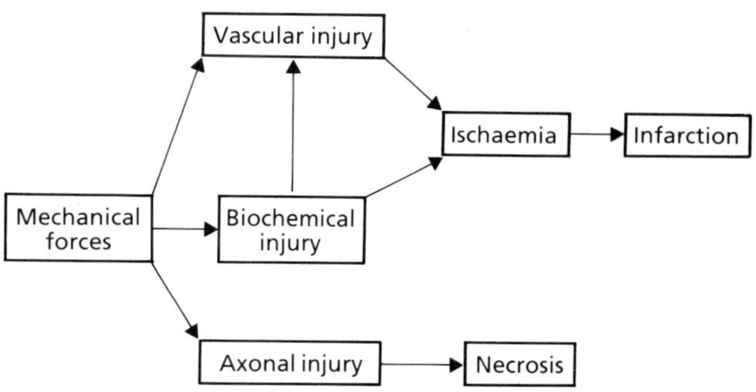

Fig. 60.5 Hypothesis for pathophysiology of acute spinal cord injury indicating the role of post-traumatic oedema and infarction. After Tator & Rowed (1979).

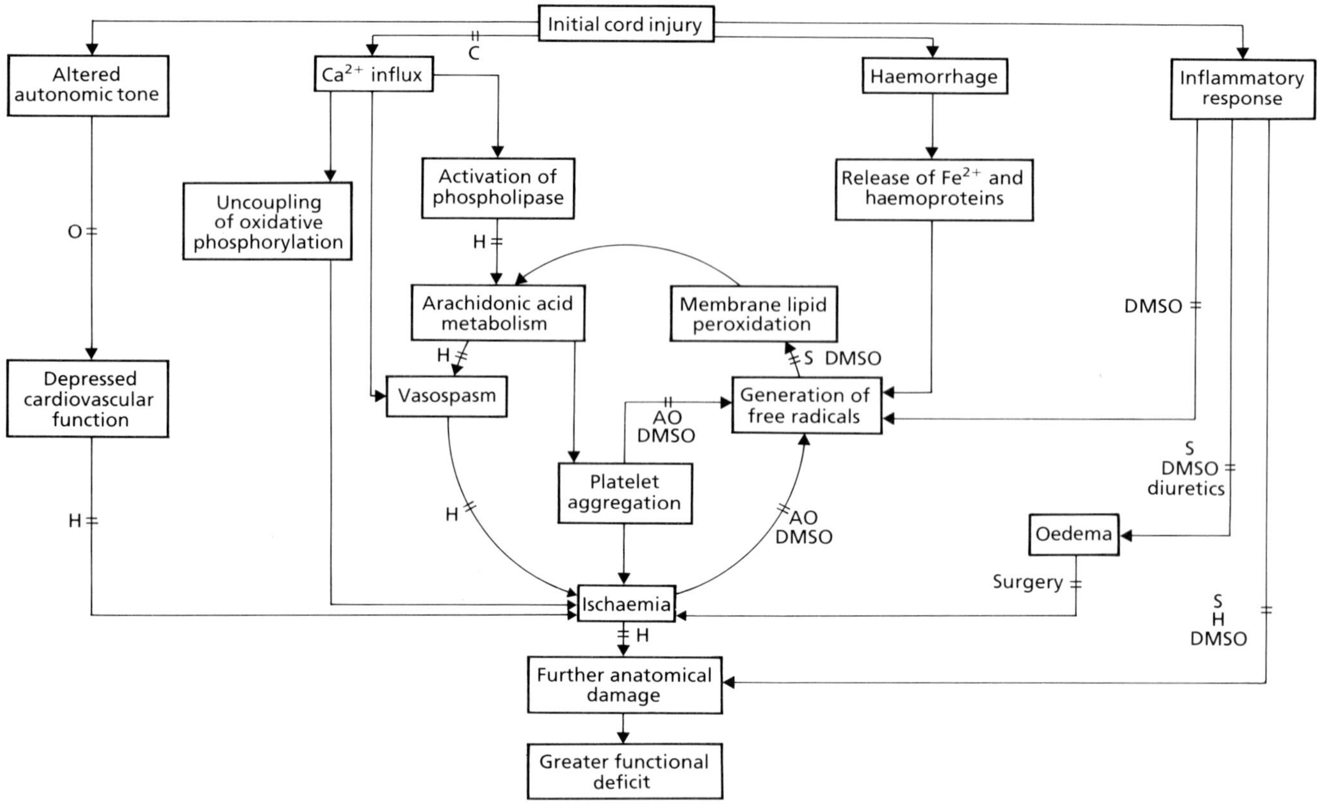

Fig. 60.6 Proposed mechanism(s) of delayed spinal cord injury, and possible effects of currently practised treatments. AO, antioxidants; C, calcium channel blockers; DMSO, dimethylsulphoxide; H, hypothermia; O, opiates; S, steroids. After Janssen (1989).

adenosine diphosphate and glucose. Overall, the picture is described as reflecting ischaemia/hypoxia-induced uncoupling of oxidative phosphorylation and a shift to anaerobic glycolysis (Janssen & Hansebout, 1989).

Other investigators have reported an accumulation of a variety of neurotransmitters including norepinephrine, dopamine, histamine, substance P, and serotonin. The possible effects of these and other substances on the secondary response of the injured cord have been illustrated diagrammatically (Fig. 60.6) and have led to the search for chemical as opposed to physical methods of treatment.

The new neuroanatomy and therapeutic theory

Over the decades discoveries concerning the biochemical changes following experimental SCI have led to a number of suggested lines of medical treatment.

Important advances in neurochemistry in the past 10 years, with the discovery of monoclonal and polyclonal antibodies to central nervous system proteins, have led to the discovery of about 40 active neuropeptides in addition to the seven classical neurotransmitters (Hughes, 1989). More detailed knowledge of the nature of the anatomy and physiology of the cord may lead to more sophisticated attempts to modify the behaviour of the injured cord by chemical means. Up until now such attempts have been limited to a small number of substances which have been shown to be of some value experimentally, but have been found wanting in clinical practice.

The preliminary results of Professor Wise Young working on cats indicated that the salvage rates of the long tracts could be improved using methylprednisolone, naloxone, gangliosides, or pulsed magnetic energy 4 hours after injury (Kakulas & Dimitrijevich, 1987).

Hitchon *et al.* (1989) found methylprednisolone to have no effect on SCBF or sensory evoked potential in cord-compressed lambs although other workers have shown increased SCBF following injury to cats and decreased neurofilament degradation with restoration of membrane function following the use of this drug. However, a national US trial on the benefit of high-dose as opposed to low-dose methylprednisolone (Bracken, quoted by Janssen & Hansebout, 1989) found no difference between the two. Unfortunately this study was not controlled with patients given no prednisolone.

Other proposed medical treatments have included opiate antagonists (naloxone, thyrotropin-releasing hormone, which lead to a rise in mean arterial blood pressure and an increase in SCBF with a possible effect on membrane lipid peroxidation), also dimethyl sulphoxide and other diuretics, 6-hydroxydopamine (leading to chemical denervation of norepinephrine and serotonin-dependent neurones), and other noradrenergic blocking agents.

While some experimental evidence exists in support of all of these substances, none has been proven effective in clinical practice. In particular steroids, until recently, had never been shown to be of value in human SCI. In 1990, however, Bracken *et al.* published the results of a multicentre trial indicating that methylprednisolone given within 8 hours of injury improves neurological recovery. The study did not indicate whether the improved neurological recovery was of functional significance, and independent confirmation of these results is awaited.

Current research includes studies of calcium channel antagonists in view of the dramatic changes in intra- and extracellular calcium following injuries (Simpson, 1991).

Hyperbaric oxygen has been shown to increase local tissue $P\text{O}_2$ following SCI, although without increasing SCBF (Ducker, 1976). Encouraging results in the treatment of experimental SCI in sheep led to its introduction into clinical practice in a limited series with some encouraging results (Yeo, 1978). However, its value remains unproven and there are practical problems in its use, requiring as it does the nursing of an acutely injured and seriously ill patient in a hyperbaric oxygen chamber.

Spinal cord cooling, following encouraging experimental results, was reported as proving beneficial in some clinical trials (Janssen & Hansebout, 1989) but was used in combination with steroids in some cases, and in general the results have not been sufficiently convincing to lead to its widespread adoption.

There are a number of reasons for the discrepancy in the results of animal as opposed to human trials, including the nature of the experimental injury which tends to be uniform, moderate and limited in animals; the lack of complications in the injured animals as opposed to humans where the injury is associated with shock, blood loss and commonly other injuries; the fact that only the most severe cases of human spinal cord injury tend to be treated with the newer experimental methods; and finally the timing, in that treatment, if it is to be helpful, should be commenced ideally well within four to eight hours following injury.

The compression conundrum

To what extent is the ultimate neurological deficit the result of initial mechanical neural damage, of vascular disruption, or of ischaemic change brought about by toxic metabolites? What part is played by compression and other pathophysiological mechanisms including oedema?

The initial impact leads to shearing of axons, rupture of the veins, haemorrhage and oedema, and there is no doubt that the major determinant of the neurological outcome is the force of the initial injury. However, there is little correlation between neurological deficit and the extent of pathological changes after experimental SCI, and even a small amount of surviving tissue is compatible with considerable surviving neurological function (Eidelberg, 1976, quoted by Guha *et al.*, 1987).

While studies of the effect of force and duration of compression on neurological recovery have indicated that there is a relationship, this has been found to be true for very light compressive forces only, with follow-up limited to eight weeks (Guha *et al.*, 1987). Tarlov & Klinger (1954), in spinal cord compression studies with balloons, concluded from the instantaneous onset of paralysis and delayed recovery after release of compression that loss of function was initially mechanical and not secondary to ischaemia. They found the cauda equina to be much more resistant to compression of this type. More recently Garvin *et al.* (1990) have demonstrated that hypotension increases significantly the effect of compression of the cauda equina nerve roots in pigs. The changes were most marked with a relatively minor degree of compression, a pressure having no effect on nerve function of normotensive animals.

Clip compression studies of the lower cervical cord in rats (Rivlin & Tator, 1978) revealed that after five minutes compression there was extremely low SCBF for up to 24 hours (the end of the experiment) and that the changes extended proximally and distally for at least 5 mm (the experimenters did not reach normal cord). This emphasizes once again the longitudinal nature of the cord damage, while the demonstration of diminished SCBF for so long may serve as a counter to the argument of Tarlov & Klinger (1954) that loss of function is mechanical.

In summary, while these and other experiments confirm that the severity of the initial injury is the main determinant of the ultimate deficit, there is abundant work to show that for the spinal cord rather than the cauda equina, and with very light forces particularly, early relief of compression may improve recovery. The techniques employed are so artificial, however, and the times of both compression and follow-up so short, that it is difficult to relate these conditions to that of the patient who arrives in hospital suffering from the local and systemic effects of high-velocity trauma occasioned some hours earlier.

In clinical practice posterior decompression of the injured cord by laminectomy has been proven to be ineffective. Myelotomy was reported to lead to improvement in 50% of cases, but had a mortality of up to 42% (Janssen & Hansebout, 1989). Nonetheless a recent report indicates that it is still practised for the radiologically proven swollen cord (Koyanagi *et al.*, 1989).

Anterior decompression is in vogue at present for cases where there is radiological evidence of bone and/or disc encroaching on the spinal canal. Evidence for its effectiveness remains anecdotal (Donovan & Dwyer, 1984) and the experimental evidence in its favour must be weighed against the rarity of compression at post mortem (Kakulas, 1988) and the absence of correlation between radiological spinal canal compromise and neurological deficit (Keene *et al.*, 1986; Gertzbein *et al.*, 1988) Clearly the presence of extraneous material in the spinal canal does not mean that it is necessarily compressing the cord, or is a factor in the continuing evolution of the pathological process.

Repair and regeneration

As all forms of treatment to date have been shown to have very little effect on the degree of neurological recovery, attention is turning increasingly to the possibility of influencing the repair and regenerative processes in the injured cord.

Humans are more complex than the lower species, and regeneration of nervous tissue is therefore less complete (Hughes, 1984). However, it does occur in the meninges, in the spinal vessels, in the connective tissue, and incompletely in the glial tissue. Small tears in the meninges heal normally, but large and displaced tears heal with a connective tissue scar. Vessels regenerate essentially to normal size but with some histological change. Connective tissue healing with astrocytes and fibrous processes leads to a glial scar in less severe cord injuries, but in the more severe injuries with massive haemorrhage and necrosis there is a connective tissue scar with glial tissue on either side. Possibly the problem with regeneration is not the scar itself but the lack of glial tissue in it, and particularly the lack of central-type myelin sheaths developed from such tissue.

Complete loss of neurones is irrecoverable in the adult human spinal cord. Spinal motor neurones which travel only a short distance in the cord do regenerate, but may get lost. The central processes of the neurones of peripheral sensory nerves may regenerate in a disorderly way, but the long intraspinal neurones are not replaced after trauma and show not even abortive regeneration. It is not known whether internuncial neurones regenerate, but synapses can be reformed and new ones made. Intramedullary sprouts from posterior root ganglia and posterior and/or anterior nerve roots are probably the most important source of regenerating fibres, while others are derived from perivascular nerve fibres (Jellinger, 1976).

Following hemisection of the rat's spinal cord 90–95% of the neurites that reinnervate neurones rostral to the site of the lesion appear to be sprouts of normal intact nerves, whereas only 5–10% are derived from severed neurites (Jellinger, 1976).

Experimentally, following SCI in mature animals, injured axons fail to regenerate, while regeneration in the transected spinal cord or nerve tracts has been shown to last up to two weeks, but to travel short distances only (de la Torre, quoted by Mizrachi *et al.*, 1983). However, axonic growth can be enhanced dramatically by a peripheral nerve graft providing a substrate (Jansen, 1986). Aquayo's classic experiments (1983 quoted by Fawcett, 1991) demonstrated that all axons can regenerate, given the right environment, and that CNS tissues are inhibitory. Schwab (1991) identified two specific proteins (NI 35 and NI

250), on oligodendrocyte cell bodies which arrested axon regeneration, and he was able to reverse this effect with specific antibodies.

Wilson (1984), in his work on cats, also demonstrated that following partial resection of a segment of cord autogenous peripheral nerve graft helped regeneration, presumably by acting as a substrate. Functional, sensory evoked potential, and histological proof of regeneration was given.

In another study minced peripheral nerve autograft inserted immediately following hemicordotomy showed microscopic evidence of regeneration and diminished degeneration distally in the treated as compared with control animals (Hadi Khalili & Hamash, 1988), but no functional assessment was carried out.

Other work on spinal cord regeneration includes studies with nerve growth factor, with trophic central nervous system (CNS) factors, with Schwann cell factor, fibroblast and epidermal growth factor, and electromagnetic fields (Kakulas, 1988). Components inducing neuronal sprouting have been demonstrated in normal human sera. However, 86% of patients with SCI have been shown to have antibodies to brain gangliosides and/or myelin basic proteins (as compared with 32% of controls) and sera from these patients have markedly reduced trophic effect for sprouting from chick dorsal root ganglia *in vitro* (Mizrachi *et al.*, 1983).

The future

Molecular neurobiology may lead to the identification of the genes controlling CNS growth, regeneration and maturation, which in turn may lead to the use of autografts to replace lost spinal tissue. Perhaps such grafts could be 're-educated' once the molecular basis of plasticity becomes known (Kakulas & Dimitrijevich, 1987). Perhaps 'The cure for spinal cord injury is a matter of derepressing the genes responsible for multiplication of neuroblasts, the sprouting of neurites, and the regrowth of axons and collaterals with the restoration of physiological connections and functionally useful reflexes by means of guided plasticity and synaptogenesis' (Kakulas, 1988).

Or perhaps the answer will be electrophysiological or other technology as yet undreamt of. What does seem certain is that for the foreseeable future, as for the past century, the pendulum of management of spinal cord injury will continue to swing among the range of conservative, medical and surgical management presently available, creeping fractionally over new ground as it does so.

In the past 4000 years our knowledge of spinal cord pathology following injury has become increasingly detailed, yet in some ways our ability to influence the process is no more advanced than in the days when the Edwin Smith papyrus was inscribed.

Chairman Mao ended his parable of the mountains with the statement that 'God looked kindly on the old man and sent two angels and demolished the mountains for him.' The angels to demolish the mountains of spinal cord injury have yet to appear.

REFERENCES

Braakman, R. & Penning, L. (1976) Injuries of the cervical spine. In Vinken, P.J. & Bruyn, G.W. (eds) *Handbook of Clinical Neurology*, vol. 25, chap. 13. North-Holland, Amsterdam.

Bracken, M.B., Shepard, M.J., Collins, W.F., Holford, T.R., Young, W., Baskin, D.S., Eisenberg, H.M., Flamm, E., Leo-Summers, L., Maroon, J., Marshall, L.F., Perot, P.L., Piepmeier, J., Sonntag, V.K.H., Wagner, F.C., Wilberger, J.E. & Wynn, H.R. (1990) A randomised controlled trial of Methylprednisolone or Naloxone in the treatment of acute spinal cord injury. *N. Engl. J. Med.*, **322**, 1403–1411.

Bohlman, H.H., Freehafer, A. & Dejak, J. (1975) Late anterior decompression of spinal cord injuries. *J. Bone Jt. Surg.*, **57A**, 1025.

Bramwell, B. (1884) *Diseases of the Spinal Cord.* Young J. Pentland, Edinburgh.

De La Torre, J.C. (1981) Spinal cord injury, review of basic and applied research. *Spine*, **6**, 315–335.

Dimitrijevic, M.R. (1987) Neurophysiology in spinal cord injury. *Paraplegia*, **25**, 205–211.

Donovan, W.H. & Dwyer, A.P. (1984) An update on the early management of traumatic paraplegia (non-operative and operative management). *Clin. Orthop.*, **189**, 12–21.

Ducker, T.D. (1976) Experimental injury of the spinal cord. In Vinken, P.J. & Bruyn, G.W. (eds) *Handbook of Clinical Neurology*, vol. 25, chap. 2. North-Holland, Amsterdam.

Fawcett, J.W. (1991) Factors influencing the regeneration of axons in the central nervous system. *Paraplegia*, **29**, 287–293.

Garfin, S.R., Cohen, M.S., Massie, J.B., Abitbol, J.J., Swenson, M.R., Myers, R.R. & Rydevik, B.L. (1990) Nerve roots of the cauda equina. The effect of hypotension and acute graded compression on function. *J. Bone Jt. Surg.*, **72A**, 1185.

Gertzbein, S.D., Court-Brown, C.M., Marks, P., Martin, C., Fazl, M., Schwartz, M. & Jacobs, R.R. (1988) The neurological outcome following surgery for spinal fractures. *Spine*, **13**, 641–644.

Goldsmith, H.S., Nell-Dwyer, G. & Barsoum, L. (1986) Omental transposition to the acute and chronically injured spinal cord. Presented at the International Medical Society of Paraplegia Annual Scientific Meeting, Oslo, 26–28 June.

Goodkin, R. (1976) Experimental injuries of the spine. In Vinkin, P.J. & Bruyn, G.W. (eds) *Handbook of Clinical Neurology*, vol. 25, chap. 1. North-Holland, Amsterdam.

Guha, A., Tator, C.H., Endrenyi, L. & Piper, I. (1987) Decompression of the spinal cord improves recovery after acute experimental spinal cord compression injury. *Paraplegia*, **25**, 324–339.

Hadi Khalili, A. & Hamash, H.M. (1988) Spinal cord regeneration: new experimental approach. *Paraplegia*, **26**, 310–316.

Hitchon, P.W., McKay, T.C., Thornton Wilkinson, T., Girton, R.A., Hanson, T. & Dyste, G.N. (1989) Methylprednisolone in spinal cord compression. *Spine*, **14**, 16–22.

Hughes, J.T. (1978) *Pathology of the Spinal Cord.* Lloyd-Luke Medical Books, London.

Hughes, J.T. (1984) Regeneration in the human spinal cord: a review of the response to injury of the various constituents of the human spinal cord. *Paraplegia*, **22**, 131–137.

Hughes, J.T. (1988) The Edwin Smith surgical papyrus: an analysis of the first case reports of spinal cord injuries. *Paraplegia*, **26**, 71–82.

Hughes, J.T. (1989) The new neuroanatomy of the spinal cord. *Paraplegia*, **27**, 90–98.

Jansen, J. (1986) Repair after experimental injuries to the spinal cord. Presented at the Annual Scientific Meeting of the International Medical Society of Paraplegia, Oslo, 26–28 June.

Janssen, L. & Hansebout, R.R. (1989) Pathogenesis of spinal cord injury and newer treatments—a review. *Spine*, **14**, 23–32.

Jellinger, K. (1976) Neuropathology of cord injuries. In Vinken, P.J. & Bruyn, G.W. (eds) *Handbook of Clinical Neurology*, vol. 25, chap. 4. North-Holland, Amsterdam.

Kakulas, B.A. (1988) The applied neurobiology of human spinal cord injury: a review. *Paraplegia*, **26**, 371–379.

Kakulas, B.A. & Bedbrook, G.M. (1976) Pathology of injuries of the vertebral column—with emphasis on the macroscopical aspects. In Vinken, P.J. & Bruyn, G.W. (eds) *Handbook of Clinical Neurology*, vol. 25, chap. 3. North-Holland, Amsterdam.

Kakulas, B.A. & Dimitrijevich, M.R. (1987) The contribution of neuropathology to the restorative neurology of spinal cord injury: acute, sub-acute and chronic: a review of existing and possible new interventions. *Paraplegia*, **25**, 409–410 (abstract).

Keene, J.S., Fischer, S.P., Drummond, D.S. *et al.* (1986) The neurological consequences of post-traumatic neural canal impingement. *Paraplegia*, **24**, 45–46 (abstract).

Koyanagi, I., Iwasaki, Y., Isu, T., Akino, M. & Abe, H. (1989) Significance of spinal cord swelling in the prognosis of acute cervical spinal cord injury. *Paraplegia*, **27**, 190–197.

Mao Tsetung, Chairman (1972) *Quotations.* Foreign Languages Press, Peking.

Mizrachi, Y., Ohry, A., Aviel, A., Rozin, R., Brooks, M.E. & Schwartz, M. (1983) Systemic humoral factors participating in the course of spinal cord injury. *Paraplegia*, **21**, 287–293.

Panjabi, M. & Wrathall, J.R. (1988) Biomechanical analysis of experimental cord injury and functional loss. *Spine*, **13**, 1365–1370.

Rivlin, A. & Tator, C.H. (1978) Regional spinal cord blood flow in rats after severe cord trauma. *J. Neurosurg.*, **49**, 844–853.

Shwab, M.E. (1991) Regeneration of lesioned CNS axons by neutralisation of neurite growth inhibitors: a short review. *Paraplegia*, **29**, 294.

Simpson, R.K., Hsu, C.Y. & Dimitrijevich, M.R. (1991) The experimental basis for early Pharmacological intervention in Spinal Cord Injury. *Paraplegia*, **29**, 364.

Tarlov, I.M. & Klinger, H. (1954) Spinal cord compression studies. *Arch. Neurol. Psychiatry*, **71**, 271.

Tator, C.H. & Rowed, D.W. (1979). Current concepts in the immediate management of acute spinal cord injuries. *CMA J.*, **121**.

Toscano, J. (1988) Prevention of neurological deterioration before admission to a spinal cord injury unit. *Paraplegia*, **36**, 143–150.

Wilson, D.H. (1984) Peripheral nerve implants in the spinal cord in experimental animals. *Paraplegia*, **22**, 230–237.

Yeo, J.D. (1978) Preliminary report on ten patients with spinal cord injuries treated with hyperbaric oxygen. *Med. J. Aust.*, **2**, 572–573.

61 · Systemic Effects of Spinal Cord Injury

By J.R. SILVER and S.J. WILLIAMS

Spinal cord injuries have been known since antiquity. They have a high initial mortality and morbidity. Thompson Walker, writing in 1917 and 1937, found that of 339 patients with spinal injury admitted to the King George V Military Hospital from 1915 to 1919, 160 (47.2%) died from urinary infection within eight to 10 weeks of admission. Connors & Nash (1934) and Kennedy (1946) found that of US Army paraplegics, fully 80% of them died in the first few weeks in consequence of infection from bedsores and catheterization. Until Donald Munro (1943) and Sir Ludwig Guttmann (1949) devised modern methods of treatment all patients died within weeks of injury. By the use of antibiotics and the rapid transfer of patients to specialized centres, the patient with a low spinal cord injury survived and could be successfully returned to a working life.

However, patients with cervical injuries still had a very high mortality. Durbin in 1957 recorded his experience of 75 patients with cervical injuries. Of these 15 with complete cord transections 14 died within days of injury, death occurring from bronchopneumonia and hyperpyrexia. Silver (1967/8) recorded his experience of 50 patients between 1965 and 1967 at a regional paraplegic centre; of these 29 had cervical injuries. There were eight deaths, and seven of these were among cervical patients. They died of respiratory failure and bronchopneumonia. Thus there is a significant difference in the initial mortality between tetraplegic patients and paraplegic patients.

Scope of the problem

Each year about 300 patients with acute spinal cord injury are admitted to hospital in the UK (although there are many more injuries to the spinal column where the spinal cord is not involved). The majority of patients are initially admitted to a district general hospital before they are referred to a specialized centre.

The distribution of these injuries is similar to that in other western countries. The majority are young males and about 50% of the injuries will be in the cervical region; of these about 50% will have a complete interruption of the cord (Fig. 61.1). Road traffic accidents cause about 50% of these injuries. These are mainly to the driver and passengers of the vehicle, although recently motor-cycle accidents have begun to increase. It is almost impossible to injure the spinal column in isolation, and such injuries occur as part of a major accident. About 75% of the victims have major injuries to the rest of their body.

Table 61.1 Comparison of mortality in three series of cervical injuries. From Cheshire (1963)

	Durbin (1957)	Norton (1962)	Cheshire (1964)[a]
Period of time (years)	9	9	4
Number of cases of cervical injury	75	88	100
Neurological involvement	42	41	100
Roots only	16	6	9
Cord lesions	26	35	91
Complete	15	21	39
Incomplete	11	14	52
Deaths	15	4	17
Number of complete lesions	15	21	39
Acute respiratory deaths	14	3	7

[a] Over the period 1959–1963.

Table 61.2 Analysis of 50 traumatic cases. From Silver (1967/8)

Sex	40 males, 10 females	
Age	12–77 years	
Deaths	8	
Levels	Cervical 29 Thoracic 15 Lumbar 6	
Causes	Road traffic accidents	25
	Falls (two suicides, one hysteria)	19
	Blows on the back	4
	Diving	1
	Pathological (multiple myeloma)	1
		50

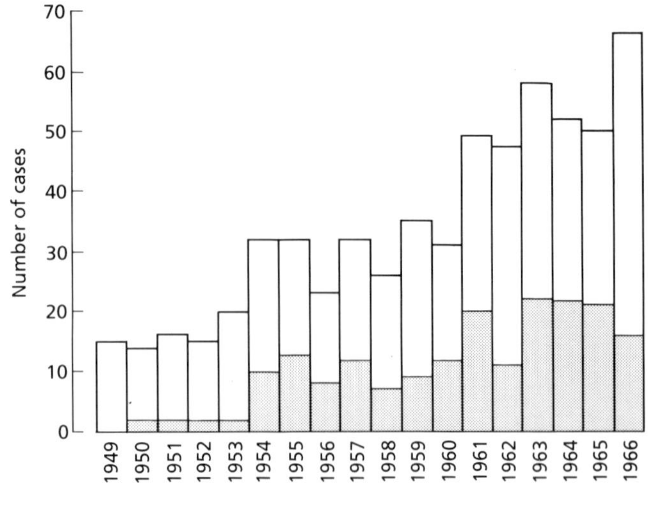

Fig. 61.1 Total tetraplegics admitted year by year compared with total admissions. Year average is 30%. From Silver & Gibbon (1968).

In view of their relative rarity the surgeon at the receiving hospital, confronted with a patient with such an injury to the spinal cord, has a series of difficult decisions to make in the management of the patient. He is anxious to treat any remediable injury to the spinal column and cord and to prevent the patient's neurological condition deteriorating, but an injury to the spinal cord also produces significant changes in the rest of the patient's body. The serious concurrent injuries may well be life-threatening, such as a tension pneumothorax or rupture of an abdominal organ, and must be dealt with before the spinal injury can be managed. Thus the planning and timescale of the treatment of the spinal injury is a matter of careful judgement.

We wish to present our experiences in a large and well-established spinal unit in the UK, to which patients are transferred early from district and specialist hospitals shortly after injury. It is part of a district general hospital where all the facilities of surgery, orthopaedics and an acute intensive-care unit for patients on ventilators are available. This is the combined experience of a spinal injury consultant working in the field, and a consultant physician who has had responsibility for many of the medical problems in the spinal centre and for all the spinal patients (100) admitted to the intensive-care unit for the past 10 years.

Table 61.3 Analysis of the cause of death in eight fatalities. From Silver (1967/8)

Level	Age (years)	Number of days between injury and death	Associated injuries	Cause of death
C4	57	7	Head injury	Respiratory failure
C4	53	3	Nil	Respiratory failure
C4	40	2	Head injury, tibia and fibula	Respiratory failure
C4	66	17	Head injury	Respiratory failure
C4 inc.	68	101	Nil (bronchitis)	Bronchopneumonia
C5 inc.	60	272	Head injury, ribs (bronchitis)	Bronchopneumonia
C6	52	8	Head injury, femur	Respiratory failure
T12	62	19	Head injury, heart failure, ribs and sternum	Pulmonary embolism

Introduction

In order to understand the principles of spinal cord injury management it is necessary to appreciate that the basis of rehabilitation is to develop the functions of the body which remain normal and to compensate for those that have been lost by the injury. A cord transection produces negative factors due to this loss; also the paralysed parts can produce positive harmful effects upon the normal parts of the body. In addition the trauma of the initial injury will produce its own deleterious effects; all these factors will be compounded by the psychological effects.

Negative (loss of function)

Depending on the level and severity of cord transection there is a loss of function below the level of damage. A loss of muscle power and sensation, also impairment of the autonomic system, lead to impairment of bowel, bladder and sexual function, temperature regulation and vascular control.

Positive (harmful effects)

The positive harmful effects are that the patient is confined to bed while the fracture stabilizes and the muscles are paralysed; this immobilization causes deossification of the skeleton. In children this is manifested by a raised serum calcium level leading to hypercalcaemia, particularly in tetraplegics. In adults, while the serum calcium is not raised, stone formation in the kidney and bladder can occur within weeks of injury. Muscle tissue also wastes and breaks down, leading to a raised blood urea and an increased load upon the kidneys.

The immobility of the legs leads to deep vein thrombosis and pulmonary embolism.

The loss of sensation means that painful stimuli do not reach consciousness, and pressure sores develop, resulting in toxicity and septicaemia. Loss of bowel function results in distension of the abdomen and paralytic ileus. Loss of bladder function leads to impaired emptying of the bladder, retention of urine, with ascending infection to the kidneys causing pyelonephritis. The combination of pressure sores and pyelonephritis led to the high morbidity and mortality of the First World War.

Abnormal reflex responses of the striped muscle cause spasms. Abnormal autonomic response can result in paroxysms of raised blood pressure; these usually take some weeks to develop but can be present within a week of injury.

Associated trauma

About 75% of patients suffer from associated trauma. Fracture or dislocation of the cervical vertebra is frequently associated with a severe head injury. This can be of such severity as to mask, or to lead to failure to diagnose, the cervical injury.

The resultant depression of consciousness leads to difficulties in managing a patient's chest condition, and causes a lack of the cooperation which is so necessary to the success of turning and nursing regimes in the early stages.

Later, the head injury can lead to behavioural disturbance which again makes rehabilitation impossible.

It is not possible to fracture the thoracic spine without suffering injury to the chest wall, lungs or ribs. In consequence haemopneumothorax with ventilatory impairment frequently occurs. A patient with lumbar or pelvic fractures will have a significant retroperitoneal haemorrhage which will lead to a paralytic ileus of long duration. In thoracic spinal injury, fracture of the scapula, clavicle and upper limbs frequently occurs, associated with a brachial plexus lesion. This can lead to difficulties in diagnosis.

Lumbar and pelvic fractures are also associated with fractures of the femur. These fractures should be treated early with internal fixation, since traction and plaster immobilization lead to difficulties in turning and can give rise to pressure sores and problems in draining the chest. Any of the foregoing fractures will have a significant blood loss and give rise to surgical shock even in the absence of spinal injury.

Psychology

A patient with a spinal injury admitted to a spinal unit will be terrified. He or she is ignorant of the implications of the injury and is frightened.

Later, when the severity of the injury is realized, the patient may well be justifiably depressed. He or she is fearful of the effects of the injury on family, the future and ability to earn. Relationships and sexuality are major areas of anxiety and this is intensified by

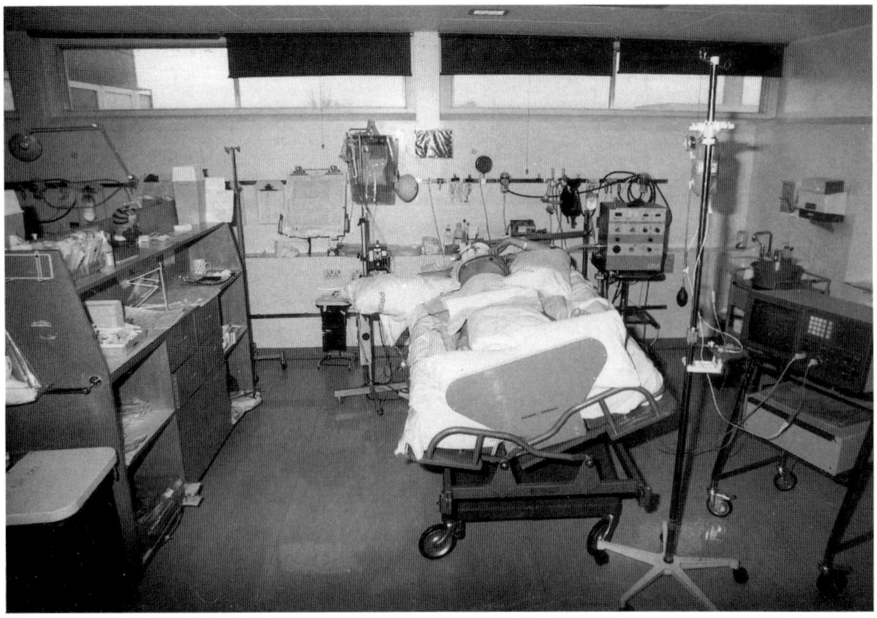

Fig. 61.2 Patient in an intensive-care unit. It can be seen that monitoring equipment and numerous lines makes turning and nursing extremely difficult.

the patient's isolation, perhaps because of an inability to speak following a tracheotomy or because of the effect of drugs being administered. The patient may have irrational fears that the injury may ascend and that he or she will become totally paralysed. This is also compounded by drugs administered for sedation purposes. Drugs that are given to the patient, such as opiates or steroids, may cause confusion, thus contributing to the patient's unhappiness. He or she may become resentful and aggressive, or guilty, depending on the circumstances of the accident. The patient may have been the driver of the car in which people were killed. Unfortunately many of these accidents are alcohol-related and it is not uncommon to see the effects of delirium tremens due to alcohol withdrawal. Sepsis from pressure sores can lead to a toxic psychosis or justifiable depression or resentment against the staff whose treatment has created the pressure sore.

Another major factor contributing to the patient's unhappiness is pain from the fracture site, the associated injury, and pain of spinal origin such as root pain which usually takes some six weeks to develop but can be apparent much earlier.

Thus it is good and necessary medical practice to explain to the patients and their relatives the nature and implications of the injury, and to keep them informed of their progress by means of frequent multidisciplinary case conferences.

Anatomy

Phylogenetically, because of the contribution the spinal cord makes to the arms and legs, the spinal cord is shorter than the spinal column which encloses it. The vertebral level does not correspond to the cord level. The result is that the eighth spinal segment is located at the level of the sixth/seventh disc space, the twelfth spinal segment at the level of the tenth thoracic vertebra, and the cord ends at the lower border of the first lumbar vertebra. It follows that the nerve roots pursue an oblique course downwards. Therefore injury to a vertebra damages the cord and roots at a different level.

Pathology

An injury to the cord is rarely a clear-cut transection and there is usually longitudinal damage to the tissues extending several segments above and below the site of maximal damage. Any neural tissue involving the cord that is destroyed will not recover; but cells may be temporarily inhibited by oedema. Other mechanical factors such as pressure and stretching will also cause inhibition. Usually the maximal neurological deficit will be seen at the moment of injury, but the injury can be made worse by inappropriate handling when further damage can be inflicted to the cord and oedema develops. Subsequent recovery is due not to regeneration but to the partial recovery of damaged cells.

Prognosis

In general any cord lesion that is complete at the outset and shows no sign of becoming incomplete by 48 hours after injury will not show any useful recovery of function.

Cauda equina

An injury to the cauda equina is a lower motor neurone lesion. Regeneration may take place as in other peripheral nerve lesions, but if regeneration takes place the advancing neural tissue has a greater distance to travel to the neuromuscular junction and therefore recovery is usually incomplete and painful.

Loss of motor function

The impairment of motor function is not life-threatening unless it involves the respiratory muscles; however, the loss of movement will result in contractures and ectopic calcification. It is necessary that regular passive movement takes place to prevent this happening and to reduce the possibility of deep vein thrombosis. Contractures of the shoulders, elbows and fingers are particularly disabling and unless prevented (by nursing in the crucifixion position) frozen shoulders and painful contractures will occur. These can take many months to eliminate and will prevent successful rehabilitation later.

Cardiopulmonary and thoracic implications

In view of the high mortality associated with cervical injuries, due largely to chest injuries in association with the paralysis, it is necessary to dwell on the former in some detail. The cardiorespiratory effects of acute spinal injuries are mainly the result of:

1 respiratory muscle paralysis;
2 direct injury, particularly to the chest;
3 alteration in the function of the autonomic nervous system.

There is also an increased risk of pulmonary oedema and of deep venous thrombosis with pulmonary embolism, unless preventive measures are taken.

Respiratory muscle paralysis

The muscles of respiration can be divided into four groups: the abdominals, intercostals, diaphragm and accessory muscles. In a complete spinal injury below C5 there is sparing of the diaphragm and accessory muscles but paralysis of the intercostals and abdominals. The intercostal muscles can have both inspiratory and expiratory function. When they contract at low lung volumes they promote inspiration, and at high lung volumes, expiration (De Troyer *et al.*, 1983). Thus if their function is impaired both inspiration and expiration are reduced. Normally the body selectively alternates the use of respiratory muscles when they are under stress, in order to delay the onset of fatigue, just as we change hands with increasing frequency when carrying a heavy load. For example, inspiration can be achieved by contraction of the intercostal muscles for a period to allow the diaphragm to rest when fatigue is imminent. The ability to do this is severely impaired if the intercostal muscles are paralysed, reducing the respiratory muscle reserve and making the system far more liable to fail.

Intercostal muscles also contract during full inspiration to prevent the intercostal spaces being sucked in by negative intrathoracic pressure produced by contraction of the diaphragm. If they are paralysed the chest wall will be sucked in paradoxically on inspiration, reducing the efficiency of inspiration. A considerable part of the contraction of the diaphragm may be wasted in some spinal patients by this insuction of the intercostal spaces (Morgan *et al.*, 1985). There may be considerable variation in the degree of paradox between patients with similar vital capacities. The greater the intercostal paradox the

Table 61.4 Functions of respiratory muscles

Muscle group	Spinal nerve supply	Main respiratory function
Abdominals	T2–L1	Forced expiration
Intercostals	T1–T11	Inspiration and expiration Stabilization of intercostal spaces
Diaphragm	C3–C5	Inspiration
Accessory muscles	C1–C8	Inspiration

more the patient has to work to produce a given vital capacity. Monitoring these patients by vital capacity alone may therefore be misleading.

A complete cervical lesion will also cause paralysis of the abdominal muscles. The main respiratory function of these muscles is to produce a forced expiration or cough. Patients with paralysed abdominal muscles therefore have difficulty in clearing secretions which may result in collapse of segments, a lobe or even a whole lung. Frequent chest physiotherapy with regular changes of position must be instituted early on in these patients (Brownlee & Williams, 1987). It is also important to nurse the patients on both sides despite the presence of rib fractures. In patients with long-standing paralysis a simple respiratory infection may cause similar problems of sputum retention, and vigorous physiotherapy should be started immediately. If the patient has difficulty in clearing secretions from the trachea because of a poor cough, a mini-tracheostomy is sometimes useful. An alternative is nasal and pharyngeal suction, but in our experience this is not so effective and is less well tolerated by the patient. It is also more likely to produce reflex bradycardia. If major airways collapse and cannot be cleared by intensive physiotherapy then bronchoscopy using a fibreoptic bronchoscope will be needed. It is our practice to perform this through an indwelling endotracheal tube. We have found that most spinal patients who have a collapsed lobe or lung requiring ventilation for a short period should not be immediately extubated after bronchoscopy. Sputum retention with or without major lobar lung collapse has been the most common reason for ventilating acute spinal patients in our experience.

The diaphragm is normally shaped like a dome above the lower ribs. It is maintained in this position in the erect posture because of the effects of abdominal tone on the incompressible abdominal contents pushing the diaphragm upwards. If the abdominal muscles are paralysed the abdominal contents fall downwards and forwards when the patient is moved into the erect position. The diaphragm will then descend into the abdominal cavity and may lie at or below the level of the lower ribs at the start of inspiration. Contraction of the diaphragm will then pull the lower ribs inwards, reducing and not expanding the lower part of the chest. Within certain limits the contraction of a muscle is greater when it is stretched. The intra-abdominal pressure caused by abdominal muscle contraction maintains the degree of stretch in the diaphragm, improving its efficiency. These beneficial effects are lost in patients with high spinal injury. Their vital capacity may fall by as much as 45% when they are tipped vertically. This can be corrected to some extent by the use of abdominal binders (Goldman *et al.*, 1986). The main inspiratory muscle is the diaphragm. Its function can be assessed at the bedside by inspecting or palpating the upper part of the abdomen during full inspiration. Normally both the chest and upper abdominal walls move outwards during inspiration. If the diaphragm is paralysed or weak the negative intrathoracic pressure during inspiration sucks the diaphragm into the thorax, and the upper part of the abdomen will then move in and not out during inspiration.

In a complete lesion above C3 the diaphragm is paralysed, leaving only the accessory muscles, especially sternocleidomastoid (C1, C2 and C3) and trapezius (C1–C4) available for inspiration. These muscles can sometimes produce a vital capacity of several hundred millilitres, and the patients can sometimes be weaned off the ventilator at least during the day. However, the muscles frequently prove inadequate for prolonged ventilation and may fail if respiration is depressed for any reason, or during sleep. Such patients need long-term ventilation either by a positive-pressure ventilator or, if the cell bodies of C3, C4 and C5 of the spinal cord are viable, by a diaphragmatic pacing device (Glenn *et al.*, 1980). Negative-pressure ventilators are not useful in these patients, mainly because of the problem of pressure sores in areas without any sensory appreciation.

In patients with an acute high cervical injury the vital capacity is reduced because of the paralysis of some of the respiratory muscles, paradoxical movement of the chest wall and possibly an abnormal, inefficient position of the diaphragm. In a cervical lesion at C5–C6 the vital capacity may fall to 30% predicted immediately after injury (McMichan *et al.*, 1980). In the first few hours or days the respiratory function may fall even further due to fatigue, collapse of part of the lung, sputum retention or ascent of the neurological lesion due to oedema. In our experience most of the patients who require ventilation with high spinal lesions do so within 36 hours of the injury. In patients with unstable cervical injuries extreme care must be taken during intubation to reduce movement of the neck to a minimum. In difficult cases a fibreoptic bronchoscope may be used as an introducer for the endotracheal tube. If major complications do not develop the vital capacity usually improves gradually. Most of the improvement occurs during the first five to six weeks, and by the fifth month is usually stable at about 50% of the predicted normal. This improvement may be due to resolution of oedema in the spinal cord with descent of the spinal level, increased tone in the paralysed intercostal muscles reducing the degree of chest wall paradox and possibly some reinnervation of partly paralysed muscles. Because of sputum retention and reduced vital capacity which occurs in patients with high spinal injury, microatelectasis following small airways obstruction is common. This results in ventilation and perfusion mismatch with hypoxia and a normal or low arterial carbon dioxide. Significant hypoxia occurs in about half the patients with acute cervical injury and it does not correlate closely with the impaired vital capacity (Ledsome & Sharp, 1981), so that arterial blood gases should be monitored closely in all patients with acute cervical and thoracic injuries. We use an oximeter for constant monitoring of oxygen saturation in these patients; this enables the saturation to be monitored during sleep, which is a particularly vulnerable time. Added oxygen can be given if necessary.

Haemopneumothorax

Most patients with a thoracic spine injury will usually have suffered major trauma to the chest wall. Over 50% have fractured ribs with a haemothorax and/or pneumothorax. These patients are nursed horizontally; therefore the detection of blood or air in the thorax may be difficult. A considerable amount of fluid may be contained in the thorax of a patient nursed in the supine position, and the chest films show only a general slight haze. This is especially difficult to detect if it occurs on both sides of the chest. Sometimes the fluid is easier to see at the apex, and in doubtful cases the patient may be tilted head down or X-rayed on the side. Fluid should be removed from the chest with an intercostal drain if the lung function is severely depressed, or if it is heavily bloodstained, to prevent significant pleural scarring which may impair lung function in the future; also for diagnostic reasons, especially if the patient has an unexplained pyrexia.

The signs of a pneumothorax in a supine patient include relative transradiency of the lower chest and upper abdominal region, together with deepening of the lateral costophrenic sulcus. Sometimes the diaphragm and cardiac border are more sharply visible and lobular opacities of apical pericardial fat pads may be seen. In doubtful cases a computerized tomography (CT) scan of the chest is often very helpful, but difficult to perform.

Flail segment and pulmonary contusion

If several ribs are fractured in more than one place there may be a flail segment resulting in paradoxical chest movements or absence of movement in part of the chest during inspiration. This may be especially difficult to detect in spinal patients, who normally have reduced chest wall movement. A slight degree of paradox can critically reduce lung function, and in our experience such patients frequently need ventilation. A flail segment is associated with significant contusion of the lung underneath (Trinkle, 1977). This may also occur in the absence of a flail segment, and is usually associated with considerable pulmonary oedema due to capillary leakage in the lung involved. It is especially important not to overload these patients with fluid; rapid deterioration of lung function may occur. Rupture of the diaphragm has also been reported in patients with spinal cord injury (Hall *et al.*, 1981) and this may result in further deterioration of lung function. Surgical repair of these lesions is necessary as spontaneous healing is unlikely.

Mediastinal widening

Frequently in a thoracic injury the mediastinum appears widened. This is usually caused by bleeding around the site of the injury, but always raises the question of a dissection of the arch of the aorta. These patients obviously need to be examined and monitored carefully, and in any doubt a CT scan with contrast has proved a very useful investigation. If a dissection is found at CT scan, or if there is any doubt, then an angiogram may be necessary. Cardiac contusion and pericardial bleeding may also occur in these patients who need continuous electrocardiographic (ECG) monitoring and regular physical examination with monitoring of the pulse and blood pressure (BP). If pericardial bleeding with cardiac tamponade is suspected an echocardiogram should be performed, and the fluid drained if necessary.

Pulmonary oedema

Patients with high spinal injuries have a significant risk of developing pulmonary oedema (Poe *et al.*, 1978). There are a number of factors involved: the BP may be low and the patient may be incorrectly given too much fluid in an attempt to raise the pressure. Patients may have other major injuries and be at risk of developing pulmonary capillary leakage and the adult respiratory distress syndrome. Pulmonary contusion and neurogenic factors may also increase the risk of pulmonary oedema. It is therefore important that the fluid balance in these patients is carefully monitored. This can be especially difficult because the absence of sympathetic tone to the venous capacitance vessels may make the interpretation of central venous pressure difficult. Normally a BP of 90 mm systolic and a urine output of 0.75–1 ml/kg per hour indicates good fluid balance in these patients.

Tracheal stenosis

If the patient develops respiratory problems several weeks or months after a tracheostomy, the development of tracheal stenosis should always be considered. Inspiratory stridor may be present and a flow volume loop may show the classical appearance of severe reduction of peak expiratory and inspiratory flow rates with relative preservation of expiratory flow at low lung volumes. However, if ventilation is severely reduced these signs may be difficult to detect, and special X-rays such as CT scan or tomograms of the area or direct inspection, usually with a flexible bronchoscope or laryngoscope, may need to be performed.

Respiratory monitoring

It is obviously important that the respiratory state of the patient is monitored carefully. The respiratory rate and depth is a very important indicator of the respiratory state, and should be observed frequently in all cases of high spinal injury. The muscles which the patients are using to breathe should also be noted. If patients are relying to any great extent on their accessory muscles for ventilation then they will need very careful observation. Contraction of the sternomastoid muscles and trapezius can easily be seen and felt at the bedside. Diaphragmatic function can be estimated by observing the upper part of the abdomen during inspiration and the diaphragm can be screened by X-ray or ultrasound if necessary. The chest wall should be examined for paradoxical movement of the intercostal spaces and also of the ribs. The efficiency of the patient's cough should be assessed, and the chest should be examined to detect any retained secretions, collapsed portions of lung or abnormality of air entry. The vital capacity should be measured regularly, and it is especially important that it is measured in every position in which the patient will be nursed, as it may change significantly and sometimes catastrophically when the patient is moved into a different position (Silver *et al.*, 1980). Chest X-ray and blood gases should be performed, and the oxygen saturation monitored continuously by an oximeter if possible.

Table 61.5 Respiratory assessment

Respiratory rate and depth
Muscles used in ventilation
Diaphragm function
Chest wall movements
Intercostal paradox
Rib paradox
Cough
Auscultation
Vital capacity
Chest X-ray
Blood gases

Anaesthetic problems

The importance of ensuring minimum movement of the neck during intubation, and the likelihood of bradycardia due to laryngeal stimulation, have already been mentioned. Shortly after the spinal injury, muscle cells become hypersensitive to acetylcholine and depolarizing muscle relaxants. Administration of such relaxants results in the release of large amounts of potassium into the circulation, and this can cause severe cardiac problems. Non-depolarizing muscle relaxants should be used and the dose reduced in patients with cervical and thoracic lesions. The drugs used should have minimum effects on the cardiovascular system.

Pulmonary embolism

There is a high risk of phlebothrombosis and subsequent pulmonary embolism in patients with spinal cord injuries, due to the loss of movement in the paralysed lower extremities and the severe associated trauma at the time of the accident. The deep veins of the legs in a normal person become thrombosed within a week in 15% of patients confined to bed, and in 77% by the second week (Gibbs, 1957). Pulmonary embolus arises as a result of the detachment of thrombi from the veins in the pelvis and the lower limbs. To be effective, treatment must commence before these become thrombosed and continue after the risk period has passed. The high risk of thromboembolic complications makes routine prevention in paraplegics highly desirable. A regime of prophylactic anticoagulant therapy has been adopted at various spinal injury centres during the time that the patients are at risk. It has still not been defined how long this treatment should be administered and what regime is most effective, since none of the studies has been prospective, randomized or subjected to objective assessment. In view of the observation that a spinal injury is part of a major injury with a high risk of associated gastrointestinal bleeding we prefer waiting until the patient has been assessed in the unit for 48 hours and can take food by mouth before commencing major anticoagulant therapy.

Anticoagulants

When started, oral anticoagulants are not immediately effective. These drugs act by reducing the synthesis of various clotting factors, factor VII initially and eventually factors V, IX and X. The reduction of factor VII at an early stage does not ensure effective anticoagulation and it may take a week for factors V, IX and X to be sufficiently reduced. Prophylactic anticoagulant therapy must therefore be commenced at the earliest possible moment after injury, bearing in mind the proviso previously stated.

Therapy is discontinued at three months, since by this time the risk period is thought to have passed. Some patients, however, have pulmonary emboli following cessation of therapy at, or after, this time. There is therefore a need for prophylactic anticoagulant to be continued for a longer period in high-risk patients (those with obesity or previous deep vein thrombosis or pulmonary embolus) and all those who have not been anticoagulated within two weeks of injury. It is now our practice to continue if possible for up to six months in such cases (El Masri & Silver, 1981).

A disadvantage of full anticoagulation is that regular blood sampling for determination of prothrombin index is necessary. Haemorrhage from the gastrointestinal tract and the bladder can prove troublesome, and has necessitated discontinuation of treatment in a small number of patients. The use of low-dose heparin therapy does not significantly prevent deep vein thrombosis in patients with fractured necks of femur, or in patients with spinal injuries, since in these patients presumably damage has occurred to the tissues and veins at the moment of injury.

Autonomic regulation

In normal people heating of the trunk and lower limbs leads to reflex dilation and sweating of the whole body. This reflex is probably initiated in the central nervous system and mediated by the spinal cord and sympathetic efferents which exit between T1 and L2; the stimulus being a rise in skin and blood temperature. As a result of this compensatory mechanism there is no rise in the central temperature. In contrast, a patient with traumatic tetraplegia, when heated in identical conditions, cannot increase the blood flow to the peripheral areas, sweating does not occur, so the temperature rises (Guttmann *et al.*, 1958). When a normal subject is cooled the response is reflex vasoconstriction so that further heat loss is reduced and the body generates further heat by muscular activity, and shivering. However, when a patient with a complete cervical cord transection is cooled, because of sympathetic paralysis there is no vasoconstriction and heat loss continues, the patient's central temperature falls and hypothermia results. Shivering does not occur in the paralysed part of the body, only in the normally innervated parts, such as the masseters and temporalis muscles above the cord transection. The practical implications are that a tetraplegic patient is unable to regulate his or her temperature independently of the environment, i.e. the patient is poikilothermic.

Environmentally induced hyperpyrexia in temperate climates is rare, but in South Africa, Australia or the USA it is necessary to have specially air-conditioned wards to prevent patients becoming hyperpyrexial during the summer months. In consequence problems arise in the management of patients with acute spinal injury, in that they are liable to be transferred on long journeys in unheated ambulances and become hypothermic, or conversely small infections due to blood in the chest or spinal cord can lead to

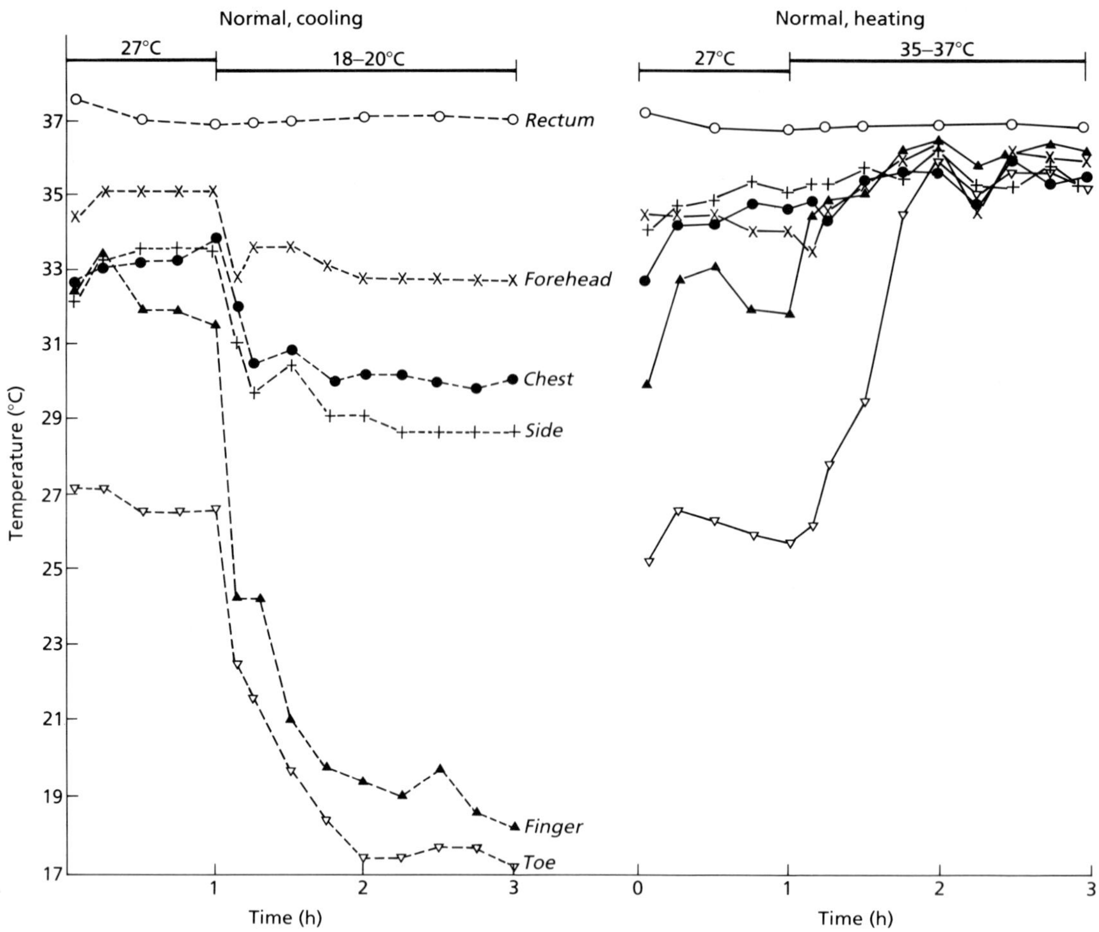

Fig. 61.3 Response of a normal person to cooling. There is a fall in the blood flow due to vasoconstriction in the fingers and toes, and the central temperature is preserved. From Guttmann *et al.* (1958).

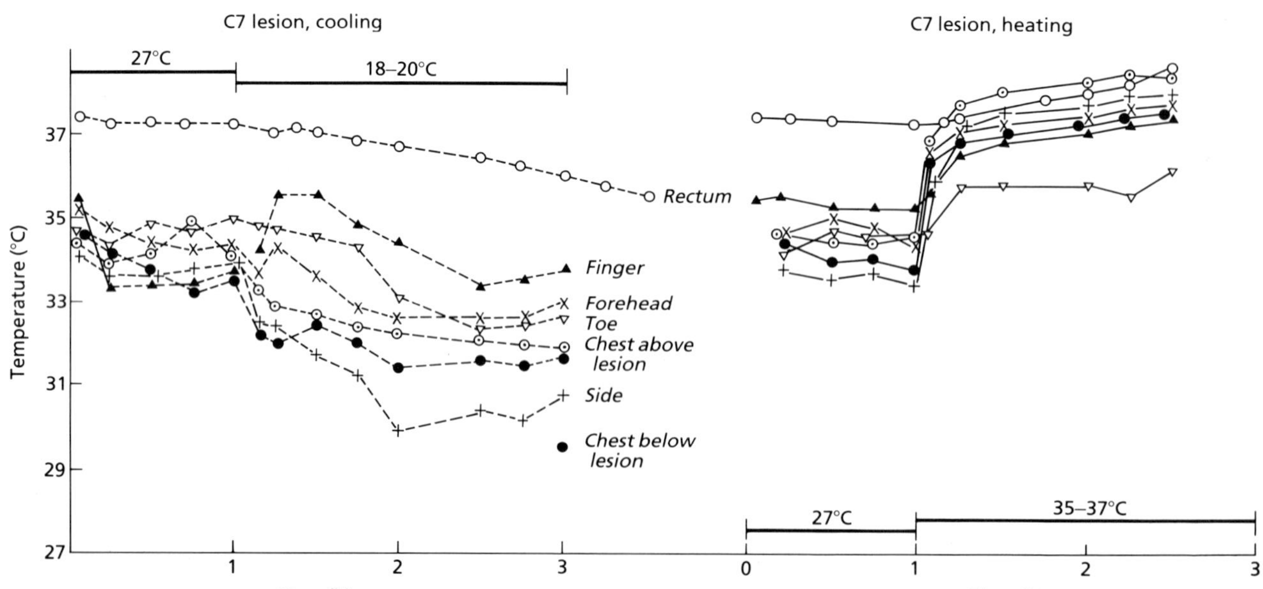

Fig. 61.4 In contrast to Fig. 61.3, a patient with a C7 lesion does not vasoconstrict his fingers or toes. Central temperature drops. From Guttmann *et al.* (1958).

hyperpyrexia. Tetraplegic patients are particularly liable to develop hypothermia immediately after injury while they are in a state of spinal surgical shock, or if infection develops. This condition may be missed unless a special recording thermometer is used. The clinical condition is similar to that seen in hypothermia in elderly people. The patient is confused, has a low temperature, bradycardia, cardiac arrhythmia, low blood pressure and possibly peripheral oedema, particularly around the eyelids.

It is of interest that terminally ill patients who suffer from hypothermia, and tetraplegic patients, may have raised serum amylase levels, and the pancreas is found to be necrotic at post-mortem.

Regulation of blood pressure

The loss of sympathetic tone to the arteries and arterioles results in decreased systemic vascular resistance and hypotension. A systolic BP of 90 mmHg is quite common in acute spinal injury shortly after the accident, and is usually quite adequate for tissue perfusion. If, however, the patient is tilted from a horizontal to head-up position there can be marked postural hypotension. After the acute stage, improved cardiovascular response follows repeated tilting in tetraplegic patients, but postural hypotension may still seriously limit rehabilitation.

Dilation of the capacitance veins reduces the preload, and this can dramatically reduce cardiac output. Normal inspiration results in negative intrathoracic pressure which improves venous return. If a patient is ventilated using positive pressure, the positive intrathoracic pressure can reduce venous return. The normal response is sympathetically induced constriction of the capacitance veins restoring cardiac output, but this mechanism is absent in patients with high spinal injury. Patients may become severely hypotensive when positive-pressure ventilation is commenced. It is therefore important that any fluid deficit is corrected and the BP is adequate before such patients are commenced on a ventilator. They also need to be observed closely shortly after ventilation has been started, and if they become hypotensive careful addition of intravenous fluids and possibly vasopressive agents may be necessary. These patients may have increased sensitivity to vasopressive agents; therefore these agents must be used with caution. In difficult cases measurements of pulmonary wedge pressure using a flotation catheter can be invaluable.

Tracheal stimulation in normal humans results in hypotension and tachycardia. These reflexes are probably dependent on intact sympathetic pathways. In patients with high spinal injuries bradycardia and even cardiac arrest may occur during tracheal suction when the patient is hypoxic (Frankel *et al.*, 1975). It appears to be due to unopposed vagal activity and may be abolished by adequate doses of atropine. Atropine should always be readily available and the pulse carefully monitored during suction of the pharynx and manipulation of the larynx. Before such procedures are undertaken the patient should be adequately oxygenated and the procedures performed as smoothly and quickly as possible. If atropine has to be given frequently, because of bradycardia, thickening of the bronchial secretions and other anticholinergic side-effects may result. In these circumstances the incidence of bradycardia may be reduced by using a β-stimulant such as orciprenaline, but these patients may be quite sensitive to a β-stimulant and therefore a low dose should be used in the first instance.

The cardiovascular effects of sympathetic paralysis are usually evident in the first few weeks or months following a spinal injury. After the resolution of spinal shock, autonomic and somatic hyperreflexia may occur. This results in hypertension, bradycardia, profuse sweating, facial flushing and headache in response to visceral and other stimuli below the level of the spinal injury. A common visceral stimulus causing hyperreflexia is bladder distension. Treatment of autonomic dysreflexia involves identification and removal, if possible, of trigger stimuli, tilting the patient head-up to induce venous pooling in the legs, and antihypertensive medication.

Management of the bladder (see also Chapter 8)

Immediately following an acute cord transection there is a decreased excretion of urine and it may appear that the patient is suffering from acute tubular necrosis of the kidney. However, the urine that is excreted has a high specific gravity and a low sodium content, which excludes this diagnosis.

As a result of acute cord injury, unless the damage is minimal there will be paralysis of the bladder, and it will be necessary to drain it by some means after a few hours, otherwise the bladder will become overdistended.

There is considerable controversy as to the best

means of draining the bladder. Attempts have been made to express the bladder manually, to avoid introducing infection by catheter, but in a shocked ill patient with other injuries this is not to be recommended outside specialist centres.

Intermittent catheterization is undoubtedly the best method, but unless there is a regular team of doctors and nurses trained in this method, and able to carry it out, it can be dangerous due to unskilled catheterization damaging the urethra, resulting in a combination of infection and distension. The alternative choices are the use of an indwelling catheter, which may cause infection within 48 hours of its insertion, or the use of a fine-bore suprapubic catheter. This is a method to be favoured in young female patients, to save them the inevitable embarrassment of repeat catheterization. In male patients it is also a treatment of choice where there are major injuries, since it eliminates sepsis in the bladder and urethra and also such complications as orchitis and the effects of unskilled urethral catheterization.

If a urethral catheter is inserted it should be strapped to the anterior abdominal wall to prevent angulation at the penile scrotal junction in males where a urethral and periurethral abscess, leading to fistulae, can occur. It must be checked every four hours to see that it is draining, since blockage will lead to retention of urine and back-pressure within the genito-urinary (GU) tract, giving rise to hydronephrosis, orchitis and overdistension of the bladder with secondary atony of the bladder wall due to the stretching of the muscles and nerve fibres, also infection. Provided the urine is allowed to drain freely, routine antibiotics should not be given as they will lead to the emergence of resistant organisms. Antibiotics should be reserved for episodes of acute sepsis.

When the patient has begun to pass urine the residual urine must be frequently checked by the use of a catheter or ultrasound. It is easy to fail to empty the bladder completely and to develop a sump of infected urine.

Abdominal complications

It is impossible to deal adequately with the important abdominal complications of spinal injury in this chapter; however, there are some points which should be considered.

Gastric dilatation and paralytic ileus are frequently seen in cervical and high thoracic spinal injury. They may be life-threatening if unrecognized and inadequately treated (Gore *et al.*, 1981). Acute gastric dilatation may be associated with the loss of large amounts of fluid into the stomach, and this can result in profound hypovolaemic shock. Gastric dilatation may also limit diaphragmatic movement, impairing respiratory function even further. The contents of the stomach can be regurgitated in those patients who are nursed supine, resulting in aspiration pneumonia. Prompt decompression of the stomach is essential with nasogastric suction and intravenous fluid replacement. Because of the gastrostasis and paralytic ileus seen in patients with high spinal injury the administration of oral fluids and feeding should be delayed until bowel sounds can be clearly heard, and even then be introduced cautiously.

Compression of the third or fourth part of the duodenum by the superior mesenteric artery or one of its branches is one cause of upper intestinal obstruction in these patients. It is especially liable to occur if the patient is nursed in a position of marked hyperextension. A reduced degree of hyperextension, together with nasogastric suction, may completely relieve the obstruction, but sometimes surgery is necessary. Peptic ulceration may occur in patients with high spinal injury. Acute ulceration has been reported in up to 22% of patients with spinal cord injury. The use of H_2 blockers such as cimetidine or ranitidine in the prophylactic treatment of such cases remains controversial. Gastrointestinal bleeding is common in cervical patients and usually occurs within three weeks of injury. It presents with melaena or haematemesis, and may be due to the development of a stress ulcer or exacerbation of a chronic ulcer. The misguided use of steroids given in the hope of preserving spinal cord function can exacerbate this problem, as can the use of anticoagulants which are necessary to prevent pulmonary emboli. Early gastroscopy should be performed to exclude bleeding from a large chronic ulcer that may not heal by conservative means.

The impaired sensory output from the parietal peritoneum makes evaluation of intra-abdominal problems difficult. These patients frequently do not manifest the usual symptoms and signs; their compensatory response to an acute abdominal problem is also impaired. In one study the appendix was found to have perforated so that in patients with spinal cord injury a high index of suspicion is necessary, especially in those who feel generally unwell, or who have an abnormally raised or low temperature, tachycardia, shoulder-tip pain or abnormal abdominal distension.

Straight X-rays of the abdomen to detect gas under the diaphragm can be diffícut to interpret because of the problems of positioning. We have found that abdominal ultrasound is a very useful investigation in such circumstances. The abdominal viscera may also be injured at the time of the original accident (Carey *et al.*, 1977). Again the spinal injury may make assessment more difficult and a high index of suspicion, frequent examination and early investigations such as abdominal ultrasound and CT scan are important.

Sensory loss

Sensory loss varies with the level and completeness of the cord lesion. It does not correspond to a peripheral nerve distribution but rather to a segmental distribution akin to section of the posterior roots. It may be dissociated, depending on which tracts are lost and which are preserved. The most striking manifestation of the loss of appreciation of painful stimuli is the pressure sore; this is caused by an inability of the patient to feel painful stimuli and to move in response. The sore is not caused by the bed but is caused by pressure that the body exerts on the vulnerable tissues overlying the prominent bony points. This leads to ischaemia involving tissue at all levels; skin, fat, muscle and bone, resulting in tissue necrosis. The areas subject to excessive pressure are the feet when the subject stands, the back of the heels and sacrum when lying on his or her back, the greater trochanter, lateral malleoli and shoulder tips when lying on his or her sides, and the ischial tuberosities when sitting. Inevitably the tissues overlying these areas will be rendered avascular unless the subject moves and the blood supply is restored. Initially, there is transient erythema and then vesiculation, oedema and tissue induration if the pressure continues. This stage is reversible provided the pressure is relieved. The surface may be excoriated exposing the cutis vera, or haemorrhagic blisters may be observed. If the process is not arrested at this stage, deep penetrating necrosis of the subcutaneous tissue, fascia, muscle and bone develops, leading to gangrene, osteomyelitis and septicaemia.

Pressure sores, however, do not always present in this way, since the skin has a better blood supply than the deep tissues beneath; fat, fascia and bone. Thus devitalization of these tissues can occur while the skin remains healthy. The fatty tissues may be absorbed, giving rise to loss of subcutaneous resilience, so the skin and tissues become fibrous and more brittle. Fibrous tethering of the skin to the underlying bone causes abnormal sheering pressures so that the tissues may again break down. Fatty necrosis, due to prolonged pressure, can result in bursa formation. These bursae can become infected and fill with pus, so that the patient may present with blushing of the skin and an infected bursa beneath.

As tissues are rapidly rendered anoxic and are quickly destroyed if load blood flow is compromised, it is necessary that whatever the patient's spinal condition, or whatever surgery is contemplated, regular turning must continue, otherwise the patient will develop a sore which becomes infected, resulting in toxic absorption which may take months to heal. When a sore develops it precludes further surgery and holds up the patient's further rehabilitation. A full-thickness sore can develop in a patient in spinal shock within six hours if the patient is not turned. It is thus vital that regular turning takes place, taking into account the other injuries and the management of the chest. No patient is too ill to be turned. A proper regime of turns can be devised supported by the provision of low-air-loss beds and, as explained earlier, adequate fixation of associated fractures can facilitate this. Finally the doctor must himself regularly check that the skin is intact.

Conclusion

The way ahead

This chapter started by reviewing the mortality figures which 30 years ago were extremely high, few cervical injury patients surviving outside specialist centres. Even in specialist centres, until the lessons elucidated here were learnt, the mortality rate remained unacceptably high.

By the 1970s there were significant advances. A personal series reported prior to the opening of the intensive-care unit at the authors' unit showed that of 166 tetraplegic patients admitted from 1970 until 1981, only four died within four months of paralysis (Ravichandran & Silver, 1982). Subsequent to opening the unit facilities to treat much sicker patients were available, and the mortality of patients with acute

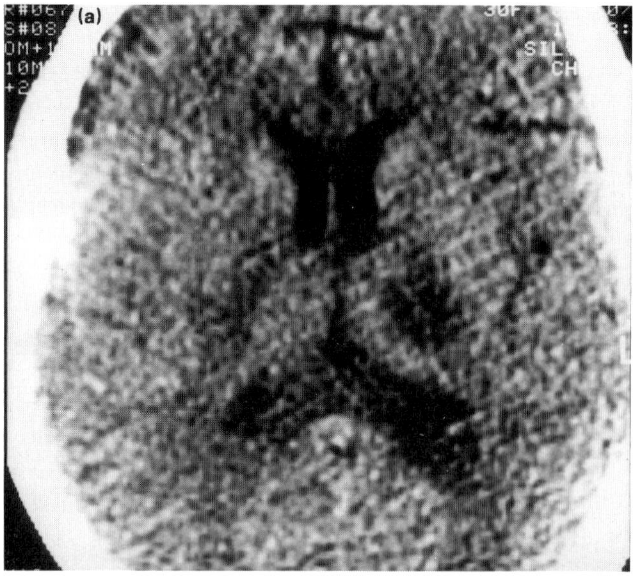

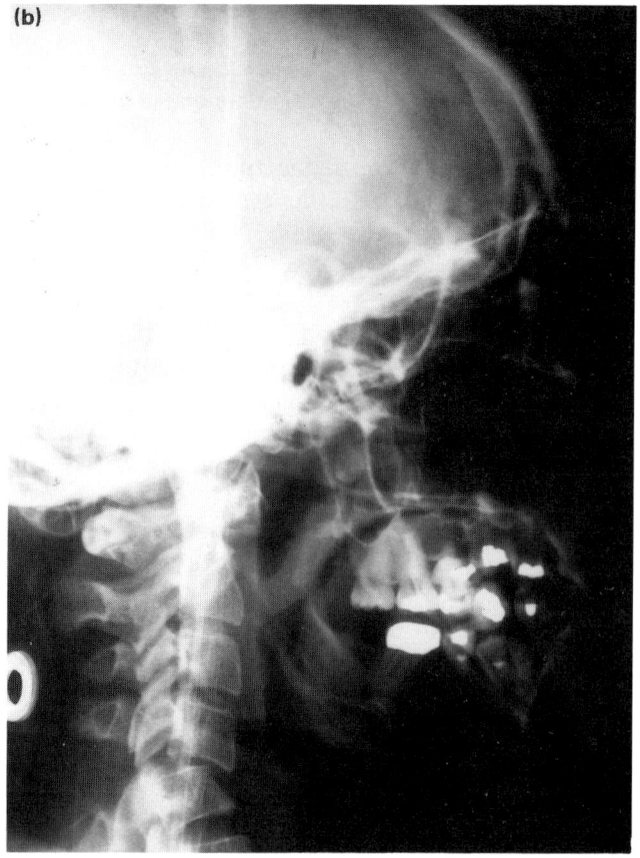

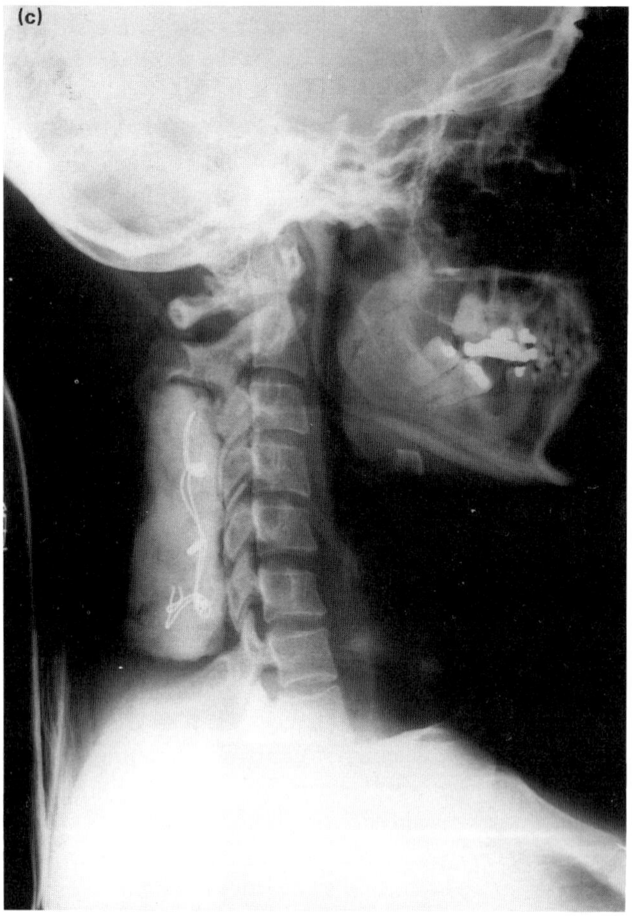

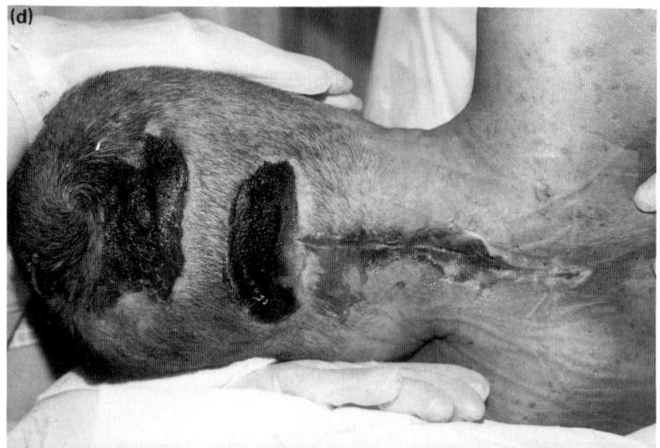

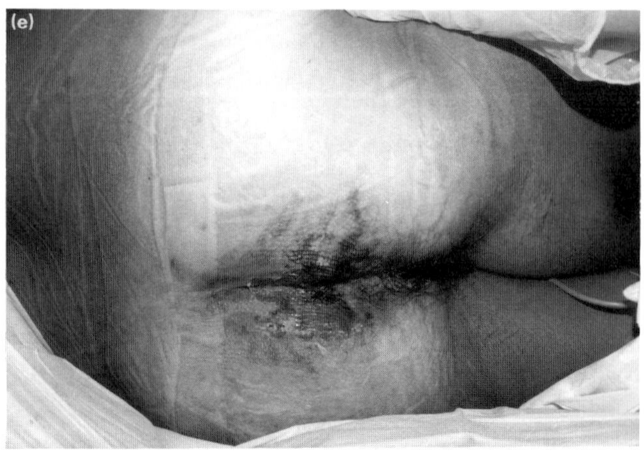

Fig. 61.5 This young woman sustained head injury with dislocation of the cervical spine while she was abroad. There is intracerebral bleeding shown by CT scan (a) and marked dislocation (b). The dislocation required fixation; this was carried out with a wire-and-cement cast (c). The patient was sat up and immediately developed severe pressure sores of the back, head and buttocks (d,e), the whole area became infected and the cast had to be removed, the area then took many months to heal.

spinal injury ventilated over the past 10 years has been 19%, with 75% completely independent of the ventilator six months after injury.

These figures for mortality are open to criticism since they depend on the time of admission. If patients are admitted to a centre late, the immediate mortality for that centre will be falsely lowered. Many very sick patients will have died before transfer and these deaths will not be recorded. Nevertheless the figures do represent a significant improvement, and the main lesson to be learnt if early mortality and morbidity is to be improved is that the injury does not occur in isolation. It is part of major organ trauma and a plan for treatment covering all the injuries must be drawn up involving all medical and paramedical staff.

Certain combinations of injury are particularly lethal.

1 A head injury in combination with a complete cervical lesion, the central respiratory depression due to the head injury being added to respiratory muscle paralysis from the cervical injury.

2 An injury to the chest wall combined with mid-thoracic spine injury will lead to impairment of ventilation due to paralysis of the intercostal muscles and direct trauma to the lungs.

3 Multiple injuries to the limbs and spine cause difficulties in the turning regime.

4 Multiple bone and soft tissue injury combined with a spinal injury requires expert management and teamwork.

Unfortunately medical mismanagement may contribute significantly to the morbidity and mortality of these patients:

1 A spinal injury where the patient's condition has been mismanaged resulting in pressure sores, renal sepsis due to inadequate bladder drainage, and clumsy catheterization leading to rupture of the urethra.

2 Inappropriate drug use: peptic ulcers created or aggravated by steroids; depression of consciousness of patient with head and spinal injury by overdose of opiates so that it is impossible to assess the patient's condition on arrival at the spinal centre.

3 Inappropriate transfer of patients whose condition is rapidly changing with inadequate notes and medical and nursing escort. Specifically, if a patient in respiratory distress is to be transferred, that patient must be accompanied by an anaesthetist and possibly moved by helicopter if travelling considerable distances. A patient with an extradural or a subdural haemorrhage should not be transferred from a neurological centre to a spinal centre until this condition has been evaluated. These are very sick patients and their transfer requires careful and exact management.

Thus it is clear that human beings are not just the sum of their parts, 'The whole is greater than the sum of its parts', and that all factors interact together. Unless this analysis is made we miss the key to this situation.

REFERENCES

Brownlee, S. & Williams, S.J. (1987) Physiotherapy in the respiratory care of patients with high spinal injury. *Physiotherapy*, **73**, 148–152.

Carey, M.E., Nance, F.C. & Kirgis, H.D. (1977) Pancreatitis following spinal cord injury. *J. Neurosurg.*, **47**, 917–922.

Cheshire, D.J.E. (1963) Respiratory management in acute traumatic tetraplegia. *Paraplegia*, **1**, 252–261.

Connors, J.F. & Nash, I.E. (1934) Management of urologic complications in injuries to spine: report of 54 cases without single infection in urinary tract. *Am. J. Surg.*, **26**, 159–167.

De Troyer, A., Kelly, S. & Zin, W.A. (1983) Mechanical action of the intercostal muscles on the ribs. *Science*, **220**, 87–88.

Durbin, F.C. (1957) Fracture–dislocations of the cervical spine. *J. Bone Jt. Surg.*, **39B**, 23–38.

El Masri, W.S. & Silver, J.R. (1981) Prophylactic anticoagulant therapy in patients with spinal cord injury. *Paraplegia*, **19**, 334–342.

Frankel, H.L., Mathias, C.J. & Spalding, J.M.K. (1975) Mechanism of reflex cardiac arrest in tetraplegic patients. *Lancet*, **2**, 1183–1185.

Gibbs, N.M. (1957) Venous thrombosis of the lower limbs with particular reference to bedrest. *Br. J. Surg.*, **XLV**, 209.

Glenn, W.W.L., Hogan, J.F. & Phelps, M.L. (1980) Ventilatory support of the quadriplegic patient with respiratory paralysis by diaphragmatic pacing. *Surg. Clin. N. Am.*, **60**, 1055.

Goldman, J.M., Rose, L.S., Williams, S.J., Silver, J.R. & Denison, D.M. (1986) Effect of abdominal binders on breathing in tetraplegic patients. *Thorax*, **41**, 940–945.

Gore, R.M., Mintzer, R.A. & Calenof, L. (1981) Gastrointestinal complications of spinal cord injury. *Spine*, **6**, 538–544.

Guttmann, L. (1949) Paralysis—management of. *Br. Surg. Pract.*, **6**, 445–466.

Guttmann, L., Silver, J.R. & Wyndham, C.H. (1958) Thermoregulation in spinal man. *J. Physiol.*, **142**, 406–419.

Hall, J.C., Douglas, M.C. & Burke, D.C. (1981) Rupture of the diaphragm associated with spinal cord injury. *Austral. N.Z. J. Surg.*, **51**, 594–597.

Kennedy, R.H. (1946) New viewpoint toward spinal cord injuries. *Ann. Surg.*, **124**, 1057–1065.

Ledsome, J.R. & Sharp, J.M. (1981) Pulmonary function in acute cervical cord injury. *Am. Rev. Resp. Dis.*, **124**, 41.

McMichan, J.C., Michel, L. & Westbrook, P. (1980) Pulmonary disfunction following traumatic quadriplegia. *J. Am. Med. Assoc.*, **243**, 528–531.

Morgan, M.D.L., Goutlay, A.R., Silver, J.R., Williams, S.J. & Denison, D.M. (1985) The contribution of the ribcage to breathing in tetraplegia. *Thorax*, **40**, 613–617.

Munro, D.J. (1943) Thoracic and lumbosacral cord injuries; study of 40 cases. *J. Am. Med. Assoc.*, **122**, 1055–1063.

Norton, W.L. (1962) Fractures and dislocations of the cervical spine. *J. Bone Jt. Surg.*, **44A**, 115.

Poe, R.H., Reisman, J.L. & Rodenhouse, T.G. (1978) Pulmonary oedema in cervical spinal cord injury. *J. Trauma*, **18**, 71–73.

Ravichandran, G. & Silver, J.R. (1982) Survival following traumatic tetraplegia. *Paraplegia*, **20**, 264–269.

Silver, J.R. (1967/8) Chest injuries and complications in the early stages of spinal cord injury. *Paraplegia*, **5**, 226–243.

Silver, J.R., Morris, W.R. & Oefinowski, J.S. (1980). Associated injuries in patients with spinal injury. *Injury*, **12**, 219–224.

Trinkle, J.K. (1977) Flail chest—facts and fantasies. In Williams, W.G. & Smith, R.E. (eds) *Trauma of the Chest*, pp. 39–50. John Wright, Bristol.

Walker, J.W.T. (1917) Hunterian lecture on the bladder in gunshot and other injuries of the spinal cord. *Lancet*, **1**, 173–179.

Walker, J.W.T. (1937) Treatment of bladder in spinal injuries in war. *Br. J. Urol.*, **9**, 217–230.

62 · Management of the Neuropathic Bladder

By K.F. PARSONS

Recent advances in the understanding of vesico-urethral physiology have helped provide a rational basis for treatment of the neuropathic bladder whatever the cause. The incidence of bladder dysfunction in spinal disease seems very variable and, excluding trauma, the three conditions in which it is commonly seen are meningomyelocele (97%), lumbar disc disease (6–18%) and spinal neoplasia in which the incidence is less well defined.

Much of the management of vesico-urethral neuropathy has evolved from the treatment of spinal cord injury patients, and these cases do pose rather specific problems for which a system of care has been worked out, even though the mechanisms of abnormal bladder function now seem more complex than had previously been supposed.

In these cases, satisfactory micturition differs from that in neurologically intact individuals because the emphasis shifts from a function which has to be socially acceptable, to that which is mandatory for preservation of the upper urinary tracts and avoidance of urinary infection.

There is no doubt that the attention paid to the urinary tract has improved the survival of spinal cord injury patients, by the prevention of urosepsis. This gratifying change in the mortality has been carefully recorded over the past 30 years. In 1961 it was found to be around 50% (Breithaupt *et al.*, 1961); by 1968 it had dropped to 36% (Jousse *et al.*, 1968) and yet a further drop was found in 1973 (Geisler *et al.*, 1977). The marked decrease in renal deaths continued when in 1983 it stood at 15.3% (Geisler *et al.*, 1983). The concurrent advent of renal replacement therapy which is available to spinal cord injury patients, will have had a significant effect on mortality figures, but nonetheless careful urological management has had a substantial impact to the point where in the 1990s, renal compromise is a rarity, possibly no more prevalent than 1% of cases and certainly not the common cause of death that it once was.

Recent developments have allowed a further dimension to be added to the management of the neuropathic bladder. Whereas previously continence might have been sacrificed for the preservation of renal function and urinary sterility, the current aim of treatment should always include consideration of techniques which preserve or restore continence, providing that they neither provoke infection nor put the upper urinary tracts in jeopardy.

THE BLADDER IN ACUTE SPINAL TRAUMA

Acute injury to the spinal cord induces a period of spinal shock during which all reflex activity below the level of the lesion is absent or markedly reduced. While reflex function is absent, the closure pressure at the bladder neck is maintained and some method of bladder drainage is essential and urgent. The longer that this is delayed, the more the detrusor is overstretched and the more prolonged will be the recovery period before it will function. This may extend to up to 12 months after the initial injury, which underscores the importance of immediate bladder decompression in this circumstance.

Catheterization

The options for catheterizing the bladder in the acute situation are threefold: per urethram and indwelling, per urethram and intermittent, or suprapubic. Each has its advocates but, because of associated injuries and the need to monitor urinary output, the most convenient method of bladder drainage is usually by indwelling Foley catheter for the first 48–72 hours. This is especially so in those patients requiring neurosurgical, orthopaedic or other surgical procedures.

Indwelling urethral catheterization

Fine-diameter catheters should always be used, with a high ratio of internal to external diameter. Thought must be given to the time that the catheter is likely to be in place, and if this is to be prolonged, a silicone catheter should be used. Unfortunately these catheters do not have a particularly large internal diameter, but the diminished reaction which they provoke within the urethra, when compared to latex catheters, provides a great advantage. It is as well to remember that silicone-coated latex catheters, produced in an attempt to match the properties of a pure silicone catheter, lose the coating within 24 hours within the urethra, negating any advantage which the silicone coating may have (Blacklock, 1986).

The weight of the tubing and the drainage bag must always be supported, especially in females. If attention is not paid to this simple detail, damage by pressure necrosis at the bladder neck in females, progressing ultimately to complete destruction of the whole urethra, will occur. In males, if the catheter and tubing are not supported, a 'bow-string' of the urethra will produce a urethral stricture at the site of maximum pressure against the urethral wall.

It must be accepted that the intravesical foreign body of an indwelling catheter will provoke lower urinary tract infection if present for more than three days or so, but antibacterial therapy should be withheld unless systemic effects of the infection become manifest. It is likely, however, that in the acute phase, antibacterial agents will be administered for other indications.

It is possible that efficient bladder emptying may be achieved even in the acute stage by Crede expression of the bladder. This will apply only to those male patients who have previously had a prostatectomy and in whom the urethral outflow resistance is solely constituted by muscle activity in the region of the external urethral sphincter. This resistance inevitably is reduced in acute spinal injury allowing, when appropriate, Crede expression of the bladder to be used. In all other cases the bladder neck closure mechanism precludes Crede expression as a treatment option.

Intermittent catheterization

It is relatively easy to implement intermittent catheterization in patients with lesions at or below T12, even in acute spinal injury. The benefit of this method of drainage was realized when it was appreciated that urinary infection was rendered less likely when the bladder was drained regularly and completely (Guttman & Frankel, 1966), in the absence of an indwelling foreign body. Furthermore, it was realized that, when these prerequisites were met, it was unnecessary always to use a sterile catheter passed under aseptic conditions but that a clean intermittent self-catheterizing (CISC) technique could be adopted (Lapides *et al.*, 1972). In patients with higher lesions the technique may still be used, but will involve organizational problems as these patients are unable to catheterize themselves. As the spinal cord injury evolves, these patients develop peculiar urinary output patterns which make it more difficult to adhere to a rigid timed schedule of catheterization.

The technique, though simple in concept, has to be carefully taught and practised with great diligence. Once adopted there can be no respite, for the bladder must be emptied regularly with adjustment of the schedule to prevent volumes in excess of 600 ml. In tetraplegics typically the urinary output is small during the day when the patient is upright in a chair, and the interval between catheterization can be increased, but on assumption of the supine position a diuresis occurs which may require hourly catheterization.

Suprapubic catheterization

Suprapubic catheterization might appear a logical solution to the acutely paralysed bladder because it will leave the urethra uninstrumented and theoretically uncontaminated. However, it requires skill to perform and carries with it a certain morbidity. The colon and peritoneum are both vulnerable to perforation, yet serious damage is fortunately rare.

Frustratingly, a suprapubic tube may not always keep the bladder entirely empty and as a result some small quantity of urethral leakage may occur. Finally, theoretically at least, the tract may reopen if, once voiding is re-established, the bladder develops outflow obstruction as it may potentially do in a spinal injury patient.

Extended intermittent catheterization

It is perfectly practical to continue intermittent catheterization indefinitely in many patients (Herr, 1975; McGuire & Brady, 1979). However, with recovery of reflex activity as spinal shock recedes, both sphincteric and bladder pressure increases in virtually all patients with spinal cord or spinal root lesions. Urodynamic assessment should therefore be undertaken to answer the simple question whether urine is stored to those volumes recorded at catheterization at low pressure. Absolute pressure values are relatively arbitrary but should be less than 20 cmH_2O. If so, intermittent catheterization can be continued. If not, some means of decreasing intravesical pressure is needed. In those cases with detrusor areflexia an important observation is the pressure at which leakage occurs. This leak point pressure is governed by the urethral resistance, which will need to be reduced if the leak point pressure is high. In practice, in patients with sacral spinal cord or root lesions the intravesical pressure rises only as high as the urethral resistance will allow.

The same principles of pressure relationships govern the adequacy of intermittent catheterization in patients with suprasacral lesions. In these cases reflex vesical activity returns and this is frequently associated with discoordinate urethral activity producing 'detrusor–sphincter dyssynergia'. In this circumstance it is necessary to reduce detrusor activity by medication and then to judge the safety of intermittent catheterization by assessing the peaks of intravesical pressure urodynamically to ensure that they remain within the safety limits.

MANAGEMENT OF LONG-TERM VESICO-URETHRAL NEUROPATHY

There are in simple terms four particular areas of abnormality of vesico-urethral function produced by chronic neuropathy which may or may not coexist, and to which treatment must be addressed. A functional classification of the neuropathic bladder can be based upon them, and this can be correlated to the level of neurological lesion. The bladder may be (a) hyperactive, producing high pressures or (b) hypoactive, at low pressure and acontractile and the urethra or outlet may be (c) hyperactive, increasing outlet resistance or (d) hypoactive, reducing the resistance.

Clearly, the diagnosis of these abnormalities can be made only by a careful urodynamic assessment and, bearing in mind the delicate balance which pertains between the detrusor and the outflow in neuropathic states and indeed the potential for any subtle change in the neurological condition profoundly to upset this balance, urodynamic assessments should be repeated regularly.

Correction of vesico-urethral functional abnormalities can be medical or surgical.

Pharmacological management of the neuropathic bladder

The concept of using drugs to control neuropathic vesico-urethral dysfunction is not new, but new pharmacological agents which are now available broaden the treatment options. These agents have specific target sites and a combination of therapeutic modalities may be necessary in order to achieve the desired effect.

Drugs which inhibit detrusor activity

These agents can be used to reduce unwanted detrusor pressure; increase capacity; or inhibit uninhibited reflex activity. Pure anticholinergic agents can be subdivided into: (a) belladonna alkaloids (tincture of belladonna); (b) quaternary ammonium derivatives of the belladonna alkaloids (meth scopolamine bromide); and (c) synthetic substitutes (propantheline, methantheline and emepronium bromide). They all block the effect of acetylcholine at postganglionic cholinergic nerve endings yet have to be given in relatively high doses for a significant effect to be recorded and at a level at which side-effects are often noticed.

Anticholinergic/antispasmodic agents are perhaps better suited to control uninhibited detrusor contractions (Vinson & Diokno, 1976), of which oxybutinin hydrochloride and dicyclomine chloride are both antimuscarinic and have an additional direct effect on the detrusor smooth muscle membrane.

All the anticholinergic agents have similar side-effects of which a dry mouth and blurred vision are the commonest.

Not all the 'bladder relaxants' work equally well, but in practice oxybutinin will have the greatest beneficial effects.

Drugs which enhance detrusor activity

Cholinergic agents may improve bladder emptying by increasing the efficiency of detrusor contractility. If they are to be used where detrusor dyssynergia is present then some method of reducing sphincteric activity must also be employed, for potentially they might increase urethral resistance in addition to increasing detrusor contraction.

Bethanechol hydrochloride is a choline ester that acts directly on the effector cells and probably is the most potent cholinergic agent available.

Distigmine bromide is an anticholinesterase which relies upon enhancement of endogenous acetyl choline to exert its effect.

Recent reports of the use of prostaglandin F2α in patients with neuropathic bladder dysfunction have shown that the drug given intravesically produces contractions that can induce voiding in patients with suprasacral lesions but not in patients with complete denervation, detrusor–sphincter dyssynergia or spinal shock (Vaidyanathan *et al.*, 1981)

Drugs which reduce outlet resistance

Outlet resistance in the neuropathic bladder is composed of a striated and an intrinsic muscular element. Skeletal muscle relaxants can therefore be utilized and are grouped according to the site of action. Centrally acting benzodiazepines such as diazepam or GABA-mimetic agents such as baclofen have both been shown to enhance bladder emptying by reducing outlet resistance (Leyson *et al.*, 1980) whereas dantrolene can produce a similar effect by a direct action on skeletal muscle (Pedersen *et al.*, 1978).

Intrinsic urethral muscle can be relaxed by α-adrenolytic agents and of all the pharmacological manipulations this is probably the most reliably effective. Phenoxybenzamine was the first used and was shown to be effective alone in reducing residual urine (Krane & Olsson, 1973), or in combination with cholinergic agents (Khanna, 1976). Unfortunately, subsequent studies have shown a tiny carcinogenic potential of this agent in mice and thus its use has been curtailed but other α-blocking agents such as prazosin and indoramin have more specific α_1-receptor blocking effect and do not block presynaptic receptors so they are more specific to urethral responses (Anderson *et al.*, 1981) and produce fewer cardiovascular side-effects.

Drugs which increase urethral resistance

Urethral intrinsic muscular tone can be increased by α-adrenergic stimulants, of which two are commonly prescribed for this purpose, but both are contraindicated in patients with hypertension and thus should be avoided in cases where autonomic dysreflexia is a possibility.

Ephedrine has both α- and β-adrenoreceptor stimulating properties. In addition to a direct effect on receptors it has the ability to release noradrenaline from storage sites in the sympathetic nerves. The primary use is to control sphincter weakness incontinence, and in mild to moderately severe cases this can be achieved in perhaps 73% (Diokno & Taub, 1975).

Phenylpropanolamine hydrochloride has similar pharmacological effects to ephedrine yet causes fewer central stimulant effects (Awad *et al.*, 1978). These two agents are often found in proprietary cold cures, and are worth using particularly in patients with neuropathic bladder secondary to spina bifida where the outlet is paralysed yet some reasonable expulsive force can be generated.

Theoretically at least, β-adrenoreceptor blockers should increase urethral intrinsic muscle tone and thus increase urethral outflow resistance. In practice, however, this proves not to be the case, and in any event their cardiovascular side-effects militate against their use (Khanna, 1976).

SURGICAL MANAGEMENT OF THE NEUROPATHIC BLADDER

Surgical intervention in vesico-urethral neuropathy can be grouped into three categories. Firstly, there are a selection of procedures designed to modify vesico-urethral dysfunction indirectly; secondly operations to relieve functional outflow obstruction and finally, cutaneous urinary diversion which perhaps is indicated when attempts to achieve voiding have failed and an indwelling catheter is contra-indicated, or when hopeless incontinence is present in the female.

Procedures which modify vesico-urethral dysfunction

Inhibition of detrusor contractility

In those cases where the detrusor is shown urodynamically to be uninhibited and hyperreflexic a procedure to inhibit the contractility might be considered. Ablation of the vesical pelvic nerves is an attractive option and pudendal neurectomy, sacral rhizotomy, intrathecal phenol injection or conectomy have all been advocated and should be considered particularly when the exaggerated bladder activity is associated with peripheral mass somatic spasms. In the male, impotence is invariably produced by these operations. A more peripheral denervation, or more correctly decentralization procedure, has been tried and transvaginal neurotomy seems excellent in controlling idiopathic detrusor instability in women, but strangely proves to be ineffective in neuropathic cases. Similarly, transtrigonal injection of phenol should produce a satisfactory neurotomy in neuropathic cases but fails to do so, except in demyelinating disease (Ewing *et al.*, 1983). Bladder transection (Gibbon *et al.*, 1973), which is a procedure designed to reduce detrusor contractility in neurologically intact patients also seems ineffective in neuropathic cases.

Interpositional cystoplasty is perhaps the most effective operation to increase bladder capacity and to reduce contractility. A segment of ileum, isolated upon its mesentery, is laid into the bladder opened coronally, in the 'clam' operation (Bramble, 1982, 1990) or sagitally. The very presence of the bowel segment increases bladder capacity, but has the added benefit of preventing transmission of a contractile wave from bladder base to fundus, whilst presenting also a barrier to potential reinnervation.

This procedure is particularly effective in increasing compliance in the congenital neuropathic bladder seen in patients with meningomyelocele (Parry *et al.*, 1990). It is important to ensure that, in any neuropathic vesico-urethral dysfunction, the intrinsic bladder pressure is not elevated for prolonged periods, for this will adversely affect the upper urinary tracts. Interpositional cystoplasty can be used in combination with a procedure to increase outflow resistance (see later) in those cases who are able thereafter to catheterize intermittently (Rickwood *et al.*, 1982; McRae *et al.*, 1987). Interestingly, however, it is unusual if not exceptional for this type of combined procedure ever to be needed in spinal injury patients, which is perhaps a reflection that the growing, decentralized bladder exhibits different viscoelastic properties than does the normal bladder deprived acutely of its innervation.

Relief of midline outflow obstruction

Suprasacral lesions

Detrusor contractility in these cases is usually regained in an uninhibited and hyperreflexic fashion. Urine is thus only retained within the bladder if the midline outflow resistance exceeds the intravesical pressure. This midline resistance is exerted at the level of the bladder neck, at the level of the membranous urethra, or both. Bladder neck closure may be maintained despite a powerful detrusor contraction; thus it is important always to determine whether this is the case. The forces which produce the pressure resistance at the level of the membranous urethra comprise intrinsic urethral muscle contractility, dyssynergic pelvic floor striated muscle activity or a combination of the two.

The level of obstruction therefore has to be determined and the contribution of each potential obstructing element assessed so that appropriate surgical correction can be undertaken.

In female patients it is unusual to be able satisfactorily to reduce outflow resistance without provoking incontinence and thus high lesions are probably best treated by long-term catheterization. Similarly, bladder neck resection in the female with an acontractile bladder should not be countenanced because of the risk of incontinence (Delaere *et al.*, 1983), but fortunately the option of intermittent catheterization makes this operation obsolete in these cases.

In males the treatment options are greater, but a fundamental decision must first be taken whether to leave the midline vesico-urethral apparatus untouched and artificially to provoke micturition using a sacral anterior root stimulator (Brindley *et al.*, 1986) or whether to reduce or ablate the midline resistance and produce unobstructed, uninhibited voiding per urethram into a condom collecting device.

When the latter is chosen, there are three surgical options: incision or resection of the bladder neck, incision of the distal urethral mechanism (external sphincterotomy), or both.

BLADDER NECK RESECTION

The correction of bladder outflow obstruction should be undertaken only by surgeons well-practised in endoscopic surgical techniques and all the usual prerequisites for this type of surgery are mandatory. Antibacterial prophylaxis should always be used whether or not preoperative urine cultures are positive because patients with vesico-urethral neuropathy who have had any type of instrumentation whatever, at any stage, seem always to have a significantly higher tendency to bacteraemia, endotoxaemia or septicaemia following endoscopic surgery. The patient should be placed in the relaxed lithotomy position, which usually means that paralysis under anaesthesia with positive-pressure ventilation will be needed. In some circumstances controlled hypotension can be useful.

Ablation of bladder neck resistance can be either by incision or resection. Bladder neck incision, however, does not seem totally to relieve obstruction in neuropathic cases and a formal resection is preferable. Furthermore, though uncommonly seen in spinal injury cases, prostatic hyperplasia may also be present and any obstructing adenoma also needs to be resected.

A circumferential resection of the bladder neck is unnecessary and will increase the incidence of postoperative bladder neck sclerosis. An anterior mucosal bridge should thus be retained to prevent this tedious complication. The resection should be deep, leaving only a thin rim of circumferentially orientated bladder neck fibres without a prominent ridge on which a catheter may catch.

Postoperative catheterization with irrigation, either by a three-way catheter or augmented diuresis, should be used because it is vital that blockage by clots should never occur for this may induce autonomic dyssreflexia.

On removal of the catheter, the output from the bladder must be monitored carefully and the residual urine checked, preferably by ultrasound examination. If a satisfactory voiding pattern is not quickly established the catheter should be replaced for a day or two.

INCISION OF THE DISTAL URETHRAL MECHANISM—EXTERNAL SPHINCTEROTOMY

This operation is designed to abolish any obstructing element at the level of the distal urethral mechanism whether it is due to overactivity of the intrinsic urethral muscle, or due to a hyperreflexic striated pelvic floor, or both. Antibacterial prophylaxis is mandatory, and the patient crossmatched for a blood transfusion, for the area at which the operation is done is exceptionally vascular and replacement of blood may be necessary. As with bladder neck surgery this operation is not for the occasional operator.

The 'external urethral sphincter' presents itself to the endoscopic operator as a circular ring below the level of the prostatic verumontanum. Incision can therefore be single or multiple, and in various anatomical orientations. If a single incision is to be used it is preferable not to orientate it posteriorly or posterolaterally, for this seems to encourage restoration of sphincteric activity perhaps by encouraging early healing of the disrupted muscular ring. Incision at the midline, 12 o'clock, position avoids this complication (Madersbacher & Scott, 1976; Whitmore *et al.*, 1978).

Posterobilateral incisions are effective in totally abolishing sphincteric activity and relieving obstruction (Gibbon, 1973), but carry the disadvantage that the incisions are precisely at the point where the nerves to the corpora cavernosa traverse the membranous region (Walsh & Donker, 1982) and thus erectile failure is a potential complication. Median sphincterotomy is therefore preferable in the younger male patient.

The surgery is relatively simple but requires accurate and confident identification of endoscopic landmarks. All the muscle layers of the urethra must be divided from a point just above the verumontanum to some 2–3 cm below it. The incision is made with a 'Collins' diathermy electrode in a resectoscope using the cutting current. Care has to be taken not to cut too deeply at the distal end of the incision, for at this point the corpus spongiosum of the urethra is close by, and if opened will bleed alarmingly and persistently despite all endoscopic attempts to stop it. The haemorrhage can be arrested relatively easily utilizing tamponade by a large-diameter (24Ch) urethral catheter, augmented if needed by compression through the perineum.

The indwelling catheter should be retained for six or seven days, and upon removal strict attention should be paid to the adequacy of voiding.

Sacral lesions

The first cases of external sphincterotomy were performed on patients with sacral neuropathy and an acontractile detrusor in whom micturition by straining was obstructed within the urethra (Ross *et al.*, 1957). The cause of the obstruction was not realized, but subsequently it has been recognized that in these cases the urethral obstruction is due to activity in the intrinsic urethral muscle. Bladder emptying was satisfactory once this obstruction had been dealt with by sphincterotomy.

In adult female patients, and in children both male and female with sacral neuropathy, unwanted excess pressure generated by the intrinsic urethral mechanism can be modified by simple urethral overdilatation or urethrotomy (Rickwood, 1982). The physical overdistension disrupts the integrity of the intrinsic urethral spiral muscle fibres and thus reduces the resistance which they impart. If the bladder neck is competent this will not provoke incontinence, but paradoxically may cure stress-induced leakage from a chronically overdistended bladder in which the bladder neck is constantly pulled open by the excessive volume by allowing complete emptying by abdominal straining.

Endoscopic resection of the bladder neck of incision of the distal urethral mechanism is designed to reduce the outflow resistance pressure. This can theoretically at least be achieved by stenting the urethra open. Early work has shown that this is a realistic treatment option and a recently introduced 'Wallstent' (AMS Medical, UK), designed for the treatment of urethral strictures, has been successfully used to maintain an open urethra in vesico-urethral neuropathy (McInerney *et al.*, 1990; Shaw *et al.*, 1990).

DETRUSOR STIMULATION/URETHRAL RELAXATION

A logical method of provoking micturition in patients with vesico-urethral neuropathy would be to stimulate the bladder artificially. Direct stimulation by electrodes implanted into the bladder wall was first reported in 1964 (Boyce *et al.*, 1964) and several others tried the technique which failed, however, to gain clinical acceptance. Movement often led to fractured cables, infection was common, electrodes tended to erode into the bladder, and current spread led to pain and stimulation of the outlet resistance during voiding.

As an alternative, nerve stimulation techniques have been developed designed to provoke detrusor contraction. Conus medullaris electrodes positioned in the intermediolateral grey columns of the cord at S1 or lower has produced successful long-term results in three of five paraplegics (Nashold *et al.*, 1972).

THE SACRAL ANTERIOR ROOT STIMULATOR

The most efficient electrostimulation of micturition in patients with complete spinal cord section and neuropathic bladder dysfunction has been by the sacral anterior root stimulator popularized by Brindley (1973, 1977).

Stimulation of the S2, S3 or S4 anterior root causes contraction of the pelvic floor producing unwanted outflow resistance. To overcome this, intermittent bursts of stimulation are used whereby the detrusor and pelvic floor initially contract in unison. When stimulation ceases, pelvic floor relaxation is instantaneous, whereas the detrusor pressure decays much more slowly such that during this period of pressure differential poststimulation voiding occurs. Thus good bladder emptying is achieved whilst continence is often maintained.

An intradural approach via laminectomy is required. The anterior roots of S2, S3 and S4 are identified on each side in the cauda equina and the function of each is ratified by electrical stimulation monitoring bladder, rectal and pelvic floor activity. The anterior is separated from the posterior root and each is laid within the stimulator booklet. From it, cables are led subcutaneously to a radio receiver buried in the subcutaneous tissues of the anterolateral chest wall. Within the buried receiver there are three radio receivers of differing frequency tunings, one for each pair of nerve roots.

Following operation when voiding is required, a small triradiate transmitter is placed over the receiver so that its three coils correspond to those which stimulate the nerve roots. The transmitter can then be tuned to stimulate whichever nerve root has been shown predominantly to effect micturition. It can also be used to stimulate erection, largely a function of the S2 root, or assist bowel emptying by S4 root stimulation.

In order to abolish uninhibited detrusor contraction the posterior roots of S3 and S4 are divided. This has the advantage of increasing functional bladder capacity and enhancing continence, and will also abolish pain associated with electromicturition.

The advantage of this type of implanted device is that satisfactory micturition can be achieved with reasonable continence and no need for an external collecting device. The incidence of urinary infection is reduced because residual urine is reduced to virtually nil, and the self image and dignity of the patient is greatly enhanced.

RESTORATION OF URETHRAL RESISTANCE

Loss of support of the pelvic floor, which will allow transmitted abdominal pressure to be deflected away from the urethra, may in time render the closure mechanism in the urethra incompetent and stress-induced leakage of urine will occur. This is especially prevalent in congenital neuropathy, and in this circumstance may be associated with persistence of detrusor contractility. In these cases it is necessary to reduce detrusor pressure prior to restoring urethral resistance.

In females, surgical repositioning of the bladder neck and proximal urethra, to ensure that the compressive influence of abdominal pressure is maintained, can be achieved by an open suprapubic colposuspension operation. A simple 'Stamey' endoscopic needle suspension is an attractive alternative which achieves a similar elevation of the bladder neck and can be used in neuropathic cases (Kato *et al.*, 1987; Lawrence & Thomas, 1987).

A sophisticated and useful option to restore urethral competence and thus produce continence is by implantation of an artificial urinary sphincter (AUS; AMS Medical, UK). This device works by utilizing a compressive cuff implanted either around the bladder neck or the bulbar urethra, inflation of which is maintained at all times by connection to a pressure-regulating reservoir, implanted suprapubically, and thus under the influence of abdominal pressure. Micturition can occur by deflation of the cuff by activating a small pump implanted in the scrotum in males and the labia in females. This allows fluid to be pumped out of the cuff and into the reservoir. Some 90 seconds later the valvular mechanism automatically reverses returning fluid from the reservoir to reinflate the cuff.

It is important always to be sure that detrusor pressure is never consistently elevated when an obstructing mechanism such as this is employed (Murray *et al.*, 1988).

The predominant use of the AUS in neuropathic incontinence is in cases of meningomyelocele where a prior sphincterotomy to abolish any dyssynergic urethral sphincteric activity may be needed, together with an interpositional cystoplasty if compliance is low (Stephenson & Mundy, 1985), and clean intermittent catheterization used in those patients unable to empty the paralysed bladder by straining.

Cutaneous urinary diversion

Despite the application of a multitude of procedures designed to correct neuropathic vesico-urethral dysfunction occasionally it is necessary to divert the urine to the skin when all else fails. A classical ileal diversion can be performed, remembering that the purpose of the procedure is to transmit urine to the collecting bag as efficiently and quickly as possible. The procedure therefore in no way is meant to construct an 'ileal bladder'.

Newer methods of urinary diversion, however, do set out to achieve just this aim by construction of an intra-abdominal urinary pouch which can be emptied by catheterization of a narrow-tubed access pipe so that the diversion is continent. The principle of the surgery was first proposed by Mitrofanoff (1980), who suggested that the atonic orthotopic bladder should form the pouch. The catheterizable narrow-tubed access was formed either by the appendix isolated on its mesentery, inverted with the distal end cut off, and implanted into the bladder by a non-refluxing submucosal tunnel with the caecal end brought to the skin as a catheterizable stoma; or, alternatively, by a ureter transected and anastomosed to its contralateral mate to allow the proximal end of the distal third to be brought to the skin.

Adaptations of the Mitrofanoff principle have been suggested, constructing an intra-abdominal pouch of bowel to form the reservoir, and using similar techniques of construction of a catheterizable stoma.

These techniques are still in their infancy, but no doubt will mean a greatly enhanced quality of life for patients who do require a cutaneous urinary diversion, and will be rid of the need for a collecting bag to be stuck to the skin.

COMPLICATIONS OF THE NEUROPATHIC BLADDER

The upper urinary tracts are always threatened by lower tract dysfunction. By the very nature of the neuropathy these complications can be entirely asymptomatic and discovered by routine urological follow-up.

Chronic bacterial infection is always a potential hazard and thus patients with vesico-urethral neuropathy should have regular bacteriological surveillance. By paralysing ureteric smooth muscle with toxins the infected neuropathic urinary tract is prone to upper tract dilatation, and compromised renal function.

Vesico-ureteric reflux may be transient or permanent and therefore more sinister, especially in the presence of chronic infection. It is more common in higher lesions, and more prevalent the longer after spinal injury.

Reimplantation of a refluxing ureter into a grossly trabeculated neuropathic bladder is beset with difficulties, and it is mandatory to ensure before embarking on such surgery that there is no persistent midline bladder outflow obstruction. Nipple valve reimplantations are best avoided, because as the bladder distends the nipple is distracted and loses its antirefluxing properties. Perhaps the easiest solution to the problem of vesico-ureteric reflux in a neuropathic bladder will be the use of submucosal Teflon injected into the orifice (Puri & O'Donnell, 1984, 1987). This relatively simple technique is effective in correcting reflux without the risk of ureteric obstruction or the need for an open operation, and if unsuccessful at the first attempt may readily be repeated (Dewan & Guiney, 1990).

Intramural ureteric obstruction may occur as the ureter passes through a grossly thickened detrusor, and is more likely in those cases with excessive fibrosis of the bladder wall. Scarring of the mucosal orifice itself as a result of chronic infection is a further cause of this type of upper tract obstruction in neuropathic bladder dysfunction. The condition surprisingly can occur rapidly and bilaterally, producing acute renal failure and requiring decompression of the upper tracts by percutaneous nephrostomy. Ureteric reimplantation is required in those cases which do not respond to intensive antibacterial therapy after decompression.

Urinary calculi are more common in both the upper and lower tracts in neuropathic bladder dysfunction. Approximately 6% of patients with spinal injuries will form upper tract stone compared with 2% of the general population. The genesis of the stones relates to more than just recumbency as a result of the injury, for over two-thirds will form after the first two years following injury. Intriguingly, though no correlation exists between the neurological level and the incidence of stones, they are never seen in spinal cord injury patients with a neurological level below L1, yet are depressingly common in congenital neuropathic patients, largely secondary to infection.

With the development of modern urological stone management all calculi should be treated aggressively (Bush *et al.*, 1984; Brannen *et al.*, 1985; Marberger *et al.*, 1985; Mayo *et al.*, 1985). Modern percutaneous lithotriptors, whether electrohydraulic or ultrasonic, will disintegrate stones without significant morbidity (Wickham *et al.*, 1983) and rigid ureterorendoscopy allows access to the ureter endoscopically for intraureteric lithotripsy and stone retrieval (Ford *et al.*, 1983; Watson *et al.*, 1983).

External shockwave lithotripsy can also be employed, provided that access is not hindered by spinal deformity.

All patients with vesico-urethral neuropathy must thus be on a programme of follow-up whereby these potential complications are excluded on a regular basis. The system of investigation should include a regular morphological study, best performed by ultrasonographic scanning rather than intravenous urography, together with functional studies by radionuclide renography and biochemical assessment. Each patient should be studied at least every six months in the early years following the neuropathy until a stable state is achieved.

REFERENCES

Anderson, K-E., Ek, A., Hedlund, H. & Mattiasson, A. (1981) Effects of prazosin on isolated human urethra and in patients with lower motor neuron lesions. *Invest. Urol.*, **19**, 39–42.

Awad, S.A., Downie, J.W. & Kiruluta, H.G. (1978) Alpha-adrenergic agents in urinary disorders of the proximal urethra. II. Urethral obstruction due to 'sympathetic dyssynergia'. *Br. J. Urol.*, **50**, 336–339.

Blacklock, N.J. (1986) Catheters and urethral strictures. *Br.*

J. Urol., **58**, 475–478.
Boyce, W.H., Latham, J.E. & Hunt, L.D. (1964) Research related to the development of an artificial electrical stimulator for the paralysed human bladder. *J. Urol.*, **91**, 41–51.
Bramble, F.J. (1982) The treatment of adult enuresis and urge incontinence by enterocystoplasty. *Br. J. Urol.*, **54**, 693–696.
Bramble, F.J. (1990) The Clam cystoplasty. *Br. J. Urol.*, **66**, 337–341.
Brannen, G.E., Bush, W.H., Correa, R.J., Gibbons, R.P. & Elder, J.S. (1985) Kidney stone removal: percutaneous versus surgical lithotomy. *J. Urol.*, **113**, 6–12.
Breithaupt, D.J., Jousse, A.T. & Wynne-Jones, M. (1961) Late cause of death and life expectancy in paraplegia. *Can. Med. Assoc. J.*, **85**, 73–77.
Brindley, G.S. (1973) Emptying the bladder by stimulating ventral sacral roots. *J. Physiol.*, **237**, 15–16P.
Brindley, G.S. (1977) An implant to empty the bladder or close the urethra. *J. Neurol. Neurosurg. Psychiatry*, **40**, 358–369.
Brindley, G.S., Polkey, C.E., Rushton, D.N. & Cardozo, L. (1986) Sacral anterior root stimulation for bladder control in paraplegics—the first 50 cases. *J. Neurol. Neurosurg. Psychiatry*, **49**, 1104–1114.
Bush, W.H., Brannen, G.E., Gibbons, R.P., Correa, R.J. & Elder, J.S. (1984) Radiation exposure to patient and urologist during percutaneous nephrostolithotomy. *J. Urol.*, **132**, 1148–1152.
Delaere, K.P.J., Debruyne, F.M.J. & Moonen, W.A. (1983) Bladder neck incision in the female: a hazardous procedure. *Br. J. Urol.*, **55**, 283–286.
Dewan, P.A. & Guiney, E.J. (1990) Endoscopic correction of vesicoureteric reflux in children with spina bifida. *Br. J. Urol.*, **65**, 646–649.
Diokno, A.C. & Taub, M. (1975) Ephedrine in the treatment of urinary incontinence. *Urology*, **5**, 624–625.
Ewing, R., Bultitude, M. & Shuttleworth, K.E.D. (1983) Subtrigonal phenol therapy for incontinence in female patients with multiple sclerosis. *Lancet*, **1**, 1304–1305.
Ford, T.F., Watson, G.M. & Wickham, J.E.A. (1983) Transurethral ureteroscopic retrieval of ureteric stones. *Br. J. Urol.*, **55**, 626–628.
Geisler, W.O., Jousse, A.T. & Wynne-Jones, M. (1977) Survival in traumatic transverse myelitis. *Paraplegia*, **14**, 262–275.
Geisler, W.O., Jousse, A.T., Wynne-Jones, M. & Briethaupt, D.J. (1983) Survival in traumatic spinal cord injury. *Paraplegia*, **21**, 364–373.
Gibbon, N.O.K. (1973) Division of the external sphincter. *Br. J. Urol.*, **45**, 110–115.
Gibbon, N.O.K., Jameson, R.M., Heal, M.R. & Abel, B.J. (1973) Transection of the bladder for adult enuresis and allied conditions. *Br. J. Urol.*, **45**, 306–310.
Guttman, L. & Frankel, H. (1966) The value of intermittent catheterisation in the early management of traumatic paraplegia and tetraplegia. *Paraplegia*, **4**, 63–84.
Herr, H.W. (1975) Intermittent catheterisation in neurogenic bladder dysfunction. *J. Urol.*, **113**, 477–479.
Jousse, A.T., Wynne-Jones, M. & Briethaupt, D.J. (1968) A follow-up study of life expectancy and mortality in traumatic transverse myelitis. *Can. Med. Assoc. J.*, **98**, 770–772.
Kato, K., Kondo, A., Takita, T., Gotoh, M., Tanaka, J. & Mitsuya, H. (1987) Incontinence in female neurogenic bladders, resolution by endoscopic bladder neck suspension. *Br. J. Urol.*, **59**, 523–525.
Khanna, O.P. (1976) Disorders of micturition: neuropharmacologic basis and results of drug therapy. *Urology*, **8**, 316–328.
Krane, R.J. & Olsson, C.A. (1973) Phenoxybenzamine in neurogenic bladder dysfunction. II. Clinical considerations. *J. Urol.*, **110**, 653–656.
Lapides, J., Diokno, A.C., Silber, S.J. & Lowe, B.S. (1972) Clean intermittent self catheterisation in the treatment of urinary tract disease. *J. Urol.*, **107**, 458–461.
Lawrence, W.T. & Thomas, D.G. (1987) The Stamey bladder neck suspension operation for stress incontinence and neurovesical dysfunction. *Br. J. Urol.*, **59**, 305–310.
Leyson, J.F.J., Martin, B.F. & Sporer, A. (1980) Baclofen in the treatment of detrusor–sphincter dyssynergia in spinal cord injury patients. *J. Urol.*, **124**, 82–84.
Madersbacher, H. & Scott, F.B. (1976) The twelve o'clock sphincterotomy. Technique, indications, results. *Paraplegia*, **13**, 261–267.
Marberger, M., Stackl, W., Hruby, W. & Kroiss, A. (1985) Late sequelae of ultrasonic lithotripsy of renal calculi. *J. Urol.*, **133**, 170–173.
Mayo, M.E., Kriegger, J.N. & Rudd, T.G. (1985) Effect of percutaneous nephrostolithotomy on renal function. *J. Urol.*, **133**, 167–169.
McGuire, E.J. & Brady, S. (1979) Detrusor sphincter dyssynergia. *J. Urol.*, **121**, 774–777.
McInerney, P.D., Vanner, T.F., Harris, S.A.B. & Stephenson, T.P. (1990) Permanent urethral stents for detrusor sphincter dyssynergia. *Br. J. Urol.*, **67**, 291–294.
McRae, P., Murray, K.H.A., Nurse, D.E., Stephenson, T.P. & Mundy, A.R. (1987) Clam enterocystoplasty in the neuropathic bladder. *Br. J. Urol.*, **60**, 523–525.
Mitrofanoff, P. (1980) Cystostomie continente transappendiculaire dans le traitement des vessies neurologiques. *Chir. Pediatr.*, **21**, 297–305.
Murray, K.H.A., Nurse, D.E. & Mundy, A.R. (1988) Detrusor behaviour following implantation of the Brantley Scott artificial urinary sphincter for neuropathic incontinence. *Br. J. Urol.*, **61**, 122–128.
Nashold, B.S., Friedman, H., Glenn, J.F., Grimes, J.H., Barry, W.F. & Avery, R. (1972) Electromicturition in paraplegia. *Arch. Surg.*, **104**, 195–202.
Parry, J.R.W., Nurse, D.E., Boucaut, H.A.P., Murray, K.H.A. & Mundy, A.R. (1990) Surgical management of the congenital neuropathic bladder. *Br. J. Urol.*, **65**, 165–167.
Pedersen, E., Harving, H., Klemar, B. & Torring, J. (1978) Human anal reflexes. *J. Neurol. Neurosurg. Psychiatry*, **41**, 813–818.
Puri, P. & O'Donnell, B. (1984) Correction of experimentally produced vesicoureteric reflux in the piglet by intravesical injection of teflon. *Br. Med. J.*, **289**, 5–7.

Puri, P. & O'Donnell, B. (1987) Endoscopic correction of grades IV and V primary vesicoureteric reflux: six to 30 month follow-up in 42 ureters. *J. Paed. Surg.*, **22**, 1087–1091.

Rickwood, A.K.M. (1982) Use of internal urethrotomy to reverse upper renal tract dilatation in children with neurogenic bladder dysfunction. *Br. J. Urol.*, **54**, 292–294.

Rickwood, A.K.M., Thomas, D.G., Philp, N.H. & Spicer, R.D. (1982) A system of management of the congenital neuropathic bladder based upon combined urodynamic and radiological assessment. *Br. J. Urol.*, **54**, 507–511.

Ross, J.C., Gibbon, N.O.K. & Damanski, M. (1957) Resection of the external sphincter in the paraplegic—a preliminary report. *Trans. Am. Assoc. Genito. Surg.*, **69**, 193–198.

Shaw, P.J.R., Milroy, E.J.G., Timoney, A.G., El Din, A. & Mitchell, N. (1990) Permanent external striated sphincter stents in patients with spinal injuries. *Br. J. Urol.*, **66**, 297–300.

Stephenson, T.P. & Mundy, A.R. (1985) Treatment of the neuropathic bladder by enterocystoplasty and selective sphincterotomy or sphincter ablation and replacement. *Br. J. Urol.*, **57**, 27–31.

Vaidyanathan, A., Rao, M.S., Mapa, M.K., Bapna, B.C., Chary, K.S.N. & Swamy, R.P. (1981) Study of intravesical instillation of 15-(S)-15 methyl prostaglandin F_2a in patients with neurogenic bladder dysfunction. *J. Urol.*, **126**, 81–85.

Vinson, R.K. & Diokno, A.C. (1976) Uninhibited neurogenic bladder in adults. *Urology*, 7, 376–378.

Walsh, P.C. & Donker, P.J. (1982) Impotence following radical prostatectomy: insight into etiology and prevention. *J. Urol.*, **128**, 492–497.

Watson, G.M., Wickham, J.E.A., Mills, T.N., Bown, S.G., Swain, P. & Salmon, P.R. (1983) Laser fragmentation of renal calculi. *Br. J. Urol.*, **55**, 613–616.

Whitmore, W.F. III, Fam, B.A. & Yalla, S.V. (1978) Experience with anteromedian (12 o'clock) external urethral sphincterotomy in 100 male subjects with neuropathic bladder. *Br. J. Urol.*, **50**, 99–101.

Wickham, J.E.A., Kellett, M.J. & Miller, R.A. (1983) Elective percutaneous nephrolithotomy in 50 patients: an analysis of the technique, results and complications. *J. Urol.*, **129**, 904–906.

63 · Soft Tissue Injuries of the Cervical Spine

By J. DVORAK

Evaluation of the patient with cervical spine injury, particularly with only apparent soft tissue injury, is very difficult (Hohl, 1974; Pearce, 1989). In Switzerland (population approx. 6 million), 5000 patients with cervical spine injuries are registered annually. Based upon a survey (Dvorak *et al.*, 1987c; Dvorak & Valach, 1989) it was found that a majority of the registered injuries of the cervical spine were only so-called 'soft tissue injuries' (Fig. 63.1). Only 13% out of the 11 000 injured suffered cervical spine fracture with or without a spinal cord lesion, while in 87% no bony lesion was detected. In such cases a morphological substrate which could be considered responsible for the patient's complaints is often not evident. The attending physician as well as the independent consultant have to base their decisions upon other information, including the functional radiological assessment of the cervical spine. It is well known that injured patients of this type describe their pain subjectively as related to the injury. Quite frequently the question of the degree of objectiveness of those injured, and the reality of their complaints, becomes the most decisive factor in the assessment.

Based upon earlier work dealing with cervical spine injuries, particularly on 'whiplash' (Kuhlendal, 1966; Hinz, 1970; Erdmann, 1973), it was assumed that the consequences of soft tissue injury of the cervical spine would fade by, at the latest, two years after the injury. This belief was refuted in later papers (Wiesner & Mumenthaler, 1975; Suter & Mumenthaler, 1977). No unified opinion exists for the diagnostic assessment or for the initial therapeutic intervention, nor is there agreement on the treatment of chronic complaints. However, a soft or hard collar is generally recommended initially to restrict movements. The possibility of early mobilization or chiropractic adjustment in the treatment of acute cervical spine injury has also been addressed.

Several authors (Hohl & Baker, 1964; Hinz, 1970; Erdmann, 1973; Ommaya, 1985; Walz, 1987; White, 1990) have unsuccessfully analysed the relationship between the mechanism of a motor accident and its repercussions on the cervical spine. In this respect, the *in vitro* studies are of limited value, as the important factors, such as the time for the impact, the muscle tone and voluntary innervation of the neck muscles, are missing. Obviously, the extent of the car damage does not automatically correlate to the seriousness of the injury the passenger or the driver may suffer.

Studies by Saternus & Thrun (1987), who analysed cervical spines from patients who died as a result of the severe injuries, found a high percentage of damaged soft tissues of the cervical spine, mainly the ligaments. In particular, the fact that this series included ruptures of the alar ligaments in patients without direct head and neck injury, brought new possibilities to the validation of patient's symptoms, clinical findings and the analysis of functional radiographs. As no prospective or long-term studies have been performed on a non-selected population of the course of the development after injuries concerning the cervical spine, some conclusions may be presently drawn from a comparison between the injured who later are complaint-free, and those who exhibit therapy-resistant complaints or later receive a disability compensation.

Based upon the retrospective studies by Dvorak *et al.* (1987c) and Dvorak & Valach (1989), it was found that 55% of the whiplash patients were injured in a car accident, while 45% were injured by other means. In the later group, sport injuries, falls, direct cervical

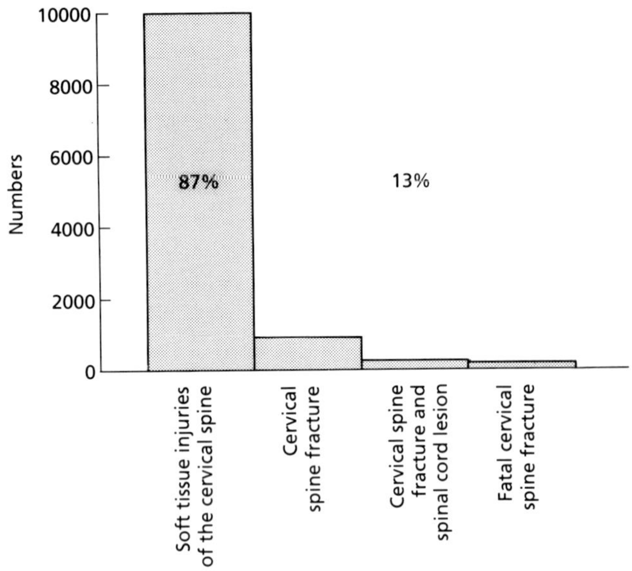

Fig. 63.1 Cervical spine injury combined with a fracture in Switzerland in the years 1978–1981. Based on Dvorak *et al.* (1987c).

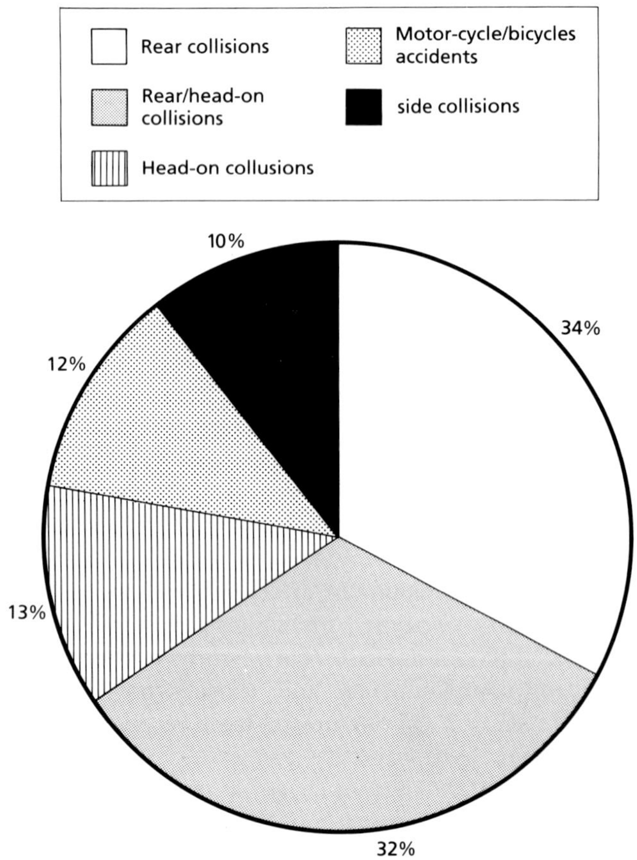

Fig. 63.2 Mechanism of the motor vehicle accident. Based on Dvorak *et al.* (1987c).

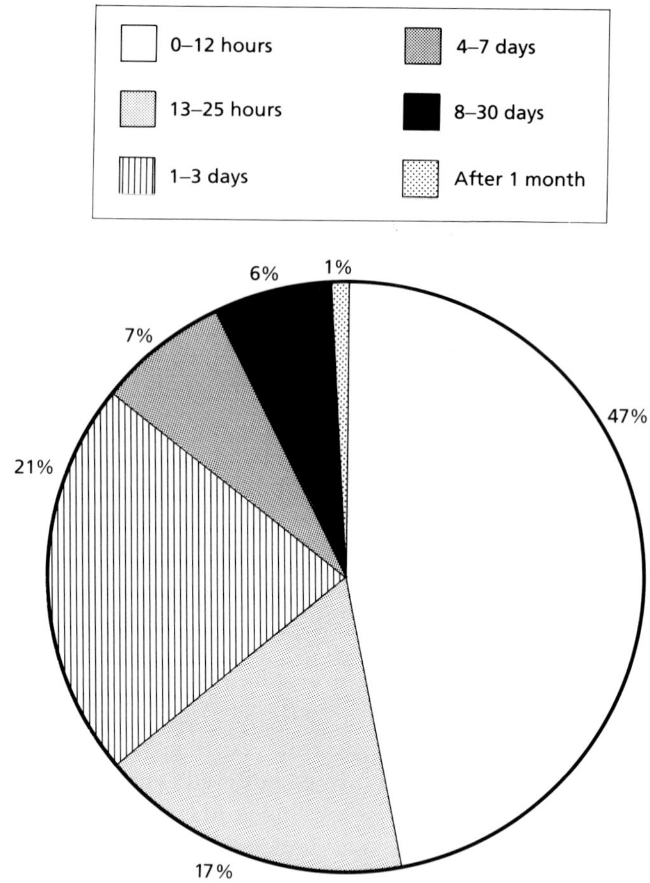

Fig. 63.3 Time interval until the first medical consultation. Based on Dvorak *et al.* (1987c).

spine trauma, etc. were included. The car accident group was split into five classes. The most common class was the head on and rear end collisions (Fig. 63.2). In retrospectively analysing the different classes of car accidents, a significant difference between the groups as related to long-term symptoms was not found. The majority (75%) became pain-free within four to six weeks. Only 1% of all injured patients with soft tissue injuries later received a disability pension; however, 25% of the soft tissue injured patients reported neck and arm pain years after the injury. Degenerative changes of the cervical spine have been determined to be a significantly unfavourable factor for the long-term prognosis.

HISTORY, INITIAL SYMPTOMS AND FINDINGS

Almost half of the injured patients consulted the physician within the first 12 hours, and another 40%

within the first three days (Fig. 63.3). In the majority of cases the first consultation was performed by either the general practitioner or by local specialists. Only a small group (9%) were initially referred to a specialist centre (Fig. 63.4). This fact stresses the importance of the general practitioner as related to this particular problem, as the first assessment may elicit prognostic values of great importance. Almost 70% of the injured patients reported immediate occurrence of symptoms after the injury. The most frequent complaints were cervical spine pain and painful spinal rotation. Shoulder pain and pain of the lumbar spine were also reported quite frequently, and disturbance of consciousness, as well as dizziness, were also common symptoms. Paraesthesia and muscle weakness of the upper extremities, as well as radicular deficits, found during initial clinical investigation, were found to be unfavourable symptoms (Fig. 63.5).

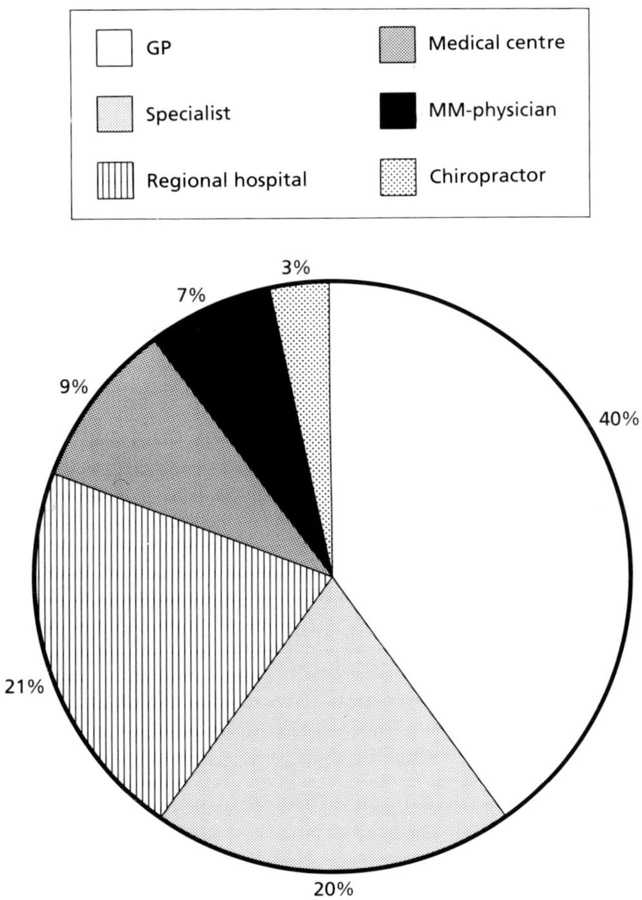

Fig. 63.4 First medical institution. Based on Dvorak *et al.* (1987c).

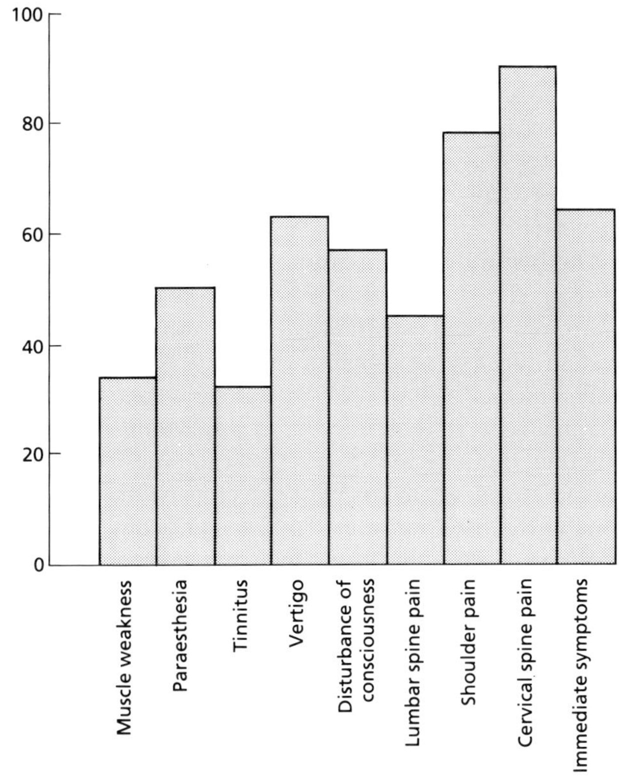

Fig. 63.5 Initial symptoms in patients with soft tissue injuries (n = 320). Based on Dvorak *et al.* (1987c).

On examination painful rotation of the head, as well as neck stiffness, were observed most frequently.

Psychosocial symptoms or neuropsychological deficits were found in 79% of patients who were later compensated, but the problems occurred in only 10% of other patients who suffered from pain. The neuropsychological deficits were present in 12% of the compensated patients immediately after the accident, and in 30% several months later. The most common were: loss of general and occupational achievement ability, a depressive frame of mind, decreased vitality, lack of concentration, and sleep disturbance.

Of the group of patients who later received a disability pension, 70% were receiving some kind of medical or physiotherapeutic treatments related to their injuries. In the group who suffered pain related to injury after several years, 25% were receiving medical treatment. The most common complaints were neck and head pain, pain in the shoulders and arms, dizziness during head rotation as well as constant dizziness.

DIAGNOSIS AND MANAGEMENT

Based upon the results of these studies and the experience with the evaluation of the medical records of the Swiss National Insurance Company (SUVA) the following diagnostic and therapeutic procedures for patients with cervical spine soft tissue injuries are suggested.

The history of the injured patient before the accident as related to absence from work and necessity of treatment due to disturbances of the musculoskeletal system must be recorded in the medical history.

The mechanism of the accident should be recorded as precisely as possible. It is important to note whether the patient was prepared for the impact or was unaware, as the effect of the preparedness on the tone of the neck muscles may be significant. Krämer (1983) suggested that there were three groups of significance, depending on the type of head and neck injury. These groups comprise patients with: direct injuries to the neck and the head, an indirect injury to the cervical spine with a direct head injury, and cases where the injuries to both the head and the neck are indirect.

With regard to the biomechanics of the accident, not only is the speed important, but also the movement of the head, described as pure flexion–extension, bending (mainly due to side-collision) or whether the head was rotated during the impact. The last is biomechanically probably the most vulnerable position of the head, as the alar ligaments are already stretched during rotation and through additional flexion it is possible that the ligaments could be irreversibly overstretched or even ruptured (Dvorak & Panjab, 1987; Dvorak *et al.*, 1987, 1988c).

Initial investigation

The primary care physician should perform a complete functional examination of the cervical spine (Dvorak & Dvorak, 1990). A complete neurological assessment should also be performed and documented in the medical records. Important signs are dermatomal sensory loss, reflex loss or muscle weakness.

An AP and lateral radiograph of the entire cervical spine should always be performed. If an injury to the upper cervical spine is suspected a special X-ray, focusing on the odontoid, should additionally be made. The X-rays are of value in determining pre-existing degenerative changes of the cervical spine and can help later on in comparison of reactive changes following a segmental instability for example.

Initial therapy

The most appropriate initial management is to provide a soft or semi-hard collar during the first days. The collar may be taken off and treatment such as hot packs or ultrasound may be appropriate, combined with anti-inflammatory medication. In the initial four to six weeks after the accident any kind of manipulation or chiropractic adjustments should be avoided (Dvorak *et al.*, 1990b).

Further investigation

If the patient does not improve in the first six weeks some kind of soft tissue damage should be suspected. In addition to a complete functional, clinical and neurological assessment, functional X-rays in AP and lateral projection should be performed. If there is a suspected segmental dysfunction of the upper cervical spine, the AP projection, focusing on the odontoid peg during lateral bending, can offer additional information.

The flexion–extension X-rays, passively performed, give information about the segmental function throughout the whole cervical spine as related to the rotation above the *x* axis of the three-dimensional system. For routine measurements a method described by Penning is the most suitable and reliable (Dvorak *et al.*, 1988b).

If a nerve root or a plexus lesion is suspected, a neurophysiological examination may offer additional data to aid the diagnosis. Electromyography of the segmental muscles may show denervation, and nerve conduction studies will exclude compression of peripheral nerves. The motor pathways can be evaluated by using the transcranial magnetic stimulation of the vertex, the spinal cord and plexus. With this new method the central conducting time for motor pathways can be determined (Merton & Morton, 1980; Barker *et al.*, 1986; Dvorak *et al.*, 1990a,c).

For patients who show psychological symptoms such as lack of concentration and increased tiredness combined with the disturbance of the sleeping cycle, a neuropsychological assessment might be helpful to exclude psycho-organic syndromes. It is advisable to perform the neuropsychological evaluation in a somatic surrounding in order not to reduce the compliance of the patient by referring the patient to a psychiatrist.

Therapy after seven weeks

If segmental hypermobility and bony lesions are excluded, and the patient is suffering from segmental dysfunction and no radicular signs occurred, mobilization should be initiated by using direct muscle force or postisometric relaxation combined with muscular rehabilitation, as there is stretching of the shortened postural muscles and strengthening of the phasic weak muscle groups. At this time the patient should be instructed in home-training and self mobilization, including instructions for back school. Within the following weeks there should be a maximal therapeutic effort in order to reintegrate the patient to normal activities before a time period of six months. Dvorak & Valach (1989) found that patients who did not return to work before six months tended to remain out of work even after a period of two years.

Late investigation and treatment

As mentioned above, it is important to exclude any kind of organic lesions before the period of six months. In this phase the patient should be referred to an interdisciplinary spine unit, where trained neurologists, orthopaedic surgeons, psychiatrists, neurosurgeons, neuroradiologists and neuropsychologists can evaluate the possible reasons for the resistance of the patient's symptoms to therapy.

In patients with persistent symptoms, functional computer tomography, Doppler sonography and functional electronystagmography can be particularly useful in determining the rotatory instability of upper cervical spine (Dvorak *et al.*, 1987a, 1988c).

If a properly performed mobilization/manipulation of the cervical and thoracic spine does not show any results after 10–12 treatments there is no logical reason for continuing with this therapeutic approach.

In resistant cases additional invasive examinations such as discography, diagnostic infiltration of the apophyseal joints or trial stabilization by Minerva cast or a stiff brace may be tried. These procedures might be used to reveal a suspected segmental instability and a possible indication for a segmental fusion.

REFERENCES

Barker, A.T., Freeston, I.L., Jalinous, R. & Jarratt, J.A. (1986) Clinical evaluation of conduction time measurements in central motor pathways using magnetic stimulation of the human brain. *Lancet*, **1**, 1325–1326.

Dvorak, J. & Dvorak, V. (1990) *Manual Medicine: Diagnostics*, 2nd rev. edn, pp. 1–346. G. Thième, Stuttgart.

Dvorak, J. & Panjabi, M. (1987) Functional anatomy of the alar ligaments. *Spine*, **12**, 183–188.

Dvorak, J. & Valach, L. (1989) Cervical spine injuries in Switzerland. *J. Manual Med.*, **4**, 7–16.

Dvorak, J., Hayek, J. & Zehnder, R. (1987b) CT-functional diagnostics of the rotatory instability of the upper cervical spine. *Spine*, **12**, 726–731.

Dvorak, L., Valach, L. & Schmid, S. (1987c) Verletzungen der Halswirbelsaule in der Schweiz. *Orthopade*, **16**, 2–12.

Dvorak, J., Panjabi, M.N., Gerber, M. & Wichmann, W. (1987a) CT-functional diagnostics of the rotatory instability of upper cervical spine. *Spine*, **12**, 197–205.

Dvorak, J., Penning, L. & Panjabi, M. (1988a) Functional diagnostics of the cervical spine using computer tomography. *Neuroradiology*, **30**, 132–137.

Dvorak, J., Dvorak, J., Frohlich, D., Penning, L., Baumgartner, H. & Panjabi, M.N. (1988b) Functional radiographic diagnosis of the cervical spine: flexion/extension. *Spine*, **13**, 748–755.

Dvorak, J., Dvorak, J., Schneider, E., Saldinger, P. & Rahn, B. (1988c) Biomechanics of the craniocervical region. *J. Orthop. Rel. Res.*, **6**, 452–461.

Dvorak, J., Herdmann, J. & Theiler, R. (1990a) Magnetic transcranial brain stimulation: painless evaluation of central motor pathways: normal values and clinical applications in spinal cord diagnostics. I: Upper extremities. *Spine*, **15**, 155–160.

Dvorak, J., Herdmann, J. & Theiler, R. (1990b) Motor evoked potentials: evaluation of central motor pathways in patients with cervical spine disorders. *Spine*, **15**, 1013–1016.

Dvorak, J., Janssen, B. & Grob, D. (1990c) The neurological work-up in patients with cervical spine disorders. *Spine*, **15**, 1017–1022.

Erdmann, H. (1973) *Schleuderverletzungen der Halswirbelsäule, Erkennung und Begutachtung.* Hippokrates, Stuttgart.

Hinz, P. (1970) Die Verletzung der Halswirbelsäule durch Schleuderverletzung und durch Abknickung. In Junghans, K. (ed.) *Die Wirbelsäule in Forschung und Praxis*, p. 47. Hippokrates, Stuttgart.

Hohl, M. (1974) Soft tissue injuries of the neck in automobile accidents: factors influencing prognosis. *J. Bone Jt. Surg.*, **56A**, 1675–1682.

Hohl, M. & Baker, H.R. (1964) The atlanto-axial joint. *J. Bone Jt. Surg.*, **46A**, 1739–1752.

Krämer, G. (1983) HWS-Schleudertraumen. Zur Pathogenese der zerebralen Beteiligung und persistierender posttraumatischer Störungen. *Medwelt*, **34**, pp. 1134–1140.

Kuhlendal, H. (1966) Schleudertrauma der Halswirbelsäule. Neurochirurgische Probleme. *Langenbecks Arch. Klin.*

Chir., **316**, 470–475.

Merton, P.A. & Morton, H.B. (1960) Stimulation of the cerebral cortex in the intact human subject. *Nature*, **285**, 227–228.

Ommaya, A.R. (1985) The head: kinematics and brain injury mechanisms., In Aldman, B. & Chapon, A. (eds) *The Biomechanics of Impact Trauma*, pp. 117 138. Elsevier, Amsterdam.

Pearce, J.M.S. (1989) Whiplash injury: a reappraisal. *J. Neurol. Neurosurg. Psychiatry*, **52**, 1329–1331.

Saternus, K.-S. & Thrun, C. (1987) Traumatology of the alar ligaments. *Aktuel Traumatol*, **36**, 214–218.

Suter, J. & Mumenthaler, M. Gutachterliche Aspekte bei Schueuderverletzungen der Halswirbelsäule. Eine Studie von Fällen, die eine Rente oder Kapitalabfindung erhielten. *Arch. Orthop. Unfall-Chir.*, **90**, 325–342.

Walz, F. (1987) Das Schleudertrauma der Halswirbelsäule im Strassenverkehr: biomechanische und gutachterliche Aspekte. *Schweiz. Med. Wochenschr.*, **117**, 619–623.

White, A. (1990) *Clinical Biomechanics of Spine*, 2nd edn. Lippincott, Philadelphia, PA.

Wiesner, H. & Mumenthaler M. (1975) Schleuderverletzung der Halswirblesäule. *Arch. Orthop. Unfall-Chir.*, **81**, 13–36.

64 · Penetrating Spinal Injuries

By S.M. EISENSTEIN

One of the functions of the spinal column is to protect its most important contents, the spinal cord and cauda equina. The difficulties associated with surgical exposure of the spinal neural tissues testify to the success with which the spinal column performs this function. Penetrating injuries of the spine sufficient to cause neurological deficit are appropriately uncommon, requiring either ingenuity or high velocity. The two most common penetrating injuries are therefore those effected by a carefully directed skewer or by gunshot, and mostly the result of evil intent. Singular misfortune may also be implicated, as in the very rare impalement injuries.

Penetrating injuries include those in which foreign bodies penetrate and lodge in the hard and soft tissues of the spinal column, but not necessarily within the spinal canal. These injuries may not cause paralysis but produce other complications associated with injuries penetrating to the spine.

The questions that bedevil the management of penetrating spinal injuries arise only because very few surgeons have sufficient experience to be able to treat with the confidence that experience brings. Thus, in the management of a single case, several dilemmas exist. For example, how radical should be the search for every penetrating fragment, or is mere debridement of the surface wound sufficient? Do retained bullets really cause lead poisoning, or will radical exploration reduce or increase the degree of neurological deficit? Uncertainty is compounded by the fact that the penetration can transgress so many different anatomical fields on its way to the spine, and the surgeon operating alone may feel inadequate in some of these areas. Finally, there may be medicolegal implications related to the matter of survival, or the lack of it, to raise the stakes in treatment success and failure.

PREVALENCE AND MODE OF INJURY

For many years the major civilian experience in penetrating injuries of the spine worldwide, was to be found in South Africa, because of the preference for stabbing by bicycle spoke and a wide variety of knives, in a reign of terror by ghetto gangsters (Lipschitz, 1967, 1976; Key & Retief, 1970). The ingenuity demonstrated by these individuals is all the more remarkable in the light of the fact that they usually paralysed their victims in crowded trains or in darkness, through clothing; and in the light of an early report on stab wounds of the spinal cord which concluded that 'One could almost never deliberately pierce a spinal cord with a sharp instrument' (Rand & Patterson, 1929). In South Africa, gunshot injuries of the spine were uncommon in the 1960s, but this situation appears to have been reversed dramatically in recent years (S. Govender, personal communication, 1989), probably reflecting increasing accessibility to firearms. In the United States, gunshot injuries are increasing in proportion to other causes of spinal cord injury and are now second only to road traffic accidents as the major cause of traumatic quadriplegia and paraplegia (Morgan *et al.*, 1971; Stauffer *et al.*, 1979). Conversely, the rarity of gunshot injuries of the spine in the United Kingdom must be a reflection of the severe restrictions on firearm possession.

It is almost certainly the case that many instances of gunshot penetrating the spine are never reported because spine penetration was only one of many injuries causing death. Every level of the spine is vulnerable to gunshot, including the odontoid process (Pattisapu & Al-Mefty, 1987).

One might expect military conflict to provide the ultimate experience in penetrating gunshot injuries of the spine, but the war in South-East Asia did not support this expectation: in the United States Armed Forces, penetrating injuries were 13% lower in Vietnam than in the United States (Myers, 1973). On the other hand, the devastation wrought by the high velocity of missiles in battle is unusual in civilian gunshot injuries (Myers, 1973; Yashon, 1973).

Missile injuries are generally divided into low-velocity, and high-velocity (the bullet or fragment moving at 1000 m/s or more) because of the contrasting modes of injury. Low-velocity missiles injure by direct contact, crush, contusion, laceration and haemorrhage; high-velocity missiles can produce massive necrosis and paralysis merely by the dissipation of enormous energy throughout the soft tissues and without any naked-eye evidence of viscous or cord injury (Morgan *et al.*, 1971; Myers, 1973). Bullets and fragments which 'tumble', rather than spin, produce greater tissue destruction.

Impalement injuries are rare. Horowitz *et al.* (1985) reported a motorcyclist who was catapulted onto a building site and pierced by a reinforcing rod set in concrete. In a domestic injury a patient sustained penetration by a glass fragment when a glass-topped table shattered under his weight (Baghai & Sheptak, 1982). Two patients in the timber industry sustained penetration to the spine by wood splinters entering the abdomen anteriorly (S. Govender, personal communication, 1989).

Iatrogenic impalement of the spinal dura has been reported following sublaminar wiring for fracture of the odontoid process (Dunn *et al.*, 1987). It is expected that similar injuries lower down the spine at thoracic and lumbar levels will increase in number as Luque segmental sublaminar wiring increases in popularity, and as the need for subsequent removal of wire inevitably increases.

CLINICAL FEATURES

The most obvious primary grouping of patients presenting with penetrating spinal injuries is that they will have, or will not have, some degree of paralysis. Neurological deficit is certainly the spinal surgeon's greatest concern. The problem is that some degree of paralysis may be present but remain undiscovered because of associated head injury, or because of greater concern for associated injuries of life-threatening severity. In unconscious patients a clue to the presence of a severed spinal cord is the combination of 'cold nose and warm feet', where vasodilatation of the lower limbs has followed a spinal injury (Lipschitz, 1967).

The neurological deficit below the level of injury may be complete or incomplete; upper motoneurone or lower motoneurone, unilateral or bilateral. A complete bilateral upper motoneurone deficit carries a poor prognosis; a partial lower motor neurone deficit, on one side only, carries a good prognosis for some (unpredictable) degree of recovery.

The spinal surgeon's concern is that a partial deficit may become complete, or that a neurological deficit may develop in a patient who presented initially without one. The importance of early and detailed charting of neurological status is self-evident. A progressive loss of neurological function constitutes a surgical emergency. An incomplete deficit can present with any combination of motor and sensory loss, but a characteristic incomplete deficit of stab injuries of the spine is the Brown–Séquard syndrome. Here it is assumed that the penetrating implement has produced a hemilateral cord injury, resulting in motor and proprioceptive loss on the injured side with loss of pain sensibility and temperature perception on the opposite side (Rosenberg, 1957; Heiden *et al.*, 1975; Lipschitz, 1976).

A patient with a stab wound and marked loss of function in all spinal tracts other than posterior columns, has probably suffered 'contre-coup' spinal cord concussion or 'contusion'; the cord is not damaged at the site of penetration or impact but has been carried forwards by the force of impact, to be injured against the bony walls of the spinal canal on the side opposite to the point of entry (Lipschitz & Block, 1962).

There may be multiple stab wounds or gunshot wounds and clinical examination alone will suggest which wound probably caused the spinal injury. One or more of the stabs or shots may have produced associated injuries to major thoracic and abdominal viscera which may be life-threatening. High-velocity bullet or shrapnel injuries may present with extensive paralysis but without any naked-eye evidence of injury to the spinal cord and dura: passage merely close to the cord can produce complete and permanent paralysis through neural tissue necrosis produced by the 'shock wave' (Myers, 1973). At the other extreme it is remarkable that some penetrating injuries, with a potential for causing major neurological loss, have caused none at all. A glass shard completely traversed the lumbar canal but the relatively slow rate of penetration must have allowed the neural tissue to give way ahead of the penetrating object (Baghai & Sheptak, 1982). Harmit *et al.* (1985) reported a case of low-velocity penetration into the spinal canal in a stabbing injury which did not produce any neurological deficit because the knife-point passed alongside the dura without entering it. Any penetration of the spinal meninges may present with a leak of cerebrospinal fluid from the wound and a late presentation may include meningitis or an abscess (Lipschitz, 1976).

COMPLICATIONS OF THE INJURY

The spine-related complications of penetrating injuries are the obvious ones of neurological deficit, infection, and leakage of cerebrospinal fluid. Less obvious and much less frequent complications are those of lead poisoning in gunshot, migration of the penetrating foreign bodies, arteriovenous fistulae and discitis. The injury may frequently be associated with major extraspinal complications.

Occasionally, complications may develop years after the injury. Wu (1986) described a case where a bullet lodged in the vertebral body of L3 produced a cauda equina deficit 28 years after injury, as a result of proliferation of bony callus in the spinal canal adjacent to the bullet. An intradural shell fragment in the cervical spine caused a cervical myelopathy 29 years after injury, possibly the result of extradural fibrous tissue (Amitani *et al.*, 1976). Jones & Woosley (1981) blamed rust and fibrous tissue for the development of myelopathy eight years after a stab injury to the thoracic spine with retention of the knife-tip in the spinal canal. A bullet in the vertebral body of L4 produced a radiculopathy of the L4 root indirectly by forcing disc material from the L4–L5 space into the root canal (Mariottini *et al.*, 1984).

Any projectile penetrating to the spine can be expected to cause spinal or paraspinal infection, but it is interesting to note how unusual is this complication whether in stabbing or in gunshot injuries (Lipschitz, 1967; Yashon *et al.*, 1970; Heiden *et al.*, 1975; Stauffer *et al.*, 1979; Craig, 1986). The reason is probably to be found in the routine early administration of antibiotics. Infection emerges more as a complication of spinal surgery than of the penetrating injury. An important distinction is made between gunshot injuries which perforate colon before spine, and those which perforate stomach and small bowel: colon perforations carry a high risk of spinal infection by *Escherichia coli* and a variety of other organisms (Romanick *et al.*, 1985; Roffi *et al.*, 1989). Transpharyngeal injuries are associated with the late complication of streptococcal cervical spine osteomyelitis (Schaefer *et al.*, 1981; Craig, 1986). In 252 stab wounds of the spinal cord there were two cases of Brodie's abscess of vertebral bodies, two cases of chronic epidural granuloma, and four cases of meningitis (Lipschitz, 1967). Lipschitz also reports nine cases of chronic leakage of cerebrospinal fluid ascribed to inadequate dural suture at initial treatment. Both of the patients who suffered transabdominal penetration of lumbar discs by wood splinters developed infective discitis with a mixture of organisms (S. Govender, personal communication, 1989).

Lead poisoning from retained bullet or shrapnel fragments elsewhere in the body has been reported in a small number of cases (Linden *et al.*, 1982), but only once from a bullet retained in the spine (in a lumbar disc), the patient presenting with typical plumbism 12 years after injury (Grogan & Bucholz, 1981).

Migration of the penetrating material within the spinal canal is rare. Movement of bullets within the spinal canal is reported as possible only below T10 because the canal is too narrow higher up (Ledgerwood, 1977), but a pellet in the cervical spine canal of a 10-year-old boy migrated to sacral levels within three months of injury (Tanguy *et al.*, 1982). A glass fragment from a shattered table-top came to rest in a lumbar interlaminar space without causing any neurological deficit. It is alleged that the fragment migrated under the influence of the patient's ambulation during the following day and severed a lumbar nerve root (Wu, 1986).

Arteriovenous fistulae of the vertebral artery have been described in two patients suffering high cervical gunshot injuries (Leape & Palacios, 1971; Sherk *et al.*, 1974).

Extraspinal complications

Penetration to the spine from a posterior direction is likely to produce a neurological deficit prior to doing damage to any other anatomy. Penetration from anteriorly or laterally is likely to produce any number of associated injuries before the spine is reached. Virtually every nameable structure in the body has been injured at one time or another in association with penetrating injuries to the spine. In 252 stab injuries of the spinal cord there were 86 associated extraspinal injuries (Lipschitz, 1967). This remains the best published account of injuries associated with stabbing. There were 12 patients admitted unconscious because of separate head injury administered as part of an assault. In such cases it may be very difficult to decide whether the neurological deficit is related to the spinal injury or to that of the head.

Major vessels in the neck and thorax have been injured, as well as the heart. The intercostals and internal mammary arteries are also potent sources of haemorrhage. The brachial plexus, trachea and oesophagus, diaphragm, lung, thoracic duct and all organs in the abdomen have been injured, resulting variously in peritonitis, surgical emphysema, diaphragmatic hernia, haemopneumothorax and chylothorax, amongst others. An unusual case where the trachea and the oesophagus were transfixed to the cervical spine by an embedded knife was described by Das (1976).

Widespread associated injury in high-velocity gunshot is associated with major tissue damage and high mortality. In low-velocity gunshot injury, visceral damage is less extensive but the consequences may be severe, particularly with regard to infection (Romanick *et al.*, 1985; Roffi *et al.*, 1989).

MANAGEMENT

Life-threatening injury to major extraspinal structures within the skull, neck or the thoracic and abdominal cavities requires urgent resuscitation, assessment and appropriate management as a priority.

Once the patient has been stabilized, attention can then be turned to the spinal injury. As in all types of spinal injury, the first priority is to perform a thorough neurological assessment which is in turn followed by repeated assessments to identify any deterioration.

Radiographic assessment is required to locate retained fragments and to assess any damage to the structural integrity of the spinal column. Plain radiography of the spine, in the area of suspected injury, is the most obvious early investigation to arrange from the point of view of usefulness and availability. Views in two planes will give an idea of the location and spread of retained metal fragments, whether bullet, shrapnel, or knife-point. Plain radiography however, gives only limited information about bony injury (unless it is gross), or paraspinal soft tissue injury; and computerized tomography is necessary for complete assessment. The high-definition axial views of the spine can accurately locate all retained metal and glass fragments, whether in bone or in spinal canal or in paraspinal soft tissues. Alteration of the window settings will reveal the wound track, and haemorrhage, oedema or abscess.

Sagittal reconstructions can show the precise relationships between fragments and spinal segmental levels (Patricolo *et al.*, 1981; Plumley *et al.*, 1983; Kaiser & Capesius, 1985). Zigler *et al.* (1986) found that computer-assisted digital analysis of plain radiographs in two planes was more useful even than computerized tomography in localizing each of a profusion of pellets in the spine.

Computerized tomography unfortunately also has areas of difficulty. It provides little information about the degree of damage to the spinal cord and cauda equina and the artifacts produced by metal also may hamper interpretation.

Magnetic resonance imaging (MRI) is ideally suited to the demonstration of soft tissue injury, including injury to the spinal cord, but there is some concern as to the consequences of applying intense magnetic fields to intraspinal metallic fragments. These may be ferromagnetic, producing major artifact, and they may be converted to projectiles once again (New *et al.*, 1983; Bore, 1985). Some recent experience suggests that this concern may be unnecessary (Tracy *et al.*, 1989) but much experimental work remains to be done.

Water-soluble myelography must still have its uses when computerized tomography and MRI are simply not available. It is at least possible then to determine which fragments of metal or bone are producing neural compression, when planning surgery to relieve compression.

Treatment and prognosis

The prognosis for the patient's life depends on the severity of the associated injuries, the energy with which they are treated, and the severity of complications of the spinal cord injury. The prognosis for recovery of spinal cord function is poor when the initial presentation is that of a total loss of function below the level of injury. This situation is no different from that applying to spinal cord injury by any other means, and applies in the present context to both gunshot and stabbing. In his classic paper, Taylor (1941) said 'When ... we remember how narrow a bottle neck is the cord in the pathways from the relatively enormous brain to the vast periphery, we have the explanation of two salient facts: first that injuries of the cord most commonly cause permanent paralysis, second that a small volume of trauma has disastrously extensive consequences.'

However, there is hope for some recovery, of unpredictable degree, in partial or incomplete injuries of the cord but here a distinction must be drawn between gunshot and stabbing. In the partial cord injuries of gunshot, little or no recovery occurs (Taylor, 1941; Morgan *et al.*, 1971; Heiden *et al.*, 1975; Waters, 1984; S. Govender, personal communication, 1989), but in the incomplete or Brown–Séquard deficit of stabbings, considerable recovery can be expected (Rosenberg, 1957).

There is little disagreement that deteriorating neurological function in the early postinjury period constitutes a surgical emergency, possibly the result of intraspinal bleeding. Even so, the results of surgical clearance and toilet, in these circumstances, are disappointing. The treatment of the spine penetration itself is a matter of great controversy, where philosophical differences rather than statistical evidence separate clinicians into enthusiastic surgical activists (Rand & Patterson, 1929; Meirowsky, 1963; McFadden, 1972; Myers, 1973; Lipschitz, 1976) ranged against equally enthusiastic conservatives (Yashon *et al.*, 1970; Heiden *et al.*, 1975; Stauffer *et al.*, 1979; Waters, 1984; Romanick *et al.*, 1985).

Close examination of the evidence reveals that those who suggest complete and wide debridement of the whole wound and removal of metal fragments in every case, were published less recently than those who propose a superficial debridement plus antibiotics. The more radical approach was also more usually related to war injuries rather than to civilian injuries.

The hope for radical surgery (usually including laminectomy) is that it will relieve pressure on neural tissue, prevent infection by removal of the contamination, and allow a direct visual assessment of the physical damage done. This philosophy has withstood the test of time and countless wars, but the modern conservatives have the statistical evidence in their favour, at least as regards civilian injuries, and with exceptions in special circumstances. There is a 10% risk of complication from surgery, resulting in the very problems surgery was intended to prevent: infection, spinal fistulae, and spinal instability (Stauffer *et al.*, 1979). The degree of neurological recovery in those with incomplete cord injuries was greater where surgery was not performed.

However, there are certain situations where a more radical approach is necessary. Transpharyngeal and transoesophageal penetrations, whether by stab or gunshot, carry such a high risk of vertebral osteomyelitis from continuing contamination that it is indeed advisable to perform a good debridement and mucosal repair (Schaefer *et al.*, 1981; Craig, 1986; Pattisapu & Al-Mefty, 1987). Roon & Christenson (1979) suggested exploration of all cervical penetrating injuries in order to minimize morbidity and mortality, because the degree of injury was frequently underestimated. Major disruption of a lumbar disc, with residual lead or wood fragments, appears to produce a 'discitis' with chronic pain and disability until anterior discectomy and strut grafting are carried out (S. Govender, personal communication, 1989).

The reported high rate of spinal infection when the colon is perforated is considered an indication for debridement (Romanick *et al.*, 1985), but even this apparently reasonable indication has been contested, provided adequate antibiotic treatment is given (Roffi *et al.*, 1989). Reports that intraspinal fragments of bullet and glass may result in delayed myelopathy have been used as justification for early removal of intraspinal fragments (Amitani *et al.*, 1976; Jones & Woosley, 1981; Wu, 1986). The fact remains that such cases of delayed myelopathy are extremely rare, and the case for early surgical removal on that basis has not been conclusively established.

In summary, therefore, it seems that treatment for the spinal component of a low-velocity penetrating spinal injury, by any means, need consist only of early debridement of the superficial wound and a full course of broad-spectrum antibiotic, with careful follow-up for the recognition of late complications. However, high-velocity injuries and injuries with anterior cervical or colonic penetration require wide exploration, debridement, and repair where possible. Persistent cerebrospinal fluid leakage requires repair, and it is possible that retained fragments within a lumbar disc may possibly require discectomy and fusion.

REFERENCES

Amitani, K., Tsuyuguchi, Y. & Ilukuda, S. (1976) Delayed cervical myelopathy caused by bombshell fragment. *J. Neurosurg.*, **44**, 626–627.

Baghai, P. & Sheptak, P.E. (1982) Penetrating spinal injury by a glass fragment: case report and review. *Neurosurgery*, **11**, 419–422.

Bore, P.J. (1985) Safety of NMR. *Lancet* (letter), **1**, 1107–1108.

Craig, J.B. (1986) Cervical spine osteomyelitis with delayed onset tetraparesis after penetrating wounds of the neck. *S. Afr. Med. J.*, **69**, 197–199.

Das, P.B. (1976) Simultaneous penetrating injury of the trachea and esophagus by a knife jammed into the vertebral body. *Int. Surg.*, **61**, 160–161.

Dunn, V., Smoker, W.R.K. & Menezes, A.H. (1987) Transdural herniation of the cervical spinal cord as a complication of a broken fracture-fixation wire. *AJNR*, **8**, 724–726.

Grogan, D.P. & Bucholz, R.W. (1981) Acute lead intoxication from a bullet in an intervertebral disc space. *J. Bone Jt. Surg.*, **63A**, 1180–1182.

Harmit, S., Singhal, V. & Bansal, V.P. (1985) Intraspinal, extradural stab injury of the spine without neurological deficit: a case report. *Int. Orthop.*, **9**, 277–278.

Heiden, J.S., Weiss, M.H., Rosenberg, A.W., Kurze, T. & Apuzzo, M.J.L. (1975) Penetrating gunshot wounds of the cervical spine in civilians. *J. Neurosurg.*, **42**, 575–579.

Horowitz, M.D., Dove, D.B., Eismont, F.J. & Green, B.A. (1989) Impalement injuries. *J. Trauma*, **25**, 914–916.

Jones, F.D. & Woosley, R.E. (1981) Delayed myelopathy secondary to retained intraspinal metallic fragment. *J. Neurosurg.*, **55**, 979–982.

Kaiser, M.C. & Capesius, P. (1985) Gunshot wounds to the spine as evaluated by CT-scanning. Two illustrative case reports. *Comput. Radiol.*, **9**, 121–124.

Key, A.G. & Retief, P.J.M. (1970) Spinal cord injuries. *Paraplegia*, 243–249.

Leape, L.L. & Palacios, E. (1971) Acute traumatic vertbral arteriovenous fistula. *Ann. Surg.*, **174**, 908–910.

Ledgerwood, A.M. (1977) The wandering bullet. *Surg. Clin. N. Am.*, **57**, 97–109.

Linden, A., Manton, W.I., Stewart, R.M. & Thal, E.R. (1982) Lead poisoning from retained bullets. Pathogenesis, diagnosis, and management. *Ann. Surg.*, **195**, 305–313.

Lipschitz, R. (1967) Associated injuries and complications of stab wounds of the spinal cord. *Paraplegia*, 75–82.

Lipschitz, R. (1976) Stab wounds of the spinal cord. In Vinken, P.J. & Bruyn, W. *Injuries of the Spine and Spinal Cord*, Part 1, pp. 197–207. North-Holland, Amsterdam.

Lipschitz, R. & Block, J. (1962) Stab wounds of the spinal cord. *Lancet*, **1**, 169–172.

Mariottini, A., Delfini, R., Ciapetta, P. & Paolella, G. (1984) Lumbar disc hernia secondary to gunshot injury. *Neurosurgery*, **15**, 73–75.

McFadden, J.T. (1972) Tissue reactions to standard neurosurgical metallic implants. *J. Neurosurg.*, **36**, 598–603.

Meirowsky, A.M. (1963) Penetrating wounds of the spinal canal. *Clin. Orthop.*, **27**, 90–107.

Morgan, T.H., Wharton, G. & Stuart, F. (1971) Spinal cord injuries secondary to gunshot wounds. *Proc. Veterans Admin. Spinal Cord Inj. Conf.*, **18**, 220–223.

Myers, P. (1973) Open injuries of the spine and spinal cord: missile wounds and shell fragments. *Proc. Veterans Admin. Spinal Cord Inj. Conf.*, **19**, 157–160.

New, P.F.J., Rosen, B.R., Brady, T.J., Buonanno, F.S., Kistler, J.P., Burt, C.T., Hinshaw, W.S., Newhouse, J.H., Pohost, G.M. & Taveras, J.M. (1983) Potential hazards and artifacts of ferromagnetic and nonferromagnetic surgical and dental materials and devices in nuclear magnetic resonance imaging. *Radiology*, **147**, 139–148.

Patricolo, A., Delitala, A., Esposito, S. & Biasibetti, G. (1981) Computerized tomography in diagnosis of bullet cervical injuries. *J. Neurosurg. Sci.*, **25**, 131–134.

Pattisapu, J.V. & Al-Mefty, O. (1987) Gunshot wound to the odontoid process. A case report. *Spine*, **12**, 1052–1054.

Plumley, T.F., Kilcoyne, R.F. & Mack, L.A. (1983) Computed tomography in evaluation of gunshot wounds of the spine. *J. Comput. Assist. Tomogr.*, **7**, 310–312.

Rand, C.W. & Patterson, G.H. (1929) Stab wounds of the spinal cord. *Surg. Gynecol. Obstet.*, **48**, 652–661.

Roffi, R.P., Waters, R.L. & Adkins, R.H. (1989) Gunshot wounds to the spine associated with a perforated viscus. *Spine*, **14**, 808–811.

Romanick, P.C., Smith, T.K., Kopaniky, D.R. & Oldfield, D. (1985) Infection about the spine associated with low-velocity-missile injury to the abdomen. *J. Bone Jt. Surg.*, **67A**, 1195–1201.

Roon, A.J. & Christensen, N. (1979) Evaluation and treatment of penetrating cervical injuries. *J. Trauma*, **19**, 391–397.

Rosenberg, A.W. (1957) Stab wounds of the spinal cord. Report of three cases. *Bull. Los Angeles Neurol. Soc.*, **22**, 79–84.

Schaefer, S.D., Bucholz, R.W., Jones, R.E. & Carder, H.M. (1981) The management of transpharyngeal gunshot wounds to the cervical spine. *Surg. Gynecol. Obstet.*, **152**, 27–29.

Schaefer, S.D., Bucholz, R.W., Jones, R.E., Anderson, R.G. & Carder, H.M. (1981) Treatment of transpharyngeal missile wounds to the cervical spine. *Laryngoscope*, **91**, 146–148.

Sherk, H.H., Giri, N. & Nicholson, J.T. (1974) Gunshot wound with fracture of the atlas and arteriovenous fistula of the vertebral artery. Case report. *J. Bone Jt. Surg.*, **56A**, 1738–1740.

Stauffer, E.S., Wood, R.W. & Kelly, E.G. (1979) Gunshot wounds of the spine: the effects of laminectomy. *J. Bone Jt. Surg.*, **61A**, 389–392.

Tanguy, A., Chabannes, J., Deubelle, A., Vanneuville, G. & Dalens, B. (1982) Intraspinal migration of a bullet with subsequent meningitis. *J. Bone Jt. Surg.*, **64A**, 1244–1245.

Taylor, J. (1941) Discussion on war injuries of the spine. *Proc. R. Soc. Med.*, **34**, 447–454.

Tracy, P.T., Wright, R.M. & Hanigan, W.C. (1989) Magnetic

resonance imaging of spinal injury. *Spine*, **14**, 292–301.
Waters, R.L. (1984) Gunshot wounds to the spine: the effects of bullet fragments in the spinal canal. *J. Am. Paraplegia Soc.*, **7**, 30–33.
Wu, W.Q. (1986) Delayed effects from retained foreign bodies in the spine and spinal cord. *Surg. Neurol.*, **25**, 214–218.
Yashon, D. (1973) Missile injuries of the spinal cord. *Proc. Veterans Admin. Spinal Cord Inj. Conf.*, **19**, 160.
Yashon, D., Jane, J.A. & White, R.J. (1970) Prognosis and management of spinal cord and cauda equina bullet injuries in sixty-five civilians. *J. Neurosurg.*, **32**, 163–170.
Zigler, J., Bahniuk, E., Van Dyke, C. & Bohlman, H. (1986) Localization of foreign bodies in the spinal canal by computer-assisted biplanar digitizer. *Spine*, **11**, 892–894.

65 · Injuries to the Upper Cervical Spine

By T. McSWEENEY

Injuries to the upper cervical spine differ in many respects from vertebral injuries at a lower level. More often than not the injuring force is applied directly through the base of the skull, in contrast to injuries at other levels where indirect forces are transmitted through the lever arm of several segments above or below the major site of injury. With the exception of certain fractures of the odontoid process, the bony injuries tend to stabilize quickly and surgical intervention is seldom required. Primary ligamentous and capsular injuries often require early or late surgical stabilization.

The consequences of upper cervical injuries vary immensely. While many of the injuries are associated with serious intracranial or brain stem lesions, and are immediately fatal, other patients usually survive and present a variety of uncommon neurological symptoms. These include coma vigil, sleep apnoea (Ondine's curse) and the 'locked-in syndrome' in which there is loss of all motor and sensory modalities up to the level of the oculomotor nerves.

Assuming that the patient quickly recovers from the effects of any head injury then the overall prognosis is good. There is usually a low incidence of serious permanent neurological impairment in survivors. Absent intercostal function and a flaccid paralysis with loss of the deep tendon reflexes are more in keeping with a cord injury irrespective of the patient's state of consciousness. There is no set pattern of motor or sensory loss and the picture may change quickly. There may be no neurological deficit; this may be partly explained by the configuration of the spinal canal, the cushioning effect of the extradural soft tissues and the ratio of cord to canal at this level (Fig. 65.1). Some patients may have few physical signs or symptoms, so that many injuries in this region remain unrecognized until the onset of pain, neck stiffness or gradual neurological impairment some time later. In the more serious cases, usually the result of traffic accidents, impairment in cord conduction, intracranial lesions and associated limb or visceral injuries compound the problem. These patients present a considerable challenge requiring expert resuscitation and a multidisciplinary approach under the direction and guidance of a surgeon familiar with all aspects of trauma care. It has been emphasized that in many patients the neurological impairment gradually lessens, but the time interval varies. Accompanying paralysis or sensory loss should not be regarded as an isolated phenomenon; the dysfunction of the autonomic nervous system with its effects on existing respiratory, cardiovascular and metabolic problems must be recognized and treated appropriately. For these reasons the principles applicable to the overall management of spinal cord-injured patients apply (McSweeney, 1983).

In addition to injuries in an otherwise normal spine, the effects of relatively minor trauma to a pathological upper cervical spine form a fascinating and important study. Rheumatoid disease and other inflammatory arthropathies are commonly associated with ligamentous laxity, especially of the atlanto-axial joint. The ligamentous softening favours subluxations, either spontaneous or precipitated by a relatively minor injury. Pharyngeal infections and infiltrating neoplasia are less common causes with a similar effect.

There are a number of bony anomalies in the occipitocervical region which may be brought to light following radiography for injury or because of a slowly developing myelopathy. These include developmental abnormalities and those associated with

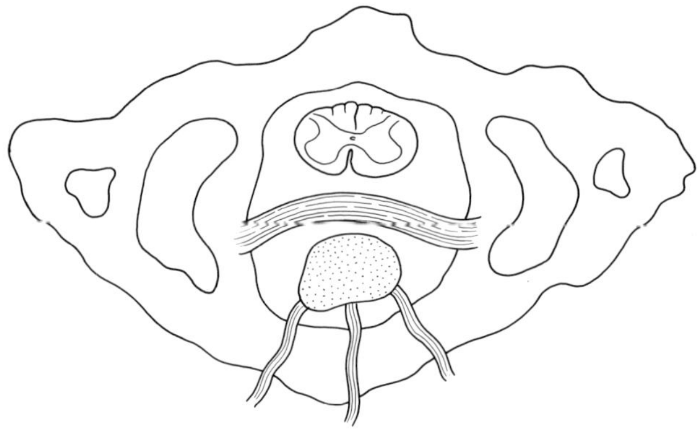

Fig. 65.1 The spinal cord occupies one-third of the space in the spinal canal at the level of the atlas and axis. This area represents a safety zone (Steel, 1986) in which displacement may occur without neurological compression.

generalized skeletal diseases, notably the mucopolysaccharide disorders and Down's syndrome. The importance of recognizing these anomalies is that acute neurological impairment may follow on comparatively trivial injury (see Chapter 15).

Initial management and assessment

The early care of the severely injured, for example the victims of road traffic accidents, has improved dramatically following the experience gained by accident and military surgeons, together with the advances in anaesthesia and emergency medicine developed in specialized trauma centres. Not all patients with injuries of the upper cervical spine fall into this category. The potential hazards of domestic and athletic injuries, however, are such that specialized care is essential. The radiological facilities of smaller hospitals seldom meet the requirements; a round-the-clock consultant service is rarely provided so that transfer to a designated centre is in the patient's best interest. It is not the purpose of this chapter to detail the various advances in primary care, but certain points pertinent to the management of patients suspected of having sustained an injury in the upper cervical spine are stressed.

Transportation

The correct care begins at the site of the accident, and gentle head traction is sustained during all manoeuvres until more efficient temporary splintage can be applied. Many splinting devices are available and ambulance crews usually have a local preference. In default of a manufactured splint, good protection can be achieved by resting the head on a padded backboard. Movements are minimized by securing the head with adhesive tape or velcro fasteners, with sandbags on each side. Neurological deterioration during transportation and after admission to hospital has long been recognized (Geisler *et al.*, 1965), but the precise role of injudicious movement in such cases is often open to question. Pringle reviews this and other aspects of spinal cord pathology in Chapter 60. Neurological deterioration after injury may be caused by a number of factors of which poor oxygenation is a crucial element. Baker (1989) has shown that in the early days after spinal cord injury, the vertical position ('sitting up') has resulted in severe hypotension and increasing neurological impairment. From personal experience the author can confirm his findings and has often been surprised at the dramatic improvement once the patient has been placed in the recumbent position. While these observations have important medicolegal implications the responsibility for meticulous care in transportation and adequate oxygenation cannot be overemphasized.

Respiratory and circulatory problems

Ambulance crews are usually aware of the possibility of a neck injury in accident victims, and should be prepared to modify the principle of immobilizing the neck in a fixed position if an obstructed airway or vomiting is present. Most ambulances are now fitted with suction apparatus and a face mask with oxygen supply. Insertion of an airway is vital. After admission to hospital an experienced anaesthetist must be available with the full range of fibreoptic instrumentation and armoured nasoendotracheal tubes. Tracheostomy is not advised as endotracheal intubation and nasogastric suction will tide the patient over the early critical period. Bronchial and nasopharyngeal suction are performed with caution; ill-understood alterations in reflex activity may cause sudden respiratory or cardiac arrest (Frankel & Matthias, 1975). Prophylactic atropine and humidification are helpful.

It should be remembered that any neurological impairment will involve the autonomic nervous system so that hypotension and bradycardia (vagal inhibition) are common presenting features. Other injuries with blood loss will lower the blood pressure causing an increase in pulse rate; cord perfusion is diminished. Fluid replacement is essential but is approached with caution as overloading of the labile circulation is easily produced. The administration of corticosteroid preparations has been popular but the beneficial effects are disputed. A multicentre double-blind randomized clinical trial (Bracken *et al.*, 1985) showed no significant neurological recovery in patients examined a year later. A second trial (Bracken *et al.*, 1990) using higher doses of corticosteroids, has now been reported. Methylprednisolone in an initial dose of 30 mg/kg was administered intravenously over a 15-min period followed by a 45-min pause. A maintenance infusion was continued using 5.4 mg/kg per hour for 23 h. An improvement in motor function, sensation to touch and pinprick at six months was recorded. Meanwhile, Geisler *et al.* (1991) report on an enhancement in the recovery of neurological function using monosialotetrahexosylganglioside (GM-1). The increased recovery in the GM-1 group was attributed to an effect on initially paralysed muscles.

Resuscitation, assessment and diagnosis are a continuous process in which the patient's apprehension and the relatives' anxiety should not be forgotten. Light skull traction is required in almost every case. Gardner–Wells tongs are generally satisfactory and do not require predrilling; scalp wounds may preclude their use, in which instance Crutchfield calipers may be used as a temporary measure. Halter traction is condemned as it quickly produces pressure sores on the chin or occiput. Short periods of carefully monitored halter traction are permissible in the management of certain neck injuries to be mentioned later.

The incidence of cervical injuries is governed by social, industrial and environmental factors in which road traffic accidents and recreational activities play a major part. Alcohol and drug abuse are compounding factors. There is an obligation on the medical profession to consult with the information services so that the public are made aware of these risks.

The more important injuries of the upper cervical spine are now considered, realizing that every case is an individual patient and that an eclectic approach is paramount.

Injuries of the occipito-atlantal area

Injuries of this region vary in severity but are usually accompanied by a profound intracranial lesion with respiratory embarrassment and unconsciousness. The injuring force is transmitted through the occipital condyles to the complex occipito-atlanto-axial joint. Gunshot and stab wounds in the area may also result in ligamentous disruptions. The craniovertebral joints are best considered as a single unit. Nodding movements and some lateral flexion occur at the occipito-atlantal joints but rotation is prevented by the configuration of the articular surfaces.

Condylar fractures

These often occur in association with fractures at the base of the skull extending towards the foramen magnum, and as such are rarely recognized. These fractures are stable because the alar ligaments and tectorial membrane are usually intact. The proximity of the hypoglossal nerve to the fracture site should be noted.

Axial loading may produce comminution of the occipital condyles and associated damage to the lateral masses of the atlas, as in the Jefferson injury. Forcible rotation and lateral flexion, as may follow a blow to the side of the head, can result in avulsion of a small bony condylar fragment attached to an alar ligament. The presence of a bony fragment in the foramen magnum should arouse suspicion of an avulsion injury and of potential instability because of a defunctioned alar ligament. It will be appreciated that patients surviving these injuries are usually unconscious on admission to hospital and that neurological assessment may not be feasible for many hours. Conventional radiography may be equally unhelpful. Nuclear magnetic imaging or computerized tomography (CT) with coronal reconstruction will quickly establish the diagnosis.

Occipito-atlantal dislocation

This is a rare and usually fatal injury; the precise incidence is unknown but Bucholz & Burkhead (1979) reported nine occipito-atlantal dislocations in the post-mortem examination of 112 victims of multiple trauma. The high incidence of facial injuries and lacerations of the posterior pharyngeal wall suggested a hyperextension (deflexion) mechanism but Alker *et al.* (1975), in a post-mortem radiological study, thought that it was a hyperflexion injury. In a fatal case observed by the author there was a large haematoma over the occiput suggesting a flexion or

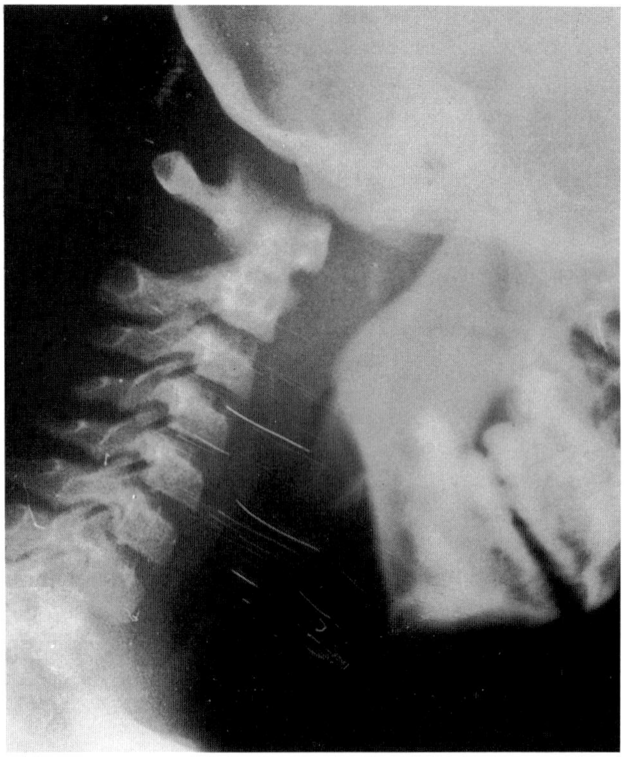

Fig. 65.2 Occipito-atlantal dislocation. The victim of a motorway accident, died shortly after admission to hospital.

translational injury (Fig. 65.2). It seems likely that in bilateral dislocations all the ligaments are disrupted as was shown in the Bucholz & Burkhead study. When halter traction was applied the disruption was immediately apparent on lateral radiographs of the cadaver. We have seen a child in whom only one occipito-atlantal joint was dislocated; at operation the corresponding joint was intact and apparently stable.

Gabrielson & Maxwell (1966) reported the case of a 41-year-old man who survived the injury. Conservative measures were adopted for a year after the accident, followed by operative fusion of the occiput to the upper cervical spine. They were unable to trace any other well-documented case, but Evarts (1970) described a personal case of an 11-year-old boy admitted following a car accident, with a hemiparesis and cranial nerve palsies. Radiographs had shown an occipito-atlantal dislocation. Occipitocervical fusion in a halo apparatus was performed a month later with almost complete recovery. Evarts referred to the case of a six-year-old child described by Farthing (1948), in the *North Carolina Medical Journal*. The child had been struck by a car and had sustained an anterior dislocation. Great irregularities of pulse and respiration were noted on admission, but these quickly disappeared on extending the head. Neurological examination was normal; the child was treated conservatively and made a full recovery. More recently Ramsay *et al.* (1986) reported a patient who survived the injury, and mentioned that review of previously reported cases included 22 survivors.

Most patients are unconscious on admission and in respiratory arrest or grave respiratory impairment. Prompt resuscitation and ventilatory support are lifesaving. Cranial nerve palsies may become apparent. The patient in respiratory arrest and complete tetraplegia with no bony injury on a 'spot' lateral radiograph of the cervical spine is always suspect. Good-quality lateral radiographs may show widening of the prevertebral shadow due to the retropharyngeal haematoma. This should always arouse suspicion of a cervical injury and, in the context of an occipito-atlantal injury, to the need for CT scan or magnetic resonance investigations of the upper cervical spine.

It has to be said that diagnosis may be extremely difficult and easily overlooked in the patient who quickly recovers consciousness, and who presents with minimal neurological signs. One of our patients involved in a frontal collision was struck on the back of his head by an unrestrained toolbox which had been placed on the rear seat of his car; he complained merely of occipital discomfort and transient diplopia. Later investigation showed an anterior occipito-atlantal dislocation which was easily reduced on minimal traction and extension. He died of a massive pulmonary embolus 10 days after an attempted occipitocervical fusion.

Treatment

Once control of respiratory problems has been achieved it may be possible to reduce the dislocation by gentle manual traction, failing which skull calipers are applied. Traction should not exceed 2 kg with careful radiographic monitoring of the space between the occiput and the atlas. Token traction is continued for a few weeks followed by immobilization in a halo vest. Dynamic radiographs at four months help to establish the need for surgical stabilization.

The timing of surgery is important. It seems likely that most adults will require occipitocervical fusion and that there is an advantage in postponing this until respiratory and cardiovascular functions have returned to normal. The long-term neurological recovery is good.

Fractures of the atlas

Fractures of the atlas are generally expected to follow a benign course. This is true provided that there are no associated injuries, and that the troublesome and often persistent dysaesthesia of the scalp following injury to the great occipital nerve is recognized. The mechanism of injury and the clinical features have generated a considerable literature following the introduction of radiography and the increase in road traffic accidents. Jefferson (1920), whose name is rightly associated with these injuries, described two clinical cases and two pathological specimens with a review of 46 previously reported examples. In later papers he described the historical background and treatment of these injuries (Jefferson, 1940, 1960). More recently Sherk & Nicholson (1970) have discussed the management of atlantal fractures noting that the most frequently encountered injury involves the posterior arch.

The injuring force is transmitted through the occipital condyles and converted into a more or less horizontal force so that the lateral masses are separated, leading to one or more fractures of the atlantal ring. Primary fractures of the skull are uncommon but a period of unconsciousness following the injury is the rule. Vertical compression is the major injuring force but the high incidence of associated injuries (almost 50%) suggests that more complex forces are often involved. Most of these fractures result from high-energy injuries to the skull, as in falls from a height and from car accidents. Traditionally, blows to the head by a semicompressible object, or falls on to sand have been described.

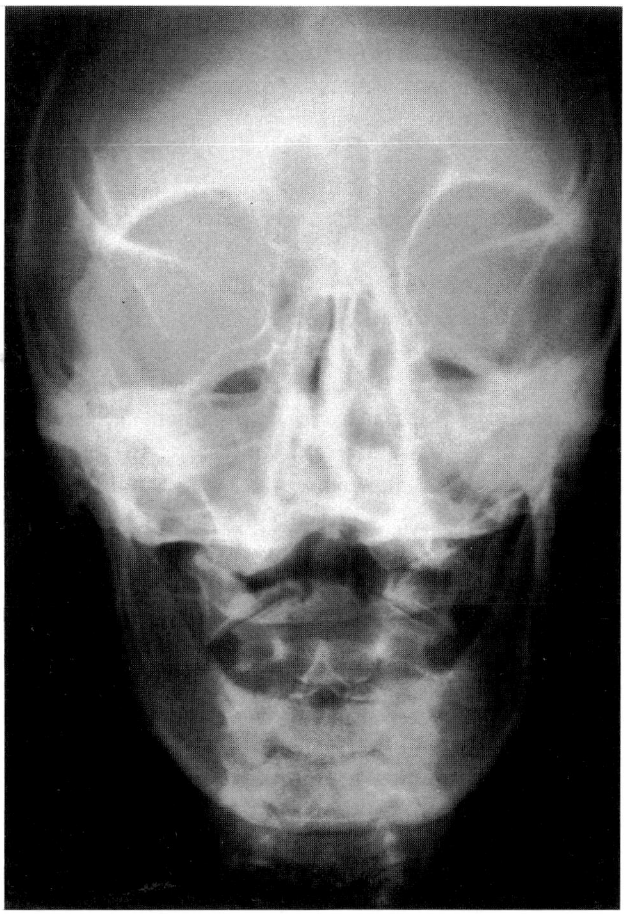

Fig. 65.3 Four-part Jefferson fracture. No associated injuries. Treated conservatively with satisfactory outcome.

Patterns of injury

The fracture may be confined to a single arch, or fractures may occur in both anterior and posterior arches as in the classical four-part fracture (Fig. 65.3). Fractures of one or both lateral masses are less common.

Concomitant injuries include fracture of the odontoid process, fractures of the pedicles of the axis, injuries at lower levels in the cervical spine, and widely displaced bursting injuries which may be associated with rupture of the transverse ligament. Confusion may arise with congenital anomalies (Fig. 65.4).

Symptoms

Pain in the upper part of the neck with selective restriction of rotation and anaesthesia or dysaesthesia of the scalp over the occipital region are the presenting symptoms. Difficulty in swallowing may occur. Damage to the spinal cord is unusual because the fragments are centrifugally displaced. Long tract signs should suggest an associated injury.

Diagnosis and treatment

Lateral and transoral radiographs will display most of these injuries and, in suspicious cases, two-plane

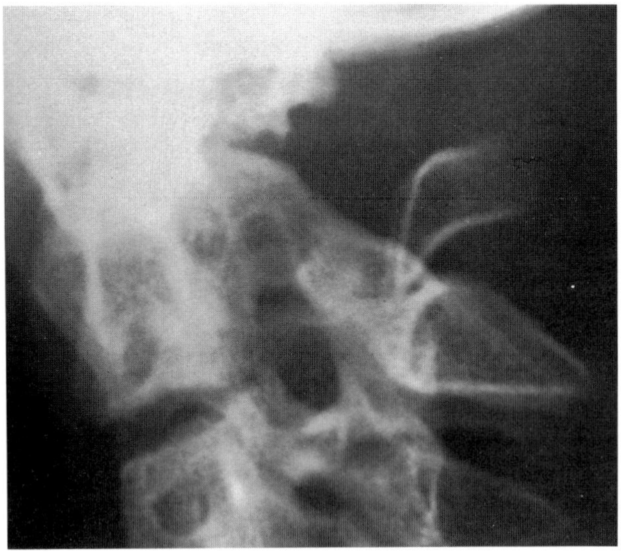

Fig. 65.4 Common congenital anomaly, sometimes mistaken for fracture.

tomography or a CT scan will clarify the diagnosis and reveal any associated injuries.

Isolated fractures of the posterior arch are stable injuries which result from compression–hyperextension forces. Some may follow direct compression between the spinous process of the axis and the occiput, but Jefferson was not disposed to accept this as the usual mechanism. Such injuries may be adequately treated by immobilization in a collar.

Most of the other bursting-type injuries require more careful assessment and stricter immobilization. Our practice is to apply light skull traction for eight weeks during which time a precise radiological diagnosis is reached: a programme appropriate to the patient and the injury can then be made. The action of the regional muscles tends to exaggerate the lateral displacement of the fragments and the amount of traction should be balanced accordingly. Progress is monitored radiologically and many patients can be successfully managed in a well-fitting collar after the initial period of recumbency. Some surgeons favour immobilization in a halo vest or Minerva jacket for the final period of six to eight weeks. Both devices have inherent disadvantages. The art of applying a satisfactory Minerva jacket is not easily learned. The immobilizing effect is quickly lost when too much mandibular movement is permitted. The halo vest may offer more effective immobilization and despite a number of potential dangers it has become increasingly popular.

Most of these fractures unite following conservative management but the presence of related injuries often demands later surgical intervention. For example, a displaced fracture near the waist of the odontoid process may fail to unite and thus require posterior atlanto-axial fusion. It would be unwise to attempt this until the arch fracture is united.

Rupture of the transverse ligament is rarely encountered except in extreme examples of the bursting injury. Spence *et al.* (1970) described a case in which the initial spreading of the lateral masses measured 10 mm. Persistent forward subluxation at the atlanto-axial joint at six weeks was reduced by gravitational hyperextension, and was followed by a successful atlanto-axial fusion. Ten post-mortem specimens were examined to establish the safe margin of displacement, beyond which the transverse ligament would fail. Each specimen was examined in an Instron device, having cut the anterior and posterior arches to duplicate a bursting fracture. Steel pin markers were placed in each lateral mass. Tension was then applied to the specimen to remove all slack from the transverse ligament. The transverse diameter of the atlas was again measured and compared with the intact measurement. The difference between the measurements represents the permitted excursion with a simulated bursting fracture before major stress is applied to the ligament. The stress necessary to rupture the ligament was then applied, and ranged from 38 to 104 kg. The total separation of the lateral masses from resting width to ligament rupture ranged from 4.8 to 7.6 mm. Analysis of the data suggested that the ligament is intact when the spread of the lateral masses is less than 5.7 mm, and that a spread greater than 6.9 mm indicates rupture of the transverse ligament.

Rupture of the transverse ligament

Rupture of this immensely strong ligament without fracture of the dens allows forward luxation of the atlas and endangers the spinal cord. Watson-Jones (1955) pointed out that the injury is less dangerous when accompanied by a fracture of the odontoid process which is carried forwards with the atlas. Primary rupture may follow a heavy blow to the occipital region, or when other forces of considerable magnitude are applied to the head. This is in contrast to secondary rupture associated with inflammatory processes where minimal trauma may result in atlanto-axial subluxation.

Bruising of the scalp and marked muscle spasm are the presenting physical signs; neurological features tend to improve when the neck is extended thus reducing the forward subluxation. For this reason lateral radiographs made with the neck in neutral or slightly extended will fail to demonstrate the lesion. As previously mentioned, unexplained widening of the prevertebral shadow or the presence of a small bony avulsion fragment in transoral views should alert the clinician to the need for further radiographic investigation under careful supervision. The normal joint space between the dens and the posterior aspect of the anterior arch of the atlas does not exceed 3 mm in adults. Displacement of over 5 mm is generally accepted as an indication for stabilization.

Treatment

The luxation is reduced on skull traction which maintains the neck in slight extension during subsequent procedures. Early or late surgical stabilization is advised and in reported cases the results of posterior atlanto-axial fusion have been satisfactory.

Fractures of the odontoid process (dens)

Earlier accounts of the odontoid fractures make gloomy reading, presumably because the less severe cases were not recognized, and fatal cases were often complicated by life-threatening associated injuries

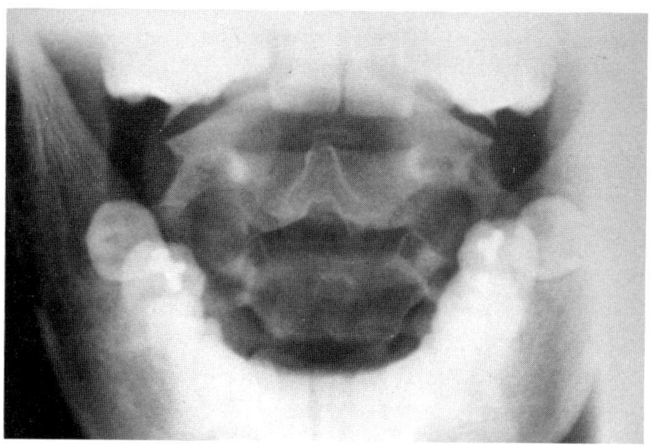

Fig. 65.5 Overlap of incisor teeth may mask fracture of dens.

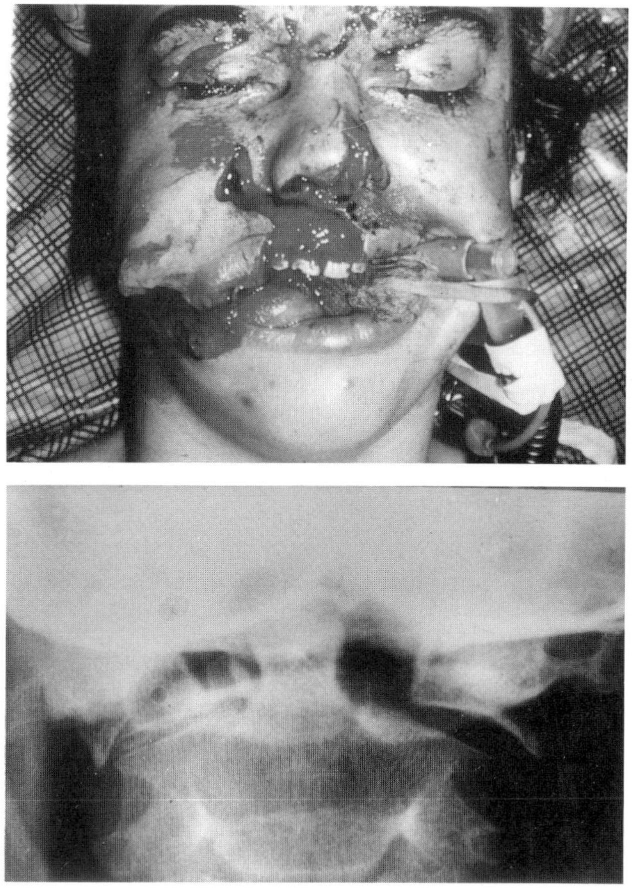

Fig. 65.6 Severe facial and associated injuries may delay diagnosis of vertebral injury.

in the upper cervical spine. Osgood & Lund (1928) reviewed the literature and found a 50% mortality in 55 cases reported to that date. Contemporary experience suggests a mortality of less than 8% and a significant reduction in the incidence of non-union. The real incidence of the injury has probably increased in parallel with traffic accidents; with improved technique its radiological recognition is now a relatively simple matter (Fig. 65.5). Nevertheless, diagnosis is often delayed because symptoms may be mild, or overshadowed by other injuries (Fig. 65.6).

Mechanism of injury

It is generally accepted that in adults high-velocity forces are involved and that fractures of the dens may follow flexion–extension or rotation of the head. It is probable that lesser forces are required to produce the injury in young children. The isolated odontoid injury is not normally associated with immediate neurological impairment. Wide displacement or angulation, and late recognition of the injury invites failure of union leading to atlanto-axial instability. Robert Debenham (quoted by Hutchinson, 1868) described the gradual onset of paralysis following a displaced fracture of the odontoid process. Delayed myelopathy associated with atlanto-axial instability is described under that heading.

A significant advance in the understanding and classification of these injuries was made by Anderson & D'Alonzo (1974). They described an avulsion fracture at the tip of the dens (Type I) which is regarded as a benign injury but it is important to exclude an occipito-atlantal disassociation.

Type II fractures occur above the junction of the body of the axis and the base of the odontoid and therefore above the level of the atlanto-axial joints. Fractures at this level are prone to non-union. Schiff & Parke (1973), prompted by the high rate of non-union, made a detailed study of the regional blood supply. They noted its tenuous nature and the lack of vascular communication between the dens and the body of the axis. Later observers (Appuzo *et al.*, 1978) commented on the intimate vascular relationship with the supporting alar and cruciate ligaments.

In Type III the fracture line extends downwards into the cancellous body of the axis; failure of union is uncommon except in grossly displaced fractures.

Treatment

Our practice is to immobilize odontoid fractures on skull traction until a precise radiological diagnosis has been made. The initial traction should be just sufficient to counterbalance the weight of the head and should seldom exceed 2.5 kg. Overdistraction invites failure of union and is monitored on serial radiographs.

Apical fractures (Type I) are stable and sufficient immobilization is provided by a four-poster collar which is worn for three months. Basal fractures (Type III) usually unite promptly; the traction is removed after two weeks. For undisplaced fractures a well-fitting orthosis of the sternal occipitomandibular type (SOMI collar) is used for three months. Displaced fractures require frequent radiological control and are probably safer when immobilized in a Minerva jacket or in a halo vest. Bony stability is assessed by dynamic flexion–extension views at three months.

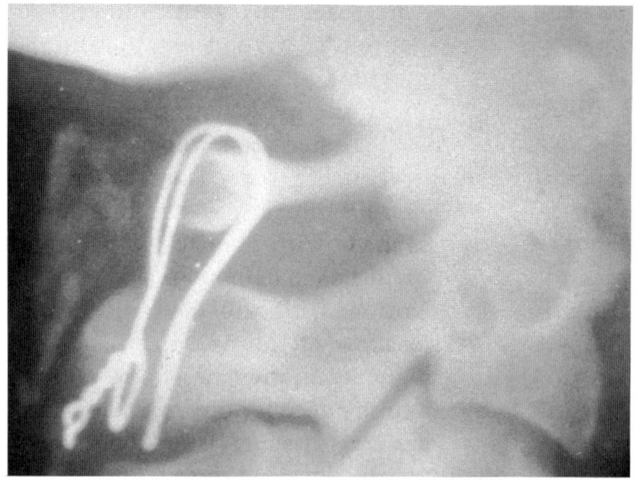

Fig. 65.7 Posterior atlanto-axial fusion for delayed union of Type II odontoid fracture.

Type II fractures are prone to non-union; the failure rate has been variously reported, so much so that many surgeons advise primary fusion. The author favours an initial period of carefully adjusted traction in recumbency for four weeks in undisplaced fractures and for two months when there is displacement or angulation. Immobilization in a Minerva jacket or halo vest is continued for a further month, during which time the patient may gradually increase activities. Dynamic radiographs are made at the end of the 12th week. At this time some fractures will have united. Others may show no signs of instability but bony trabeculation across the fracture site is incomplete. Here it is advised to continue immobilization even as long as six months from the time of injury. Manifest instability or pain is the indication for surgical fusion. Where surgery is required we have found a posterior atlanto-axial fusion entirely satisfactory (Fig. 65.7). Screw fixation (Fig. 65.8a) and anterior stabilization procedures have been described. These are not recommended for the occasional operator and in our opinion carry a significant morbidity (Fig. 65.8b).

This regimen has been criticized by those who favour early surgery for Type II fractures, and for displaced Type III injuries. Non-union rates of 30% or more for Type II injuries with a 13% failure of union in basal fractures have been reported in a multicentre survey (Clark & White, 1985) and must surely merit careful consideration. It should be recognized, however, that the fusion will restrict rotatory movements and may be associated with some morbidity.

The management of odontoid fractures remains controversial, but there is no dispute about the potential hazards of non-union and the accompanying atlanto-axial instability. The concept of a firm fibrous union, especially in older patients, is yet another area open to discussion. Pringle (1974) believed that a stable fibrous union was probably a safe situation, and reminds us that prolonged immobilization is not well tolerated by older patients. Ryan & Taylor (1982) have commented on the dangers of skull traction and advise fixation in a halo cast for male patients and in a Minerva jacket for women. They emphasize the need for adequate reduction and a cast which does not rest on the pelvic brim.

Atlanto-axial instability

The first reported case of spontaneous atlanto-axial instability is attributed to Sir Charles Bell (1830), and the earliest attempt at classification of cervical spine injuries was by Joseph Francois Malgaigne. Malgaigne (1855) believed that luxation of the atlas on the axis was possible, but he had not encountered a case, nor had he been able to produce a pure luxation in a cadaver. Pilcher (1910) described his unsuccessful attempt to reduce a subluxation by open operation. Many of the earlier reports of atlanto-axial instability with chronic compression of the upper cervical spinal cord were associated with un-united fractures of the odontoid process. The remarkable case of a man who had survived four episodes of cord compression over a period of 35 years was recorded in a detailed report by Elliot & Sachs (1912). The complexity of the resulting neurological picture was recognized in many studies including those of Kahn & Yglesias (1935), Bachs *et al.* (1955) and Wadia (1967). Vascular complications were reviewed by Schneider & McGillicuddy (1976) and by Dyck (1978).

The atlanto-axial joint permits rotation, some slight anteflexion and retroflexion, but little or no lateral flexion. Stability depends on age (less in the child), on whether the regional muscles are 'on guard' or relaxed at the time of injury, but primarily on the strength of the joint capsules and ligamentous structures. The reader is referred to Chapter 3 of this book, and to the studies of Werne (1957) and White & Panjabi (1978) for more detailed information.

Anterior subluxation is more frequently encountered than the other varieties. Posterior displacements may occur in association with fractures and anomalies of the dens, while lateral and severe rotatory luxations are late developments of the primary anterior type.

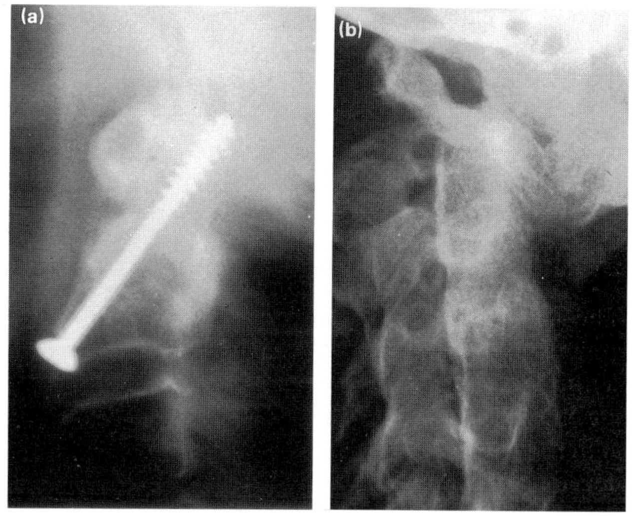

Fig. 65.8 (a) Screw fixation for odontoid fractures requires familiarity with the procedure. Failure of union may occur because of technical mistakes and osteoporosis.
(b) Unsuccessful anterior fusion presents a difficult problem.

Clinical features

Abnormal postures of the head with pain over the occipital region may be the only presenting features. A host of neurological symptoms and signs have been described, varying from easy fatigue to tetraparesis. Respiratory impairment, sleep apnoea, tinnitus and nystagmus have been attributed to brain stem involvement. Symptoms associated with vascular complications because of repetitive injury or intermittent obstruction of the vertebral vessels following abnormal mobility at the atlanto-axial joint have been noted. While it is difficult to show angiographic evidence, a temporary alteration in the level of consciousness, transient loss of vision and episodic hemiparesis point to a vascular basis. Schneider & Johnson (1971) and Schneider *et al.* (1972a,b) reported various cranial nerve palsies in atlanto-axial luxations. One of our patients presented with paralysis involving the sixth to the twelfth cranial nerves; there was a gradual recovery in all but the left abducent nerve (Grundy *et al.*, 1984). Perhaps the commonest clinical manifestation is a recovering tetraparesis but minor compression of the anterior surface of the lower medulla may result in paralysis or paresis of the upper limbs without weakness of the lower extremities (Bell, 1970). Confusion with multiple sclerosis or other demyelinating disease may arise when the compression is chronic or intermittent.

Diagnosis

The circumstances of the accident and the radiographs will lead to the correct diagnosis in the injured normal spine. Difficulties in diagnosis and interpretation often arise following lesser injuries in patients suffering from rheumatoid arthritis and in those with developmental abnormalities in the region of the foramen magnum. The latter include variants of the Klippel–Feil syndrome, occipitalization of the atlas and basilar impression. These anomalies are occasionally associated with atlanto-axial instability and often remain relatively symptomless until a minor injury precipitates dysaesthesiae of the hands or a major paralysis. Important contributions to this often perplexing problem were made by List (1941), Spillane *et al.* (1957) and Wadia (1967). The radiological features were described by McRae in his Caldwell Lecture (McRae, 1960).

Treatment

The decision to fuse the upper cervical spine is often extremely difficult; especially so when there are no neurological features and only minor symptoms. It is made in the light of the pre-existing pathology and its natural history, on the patient's age, on the severity of pain and on the degree of neurological impairment. There is no orthosis which effectively controls atlanto-axial instability, and in many cases operative stabilization is advised, having discussed the lack of a reasonable alternative with the patient and relatives.

Post-traumatic atlanto-axial instability in the otherwise normal adult spine is an indication for posterior atlanto-axial fusion. Screw fixation (Fig. 65.9) has been recommended, but it is not an easy procedure. The place for operative intervention in rheumatoid disease is discussed by Crockard & Ransford in Chapter 52. Many of the abnormalities of the craniovertebral junction require decompression of the foramen magnum, often combined with decompression of the upper cervical vertebrae. The resulting instability is treated by occipitocervical fusion. The subject is considered by Jeffreys in Chapter 15.

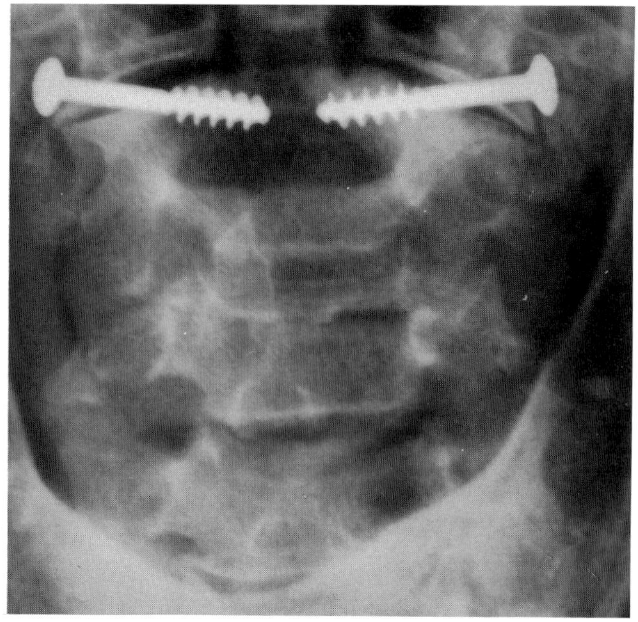

Fig. 65.9 Screw fixation as a method of atlanto-axial fusion has its advocates.

Atlanto-axial rotatory injuries

The distinction between congenital muscular torticollis (sternomastoid 'tumour') and other causes of wry neck has been recognized for many years. Malgaigne (1855) described traumatic and inflammatory causes, and Walton (1892, 1899) reviewed a number of cases of rotatory dislocations of the atlas and suggested a method of manipulative reduction.

The primary function of the atlanto-axial joint is to allow rotation; more than half of all the rotatory movement of the head and neck occurs at this articulation. The joint surfaces are almost plane, the joint capsules are lax and stability depends largely on the tone of the neck muscles. When the muscles are off guard luxations may occur—a feature well known to anaesthetists. Corner (1907) believed that the injury was often overlooked; he mentioned two personal cases and 18 others gathered from earlier reports. He made the point that when muscles are relaxed any force applied to the head has a 'flying start' before it meets resistance. Forces of greater magnitude result in rupture of the capsular ligaments of one or both atlanto-axial joints allowing an abnormal degree of rotation, and in the more severe injuries a varying degree of atlanto-axial instability. It will be appreciated that all gradations of rotatory displacement may be encountered between the mild rotatory subluxations of childhood and the incorrigibly fixed rotatory deformities described by Fielding & Hawkins (1977). Since Corner's description, many accounts of rotatory luxations have appeared; most of these were concerned with uncomplicated cases. Of special interest are those of Mixter & Osgood (1910), Jackson (1927), Greeley (1930) and Coutts (1934). Wortzman & Dewar (1968) undertook a detailed anatomical, radiological and clinical study. They noted that in the early phase many of their patients held the head looking to one side. They likened this to a bird with its head cocked listening for a worm. Fielding and his associates recognized that rupture of the transverse ligament might rarely complicate these injuries, leading to an associated atlanto-axial instability and a much more critical situation (Fielding & Hawkins, 1977; Fielding *et al.*, 1978). From their study of 17 patients they described four types of fixed rotation. In Type I the transverse ligament is intact so that anterior subluxation of the atlas does not occur. The dens acts as a pivot permitting rotation within the normal range of motion. Reduction is usually achieved on traction and sedation. Type II is associated with anterior atlanto-axial instability because of deficiency of the transverse ligament. Unilateral anterior displacement occurs while the opposite atlanto-axial joint remains intact and acts as a pivot. This is a dangerous injury requiring surgical stabilization. Type III is a rare injury characterized by deficiency of both the transverse and capsular ligaments. Both joints are displaced—one more than the other, producing a rotated position. Rotatory fixation with posterior displacement (Type IV) implies a deficient odontoid process and consequently is extremely rare.

Diagnosis

This is often delayed because the initial symptoms are not always remarkable and the appearance of the wry neck deformity may be delayed and is often overlooked. Delay in restoration of the normal anatomy leads to reactive fibrosis and increasing fixity. The evolution of the clinical features is variable and depends on the severity of the initial injury. In this respect one must contrast the often self-correcting deformity in young children with the almost irredeemable Stage II and III deformities described by Fielding and associates.

Most patients will recall an unguarded and forcibly twisting movement or a glancing blow to the head. The more severe injuries accompanied by atlanto-axial subluxation follow on road traffic accidents or other major trauma. With minimal luxations the patient may not complain of discomfort until spasm of the sternomastoid muscle on the side opposite to the direction of rotation becomes intrusive. Difficulty in swallowing, and inability to open the jaw fully, may be early signs before tilting of the head and deviation of the chin is noticed by the patient or relatives. Transoral palpation of the back of the throat may offer useful information but we have not found this a practical test.

Radiology

An open-mouth view is not always feasible in the acute phase but it may show deviation of the spinous process of the axis and that the forwardly rotated lateral mass of the atlas is closer to the dens (medial offset). Such appearances do not confirm fixation, but indicate rotation of the atlas and the need for further investigation. Wortzman & Dewar (1968) advised a transoral view with the neck in 10–15° rotation. They suggested that a persistent asymmetrical relationship of the dens to the articular mass of the atlas not correctable by rotation is the basic diagnostic sign. A lateral view is essential to exclude atlanto-axial instability. Cine-radiography is a more useful investigation: fixation is confirmed when the posterior arches of the atlas and axis are seen to move as a unit when the neck is rotated. Tomography and CT scanning (Fig. 65.10a,b) are very helpful and less distressing for the patient.

Treatment

Intermittent and carefully monitored halter traction is usually successful in reducing uncomplicated rotatory deformities seen within a few weeks of injury, and almost invariably so in children. Skull traction is advised for late cases. The rotatory deformity may respond to gentle manipulation under appropriate light sedation but recurrence is not

(a) (b)

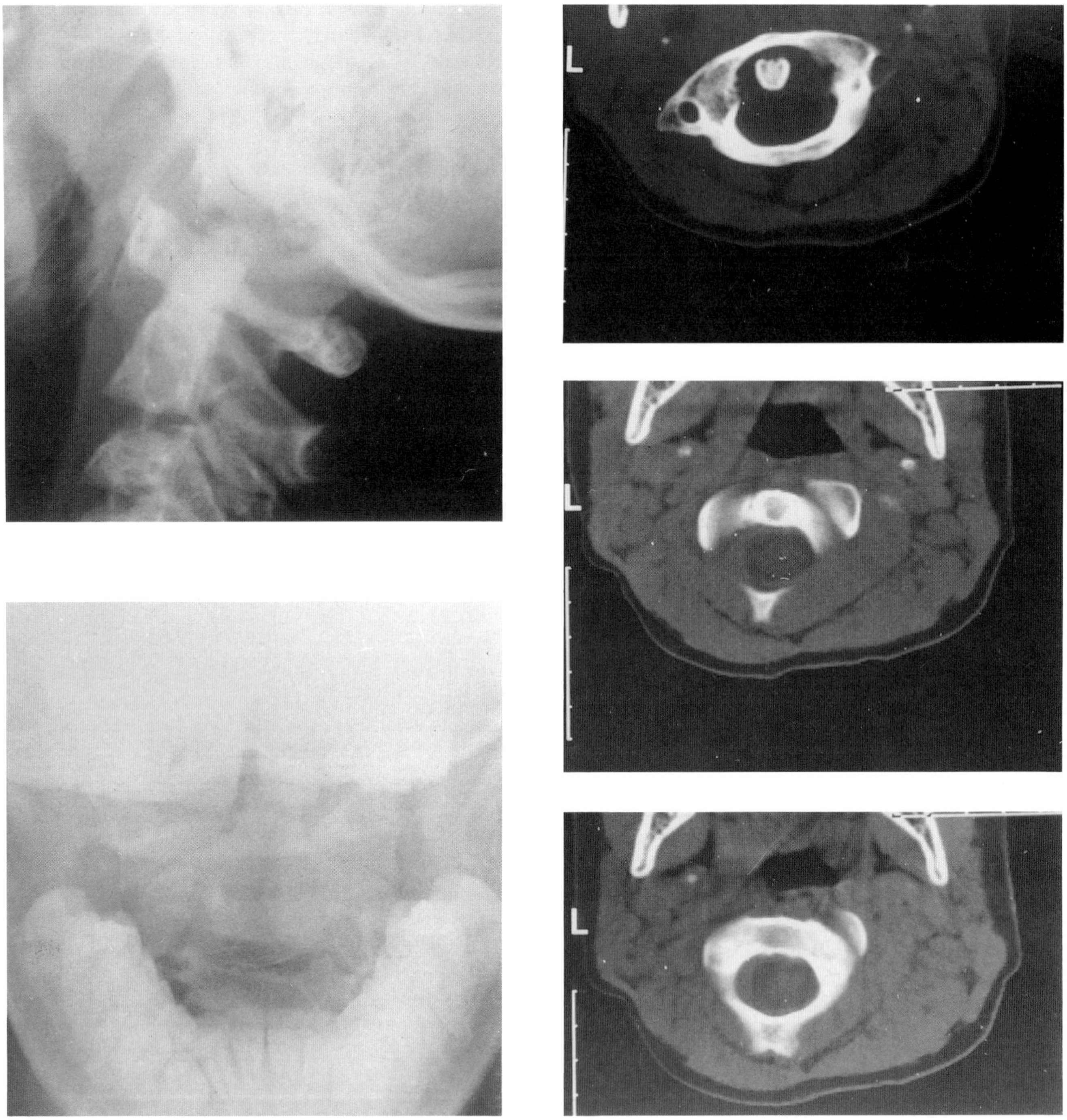

Fig. 65.10 (a) Rotatory atlanto-axial subluxation following glancing blow on the head. (b) CT scans showing rotation of the atlas on the axis with overlap on the facet on the right.

uncommon. Some surgeons have commented favourably on the use of oropharyngeal topical anaesthesia to facilitate direct manipulation of the displaced atlantal arch. Assuming a successful reduction, then immobilization in a Minerva cast or a halo vest should be continued for three months. We have not encountered fixed rotatory deformities with atlanto-axial instability or the severe cases described by Fielding and others. We endorse the recommendation that if conservative treatment fails, or is followed by recurrence, then posterior atlanto-axial fusion should be considered. A preliminary period of traction is always advised and may improve the cosmetic appearance. In the unreduced case the deformity tends to lessen with time, presumably by compensatory changes below the level of injury.

Traumatic spondylolisthesis of the axis—fractures through the pedicles

This injury, with its emotive eponym of hangman's fracture, is associated with an engrossing historical background quite apart from its clinical interest. Wood Jones (1908), discussing the findings in the bodies of men executed in Roman times, described a peculiar fracture pattern in the base of the skull. In comparing these specimens from the Nubian Survey collection and the skull of a poisoner executed by hanging in 1865, he felt justified in assuming that the knot had been placed far back upon the jaw (subaural), as it clearly seemed to have been in the Nubian cases. He speculated that in such circumstances as many died from suffocation as from the effects of the skull fracture, which he believed was caused by direct leverage on the temporal bone. Wood Jones (1913) later described the 'ideal lesion' produced by judicial hanging, basing his findings on five cases of medically supervised hangings from Rangoon jail. A submental or near-submental knot was used in these cases. The lesion is produced by the violent jerk which throws the head backwards and snaps the pedicles of the axis. Death is instantaneous because of the extreme distraction of the spinal cord, which is often severed. Grogono (1954) commented on the radiological similarity between the 'ideal lesion' and a bilateral pedicle fracture in a patient who suffered a transient tetraparesis following a car accident. Schneider and Livingston, with their anatomist colleagues Cave and Hamilton, after a detailed clinical and anatomical study accepted the close resemblance between the neural arch fractures sustained in certain road traffic accidents and the symmetrical pedicular fractures of the axis produced by a properly conducted judicial hanging (Schneider *et al.*, 1965). They described the distinctive bony injury and from their extensive historical review introduced the title 'hangman's fracture'. (Critics have since suggested that 'the hanged man's fracture' is more appropriate, but such pedantry seems unnecessary.)

The differing mechanisms of injury were discussed by Garber (1964), Cornish (1968) and Williams (1975). The commoner injury is associated with road traffic and diving accidents, and is caused by hyperextension and axial compression. Bruise marks or abrasions are found on the scalp or forehead. The fractures occur bilaterally through the narrowest part of the pedicles and may rarely extend across the posterior part of the body of the axis. Hyperextension causes rupture of the anterior longitudinal ligament, often with avulsion of a small triangular fragment from the anterosuperior margin of the third cervical vertebral body. More violent hyperextension separates the intervertebral disc from the adjacent vertebra with damage to the posterior longitudinal ligament. These severe forms are accompanied by forward displacement of the body of the axis and relative enlargement of the spinal canal.

The civilian counterpart to hangman's fracture is an uncommon injury where hyperextension is accompanied by distraction. This may occur when the moving body is abruptly restrained by contact with an object under the chin (as in the submental knot) or across the front of the neck. In one of our cases a motorcyclist was caught under the jaw by a rope which had been stretched across the road (Edgar *et al.*, 1972). There was a friction mark across the front of his neck: he had sustained a distraction fracture through the pedicles of the axis with a recovering tetraplegia.

Clinical features

Suboccipital pain and reluctance to turn the head because of muscle spasm are usually found. The fracture is often overlooked because attention is centred on the facial or other injuries. Neurological impairment is uncommon except in extension–distraction injuries.

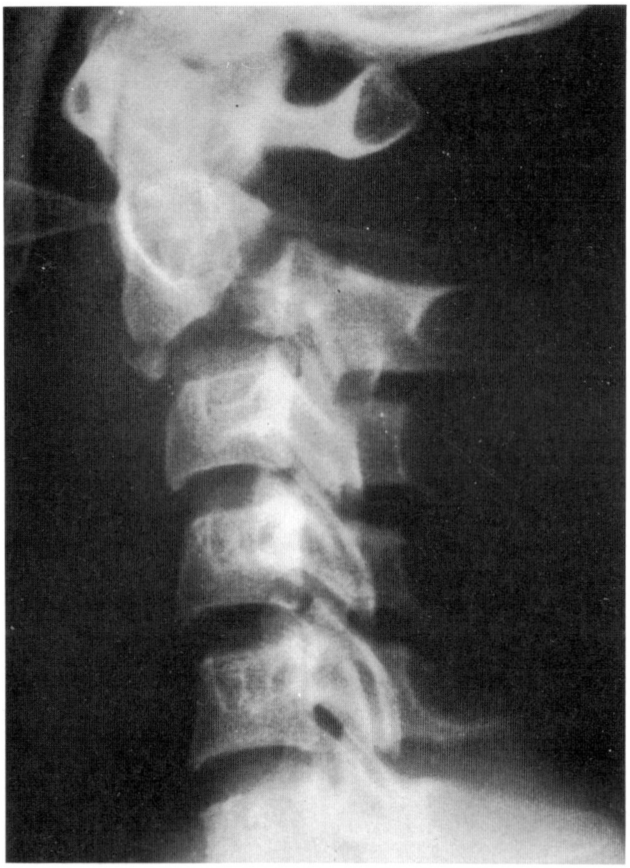

Fig. 65.11 Typical fracture through the pedicles of the axis. Further views to include the entire cervical spine are essential.

Radiological examination

Lateral radiographs centred on the upper cervical spine will normally display the bony lesion which is similar in appearance irrespective of the mechanism of injury (Fig. 65.11). It is important to obtain radiographs of the whole cervical spine as hyperextension–compression injuries are often accompanied by fractures at a lower level.

Treatment

Most of these fractures unite within three months with little or no residual disability. Undisplaced stable fractures may be treated in a SOMI collar or similar orthosis. More severe injuries with displacement and instability require a few weeks skull traction. Extra caution is required to prevent over-distraction, particularly when the injury follows extension–distraction forces, lest the patient be 'hanged by mistake'. Immobilization is continued in Minerva or halo jacket in which the patient may resume most normal activities.

Operative intervention may exceptionally be required for late instability or chronic pain of discogenic origin. Anterior interbody fusion is preferred in that it does not interfere with rotation.

(Readers interested in the historical aspects of this injury may refer to Haughton, S. (1866) On hanging, considered from a mechanical and physiological point of view. *Phil. Mag. J. Sci.*, 4th series; **32**, 23–34; Judicial hanging (an annotation) (1913) *Lancet*, **1**, 629; Marshall, J.J. (1913) Judicial hanging. *Lancet*, **1**, 639; and Judicial hanging (Any Questions) (1947) *Br. Med. J.*, **2**, 160.)

Paediatric injuries

The child's spine is more mobile than the adult spine so that injuring forces are more easily absorbed. Spinal injuries in children are mercifully rare, and in most instances involve the upper cervical spine. Underlying anomalies and the relatively large skull compared to the rest of the body proportions, are significant factors.

Birth injuries

These have been recognized for many years, and to a large extent reflect the standard of obstetric practice. Weak musculature and ligamentous laxity permits an injudicious longitudinal force to separate the vertebral bodies and elongate the spinal column. Following temporary elongation the spinal column returns to normal, but the overstretched spinal cord may have suffered varying degrees of permanent damage. Similarly, elongation or pathological angulation during delivery of a 'star-gazing' fetus (Russel & Aird, 1976) may cause neural damage or ischaemia in the vertebrobasilar circulation (Yates, 1959). The true incidence is unknown; most of the infants who sustain a serious spinal cord injury die shortly after birth or are stillborn.

Others may survive and present a variety of incomplete neurological syndromes. The differential diagnosis includes amyotonia congenita and infantile spinal muscular atrophy. The continuing presence of autonomic and sensory dysfunction in the older child may help to distinguish such cases from the rare familial myopathic disorders. Allen (1976), in a masterly review of the subject, concluded that misdiagnosis of birth injury to the spinal column is more common than is generally appreciated, and that most post-mortem examinations following neonatal deaths are incomplete.

Fractures

Bony injuries are decidedly uncommon and the few young patients whom the author has seen made a good recovery, including those associated initially with some neurological impairment. A custom-made plastic collar usually suffices until bony union is secured. Fracture of the dens in children less than seven years of age requires special mention. The antecedent injury is often a comparatively trivial one, and radiographs shortly after may fail to reveal the fracture. Other cases are associated with severe displacement and atlanto-axial instability (Fig. 65.12). We have seen seven such cases as a result of traffic accidents in which the children were securely harnessed in front-facing seats. Three of these children were tetraplegic at a lower cervical level on admission to hospital. In less severe injuries, intermittent neck pain and a mild torticollis should suggest the diagnosis. Seimon (1977) attached great significance to the crying and pain experienced when the child is sat up without active support of the head from behind.

Blockey & Purser (1956) described these injuries in young children as epiphyseal separations, and pointed out that imperfections of reduction are smoothed off in time. The epiphyseal nature of the injury has failed to find general acceptance. Ewald (1971) does not regard the radiotranslucent area

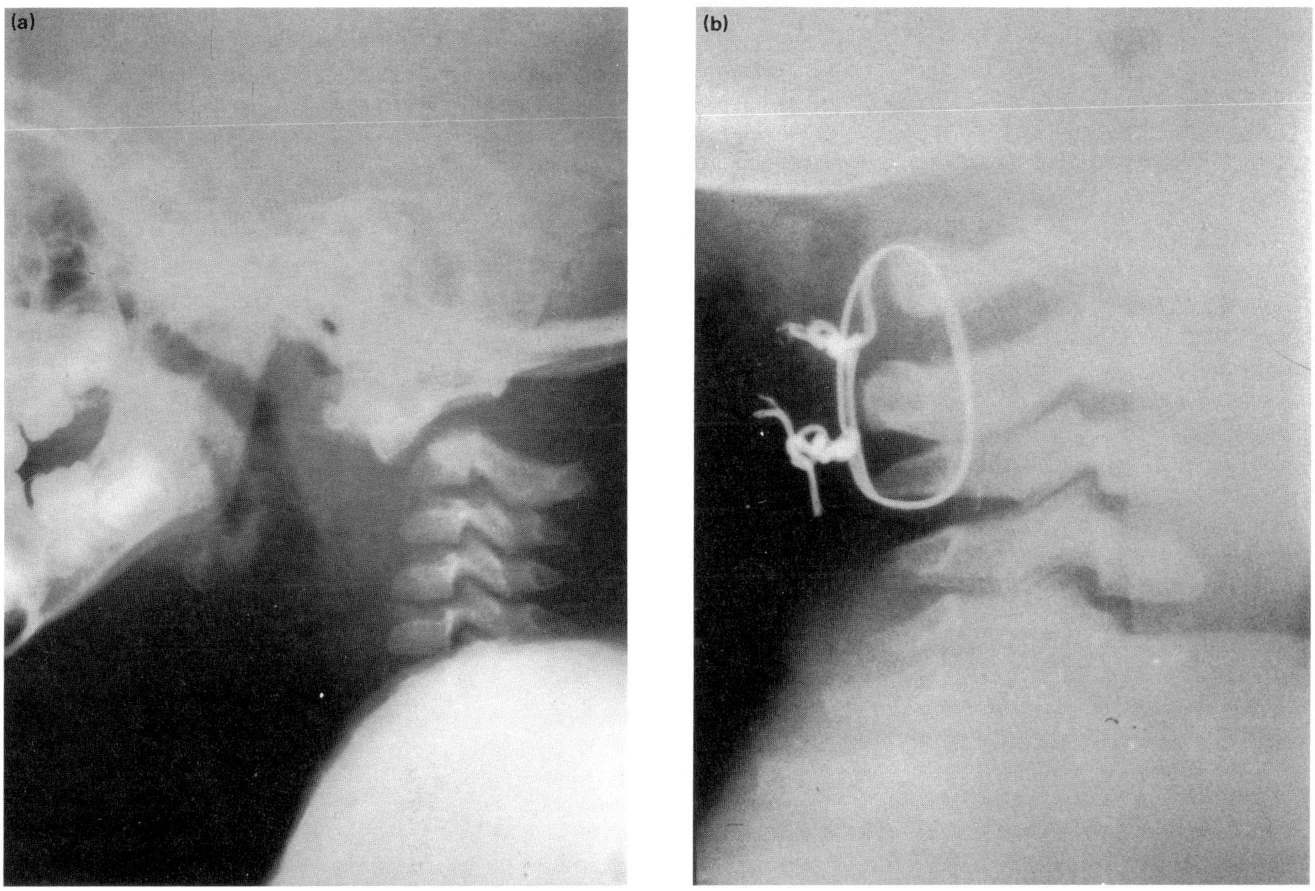

Fig. 65.12 Fracture of the dens with atlanto-axial dislocation. Child was rendered tetraplegic at a lower level. Considered as a valid indication for open reduction and fixation.

between the dens and the body of the axis as an epiphyseal plate. From his study of a two-month-old infant who died from gastroenteritis he believes that the junctional area is a cartilaginous plate between two advancing areas of endochondral ossification, and that it lacks the strength of a linear epiphyseal plate. The observation would appear to give some support for the traumatic theory for the genesis of os odontoideum. A short period of recumbency followed by immobilization in a collar is sufficient to secure bony union in most cases. When diagnosis is delayed, immobilization in a plexoloid Minerva jacket is advised. Open reduction and posterior fusion merits consideration when there is an atlanto-axial subluxation or other complicating factors such as a cord injury at a lower level.

Ligamentous injuries

Awareness of the variations in the normal radiological appearance of the cervical spine helps to prevent overtreatment. An apparent forward displacement of the second on the third cervical vertebra is frequently observed in children following injury. Bailey (1952) described this as a 'pseudo-subluxation' without sinister significance. Dunlap *et al.* (1958) surveyed the radiographs of uninjured children and reported similar appearances in many of their cases. Cattell & Filtzer (1965) gave an account of other normal bony and ligamentous variations. Two of these continue to confuse the unwary. Overriding of the arch of the atlas on the dens with the neck in extension occurred in 20% of the radiographs of normal children. Overriding was present when more than two-thirds of the visible anterior arch lay above the superior margin of the dens. Apparent widening of the space between the dens and the anterior arch of the atlas in flexion radiographs often exceeded the 3 mm accepted as the upper limit of normal in adults.

True traumatic subluxation does occur as a result of severe violence, notably in road traffic and athletic injuries. The subluxation may additionally involve the third and fourth cervical vertebrae with major disruption of the corresponding interspinous ligaments. It is characterized by continued neck pain and muscle spasm. Early radiographs show marked subluxation or borderline dislocation in flexion views. Subsequent radiographs often reveal calcification or commencing ossification in the damaged interspinous ligament and reduction is not secured on hyperextension of the neck. Continued pain and apprehension requires a localized posterior fusion (Fig. 65.13a,b).

Pseudo-subluxation may be discovered following a minor neck injury. An accurate history and evaluation of the injuring force is essential. If doubt persists, a few days of intermittent halter traction in recumbency will lead to disappearance of muscle spasm. Radiographs in hyperextension will then show a normal appearance, and further immobilization is not required. Repeat radiographs after three months should dispel any lingering doubts.

A further consideration in ligamentous injuries is the hyperaemic softening which accompanies infective lesions in the oropharynx. Grisel (1930) described this phenomenon, which Lippman (1953) likened to the ligament softening accompanying septic dislocation of the hip in childhood. Watson-Jones (1932) did not accept the importance of the traumatic factor, believing that most cases occurred spontaneously. The incidence has decreased since the introduction of antibiotic therapy, and rheumatoid disease is now the commonest cause of ligamentous softening. Tuberculosis and tumour formation may cause a similar hyperaemic effect.

Other conditions often accentuated by injury

Reference has been made to bony abnormalities at the base of the skull and to other anomalies in the upper cervical spine which may be recognized for the first time following injury. Two other conditions, namely Down's syndrome and os odontoideum, merit further attention.

Down's syndrome

The generalized ligamentous laxity in Down's syndrome and other genetically determined collagen disorders has been recognized for many years. The significance of symptomless atlanto-axial instability has been variously assessed and an incidence of 12–15% is generally accepted. Martel & Tishler (1966) found 14 cases of asymptomatic atlanto-axial dislocation in 70 children with Down's syndrome. More importantly, we do not know the true incidence of neurological impairment or the precise role of injury in the production of symptoms in such cases. Certain it is that many individuals complain of neck discomfort, transient weakness of a limb and in-

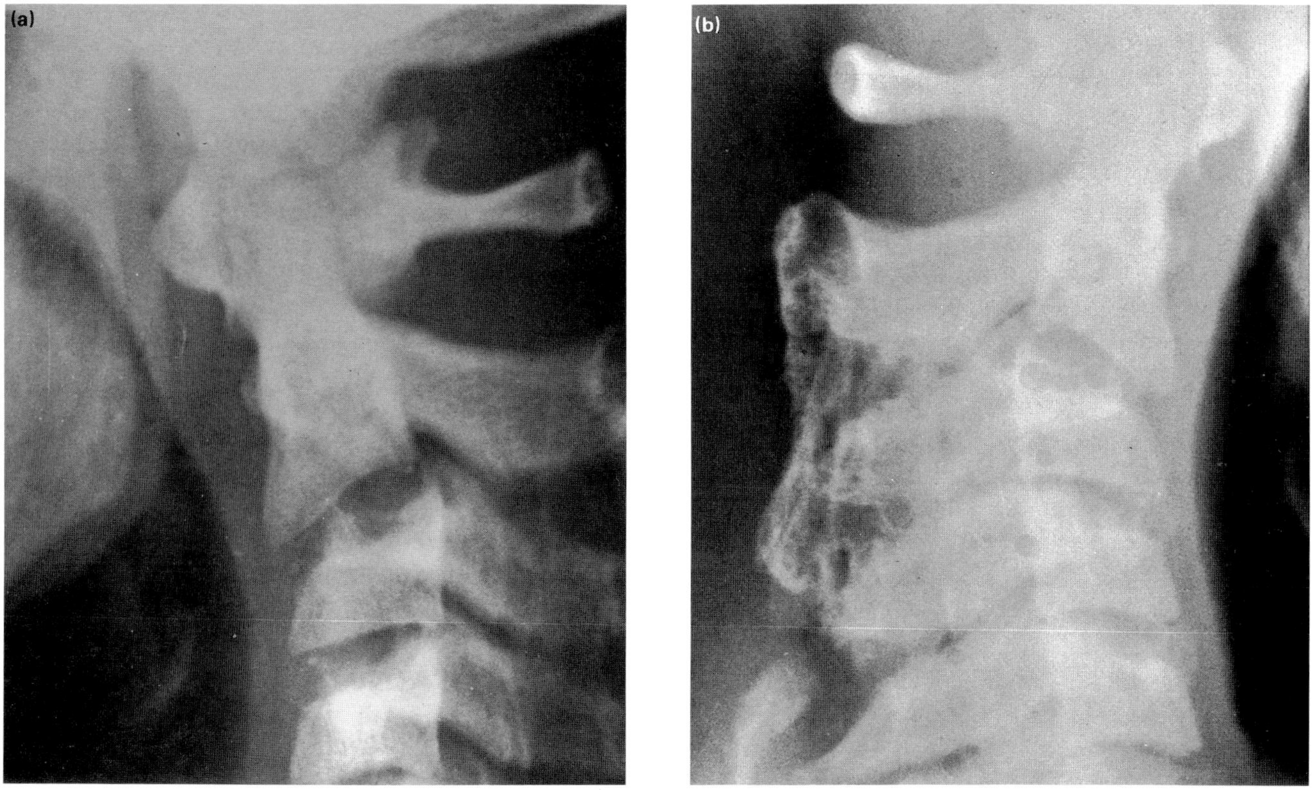

Fig. 65.13 (a) True traumatic subluxation of C2 on C3 in a boy aged 12 years. (b) At operation the interspinous ligament between C3 and C4 was also disrupted, hence the extended fusion.

termittent impairment of grip, and that an injury may be followed by major neurological disabilities. Pulschel & Scola (1987) observed that in some patients the ligamentous laxity decreased with age.

Advice from the Department of Health and Social Security in the United Kingdom (Acheson, 1986) is that while those patients with Down's syndrome are at risk from deceleration injuries in day-to-day activities, they should not be deprived unnecessarily of the reasonable activity they enjoy. Davidson's (1988) findings would appear to support this contention, and he stresses the point that prodromal clinical signs should alert the clinician. It would seem reasonable to warn parents of such individuals about the possible dangers of competitive sports, advising that they should report any unusual symptoms.

Prophylactic fusion in symptomless cases is not indicated. In those with minor and non-progressive neurological symptoms operative intervention is rarely justified, and in our opinion should be discouraged. Relief of symptoms in such cases is seldom an unqualified success, and the operative risks are considerable. In a minority of patients presenting progressive cord compromise, early stabilization must be carefully considered.

Os odontoideum

The os odontoideum is a rare bony abnormality which has given rise to much discussion as to its origin, its clinical significance and the indications for treatment. Minderhoud *et al.* (1969) reviewed the extensive literature then available, and proffered a classification based on their experience of 13 cases. They discussed the vexed question of causation, noting the not-infrequent association with other congenital skeletal anomalies. The authors also referred to a case report by Freiberger *et al.* (1965) in which a normally developed odontoid process, demonstrated radiologically at the age of two years, subsequently disappeared, producing a radiographic appearance similar to that of congenital absence of the odontoid. It is interesting to note that Fielding (1965) reported a similar case in the same volume of the *Journal of Bone and Joint Surgery*. Since then a number of well-authenticated cases who had a previously normal odontoid process documented radiologically, and who later presented as an os odontoideum, have been reported. The traumatic origin is supported by Fielding & Griffin (1974), Hawkins *et al.* (1976) and Fielding *et al.* (1980). Perhaps the two theories are not mutually exclusive (see Chapter 15).

The size of the ossicle varies, and at times the odontoid process appears to be hypoplastic. The anomaly is associated with differing degrees of instability of the atlanto-axial joint, but the crucial factor is the accompanying narrowing of the spinal canal between the posterior arch of the atlas and the posterior border of the body of the axis on forward flexion of the neck. Spierings & Braakman (1982), when evaluating 37 cases, undertook a detailed radiological study of 21 patients. They found that the sagittal diameter of the spinal canal between the posterior border of the axis and the posterior atlantal arch in flexion views was reduced in the five patients who developed permanent cord signs. The minimum diameter ranged between 7 mm and 13 mm, and they regarded 13 mm as the threshold measurement. This would appear to be in accord with the earlier studies of Greenberg (1968), who suggested that cord compression behind the odontoid occurred with a sagittal diameter of 14 mm or less.

The abnormality may present because of discomfort in the neck or across the shoulder girdles, and rarely because of overt neurological signs. We are concerned here with the features following injury. Two of our patients were involved in minor road traffic accidents and five in athletic injuries. There had been no premonitory symptoms, and in so far as

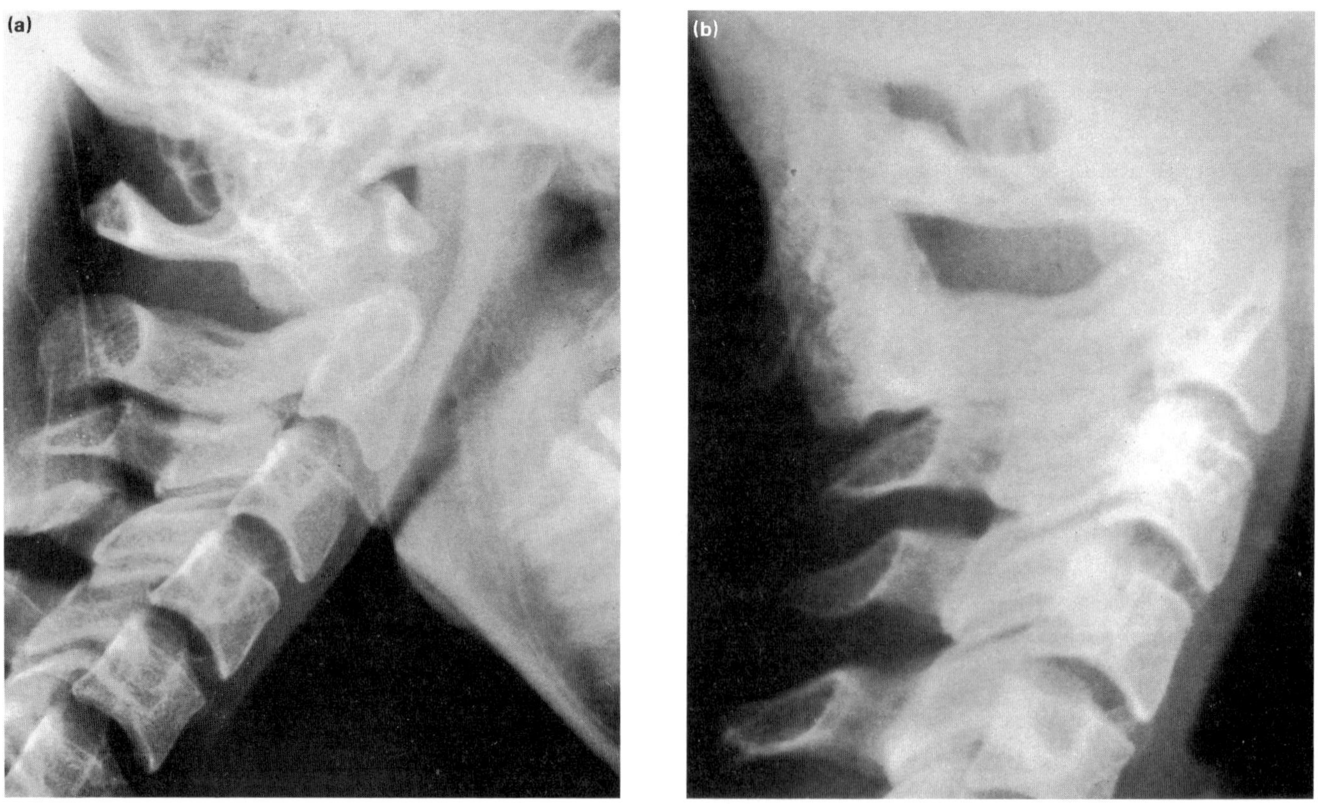

Fig. 65.14 (a) Os odontoideum, noted following a trampoline accident. Patient remained tetraplegic for two weeks but gradually improved on skull traction. Made a complete neurological recovery following upper cervical fusion. (b) Occipitocervical fusion. The arch of the atlas was so attenuated as to make atlanto-axial fusion inappropriate.

could be ascertained no history of neck injury in infancy. Three patients complained of severe neck pain and had a transient paresis of the upper limbs. These patients were treated conservatively and advised about their work and sporting activities. Their follow-up has been uneventful. Four patients were almost completely tetraplegic on admission; the paralysis lessened on skull traction. Two were treated by posterior atlanto-axial fusion. In the other two patients an occipitocervical fusion was performed because of a much-attenuated posterior atlantal arch (Fig. 65.14a,b). All made a complete neurological recovery.

Spierings & Braakman (1982) are opposed to operative intervention for local symptoms. They believe that the degree of instability of itself bears no relationship to the presence or development of cord signs. They attach paramount importance to the accurate measurement of the smallest diameter of the spinal canal at the critical level, using 13 mm or less as the decisive figure.

Conclusion

Most bony injuries in the upper part of the cervical spine, with the notable exception of fractures through the waist of the odontoid process, can be treated conservatively. Ligamentous injuries do not heal well if at all, and often require surgical stabilization. A preliminary period of carefully monitored skull traction will realign the spinal column and allow for precise diagnosis.

There may be no neural damage, or a cascade of confusing neurological features may develop. Diagnosis is often difficult and the temptation to use the label hysteria must be resisted.

Operative intervention is supported by skilled nursing and general medical care, with early emphasis on the rehabilitation of those who have suffered neurological impairment. The posterior approach with skull traction and intraoperative radiological monitoring is satisfactory in most instances. The anterior approach has special merits in complex odontoid problems but many surgeons may feel unfamiliar and uncomfortable in this area. Lateral approaches are well established.

Operations in the upper cervical spine are associated with a significant mortality and morbidity, and surgeons are well advised to use the methods with which they and their supporting staff are most familiar.

REFERENCES

Acheson, E.D. (1986) Atlanto-axial instability in people with Down's syndrome. Department of Health and Social Security (circular letter CMO (86): 9; London).

Alker, G.J., Young, O.S., Leslie, E.V., Lehotay, J., Panaro, V.A. & Eschner, E.G. (1975) Post mortem radiology of head and neck injuries in fatal traffic accidents. *Radiology*, **114**, 611–617.

Allen, P.J. (1976) Spinal cord injury at birth. In Vinken, P.J. & Bruyn, G.W. (eds), *Handbook of Clinical Neurology*, vol. 25, pp. 155–173. North-Holland/Elsevier, Amsterdam.

Anderson, L.D. & D'Alonzo, R.T. (1974) Fractures of the odontoid process of the axis. *J. Bone Jt. Surg.*, **56A**, 1663–1674.

Appuzo, M.L., Heiden, J.S., Weiss, M.H., Ackerson, T.T., Harvey, J.P. & Kurze, T. (1978) Acute fractures of the odontoid process. *J. Neurosurg.*, **48**, 85–91.

Bachs, A., Barraguer-Bordas, L., Barraguer, L., Candell, J.M. & Modollel, A. (1955) Delayed myelopathy following atlanto-axial dislocation by separated odontoid process. *Brain*, **78**, 537–553.

Bailey, D.K. (1952) The normal cervical spine in infants and children. *Radiology*, **59**, 712–719.

Baker, J.H.E. (1989) The first aid management of spinal cord injury. *Sem. Orthop.*, **4**, 2–14.

Bell, C. (1830) *The Nervous System of the Human Body*. Longman, Rees, Orme, Brown & Green, London.

Bell, H.S. (1970) Paralysis of both arms from injury of the upper portion of the pyramidal decussation. *J. Neurosurg.*, **33**, 376–380.

Blockey, N.J. & Purser, D.W. (1956) Fractures of the odontoid process of the axis. *J. Bone Jt. Surg.*, **38B**, 794–817.

Bracken, M.B., Shepard, M.J., Hellbrand, M.P.H., Collins, W.F., Leo, L.S., Freeman, D.F., Wagner, F.C., Flamm, E.S., Eisenberg, H.M., Goodman, J.H., Perot, P.L., Green, B.A., Grossman, R.G., Meagher, J.N., Young, W., Fisher, B., Clifton, G.L., Hunt, W.E. & Rilkinson, N. (1985) Methylprednisolone and neurological function one year after spinal cord surgery: results of the National Acute Spinal Cord Injury Study. *J. Neurosurg.*, **63**, 704–713.

Bracken, M.B., Shepard, M.J., Collins, W.F., Holford, T.R., Young, W., Baskin, D.S., Eisenberg, H.M., Flamm, E.S., Leo, L.S., Maroon, J., Marshall, L.F., Perot, P.L., Piepmeir, J., Sonntag, V.K.H., Wagner, F.C., Wilberger, J.E. & Winn, R.H. (1990) A randomized, controlled trial of methylprednisolone or naxolone in the treatment of acute spinal cord injury. Results of the Second National Acute Spinal Cord Injury Study. *N. Engl. J. Med.*, **322**, 1405–1411.

Bucholz, R.W. & Burkhead, W.Z. (1979) The pathological anatomy of fatal atlanto occipital dislocations. *J. Bone Jt. Surg.*, **61A**, 248–250.

Cattell, H.S. & Filtzer, D.L. (1965) Pseudo subluxation and

other normal variations in the cervical spine in children. *J. Bone Jt. Surg.*, **47A**, 1295–1309.
Clark, C.R. & White, A.A. (1985) Fractures of the dens: a multicentre study. *J. Bone Jt. Surg.*, **67A**, 1340–1348.
Corner, E.M. (1907) Rotatory dislocation of the atlas. *Ann. Surg.*, **45**, 9–26.
Cornish, B.L. (1968) Traumatic spondylolisthesis of the axis. *J. Bone Jt. Surg.*, **50B**, 31–43.
Coutts, M.B. (1935) Atlanto-epistropheal subluxation. *Arch. Surg.*, **29**, 297–311.
Davidson, R.G. (1988) Atlanto-axial instability in individuals with Down's syndrome: a fresh look at the evidence. *Paediatrics*, **81**, 857–865.
Dunlap, J.P., Morris, M. & Thompson, R.G. (1958) Cervical spine injuries in children. *J. Bone Jt. Surg.*, **40A**, 681–686.
Dyck, P. (1978) Os odontoideum in children: neurological manifestations and surgical management. *Neurosurgery*, **2**, 93–99.
Edgar, M.A., Fisher, T.R., McSweeney, T. & Park, W.M. (1972) Tetraplegia from hangman's fracture: report of a case with recovery. *Injury*, **3**, 199–202.
Elliot, G.R. & Sachs, E. (1912) Observations on fracture of the odontoid process of the axis with intermittent pressure paralysis. *Ann. Surg.*, **56**, 876–882.
Evarts, C.M. (1970) Traumatic occipito atlantal dislocation. Report of a case with survival. *J. Bone Jt. Surg.*, **52A**, 1653–1660.
Ewald, F.C. (1971) Fracture of the odontoid process in a seventeen month old infant treated with a halo. *J. Bone Jt. Surg.*, **53A**, 1636–1640.
Farthing, J.W. (1948) Atlanto cranial dislocation with survival. A case report. *N. Carolina Med. J.*, **9**, 34–36.
Fielding, J.W. (1965) Disappearance of the central portion of the odontoid process: A case report. *J. Bone Jt. Surg.*, **47A**, 1228–1230.
Fielding, J.W. & Griffin, P.P. (1974) Os odontoideum: an acquired lesion. *J. Bone Jt. Surg.*, **56A**, 187–190.
Fielding, J.W. & Hawkins, R.J. (1977) Atlanto-axial rotatory fixation. *J. Bone Jt. Surg.*, **59A**, 37–44.
Fielding, J.W., Hawkins, R.J., Hensinger, R.N. & Francis, W.R. (1978) Atlanto-axial rotatory deformities. *Orth. Clin. N. Am.*, **9**, 955–967.
Fielding, J.W., Hensinger, R.N. & Hawkins, R.J. (1980) Os odontoideum. *J. Bone Jt. Surg.*, **62A**, 376–383.
Frankel, H.L. & Matthias, C. (1975) Mechanisms of reflex cardiac arrest. *Lancet*, **2**, 1183–1185.
Freiberger, R.H., Wilson, P.D. & Nicholas, J.A. (1965) Acquired absence of the odontoid process: A case report. *J. Bone Jt. Surg.*, **47A**, 1231–1236.
Gabrielson, T.O. & Maxwell, J.A. (1966) Traumatic atlanto-occipital dislocation, with case report of a patient who survived. *Am. J. Roentgenol.*, **97**, 624–629.
Garber, J.N. (1964) Abnormalities of the atlas and axis vertebrae—congenital and traumatic. *J. Bone Jt. Surg.*, **46A**, 1782–1791.
Geisler, F.H., Dorsey, F.C. & Coleman, W.P. (1991) Recovery of motor function after spinal cord injury—A randomized, placebo-controlled trial with GM-1 ganglioside. *N. Engl. J. Med.*, **324**, 1829–1838.
Geisler, W.O., Wynne Jones, M. & Jousse, A.T. (1965) Early management of patients with trauma to the spinal cord. In de Vet, A.C., Kennedy, W.F.C. & Vinken, P.J. (eds), *Proceedings, Third International Congress of Neurological Surgery of the World Federation of Neurosurgical Societies 1965*, pp. 331–339. ICS 110, Excerpta Medica, Amsterdam.
Greeley, P.W. (1930) Bilateral (90 degree) rotatory dislocation of the atlas upon the axis. *J. Bone Jt. Surg.*, **12**, 958–962.
Greenberg, A.D. (1968) Atlanto-axial dislocation. *Brain*, **91**, 655–684.
Grisel, P. (1930) Enucleation de l'atlas et torticollis naso pharyngien. *Presse Med.*, **38**, 50–53.
Grogono, B.J.S. (1954) Injuries of the atlas and axis. *J. Bone Jt. Surg.*, **36B**, 397–410.
Grundy, D.J., McSweeney, T. & Jones, H.W.F. (1984) Cranial nerve palsies in cervical injuries. *Spine*, **94**, 339–343.
Hawkins, R.J., Fielding, J.W. & Thompson, W.J. (1976) Os odontoideum: congenital or acquired. *J. Bone Jt. Surg.*, **58A**, 413–414.
Hutchinson, J. (1868) Case of fracture of the odontoid process with peculiar symptoms: Notes of the case by Robert Debenham. *London Hospital Review*, pp. 210–212.
Jackson, R.H. (1927) Simple uncomplicated rotatory dislocation of the atlas. *Surg. Gynecol. Obstet.*, **45**, 156–164.
Jefferson, G. (1920) Fracture of the atlas vertebra. Report of four cases and a review of those previously recorded. *Br. J. Surg.*, **20**, 407–421.
Jefferson, G. (1940) Discussion on fractures and dislocations of the cervical spine. *Proc. R. Soc. Med.*, **33**, 657–660.
Jefferson, G. (1960) In *Selected Papers*, pp. 213–231. Pitman Medical, London.
Kahn, E.A. & Yglesias, L. (1935) Progressive atlanto-axial dislocation. *J. Am. Med. Assoc.*, **105**, 348–352.
Lippman, R.K. (1953) Arthropathy due to adjacent inflammation. *J. Bone Jt. Surg.*, **35A**, 967–979.
List, C.F. (1941) Neurological syndromes accompanying developmental anomalies of the occipital bone, atlas and axis. *Arch. Neurol. Psychiatry*, **45**, 577–616.
Malgaigne, J.F. (1855) *Traite des Fractures et des Luxations*, Tome II, pp. 334–338 and 1108. J.B. Baillière, Paris.
Martel, W. & Tishler, J.M. (1966) Observations on the spine in mongolism. *Am. J. Roentgenol.*, **97**, 630–638.
McRae, D.L. (1960) The significance of abnormalities of the cervical spine. *Am. J. Roentgenol. Rad. Ther. Nucl. Med.*, **84**, 3–25.
McSweeney, T. (1983) Management of tetraplegia and paraplegia. In Harris, N.H. (ed.), *Postgraduate Textbook of Clinical Orthopaedics*, vol. 31, pp. 944–978. Wright, Bristol.
Minderhoud, J.M., Braakman, R. & Penning, L. (1969) Os odontoideum: Clinical, radiological and therapeutic aspects. *J. Neurol. Sci.*, **8**, 521–544.
Mixter, S.J. & Osgood, R.B. (1910) Traumatic lesions of the atlas and axis. *Ann. Surg.*, **51**, 193–207.
Osgood, R.B. & Lund, C.C. (1928) Fractures of the odontoid process. *N. Engl. J. Med.*, **198**, 61–71.
Pilcher, L.S. (1910) Atlanto-axoid fracture dislocation. *Ann.*

Surg., **51**, 208–211.

Pringle, R.G. (1974) Fractures of the dens (odontoid process) of the axis. In Proceedings of the British Orthopaedic Association. *J. Bone Jt. Surg.*, **56B**, 200–201.

Pulschel, S.M. & Scola, F.H. (1987) Atlanto-axial instability in individuals with Down's syndrome: epidemologic, radiographic and clinical studies. *Paediatrics*, **80**, 550–560.

Ramsay, A.H., Waxman, B.P. & O'Brien, J.F. (1986) A case of traumatic atlanto-occipital dislocation with survival. *Injury*, **17**, 412–420.

Russel, T.G.B. & Aird, M.R.C. (1976) Fetal hyperextension in breech presentation. *Br. J. Radiol.*, **49**, 580–582.

Ryan, M.D. & Taylor, T.K.F. (1982) Odontoid fractures: a rational approach to treatment. *J. Bone Jt. Surg.*, **64B**, 416–421.

Schiff, D.C.M. & Parke, W.W. (1973) The arterial supply of the odontoid process. *J. Bone Jt. Surg.*, **55A**, 1450–1456.

Schneider, R.C., Livingston, K.E., Cave, A.J.E. & Hamilton, G. (1965) 'Hangman's fracture' of the cervical spine. *J. Neurosurg.*, **22**, 141–154.

Schneider, R.C. & Johnson, F.D. (1971) Bilateral traumatic abducens palsy. A mechanism of injury suggested by the study of associated cervical spine fractures. *J. Neurosurg.*, **34**, 33–37.

Schneider, R.C. & McGillicuddy, J.E. (1976) Concomitant craniocerebral and spinal trauma with special reference to the cervico medullary region. In Vinken, P.J. & Bruyn, G.W. (eds), *Handbook of Clinical Neurology*, vol. 24, pp. 141–179. North-Holland/Elsevier, Amsterdam.

Schneider, R.C., Gosch, H.H. & Taren, J.A. (1972a) Blood vessel trauma following head and neck injuries. *Clin. Neurosurg.*, **19**, 312–354.

Schneider, R.C., Crosby, E.C., Russo, R.H., Gosch, H.H. (1972b) Traumatic spinal cord syndromes and their management. *Clin. Neurosurg.*, **20**, 424–492.

Seimon, L.P. (1977) Fracture of the odontoid process. *J. Bone Jt. Surg.*, **59A**, 943–947.

Sherk, H.H. & Nicholson, J.T. (1970) Fractures of the atlas. *J. Bone Jt. Surg.*, **52A**, 1017–1024.

Spence, K.F., Decker, S. & Sell, K.W. (1970) Bursting atlantal fracture associated with rupture of the transverse ligament. *J. Bone Jt. Surg.*, **52A**, 543–549.

Spierings, E.L. & Braakman, R. (1982) The management of os odontoideum: analysis of 37 cases. *J. Bone Jt. Surg.*, **64B**, 422–428.

Spillane, J.D., Pallis, C. & Jones, A.M. (1957) Developmental anomalies in the region of the foramen magnum. *Brain*, **80**, 11–48.

Steel, H.H. (1968) Anatomical and mechanical considerations of the atlanto-axial articulations. *J. Bone Jt. Surg.*, **50A**, 1481–1482.

Wadia, N.H. (1967) Myelopathy caused by atlanto-axial dislocation: a study of 28 cases. *Brain*, **90**, 449–471.

Walton, G.L. (1892) Dislocation of cervical vertebrae. *Int. Clin.*, **2**, 207–216.

Walton, G.L. (1899) Dislocation of cervical vertebrae: five cases; recovery without operation. *Boston Med. Surg. J.*, **120**, 277–281.

Watson-Jones, R. (1932) Spontaneous hyperaemic dislocation of the atlas. *Proc. R. Soc. Med.*, **25**, 586–590.

Watson-Jones, R. (1955) *Fractures and Joint Injuries*, vol. 2, 4th edn, p. 983. E. & S. Livingstone, Edinburgh.

Werne, S. (1957) Studies in spontaneous atlas dislocation. *Acta Orthop. Scand.*, Suppl. 23.

White, A.A. & Panjabi, M.M. (1978) *The Clinical Biomechanics of the Spine*. J.B. Lippincott, Philadelphia.

Williams, T.G. (1975) Hangman's fracture. *J. Bone Jt. Surg.*, **57B**, 82–88.

Wood Jones, F. (1908) The examination of the bodies of 100 men executed in Nubia in Roman times. *Br. Med. J.*, **1**, 736.

Wood Jones, F. (1913) The ideal lesion produced by judicial hanging. *Lancet*, **1**, 53.

Wortzman, G. & Dewar, F.P. (1968) Rotatory fixation of the atlanto-axial joint: rotational atlanto-axial subluxation. *Radiology*, **90**, 479–487.

Yates, P.O. (1959) Birth trauma to vertebral arteries. *Arch Dis. Child.*, **33**, 436–441.

66 · Conservative Management of Spinal Injury

By J.R. SILVER and N.J. HENDERSON

This chapter represents the views of a physician with many years of experience in treating spinal injuries, initially trained by the late Sir Ludwig Guttmann who was his colleague, mentor and friend. Latterly his philosophy of management has changed in emphasis, providing the best of conservative management augmented where appropriate by contemporary surgical techniques, in collaboration with the second author.

The treatment of spinal injuries has always been controversial. From the first written records there has been argument as to the place of surgery in reducing the dislocated spine and the role of operations to decompress the spine.

However, the belief that there is some conflict of approach between the conservative and operative management of spinal injuries should be resisted. The misconception emanates in part from the unfortunate use of the term 'conservative management', which may imply, to some, that this is inactive management. On the contrary, in the context of spinal injuries with neurological involvement, surgery should be seen as one possible approach in the management of one aspect, admittedly an important one, during the treatment of the disease process which may last the rest of the patient's life. With the recent evolution of dedicated spinal surgical techniques we are now in an exciting phase, exploring the possibility of improving the outlook of the skeletal injury itself within the setting of appropriate 'conservative management' of the patient as a whole.

HISTORICAL BACKGROUND

In order to consider the relationship of conservative management to the more aggressive surgical approach it is valuable to appreciate that controversies have existed since medicine first became recognized as a discipline independent from religion, and to accept that there is nothing new in the world.

In Egypt, paraplegia due to injury of the spine was first described in the Edwin Smith surgical papyrus in Egypt about 3000 BC (Breasted, 1930). The Egyptian surgeons carefully distinguished between patients with open wounds or sprains of the cervical vertebrae in whom the spinal cord was not involved, and patients with dislocations and fractures of the spine who had lost power and sensation in all four limbs. They noted that the patient would have priapism, and incontinence of urine and semen. They also described bloodshot eyes, no doubt due to involvement of the sympathetic nervous system. Surgeons were unwilling to treat patients with paraplegia because of its poor prognosis. Doctors then, as now, were unwilling to be associated with a hopeless case.

After the decline of the Egyptian Empire the next to leave a record of their medical practice were the Greeks, foremost among them Hippocrates. He dissociated medicine from religion and presented a systematic record of practice. He made no distinction between fractures and dislocations of the spine, but he was the first to describe traction in the treatment of these injuries. He even attempted to reduce the dislocation by means of hyperextension, placing the patient on his back with a bladder beneath his spine, inflating it by means of a pipe. Greek thought spread throughout the ancient world, particularly to Alexandria, and was eventually incorporated into Roman philosophy. The Romans had little original to contribute in this sphere and Galen (AD 129–199) merely repeated the teachings of Hippocrates.

The next significant discovery was that of Paul of

Aegina (625–690), who employed a windlass for traction of the spine; after he had achieved reduction he used a piece of wood to splint the bones. He was the first to describe the operation of laminectomy. This he recommended when there was a fractured spine with compression of the cord. He suggested that an incision should be made above the site of injury, and that the piece of bone compressing the cord should be removed if possible. He also advised removal of a fractured spinous process if this was causing pain. It would appear that he actually carried out this operation, or knew of surgeons who had. He was aware of the serious nature of the operation and admonished his readers to warn those concerned about the full dangers of the operation.

The fall of the Roman Empire led to an almost total abolition of the practice of medicine in Western Europe. Greek and Roman traditions were preserved in the Eastern Empire and in the Arabian Empire by Christian, Jewish and Moslem physicians. Avicenna (980–1037) followed the teachings of Paul of Aegina and maintained that a fracture of the body of the vertebra was fatal when accompanied by paralysis. At that stage a significant but retrograde development occurred. Galen taught that 'surgery is only a mode of treatment'—the surgeon lost his position of equal status with the physician.

In Europe prior to the Renaissance, medical schools associated with the universities were gradually re-established, the first at Salerno, where Roland of Parma studied. He used manual extension for the treatment of fractured spines and was the first to emphasize one of the keystones of modern practice: the necessity for early treatment. Following this important pre-Renaissance school, several Italian surgeons wrote textbooks on treatment, one of which (by Lanfranc) was translated into English. He repeated the earliest advice given by the Egyptian surgeon with regard to paralysis: 'If thou seest evil signs in that case, go away therefrom'.

The Renaissance brought about the beginning of medicine as we recognize it today. Accurate dissections of the human body, initially by Leonardo DaVinci (1452–1519), whose anatomical studies were lost sight of, and Vesalius (1514–1564), whose anatomical studies enabled Harvey and others to think rationally about their work, laid the scientific basis for the practice of surgery.

Ambrose Pare (1564–1598) was the first modern surgeon. Although a barber surgeon by training he rose to be head surgeon to the army and head physician to four kings of France. He wrote a textbook of surgery and recommended laminectomy for spinal compression. However, contrary to Paul of Aegina, he stated that the fractured spinous process should not be removed if it was still attached to the periosteum. He clearly described and illustrated methods of reducing the dislocated spine, advising initial manual reduction and then the use of pieces of wood to achieve a more satisfactory reduction. He was aware of the fatal nature of this injury, but did not specify the cause of death.

There was little progress in treatment following Pare's work. Such advances as were made were stimulated by the wars that necessitated having a large number of surgeons to treat the wounded throughout Europe. Fabricius Ab Aquapendente (1661), in Germany, suggested open reduction for fracture dislocation of the spine, pointing out the practical difficulties of intractable haemorrhage that could be arrested by the use of twisted oakum steeped in tow. In France, Jean Louis Petit (1705) recommended hyperflexion to disengage the locked facets of the vertebral column; while this manoeuvre would relieve the vertebral problem it would only damage the spinal cord still further (Figs 66.1 & 66.2).

In the United Kingdom Sir Astley Cooper, the doyen of British surgeons, was very interested in the management of spinal injuries, a popular teacher and author of many textbooks. In 1824 he described how a violent blow to the loins could produce paralysis of the lower extremities. This paralytic state could be dealt with by cupping, but if at the end of a week or 10 days the paralytic state still continued, blisters should be applied. However, if there was extravasation on the spine, then he described how cupping should be performed. He went on to describe an instructive case when he was living, presumably as a pupil, with Mr Cline:

> A girl received a severe blow in the neck, and after this it was found that, whenever she attempted to look at any thing above her head, she was under the necessity of putting her hands behind it, and gradually elevating it to the object. When she wanted to look at any thing beneath her head, she put her hands under her chin and lowered her head to the object.

This presumably was a case of instability of the atlas with some cord involvement produced whenever the head was moved.

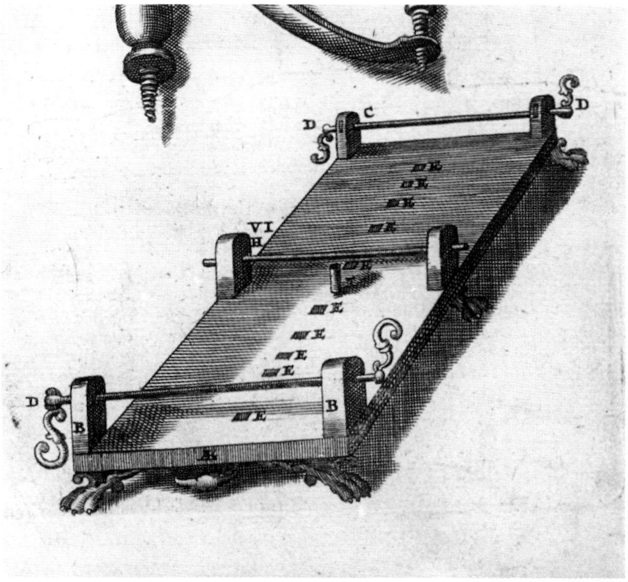

Fig. 66.1 Equipment for reducing dislocated spine. From Scultetus (1674).

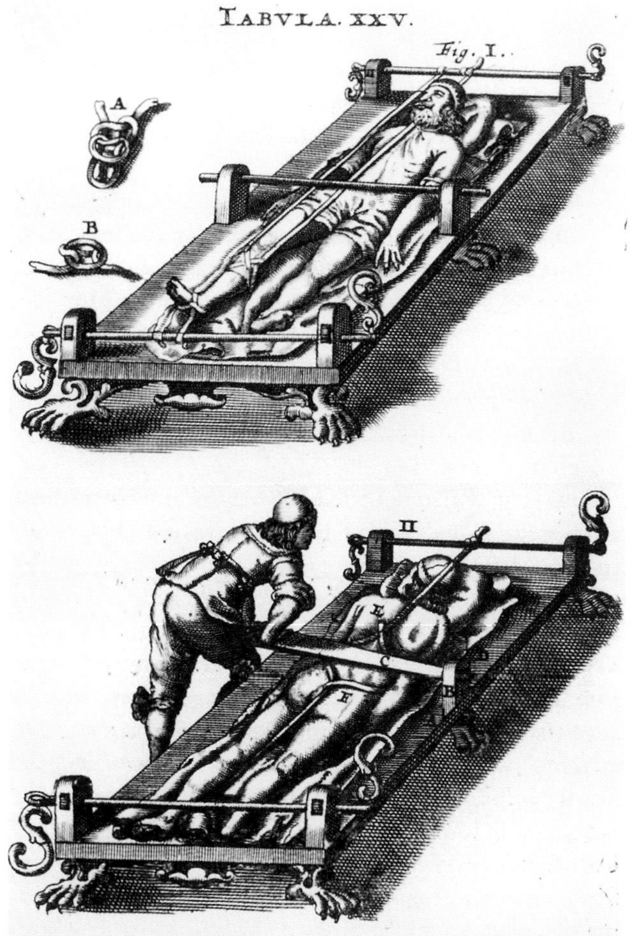

Fig. 66.2 Manual reduction of dislocated spine. From Scultetus (1674).

> The child lived twelve months after the accident. On examination of the body after death, Mr Cline found the atlas broken through; there was a transverse fracture of the atlas, but no displacement. When she endeavoured to raise her head, the dentiform process quitted its natural situation, and carried back a portion of the atlas; when her head inclined forward, pressure was produced upon the spinal marrow, as it was likewise when the body was agitated.
>
> Mr Henry Cline was the first person who attempted to give relief in this accident. Being an excellent anatomist and a most reasonable surgeon, he saw no reason why cases of this kind should not be treated as cases of fracture with depression of the skull. Accordingly he cut down upon the arch of the spinal marrow, where the compression was greatest, and with a small trephine of his own invention he sawed through the arch of the spinous process, and took off the pressure on the spinal marrow, by raising the depressed portion of the arch. It is well known, that in cases of fracture where the displacement has been slight, union of the bone has been produced.

Astley Cooper went on to discuss the difficulties of the operation, pointing out that:

> In many of these cases the spinal marrow is itself torn through. In some cases of fracture, with displacement, it is completely torn.

He then pointed out that Mr Tyrrell had attempted the operation since Mr Cline, but that

> Both cases have terminated unfavourably. Whether future experiments may be attended with better success it is impossible to say. The proposal was plausible; the operation was easily performed, and as to the result, if the spinal marrow were not torn, there seems no reason why a person should not recover after such an operation.

He was not a blind advocate of laminectomy.

> We are obliged, however, to speak doubtingly on this subject, since the first experiments have been unsuccessful. If you could save one life in

> ten, aye, one in a hundred, by such an operation, it is your duty to attempt it, notwithstanding any objections which some foolish persons may have urged against it.

He advocated Cline's operation in the following words:

> He was blamed for making this trial, I am not sure he would have been ultimately successful; but in a case otherwise without hope, I am certain such an attempt was laudable. Nothing is so easy as to condemn others; but let it be mentioned that the disposition to do so, is proof of a weak head and a bad heart and that it ought always to be discouraged in a profession in which character is all in all.

Cooper (1823) also described the signs and symptoms of paraplegia at different levels, stressing the incontinence of urine and faeces, and making interesting observations on the preservation of circulation and inflammatory responses in the paralysed limbs.

At that stage surgical and nursing care must have been developed to quite a high degree of skill: not all patients with traumatic paraplegia died immediately. Patients with lumbar fractures died within one month, but Cooper recorded patients living as long as two years before dying of pressure sores. One patient was successfully rehabilitated so that he was able to dress and undress himself. Patients with cervical injuries died within one week of injury—and it was recognized that in general these cases were fatal.

Unfortunately Cooper's observations of the physical signs and prognosis in paraplegia were lost sight of because of his views on treatment by laminectomy. He accused anyone who opposed him of being a blockhead, and this led to the celebrated controversy with Sir Charles Bell, a highly cultured scientist, artist, philosopher, physiologist and anatomist, who wrote a textbook (Bell, 1824) discounting Sir Astley Cooper's views. In his introduction he asked pertinently:

> What shall be said of the recommendation clearly given to students in our own times, who are taught to despise the study of books, and to neglect all authority but that of the person who is addressing them, and all practice or example, but that of the hospital to which chance has led them.

His approach was modern, pointing out that the damage to the spinal cord occurred at the moment of injury, and that it was not continuing pressure that damaged the cord. He emphasized that all the efforts of the surgeons should be devoted to making an accurate diagnosis in the first instance, and that operation on the spinal column was both dangerous and useless. He also pointed out that, in cases of paraplegia, death was attributable to the retention of urine and subsequent inflammation—the first mention of renal failure being a cause of death.

His words in the debate with Astley Cooper are profound, stimulating and still relevant today:

> For it must be acknowledged, that what are professionally called facts, are for the most part only those notions which a man insensibly adopts in the course of his practice, and which takes colour from his education and previous studies. It is this which makes the facts of one age differ from the facts of another age: and the opinions of men differently educated to vary on what they are inconsistent enough to call matters of fact (Bell, 1824).

Bell's views received wide acceptance in Britain. He made a lasting contribution to our knowledge of neurology, and there is a fascinating and beautiful description of an early case of missed injury of the spinal cord, which unfortunately has echoes today.

> March 29, 1816—Marshal, a coal waggoner, was brought into the hospital from Edgeware; the account given by the people who had brought him was rather confused. They agreed that he had been riding on the foreshaft of his cart, and, by a sudden jerk, was thrown off, and pitched on the back of his neck and shoulders. The man was somewhat intoxicated, and could not give a distinct description of what befell him. When carried into the hospital he was put up on his legs but he could not stand; and when supported by the shoulders, he dragged his legs after him. At this time he complained of pain in his loins but no injury was perceptible there. Between his shoulders, however, there was a degree of swelling and discolouration. Some of the people who were with him said that the wheel of the cart, which was empty, had gone over the small of his back; but after the first day he never complained of that part. Leeches were applied to the spine betwixt the shoulders and his bowels were opened (Bell, 1838).

When he died, this man was found to have a complete separation of his last cervical from the first thoracic vertebra.

There was little advance in the treatment of renal failure as a cause of death throughout the 19th century, but there was a better understanding of the pathological sequelae. Curling (1833, 1836) described the suppurative consequences of paralysis of the bladder on the kidneys, and pointed out that the survival time was proportional to the severity of the infection. Gull (1856, 1858), Thorburn (1889) and Fagge (1891) also drew attention to renal pathology in this condition.

There seems to have been a great deal of interest in spinal injuries and their management at the London Hospital, and in a little-known paper by Hutchinson (1866) there is a series of accounts of the clinical manifestations, treatment and pathological findings of those patients with spinal injuries. It is interesting that many cases survived and left the hospital ambulant, having sustained severe injury of the spinal cord; the patients were treated with intermittent catheterization. Hutchinson stated categorically that injury to the spinal cord was due to direct trauma and not to haematoma. He reiterated the views of Sir Charles Bell on the dangers of carrying out laminectomy, he recorded the dangers of pressure sores and recommended the use of a water-bed to prevent them. His views are extraordinarily modern, and he draws attention to how badly patients are examined and how one should be sceptical of the clinical observations.

> Another source of fallacy is the difficulty of accurate observations. A man tells you; 'I cannot move my legs' and you are unable to prove the contrary, though it is still possible that a very vigorous exertion of will might be able to set certain muscles in action; in other words, that voluntary motion, although seemingly in abeyance, is not absolutely lost. The same patient tells you that he 'can feel well' yet very probably, if you try accurate tests, such as the compasses or drawing a hair or a feather over the surface, you will find that his sensory function is very far from perfect. On account of our frequent neglect of such tests we are compelled to receive with much qualification, recorded statements as to 'perfect sensation' being retained after these accidents.

The association of the London Hospital with the management of spinal injuries was maintained by Head and Riddoch, who were both physicians to the hospital.

First World War

During the First World War there was a superb series of clinical observations by Head & Riddoch (1917) and Gordon Holmes (1915). They served as officers in the casualty stations, examining the patients soon after injury, and produced beautiful accounts, that can be read with profit today, of the clinical manifestations of spinal cord injury at various levels, and describing for the first time autonomic dysreflexia and giving the first modern account of the pathophysiology of bladder function following spinal injury. Gordon Holmes described pathological findings, at post mortem, where cores of tissue that he thought were damaged tissue from the spinal injury, like toothpaste, were found at the base of the posterior column of the spine, which may be the cause of post-traumatic syringomyelia.

Although the clinical descriptions could not be bettered, although medicine, surgery and nursing had reached a high level of technical skill and the significant causes of death from pressure sores and renal infection were now appreciated, no satisfactory programme of treatment was achieved; the outlook was just as hopeless as 5000 years previously when the Egyptian physician first described this condition.

Walker, writing in 1917 and 1937, found that of 339 patients with spinal injury admitted to King George V Military Hospital from 1915 to 1919, 160 (47.2%) died of urinary infection eight to 10 weeks later. He estimated that the total mortality rate due to urinary sepsis in British soldiers in the First World War was 80%. Not all the First World War veterans died, and one of the authors (J. R. S.) has seen a small number of survivors, but the striking feature was that they had had minimal interference with their bladders.

The experiences of other allied forces with the spinally injured was identical:

> These did very badly throughout, as was anticipated. Most of them were immediately evacuated to base hospitals and fully 80% died in the first few weeks in consequence of infection from bed sores and catheterization. The conditions were such, owing to pressure of work, as to make it almost impossible to give these unfortunate men the care their condition required. No water beds were available, and each case demands the almost undivided attention of a nurse trained in the care of paralytics. Only those

cases survived in which the spinal lesion was a partial one. (Woodhall, 1959)

The results of spinal injuries were described as extremely discouraging, and the mortality as very high. In one series of 32 cases reported by Col. Harvey Cushing (1927), eight were inoperable and there were 23 deaths (71.8%). Of the 24 patients operated on, 15 died (62.5%). All of these patients were cared for in forward areas, and the follow-up was inadequate because casualties with spinal cord injuries were evacuated promptly if they were regarded as at all transportable.

Another of the neurosurgeons who looked after these servicemen was Frazier. He was a pioneer; one of the founders of neurosurgical tradition in the United States of America, and had a particular interest in traumatic paraplegia. He wrote a monumental textbook, wholly devoted to surgery of the spine and spinal cord (Frazier & Allen, 1918). It is thoroughly modern in its approach, with a section given to trauma of the spinal cord, including a separate section on gunshot wounds. He compared the results of 499 cases treated prior to 1911, and 314 treated between 1911 and 1915. Those treated before 1911, many of whom had immediate operation, had a mortality of 67.9% compared with 1911–1915, who had a mortality of 26.8%.

He discussed the place of a decompressive laminectomy, and felt that:

> The fact remains that in my clinical experience there are records of function recovered that without operation would not have been anticipated.

The natural history of a spinal injury, if treated conservatively, is that there is a tendency to recover. The view that he advanced, since there were no controls and few patients survived, subsequently made rational evaluation of the role of surgery versus conservative treatment extremely difficult to this day.

He was a forerunner, and the teacher of Munro. He made clear the primacy of the prevention of bed sores and the preservation of renal function.

> Regarding the care of the patient surviving the immediate effects of an injury to the spinal cord, attention is required principally for the prevention of bed sores, for protection of the urinary tract against secondary infection.

He recognized the probability of infection of the bladder, and described how in many circumstances the paralysis could increase. He described how a fatal

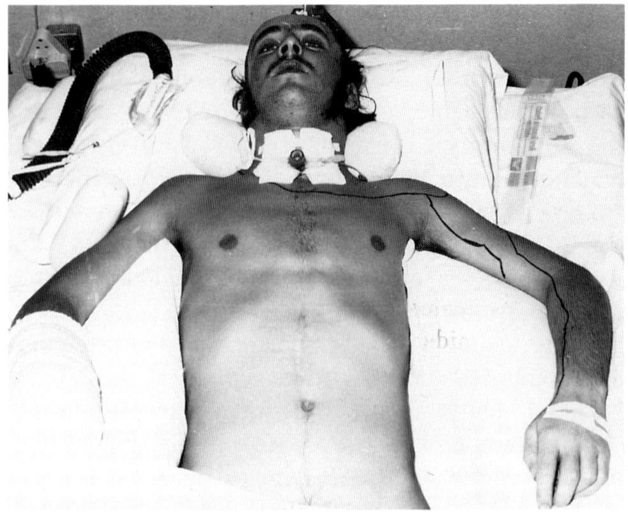

Fig. 66.3 As a result of a fall, this patient sustained fracture dislocation of C5 and C6, with a sensory level at C3 on the left, C2 on the right. His vital capacity on his back was 750 but when he was turned on his right side it dropped to 450 and he had to go on to a respirator.

attack of respiratory embarrassment could follow the turning of the patient on his side. No doubt this was due to paralysis of the diaphragm on one side, where the vital capacity can vary in the different positions in which the patient is nursed, being adequate when the normally innervated leaf of the diaphragm is uppermost, and inadequate when the paralysed leaf is uppermost. (Silver, 1980; Fig. 66.3)

He analysed the prognosis in injuries, and he followed up 75 cases who had been operated on. He found that, 10 years after the accident, one in nine had entirely recovered, one in three were partially self-supporting, and one in seven were entirely incapacitated.

The modern era

Donald Munro was trained by Frazier at Philadelphia. He was the pioneer of the treatment of traumatic paraplegia in the United States. In 1936 he set up a spinal centre at the Boston City Hospital. He started publishing on the management of spinal injuries in 1936, but his paper in 1943 was a landmark, laying the foundation for the whole of the modern treatment of spinal injuries. His views were quite dogmatic and forceful, and he maintained that, by meticulous care of the patient and prevention of pressure sores, if the patient had a good pair of arms he or she could be returned to a useful independent existence.

He believed that the treatment of the patient's spine was of only secondary importance, and that no effort should be made to reduce a fracture by operation, but that gentle traction should be used to replace the vertebrae. He recommended that constant X-ray checks should be made of the bone injury until such time as the physician was certain that it was completely healed and capable of bearing body weight without the aid of a splint. He was not in favour of a decompressive laminectomy, stating that it should not be undertaken lightly. He showed a drop of 30% in the mortality of cervical cases after laminectomies were abandoned.

He recognized that care of the bladder was paramount; he established a system of tidal drainage to protect the bladder, and would not countenance genito-urinary sepsis in his service. He stated that:

> Regardless of any other causes of death, kidneys, ureters and bladders removed at autopsy should show no more than a very superficial cystitis.

He emphasized that:

> Pressure sores always antedate bed sores. The former develop because of prolonged weight bearing on bony prominences and of maceration of the horny layers of the skin. The latter follow because of interference with the skin-vascular reflexes. The best treatment of bed sores is prevention.

He insisted that this should be accomplished by keeping patients constantly dry and never allowing them to lie in a wet bed for even as little as 15 minutes. The patient should be turned every two hours day and night so long as he or she is bedridden. Serum protein levels must be maintained. He felt it best to refrain from surgery to the bed sore, and recommended that it be dressed only once a day by sterile dressing. He set himself against the application of plaster of paris in paraplegic patients.

His views were widely adopted and followed in the treatment of American servicemen in the Second World War. Reviewing the experiences of the American forces, Prather (1959) devoted considerable space to Munro's methods of tidal drainage in spinal patients. He acknowledged Munro's contribution by saying:

> Most of the diagnostic and therapeutic procedures employed in Army hospitals had previously been tested in civilian clinics. World War II simply supplied the opportunity for their trial on a mass scale.

His views gained wide acceptance in Canada, where spinal centres followed his methods, and clearly led the way in the United Kingdom, where Watson-Jones, writing an editorial in 1949 said, quoting Nicoll, that:

> A group of surgeons are trying to achieve in Great Britain a general and unified paraplegia service, comparable in efficiency with the magnificent paraplegic units of Canada and the United States of America which have proved beyond doubt the possibility of restoring the victims of paraplegia to happy and useful lives.

At the beginning of the Second World War Ludwig Guttmann, a distinguished neurosurgeon, research worker and assistant to Foester, the dominant neurologist and neurosurgeon in Europe between the World Wars, fled to England. He continued neurological research work at Oxford but he was unable to carry out his clinical practice as a neurosurgeon. However, just as Frazier had trained and influenced Munro, Riddoch—a surgeon in charge of neurological services in the British Army—offered Guttmann the directorship of a new spinal unit that was to be opened in time for the casualties expected from the invasion of Europe in 1944. This was part of a chain of specialized spinal, head injury and burns units. The unit was located at Stoke Mandeville Hospital where during the next 22 years Guttmann's dynamic approach dominated attitudes to spinal injury management.

The two great dangers were from bed sores and urinary infections. Guttmann studied Munro's methods, paid tribute to his ideas and followed them very closely in the United Kingdom. Guttmann, like Munro, gave orders that the patients were to be turned prone to supine and back, or from side to side every two hours, night and day, waking or sleeping. In suitable cases the process of healing of bed sores was accelerated by cleaning and application of skin grafts. He also instituted a method of intermittent catheterization, recognizing the dangers of indwelling catheterization and suprapubic cystotomy. He considered that an immediate operation upon the spinal cord was irresponsible meddling, and by administering a superb standard of treatment, reaffirmed the views of Bell and Hutchinson. In United Kingdom practice as a result immediate laminectomy has virtually ceased. He paid particular attention to the psychological handling of the patients, and stressed that the only way the patient could be correctly and completely rehabilitated was by management in a centre where staff understood all aspects of the treatment of patients.

It is depressing that, while lip service is paid to Guttmann's methods, it either takes the form of uncritical repetition of dogma, or alternatively an iconoclastic attack. In neither case are his concepts and ideas appreciated and understood. For this reason it is valuable to state what the situation was at the time of his contribution. It is thus necessary to consider the state of medical knowledge and the organization of medical care at the time Munro and Guttmann introduced, pioneered and revolutionized the treatment of spinal injuries.

It must be appreciated that, prior to the opening of spinal centres in the United Kingdom during the Second World War patients with spinal cord injuries died rapidly, and an unfortunate distinction was made between the patients with fractures of the spinal column without neurological involvement, and those with spinal cord injuries. This was unfortunate in that it led to a poor understanding of the mechanics of spinal injury. Thus it is necessary to consider what was the state of knowledge of spinal fractures at that time.

The majority of paraplegics were servicemen and had suffered open wounds of the spinal cord. Clearly, for these patients a debridement was necessary, but whether an immediate laminectomy should be performed to inspect a closed injury of the spinal cord was controversial. It was believed at the time that it might be appropriate, and Guttmann himself acknowledges that he had initially thought so (Guttmann, 1973).

Frazier believed that surgical intervention might be indicated, but it carried a high mortality, and Munro, while recognizing in specialized circumstances a laminectomy might be valuable, accepted that in the early stages it carried an unacceptably high mortality for patients with injuries of the cervical cord.

The American experience in the Second World War was conflicting:

> While the great majority of patients with immediate and complete paralyses could be expected to recover little if any function after the operation, there were numerous exceptions. For this reason, if the patient's general condition were satisfactory and if other high-priority casualties with better chances of recovery were not thereby denied operation, debridement and laminectomy were performed even in apparently hopeless cases.
>
> In general, there were two reasons for attempting decompression of the cord: (1) the necessity for debridement of the wound, which was just as valid in this region as anywhere else in the body, and (2) an attempt to relieve pressure upon the cord. Debridement was regarded as particularly essential if the wound of entrance or of exit was in the back. (Campbell, 1959)

> Neurosurgeons, at least early on, were not in agreement about the value of surgical exploration of spinal cord injuries. The dictum that very few injuries of the spine in which the cord was involved would be improved by operation had been carried over from civilian into military practice, and for a time it seriously handicapped military neurosurgeons. As a matter of fact, the attempt to correlate the two types of injuries was as fallacious as it was misleading. The 'broken back' of civilian practice is usually a lesion which affects the vertebral body primarily. The major lesion in a gunshot wound of the spine was likely to be in the vertebral arches.
>
> Paraplegia proved the most distressing of all military neurosurgical conditions and the most difficult to benefit. It was fully realized that in only a very small proportion of these cases could surgery improve the patient's lot, but it was also realized, with equal clarity, that in an occasional case, particularly the type of case in which the bony injury was limited to the vertebral arches, debridement of the spinal canal might occasionally result in dramatic improvement. (Spurling, 1959)

Despite the reports of experienced surgeons on the dangerous effects of laminectomy, during the 1950s routine posterior laminectomy to decompress the spinal cord and cauda equina was practised as the standard of care. However, analysis of these injuries shows that posterior laminectomy does not decompress the spinal canal, since most of the compression is usually anterior. Moreover, by destroying the posterior column completely the spine is further destabilized, resulting in increased kyphosis in the short—and often the long—term, placing more pressure on the anterior part of the spinal cord and nerve roots. Decompression by means of a laminectomy alone has been shown to be of no value (Comarr, 1959) and has been generally abandoned, though in our experience patients are still quite frequently admitted following laminectomy at the receiving hospital.

In view of the high mortality that had been experienced in these patients in the First World War, doctors who saw them were very pessimistic, and thought that any treatment for paraplegics would only prolong a useless life, so they should be given large doses of morphine and left to die as quickly as possible. It was even thought that where the legs were useless and paralysed they should be amputated, as they were too heavy to help transfers, and could only be the source of pressure sores. It had been thought that these were useless cripples; those who survived had been immobilized for many years in bed and had developed stones, pressure sores and a 'cripple' mentality. This pessimism was compounded by the fact that patients arrived very late at specialized facilities, and with many severe complications.

Bladder management

The cause of death in spinal patients was either overwhelming sepsis from pressure sores or acute ascending pyelonephritis. Intermittent catheterization had proved disastrous in the First World War. It had been thought that a suprapubic catheter offered the best chance of preventing infection, and this practice was followed during the Second World War by the United Kingdom medical services (Riches, 1943), whilst the United States forces followed Munro's approach, favouring tidal drainage.

Management of the fracture

Watson-Jones (1949) had shown that a dislocated spine could be reduced by hyperextension and then immobilized in a plaster jacket, and he believed that by achieving an anatomical reduction of the fracture, and by the early institution of active exercises for the spinal musculature, pain could be reduced and disability could be avoided. However, he readily admitted, following his experience in the Second World War, that it was not necessary to achieve reduction of the fracture and a perfect anatomical result to achieve satisfactory rehabilitation, and he thought the best treatment for a spinal fracture was to send the servicemen to a rehabilitation centre as soon as the pain had subsided, to give them an active programme of exercises and to return them to duty. The significant advance was the institution of active exercises.

Nicoll studied (1949) 166 coal miners and followed up Watson-Jones' work. He made a fundamental distinction between stable and unstable fractures of the thoracolumbar spine. The stable fracture could be treated in the way that Sir Reginald Watson-Jones had outlined by early mobilization, but the unstable fractures required a different form of treatment. Nicoll showed that the fulcrum of movement was the nucleus pulposus and that the three most important factors concerned in the redisplacement of a spinal fracture were:

> Comminution of the vertebral body, crushing of the invertebral disc and rupture of the interspinous ligament. (Nicoll, 1949)

Holdsworth (1963), in charge of the Spinal Centre at Sheffield, showed clearly that the best solution was to admit the patients immediately to a spinal centre, where they could receive expert treatment. They did not need to develop complications; renal sepsis could be avoided and any pressure sores developed elsewhere could be healed and worthwhile rehabilitation could proceed.

Holdsworth made an important contribution by showing that fractures of the whole spine were subject to the same rules for stability as Nicoll had postulated for the lumbar spine, and he considered that the stability largely depended upon the integrity of the posterior spinal ligament. When the fractures were unstable he believed they should be fixed by a plate, though he did not use a bone graft. By this means early mobilization could be achieved, which would facilitate nursing. Follow-up studies showed that the operation was technically difficult. Though in his hands it worked well, unfortunately some patients were mobilized too early, and many of the plates fractured. It was difficult to predict which cases were suitable except by manipulating the spinous processes at operation, and many stable fractures were fixed unnecessarily.

In 1965 Hardy, who was Holdsworth's colleague, reviewed all the cases that had been plated and those treated conservatively at the Sheffield unit. He realized that they were not matched cases, but could see little difference in the outcome of the results between the two groups.

Subsequently, emphasis was placed on developing better plates, and Meurig-Williams devised another plate for fixation of spinal fractures. Sixty-four of his patients with spinal fractures were admitted to the Cardiff Royal Infirmary, where they were fixed with plates prior to being transferred to the spinal centre. The remaining 29 patients were admitted directly to the spinal centre, and were treated conservatively without plating. Once at the centre, all patients received the same treatment. The results of the two groups of patients were compared by Lewis and McKibbin in 1974. Their conclusions were that open reduction and internal fixation did not improve the chances of neurological recovery, and that patients with the most severe spinal deformity were the least likely to recover. They showed that there was a tendency for all the patients to improve their neurological function with time, and some patients who were completely paralysed on admission did make a considerable degree of recovery. Those patients treated by plating did not develop residual deformity or pain.

Guttmann popularized the method of conservative management of spinal injuries following Munro's pioneering work. This method gained increasing acceptance in spinal injury centres throughout the world, and it is worth looking at what Guttmann actually believed and practised. The senior author practised Guttmann's regime over many years, gaining considerable experience of the method both at Liverpool and Stoke Mandeville.

In 1944 Guttmann introduced and developed the method of graduated reduction of fractures and fracture–dislocations of the spine and immobilization of pillow-packs combined with two-hourly turning of the paralysed patient, day and night. The original pillow-packs were later replaced by the more suitable and more hygienic sorbo rubber packs. The patient was placed, by three orderlies, on a prepared bed consisting of sorbo packs which lay on a hard surface to prevent sagging. An additional pillow or roll was placed underneath the fracture to ensure the normal contour of the spine. The patient's hips, buttocks and sacrum, as well as the heels, were completely free from pressure. From the initial supine position the patient was carefully turned by the orderlies in one piece, at two-hourly intervals to the sides and later back to the supine position, whereby the hyperextended position of the spine was secured by a heavy sandbag in the lateral positions. Reduction of the broken spine was monitored by repeated control X-rays commencing on the first day in order, if necessary, to correct and modify the position of the broken vertebra. Latterly, sorbo packs were replaced by a turning table, facilitating turns during the day.

He believed that the position of the vertebra could be corrected. Thus in compression fractures the compressed vertebral body, whether wedged or completely flattened, could be re-expanded and remain more or less so. He did not share the view that simple wedge fractures do not require reduction.

Some idea of the Guttmann approach can be gleaned from the following quotes taken from his textbook published in 1973.

> To leave the impacted anterior part of the wedged vertebra unreduced means ignoring the damage to the anterior longitudinal ligament, which in such a case is crumpled up. If the wedged vertebra is re-expanded by postural reduction the straightened anterior ligament helps to keep the reduced vertebral body, if not permanently completely expanded, at least in a better position, thus preventing severe angulation later.

> Dislocations and fracture dislocations of various types, including those of the most severe burst fractures with avulsion of parts of the vertebral body and regardless whether stable or unstable, can be successfully reduced and stabilised.

> Atrophy of the back muscles which is the rule following long-term conservative fixation in plaster casts, plaster beds and following operative procedures, can be absolutely avoided, which is so important for the later physical readjustment of the paralysed.

> Pressure sores, which hitherto were considered as inevitable, can be completely avoided, thus preventing sepsis and avoiding long-term and costly conservative and surgical treatment afterwards.

> The continual change of posture counteracts stagnation in the urinary tract, thus preventing the dreaded complications of ureters and kidneys following infection.

> The constant change of posture has proved beneficial in restoring the disturbed vasomotor control and thus better blood circulation, especially in the high lesions.

Table 66.1 Time in bed. The average time that the patients were kept in bed before sitting up is noted, but patients who were kept in bed for reasons other than the vertebral injury, e.g. associated fractures, were excluded. From Frankel *et al.* (1969)

Cervical fractures, 10.8 weeks
Cervical fracture–dislocations, 12.0 weeks
Cervical: no visible fracture, 10.0 weeks
T1–T10 fractures, 9.8 weeks
T1–T10 fracture–dislocations, 11.1 weeks
T1–T10 no visible fracture, 11.0 weeks
T11, T12–L1 fractures, 11.3 weeks
T11, T12–L1 fracture–dislocations, 12.0 weeks
T11, T12–L1 no visible fracture, 6.6 weeks
Lumbar fractures, 13 weeks
Lumbar fracture–dislocations, 12.2 weeks

He was thus in favour of obtaining a good anatomical result, and as early mobilization as was compatible with a pain-free situation and a lack of deformity. It is important that any analysis of results be on an identifiable group of patients—namely those admitted soon after injury before they have had surgery or developed complications elsewhere.

The Stoke Mandeville results were documented in 1969 by Frankel *et al.* Between 1951 and 1968 682 patients, divided into four groups on the basis of their initial skeletal injury, were admitted all within 14 days of injury. All the patients were immobilized in bed for about 12 weeks. The results were analysed in terms of neurological recovery, time in bed and stability. The patients who died in the first three months were excluded from the analysis, which is unfortunate, and the results are given in terms of stability, reduction and the time in bed. There is no account of pain or deformity.

They found that many of the fractures could be reduced with a low incidence of instability. Only four patients developed instability of their fracture site, and it was found that, throughout, a small number of initially complete neurological lesions became incomplete and a larger number of incomplete lesions improved. There was, however, no clear correlation between the types and degree of the vertebral injury and the severity of the neurological lesion, nor was there any correlation between the degree of reduction achieved and neurological recovery (Table 66.1).

This work was followed up by Frankel *et al.* (1987), in which they studied the conservative treatment of thoracic fractures, giving a rather shorter time in bed for the thoracic injuries than in the initial study, and finding a considerable degree of neurological recovery (Table 66.2). Unfortunately, no information is given about pain or deformity in these studies.

Table 66.2 Average number of days of bed rest and average number of days in hospital for patients at different levels. The results of the Stoke Mandeville figures and the Oswestry figures (in parentheses) on conservative treatment are compared. The length of time that the patients were kept in bed has been reduced from the previous study. From Frankel *et al.* (1987)

	Days bed rest	Days in hospital
D1–D6	49 (51)	192 (145)
D7–D10	62.5 (54)	177 (151)
D11–L1	77 (58)	182 (139)
Below L1	89 (63)	170 (127)

Subsequent progress

Guttmann placed great emphasis on taking frequent X-rays of the patient and he strove to achieve satisfactory reduction of the fracture, which he believed was achievable. Holdsworth, from his similar experience but backed up by his findings at operation, thought that you could tell little from the X-ray of the state of the fracture. Holdsworth's views have been vindicated by the development of computerized tomography (CT) scanning, and it would appear that many plain X-rays give limited information about the nature of the bony injury. With the development of the CT scanner, which has revolutionized our insight into fracture management, it seemed inappropriate to attempt to manage the spinal fracture without this facility.

Furthermore, many patients admitted to our centre, having already received internal fixation elsewhere (some from abroad), were assessed, and if fixation had been adequately performed and the spine was thought to be in a satisfactory condition, a programme of early mobilization was instituted. There were thus at our centre two populations of patients—those who had been fixed and were being mobilized early, and those who were admitted who followed a regime of conservative treatment. Early mobilization following fixation was not to the detriment of the patient, the ultimate prognosis depending more on the personality of the patient than on the method of initial treatment.

With this background, a change of emphasis has emerged in our unit, whereby patients are now jointly evaluated by physician and surgeon, and if appropriate are operated on. The principles underlying this combined approach are as follows.

PRINCIPLES OF MANAGEMENT

Primary spinal cord damage

The main damage to the spinal cord is due to displacement or impact at the moment of injury. It is important to distinguish this primary damage, about which nothing can be done, from secondary damage which we may be able to influence (see below). The primary damage may be due to the direct trauma of bone or disc intrusion into the canal, or by distraction. The position of the spinal cord and the hard tissues around it at the moment of impact may be very different from the position of rest which they adopt when studied on X-rays some time later. This is one factor which can account for the widely varying neurological involvement consequent on different degrees of skeletal injury and displacement. It may also account for the controversy that surrounds the presence of disc or bone within the canal, and their relevance to the indications for decompression or potential for neurological recovery after their removal.

Secondary spinal cord damage

A considerable amount of deterioration or improvement following injury is due to secondary effects on the spinal cord. There is scope here for improving the prognosis or precipitating deterioration according to management.

The majority of secondary neurological damage is due to swelling and vascular effects. The role of steroids is still controversial (Bracken *et al.*, 1990; see also Chapter 60). There is some evidence that appropriate doses, given early enough within the first eight hours of injury, may influence the outcome. Important secondary damage may also arise from poor mechanical handling of the patient, and continued irritation of the cord directly and through vascular compromise. A cornerstone of management is to avoid the following, which we believe to be injurious to the cord.

1 *Stretching.* The work of Breig *et al.* (1989) has shown that inappropriate traction of the spinal cord will cause neurological deterioration. The effect of gross overdistraction with large weights is obvious, but even quite small amounts of distraction have deleterious effects on the cord, or stretch the cord over impinging bone fragments of kyphotic segments. Thus traction should be applied only with the greatest of care, and under medical supervision, with monitoring of the neurological condition in the conscious patient. There is no place for the use of excessive traction to splint the spinal cord once reduction has been achieved.

2 *Compression.* Compression may be obvious on plain radiographs due to dislocations, acute kyphos or bone fragment. However, compression can also arise from soft tissue intrusion, such as disc prolapse or ligamentum flavum folding. This should be considered, and may be evident only on sophisticated radiological investigation. Bohlman (1979) has shown that 50% of spinal injuries are accompanied by massive disc protrusion, and recent studies confirm this reference.

3 *Undue movement after injury.* It is recognized that unsupervised movement of a fracture can cause neurological deterioration. Great care must be taken at the site of the incident, when transporting the patient and within hospital, that the fracture is supported. Deterioration has been shown by Toscano (1988) and by Ravichandran & Silver (1982).

4 *Hypotension.* The injured spinal cord is sensitive to low blood pressure, and one of the most potent means of preventing secondary damage is rapid effective resuscitation (see Chapter 60). This must be taken into account during anaesthesia for spinal or any other surgery that the patient may undergo, particularly in the very early stages after injury. Varying degrees of hypotensive anaesthesia are sometimes employed during surgery on the spine and central nervous system, and the anaesthetist unfamiliar with these patients may exacerbate the neurological deficit by infarcting the cord (Silver & Buxton, 1974).

5 *Inappropriate surgery.* Inappropriate surgery on the spinal cord in the early stages has been recognized to carry a high morbidity and mortality from the time of Frazier and Munro. Manipulation of the fracture or dislocation is recognized as causing deterioration. The saddest group of all are patients with dislocation of the cervical spine who have no neurological deficit prior to surgery and wake up tetraplegic. The exact factors causing this are ill-understood.

6 *Infection.*

These factors seldom occur in isolation, and inevitably several deleterious factors occur together and are cumulative. It is a frequent observation that the patient with an undiagnosed spinal injury can become completely paralysed as a result of mistreatment. It is often difficult to isolate the precise causative factor. For example, since the patient with an unstable midthoracic fracture will almost inevitably have a haemopneumothorax and be surgically shocked: was the causative factor bringing about neurological deterioration inappropriate movement or hypotension leading to infarction of the cord?

It is not unusual for there to be transient deterioration in the neurological situation of the patient over the first hours and days following injury, though this effect is usually reversible. This may be due to oedema of the cord. A recent review of 1300 cervical injuries has shown that of a subgroup of 50 patients with unreduced dislocations, 13 who were not initially paralysed developed a delayed paralysis due to swelling of the cord (Mahale & Silver, 1992).

Medical aspects of care

The cornerstone of management is to deal with any associated injuries, and to maintain the patient's general condition (see Chapter 61). In the early stages, resuscitation and monitoring of the respiratory status are vital, and care must be taken with abdominal assessment, given associated paralytic ileus and potentially silent intra-abdominal injuries in the paralysed patient. Prevention of complications is vital, in particular paying attention to urinary tract infection, pressure sores and thromboembolic complications.

The physician frequently has to pick his way through a difficult situation, given that 75% of patients have associated injuries. Head injury, fractured ribs and pelvis in particular complicate general care.

Surgical care of the patient

There are several aspects to surgical care. The spinal injury is part of a general trauma scenario. General surgical and other specialist surgical input may be required at an early stage, depending on the range of associated injuries. There is a frequent requirement for specialist neurosurgical procedures at a later stage. Orthopaedic surgery, skilled orthopaedic assessment and management of associated skeletal injuries is vital, since in the paralysed patient the arms will be needed for transfers. Consequently meticulous treatment of upper limb fractures is required to preserve as much function as possible. It may be too early at the time of injury to assess whether there is potential for standing and walking, and it should be presumed in all patients that at least standing will be achieved and the lower limb fractures must be managed with this goal in mind.

A surgeon with an understanding of spinal injuries is an integral part of the team, and should see all the patients from the outset so that a combined evaluation of the best method of treatment can be made with the physician. The surgeon must be able to examine the patient neurologically as well as orthopaedically, and will require accurate information in the form of plain X-rays and CT scans. Magnetic resonance imaging (MRI) is desirable. The role of tomography and myelography is being reviewed in conjunction with the availability of MRI.

Nursing care

The nursing regime must protect the skin, respiratory and urinary function. Without this, all other attempts at management will flounder. Not least of the nursing duties is reassurance and counselling for these frightened patients whose world has suddenly become horizontal.

Rehabilitation

Rehabilitation commences from the moment of injury as a central and evolving aspect of the management of the whole spinal fracture condition, whatever intercurrent surgical or medical events may be happening (see Chapter 69). Physiotherapists, occupational therapists, psychologists, social workers and others who will construct the framework of a new existence must be involved from the outset.

Immobilization should be minimized. Whilst the patient may have to be recumbent as part of the management of the spinal, pelvic or other fractures, muscular exercise, particularly to develop the respiratory muscles and those above the level of the lesion, should be as vigorous as possible to combat the well-recognized deleterious effects of prolonged immobilization. Indeed, many of the supposed effects of spinal injury and paralysis, such as osteoporosis, hypercalciuria with stone formation and renal and bladder calculosis, deconditioning of the sympathetic nervous system, urinary tract stagnation and psychological problems from boredom, are contributed to in large part by simple immobilization.

Environment

We believe that a patient should be under the care of a single physician who supervises and coordinates the medical, surgical and rehabilitation disciplines from the time of injury until discharge. The patient can be looked after properly only in a unit with access to intensive care, imaging facilities and the full range of specialist services. Furthermore, it is less than ideal for a patient to be admitted to one hospital for treatment for acute injuries, then be transferred to a specialist spinal unit, as this breaks the continuity of rehabilitation. This may conflict with the geographical position of spinal injuries centres as some rehabilitation units are remote from the latest technical and specialist facilities. Whatever facilities are available, simple conservative measures are lifesaving and can give excellent results. More adventurous techniques should be applied only when facilities allow.

Objectives of spinal management

The function of the spinal cord cannot be influenced directly, and our objective should be to achieve the best situation for any residual function to recover. This should be brought about by achieving the best anatomical situation to prevent traction, compression and undue movement at the fracture site with the least associated risk. Concurrently the rest of the body must be maintained in the best state of health and nutrition to allow the area to recover, i.e. prevent anoxia, hypotension, toxicity from urinary infection and pressure sores. From the historical survey it is clear that there has been a great deal of controversy from the outset about the role of operation in spinal injuries. We believe that, having practised conservative treatment for many years, the modern concepts of stability have to be addressed in the context of the overall management of the injury, if the best result is to be achieved for the patient.

Stability

The question of stability remains a central issue in consideration of spinal fractures and their treatment. It is a widely used term which has different meanings to anatomists, bioengineers and clinicians. It is on occcasions an abused term adapted to justify an approach or dogma. White & Panjabi (1978) introduced the concept of 'clinical instability', defining this as the loss of the ability of the spine under physiological loads to maintain relationships between vertebrae in such a way that there is neither damage nor subsequent irritation to the spinal cord or nerve roots, and in addition that there is no development of incapacitating deformity or pain due to structural changes. This stresses the concept that the importance of stability is functional outcome, and does not mention the anatomical shape of the skeleton. The functional outcome is measured in terms of the avoidance of damage to the spinal cord and nerve roots, and in terms of the integrity of the bony support. However, whilst the precise anatomy at the region of the fracture after healing may not be important as long as it supports the body and is painfree, it is important to consider the residual deformity in terms of the stresses and strains placed above and below the level of injury. For example kyphosis in a paraplegic patient with a fracture of the thoracolumbar region will cause the patient to sit on the sacrum and develop pressure sores, even though the spine has not given rise to problems.

Holdsworth (1963) stated that: 'The object of treatment of any fracture or fracture–dislocation of the spine is to restore a painless, powerful, mobile back.' The classification proposed by Holdsworth, which had a major impact on the understanding of thoracolumbar injuries, subdivided the spine into two columns. This was useful in predicting the complexity of spinal injuries, although he insisted that rupture of the posterior column was sufficient to create instability of the spine. Several subsequent experimental studies demonstrate that instability or the ability to subluxate or dislocate appears only after additional rupture of the posterior longitudinal ligament and of the annulus fibrosus. Holdsworth did not acknowledge flexion distraction injuries as reported by Chance in 1948.

A new biomechanical concept and classification was proposed by Denis (1983) following a retrospective study of 412 thoracolumbar injuries. The concept of a middle column or middle osteoligamentous complex, between the traditionally recognized posterior osteoligamentous complex and anterior column, was introduced (see Chapter 68). These proposals highlight the susceptible nature of the thoracolumbar junction area of the spine to injury, given its lack of external support and the changing anatomy, in particular of the facet joints. Fractures in the upper thoracic region are probably the result of much greater forces, reflecting the stability afforded by the rib cage in lesser trauma. This is demonstrated by the frequent association of rib and sternal fractures, together with parenchymal damage. The ribs increase the stability of the thoracic spine in two ways: firstly, the ligamentous complex at the head and neck of the rib and secondly, the rib cage as a unit, which effectively increases the transverse dimensions of the spine. Andriacchi *et al.* (1974) showed that these increase resistance to bending in the sagittal and frontal planes, as well as axial rotation. Not only does the presence of the rib cage dictate a different pattern of injury, but it may also contribute to the different outcomes following fractures. For example, Leidholt *et al.* (1967) noted that complications such as pain and increasing deformity were much less common in the higher thoracic vertebrae than at the thoracolumbar junction.

While the concept of stability in acute injuries concentrates on the potential for damage and the inherent integrity of the spine, scant attention is given to the situation in which that spine is being treated. A structurally unstable spine may unite in an acceptable position with no increased neurological damage when nursed in a skilled fashion by trained nursing staff with adequate time and facilities. The necessity to stabilize such a spine is much more pressing when facilities for conservative treatment are inadequate although, unfortunately, the facilities for proper surgical intervention are then frequently lacking also.

Relationship between surgical and conservative management

The evil effects of the mistreatment of spinal injuries—with the inevitable development of pressure sores, severe urinary sepsis and the abandonment of these patients—gave rise to high morbidity and mortality, and consequently any surgery that was carried out shared this fate. The enthusiasm and self-confidence of those practising conservative management of spinal injuries, and the stature of the early exponents such as Munro and Guttmann, grew during the 1940s, and demonstrated that excellent rehabilitation could be achieved. This led to the adoption in large parts of the United Kingdom and Europe of a conservative regime, which became the mainstream approach, as it was clear that the only satisfactory way that patients with spinal injuries could be looked after was in a well-organized spinal service. Similarly, with the development of spinal services in the United States of America, patients could be looked after without detriment to their condition. The potential role of surgery as an adjunct to this mainstream approach was almost eclipsed. This situation arose for several reasons.

At this time surgical techniques were found wanting. There had been attempts at internal fixation of spinal fractures more than a century previously, by wiring together fractured vertebrae. Almost 100 years later the concept of fixation of the posterior elements behind an unstable injury was advanced by the application of Meurig–Williams plates. Whilst some reports (Lewis & McKibbin, 1974) suggested that there was less deformity and pain after such fixation, others (Burke & Murray, 1976) indicated that those who had been treated surgically fared worse. Guttmann received many patients whose stability had not been enhanced by fixation, and in whom there had been plate cut-out. This served to reinforce his view that surgery was very seldom indicated.

Certainly in the United Kingdom, and in many other countries, the geographical location of spinal injuries rehabilitation centres at some distance from teaching and university hospitals served to isolate them from the advances in spinal surgery. Frequently, those who operated on patients with spinal fractures were utilizing techniques and training founded in surgery of spinal deformity. There was a failure to understand the specific requirements of patients with spinal injuries, particularly those who were paralysed. They did not necessarily follow the patients through into the spinal rehabilitation centres, and did not realize that much of what they achieved technically was inappropriate to the patients' needs. For example, lumbar mobility is fundamental to the independence and rehabilitation of paraplegic patients, and it is generally a disservice to immobilize several lumbar segments if this can possibly be avoided.

Recent techniques

Until very recent times the evolution of spinal stabilization techniques for spinal fractures has paralleled the evolution of techniques used in spinal deformity surgery from where they have been borrowed. Enthusiasm was rekindled following the introduction of Harrington instrumentation for the scoliotic spine in the 1950s. This system of rod and distraction hooks was the mainspring for many techniques that followed, and it was not long before it was being applied to spinal injuries. The principle of this system involved posterior distraction against an intact anterior longitudinal ligament. Reduction was thus achieved by three-point fixation. Whilst an excellent reduction of the involved segment could frequently be achieved, there were disadvantages of this technique more obvious to the nursing and physiotherapy staff who had to mobilize patients and achieve their independence than to the surgeon.

The technical principle involves setting hooks at least two segments above and two segments below the involved level in order to achieve mechanical stability. If the injury is, for example, at L1 then L3 will be incorporated in the stabilization, leaving only three motion segments free below. Moreover, classical Harrington rods with round ends have to be straight, though the square-ended modifications allow contouring and restoration of lumbar lordosis. The principal problem has been the requirement for postoperative bracing to continue for up to six months, which for activities such as long sitting and some transfers, actually delayed rehabilitation.

There were some modifications to this technique, such as those involving short fusion with long rodding, allowing later removal of rods with the idea of the restoration of motion segments. However, immobilization of motion segments, particularly under distraction for several months, results in facet joint and disc degeneration (Kahanovitz *et al.*, 1984).

Following the emergence of Luque sublaminal wiring techniques, the stability of the Harrington distraction system could be greatly enhanced by sublaminal wiring of additional segments. This reduced the requirement for prolonged postoperative bracing, and was a significant advance. For fracture dislocations or subluxations, with intrinsic stability under compressive load when reduced, the use of Luque rods offered a high degree of immediate stability, obviating the necessity for postoperative bracing. However, it is still necessary to incorporate at least two levels above and two below the plane of injury (this may include the vertebra immediately below a dislocation).

For these short fusions, rectangles such as the Hartshill rectangle are superior to the classical double 'L' rod of Luque, having greater torsional stability. Moreover the implant can readily be contoured, improving reduction by the three-point principle. The philosophy of both segmental fixation and posterior vertebral hold with possible distraction has evolved further with the Cotrel–Dubousset instrumentation.

It has been proposed that decompression can be achieved by distraction, in particular with the use of Harrington rods. The theory is that the posterior longitudinal ligament remains intact, and when distracted is pulled straight, thus projecting fragments of vertebral body forward like a bowstring. While some series demonstrate this to be true, others are less convincing, and it is yet to be shown that such a manoeuvre actually improves neurological outcome.

Principles of surgery

The imperfections of these techniques perpetuated the reluctance of physicians convinced by the efficacy of conservative techniques to consider a surgical solution to the fracture itself. An ideal method of fracture stabilization should incorporate the following features.

1 Short segment fusion. Stabilization should only involve the injured level if possible (Fig. 66.4).

2 The fixation should not require postoperative immobilization.

3 Techniques should not increase the risks of secondary damage.

4 Sitting up and early mobilization and an accelerated rehabilitation programme should be achieved.

There will always be a complication rate, but this should be sufficiently low that the problems provoked by surgery in the few should not outweigh the advantages for the majority. It was the realization that the pedicle can be used as a fixation site that moved us towards such a technical solution to fracture fixation, and is making this option attractive. Roy-Camille had been using pedicular screw fixation through internal plates for some time, but there was no intrinsic stability between the screw and the plate itself. Current systems used in fracture surgery have evolved from the external fixation device of Magerl (1984), first used in 1977. Schanz screws were passed through the pedicles into the vertebral bodies and were clamped to an external fixation frame, allowing distraction and reduction of thoracolumbar injuries.

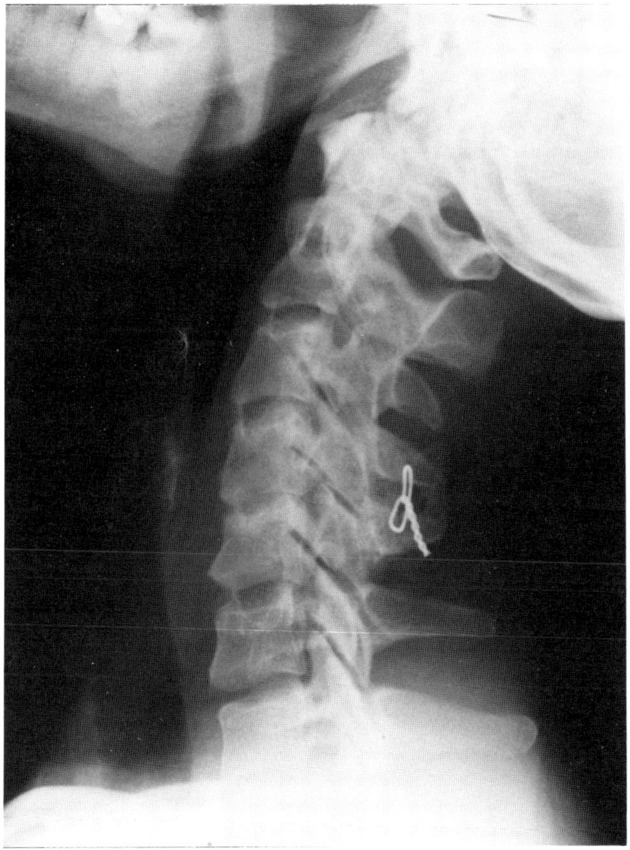

Fig. 66.4 Stabilization should, if possible, involve only the injured segments. Preservation of cervical spine mobility is particularly important in high cervical lesions as head movement may be a means of communication, through writing and computers, and mobility by means of a wheelchair joy stick.

It was a short step in logic to provide an internal frame, and there are now a variety of such *fixateur internes*, in particular those developed by Dick, Kluger and Olerud. Moreover, Cotrel and Dubousset have also adapted their instrumentation to use pedicle screw constructs.

Whatever system of fixation is used, proper techniques of bone spinal fusion must not be overlooked. Facet joint excision, decortication and application of bone graft are essential, otherwise metalwork failure is likely.

Other techniques of anterior stabilization, anterior decompression and combined anterior and posterior surgery are discussed in Chapter 68.

Surgery is an option in the management of spinal injuries. Both the decision whether to operate and the nature of the surgery itself are matters of judgement. Surgery can be more or less aggressive, and it may in many cases be prudent to stop short of the most technically adventurous intervention in a particular patient. Decisions on the nature of the operation may depend upon:

1 local circumstances,
2 the surgical expertise,
3 the equipment and implants available,
4 availability of high-quality standard X-rays, special views, tomograms, CT scans and MRI scans.

Specific surgical techniques are discussed in detail in other chapters, but a brief mention of general principles is appropriate here.

Cervical spine

BIFACETAL DISLOCATION

A bifacetal dislocation should be reduced as quickly as possible at the receiving hospital. In the majority of cases there will be severe neurological damage from the initial trauma, probably caused by the immediate destruction of the cord by a violent dislocation, but further neurological damage will occur because of swelling. When the canal diameter is jeopardized by a bifacetal dislocation these changes will be accentuated, and there will also be severe pain at the level of the dislocation. The method of reduction is controversial, but it would appear that there is no need to wait for graduated reduction over 48 hours. It should be done rapidly under image intensification with frequent sequential increase in weight to a maximum of 24 kg depending on the level, monitored by a regular neurological examination. If the reduction cannot be achieved within six hours or less, then one manipulation can be performed, but the surgeon should be prepared to proceed directly to open reduction, accompanied by wiring plus bony fusion. Wiring alone is inadvisable, since wires have been seen to cut out subsequently. The first few hours are critical, and patients should not have the diagnosis or treatment delayed. They should not be subjected to repeated manipulations, nor should they be transferred with an unreduced dislocation. If more than 12 hours are allowed to elapse after dislocation the pathological changes and increased swelling make the reduction difficult and the outcome poor.

The method of reduction is controversial. Walton (1893), and subsequently Evans (1961), introduced the method of reduction by manipulation. A comparison between two units in Australia (Osti *et al.*, 1989) has shown that there is a lower morbidity in bifacetal dislocation if manipulation is carried out rather than an open reduction in the first instance. In a small number of cases there may be no or minimal neurological damage at the outset, but after a period of hours if the dislocation is left unreduced, swelling, cord changes and a delayed paralysis appear (Mahale & Silver, 1992). It is vital in these cases that reduction be achieved as quickly as possible.

UNIFACETAL DISLOCATION

The same principles apply as in a bifacetal dislocation except that the chances of missing the diagnosis are much higher, even when adequate X-rays are taken. Ideally, the dislocation should be reduced in the same way and as quickly as a bifacetal dislocation. The problem arises in the cases that are seen late with little neurological impairment and often minimal pain. Each case must be assessed individually, but in general it may be desirable to accept some deformity and fuse the vertebrae *in situ* (if they have not fused spontaneously) rather than attempt to reduce the dislocated spine.

EXTENSION INJURIES

There is a group of cases who present with a tetraplegia of the cervical spine without bony injury. There are various suggestions as to the pathology. The majority of these occur in elderly people and are due to a transverse tear to a disc. It is impossible to determine without sophisticated radiology whether they are stable or unstable. The situation becomes apparent only later, after the patient has been sat up, when there has been disc narrowing or the vertebrae have slipped. These patients should be immobilized between sandbags for six weeks, flexion/extension radiographs carried out, and then cautiously mobilized in a firm collar. Should they prove to be unstable they will require fusion as in any other group.

There is another group of patients, much smaller, where there is unquestionably no injury to the spinal column, and this can only be determined by CT scans, MRI and dynamic views. These patients can be mobilized straight away but there can be no *a priori* views as to the stability of these fractures based on limited radiographical findings.

Thoracic injuries

The view that the upper thoracic spine is supported by the rib cage, and the view that fractures in this region are splinted by the ribs, is debatable. Many of the injuries in this region, whether they be burst fractures, anterior wedging, or full fracture dislocations, give rise to a severe kyphosis. Fifty per cent of patients with upper thoracic fractures have fractured ribs and a haemothorax, and some have widening of the mediastinum; so that the major thrust of management is directed at the visceral chest injury. Consequently the patient is frequently too ill to sustain early surgery irrespective of whether the cord is involved. Improvement in the spinal alignment can frequently be achieved by postural reduction. However, this must be maintained for eight to ten weeks, followed up by three-point extension brace to prevent secondary collapse back to the position on presentation. This regression is frequently seen. It is questionable whether such fractures can ever be permanently controlled.

INJURIES WITH MINOR DISPLACEMENT

Whether there is neurological involvement or not, these injuries are well treated by conservative methods which are safe and effective. As pedicles are frequently too small to accept screws above T8 the internal fixation of upper thoracic fractures often involves extending over several levels with Harrington or Luque techniques. There is potential neurological morbidity from sublaminal wires or hooks, and late pain is seen with these methods of fixation.

FRACTURE–DISLOCATIONS

These frequently unite, but may cause late problems particularly when associated with lateral wedging. If there is a significant kyphotic segment there will be pain above and below where compensatory movements are taking place. In order to hold the head up the patient may need to sit on his sacrum, thus leading to an increase in pressure sores (Fig. 66.5). We have carried out a number of late reconstructions for this deformity. Vertebral body excision and considerable rearrangement of chest anatomy is required, with a high attendant morbidity. In order to prevent this late problem, early open reduction and fixation should be considered.

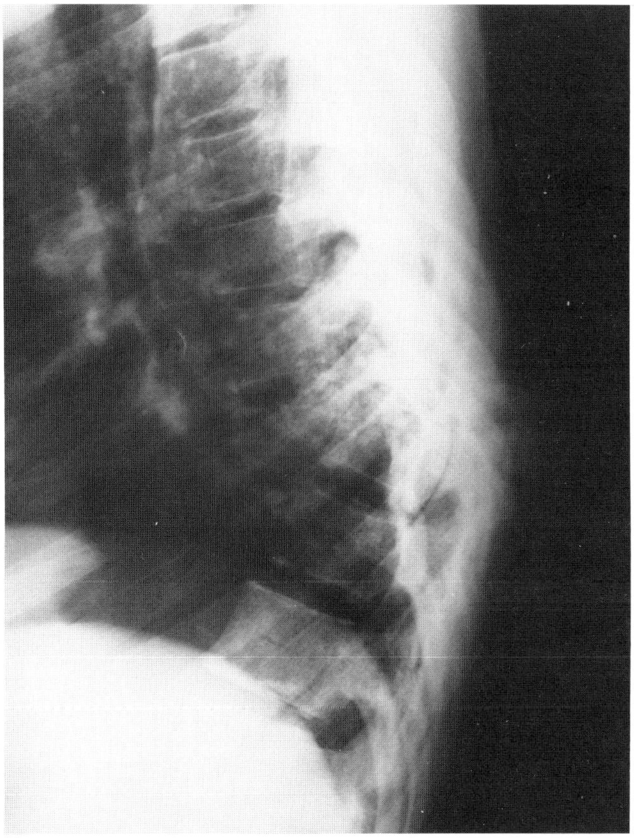

Fig. 66.5 Kyphotic deformity persists in this D8–D9 fracture–dislocation one year after injury. This was associated with a complete T6 paraplegia. Although this spinal injury, despite the deformity, was not itself causing any symptoms there were considerable difficulties in avoiding sacral sores because of sacral sitting.

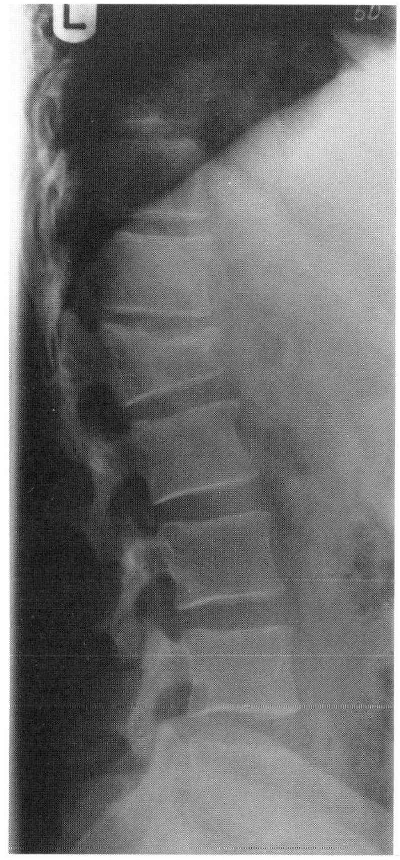

Fig. 66.6 Six months following T12–L1 burst fracture without any neurological involvement, this 42-year-old patient returned to his active light engineering employment without significant spinal symptoms.

Thoracolumbar injuries

These injuries may respond well to conservative management (Fig. 66.6). There is no clear evidence to suggest an open reduction or stabilization improves neurological recovery, but there is some evidence, particularly if there is significant kyphosis, to suggest that surgery decreases the long-term chances of pain and deformity (Fig. 66.7). However, surgery must be restricted to a very small number of segments in order to preserve lumbar mobility which is vital for the paraplegic patient. Older techniques of Harrington rod fixation, or even sublaminal wiring, which must at the very least include four vertebrae and usually five or more, have been superseded by pedicle screw fixation, which may safely stabilize as little as one motion segment and allow early mobilization. Surgery is probably of little benefit unless it allows early mobility.

Lumbar fractures

The most important consideration is preservation of lumbar mobility in the paraplegic patient, and this same principle applies to those without neurological involvement, so long as this does not compromise the neurological situation. As for thoracolumbar fractures, unless there is marked displacement, conservative approaches will still give very good results. If internal fixation is to be considered, then this really should, if at all possible, involve very short segment fusion with anterior techniques or posterior pedicle screw systems.

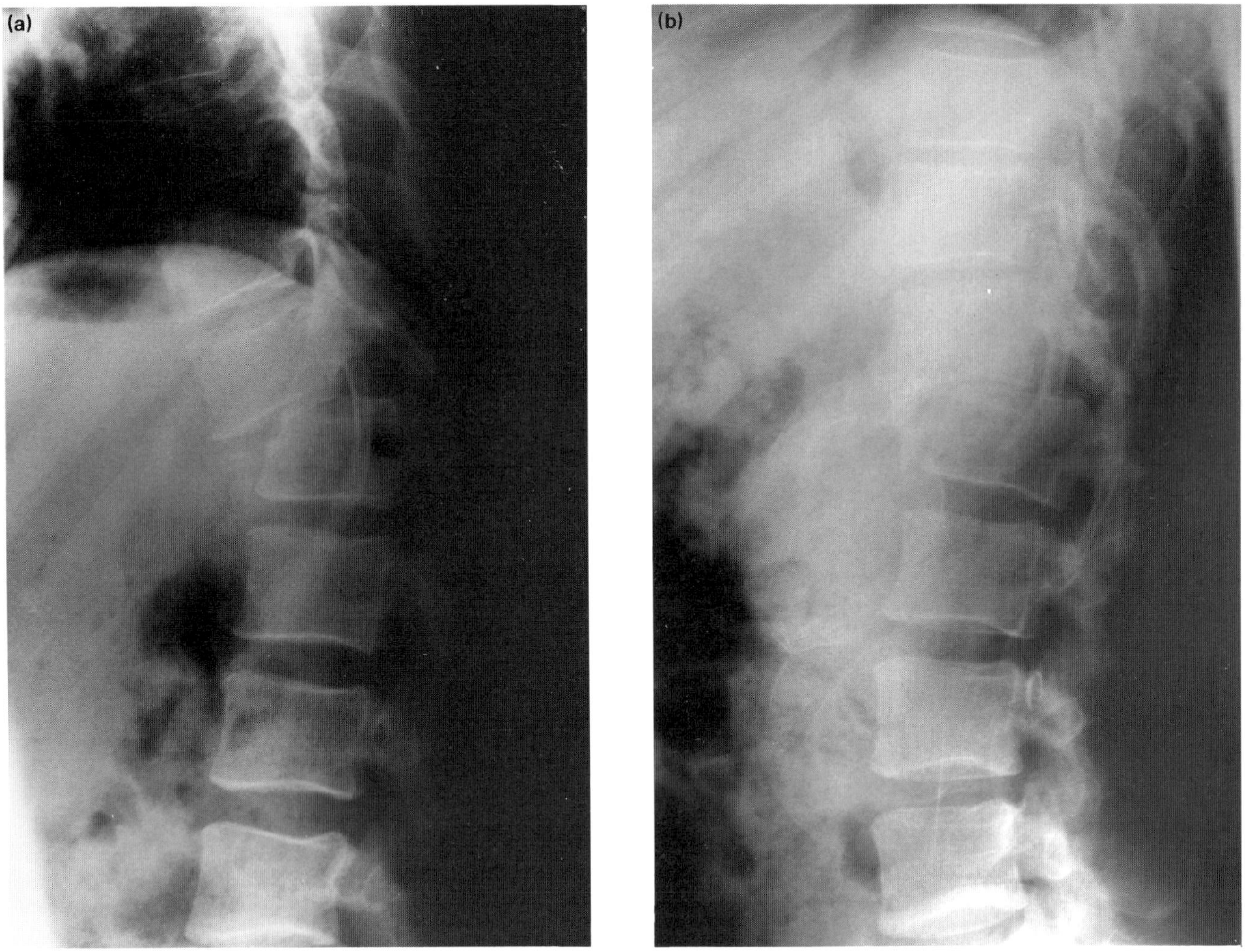

Fig. 66.7 Twelve months following T12–L1 fracture–dislocation with complete paraplegia persistent pain may arise from occult instability. Immediate flexion–extension films may not show movement, but flexion pictures (a) taken after 30 minutes sitting bent forward compared with extension pictures (b) taken 30 minutes after lying extended over a block, demonstrate clearly that movement is present.

Present approach

We have set out earlier the results of conservative management.

Since operations were rarely practised in the early years, less and less attention was paid to the position of the fracture after the initial treatment, unless pain and deformity became very obtrusive. However, in recent years we have modified our approach so that surgical techniques are now invoked in certain situations. We have analysed the results of 100 consecutive patients admitted between September 1983 and April 1989 presenting with traumatic skeletal or cord injury from C2–L5.

The patients were comparable in age, level of lesion and other parameters to those admitted to other spinal centres from western societies. Half were due to traffic accidents and half had cervical injuries. The age distribution was also similar, with 44 of the patients being under the age of 24, and 65 being under the age of 34.

In order for there to be a choice between conservative and surgical management the patients must be admitted within a week, and ideally within 24 hours of injury. This allows the associated injuries to be dealt with at the same time as the management of the spinal injury, before complications have developed which may prevent surgical management of the

Table 66.3 Associated injuries

	Patients admitted less than one month from injury	Patients admitted between one and two months from injury
Total no. of patients	68	13
No. of patients with associated injury	31	11
Injury severe enough to delay rehabilitation		
Total	20	7
Head	3	4
Chest	10	3
Abdomen	1	1
Pelvis	1	3
Brachial plexus	3	—
Limb	8	3
Additional minor injuries	7	2
Injury not severe enough to delay rehabilitation		
Total	11	4
Head	6	1
Chest	2	3
Limb	4	1

The remaining 18 patients were admitted more than two months after injury.

Table 66.4 Operative intervention summary

	Cervical	Thoracic and lumbar	No. bone injury
Total no. of patients	52	41	7
Total no. of patients operated on	20	16	
Patients operated on early:			
Prior to NSIC	4	11	
At NSIC	7	4	
Patients operated on late (at NSIC)	9	1	

spine. For example by the time pressure sores can be healed, the spine may have united in an unsatisfactory position. This was not always possible in the series, and only 48 of the patients came in within a week of injury.

In common with other series, of the patients admitted less than a month after injury, 31 had associated injuries of considerable severity, and in 20 of these they were severe enough to delay rehabilitation. The proportion of those admitted late with severe associated injuries was greater. The severely injured no doubt were not fit for transfer in the early stages (Table 66.3).

We did not have the choice of either surgical intervention or conservative management as we would have wished, since 15 patients had had surgery prior to being referred (Tables 66.4 & 66.5). Despite our inclination to a more aggressive approach, our management was essentially conservative, in that 77 patients were treated conservatively, and only 11 were operated on as a primary procedure. Ten patients following a regime of conservative management required secondary surgery, nine of which were cervical spines where the injury was found to be unstable on mobilization. This has led to more aggressive selection of cases for early surgery.

In common with the objective of surgical stabilization of lower thoracic lumbar fractures over the

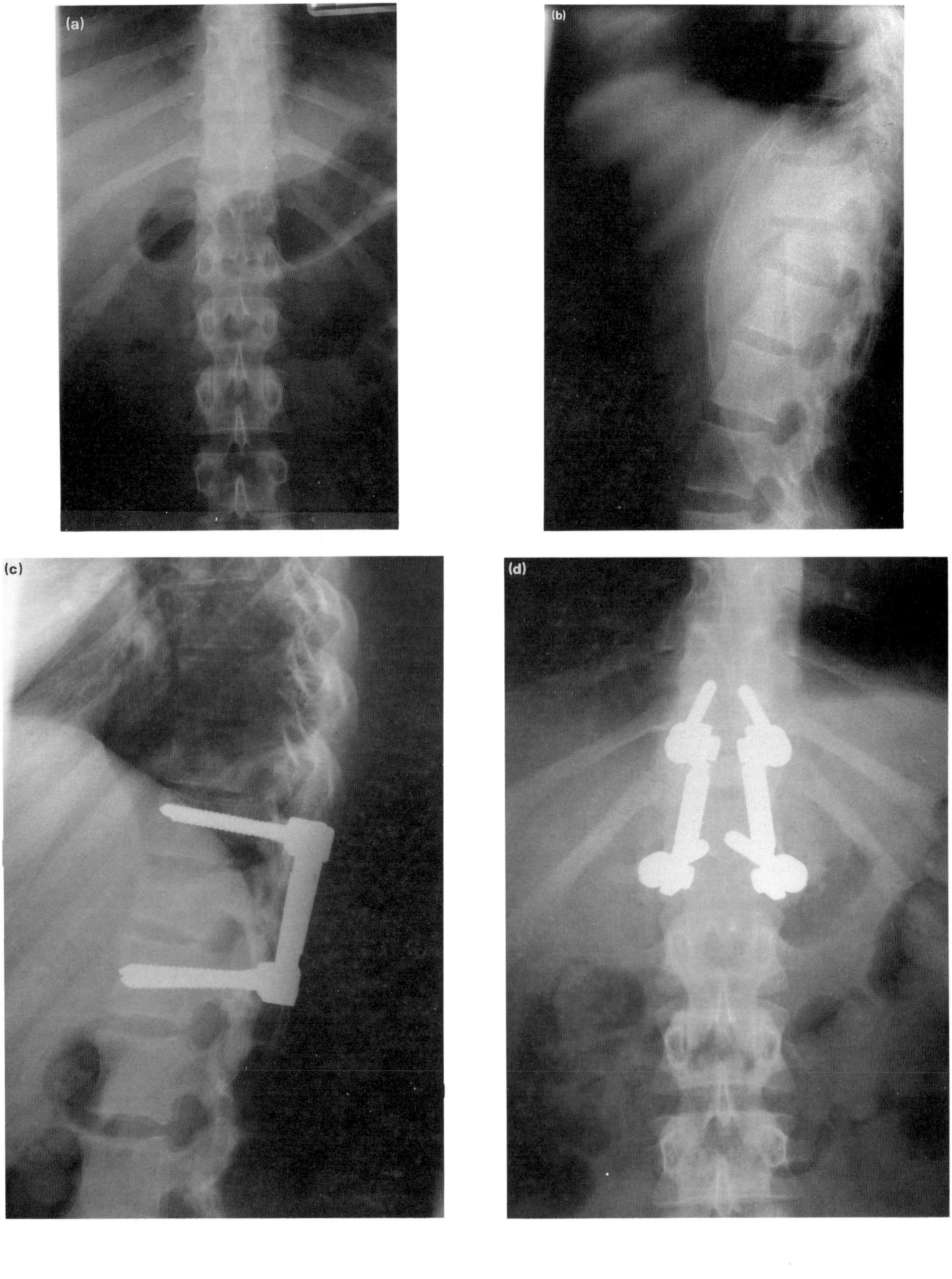
(a)
(b)
(c)
(d)

Table 66.5 This table shows the source of admission of those patients who were brought in at less than two months from injury. The source of admission is important as an indicator of the style of immediate management. Skills and facilities required for specialist spinal surgery might not be available in every district general hospital (information not available in two cases)

District general hospital	55
Teaching hospital	13
Neurosurgical unit	7
Oxford	3
Abroad	20

shortest possible segment we are now using Kluger type of *fixateur interne* (Fig. 66.8). Preliminary review of our first 10 cases with a mean follow-up of one year shows encouraging results. Excellent correction of kyphosis and alignment has been achieved except in one case where intervention was too late to achieve satisfactory reduction. This stabilization has not influenced neurological outcome but rehabilitation has been accelerated, with patients being able to sit or stand by two weeks from surgery.

The whole management of the spinal injury is teamwork. It is vital to have the input of orthopaedic surgeons, neurosurgeons and chest physicians. This is achieved by involving all these disciplines from the outset, and by regular weekly combined rounds, so that they are not just called in for crisis management when a problem has occurred. Thereby each member of the team acquires knowledge of the full spectrum of spinal injury. If the best result in terms of independence and reintegration into the community for the patient is to be achieved, the management of the spinal fracture, though important, is only part of the total management of the patient.

Unanswered questions

Many questions remain unanswered in the field of spinal injuries. For example it is known that there is a higher incidence of post-traumatic syringomyelia in patients with thoracic injuries, and that a small cyst occurs at the level of injury. How is this related to post-traumatic syringomyelia, and does the initial management alter the manifestations of the condition?

What is the role of disc protrusion in the pathogenesis of spinal cord injury, given that rupture of a disc is found in 50% of spinal injuries? (Bohlman, 1979). Does removal of this disc influence subsequent recovery? What is the place of anterior approaches for reconstruction and stabilization of a shattered vertebral body?

These and many other questions will have to be answered in the future, but the fact that we are in a position to pose such questions is a tribute to the extraordinary visionary pioneering work of Munro and Guttmann. Munro showed—by his practical approach of regularly turning the patient, stopping unnecessary operations on the spine, and preserving bladder function—that the patients could be returned to a useful life, and that rehabilitation was possible for those patients who had previously been condemned to a lingering death from pressure sores.

It is Guttmann, with his great organizing ability, vision and fundamental research training with Foester, who in the postwar years pioneered the development of a comprehensive spinal service throughout the United Kingdom, Europe and latterly the world.

This chapter has really been a tribute to these two great men, who pioneered the work and made possible a dignified life for all disabled people; since by showing how paraplegic and tetraplegic patients could be kept alive and lead full significant lives, that the paraplegic patients have served as a model for all those disabled, leading subsequently to the founding of the international sporting movement.

REFERENCES

Andriacchi, T., Schultz, A., Belytschko, T. & Galante, J. (1974) A model for studies of mechanical interactions between the human spine and rib cage. *J. Biomech.*, 7, 497–507.

Bell, Sir Charles (1824) *Observations on Injuries of the Spine and the Thigh Bone*, pp. 3–31. Kegg, London.

Bell, C. (1838) *Case of Diastasis of Subluxation of the Spine, Fatal*. Institutes of Surgery, vol. 1, pp. 150–153. Adam & Charles Black, Edinburgh.

Fig. 66.8 (*Opposite*) This 18-year-old girl sustained a complete paraplegia in association with a T11–T12 fracture–dislocation. This has been reduced and held by a Kluger *fixateur interne* and bone grafting. Considerable correction in alignment has been achieved, as demonstrated by comparing the preoperative radiographs (a) and (b) with those taken four months later (c) and (d).

Bohlman, H.H. (1979) Acute fractures and dislocations of the cervical spine. *J. Bone Jt. Surg.*, **61A**, 8. 1119–1141.

Bracken, M.B., Shepard, M.J., Collins, W.F. *et al.* (1990) A randomized controlled trial & methylprednisolone or naloxone in the treatment of acute spinal-cord injury. *N. Engl. J. Med.*, **322**, 1405–1411.

Breasted, J.H. (1930) *The Edwin Smith Surgical Papyrus*, vol. 1, pp. 316–342, 425–428. Chicago University Press, Chicago, IL.

Breig, A., Silver, J.R. & Renard, M. (1989) *Skull Traction and Cervical Cord Injury*. Springer, Berlin.

Burke, D.C. & Murray, D.D. (1976) The management of thoracic and thoracolumbar injuries of the spine with neurological involvement. *J. Bone Jt. Surg.*, **58B**, 72–78.

Campbell, E.H. (1959) The Mediterranean (formerly North African) theater of operations. Surgery in World War II. *Neurosurgery*, **II**, 19–23.

Chance, G.Q. (1948) Note on a type of flexion fracture of the spine. *Br. J. Radiol.*, **21**, 452–453.

Comarr, A.E. (1959) Laminectomy in patients with injuries of the spinal cord. *J. Int. Coll. Surg.*, **31**, 437–442.

Cooper, Sir Astley P. (1823) *A Treatise on Dislocations and Fractures of the Joints*, pp. 536–562. Longman, Hurst, Rees, Orme and Browne, London.

Cooper, A.P. (1824) Lecture 19 of Injuries of the Spine. *Lancet*, **1**, 394–398.

Curling, T.B. (1833) Essays on affections of the bladder in paraplegia. *Lond. Med. Gaz.*, **13**, 76–80.

Curling, T.B. (1836) Further observations on affections of the bladder in paraplegia. *Lond. Med. Gaz.*, **18**, 325–331.

Curling, T.B. (1842) On acute ulceration of the duodenum, in cases of burns. *Med. Chir. Trans.*, **25**, 260–281.

Cushing, H. (1927) Organisation and activities of the Neurological Service, American Expeditionary Forces. In *The Medical Department of the United States Army in the World War*, vol. XI(1), pp. 749–758. Government Printing Office, Washington.

Denis, F. (1983) The three column spine and its significance in the classification of acute thoracolumbar spinal injuries. *Spine*, **8**, 817–831.

Evans, D.K. (1961) Reduction of cervical dislocations. *J. Bone Jt. Surg.*, **43B**, 552–555.

Fabricius, Ab Aquapendente (1661) *Oeuvres Chirurgicales*, p. 633. Lyon

Fagge, C.H. (1891) *Textbook of the Principles and Practice of Medicine*, 3rd edn, vols I & II. J.&A. Churchill, London.

Frankel, H.L., El Masri, W.S. & Ravichandran, G. (1987) Non-operative treatment—rehabilitation and outcome. In Harris, P. *Thoracic and Lumbar Spine and Spinal Cord Injuries*, pp. 139–170. Springer, Vienna.

Frankel, H.L., Hancock, D.O., Hyslop, G., Melzak, J., Michaelis, L.S., Ungar, G.H., Vernon, J.D.S. & Walsh, J.J. (1969) The value of postural reduction in the initial management of closed injuries of the spine with paraplegia and tetraplegia. *Paraplegia*, **7**, 179–192.

Frazier, C.H. & Allen, A.R. (1918) *Surgery of the Spine and Spinal Cord*. Appleton, New York.

Gull, Sir W.W. (1856) Causes of paraplegia (with autopsies of Ataxic cases, showing lesions in the posterior columns of the spinal cord). *Guy's Hosp. Rep.*, **2**, 143–190.

Gull, Sir W.W. (1858) Causes of paraplegia (with autopsies of ataxic cases, showing lesions in the posterior columns of the spinal cord). *Guy's Hosp. Rep.*, **4**, 169–216.

Guttmann, L. (1949) Paralysis—management of. In Carling, Sir R., & Ross J.P. (eds), *British Surgical Practice, Malingering to Peritoneum and Peritonitis*, vol. 6, pp. 445–466. Butterworth, London.

Guttmann, Sir Ludwig (1973) *Spinal Cord Injuries, Comprehensive Management and Research*. Blackwell Scientific Publications, Oxford.

Hardy, A.G. (1965) Treatment of paraplegia due to fracture–dislocation of the dorso-lumbar spine. *Paraplegia*, **3**, 112.

Head, H. & Riddoch, G. (1917) The automatic bladder, excessive sweating and some other reflex conditions in gross injuries of the spinal cord. *Brain*, **40**, 188–263.

Holdsworth, F.W. (1963) Fractures, dislocations, and fracture–dislocations of the spine. *J. Bone Jt. Surg.*, **45B**, 6–20.

Holdsworth, F.W. & Hardy, A. (1953) Early treatment of paraplegia from fractures of the thoraco-lumbar spine. *J. Bone Jt. Surg.*, **35B**, 540–551.

Holmes, G. (1915a) The Goulstonian lectures on spinal injuries of warfare. I: The pathology of acute spinal injuries. *Br. Med. J.*, **2**, 769–774.

Holmes, G. (1915b) The Goulstonian lectures on spinal injuries of warfare. II: The clinical symptoms of gunshot injuries of the spine. *Br. Med. J.*, **2**, 815–821.

Holmes, G. (1915c) The Goulstonian lectures on spinal injuries of warfare. III: The sensory disturbances in spinal injuries. *Br. Med. J.*, **2**, 855–861.

Hutchinson, J. (1866) On dislocations and fractures of the spine. *Clinical Lectures and Reports, The London Hospital*, vol. III, pp. 357–372.

Kahanowitz, N., Bullough, P. & Jacobs, R.R. (1984) The effect of internal fixation without arthrodesis on human facet joint cartilage. *Clin. Orthop. Rel. Res.* **189**, 204–205.

Lanfranc (1894) *Science of Cirurgie*, pp. 317–318, 322–323. Early English Text Society, Berlin.

Leidhold, J.D., Young, J.Y., Hahn, H.R., Jackson, R.E., Gamble, W.E. & Miles, J.S. (1967) Evaluation of late spinal deformities with fracture–dislocations of the dorsal and lumbar spine in paraplegics. *Paraplegia*, **7**, 16–23.

Lewis, J. & McKibbin, B. (1974) The treatment of unstable fracture–dislocations of the thoraco-lumbar spine accompanied by paraplegia. *J. Bone Jt. Surg.*, **56B**, 603–612.

Magerl, F.T. (1984) Stabilisation of the lower thoracic and lumbar spine with external skeletal fixation. *Clin. Orthop. Rel. Res.*, **189**, 124–141.

Mahale, Y.J. & Silver, J.R. (1991) Progressive paralysis after bilateral dislocation of the cervical spine. *J. Bone Jt. Surg.*, **74B** (In press).

Munro, D. (1936) Activity of the urinary bladder as measured by a new and inexpensive cystometer. *N. Engl. J. Med.*, **214**, 617–624.

Munro, D. (1943) Thoracic and lumbosacral cord injuries. *J. Am. Med. Assoc.*, **122**, 1055–1063.

Nicoll, E.A. (1949) Fractures of the dorso-lumbar spine. *J. Bone Jt. Surg.*, **31B**, 376–394.

Osti, O.L., Fraser, R.D. & Griffiths, E.R. (1989) Reduction

and stabilisation of cervical dislocations. *J. Bone Jt. Surg.*, **71B**, 275–282.

Pare, A. (1564) *Dix-Livres de la Chirurgie, avec le Magasin des Instruments Necessaires a Icelle.* Jean le Royer, Paris.

Pare A. (1598) *Oeuvres*, pp. 528, 554–559. Paris.

Petit, J.L. (1705) *Traite des Maladies Os*, pp. 46–63. Paris.

Prather, G.C. (1959) Urologic aspects of spinal cord injuries. *Surgery In World War II. Neurosurgery*, II, chap. VI, pp. 67–125. US Government Printing Office, Washington, DC.

Ravichandran, G. & Silver, J.R. (1982) Missed injuries of the spinal cord. *Br. Med. J.*, **284**, 953–956.

Riches, E.W. (1943) Methods and results of treatment in cases of paralysis of bladder following spinal injury. *Br. J. Surg.*, **31**, 135–146.

Scultetus, J. (1674) *The Chyrugeons Store-House.* John Starkey, London.

Silver, J.R. (1980) The management of physical disabilities. In Nicholls, P.J.R. (ed.) *Rehabilitation Medicine*, pp. 223–250. Butterworth London.

Silver, J.R. & Buxton, P.H. (1974) Spinal stoke. *Brain*, **97**, 539–550.

Spurling, G. (1959) European Theatre of Operations, *Neurosurgery*, **II**, 66–68.

Thorburn, W. (1889) *A Contribution to the Surgery of the Spinal Cord.* Griffin, London.

Toscano, J. (1988) Prevention of neurological deterioration before admission to a spinal cord injury unit. *Paraplegia*, **26**, 143–150.

Walker J.W.T. (1937) The treatment of the bladder in spinal injuries in the war. *Brit. J. Urol.*, **9**, 217–230.

Walton, G.L. (1893) A new method of reducing dislocation of cervical vertebrae. *J. Nerv. Ment. Dis.*, **20**, 609–611.

Watson-Jones, Sir R. (1949) Fractures of the spine. *J. Bone Jt. Surg.*, **31B**, 322–323.

White, A.A. & Panjabi, M.M. (1978) *Clinical Biomechanics of the Spine.* Lippincott, Philadelphia, PA.

Woodhall, B. (1959) Historical note. *Surgery in World War II. Neurosurgery*, II, chap. I, pp. 3–4. US Government Printing Office, Washington, DC.

67 · Surgical Treatment of Midcervical Spinal Injuries

By E.B. RISKA

Midcervical spinal injuries are a potential source of prolonged and sometimes permanent disability, but the risk of neurological catastrophe and instability can often be minimized and even eliminated by prompt and judicious primary treatment and early surgery. An important maxim in this context is that neck injury is often masked in patients with multiple injuries, posing diagnostic problems and the possibility of disaster neurologically.

The pathology of spinal cord and nerve root damage following spinal trauma, also the secondary changes that ensue, especially vascular and biochemical, are adequately discussed elsewhere in this text. We believe that these deleterious changes can be greatly minimized especially in cervical trauma by prompt decompression and reconstitution of the spinal canal at the level of injury followed by surgical stabilization. We appreciate that there is still much to be learnt about the microanatomy of the cervical cord and of the metabolic disturbance to neural tissue that occurs following direct compression, distortion and torsion. Nevertheless it seems reasonable that the deleterious effects of secondary oedema and haemorrhage such as chromatolysis, necrosis and axonal death can be greatly minimized by such early surgery.

Prior to any intervention, however, a very accurate assessment of both the neurological state of the patient and the degree of neck instability is essential, although at the primary examination this may be very difficult for many reasons.

In our own unit serving a population of one million people, a substantial number of patients with midcervical spinal injuries are admitted annually, often suffering from multiple injuries. We estimate that a third of patients sustaining severe neck injuries die prior to admission, although with the advances in primary care at the site of accident and during transportation the chances of survival have much improved. Following admission we are convinced that the prospects of limiting neurological disability or even gaining full recovery are much enhanced by practising our policy of early surgical interventions in appropriate cases.

Indications for surgical treatment

The majority of midcervical spinal injuries can be treated conservatively, but if for any reason skeletal traction and manipulative reduction is unsuccessful operative reduction must be entertained early; furthermore surgical stabilization is indicated in those cases in which skull traction is not successful in maintaining the reduced position, as otherwise neurological embarrassment may ensue.

We would go further and state that all cases with unstable fractures of the cervical spine—including those with disruption of posterior ligaments, fracture–dislocations and extension and flexion injuries associated with rotational instability—should be treated by operative stabilization. Surgery in our view is indicated in those cases with compression of the spinal cord where reduction and decompression has not been achieved by conservative means (Green *et al.*, 1981). In these cases decompression should be undertaken early in order to offer the best possible chance of neurological improvement. We appreciate, of course, that this is a controversial stance and that other authorities might be more circumspect in their approach (see Chapter 66).

The mechanism of injury

The majority of severe fractures and dislocations of the midcervical spine are caused by traffic accidents. The frontal motor vehicle crash usually results in flexion–dislocation injuries, whereas the reverse involves a whiplash injury which might be unstable if rotational forces contributing to the trauma mechanism resulting in extension–subluxation. High-speed vehicular accidents associated with rotational forces may result in extremely unstable situations in the cervical spine (Stauffer, 1986). Motorcycle accidents are often associated with injuries to the lower cervical spine with vertebral body compression and fracture–dislocations of varying degrees. Diving into shallow water, or falling from heights, result in compression burst fractures and extension fracture–dislocations, especially in the lower region of the cervical spine (Bateman, 1978). Suicide attempts may have the added problem of multiple injuries; therefore, careful examination of these patients is most important and treatment should be commenced as soon as possible. By contrast, unstable neck injuries may also follow apparently simple falls, especially in the elderly.

Primary treatment at the scene of accident

Management of injured patients prior to hospital admission has improved greatly in recent times. Training of individuals working in the ambulance services in most countries has achieved a high standard, so that personnel are familiar with evaluating patients, taking care of ventilatory problems, controlling external bleeding and, if necessary, immobilizing the injured cervical spine with collars and sandbags during transportation. If necessary they will administer resuscitation by supplemental oxygen via face-mask or nasal cannulae. In some cases intubation might be necessary. Concurrently circulatory support by intravenous lines and plasma expanders might be practised (Garfin *et al.*, 1989). If spinal injury is suspected assessment and recording of motor and sensory function should be undertaken at the scene of the accident before transferring the patient, as the clinical status might change radically during transportation.

Finally transfer to a properly equipped trauma centre is essential, particularly where the spinal cord-injured patient is in need of sophisticated diagnostic and therapeutic skills *ab initio*. Transporting patients with neck injuries from one hospital to another is to be vigorously discouraged.

Clinical diagnosis

The monitoring of motor function and sensation of the extremities and taking a detailed case history is most important, because the neurological situation may be very labile. Frankel's classification is used to grade spinal cord function (Frankel *et al.*, 1969). In Group I there is complete motor paralysis and sensory loss; in Group II there is paralysis with incomplete sensory loss; in Group III there is some motor power below the injured segment but of no practical use; in Group IV there is useful motor power with incomplete sensory loss and in Group V there is normal motor and sensory function. Registering bladder function and repeated examination of the anal sphincter are important elements of routine examination, as well as noting the anal wink, bulbocavernosus, cremasteric, and the Babinski reflexes. Thus a careful clinical examination is paramount in estimating the severity of the cervical spinal injury (Osti *et al.*, 1989).

Laboratory tests such as blood gas values and the oxygen content of the arterial blood complete the picture (Garfin *et al.*, 1989). Such data concerning ventilation and oxygenation are also valuable during transportation in some cases. In patients with multiple injuries the situation is somewhat different. The ABC regime takes priority in the emergency room and subsequent operations follow in order of importance.

Radiological investigation

Plain films by anteroposterior (Fig. 67.1) and lateral projections (Fig. 67.2) are taken in all cases, together with oblique views (Fig. 67.3). Because the whole cervical spine including the first thoracic vertebra should be examined, the 'swimmers' projection (Fig. 67.4) provides useful information in visualizing the cervicothoracic junction. In many cases a lateral tomogram (Fig. 67.5) is indicated, giving precise detail of the extent of the fracture. Computerized tomography (CT) of the affected vertebra will give additional information regarding the stability of the injured segment (Fig. 67.6). This is indicated in fractures involving the middle and posterior columns. In some cases myelography (Fig. 67.7) might be required,

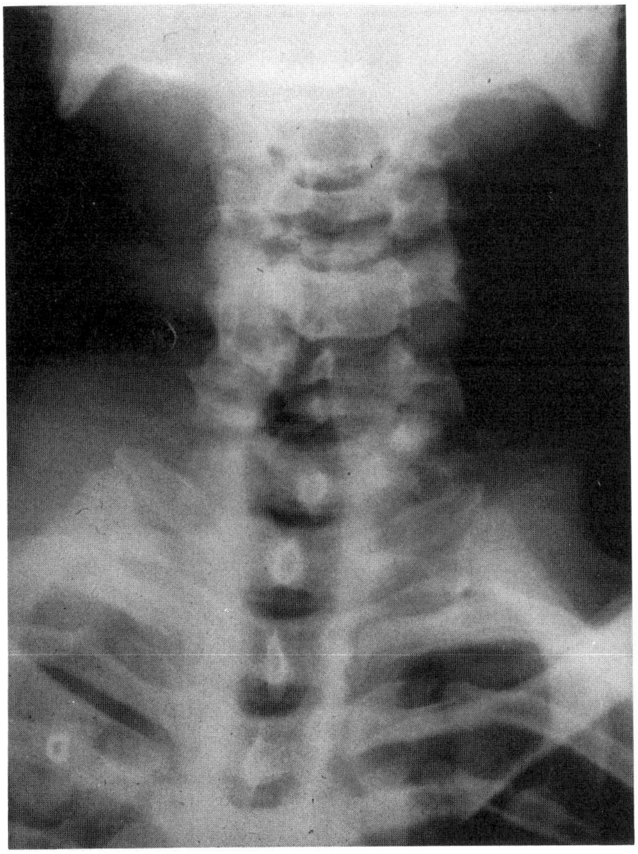

Fig. 67.1 Anteroposterior roentgenogram of a fracture of C6.

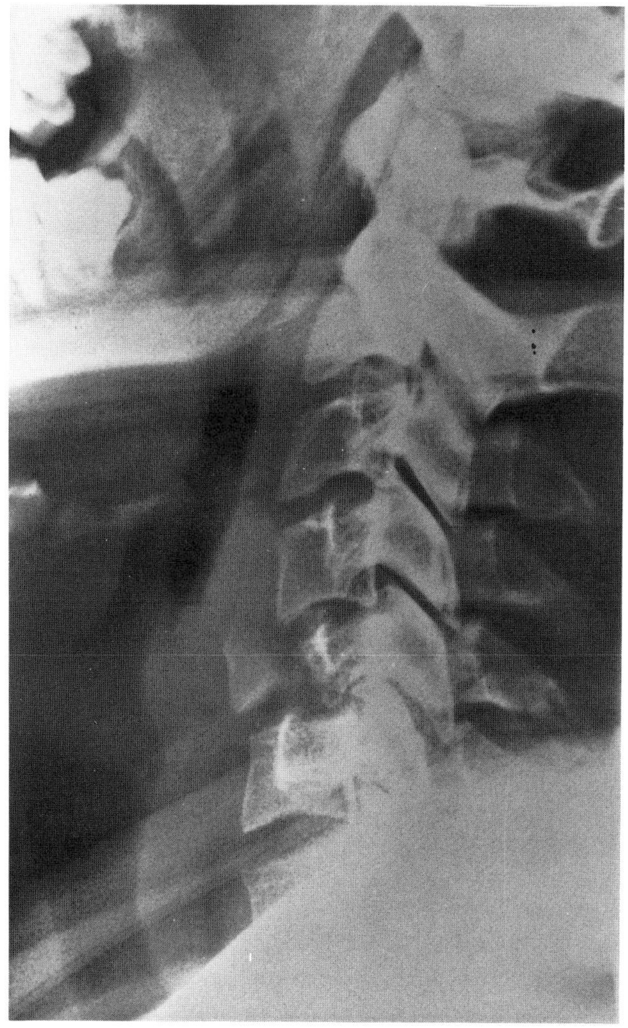

Fig. 67.2 Lateral projection of a fracture of C5 with tetraplegia.

to demonstrate encroachment on the spinal cord by intervertebral disc tissue.

Classification of fractures

Cervical spinal fractures can be classified into five groups depending on the mechanism of injury; but often it is difficult to obtain good information about the accident and reconstruction of the mechanism of the injury. Therefore radiological examination is most important, and indeed indispensable, in selecting methods of treatment (cf. Stauffer, 1989).

WEDGED COMPRESSION FRACTURES

These are classified as unstable when associated with rupture of posterior ligaments (Fig. 67.8). *Burst fractures* of the vertebral bodies are classified as stable in retrospect after consolidation of the fracture (Burke & Berryman, 1971). But in the beginning these fractures are potentially unstable and may cause additional injury to surrounding tissues, including compression of the spinal cord. Indeed these vertical compression fractures are often associated with neural involvement and need surgical treatment from the beginning (Fig. 67.5).

HYPEREXTENSION–DISLOCATION FRACTURES

These result from a force causing disruption of the anterior longitudinal ligament, and if there is a rotational element the cervical segment is further destabilized. If in addition there is a fracture of the posterior column the neck is highly unstable (Fig. 67.3).

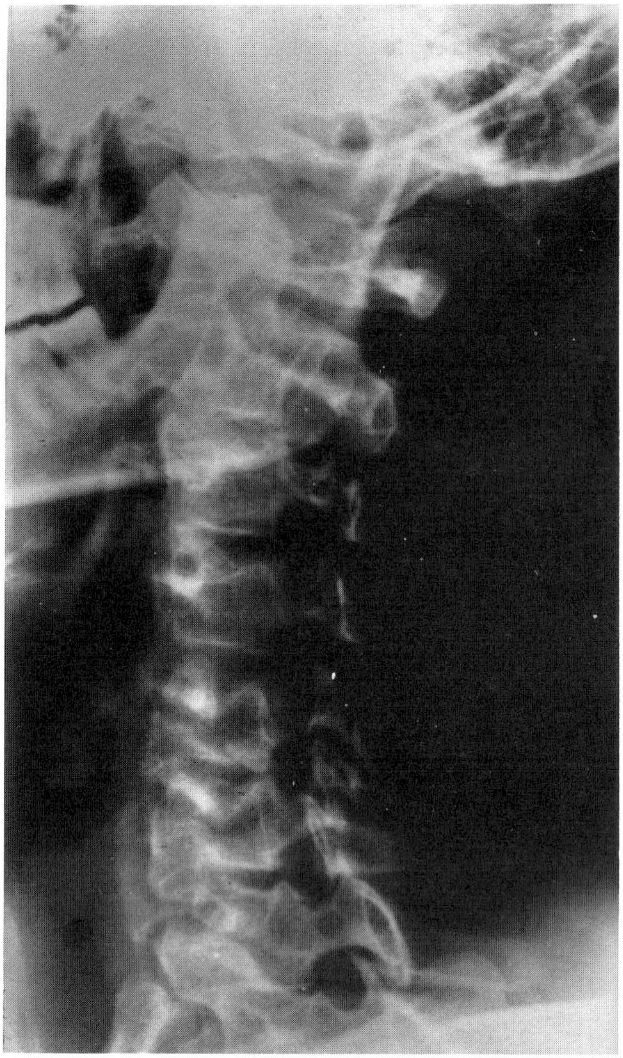

Fig. 67.3 Oblique view of a fracture of C6 with tetraparesis.

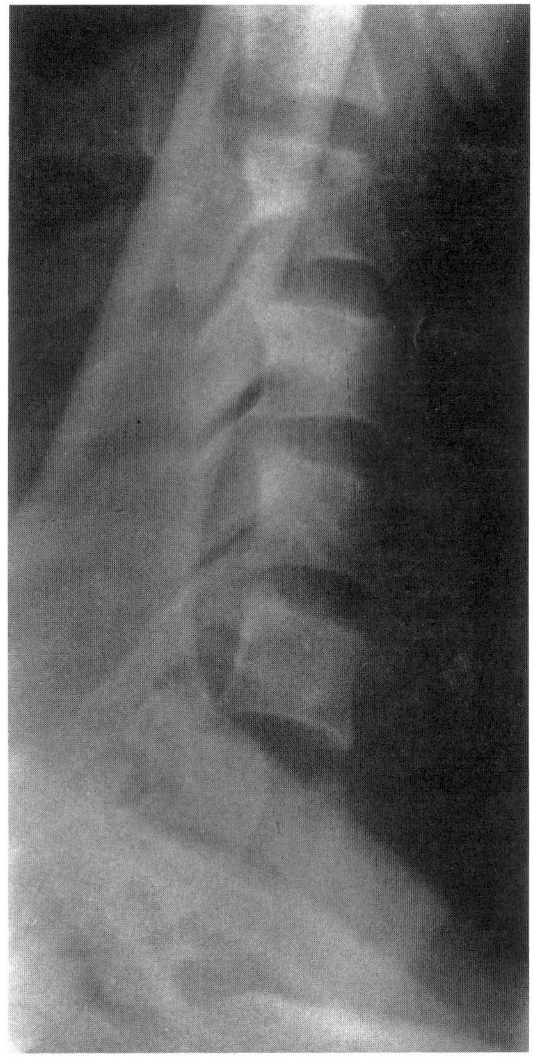

Fig. 67.4 'Swimmers' projection of a fracture of C7.

HYPERFLEXION INJURIES

These are often sustained in motor vehicle accidents, and if combined with rupture of posterior ligamentous elements (Fig. 67.9), are classified as unstable injuries. Severe fracture–dislocations with characteristic anterior displacement of the dislocated segment is seen in connection with motorcycle accidents and diving into shallow water. These associated with rupture of ligaments often result in spinal cord damage (Fig. 67.10).

In conclusion comminuted bursting type fractures and fracture–dislocations nearly always compromise the spinal cord and nerve roots. In addition fractures of vertebral laminae, pedicles and facets often damage the spinal cord, especially if there are loose bony fragments in the neural canal.

Stability of the injury

As mentioned, lateral tomography (Fig. 67.5) and CT scanning of the affected vertebra (Fig. 67.6) yield additional information regarding the stability of the injured segment. In general cases with neural involvement are almost always unstable, except rarely in patients with a severe degree of spondyloarthrosis

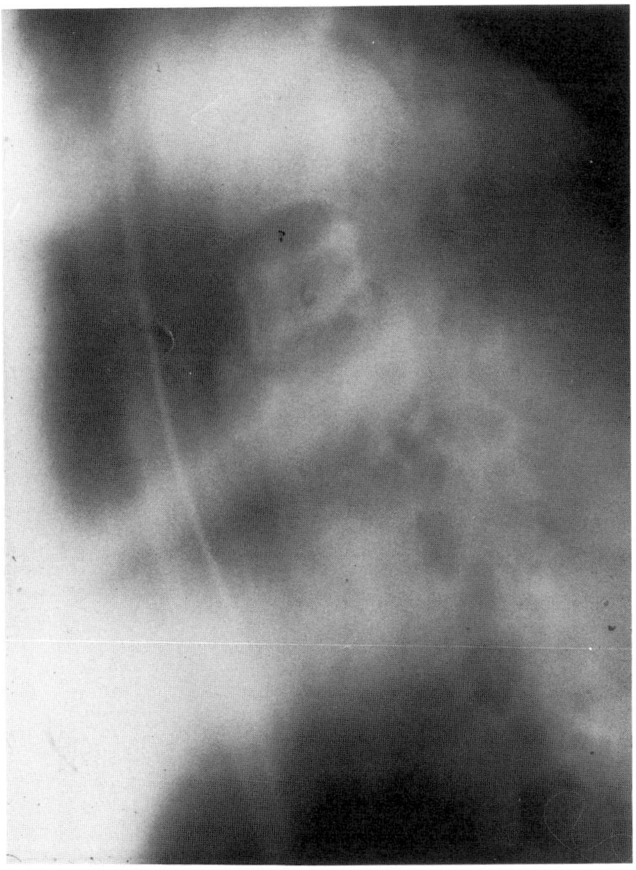

Fig. 67.5 Tomography of a burst fracture of C7 with tetraplegia.

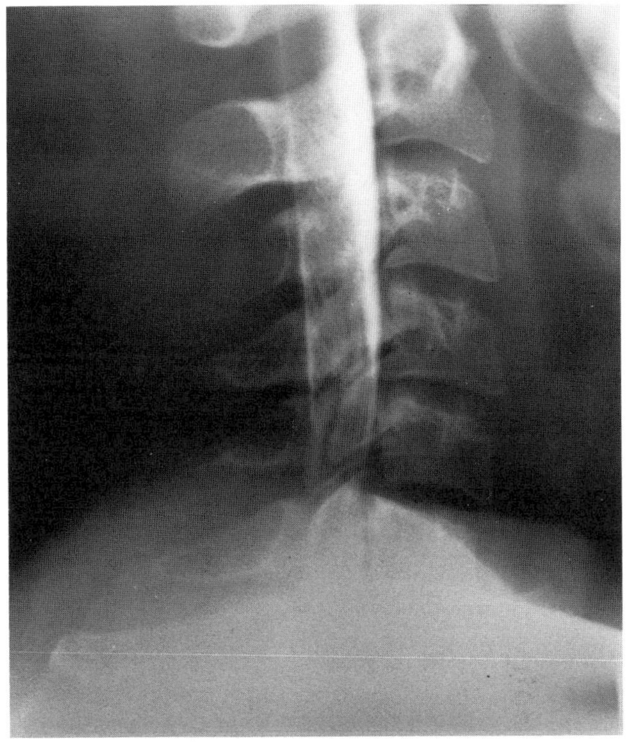

Fig. 67.7 Myelography of a fracture dislocation C5–C6 with paresis of bilateral radial nerves.

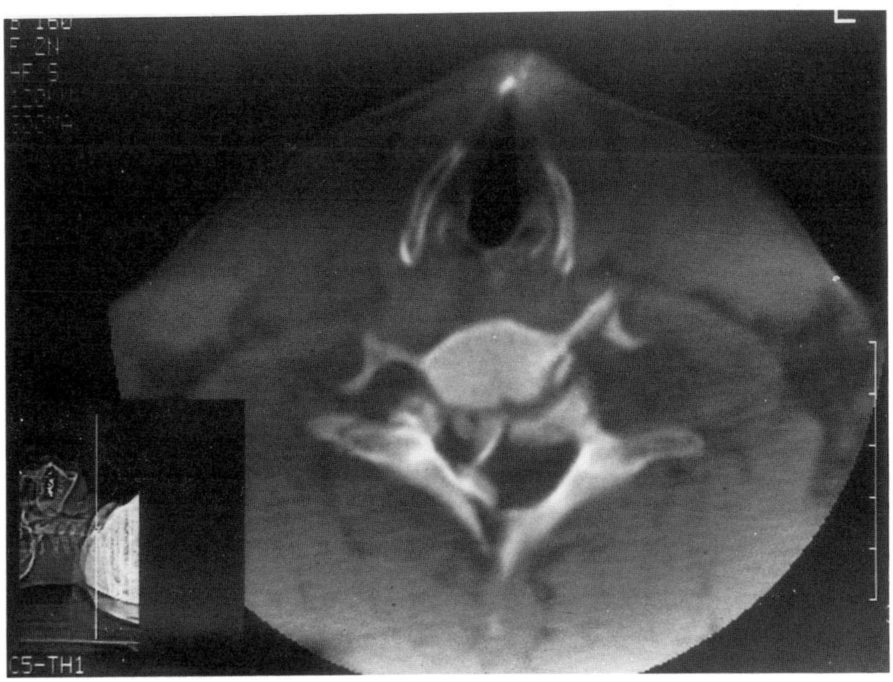

Fig. 67.6 Computerized tomography of a fracture of C6 with tetraplegia.

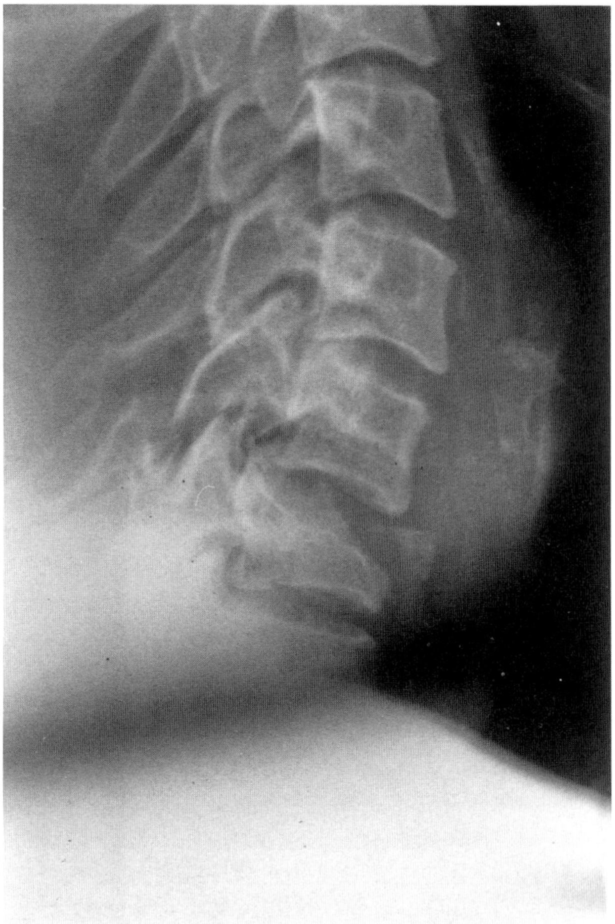

Fig. 67.8 Wedge compression fracture of C6 with tetraparesis.

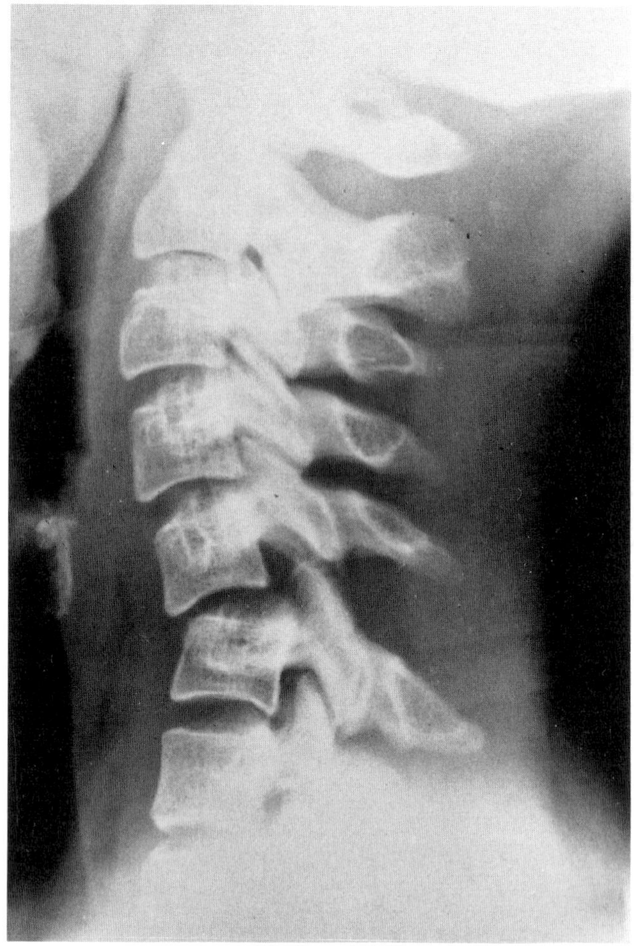

Fig. 67.9 Rupture of posterior ligaments and sublocation of C5–C6 without neural involvements.

of the cervical spine. In the latter there is possibly added encroachment on the cord from thickened soft tissues and osteophytes. Thus fracture–dislocations, most burst fractures and fractures with ruptured posterior soft tissue elements, are considered unstable injuries. Certain locked fracture–dislocations (Fig. 67.3) might be stable originally (Braakman & Vinken, 1967), but after reduction under general anaesthesia they are converted into unstable fractures. This must be taken into account in planning the next stage of treatment. A stabilization procedure might be indicated.

Primary hospital treatment

Patients with unstable injuries are placed on Gardner–Wells tong skull traction applied under local anaesthesia (Fig. 67.11). If reduction is indicated, traction is gradually increased until alignment is achieved. If the facet joints are locked reduction is undertaken under general anaesthesia by manual manipulation (Evans, 1961). Television (TV) fluoroscopy will confirm the reduction. Then skull traction is reduced to an extent corresponding to the level of the injured segment. In stable injuries the halovest ring is acceptable for

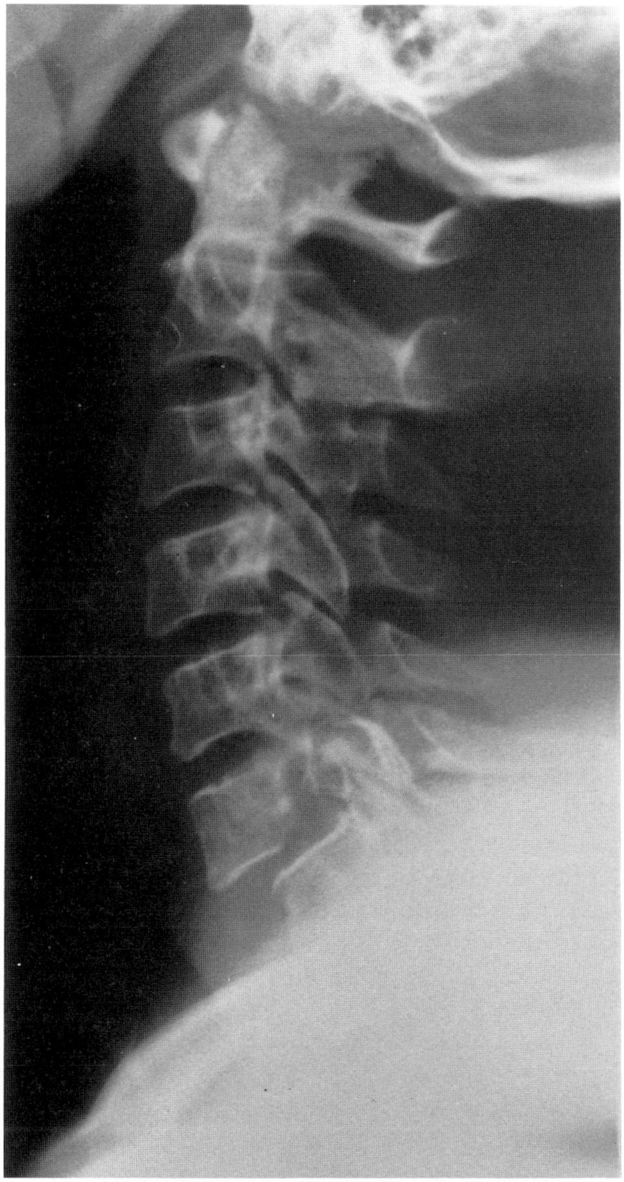

Fig. 67.10 Fracture–dislocation of C6–C7 with paresis of the left upper extremity.

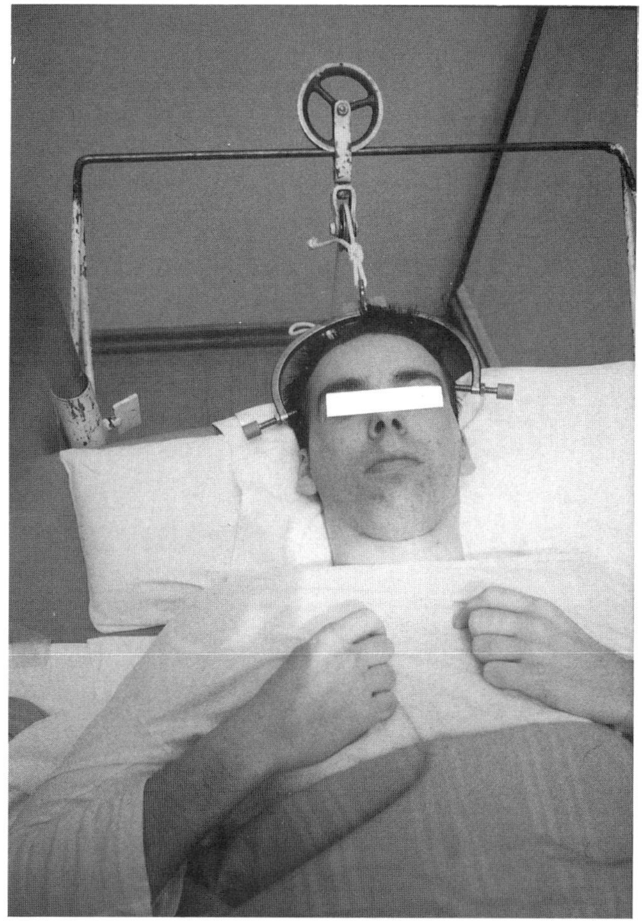

Fig. 67.11 Gardner–Wells tong skull traction.

skull traction throughout treatment (Botte *et al.*, 1989), allowing early mobilization of the patient (Fig. 67.12). Maintenance of reduction is monitored by AP and lateral X-rays. In certain cases lateral tomograms and CT scans might be necessary to visualize the spinal canal. The reduction must be completed within six hours and, if not successful, operative treatment is indicated, both in patients with locked facet joints and those with fracture–dislocations.

Operative reduction

In addition to the cases mentioned above, patients with obvious instability and those with spinal cord involvement should be considered for early surgical reduction (Capen *et al.*, 1985).

Under nasotracheal intubation–anaesthesia the patient is carefully placed on the operating table in the prone position. During turning, skull traction is maintained with the surgeon controlling the head and shoulders. Thereafter the head is controlled on the head rest in continuous traction with TV fluoroscopy in place. The appropriate area from C2 to C7 is defined by dissecting the soft tissues and muscles from the tip of the spinous processes and laminae out as far as the lateral aspects of the facet joints. Loose fragments are removed and facet joints reduced appropriately. After reduction traction is decreased, and the area surveyed by TV fluoroscopy. In case of one-

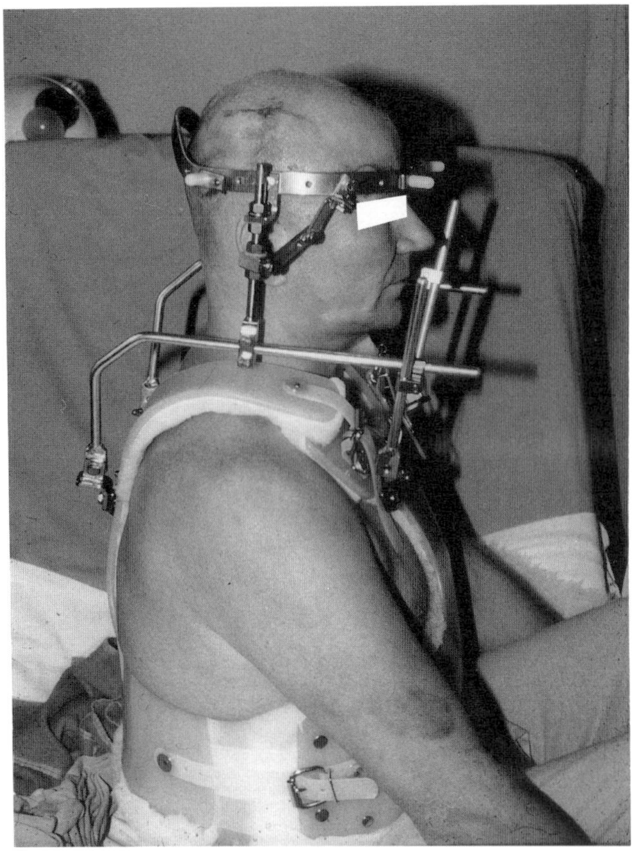

Fig. 67.12 The halo skeletal fixator.

segment locked dislocation the fracture is stabilized by the Rogers technique (Fig. 67.16). If there are two or more injured segments a modified Forsyth method (Fig. 67.17) of stabilization may be used. If laminectomy has been performed because of injury to posterior elements the Robinson & Southwick technique is preferred.

If there is a spinal cord injury with anterior bony fragments in the spinal canal (Fig. 67.13) reduction and decompression by the anterior approach is indicated.

The patient is put on the operating table in the supine position with the head in Gardner–Wells skull traction and slightly extended. The right-sided approach is favoured. A transverse incision is made in the skin and platysma or along the medial margin of the sternocleidomastoid muscle. The midcervical fascia is incised along the same margin. The carotid sheath is displaced laterally and the thyroid gland, trachea and oesophagus retracted medially. The approach is extended down to the anterior longitudinal

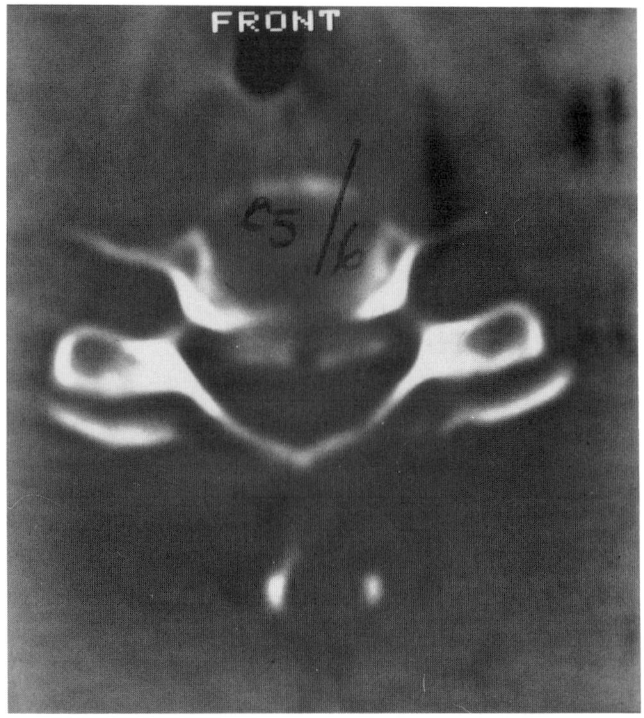

Fig. 67.13 Computerized tomography of a fracture of C5 with bone fragments in the spinal canal compressing the spinal cord, resulting in tetraparesis.

ligament, the colli muscles are defined and the injured segment identified. TV fluoroscopy is useful for accurate identification. Through a rectangular opening the spinal canal is exposed; bony fragments from the vertebra and compressing disc tissue are removed. This delicate procedure is enhanced by microsurgical techniques. Stability is established by interbody fusion using a keystone iliac bone graft as described by Simmons. The bone graft may be further secured to the adjacent vertebral bodies by two screws (Fig. 67.14) or an ASIF (Fig. 67.19) or a Caspar plate (Fig. 67.18). Usually stability is good enough following surgery to dispense with skull traction on the following days, preceded by radiographs.

Timing of stabilization procedures

Operative reduction is indicated within six hours of admission (Aebi *et al.*, 1986). If bone fragments and disc tissue are found in the spinal canal compressing the spinal cord, a decompression operation should be considered as soon as possible, at least within four days. Otherwise operative stabilization can con-

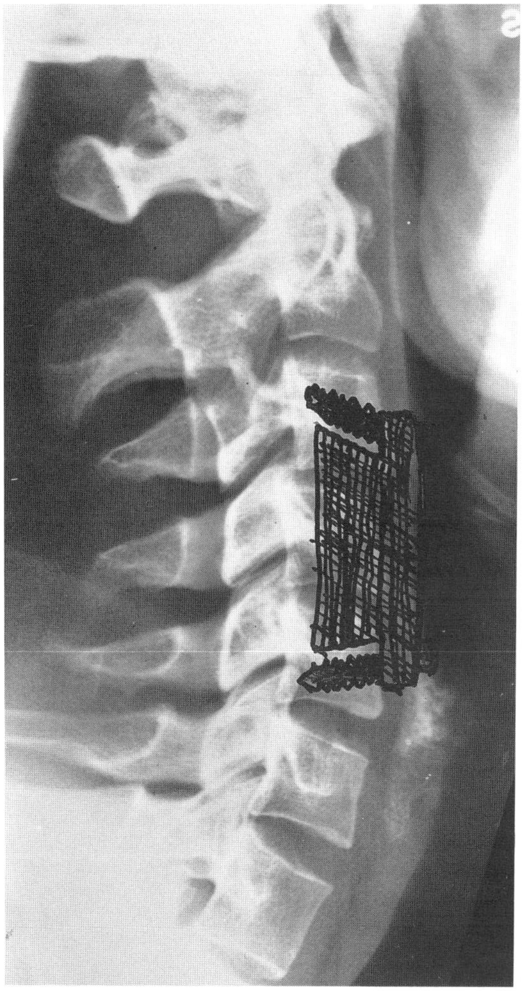

Fig. 67.14 Decompression of the spinal cord and intercorporeal fusion with keystone iliac bone graft fixed to adjacent vertebral bodies with AO screws.

veniently be postponed for three weeks or so following conservative reduction and Gardner–Wells tong traction. During these three weeks some consolidation of the fracture and healing of ligaments will have taken place. Also in cases with multiple injuries stabilization procedures might need postponing.

If the spinal cord has been transected, early reduction and internal fixation with a Daab plate is recommended with or without skull traction (Fig. 67.15). In such patients mobilization and nursing is made much easier—dispensing with prolonged use of cervical collars. Thus Roy-Camille has recommended surgical stabilization of the affected area at an early stage in all tetraplegic patients. In such circumstances protection of nerve roots immediately above the level of injury can be of special importance and late pain might be avoided.

Stabilization by the posterior approach

Locked facet joints, ruptured posterior ligaments, as well as certain fracture–dislocations need operative reduction and stabilization by the posterior approach (Stauffer & Kelly, 1977).

ROGERS TECHNIQUE

A posterior tension band system with a figure-eight loop of cerclage wire led through holes drilled at the base of the spinous process of the vertebra above and around the spinous process of the vertebra below is simple and effective (Bateman, 1978). The segment is fused by cortical cancellous grafts taken from the iliac crest pressed in between the spinous processes and the wire loops and overlaid by cancellous bone (Fig. 67.16) (Rogers, 1942). If good stability is achieved skeletal traction could be discarded after some days.

FORSYTH TECHNIQUE

If two or more segments need fusion the Forsyth technique (Forsyth *et al.*, 1959), or a modification of this (Fig. 67.17), is indicated. The relevant neck segments are carefully exposed by subperiosteal dissection as previously described. The injured segment is defined and loose fragments removed. Reduction is achieved by elevators in combination with increased skull traction. Bone grafts from the tibia or iliac crest are fixed with wire loops on each side of the spinous processes and laminae of three or four cervical vertebrae complemented by cancellous bone. If fixation is sound the skull traction can be removed after a few days, allowing early mobilization of the patient.

ROBINSON & SOUTHWICK TECHNIQUE

In cases of bilateral fracture–dislocations combined with fractures of the posterior column, limited laminectomy might be necessary in selected cases. If so posterior fusion with the Robinson & Southwick technique is indicated (Robinson & Southwick, 1960). It is necessary to extend the fusion above and below the injured segment, and bone grafts from tibia or iliac crest are preferred. The grafts are anchored with wires to the inferior articular facets with great care.

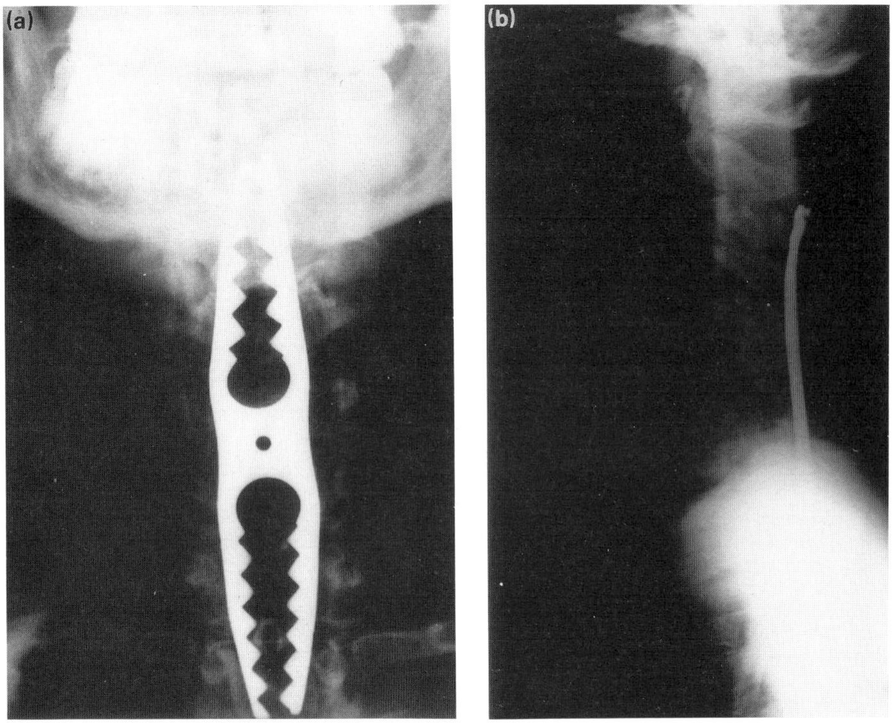

Fig. 67.15 Internal fixation with a Daab plate of a fracture dislocation of C6–C7 with transection of the spinal cord.

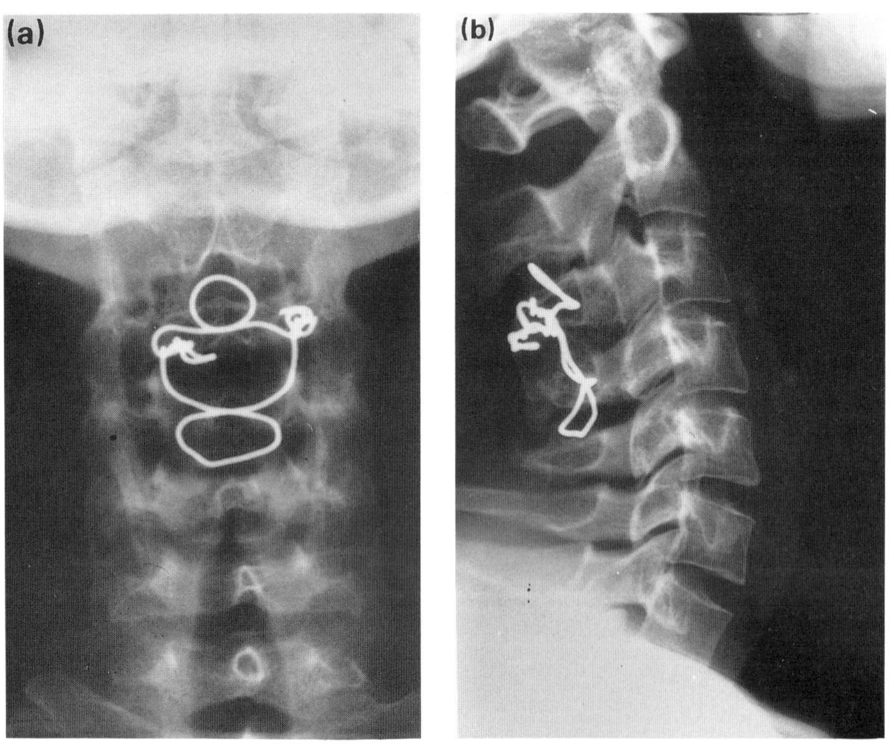

Fig. 67.16 A fracture–dislocation of C4–C5 fixed with a posterior tension band system with a figure-eight loop of cerclage wire according to the Rogers technique after operative reduction.

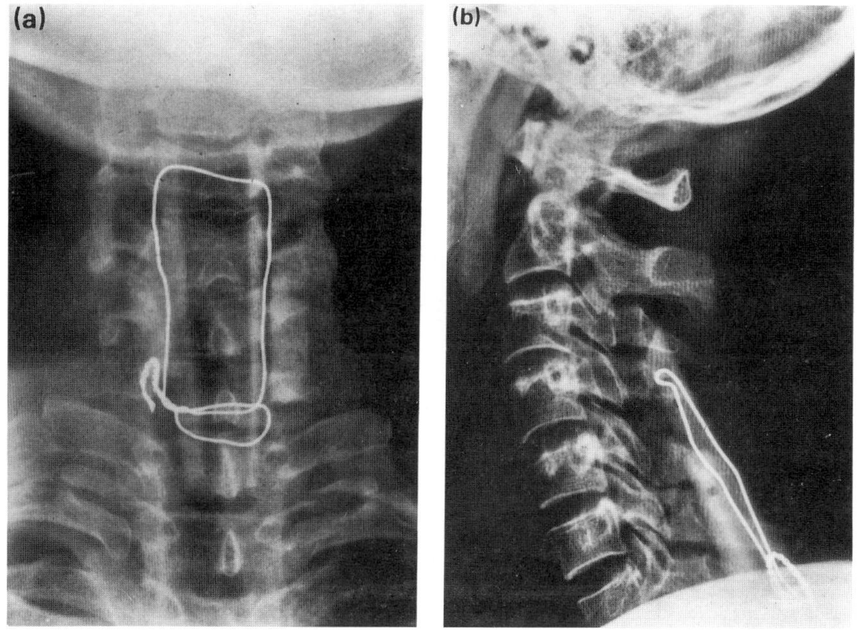

Fig. 67.17 Fracture–dislocation C5–C6 with tetraparesis treated with operative reduction and stabilized with tibial bone grafts according to a modification of the Forsyth technique.

Drill holes into the graft can be made before detaching the bone. Great care should be observed in preparing the bed for the fusion. Reduced skeletal traction is continued during the period of bed rest. If the cord is intact, the patient should remain in bed for four to six weeks and a cervical collar used until fusion is complete (Figs 67.20 & 67.21).

DAAB TECHNIQUE

In tetraplegia operative reduction and internal fixation without bone grafting is indicated. Fixation with a Daab plate (Fig. 67.15) is easily performed after reduction of the fracture–dislocation (Daab & Gluch, 1977). Three different plate lengths are available. As these are sufficiently malleable they can be adapted to the shape of the spinous processes prior to being secured. After surgery skull traction is removed, and external support is not necessary.

ROY-CAMILLE TECHNIQUE

Nursing is made easier after stabilization of the cervical spine. Roy-Camille practises posterior plating of the injured neck in all tetraplegic patients (Roy-Camille, 1988). Pedicle screw plates are preferred for stabilizing the lower reaches of the neck (Murphy *et al.*, 1986). These are also effective in actually achieving reduction, because they can be premoulded and will conveniently span the cervical segments as the distance between the pedicles corresponds with the plate's screw apertures. Again bone grafting is not essential though many surgeons would prefer to augment the instrumentation with fusion.

Stabilization by the anterior approach

The anterior approach is mainly used in injuries involving the anterior column of the spine, that is those concerning the vertebral bodies and intervertebral discs as well as some elements of the facetal vertebral joints. These injuries include wedge compression fractures, flexion and burst fractures of the vertebral bodies as well as ruptures of the intervertebral discs, also the anterior longitudinal ligaments, by hyperextension forces. In addition decompression is occasionally performed in selected cases as a second-stage procedure following posterior operative reduction.

The surgical approach is as described on page 1106. On this occasion the surgical field is enlarged to expose the endplates of adjacent vertebral bodies and as previously a keystone bone graft is taken from the iliac crest and slotted under tension into the prepared intervertebral bed (Simmons & Bhalla, 1969). The bone graft can be fixed to the adjacent vertebrae with

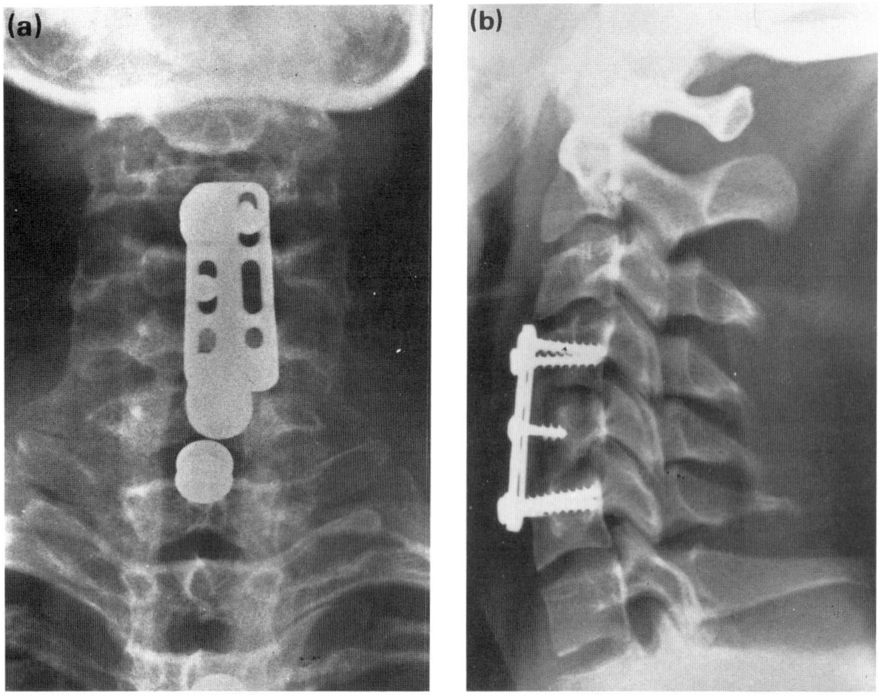

Fig. 67.18 Decompression of the spinal cord and intercorporeal fusion of C4–C6 with Caspar plate and iliac bone graft.

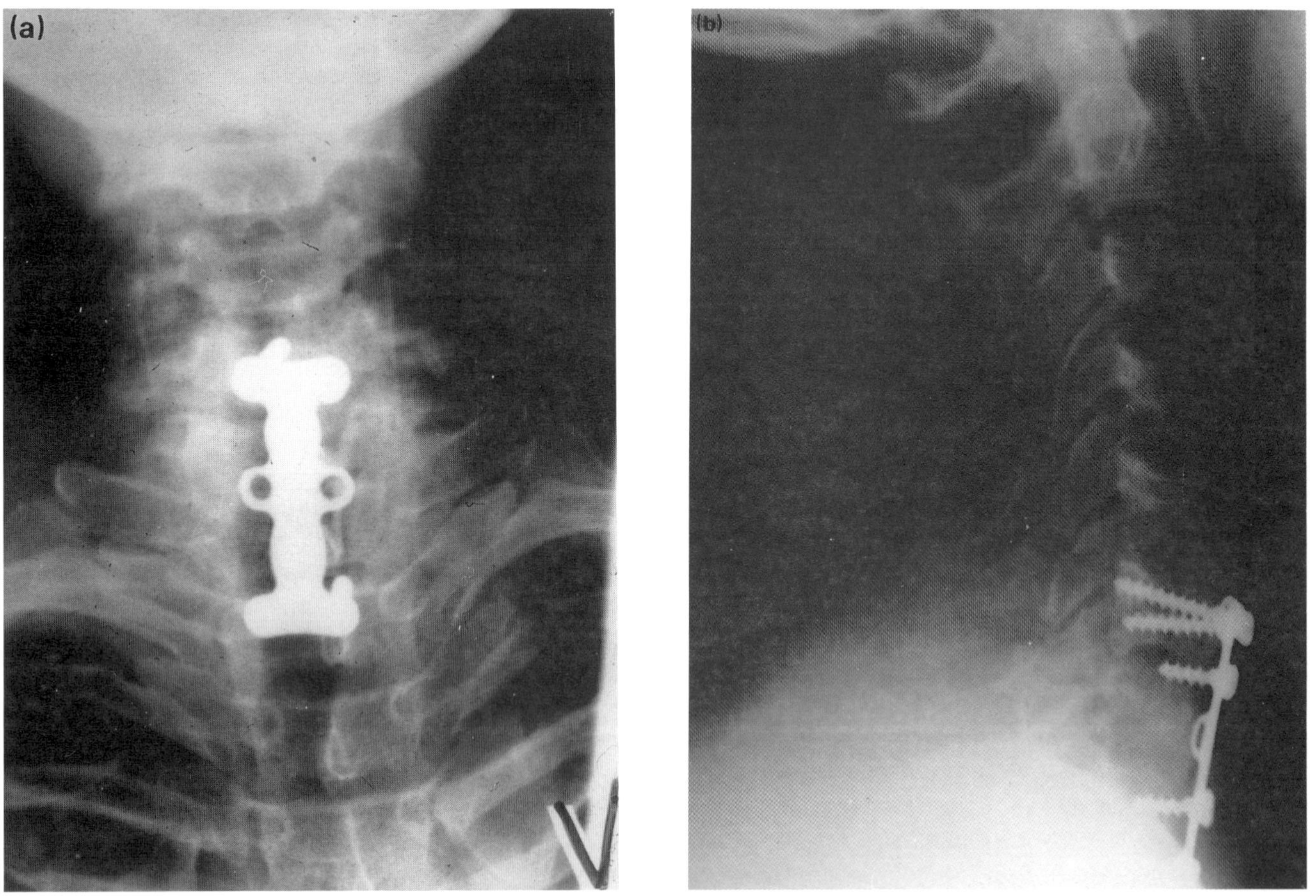

Fig. 67.19 A burst fracture of C7 with tetraplegia treated with decompression and intercorporeal fusion. Internal fixation with a ASIF plate: (a) anteroposterior view, (b) lateral view.

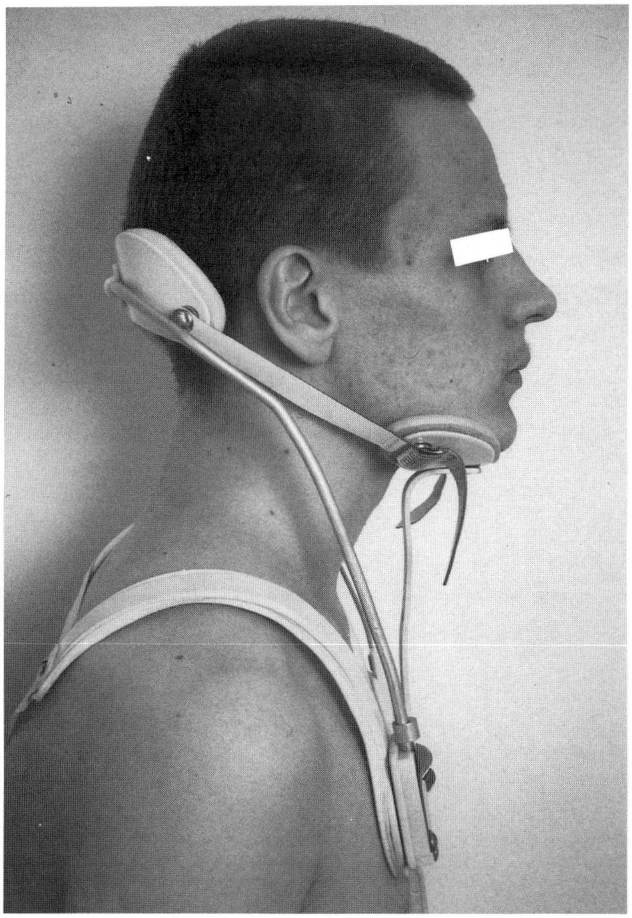

Fig. 67.20 External support after surgery.

AO screws (Fig. 67.14), or Caspar plate (Fig. 67.18). ASIF (Fig. 67.19) plates may be equally effective as described by Böhler (Böhler & Gaudernak, 1980); these are secured by screws to the vertebral bodies and graft. Stability following surgery is usually good and the skull traction can be removed.

In selected cases internal ASIF plate fixation without bone grafting is sufficient to achieve good stability provided normal anatomical alignment of the spine has been achieved. After surgery the patient is mobilized early with a Halovest skeletal fixator for one month or so, followed by a cervical collar (Fig. 67.20). In these cases the duration of hospital treatment is short.

Stabilization by the posterior and anterior approach

If following posterior operative reduction, radiological examination—including lateral tomography and in selected cases myelography and CT scan—demonstrate fragments in the spinal canal with encroachment on the spinal cord, or if posterior stabilization is inadequate, early additional anterior decompression might be necessary. Decompression is combined with intercorporeal fusion with a keystone bone graft as previously described, with or without screw or plate fixation. Alternatively the anterior operation can be undertaken immediately after posterior surgery at the same sitting. This is especially indicated in cases where all three spinal column elements are affected (McAfee & Bohlman, 1989).

Postoperative care

Patients are kept in bed for one to six weeks depending on the duration of skull traction. Follow-up examinations are routine and in selected cases further CT scanning may help. The duration of skull traction is dependent on the stability of the injured segments. In cases with multiple injuries this may well extend to many weeks, especially if prolonged intensive care is needed. After surgery and the application of external support (Fig. 67.20), patients participate in a full rehabilitation programme either locally or in special departments. A cervical collar is used during the day for two to four months, after which the patient is normally able to return to former work. If not, a new training programme might be designed, especially in cases with spinal cord injuries and persisting neural deficits.

Conclusion

In cases with instability of the cervical spine with neural involvement, especially when some motor function and sensibility remains below the injured segment, reduction with skull tong traction and/or manual manipulation is indicated within the first six hours. If this is not successful, operative reduction is indicated. Stabilization of the fracture may be performed at the time of the operative reduction, or if manual manipulation has been successful after three weeks. Internal fixation and bone grafting is performed. If there appears to be compression of the spinal cord with bone fragments in the spinal canal, decompression is undertaken via the anterior approach together with intercorporeal fusion (Fig. 67.21). In transection of the spinal cord with tetraplegia, internal fixation without bone grafting is indicated.

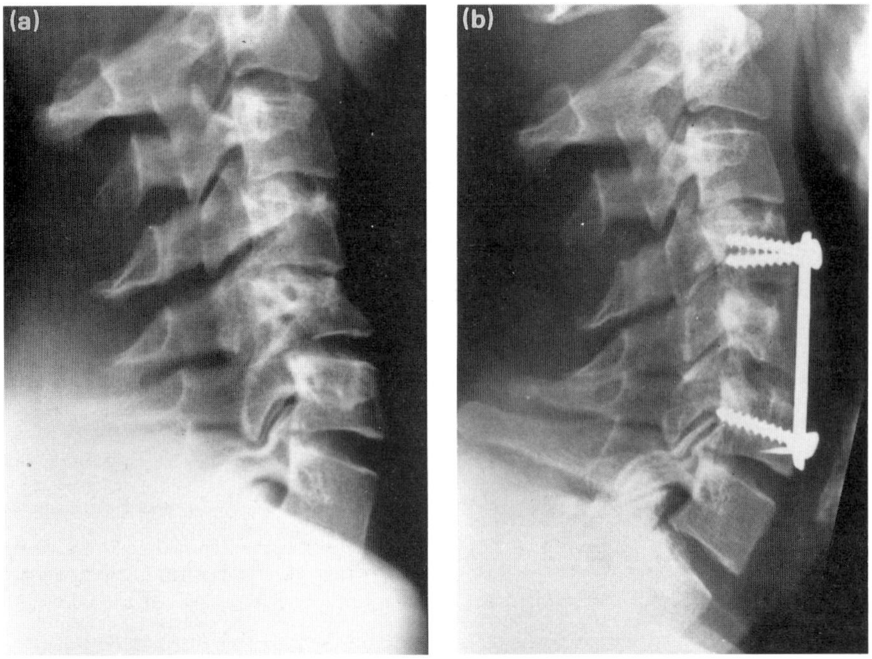

Fig. 67.21 A wedge fracture with compression of the spinal cord and tetraparesis treated with decompression and intercorporeal fusion and Caspar plate fixation. The recovery was complete: (a) before surgery, (b) after surgery at follow-up examination.

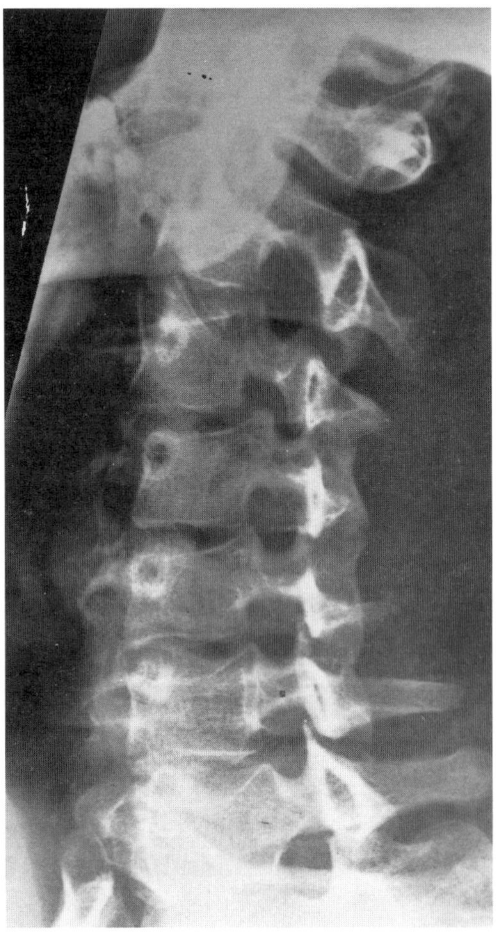

Those who deal with cervical spine injuries know that prior to treatment it is difficult to estimate the real extent of damage to the spinal cord, especially if spontaneous reduction of the vertebral fractures has taken place immediately after the accident (Fig. 67.22). It might also be difficult to localize the exact level of the injury. Thus reconstruction of the spinal canal and stabilization is in our view important.

How long is it possible to postpone a decompression procedure in cases with cervical fractures? This is difficult to answer, though in our series the results of treatment seem better if the operation is undertaken early. On the other hand, several other factors, such as the type of vertebral fractures and the grade of spinal cord injury, have a bearing on the final result of treatment.

Fig. 67.22 (*Left*) A fracture–dislocation of C4–C5 with severe neural involvements. Spontaneous reduction might have taken place because severe neural involvement did not correspond to the radiological findings. Operative reduction and internal fixation was undertaken, with complete recovery.

REFERENCES

Aebi, M., Mohler, J., Zäch, G.A. & Morscher, E. (1986) Indications, surgical technique and results of 100 surgically-treated fractures and fracture–dislocations of the cervical spine. *Clin. Orthop.*, **203**, 244–257.

Bateman, J.E. (1978) Trauma to the neck and shoulder. In Bateman, J.E. (ed.) *The Shoulder and Neck*, pp. 413–616.

Böhler, J. & Gaudernak, T. (1980) Anterior plate stabilization for fracture-dislocations of the lower cervical spine. *J. Trauma*, **20**, 203–205.

Botte, M.J., Grafin, S.R., Byrne, T.P., Wood, S.L.Y. & Nickel, V.L. (1989) The halo skeletal fixator. *Clin. Orthop.*, **239**, 12–18.

Braakman, R. & Vinken, P.J. (1967) Unilateral facet interlocking in the lower cervical spine. *J. Bone Jt. Surg.*, **49B**, 249–257.

Burke, D.C. & Berryman, D. (1971) The place of closed manipulation in the management of flexion–rotation dislocations of the cervical spine. *J. Bone Jt. Surg.*, **53B**, 165–182.

Capen, D.A., Garland, D.E. & Waters, R.L. (1985) Surgical stabilization of the cervical spine. *Clin. Orthop.*, **196**, 229–237.

Daab, J. & Gluch, H. (1977) Indications and clinical evaluation of stabilization by means of Daab's plate in spine fractures. *International Symposium on Acute Management and Rehabilitation after Spinal Cord Injuries, Konstancin, Warsaw, Poland*, pp. 26–46.

Evans, D.K. (1961) Reductions of cervical dislocations. *J. Bone Jt. Surg.*, **43B**, 552–555.

Forsyth, H.F., Alexander, E. Jr, Davis, C. Jr & Underdal, R. (1959) The advantages of early spine fusion in the treatment of fracture–dislocation of the cervical spine. *J. Bone Jt. Surg.*, **41A**, 17–36.

Frankel, H.L., Hancock, D.O., Hystop, G. *et al.* (1969) The value of postural reduction in the initial management of closed injuries of the spine with paraplegia and tetraplegia. *Paraplegia*, **7**, 179–192.

Garfin, S.R., Shackford, S.R., Marshall, L.F. & Drummond, J.C. (1989) Care of multiple injured patients with cervical spine injury. *Clin. Orthop.*, **239**, 19–29.

Green, B.A., Callahan, R.A., Klose, K.H. & DeLa Torre, J. (1981) Acute spinal cord injury: current concepts. *Clin. Orthop.*, **154**, 125–135.

McAfee, P.H. & Bohlman, H.H. (1989) One-stage anterior cervical decompression and posterior stabilization and circumferential arthrodesis. *J. Bone Jt. Surg.*, **71A**, 78–88.

Murphy M.J., Daniaux, H. & Southwick, W.O. (1986) Posterior cervical fusion with rigid internal fixation. *Orthop. Clin. N. Am.*, **17**, 55–65.

Osti, O.L., Fraser, R.D. & Griffits, E.R. (1989) Reduction and stabilization of cervical dislocations. *J. Bone Jt. Surg.*, **71B**, 275–282.

Robinson, R.A. & Southwick, W.O. (1960) Indications and technics for early stabilization of the neck in some fracture dislocations of the cervical spine. *South. Med. J.*, **53**, 565–579.

Rogers, W.A. (1942) Treatment of fracture–dislocations of the cervical spine. *J. Bone Jt. Surg.*, **24**, 245–258.

Roy-Camille, R. (1988) In Roy-Camille R. (ed.) *Rachis Cervical Inférieur*. Masson, Paris, pp. 91–125.

Simmons, E.H. & Bhalla, S.K. (1969) Anterior discectomy and fusion. *J. Bone Jt. Surg.*, **51B**, 225–237.

Stauffer, E.S. (1986) Management of spine fractures C3 to C7. *Orthop. Clin. N. Am.*, **17**, 45–53.

Stauffer, E.S. (1989) Subaxial injuries. *Clin. Orthop.*, **239**, 30–39.

Stauffer, E.S. & Kelly, E.G. (1977) Fracture–dislocations of the cervical spine. *J. Bone Jt. Surg.*, **59A**, 45–48.

68 · Surgical Management of Injuries to the Thoracic and Lumbosacral Spine

By M.J. BOLESTA and H.H. BOHLMAN

The goal of all treatment of spinal injury, operative and non-operative, is the maximal restoration of function possible, which begins at the scene of the accident. Emergency medical technicians are trained to have a high index of suspicion for spinal injury when a person sustains a major traumatic injury. Although they must address life-threatening conditions first, the entire spine is immobilized and protected. Transport is facilitated by the use of back boards, cervical collars, sand bags and special stretchers.

Once the patient arrives at hospital, an initial assessment is made, searching for injuries which may result in rapid demise. Subsequent examinations look for all other important but less urgent injuries. It is assumed that spinal column injury is present until proven otherwise. In the conscious patient one can elicit complaints of pain, its location, and character. The entire spine is palpated looking for regions of tenderness and blunt trauma. A careful neurological examination of the entire body is performed, and the cause of any deficit is analysed. The task is more difficult in the multiply injured patient, especially with head injury, where there will be a heavier reliance on imaging techniques. External protection of the spine should continue until any suspicion of spine or neurological injury is allayed.

Following clinical assessment, anteroposterior and lateral radiographs of the spine are obtained initially. Oblique views are helpful, particularly in assessing subluxations, and dislocations. Generally the plain radiographs will allow one to localize the injured spinal segments, infer the mechanism of injury, classify them, and plan early management.

Tomography is used less frequently with the advent of newer technologies, but remains an excellent technique for defining osseous pathology, particularly in the posterior elements. It can delineate fractures in the transverse plane that can be missed by computerized tomography.

Myelography remains quite useful in localizing neural compression in those cases without obvious fracture or dislocation. Its major disadvantage is that it is invasive and requires some manipulation and positioning of the patient which may be difficult because of injuries to other organ systems.

Computerized tomography (CT) with intrathecal contrast provides essential information about the shape of the spinal canal and any alterations, especially bony impingement. High-resolution CT, occasionally supplemented with reconstructions, can sometimes provide sufficient information even without myelography; however, the use of intrathecal contrast is still favoured. It allows accurate assessment of the spinal cord and nerve roots and contrast also allows one to identify dural disruption, common in thoracolumbar junction injuries (Cammisa *et al.*, 1989).

Magnetic resonance imaging (MRI) produces direct images in the sagittal and transverse planes. Oblique and coronal views are also available. Different pulse sequences can be used to modulate the contrast between the spinal cord, cerebrospinal fluid, and surrounding structures. Early studies suggest that images of the cord itself may be of prognostic value in spinal cord-injured patients (Fasano & Stauffer, 1988; Bondurant *et al.*, 1989; Kitchel *et al.*, 1989). The utility of MRI is compromised by lengthy scan times and the relative inaccessibility of the recently injured patient. It does provide excellent soft tissue definition but it is inferior to CT in displaying the bony injury. It is uniquely useful in determining the integrity of the interspinous ligaments (McArdle *et al.*, 1986; Emery *et al.* 1989).

With the impressive array of imaging technologies available, it seems likely that a combination of modalities, rather than a single test, should be used to obtain an accurate diagnosis of spine and spinal cord pathology to plan optimal management of the patient. Intraoperative findings will still alter the plan at times, but there is now no longer any need for exploratory surgery.

THE RATIONALE FOR OPERATIVE TREATMENT

The normal spinal column provides a protective conduit for the spinal cord and its roots, allowing structural support and mobility. When the spine is disrupted by trauma, the extent and nature of the injury must be assessed. Some injuries are stable and do not require operative intervention whereas others are mechanically unstable. Under physiological loading, an unstable spine will deform beyond the usual constraints. This mechanical instability can vary in its severity depending on the level of spinal injury and the extent of osseoligamentous disruption. Spinal injuries may be subdivided into acute and chronic. For example, predominantly osseous injuries may allow potentially dangerous movements shortly after the insult, but become stable with healing. Injuries with significant ligamentous damage may be both acutely and chronically unstable as scar does not adequately reconstitute the ligaments.

One may also speak of neurological stability. A lesion is neurologically unstable if normal activity results in compression of neural elements. The significance of this lies in the extent of this compression, as well as the nature of the initial insults.

In patients who are neurologically normal it is essential to prevent secondary neurological deficit and to restore stability. Normal function in the face of demonstrated neural impingement may require decompression. This is an area of controversy, but most would agree on the need for decompression in these individuals if there is persistent pain or increasing neurological deficit.

Cases of incomplete neural deficit with persisting canal compromise are more clear. Neural decompression maximizes the potential for neurological recovery, as has been demonstrated in both the acute and chronic situation (Larson *et al.*, 1976; Bohlman *et al.*, 1985b; McAfee *et al.*, 1985a; Benzel & Larson, 1986). Stabilization is added if the initial insult or the decompression results in instability.

In individuals with complete cord injury between the first and eleventh thoracic levels, mechanical stability is generally not an issue. Decompression does not result in return of cord function, and root recovery is not meaningful.

CLASSIFICATION OF SPINAL INJURIES

Many schemes have been proposed to classify spinal injuries. One of the more widely used was that of Holdsworth, which was based on a two-column concept (Holdsworth & Hardy, 1953; Holdsworth, 1970; Bohlman, 1985). Based on more recent biomechanical studies, as well as the additional clinical information generated by CT scanning, Denis proposed a three-column model with a mechanistic classification of thoracic and lumbar injuries (Denis, 1983, 1984). The posterior column is formed by the posterior arch and the posterior ligamentous complex, including supraspinous and interspinous ligaments, facet capsule, and ligamentum flavum. The middle column is formed by the posterior longitudinal ligament, the posterior annulus fibrosus, and the posterior third to half of the vertebral body. The anterior column is formed by the anterior longitudinal ligament, the anterior annulus fibrosus, and the anterior half to two-thirds of the vertebral body. Based on his retrospective review, Denis divided the injury patterns into major and minor. Minor injuries included articular process fractures, transverse process fractures, spinous process fractures, and pars interarticularis fractures. Major injuries were compression fractures, burst fractures, seatbelt-type injuries, and fracture–dislocations.

Compression fractures occur with either anterior or lateral flexion, producing anterior or lateral compression respectively. There is failure of the anterior column in compression with an intact middle column. Most compression fractures have an intact posterior column and are stable unless it is severe, in which case there may be posterior disruption.

Burst fractures result from axial loading which can occur in isolation or in combination with flexion, rotation, or lateral flexion. Denis subdivided burst injuries into five different types depending on the combination of forces and the resultant radiographic pattern. Both the anterior and the middle columns fail in compression, and the posterior column remains intact. Although this was not part of his original classification, there are burst injuries in which the posterior column is disrupted, the so-called unstable burst injury.

The seatbelt injury occurs with flexion and distraction, with the fulcrum anterior to spinal column. Both the middle and posterior columns fail in distraction; the anterior column may be intact or may fail in compression. This may be a purely bony injury as in the Chance fracture, purely ligamentous, or a combination of the two.

Fracture–dislocations are a result of flexion rotation, shear, or flexion distraction. In shear injuries, failure is shear in all three columns. With flexion and distraction the anterior column fails in compression and the middle and posterior columns in distraction; with flexion rotation the anterior column fails in compression and rotation and the remaining columns in distraction and rotation.

Although most thoracolumbar fractures can be placed into these categories, other patterns have also been described. For example, Bohlman has reported thoracic sagittal slice fractures in which a vertebral body is split in the sagittal plane, as though the cranial vertebra is driven through the subjacent body (Bohlman *et al.*, 1985b). The experienced spine surgeon will recognize these variations and apply the three-column concept to them. Decisions may then be made about stability and the need for decompression.

THORACIC INJURIES (T1–T10)

The spinal canal in the thoracic region is ovoid and smaller in cross-sectional area than in the cervical or lumbar region. The spinal cord occupies a greater percentage of the canal. Hence any displacement of the vertebral bodies or soft tissues is likely to result in neural damage. However, the thoracic spine is a relatively rigid portion of the spine as compared to the cervical and lumbar regions with the strong ligamentous attachments to the rib cage resulting in a very stable structure.

It has previously been felt that the supposed paucity of vascular anastomotic channels in the thoracic region, placed the cord at increased risk (Domisse, 1974). However, refined injection techniques by Crock & Yoshizawa (1977) demonstrated smaller vessels which were consistently present at each level, disputing the notion of vascular fragility.

Somatosensory evoked potentials provide early identification of potentially serious neurological complications (Meyer *et al.*, 1988), but may miss both subtle and more profound alterations. Motor evoked potentials are currently under investigation (Machida *et al.*, 1988; Owen *et al.*, 1988). The place of such electrophysiological tests outside the operating room is not yet clear.

Compression fractures

Compression fractures are commonly encountered in the thoracic region and can occur with trivial trauma in the presence of osteopenia. The middle column is intact, and generally the posterior column is too. Neurological injury does not occur unless there is concomitant disc herniation (Fig. 68.1).

These injuries are quite stable, and seldom require operative intervention. One could consider fusion in the case of severe compression with disruption of the posterior elements resulting in a progressive kyphosis. With a kyphosis of less than 50°, posterior instrumentation and fusion is adequate but a more severe kyphosis may require an anterior approach. Patients with persistent pain or an incomplete spinal cord syndrome secondary to a herniated disc may benefit from a transthoracic anterior discectomy (Bohlman & Zdeblick, 1988).

Burst fractures

These are more severe injuries resulting from axial loading, with or without other forces. In the thoracic region these will stabilize after a period of bed rest or external support in a moulded orthosis. Most are associated with a complete spinal cord injury. The less common incomplete syndrome is thoroughly evaluated as described in the imaging section. Should decompression be necessary, a costotransversectomy or a transpedicular approach (Larson *et al.*, 1976) can be used, but the excellent visualization and safety of the transthoracic approach described above makes anterior corpectomy and strut fusion the procedure of choice. A moulded orthosis is used until the fusion is solid. Bohlman and others have shown excellent results in both early and late decompressions using this technique in patients with incomplete cord lesions (Bohlman & Eismont, 1981; Johnson *et al.*,

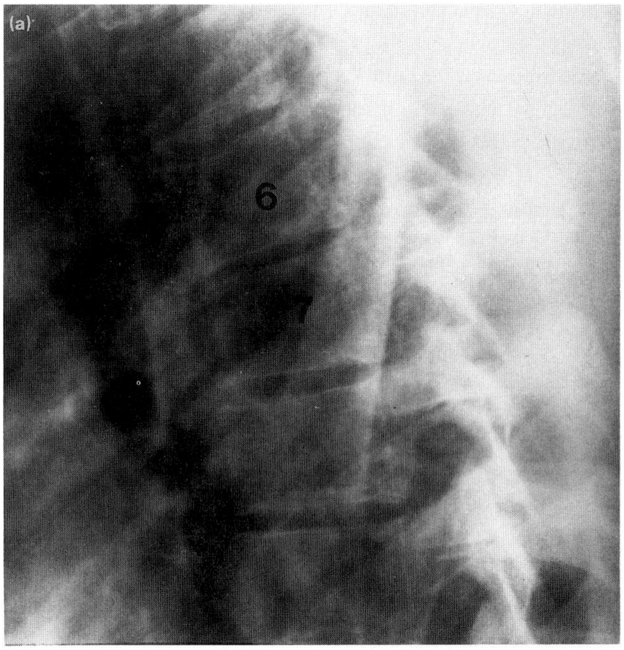

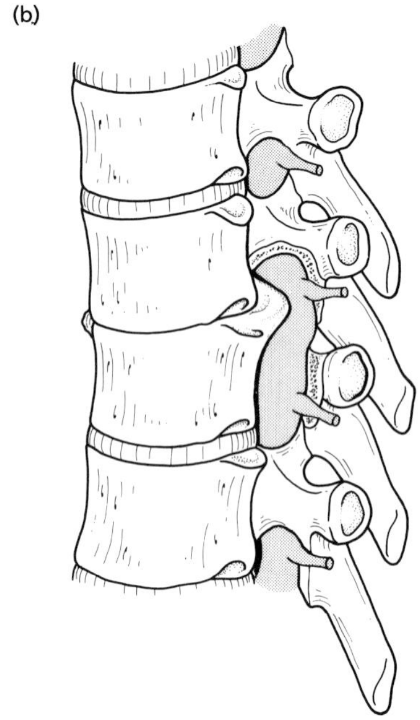

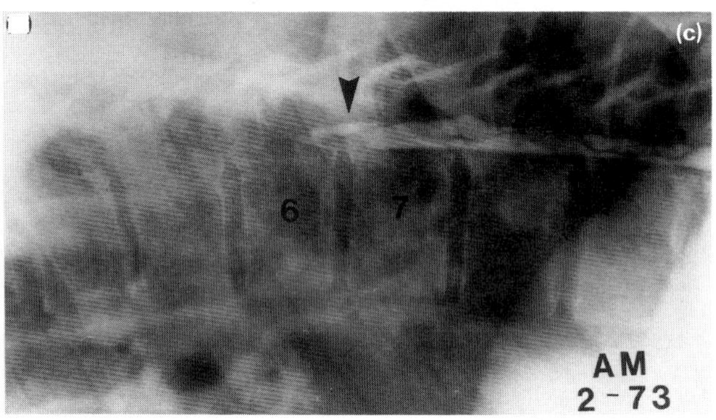

Fig. 68.1 Thoracic disc herniation. Radiograph (a) and drawing (b) of patient with complete neurological deficit and no significant fracture. (c) Pantopaque myelogram demonstrating thoracic disc herniation.

1983; Bohlman *et al.*, 1985b; Riska *et al.*, 1987). This is in contrast to those with complete paraplegia who do not recover neural function regardless of the operative approach. In the rare individual who is neurologically intact with a burst fracture, there is some evidence that remodelling will take place and decompression may not be necessary (Edwards *et al.*, 1989). Severe pain, or increase in the neurological deficit, or degree of kyphosis should prompt the surgeon to consider decompression and fusion.

Operative technique of anterior transthoracic decompression and fusion

The thoracotomy is made in the intercostal space below the rib articulating with the disc which has ruptured (Fig. 68.2a). Generally the entire rib need not be excised. If this is necessary, however, the chest is entered through the rib bed. In either case the corresponding nerve is identified and traced proximally. The parietal pleura is reflected away from the disc and bodies. The segmental vessels of both vertebral bodies are identified, ligated, and divided (Fig. 68.2b). The head and neck of the rib are excised to expose the pedicle and the intercostal nerve is used to find the foramen. The pedicle of the caudal vertebra is then excised (Fig. 68.2c) followed by the interior portion of the disc. The posterior half of the inferior portion of the superior vertebra, and the cranial aspect of the inferior vertebrae, are removed using a high-speed burr when the fracture is healed or curettes in a fresh fracture. This is carried out across the width of the vertebral body, staying out of the spinal canal until the trough is complete. In an intact vertebra or healed fracture, a diamond burr is used to thin the bone posteriorly at the cranial and caudal aspects of the trough as well as on the contralateral side. The impinging bone and disc are then pulled away from the dural sac (Fig. 68.2d). The fractured vertebra must be stabilized by the insertion of an iliac crest strut graft placed under distraction

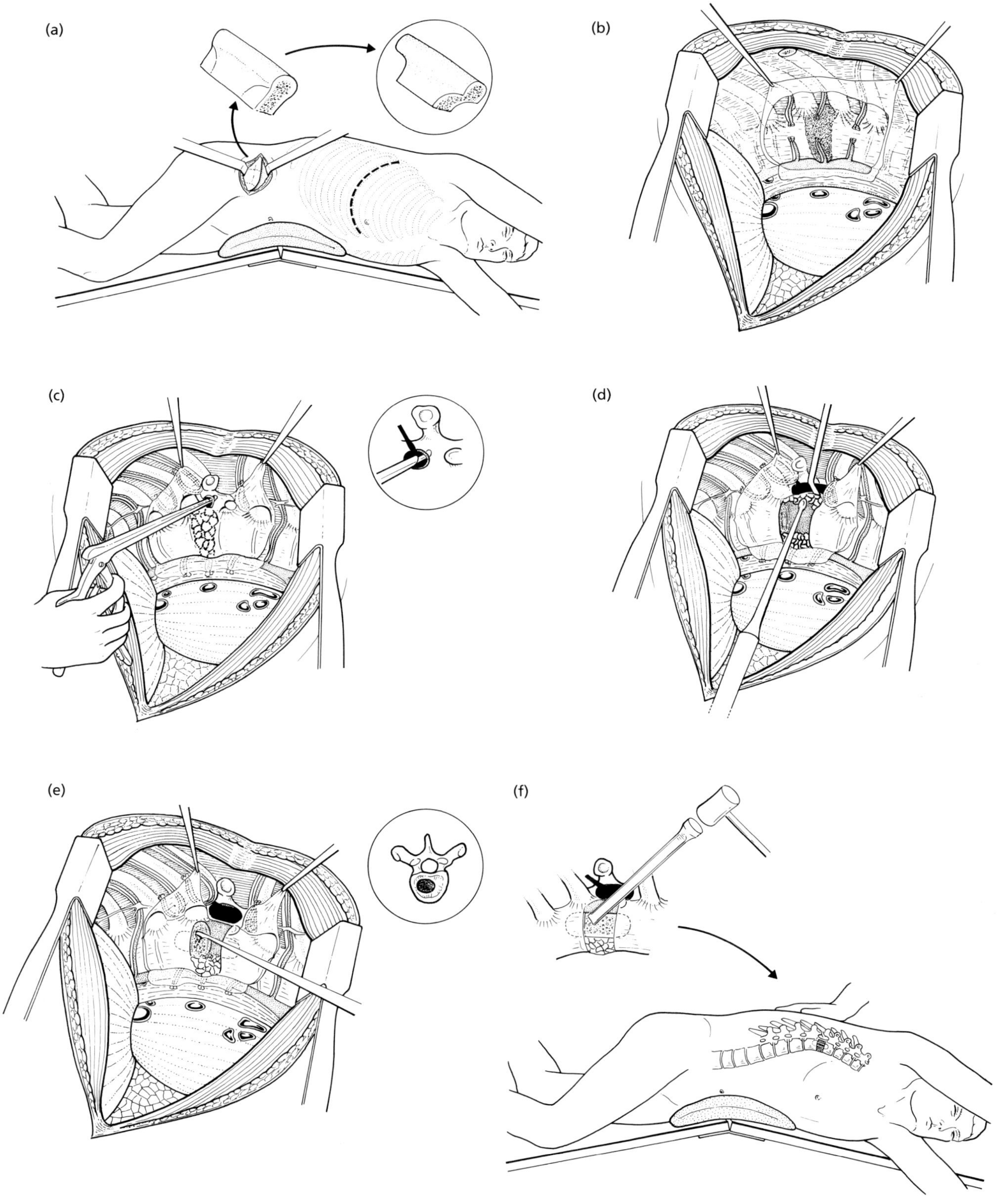

Fig. 68.2 Transthoracic anterior decompression and fusion. (a) Surgical position; (b) burst fracture seen through periosteum; (c) removal of pedicle; (d) dural compression by removal of bone and disc fragments; (e) preparation of beds to receive graft; (f) graft inserted under distraction achieved by pressure from posteriorly. Redrawn with permission from Bohlman *et al.* (1991).

between the intact vertebrae (Fig. 68.2e,f). The chest is closed over a thoracostomy tube. The patient can be mobilized in a thoracolumbar orthosis as soon as the other injuries allow. Some modification of the approach has to be made when necessary from the first to the third thoracic body region (Turner & Webb, 1987; Charles & Govender, 1989) Alternatively, a costotransversectomy could be performed, but visualization is not as good (Bohlman & Eismont, 1981) and there may be unwanted manipulation of the cord itself.

Laminectomy does not decompress the cord and destabilizes the spine (Tencer *et al.*, 1985a,b). If laminectomy is used to provide access to the anterior structures, there is a high rate of increased neurological deficit from the manipulation of the dural contents. The use of laminectomy is to be strongly condemned (Stauffer, 1984; Bohlman *et al.*, 1985b).

Fracture dislocation

Because of the intrinsic stability of the thoracic spine, these injuries are the result of high-energy violence. Most are associated with complete paraplegia, and they can be treated non-operatively (Fig. 68.3). One indication for surgery would be complete dislocation with 80–100% displacement of the vertebrae. The recommended approach would be posterior reduction, instrumentation, and fusion. The type of instrumentation is a matter of the surgeon's preference (McAfee *et al.*, 1985b; Keene *et al.*, 1986; Gurr *et al.*, 1988), though one should avoid excess distraction in these mechanically unstable injuries. It should be noted, however, that after a period of one week or more, even injuries resulting in complete translation of one vertebral body relative to another will become very difficult to reduce because of callus formation and will normally stabilize with conservative therapy.

However, in the rare instance where there is no or partial neurological deficit, open reduction and internal fixation via a posterior approach may be advised (Sasson & Mozes, 1987). Again, instrumentation type is a matter of surgeon preference, and one should achieve stability by instrumenting two or three segments proximal and distal to the damaged segment. After the reduction, the patency of the canal should be ensured either by intraoperative ultrasonography or immediate contrast myelography.

Sagittal slice fractures

These severe injuries are invariably associated with complete paraplegia and do not require operative management (Fig. 68.4). They are treated with bed rest for two weeks then mobilization in a moulded orthosis.

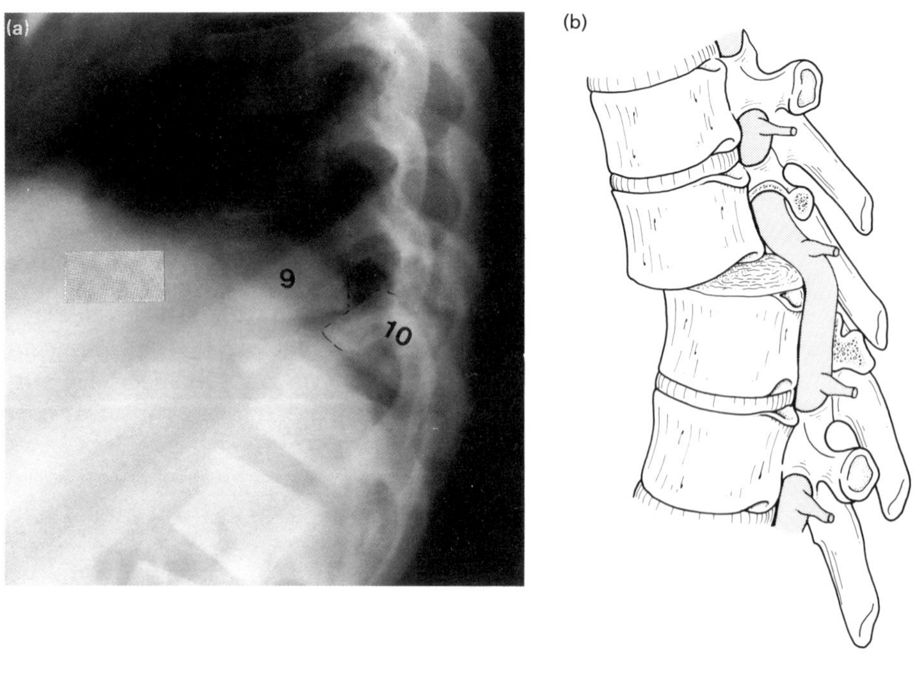

Fig. 68.3 Thoracic fracture dislocation. Radiograph (a) and drawing (b) of patient with complete paraplegia who was treated non-operatively. From Bohlman and Ducker (1991).

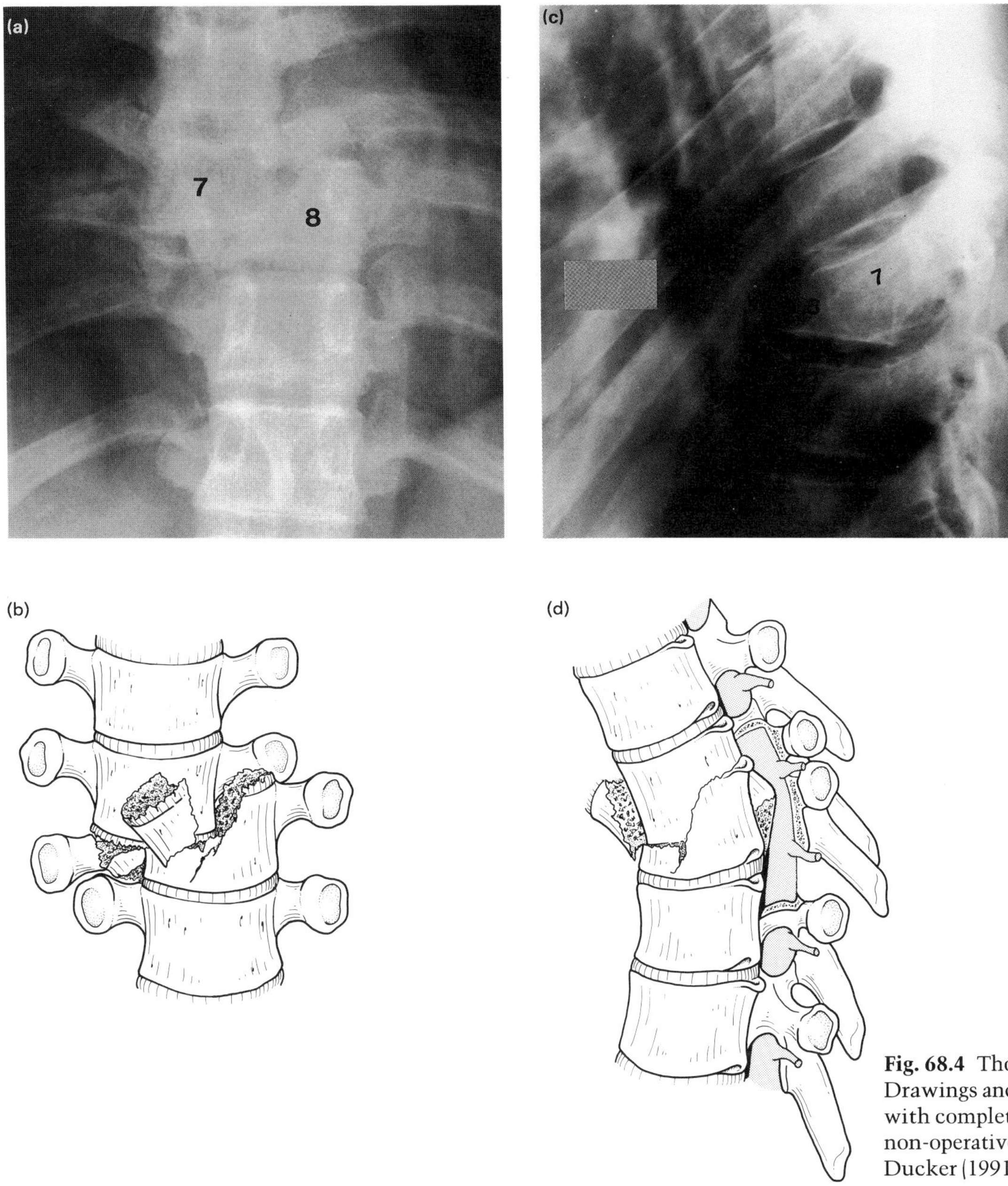

Fig. 68.4 Thoracic slice fracture. Drawings and radiographs of patient with complete paraplegia, treated non-operatively. From Bohlman and Ducker (1991).

Traumatic thoracic disc herniation

Unless there is disc space narrowing, the location of the injury may not be apparent except with the more sophisticated imaging modalities (Fig. 68.1). Disc excision as described above is indicated in patients who are neurologically normal but have persistent pain, and in individuals with incomplete cord injury syndromes. External support postoperatively is not necessary.

THORACOLUMBAR AND LUMBAR INJURIES

Regional considerations

The lower thoracic and lumbar vertebrae are larger than those found in the cervical and thoracic region. The vertebral canal can vary from ovoid to triangular depending on developmental factors and coexistent degenerative disease. In the thoracolumbar and upper lumbar region the canal contains the spinal cord and its tip, the conus medullaris. Distal to L2 in most individuals the vertebral canal contains only the cauda equina. Hence injuries in this region can produce varying degrees of cord and/or root injury with variable prognosis for recovery. When present, neurological deficit is more likely to be incomplete.

The thoracolumbar junction provides greater mobility than that seen in the upper thoracic spine, therefore stability is more of an issue. The thoracolumbar junction is a transition zone not only in the morphology of the vertebra but also mechanically. The high incidence of injury seen in this region is attributed to the transition of the relatively rigid thoracic spine to the more mobile lumbar spine. There is a trend to attempt to preserve lumbar lordosis and to limit fusion to as few motion segments as possible, to avoid increased stress at the remaining normal levels. Many of these concepts have developed from long-term follow-up of long instrumented fusions in adolescents for scoliosis, but are now also appreciated in other types of patients (Kostuik *et al.*, 1988; Lagrone *et al.*, 1988).

Compression fractures

These are common injuries and may occur with forward or lateral flexion. As an isolated injury, most are not associated with neurological deficit. Unless there is severe compression with disruption of the posterior ligamentous complex producing a three-column injury or significant kyphosis, these injuries can be treated non-operatively.

Burst fractures

These injuries are also quite common particularly at the thoracolumbar and midlumbar regions. The assessment of stability in these lesions is of critical importance and the Denis classification is of great help (Denis, 1983, 1984). Alternatively they may be thought of as stable or unstable with the latter implying disruption of the posterior bony and ligamentous structures. This is best assessed by CT and MRI. In the absence of surgical stabilization the stable burst, which may exhibit acute mechanical instability, will heal with late stability. The unstable burst fracture may not achieve mechanical stability late, even with osseous union, because of the posterior ligamentous damage (McAfee, 1982).

Burst fractures associated with complete paraplegia are uncommon, but could be treated conservatively, unless there is posterior column disruption and severe kyphosis. In that case one would consider posterior instrumentation and fusion without decompression to achieve stability.

More commonly, one encounters no deficit or an incomplete lesion. In the latter case this is a result of root injury or mixed root and cord injury. Except in cases of complete nerve disruption, root lesions have a better prognosis for recovery, but incomplete cord lesions may well benefit from anterior decompression (Clark, 1981; McAfee, 1985a). It is, however, essential that such surgical decompression and stabilization should be performed by very experienced teams as skilled conservative management can also produce good clinical results. It is important that operative intervention does not jeopardize the chance of recovery but experience does suggest that appropriate surgical decompression in a patient with an incomplete neurological deficit and significant canal compromise can result in immediate neurological improvement. Conus lesions often have a good prognosis (Coolican *et al.*, 1983).

Operative technique of retroperitoneal anterior decompression and fusion

As the pathological entity causing the cord compression is anterior, the anterior approach is the favoured technique (McAfee *et al.*, 1985a; Riska *et al.*, 1987). Posterior techniques requiring manipulation or the removal of anterior placed fragments are not only less controlled but also less reliable. The procedure is performed in the lateral decubitus position (Fig. 68.5). Generally the left side is entered to avoid the liver and the inferior vena cava. The latissimus dorsi and the abdominal muscles are divided over the twelfth rib, which is excised subperiosteally. The retroperitoneal space is entered through the bed of this rib and the subcostal nerve is identified and traced to its foramen. The paralumbar musculature is preserved and neither the pleura nor diaphragm are violated. With this approach an exposure from T11 to L3 and occasionally L4 can be achieved, though injuries at L3 and L4 are best approached via a lower incision between the rib cage and iliac crest. The appropriate transverse process is excised. Proximally a portion of

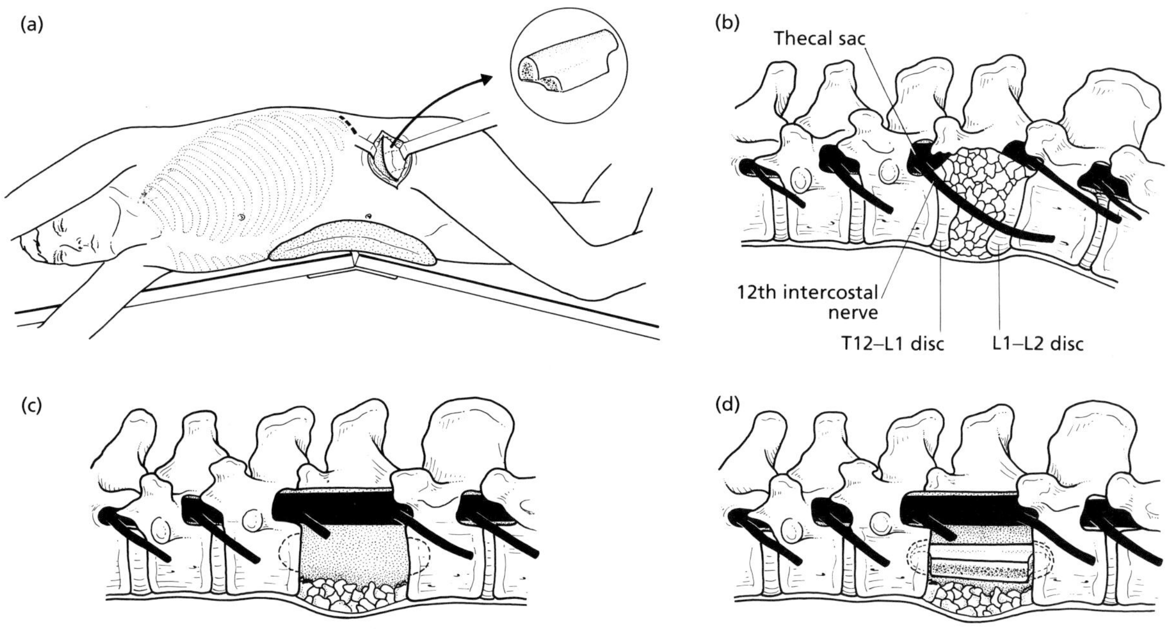

Fig. 68.5 Operative technique for retroperitoneal anterior decompression and fusion. Redrawn with permission from McAfee *et al.* (1985a).

the diaphragmatic crus may need to be taken down. The psoas is reflected anteriorly at the appropriate level. The segmental vessels of the appropriate vertebral body are identified, ligated, and divided as close to the aorta as possible. The nerve root corresponding to the vertebral body is identified and traced to the foramen. The pedicle is identified and excised, thus defining the spinal canal. The central portion of the disc proximally and distally is removed. A trough is made in the lateral aspect of the body and a midportion removed with high-speed burr or in the fresh fracture with a curette. In the fresh fracture, curettes can be used to pull bony fragments out of the canal, away from the dura. In a healed fracture the diamond burr is used to thin the bone to the point that it is possible to pull the protruding bone into the cavity created, away from the thecal sac. It is usually necessary to sharply divide the remaining fibres of the annulus fibrosus and posterior longitudinal ligament. Care is taken to decompress the entire width of the spinal canal. In the acute fracture an iliac crest strut graft is placed. In thin patients it may be possible to harvest this through the same incision by subcutaneous dissection. Other authors prefer to use fibula, but this rigid strut tends to sink into cancellous bone, increasing the kyphosis; also revascularization is slower. In the absence of osteopenia the iliac crest provides sufficient mechanical stability. In late decompressions the residual anterior body may provide sufficient stability to obviate fusion. In the acute situation an unstable burst fracture will require either anterior instrumentation or a separate posterior instrumentation and fusion. The patient is mobilized in a moulded TLSO.

Other authors favour a posterior approach to these fractures (Larson *et al.*, 1976; Garfin *et al.*, 1985; Benzel & Larson, 1986). After the standard midline incision and exposure, laminectomy is performed. The pedicle of the involved vertebra is identified and curettes and burrs are used to enter the vertebral body through the pedicle. The inner body is removed, creating a cavity. Curved instruments are then used to push protruding bone and disc fragments into this cavity. Intraoperative ultrasonography is used in some centres to confirm the adequacy of the decompression (Eismont *et al.*, 1984). Posterior instrumentation and fusion is then performed. This method has the advantage of allowing for immediate stabilization of unstable burst fractures with a single surgical approach. If there is an associated posterior dural tear this approach provides good visualization. This technique is attractive to surgeons unaccustomed to anterior spinal approaches. Its major disadvantage is the increased manipulation of the dura and its contents, and poorer visualization of the anterior aspect of the dura. Dall & Stauffer (1988) correlated recovery to kyphosis and canal compromise.

The posterior approach may be used with distraction instrumentation to effect indirect reduction of burst fractures. To be effective this must be performed early, within days of injury (Willen *et al.*, 1984). Complete reduction is generally not achieved, but this may not be necessary, particularly in the neurologically normal individual.

There has been a resurgence of interest in transpedicular fixation (Aebi *et al.*, 1987, 1988; Dick, 1987; Olerud *et al.*, 1988). The putative advantage is the ability to immobilize a single vertebral body above and below the fracture, preserving motion segments and lumbar lordosis. Although promising, these techniques are technically demanding and carry the risk of root injury, great vessel injury, and instrumentation failure. Long-term results are as yet unknown. In any case transpedicular fixation should be used only by those surgeons trained and experienced in its application.

Similarly, a variety of anterior devices are under investigation (Dunn, 1984; Kaneda *et al.*, 1984). Their use should probably be restricted until their long-term safety has been established. Burst fractures in the lower lumbar region (fourth and fifth lumbar) may be difficult to approach retroperitoneally, and can be decompressed by laminectomy and dural retraction or transpedicular decompression as described above.

It is essential to stress that all such instrumentation techniques must be accompanied by bone grafting and most surgeons favour the use of some form of external support until the fusion mass consolidates.

Somewhat more controversial is the individual with a burst fracture who is neurologically normal. Investigators have recently reported data suggesting that there is some remodelling of burst injuries (Edwards *et al.*, 1989) suggesting that a neurologically intact patient might be treated conservatively and followed for the development of late neurological loss or pain. The stable burst with severe kyphosis or an unstable burst may benefit from posterior instrumentation with attempted correction and fusion. Again close follow-up would be needed to detect late pain or deficit. The extent to which one can depend on remodelling is unknown. Experimental cauda equina compression as reported by Delamarter *et al.* (1989), suggests that compression in excess of 50% will produce alterations in electrophysiology, vascularity, and histology which can improve with decompression. Not all patients exhibit the remodelling phenomena. Neurologically intact patients who later develop a deficit or pain will benefit from anterior decompression and stabilization. Except in the less common lower lumbar burst injury, the approach of choice is anterior retroperitoneal decompression to minimize manipulation of the neural elements.

Seatbelt injuries

Seatbelt injuries were initially described by Chance (1948). He described the bony injury which can generally be treated non-operatively (Fig. 68.6). Although it can exhibit acute mechanical instability, osseous healing ultimately results in stability.

Those seatbelt injuries occurring at a single level purely through ligamentous structures are more likely to be chronically unstable and should be treated with posterior compression instrumentation and fusion. The number of levels fused necessarily depends on the type of instrumentation, the choice of which is partially a matter of surgeon preference. Distraction should not be used.

Mixed bony and ligamentous two-level injuries may or may not require operative stabilization depending on which structures are injured.

Neurological deficit is uncommon in this type of injury. When there is a deficit, one must search for occult neural compression.

Fracture–dislocation

These severe injuries are always mechanically unstable and have a high rate of concomitant neurological injury. As in the thoracic spine, complete reduction is possible only in the acute period. If this is not feasible, stabilization is usually indicated to avoid chronic instability which may threaten remaining neurological function.

Preoperative imaging will help evaluate the extent of the posterior column injury which may be incompletely appreciated on plain radiographs. MRI can identify posterior ligamentous disruption. Bone or extruded discs within the vertebral canal can also be identified (Fig. 68.7).

Generally these injuries require posterior instrumentation and fusion (Jacobs *et al.*, 1980; Willen *et al.*, 1985). Because of their instability, two or three

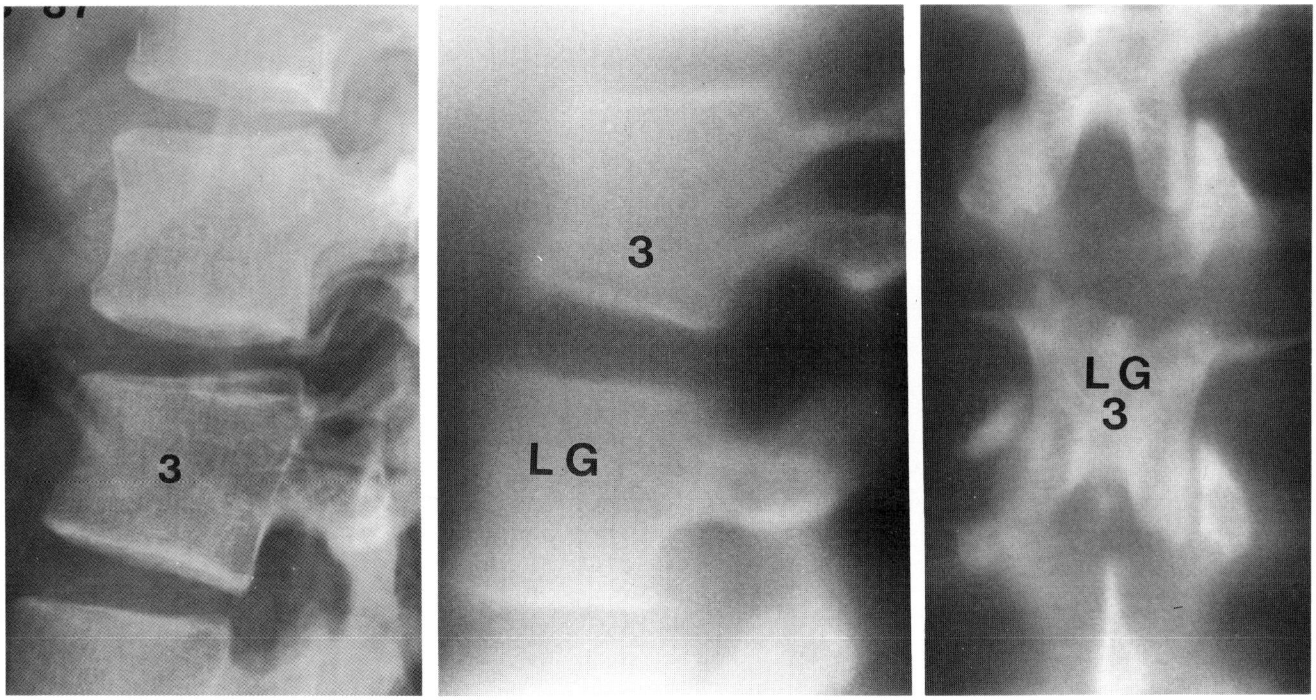

Fig. 68.6 Seatbelt fracture. Radiographs of an adolescent with L3 seatbelt injury and decreased sensation over the anterior thigh but no motor deficit. She recovered in a brace.

segments proximal and distal to the disruption should be included in the construct. Care must be taken to preserve lumbar lordosis. It is not yet clear whether the pedicular systems are rigid enough to allow short fusions in this type of injury. External support should be used postoperatively. Generally, reduction and stabilization will effect decompression, but this should be assessed by postoperative imaging.

Fractures of the spinous processes, transverse processes, articular processes, and pars articularis are often seen in conjunction with major injuries. As isolated entities they generally do not require operative treatment.

SACRAL INJURIES

Classification

The sacrum is intrinsically stable and is firmly attached to the pelvis by strong ligaments. The sacral canal transmits the sacral and coccygeal nerve roots. Injuries to these structures are uncommon, accounting for less than 1% of reported spinal injuries. They are often the result of high-energy trauma and are associated with pelvic injuries. They are often missed initially because of suboptimal plain radiographs. Furthermore, sacral root dysfunction may be missed if the bladder is catheterized, as is generally the case, and rectal tone is not determined (Dowling *et al.*, 1985; Denis *et al.*, 1988).

The injuries can be divided into transverse and parasagittal.

The transverse fracture is analogous to a shear fracture in other areas. There is failure of the anterior and middle columns which is entirely bony. The dural sac is draped over the kyphosis. If imaging demonstrates root compression, decompression can be performed through a sacral laminectomy with gentle retraction of the sac, and removal of the bone within the canal. Recovery of bladder and bowel function is uncertain but possible (Ferris & Hutton, 1983; Roy-Camille *et al.*, 1985).

The parasagittal fracture through the sacral foramina is associated with vertical shear pelvic injuries. In this instance failure is through the sacral ala rather than the sacral–iliac joint. Disruption of the roots of the sacral plexus carries a poor prognosis. Since this is a bony injury there is good prognosis for healing

(a)

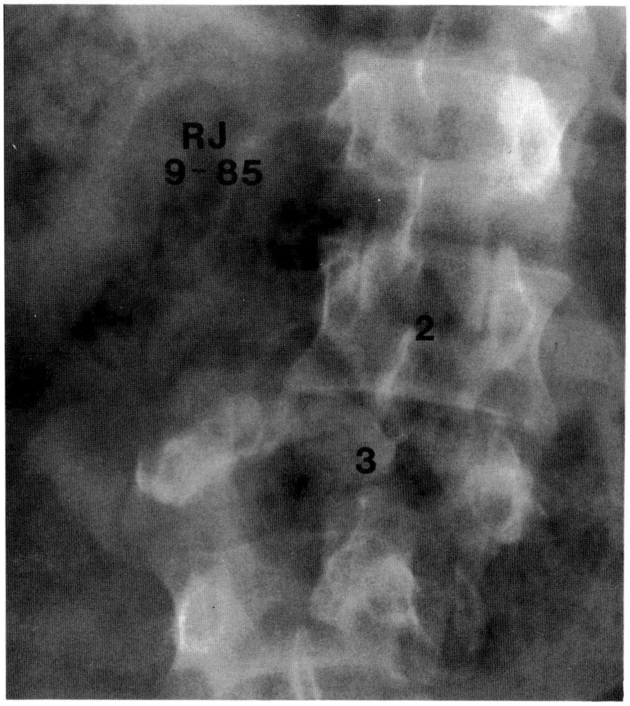

(b)

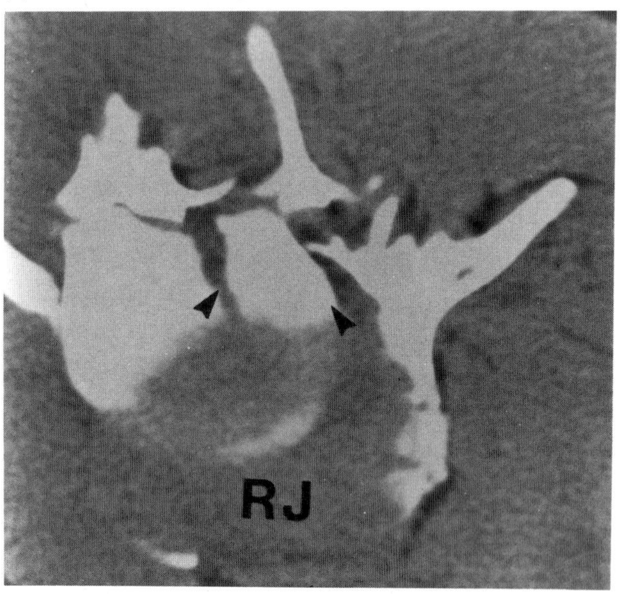

(c)

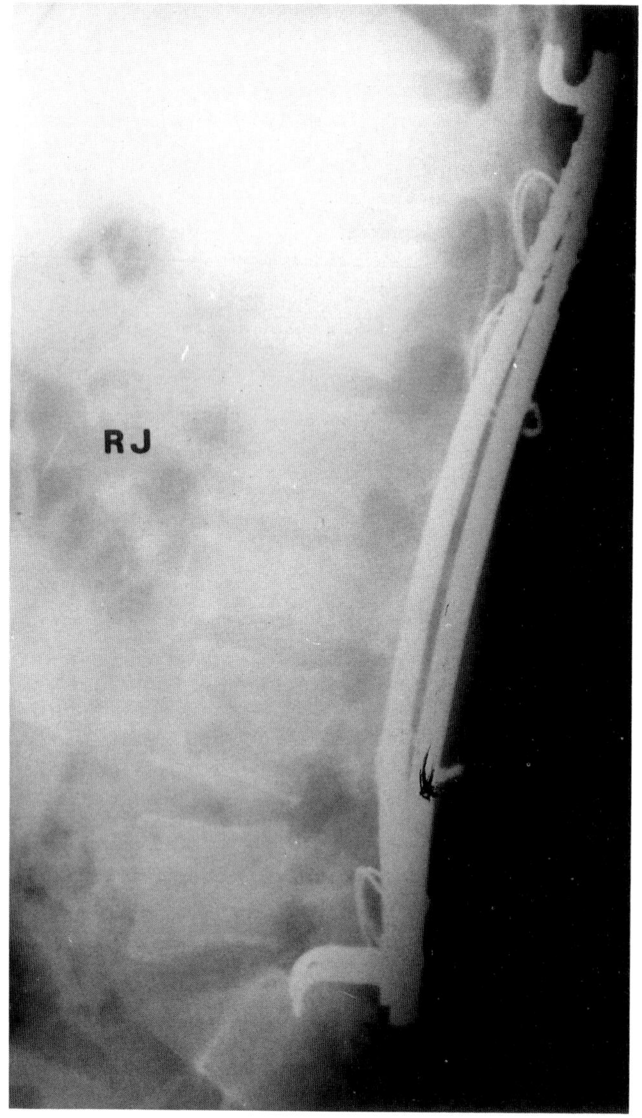

Fig. 68.7 Lumbar fracture–dislocation. AP radiograph (a) and CT scan (b) of a patient with L3–L4 fracture–dislocation; (c) shows the position following open reduction, instrumentation and fusion.

with stability unless there is gross displacement. If there is a single root compression by a bone fragment, especially the first or second root resulting in radiculopathy and pain, then a posterior foraminotomy should be performed (Fig. 68.8). Increasingly the associated pelvic fractures are being treated aggressively by either open reduction and internal fixation or external fixation.

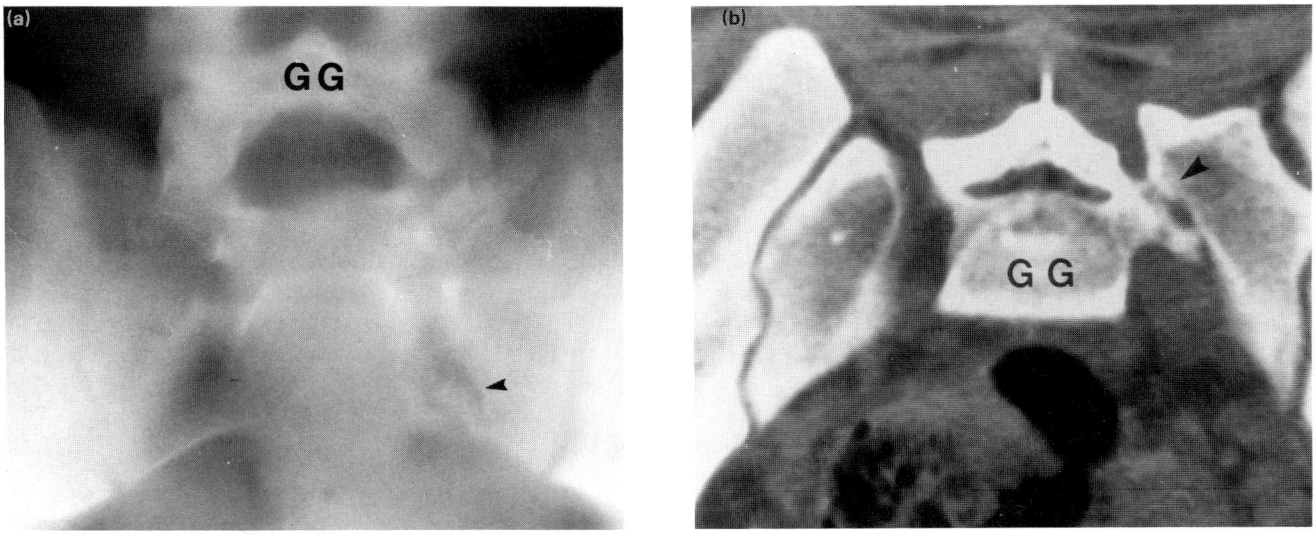

Fig. 68.8 Sacral fracture. Radiograph (a) and CT scan (b) of a patient with longitudinal right sacral fracture and S1 radiculopathy from root entrapment. He was successfully treated with a foraminotomy.

REFERENCES

Aebi, M., Etter, C., Kehl, T. & Thalgott, J. (1987) Stabilization of the lower thoracic and lumbar spine with the internal spinal skeletal fixation system: indications, techniques, and first results of treatment. *Spine*, **12**, 544–551.

Aebi, M., Etter, C., Kehl, T. & Thalgott, J. (1988) The internal skeletal fixation system. A new treatment of thoracolumbar fractures and other spinal disorders. *Clin. Orthop.*, **227**, 30–43.

Benzel, E.C., Larson, S.J. (1986) Functional recovery after decompressive operation for thoracic and lumbar spine fractures. *Neurosurgery*, **19**, 772–778.

Bohlman, H.H. (1985) Treatment of fractures and dislocations of the thoracic and lumbar spine. *J. Bone Jt. Surg.*, **67A**, 165–169.

Bohlman, H.H. & Eismont, F.J. (1981) Surgical techniques of anterior decompression and fusion for spinal cord injuries. *Clin. Orthop.*, **154**, 57–67.

Bohlman, H.H. & Zdeblick, T.A. (1988) Anterior excision of herniated thoracic discs. *J. Bone Jt. Surg.*, **70A**, 1038–1047.

Bohlman, H.H. & Ducker, T.B. (1991) Spine and spinal cord injuries. In Rothman, R.H. & Simeone, F.A. (eds), *The Spine*, pp. 720–722. W.B. Saunders, Philadelphia.

Bohlman, H.H., Freehafer, A. & Dejak, J. (1986) The results of treatment of acute injuries of the upper thoracic spine with paralysis. *J. Bone Jt. Surg.*, **67A**, 360–369.

Bondurant, F.J., Kulkarni, M.V., Cotler, H.B., Harris, J.J., Kopaniky, D.R., Miner, M., Donovan, W.H. & Carter, E. (1989) Magnetic resonance imaging in acute spinal cord injury. Federation of Spine Associations Program, 12 February, pp. 22–23.

Cammisa, F.J., Eismont, F.J. & Green, B.A. (1989) Dural laceration occurring with burst fractures with associated lamina fractures. Federation of Spine Associations Program, 12 February, pp. 17–18.

Chance, C.Q. (1948), Note on a type of flexion fracture of the spine. *Br. J. Radiol.*, **21**, 452.

Charles, R. & Govender, S. (1989) Anterior approach to the upper thoracic vertebrae. *J. Bone Jt. Surg.*, **71B**, 81–84.

Clark, W.K. (1981) Spinal cord decompression in spinal cord injury. *Clin. Orthop.*, **154**, 9–13.

Coolican, M., Taylor, T.K.F., Ryan, M.D., Yeo, J.D. & Rutkowski, S. (1983) Prognosis of conus lesions due to fractures and fracture-dislocation of the lumbar spine. *J. Bone Jt. Surg.*, **65B**, 670.

Crock, H.V. & Yoshizawa, H. (1977) *The Blood Supply of the Vertebral Column and Spinal Cord in Man*. Springer, Vienna.

Dall, B.E. & Stauffer, E.S. (1988) Neurologic injury and recovery patterns in burst fractures at the T12 or L1 motion segment. *Clin. Orthop.*, **233**, 171–176.

Delamarter, R.B., Bohlman, H.H., Dodge, L.D. & Biro, C. (1990) Experimental lumbar spinal stenosis. Analysis of the cortical evoked potentials, microvasculature and histopathology. *J. Bone Jt. Surg.*, **72A**, 110–120.

Denis, F. (1983) The three column spine and its significance in the classification of acute thoracolumbar spinal injuries. *Spine*, **8**, 817–831.

Denis, F. (1984) Spinal stability as defined by the three-column spine concept in acute spinal trauma. *Clin. Orthop.*, **189**, 65–76.

Denis, F., Davis, S. & Confort, T. (1988) Sacral fractures: an important problem. Retrospective analysis of 236 cases. *Clin. Orthop.*, **227**, 67–81.

Dick, W. (1987) The 'fixateur interne' as a versatile implant for spinal surgery. *Spine*, **12**, 882–900.

Domisse, G.F. (1974) The blood supply of the spinal cord. A critical vascular zone in spinal surgery. *J. Bone Jt. Surg.*,

56B, 225–235.

Dowling, T., Epstein, J.A. & Epstein, N.E. (1985) S1–S2 sacral fracture involving neural elements of the cauda equina. *Spine*, **10**, 851–853.

Dunn, H.K. (1984) Anterior stabilization of thoracolumbar injuries. *Clin. Orthop.*, **189**, 116–124.

Edwards, C.C., Rosenthal, M.S., Gellad, F. & Levine, A.M. (1989) The fate of retropulsed bone following thoracolumbar burst fractures: late stenosis or resorption? *Orthop. Trans.*, **13**, 32–33, 49–50, 119.

Eismont, F.J., Green, B.A., Berkowitz, B.M., Montalvo, B.M., Quencer, R.M. & Brown, M.J. (1984) The role of intraoperative ultrasonography in the treatment of thoracic and lumbar spine fractures. *Spine*, **9**, 782–787.

Emery, S.E., Pathria, M.N., Wilber, R.G., Masary, T., Bohlman, H.H. (1989) Magnetic resonance imaging of post-traumatic spinal ligament injury. *J. Spinal Disorders*, **2**, 229–233.

Fasano, F.J. & Stauffer, E.S. (1988) Traumatic division of the spinal cord demonstrated by magnetic resonance imaging. *Clin. Orthop.*, **233**, 168–170.

Ferris, B. & Hutton, P. (1983) Anteriorly displaced transverse fracture of the sacrum at the level of the sacroiliac joint. *J. Bone Jt. Surg.*, **65A**, 407–409.

Garfin, S.R., Mowery, C.A., Guerra, J. & Marshall, L.F. (1985) Confirmation of the posterolateral technique to decompress and fuse thoracolumbar spine burst fractures. *Spine*, **10**, 218–223.

Gurr, K.R., McAfee, P.C. & Shih, C. (1988) Biomechanical analysis of posterior instrumentation systems after decompressive laminectomy. *J. Bone Jt. Surg.*, **70A**, 680–691.

Holdsworth, F.W. (1970) Fractures, dislocations and fracture–dislocations of the spine. *J. Bone Jt. Surg.*, **52A**, 1534–1551.

Holdsworth, F.W. & Hardy, A. (1953) Early treatment of paraplegia from fractures of the thoracolumbar spine. *J. Bone Jt. Surg.*, **35B**, 540–550.

Jacobs, R.R., Asher, M.A. & Snider, R.K. (1980) Thoracolumbar spinal injuries. A comparative study of recumbent and operative treatment in 100 patients. *Spine*, **5**, 463–477.

Johnson, J.R., Leatherman, K.D. & Holt, R.T. (1983) Anterior decompression of the spinal cord for neurological deficit. *Spine*, **8**, 396–405.

Kaneda, K., Abumi, K. & Fujiya, M. (1984) Burst fractures with neurologic deficits of the thoracolumbar spine. Results of anterior decompression and stabilization with anterior instrumentation. *Spine*, **9**, 788–795.

Keene, J.S., Wachwitz, Drummond, D.S. & Breed A.L. (1986) Compression–distraction instrumentation of unstable thoracolumbar fractures: anatomic results obtained with each type of injury and method of instrumentation. *Spine*, **11**, 895–902.

Kitchel, S.H., Eismont, F.J., Quencer, R.A. & Green, B.A. (1989) Evaluation of acute thoracolumbar fractures with MR imaging. Federation of Spine Associations Program, 12 February, pp. 29–30.

Kostuik, J.P., Maurais, G.R., Richardson, W.J. & Okajima, Y. (1988) Combined single stage anterior and posterior osteotomy for correction of iatrogenic lumbar kyphosis. *Spine*, **13**, 257–266.

Lagrone, M.O., Bradford, D.S., Moe, J.H., Lonstein, J.E., Winter, R.B. & Ogilvie, J.W. (1988) Treatment of symptomatic flatback after spinal fusion. *J. Bone Jt. Surg.*, **70A**, 569–580.

Larson, S.J., Holst, R.A., Henny, D.C. & Sances, A. (1976) Lateral extracavitary approach to traumatic lesions of the thoracic and lumbar spine. *J. Neurosurg.*, **45**, 628–637.

Machida, M., Weinstein, S.L., Yamade, T., Kimura, J., Itagaki, T. & Usui, T. (1988) Monitoring of motor action potentials after stimulation of the spinal cord. *J. Bone Jt. Surg.*, **70A**, 911–918.

McAfee, P.C. (1982) The unstable burst fracture. *Spine*, **7**, 365–373.

McAfee, P.C., Bohlman, H.H. & Yuan, H.A. (1985a) Anterior decompression of traumatic thoracolumbar fractures with incomplete neurological deficit using a retroperitoneal approach. *J. Bone Jt. Surg.*, **67A**, 89–104.

McAfee, P.C., Werner, F.W. & Glisson, R.R. (1985b) A biomechanical analysis of spinal instrumentation systems in thoracolumbar fractures. *Spine*, **10**, 204–217.

McArdle, C.B., Crofford, M.S., Mirtakhraeem Amparo, E.G., Calhoun, J.S. (1986) Surface coil MR of spinal trauma: preliminary experience. *Am. J. Neurorad.*, **7**, 885–893.

McEvoy, R.D. (1985) The management of burst fractures of the thoracic and lumbar spine. Experience in 53 patients. *Spine*, **10**, 631–637.

Meyer, P.R., Cotler, H.B. & Gireesan, G.T. (1988) Operative neurologic complications resulting from thoracic and lumbar spine internal fixation. *Clin. Orthop.*, **237**, 125–131.

Olerud, S., Karlstrom, G. & Sjostrom, L. (1988) Transpedicular fixation of thoracolumbar vertebral fractures. *Clin. Orthop.*, **227**, 44–51.

Owen, J.H., Laschinger, J., Bridwell, K., Shimon, S., Nielson, C., Dunlap, J. & Kain, C. (1988) Sensitivity and specificity of somatosensory and neurogenic-motor evoked potentials in animals and humans. *Spine*, **10**, 1111–1118.

Riska, E.B., Myllynen, P. & Bostman, O. (1987) Anterolateral decompression for neural involvement in thoracolumbar fractures. *J. Bone Jt. Surg.*, **69B**, 704–708.

Roy-Camille, R., Saillant, G., Gagna, G. & Mazel, C. (1985) Transverse fracture of the upper sacrum. *Spine*, **10**, 838–845.

Sasson, A. & Mozes, G. (1987) Complete fracture–dislocation of the thoracic spine without neurologic deficit. A case report. *Spine*, **12**, 67–70.

Stauffer, E.S. (1984) Internal fixation of fractures of the thoracolumbar spine. *J. Bone Jt. Surg.*, **66A**, 1136–1138.

Tencer, A.F., Allen, B.L. & Ferguson, R.L. (1985a) A biomechanical study of thoracolumbar spinal fractures with bone in the canal. Part I. The effect of laminectomy. *Spine*, **10**, 580–585.

Tencer, A.F., Allen, B.L. & Ferguson, R.L. (1985b) A biomechanical study of thoracolumbar spinal fractures with bone in the canal. Part III. Mechanical properties of the dura and its tethering ligaments. *Spine*, **10**, 741–747.

Turner, P.L. & Webb, J.K. (1987) A surgical approach to the upper thoracic spine. *J. Bone Jt. Surg.*, **69B**, 542–543.
Willen, J., Lindahl, S., Irstam, L. & Nordwall, A. (1984) Unstable thoracolumbar fractures. A study by CT and conventional roentgenology of the reduction effect of Harrington instrumentation. *Spine*, **9**, 214–219.
Willen, J., Lindahl, S. & Nordwall, A. (1985) Unstable thoracolumbar fractures. A comparative clinical study of conservative treatment and Harrington instrumentation. *Spine*, **10**, 111–122.

69 · Rehabilitation and the Paralysed Patient

By H.S.Y. FANG and G.M. BEDBROOK

HISTORICAL

The spinally injured man, or 'the spinal man', has been known to exist and has been carefully recorded as early as over 4000 years ago in the Egyptian papyri (Hughes, 1988). In one set of these translated papyri, *The Edwin Smith Surgical Papyrus*, there were six selected case reports of spinal cord injuries among 48 medical case reports (Bedbrook, 1987a). The most illustrative one is Case 31:

Examination: If thou examinest a man having a dislocation in a vertebra of his neck shouldst thou find him unconscious of his two arms, his two legs on account of it, whilst his phallus is erected on account of it, urine drops from his member without his knowing it.

Diagnosis: Thou shouldst say concerning him, One has a dislocation in a vertebra of his neck, while he is unconscious of his two legs and his two arms and his urine dribbles.

Treatment: An ailment not to be treated.

Despite these early records, medical practice over the centuries yielded very few advances in the treatment of the spinally paralysed because it was felt that little could be done. Just before and during the Second World War, however, attitudes changed; largely because of the dynamic influence of Guttman and others. The development of treatment and rehabilitation of the spinally paralysed can therefore be considered chronologically and divided into three clearly defined periods: the Pre-Guttman, the Guttman, and the Post-Guttman Eras.

The Pre-Guttman Era (before 1944)

This period spans many centuries in time. Progress in the understanding of the spinal cord and its disorders was slow until the 17th century. Because of the work of Harvey, Lasuus, Stenson, Haller and Morgagni, many advances in neuroanatomy and neurophysiology were made. The specialities of clinical neurology and neuropathology began in the 18th century and expanded into the 19th century, during which time many lesions affecting the spinal cord were recognized and accurately recorded. However, this was not accompanied by any notable improvement in treatment (see Chapter 66).

The treatment of spinal cord lesions, however, improved during the First World War when advances in modern neurological diagnosis and assessment were made, but there was not much progress in long-term treatment and care of the paraplegic person. Between 1918 and 1944 the only development was the understanding of fundamental neurology and urinary drainage. No commitment to patient care prevailed despite advances in orthopaedics, nursing care, physical rehabilitation and aftercare facilities (Bedbrook, 1987b). Although the importance of urinary care and the prevention of contractures and bedsores were emphasized, application of these principles was not diligently applied to spinally paralysed patients. Well over 80% of patients died of complications of ascending urinary tract infection and decubitus pressure sores within 3 years from injury. Many patients drank heavily out of desperation. The general pessimism was clearly revealed in the Report of the Medical Research Council of 1924.

The Guttman Era (1944–80)

The Guttman Era began when Sir Ludwig Guttman (Fig. 69.1) was appointed Director of the Stoke Mandeville Spinal Injuries Centre in the United Kingdom in 1944. He organized specialist departments

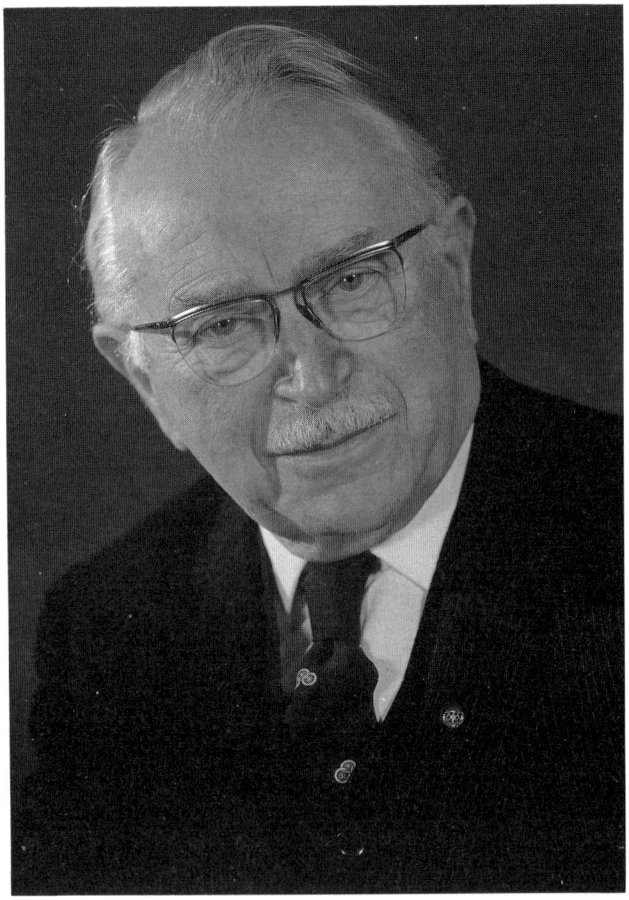

Fig. 69.1 Sir Ludwig Guttman.

for the treatment and extended care of paraplegic and quadriplegic patients. With a multidisciplinary team approach and personal attention he was able to heal neglected decubitus ulcers, correct contractures of joints and diminish limb spasticity in long-standing paraplegics. Above all, he inspired such people with new faith and hope. At the same time, Munro of Boston, Botterall of Montreal, Bedbrook of Perth, amongst others, established similar centres in North America, Australia and Europe.

This concept of comprehensive service for paraplegics and tetraplegics encompassing the initial, as well as long-term, treatment and rehabilitation was refreshing. The essence of his approach was:

1 The supervision of such units by an experienced physician or surgeon who is prepared to give up some of his or her own specialty in order to devote full attention to work in this multidisciplinary specialty. This demands meticulous attention to detail, planning and organizing the management of individual patients, and correlating the often conflicting interests of visiting specialists concerned with special aspects of management.

2 The dedication of nursing and other paramedical staff, such as physiotherapists and occupational therapists, to cope with the many details involved in the work, and avoidance of frequent staff changes.

3 Adequate technical facilities such as workshops for social rehabilitation and prevocational training.

4 Attention to social, domestic and industrial resettlement.

5 Regular aftercare or extended care over the lifetime of each individual.

As a result of this specialized care many spinally paralysed patients survived a near-normal lifespan. A majority returned to work and lived at home.

The post-Guttman era (after 1980)

Following Guttman's death in 1980, the case of 'spinal man' has advanced further. The last decades have seen significant developments in:

1 more comprehensive spinal centres—it was reported in 1968 that over 100 new centres had emerged all over the world (Kakulus, 1987);

2 advances in research, medical science and computer technology;

3 prevention of injuries (prophylaxis);

4 provisions of community activities for the disabled.

With better understanding of the underlying pathology and correlation with the clinical findings, the treatment and rehabilitation process has made further progress. Significant advances in computer technology have helped not only in improving diagnosis and prognosis but also in the quality of life for the patient.

Research into spinal cord regeneration and repair is under way in a number of centres. Major campaigns are being launched worldwide on prevention or diminution of unnecessary sports, traffic and work accidents that cause spinal injuries.

PATHOLOGY

A clear understanding of the pathological changes and their relationship to the clinical picture in spinal injuries should provide a sound basis for rehabilitation.

Spinal cord injuries result in a variety of morbid anatomical changes ranging from haemorrhages within and outside the cord to gross destruction of the cord and shredding and avulsion of the nerve roots. Kakulus & Donovan (1987) showed that in the first 24 hours after injury, little neural damage was not infrequently found at necropsy. This probably accounts for the syndrome of concussion or spinal shock associated with good recovery. Also at necropsies, the spinal cord is usually intact even in the presence of severe bony injuries. This emphasizes the importance of careful initial handling after the accident diminishing the likelihood of post-accident spinal cord damage and paralysis. Any neurological sparing in the beginning is a manifestation of an incomplete lesion which is salvageable. Careful and repeated clinical neurological examination is therefore essential in initial management and in planning rehabilitation.

Thus appreciation of cord pathology has increased our understanding of tissue healing and of scars and cyst formation in the injured spinal cord. Some of these are found to be treatable by surgery, and this may enhance further improvement in functional rehabilitation.

DIAGNOSIS

As mentioned, it is of paramount importance to make an accurate diagnosis by systematic and meticulous history-taking, physical examination and repeated regular charting of sensory and motor changes; reflexes must also be tested carefully. This will assist tremendously in the planning of treatment and rehabilitation. The level and extent of the lesion will determine the ultimate functional disabilities and the physical limitation of activities and daily living, which include personal hygiene, ambulation, ability of transfer, dressing, eating, and communication, etc. The reappearance of the slightest voluntary movement, and of sensation below the level of spinal cord injury, is evidence of some spinal cord or nerve root continuity heralding a better prognosis. If the paralysis is total after 8 hours, together with return of reflexes and priapism in the male, a complete lesion is likely with an unfavourable prognosis. Advances in modern technology are also helpful in planning short-term and long-term management. This particularly applies to computerized tomography (CT) scans and magnetic resonance imaging (MRI), whereas myelography in the acute stage has been found of little benefit.

REHABILITATION

Early management

Rehabilitation is no longer regarded as the third phase of management. It starts from the time of injury.

First aid and emergency care

When the patient is found after an accident the earliest responsibility usually falls on the person rendering first aid. Apart from the emergency measures of preserving life, the injured person should be moved with great gentleness with the spine in neutral position and the head and neck supported. The conscious patient must be consulted with every move and transported to a comprehensive spinal injury centre at the earliest possible moment as delay will result in increased morbidity and often neurological deterioration (see Chapter 67). Recent research in Australia has shown that as much as 26% of spinal paralysis cases were made worse by poor handling, splintage and transportation, both from the site of accident and during admission to hospital (Toscano, 1988).

Standard care in spinal centres

Following admission, besides resuscitation, the key word in management should be 'prevention'—of contractures and deformity, of urinary infection, of pressure sores, of debilitation and other complications. Prevention and rehabilitation are inseparable and must proceed together.

POSTURE

The patient is nursed in a supine position and turned laterally at regular 2-hourly intervals around the clock, either by a spinal turning team or a spinal turning bed (Guttman, 1977a). No pressure sores should be allowed to develop. Most cases of dislocation and unstable fractures of the lower thoracic or lumbar spine are capable of being reduced with traction, positioning and gentle manipulation, with or without general anaesthesia.

NURSING

Good nursing care is all-important, especially in the prevention of pressure sores, maintaining reduction, preventing contractures, and caring for the neurogenic bladder and bowel, as well as in the early detection of cardiopulmonary problems.

Ensuring an adequate diet, a bright environment and giving much-needed psychological support is routine. The care of the paralysed bladder is covered in Chapter 62, but it must be emphasized that sterile catheterization in the early stages of management is essential and that long-term use of an indwelling catheter should be avoided whenever possible.

CARE OF THE NEUROGENIC BOWEL

In cauda equina lesions the bowel becomes atonic. Bowel training is enhanced by the regular use of faecal softeners, enemas and manual evacuation. In higher spinal cord lesions where there is a return of reflexes, evacuation is assisted by the use of suppositories, aperients and the physiologically stimulated reflexes such as the gastrocolic reflex and anal canal dilatation by digital insertion. Toilet training of the bowel requires diligence and reassurance as in the case of the bladder.

Prior to the return of bowel sounds no attempt should be made to stimulate evacuation. However, if the rectum is full, a gentle normal saline or oil enema is helpful, combined with manual evacuation. After bowel sounds have fully returned, and solid food has been consumed, the patient is placed on a bowel programme so that the bowel empties at a specific time each day; thus soiling and faecal incontinence is minimized or prevented. Three factors are important in this regard; namely (1) timing, (2) use of reflexes, and (3) dietary consistency.

Timing

The bowel programme works best when it is performed at the same time each day. Even if no results are achieved initially, and even if incontinence occurs, perseverance is essential.

Use of reflexes

The most important reflex is the gastrocolic reflex. Normally, after the stomach fills, reflex peristaltic movement of the colon is induced, filling the rectum and inducing the defaecation reflex. Therefore, the bowel programme is performed 30–60 minutes after either the morning or evening meal. To further assist reflex emptying a suppository, usually containing glycerin or bisacodyl, is employed. It is lodged against the rectal wall, acting as a stimulant and automatically inducing peristalsis in the lower gut within 15–30 minutes. If, however, emptying is not complete the bowel is further stimulated by the insertion of a lubricated, gloved finger high up into the rectum followed by three circular movements, which further stimulates peristalsis and in some cases relaxes the external sphincter. This may be repeated again in 15 minutes to assure complete emptying. Care must be taken not to irritate or overstretch the delicate mucous membrane which might result in fissures or cause haemorrhoids to bleed. In patients with suprasacral or upper motor neurone lesions, reflexes of the perineal floor are intact or hyperactive. The sphincter area is in tonic contraction as in normal individuals, contributing to the maintenance of continence once defaecation has occurred (Green, 1983).

Patients who have a lax perineal floor due to a cauda equina or conus lesion, however, will find that stimulation by suppository or finger is often ineffective and the suppository may simply fall out. Such patients usually have their abdominal muscles intact and are capable of aiding defaecation by straining. However, this is not always effective due to the flaccidity of the pelvic floor, and manual removal is sometimes the only way to evacuate. These patients will usually have a patulous anus and be liable to faecal incontinence, particularly when straining. This is especially noticeable when transferring or using braces. In these cases it may be unwise to prescribe stool softeners.

DIETARY CONSISTENCY

It is well known that the type of food one consumes has a direct effect on the frequency of bowel movements. Spicy foods which contain laxative irritants can result in more than one bowel movement per day. Therefore, it is important to adhere to a policy of consistency of diet relative to quantity and character of food. Patients are encouraged to consume a reasonable amount of fibre in the form of fruit and vegetables, since the added bulk will hasten the transit time and ensure soft stools.

Early physical rehabilitation

The physiotherapist, occupational therapist and the ward nurse should stimulate any remaining muscular function in the limbs by active and assisted exercises whilst the patient is in bed in the very early days. This includes the use of simple static and dynamic splints, graded weights and pulley systems. Maintenance of morale, persistence and hard work will encourage independence within days of the accident, while gentle passive movements and splints prevent joint stiffness and contractures. Any delay in this regard will result in extensive muscle wasting and stiffness. Repeated acts of small activities of daily living made as interesting as possible are vital. Most patients with spinal injuries and paralysis after 6–8 weeks in bed, or much earlier if effective internal fixation of the spine has been achieved, can be mobilized out of bed into a wheelchair or into an exoskeleton brace. By 3 months the majority of spinal fractures will be well healed and stable. A formal regime of more vigorous physical and occupational therapy is then carried out in respective departments with proper equipment, to restore function and develop residual muscles (Table 69.1). Such activities include individual and group exercises as well as gymnasium work, activities of daily living and toilet training. The wheelchair must fit the patient in dimension and usage. The chair cushions must be custom-made in order to prevent decubiti.

As the tempo of physical activities increases, the patient is encouraged to do more in areas of interest, in prevocational education and training of skills. These are aided as required by professional bodies, special agencies as well as vocational counsellors. Most patients will eventually come around to accepting their disability. This will greatly enhance the process of rehabilitation. The assistance of a psychologist will on occasion be required.

When the patient fully cooperates with the professional team, his or her residual functions can be developed to maximum potential. Many disabilities can be partially or completed circumvented through adaptive techniques, the use of technical aids and retraining. The level of performance can be graded as: (a) complete dependence, (b) requiring partial physical

Table 69.1 Functional goals in spinal cord lesions. Data from Bedbrook (1981)

Spinal cord lesion	Neurological key muscle control	Functional goals
C5	Neck Upper trapezius	Manipulated electric wheelchair with mouth stick. Limited self-care (feeding, make-up) using arm supports and externally powered hand splints.
C6	Shoulder muscles Elbow flexors	Turn self in bed with overhead arm slings. Transfer to and from bed with assistance. Propel wheelchair with handrim projections. Self-feeding with externally powered hand splints or clip-on equipment. Light hygiene (make-up, brushing teeth). Dress upper trunk.
C7	Wrist extensors Supinators	Transfer to and from bed and into car without assistance. Transfer to commode chair with assistance. Propel chair with projections. Self-feeding, hygiene (shaving and grooming hair), dressing, writing, and skin inspection, using wrist-driven flexor hinge hand splints where prehension is required. Drive car with hand controls.
C8	Elbow extensors Weak hand	Transfer independence—bed, car, toilet. Propel wheelchair without hand projections. Wheelchair in and out of car. Independent in all self-care without hand splints or adapted equipment. Household activities from wheelchair.
T1–T8	Hand muscles	Wheelchair up and down kerb. Transfer to and from bath. Wheelchair to floor and return. Therapeutic standing with posterior leg splints.
T9–T12	Trunk stability	Wheelchair independence. Physiological ambulation with bilateral long leg braces and crutches. Complete self-care.
S1–S2	Knee extension Hip flexion	Ambulation with short leg braces, crutches, or canes.
L1–L5	Pelvic stability	Ambulation with bilateral long leg braces and crutches.

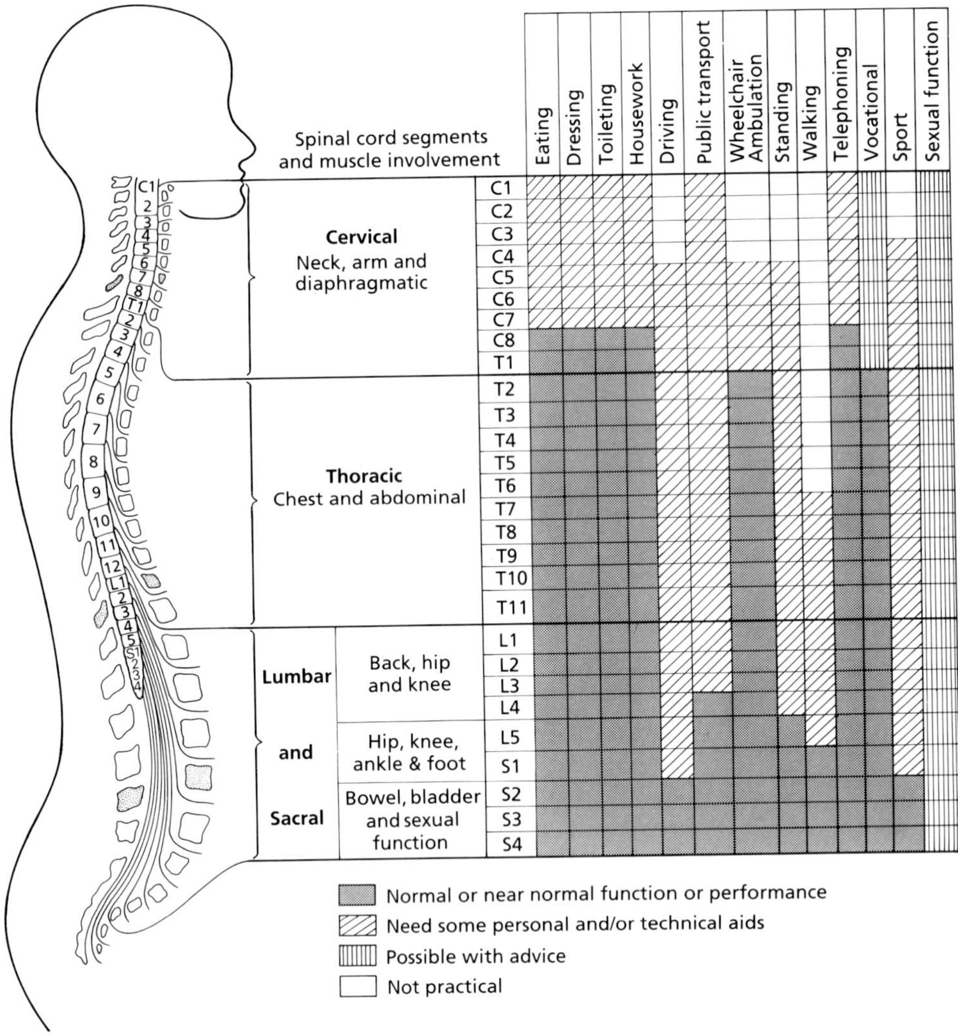

Fig. 69.2 Graphic summary of functional activities at different levels of spinal cord lesions. Variation of chart produced by Harmarville Rehabilitation Center (1987).

assistance, (c) requiring standby assistance, (d) total independence. This grading can be used in tabulated form to monitor residual function at various levels (Fig. 69.2).

Role of surgery

The role of surgery in the early management of spinal injuries in paraplegia and tetraplegia has been controversial for half a century. The protagonists are of the view that surgery will correct the deformity of the spinal column, salvage the partially damaged spinal cord and nerve roots, as well as provide stability. The antagonists say that surgery is unnecessary and that there is no proof that surgery has helped in greater neurological recovery. They claim that there is a definite risk of further damaging the precariously injured cord and nerve roots, as well as adding to complications and that surgery for stability is not essential (see Chapter 68).

The debate continues, but on balance when considering the dorsal and dorsolumbar areas, surgery in the early management of paralysis should be selective. However, with safer surgical environments the advent of CT scans and MRI, improved surgical skills and the added assistance of electronic cord monitoring, well-planned surgery might be considered in cases found to have large bony fragments directly compressing the cord and nerve roots. Surgery should also be considered in late cases of bony deformity where the salvaging of a nerve root or part of the cord may make a tremendous difference, as between a permanent wheelchair existence and a more vigorous life of standing and walking. Laminectomy has no place in the injured spine except when there is a large displaced posterior laminal fragment causing direct compression. When the canal is encroached upon from in front, the surgery of choice is by the anterior approach (Fang *et al.*, 1964; Hodgson & Yau, 1969).

Cardiopulmonary complications

The spinally paralysed, depending on the level and extent of the spinal cord injury, will face a variety of cardiopulmonary complications both in the immediate phase and later. As a result of interference with the autonomic nervous system there may be a sudden loss of peripheral vascular tone leading to hypotension, bradycardia, venous thrombosis, lung embolism and cardiac failure (see Chapter 61).

Impaired breathing and reduced vital capacity will result from paralysis involving the thoracic muscles and the diaphragm, endangering life. Emergency medical resuscitation measures may be required. A permanent tracheostomy should be avoided if possible, because it increases the patient's susceptibility to respiratory infection, reduces communication and social interaction and increases the patient's dependence on the attendants. Postural hypotension and fainting is countered by graduated tilting.

The caring team will ensure that the patient's lungs are adequately filled and emptied, supported by postural drainage. The patient is encouraged to cough and expectorate with manual assistance by fixing the lower thoracic cage to assist diaphragmatic activity. The patient and staff must also be familiar with the use of the intermittent positive pressure ventilator. Building up the residual accessory respiratory muscles will prevent stiffness of the thoracic cage and atelectasis. Many patients have learned effective compensating mechanisms consisting of elevation of the thoracic cage, tilting the trunk forward and coordinating contractions of the latissimus dorsi and pectoralis major, to achieve relatively good expiratory airflow.

Long-term management

Physical rehabilitation

SPASTICITY

Most spinally injured patients have spasms of their limb muscles due to spinal cord isolation, giving rise to uncontrolled muscle contractions. These may be painful, frustrating and tend to impede the process of rehabilitation. Patients may respond to a variety of measures which include medication, educated voluntary control with physical and psychotherapy, conductive education (Hari & Akos, 1988), acupuncture (Nan Deng Kun, personal communication) and functional electrical stimulation (Kanak, 1988) with varying degrees of success. Epidural injections of phenol and alcohol have yielded partial success. Intrathecal infusions of baclofen (Penn & Kroin, 1987) and microamounts of morphine (Kakulus & Donovan, 1987) are thought to provide dramatic relief. However, reports of long-term benefit are awaited.

THE WHEELCHAIR

In most advanced countries the wheelchair is custom-made for individual requirements. This includes the chair cushion which enables the patient to sit comfortably when out of bed. The patient learns to change posture regularly to avoid pressure sores of the anaesthetic skin. The propelling rims and detachable arms are adapted to allow ease of independent wheelchair ambulation and transfer. Specially designed chairs are made of light metal to cater for the keen sportsman, as well as automated electrical chairs for the tetraplegic patient.

ORTHOTIC DEVICES

The therapists make extensive use of plastic splints which are easy to apply. These prevent deformity, and enhance functional activities of the limbs. External bracing of the spine is designed to give additional stability to the spine and to get patients out of bed at the earliest possible time, usually within 6–8 weeks. For the cervical spine injury a halo and extension rods are incorporated into the spinal brace. In lesions below the neck, calipers and lower limb braces are used to assist patients to assume the erect position and in walking.

Sexual rehabilitation

All patients, particularly the young, are concerned about their sexual responses and function. They should be reassured at the earliest opportunity that an active sex life is possible and help is available. The non-physical side of sexuality must be encouraged through real affection and love.

After the neurological state has stabilized, a careful

assessment will reassure the female that intercourse and conception is possible. Sexual orgasm may be experienced via other orgogenic areas of the body if perineal sensation is lost. In due time, with practice, some females may indeed recover cervical vaginal orgasm by sympathetic neural pathways. In the male, reflex erection in those with spinal cord isolation becomes more intense as the lesion proceeds cephaladwise, and thus intercourse is possible with positioning and help from the partner. Normal orgasm is not experienced, but abnormal orgasm may occur. Ejaculation is rare. Flaccid lesions have only a small chance of psychogenic erection, thus coitus may only be achieved by the stuffing technique or other prosthetic devices (Kakulus & Donovan, 1987).

Substantial advances have been made in counselling, in regard to sexual techniques and devices that disabled couples can resort to (Neistadt, 1987). Every patient must be treated individually. There are now special clinics helping greatly with disordered sexual functions.

Social rehabilitation

In the case of the spinally paralysed, psychological trauma is tremendous. The injured patients pass through a period of shock, anguish and apathy. It is important that the whole professional team pays special attention in this respect with compassion on the one hand, and firmness on the other. The true picture and prognosis need to be fully explained by the doctor in charge to patients and their family when the neurological deficit is stabilized. The patients have to be taught and made to understand all procedures in detail, if they are to gain independence.

As patients' physical functions improve, the aim is to assist them to return and live in the society or the community, and to get involved in all normal social activities. Structural alterations need to be made to their homes, also provision for access. Transport needs to be provided. Some patients may prefer to drive themselves, with specially fitted hand controls. It should be impressed upon them that, apart from facing the world in a sitting position, they are just as normal and have the same rights and obligations as able-bodied individuals.

In most advanced countries, architectural barrier-free designs for public buildings and houses of entertainment, and restaurants exist, and more legislation is being adopted to provide increasing facilities for access. International campaigns in the past two decades have helped in achieving a better understanding of the problems of the disabled, in improving the public attitude and a stronger commitment on the part of governments. These include the International Year of the Disabled, pronounced by the United Nations in 1981; the Movement of the Right of the Physically Disabled in 1975 (WHO, 1976) and the Right of the Mentally Disabled Persons in 1978. The World Health Organization quoted figures indicating that 10% of the world population is disabled. The paralysed patients are not isolated or alone in facing their problems. There is every indication that more and more is being provided for the disabled in all countries in the world.

QUALITY OF LIFE

The ultimate goal is to restore and resettle the spinally paralysed into the community. Ninety per cent of these patients can return to their own homes, suitably adapted, and having access to community facilities (Guttman, 1977). Patients can be trained to drive, or alternative means of transport should be arranged.

EXTENDED CARE

Rehabilitation of some patients is a lifelong process. Extended nursing, therapy and care services are important. Patients who develop complications are followed at day specialist clinics or are admitted for short periods of treatment when required.

Ten per cent of patients, mostly tetraplegics, who would need more nursing care, and those who are totally dependent, may require to stay in a hostel or a permanent nursing home setting where care and therapy, as well as work activities, are provided in a dynamic and cheerful environment. This type of hostel within the community for dependent living for the spinally paralysed is being established in the United Kingdom, Europe, Australia and North America. The aim of these centres is to achieve an optimum lifestyle adapted to the individual rather than the need for absolute dependence.

RECREATION

As part of physical restoration, sport plays a prominent part. Participation in sport gives inspiration, confidence and great encouragement to disabled individuals in readjusting themselves into society. Organization of competitive local, national and international sporting events gives further impetus, assurance, pride and dignity to the disabled. The Stoke Mandeville Games and the Paralympics were founded by Guttman in the 1960s; other events include the Far East and South Pacific Games (FESPIC) in the Asian region founded by Nakamura in 1973. Wheelchair marathons and world championship events developed in the 1980s not only engendered great enthusiasm and added aspirations to disabled athletes, but also helped tremendously in changing the attitudes of people and governments.

Vocational rehabilitation

Prevocational education should be commenced and work interest developed as soon as the patients are up and about, centred on the occupational therapy department. The goal is set to help them to return to their previous job. If that is not possible, the patients would be helped to choose an area of interest or profession, and training arranged through the assistance of vocational counsellors and special agencies. If necessary, further schooling or special education should be arranged.

The advancement of computers has opened up a wide variety of new work opportunities which will allow disabled individuals to be gainfully employed or self-employed working at home. In a number of countries, governments exert direct influence on industry and commerce to enable placement of the disabled. Introduction of the quota system of disabled workers in factories practised in some countries has its advantages and disadvantages (Marano, 1986; Matsui, 1988). The most successful example is that run in Japan, where the Government imposes a 1.5% quota on all employment. Companies and organizations that do not reach the quota pay a fine to a statutory body—the Work Compensation Authority. The collected fines, which run into huge sums of money every year, are used to expand rehabilitation facilities and activities, and the development of sheltered workshops run for and by the disabled. As this is run as a strictly self-disciplined system, the administration has been made simple and effective (Kulkarni, 1984; Japan Association for Employment of the Disabled (JAED), North Tower, New Pier Takeshiba, 1-11-1 Kaigan, Minato-ku, Tokyo 105, Japan.

The quest for more work opportunities for the disabled is still very much dependent on the motivation of the disabled individuals themselves, the public attitude, and an understanding and determined government.

Recent advances

Functional electrical stimulation

Functional electrical stimulation (FES), also known as functional neuromuscular stimulation (FNS), is a system of electrical stimulation applied to paralysed muscles, with intact lower motor neurones, in paraplegic and tetraplegic patients. With the use of such sequential stimulations, controlled by computer, useful functions can be restored to paralysed hands to grip and grasp, and legs to straighten, to enable patients to stand and walk. Although a number of research centres can demonstrate the usefulness of this simple FES systems, it is still in the experimental stages of development. Further refinements are necessary before it can be converted into a practical piece of equipment with regard to actual level of function, ease of use, amount of energy spent, safety and cosmesis; as, for example, the pacemaker for the heart. As Marsolais (1988) put it:

Functions: must include standing for 1 hour with no break, getting up from a chair, getting up from a fall, walking on ramps and uneven surfaces, negotiating steps and escalators, exercise and recreational activities independently.

Ease of use: the system should require no more than 15 minutes to connect and 5 minutes to disconnect from the stimulator, and no more than 15 minutes for donning. It should require checking and maintenance no less than once a month.

Energy requirement: must not exceed 50% of maximum aerobic capacity.

Cosmesis: do not make abnormal sounds or have an unusual appearance that draws attention.

Safety: no catastrophic failure, and non-catastrophic failure rate of less than twice every month.

It is believed that existing technology can eventually achieve these goals to produce a radio-controlled wireless FES implant. Meanwhile, FES systems are adopted in the form of equipment such as bicycles which help the paraplegic patient to build up muscle bulk and prevent muscle atrophy. They are also employed to supplement existing orthosis for the tetraplegic hand and, for the incomplete paraplegic, in walking without braces.

Electromyographic biofeedback studies

Brucker and co-workers (Barth *et al.*, 1987) used electrodes anchored to patients' bodies at the site of the paralysed muscle, and connected these to a computer which projects onto a screen, registering the state of the paralysed muscle. The patient is then asked to try to move the muscle by performing an action. There is often residual function which is registrable on the screen on which the patient is asked to focus. With an increasing effort the amplitude is reflected on the screen, giving the patient a visual record of what his/her muscles can achieve.

This is, in a way, re-educating the uncontrolled muscles through the patient's conscious effort. This programme is exceptionally useful in cases of cerebral palsy, where patients learn to relax certain groups of muscles while others are in contraction.

The visual experience, once gained, is stored in the memory. The patient is able to recall this memory, as shown at later sessions of treatment.

We were able to see patients improve dramatically after only a few sessions. Brucker's view is that, in addition to promoting residual function, there could be dormant cells in the cortex or other neuronal pathways being activated in the process of such EMG biofeedback.

Extensive research is taking place in this respect in North America and Europe. Its clinical application is being critically examined (Vodovnik, 1981; Green & Brucker, 1987).

Acupuncture

For over 2000 years the Chinese have practised acupuncture, with successes claimed in the treatment of a wide range of ailments; nevertheless its therapeutic value is still debatable.

The technique has in the past 20 years or so been refined. Of the 300 acupuncture points covering the whole body, only some 30 points are in common usage and needling by hand is being modified by the use of electric stimulation.

Using the modern technique, trials of treatment for hemiplegic and paraplegic patients are being carried out at many centres in China, including the Tongji Medical University Hospital (TGUH) in Wuhan, known to the author.

At the TGUH rehabilitation department, acupuncture is used on paraplegics for relief of spasm and promotion of cord and root recovery. The following acupuncture points are often used:

Huat'ochiachi (Extra 21) and several back *Shu* points, as the main therapeutic points for restoring or improving the function of the spinal cord and nerves (Figs 69.3 & 69.4); *Wushu* (GB 27), *Shusi* (Extra),

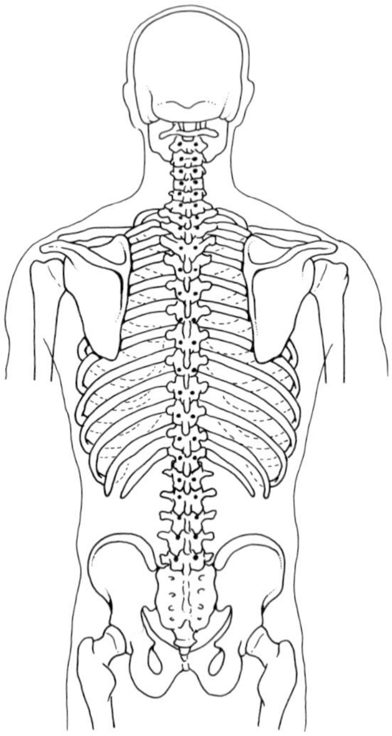

Fig. 69.3 Huat'o chiachi points.

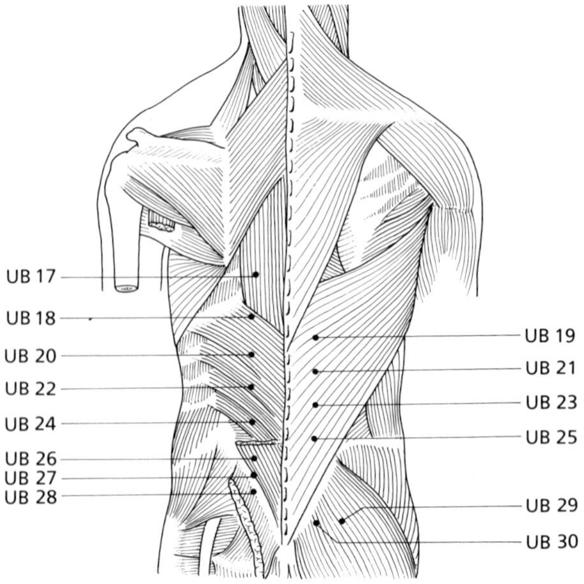

Fig. 69.4 Back *Shu* points (UB 17–30).

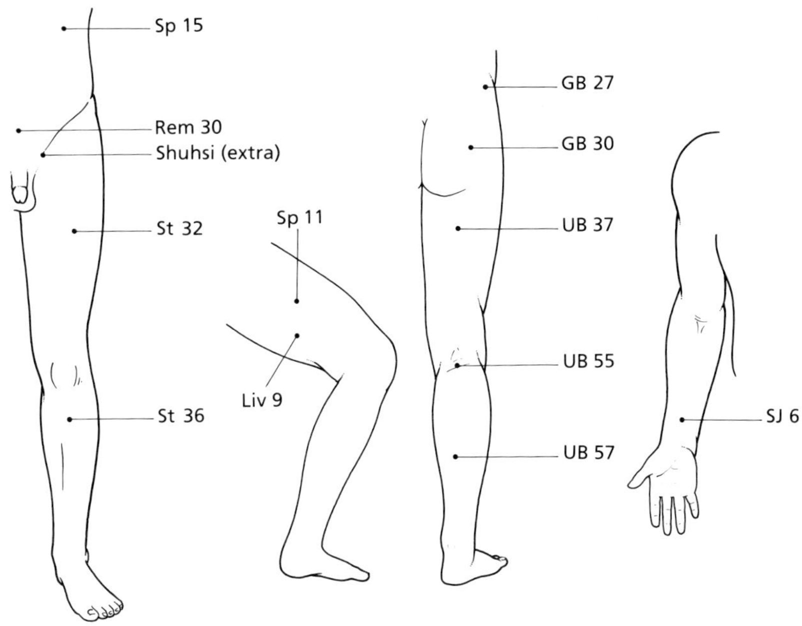

Fig. 69.5 Some related points.

*Huant'iao*PS (GB 30), *Yinmen* (UB 30), *Chimen* (SP 11), *Yinbao* (Liv 9), *Fut'u* (St 32), *Hoyang* (UB 55), *Ch'eng-shan* (UB 57), *Tsusanli* (St 36) for the paralysed muscles of the lower legs respectively; some spasmolytic points usually located in the distal parts of spastic muscles for relaxing the spasm; and points *Paihuanshu* (UB 30), *Chungchi* (Ren 30), *Yinpin* (Extra), *Taheng* (Sp 15), *Chikou* (SJ 6) for improving both urine and stool excretion (Fig. 69.5).

Moxibustion (the burning of special therapeutic herbs) is used in acupuncture, and moxibustion is carried out 20–30 minutes once or twice daily in a course of 20–30 days.

These techniques need further scrutiny and unbiased longer-term assessment, especially in the fields of spinal paralysis and post-traumatic root pain. They could be studied on a multicentre basis in selected spinal surgery units internationally.

COMMUNITY-BASED REHABILITATION

Much is said about the care and rehabilitation of the spinally paralysed in advanced countries. Such services and facilities are being developed piecemeal, and to a very limited extent, in most developing countries. It is fair to state that in the vast majority of developing countries there are no organized services, no matter how basic, for the spinally paralysed. Most developing countries are still waiting for increase of national resources and development for the eventual establishment of comprehensive spinal centres. In addition to rehabilitation institutions being costly there is also a lamentable lack of trained personnel. It is vital that some such services be established in the near future. Fifteen years ago the United Nations World Health Organization promoted the concept of community-based rehabilitation using available local resources and community effort to care for the disabled in their own families.

The World Health Organization has produced a practical manual with detailed illustrations and easy-to-follow instructions for the lay helper (WHO, 1983). The idea is to mobilize and train a whole army of non-professional volunteers working with guidance from the book, and instructed by someone who has acquired experience. The lowest-ranking worker is called the trainer, who is either the patient's relative or neighbour, who receives 3 weeks of training to learn how to use the book of 30 chapters. Each chapter of the manual deals with the care needed for specific situations. The trainer normally looks after one patient and helps with his or her needs, entering the patient's daily progress in an evaluation sheet and reporting to a local supervisor who has had 3 months' training and who looks after 10 trainers. The local supervisor, in turn, reports to an intermediate supervisor who is in charge of 30 local supervisors. This intermediate supervisor is usually medical, with direct access to a district medical station or hospital. Although the system is very primitive and basic, it has been field-tested and proven. It is presently being effectively practised in over 60 developing countries.

As Frankel (1987) rightly points out, the treatment of spinal cord injuries is labour-intensive, and in countries where semi-skilled labour and family help are easily found there are opportunities to develop an effective service (Green & Brucker, 1987). The absence of sophisticated diagnostic and therapeutic facilities is not a great disadvantage; but there is still a gross lack of trained medical and other paramedical personnel. The International Medical Society of Paraplegia is trying to assist in such training. In China a new course was established for this purpose, in 1989, at the Tong-Ji Medical University in Wuhan under the auspices of the World Health Organization (S. Purves, personal communication). As more resources are made available in the various countries, it is hoped that 'spinal man' will get his fair share of attention.

CONCLUSIONS

Rehabilitation should be considered as a continuous and comprehensive process from the early days of the accident, even for a lifetime for some of the more seriously injured. The secret of successful rehabilitation of the spinally paralysed is to ensure undivided attention from all professionals and staff. Comprehensive spinal centres are paramount for immediate care. Long-term rehabilitation and services are dependent on availability of trained personnel, financial resources, mobilization of public and government attitudes. Given the necessary care, 'spinal man' is capable of living a normal span of life. Further enrichment and fulfilment are entirely dependent on the quality of rehabilitation services. The right of the disabled must be respected, and equal opportunities provided.

The authors wish to end by quoting Guttman, from one of his last communications:

> As long as civilisation and humanity remain the basic principles of community life, no country can be so poor that it cannot afford to give to the severely disabled citizens their rightful place in society, the more so as thousands of spinally paralysed are today playing their part in contributing to the wealth of nations. To be able to do what they had to to overcome seemingly insurmountable obstacles caused by one of the greatest catastrophes which can befall mankind. (Guttman, 1977).

REFERENCES

Bedbrook, G.M. (ed.) (1984) *Lifetime Care of the Paraplegic Patient*, pp. 149–161. Churchill Livingstone, Edinburgh.

Bedbrook, G.M. (1987a) The development and care of spinal cord paraplegics 1918–1986. *Paraplegia*, **25**, 172–184.

Bedbrook, G.M. (1987b) The Development and care of spinal cord paralysis. *Paraplegia*, **25**, 176–183.

Fang, H.S.Y., Ong, G.B. & Hodgson, A.R. (1964) Anterior spinal fusion: the operative approaches. *Clin. Orthop.*, **35**, 16–33.

Frankel, H. (1987) Spinal cord injuries units. *Paraplegia*, **25**, 239–240.

Green, B.A. (1983) Kinetic therapy for spinal cord injury. *Spine*, **8**, 722–728.

Green, B.A. & Brucker, S. (1987) Functional electrical stimulation, *Rehabil. R & D Progress Report 1987.*

Guttman, L. (1977) Spinal paraplegia and tetraplegia. *Commun. Health*, **8**, 198–200.

Guttman, L. (1977a) On health deviation and rehabilitation in spinal paraplegia and tetraplegia. *Commun. Health*, **8**, 193.

Guttman, L. (1977b) Spinal paraplegia and tetraplegia. *Commun. Health*, **8**, 186–208.

Hari, M. & Akos, K. (1988) *Conductive Education* (translated from Hungarian by N.H. Smith and J. Stevens. Routledge, London.

Hodgson, A.R. & Yau, A.C.M.C. (1969) *Surgical Approaches to the Spinal Column*, pp. 289–323. Churchill Livingstone, London.

Hughes, J.T. (1988) The Edwin Smith Surgical Papyrus: An analysis of the first case report of spinal cord injuries. *Paraplegia*, **26**, 71–82.

Kakulus, B.A. (1987) Pathology of spinal injuries. *Central Nerv. Syst. Trauma*, **1**, 117.

Kakulus, B.A. & Donovan, W.H. (1987) Review and research. Menzies Technical Report No. 1, pp. 87–104.

Kanak, T.S. (1988) Paper presented at 27th Annual Scientific Meeting, International Medical Society of Paraplegia.

Keogh, E.J. (1986) Impotence following spinal injury. *J. Neurol. Neurosurg. Psychiatry*, **49**, 1104–1114.

Kulkarni, M.R. (1984) *Quota System and the Employment of Handicap; Experience in Three Countries.* University Centre for International Rehabilitation, Michigan State University.

Marano, A. (1986) Book on Vocational Rehabilitation Services for the Disabled in Japan. Published by the National Vocational Rehabilitation Centre for the Disabled.

Marsolais, E.B. (1988) Paper on Criteria for Practical FNS Systems presented at 27th Annual Scientific Meetings, International Medical Society of Paraplegia.

Matsui, R. (1988) Rehabilitation in Japan 1988. Japanese Society for Rehabilitation of Disabled. *Proceedings of the 16th World Congress of Rehabilitation International.*

MRC (1924) Report of the Medical Research Council of 1924 in the United Kingdom.

Neistadt, M.E. (1987) Choices: a guide to sex counselling with physically disabled adults, Krieger.

Penn, R.D. & Kroin, J.S. (1987) Long-term intrathecal baclofen infusion for treatment of spasticity. *J. Neurosurg.*, **66**, 181.

Shanghai College of Traditional Chinese Medicine (1974). *A Textbook of Acupuncture and Moxibustion*, pp. 417–474. People's Medical Publishing House, Beijing.

Toscano, J. (1988) Prevention of neurological deterioration before admission to a spinal cord injury unit. *Paraplegia*, **26**, 143–150.

Vodovnik, I. (1981) Edward Kardelj University, Kjubligana, Yugoslavia. *Critical Reviews in Bioengineering*, vol. 6, p. 63. CRC Press, Boca Raton, Florida, FL.

Wang Yunkai, *et al.* (1988) *Pocket Book of Acupuncture and Moxibustion*, pp. 324–325. Hebei Scientific and Technical Books Publishing House, Shijiazhang.

WHO (World Health Organisation) (1976) Resolution 29.68 adopted 20 May 1976, entitled 'Disability Prevention and Rehabilitation'.

WHO (World Health Organization) (1983) *Manual*. WHO, Geneva, Switzerland.

Zhang Zhenhuan (1985) *A Collection of Experiences in Acupuncture and Moxibustion*, pp. 1–7. People's Medical Publishing House, Beijing.

Zhu Lian (1980) *Acupuncture and Moxibustion*, pp. 1–4, 177, 194. Guangxi People's Publishing House, Nanning.

Index